360
24
$$\begin{array}{r} 360 \\ \times 24 \\ \hline 1440 \\ 720 \\ \hline 8640 \end{array}$$

Frieda A. De Muccio

Textbook of
MEDICAL-SURGICAL NURSING

Lillian Sholtis Brunner

R.N., B.S., M.S., *Consultant in Medical-Surgical Nursing, Bryn Mawr Hospital School of Nursing; formerly Assistant Professor of Surgical Nursing, Yale University School of Nursing; Supervisor of Operating Rooms, Hospital of the University of Pennsylvania.*

Charles Phillips Emerson, Jr.

A.B., M.D., *Associate Professor of Medicine and Chief of Hematology Section, Department of Clinical Research, Boston University School of Medicine; Senior Visiting Physician and Director of Clinical Laboratories, Massachusetts Memorial Hospital, Boston University Medical Center; Hematology Consultant, U.S. Public Health Service.*

L. Kraeer Ferguson

A.B., M.D., F.A.C.S., *Professor of Surgery, School of Medicine and Graduate School of Medicine, University of Pennsylvania; formerly Chairman of the Department of Surgery, Woman's Medical School of Pennsylvania and Graduate School of Medicine of the University of Pennsylvania.*

Doris Smith Suddarth

R.N., B.S.N.E., M.S.N., *Coordinator of the Curriculum, Alexandria Hospital School of Nursing, Alexandria, Virginia; formerly Instructor in Nursing, Alexandria Hospital School of Nursing, Alexandria, Virginia.*

Textbook of

Medical-Surgical Nursing

Brunner
Emerson
Ferguson
Suddarth

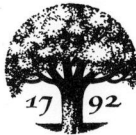

J. B. LIPPINCOTT COMPANY

Philadelphia and Montreal

Preface

This volume, newly published, stems from the fusion of two texts long familiar to the nursing profession. The direct descendant of ESSENTIALS OF MEDICINE and SURGICAL NURSING, their offspring boasts a lineage which includes 29 antecedent editions and spans a combined total of 90 years' continuous publication. The selection, modernization, amplification and amalgamation of pertinent portions of the parent texts and the incorporation of new material reflect the very close collaboration of two nursing educators, an internist and a surgeon.

The authors of MEDICAL-SURGICAL NURSING, in the course of multiple conferences, have considered at length various alternative methods of presenting and teaching this extensive subject. The choice of teaching method, they propose, is the prerogative of the teacher and student. This is an individual matter, just as care planned for the patient is individualized to satisfy his particular needs. Regardless of the approach pursued, be it symptomatic, problematic, physiological, disease oriented, etc., this text can be adapted readily to any program.

The product is designed for the nursing student to promote an intelligent understanding of each patient from the standpoint of his altered physiology, the symptoms he experiences and the signs he exhibits; the management of his condition; and his rehabilitation. The responsibilities of the nurse in relation to the protection and restoration of health have been delineated at length and in detail throughout the text. Organization of the latter, including the sequence of presentations, reflects the authors' intent to develop as early and as effectively as possible a keen *clinical awareness* on the part of the student, and to present in comprehensible and assimilable form the formidable mass of factual information which the nursing candidate must acquire.

Factual completeness and accuracy, comprehensiveness of scope and practical usefulness have been the guiding considerations of its authors; and the style in which it is composed, designed for maximum lucidity of presentation and readability, has been of equal concern. Technical discussions and data relating, for example, to applied pathologic physiology and therapeutic procedures, have been incorporated to an extent that is unusual, if not unprecedented in a publication of this type, for knowledge in this area is the key to nursing competence. The professional nurse, prime confidante and educator of her patient, as well as key intermediary between him, his physician and all paramedical personnel who contribute to his investigation and care, can scarcely afford to disregard this aspect of his problem. So oriented, this volume hopefully will serve primarily as a comprehensive text for the student who is enrolled in a professional nursing program, thus providing her with an authoritative background to assure graduate practice at a high level of clinical competence.

Part One of TEXTBOOK OF MEDICAL-SURGICAL NURSING, comprising 7 major units and 21 chapters, is directed to the "core problems" of medical and surgical nursing. Unit I discusses the person as a patient: his problems and his needs in a situation occasioned by illness. Unit II is concerned with the preventive aspects of medical and surgical nursing, specifying, among other things, prophylactic measures which are applicable to communicable infections, and describing the technical aspects of antisepsis and asepsis. Unit III presents the clinical evaluation of the patient, emphasizing the role of the nurse in the elicitation, detection and interpretation of signs and symptoms. A chapter is devoted to laboratory, radiologic and other diagnostic procedures, discussing these from the standpoint of general methodology, interpretation and the specific nursing responsibilities that attach to their performance. The seven chapters of Unit IV deal with specific supportive and symptomatic treatments in the care of the patient. Measures for the promotion of physical comfort and for the relief of psychologic distress are described in detail. Unit V addresses itself to "the patient with a surgical problem": in the course of 5 chapters a patient is followed to the operating room, under general anesthesia, through an operative procedure, into and out of the gamut of postoperative complications, through various stages of convalescence and through a series of rehabilitation programs, characteristic nursing problems being featured throughout this sequence. Unit VI is devoted to patients, both medical and surgical, who pose in common special problems relating to a specific situation: problems, for example, that are peculiar to adolescence or advanced age; problems dictated by chronic, as opposed to acute, illness; and problems that commonly arise in relation to malignant disease.

The principles and practice of rehabilitation nursing are discussed in Unit VII, with special heed to the characteristic needs of patients with various specific illnesses or disabilities and emphasizing the role of the nurse as an educator dedicated to the task of teaching the patient with chronic—perhaps incurable—disease or disability to compensate effectively for his handicap. Rehabilitation, an extension of convalescence, should be a wholesome, constructive, and optimistic experience for the patient as he moves on to independence and self-sufficiency. Even though this chapter is set apart in this book for emphasis and learning expediency, it must be clarified that the principles presented are integrated throughout the book as a vital part of the total medical or surgical experience of the patient.

Part Two, which includes 27 of the 49 chapters of the book, is concerned with patients with specific medical and surgical disorders. This material is presented in 11 units, based either on anatomic and physiologic considerations, i.e., in accordance with the particular organ system involved, or on the basic nature of the disease process under consideration. These conditions are discussed in depth from the standpoint of the nurse's role in the recognition and prevention of each; its symptomatology; relevant diagnostic procedures, the therapeutic measures that are likely to be employed and special nursing problems to be anticipated.

Examples of criteria which have given guidance are: Is this subject generally taught in Fundamentals of Nursing? If so, it should not be in this textbook. Is the condition one which is best studied in Nursing of Children? Then perhaps it should be placed there. Is content organized so that it goes from the simple to the complex, building on previously presented material? Some aspects of patient care may be too difficult for a beginning student. Here the answer depends upon the learning situation. For example, in the unit on the care of female patients with conditions of the reproductive system, a beginning student may care very effectively for a woman who has had a dilatation and curettage but would be overcome by the needs of the patient who has had a pelvic exenteration.

Even though we have given careful consideration to presentation, there will properly be differences of opinion from faculty to faculty. The important point is that the subject in question be taught or learned where it best fits into the local learning situation at that time.

The authors are convinced of the importance of proper teaching, direction and referral of the patient which will permit his becoming increasingly independent. These functions are an integral part of nursing. For this reason, a list of the most helpful pamphlets, booklets and brochures is given at the end of each chapter in Part Two. Likewise, a listing of related voluntary agencies and their addresses is offered from which the nurse or patient may secure additional valuable information.

As a means of review or a check on learning, clinical situations are given at the end of each chapter in Part Two.

The successful practice of nursing, especially in an emergency or disaster, depends upon a knowledge and application of principles. The broad principles of patient care are presented in Parts One and Two. In *Part Three,* principles are reemphasized and applications stated in relation to situations of unusual urgency. Integration then takes place in the learner, permitting her to perform effectively in stress situations. Medical and nursing management is presented on the basis of an individual emergency; in some conditions in which mass casualties are likely to be encountered, mass management is included. The authors wish to make clear that as with principles of rehabilitation, the principles of emergency and disaster care, ideally, are correlated throughout the study of medical and surgical nursing and are merely separated out as an independent unit for emphasis. When assigned to the Emergency Room, the student may find it helpful to review this section.

The authors have been aided materially in their efforts to render a complete and up-to-date text by many friends and associates. We are particularly indebted to Dr. H. R. Stone and Dr. Robert Dripps, professors of anesthesiology at the University of Pennsylvania, who have rewritten the chapter on anesthesia; to Dr. Bernard Ronis, professor of otolaryngology at Temple University, who has added a chapter to include the many important treatments now available for the correction of deafness; to Dr. C. M. Luce for his contributions to the section on ophthalmology; to Mrs. Thomas Royle Dawber of the Simmons College faculty and Newton-Wellesley Hospital staff, who is responsible for the chapter on nutritional needs and problems; and to Dr. Gloria Green for her effective drawings and diagrams.

For their assistance in the rehabilitation nursing portions of the manuscript, we wish to thank Josephine Buchanan, M.D.; Glenn G. Reynolds, M.D.; Robert D. Becker, R.P.T.; Marie Hansen, R.N., M.S.N.; Mary Slaughter, O.T.R.; and Miriam Zumwault, R.T.T. Also our thanks are tended to Colonel Kathleen Phillips, A.N.C., for help with the Emergency and Disaster Section. In addition, we acknowledge the help given by Ira Green, M.D.; Richard C. Rhame, M.D.; and H. Millard Smith, M.D. We are especially grateful to Mr. Bart Lippincott whose concept it was to consolidate the two parent texts and whose tact and experienced editorial guidance have been major factors in its achievement.

THE AUTHORS

Contents

PART ONE   Fundamentals of Medical and Surgical Nursing

UNIT I. The Patient: His Problems, His Needs and His Care   3

  1. The Patient and His Problems   3
    Problem-Solving   7
    The Team Approach to Patient Care   8
    Specific Areas of Nursing Responsibility   10
    The Planning of Patient Care   14

UNIT II. Preventive Aspects of Medical and Surgical Nursing   15

  2. Prevention of Disease   15
    Accomplishments and Challenges   15
    The Nurse's Role in Disease Prevention   15
    Environmental Health   17

  3. Defense of the Patient Against Infection   18
    The Reticuloendothelial System   18
    Immune Antibodies   19
    Inflammation   20
    Nursing Care of Local Inflammation   24
    Nursing Care of General Inflammation   29
    Wound Infections   31
    Staphylococcosis (Staphylococcus Infections)   33

  4. Antisepsis and Asepsis   36
    Development of Asepsis   36
    Principles of Sterilization—Definitions   37
    Heat Sterilization   37
    Radiant Energy Sterilization   45
    Gaseous Sterilization   45
    Chemical Methods of Disinfection—Antiseptics   45

UNIT III. The Clinical Study of the Patient   50

  5. Observation of the Patient   50
    Symptoms and Their Significance   50
    Detection and Recording of Physical Signs   51

  6. Diagnostic Studies in Clinical Evaluation   65
    The Nurse's Role in Diagnostic Procedures and Tests   65
    Examination of the Urine   65

6. Diagnostic Studies in Clinical Evaluation (*Continued*)
   Blood Chemistry: Proteins, Electrolytes, Absorbates
       and Metabolites   77
   Hematology: Examination of the Formed Blood Elements
       and Evaluation of Hemostasis   85
   Measurements of Cardiac and Pulmonary Function 94
   Stool Examination and Gastric Analysis 95
   Examination of the Cerebrospinal Fluid and Other
       Extravascular Fluids   97
   Roentgenologic Studies   100
   Radioisotope Tests   106

UNIT IV. **Therapeutic and Supportive Measures** 115

7. Promotion of Comfort and Relief of Symptoms   115
   Relief of Pain and Discomfort   115
   Therapeutic Rest   123
   The Patient in Pain   125

8. Psychological Considerations   129
   Effective Nurse-Patient Interaction   128
   Psychopharmacology   134
   Patients With Mental and Emotional Problems   136
   The Nurse and the Disturbed Patient   140

9. Nutritional Needs and Problems   145
   Food Guide ("The Basic Four")   143
   The Major Food Components   143
   Therapeutic Diets   150
   Patients With Nutritional Problems   151
   Problem Solving Activity   157
   Sources for Nutrition Education   157

10. Parenteral Therapy   159
    Body Water   159
    Methods of Administering Parenteral Fluids   169
    Pyrogenic Reactions to Fluid Therapy   171
    Nursing Supervision of Parenteral Therapy   172

11. Blood Transfusion   174
    The Nurse in the Donor Clinic   174
    Blood Groups and Blood Group Compatibility   177
    Transfusion Therapy   179
    Transfusion Complications   180
    Summary of the Problems of the Transfusion Recipient . . 184

12. Oxygen Inhalation Therapy   186
    Indications for Use   186
    Precautions to Observe in Handling Oxygen   186
    Methods of Oxygen Administration   187
    Complications and Hazards   190

13. Antimicrobial Chemotherapy   192
    Antibiotics   192
    Sulfonamides   196
    Isoniazid and Para-Amino-Salicylic Acid   197
    Quinolines, Emetine and Stilbamidine   198

UNIT V. The Patient With a Surgical Problem 201

   14. The Preoperative Patient 201
      Surgery in the Past 201
      Surgery at Present 201
      The Nurse and the Surgical Patient 204
      Preoperative Care 204
      The Patient's Family 215

   15. The Patient in the Operating Room: Anesthesia 219
      Reception and Greeting of the Patient 217
      The Anesthetist and the Patient 217
      Types of Anesthesia 220
      Position on Operating Table 231

   16. Operating Room Nursing 234
      Teamwork in the Operating Room 235
      Maintenance of Surgical Asepsis 235
      Technic of Scrubbing, Putting on Gown and Gloves 236
      Outline of Principles and Applications 238
      Surgical Draping 242
      Handling of Sterile Equipment by the Circulating Nurse 244
      Preparation of Tables for the Operation 246
      Ligatures and Sutures 249
      Immediately Before the Operation 251
      During the Operation 251
      Between Operations 258
      At the End of the Operative Schedule 259
      Safety Practices in the Operating Room 260
      Sterilization and Care of Various Articles 261

   17. The Postoperative Patient 271
      Recovery Room 271
      Removing Patient From Operating Table 272
      Principles of Immediate Postoperative Nursing Care 272
      Needs of the Patient Returning to Complete Consciousness 278
      Body Alignment and Good Body Mechanics 280
      Early Postoperative Ambulation 281
      Postoperative Diet 282
      Care of the Wound 283
      Charts and Nurses' Records 288

   18. Postoperative Discomforts, Complaints and Complications 291
      Postoperative Discomforts and Complaints 291
      Postoperative Complications 295

UNIT VI. Special Problems Common to Medical and Surgical Nursing . . . 309

   19. Cancer Nursing 309
      Introduction 309
      Classification of Cysts and Tumors 309
      Incidence of Various Malignancies 315
      The Nurse and the Cancer Patient 315
      Treatment of Neoplasms 316
      Psychological Aspects of Nursing the Cancer Patient 325
      Terminal Nursing Care 326
      The Follow-Through 328

20. Problems Associated With Aging and Long-Term Illness   330
   Modifying Factors   330
   Sociologic and Health Problems of the Aging   331
   The Nurse and the Elderly Patient   334
   Significant Characteristics of the Older Patient   335
   Surgery of the Elderly Patient   340
   Convalescence, Rehabilitation and Recreation   343
   Long-Term Illness   345
   Gravity of Prognosis   345

UNIT VII. Rehabilitation Nursing Concepts   349

21. Principles and Practices of Rehabilitation Nursing   349
   Philosophy of Rehabilitation   349
   The Rehabilitation Team   350
   Psychological Implications of a Disability   351
   Principles and Practices of Rehabilitation Nursing   351
   Clinical Situation   372

**PART TWO   Nursing Care of Patients With Specific Medical
           and Surgical Problems**

UNIT VIII. Patients With Conditions of the Respiratory Tract   376

22. Nursing in Conditions of the Nose and the Throat   376
   Anatomy of the Upper Respiratory Tract   376
   The Patient With Problems of the Nose   377
   The Patient With Sinusitis   381
   The Patient With Problems of the Pharynx and the Tonsils   382
   The Patient With Problems of the Larynx   386
   Specific Infections of the Upper Respiratory Tract   392
   Clinical Situation: The Patient With a Tracheostomy   395

23. Patients With Medical and Surgical Conditions of the Chest   397
   Anatomy and Physiology of the Lungs   397
   Pathologic Physiology of Respiration   399
   Diagnostic Studies in Thoracic Conditions   401
   Problems of Patients With Pulmonary Disorders   403
   Nursing Care of the Patient With Chest Surgery   408
   The Patient With a Pulmonary Infection   419
   The Patient With Pulmonary Emphysema   432
   The Patient With a Pulmonary Embolus   436
   Patients With Tumors of the Chest   438
   The Patient With an Aspirated Foreign Body in the Lung   440
   The Patient With Chest Injuries   441
   Clinical Situations   443
   Plan of Nursing Care   444
   Appraisal of Patient Needs   444

24. Patients With Pulmonary Tuberculosis   446
   Clinical Manifestations   446
   Miliary Tuberculosis   447
   Chronic Pulmonary Tuberculosis   447
   Clinical Situation   457

UNIT IX. Nursing Care in Hematologic and Cardiovascular Disorders . . . 459

    Orientation 459

25. Patients With Hematologic Disorders 460
    The Cellular Components of Normal Blood 460
    The Anemic Patient 461
    Hemolytic Disorders 466
    Hemoglobinopathies 468
    The Patient With Toxic Bone Marrow Depression 469
    The Patient With Polycythemia 471
    Patients With Leukemia and Lymphoma 471
    The Patient With a Bleeding Disorder 475
    Splenectomy 479
    Clinical Situations 481

26. Patients With Vascular Disorders 483
    Vascular Anatomy and Physiology 483
    Patients With Disorders of the Arteries and the Veins 485
    Nursing Care of the Patient With a Peripheral Vascular Problem . . 500
    The Patient With a Lymphatic Condition 503
    Clinical Situation 505

27. Patients With Conditions of the Heart 507
    The Nurse and Her Cardiac Patient 507
    Anatomic Features of the Heart and Normal Cardiac Function . . . 507
    Tests of Cardiac Function and Diagnostic Aids in Cardiac Disease . 508
    Cardiac Arrhythmias 508
    Patients With Coronary Artery Disease 518
    Patients With Endocardial Disease 523
    Patients With Myocarditis 532
    Patients With Pericarditis 533
    Patients With Aortic Disease 534
    The Patient in Congestive Heart Failure 540
    The Patient With Acute Pulmonary Edema 545
    Cardiovascular Surgery 548
    Cardiovascular Surgical Nursing 554
    Role of the Nurse in Preventing Heart Disease 561
    Clinical Situations 562

UNIT X. Nursing Care of Patients With Digestive Disorders 565

    Orientation 565

28. Patients With Conditions of the Lips, the Mouth and the Esophagus . . 571
    Conditions of the Lips 570
    Conditions of the Mouth 571
    Clinical Situation 584

29. Patients With Gastric and Intestinal Problems 586
    Terminology and Topography 586
    The Role of the Nurse in Gastrointestinal Diagnosis 588
    Gastric and Intestinal Intubation 591
    Problems Related to the Stomach and the Duodenum 594
    Problems Involving the Small and the Large Bowel 612
    Clinical Situations 643

30. Patients With Disorders of the Liver and the Biliary Tract 646
    Normal Structure and Function 646
    The Jaundiced Patient 649
    Special Problems of Patients With Disorders of the Liver 650
    Viral Hepatitis 653
    Toxic Hepatitis 654
    Liver Abscesses 654
    Hepatic Cirrhosis 655
    Hepatic Tumors 659
    The Patient With Gallbladder Disease and Biliary Obstruction . . . 662
    Clinical Situations 666
31. Patients With Disorders of the Pancreas 668
    The Patient With Acute Pancreatitis 668
    The Patient With Chronic Pancreatitis 669
    The Patient With Prancreatic Cysts 670
    The Patient With Pancreatic Tumors 670

UNIT XI. **Nursing in Conditions Involving the Kidneys, the Urinary Tract and the Reproductive System** 674
    Orientation 674
32. Patients With Renal and Genitourinary Problems 676
    Normal Structure and Function 676
    Examination of the Patient 678
    Problems Encountered 680
    Nursing Responsibilities 681
    Problems Affecting the Kidneys 683
    The Patient Having Kidney Surgery 697
    Problems Affecting the Bladder 699
    The Patient With Urinary Diversion 700
    Problems Affecting the Urethra 705
    Problems Related to the Male Reproductive System 706
    Clinical Situation 715
33. Female Patients With Conditions of the Reproductive System 717
    The Female Organs of Reproduction 717
    Gynecologic Examination of the Patient 719
    Disturbances of Menstruation 724
    The Menopausal State 724
    The Patient With a Gynecologic Problem 725
    Conditions of External Genitalia and Vagina 727
    Conditions of the Uterus 731
    Conditions of Ovaries and Broad Ligaments 738
    Conditions of Fallopian Tubes 738
    Pelvic Exenteration 740
    Clinical Situation 741
    Problem-Solving Activity 741

UNIT XIII. **Nursing in Conditions of the Integumentary System** 743
34. Patients With Dermatologic Problems 743
    Normal Skin 743
    Problems of the Dermatologic Patient 744
    Nursing Responsibilities in Dermatology 745

34. Patients With Dermatologic Problems (*Continued*)
Pigmentary Disorders 747
Secretory Disorders 750
Seborrheic Dermatoses 752
Traumatic Dermatoses 753
Infections and Infestations of the Skin 755
Dermatoses of Unknown or Nonspecific Etiology 762
Systemic Diseases With Dermatologic Manifestations . . . 765
Congenital Disorders of the Skin 768
Ulcers and Tumors of the Skin 768
Disorders Involving the Hair 771
Dermatologic Surgery and Plastic Reconstructive Surgery . . 772
Clinical Situation 780
35. Patients With Problems of the Breast 782
The Development of the Breast 782
Diseases of the Female Breast 782
Nursing Care of the Patient Having a Breast Operation . . 787
Clinical Situation 790
36. Patients With Burns 793
Problems of Burns 793
Causative Factors 793
Classification of Burns: First Aid Treatment 793
Medical and Nursing Management of the Burn Patient . . . 794
Clinical Situation 798

UNIT XIII. Nursing in Allergic Disorders 800
Orientation 800
37. Patients With Allergic Disorders 802
Hay Fever 802
Vasomotor Rhinitis 802
Bronchial Asthma 803
Anaphylactic Shock 805
Allergic Dermatoses 806
Gastrointestinal Allergy 809
Desensitization, Antihistaminics and Hormones in Allergy . . 811
Clinical Situations 811

UNIT XIV. Nursing in Metabolic Disorders 814
Orientation 814
38. Patients With Endocrine Conditions 816
The Thyroid Gland 816
The Parathyroid Glands 824
The Pancreas 826
The Adrenal Gland 838
The Pituitary Gland 845
Clinical Situations 848

UNIT XV. Nursing in Conditions of the Eye and the Ear . . . 850
39. Patients With Problems of the Eye 850
The Nurse and Eye Health 850
Anatomy and Physiology 851
Examinations and Diagnostic Procedures 853

39. Patients With Problems of the Eye (*Continued*)
  "Eye Glasses" and Contact Lenses 854
  Drugs Used Frequently in Eye Conditions 855
  Psychological and Physical Needs of the Eye Patient 857
  The Patient With Trauma to the Eye 860
  The Patient With an Inflammation of the Eye 864
  The Patient Having Eye Surgery 866
  The Nurse and the Newly Blind 872
  Clinical Situation 872

40. Patients With Problems of the Ear and the Mastoid 875
  Anatomy and Physiology 875
  General Hygiene of the Ear 876
  Patients With Problems of the External Ear 877
  Patients With Problems of the Middle Ear 878
  Patients With Problems of the Inner Ear 888
  Hearing Aids 888
  Communicating With a Person Who Has a Hearing Impairment . . 890

UNIT XVI. Nursing in Conditions of the Nervous System 892

  Orientation 892

41. Patients With Neurologic and Neurosurgical Problems 893
  Normal and Abnormal Anatomy and Physiology 893
  Assisting With the Neurologic Examination 907
  Special Problems of Neurologic and Neurosurgical Patients 913
  The Patient With a Headache 916
  The Patient With Increased Intracranial Pressure 920
  Febrile and Hypothermic Patients 921
  The Unconscious Patient 922
  Patients With Cranial, Spinal and Peripheral Neuropathies 923
  The Patient With A Cerebral Vascular Accident 931
  Patients With Brain Tumors and Aneurysms 941
  The Patient With Multiple Sclerosis 946
  Patients With Extrapyramidal Disease 949
  Patients With Cerebral Infection 951
  The Epileptic Patient 954
  Patients With Injuries of the Central Nervous System 959
  The Patient With Intractable Pain 976
  Clinical Situations 976

UNIT XVII. Nursing in Musculoskeletal Conditions 980

  Orientation 980

42. Patients With Musculoskeletal Problems 981
  Musculoskeletal Structures and Functions 981
  Patient Problems and Nursing Solutions 981
  Patients With Musculoskeletal Trauma 984
  The Patient With an Amputation 1013
  Patients With Bone and Joint Infections 1017
  Patients With Arthritis 1022
  The Patient With a Bone Tumor 1033
  Congenital Deformities 1035
  Developmental Defects 1039
  Osteomalacia and Osteoporosis 1042

42. Patients With Musculoskeletal Problems (*Continued*)
    Osteitis Deformans: Paget's Disease 1043
    Primary Muscular Dystrophies 1044
    Mysasthenia Gravis 1044
    Nursing Care of the Orthopedic Patient 1046
    Clinical Situations 1048

UNIT XVIII. Nursing in Communicable Infections 1051
    Orientation 1051
    Scope of Nursing Responsibilities 1051
    Immune Prophylaxis 1051
    Immune Therapy 1054
    Communicable Disease Nursing 1055
    Epidemiology of the Prevailing Communicable Infections 1060

43. Patients With Specific Bacterial Infections 1065
    Types of Bacteria 1065
    Scarlet Fever 1065
    Erysipelas 1068
    Diphtheria 1068
    Pertussis 1071
    Typhoid Fever 1072
    Paratyphoid Fever 1077
    Bacillary Dysentery (Shigellosis) 1078
    Brucellosis 1079
    Botulism 1079
    Gonorrhea 1080
    Meningococcal Meningitis 1081
    Influenzal Meningitis 1083
    Tularemia 1084
    Anthrax 1085
    Glanders 1085
    Asiatic Cholera 1085
    Bubonic Plague 1087
    Leprosy 1087

44. Patients With Viral Infections 1090
    Nature of Viruses 1090
    Measles 1090
    German Measles 1092
    Chickenpox 1093
    Smallpox 1094
    Mumps 1095
    Infectious Mononucleosis 1096
    Influenza 1097
    Poliomyelitis 1099
    Other Enteroviral Infections 1104
    Epidemic Pleurodynia 1105
    Epidemic Encephalitis 1105
    Lymphocytic Choriomeningitis 1108
    Rabies 1108
    Lymphogranuloma Inguinale 1109
    Dengue 1110
    Yellow Fever 1110

44. Patients With Viral Infections (*Continued*)
    Psittacosis 1111
    Foot-and-Mouth Disease 1112
45. Patients With Rickettsial Infections 1113
    Rickettsiae 1113
    Typhus Fever 1113
    Rocky Mountain Spotted Fever 1115
    Q Fever 1116
    Rickettsialpox 1116
    Trench Fever 1117
46. Patients With Protozoan Infections 1118
    Protozoa 1118
    Spirochetal Infections 1118
    Malaria 1126
    Amebiasis 1129
    Kala-azar 1130
    African Sleeping Sickness 1130
47. Patients With Systemic Mycoses 1131
    Actinomycosis 1131
    Histoplasmosis 1131
    North American Blastomycosis 1133
    Coccidiomycosis 1133
    Sporotrichosis 1133
    Cryptococcosis 1133
    Aspergillosis 1133
48. Patients With Parasitic Infestations 1135
    Filariasis 1135
    Trichinosis 1135
    Hookworm 1136
    Roundworm 1137
    Pinworm 1137
    Tapeworm 1137
    Hydatid Disease 1138
    Fluke Infestations: Distomiasis 1139
    Clinical Situation 1142

PART THREE   Nursing Care of Patients Under Emergency and
             Disaster Conditions

49. Emergency and Disaster Nursing 1149
    Orientation 1149
    The Meaning of Disaster 1149
    Nursing Responsibilities in Relation to Wartime Emergencies . . . 1149
    Psychological Management of Patients in
        Emergency-Disaster Situations 1150
    Principles of Emergency Care 1151
    Accident Prevention 1166
    Improvisation and Resourcefulness 1170
    Clinical Situation 1170

APPENDIX 1175

INDEX 1181

PART ONE

Fundamentals of Medical
and Surgical Nursing

1

The Patient and His Problems

Nursing is a service devoted to the prevention and the relief of physical suffering. Inherent in nursing is the control of disease, the care and rehabilitation of the sick and the promotion of health through teaching and counseling. The nurse, applying her technical knowledge, experience and skill, combats the physical disabilities of her patients; and through the contribution of her wisdom and insight, she assists them to overcome their emotional difficulties.

The central figure in and the principal object of these services is, of course, the patient. The patient comes to the hospital as an individual, a member of a family and a citizen of the community. He comes with a health problem and is laden, in addition, with a number of personal concerns that have been exaggerated and compounded by illness. Confronting him, perhaps, are problems that he feels are at once inescapable and insurmountable; problems that demand a solution but are incapable of solution; problems for which he feels solely responsible, which he is reluctant to share and refuses to delegate. He may be wholly absorbed in problems that are of minor consequence while dismissing others that truly are of paramount importance relative to his illness, which may bear, for example, on the prevention of complications or recurrences of his disease, or on the pursuit of his rehabilitation. As a potential source of frustration and anxiety and as an impediment to recovery, these personal problems naturally are of concern to the nurse; and to help her patient to sort them out, reduce them to their essentials, place them in proper perspective and cope with them effectively is one of her important functions.

The nurse, by virtue of her proximity and accessibility to the patient, is in a position to discover and identify his problems, to establish his needs and to plan his care appropriately. And while directing her attention to the problems of immediate importance—the overt problems—she must be ever alert to sense the subtle, unexpressed needs of her patient, needs that may be influencing his behavior and may be producing, or at least modifying, his symptoms.

The Patient's Symptoms

From the standpoint of the symptomatic patient, the most important problem confronting him is his major symptom. If he is gasping for breath, his most pressing need is to be relieved of his respiratory distress. Dyspnea is his primary problem. The nurse must undertake to evaluate this symptom and alleviate it.

If she is to deal with this problem effectively she must understand correctly the pathologic physiology underlying her patient's dyspnea. Is it caused by pulmonary congestion? by pneumonia? by pleurisy? or by asthma? Does the patient have respiratory obstruction? Should he be placed in an orthopneic position? or in low Fowler's position? or should he lie flat? Should he be receiving oxygen? Is he in need of tracheal suction? Is a tracheotomy likely to be required? Should a sedative be administered, or is sedative medication strictly contraindicated in this patient? Close scrutiny of an occasional patient might convince the nurse that his breathing, although abnormally rapid and deep, is not attended by discomfort and does not involve undue effort. In other words, this particular patient is not dyspneic but hyperpneic. Hyperpnea is a different symp-

3

TABLE 1. Estimated Death Rates for the 10 Leading Causes of Death: United States, 1961*

Rank	Cause of Death	Death Rate per 100,000 Population	Per Cent of Total Deaths
	ALL CAUSES.........................	930.3	100.0
1	Diseases of the heart....................	365.2	39.3
2	Malignant neoplasms, including those of lymphatic and hematopoietic tissues.......	147.5	15.9
3	Vascular lesions affecting central nervous system...............................	105.1	11.3
4	Accidents............................	50.7	5.5
5	Certain diseases of early infancy...........	36.6	3.9
6	Influenza and pneumonia, except pneumonia of the newborn......................	29.8	3.2
7	General arteriosclerosis..................	19.0	2.0
8	Diabetes mellitus.......................	15.8	1.7
9	Congenital malformations................	11.5	1.2
10	Other diseases of the circulatory system......	11.4	1.2
	All other causes........................	137.7	14.8

* U. S. Department of Health, Education, and Welfare, Monthly Vital Statistics Report, Annual Summary, 1961, vol. 10, no. 13, Washington (D.C.), U. S. Government Printing Office, 1962.

tom altogether, and the problems it entails are quite different from those of dyspnea. Is this a case of hysterical hyperventilation? or diabetic acidosis? or has this patient been poisoned? On the appropriate answers to these and to a host of other pertinent questions may hinge the correctness of diagnosis, the effectiveness of treatment and, in many instances, the very survival of such a patient.

Every step in the care of the patient represents a team effort, as will be discussed later; and a key member of the medical team that is charged with this responsibility is the professional nurse. Among the most important of her contributions to this joint effort are her clinical observations. To what extent these observations are significant, informative and helpful depends on how well she knows and understands symptoms. Confronted with one, she must be able to recognize it as a pathologic deviation from the normal. Moreover, she should be able to relate the abnormal manifestation to the particular organ system whence it is likely to have originated and accordingly which might be the site of disease. Details concerning the nature, the mechanism and the significance of specific symptoms and other nursing observations are discussed in later chapters of this text.

Her knowledge of symptomatology and of causative factors, treatment and prevention as well should extend to all of the common medical and surgical conditions. Most of the serious illnesses she will encounter will represent various stages of the diseases listed in Table 1, specifying the leading causes of death in the United States. Table 2, listing the principal causes of death in 14 countries with comparable health programs, demonstrates that similar diseases challenge health workers throughout the world.

The Patient's Basic Needs

Common to all human beings are certain needs that are basic and demand satisfaction. Unfulfilled needs in this category are among the patient's most pressing problems. These differ in their urgency; as each is satisfied, a "higher" one emerges and takes precedence. Ranked in order of priority* they include the following: physiologic needs; safety needs; the need to belong; need for recognition, esteem and affection; the need to create; need for knowledge and comprehension; and aesthetic needs.

Physiologic Needs. These needs predominate in the motivation of human behavior and drive the mechanisms that maintain *homeostasis*—the constancy of the internal environment of an organism. It involves the

* Maslow, A. H.: Motivation and Personality, New York, Harper, 1954.

TABLE 2. Ten Principal Causes of Death in the Modern World

	U. S.	Canada	Germany	Denmark	Finland	France	Norway	Nether- lands	England & Wales	Scot- land	Northern Ireland	Sweden	Switzer- land	Australia
Heart diseases..........	1	1	1	1	1	1	1	1	1	1	1	1	1	1
Malignant neoplasms.....	2	2	2	2	2	2	2	2	2	2	2	2	2	2
Vascular lesions.........	3	3	3	3	3	3	3	3	3	3	3	3	3	3
All accidents...........	4	4	4	4	4	4	4	4	6	4	6	5	4	4
Pneumonia.............	5	5	5	6	6	5	5	5	5	6	4	4	5	5
Birth injuries...........	6	6		7	9		10	8		9	9			10
Diabetes...............	7	9	10			10		7						8
Congenital malformations...	8	7		9	10	9	9	6		10	7	9	9	9
Nephritis and nephrosis....	9	8			8	7	8	10	10			7		6
Cirrhosis of liver........	10		9			6	6						10	
Tuberculosis...........		10	6		5	8				7	8	8		
Suicide...............			7	5	7				9			6	7	
Bronchitis.............			8					9	4	5	5		6	
Hyperplasia of prostate.....				8										
Hypertension without mention of heart..............							7		7					7
Ulcer of stomach and duodenum.............									8	8	10	10		
Influenza..............													8	
Benign neoplasms.........				10										

World Health Organization, Division of Public Information, Palais des Nations, Geneva, Switzerland, Jan.-Feb., 1960.

regulation of respiratory, nutritive and excretory functions, as well as maintenance of the water content of tissues, adjustments of body temperature and the operation of numerous protective mechanisms. These needs are powerful; unless satisfied, they dominate the conscious mind. For example, if, a patient is obliged to restrict his fluid intake for therapeutic reasons, thirst will absorb his thoughts. He may discuss nothing but drinking, complain incessantly of thirst and repeatedly question his nurse and physician as to when fluids will be forthcoming. During this period he is not likely to be too concerned about the aesthetic features of his environment. As soon as his thirst is quenched he becomes aware of other needs; now he may be disturbed by the absence of privacy.

Safety Needs. If the physiologic needs are satisfied, the concern for safety emerges. The normal adult is able to protect himself and usually does not feel endangered. He is relatively "safe" from death. His job is "safe." His insurance program and his savings account furnish a sense of economic security.

Illness naturally poses a threat. The sick person may be apprehensive in response to the many different persons with unfamiliar functions who enter his room. Diagnostic tests and therapeutic procedures may contribute to his fears. He wants to feel safe and secure. Although he may not express his feelings in these terms, he wants the health team to be aware of his insecurity. In order to help to protect the patient from danger the nurse must know the nature of his illness and be cognizant of its possible complications, so that she may be in a position to forestall the latter, if they are preventable, and to supply intelligent care if they should occur. The nurse's role in promoting the psychological safety of the patient is discussed in Chapter 8.

Need for Affection and Recognition. His physiologic and safety needs having been satisfied, the patient's need for affection will become apparent. Every individual, sick or well, desires the companionship and recognition of others. A sick person wants and needs his family or, in its absence, friends, or even just friendliness. The wise nurse is constantly aware of this need and of its importance in relation to her patient's morale. She

will help the family members to feel that they have a definite contribution to make to his recovery. She will seek relevant information from them concerning his habits, his preferences and his antipathies, and will be guided by this information to whatever extent may be possible.

Man is by nature a social being, abhorring isolation. Illness removes him from his relatively convivial world and transplants him into a strange environment, an environment that is entirely unsought and unfamiliar, one in which he feels incompetent and alone. Previously an actively contributing member of society, he now must accept a position of useless dependency with the risk of becoming a nonentity. This patient needs to preserve his self-esteem. He needs to be recognized as an individual, a distinct personality. The professional nurse, imbued with the concept of the individual worth and the dignity of man, sees to it that this need is fulfilled. She takes time to listen to her patient. To the extent that he desires it and opportunity permits it she joins him in conversation. She exhibits interest, not only in matters that concern her, but also in all matters that seem important to him — her attentiveness, thoughtfulness and kindliness conveying the conviction that he is held in esteem and affection, and that his needs and problems are recognized.

The Creative Impulses. His physiologic needs having been compensated, feeling secure, esteemed and wanted, the patient's creative impulses may now emerge. During the course of a short hospital stay this need is not likely to be frustrated. However, the patient with a protracted illness must be assured an opportunity to express himself creatively and to be, or at least feel, useful.

The Need to Know and to Understand. This need is a strong drive. The intelligent person seeks information, organizes it, analyzes it and searches for its meaning. In general, patients want to know what is in store for them, and they are thwarted by explanations that are too brief or vague. Many have studied and know a surprising amount concerning the bodily functions. However, while some of their information may be factual more of it is likely to be erroneous, and correction or clarification is usually necessary.

Their instruction is the responsibility of the nurse, and the teaching of patients, one of the most responsible functions of her profession. To teach correctly and effectively the nurse must have a thorough knowledge of her subject, be skilled in communication and cognizant of the basic mechanisms of learning. Her explanations, while simple for the sake of comprehension, at the same time must be meaningful if they are to be accepted.

Much of her instruction will refer to specific tests or treatments that are in prospect, describing the technical steps that are involved, the sensations likely to be experienced and the after-effects to be anticipated, and specifying what the patient can do to facilitate the procedure, minimize his discomfort and reduce complications. Of course, when discussing anything with her patient the nurse must take into consideration his physical and emotional status, his intelligence, his experience as a patient and his awareness of the situation, as well as the urgency of his need to know and understand. She also must consider the possible implications of her intended remarks and guard with equal care against inaccuracies on her part and misunderstandings on the part of the patient.

Aesthetic Needs. These needs vary in importance from individual to individual, but for all patients the most salutary environment is one that is orderly and one in which there is beauty. The patient with acute aesthetic sensibilities will be acutely distressed by unpleasant sights, sounds and odors, and intolerant of disarray. He may crave flowers, books or music, and when supplied, these amenities add immeasurably to his well being.

Concluding this discussion, it may be pointed out that most of the needs of the average individual, ill or well, can be satisfied only in part. Moreover, the nurse whose responsibility and privilege it is to help the patient to meet his problems must recognize the fact that some problems can be neither eliminated nor solved. In relation to the patient with such a problem her role is to help him to make a mature, objective and compensatory adjustment to its continued existence or to its imperfect solution, if this solution is the best that can be achieved.

PROBLEM-SOLVING

The following are the basic steps in the solution of problems:

Identification of the Problem. The nurse should learn everything possible about the patient before she makes her initial contact. While caring for him she should heed his remarks attentively, observe him closely for symptoms, note his reactions in response to each therapy and ferret out his needs, including those that are unexpressed but that his behavior may reflect.

Collection of Data. All information pertaining to the patient and his illness should be assembled and organized for analysis. Relevant data are likely to be available in the clinical chart, recorded in the patient's medical, social and family history, the description of physical findings, the physician's progress notes, the nurse's records and the laboratory reports. Every member of the health team is in a position to contribute personal observations that may bear on the problems under consideration. All possible sources of information should be utilized.

Establishing the Hypothesis. The hypothesis refers to a proposed solution to a specific problem—a solution that is tentative and that is put to the test. For example, if an elderly patient reportedly becomes confused and noisy each night, and only at night, the health team might postulate that this individual is stirred to apprehension in response to the dark and unfamiliar environment of his hospital room. The solution of the problem may depend on improved illumination. Accordingly, it is recommended that an extra night light be installed. This device may fail; the patient may continue to exhibit panic and struggle to get out of bed. In this event it may be planned that the night nurse will assist him from bed, install him in an arm chair, make him comfortable with feet and legs supported on a stool and remain in attendance until he has become adjusted to his new situation. Should his agitation persist notwithstanding, a member of his family might then be contacted and urged to stay with him during the night. Meanwhile, the physician will explore the possibility that the patient may be reacting atypically and adversely to some drug he has been receiving —perhaps a hypnotic that has been prescribed at bedtime. Thus, instead of resorting to a temporary and, possibly, dangerous expedient, such as the application of restraints or the administration of heavy sedation to control this patient's nocturnal agitation, a solution to his problem is sought that will correct his basic need and therefore be most likely to achieve permanent success—a solution, in short, that is based on imaginative planning and constructive nursing action.

Evaluation of Hypothetical Solution. The final step in problem solving is to test the hypothesis, translating it into action, observing its effectiveness and thereby establishing its validity. Have the proposed actions influenced the situation in any way? Have they solved the problem? Has the solution proved beneficial? The observations and the conclusions of the nurse may be analyzed and the situation as a whole explored most fruitfully in a team conference.

Problem Exercise

Select a patient for study. While caring for him, converse with him; listen to him closely; observe him carefully.

1.   What are his major symptoms?
2.   What complaints does he voice? How are they expressed?
3.   What needs does he express? What needs, although unexpressed, do you surmise are present in addition?
4.   Summarize the patient's primary problem, or problems, according to your analysis of the situation.
5.   What could be done or said that might help to fulfill this patient's needs?
6.   What nursing activities might be suggested to support the patient?

THE TEAM APPROACH TO PATIENT CARE

The professions devoted to healing constitute an organized team in which numerous and diverse arts, sciences and industries function in co-ordinated and mutually dependent roles. Those individuals and institutions engaged in the health professions serve in the greatest of all enterprises—the relief

and the prevention of suffering, the improvement of human effectiveness, both social and economic, and the prolongation of life. Key personnel are the practicing nurses and the physicians who, for the furtherance of these objectives, have elected to accept responsibilities of the gravest sort. Few disciplines are as demanding. The labors of nursing and medicine are extremely taxing; many of their problems are not solved easily, but the rewards are correspondingly great. Opportunities for effective contributions never end, and the value of each successful accomplishment is immediately or eventually obvious.

The Health Team

Whether a particular project is designed to provide relief from intractable pain suffered by one individual or to protect an entire population from a variety of communicable diseases, its success depends on the contributions of innumerable practitioners, past as well as present, representing many areas of endeavor.

Those responsible for actually executing the mission of the entire vast medical organization are, however, members of the health team, or, more specifically, the professional nurses, the practicing physicians, the occupational therapists, the physical therapists, the nutritionists, the social workers, the practical nurses and the auxiliary employees. Through their teamwork the fruits of scientific investigation and the technical achievements are distributed. On them depend the successful accomplishments of the medical profession as a whole. Obviously, were it not for the endeavors and the accomplishments of these members, medical science could be classed as little more than an academic exercise, devoid of any acute sense of obligation or high responsibility—a sterile pursuit motivated by intellectual curiosity, perhaps, but certainly not by compassion.

The responsibility for patient care is a communal one, whether shared by many, as in hospital practice, or by few. The principal participants are the professional nurse and the physician; their roles are interdependent and mutually complementary, each bearing a well-defined portion of the responsibility. The physician evaluates each individual case on the basis of the medical history, the

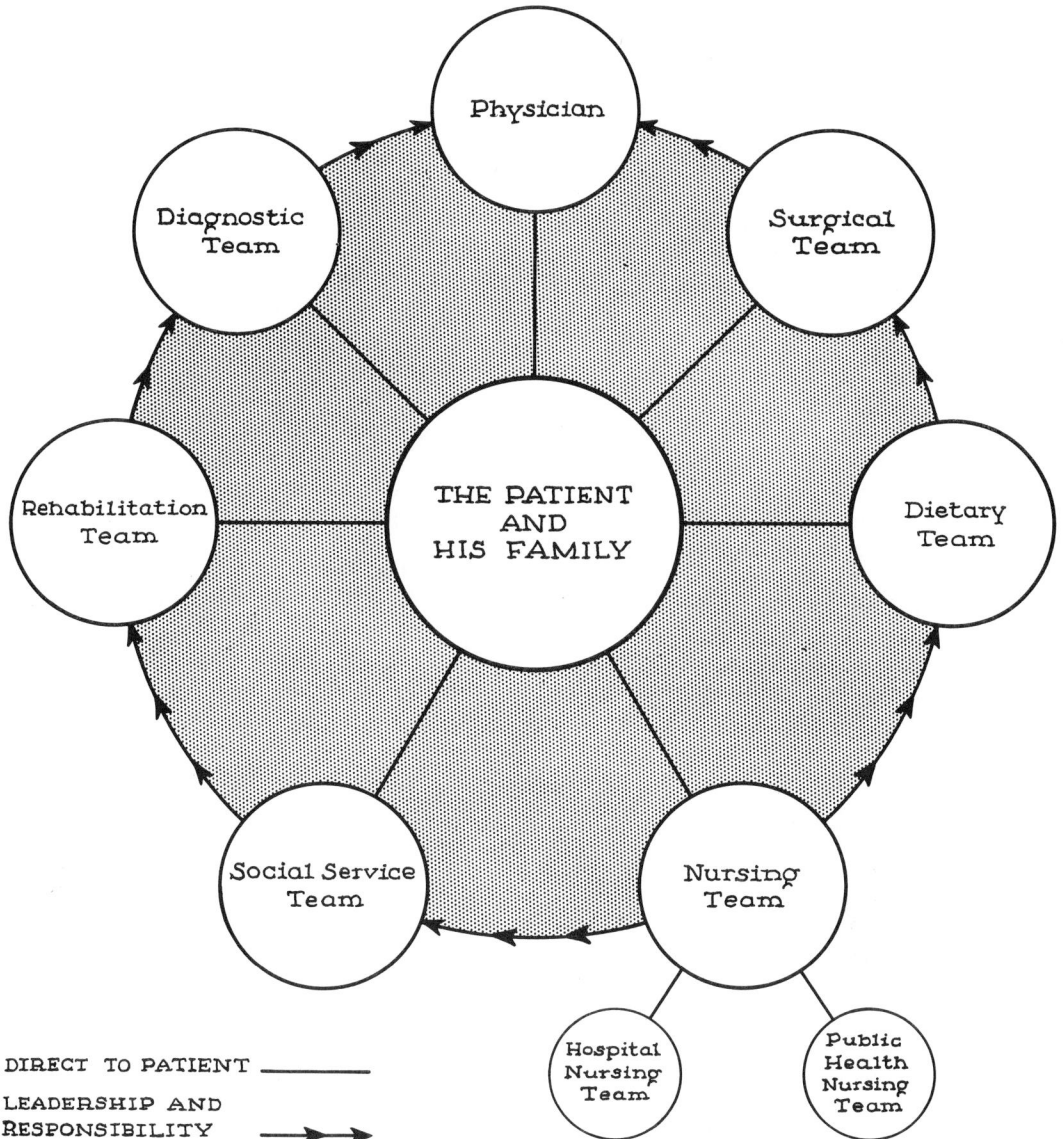

DIRECT TO PATIENT _____

LEADERSHIP AND
RESPONSIBILITY ⟶

FIG. 1. The team approach to patient care.

course of the disease, the physical examination of the patient and a laboratory investigation. He then outlines the therapeutic program which he considers is indicated and performs whatever technical procedures may require his personal participation. The physician's decisions regarding treatment require implementation, of course, or they are worthless. Implementation, through the actual performance of the prescribed treatment, is one of the functions of nursing.

The Nursing Team

Team nursing, as the term implies, refers to the care of patients by an organized group of nursing personnel, rather than by an individual nurse. Nursing duties are apportioned among a team, the members of which represent various levels of training and competence, and which is so constituted as to provide optimum nursing care with maximum efficiency. Comprising the team are professional nurses, nursing students, nursing aides and orderlies. To each of these individuals specific responsibilities are delegated that are in keeping with his or her educational background and experience.

The *team leader* is responsible for planning and evaluating the care of each patient. She delegates responsibilities and assigns specific duties to the personnel in her charge. She guides and supports the activities of every team member. The major decisions are hers.

The functions of the *professional nurse* are determined largely by the needs of the patient and the nature of his problems. She undertakes the care of patients whose conditions are complex, requiring judicious decisions, experienced teaching or advanced nursing skills. In addition, she assists the other team members in the care of their patients.

The *nursing student* participates to an extent commensurate with her education and in a manner that should prove of mutual benefit to her and to the patients whose care she is assigned.

The role of the *practical nurse* is dictated by her educational background, clinical experience and individual competence, and by the needs of the team. The *aides* and *orderlies* perform the functions for which they are trained. Each member has a distinctive contribution to make to the patient's care and to the smooth functioning of the team.

For each patient a *nursing-care plan* is composed and written, the purpose of which is to co-ordinate all activities of the team that relate to him. Such a plan provides complete assurance that no facet of his care will be overlooked, that he will receive individualized care from nursing personnel at all levels and that there will be continuity of care from hour to hour, and from day to day. Incorporated in the plan are all relevant nursing observations and judgments. Problems and their solutions are described. Relevant information from the patient and his family is included. Supplemental data are inscribed by the team leader on each tour of duty. Serving, as it does, to facilitate communications between members of the team and to acquaint them thoroughly with their patient, his problems and his needs, the care plan proves a tremendous asset to the nursing

personnel, and a device that is correspondingly advantageous for the patient.

The *team conference* serves as a "clearing house" for the exchange of information concerning each patient. Such a conference is scheduled daily, and usually is held as soon as possible after the completion of the major portion of the patient's care. The team leader inscribes pertinent notations on the nursing-care plan, revising the latter according to the suggestions offered and the solutions proposed at the conference. Thus, the patient benefits promptly and directly from the combined observations, the cumulative knowledge and the joint problem-solving ability of the several team members, all of whom are operating in concert to provide nursing care of the highest possible quality.

SPECIFIC AREAS OF NURSING RESPONSIBILITY

The scope of nursing responsibility includes far more than the conduct of prescribed technical therapeutic maneuvers and hygienic procedures. By virtue of her intimate contact with the sick, the voice of the nurse, so far as her patients are concerned, is likely to be interpreted by the patient as the voice of the medical profession. Therefore, she must be competent to serve as a coeducator. The psychological aspects of illness may present complex problems of far-reaching significance. The nurse can often facilitate the recognition, hence the solution, of such problems. Being in the most favorable position to make prolonged and close observations of the patient, and being skilled in the recognition and the reporting of clinical signs, the nurse can make a valuable contribution to the treatment of the patient in accurate observation and intelligent reporting.

These are responsibilities of a very high order, presupposing a formidable mass of factual information in the possession of the nurse who undertakes them. Disease states are understandable only when considered in relation to normal structures and processes, and clinical signs and symptoms can be interpreted reliably only if one is aware of the mechanisms responsible for their production. Reliable clinical observation depends on a working knowledge of the basic physical and social sciences, as well as experience in the nursing arts. Because of their importance in relation to the quality of nursing care, considerable data of morphologic, physiologic, biochemical and psycho-social significance have been incorporated in this text, in conjunction with discussions of specific clinical problems.

Observing the Patient

One of the most important of the nurse's duties is the accurate recording of all pertinent data relating to the patient, the course of his illness and his responses to treatment. Many of these data are secured as a matter of routine — for example, measurements of the body temperature, pulse and respiratory rates, and the timing of defecation. In connection with particular patients, additional information may be requested relative to the body weight, the arterial blood pressure, volumes of fluid ingested and voided, or the volume of sputum expectorated each day. Unusual and unpredicted developments, such as the onset of vomiting, stupor or disorientation, the appearance of a skin rash, blood in the urine or stool, or jaundice, are invariably important and must be recorded in complete detail. Indeed, any unusual observation should be regarded as potentially significant and therefore deserving of a full and accurate description.

Detailed observation of the patient at the time of admission and continually thereafter is the responsibility of the nurse. She must be acutely aware of this responsibility, recognizing the importance of observing and recording not only symptoms and physical signs but the patient's emotional reactions as well. She may find it appropriate to question certain patients and discuss with them specific aspects of their illness or their general situation that might affect their current progress or impede their convalescence. Any new information of possible pertinence so uncovered should be relayed promptly to the attending physician and incorporated in the patient's record.

Promoting a Therapeutic Nurse-Patient Relationship

An understanding of one's self, what one means to the patient and what the patient means to the nurse is basic for satisfactory interaction. Very early in her contact with the patient, the nurse needs to know the effect of illness and hospitalization on the patient. C. R. Rogers, Professor of Psychology, University of Chicago, expressed his hypothesis of human relationships in this manner:

If I can create a relationship characterized on my part:

By a genuineness and transparency, in which I *am* my real feelings,

By a warm acceptance of and liking for the other person as a separate individual,

By a sensitive ability to see his world and himself as he sees them,

Then the other individual in the relationship:

Will experience and understand aspects of himself which previously he has repressed,

Will find himself becoming better integrated, better able to function effectively,

Will become more similar to the person he would like to be,

Will be more self-directing and self-confident,

Will become more of a person, more nearly unique, and more self-expressive,

Will be able to cope with the problems of life more adequately and more comfortably.*

Teaching the Patient

The attitudes accompanying simple comfort skills are needed for therapy, too, but in addition there is needed in therapy an important attitude of expectation—expectation that the patient will purposefully participate in his own recovery, will focus his own energy and spirit on the goals of therapy.

The patient is informed of the therapeutic goals and his co-operation sought in attaining them. Here, too, the nurse needs facts to impart, judgment as to what and when to inform, and the proper accompanying attitude.†

In the past one of the weaknesses with regard to the care of the patient has been in offering him the kind of assistance necessary to carry on when he leaves the hospital environment. Throughout this text a concerted

* Rogers, C. R.: A counseling approach to human problems, Am. J. Nursing **56**:997, 1956.
† Leone, L. P.: Design for nursing, Am. J. Nursing **54**:731, 1954.

effort has been made to emphasize this important aspect of care. At the end of the chapters on the clinical areas, a list of patient teaching aids are given; however, it must be understood that merely to hand a patient a list of instructions or a brochure is not enough. He must be prepared to absorb and practice that which he needs to know. The following guide is offered to assist in the nurse's instruction of patients.

*A Guide to Teaching the Patient**

A. Approaching the Learning Situation.
  1. Readiness for learning.
    a. The need to learn exists, but does the patient recognize this need?
       (a) Is the patient ready physically from the physician's point of view?
       (b) Is he psychologically ready?
    b. Are there other problems more important to him at this time that take priority?
  2. Content.
    a. What do I know or need to know about this patient and his disease or condition?
    b. How much does the patient already know and what more does he need to know? (Consult with physician.)
  3. Factors affecting the patient's learning ability.
    a. How does his educational experiences or occupation affect or influence the learning process?
    b. What adaptations must be made because of his cultural or religious background?
    c. What economic factors should be considered?
    d. Will his illness affect his ability to learn?
    e. Where would be the best place for the patient to learn? Is this place optimal?

B. Selection of Teaching Methods.
  1. To begin with, ascertain from the patient his understanding and needs regarding the problem.

* In collaboration with Martha E. Warstler, formerly Dir. School of Nursing, Reid Memorial Hospital and School of Nursing, Richmond, Ind.

  2. Select materials and methods appropriate to the level of the particular patient.
    a. Discussion.
    b. Demonstration and use of equipment.
    c. Charts, pamphlets and other visual aids.
    d. Return demonstration.
    e. Consider modifications necessary for patient in order to perform effectively in his own environment with his own equipment. Suggest improvisations.
  3. What other resources, such as dietitian, physical therapist and so forth, might be helpful?
  4. Ascertain how much can be taught in a given period of time.
  5. Provide time for questions and offer encouragement.
  6. Learning is facilitated if the patient knows "why" he is doing something as well as "how" to do it.

C. Evaluation and Referral.
  1. Provide opportunity for the patient to practice and to ask questions.
  2. If he has problems or questions when he is at home, provide him with the sources he can contact, e.g., visiting nurse association, his physician, voluntary agencies, the hospital clinic.

Communicating With Others

In order to communicate effectively with patients, the nurse needs to know how and when to listen, to recognize and evaluate patient's feelings, to communicate supportive attitudes, to ask and answer questions, to manipulate conversation into desired channels and to recognize the high communication value of touch, manner, expression and attitude. The nurse will recognize that when an ill person moves from the routine activities of a busy world into the very different atmosphere of a hospital, in many instances he tends to exaggerate what he feels, sees and hears. Fears often are responsible for this change. By communicating effectively with the patient, the nurse assures that his understanding will be broader and his misconceptions and fears will be reduced.

SAMPLE NURSING CARE PLAN

Name: JONES, MRS. J.J.   Marital Status: MARRIED   Age: 56

Admission Date: 2/23   Occupation: CLERK (PART TIME)   Religion: PROTESTANT

Diagnosis: PULMONARY EDEMA
CONGESTIVE HEART
FAILURE
    Hospitalization
Insurance: YES - #CN2264   Physician: DR. JAMES GRAY

DATE	PATIENT'S PROBLEMS	NURSING MANAGEMENT
2/23	DYSPNEA	ORTHOPNEIC POSITION. WELL SUPPORTED ABSOLUTE BED REST — INCLUDING BATHING AND FEEDING
	EXTREME APPREHENSION AND RESTLESSNESS	O₂ (POSITIVE PRESSURE) DISCONTINUED AT 7:30 P.M.
		ROTATING TOURNIQUETS DISCONTINUED AT 7:45 P.M. NOTE REACTION AFTER SEDATION IS GIVEN (q. 4 H.) CALL DR. GRAY IF RESTLESSNESS CONTINUES.
2/24	COMPLAINING OF DRY MOUTH	ORAL HYGIENE q. 3H. (ALTERNATE DOBEL'S SOL, HYDROGEN PEROXIDE AND LAVORIS — AS MOUTH WASH)
	ASKING FOR NURSE TO "STAY WITH ME"	REQUEST VOLUNTEER TO READ TO PT. DURING AFTERNOONS (FAMILY UNABLE TO COME DURING AFTERNOON VISITING HOUR).
		T.V. SET TO BE BROUGHT FROM PT'S HOME TONIGHT (PERMISSION HAS BEEN OBTAINED FROM DR. GRAY)
		"VISIT" WITH PT. AS FREQUENTLY AS POSSIBLE.
2/25	TENDERNESS OF RT. CALF NOTED DURING BATH.	ELASTIC COMPRESSION BANDAGES TO BOTH LEGS (RE-WRAP 9 A.M. AND P.M)
		PASSIVELY / ACTIVELY MOVE LEGS QUADRICEPS SETTING EXERCISES — q.I.D. ENCOURAGE DEEP BREATHING 5-10 TIMES q.H.
2/26	VERBALIZING THAT "I'M AFRAID I'LL HAVE ANOTHER ATTACK WHEN I GO HOME" — FEARS THAT TAKING "SO MANY PILLS WILL BECOME A HABIT".	REASSURE PT. THAT THE FOLLOWING WILL HELP PREVENT FUTURE "ATTACKS" A. TAKING DIGITALIS DAILY AS ORDERED B. TAKING DIURETIC AS ORDERED C. KEEPING WEIGHT GRAPH D. REPORTING TO DR. GRAY'S OFFICE WEEKLY AS SCHEDULED DIETITIAN TO REVIEW LOW SODIUM DIET WITH PATIENT VISITING NURSE TO SEE PT. TWICE WEEKLY.
		REFERRED TO HOME MAKER SERVICE. (FAMILY HAVE TALKED WITH DR. GRAY AND DIETITIAN. SEEM TO UNDERSTAND PT.'S CONDITION.)

Directing the Work of Others

Because of the central position which the nurse occupies in the many-faceted attentions which the patient receives, it is essential that the nurse learn how to direct the work of others and how to act in a liaison position as all efforts are coordinated. This involves experience in planning, assigning, teaching, supervising and evaluating.

THE PLANNING OF PATIENT CARE

The essential elements of nursing that must be considered in planning the care of every patient include the following:

1. Identification of the patient's problems and needs;
2. The provision of safety and comfort;
3. The maintenance of proper hygiene, adequate nutrition, correct fluid and electrolyte balance, and satisfactory elimination;
4. Suitable control of physical activity with optimum apportionment of exercise, rest and sleep;
5. The prevention of deformities and assisting in their correction;
6. The recognition and the modification of undesirable emotional reactions;
7. The arranging and utilization of effective communications; and,
8. The promotion of a therapeutic nurse-patient relationship.

BIBLIOGRAPHY AND SELECTED READING

Books

Abdellah, F., Beland, I., Martin, A., and Matheney, R.: Patient-Centered Approaches to Nursing, New York, Macmillan, 1960.

Kron, T.: Nursing Team Leadership, Philadelphia, Saunders, 1961.
Lambertson, E. C.: Nursing Team Organization and Functioning, New York, Bureau of Publications, Teachers College, Columbia University, 1953.
Maslow, A. H.: Motivation and Personality, New York, Harper, 1954.
Newcomb, D. P.: The Team Plan, New York, Putnam, 1953.
Peplau, H.: Interpersonal Relations in Nursing, New York, Putnam, 1952.

Articles

A.N.A. Committee on Allied Nursing Personnel: Auxiliary personnel in nursing service, Am. J. Nursing 62:72-73, July, 1962.
Brooks, E. A.: Team nursing—1961, Am. J. Nursing 61:87-91, April, 1961.
Brozenhard, J., and Fitt, W.: The staff nurse speaks for the nursing team, Am. J. Nursing 53:425-426, 1953.
Holmes, M.: The need to be recognized, Am. J. Nursing 61:86-87, Oct., 1961.
Ingles, T.: Do patients feel lost in a general hospital? Am. J. Nursing 60:648-651, 1960.
Ingles, T.: Understanding the nurse-patient relationship, Nursing Outlook 9:698-700, 1961.
Johnson, D. E.: The significance of nursing care, Am. J. Nursing 61:63-66, Nov., 1961.
Larsen, V. L.: What hospitalization means to patients, Am. J. Nursing 61:44-47, May, 1961.
Sawyer, J.: The nursing team and student education, Am. J. Nursing 54:953, 1954.
Wasson, E. E.: A team leader's day, Am. J. Nursing 55:1470-1471, 1955.

Periodicals:

World Health, Columbia University Press, International Documents Service, 2960 Broadway, New York 27, New York.

2

Prevention of Disease

ACCOMPLISHMENTS AND CHALLENGES

Since the turn of the century the mortality rate throughout the world has declined steadily and the average life span has increased, largely due to the successful control of many infectious diseases. Improvements in nutrition likewise have contributed significantly to the well-being of populations everywhere. Our environment unquestionably has become safer and more healthful. However, new problems are arising constantly. For example, traumatic accidents have become a major cause of death between the ages of 1 and 34 years.

As the average life span has increased, there has been a corresponding increase in the prevalence of chronic diseases. Cardiovascular disease and cancer now are responsible for over 70 per cent of the deaths in the United States. Ten per cent of this country's population are afflicted with chronic disease of one type or another. The resultant drain on individual economic and community resources is tremendous.

More than 50 per cent of the hospital beds in this country are occupied by patients with mental illness, and an estimated 6 per cent of the total population currently are in need of psychiatric care.

Public health problems confront us as a result of rapid industrial expansion and the development of large and overcrowded urban centers. The pollution of water, air and food by industrial waste products and the threat of damaging radiation from artificial sources are problems of great magnitude and long-range importance.

During the past several decades medical research has advanced our knowledge at a fantastic pace. Among the most brilliant accomplishments have been those in the field of preventive medicine. But between the acquisition and the application of medical knowledge there may be unfortunate time lags. For example, although rheumatic fever is largely preventable by the prompt and vigorous treatment of streptococcal pharyngitis, nevertheless rheumatic fever and rheumatic heart disease still are responsible for more than 20,000 deaths in this country each year. Glaucoma and diabetes remain the leading causes of blindness, solely because these diseases, although readily detectable even in their early stages, if detection is sought, have escaped detection too often and too long, and the benefits of early treatment have been missed. Were all individuals over the age of 40 to undergo regularly a competent health examination, much human misery might be spared.

THE NURSE'S ROLE IN DISEASE PREVENTION

Powerful ammunition for the battle against disease has been provided through the contributions of many basic sciences, including epidemiology, immunology, nutrition, sociology, psychology and biochemistry. However, the effectiveness of these weapons is dependent not only on their general availability but also on a wide knowledge of their application. *Education of the public, therefore, may be counted as the most important single aspect of this defense program.* Of all the agencies concerned with public health education, one of the most effective is the nursing profession.

Early in the nurse's professional career the significance of disease prevention becomes apparent and she becomes aware of her responsibilities in relation to its accomplishment. Throughout the period of her basic course she is instructed in the close relationships existing between individual health and group health, between health and economics, health and the physical environment, health and group immunization, standards of nutrition, sanitation and a host of other factors that mutually affect the public health.

There is a relationship between the status of an individual in his community and his attitude toward health practices. Patients in the lower socioeconomic groups are inclined to disregard their symptoms unless these prevent them from working or unless emergencies arise. These persons usually do not seek treatment early. Social scientists have observed that the behavior of an individual in relation to his health conforms to that which he considers acceptable to, and prevalent in, his social group. Moreover, it depends upon the importance that he and his family attach to health. Other factors that may have a

bearing on attitude and behavior in this regard include the intellectual and the educational level, the age, the race and the sex of the patient.

In order to teach her patient effectively, the public-health nurse must familiarize herself with his concepts and system of values pertaining to illness and health. It may be her mission to convince him that he is not invulnerable, that he probably is susceptible and might well acquire a given disease, and that the preventive measures she is advocating are both safe and effective.

The instruction of patients and their families in the principles of health and disease prevention can be among the most valuable contributions of the nurse. If her instructions are to be realistic, she must evaluate her patients correctly with respect to their intelligence, physical capacity and handicaps—factors that determine the degree of responsibility they can accept for the protection of their own health and the extent to which this responsibility must be consigned to their families or to social agencies in their communities.

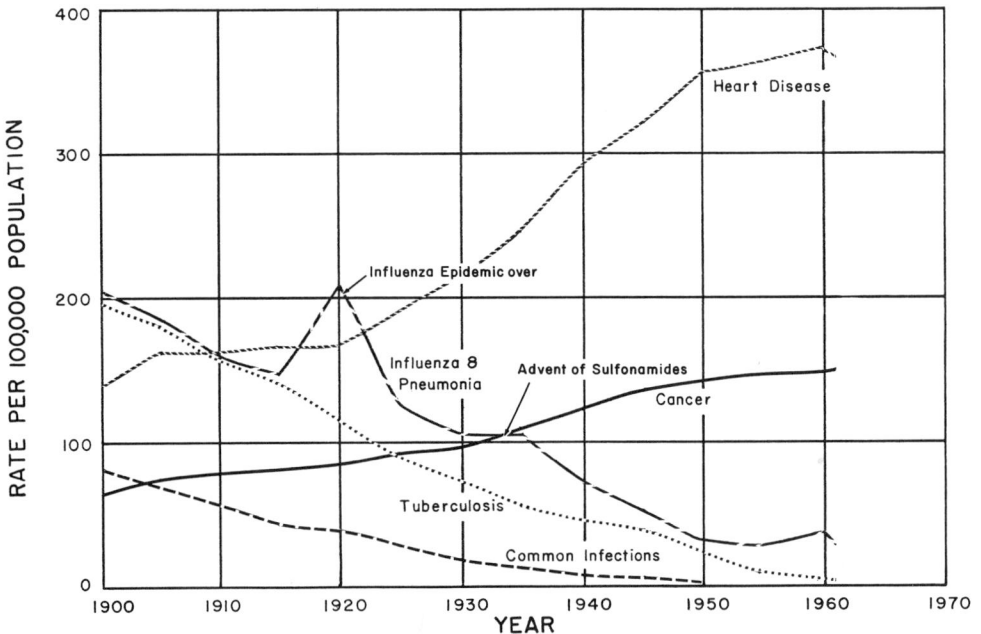

FIG. 2. Death rates of selected diseases in the United States for the period between 1900 and 1960. These trends indicate the importance of past achievements and the importance of current problems. (Adapted from American Cancer Society)

ENVIRONMENTAL HEALTH

In addition to health teaching, the nurse has numerous other functions in relation to preventive medicine. She must be cognizant of the environmental factors that pertain to each of the illnesses with which she deals—factors such as housing and sanitation, which, if defective, predispose to their onset, progression, recurrence and spread. Such factors obviously are of importance, not only to the patient and his family, but also to the community as a whole.

In every home she visits, the nurse is a potential "case finder." People frequently will voice their complaints and describe their symptoms to her. They may mention casually a problem that to them seems minor, but that the nurse recognizes as a potential clue to disease. She finds many opportunities to convince reluctant sufferers to report to a physician or clinic for attention that they have sought to avoid.

Through direct referrals, the hospital nurse is able to assure continuity of patient care between the hospital and the community health and welfare agencies. The public health nurse represents the long arms of the hospital and the clinic. Not only is she herself familiar with the principles and the practice of preventive medicine, but she also knows the agencies, official and voluntary, that are accessible and whose services are available, to the patient.

As agents of public health services, nurses are active in the schools, industries, recreation centers and homes, serving as skilled observers, professional advisers, administrators of prescribed therapy. The improvements in health and living conditions in every department of community life in which they serve bear witness to their far-reaching accomplishments and professional influence.

BIBLIOGRAPHY AND SUGGESTED READING

Books

Anderson, G. W., Arnstein, M. G., and Lester, M. R.: Communicable Disease Control, New York, Macmillan, 1962.

Hilleboe, H. E., and Larimore, G. W.: Preventive Medicine, Philadelphia, Saunders, 1959.

Maisel, A. Q.: The Health of People Who Work, New York, National Health Council.

Turner, C. E.: Personal and Community Health, St. Louis, Mosby, 1959.

Articles

Chambers, W.: Nursing diagnosis, Am. J. Nursing **62**:102-104, Nov., 1962.

Kariel, P. E.: The dynamics of behavior in relation to health, Nursing Outlook **10**:402-405, 1962.

Journal

American Journal of Public Health, American Public Health Association, Inc., 1790 Broadway, New York 19, N. Y.

3

Defense of the Patient Against Infection

THE RETICULOENDOTHELIAL SYSTEM

The human body is protected against microbial invasion by the integrity of its surface coverings, namely the skin, the mucous membranes and the epithelial lining of the respiratory, the gastrointestinal and the genitourinary tracts, all of which are covered and fortified by bacteriostatic secretions. Organisms that succeed in penetrating the surface are confronted by the internal defenses of the body, including mechanical barricades designed to immobilize any microbes that enter; chemical weapons, capable of neutralizing their toxic products or ingredients and of forcing these organisms into clumps; and scavenger units, both stationary and mobile types, that are prepared to entrap, engulf and liquefy these invaders. The source of all this defensive activity is the *reticulum cell.*

The reticulum cell is the progenitor of several varieties of cells, each type differing from the others in appearance, activity and function. The entire family is represented in the bone marrow; a partial assortment is to be found in lymph nodes and in the spleen; and one variety is stationed as individual units at various strategic sites throughout the body. All of these various components, regardless of location, together comprise the so-called *reticuloendothelial system.* The reticulum cells of the marrow produce, in addition to erythrocytes and megakaryocytes (which play no direct role in defense), polymorphonuclear neutrophils, histiocytes and plasmacytes. Reticulum cells outside the marrow generate lymphocytes, histiocytes and monocytes.

Cellular Defenses

Polymorphonuclear leukocytes, histiocytes and monocytes are actively phagocytic, engulfing and digesting particulate matter of all types. The function of these units is to check the invader at the point of invasion in the tissue itself, before it has had an opportunity to reach any lymph or blood channel. Within a few hours from the time a germ or any foreign substance becomes implanted in the tissue, it finds itself surrounded by these phagocytes attempting to eat it. It is the accumulation of these guardian leukocytes that we describe by the term *pus.*

Polymorphonuclear neutrophils, histiocytes and monocytes are contained in the circulating blood where they are constantly available and from whence they can be marshaled for immediate defensive action in any tissue. Histiocytes and monocytes also are contained in the spleen and in the lymph nodes, which serve as filter beds for the purification of the circulating blood and lymph, respectively. Most of the lymphocytes and tissue macrophages do not circulate but operate as stationary units, or permanent traps, in the spleen, the liver, the lymph nodes, the lungs, the walls of the respiratory and gastrointestinal tracts, the subcutaneous tissue and elsewhere.

Lymph Nodes

Lymph nodes consist of pea-sized to bean-sized accumulations of lymphocytes, plasma cells and histiocytes, all held together by a loose network of reticulum cell fibers and contained within a fibrous capsule. The bulk of the cell population consists of lymphocytes which are produced *in situ* by lymphoblasts in their center. Each node is equipped with its own vascular communications and has multiple connections with lymph vessels. These channels, draining all surfaces and all organ tissues, eventually join to form the thoracic duct, through which their contents are returned to the circulating blood. Before this juncture, however, each lymph vessel passes through one or several lymph nodes, and, with the extraordinary cells of the latter, its contents must perforce come into intimate contact. The function of the lymph nodes is to furnish facilities for the filtration of lymph and the removal of particulate matter and cellular aggregates of all sorts, including bacteria. Therefore, if any organism succeeds in forcing an entrance through the natural barriers of a mucous membrane surface, for example, in all probability it will find its way into a lymphatic vessel and on the way to confinement in a lymph node. Aside from their trapping function, lymph nodes serve as a device for exposing plasmacytes to any foreign substances that may be dissolved in the lymph. Such contact is essential, since these cells are responsible for fashioning gamma globulin into specific antibodies capable of clumping or lysing bacteria and neutralizing their toxic products.

Nodes are to be found in profusion in the anterior and posterior regions of the neck, as well as in the nasal and oropharynx, there designed to trap any organism penetrating into the tissues of the nose, the throat, the gums, the scalp or the face. There are many nodes located in the thorax, and through these drain secretions from the lower respiratory tract, the trachea and the bronchi. Similar lymphoid tissue is distributed in patches throughout the length of the intestine, should any living bacteria find their way into the bowel wall. The tissue lymph from the extremities is strained through chains of nodes, some of which are located about the elbow and the shoulder, in the axillae, in the groin and posterior to the knee. These make their presence known, by swelling and tenderness, should infection involve the tissue area from which the lymph filtering through them is derived.

Lymph nodes are designed and situated to clear the lymph stream but afford no direct protection to the circulating blood. However, in the spleen, the liver, the lungs, the bone marrow and the adrenal glands, directly on the course of the blood stream, are located large phagocytic cells called *tissue macrophages,* which in appearance and function are quite analogous to certain of the lymph node cells. Usually, macrophages are distributed singly throughout the organs mentioned, in the structure of which they form an integral part. The engulfing and digestion of blood-borne organisms, as well as of dead cells and foreign particles in general, appear to represent their prime function.

The Spleen

The spleen combines in a single organ all of the defensive functions that are known to be associated with the reticuloendothelial system. In addition, the spleen is adapted for the sequestration of formed blood elements which, although of native origin, are of odd size or shape, such cells being trapped and eliminated within the spleen. Moreover, any tendency to aggregate on the part of any particulate matter, including red cells, white cells and platelets, as well as bacteria, is enhanced within the splenic sinusoids. Such particles, once clumped, never make their exit from that organ, being ingested by phagocytic cells which are present in abundance. Within the spleen, plasma and any foreign material that might be dissolved in it come into relatively prolonged contact with plasmacytes, setting the stage for the production of specific antibodies. So far as is known, no important defensive function is served by the spleen that is not duplicated elsewhere in the reticuloendothelial system. With respect to the contribution of the spleen to immunity, evidence has been cited which suggests that children and adolescents whose spleens have been removed might be more prone to acquire bacterial infections than are individuals whose spleens are intact.

IMMUNE ANTIBODIES

Antibodies are produced in the course of all infectious disease, and on recovery the patient possesses an immunity against the organism which caused it; this immunity will persist as long as the antibodies continue to be produced—perhaps for the rest of his life. Immunity against one organism may carry with it some measure of protection against other organisms whose chemical products are related closely. Therefore, one need not necessarily have been exposed to a certain variety of organism in order to possess an immunity to it. But, in general, these antibodies are quite specific, and the antibody produced in response to the products of one organism will react with these and to the products of no other.

Animals can be stimulated to produce, and accumulate in their blood, specific antibacterial antibodies or antitoxins by injecting into them the corresponding organisms or toxins. By this means we obtain serums containing these protective substances that can be given to patients before their powers of protection have developed or when they are insufficient to combat the disease. The sera produced by injection of toxins are called *antitoxins;* those formed by injection of dead or living bacteria are called *antisera.* Those used most often in surgery are tetanus antitoxin, gas-gangrene antitoxin, streptococcus antitoxin and streptococcus antiserum. Other immune agents that are clinically important include an antiserum that is specific for diphtheria toxin; antiserums against the toxins of *Staphylococcus aureus,* the bacillus of Shiga dysentery and the organism responsible for one type of food poisoning (botulism); and antitoxins against certain snake venoms. Also available, but used relatively little in this era of antimicrobial chemotherapy, are certain antibacterial antibodies, including antiserums that are specific for various types of pneumococci.

The injection of any heterologous serum (serum from another species, from some source other than human), including an antitoxin or an antibacterial serum, invariably is attended by the risk of an immune reaction occurring in the recipient in response to the animal proteins. Such a reaction may take place immediately (anaphylactic shock) or have its onset after an interval of several days following the injection (serum disease). These complications are described in Chapter 37.

INFLAMMATION

By *inflammation* we mean the reaction of the body tissues to an injury. The reactions may be rapid in appearance, producing marked and significant signs and symptoms that often require early surgical intervention. Such an inflammation is spoken of as *acute;* for example, a sudden inflammation of the appendix is spoken of as acute appendicitis. When the tissue reaction is insidious and continues over a long period of time, the inflammation is said to be *chronic.*

The Injuring Agent

This may be any one of several kinds. Physical agents, such as a blow, or even a surgeon's sterile knife, excite a typical inflammation. Chemicals, especially acids and caustic alkalies, electricity, heat and cold— all cause reactions when they are applied to body tissues. Bacteria are by far the most common and the most serious of the injuring agents; they invade and become a secondary factor in a large majority of inflammations that may have been started by physical, chemical or thermal agents.

Local Symptoms of Inflammation

Perhaps the simplest kind of inflammation may be found in an injury inflicted by the sterile knife of a surgeon. However sharp the knife, millions of tiny cells are damaged, blood vessels are cut, and lymphatics are crushed. Even if the wound is sutured accurately, the tissues show their resentment by progressing through all the stages of a mild inflammation. In a very short time the edges of the wound will be found to be redder than the surrounding skin, and the tissues will feel somewhat more tense and slightly warmer near the wound. The area about the wound will appear to be somewhat raised; it will be painful, and movement of the cut tissues will increase the pain. From these observations we discover the *cardinal signs of an inflammation:* redness, swelling, heat, pain and loss of function.

In order to understand the cause of the appearance of these signs, we must examine these tissues microscopically. The first reaction of the injured tissues is to increase their blood supply. The capillaries and the veins dilate widely, and the blood, flowing rapidly at first, slows gradually because it is flowing from a smaller to a larger area. This increase in the blood supply accounts for the redness and the heat associated with an inflammation.

As the capillaries dilate, their walls become permeable, so that serum and white blood cells—and red blood cells to a lesser degree—escape into the surrounding tissues. This movement of fluid is called *exudation.* A clear fluid discharge is *serous;* a cloudy, creamy exudate is *purulent;* one containing blood is *hemorrhagic* or *sanguineous.* This increase of fluid and blood cells extending into the tissues accounts for the swelling observed above, and, by causing pressure on the delicate nerve endings, it produces pain.

If the wound is sterile, the inflammation goes no farther. The white blood corpuscles, called leukocytes, having the power of independent movement, seek out and literally devour all fragments of dead cells while the serum is being reabsorbed into the blood vessels and the lymphatics. Soon the wound edges are united by delicate long cells (fibroblasts) that are the forerunners of the strong fibrous network called connective tissue. The hemorrhage is absorbed, and the superficial layers of cells bridge the gap to close the wound. Such healing is called *healing by primary union, per primam* or *by first intention.* Every surgeon strives for this type of union. When primary union does not take place because of infection or loss of tissue, healing occurs by *secondary intention* or by *granulation* (discussed in detail on page 23).

If there are bacteria in the wound, the reaction of the tissues to these minute organisms is of the same character as described above but to a more marked degree. The bacteria that make their way into the tissues find food, moisture and warmth—an environment in which they can multiply very rapidly. Substances toxic to the tissues about them are formed, and an inflammation occurs. The increased blood supply produces a redness and an increased temperature of the tissues for some distance about the area of infection, and the fluid that leaks out of the dilated capillaries causes a swelling. This hot area of red, swollen tissue about an area of inflammation is called a *cellulitis.* The white blood cells reaching the area attempt to devour and kill the offending organisms. The blood serum that has escaped contains antitoxins and other immune substances that are believed to make the bacterial toxins harmless and inert or to make the bacteria more easily digested by the phagocytes. If these defensive measures are sufficient, the bacteria are killed, and the inflammation subsides. However, more often the rapidly forming toxins are too much at first for the early defense measures, with the result that many white blood cells are killed, along with the cells of the tissue in which the inflammation is taking place. These dead leukocytes and tissue cells and dead and living bacteria, with the blood and tissue fluids around them, form what is called *pus.* As a result of the action of bacterial toxins, tissue cells are killed. These cells lose their characteristics and separate from the living tissue, becoming a yellow mass of soft dead tissue called *slough.* Through the action of enzymes the dead tissue undergoes a gradual liquefaction. This process is called *necrosis,* and the tissue is said to be *necrotic.*

Around this area of dead cells the body attempts to build a protective wall composed of tissue and white blood cells, firmly packed together by the coagulation of the blood and tissue fluids about them. When pus is enclosed by such a wall, an *abscess* is formed. The abscess, at first small, grows larger gradually, advancing in the direction in which there is the least resistance to its progress.

If the abscess approaches the skin, its outer wall grows weaker because the pressure of the abscess closes the tiny capillaries that bring the cells to strengthen it. The weakest point appears often as a small, raised yellow dot on the skin surface, and the abscess then is said to "point" or to "come to a head." As these skin cells die and disintegrate, the pressure inside the abscess pushes them out and they are followed by the pus from its cavity. Often the surgeon must aid nature, save many cells from death and relieve the patient of much pain and discomfort by making an incision in the abscess wall and allowing the pus to escape. (Furuncles, carbuncles, felons, and so forth are discussed in Chapter 34.)

Constitutional Symptoms of Inflammation

These symptoms are caused by the absorption of toxic substances by the blood from the inflamed area. Their severity depends upon the amount and the degree of toxicity of the absorbed substances. Some bacteria—for example, streptococci—form pus that is much more toxic than other varieties.

The usual symptoms are fever, increase in pulse and respiratory rates, headache and general malaise, hot dry skin, flushed cheeks, loss of appetite, thirst, coated tongue, constipation and highly colored, scanty urine. When the toxic absorption is rapid, there may be chills, followed by sweating, and even delirium. An examination of the blood usually shows an increase in the number of white cells (leukocytes), and there is said to be *leukocytosis*.

When the inflammation is mild or when

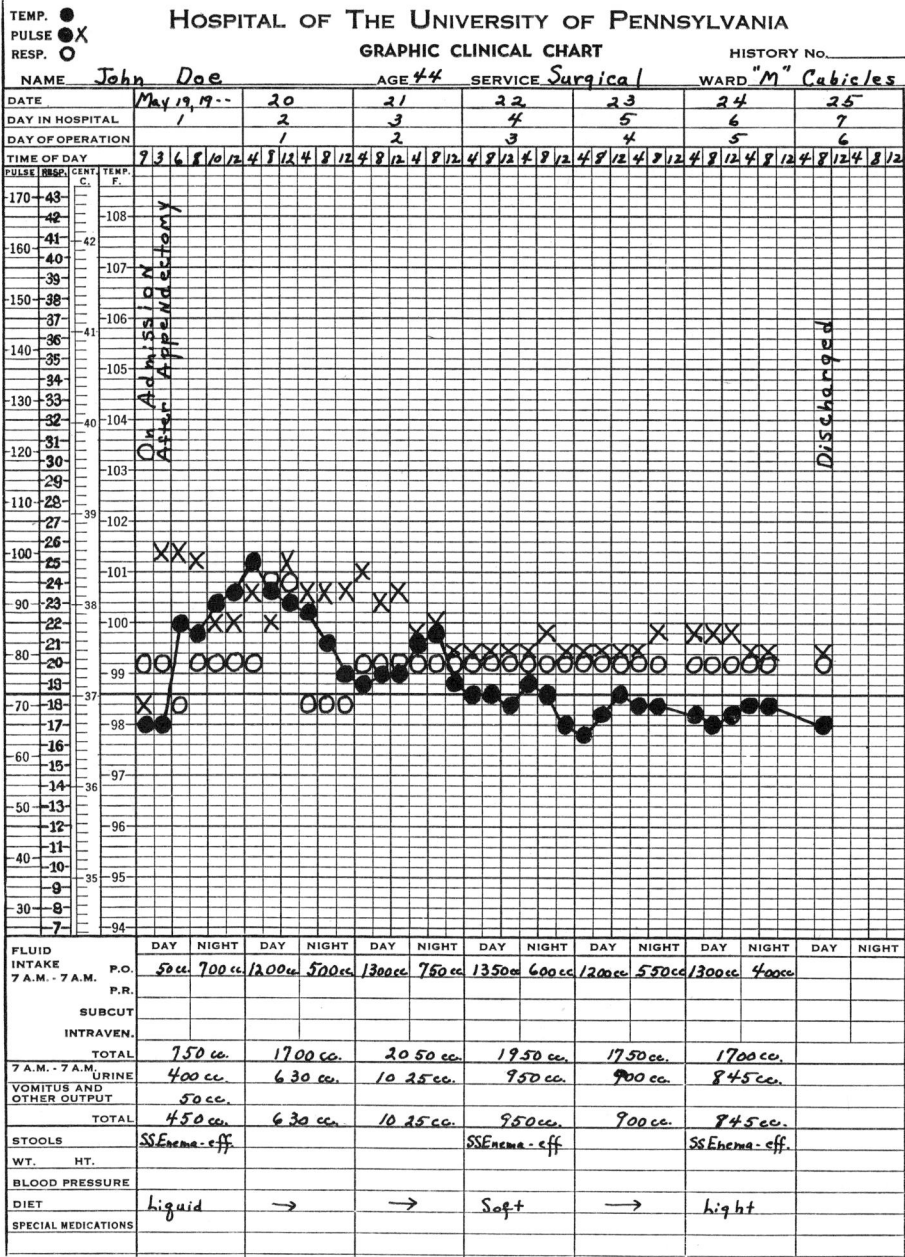

FIG. 3. Chart showing temperature, pulse and respiratory rate in a mild inflammation. Crosses indicate pulse; dots indicate temperature; circles indicate respirations.

the resistance of the individual is low, the leukocyte count may have changed little. Hence, we may regard the variation of the number of white cells in the blood as somewhat of an indication of the patient's natural resistance to disease and of the severity of the inflammation. There are some inflammations, one of which is due to the tubercle bacillus, that cause a lowering of the number of leukocytes and produce a *leukopenia.*

The constitutional symptoms of an inflammation may be much more marked in children than in adults. Besides the symptoms mentioned above, nausea and vomiting are frequent, even with moderately severe inflammation. The child often may show distressing nervous symptoms, such as convulsions or delirium. These reactions are not so pronounced in the aged. The patient does not complain very much; often he is listless and indifferent, the temperature is lower, the pulse has increased only slightly, and the leukocyte count is lower or shows no increase. Frequently, he will not swallow even water, and often he is incontinent. The whole picture is that of an acutely sick patient apparently without acute symptoms.

Reparative Processes

Healing by First Intention (Primary Union). Wounds made aseptically and with a minimum of tissue destruction heal with very little tissue reaction "by first intention."

Healing by Second Intention (Granulation). In cases in which pus formation (suppuration) has occurred, the process of repair is less simple and delayed longer. When an abscess is incised, it collapses partly, but the dead and the dying cells forming its walls are still being thrown out into the cavity. For this reason rubber tubes, rubber tissue or gauze packing often is inserted into the abscess pocket to allow the pus to escape easily. Gradually the necrotic material disintegrates and escapes, and the abscess cavity fills with a red, soft, insensitive tissue that bleeds very easily. It is composed of minute thin-walled capillaries, growing off from the parent vessels, each bud surrounded by cells that later form connective tissue. These buds, called granulations, enlarge until they fill the area of the tissue destroyed. The cells surrounding the capillaries change their round shape; they become long and thin, intertwining with

each other to form a *scar* or *cicatrix.* Healing is complete when skin cells (epithelium) grow over these granulations. This method of repair is called *healing by granulation,* and it takes place whenever pus is formed or when loss of tissue has occurred for any reason.

Healing by Third Intention (Secondary Suture). If a deep wound has either not been sutured early or breaks down and then is resutured later, two apposing granulation surfaces are brought together. This results in a deeper and wider scar.

Factors Affecting Wound Healing

In healthy tissue a wound heals at its normal optimal rate. There is no way in which this rate can be accelerated. In less healthy tissue certain aids can be introduced to assist the reparative process. This is brought about by providing an adequate nutritional level in the individual through proper diet. Protein elements and vitamin C are examples of essential needs. Whole blood may be given, since it is necessary to maintain the red blood cell count as near normal as possible; the wounds of anemic patients are known to heal less well than normally. Edema also interferes with the healing process. Tissues heal more readily in the younger patient; hence, age is a factor.

Complications of Inflammation

The body makes every effort to localize an inflammation and to prevent the absorption of its toxic products. When the patient is in good physical condition, his natural powers to resist inflammation are great. His blood rapidly supplies increasing numbers of vigorous leukocytes, immune substances are added quickly to those present naturally in his blood, and the protective wall forms fast and strong about the area of inflammation.

Occasionally, the defensive measures are inadequate to cope with the virulent organism causing the inflammation. The process of walling-off is incomplete, or the formation of immune substances is slow, with a consequent absorption into the blood of a large amount of very poisonous products.

Toxemia, Septicemia and Pyemia. If only the toxins are absorbed, the condition is called a *toxemia.* When the bacteria and their toxins are absorbed into the blood, we have a *septicemia,* and, if pus is discharged into the blood stream, a *pyemia* has occurred. Such complications are often called *blood poisoning.*

These conditions are somewhat similar in their symptoms. There is an increasing severity of the constitutional symptoms, associated with an inflammation. To these are added chills, sweats, a temperature that shows abrupt rises and rapid falls once or oftener daily, a very rapid pulse and a very high leukocyte count. A toxic delirium often occurs.

When a smear of the white cells is examined under the microscope, it is noted often that some of the cells are immature. This is the result of the action of the toxic substances upon the bone marrow. Frequently, the severity of the toxemia may be judged by noting the number of immature leukocytes in relation to the number of mature cells. When the number of immature cells is high, the infection is severe and the prognosis is more grave.

In septicemia, and especially in pyemia, the bacteria floating in the blood stream lodge often at points far distant from the original inflammation and there set up secondary or metastatic abscesses.

Chronic Inflammation. This differs from an acute inflammation in that the injuring agent is weak, but its action continues over a long period of time. Consequently, the reaction of the tissues is less, and the cardinal symptoms of an inflammation may be hard to demonstrate. Swelling usually is present, pain often is moderate or slight, redness usually is indistinct, and heat may be absent. The process may go on to pus formation. The most common organisms causing chronic inflammation are those of tuberculosis and syphilis. The treatment indicated is that for acute inflammation plus the specific measures for the diseases mentioned. Chronic diseases usually require prolonged care.

NURSING CARE OF LOCAL INFLAMMATION

The nursing care of a patient with a local inflammation consists of the following: (1) rest of the inflamed part, (2) elevation of it, (3) the application of heat, or cold.

These measures all are directed toward the relief of the local pain and the hastening of the termination of the inflammation.

Often it may be necessary to add to the above (4) incision and drainage of the inflamed area, which procedure is a duty of the surgeon.

Rest of the Inflamed Part

Rest of the inflamed part is indicated for two reasons: first, because it allows all the forces of nature to be directed to combating the inflammation, which tends to hasten the walling-off process and thereby lessen the absorption of toxin; second, because any movement of the inflamed part is painful to the patient. The painful smile of the patient with cracked lips is a common example of the discomfort caused by even a slight movement in the case of a mild inflammation. The delayed healing of a wound over a finger joint is an illustration of how movement hinders the delicate healing processes. To ensure absolute rest, splints, bandages, plaster casts or plaster splints are applied when possible. In inflammations of the head, the trunk and the lower extremities, rest in bed often is a necessity.

Elevation of the Inflamed Part

Elevation of the inflamed part is one of the procedures for which the patient will be most grateful. In this manner the throbbing pain and the swelling may be relieved greatly; the force of gravity helps to drain the engorged blood vessels and tissue spaces and at the same time permits an increased arterial circulation that brings new forces in greater numbers to combat the inflammation. The almost immediate relief obtained by elevation of the hand in cases of fingertip infection is a familiar example of this.

This procedure cannot be practiced when the inflammation is of the chest or the abdomen, but it can be used to advantage in inflammation of the head, the neck and the extremities. The degree of elevation (above the heart level) will vary according to the site of the inflammation. In cases of the extremities, it is better to elevate the whole part. Thus, in elevating the arm, the hand should be higher than the elbow and the elbow higher than the shoulder. The same would apply to the leg.

Elevation can be accomplished best by pillows when the patient is in bed or by a sling when the patient is ambulatory. The pillows should be protected with rubber or plastic pillowcases or sheeting and should support the extremities completely. The areas which do not come in contact with the pillow—for example, the knee joint—can be made more comfortable by placing small pillows or cotton pads underneath them. A bed cradle should be used to relieve pressure of the bedclothes on the elevated part.

The Application of Heat

Very frequently applications of heat are valuable aids in the treatment of surgical diseases. The heat causes a local hyperemia (increased blood supply), a function that may be used to advantage in the treatment of inflammation, especially after the stage of extravasation of cells and serum has taken place. Heat often relaxes the spasm of involuntary muscle, especially that occurring in cases of renal, biliary or intestinal colic.

Pain often is completely relieved by heat applications, especially in cases of acute infective inflammations and in the later stages of many traumatic conditions. However, at times heat actually increases the amount of pain. In such cases cold applications usually give some measure of relief.

Heat may be applied in the dry or the moist form.

Dry Heat

Dry heat may be applied in the following ways:

Hot-water Bottle. This probably is the form in most common use by the laity. The bottle always should be covered with a layer of flannel cloth before being applied to skin surfaces, and the temperature never should exceed 130° F. Heat may be applied in this manner (1) to relieve "deep" pain; (2) to supply heat when the temperature of the patient becomes subnormal in cases of shock and hemorrhage and after operation; and (3) to retain heat in various forms of moist dressings. Special care is necessary to prevent burns from hot-water bottles when they are used to supply heat to unconscious patients or those still under the effect of an anesthetic.

Electric Pad. This appliance is a source of great comfort to patients when heat is to be applied over large surfaces for a long

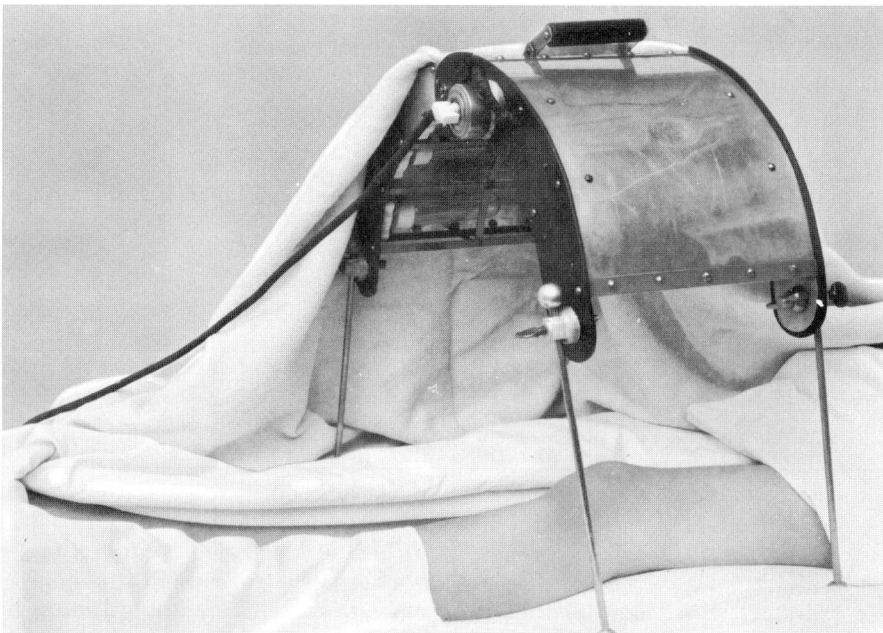

Fig. 4. Dry heat being applied in traumatic arthritis of the knee.

time. The pad should not be allowed to get wet, because of the danger of causing a short circuit. Therefore, unless it is covered with rubber or very well protected by oiled silk or waxed paper, the electric pad should not be used with moist dressings.

Bake Oven. This apparatus is made in many shapes and sizes adaptable for the application of heat to various parts of the body. The heat usually is generated by electric-light bulbs. The part to be baked is wrapped well in cotton or flannel to prevent blistering. This method of heat application is useful in the treatment of the more chronic inflammation of bones and joints—for example, arthritis, after fractures and bursitis (Fig. 4).

The chief hazard associated with the application of dry heat is the danger of burning the patient. For this reason the nurse should keep under observation the area to which the heat is being applied, and at the first signs of burning—pain to the patient or marked redness of the part—the application must be discontinued. The pain sense in extremely ill, toxic, shocked or aged patients often is markedly dull, so that these patients, and also those who are unconscious, must be watched with extreme care.

Diathermy. Heat may be induced in the tissues by the passage through them of high-frequency electric currents. The resistance offered by the tissues to the passage of the current generates heat in the same way that the filament of a light bulb becomes hot when the electricity is turned on. The current is applied to the part to be treated through two metal electrodes fixed firmly in place. Usually either the electrodes or the skin is moistened to give a better contact to the skin surface. The amount of heat generated in the tissues is regulated by the amount of current used, and the greatest intensity of heat is in the area between the electrodes, through which the current passes. By this method of application, heat may be induced deep in the tissues and directly at the site of the lesion to be treated. Diathermy is valuable especially in the treatment of traumatic inflammations of soft tissues, such as sprains and bruises, and of low-grade or chronic inflammations of muscles, joints or bursae.

Electric Warmers with Controlled Circulation of Warm Air. Electric warmers made to furnish controlled circulation of warm air are available. These are very convenient for drying plaster-of-Paris casts, for warming beds for patients in shock and for taking the place of hot-water bottles and heat lamps in the other treatments.

Moist Heat

Moist heat probably is the most valuable application that can be made to an acute inflammation, especially inflammation at or near the skin surface. Other uses of moist heat are indicated below with descriptions of the various methods of application.

Hot Compresses — Hot Wet Dressings. These dressings may be applied by frequent changing of gauze compresses wrung out of hot solutions, or by application of hot solutions to dressings already bandaged to a part. The solutions in common use are physiologic salt solution and antiseptic solutions, such as boric acid, or hypertonic salt solutions, such as saturated magnesium sulfate solution or Wright's solution.

When the compress is bandaged in place, care should be taken that the solution is not too hot. If there is no thermometer at hand, the nurse should draw the solution into a dressing syringe and expel a little on the back of her hand or arm to test its temperature before she applies it slowly to the dressings. (See Fig. 5 A, B, and C.)

The moisture will be retained if the dressings are covered with waxed paper, thin rubber, heavy toweling or plastic. The heat can be kept fairly constant if hot-water bottles are applied; however, the weight of the hot-water bottles should be considered in placing them. A much more constant heat can be applied by the use of rubber-covered electric pads. A cradle with electric lights also may be placed over the dressings to keep a constant elevated temperature about the part (Fig. 5 B). If the solution is used from about 105° to 110° F. and the hot-water bottles from 115° to 120° F., there is little chance of burning the patient. Because moist heat burns more readily than dry heat, the area should be inspected frequently.

The nurses should not forget that hot solutions applied to compresses on a bandaged part are more likely to burn the patient than when applied to the open skin because of the

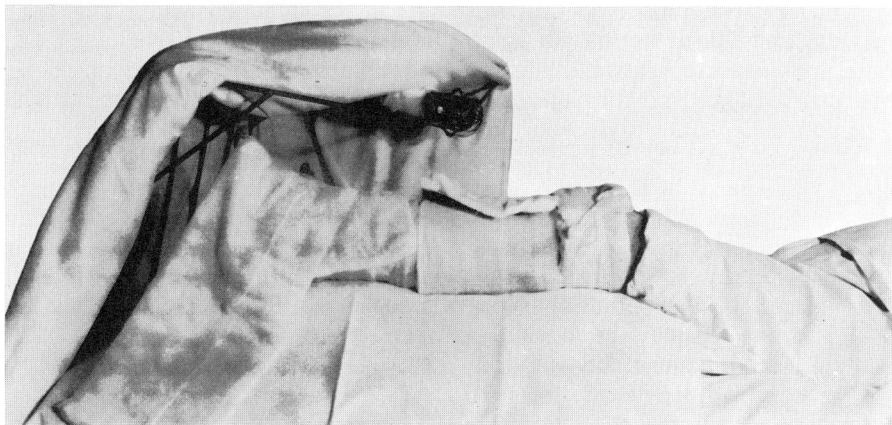

FIG. 5A. Application of hot moist dressings to the lower extremity. The leg is elevated, and the entire foot and leg are swathed in gauze compresses, lint or commercial pads in 3-foot lengths. A folded pad is tied round the upper part of the dressing to prevent leakage of the solution.

fact that evaporation cannot take place and cool the dressings. Therefore, extreme care should be taken that burning does not occur. This is especially important in treating aged and debilitated or paralyzed patients. Excessive heat in extremities with disturbed metabolism, such as exists in arteriosclerosis or diabetic gangrene, does more harm than good. Moist heat in the form of hot baths is frequently used in the treatment of infections of the hands and the feet.

Douches. The application of heat by a current of warm solution is a valuable method of treatment in inflammations of the ear, the vagina and the pelvis. The solutions should be as warm as the patient can tolerate with comfort. Those employed most commonly are saline for the ear and various other antiseptic solutions for the vagina.

Baths. SITZ BATH. The patient sits for from 15 to 20 minutes in a bath of water heated to a temperature of from 105° to 110° F. There should be just enough water to cover the patient's hips. The bath is useful for treating acute pelvic inflammatory disease and for producing relaxation of the bladder sphincters in cases of urinary retention. It may be tried at times as a means of

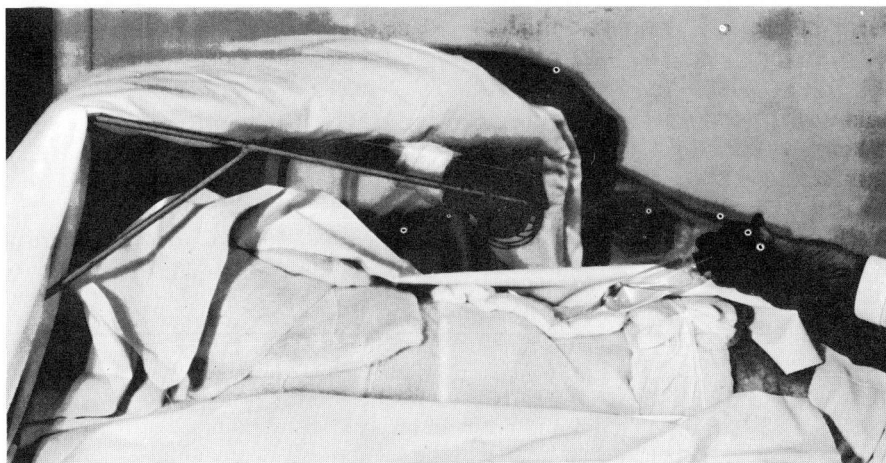

FIG. 5B. The compresses are moistened with warm solution.

producing sufficient relaxation to permit the reduction of a strangulated hernia. It is of special value in the postoperative treatment of lesions about the anus and the perineum, such as hemorrhoids, fissure in ano and ischiorectal abscess.

Warm baths for parts of the body often are indicated in the treatment of acute infections, sprains and severely traumatized wounds when there is a threat of sloughing. The part is placed in the solution at the ordered temperature—usually as warm as the patient can stand comfortably—and is kept there the specified length of time. If there is an open wound, the basin and the solution should be sterile. The temperature of the solution must be kept constant by adding warmer solution as necessary, but this must be done with care to avoid burning.

Warm Bath, Entire Body. The body is submerged in a tub of warm solution, preferably physiologic saline solution at from 95° to 100° F. This is useful in cases of severe superficial burns.

The Application of Cold

Cold is used in treatment of recent inflammations. It causes a constriction of the vessels in the inflamed zone. This results in a lessening of serum and cellular leakage into the tissues. There is also an inhibition of bacterial growth. If the application is continued for a sufficient time, a paralysis of the vessels occurs, so that, when the cold is removed, it increases the hyperemia. Therefore, the result is an inhibition of the inflammatory process. In addition, cold causes a sensation of comfort to an inflamed part and, if continued, produces an anesthesia of the skin.

Dry Cold

Icebags. Dry cold is applied best in the form of icebags (rubberized bags filled with cracked ice). These are made in several forms for ease of application to different parts of the body. Care should be taken that the cap is water-tight, and a layer of fabric should be interposed between the skin and the icebag to prevent too great cooling of the skin.

Moist Cold

Moist cold is used most logically in the treatment of recent traumatic inflammation.

Moist Cold Compresses. These may be

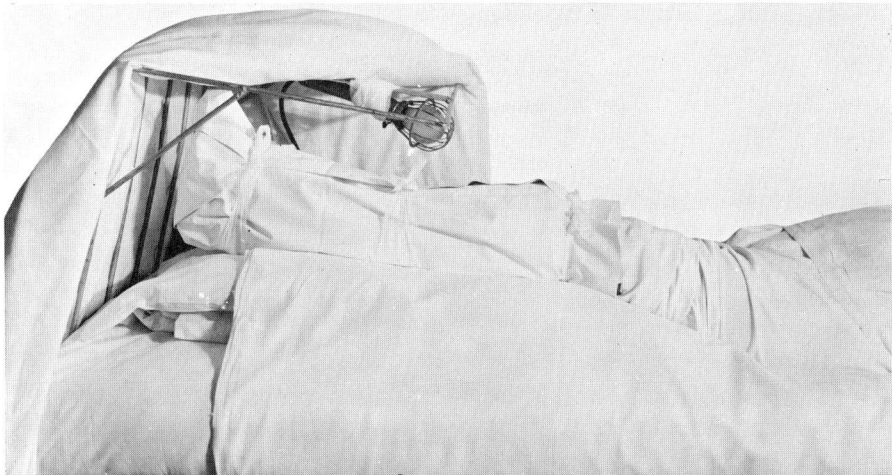

FIG. 5C. The entire leg then is enclosed in Pliofilm, oiled silk, waxed paper or a light mackintosh. This waterproof dressing should be held in place by bandage ties. If it is desired to apply heat externally by hot-water bottles or an electric pad, these are placed outside the Pliofilm and are held in position by pinning a towel around them. Note elevation of the extremity with protection of bed and pillows by Pliofilm covered with a sheet. Heat is applied in this case by a guarded electric light attached to the bed cradle.

applied best in the form of moist compresses wet with saline or boric acid solution. The solutions are kept cool by placing the vessel containing them in a basin of ice and water or by placing the compresses on a block of ice. The compresses require changing every 3 or 4 minutes, and they should not be applied for more than 10 minutes at a time. If bluish discoloration of the skin appears, the compresses should be discontinued, and the circulation stimulated by rubbing.

Cold compresses are specially useful in the prevention of swelling and inflammation after operations on the eye, and in the treatment of other traumatic inflammations—for example, sprains, bruises and contusions.

Evaporating Lotions. Evaporating lotions are of special value in the treatment of sprains and other injuries of joints. Several layers of gauze are bandaged to the part and kept moist with solution. Evaporation is allowed to take place; therefore, no effort should be made to cover the dressing with waxed paper or plastic materials.

Solutions of normal salt, boric acid, Epsom salts (1 tablespoonful to a pint of water) and alcohol (50%) are in common use.

NURSING CARE OF GENERAL INFLAMMATION

The nursing care of a patient with a general inflammation often is as important as the measures used locally. This consists of: constitutional rest (of heart, lungs, alimentary tract and the mind); promoting elimination (encouraging the intake of fluids and giving laxatives); increasing the patient's resistance (by sera, antitoxins, vaccines, transfusions, chemotherapy and antibiotics); and the relief of pain.

Promoting Constitutional Rest

Rest of Heart and Lungs. Constitutional rest is imperative in most inflammations of more than a mild nature, and this is especially the case in inflammations of the abdominal organs. By keeping the patient in bed, the least possible strain is placed upon the heart and the lungs, and all the body

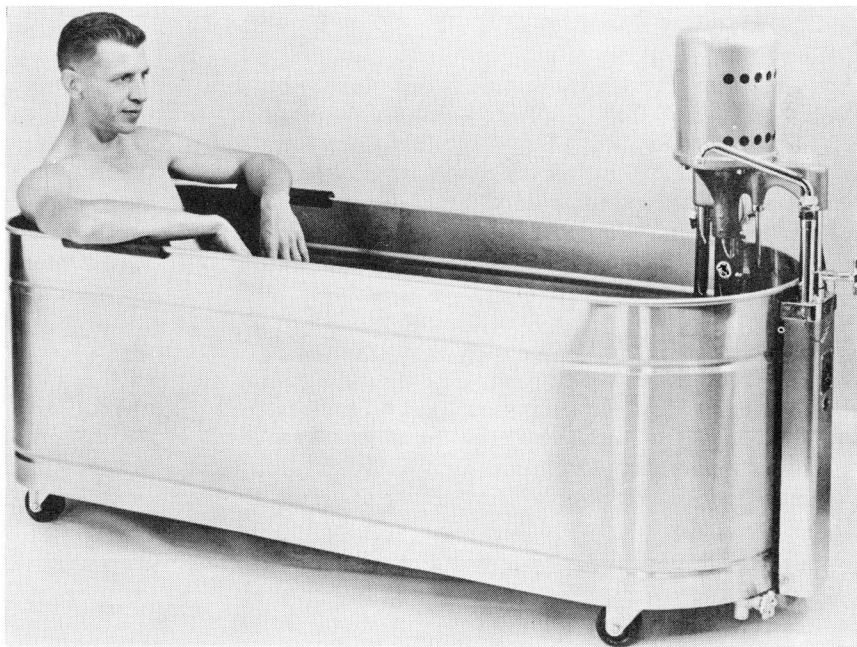

FIG. 6. The whirlpool bath may be used for the entire body with the temperature of the fluid never exceeding 110° F. Smaller whirlpool tubs are available for the extremities. (Ille Electric Corp., Williamsport, Pa.)

activities may be turned toward overcoming the inflammation. In desperate cases, a daily bath often is too exhausting.

Rest of the Alimentary Tract. The diet usually should be soft or liquid and easily assimilated. Milk, fruit juices, broths and so forth may be given while fever is present, and soft foods (eggs, milk toast, junket, chicken, baked potatoes and so forth) may be added as the temperature decreases.

Mental Rest. Finally, it should not be forgotten that rest of the mind, as well as of the body, is necessary. Every effort should be made to prevent undue disturbance and mental anxiety in a patient who is very ill.

Promoting Elimination

Administration of Fluids. The elimination of the toxic materials absorbed during the course of an inflammation is largely the function of the kidney. This organ often shows the effects of this work in the form of a nephritis. It is believed that we can dilute the circulating toxins, lessen their effect upon the kidneys and increase their elimination by administering fluids to the patient. Fluids may be given in any form by mouth in all cases of inflammation, except those involving the abdominal organs, when often it is best to give the fluid by vein. In order to increase elimination via the urine, the patient should receive between 3,000 and 5,000 ml. of fluid daily.

Laxatives may be of use in the early stages of inflammations, except those of the abdomen. This treatment overcomes the constipation and promotes elimination by the bowel. Enemas may be used thereafter.

Increasing the Patient's Resistance

Body Defense Forces. Every measure employed in the treatment of an inflammation is, or should be, simply an effort to aid nature. Some inflammations could be cared for by body defense forces with no treatment at all; others are combated with more difficulty. A great deal can be known about the severity of the inflammation if we identify the infecting organism. This can be done easily by culture, by staining smears and by the symptoms which they produce. Thus, when a patient develops stiffness of the jaw several days after a rusty nail has punctured his foot, we recognize the tetanus organism by its symptoms. Or, if we culture the blood in a septicemia, we can identify the infecting bacteria as a staphylococcus or a streptococcus. Knowing the organism, we know whether the body needs aid in combating the infection, because we know the usual course of that disease.

Conferred Immunity. We are fortunate in the knowledge that present-day science has given us ways of combating these infections. We can supply immune substances in the form of antitoxins and antisera until the body is able to develop an immunity. Thus, we give tetanus antitoxin to patients with tetanus.

The earlier these sera are given in the course of the disease, the more beneficial they are. Knowing this, we often try to steal a march on certain diseases. Thus, tetanus antitoxin is given to every patient who has received a contaminated wound, because we know that *Clostridium tetani,* the tetanus bacillus, often infects such wounds. This treatment has reduced the incidence of tetanus to a comparatively few cases and, when it does develop, usually it is of very moderate severity. Such measures used to anticipate infection and prevent disease are called *prophylaxis.*

Induced Immunity. By the hypodermic injection of toxins which have been treated to reduce the toxic effects, the body may be forced to develop an active immunity. This is used most commonly in the prevention of tetanus. Three injections of chemically processed and relatively weak tetanus toxin, or "toxoid," are performed a few weeks or months apart. These injections induce in the patient a reasonably protective and long-lasting immunity to tetanus. Immunity may be elevated further by the injection of a small "booster" dose if a wound occurs in which tetanus may be a contaminating organism. This method of preventing tetanus was used during World War II so successfully that even though many of the wounds were wide and deep, the appearance of tetanus was relatively rare.

Antimicrobial Chemotherapy. We have at our command, in addition to the various defense mechanisms of the body, a group of drugs which have proved to be of value in the treatment of infection. These drugs, frequently called the sulfa drugs, are used perhaps less frequently since the appearance of antibiotics, but they still offer considerable help in the treatment of infection.

The Antibiotics are a group of drugs which have been developed during and since World War II. They are powerful bactericidal agents producing rapid results which are much superior to those that are obtained by any other form of treatment. These drugs will be discussed fully in Chapter 13.

Relieving Pain

Analgesics often are necessary to relieve the pain associated with an inflammation. The salicylates and other coal-tar drugs frequently are adequate, but for pain that cannot be relieved otherwise, to quiet the patient and to allow sleep, morphine or Demerol should be used. Since opium so easily may cause an addiction, it is best to withhold it until other measures are given a fair trial. However, its benefits far outweigh its disadvantages, and a suffering patient is most grateful for its effects.

WOUND INFECTIONS

Tetanus (Lockjaw)

Etiology. Tetanus is a disease caused by *Bacillus tetani (Clostridium tetani).* The bacillus cannot live in the presence of oxygen (air) (anaerobe). It is found most commonly in wounds with small external openings. It may occur in any deep wound that is contaminated with soil or harbors foreign bodies. It happens not infrequently that the wound of entrance is so insignificant that it cannot be found.

Signs and Symptoms. The toxins formed in this disease have an especial affinity for nervous tissue. They are absorbed by the peripheral nerves and carried to the spinal cord, where they produce what amounts to a stimulation of the nervous tissue. The sensory nerves become sensitive to the slightest stimuli, and the hypersensitive motor nerves carry impulses that produce spasms of the muscles that they supply.

The muscle group first affected is that of the jaws, and the patient is unable to open his mouth. This characteristic symptom has given the name *lockjaw* (trismus), which is used commonly by the laity.

Other groups of muscles are included rapidly in the spasms, until the whole body is involved. The spasm of groups of muscles is continuous, but the least stimulus—a door banging or a loud voice—may add a generalized convulsion, with every muscle in violent contraction. Because the extensor muscles are stronger than the flexors, the head is retracted, the feet are extended fully, and the back is arched, so that during a convulsion the whole body may be supported on the back of the head and the feet. This condition is called *opisthotonos* (Fig. 7).

The spasms of the facial muscles produce a so-called sardonic grin, which is quite char-

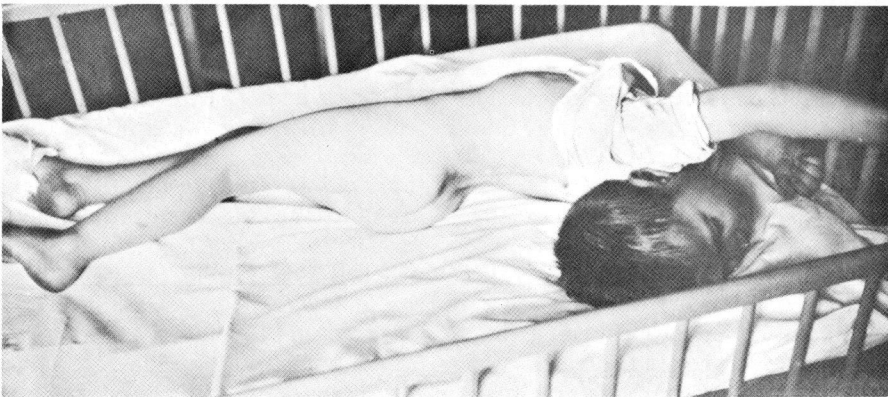

FIG. 7. Opisthotonos of tetanus. (Blake and Wright: Essentials of Pediatric Nursing, ed. 7, Philadelphia, Lippincott)

acteristic for this disease and persists even during convalescence (Fig. 8).

Death may occur from asphyxia due to spasm of the diaphragm and, more frequently, from exhaustion due to loss of sleep and lack of nourishment, and excessive fatigue due to the constant muscle spasms.

Preventive Measures. Routine immunization with tetanus toxoid is recommended in all child health, industrial or other immunization programs, especially in an environment, situation or occupation in which the incidence of the disease or exposure is increased. Booster doses are given preferably every 4 or 5 years.

Every primarily infected wound, especially a septic puncture wound, should be treated as if it were infected with the tetanus organism. Thorough cleansing of the wound, usually with wide incision, and removal of foreign bodies are the important procedures in the primary treatment of the wound. In addition, a prophylactic dose of 1,500 to 3,000 units of tetanus antitoxin should be given hypodermically. (See Serum Reaction and Treatment, p. 805.) Pencillin is often given also in larger doses (300,000 units).

Treatment and Nursing Care. If the disease already has developed when the patient is first seen, the same care of the wound is indicated. To neutralize the toxins that have formed, large doses (as much as 100,000 units daily) of the antitoxin are given around the wound, by intramuscular and by intravenous injection. Usually, penicillin is given intramuscularly in a dosage of 600,000 units or more each day. Adult patients may receive in addition one of the broad spectrum antibiotics such as terramycin, prescribed in 500 mg. doses every 8 hours.

These measures are to be supported by most careful nursing of the patient. Since the slightest stimulation may excite convulsions, absolute silence must be enforced. Even such apparently insignificant disturbances as a draught of cold air, the jarring of the bed, bright lights, squeaky doors and cold hands are to be avoided.

One of the important problems of tetanus is the maintenance of an adequate airway. Convulsive spasms, especially those involving the respiratory muscles, interfere with normal breathing, so that in many hospitals

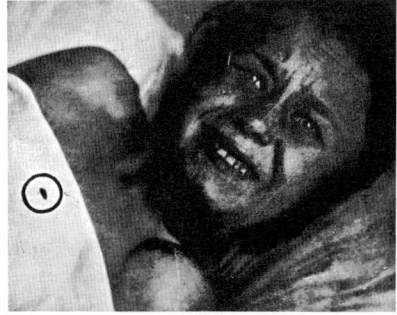

FIG. 8. Tetanus in an 11-year-old girl. The wound between the toes contained pieces of decayed wood. Mouse inoculation with this wood produced tetanus. (Pfaundler and Schlossmann: The Diseases of Children, Philadelphia, Lippincott)

tracheotomy is done routinely. This makes the nursing care the most important aspect of the patient's treatment. (See Tracheotomy Care, p. 389.)

Efforts are made to control the muscular spasms with various drugs, sedatives, anticonvulsants, and muscle relaxants. Some of these may be given by mouth or intramuscularly. Meprobamate (Miltown), secobarbital (Seconal), pentobarbital, (Nembutal), methocarbomal (Raboxin), and chlorpromazine (Thorazine) seem to be the best of these drugs.

Gas Bacillus Infection (Gas Gangrene)

Etiology. Gas bacillus infection is observed frequently as a complication of severe contusions, often associated with compound fractures, and it may be found in supposedly clean wounds, especially after amputations for gangrene. The gas bacillus—*Bacillus welchii (Clostridium welchii), B. oedematiens (Clostridium oedematiens),* and vibrion septique *(Clostridium septicum)*—like the bacillus of tetanus, is an anaerobe, and a spore former; therefore, it occurs in wounds in which the oxygen supply is reduced by reason of injury or disease of the blood vessels.

Signs and Symptoms. The wounds infected by the gas bacillus are characterized by an extreme tenderness, swelling and a bronzed discoloration of the surrounding skin. These signs are associated with a rapid pulse and respiration and some temperature elevation. As the disease progresses, gas forms in the tissues due to the action of the bacteria on the tissues, and the area about the wound crackles (crepitation) under the fingers. If the wound is opened, a frothy fluid and malodorous gases escape, and the muscles form a purple pultaceous mass. Death from toxemia usually results if the process is at all advanced.

Treatment and Nursing Care. The prophylactic treatment here, as in tetanus, is most important. Early excision (débridement) of all devitalized and infected tissue with wide incisions will prevent the disease in most traumatic cases. Once the infection has developed, extensive incisions are made in the affected part to allow air to inhibit the growth of the anaerobic organisms. This, plus excision of gangrenous tissue and the use of antibiotics (particularly the tetracyclines), may prevent the spread of infection. Supportive therapy is essential to maintain fluid and electrolyte balance.

Because the gas bacillus is an inhabitant of the human intestinal tract, it is likely to be the infecting organism in wounds of thigh amputations, especially if the patient is incontinent. Gangrene, incontinence and debility often are combined in patients with diabetes, and it is in the amputation stump of diabetic patients in which gas gangrene is most prone to occur.

The disease is important from the nursing point of view because of the extreme care that is necessary. The danger, of course, is the spread of the infection to other wounds. To guard against this, strict aseptic technic is practiced and all dressings are disposed of by incineration. It is advisable to isolate the patient and to keep a single dressing tray for that patient alone.

Gas bacillus infection produces an intense toxemia. The essentials in nursing care are the adequate administration of fluids, either by mouth or intravenously, and an easily assimilated high caloric diet.

STAPHYLOCOCCOSIS (STAPHYLOCOCCUS INFECTIONS)

The staphylococcus is responsible for most of the abscesses that mar the human skin. The furuncle, or common boil, is almost always a staphylococcal abscess, and the familiar carbuncle on the back of the neck is a coalition of staphylococcal abscesses. The vast majority of staphylococcal abscesses are located in superficial subcutaneous tissues and do not extend beyond the original site. Eventually, their purulent contents, under mounting pressure, perforate the overlying skin and are evacuated externally, leaving the empty cavities to fill in with granulation tissue, close over and heal.

This sequence of events, so common, usually so benign, might be misconstrued as evidence that the staphylococcus is a relatively innocuous microbe. Far from it! From the standpoint of aggressiveness, destructiveness, tenacity and talent for survival, this organism has few equals. The prevalence of the common boil is a tribute to its ability to penetrate the body's first line of defense and a reflection of its ubiquitous presence. The tendency of the organism to localize in superficial areas of the body merely establishes its potency as an antigen, one which rouses the defense to feverish activity; and the voluminous pus that typifies its lesions demonstrates the lethal effect which it has on tissue cells and the defending leukocytes.

Systemic Staphylococcal Infections

Whenever the peripheral defenses are unable to contain the staphylococcus, its vicious qualities soon become manifest through signs and symptoms which reflect acute tissue necrosis, profound toxemia and organ dysfunction of one type or another, depending on the localization of the infection. Invasion of the lymphatics may result in axillary, cervical, mediastinal, retroperitoneal or subdiaphragmatic abscesses. Blood stream invasion may produce acute ulcerative endocarditis, staphylococcal pneumonia, empyema, perinephric abscess, hepatic abscess, staphylococcal enteritis, pyogenic arthritis, meningitis, osteomyelitis or generalized sepsis. Constitutional symptoms are extremely severe, attesting to the potency of the exotoxin produced by this organism. Irrespective of location, staphylococcal lesions possess many characteristics in common, including extreme degrees of necrosis, a tendency to localize and a tendency to persist, despite intensive chemotherapy, until the exudate finds an escape route and is evacuated. Their resistance to therapy is explained in part by the extraordinary ability of the staphylococcus to adapt itself to an unfavorable environment, for example, one containing a bactericidal drug. Given an opportunity to metabolize for a brief period in its presence, this organism develops an immunity which enables it to grow and thrive in the face of high concentrations of the drug. Thus, responsiveness to antibiotic chemotherapy, however gratifying at the outset, may diminish to the point of true refractoriness. This adaptation phenomenon becomes apparent when one compares a strain of staphylococcus recovered from a patient who has acquired an infection in the hospital with one that has been isolated elsewhere; to three antibiotics most used in hospitals, namely, penicillin, streptomycin and tetracycline, the hospital strain is almost certain to show resistance.

Hospital Staphylococcal Infections

During recent years many hospitals throughout the world have experienced serious outbreaks of staphylococcus infection which have been responsible for a number of fatalities, especially among infants. The problem is not diminishing in magnitude, but growing, and is the source of immense concern. Many factors have conspired to produce this situation. Among these doubtless are included the capacity of the staphylococcus to develop resistance to most antibiotics, the ability of this organism to penetrate skin and destroy tissue and the prevalence of the staphylococcus, especially in hospitals, where its presence is ubiquitous.

Control Measures. The elimination and the prevention of hospital staphylococcosis require the combined and co-ordinated efforts of many individuals, from all departments of the hospital. Housekeeping practices which need special review, since they are potential vectors of infection, include all operations tending to disperse dust. Vacuum cleaning and the use of rotary buffs must not be permitted. Dry mopping and dry sweeping, if practiced, likewise must be discontinued and supplanted by wet mopping. Germicidal solutions should be applied liberally to the floors, and mops should be autoclaved regularly. Containers for the disposal of waste should be equipped with disposable liners, and the receptacle themselves should be autoclaved frequently. Bedpans likewise should be equipped with disposable covers and should be sterilized frequently. Garbage removal carts should be covered with a sterile cover. Soiled linens should be packaged in a special bag which is kept separate from other hospital linen until autoclaved. Mattresses should be protected by a plastic cover. Intensive antiseptic scrubdowns should be carried out in the nurseries, the operating room and the recovery room. Effective measures for controlling flies and other pests should be adopted as needed.

Nursing Policies and Practices. Cross-traffic between hospital areas housing infected patients and those in which noninfected patients are quartered should be reduced to a minimum. None but authorized personnel should be allowed entry into isolation units. Devices which permit the immediate detection of persons who are "off-limits" should be worn by all personnel. For example, personnel attached to the operating room, the obstetric department and the nursery might be distinguished by the color of their scrub clothes. Visitors from outside should be allowed only limited, infrequent and carefully supervised access to isolation areas. Visits between patients are likewise to be discouraged. Isolation technics should be reviewed and demonstrated for the benefit of the nursing staff and rehearsed by every nurse in the institution.

Chemotherapy of Hospital Staphylococcal Infections. Treatment is selected which is most apt to eradicate the infection rapidly. Oxacillin, methicillin and vancomycin are among the most efficacious of the antistaphylococcal drugs currently available. Oxacillin (Prostaphlin) is given by mouth in the amount of 50 to 100 mg. per kilogram of body weight per day, one sixth of the total daily dose being ingested every 4 hours. Methicillin (Staphcillin) must be received parenterally; for adults the dose is 1 Gm. by intramuscular injection every 4 hours, or 6 to 8 Gm. daily by continuous intravenous infusion; for infants, half of these amounts are prescribed. Vancomycin (Vancocin) is administered by intravenous injection in 2 to 4 divided doses totaling 2 to 4 Gm. each day.

Infectious reservoirs responsible for endemic staphylococcosis in hospitals are sustained both by infected patients and infected personnel. Personnel should be urged to report all skin lesions, which, if discovered and identified as staphylococcal in origin, should be treated vigorously, the individual meanwhile being barred from contact with patients. Newborn infants are to be regarded both as vulnerable targets and as potential sources of infection. Occupants of the nursery must be protected from all unnecessary contacts, and whoever is in contact with these infants should observe meticulously all the precautions that are entailed in communicable disease nursing.

BIBLIOGRAPHY AND SUGGESTED READING

Books

Fuerst, E. V., and Wolff, L.: Fundamentals of Nursing, Heat, Cold and Counterirritants as Comfort and Therapeutic Agents, ed. 2, Unit 12, pp. 399-420, Philadelphia, Lippincott, 1959.

Harkins, H. N., Moyer, C. A., Rhoads, J. E., and Allen, J. G.: Surgery: Principles and Practice, Chap. 2, Wound Healing, pp. 7-32; Chap. 3, Applied Surgical Bacteriology, pp. 33-45; and, Chap. 4, Surgical Infections, pp. 46-70; ed. 2, Philadelphia, Lippincott, 1961.

Articles

Altemeir, W. A., Culbertson, W. R., Vetto, M., and Cole, W.: Problems in the diagnosis and treatment of gas gangrene, A.M.A. Arch. Surg. **74**:839-845, 1957.

Barton, J.: What to do about hospital infections, Mod. Hosp. **90**:51-54, 1958.

Caswell, H. T.: Staphylococcal infections among hospital personnel, Am. J. Nursing **58**:822-823, 1958.

Cirksena, W. J.: Tetanus, Am. J. Nursing **62**:65-69, April, 1962.

Creech, Jr., O., Glover, A., and Ochsner, A.: Tetanus: evaluation of treatment at Charity Hospital, New Orleans, Louisiana, Ann. Surg. **146**:369-383, 1957.

Dull, H. B., and Rakich, J. H.: Tetanus today, Nursing Outlook **7**:464-466, 1959.

Lester, M. R.: Staphylococcal infections, Am. J. Nursing **59**:1805-1828, 1959.

McCray, P., Nutrition and wound healing, Am. J. Clin. Nutri. **3**:461-465, 1955.

Rakich, J. H., Thomas, M. W., and Lester, M.: Nurses are asking about staphylococcal infections, Am J. Nursing **60**:1766-1769, 1960.

Ravenholt, R. T., and Nixon, M.: The telephone in epidemiology of staphylococcal disease, Am. J. Nursing **61**:60-64, Aug., 1961.

Rogers, D. E.: Staphylococcal disease on general medical services, Am. J. Nursing **59**:842-844, 1959.

Sheldon, N. S.: Sterile warm wet compresses, Am. J. Nursing **59**:982-984, 1959.

Staphcillin, Am. J. Nursing **61**:58-59, March, 1961.

Prevention and control of infection, Am. J. Nursing **60**:657, 1960.

4

Antisepsis and Asepsis

Surgery as practiced up to the 19th century was a discouraging and distressing branch of medicine. Pus formed in a majority of all open wounds whether accidental or as a result of operation. Many patients developed more serious complications, such as septicemia (blood poisoning), hemorrhage and gangrene. As a consequence, amputations were frequent, prolonged illness with crippling disability often resulted and, only too often, death occurred.

The first advance toward the present-day practice of surgery was made by a chemist, Louis Pasteur. In 1857, while studying the phenomena of fermentation, he demonstrated the presence and the activity of micro-organisms or bacteria. Later, he showed that "putrefaction was a fermentation caused by the growth of microbes." These organisms, he found, were killed by heat, and putrefaction could be avoided by preventing further entrance of the germs, the present-day concept of prophylaxis in surgery.

A short time later, an English surgeon, Joseph Lister, directed his attention to Pasteur's work. He attempted first to prevent putrefaction and pus formation in wounds infected with microbes by destroying the germs with carbolic acid, a solution of which, he had found, would kill bacteria. Later, he developed an elaborate technic for operation on clean wounds, with the carbolization of the patient's skin and wound, the surgeon's hands and all the materials used at the operation. He even attempted to destroy the germs in the surrounding air by the use of a carbolic acid spray.

DEVELOPMENT OF ASEPSIS

Surgery has made great strides since Lister's time. The principles that he laid down are still adhered to, but with fuller knowledge and added experience his methods have been modified. It is known now that the materials used in the treatment of wounds may be freed from living organisms by heat, thus largely replacing chemical disinfection. It has been found unnecessary to attempt to rid the air of bacteria because, when germs are excluded from entrance to the wound by other paths, healing occurs usually without infection. Experience has shown that tissues have a natural power of self-protection against the action of bacteria. The power is lessened markedly by the application of strong antiseptics but, in most cases of clean wounds, is sufficient in itself to kill organisms that gain entrance to the wound during an operation.

For these reasons, surgical procedures have been changed largely from the *antiseptic* (against putrefaction) methods of Lister to the *aseptic* (without infection) technic of today. An effort is made to operate without any initial entrance of bacteria into the wounds. This object is gained by *sterilizing* (killing the bacteria in) all materials used in the operation.

Principles of Aseptic Surgery

The successful practice of aseptic surgery requires a strict observance of preoperative sterilization of the surgical materials, of rigid precautions against infection during the course of the operation, and of guarding the wound from infection afterward until such time as it is healed.

Preoperative Treatment. This comprises sterilizing and keeping sterile (free from micro-organisms) all surgical materials that are to come in contact with the wound and exposed tissues or that are to be handled by the surgeon or his assistants. These include all instruments, needles, sutures, dressings, gloves, covers and so forth. In addition, the surgeon and his assistants and nurses must prepare themselves before touching any of these materials. While their hands and arms cannot be rendered absolutely sterile, they must be made as clean as possible by the use of soap, water and chemicals, and then covered with sterile rubber gloves. A cap is used to cover the head and enclose the hair. Masks covering the nose and the mouth are employed to prevent bacteria from the upper respiratory system from entering the wound. A long-sleeved sterile gown must be worn over the clothing. The patient's skin, over an area considerably larger than that requiring exposure during the course of operation, also demands the highest possible degree of cleanliness and the application of some chemical agent. The rest of the patient's body is covered with sterile drapes.

During Operation. During the operation neither the "scrubbed" surgeon nor his nurses or assistants touch anything that has not been rendered and kept sterile. "Nonscrubbed" assistants refrain from touching or infecting anything that is sterile.

After Operation. After the operation the wound is protected from possible infection by means of sterile dressings and by an occasional disinfection of the surrounding skin with chemical agents. Particular care is taken to prevent contact of anything that is not sterile with the unhealed wound. In most cases not previously infected, this aseptic regimen is all that is necessary to ensure rapid aseptic healing. In recently infected wounds, it is necessary to remove and destroy such micro-organisms as are already in the tissues, and also to prevent subsequent infection from without. The first condition is affected by the removal of foreign bodies and devitalized tissues from the wound (*débridement*). The second condition is fulfilled by the use of a rigid aseptic technic during the course of the treatment.

When infection already has developed in the tissues, the chief indication is to help the body to eliminate the organisms by incision and to prevent the entrance of further infection from without.

It must be recognized then that, although the surgical technic of today is said to be aseptic, there are still many uses for chemical disinfection in the treatment of infected, and even of aseptic, wounds.

PRINCIPLES OF STERILIZATION— DEFINITIONS

Sterilization, in surgery, means the destruction of all organisms, including spores.

Disinfection is the act of destroying all non-spore-bearing pathogenic organisms, i.e., those responsible for the communicable diseases. This method would be applicable for the disinfection of clothing, bedding, bedpans, and so forth.

Disinfectants are agents, usually a chemical, that destroy disease-producing organisms.

Antiseptics are agents that prevent the growth of micro-organisms without necessarily destroying them.

Germicides or **bactericides** are agents that kill micro-organisms.

Deodorizers or deodorants are agents employed to destroy or prevent offensive odors.

Mechanical Disinfection. When a physician or a nurse "scrubs" or prepares the skin of the operative site, it is an effort to cleanse mechanically the skin surfaces that may be exposed during the operation. This means removal of the surface dirt and fat and the organisms that are found normally on the skin. Usually, this is accomplished by the use of warm water and a soap that produces an abundant lather. Some surgeons prefer soaps containing antiseptics that appear to be more efficient in reducing the bacterial habitants of the skin surface. Others use detergents containing antiseptics for the same purpose (see Technic of Scrubbing, p. 236).

A further method of mechanical disinfection is utilized in recently infected traumatic wounds. Under sterile conditions an effort is made to cut away all the devitalized tissue, so as to remove foreign materials and contaminating bacteria. This procedure is known as *débridement*.

HEAT STERILIZATION

Sterilization by heat ensures the destruction of micro-organisms and their spores. It is the method to be chosen for all materials, except those that suffer damage from re-

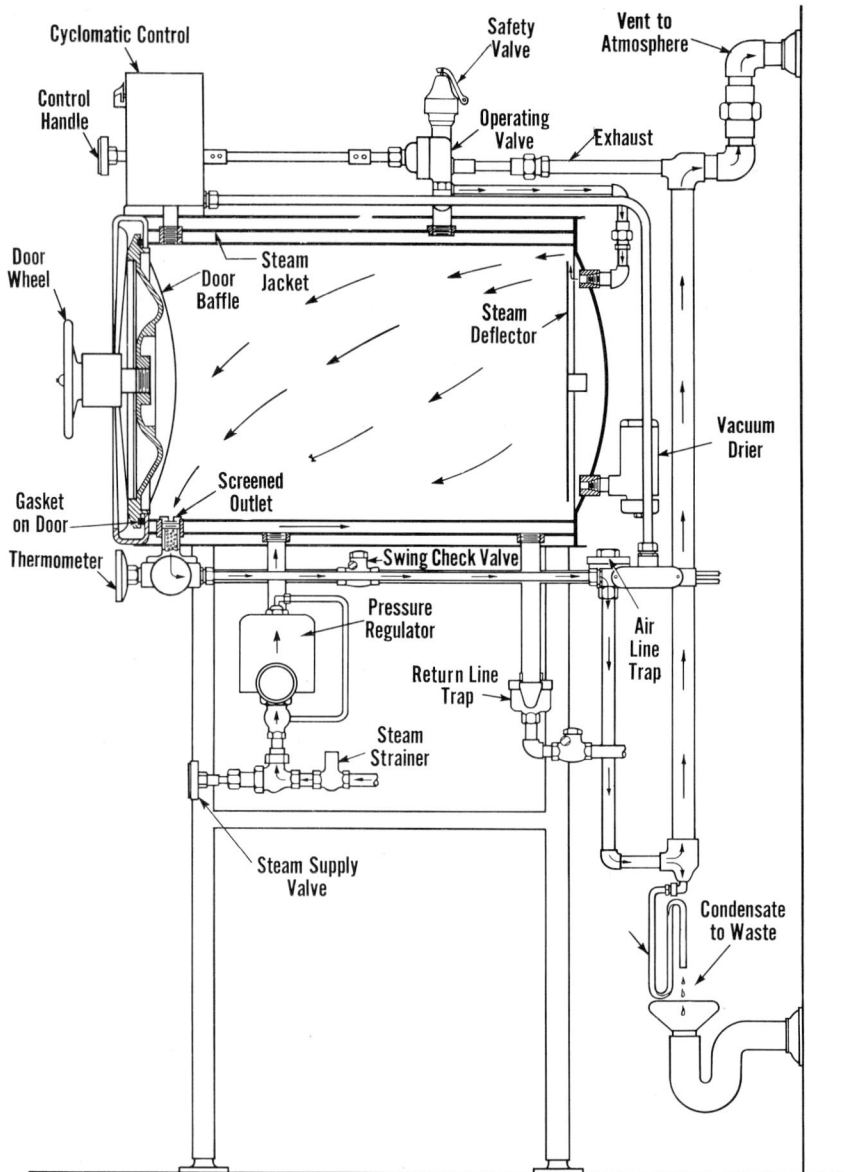

FIG. 9. Longitudinal cross section of steam-heated pressure steam sterilizer. Steam is delivered from source to steam jacket through a pressure regulator that maintains automatically the desired range. The same principle applies for steam heat (as shown) or for sterilizers heated by gas or electricity. Jacket steam then is admitted through operating valve to chamber at back end behind a deflector. Arrows indicate passage of air and steam through chamber to screened outlet drain at front end. Drainage system includes thermometer and thermostatic valve. All discharge flows to the vertical riser, which drains water through the open air break to the waste system. Steam or vapors are exhausted to atmospheric vent. (The Surgical Supervisor, American Sterilizer Co., Erie, Pa.)

peated exposure to heat. Before subjecting a material to sterilization by heat, it is essential that it be clean and free from any dirt, threads, ravelings and so forth that might remain as foreign bodies in the wound. The mode of applying heat varies with the nature of the material to be sterilized and with the circumstances under which the sterilization is to be carried out. The two main forms of heat are: moist heat and dry heat.

Moist Heat

Moist heat may be applied as steam or boiling water.

Steam Under Pressure.

This is the most desirable method of sterilizing nearly all surgical supplies. The sterilizer or *autoclave* (Fig. 9) is built in such a manner that steam enters the sterilizing chamber under pressure for the purpose of attaining high temperatures. Materials thus sterilized are subjected to a temperature of from 115° to 123° C. (240° to 254° F.). The steam of the autoclave at these temperatures destroys all vegetative bacteria, and even the most resistant pathogenic spores, in a relatively brief interval of time. Tests have proved that the spores of *Cl. oedematiens, Cl. tetani* and *Cl. welchii* are destroyed in direct contact with steam at 121° C. (250° F.) in 1 minute, at 115° C. (240° F.) in 4 minutes and at 110° C. (230° F.) in 10 minutes. Since these are the absolute minimum requirements, a considerably longer period of time is necessary in order to provide for the steam to permeate the mass, whatever it is. Surrounding the sterilizing chamber is a steam jacket, where from 15 to 17 pounds of pressure is maintained before, during and after the sterilization period. One purpose of the jacket is to prevent condensation of the water vapor, with consequent wetting of the supplies.

The principle of sterilization by the use of steam is the same as in other methods of sterilization—the coagulation of the proteins in the bacterial body, which destroys the bacteria. It has been found by experiment that coagulation occurs at a much lower temperature with moist heat than with dry heat, which is the reason for the use of boiling water and of steam under pressure as sterilizing agents. Steam at atmospheric pressure can transmit a temperature of only 212° F. (100° C.). This temperature is able to kill all living or vegetative forms of bacterial life, but many spores are resistant to this temperature and are not killed.

Removal of Air. In order to reach such high temperatures, it is necessary that the air be removed as completely as possible from the sterilizing chamber. The temperature can be gauged by the pressure indicator only when the pressure represents that of steam and not that of steam plus air in the sterilizing chamber. Therefore, an attempt is made in all types of sterilizers to remove the air from the sterilizing chamber. This is accomplished best by permitting the air to escape through a drain controlled thermostatically from the bottom of the chamber, including an accurate mercury thermometer that indicates consequently the temperature of the coolest medium surrounding the load, since air or steam mixed with air will gravitate unfailingly below pure steam in the chamber. The thermostatic valve remains open and permits air and condensate to escape freely. It closes only after the air has been driven out, and relatively pure steam follows. This thermometer thus becomes the one gauge (rather than the pressure indication) under which all sterilization is controlled. Every performance is timed when the thermometer indicates 240° F. (115° C.) in its advance toward the regulated maximum of 254° F. (123° C.).

The importance of withdrawing the air is due to the fact that the presence of air reduces the ultimate temperature of the steam at any given pressure, because steam and air do not blend; therefore, the materials at the top of the sterilizer, heated by pure steam, become sterilized easily and rapidly, and those at the bottom of the sterilizer, where most of the air accumulates, are heated by a mixture of warm air and steam, and the temperature does not rise to the point which will produce sterilization for a considerable period of time. Furthermore, the presence of air in the sterilizer reduces very materially the power of the steam to penetrate and sterilize large packages of materials, because the penetration of steam into these packages depends upon the displacement of air due to gravity. If the chamber is two-thirds filled with air, there is no displacement by gravity and, therefore, poor penetration of the materials by steam.

In the operation of the sterilizer, no matter what type, the process by which sterilization is accomplished is much the same. In the stage of preparation, steam is admitted to the outer or steam jacket until the pressure of from 15 to 17 pounds is reached. In this way the sterilizing chamber is heated and is prepared for the reception of the materials to be sterilized. After the materials have been introduced into the chamber, air is evacuated from the chamber by gravity, as explained above. The operator should keep close watch until the thermometer indicates 240° F. (115° C.); then the period of exposure, which is governed by the particular load, is timed.

At the close of the period of sterilization, the operating valve is turned to "exhaust" until chamber pressure has reduced to "zero." Jacket pressure is maintained until drying is complete. When chamber pressure has reduced to zero, the operating valve (for dry loads only) is turned to the "vacuum" or "dry" position, in which a partial vacuum is created in the chamber, rarefying the vapor and hastening drying to some extent. This position is maintained for not more than 3 to 5 minutes, and the operating valve is turned to the "off" position until the chamber gauge again indicates zero pressure.

Then the door is unlocked and loosened slightly but opened not more than ½ inch for about 10 minutes, depending upon the size and the density of the load. Vapor will escape into the room from the top of the door, and drying results.

For cooling down solution loads—any aqueous solution in bottles or flasks—exhaust of the chamber steam must be controlled precisely or blown stoppers and undue loss of fluid will result. Steam exhaust can be controlled easily in the following way:

At the close of the period of sterilization, turn the operating valve toward the exhaust position so that the steam from the chamber will escape very slowly. Exhaust to the zero pressure should occur in not less than from 6 to 10 minutes, and the door must not be unlocked until all pressure has been exhausted completely. This will permit the fluid in the flasks or the bottles to lose its heat without violent ebullition down to the boiling point.

Packaging.

1. All articles must be absolutely clean and freshly laundered (or hydrated) to guard against superheating with resultant injury to the fabric.

2. All linens are checked for holes and tears; these can be mended. Threads and ravelings must be removed.

3. Sheets and covers are folded to facilitate their use, such as fanfolding, etc. Such

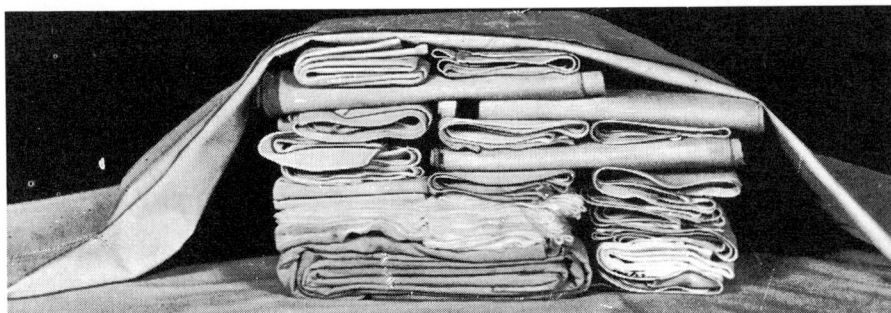

FIG. 10. A model heavy pack arrangement. None should be larger than 12"x12"x20", or more densely arranged than illustrated. Note how alternate layers are crossed to promote free circulation of steam through the mass. Note also that gauze sponges are located near the center of the pack to break up close contact between masses of more tightly woven fabrics. (The Surgical Supervisor, American Sterilizer Co., Erie, Pa.)

foresight will prevent undue handling and flourishing of sterile drapes. Covers and towels should be folded, so that the edges and not the center part will be handled when opened. Gowns must be folded wrong side out, so that the inner side only is touched by the ungloved hand when they are put on by the surgeon and his assistants. This is accomplished very easily by first folding the gown lengthwise and then, starting at the hem, rolling it into a compact bundle. A 5-inch length of 2-inch stockinet makes a very comfortable cuff for operating gowns and also one that is folded in more readily under the cuff of rubber gloves.

4. The contents of a pack are arranged in such a way that the articles which are used first appear on top. The arrangement should facilitate steam penetration (Fig. 10). Basins should not be included with fabrics in one package, since basins interfere with steam permeation and retard drying after sterilization.

5. The size of any pack should not exceed the dimensions of 12″ x 12″ x 20″. Such a package, arranged as described in

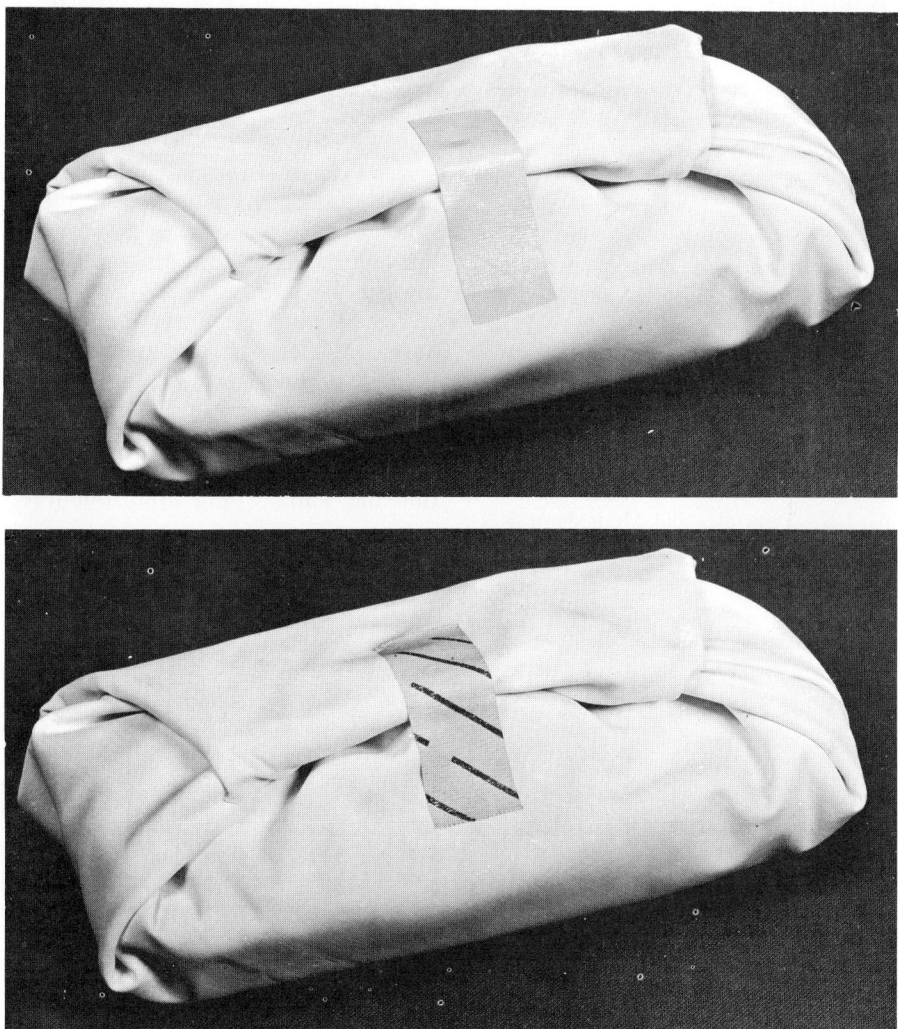

Fig. 11. Pressure-sensitive (autoclave) tape before and after sterilization. Dark striped lines appear on the tape when it is autoclaved. (Minnesota Mining and Manufacturing Co.)

Figure 10, can be sterilized in 30 minutes at 250° F. "A properly packaged and arranged kit will provide a sterile wrapper for the table, enough supplies for a procedure arranged in the order of use and a wrapper which allows prompt penetration by steam."*

6. Two double-thickness muslin wrappers are ideal to wrap supplies. These are more popular than other kinds of wrapping materials. Parchment and flat Kraft brown paper appear to have no particular advantages; their disadvantages are that they tear easily, are difficult to wrap and are noisy to handle. Two-way crepe paper appears to be easy to use and is durable. Densometer readings (a measure of porosity indicating time required for a given volume of air to pass through the sheet) are much more favorable for 2-way crepe than for parchment or brown paper.† Canvas covers or heavy woven fabric retard the passage of steam and, therefore, are not recommended. "At the present time there is insufficient evidence to warrant the use of paper as a substitute for muslin, especially for wrapping of those supplies destined for use in the operating room."‡

* Walter, C. W.: Aseptic Treatment of Wounds, New York, Macmillan, 1949.

† Christie, J. E.: Muslin vs. paper autoclave wrappers—a hospital study, Hospital Topics **35:** 117, 1957.

‡ Perkins, J. J.: Principles and Methods of Sterilization, p. 101, Springfield, Ill., Thomas, 1956.

7. Packages must be wrapped securely and fastened with cord, twill tape or pressure-sensitive tape. (See Fig. 11.) Pins should not be used, since they cause excessive wear on linen, increase the tendency of tight wrapping, and the holes they produce may permit contamination of the contents.

8. All packages should be marked legibly to identify contents and date of sterilization. When pressure-sensitive tape is used, this information can be written on the tape. (See Fig. 11.) To facilitate removal of tape, slightly invert one corner.

9. Drums are not recommended for several reasons: they are expensive, noisy to handle and encourage overloading. In addition, the metal surface of the drum retards passage of steam to the contents.

Loading of Sterilizer.

1. Prepare all packs and arrange the load in the sterilizer so as to present the least possible resistance to the passage of steam through the load, from the top of the chamber toward the bottom. (See Fig. 12.)

2. All jars, test tubes and other non-porous containers of dry material should be loaded in the sterilizer, with a horizontal path for the escape of air. "Imagine that the container is filled with water. Then place it in the sterilizer in a horizontal position so that the water would drain out freely."§

§ Perkins, *ibid.,* p. 108.

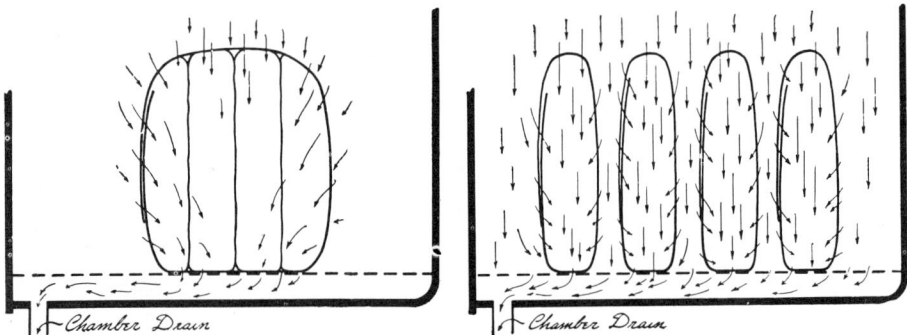

FIG. 12. *(Left)* One large pack. *(Right)* Same pack broken down into four small packs, and these are separated slightly from each other in the sterilizer. The single large pack shows why there is oversterilization of the outer portions when exposure has continued long enough to permit steam to penetrate adequately to the interior for sterilization. In the smaller packs, steam permeates the entire mass quickly, and a much shorter period of exposure is needed.

Period of Exposure.

1. Establish a period of exposure that will provide for complete penetration of the load and ensure destruction of microbial life with a liberal margin of safety.

2. Time the sterilizing period from the moment that saturated steam at 250° F. fills the chamber as indicated by the thermometer located in the chamber drain line.

Drying of Load.

1. Provide a minimum drying period of 15 minutes for all bulk loads of supplies.

2. Do not place freshly sterilized packages on cold surfaces, since condensation and wetting will take place, which results in contamination.

Nursing Responsibility. Of all the sterilizers the autoclave is probably the most important. The principles just described apply to any autoclave, be it small, large, round or square. This sterilizing unit is found in the central supply division, the operating and the delivery rooms and even in the utility or treatment rooms on the patient divisions. It is important that such a vital piece of equipment be kept in excellent working order, be kept clean and be checked frequently for its effectiveness in sterilizing. The nurse should learn how to operate the autoclave and to recognize her responsibility for supervising non-professional workers as they use it. Sterilization must be timed accurately. No guess work can be sanctioned when a patient's life may depend upon the sterility of a dressing or an instrument. To avoid error some central clock should be used and not an individual's wrist watch, which may allow timing discrepancies to occur.

Boiling Water

The once widely used technic of boiling instruments for surgery is open to question today. The boiling process should be discouraged,* and used only when steam under pressure is not available.

Boiling water (212° F. or 100° C.) will destroy all living bacteria in a few seconds, but the spores of some organisms are very

---

* Perkins considers it more appropriate to designate the boiling water process as one of disinfection or sanitization, rather than sterilization.

resistant and require boiling for a longer time (at least 30 minutes) to ensure their destruction. Some of the most difficult spores to kill, such as tetanus and gas gangrene organisms, resist many hours of boiling. The disadvantage of boiling is that it dulls the edge of cutting instruments—scalpels and so forth; also, the usual tap water leaves a deposit of scale (lime) in the joints and on the surfaces of instruments and utensils that can be removed only by vigorous scouring.

The usual technic for sterilization of instruments requires that they boil in plain water for 30 minutes or in water containing 2 per cent of sodium carbonate (from 3 to 4 teaspoonfuls to the quart of water) for not less than 15 minutes. The addition of sodium carbonate brings about the destruction of the more resistant spores in a shorter period of time than is possible in plain water. The following are important points for the nurse to remember when boiling articles: *The article must be clean.* Blood, pus, oils, grease and so forth hinder the sterilizing process. The timing of sterilization is started when the water begins to boil. *All articles must be submerged completely.* The speed at which the water boils does not change the time element; therefore, it is better to have the water boiling quietly.

Specialty Sterilizers

In addition to the autoclave, described in detail on pp. 38-40, there are specialty sterilizers.

Instrument Washer Sterilizer. Instruments can be washed by means of a vigorously agitated detergent bath. Blood, grease and tissue debris is loosened and is drawn off the top of the container and directed to an overflow valve. In the operating process the temperature reaches 270° F. (132° C.) in about 12 minutes. Upon release of water and steam, instruments are thoroughly dried and ready for use or storage.

Instrument Sterilizer. This is similar in construction to the autoclave described on p. 38 but smaller. In sterilizing instruments a layer of muslin is placed on the bottom of a wire meshed or perforated tray. Instruments are then arranged in the manner in which they will be used later. All jointed instruments must be open or unlocked to allow steam to come in contact with all surfaces. A top muslin cover is added if the tray is eventually to be carried a distance. Sterilizing time is 15 minutes at 250° F. (121° C.) or 7 minutes at 270° F. (132° C.). For emergency use a single instrument or two can be sterilized at 270° F., 27 lb. pressure in 3 minutes.

Water Sterilizer. There is a trend away from the water sterilizer (water is sterilized at 250° F. under pressure every 12 hours) to individual flasks of sterile water or isotonic solutions. The reasons are several: (1) one of the problems is to maintain the sterility of water in the large tank (there is danger of air-borne, insect and contact contamination, especially at the outlet or draw-off point; (2) the pitcher used to transfer sterile water from the tank to the sterile basin is a receptacle which is difficult to keep sterile because of the human element in handling it over and over again; and (3) surgeons are preferring isotonic autoclaved solutions for sponges and irrigation of wounds.

Testing for Sterility

Because of the probability of human error in operating a sterilizer and the possibility of mechanical failure within the equipment itself, sterilization failures may occur. There are several ways of checking proper function and adequate sterilization.

The Recording Thermometer. This instrument contains a clock, mechanically operated, which revolves an 8-inch diameter chart once in 24 hours. The chart records the temperature in the discharge outlet and also the duration of each exposure. It is a valuable means of checking when it is properly installed and used.

Sterilization Indicators. These indicators are of many types, varying from simple paper strips which change color to hermetically sealed glass tubes containing a pellet that melts and changes color when sterilization temperatures are reached. Perkins has observed "that all sterilization indicators possess the same general disadvantage, to a greater or lesser degree, in that a percentage will be found to react to a time-temperature ratio inadequate for sterilization or that the end points are not sufficiently clear so as to permit accurate interpretation of the results. These controls do not indicate the actual build-up of temperature in the test pack nor do they indicate how much over-exposure may have been applied."*

Culture Tests. The best way of determining the sterility of an article is to perform a bacteriologic culture test. Periodic check on a bimonthly basis is recommended. The sporebearing organisms used in culture tests are *Bacillus subtilis* and *Bacillus stearothermophilus*.

Perkins describes an effective and simple means by using bacterial spore strips. These are small strips (2″ x ½″) of filter paper upon which a specific number of dry bacterial spores of established heat resistance are placed. They are dried, and then 2 strips are placed side by side in a steam-permeable paper envelope. Then this is placed in the center of the most densely packed package; this in turn is placed in the front bottom portion of the sterilizer. Following the usual sterilizing and drying process, the envelope is sent to the laboratory where, under sterile procedure, the strips are removed and placed in sterile medium to incubate for 7 days.

Dry Heat

Cautery. This is used to sterilize cut tissue surfaces—for example, the base of the appendix in an appendectomy.

Hot Air. Some surgical supplies, such as various forms of oil, bone wax and talcum powder in bulk, cannot be sterilized properly by any method other than prolonged exposure to dry heat in the hot-air oven. The moist heat of the autoclave is inadequate because the moisture factor of the steam, essential to autoclave sterilization, does not permeate such masses. Such materials should be sterilized in a dry-heat sterilizer at a temperature of 320° F. (160° C.) for 1 hour or at 250° F. (121° C.) for 4 hours. Usually it is not advisable to attempt sterilization of such materials except in relatively small quantities; that is to say, in small jars or containers.

Another advantage of dry heat is that it does not destroy finely polished cutting edges of instruments, such as scissors, knife blades,

* Perkins, *op. cit.*, p. 231.

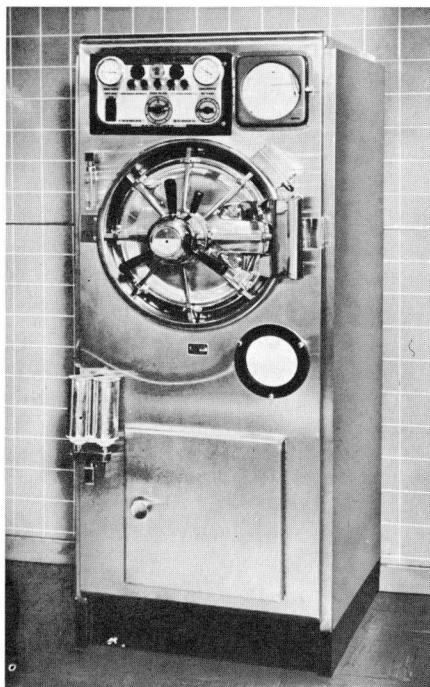

FIG. 13. Ethylene oxide sterilizer (Steroxide Gas Sterilizer). This is a self-contained unit requiring a 20-ampere electric supply and a vent to outdoors. The control panel is at the top right; a dual recorder for pressure and temperature is at top left. The glass tube below the controls contains water for humidification. On the lower left, disposable cans of inerted ethylene oxide are fastened ready for use. A circular air filter can be noted above the storage compartment. The unit is operated automatically. (Wilmot Castle Co., Rochester, N. Y.)

osteotomes, etc. It is also a desirable method for syringes, since dry heat does not attack the ground surfaces as moist heat does.

A hot-air oven can be created in the ordinary autoclave. Steam is allowed to enter the jacket but not the chamber; in this way, syringes, needles, sharp-edged instruments, etc., can be adequately sterilized overnight or for a minimum of 4 hours at 250° F. (121° C.).

RADIANT ENERGY STERILIZATION

Ultraviolet Light. There are many limitations to the use of ultraviolet light in the operating room. Since radiation does not penetrate the surface of liquids because the light is reflected, droplets are not sterilized. Every surface must be exposed for sterilization; bacteria are protected in the shadows. Sufficient time must be provided for sterilization, since it is not instantaneous. Prolonged exposure will injure skin, tissues and eyes; therefore, the head and the neck of operating room personnel should be protected if ultraviolet light is used.

GASEOUS STERILIZATION

Ethylene Oxide. C_2H_4O is a moderately toxic gas which is able to sterilize effectively many items that are sensitive to heat and moisture, such as telescopic instruments, electric cords, rubber goods and so forth. In an ethylene oxide sterilizer (Fig. 13), several conditions must obtain for proper sterilization: 1. Air must be evacuated from the chamber. 2. A relative humidity of between 25 and 50 per cent is then created, using vaporized distilled water. 3. Temperature between 100° and 140° F. is provided. 4. A concentration of 760 mg./L. of ethylene oxide is introduced. At 140° F. the exposure time is 3 hours. For a lower temperature, the time is increased. 5. Ethylene oxide is evacuated mechanically. 6. Air, sterilized by filtration and exposure to ultraviolet radiation, is admitted.

CHEMICAL METHODS OF DISINFECTION—ANTISEPTICS

Since many chemical agents are not capable of destroying all forms of microbial life, e.g., tubercle bacillus, bacterial spores and the filterable viruses, it is more nearly accurate to refer to the process as "chemical disinfection" rather than "chemical sterilization." (See Definition, p. 37.)

Chemical disinfection is used only when it is not feasible to sterilize an article by heat. Chemical disinfectants tend to congeal proteinaceous material such as blood, and organisms contained within this protein precipitate may well survive. Accordingly, chemical disinfection should not be used for instruments contaminated with blood or tissue fluid.

Factors Which Influence Disinfectant Action

1. **Cleanliness.** The presence of blood, pus, oil or grease interferes with the action

of all germicides. The effective use of soap and water for cleansing is a necessary preliminary step to ensure optimum effectiveness of a disinfectant.

2. **Concentration.** Usually a weak solution is not as effective as a strong solution of the same disinfectant. An exception is ethyl alcohol; 70 per cent aqueous solution is more germicidal than absolute alcohol.

3. **Time.** This factor varies from seconds to hours, depending on the kind of disinfectant, the strength of the disinfecting agent, and the characteristics of the organisms to be eliminated. Vegetative organisms may be destroyed in 30 minutes by some of the chemical disinfectants, whereas no amount of time (hours or days) by the same agent would result in sporicidal action.

4. **Type of Organism.** Some organisms are killed more readily than others. Examples of the resistant forms are the virus of serum hepatitis, tubercle bacillus and certain bacterial spores.

5. **Temperature.** Usually, room temperature is used; however, most chemical agents are more effective if the temperature is raised.

The Use of Disinfectants

1. **Skin Application.** Disinfectants are used to remove as many resident and transient organisms of the skin as is possible. In surgery the preoperative preparation of the skin is necessary to prevent unnecessary contamination of the surgical wound. The hands and the arms of the surgical team likewise must be prepared by scrubbing and the application of appropriate disinfectants.

2. **Application to Tissues.** Antiseptics are applied to tissues that are or may be the seat of infection, in order to assist them to destroy the germs and their products rapidly and completely. When used in this way "the ideal antiseptic should effect complete sterilization within its sphere of action without causing any damage to tissue cells" (Dakin). However, the disadvantage of most antiseptics is that in killing the bacteria they tend also to destroy tissue cells. For this reason they should be used in wounds in weak solutions, and for only a short period of time. Many antiseptics have been suggested and used in tissues, and their very multiplicity would indicate that the ideal antiseptic has not been found yet. It is being recognized

more and more that the body tissues have a natural resistance to infection, and that antiseptics are of value only occasionally in the treatment of certain specific types of infection, especially those on the surface of the body.

3. **Disinfection of Instruments and Materials.** Chemicals are used to disinfect certain instruments and materials that cannot be sterilized by heat; for example, cystoscopes, bougies and cataract knives must be immersed in a germicide. Most of the chemicals are used in the form of solutions, being dissolved in water or in alcohol. From time to time new chemical compounds appear on the market, all of them with certain advantages and disadvantages.

Groups of Disinfectants

Disinfectants are classified as follows for discussion: (1) alcohols, (2) phenols and cresols, (3) quaternary ammonium compounds, (4) aldehydes and acids, (5) oxidizing agents, (6) halogen compounds, (7) furan derivative and (8) ointments.

Alcohols

Ethyl Alcohol. This is one of the most useful disinfectants. It has a high degree of antiseptic power and has the advantage of being a fat solvent, dissolving out the fat on the surface and in the follicles of the skin, thus permitting the antiseptic to act on the more deeply situated organisms. In 70 per cent solution by weight (81.5 per cent by volume), it is used frequently in disinfection of the patient's skin and as an evaporating lotion. Because it is a fat solvent, it is used frequently in combination with other antiseptics.

Disadvantages. Alcohol causes considerable pain when applied to raw tissues and produces irritation of mucous surfaces; therefore, it should not be used in fresh, open wounds, for the eye, the urethra and so forth.

As a disinfectant for instruments, it must be remembered that they must be cleansed thoroughly because of the protein-coagulating action of alcohol. Greater effectiveness is brought about when alcohol is combined with other disinfectants.

Isopropyl Alcohol is displacing ethyl alcohol in many instances, since it exhibits slightly greater germicidal action, has a lower surface tension, is a better fat solvent and is less expensive. The dilution need not be as stable as ethyl alcohol.

Phenols and Cresols

Phenol or carbolic acid probably was the first recognized antiseptic. About a 95 per cent solution ("pure phenol" or "pure carbolic acid") is used by many surgeons to sterilize and cauterize the cut edges of intestinal mucosa; for example, the stump of the appendix is often touched with "pure phenol" before it is inverted into the cecal wall.

Disadvantages. Phenol is extremely toxic and highly destructive to tissues. Even in germicidal concentrations, it is an irritant to the skin. It is not effective against spores, and as a practical disinfectant its use is limited.

Cresols are derivatives of phenol, which they have largely replaced. They are much more effective germicides than the phenols; however, they are not effective against spores.

Hexachlorophene (G-11) is a phenol derivative which, when incorporated into soaps, detergent creams, etc., is one of the most effective agents for the preoperative preparation of the skin. (See p. 211.)

Quaternary Ammonium Compounds
(Zephiran, Phemerol, Ceepryn)

The chief property is that of lowering the surface tension of solutions. They are stable and nonirritating.

Disadvantages. These compounds are incompatible with soap, and they are not effective against tubercle bacillus and spores.

Aldehydes and Acids

Formaldehyde is a gas with high disinfecting properties. A 40 percent solution of the gas in water is known as **formalin.** Since it is too irritating for living tissue, it is mainly used as a preservative of specimens.

A solution of 20 per cent formalin and 70 per cent isopropyl alcohol solution is an effective chemical disinfectant and sporicide (exposure time, 30 minutes immersion) for clean instruments that cannot be exposed to steam under pressure sterilization, and are of a material or property that will not be destroyed by the solution.

Oxidizing Agents

The antiseptic properties of this group are due to their property of liberating oxygen that has a mild germicidal action.

Hydrogen Peroxide. This is a clear, watery solution that decomposes readily in the light or on heating. When applied to wound tissues, there is an immediate effervescence that marks the liberation of gaseous oxygen.

Its chief value lies probably in the mechanical effect of its effervescence, in loosening necrotic tissues and dressings and in breaking up thick adherent masses of pus that float to the surface in a sort of foam. Because of this property and its ability to give off oxygen, it is of special value in the treatment of anaerobic infections, such as those caused by the gas bacillus.

Hydrogen peroxide decomposes rapidly unless protected from light, heat and air.

Potassium Permanganate. This occurs as purple crystals, is soluble easily in water and gives a wine-colored solution.

Special Uses. In solution of 1:1,000 to 1:10,000 in sloughing wounds, as an antiseptic and deodorant.

Disadvantages. The solutions decompose rapidly, losing their antiseptic power on contact with dead organic material, rubber or rusty metal, as in chipped enamel ware. The change is accompanied by a conversion of the purple to a brown color.

Halogen Compound

Iodine. This antiseptic ordinarily is used as a tincture. It is one of the most useful when conditions are such that rapid and complete disinfection may be effected by a single application.

Special Uses. (1) As a 3 to 5 per cent solution in the preparation of the skin of the patient for operation.

(2) As a 2 per cent solution for the emergency treatment of contaminated wounds.

(3) An iodine solution of 0.5 to 1 per cent in 70 per cent alcohol is the agent of choice for the disinfection of clinical thermometers.

Disadvantages. (1) Iodine solutions often irritate the skin.

(2) On wet skin, iodine loses much of its

effectiveness as a skin disinfectant and frequently causes blisters or vesicles. For this reason it is used only on dry surfaces, never on the palms of the hands, the soles of the feet, the armpits and the perineum. During the summer months, when profuse sweating occurs, iodine should not be used on the face, the scrotum and any other tender parts of the skin.

(3) The strength of iodine solutions increases on standing. This is due to evaporation of the alcoholic solvent. Therefore, they should be kept tightly corked and renewed frequently.

Ioprep.* This preparation utilizes the rapid and complete killing-power of iodine against all species of bacteria in a nonstaining and nonirritating solution. A 3-minute application to the operative site, after a thorough cleansing, is recommended and has been used with good results.

Betadine. This chemical agent has been used successfully in the preoperative preparation of the skin, both as a scrubbing agent for the hands of the operating team, and for the skin disinfection of the patient. It is an aqueous solution of povidone-iodine (N.N.D.), a nonstinging and nonstaining soluble iodine complex. It is not irritating to skin or mucous membranes; and unlike tincture of iodine, it can be safely bandaged with no undesirable effects. It kills on contact fungi, viruses, protozoa and yeasts, and has a more prolonged germicidal action than ordinary iodine solutions.

Iodoform. Its chief use is in the form of "iodoform gauze"—gauze impregnated with a 10 to 20 per cent emulsion of iodoform. It is used especially for packing in foul discharging wounds. It is now seldom used.

Furan Derivative

Nitrofurazone, N.N.D. (Furacin). An effective agent against many gram-positive and gram-negative bacteria, Furacin is used in the form of a solution in the local treatment of infections and may be applied in the form of an ointment for surface lesions.

Ointments

These are used in surgery when it is inad-

* A product of Johnson & Johnson.

visable to apply watery lotions and when it is desired to protect the surrounding skin from the irritating discharges of a wound. They are used also as mildly antiseptic applications in superficial wounds and ulcers, as stimulating applications to sluggish wound surfaces and as a means of administering medicines.

The bland ointments, such as petrolatum, lanolin and cold cream, are used to soften dry and scaly skin and to prevent dressings from adhering to secreting wounds. Mildly antiseptic ointments, such as the ointments of boric acid or zinc oxide, are used in much the same manner. The zinc oxide ointment is useful especially in the treatment of the irritating excoriation of the skin that surrounds a wound having secretion. Ointments containing scarlet red and balsam of Peru have a reputation for stimulating granulation tissue and epithelial growth. They are applied to wounds that seem to be slow in healing.

Few ointments are used in surgery as a means of administering drugs. However, there are some notable exceptions to this statement. Mercury is given in the form of mercurial ointment (blue ointment). This ointment is useful also in the early treatment of local superficial infections, such as boils, infected sebaceous cysts and so forth. Methylsalicylate ointment is useful in the treatment of joint and muscle affections. It produces a local hyperemia, and its effectiveness may be due more to a local counterirritant than to its absorbed drug. Ichthyol ointment is a black, bland, oily mixture that has been used for years as a local application by the laity and the medical profession to "draw" an infection "to a head." It is probable that the only action is to keep the superficial layers of skin soft, thus making pointing somewhat easier.

Antibiotics and certain sulfonamides in the form of ointments also are used as local antiseptics for infected wounds, burns and so forth. The antibiotic ointments may produce local sensitivity. Those which are least apt to give local skin reaction are ointments of neomycin and bacitracin. Ointments particularly effective in the treatment of skin infections such as dermatitis and pruritus are the corticosteroids.

BIBLIOGRAPHY AND SUGGESTED READING

Books

Perkins, J. J.: Principles and Methods of Sterilization, Springfield, Ill., Thomas, 1956.

Reddish, G. F. (ed.): Antiseptics, Disinfectants, Fungicides, and Chemical and Physical Sterilization, ed. 2, Philadelphia, Lea & Febiger, 1957.

Spaulding, E. H.: Chemical disinfection of medical and surgical materials (in) Reddish, G. F. (ed.) *op. cit.*

Walter, C. W.: Aseptic Treatment of Wounds, New York, Macmillan, 1948.

Articles

Caswell, H. T., *et al.*: Bacteriologic and clinical experiences and the methods of control of hospital infections due to antibiotic-resistant staphylococci, Surg., Gynec., Obst. **106**:1-10, 1958.

Christie, J. E.: Muslin vs. paper autoclave wrappers—a hospital study, Hosp. Topics, Part I **35**:117-120, March, 1957; Part II **35**:111-116, April, 1957.

Errara, D. W.: Proper positioning of supplies in the autoclave, Hosp. Topics **34**:123-127, Sept., 1956.

Spaulding, E. H., Emmons, E. K., and Guzara, M. L.: Ethylene oxide sterilization, Am. J. Nursing **58**:1530-1531, 1958.

Vesley, D., and Brask, M.: Environmental implications in the control of hospital acquired infections, Nursing Outlook **9**:742-745, 1961.

5

Observation of the Patient

The initial step in the evaluation of any patient is the securing, by skillful questioning and careful listening, of a detailed historical account of all subjective symptoms that might conceivably pertain to his present illness. The second component of the clinical examination is the eliciting of physical signs, an exercise in trained observation involving a systematic and exhaustive search for any significant physical deviations from the normal. The history and the physical examination together furnish a quantity of information containing clues of diagnostic value, and on the basis of this a provisional program of therapy is adopted.

The eliciting of symptoms and signs is not concluded with the first clinical examination, nor is it solely the prerogative of the examining physician. Symptoms which were forgotten by the patient may be recalled later and described to the nurse; symptoms may change or may disappear, and physical signs may become altered in their character under her observation. Entirely new symptoms and signs may come to her attention first. In view of her opportunities for clinical observation, which are exceptionally great, it is important that she familiarize herself with the character and the significance of the cardinal signs and symptoms, for as a competent reliable observer, her contributions to the diagnosis and the treatment of her patients can be of inestimable value.

SYMPTOMS AND THEIR SIGNIFICANCE

Symptoms and Their Significance

Early in her experience, the nurse should learn to draw a sharp distinction between the patient's *subjective symptoms,* such as his sensations of pain, numbness, dizziness or nausea, which he alone can reveal, and those objective evidences of disease called *physical signs,* which are visible, audible, can be smelled or felt by the examiner and can be elicited by means of a laboratory procedure or some technical diagnostic aid. Skin rashes, lymph node enlargements, abdominal masses and sounds from the heart and the lungs heard with the stethoscope are examples of physical signs; concerning these, the examiner, with little or no assistance from the patient, can form a judgment.

The eliciting and the reporting of symptoms are very definitely within the scope of nursing care. Indeed, of all members of the professional team, the nurse may be the only one to whom some of these data are completely and readily accessible. In order for her to perform her functions as clinical observer, it is essential that the patient's complaints be described fully and with care, evaluated with discrimination and recorded as nearly as possible in the patient's own words.

The Nurse's Role in Evaluating Symptoms

The nursing student quickly learns that a patient may have a serious disease and yet express but few complaints of a relatively minor character, or he may be altogether symptom free. This is the situation in several serious disorders during most of their clinical course and in many ultimately fatal diseases during their early, curable stages.

Some patients tend to be uncommunicative regarding their discomforts and disabilities; they must be "drawn out" and questioned with persistence and persuasiveness lest in-

50

formation of diagnostic value escape the examiner. In the majority of instances, however, this problem does not exist or is overcome readily, overzealous questioning being not only unnecessary but also distinctly disadvantageous for the patient's morale. Patients with certain types of neuroses may express their anxiety predominantly in the form of multiple complaints, all of which would seem to imply serious disability but which merely represent an acute awareness of normal bodily sensations. Inasmuch as therapy in such cases often is designed to de-emphasize the importance of these symptoms and to distract the patient from his subjective discomforts, it behooves the nurse to desist from persistent questioning, which can serve only to reinforce the patient's psychogenic disability.

The following generalizations are often helpful in evaluating symptoms with respect to their importance and severity. If a patient exhibits abnormal lack of concern in connection with a disability that is obviously serious, or if he displays a high-spirited optimism that is unwarranted in circumstances that are obviously grave, he is apt to be relatively uncommunicative as regards his subjective discomforts and, if he discusses them at all, they may be minimized to a misleading extent. Conversely, if a patient describes a multiplicity of complaints for which there is relatively little or no confirmatory objective evidence in the form of physical signs or manifest incapacity, the observer must reserve judgment in attempting to grade the discomfort.

Finally, it should be observed that individuals with neurotic tendencies are quite as susceptible to organic disease as are individuals without neuroses, but they are in far greater danger of medical neglect because of the suspicious nature of their complaints, which may color the judgment of their family, associates and professional advisors.

The Nurse's Role in Reporting Symptoms

The nurse should become practiced in the description of symptoms, learning to specify their characteristics according to a definite pattern. The following attributes, if possible, should be elicited and reported in connection with each: total duration, time of onset or first occurrence, constancy since onset, character of onset, location and degree of severity. In describing pain, the presence or absence of "radiation," i.e., spread of the pain from its point of origin or greatest intensity, should be specified, and the pain itself should be described in terms as informative as the patient can supply, such as "knifelike," "dull," "boring," "pressurelike," "steady," "wavelike," "crampy," "spasmodic," etc.

The final interpretation of symptoms is, of course, the responsibility of the physician, the nurse's role in diagnosis being chiefly that of observer and recorder. It is an essential role, however, and one requiring knowledge that can be derived only from study, from judgment based on clinical experience and, above all, from keen interest in the problems of her patients.

DETECTION AND RECORDING OF PHYSICAL SIGNS

General Appearance

Certain features of the patient's appearance are invariably important in diagnosis and never should escape the attention of the nurse. These signs include, in addition to the quality of his physical development and the degree of nourishment, manifestations indicative of the patient's physical comfort and mental state, his facies, posture and, if ambulatory, his gait.

The observing nurse soon learns to judge the mental and emotional status of her patient. Is he comfortable? If not, what is the apparent source of his discomfort? Is he alert? Is he stuporous or comatose? Is he accurately oriented, aware of his present location and identity? Does he recognize his visitors and attendants? Does he know what hour of the day, what day of the week, what month and what year it is? Does he appear to have adequate insight into his situation? Is he unduly depressed and anxious or is he euphoric, experiencing an abnormal sense of well-being and prowess? Does he describe hallucinations (visual, auditory or tactile sensations not founded in reality) or delusions (gross misinterpretations of true perceptions)? Can he move all four extremities?

Evidence of mental aberrations should be detected and recognized speedily so that close observation, active therapy and, if necessary, protective measures can be instituted in time to forestall any unfortunate developments. Any suggestion that the patient is suffering from ideas of persecution or any sign of delirium should put the nurse on her guard at once. Abnormalities of mood, unusual behavior and defective orientation may be the result of drug toxicity, uremia, severe infection or a metabolic disorder, as well as of a primary psychosis. Whatever the cause of the mental disturbance, the consequences of neglect in reporting or failure to realize the true gravity of the situation may be extremely serious.

Facies, Posture, Movements and Gait

Facies

The patient's facial color and expression should be noted carefully, for they often contribute greatly to the formulation of a correct diagnosis.

Anemia and Edema. Pallor is suggestive of anemia but is by no means diagnostic of that condition. A pale, puffy complexion may indicate the presence of edema, i.e., excessive accumulation of water in the subcutaneous tissues; therefore, it is encountered in nonanemic patients with nephritis and other disorders complicated by edema formation. In anemic individuals, pallor involves not only the skin but the lips and the conjunctivae as well. This is important, inasmuch as pallor of the skin, even in severely anemic individuals, may be obscured by skin pigmentation.

Facies in Cachexia. This is characterized by the appearance of marked wasting of the soft tissues of the face; the eyes are sunken and the cheek bones prominent. This type of facies is indicative of severe, long-standing malnutrition, due, for example, to a far-advanced neoplastic disease.

Facies in Dehydration. This condition likewise contributes the appearance of thinness, hollowness of cheeks and temples and sunken eyes, but in addition there are a lead-colored or grayish discoloration of the skin, a relaxation of the muscles about the mouth and the lips, the latter being parched and loosely apposed, and a dry, thick coating on the tongue. This, the "hippocratic facies," is observed in patients with advanced peritonitis, fluid being lost into the abdominal cavity, and in diarrheal diseases such as dysentery and cholera, voluminous and frequent liquid stools being responsible for rapid and severe dehydration.

Facies in Thyroid Disease. Often thyroid disease is suspected from the facial configuration and expression. The physiognomy of the patient with myxedema, which may be described as "moon face," with puffy lids and lack of expression, betrays his sluggish metabolism and retarded psychomotor activity. On the other hand, the patient with hyperthyroidism exhibits characteristically a staring expression suggesting "crystallized fear"; this is attributable to exophthalmos and to retraction of the eyelids, exposing the white sclerae, as well as to the smoothness of the forehead and the evident tension of all the facial muscles.

Facies in Liver Disease. The hepatic facies, encountered in patients with cirrhosis of the liver, may be recognized by the thinness of the face and the neck, the muddy, yellowish discoloration of the skin and the sclerae, the sunken eyes and the localized dilatations of small blood vessels arranged in spiderlike configurations ("spider angiomata") on the face and the neck.

Posture

The positions in which patients lie or sit and the bodily attitudes adopted when standing are of diagnostic importance.

In Congestive Heart Failure. The patient with congestive heart failure, particularly when there is fluid accumulation in the chest or the abdomen, sits propped up in bed, breathing being easiest in that position. The greater the respiratory distress, the more erect the posture (*orthopnea*). He may lean forward and elevate his shoulders by bearing down with his hands on the bed or on the arms of a chair, thereby increasing to an even greater extent the capacity of his thorax.

In Arthritis. Patients with acute arthritis of the spine, as a result of which each breath is painful, usually lie in such a fashion that the weight of the body keeps the inflamed costovertebral joints as motionless as possible, that is, in the supine position with the back hyperextended. Those with acute arthritis involving one or more peripheral joints hold the latter in the position of semi-flexion, which affords the greatest capacity to the synovial sac distended with fluid and reduces to a minimum the tension of the surrounding muscle groups.

In Intra-abdominal Disease. When caused by an inflammatory process involving the peritoneum, abdominal pain is aggravated by pressure; therefore, persons with acute appendicitis, an infection of the gallbladder or peritonitis tend to lie supine with knees flexed in order to relax the abdominal muscles.

Movements

Tremors. These may be rhythmic or arrhythmic, their speed slow or rapid, and their quality coarse or fine. In cases of hyperthyroidism, the tremor may be so rapid and its excursion so small that it may not be apparent until the examiner places a sheet of paper on the back of the patient's extended hand. The "intention tremor" of multiple sclerosis appears only in the course of directed movements of the extremities; when the patient attempts to place a finger on a specific object or point, the excursion of the tremor increases in amplitude as the finger approaches its goal. Parkinson's disease often is accompanied by a tremor involving the hands; the presence of this tremor is quite unrelated to voluntary muscular activity. This type of tremor is repetitive and stereotyped in quality, and the movements suggest "pillrolling."

Peculiar to patients with impending liver coma is the so-called "liver flap," characterized by irregular bursts of rapid, arrythmic movements of the wrist in flexion and extension, appearing as the patient attempts to hold his arm and hand in rigid extension. Comparable movements may be exhibited by the elbows and shoulder girdles, the protruded tongue and the retracted lips.

Tics. "Habit spasms" are involuntary muscular contractions involving whole groups of muscles; they result in a coordinated,

stereotyped movement of the head or an extremity or cause a facial contortion. They seem to be devoid of purpose and serve no useful function. Common varieties of tics include a sudden jerking or twisting of the head to one side (torticollis), the winking of an eye and particular types of facial grimaces. Although clearly involuntary, tics are replicas of perfectly natural, although perhaps unusual, voluntary movements and occasion no disability.

Chorea. Choreal movements are irregular, jerky, purposeless, involuntary and unpredictable muscular movements which may involve all extremities and the entire trunk as well. This sign occurs as a transient complication of acute rheumatic fever, when it is referred to as "Sydenham's chorea," and is displayed persistently in one specific degenerative disease of the nervous system designated as "Huntington's chorea."

Athetosis. This term is applied to involuntary, more or less constant, slow wormlike twistings and bendings of the fingers and alternate flexion and extension of wrists, arms and feet, with coarse, jerky choreal movements affecting the entire limb. The appearance of athetosis signifies the presence of a serious organic disease of the brain.

Convulsions. Such movements may be described as spontaneous paroxysms of involuntary, purposeless muscular contractions. The implications of this sign, diagnostically and therapeutically, are invariably important. There are several possible causes to be considered, and, since the character of the convulsion is usually the most helpful diagnostic clue, an accurate description of the seizure is essential. The nurse must be prepared to take advantage of every opportunity that may present itself to serve as expert observer and witness in such cases. Her observations at the time of the convulsive seizure should enable her to report the following pertinent information: the duration of the episode; the character of the onset, including the presence and the character of antecedent and associated signs (for example, the appearance of pallor, flushing, changes in facial expression, mental confusion, instability of gait, irregularity of respirations and pulse); the portions of the body involved and the sequence in which they are involved; the position of the eyes and their movements, if any, during the episode; the onset of stupor or coma; the occurrence of involuntary micturition or defecation; and, finally, signs and symptoms displayed following the seizure.

Convulsions may be "tonic" or "clonic" in type, the former being characterized by generalized muscular rigidity and the latter by rhythmic but violent flexion-extension jerkings. Characteristic types of seizures are observed as the predominant manifestation of epilepsy, neoplastic, vascular and infectious diseases involving the brain, eclampsia, uremia, hypoglycemia, calcium deficiency, tetanus, toxic states attributable to certain drugs and conditions resulting in gross interference with the oxygen supply to the brain.

Gait

Disorders involving the nervous and the musculoskeletal systems may be quite apparent and their diagnoses suspected on the basis of the gait.

Limping Gait. A limp may be attributable to pain on walking, to inequality of length or strength of the legs or to the limitation of motion of one or more joints in the lower extremities. Patients with partial hemiplegia, with motor weakness affecting one leg and the corresponding arm, tend to drag the affected leg when walking, characteristically supporting the arm on the affected side stiffly and in a position of slight flexion. Patients with impaired position sense due, for example, to combined system disease or tabes dorsalis, characteristically walk with a slapping or flail-like gait, fixing their gaze on the ground, keeping their feet well apart and raising their legs high between steps.

Propulsive Gait. Patients with Parkinson's disease, or "paralysis agitans," typically walk with the so-called propulsive gait. Head and body forward, the patient trots toward his goal, the tempo of his gait progressively increasing until the objective is reached or until he is able to check his forward movement and resume at a slower pace.

Spastic Gait. The spastic gait, encountered in patients with multiple sclerosis and other disease affecting the central nervous system, may be described as a slow, stiff, choppy walk, obviously entailing considerable effort.

Other Abnormal Gaits. Other abnormal gaits characteristic of specific diseases include the *waddling* gait of patients with congenital dislocation of the hips; the slow, clumsy, *high-stepping* gait seen in cases of peripheral neuritis and related to the presence of numbness or acute pain affecting the feet; and the grossly irregular, reeling, *swinging* gait of the patient suffering from ataxia due to cerebellar disease. This last gait results from the patient's inability to place his feet in their intended location, a problem of faulty regulation of muscular movement rather than lack of position sense.

Body Temperature

The heat which maintains body temperature is generated as a result of biochemical reactions associated with metabolic activities constantly in progress throughout the body.

The constancy of the body temperature is explained by the activity of nerve centers located at the base of the brain. These centers control all of the physiologic mechanisms that are concerned with the control of heat production and heat loss, including the volume of blood flow through the skin and the respiratory mucosa and the phenomena of sweating, shivering and panting. The precision by which this regulation is accomplished is attested to by the fact that in normal individuals the body temperature rarely fluctuates beyond a range of 2° F., day or night, despite extreme variations of the surrounding temperature. A progressive accumulation of body heat, resulting in fever, normally is prevented by an increased volume and rate of blood flow in the skin and the subcutaneous tissues. This increased blood flow permits a greater volume of blood to be cooled in a given period of time as a result of radiation. Sweating increases the cooling effect of vaporization on the skin, and panting produces a similar result in the respiratory tract. These mechanisms effectively increase the rate of heat loss and protect against fatal overheating in hot weather and in the course of muscular exertion. Cooling of the body to subnormal temperatures in cold environments is prevented chiefly by two mechanisms. One of these constricts the peripheral blood vessels, decreasing the blood flow in the skin and the respiratory tract, and the other mechanism stimulates vigorous muscular exertion in the form of voluntary activity or involuntary shivering.

Normal Temperature Variations

The course of the normal body temperature is by no means constant, as is evident from the inspection of a 24-hour chart (Fig. 14). At 4 A.M. the temperature of normal individuals may be as low as 97.0° F.; between 9 and 10 A.M. it attains a peak of approximately 98.6° F. and then it declines to about 98.2° F. before the noonday meal. Afterward it rises slowly, reaching its maximum, between 98.7° and 98.9° F., during the early evening hours and thereafter falls slowly until 4 A.M. the following morning. The temperature charts characteristic of individuals working during the night, although similar in form, are quite different with respect to the timing of the fluctuations; the maximum peaks occur not during the late afternoon or the early evening hours but early in the morning.

The maximum degree of body temperature that is customarily regarded as normal is 99.0° F. Values in excess of 99.0° F. are considered indicative of fever, although individuals are encountered who habitually exhibit oral temperatures as high as 99.4° F. without other evidence of ill health. Normal variations in the lower temperature ranges are much greater; the lowest temperature recorded in most individuals is 97.0° F., but readings as low as 96.0° F. are not uncommon.

Hypothermia

Abnormal conditions responsible for an unusual reduction of body temperature are relatively few. Hypothermia is attributable either to a lessened production of body heat, as in hypothyroidism, or to excessive heat loss resulting from prolonged exposure to cold or from profuse sweating (diaphoresis). It is observed in circulatory failure due to severe blood loss (oligemic shock), in patients who have ingested large doses of antipyretic drugs such as aspirin and as a complication of diseases which involve the temperature-regulating centers in the brain or the nerve pathways through which these exercise their physiologic functions.

Fever

An abnormal elevation of temperature is one of the most valuable of all clinical

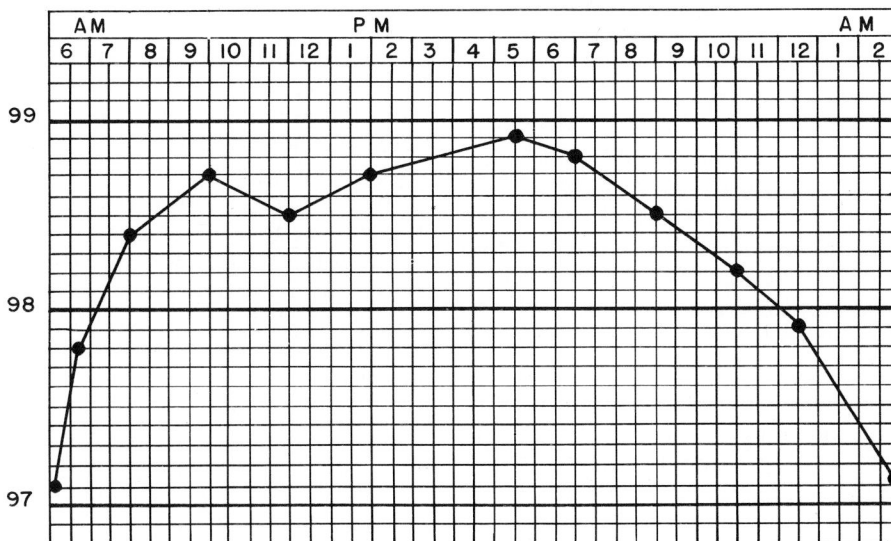

FIG. 14. Course of normal body temperature, measured orally, for 24 hours.

signs, not only because it occurs with great regularity in a large proportion of disease states, but also because of its specific characteristics in many types of disorders. By the same token, the absence of fever is equally important because of its usefulness in the exclusion of diagnostic possibilities.

Symptomatology of Fever. The onset of fever may be accompanied merely by a subjective sense of malaise, fatigue, loss of appetite, headache and generalized aches and pains of a mild degree. If, on the other hand, the onset is rapid and the elevation is of marked degree, the accompanying symptoms are correspondingly severe; the symptoms usually include the appearance of rigor (chills), severe malaise, occasionally nausea, vomiting and mental changes ranging from mild confusion to frank delirium or deep stupor. Convulsive seizures, rather than chills, may mark the onset of fever of this type, particularly in young children.

During an episode of rigor, all of the mechanisms described as contributory to the production of fever are manifest, and all are operating at full capacity, which explains the speed with which the temperature peak is attained. The peripheral skin vessels become markedly constricted; as a result, the circulating blood is shunted away from the superficial tissues, and the heat-producing organs are cooled less efficiently. Moreover, because of the accompanying muscular contractions, which may be so vigorous as to shake the entire bed, the total heat production in the body is greatly increased.

The abatement of fever, or "defervescence," may occur very abruptly, within a few hours, or gradually over a period of many days. In the former instance, the temperature is said to fall by "crisis" and in the latter by "lysis." Symptomatic improvement occurs at a corresponding rate, preceded, in rapid defervescence, by the appearance of profuse sweating.

Interpretation of Fever. Fever most often denotes the presence of an active infection, and, when attended by chills, a bacterial infection is the probable diagnosis. Alternate possibilities include various neoplastic diseases, especially carcinoma of the kidney or the lung, and tumors of the lymphoma group; immune reactions of many types, including those which follow the administration of vaccines or prophylactic serums of animal origin; toxic reactions to certain drugs; and conditions in which the temperature-regulating centers are directly damaged by heat (heat stroke), trauma or a disease involving the central nervous system.

The nurse can be extremely helpful in the diagnosis of obscure fever, not only by routinely recording the vital signs, but also as a clinical observer. She must be constantly on the alert for novel and significant developments in her patients—for example, the onset of cough, headache, nausea, pain, mental changes or skin rash, and she should maintain the attitude that any unusual phenomenon deserves reporting.

Factitious Fever. Sooner or later in the course of her professional career, the nurse is very likely to become the victim of deception at the hands of a psychopathic patient who appears to be running a febrile course but whose "fever" is, in fact, spurious and fraudulent. These individuals, in order to attract attention, create concern and prolong their hospitalization, falsify their temperature charts by manipulating thermometers, warming them adjacent to incandescent bulbs or cigarette lighters, or by applying friction, before they are retrieved and read by the nurse. A more sophisticated method involves the possession of one or more extra thermometers which can be manipulated at opportune times and substituted for those actually placed by the nurse. Most patients in this category have had some medical background, either as patients or hospital employees in the past.

The alert nurse is aware of the possibility of factitious fever, and is not likely to be deceived for long. Her suspicions will be aroused by the exhibition of fever by a patient solely when his temperature is recorded in her absence, i.e., when she is not in his immediate vicinity throughout the procedure, or by a patient's refusal to permit his temperature to be taken in her presence. (However, expert prestidigitators have been encountered with an uncanny ability to substitute thermometers undetected, under the very noses of suspicious doctors and nurses!) She will become suspicious on observing certain discrepancies in the patient's clinical chart, particularly the absence of the expected diurnal temperature variation and the lack of correlation between pulse rates and temperature readings.

In the event of suspicion, steps must be taken immediately to establish or exclude fraudulence. With no indication of distrust, she should place a thermometer in the patient's mouth or rectum in the usual manner and at the scheduled time, having first noted the serial number of that thermometer. While the temperature is registering, he should be observed no more, but less, closely than usual. If the instrument which she retrieves and reads bears a different serial number, the deception is unmasked; if it is the correct thermometer and records an elevation, it should be readjusted to a normal reading, replaced immediately in mouth or rectum and read again after 3 minutes, during which period the nurse will be standing by and observing closely.

If the serial numbers check and the reading is the same, the latter is obviously valid and has been so proved without embarrassment to patient or nurse. Otherwise, if the temperature proves to be normal or a thermometer substitution is discovered, the attending physician is to be notified at once, without preliminary comment to the patient. An elaborate, expensive and time-consuming investigation of F.U.O. (fever of unknown origin) is thus concluded, and one problem is replaced by another that is likely to prove even more difficult—one having profound psychiatric implications and beyond the scope of internal medicine.

Respiration

Aspects of breathing which are of clinical importance and which should be noted by the nurse as routine in all patients are its rate, rhythm and depth; the effort it involves and the discomfort it causes; the position which the patient adopts in order to breathe most comfortably; the sounds which accompany it and the presence or the absence of cyanosis.

Respiratory Rates

The normal rate of respiration in adults is from 16 to 20 per minute; in children, from 20 to 40, depending on age and size; and in infants, 40 or over. *Hyperpnea* and *polypnea* indicate a very rapid respiratory rate, and *oligopnea,* one that is abnormally slow; *apnea* signifies the temporary cessation of breathing.

Hyperpnea. A rapid respiratory rate is normal in children and young adults, occurring in response to exercise, painful stimuli or emotional distress. Although deep, hyperpnea requires no unusual effort, a feature distinguishing this type of respiration from dyspnea. Hyperpnea is as much a part of the fever syndrome as are the elevations of body temperature and pulse rate. The rate of respiration increases on the average about 5 per minute for each degree of temperature elevation, except in patients with pneumonia and infarcts of the lung which are accompanied by increases in the respiratory rate which are relatively much greater. Hyperpnea is also a common manifestation of hysteria; in some cases the rate approximates 50 to 60 per minute, and each breath is full, easy and painless. Inasmuch as hysterical hyperpnea is not stimulated by oxygen lack or carbon dioxide excess, as is hyperpnea due to exercise, it is often designated as "hyperventilation." The latter is not without effect on the physiologic state of the individual, for, as a result of "washing out" the carbon dioxide, the blood becomes abnormally alkaline, and the patient experiences spasmodic muscular contractions, as well as subjective numbness of the extremities, dizziness and faintness.

Oligopnea. Oligopnea (slow respiration) is most often attributable to toxic depression of the respiratory centers by opiates, particularly morphine and its derivatives.

Apnea. The temporary cessation of respiration is termed apnea. It is best exemplified in one of the respiratory arrhythmias termed *Cheyne-Stokes respiration.*

Cheyne-Stokes Respiration. This is a type of breathing characterized by periods of apnea, lasting from a few seconds to almost a minute, alternating with periods of similar length during which breathing is resumed (Fig. 15). Following periods of apnea the respiration is at first quiet and shallow; it then acquires a definite crescendo quality, with rate, depth and effort steadily increasing to peak intensity. After this it becomes progressively quieter and shallower until the return of apnea. This abnormality of respiration is frequently associated with increased intracranial pressure due, for example, to meningitis or cerebral tumor. It is exhibited also by patients with cerebral arteriosclerosis, who may exhibit Cheyne-Stokes breathing for periods lasting many months—usually, however, only when asleep or under the influence of sedative medication.

Respiratory Movements

When the predominant respiratory movement is confined to the ribs and the clavicles the term "costal breathing" is applied. This is in contrast to "abdominal breathing," which refers to respiration that is accomplished chiefly by the diaphragm as evidenced by the appearance of abdominal expansion and contraction, the excursion of which exceeds that of the chest movements. Normal breathing employs both types of movement, the costal component predominating in women, and the diaphragmatic in men. Excessive predominance of either, however, requires explanation.

Abdominal Respiration. This may be due to pleurisy or to acute arthritis of the costovertebral joints, motion of the chest being inhibited by pain. It also is found in patients with bilateral pleural effusion and extensive pneumonia. A long persistence of this respiratory abnormality suggests either fixation of the costovertebral joints due to chronic arthritis or bilateral paralysis of the intercostal muscles.

Costal Breathing. This may result from paralysis of the diaphragm or the abdominal musculature. It also may be related to the presence of fluid in the peritoneal cavity or to gaseous distention of the abdomen, which forces the diaphragm into an elevated position and restricts its normal excursion. Per-

sistent limitation of both costal and diaphragmatic movements indicates that the lungs have lost their normal elasticity. In pulmonary emphysema, for example, the chest becomes immobilized in a position of inspiration, with the ribs and the clavicles elevated and the costal angle widened.

Asymmetric Respiration. Unilateral predominance of respiratory movements on the right or the left side, may be indicative of acute pleurisy, the respiratory movements on the affected side being limited by pain. It also may be attributable to scarring and contracture of one lung as a late complication of chronic tuberculosis.

Dyspnea. This implies labored breathing. The respiratory rate may be rapid or reduced, the rhythm regular or irregular, each breath shallow or deep. The important characteristic is its labored quality, unusual effort being entailed in each respiratory movement. There is active participation on the part of the accessory muscles of respiration, especially the sternocleidomastoid muscles in the neck, which visibly contract, lifting the clavicles with each inspiration, while the nostrils actively dilate. The dyspneic patient appears anxious; his pupils are dilated, his mouth is held open, his tongue and lips are dry, and the entire skin is moist and usually cyanotic. Severe dyspnea almost always is accompanied by *orthopnea,* the patient maintaining an erect position or leaning forward in order to breathe with optimum efficiency and comfort.

Dyspnea may result from the mechanical obstruction of the trachea, of a major bronchus or of numerous bronchioles within the lung tissue. It also may occur as a result of a reduction in the area of functioning respiratory surface within the lungs; this may be due to an infectious process, an invading tumor or fibrous scarring. Heart failure may

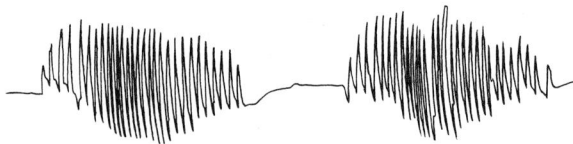

FIG. 15. Respiratory movements of a patient exhibiting Cheyne-Stokes breathing.

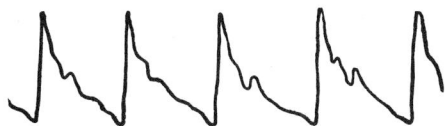

FIG. 16. Normal pulse wave.

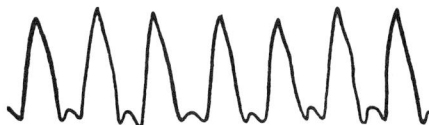

FIG. 18. Bounding pulse.

FIG. 19. Thready pulse.

cause the lung capillaries to become overdistended with blood and the alveoli, or air cells, to fill with edema fluid. A portion of the lung may be collapsed due to a fluid accumulation in the pleural cavity or the pericardial sac, or the lung may be compressed externally by air which has leaked into the mediastinal or pleural cavity.

Asthma. This is a type of breathing which is accompanied by an audible wheeze, the latter being more pronounced on expiration than on inspiration. It is due to partial obstruction of the small bronchi as a result of their spastic contraction, as in bronchial asthma. It may be attributable to the presence of fluid secretions within the bronchioles, which is the situation in asthmatic bronchitis and in congestive heart failure, when it is often referred to as "cardiac asthma."

"Kussmaul Breathing." A classic finding in diabetic acidosis, this is characterized by a continuous dyspnea in which the respiratory movements are unusually deep, although not necessarily hurried. Considerable effort may be entailed, but there is little or no evidence of discomfort. Neither cyanosis nor orthopnea is associated with Kussmaul breathing, which distinguishes it from most other types of dyspnea. The cause of the disorder is abnormal acidity of the blood which provokes a persistent and excessive stimulation of the nerve centers controlling respiration.

Noisy Respiration

Stertorous breathing, or snoring, is produced by the vibration of the relaxed soft

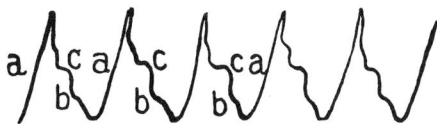

FIG. 17. A diagram of the normal pulse waves (a modified "pulse tracing"): (a) the ascent of the wave; (b) the descent; (c) the dicrotic wave.

palate when an individual breathes simultaneously through nose and mouth and is observed commonly in association with stupor and deep, normal sleep. *Stridor,* the production of harsh, whistling noises, is attributable to partial obstruction of the larynx or the trachea by an infectious inflammatory disease such as diphtheria, by a foreign body or by spasm of the laryngeal muscles. Tracheal rales, responsible for the "death rattle" in terminal cases of pulmonary edema, are gurgling, bubbling sounds which are synchronous with respiration, indicating the presence of fluid in the major respiratory passages.

Arterial Pulse

The Pulse Examination

Each beat of a normally functioning heart propels approximately 100 ml. of blood into the arterial system and simultaneously initiates a fluid wave. This wave is propagated throughout the entire extent of this system and is palpable as a vibration called the "pulse," the rate and the character of which are highly informative as regards the state of the circulation (Fig. 16). The pulse is examined by applying digital pressure over one of the large superficial arteries, preferably one which courses just beneath the skin and directly over bone and is surrounded by relatively little soft tissue. The temporal, the mandibular, the brachial and the femoral arteries fulfill these criteria, and circumstances occasionally require their selection, but the vessel that is most suitable for examination, and usually most readily accessible, is the radial artery at the wrist.

Normally, the pulse waves, when palpated from moment to moment, appear to be approximately equal in force and are separated by time intervals of equal length. In other words, the pulse is expected to be regular with respect to rate, rhythm and force, and any deviation from the normal in any of these qualities suggests the possibility of heart disease. However, as will become evident from the following discussions, abnormalities of the pulse occur in certain diseases other than cardiac, as well as in individuals who present no evidence of ill health.

Pulse Quality. The normal arterial pulsation, as observed by palpation, reaches its maximum intensity very rapidly and subsides more slowly. A small "dicrotic" impulse may be discerned as it subsides (Fig. 17); this impulse is related to the closure of the aortic valve. If unduly pronounced, the term "dicrotic pulse" is applicable.

A forceful or "bounding pulse" suggests an increase in the magnitude of the pulse wave and a high "pulse pressure" (Fig. 18). This may be associated with a decrease in the diastolic arterial pressure, the systolic pressure remaining normal, or an increase in the systolic pressure while the diastolic is normal or low. Contrariwise, when the difference between systolic and diastolic pressures is unusually small (i.e., when the pulse pressure is low), the peripheral pulse is endowed with a feeble quality. A "thready pulse" is one that is not only feeble but also rapid (Fig. 19). The "Corrigan" or "water hammer pulse" is one which strikes the palpating finger with a quick, sharp stroke. This abnormality in pulse quality, usually attributable to incompetence of the aortic valve (see p. 529), is elicited best by grasping the patient's wrist in the whole hand with the palmar surface of the fingers clasped firmly against the flexor surface of the patient's wrist and by elevating the wrist to a vertical position. A converse type of abnormality is the "slow pulse," one that is characterized by an unusually slow development of maximum force. It is encountered in patients with aortic stenosis, a condition in which, because of a reduction in the size of the aortic orifice, egress from the ventricles into the arterial system is impeded, blood being slowly squeezed with each contraction from the heart into the aorta.

Pulse Rates. The pulse rate is influenced by the degree of muscular activity. For example, that of a normal recumbent man may be approximately 66 beats per minute, slower when he sleeps, 70 while sitting or leaning and 80 while standing. During strenuous physical exercise, and for a short period thereafter, rates between 100 and 140 normally are attained, depending on the degree of exertion and the condition of the individual. Another influential factor is the emotional state; an increase in pulse rate occurs in response to anxiety, fear, displeasure, discomfort and accompanying excitement of any type.

Tachycardia, an unusually rapid heart rate, may represent either a normal response to stimuli of the types mentioned or a manifestation of some disorder.

When the heart rate is consistently less than 50 or 60 beats per minute, the condition is described as *bradycardia.*

Abnormalities of pulse rate or irregularities of pulse rhythm are described in Chapter 27.

Pulse Deficit and Its Measurement. The pulse rate in untreated patients with atrial fibrillation is usually between 100 and 120 per minute. Its value, however, may not necessarily indicate the actual ventricular rate, for, unless the fibrillation is unusually slow, a certain proportion of the pulse waves do not possess sufficient force to be palpable at the wrist. There results, therefore, a "pulse deficit," which refers to the numerical difference between the ventricular and the peripheral pulse rates. The existence of a pulse deficit is important in establishing a diagnosis of atrial fibrillation and in differentiating this type of arrhythmia from others similarly characterized by pulse irregularities, such as premature beats, sinus arrhythmia and flutter with varying degrees of block. Moreover, the amount of deficit is one of the most valuable therapeutic guides in the treatment of patients with fibrillation.

The pulse deficit is determined by the simultaneous measurement of the rate of arterial pulsation, palpated at the wrist, and the rate of ventricular contraction, determined by direct auscultation of the heart with a stethoscope applied over the cardiac apex.

Two individuals are involved in this maneuver, each making an independent count, one counting the radial pulsations and the other counting the audible heart beats, both counting from the same watch and both counts being started and completed simultaneously. A full minute of counting is required as a minimum, and a 2-minute count is preferable for accurate measurements of pulse deficit.

Arterial Pressure

The force exerted by each systolic contraction of the left ventricle is normally sufficient to increase the pressure of the blood in the aorta and in all of the major arteries to a peak between 120 and 150 mm. of mercury (or between 5 and 7 feet of water). Venous pressure, by contrast, differs widely throughout the body, being greatest in the areas which are most dependent on their relation to the heart. The normal value, calculated with reference to the position of the right atrium, is approximately 7 mm. of mercury (or 4 inches of water).

The level of arterial pressure is determined by two factors: (1) the *cardiac output,* in other words, the rate with which blood is ejected from the heart into the aorta; and (2) the ease with which blood flows from the larger arteries through the smallest arterial branches, or the *degree of peripheral resistance* to blood flow. The magnitude of cardiac output depends on the speed and the force of ventricular contractions, as well as on the volume of blood filling the left ventricle before its contraction; the peripheral resistance is determined by the caliber of the arterioles.

The measurement of the arterial blood pressure is one of the most important aspects of the clinical examination. It, together with measurements of the pulse rate, the body temperature and the respiration, should be performed routinely as an integral part of every diagnostic investigation, for these pressure values supply vital information with respect to the efficiency of cardiac function and the status of the peripheral vascular system.

Systolic Pressure

This is defined as the peak level of arterial pressure that is attained during the cardiac cycle; it coincides with the crest of the pulse wave. This pressure, in a normal adult at rest, varies between 110 and 140 mm. of mercury; in normal children it lies between 95 and 110, and in infants between 75 and 90 mm. of mercury. It is precisely equal to the degree of arterial compression that is necessary and just sufficient to halt the flow of arterial blood completely and continuously.

Diastolic Pressure

The diastolic pressure, normally between 70 and 85 mm. of mercury, is the lowest level of pressure in the cardiac cycle, occurring immediately following the subsidence of each ventricular contraction when the muculature of the heart is relaxed most completely. Its height depends, in part, on the elasticity of the arterial vessels—in other words, on the degree of compression exerted by their muscular walls as they contract from the state of stretch after each systolic wave. In part, its height also depends on the rapidity with which blood escapes from the arteries through the arterioles.

Pulse Pressure

The difference between systolic and diastolic pressure is termed the pulse pressure; normally it is about one third the value of the systolic arterial pressure. A "wide" pulse pressure, with a reduced diastolic and a normal or elevated systolic pressure, usually denotes the presence of a normal or increased cardiac output and a simultaneous reduction of peripheral arteriolar resistance; this is a situation observed in febrile states, in patients with hyperthyroidism and in normal individuals following exertion attributable both to a subnormal diastolic and an increased systolic pressure. It also is observed in certain types of heart disease affecting the aortic valve, failure of its effective closure in diastole permitting blood to flow back into the left ventricle from the aorta after each systolic contraction.

Errors in Sphygmomanometry

Transient elevations of blood pressure may be attributable solely to an increase in cardiac output caused by emotional stress or recent physical exertion. Failure to elicit audible sounds of any type may be due to malposition of the stethoscope or, in hypertensive patients, to failure of the examiner to elevate the cuff pressure high enough to exceed the systolic pressure.

The first step in determining the source of the difficulty is to palpate the radial pulse while simultaneously elevating the pressure cuff to the precise level at which the pulse is obliterated completely; this corresponds approximately with the systolic arterial pressure. If the latter is substantially above or below the range tested previously, the observer then proceeds by the auscultatory method, as indicated; otherwise the difficulty must be attributable to failure to locate the end piece of the stethoscope in correct relation to the brachial artery, assuming of course that the instrument itself is patent and functioning properly. This artery may have been obliterated as a result of disease or it may be located in an unusual position. In any event, it is necessary to establish the location of the brachial pulse by means of palpation and to repeat the determination with whatever modifications are indicated.

Erroneously high arterial blood pressure values are obtained in very obese individuals because of the excessive girth of the upper arm. Valid recordings under these circumstances require the use of an unusually broad cuff. Otherwise, the latter impinges unevenly, and the distribution of pressure is not as an even band but as a wedge. In this case, the manometric readings are recording certain components of pressure that are directed tangentially toward the shoulder and the elbow and are spreading the soft tissues rather than compressing the deeper structures of the arm.

Difficulty in determining the diastolic pressure may arise from the fact that the pulse occasionally remains audible throughout the entire reading range until the cuff pressure is reduced to zero. This situation emphasizes the importance of learning to recognize and interpret correctly the quality of sounds, for one must depend exclusively on one's ability to detect the point at which there is a transition from the sharp, snapping phase of diastole to the sounds that are characteristic of subdiastolic levels, when it has acquired a muffled and indistinct quality. This point of transition is to be interpreted as the diastolic pressure, regardless of the presence or the absence of audible sound upon further reduction of the cuff pressure.

"The auscultatory gap," a potential source of error in occasional patients with severe hypertension, is a phenomenon marked by the complete disappearance of sound between the systolic and the diastolic pressure levels. Thus, the systolic pressure may be estimated at a level of 260 mm. of mercury and, with gradual release of the cuff pressure, the sounds suddenly disappear at a reading of 220. Were the test abandoned at this point, it obviously would be interpreted as indicating an arterial pressure of 260/220. However, if the nurse is accustomed to continue auscultation until the cuff pressure has been completely released, she will note, in such cases, that sounds again become audible at a much lower level—for example, at 150 —and become muffled at 130 mm. of mercury, so that the arterial pressure should be recorded as 260/130.

Arterial Hypertension and Hypotension

Temporary elevations of blood pressure normally occur as a result of emotional excitement and muscular exertion, explainable on the base of an increased cardiac output and peripheral arteriolar resistance, for which the activities of the sympathetic nervous system and of the adrenal glands are responsible. Hyperactivity of the thyroid gland usually results in a more prolonged elevation of arterial pressure, which can be related to a marked increase in cardiac output. However, in most patients with chronic arterial hypertension the cardiac output is normal, and the abnormality is assumed to result from an increase in peripheral resistance due to sustained, generalized arteriolar vasoconstriction throughout the body, with consequences which are damaging to the kidneys, the heart and the brain.

Hypotension. The term "low blood pressure," as generally applied, has no precise significance. In many normal individuals the arterial pressure consistently ranges between 90 and 100 mm. of mercury.

On the other hand, transient acute hypotension is of great importance. It is a regular occurrence in some individuals upon arising suddenly from a reclining or sitting position ("postural hypotension") and may be accompanied by attacks of dizziness or even temporary loss of consciousness. This usually is attributable to marked loss of muscular "tone" in the lower extremities due to neurologic disease, prolonged bed rest or debility; for these muscles, instead of providing a firm support for the veins in the dependent areas or assisting them to empty in the direction of the thorax, permit them to dilate and retain an excessive volume of pooled blood. Acute hypotension also occurs in patients afflicted with carotid sinus sensitivity; nerve impulses originating in these centers produce sudden dilatation of the peripheral arterioles, with consequent loss of peripheral resistance to blood flow, or cause temporary heart block with transient cessation of cardiac output. Acute hypotension is also one of the most significant features of "shock," whether due to excessive blood loss or to "forward heart failure." Chronic hypotension is an important clinical sign of Addison's disease (see Chap. 38) and of severe cachexia, whether due to inadequate function of the pituitary gland, to prolonged infection or to severe malnutrition.

Venous Pressure

The pressure in the venous system is low in comparison with the arterial pressure, although it is quite sufficient to ensure the adequate return of blood to the right atrium. The venous pressure is elevated abnormally in patients with congestive heart failure due to myocardial or valvular disease, to compression of the heart by a scarred, inelastic pericardial membrane or by a fluid accumulation within the pericardial sac. A local increase in venous pressure in one portion of the body, i.e., in one or more extremities, is a common sequel of local venous obstruction due to mechanical causes or to incompetence of the venous valves. These structures greatly facilitate the return of venous blood to the thorax and to the right atrium by reducing the hydrostatic venous pressure in dependent portions of the body; moreover, they protect the capillary vessels in those regions from exposure to processes which would almost certainly exceed their tolerance. But for the valves in the femoral and the saphenous veins, for example, the venous and the capillary pressure in the feet would approximate the diastolic arterial pressure (i.e., 40 inches of water or about 120 mm. of mercury, instead of 2 mm. of mercury) and fluid would escape rapidly through the capillary loops into the surrounding tissues.

A local increase in venous pressure, complicated by edema formation in the dependent areas, can result from venous varicosities with valvular destruction, from malignant tumors impinging on the femoral or the iliac veins or on the vena cava, from intraperitoneal fluid accumulation (ascites) compressing the vena cava and from inflammatory diseases of the veins resulting in thrombosis and the obliteration of these channels. Obstruction of a brachial or an axillary vein or of one of the great veins in the superior mediastinum into which they drain results in edema of a single upper extremity. Edema of the upper trunk, both upper extremities, the neck and the head, the lower trunk and the limbs being edema-free, suggests obstruction of the superior vena cava.

A generalized increase in venous pressure usually is detected without difficulty upon routine inspection of the patient by observing neck vein distention when the patient is sitting or standing. Normally, in these positions, venous filling is not visible much above the clavicles. However, in cases of congestive heart failure, filling is generally seen at a much higher level, distention of the neck veins occasionally being apparent at the angle of the jaw. Another observation of similar significance is the observation of venous distention in the upper extremities when the latter are raised above the level of the chest.

SUMMARY OF NURSING ROLE

Because of her frequent and intimate contacts with the patient, the nurse is indispensable as an observer and a recorder of signs and symptoms. She has numerous opportunities daily to solicit information which is potentially of diagnostic value. The confidence of patients is readily established as they become acquainted with her in her role as their nurse. She must learn to be accurate and discriminating in her observations and must train herself to record them in complete and explicit terms for the physician.

BIBLIOGRAPHY AND SUGGESTED READING

Books

Apperly, F. L.: Patterns of Disease, Philadelphia, Lippincott, 1951.

Fuerst, E. V., and Wolff, L.: Fundamentals of Nursing, ed. 2, Philadelphia, Lippincott, 1959.

MacBryde, C. M. (ed.): Signs and Symptoms, ed. 4, Philadelphia, Lippincott, 1964.

6

Diagnostic Studies in Clinical Evaluation

THE NURSE'S ROLE IN DIAGNOSTIC PROCEDURES AND TESTS

The nurse of today needs a sound working knowledge of a great many laboratory tests from several standpoints, the extent of such knowledge correspondingly enhancing her value and effectiveness as clinical collaborator in the care of her patients. Many tests require special preparation of the patient; for the details of this preparation the nurse is responsible. The assembling of appropriate equipment may be necessary for the collection of samples that are employed in specific procedures; for this too she is responsible, and her responsibilities very often include the labeling and the disposition of these samples as well. Consequently, she is obliged to become familiar with the sampling requirements that pertain to specific tests; with appropriate methods of preserving a variety of samples; with the administrative policies governing laboratory requisitions in the hospital; with the correct procedure for labeling all types of specimens and with the method of routing each specimen safely and without delay to its proper destination.

The nurse must be prepared to serve as a communications link between the laboratory and the medical staff in the transmission and the recording of data, recognizing that an error in transmission or recording negates completely the value of a test and endangers the patient. The most important safety factor in this regard is her familiarity with laboratory data, including the precise manner in which these are designated and the units of measure in which they are expressed. She also should be familiar with normal values for the more common tests and recognize the implications of deviations outside of these ranges.

Discussions with patients and their families on matters pertaining to diagnostic procedures arise frequently and are definitely to be anticipated by the nurse. The patient may be anxious concerning the possible risk that may be involved, or the expense entailed, in a proposed test; he may resent the inconvenience or the discomfort imposed in connection with a procedure, doubt the importance of that examination and question its necessity. The nurse is in the best position to provide reassurance and thereby secure the patient's full co-operation if she can describe a test in authentic terms and can indicate clearly its importance in relation to his particular problem.

The present chapter describes the laboratory tests and the diagnostic procedures that are used most widely at the present time, and that pertain to medical and surgical problems of greatest importance to the nurse.

EXAMINATION OF THE URINE

Urinalysis provides a wealth of important clinical information and is regarded as an indispensable part of every clinical study. The following section summarizes the majority of important urine tests. Certain of these comprise the so-called "routine urinalysis," which includes the observation and the evaluation of urine color and clarity; measurement of urine acidity and specific gravity; tests for the presence of protein and sugar in the urine (proteinuria and glycosuria, respectively); and microscopic examination of the urine sediment after centrifuging for the detection of red blood cells (hematuria), white blood cells (pyuria), casts (cylindruria), crystals (crystaluria) and bacteria (bacteriuria). Numerous additional tests are described which are applicable in special situations.

Collection and Preservation of Urine Samples

All urine tests are performed ideally on fresh specimens, preferably the first voiding of the day, since most urinary constituents are present in highest concentration at that time. Random specimens are satisfactory for most analyses, however, provided that they have been collected in clean containers and have been protected adequately against bacterial and chemical deterioration. Samples collected in the home should be voided into clean, dry, wide-mouth bottles of pint or quart size, equipped with screw-tops or clamp-tops, the mouth being sufficiently large to permit the male and the female alike to void directly into them. All specimens should be refrigerated as soon as possible after they are voided and maintained at refrigerator temperatures until they are transported to the testing laboratory. If more than a few hours are to elapse between the times of collection and testing, the urine should be stabilized by the addition of a chemical preservative.

Collection bottles used in the hospital should be meticulously clean and dry. Moreover, they should be equipped with a tight-sealing closure of a type that is easily applied. Every urine sample must be labeled clearly with the patient's name and bed location; the label should also specify the date and the hour of the voiding and any other data that might pertain in an individual case, such as, for example, the occurrence of menstruation. Unless the urinalysis is to proceed at once, the specimen should be placed in a refrigerator immediately.

Fractional Collections and "Sterile-Voided" Specimens

Twenty-four-hour Urine Collections. Many quantitative analytic tests are carried out on specimens which represent the entire urinary output of a patient over a 24-hour period. The reliability of such tests rests on the assumption that the sample is, in fact, representative of the 24-hour pool. This consideration applies in all electrolyte balance studies, measurements of protein and formed element excretion, tests of radioactive vitamin B_{12} absorption, certain hormonal assays and other special tests. The receptacle accommodating the urine pool should be kept in a refrigerator or should contain a preservative. It should be labeled in such a manner as to identify the patient specifically, accurately and legibly and indicate the time that the collection was started. All voidings should be funneled promptly into this receptacle. Failure to transfer one specimen voided during the test period invalidates the test. The incidence of incomplete 24-hour collections is surprisingly and distressingly high. A successful collection requires the complete understanding and willing co-operation on the part of the patient and of numerous other individuals as well, including all ward personnel who happen to be concerned with the patient's care during the period in question. The organization and the supervision of these collections is the difficult and responsible job of the nurse in charge of the patient. Her instructions to her patient and her staff must be crystal clear and adamant.

"Two-Glass" Urine Collections. The "two-glass test" is of diagnostic value in the case of the male patient whose urine contains pus or blood; it supplies an indication as to whether these formed elements are entering the urine in the upper or the lower portion of the genito-urinary tract. The patient is required to void the first 50- to 75-ml. portion into one receptacle, and the remainder, without interruption, into a second container. The sediments of the two specimens are then examined and compared. If the first sample contains a higher concentration of cells than the second, it may be concluded that these elements had entered the urine in the lower urinary tract, the second fraction having passed through this portion after it had been flushed by relatively cell-free urine from above.

"Sterile-Voided" ("Clean-Catch") Specimens. Urine samples voided in the usual way are practically useless for bacteriologic study because of inevitable contamination of the specimen by organisms residing in the vicinity of the urethral meatus. Such contamination can be avoided by catheterizing the urinary bladder. However, since the dangers of catheterization, from the standpoint of introducing infection, have become recognized and its role in the production of chronic pyelonephritis has become understood, this procedure is no longer recommended except on the basis of very specific indications. In any event, it has been demonstrated that reliable bacteriologic studies are possible without benefit of catheterization, utilizing the so-called "sterile-voiding" technic of sampling.

The male patient is instructed to cleanse the penis with multiple applications of soap and water, employing cotton pledgets or gauze squares for that purpose. The first portion of the voiding is not collected but discarded. The next portion, which is to be the test sample, is voided into a sterile, wide-mouth bottle or large-caliber tube, which, in either case, is protected by a sterile closure of appropriate design. The female patient, before voiding, must cleanse the vulva about the urethral meatus 3 or 4 times with soapy water, each time wiping the perineum backward toward the anus, then discarding the wipe. Following the lavage a mid-stream specimen is collected in a sterile receptacle.

Color and Clarity of Urine

The color of normal urine comes ultimately from the hemoglobin of hemolyzed red corpuscles. One part of this, containing iron, is split off and saved; the rest becomes bilirubin, the coloring matter of bile. In the intestine, bilirubin is slightly modified to form urobilinogen, and some of this is reabsorbed into the blood and excreted in the urine as urobilin. The higher the specific gravity of urine, the deeper, as a rule, is its color. Bile, which is excreted in the urine in cases with obstructive jaundice, darkens the urine. Its presence is best recognized not by the color of the urine but by its foam when shaken. A yellow foam invariably indicates bile. The presence of small amounts of blood lends a smoky appearance to the urine, that is, it is turbid and has a blackish-red tint.

Fresh acid urine is clear. Soon after standing there appears a feathery cloud, composed of mucus washed by the urine from the mucous membrane lining the urinary passages. If a person has not been drinking much water, but has been eating considerable meat, and the day is cold, his urine may present a remarkable appearance. A heavy precipitate settles on the bottom of the vessel as a heavy layer of white, pink or red sediment, the so-called *brick dust sediment*. This is merely the urate sediment, that is, a precipitate of the salts of uric acid which are present in every normal urine and are deposited whenever the urine is a little concentrated and the day is cold.

If a urine is clear when voided, no later-appearing sediment has any importance. If a freshly voided urine is not clear, but contains a sediment which will not disappear on warming or on the addition of acetic acid, the sediment does indeed have significance. It usually signifies the presence of bacteria, blood, pus or casts and is referred to as an "organized sediment."

Pigmenturia from Food, Drugs and Chemicals

The ingestion of beets may result in the transient appearance of pink or red urine. Certain cathartic agents, including aloes, cascara sagrada, rhubarb and senna, cause acid urine to turn yellow-brown and alkaline urine to turn red-violet in color. Antipyrine, one of the coal-tar analgesic drugs, when ingested in large doses produces deep red urine. Pyridium, a urinary antiseptic drug, colors the urine red after ingestion. Thymol, ingested as an anthelminthic agent, produces a greenish tint. Santonin, another anthelminthic, colors acid urine deep yellow and alkaline urine pink. In cases of phenol (carbolic acid) poisoning, the urine becomes olive-green and finally blackens on exposure to air. Methylene blue, employed in the treatment of methemoglobinemia, confers a blue-green color. Phenolphthalein, contained in certain cathartic preparations, is colorless in acid urine but pink or red in alkaline urine. Phenolsulfonphthalein (PSP), used in a test of renal function (p. 76) and a procedure for measuring the residual urine volume, and Bromsulphalein (BSP), employed in a liver function test (p. 83), have the same effect as phenolphthalein on urine color.

Pigmenturia in Disease

Abnormal coloration of the urine is of diagnostic importance in a variety of disorders. Tests for the identification and the quantitative estimation of urine pigments in such cases, and the nature of certain disorders which are responsible for pigmenturia, will now be described.

Bilirubinuria. The presence of bilirubin in the urine (bilirubinuria or choluria) is an abnormal finding. It signifies that there exists an obstruction to the excretion of that pigment by the liver into the gut; that instead of escaping via the biliary tract into the intestinal lumen, dissolved in the bile, it has been regurgitated by the liver cells directly into the circulating blood; and, finally, that the liver cells have succeeded in processing this pigment into the soluble glucuronide salt, the only form in which it can diffuse from the blood into the urine. Therefore, bilirubinuria is regarded as being a sign of biliary obstruction, and jaundiced patients with bilirubin in their urine are presumed to have obstructive jaundice rather than jaundice due primarily to liver failure.

Urine containing bilirubin varies from deep yellow to light brown in color. A more specific indication of its presence in the urine is the appearance of yellow foam when the sample is shaken in a glass container, the basis of the so-called "foam test." In the absence of bilirubin, urine foam is white or straw colored; if its color is yellow or brown, the presence of bilirubin is presumed. A sensitive, semiquantitative test for urine bilirubin can be accomplished with a reagent which is supplied in the form of a tablet (Ictotest). This test is performed by placing 5 drops of urine on a small square mat which is supplied together with the reagent tablet. The latter is placed on the mat, and 2 drops of water are allowed to flow over the tablet. A positive result is indicated by the appearance, within 30 seconds, of a bluish-purple discoloration of the mat in the vicinity of the tablet, the speed and the intensity of the color reaction being proportional to the amount of bilirubin present. (See Plate 1.)

Hemoglobinuria. Minute traces of hemoglobin in the urine, as in microscopic hematuria, may escape visual detection. Oxyhemoglobin in more than trace amounts imparts a pink to dark red color to urine; reduced hemoglobin, a purple to black discoloration. Methemoglobin, an oxidation product of hemoglobin, may contribute a light- to dark-brown shade. The presence in the urine of hemoglobin or methemoglobin ordinarily reflects the presence of the corresponding pigment in the circulating plasma, i.e., hemoglobinemia or methemoglobinemia, which, in turn, signifies the rapid breakdown of red cells in the circulating blood, or "intravascular hemolysis." Hemoglobin liberated from red cells in this manner is rapidly oxidized to methemoglobin, which explains the methemoglobinemia and methemoglobinuria that is associated with certain hemolytic disorders. Intravascular hemolysis is a feature of paroxysmal nocturnal hemoglobinuria (p. 468); paroxysmal hemoglobinuria (p. 468); hemolytic transfusion reactions (p. 182); hemolytic episodes following accidental injections of distilled water or other hypotonic fluids; and it follows exposure to certain toxic agents.

The detection and the measurement of hemoglobin in the urine are possible by means of a test which depends on the appearance of a blue color when hemoglobin is mixed with benzidine and hydrogen peroxide in an acid solution. A more convenient method (Occultest) utilizes a reagent tablet containing orthotolidin and strontium peroxide. One drop of urine is placed on a piece of filter paper, the tablet is placed in the moist area of the paper, and on it are placed 2 drops of water. A positive reaction is indicated by the appearance, in less than 2 minutes, of a diffuse blue color in the vicinity of the tablet. (See Plate 1.) In both the benzidine and the orthotolidin test, the production of color is brought about as the result of the oxidation of the indicator dye by oxygen released from a peroxide by an enzymatic, peroxide-splitting (peroxidase) activity on the part of hemoglobin.

Hemosiderinuria. The presence in the urine of hemosiderin, a breakdown product of hemoglobin, is an expected finding in patients with hemoglobinuria and in hemochromatosis (p. 659). Hemosiderin is responsible for the appearance of a brown or black sediment in urine. It can be identified with certainty by mixing 1 drop of urine sediment with 1 drop of 30 per cent aqueous ammonium sulfide on a glass slide. On microscopic examination, hemosiderin is visible in the form of jet black particles (ferric sulfide) in the sediment.

Myoglobinuria. Myoglobin, a pigment contained in muscle tissue exclusively, may appear in the urine following a severe crushing injury (crush syndrome); following the rupture, obstruction or prolonged spasm of a major artery in a traumatized limb; or as a complication of spontaneous femoral artery thrombosis. Myoglobinuria also occurs in a rare disorder known as *paroxysmal myoglobinuria,* or "acute recurrent rhabdomyolysis." This condition is marked by recurring episodes of muscle weakness, pain and tenderness and by the subsequent appearance of a red pigment in freshly voided urine, which turns brown or black on standing due to oxidation of myoglobin to metmyoglobin on exposure to air. Muscle lysis rather than red cell lysis is considered to be the underlying factor in these extraordinary cases. Myoglobin can be distinguished readily from hemoglobin by spectroscopy.

Porphyrinuria and Porphobilinuria. The porphyrins and porphobilin, precursors or degradation products of hemoglobin, are excreted in the urine in certain abnormal conditions, including two specific disease entities: intermittent acute porphyria and congenital light-sensitive porphyria.

Intermittent acute porphyria is a rare and extremely serious disease which is characterized by deep red discoloration of the urine by porphobilin and certain porphyrins. These patients experience episodes of abdominal pain, psychiatric disturbances and neurologic abnormalities. Attacks may be precipitated or aggravated in severity by the ingestion of certain drugs, notably the barbiturates. A fatal outcome is anticipated in a significant proportion of cases.

Congenital light-sensitive porphyria, likewise exceedingly rare, is characterized by the excretion of pink or red urine containing certain of the porphyrins in high concentration.

Exposure to sunlight may induce vesicular lesions on the skin followed by deep scarring and pigmentation in the affected areas. The teeth (and bones) may be pink due to their high porphyrin content. Involvement of the eyes may result in blindness. Anemia is a common complication. The outlook for these patients is far better than in cases of intermittent acute porphyria. Neurologic and psychiatric complications do not occur, and if sunlight is avoided a normal life expectancy is possible. Porphyrinuria of lesser degree, usually without visible discoloration of the urine, is a common accompaniment of liver disease and is also an important diagnostic feature of lead poisoning.

The diagnosis of porphyrinuria and the specific identification of individual porphyrins in the urine depend on a combination of laboratory findings. Since some of these pigments are extremely unstable, their reliable identification requires samples of freshly voided urine.

Alkaptonuria. This term denotes an inborn metabolic defect, as a result of which certain individuals fail to metabolize one of the amino acids, namely, tyrosine, and therefore excrete homogentisic acid in the urine. Alkaline samples containing this product turn black rapidly on standing.

Melaninuria. The pigment melanin and its colorless precursor, melanogen, are excreted in the urine of patients with melanosarcoma (Chap. 34). A freshly voided sample may be normal in color or only moderately tinged with brown. Eventually, however, it darkens and becomes entirely black as melanogen is oxidized to melanin. The pigment may be detected and identified by adding a few drops of 10 per cent ferric chloride solution to a urine sample; if melanin is present, a gray precipitate forms, which turns black after it has been removed by filtration and exposed to air for 30 minutes.

Reaction (pH) of Urine

Urine acidity (pH) is estimated by immersing a strip of Nitrazine Paper in the sample and comparing the resultant color with those printed on a chart. The pH varies normally between 4.5 and 8.0 units and is usually acid, i.e., less than 7 units. As in the

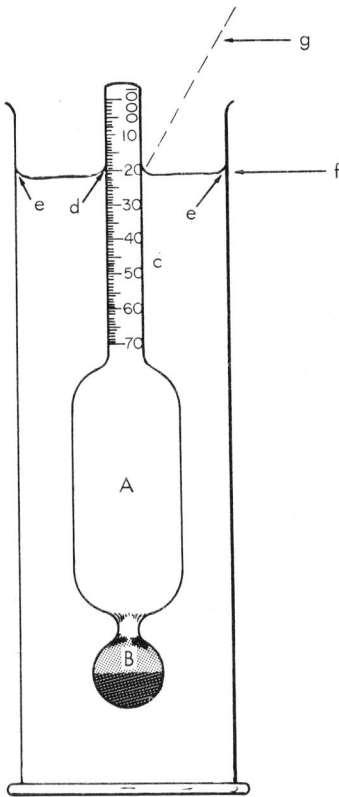

FIG. 20. Urinometer. (A) Bobbin. (B) Weight. (C) Stem. (d) Meniscus on the stem. (e) Meniscus on the walls of the glass vessel. (f) Proper line of vision. (g) Improper line of vision.

chloric acid in the stomach, a process involving the extraction of hydrogen ions from the blood. The resultant lowering of the hydrogen ion concentration in the plasma is reflected by a corresponding decrease in the urine. In cases of renal tract infection, urea-splitting organisms may alkalinize the urine before it is voided, as a product of their growth in the kidneys or the bladder. Constant alkalinity of freshly voided urine is important in such cases, not only as a diagnostic clue, but also as a factor which promotes the formation of renal and bladder stones. Renal tuberculosis represents one variety of urinary tract infection in which the urine reaction is characteristically acid; the tubercle bacillus does not split urea.

Urine Specific Gravity

Measurement of the urine specific gravity may be one of the nurse's duties. By "specific gravity of urine" is meant the ratio of the weight of a given volume of urine to that of the same volume of distilled water when these are measured at the same temperature. A liter of water at 4° C. weighs 1,000 Gm.; 1.000 is accepted as the reference value for specific gravity measurements. Suppose 15 Gm. of a soluble substance such as urea or sodium chloride were dissolved in water. The weight of the fluid would be increased correspondingly, but the volume would not change. One liter of the solution at 4° C. would weigh 1,015 Gm.; its specific gravity would be 1.015.

The specific gravity of urine is measured by the flotation of a hydrometer, or urinometer, a sealed glass bulb fitted at the upper end with a stem on which is mounted a calibrated scale and, at the bottom, with a small mercury bulb to provide ballast and to maintain the device in vertical position when immersed (Fig. 20). Urine is placed in a cylindrical receptacle and its temperature noted. The hydrometer is next introduced. The depth to which this sinks and at which its position becomes stabilized is determined in accordance with the reading on the scale at the junction of the stem and the fluid meniscus. This figure represents the specific gravity of the sample, unadjusted for temperature effect. Urinometers are usually calibrated on the basis of observations made at 20° C., and any significant deviation from

case of other urine electrolytes (see p. 74), the concentration of hydrogen ions in the urine, or the urine pH, reflects the metabolic status of the patient. The urine reaction should be tested as soon as the sample is voided, for it becomes increasingly alkaline on standing. Bacterial contaminants multiply rapidly, decomposing the urea and liberating ammonia which is a strong alkali. (Ammonia accounts for the disagreeable odor of stale urine.)

Acid urines are encountered in cases of metabolic acidosis (page 832) and sodium depletion due to diarrhea or excessive sweating. Alkaline urines are voided after ingestion of alkalizing salts, following the vomiting of acid gastric juice and in cases of respiratory alkalosis (p. 400). Transient alkalinization of the urine occurs after meals which stimulate the production of hydro-

this figure in the test sample requires an adjustment of the observed specific gravity by the addition of 0.001 for every 3° C. above, or the subtraction of 0.001 for every 3° C. below, 20° C.

Normally, the specific gravity of the total 24 hours' mixed urine is between 1.015 and 1.020, but that of a patient voiding after a heavy meal which contained little fluid may be 1.040, and that of a voiding after the ingestion of a large amount of fluid or of some food which acts as a diuretic may be as low as 1.003. A normal person's separate voidings of urine of one day could easily give these two readings, but mix all the urine voided during that whole day and night and the reading would probably lie between 1.015 and 1.020.

A specific gravity of 1.025 or more in the absence of albumin and sugar is fairly reliable evidence of normal renal function. On the other hand, if random samples from a patient consistently give specific gravity readings in the vicinity of 1.010, poor renal function is suspected.

Urine Concentration Tests

A simple, but not entirely reliable, test of renal function measures the capacity of the kidneys to concentrate the glomerular filtrate and consists in the determination of the specific gravity of urine voided from 12 to 18 hours after all fluids and food have been withheld. Concentration below specific gravity 1.015 in these circumstances is regarded as being abnormal. Whereas this test serves admirably in an ambulatory patient, it is likely to yield misleading results in persons at bed rest, for they simply do not concentrate their urine to the maximum extent in less than from 36 to 48 hours. Therefore, for reliable data, the dehydration period must be lengthened to a minimum of 36 hours. It would be highly undesirable to perform this test on any patient with high fever or with any feature predisposing to dehydration, and this would also apply to a patient in whom dehydration might be dangerous.

Abnormal Urine Constituents

Proteinuria (Albuminuria)

Normal renal cells allow a trace of albumin to pass into the urine, but this trace is so minute that it cannot be detected by the ordinary tests. If any at all can be recognized by these tests, an albuminuria is present and indicates pathology. The cause of most long-standing albuminurias is nephritis. The amount of albumin in the urine of nephritic patients varies enormously. In the acute cases, a large quantity is present, so much that when the urine is boiled it truly solidifies. The subacute cases have less, and the more chronic cases least.

One of the classic methods for the detection of albuminuria and the estimation of protein in the urine is the so-called "heat and acetic acid test." This involves filling a Pyrex test tube to approximately two thirds capacity with clear urine. If, after boiling and adding acetic acid in a certain sequence, a cloudiness is noted, the presence of protein has been demonstrated. The concentration of protein in the specimen is reflected by the degree of turbidity that develops, and it can be estimated on that basis.

Another test for the detection and semiquantitative estimation of proteinuria is based on a color reaction produced by and on a reagent tablet (Albutest). This test is carried out by placing a drop of urine on the tablet, followed after a moment by 2 drops of water. A positive reaction is indicated by the appearance of a blue-green spot on the tablet surface which persists after the addition of water, the intensity of this color being roughly proportional to the protein concentration. A modification of this procedure, employing impregnated paper strips (Uristix), is performed simply by dipping one end of a strip in urine and comparing the color of the dipped portion with a color chart. (See Plate 1.)

Bence-Jones Proteinuria. A common manifestation of multiple myeloma, occurring in approximately one half to one third of these patients, is the appearance in the urine of Bence-Jones protein, which precipitates from urine which has been heated to a temperature of 50 to 75° C., redissolves at the boiling point and again precipitates on cooling.

Glycosuria

Sugar (glucose) is present in small traces in normal urine, but not enough to be detected by ordinary tests. In certain conditions, however, notably untreated diabetes mellitus, much larger amounts are present. Also in various diseases of the nervous system—for example, after injuries to the head—there may be moderate amounts of sugar in the urine temporarily.

Each nurse, also each diabetic patient, should be able to examine the urine for sugar. The Clinitest method, currently in wide use, involves the addition of a tablet to 5 drops of urine and 10 of water, measured and delivered by a medicine dropper into a test tube. The tube is placed in a rack and left undisturbed until the solution has ceased to boil. After an interval of at least 15 seconds, the color of the material is noted, described and recorded in terms of sugar concentration in the original sample, employing a color chart.

A simple, convenient and highly specific color test for glycosuria has become available* which employs a paper strip which has been impregnated with 3 reagents: the enzymes, glucose oxidase and peroxidase, and an indicator dye, orthotolidin. The strip is merely moistened with urine, and, if the moist area turns blue, the presence (but not the quantity) of glucose is indicated.

Ketonuria

The presence of ketone bodies (acetone, acetoacetic acid and beta-hydroxybutyric acid) in the urine is characteristic of diabetic ketoacidosis and individuals who are severely dehydrated or starved. The finding is indicative of incomplete fat metabolism (see Chap. 9). One of the most reliable methods of detecting ketonuria is by means of the nitroprusside test. Approximately 1 Gm. of a powdered mixture of sodium nitroprusside and ammonium sulfate is added to 5 ml. of urine. After the reagent has dissolved, concentrated ammonium hydroxide is layered over the solution. The appearance of a red-purple ring at the junction of these layers denotes the presence of ketone bodies, and the intensity of the color provides a rough measure of their concentration. Materials which greatly facilitate the performance of this test are available commercially in the form of a powder (Acetone Test Powder)

* Tes-Tape; Uristix; Clinistix.

and a tablet (Acetest). The Acetest procedure involves the placing of 1 drop of urine on a tablet. In the event of a positive reaction, a color develops within the space of 30 seconds which varies from lavender to deep purple, depending on the concentration of ketone bodies in the sample. A paper strip test (Ketostix) is also available, which likewise is based on the nitroprusside reaction.

Phenylketonuria. This condition, otherwise known as "oligophrenia phenylpyruvica," is a rare familial metabolic disease characterized by the patient's inability to utilize phenylalanine, an essential amino acid. This substance, together with other unusual protein metabolites, are excreted in the urine. Among the serious complications of phenylketonuria are mental deficiency and faulty growth. Early recognition of this metabolic error is of the utmost importance, in view of the prophylactic value of a phenylalanine-poor diet and because of the necessity for instituting such a diet as soon as possible after birth if normal mental development and normal physical growth are to be achieved.

Diagnosis of this condition depends on the demonstration of phenylpyruvic acid in the urine, readily accomplished by means of a ferric chloride test. This test, which demonstrates other ketone bodies as well, may be performed by adding 10 per cent ferric chloride solution, drop by drop, to 5 ml. of urine. The presence of phenylpyruvic acid is indicated by the development of a dark green color which tends to fade in the course of 5 minutes. (A deep Bordeaux-red color appears in the presence of acetoacetic or beta-hydroxybutyric acid.) A paper strip test (Phenistix) is available (Plate 1) which facilitates the ferric chloride test materially and increases its availability. Capable of eliciting positive reactions on contact with diapers from affected infants, this device is applicable to screening tests which could be conducted on a massive scale, detect the disease with regularity during the first 2 to 4 weeks of life and avert its dreadful, but preventable, complications.

Formed Elements in Urine
Hematuria

Red blood corpuscles may be found in the urine—either a few, or many, or in such

FIG. 21. Casts found in the urine. (a) Epithelial casts. (b) Granular cast. (c) Hyaline casts. (d) Waxy cast. (e) Fatty cast. (Much magnified.)

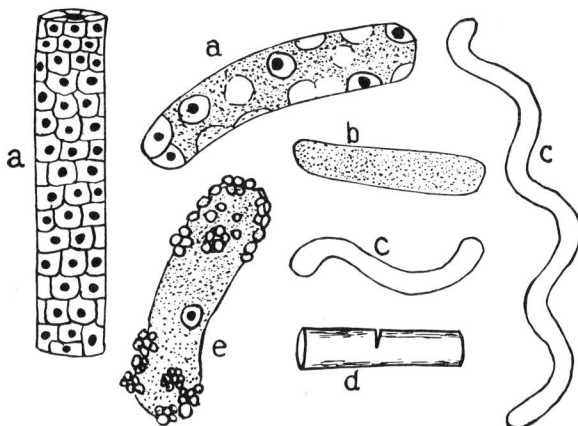

quantity that the urine appears sanguineous. When their concentration is sufficient to color the urine red, the condition is called *gross hematuria*. One practically always finds red blood cells in the urine in acute nephritis and during the acute flare-ups of chronic nephritis. In these cases the urine is often not red but more smoky in appearance.

The presence or absence of red blood cells is one of the important criteria for distinguishing a pure nephrosis, or the nephrotic stage of glomerulonephritis, from acute glomerulonephritis. Hematuria is seen in pyelonephritis, in pyonephrosis (different degrees of kidney bacterial infection) and in focal embolic nephritis such as occurs in bacterial endocarditis. It may appear as a manifestation of a hemorrhagic disease, such as thrombocytopenic purpura, or Dicoumarol toxicity. Red cells frequently are found in the urine in cases of renal stone, renal tuberculosis and carcinoma of the kidney. Hematuria is also a common complication of sulfonamide-drug therapy, due to irritation of the kidney by insoluble crystals of these drugs (excepting sulfanilamide) in patients who receive insufficient fluid and alkali with the drug.

Hematuria may also originate from sites in the genitourinary tract other than the kidney, such as the ureter, the bladder or the prostate. In all cases the source of the blood must be determined. The presence of red cells is usually detected on microscopic examination of the urine sediment. Sensitive hemoglobin tests based on the benzidine or orthotolidin reaction (pp. 96 and 68) are useful for the screening of patients for hematuria, since the latter cannot escape detection even if the red cells are hemolyzed.

Pyuria

Small numbers of leukocytes are normally present in the urine. They are observed with regularity and in quantity in the urine of patients with nephritis and other inflammatory diseases involving the urinary tract. When present in sufficient number to give the fresh urine a cloudy appearance, the condition is called *pyuria*. Pyuria of marked degree occurs in pyelitis, pyelonephritis and pyonephrosis, in tuberculosis of the kidney and, most strikingly, in cystitis and urethritis.

Cylindruria

The term "cast" owes its origin to the manner in which these elements acquire their characteristic shape, molded as they are in the renal tubules (Fig. 21). Thus, the tubular lumen becomes partially filled with a substance which hardens and forms a "cast" of their lumen. These casts are later washed out by the urine, where they can be found with a microscope.

Casts in the urine (cylindruria) have much the same clinical significance as albuminuria. As a rule, albumin and casts appear together, but for short periods either may be found alone.

It must be realized that casts deteriorate rapidly in unpreserved urine. Prolonged preservation may be accomplished, to be sure, even in unrefrigerated specimens, by means of a chemical preservative. However, this may not be uniformly effective with respect to all the formed elements, and the morphology of those that persist may be altered beyond certain recognition. The fact remains that for examination of the urine sediment there is no substitute for fresh urine.

Crystalluria

Crystals are to be found in most concentrated urine specimens, their composition and morphology dictated by the pH of the specimen. In the majority of instances, their presence denotes no metabolic abnormality or other disorder. Their identification usually can be accomplished on the basis of their microscopic appearance alone.

Cystinuria. Definite pathologic significance attaches to the finding of cystine crystals in the urine, for they are indicative of a rare familiar disorder known as "cystinuria." This is a life-long disease and represents one of the inborn errors of metabolism. Patients so affected are predisposed to the formation of renal and bladder stones composed of cystine. The crystals in question are recognized on microscopic examination as thick, highly refractile hexagonal plates. Their identity is further established from their ready solubility in hydrochloric acid and lack of solubility in acetic acid.

Leucine and Tyrosine Crystals. If either of these varieties of crystal is encountered in the urine, the other is likely to be present. This form of crystalluria has ominous implications, indicating that massive tissue autolysis is in progress. It is associated most often with severe, diffuse and advanced liver necrosis which is destined to prove lethal. Leucine crystals are yellowish, oily-looking spheres with radial and concentric striations; they are insoluble in hydrochloric acid and in ether. Tyrosine crystals appear in the form of needles, arranged in sheaves and tufts; these are soluble in hydrochloric acid and in ether.

Bacteriuria

The presence of bacteria in urine samples collected without special precautions or stored without adequate protection against contamination is of no significance. However, the demonstration, by microscopic examination or bacteriologic culture, of bacteriuria in catheterized specimens or in "sterile-voided" samples is potentially of great importance.

In order to establish the significance of bacteriuria it is necessary to perform quantitative urine cultures. This involves the dilution of urine with sterile nutrient broth and the preparation of agar pour plates from this mixture. The number of organisms per ml. of urine can be estimated from the number of bacterial colonies that are visible on the plate after 24 to 48 hours of incubation at 37° C. Counts of 5,000 or more per ml. of urine are consistent with a diagnosis of urinary tract infection.

Electrolytes and Metabolites in Urine

Urine Sodium and Chlorides

Quantitative measurements of sodium and chloride ions in the urine are useful for the evaluation and the correction of metabolic derangements such as water and electrolyte depletion by vomiting or diarrhea. These data are helpful likewise in regulating the treatment of patients with edema due to congestive heart failure, renal insufficiency or hepatic disease, and they are absolutely essential for the precise diagnosis of certain renal disorders. Urine sodium and chloride concentrations have very little significance, however, unless the patient's oral and parenteral intake of these electrolytes during the preceding day is known. Assuming that this is known, and their extrarenal losses can be estimated, the urine values provide a reliable indication as to whether or not abnormal salt retention or salt excretion is occurring.

Urine electrolytes are usually measured in 24-hour samples, although, under some circumstances, analyses of random specimens may prove to be adequate. As has been emphasized, the 24-hour excretion test depends on the certainty that the final specimen comprises all urine voided during the collection period, i.e., the total of each voiding must have been added to the total pool.

Urine chloride may be measured by a variety of technics. A simple semiquantitative method, suitable for use at the bedside and often carried out by the nurse, is known as the *Fantus test*. Ten drops of urine are introduced into a test tube with a medicine dropper. The latter, after rinsing, is used again for the addition of 1 drop of 20 per cent potassium chromate solution. The dropper is rinsed once again, and with it is added, drop by drop, 2.9 per cent silver nitrate solution. During this step, the mixture is agitated constantly and the drops are counted until the end-point is reached. This is recognized from an abrupt change in the color of the mixture, i.e., from yellow to red-brown, due to the formation of red silver chromate. The number of drops of silver nitrate that have been added at the end-point can be translated directly into a figure representing the chloride concentration in the urine sample, expressed as "sodium chloride, grams (or "milli-equivalents") per liter."

The measurement of sodium in urine is performed readily and accurately by means of the flame photometer.

Urine Potassium

Measurements of potassium in the urine are informative only to the extent that the rates of potassium intake and loss from the gastrointestinal tract are known. As in the case of urinary sodium, potassium excretion is measured on the basis of 24-hour urine collections. The method of analysis is likewise a technic of flame photometry.

Urine Calcium

The concentration of calcium in the urine is important in the evaluation of bone disease. Associated with rapid decalcification of the skeleton, such as occurs in hyperparathyroidism (Chap. 38) and following the sudden cessation of normal physical activity, the urinary excretion of calcium is increased. A decrease in urine calcium may indicate an abnormal decrease in the blood calcium level, due, for example, to hypoparathyroidism (Chap. 38) or to vitamin D deficiency (Chap. 38). A simple semiquantitative method for the estimation of urinary calcium is the *Sulkowitch test,* based on the precipitation of calcium as the insoluble oxalate salt. The Sulkowitch reagent is added to the urine, and, if no precipitation appears, it may be presumed that the concentration of urinary calcium is less than normal. Faint turbidity, visible only when viewed against a dark background, is recorded as a 1-plus reaction; this is the usual finding in normal subjects. Greater degrees of turbidity, or the appearance of frank flocculation (a 4-plus reaction), are indicative of abnormally high calcium concentrations. Since the dietary intake exerts a profound influence on calcium excretion, the patient should be instructed to adhere to a low-calcium neutral-ash diet for at least 3 days prior to the test.

Urine Urobilinogen

Urobilinogen is a substance formed by the action of intestinal bacteria on the bilirubin in the bile. A portion of this urobilinogen is reabsorbed through the intestinal wall into the blood stream and appears in the urine, the basis of the *urine urobilinogen* test. Normally there is always a certain amount present in the urine. If it is absent, it may be concluded that there is no bilirubin, hence no bile, reaching the intestine, due either to biliary tract obstruction or to failure of the liver to secrete bile. Blood containing urobilinogen is cleared of this substance as it passes through the liver, for the liver handles urobilinogen as it handles bilirubin, namely, by excreting it into the bile. If the liver cells are not functioning adequately, urobilinogen is retained in the blood, where its concentration becomes increasingly elevated. This high blood level of urobilinogen, in turn, is reflected by an abnormal increase in the urine urobilinogen. An increased urine urobilinogen is often one of the earliest signs of acute liver cell damage. Increased levels are also characteristic of patients with hemolytic anemia, whose bilirubin (hence urobilinogen) production is abnormally high as a result of rapid red cell destruction.

A simple test for urine urobilinogen entails the serial dilution with tap water of a fresh urine sample and the addition of Ehrlich's reagent. Fresh urine from a normal subject gives a pink color in a dilution of 1:8 to 1:32. If color develops only in the urine sample diluted with equal parts of water and/or an undiluted sample, or if no reaction whatever can be discerned, urobilinogen excretion is considered to be decreased. The appearance of color in urine dilutions of 1:64 or higher is presumptive evidence of increased urobilinogen.

Hormone Assays in Urine
Chorionic Gonadotropin

Gonadotropic hormone, also called anterior pituitarylike substances (APL), is produced by placental tissue in the pregnant uterus. Its demonstration in the urine may provide the earliest indication of pregnancy, positive results being obtained in 98 per cent of pregnant women tested 10 days after the first amenorrhea. Urine tests for this substance may also be positive in patients with tumors containing chorionic tissue, such as testicular teratoma and chorioepithelioma, and in cases of retained placenta following obstetric delivery. Various procedures that are available for the detection of this hormone include the Friedman test, which employs a rabbit, the Aschheim-Zondek test, utilizing a mouse, and the African frog test. Each of the above tests is based on the observation of characteristic changes in ovarian structures following the injection of gonadotropic hormone. The procedure most widely used at present utilizes a male frog belonging to the species *Rana pipiens,* commonly known as the Leopard Frog, Grass Frog or Meadow Frog. One of these amphibians is injected with a sample of urine representing the first voiding of the day. One half to 1 hour after the injection, a drop of urine is secured from the frog. This specimen is examined for the presence or absence of spermatazoa, the former indicating a positive reaction. The validity of this procedure is enhanced by imposing a 24-hour period of fluid restriction prior to the voiding of the test sample, during which drugs of all types should be withheld, especially salicylates, barbiturates and hormones.

17-Ketosteroids

The concentration of 17-ketosteroids in the urine reflects the secretory activity of the adrenal cortex. Elevated levels are characteristic of patients with Cushing's disease and functioning adrenocortical tumors, whereas decreased levels are indicative of depressed adrenal function, as in Addison's disease or panhypopituitarism (see Chapter 38). Quantitative measurement of 17-ketosteroids requires the collection of a 24-hour urine sample. This is acidified throughout the collection period by the preliminary addition of 10 ml. of concentrated hydrochloric acid (or, if chlorides are also to be measured, of sulfuric acid). The urine should be refrigerated

immediately after voiding and the analysis carried out as soon as possible following completion of the collection. The test itself is based on a color reaction produced by the addition of m-dinitrobenzene to an alcohol-ether extract of urine previously subjected to acid hydrolysis. A red chromogen is produced by this reaction which is measured quantitatively by means of a spectrophotometer. Normal excretion values for adult males range from 8 to 20 mg. and for adult females from 5 to 15 mg. of 17-ketosteroids per 24 hours.

Catecholamines

Epinephrine and norepinephrine, representing the catecholamines, are hormones which are produced mainly by the adrenal medulla and serve as the chemical mediators of the sympathetic nervous system. Excessive quantities are produced by certain tumors, specifically pheochromocytoma (Chap. 38). Urine tests in such cases demonstrate as much as a tenfold increase above normal. The catecholamines are measured by photofluorometric methods. Normal individuals excrete up to 200 micrograms of catecholamines per 24 hours, approximately one half of which is accounted for by derivatives of norepinephrine produced previously at sympathetic nerve endings. The excretion of more than 200 micrograms per day is indicative of pheochromocytoma.

Phenolsulfonphthalein (PSP) Excretion Test

PSP Test of Renal Function

The easiest, quickest and, hence, most popular test of renal functional efficiency has been for years one which requires no blood chemistry but uses phenolsulfonphthalein, a harmless dye eliminated solely by the kidneys. After having emptied his bladder, the patient, in order to promote a free secretion of urine, drinks 400 ml. of water, cold but not iced, and 20 minutes later is given an intravenous injection of 1 ml. of a sterile solution containing 6 mg. of phenolsulfonphthalein. The patient is required to empty his bladder completely at intervals of 15 minutes, 30 minutes, 1 hour and 2 hours after the injection. Additional water is given to ensure an adequate output of urine. The amount of dye present in these specimens is then estimated by a simple colorimetric method. Normally, the first specimen will contain from 20 to 40 per cent, and the remainder enough so that the total amount of dye eliminated in 2 hours is from 60 to 90 per cent of the amount injected. Interpretation of this test is not considered to be reliable unless the volume of each urine sample is 50 ml. or more.

BLOOD CHEMISTRY: PROTEINS, ELECTROLYTES, ABSORBATES AND METABOLITES

The present section is concerned with the quantitative measurement of various normal and abnormal substances that are contained in blood, including some that are introduced by design for the purpose of measuring specific organ functions. Most normal blood ingredients are found in concentrations that are predictable, when measured under standard conditions, and that vary within narrow limits. Deviations from the normal range are generally significant, attributable perhaps to an inadequate or excessive supply, a defect in absorption, impaired utilization, reduced or excessive elimination or abnormal metabolism of the substance in question. A marked increase in the concentration of certain substances, notably enzymes, may reflect tissue necrosis with liberation of materials that normally are retained within cells. The finding of abnormal ingredients, i.e., components which are not characteristic of normal blood, may supply a valuable diagnostic clue, as in the case of the cryoglobulins and "M-protein." The interpretation of abnormal chemical data is discussed briefly in conjunction with each test that is described.

Blood Sampling for Chemical Analysis

Venous Samples

The majority of chemical tests require specimens of venous blood, obtained either in the form of unmodified clotted blood as a source of serum or blood that has been collected with an anticoagulant for plasma or whole blood analysis. Relative to the collection procedure itself, certain technical considerations are pertinent:

1. The collection of blood for most chemical tests is carried out preferably 4 hours or longer after a meal and ideally before the first meal of the day. For certain tests, fasting samples are an absolute requirement.

2. Excessively prolonged stasis in preparation for venipuncture is to be avoided, since stasis promotes dehydration and increases the acidity of venous blood in the extremity distal to the tourniquet.

3. Syringes and needles used in blood collection must be chemically clean and dry, as well as bacteriologically sterile, in order to avoid chemical contamination and hypotonic hemolysis.

4. The individual who undertakes to collect the specimen should be acquainted with the sample volume that is required and with the variety of container that is appropriate for the contemplated analysis.

5. Every possible precaution must be taken to ensure that the patient whose blood is to be sampled has been identified correctly and that the specimen container has been labeled accurately, completely, legibly and securely.

Serum tests require samples that have been collected in empty tubes that are chemically clean, free of moisture and equipped with a secure closure. Samples for plasma or whole blood analyses should be placed in tubes or bottles, similarly clean and dry, which contain potassium oxalate as an anticoagulant. One mg. of potassium oxalate will bind the ionized calcium and prevent clotting in approximately 1 ml. of blood; accordingly, containers which are expected to accommodate 10 ml. of unclotted blood are prepared in advance by introducing and evaporating to dryness 0.5 ml. of a 2 per cent solution of potassium oxalate.

A third variety of blood sample is one that is collected anaerobically and requires a chemically clean dry tube containing 1 to 3 ml. of mineral oil. Such tubes may be equipped with cork stoppers or plastic screw-caps, but not with rubber stoppers because of instability of rubber in the presence of any petroleum product. Prior to an anaerobic collection, a trace of oil is aspirated into the syringe in order to seal effectively the interface between the barrel and the plunger and avoid the escape of carbon dioxide via that route. The blood, having been aspirated with minimal stasis into the syringe, is introduced without turbulence into the tube under the surface of the oil, then transported immediately to the chemistry laboratory. Collections of this type are required for the measurement of chloride and bicarbonate ions. Whole blood pH is measured in samples of unclotted blood collected anaerobically, and sealed anaerobically, in a syringe that has been moistened previously with a solution containing heparin, 100 mg., and sodium fluoride, 4 Gm., per 100 ml., the heparin serving as the anticoagulant and the sodium fluoride as an inhibitor of glycolysis and lactic acid production in the sample. After collection, the syringe containing the sample is sealed at the tip by removal of the needle and substitution of a tight-fitting metal cap or some similar device.

Capillary Blood Specimens for Ultramicroanalysis

Numerous tests can be performed reliably on samples that are relatively minute, e.g., within the volume range of 0.02 to 0.10 ml. Samples for microanalysis are obtained from an ear lobe or a finger and collected in capillary tubes measuring approximately 10 cm. in length and 4 mm. in outside diameter. Serum is separated from such samples after rapid sedimentation in a microcentrifuge by breaking the tube at the serum-cell interface and ejecting the cell-free portion with the aid of a small rubber bulb.

Plasma Proteins

Plasma contains between 6.5 and 8.0 Gm. of protein per 100 ml., of which 4 to 5 Gm. are in the form of albumin and approximately 3 represent a mixture of globulins. Plasma albumin rarely is elevated, except as a result of dehydration. A reduction of albumin (hypoalbuminemia), on the other hand, commonly occurs as a consequence of an inaedquate diet. It may be due to a reduced rate of albumin production by the liver; or to albumin depletion caused by the escape of this protein into the urine, as in nephrosis; or into ascitic fluid, as in cirrhosis; or from the body surface, through a decubitus ulcer. Any alterations involving the globulin fraction is usually in the direction of an increase, or "hyperglobulinemia."

Methods of Assay. A simple procedure providing a rapid and reasonably reliable estimate of plasma protein concentration is the familiar copper sulfate test. A drop of plasma or serum is introduced into a series of bottles containing copper sulfate in graded concentrations, each solution of known specific gravity. The specific gravity of the particular solution which holds the sample motionless in suspension corresponds exactly to the specific gravity of the specimen. This value, in turn, can be translated directly into one which represents protein concentration.

More accurate estimates of serum protein concentration are possible by means of a colorimetric test based on the biuret reaction. Separate determination of albumin and globulin involves measuring the total protein concentration in one sample and the albumin concentration in an aliquot sample, the latter having been freed of globulins by precipitation with sodium sulfate, which "salts them out." The concentration of globulins is computed from the difference between the two values.

Fibrinogen may be measured independently of the other proteins by adding thrombin to a sample of plasma. The clot so produced, incorporating all of the fibrinogen but no other protein, may then be dried and weighed, or analyzed chemically to determine the amount of clottable protein, i.e., fibrinogen, in the original sample.

Plasma and Serum Electrophoresis

The most precise method of measuring blood proteins is by electrophoretic analysis. This method is carried out by placing a drop of serum or plasma on a paper strip that is saturated with a buffer solution and given an electric charge. After a period of several hours the strip is dried, stained and examined for the location, the size and the color density of certain sharply demarcated bands that traverse the strip at several points. Each band marks the final position of an individual protein. Most distant from the point of origin is albumin which migrates the fastest, with alpha, beta and gamma globulins following in that order. The electrophoretic pattern of plasma includes also a band representing fibrinogen, least mobile of all the plasma proteins. (Serum samples do not contain fibrinogen, of course.) The width and the color depth of each band reflect the quantity of that particular protein in the sample. Quantitative analysis of the pattern is accomplished in elegant fashion by means of a "densitometer," a device which automatically passes the strip before a photoelectric "eye," draws a curve representing the variations in color density throughout its length, computes the area under each peak of the curve and translates the data into values representing the concentration of each individual protein in the sample.

Electrophoretic analysis offers a ready means of detecting and identifying certain important defects of protein metabolism. These include *agammaglobulinemia* and *afibrinogenemia,* characterized by the virtual or complete absence of gamma globulin and fibrinogen, respectively. Both of these disorders are encountered as congenital anomalies and may occur as complications of an underlying disorder. An electrophoretic pattern is marked occasionally by the presence of a band in an atypical location, signifying one type of "dysproteinemia." The appearance of "M-protein," for example, which migrates in a position between the beta- and gammaglobulins, distinguishes the dysproteinemia of myelomatosis.

Protein Flocculation Tests

A number of conditions are accompanied regularly by alterations in one or another protein constituent or by changes in the relative concentrations of individual plasma proteins that are detected by means of various turbidity and flocculation tests. For example, macroglobulins, which are proteins of great molecular size encountered most often in myeloma and its benign variant, macroglobulinemia, form a cloudy precipitate when a drop or two of plasma is added to distilled water. This change is the basis of the *Sia water test*. Cryoglobulin and cryofibrinogen tend to flocculate when serum or plasma, respectively, is chilled, redissolving when the sample is warmed. By contrast, pyroglobulins precipitate when serum is heated and redissolve when it is chilled.

Tests that are likely to be positive in chronic liver disease, and in other disorders accompanied by increased serum globulins, include the *thymol turbidity test,* utilizing a precipitating reagent in the form of a buffered thymol solution; the *cephalin flocculation test,* employing an emulsion of cholesterol and cephalin; the *Takata-Ara reaction,* producing flocculation in mixtures of pathologic serum and mercuric chloride; and the *colloidal gold test.* Similarly belonging to the general category of nonspecific flocculation reactions are certain tests that depend on the formation of precipitates in particulate suspensions when the latter are mixed with abnormal serum or plasma. The *bentonite flocculation test,* useful in the diagnosis and the evaluation of rheumatoid arthritis, is concerned with the flocculation of a colloidal clay. The *latex fixation test,* likewise of value in rheumatoid arthritis, depends on the precipitation of globulin-coated plastic beads.

Erythrocyte Sedimentation Test. As in the case of the bentonite flocculation and the latex fixation tests, the erythrocyte sedimentation rate serves to evaluate the influence of serum (or plasma, in this instance) on the tendency of particulate matter in a state of suspension to form aggregates. In this test the red cells are the particles and the aggregates are rouleaux. The rate and the extent of rouleau formation are reflected by the rapidity with which the red cells sediment spontaneously in the course of one hour in a blood sample containing mixed-oxalate anticoagulant.* The rate is increased in samples which contain an abnormally high concentration of globulin or fibrinogen in proportion to albumin, as in cases of acute and chronic infection, tissue necrosis of all types, inflammatory diseases, hyperglobulinemia or hypoalbuminemia, regardless of its cause.

Protein Metabolites in Blood

Since the function of the kidneys is to remove from the blood certain of the waste products of cellular activity, any degree of accumulation of these particular products in the blood, under controlled conditions, is a measure of the inadequacy of renal function. The substances which are measured most often for this purpose include urea (determined as urea nitrogen), uric acid and creatinine.

---

* Red cells which are grouped in rouleau formation fall more rapidly than separated cells, as an intact rock, dropped into water, sinks faster than sand.

The total concentration of the protein metabolites, including these three and others which are present in trace amounts, is often measured in the aggregate and expressed as "nonprotein nitrogen," or NPN, mg. per 100 ml.

Normally the amount of total nonprotein nitrogen in 100 ml. of blood, obtained from a vein 14 hours after the last meal, varies from 25 to 40 mg. per 100 ml. Of this total, from 12 to 15 mg. is urea nitrogen (BUN). From 2 to 5 mg. of uric acid and from 1 to 2 mg. of creatinine are present in each 100 ml. of normal blood. The determination of urea nitrogen has practically the same significance as that of the total nonprotein nitrogen, and many use it instead. In nephritis, however, the earliest signs of renal damage are the retention, first, of uric acid, and, second, of creatinine. Definite increases in both can be recognized before there is any significant rise in the urea or total nonprotein nitrogen.

Blood Sugar

The concentration of sugar in the blood of a normal fasting individual varies from approximately 70 to 100 mg./100 ml. This level fluctuates throughout the day, depending on the time and the composition of meals, the degree of physical exertion and other factors which enhance the utilization of glucose or stimulate the conversion of glycogen (storage glucose) into glucose. An elevated fasting blood sugar (hyperglycemia) is characteristic of diabetes mellitus (Chap. 38). Hypoglycemia, an abnormally low concentration of blood sugar, occurs as a manifestation of hyperinsulinism, a complication of functioning pancreatic tumors (Chap. 38). The glucose tolerance test of carbohydrate metabolism is described on page 82.

Plasma Bilirubin

Hemoglobin released from hemolyzed red cells is converted by histiocytes throughout the body into free bilirubin. The latter, present in normal plasma in a concentration of approximately 0.4 to 0.8 mg. per 100 ml., is a pigment of low solubility which, in the absence of alcohol, reacts slowly to Ehrlich's aldehyde reagent (hence the term "indirect bilirubin"). Free bilirubin is converted by liver cells into its glucuronide salt, and in this form is excreted almost entirely into the bile.

The glucuronide salt reacts promptly with Ehrlich's reagent without the addition of alcohol, hence has been designated "1-minute prompt reacting bilirubin." This is the form in which bilirubin appears in the urine. Retention in the blood of either bilirubin produces jaundice. The relative amounts of free bilirubin and bilirubin glucuronide provide an indication as to the mechanism of jaundice in various diseases, as has been discussed on page 68.

Blood Lipids and Lipid Metabolites

The concentrations of free cholesterol and cholesterol esters in the blood are of possible importance in relation to the production of atherosclerosis. Changes in the relative and absolute amounts of these metabolites are of diagnostic significance in certain hereditary derangements of lipid metabolism and as a basis for evaluating liver function. The normal ranges of concentration for free cholesterol and cholesterol esters in the plasma are from 35 to 75 mg. and from 175 to 215 mg. per 100 ml., respectively.

Blood Electrolytes

Blood pH

The hydrogen ion concentration in the blood normally is maintained within very narrow limits, i.e., within the range of from 7.40 to 7.45 pH units, values less than 7.40 units representing acidosis, those above 7.45, alkalosis.

Variations in acidity are prevented by chemical reactions in the plasma, immediately neutralizing any acid or alkaline substance that is excreted by the cells or absorbed from the gastrointestinal tract.

Direct measurement of the blood pH is performed with a "pH meter," a device incorporating 2 electrodes, 1 containing the blood sample. The affinity of the blood for free electrons (or its capacity to receive them), relative to the energy with which atoms in the other electrode attempt to expel electrons, is dictated by the concentration of hydrogen ions in the blood sample, i.e., its pH, and this is what is measured by the instrument.

Sodium, Chloride and Bicarbonate Ions

The concentration of these electrolytes in the blood provides an indication as to the presence, type and cause of many metabolic disturbances, including acidosis and alkalosis. Sodium is normally found in a concentration of 136 to 146 milliequivalents per liter; chloride ion, 100 to 106 mEq./L.; and bicarbonate ion, 25 to 30 mEq./L. In cases of metabolic acidosis, for example, the serum sodium and carbon dioxide content are markedly reduced. In alkalosis due to vomiting, chlorides are diminished and bicarbonate is increased; in alkalosis following hyperventilation, the bicarbonate level is low and the chlorides are normal or slightly elevated. Measurements of chloride and sodium are carried out on serum from clotted venous blood. Bicarbonate ion is usually measured as the carbon dioxide content of venous samples collected under oil, as described on page 77.

Serum potassium, normally from 3.8 to 5.5 mEq./L., can be dangerously affected in patients with certain metabolic disturbances. Associated with severe acidosis and alkalosis, there may be not only a deficiency of sodium, chlorides and water, but also a substantial loss of intracellular potassium, the replacement of which is particularly important in patients with diabetic acidosis. In this condition, prior to treatment, potassium leaks from the cells into the extracellular fluid, diffuses into the circulating plasma and escapes in the urine. During the early phases of treatment with insulin and parenteral fluids, the direction of potassium migration is reversed, proceeding from the extracellular fluids back into the cells, with the result that the concentration of potassium in the plasma and tissue fluids may become dangerously low, unless this element is included specifically among the materials administered by parenteral injection.

Bound Inorganic Elements in Plasma

Calcium and Phosphorus

Calcium is present in plasma, partially ionized and partially bound to albumin, its concentration totaling from 4.5 to 5.5 mEq./L. (9 to 11 mg. per cent). The normal concentration of inorganic phosphate ranges from 3.0 to 4.5 mg. per cent. Abnormally low calcium concentration (hypocalcemia) and high phosphorus values are encountered in hypoparathyroidism (Chap. 38), certain bone diseases (Chap. 42) and renal disorders (Chap. 32). Hypercalcemia and reduced phosphorus levels are characteristic of other specific bone diseases (Chap. 42), vitamin-D poisoning and sarcoidosis (p. 767).

Plasma Iron

The concentration of iron in the plasma ranges normally between 75 to 150 micrograms/100 ml. Decreased values (or hypoferremia) may indicate excessive utilization of iron relative to the supply of dietary iron, especially during periods of rapid growth; excessive depletion of iron stores as a result of hemorrhage; or a diversion of iron from the plasma to reticuloendothelial tissues, as occurs in patients with inflammatory and neoplastic lesions of all types. The plasma iron is abnormally elevated in hemosiderosis following multiple transfusions and in hemochromatosis (p. 659).

Protein-Bound Iodine

One of the most reliable and definitive indices of thyroid function is the concentration of protein-bound iodine in the blood, which reflects the amount of circulating thyroid hormone. Normal values range from 4 to 8 micrograms (0.004 to 0.008 mg.) per 100 ml. of plasma. Values exceeding 6 micrograms indicate thyroid overactivity, and concentrations of less than 4 micrograms are interpreted as evidence of hypothyroidism.

Blood Enzymes

Amylase and Lipase

Amylase, produced by the pancreas, is responsible for the splitting of starch into simple sugar. Its concentration in the blood is important clinically, due to the fact that in acute pancreatitis large amounts are secreted into the blood, the presence of a high blood amylase level providing a cardinal diagnostic sign of that disease. Measurements of amylase yield data which are expressed in terms of "milligrams of glucose hydrolyzed in 15 minutes under standard conditions from potato starch per 100 ml. of serum." Values are considered to be normal up to 150 mg. of amylase per 100 ml. of plasma.

Lipase activity, normally below 1.5 units, has approximately the same significance as the blood amylase in cases of acute pancreatitis. However, abnormally high levels may persist longer in the course of an acute attack and may also occur in chronic pancreatitis.

Blood Phosphatases

Phosphatases split organic phosphates and phosphoric esters into simpler inorganic phosphates. One type is active in alkaline solution (alkaline phosphatase) and the other at an acid pH (acid phosphatase). *Alkaline phosphatase* is increased in association with increased bone formation, whether this occurs normally, as in children, or abnormally, as in bone diseases characterized by increased osteoblastic activity, such as Paget's disease, hyperthyroidism, rickets and metastatic cancer. Alkaline phosphatase activity in blood is usually represented in terms of "Bodansky" units, and 4 units are considered to be the upper limit of normal for this enzyme. Alkaline phosphatase is excreted in the bile; in cases of obstructive jaundice, as opposed to hepatocellular jaundice, its level in the blood is increased.

Acid phosphatase is ordinarily expressed in terms of "Gutman" units. Values of less than 4 units are within the normal range. Cancer of the prostate often is attended by increased activity of this enzyme in the blood.

Transaminase

Synthesis and breakdown of protein depend in part on the activity of enzymes which transport amine (NH_2) groups from one compound to another. All amino acids are presumed to undergo transamination as they are incorporated into, or split from, protein molecules, and corresponding to each amino acid there presumably is a separate and specific transaminase. One of these is serum glutamic oxaloacetic transaminase (SGO-T), and measurements of this enzyme in the blood are potentially of diagnostic value as a quantitative reflection of tissue breakdown. Thus, the only explanation available for the presence of any SGO-T whatever in the blood is tissue cell rupture. The blood level rises rapidly, i.e., within 4 to 6 hours after myocardial infarction, whereas it is unchanged in angina pectoris. Elevated levels are also encountered in a variety of other conditions, the most important of which,

from the standpoint of its laboratory significance, are acute hepatic cirrhosis and obstructive jaundice. Up to 40 units represents the upper level of normal transaminase activity, 1 unit in this instance being defined arbitrarily in terms of optical density change in the colorimetric analysis.

Lactic Dehydrogenase (LDH)

Two to ten-fold elevations of LDH activity in the serum are found within 6 to 12 hours following an acute myocardial infarction. Accordingly, the measurement of this enzyme, as in the case of transaminase, often is helpful in establishing or excluding this diagnosis. LDH activity is increased also in patients with widespread cancer, including leukemia and lymphoma, and tends to fluctuate in parallel with the activity of the malignant process, thus providing a useful criterion of therapeutic effect in patients receiving cancer chemotherapy.

Leucine Aminopeptidase (LAP)

This peptide-splitting enzyme is present normally in all body fluids, including the blood. A pronounced increase in LAP activity is expected—and its principal diagnostic value has been—in cases of biliary obstruction due to carcinoma of the pancreas, 450 units of activity, or more, being characteristic of these patients, in contrast with values of 200 units or less in normal individuals or in patients of other types.

Absorption, Clearance and Conversion Tests
Glucose Tolerance Test

This test of carbohydrate metabolism usually is performed in the morning, as follows. The patient is asked to empty his bladder completely, this voiding being saved for a glucose test. A 5-ml. sample of venous blood is collected for a sugar determination. Then 100 Gm. of glucose (1.75 Gm. per Kg. of normal weight in children) dissolved in 300 ml. of dilute lemon juice is given by mouth, or, if the parenteral technic is preferred, 0.5 Gm. of glucose per Kg. of body weight, prepared as a 20 per cent solution in distilled water, is injected intravenously in the course of 30 minutes. One half, 1, 2 and 3 hours after the patient has received this test meal, urine and blood specimens are collected for glucose determinations. The appearance of sugar in the urine is not necessarily indicative of diabetes mellitus, especially when it occurs at a time when the blood concentration is 150 mg. per cent or less; this finding merely suggests a lowered renal threshold for glucose. The diagnosis of diabetes mellitus is based on finding a blood-sugar level that is excessively high for an unduly prolonged period of time after the administration of the test dose. Whereas the fasting blood-sugar level may be perfectly normal (70 to 100 mg. per cent), in diabetic subjects, the peak value usually exceeds 190 mg. per cent; moreover, the glucose concentration does not return to normal levels within a period of 2 hours, as is the case with patients who do not have diabetes mellitus.

Gastrointestinal Absorption Tests

D-Xylose Tolerance Test. The fasting patient receives by mouth 25 Gm. of D-xylose dissolved in 500 ml. of water. All urine specimens voided during the ensuing 5-hour period are collected and analyzed for D-xylose. The normal individual excretes between 5 to 6 Gm. of the pentose during the test period; lower values are consistent with impaired absorption. The excretion of from 1 to 2 Gm. is typical of sprue.

Vitamin A Tolerance Test. The fasting subject ingests 5 ml. of percomorph liver oil containing 300,000 international units of vitamin A. Blood samples for vitamin A analysis are collected prior to the test dose and 5 to 7 hours thereafter. Normal individuals exhibit levels of from 200 to 250 micrograms of the vitamin per 100 ml. of serum in the postprandial specimens, representing a fourfold to fivefold increase over the fasting level. In malabsorption cases, concentrations of less than 100 micrograms, i.e., no more than a twofold increase, are reported.

Butter Fat Tolerance Test. The fasting patient receives a breakfast meal which includes 30 Gm. of butter. A fasting blood specimen and 5 postprandial samples of clotted blood are collected at hourly intervals. Serum from each sample is compared quantitatively with the fasting serum with respect to turbidity, the degree of turbidity, as measured, reflecting the concentration of fat droplets in suspension. Normal individuals usu-

ally exhibit a peak concentration of serum fat (lipemia) 3 hours following the test meal, followed by a sharp decline in fat concentration. Patients with malabsorption defects fail to attain comparable degrees of lipemia and may exhibit no peak whatever in the concentration of blood fat throughout the 5-hour period of observation.

Liver Function Tests

Galactose Clearance Test. This procedure measures the ability of the liver to metabolize carbohydrates. It involves the intravenous injection of galactose in a dose of 0.5 Gm. per kilogram of body weight. Venous samples obtained before and 75 minutes following the injection are analyzed for galactose concentration. No galactose remains in the blood of normal subjects after 75 minutes. Patients with "retention" or "obstructive" jaundice show values of 20 mg. or less of galactose per 100 ml., whereas, in the presence of hepatic insufficiency and "hepatocellular" jaundice, between 20 and 80 mg. per 100 ml. may remain in the blood at the conclusion of this test period.

Hippuric Acid Conversion Test. This test permits an evaluation of another liver function, reflected in the efficiency with which the liver cell makes glycine available and conjugates this amino acid with (and thus "detoxifies") benzoic acid. The quantity of benzoic acid conjugated is determined from the amount of conjugate, i.e., hippuric acid, which appears in the urine. The fasting patient receives 6 Gm. of sodium benzoate dissolved in 250 ml. of water, or an intravenous injection of a 20-ml. sterile aqueous solution containing 1.77 Gm. of this material. In the oral test, urine is collected over a period of 4 hours, during which time a normal individual will excrete an amount of hippuric acid that is equivalent to approximately 3 Gm. of benzoic acid, the normal range being 2.50 to 3.25 Gm. Following the intravenous test dose, the hippuric acid excreted in 1 hour should represent between 0.70 to 0.95 Gm. of benzoic acid. In patients who are jaundiced due to biliary obstruction, normal excretion values are obtained, whereas in hepatocellular jaundice, as in acute hepatitis, a lesser amount is excreted.

Bromsulphalein (BSP) Test. This test is

useful for the detection of minimal and early functional impairment of the liver, especially in patients who are free of jaundice. The test dye, phenol-tetrabromphthalein (Bromsulphalein), is cleared from the blood stream after injection, due to the activity of parenchymal liver cells which extract it from the plasma and excrete it into the bile. The substance is then conveyed via the biliary duct system into the intestinal tract and is eliminated in the stool. The rate with which it is cleared from the blood is determined by a combination of factors, which include, in addition to the functional efficiency of the liver cells, the rate of blood flow through the liver and the presence or the absence, or the degree, of biliary tract obstruction. Five mg. of dye per kilogram of the patient's body weight are injected intravenously, and 45 minutes thereafter a sample of clotted venous blood is collected, which is examined colorimetrically for its Bromsulphalein content. The presence of less than 5 per cent of the injected dose in the 45-minute sample represents normal liver function.

The nurse should be aware of the fact that febrile reactions, although uncommon, have been observed following the injection of BSP dye. Rare instances of sensitization have also been described, manifested by the production of urticaria after subsequent injections of the material. She should also be familiar with the tendency of this dye to discolor the urine and the stools which, if alkaline, may turn red during the day of the test. The skin likewise may exhibit a transient local redness on contact with an alkaline soap, if such contact occurs within a period of an hour following the test injection, or longer, in the event of abnormal dye retention. The patient will not be alarmed by such phenomena if informed of these possibilities in advance.

Renal Function Tests

Clearance tests of great value in the study of renal physiology and the detection of renal pathology include the urea clearance test, which involves serial measurements of blood and urine urea, and clearance tests which entail the intravenous injection of inulin and para-aminohippurate.

Urea Clearance Test. To determine urea clearance, the urea nitrogen in the blood (removed from a vein 14 hours after the last meal) is determined. At the same time that this specimen of blood is obtained, the patient completely empties his bladder and discards this specimen. All the urine secreted during the next hour is carefully collected, and the amount of urea it contains is determined. This figure, divided by 60, is the exact amount of urea excreted per minute. From the above figures may be calculated the number of cubic centimeters of circulating blood which the kidneys are clearing of urea each minute of time. In the case of the normal person, whose kidneys secrete 2 ml. or less of urine per minute, the volume of blood cleared of urea would be at least 54 ml., and if over 2 ml. of urine per minute, at least 75 ml.

Para-aminohippurate (PAH) and Inulin Clearance Tests. If, at measured intervals of time following the intravenous injection of a given material, its concentrations in the urine and in the plasma are determined repeatedly, data are obtained from which its clearance rate can be calculated. Clearance tests which provide data of great value in studies of renal physiology and pathology are those employing inulin and para-aminohippurate (PAH), especially when these are performed simultaneously and in combination with a glucose "load test."

The clearance of PAH from the blood stream is practically complete as a result of one circulation through the kidney (partially through glomerular filtration and the remainder by tubular excretion); the clearance rate of this material provides, therefore, a measure of the total renal blood flow. Inulin, on the other hand, although filtered across the glomerular membrane, is neither excreted by the tubular cells nor reabsorbed; its clearance rate, therefore, is believed to represent the glomerular filtration rate (normally about 130 ml. per minute). Glucose is both filtered and reabsorbed; if its concentration in the blood is increased by injection to the point of causing glycosuria, at this level the capacity for its reabsorption by the tubules obviously has been exceeded, and if its clearance rate is determined at that level, together with a measurement of the filtration rate (PAH clearance), the maximum rate of tubular reabsorption can be calculated. This value, normally 300 to 400 mg. per minute, is referred to as the "tubular absorptive mass" (or glucose Tm). Finally, if a similar "load clearance" is performed with PAH instead of glucose, thereby stimulating the proximal tubules to excrete at a maximum rate, and if the filtration rate is known, one has a measure of the total excretory capacity of the tubules, namely, the "tubular excretory mass."

Congo Red Clearance Test

This test is designed specifically for the detection of amyloidosis, its basis being the affinity of amyloid tissue for Congo red dye, which surpasses that of normal tissue. This dye, 0.25 ml., is injected intravenously in a concentration of 1.2 Gm. per cent. Five, and again 65, minutes following injection, clotted venous samples are obtained and the concentration of the dye measured in each. Results are expressed in terms of the percentage of original dye remaining in the 65-minute sample, computed from the ratio of concentrations in the two samples, the 5-minute sample providing the "100 per cent" value. In normal individuals it should be possible to demonstrate between 70 and 90 per cent of the injected dose in the second sample. Values between 40 and 60 per cent are suggestive of, and values of less than 40 per cent are characteristic of, amyloidosis. Patients with marked proteinuria may excrete appreciable quantities of dye in the urine during the period of the test, with the result that the 65-minute concentration will be falsely low and possibly even suggestive of amyloidosis. On this account, all urine voided during the test should be saved for inspection in the event of an abnormal finding in the second sample, for this result may be validated and interpreted correctly in the presence of proteinuria only if the possibility of dye loss in the urine has been excluded.

HEMATOLOGY: EXAMINATION OF THE FORMED BLOOD ELEMENTS AND EVALUATION OF HEMOSTASIS

The formed elements of the blood include red cells (erythrocytes), white cells (leukocytes) and platelets (thrombocytes). The red cells, the platelets and the granulocytes (comprising approximately two thirds of the leukocytes) are bone marrow products. The remaining leukocytes, consisting of lymphocytes, monocytes and plasma cells, originate in lymph nodes, spleen and liver, as well as marrow. The characteristics of the formed blood elements constitute an important criterion of health, and cytologic changes in the peripheral blood furnish valuable diagnostic clues in many diseases. Laboratory tests for the detection, the measurement and the elucidation of these phenomena are summarized below. This is the area of "morphologic hematology."

Blood Cell Counts
Red Cell Counts (RBC)

The concentration of red cells in the circulating blood determines the presence or the absence of anemia or polycythemia, which are discussed in Chapter 25. Red cell counts are also necessary for calculating the red cell "indices" (see p. 89), which express mathematically the average size and the hemoglobin content of the red cell. The normal red cell count varies from approximately 4.5 to 5.5 million per cu. mm. of blood. The cells may be counted visually in a blood sample which has been diluted 1/200, placed in a hemocytometer chamber and examined under a microscope.

Leukocyte Counts (WBC)

Leukocytes, or "white blood cells," may be counted visually in a manner similar to that described for red cells. Unclotted whole blood is diluted 1:20 with a solution which destroys and eliminates from view the red cells (which outnumber the leukocytes 1,000 to 1). The suspension is then placed in a hemocytometer chamber and examined microscopically. The use of semiautomatic metering devices and electronic cell counters, because of their relative convenience and greater accuracy, is gradually supplanting the traditional red cell and white cell count in clinical laboratories.

Leukocytes normally are present in a concentration of between 5,000 to 10,000 cells per cu. mm. of whole blood. When the white cell count is over 10,000, the condition is called a *leukocytosis;* when it is below 5,000,

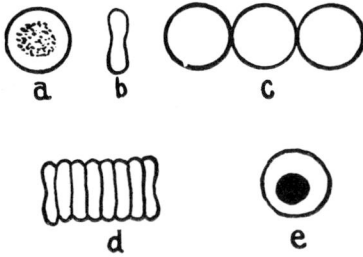

FIG. 22. Red blood cells (× 1,000). (a) The flat surface of one cell; the shadow in the center is evidence of its biconcavity. (b) One cell seen from the edge. (c) Three cells lying flat, their edges touching. (d) Several cells in a rouleau, or piled like coins. (e) A normoblast, or nucleated red blood cell.

a *leukopenia.* Inflammations anywhere in the body and diseases with abscess formation often cause a rise in the count, due to an increase in the polymorphonuclear leukocytes. In pneumonia, for example, the leukocyte count may be as high as 10,000 or more per cu. mm. In certain infections, e. g., typhoid fever, the white cells may fail to increase, and actually may become reduced in number. Not only the total count but also the relative count of these diverse varieties of leukocytes is an important aid in diagnosis.

Differential Leukocyte Counts

Leukocytes produced in the marrow, i.e., the "myeloid series," comprise about 70 per cent of all the white cells and are termed *granulocytes,* because of the abundant granules contained in their cytoplasm, or *polymorphonuclear leukocytes,* since their nuclei, when mature, are of a highly irregular configuration. The adult granulocyte containing a lobulated nucleus, the lobes of which are connected by a filament (a threadlike structure), is a "segmented" granulocyte. If the connecting structure is thicker than a thread, the cell is a "band form"; if lobulation is present but scarcely evident, it is classed as a "metamyelocyte"; if the nucleus is round or oval, a "myelocyte." The "promyelocyte," its precursor, has just begun to show granu-

lation, and the most primitive cell of this series, the "myeloblast," is neither granulated nor lobulated. Granulocytes are subdivided further according to their staining characteristics; thus, if the granules are stained by a neutral dye, it is a "neutrophil"; with an eosin dye, an "eosinophil"; with a basic dye, a "basophil." The neutrophils normally comprise about 70 per cent of all leukocytes, the eosinophils, from 2 to 4 per cent, and the basophils, only about 0.5 per cent. Eosinophilia is of great help in the diagnosis of infections by animal parasites, especially trichinosis which results from eating infected pork. The same cells, however, are increased in any parasitic infection and also in asthma and various other allergic conditions.

Lymphocytes, most numerous of the "mononuclear" cells, comprise about 25 per cent of the circulating white cells. *Monocytes,* largest of the leukocytes, account for about 5 per cent of the white count. *Plasmacytes,* distinguished from lymphocytes by their round, eccentric nuclei, normally represent less than 1 per cent of the leukocyte population.

Differential counts are carried out on stained smears of "capillary" blood obtained by finger or ear-lobe puncture or venous blood from the lumen of a hypodermic needle immediately following a venipuncture. The count represents the number of cells of each type that are encountered on a systematic scan of an area containing 100 or more leukocytes. Literally dozens of characteristic "blood pictures" have been delineated by means of differential cell counting, with the result that any deviation from the normal leukocyte destruction pattern is diagnostically important.

Platelet Counts

Blood platelets, or thrombocytes, smallest of the formed blood elements, are produced in the bone marrow by giant cells called *megakaryocytes.* There are approximately 250,000 to 400,000 platelets per cu. mm. of normal blood. An increased number (thrombocytosis) is characteristic of myeloproliferative disorders such as myelogenous leukemia and polycythemia vera. Platelets play a key role in the prevention of bleeding (hemostasis) and will be discussed later in this chapter. Platelet deficiency (thrombocytopenia) is responsible for an important hemorrhagic disorder called "thrombocytopenia purpura."

Morphologic Examination of Blood Smears and Suspensions

Rouleau Formation

The degree to which red cells tend to aggregate in rouleaux is an important observation in the blood smear. This phenomenon, as described previously, is responsible for increasing the rate of red cell sedimentation and is important as a clue to an abnormality in the distribution of plasma proteins. (A characteristic rouleau is illustrated in Fig. 22.)

Polychromatophilia, Reticulocytosis and Erythroblastosis

The rate of red cell production can be estimated from the relative proportions of immature and mature red cells in the peripheral blood. Young erythrocytes are distinguished in the smear by their size, which is 25 to 50 per cent greater than the mature cell, and by their staining properties, appearing grayish-blue in Wright-stained preparations as opposed to the reddish-brown hue typical of older cells. The term "polychromatophilia" refers to this characteristic color. Preliminary treatment of wet blood samples with brilliant cresyl blue dye (i.e., supravital staining) reveals the polychromatophil to be a "reticulocyte," so-called because of the presence of a bluish network, and, as such, it is identified as an erythrocyte which has been released from the marrow within a period of from 24 to 36 hours. The number of reticulocytes in relation to the total red count is reported as the "reticulocyte count." Counts of between 0.5 and 1.0 per cent of the total red-cell count are normal in a nonanemic individual. Since the normal response to anemia is an increase in the rapidity of red cell production (erythropoiesis), the onset of anemia should provoke a rise in the number of reticulocytes (reticulocytosis) corresponding to the degree of anemia. If the number of reticulocytes falls short of the expected value, the functional efficiency of the marrow is assumed to be faulty. Thus, the reticulocyte count is a valuable aid in the diagnosis of anemia, from the standpoint of differentiating anemias which are attributable to marrow failure from those due to hemorrhage or hemolysis.

Erythroblasts are young red cells which have not yet lost their nuclei and normally do not appear in the peripheral blood. However, in association with intense erythropoiesis, this degree of red cell immaturity may be encountered, a situation termed "erythroblastosis." The observation is customarily reported in terms of the "number of nucleated red cells per 100 leukocytes."

Defects in Red Cell Morphology

Many changes in red cell morphology are characteristic of specific disorders. Abnormally large cells are known as "macrocytes"; macrocytosis implies that the average size of red cells is increased. "Microcytes" and "microcytosis" indicate a reduction in red cell size. The term "anisocytosis" indicates an abnormal variation in the size of individual red cells. "Poikilocytosis" refers to irregularities and variations in the shape of red cells. "Hypochromia" denotes a decrease in red cell coloration reflecting a deficient hemoglobin content. The presence of "target cells" reflects an extreme degree of hypochromia, such cells containing only a rim of hemoglobin in the periphery and a small pocket in the center. "Spherocytes," as the name implies, are spheroidal in shape, small in diameter and densely colored.

Abnormal Red Cell Inclusions

Cells with abnormal inclusions that are detected on smear examination include *stippled cells,* which are dotted with stained nuclear remnants. Other nuclear inclusions may take the form of spherical blue granules (Howell-Jolly bodies) or blue rings and convolutions (Cabot rings). Such changes are indicative of abnormalities in red cell maturation. Intracellular parasites are demonstrable in cases of malaria (see p. 1126) and in cases of Oroya fever. *Heinz bodies,* visible as refractile or light blue dots in red cell suspensions and supravitally stained blood smears, appear in association with certain toxic hemolytic anemias. *"Siderocytes"* are granules of iron pigment which are demonstrable by the Prussian blue reaction in the red cells of patients with a rare hemolytic disease, congenital nonspherocytic hemolytic anemia.

Leukocyte Morphology

The sex of an individual can be ascertained from inspection of the adult polymorphonuclear leukocyte, the nucleus of which, in the case of women, exhibits a tiny, drumstick shaped projection, or lobule. The appearance of heavy granules in polymorphonuclear leukocytes and monocytes, referred to as "toxic granulation," is often associated with sepsis. Abnormally large granulocytes with nuclei that are excessively lobulated suggest B_{12} or folic acid deficiency.

Platelet Morphology

A judgment as to the adequacy of the platelet concentration can be made on smear examination. General enlargement of platelets indicates immaturity of the platelet population as a whole, i.e., enhanced platelet production. The presence of giant platelets or megakaryocytic fragments points to a fundamental derangement of marrow function due, for example, to a malignant growth. It is characteristic also of extramedullary hematopoiesis, i.e., the production of myeloid elements in tissue other than marrow, as in cases of myeloid metaplasia of the spleen.

Hemoglobinometry and Tests for Abnormal Hemoglobins

Hemoglobin is measured to establish the presence or the absence of anemia or polycythemia. A value less than 14 Gm. per 100 ml. in a woman or 15 Gm. per 100 ml. in a man represents anemia; one above 17 Gm. per cent represents erythremia or polycythemia in either sex. The coloring qualities of this pigment lend themselves to precise colorimetric measurement. The standard device for hemoglobin measurement is the spectrophotometer, which may be used to determine the optical density of hemoglobin.

Plasma Hemoglobin

Blood collected with care to avoid artifactitious hemolysis generally contains less than 5 mg. of hemoglobin per 100 ml. of plasma,

i.e., far less than the amount required to produce visible discoloration. Values in excess of 20 mg. per 100 ml. denote hemoglobinemia, an indication of intravascular hemolysis. Quantitative measurement of plasma hemoglobin concentration are generally based on the plasma benzidine reaction. Samples for these determinations require venous blood without trauma or stasis, employing a syringe which has been moistened with sterile isotonic saline and introduced into a test tube containing sodium citrate solution.

Methemoglobin and Sulfhemoglobin

These hemoglobin derivatives are encountered in certain toxic states which follow exposure to oxidizing agents. Chronic methemoglobinemia is a manifestation of a hereditary metabolic defect based on the absence of an enzyme system which normally maintains the iron moiety of hemoglobin in a reduced bivalent state.

Fetal Hemoglobin

This differs chemically and functionally from normal adult hemoglobin and is a normal constituent of fetal blood, adult hemoglobin making its first appearance after birth. Normal blood may contain a minute proportion of fetal hemoglobin. However, amounts in excess of 2 to 3 per cent of the total hemoglobin concentration are characteristic of a hereditary hemolytic disease, i.e., thalassemia. Fetal hemoglobin can be measured on the basis of its increased resistance to conversion into alkaline hematin by alkali, the basis for the "alkali denaturation test."

Hemoglobin Electrophoresis

The migration of hemoglobin in an electric field distinguishes several varieties of human hemoglobin. Electrophoretic analysis of hemoglobin has become an important hematologic procedure by virtue of the fact that several of these varieties are associated with hereditary disorders, referred to as the "hemoglobinopathies." Nine different types of hemoglobin that are of pathologic significance have been recognized to date. One of these (hemoglobin S) is the hallmark of sickle cell anemia, or "sicklemia" (see p. 468). Normal adult hemoglobin is labeled "A." Fetal hemoglobin, present in thalassemia, is designated "F." Hemoglobins C, D, E and F migrate more slowly, and hemoglobins H, I and J faster, than hemoglobin A. Mixed defects, most commonly involving hemoglobins C and S and C and F are occasionally encountered. The clinical features of these disorders are described in Chapter 25.

Sickle Cell Test

A morphologic test for hemoglobin S disease is based on the appearance of a reversible deformity, red cells containing S hemoglobin adopting the contour of a sickle when deprived of oxygen by the addition of a chemical reducing agent. A common method of testing for hemoglobin S involves the microscopic examination of a dilute red-cell suspension after adding sodium metabisulfite solution. Within a period of 15 minutes, if the test is positive, these cells will have acquired the characteristic crescentic shape.

Hematocrit Readings and Red Cell Indices

The volume occupied by red cells, white cells and platelets in a blood sample, measured in the aggregate and computed as per cent of the total volume, is defined as the "cellcritt." The term "hematocrit" refers specifically to the percentage of the total volume that is contributed by the red cells. The hematocrit reading serves as a precise measure of red cell production relative to red cell loss through hemolysis or hemorrhage. Moreover, it supplies a numerical value which is required for the calculation of three important "indices" of red cell morphology, discussed below. The Wintrobe procedure is as follows:

Blood samples for hematocrit readings are collected with an anticoagulant that causes neither swelling nor shrinking of the red cells, most commonly a mixture of potassium and ammonium oxalate salts. An aliquot sample of the unclotted blood is placed in a cylindrical tube on which is etched a 10 cm. scale graduated in millimeters. The specimen then is rotated in a centrifuge until the cell mass is thoroughly packed. The column of packed red cells and the total sample are measured with reference to the scale. The ratio between the two measurements $\times$ 100 represents the hematocrit reading, expressed in volumes per cent.

The microhematocrit technic employs a glass capillary tube containing a trace of dried heparin as an anticoagulant. This is filled to two-thirds capacity with a drop of capillary blood, plugged at one end with clay, rotated at high speed (approximately 14,000 rpm) for 5 minutes then examined with a device that permits ready calculation of the percentile red-cell mass. Although slightly greater accuracy is achieved by the Wintrobe method, this advantage is more than offset by the relative rapidity with which the microhematocrit reading can be obtained and by the fact that the latter dispenses with the need for venous samples.

The "red-cell indices" are computed on the basis of the red-cell count, the hemoglobin concentration and the hematocrit reading. The *mean corpuscular volume* (MCV) specifies, in cubic microns, the average red-cell size. The *mean corpuscular hemoglobin concentration* (MCHC), expressed in per cent, represents the concentration of hemoglobin in the red-cell mass, i.e., grams of hemoglobin per 100 ml. packed red cells. The *mean corpuscular hemoglobin* (MCH) refers to the average amount of hemoglobin, expressed in micromicrograms, that is contained in the individual red cell.

Based on the red cell indices, anemias can be classified as normocytic, microcytic or macrocytic, and as normochromic, hypochromic or hyperchromic (i.e., spherocytic). This morphologic classification is the first step in the diagnosis of any anemia. A mean corpuscular volume with the range of 82 to 92 cubic micra is normal; the red cells in such a sample, on the average, are "normocytic." Values below 82 cubic micra indicate microcytosis; over 92 they indicate macrocytosis. Mean corpuscular hemoglobin concentrations below 32 per cent signify hypochromia, i.e., less than the normal amount of hemoglobin in proportion to the volume of the average red cell, whereas an MCHC greater than 36 per cent is an expression of spherocytosis. A mean corpuscular hemoglobin content of 27 micromicrograms or less is abnormally small, characterizing the red cell population as hypochromic, microcytic, or both.

Hemolytic Tests

Specific types of hemolytic anemia are identified on the basis of one or more of the following tests.

Erythrocyte Osmotic Fragility Test

This procedure demonstrates the presence or the absence of spherocytosis, on the one hand, or hypochromia, on the other. Small aliquot samples of unclotted blood are placed in a series of test tubes containing salt solutions of graded tonicity, varying from 0.85 Gm. per 100 ml. (isotonic) to zero (distilled water), and the degree of hemolysis in that sample is estimated from visual inspection or is measured colorimetrically. Normal blood exhibits slight hemolysis when the tonicity is reduced to a level of approximately 0.5 Gm. NaCl/100ml., and most, if not all, of the red cells hemolyze at levels below 0.25 Gm. per cent NaCl. Spherocytes of the type encountered in hereditary spherocytosis (see p. 467) hemolyze at tonicities above 0.6 or 0.7 per cent saline. If osmotic hemolysis does not appear excepting in very hypotonic suspensions, e.g., at tonicity levels below 0.4 Gm. per cent salt, the red cells are presumably hypochromic, since they can accommodate a relatively large volume of fluid in addition to their original contents.

Antiglobulin (Coombs) Test

The red cells of certain patients are characterized by the presence of a globulin coating on their membrane. Demonstration of such a coating by the Coombs test is a diagnostic feature of erythroblastosis fetalis (p. 466) and of acquired hemolytic jaundice (p. 467). This demonstration depends on the agglutinating effect of antiglobulin serum (rabbit serum containing antibodies that are specific for human globulins) when this reagent is added to a suspension of saline-washed globulin-coated erythrocytes. The "indirect Coombs test" is employed for the detection, or identification, of red cell antibodies that may be present in a sample of plasma or serum. Red cells from a blood donor, for example, may be incubated with plasma from a prospective transfusion recipient. After incubation, the cells are washed and exposed to Coombs serum, as just described. If the test is positive and agglutina-tion occurs, the cells are considered to have acquired a globulin coating during incubation, comprised, it is assumed, of antibodies that were contained in the patient's plasma and were specific for the donor's red cells. Accordingly, the donor and the recipient are proved to be incompatible.

Auto-agglutinins and Hemolysins

Globulin-coated (Coombs positive) erythrocytes tend to agglutinate spontaneously when suspended in protein-containing media such as plasma. This phenomenon is the basis of auto-agglutination tests of several varieties, having the same basic significance as the antiglobulin test. *"Cold agglutinins"* represent a special type of antibody which attach themselves to red cells and cause them to agglutinate only at low temperatures. One particular hemolytic disorder called "paroxysmal hemoglobinuria" is marked by the presence of a *"cold hemolysin"* in the patient's serum, the latter hemolyzing red cells in mixtures containing complement after preliminary chilling and rewarming. The *"acid hemolysin"* test demonstrates the hemolysis of abnormal red cells from patients with paroxysmal nocturnal hemoglobinuria when suspensions of these cells are acidified and incubated in normal serum.

Blood Volume Measurements

Quantitative measurement of the circulating red cell mass occasionally is indispensable for distinguishing oligemic shock from other types of vascular collapse and for establishing a diagnosis of polycythemia vera, as opposed to other forms of erythremia. The red cell volume may be determined by reinjecting a measured sample of the the patient's own red cells after these have been labeled in vitro with radioactive chromium (Cr^{51}) (see p. 108). The radioactivity of the patient's circulating red cells after injection, relative to the radioactivity of the tagged sample, is inversely proportional to the ratio between the patient's total circulating red cell mass and the volume of injected cells. Another method of estimating the red cell mass is based on measurements of the circulating plasma volume and the plasmatocrit. The plasma volume may be computed either from measurements of plasma radioactivity following the injection of a measured sample of human albumin labeled with radioiodine (I^{131}), or from the relative color densities of the patient's plasma and a sample of Evans blue dye (T-1824) following the intravenous injection of a measured quantity of that dye.

Bone Marrow Biopsy

Practically every disorder that affects the formed blood elements is attended by changes in the bone marrow, whence most of the blood cells originate. A specific and diagnostic marrow picture is associated with a great many diseases, including the leukemias and certain other reticuloendothelial disorders; certain deficiency states, including vitamin B_{12}, folic acid, iron and pyridoxine deficiency; toxic states producing marrow depression or destruction; and neoplastic diseases in which the marrow is invaded by tumor cells.

Various sites are suitable for marrow biopsy, and a variety of technics are applicable for this purpose. By far the most commonly selected is the needle aspiration biopsy, the most frequent puncture sites including the sternum at the approximate level of the second rib interspace, the manubrium and the crest of the ilium. The items which the nurse is responsible for having in readiness include materials for shaving (if necessary), cleansing, anesthetizing and perforating the skin. These include soap solution; safety razor; procaine solution (1 or 2 per cent); an assortment of sterile hypodermic needles, gauges No. 23 to 25; sterile 5- and 10-ml. syringes; sterile Bard-Parker blades (No. 11); sterile 2- and 4-inch gauze squares; sterile gauze applicators; and adhesive tape. The rest of the equipment, including the aspiration needle and the trocar, is usually supplied by the operator. The skin at the projected site having been shaved, if necessary, cleansed and sterilized, then anesthetized with procaine and lacerated with the tip of a scalpel blade, a 12- to 16-gauge needle fitted with stylet is introduced through the periosteum and the bony cortex into the marrow cavity. The stylet is removed from the needle, a syringe is attached, and marrow fluid is aspirated. In the event that adequate marrow samples are not obtained by the aspiration method in a particular case, a surgical trephine biopsy may be required.

Bleeding and Clotting Tests

The avoidance of spontaneous or excessive bleeding depends to a large extent on the integrity of the blood vessel walls, i.e., their resistance to rupture in the face of an elevated pressure level within their lumina and their capacity to constrict in response to trauma, for example, when lacerated or bruised.

The major factor in the control of bleeding from vessels larger than capillaries is the clotting of blood inside and outside of the injured vessel. The formation of a blood clot represents the culmination of a series of enzymatic reactions in which a number of blood components are involved. The final stage of this series is the aggregation of fibrinogen molecules into an insoluble protein, *fibrin,* which forms an intricate network of fibers and causes the plasma to gel. The precipitation of fibrin from fibrinogen is attributable to the action of a proteolytic enzyme called *thrombin* which is evolved from an inactive precursor, *prothrombin.* Prothrombin, in turn, is converted into active thrombin through the agency of yet another substance, *thromboplastin.* Prothrombin conversion requires also the presence of ionized calcium, and the reaction is enhanced by three accelerator substances in the plasma, designated numerically as Factors V, VII and X.

Thromboplastin itself is not a regular constituent of the blood. It appears there only under certain circumstances, its formation requiring the participation of a factor that is not ordinarily free and available in the plasma, but confined within the platelets: namely, platelet factor 3. This substance, released into the blood from ruptured platelets, initiates the entire clotting reaction. Also required for the production of thromboplastin are several plasma components, key among which are *antihemophilic globulin* (Factor VIII), *plasma thromboplastin component* (Factor IX), *Stuart factor* (Factor X) and ionized calcium.

Many disorders are marked by episodes of spontaneous bleeding or are responsible for prolonged and excessive bleeding following vascular injury. The recognition of hemorrhagic tendencies in susceptible individuals who are candidates for surgery and the effective control of any hemorrhage in "bleeders" requires in every instance a correct analysis of the defect in hemostasis, based on a series of laboratory tests. The clinical aspects of these hemorrhagic disorders are discussed in Chapter 25. The laboratory tests on which their diagnoses depend are summarized below.

Capillary Fragility Tests

Capillary stamina, or resistance to trauma, is tested by means of the tourniquet test (Rumpel-Leeds test) which involves placing a sphygmomanometer cuff on one arm, inflating this to the standard pressure of 100 mm. of mercury, or to a point midway between the systolic and diastolic pressures. After a given period of time, e.g., 5 or 10 minutes, the pressure is released and the forearm observed for the presence and the number of minute hemorrhages called "petechiae." This count is made 5 or 10 minutes after the release of the tourniquet in a circumscribed area 1 inch below the anticubital fold measuring 1 square inch. The appearance of less than 5 petechiae following 5 minutes of stasis, or less than 10 petechiae after 10 minutes of application of a tourniquet, is considered to be normal. Another type of vascular fragility test employs a simple suction device ("petechiometer") which is applied to the forearm and exposes 1 square inch of skin to a standard low-level pressure. The number of petechiae is increased in cases of platelet deficiency and in scurvy (p. 153). The test also may be positive in arterial hypertension, not as a reflection of inadequate vascular or platelet defenses, but as a result of an increase in capillary blood pressure which becomes excessive after removal of the tourniquet.

Bleeding Time

The duration of bleeding from small lacerations has the same significance as the formation of petechiae after tourniquet stasis and pressure elevation within the capillary bed, since it is determined by the contractility of the injured capillaries and by the number of platelets available in the blood to plug these vessels. The standard procedure for measuring bleeding time involves the laceration of an ear lobe (Ivy method) or a forearm (Duke method) with the tip of a Bard-Parker blade or a special lancet, then timing the flow of blood from the wound. If the blood flows for more than 6 minutes, the bleeding time is considered to be abnormally prolonged.

Venous Clotting Time

The time elapsing before the appearance of a clot in a sample of venous blood collected in a standard 19-mm. glass tube and maintained at 37° C. (Lee-White clotting time) should not exceed 6 to 12 minutes. A normal sample collected with equipment that is completely coated with a nonwetting surface may range from 30 to 60 minutes (silicone clotting time), whereas a specimen collected from a skin puncture wound in a glass capillary tube will clot in 2 to 6 minutes. Prolongation of the clotting time beyond the expected value is indicative of thromboplastin deficiency and is characteristic of hemophilia and the hemophilic states (see p. 477). It is also consistent with a heparin effect.

Clot Retraction

The clot that forms in a normal blood sample proceeds to shrink almost at once. The occurrence and the degree of shrinkage are related to the presence and to the number of platelets in the specimen. Retraction is considered to be normal if the volume of the clot, after an interval of 2 hours following collection of the sample, has been reduced to two thirds that of the whole sample or less, or if the amount of serum remaining in the clot itself at that time is less than 15 or 20 per cent of the volume originally present.

Prothrombin Time (Activity)

Measurement of prothrombin activity, as usually performed, involves measuring the speed with which oxalated or citrated plasma clots when ionized calcium is added, together with an excess of active thromboplastin. The time interval elapsing between the addition of the latter and the appearance of a clot is normally about 12 to 14 seconds. If clotting is delayed it may be concluded that either prothrombin, one of the prothrombin conversion accelerators (Factor V, VII or X) or some combination of these is lacking. If the result is normal it follows that all four components of the prothrombin complex are present in normal amounts. If a clotting defect is discovered, an attempt is made to discover which component is involved by determining which of the following materials, added to the patient's plasma, restores its prothrombin activity to normal: normal oxalated plasma, aged in storage (containing prothrombin); fresh normal plasma, absorbed with barium sulfate (Factor V); and normal serum, aged in storage (Factor VII or X). A reduction in prothrombin activity that is restored by the addition of stored serum could represent a deficiency, either of Factor VII or Factor X. These two defects can be distinguished, however, since the latter is involved also in the production of thromboplastin, so that patients with Factor X deficiency (in contrast to Factor VII deficiency) exhibit, not only a low level of prothrombin activity, but also a prolonged venous clotting time, reduced prothrombin consumption and an abnormal thromboplastin generation test.

Prothrombin Consumption

The clotting process uses up most of the prothrombin that is present in a sample of normal blood, less than 10 or 20 per cent of the original prothrombin activity being demonstrable in the serum 1 hour after clotting has begun. In cases of thromboplastin deficiency, for example, in partially treated hemophilia, clotting may commence within the normal time span, but the amount of prothrombin consumed is considerably less than expected. This is the basis for the so-called *prothrombin consumption* test which is one of the most useful criteria of thromboplastin activity.

Thromboplastin Generation

As indicated earlier, four blood constituents are required for the normal production of thromboplastin: namely, Factor VIII (antihemophilic globulin), Factor IX (plasma thromboplastin component), Factor X (Stuart factor), and a substance contained in platelets (platelet factor 3). A defect involving one or more of these factors may result in abnormal bleeding, prolongation of the venous clotting time and other signs of thromboplastin deficiency. Effective therapy, in such a case, depends on a precise diagnosis. To this end a thromboplastin generation test may be carried out as a means of evaluating each component. A mixture is prepared that includes the following: fresh, normal, aluminum hydroxide absorbed plasma (containing Factor VIII, but not IX or X); fresh normal serum (containing Factors IX and X, but not VIII); and normal platelets. Every substance needed for the evolution of thromboplastin is present in this mixture save calcium, which remains to be added. On the other hand, prothrombin is missing, so little or no substrate is present with which thromboplastin, as it evolves, can react, become bound, inactivated or otherwise unavailable for measurement. Thromboplastin generation commences at the moment calcium chloride is added to the reaction mixture. At 1-minute intervals thereafter the mixture is sampled and tested for thromboplastic activity by measuring the speed with which clotting occurs when a sample of the mixture is added to a sample of normal recalcified plasma. A mixture such as this, comprised exclusively of normal components, is expected to generate, within a period of 6 minutes or less, sufficient thromboplastin to clot normal recalcified plasma in 8 to 14 seconds.

Four additional reaction mixtures are prepared and tested in the same manner: one that contains the patient's plasma; another, the patient's serum; and a third, his platelets (in place of normal plasma, serum and platelets, respectively). In the fourth mixture all three components are derived from the patient's blood. If thromboplastin is generated normally in this preparation, all thromboplastin components are normal; if not, one of the other mixtures will prove to be abnormal. If it is the one containing patient's plasma, he is demonstrated to have Factor VIII deficiency, i.e., hemophilia. Abnormal thromboplastin generation in the mixture containing the patient's serum could result from a deficiency of either Factor IX or Factor X; if the latter, his plasma prothrombin activity likewise is abnormal, since Factor X is required for normal prothrombin conversion as well as thromboplastin generation. Thus, by exclusion, a normal prothrombin activity test would characterize this patient as a case of Factor IX deficiency, or "Hemophilia B."

Estimation of Fibrinogen

Fibrinogen deficiency is excluded if the clot appears to be normal with respect to firmness and integrity, especially if these qualities are maintained for several hours at 37° C. The actual concentration of fibrinogen in the plasma can be determined, if indicated, by measuring the protein contained in the clot formed in a standard volume of plasma after the addition of thrombin.

MEASUREMENTS OF CARDIAC AND PULMONARY FUNCTION

Almost all components of the circulatory and respiratory systems are susceptible to precise evaluation, both structural and functional. Some of the most informative of the tests that are applicable to these systems are those that are carried out as part of every routine physical examination, namely, those described in Chapter 5. However, for definite diagnostic confirmation in certain cardiac or pulmonary cases, or for a quantitative estimation of circulatory function or pulmonary efficiency, additional tests may be required. The type of information that can be expected from these tests, and the methods by which these data are obtained, are summarized herewith.

Systemic Venous Pressure

Venous pressure is measured by means of a fluid manometer in direct communication with the lumen of an antecubital vein (or of another vein in the forearm or the hand), the manometer containing a solution of trisodium citrate to prevent clotting, the patient lying recumbent, with his arm free of stasis. The fluid level in the manometer having stabilized, the vertical distance between it and the sternum is measured at the level of the fourth interspace; the vertical distance between the sternum and the back is also measured at that level. The vertical height of the fluid above the sternum plus one third of the distance between sternum and back

(the approximate position of the right atrium) is considered to represent the venous pressure, which normally varies from 40 to 110 mm. of water.

Pulmonary Circulation Time

The pulmonary circulation time, reflecting the speed with which blood flows through the lungs, is measured on the basis of the duration of time elapsing between a rapid injection of Decholin into an antecubital vein and the earliest awareness of a bitter taste, as signaled by the patient. A variant of this test employs an injection of sodium cyanide (0.11 mg. per Kg. of body weight) instead of Decholin, the end-point in this instance being marked by an involuntary gasp by the patient. In either case, one measures the minimum time required for blood to reach the right auricle from the site of injection, enter and traverse the pulmonary circuit, return to the heart via the left auricle, enter the left ventricle, become ejected into the aorta and arrive at the point of detection, i.e., the tongue, via the lingual artery, in patients receiving Decholin, or the carotid body, via the carotid artery, in those receiving cyanide. Normal values range from 16 to 22 seconds.

Vital Capacity

The *vital capacity* represents the maximum volume of air that a person can exhale after inhaling as deeply as possible. It is measured by means of a recording bellows, of which there are numerous varieties. A normal vital capacity for a man is approximately 25 times his height, expressed in centimeters, and for a woman, her height times 20. Since it is influenced by the volume of fluid within the thorax, the vital capacity serves as a criterion with respect to the presence or the absence of excess blood volume in the pulmonary vessels and of edema fluid in the alveoli. The degree to which the pulmonary blood volume is increased and the manner in which this changes in response to therapy have great significance in patients with congestive heart failure, and measurements of the vital capacity are correspondingly important in those patients.

The *expirogram* is a graphic recording of expiration, the volume of expired air being charted automatically in relation to time. The speed at which air can be expelled from the lungs, which is indicated by this means, is dependent on the presence or the absence of obstruction in the bronchioles and the bronchi. Thus, the expirogram is a useful tool for differentiating obstructive emphysema and bronchial asthma from such nonobstructive lesions as pulmonary congestion and edema.

Arterial Oxygen Saturation

Among the laboratory procedures of special interest relative to the cardiovascular and respiratory systems is the determination of arterial oxygen saturation, which is based on gasometric measurements of the oxygen content and the oxygen capacity of arterial blood samples. The degree of saturation, expressed as per cent, is computed from the ratio of oxygen originally contained in the arterial sample to that in an aliquot sample which has been saturated fully with oxygen. Normal samples are observed to be approximately 95 per cent saturated with oxygen. Lower values indicate either a defect in pulmonary ventilation, because of interference with respiratory exchange, or the existence of a vascular communication between the systemic venous circulation (or pulmonary artery) and the systemic arterial circuit which permits blood from the vena cava to bypass the pulmonary circulation and enter the aorta with its oxygen supply unreplenished.

Electrocardiography

The electrocardiogram is a visual representation of the electrical activity of the heart, as reflected by changes in electrical potential at the skin surface, these changes being detected and recorded photographically by an electrocardiograph. Impulses generated within the heart, traveling via the conduction pathways and spreading throughout the myocardium, are depicted in the form of waves which have characteristic patterns and correspond in frequency to specific events in the cardiac cycle. Based on the direction, contour and relative location of 5, or occasionally 6, peaks in each cycle, precise information is obtainable with respect to the origin of the intial impulse, or "pacemaker," the manner of its spread and the

nature of the response throughout the heart. Therefore, precise diagnoses are possible in patients with arrythmia, conduction defects, myocardial damage of various types, including old and recent coronary occlusions, and a number of other disorders as well.

Cardiac Catheterization

Cardiac catheterization involves the passing of a small-lumen tube into the right atrium via the median basilic and subclavian veins and the superior vena cava. This is carried out under direct visualization with a fluoroscope. Pressures within the right atrium are measured and recorded, and blood samples are removed for measurements of the hematocrit and oxygen saturation. The catheter is then passed through the tricuspid valve, and similar tests are performed on the blood within the right ventricle. Finally, the tube is introduced into the pulmonary artery, i.e., through the pulmonic valve, and as far as possible beyond that point, when "capillary" samples will be obtained and "capillary" pressures recorded. Then the catheter is withdrawn.

After having made a continuous recording of the arterial pressure and of the pressures within the right atrium, the right ventricle and the pulmonary capillary bed, and intermittent recordings of the total oxygen consumption, along with measurements of the hematocrit and oxygen capacity of blood specimens as specified, it is possible to compute with accuracy the cardiac output; to estimate the pulmonary blood flow in terms of rate and resistance; to evaluate valve function with respect to all valves; and to evaluate the efficiency of pulmonary ventilation, based on the degree of equilibrium established between pulmonary capillary blood and the air in the alveoli. Most important, an accurate and precise diagnosis is possible with respect to the existence and the location of any shunt between systemic venous and arterial channels permitting the bypassing of the pulmonary circulation.

STOOL EXAMINATION AND GASTRIC ANALYSIS
Examination of the Stool

The basic examination of the stool includes an inspection of the specimen for its amount, consistency and color, and a screening test for melena. Special tests indicated in specific cases may include tests for fecal urobilinogen, fat, nitrogen, parasites, food residues and other substances. The color of stools varies from light to dark brown, depending largely on the urobilin content. (Milk-fed infants pass stools that are golden-yellow in color, due to unchanged bilirubin.) Various foods and medications affect stool color as follows: meat protein produces a dark brown coloration; spinach, a green hue; carrots and beets, red; cocoa, dark red or brown; senna and santonin, a yellowish hue; calomel, green; bismuth, iron and charcoal, black; and barium, a milky-white appearance. Blood in sufficient quantities, if shed into the upper gastrointestinal tract, produces a tarry black color; blood entering the lower portion, or passing rapidly through the gastrointestinal tract, will appear bright or dark red. Even considerable quantities of hemoglobin may fail to produce a distinctive color, in which event it is termed "occult blood." The stools in cases of steatorrhea are generally bulky, greasy, foamy, foul in odor and gray in color with a silvery sheen. The "acholic" stool of the patient with biliary obstruction is light gray or "clay-colored," due to the absence of urobilin.

Mucus or pus may be visible on gross inspection of the stool in cases of chronic ulcerative colitis (p. 623) or other ulcerative lesions of the lower bowel. Patients with constipation, obstipation or fecal impaction may pass small, dry, rocky-hard masses called "scybala." Their passage may traumatize the rectal mucosa sufficiently to cause hemorrhage, in which case these masses are streaked with red blood.

Tests for Melena

Minute quantities of hemoglobin are readily detected in the stool by a number of tests which are based on the benzidine, the gum guaiac or the orthotolidin reaction. The benzidine test involves placing a fragment of stool on filter paper, moistening it with 3 or 4 drops of benzidine base, followed by the same volume of 0.6 per cent hydrogen peroxide. A screening test with gum guaiac is similarly carried out on filter paper, add-ing, in succession, 2 drops of glacial acetic acid, an alcoholic extract of powdered gum guaiac and 3 per cent hydrogen peroxide. The specimen is observed after 1- and 5-minute intervals for the appearance of a blue color. The orthotolidin test, described on page 68, provides a rapid, simple means of detecting blood in stools as well as in urine samples.

Gastric Analysis

Examination of the gastric juice offers means of estimating the secretory activity of the gastric mucosa and of ascertaining the presence or the degree of gastric retention in cases of patients suspected of having pyloric or duodenal obstruction. A diagnosis of pernicious anemia (p. 463) is excluded by the finding of acid, and a diagnosis of gastric carcinoma may be established by the discovery of cancer cells in the gastric juice.

The fasting patient is intubated through a nostril with a Levin duodenal tube, a small rubber tube with catheter tip marked at points 45, 55, 65 and 75 cm. from the distal end. The fasting patient is placed in a sitting position, suitably draped, and given an adequate explanation of the character and the purpose of the procedure that is contemplated. Participation of the patient through active swallowing and control of gagging is essential to the success of intubation. If the tube inadvertently enters the trachea instead of the esophagus, vigorous coughing will ensue and air currents coinciding with inspiration and expiration will be felt at the proximal orifice, the signal for prompt withdrawal and reinsertion of the tube. Passage through the esophagus may be facilitated by having the patient sip small quantities of water. If neither nostril is patent, the Levin tube or the Rehfuss duodenal tube, which is equipped with a small perforated metal bulb at the tip, may be introduced through the mouth. However, the nasal route, unless barred mechanically, is preferred, since it is far less prone to stimulate gagging.

When the second marker of the Levin tube is at the point of entering the nares, the tip of the tube, 55 cm. distant, should be within the stomach. Once in place, the tube is secured to the patient's cheek by means of a small strip of adhesive tape, and the patient is placed in a semireclining position. If he exhibits any tendency to gag, he is instructed to pant gently with his mouth wide open, the effect of which is to minimize contact between the tube and the soft palate. The entire stomach contents are aspirated by gentle suction into a syringe. The color of the specimen is recorded as an indication regarding presence or absence of bile or blood. The presence or the absence of mucus and of food particles is noted. The acidity of the specimen is determined by means of an indicator dye, such as Töpfer's reagent, by indicator paper or by means of a pH meter. Other examinations in special instances may include cytologic study by the Papanicolaou technic for the presence or the absence of carcinoma cells. Tubercle bacilli may be sought by culture technics for guinea pig inoculation. Enzyme analysis of the gastric juice is sometimes indicated.

One of the most important items of information to be gained from gastric analysis relates to the ability of the mucosa to secrete hydrochloric acid. Patients with pernicious anemia secrete no acid, and patients with severe chronic gastritis or gastric cancer secrete little or no acid, whereas patients with peptic ulcer invariably secrete some acid and usually an excess amount of it. If the first sample aspirated from the stomach is found to be neutral or alkaline, 3 additional samples are obtained at 20-minute intervals and tested in similar fashion following the subcutaneous injection of histamine (0.1 ml. of a 0.5 per cent solution of histamine base) or after the intravenous injection of 10 to 20 units of regular insulin. Either of these agents is likely to stimulate maximum production of hydrochloric acid by the gastric mucosa. If, for any reason, the use of these stimulants is contraindicated, a "test meal" may be substituted in the form of 50 ml. of 7 per cent alcohol by mouth.

Tubeless Gastric Analysis. A relatively simple, convenient and reliable method for determining gastric acidity, and one that dispenses with the necessity for gastric intubation, involves the feeding of a blue dye (azure A) and subsequent examination of the urine for the presence or the absence of that dye.

The dye, when ingested, is bound to an insoluble resin from which it is released only in the presence of acid. Combined with the resin, it cannot be absorbed from the gastrointestinal tract; freed from this combination, it is absorbed and is excreted promptly in the urine. Its appearance in the urine therefore serves to indicate that the resin-dye complex has been exposed to acid.

The patient, previously fasting for 8 to 10 hours, receives 0.5 Gm. of caffeine and sodium benzoate with one-half glass of water, or an injection of histamine, to stimulate gastric secretion. One hour later, his bladder having been emptied, he ingests 2.0 Gm. of azure A granules with one-half glass of water. At the end of 2 hours he again empties his bladder, and this specimen together with all urine voided during the interim is pooled and examined for the presence and the amount of azure A.

Of course, this test provides no information except as regards the presence or absence of gastric acidity. Furthermore, its results, if they appear to show no acid, are not necessarily valid in the presence of liver disease or in patients with obstructive lesions of the gastrointestinal or the urinary tract.

EXAMINATION OF THE CEREBROSPINAL FLUID AND OTHER EXTRAVASCULAR FLUIDS

Role of the Nurse

Each of the procedures now to be described, involving a sterile entry into a tissue space or a body cavity and aspiration of its fluid contents, is one in which the nurse participates. It is her responsibility to see to it that sterile equipment and appropriate receptacles will have been made ready. Prior to the procedure the nurse will have prepared the patient for the treatment by supplying the necessary information, instructions and reassurance. During the procedure itself, the nurse will help the patient to maintain the proper posture and observe him closely for evidence of vascular collapse, such as the appearance of pallor, increase in pulse rate or a decline in blood pressure, the latter having been recorded at frequent intervals from the beginning of the procedure. The procedure having been concluded and the patient restored to his original position, recumbent, she will take the responsibility for proper disposal of the equipment and the specimen. The amount collected should be measured and recorded and samples of the fluid, properly labeled, sent to appropriate laboratories for examination of the cellular sediment, its specific gravity, protein concentration and bacterial content.

Lumbar Puncture

For the performance of the lumbar puncture, a long, sterile needle with a stylet is necessary. The procedure may be carried out with the patient sitting upright or lying on his side, knees bent and back flexed to the maximum extent possible. If the patient is unconscious, it is necessary to hold him in this position with back well arched on the edge of the treatment table or bed. A wide board sometimes is slipped between the mattress and the spring to provide more stable support.

Strict aseptic precautions are used. The proper point to penetrate the spinal column is one just on a level with a line connecting the crests of the ilium—although any interspace, if desirable, can be used. The skin at the puncture site is disinfected and anesthetized with procaine. The needle is inserted in the midline between the spinous processes at an angle such as will not strike either spinous process. After the needle has been felt to pierce the dura, the stylet is removed to see if the fluid will flow. If it does not, the chances are that the dura has not actually been pierced but has been pushed to one side. Below the second lumbar vertebra there is no danger of touching the cord, for it does not extend as low as this.

A little fluid (usually not over 5 ml. in all if the tap is solely for diagnostic purposes) is slowly collected into several test tubes and set aside for special tests. The needle then is withdrawn, the site is covered with a sterile gauze square, and the patient is kept in bed for several hours with head low. If the patient gets up and about too soon, a severe headache may result. This is probably due to spinal fluid leakage from the subarachnoid space through the needle-puncture wound into the tissue spaces, which results in a lowering of the intracranial cerebrospinal-fluid pressure, thus permitting abnormally great distention and pulsation of the cerebral arteries (the mechanism producing many types of headaches).

Spinal Fluid Pressure. From a lumbar puncture it is hoped to gain information concerning the pressure and the dynamics of the cerebrospinal fluid circulation, as well as the composition of the spinal fluid itself. The pressure is ascertained by noting at what level in the manometer the fluid finally comes to rest under conditions of the best possible relaxation on the part of the patient. A state of complete relaxation is usually difficult to attain. The patient is encouraged to loosen all his muscles and to breathe through his mouth. If the pressure remains at a high level, the operator waits for several minutes, sometimes half an hour, before manipulating the patient further. When the fluid level has become fairly constant, the pressure reading is noted. Generally it is found to be in the range between 100 to 150 mm. of water. Higher readings are obtained in patients with cerebral edema, cerebral hemorrhage (when it may even exceed 1,000 mm.) and meningitis. It is apt to be subnormal if the patient is dehydrated, if he is overbreathing (which produces alkalosis and spasm of the cerebral arteries, hence reducing the volume of the intracranial contents) or if there is some process blocking the fluid circulation somewhere between the ventricles and the lumbar canal.

Spinal Fluid Dynamics. These are tested in several ways. First, the presence of small rapid oscillations of the fluid level is sought. These are due to volume changes within the rigid bony confines of the brain and the spinal canal caused by the pulsations of the arteries coursing through the nervous system. A slower oscillation also may be observed. This occurs concomitantly with respiration and is related to rhythmic variations in intra-abdominal pressure taking place in conjunction with respiration. If the pulse and respiratory oscillations are not apparent, the patency of the needle should be questioned.

QUECKENSTEDT'S TEST. Next, pressure is applied, first over one jugular vein and then over the other. Normally this procedure causes a substantial rise in the manometer level. This is due largely to venous distention within the cranium, the effect of which is to force fluid out into the spinal canal. If this manipulation on both sides fails to raise the pressure, provided the needle is patent, one must conclude that a block exists somewhere between the point of fluid formation in the ventricles and the point of tapping. Such a block may be due to a variety of causes, the most common being inflammation (meningitis) at the base of the brain or about the cord and a tumor impinging on the spinal canal. If the expected rise in pressure occurs on compressing one jugular but not the other, it is evident that manipulation has failed in one case to cause intracranial venous distention, for which a block, involving either the jugular vein on that side or the venous sinus which it drains, must be responsible. This occurs in sinus thrombosis or thrombosis within the jugular vein itself.

Cisternal Tap

Information may be gained concerning the nature of the cerebrospinal fluid and its dynamics, when spinal block is present, by performing a cisternal tap, which involves introducing the needle into the cisterna magna (an area between the cerebellum and the superior surface of the medulla oblongata, where the subarachnoid space is much widened). The back of the neck having been shaved and an antiseptic applied, the needle is introduced just below the occipital protuberance of the skull, through the first cervical interspace, to a depth of between 4 and 5 cm.

Analysis of Cerebrospinal Fluid

The color of normal spinal fluid is water-clear, but in meningitis the fluid may exhibit cloudiness in all degrees, from faintly turbid to frankly purulent. When hemorrhage has occurred into the ventricles or into the subarachnoid space, the fluid is grossly bloody. A yellow color bespeaks the presence of a high protein concentration or of broken-down hemoglobin. This yellow color, spoken of as *xanthochromia*, is encountered in patients with tumors (especially of the cord), subdural hematomata and in patients in whom bleeding has occurred into the spinal fluid several hours or days prior to the tap. Absence of this color in the supernatant portion of a centrifuged bloody spinal fluid is assurance that the hemorrhage is no more than a day or two old at most.

Cell Count. The cell count of the fluid, for which a regular blood-counting chamber can be used, is completed as promptly as possible, the total number and relative proportions of the various cellular constituents being determined after the addition of fresh polychrome methylene blue. Normally the total number of white cells, consisting of lymphocytes and monocytes, should not exceed 10 per cu. mm. An increase in the number and also the appearance in the fluid of polymorphonuclear leukocytes indicate the presence of an inflammatory or destructive process affecting the meninges.

Spinal Fluid Protein. Normally in the vicinity of from 30 to 50 mg. per cent or lower, this can be judged roughly, so far as the presence or absence of a pathologic excess is concerned, by the addition of a drop or two of the fluid to a solution of concentrated phenol or ammonium sulfate. In each case a white cloud appears if the protein is elevated significantly. Accurate quantitative determinations of total protein, as well as nonprotein nitrogen, are made as a matter of routine.

Glucose. In the spinal fluid this ranges normally between one half and two thirds of the blood glucose level. Its determination is of value in spinal fluid studies because of the fact that its concentration is decreased in the presence of pus-forming bacteria. These hydrolyze glucose in their growth and metabolism, whereas the filtrable viruses do not. The test serves, therefore, to distinguish bacterial and virus infections of the central nervous system.

Other Tests

These include a complement-fixation test for syphilis, such as the *Wassermann test,* and the *colloidal-gold test* which is valuable in distinguishing tabes dorsalis and paresis from other forms of central nervous system syphilis and also in diagnosing multiple sclerosis. Occasionally, the quantitative estimation of chloride is performed, and, if there is any reason to suspect an infectious process, the spinal fluid is cultured and stained for bacteria. Additional bacteriologic technics, such as guinea pig inoculation for the tubercle bacillus and animal-brain injections for viruses, sometimes are employed. The character of the cerebrospinal fluid in various central nervous system diseases will be described more specifically in discussions of these diseases.

Thoracentesis

The detection of fluid in the chest by physical or roentgenographic examination is almost always followed by a diagnostic chest tap (thoracentesis) which is performed on the premise that the character of this fluid is the most direct clue as to the nature of the underlying lesion. Selection of the site of entry depends, of course, on the location of the effusion; unless the fluid is "loculated," i.e., confined in a circumscribed area, the usual approach is through the eighth or ninth rib interspace in the posterior axillary line. The patient is supported in a semirecumbent or an upright position, with neck in forward flexion and dorsal spine flexed laterally in the direction opposite that of the involved side, in order to widen the interspace to be penetrated. The skin having been cleansed with iodine or Zephiran, procaine is injected intracutaneously and into the underlying pleura. A short laceration is made with the tip of a Bard-Parker blade, and through this is introduced a needle of appropriate caliber and length which communicates via a 3-way stopcock with a 10- to 30-ml. syringe. The 3-way stopcock provides a route of exit for fluid from the pleural cavity or, if desired, from the syringe into a sterile rubber or plastic tube. The first effluent drawn into the syringe is placed in a tube containing trisodium citrate solution as an anticoagulant, and the remainder is apportioned into dry sterile tubes or bottles, depending on the number and the type of tests that are contemplated.

Data that are required in connection with most thoracenteses include the following: the volume of fluid aspirated; its color and degree of clarity; its specific gravity, a value of 1.015 or higher characterizing an exudate, as opposed to a transudate; its total protein content, as an additional criterion for differ-

entiating inflammatory exudates from transudates; and numerical cell counts, including a red cell and a differential leukocyte count. A portion of the fluid is planted in bacteria culture media, including one designed for the growth of the tubercle bacillus. Another portion may be injected intraperitoneally into guinea pigs as an additional means of excluding tuberculous infection. Finally, some or all of the remaining fluid may be rotated in a centrifuge and the sediment prepared for cytologic study as a "cell block" or examined by the Papanicolaou technic for tumor cells.

Abdominal Paracentesis

Examination of the patient with ascites, as in the case of the patient with a pleuritic effusion, must include a study of the abnormal fluid. Collection of ascitic fluid is carried out by means of abdominal paracentesis.

Preparatory to that procedure, the patient is placed in the upright position on the edge of the bed, fully supported, with his legs dangling over the side, one arm fitted with a sphygmomanometer cuff. The trocar is introduced with sterile precautions through a stab wound in the midline below the umbilicus and the fluid drained through an effluent tube into a container. *The nurse will not have neglected to have the patient void as completely as possible just prior to paracentesis.*

ROENTGENOLOGIC STUDIES

Evaluation of the ill patient very often is aided by, or may require, a roentgenologic examination, for most systemic diseases produce structural or functional changes that are of diagnostic significance and are detectable by this means alone. Basic procedures that are employed in various x-ray studies are of immediate concern to the nurse. In certain examinations she is a direct participant, their success or failure depending on the manner in which certain preliminary nursing measures have been carried out. Moreover, her familiarity with diagnostic roentgenology in general and her appreciation of the objectives of specific tests are essential to her understanding of her patients and their problems.

Any structure in the body can be visualized by roentgen rays if the molecular density of that structure differs sufficiently from that of the adjacent structures. Areas of lesser density, such as aerated lung tissue or gas-filled bowel, which transmit x-rays with less interference appear relatively "radiolucent"; those of greater density, which absorb or refract the x-rays to a greater extent, are relatively "radiopaque." In order to achieve the necessary degree of inequality in density where no such inequality exists, it may be necessary to introduce either an artificial high-density "contrast medium," which will delineate the lumen of any tube or hollow viscus containing it, or injections of air in the vicinity of the structure to be examined, after which the latter can be delineated against a relatively translucent background. Roentgenologic study of the gastrointestinal tract, the gallbladder, the bronchi, the kidneys, the spinal canal, the genitourinary tract and the blood vessels depends in each case on the ingestion or the injection of an appropriate contrast medium.

Roentgenograms. The roentgenogram, or "x-ray plate," is analogous to the familiar photographic negative, consisting of a plastic sheet which has been coated with a light-sensitive emulsion. X-rays expelled from a cathode tube are directed through whatever anatomic structure or object may be under study, through a protective casing which encloses the film and protects it from exposure to light and, finally, through the film itself. Shortly thereafter, the film is developed and studied in the form of a negative print.

Fluoroscopy. This technic involves the continuous observation of an image reflected on a screen when exposed to x-radiation in the manner of a television screen which is activated by an electrode beam. Structures of differing densities which intercept the x-ray beams are visualized on the screen in silhouette. A permanent record of a fluoroscopic image may be secured by photography. Miniature photographs of this type, called "photofluorograms," are utilized by Public Health Chest Survey Units, hospitals and other organizations as a method of excluding lung disease rapidly and economically in large numbers of individuals. Fluoroscopic images, brightened and accentuated by electronic "image intensifiers," also are capable of being recorded on motion picture film. This procedure, called *cinefluorography*, pro-

vides an unparalleled opportunity for the detailed and leisurely analysis of various phenomena—the process of deglutition, for example, and the peristaltic activity of the esophagus after a swallow of barium—which, because of their complexity, transitory nature or speed of occurrence are difficult to examine by any other means.

Angiography. This term denotes the x-ray visualization of blood vessels by a technic which entails the intravenous or intra-arterial injection of an iodide compound, such as Diodrast or Hypaque, as a contrast medium. Employing a rapid film changer a number of x-ray pictures immediately are taken in quick succession to delineate the particular vascular channels in question as these become opacified, and their caliber, integrity and degree of patency are thereby revealed. Following an intravenous injection of contrast medium it is possible to outline the chambers of the heart and to visualize the pulmonary arteries; such a study is called a *cardiopulmonary angiogram* or *angiocardiogram*. "Selective angiocardiography" involves the injection of contrast medium directly, via catheter, into the right atrium or right ventricle of the heart itself. *Trans-splenic venography* refers to a special kimographic technic involving the injection of Diodrast directly into the substance of the spleen for the detection of venous dilatations and abnormal communications between the portal and systemic circuits and in order to measure the speed of blood flow through the liver as a criterion of portal obstruction.

Laminograms. The laminogram ("planogram" or "body section roentgenogram") furnishes sharply focused silhouettes of structures that lie within one plane only, other structures being obscured. This result is accomplished by means of a mechanical device which moves both the x-ray tube and the plate through a prescribed arc during exposure, the effect of which is to blur all outlines excepting those of structures which retain their original positions relative to both tube and plate. Multiple views of a body region, focused at successively deeper layers, visualize clearly some structures that would otherwise be obscured and localize accurately any x-ray lesions that might appear, as, for example, a tumor lying deep within the mediastinum, a lesion obstructing the bronchial lumen or a small area of bone destruction in a particular portion of the vertebrae.

Roentgenographic Examination of the Chest

The posterior-anterior (P.A.) view of the chest, commonest of all roentgenologic examinations, yields a wealth of information pertaining to the lungs and the pleura, locates the trachea and the bronchi, defines the position and the dimensions of the heart and the great vessels and determines the presence or the absence of abnormal mediastinal contents. Lateral and oblique views of the lungs are obtained for more precise localization of intrathoracic lesions. A posterior-anterior view of the chest taken with the tube at a standard distance (e.g., 6 or 7 feet) from the subject permits the quantitative measurement of certain cardiac dimensions which reflect the size of each individual atrium and ventricle. As indicated above, the cardiac examination may include, in addition, fluoroscopy and kimography for the detection and the measurement of abnormal movements in its pulsating walls or to differentiate a pulsatile mass, representing an aneurysm (p. 535), from one that does not pulsate, i.e., a solid

tumor. Visualization of the small bronchi is accomplished with the aid of a contrast medium, Lipiodol, an iodized oil, which is instilled intratracheally an instant before the x-ray exposure is made. The resultant picture, called a "bronchogram," is illustrated in Figure 23.

Abdominal Roentgenograms

Anterior and posterior views of the abdomen, taken with the patient in horizontal position or sitting upright, are important in the diagnosis of intestinal obstruction. The presence, degree and location of gas and fluid levels within the intestinal lumen distinguish patients with obstruction from those with paralytic ileus. Stones (if radiopaque) in the gallbladder, the kidneys, the ureters or the bladder, as well as calcified blood vessels, lymph nodes, cysts and parasites, may be detected by this examination. Gastric or intestinal perforation may be discovered by the presence of free air under the diaphragm, observed in abdominal films. Depending on the amount of intestinal gas that is present, the spleen and one or both kidneys may be outlined in a flat abdominal film. The me-

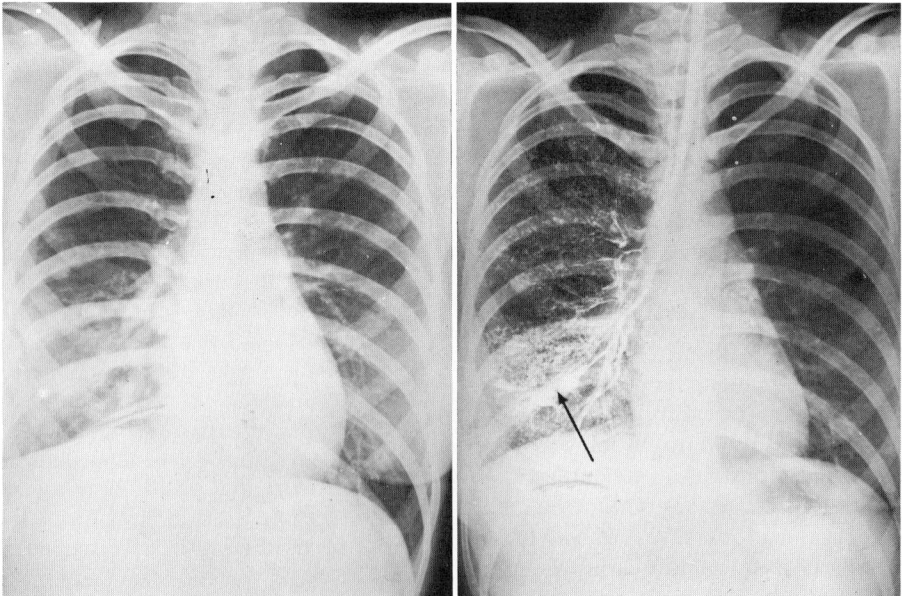

FIG. 23. Roentgenograms of chest before and after installation of contrast medium into the right main bronchus demonstrating the presence of a bronchiectatic abscess, indicated by an arrow in the right lower lobe. The cause of the lesion proved to be an accumulation of aspirated food.

dial borders of the psoas muscles are usually apparent, their characteristics and location furnishing a clue as to the presence or the absence of tumors or other lesions in the retroperitoneal space.

Skeletal Roentgenograms

The roentgenographic appearance of the skeleton is of decisive importance in establishing and excluding the diagnosis of nutritional and endocrine disorders that are complicated by derangements of calcium and phosphorus metabolism. Abnormal radiolucency of the bones, indicating demineralization of the skeleton, is a characteristic of rickets, hyperparathyroidism and myelomatosis, for example. Specific changes are characteristic of rheumatoid hypertrophic arthritis, Paget's disease, osteosclerosis and other disorders of unknown etiology. The diagnosis of lead poisoning may be established by skeletal roentgenograms. Lymphomas and metastasizing carcinomas very often manifest themselves by localized osteolytic lesions in certain areas of the skeleton, the most common sites of involvement being the skull, the pelvis, the vertebrae and the ribs, i.e., where bone marrow is proliferating actively.

Roentgenography of the Biliary System
Cholecystography

Radiologic examination of the gallbladder is carried out for the detection of gallstones, and in order to estimate the ability of the gallbladder to fill, concentrate its contents, contract and empty in normal fashion. Very few gallstones are sufficiently radiopaque to be visualized by ordinary roentgenographic technic; they must be demonstrated as negative shadows in a gall bladder filled with a radiopaque substance. To this end an iodide-containing dye which is excreted into the bile by the liver and concentrated in the gallbladder is administered to the patient, either by mouth or by intravenous injection. Drugs given as contrast media include Telepaque, Cholografin, Orabilex, Oragrafin, Priodax and Iodeikon. These preparations are given in oral doses of 2 to 3 Gm. 10 to 12 hours before x-ray study. Intravenous cholecystography involves the injection of an iodide approximately 10 minutes prior to roentgenog-

raphy. During the interval between the administration of the iodide and the x-ray study, the patient is permitted nothing by mouth lest the gallbladder be stimulated to contract and thereby expel the contrast medium.

Nursing instructions that apply to patients who are scheduled for x-ray studies of the gallbladder are:

1. One hour or more after the evening meal, and approximately 10 hours before roentgenography, the patient receives six 0.5-Gm. tablets of contrast medium by mouth.
2. These tablets are to be ingested 1 at a time, at intervals of from 2 to 5 minutes, together with a volume of water totaling at least 8 oz.
3. The patient then is to receive nothing by mouth, excepting water, until bedtime. Thereafter, until the roentgenogram is taken, not even water is permitted.
4. Laxatives must not be given during this preparation period.
5. A saline enema is to be administered early in the morning of the test.
6. Breakfast is omitted.

The right upper abdominal quadrant then is photographed by x-ray. If the gallbladder has filled and concentrated the dye normally, it will be seen as a pear-shaped shadow from 2 to 3 in. long under the right costal margin. If stones are present, there will be mottled densities within this shadow corresponding to their outlines. Next, to test the contractility of the gallbladder, the patient is fed a fatty meal containing cream, butter or eggs, and the x-ray examination is repeated at intervals until the gallbladder has expelled the dye and becomes invisible. If the gallbladder is found to fill and empty normally and to contain no stones, it is concluded that no gallbladder disease is present.

Percutaneous Transhepatic Cholangiography

The oral and the intravenous technics just described permit the visualization of the gallbladder (and occasionally the larger ducts) only if the liver cells are functioning properly and are capable of excreting the radiopaque dye into the bile. Percutaneous transhepatic cholangiography, which involves the injection of dye directly into the biliary tree itself, is effective regardless of the state of liver function. Moreover, because of the relatively large concentration of dye that is introduced into the biliary system, all components of the latter, including the hepatic ducts within the liver, the common hepatic duct throughout its length, the cystic duct and the gallbladder, are delineated with clarity.

This procedure is useful in distinguishing jaundice caused by liver disease (hepatocellular jaundice) from that due to biliary obstruction; for investigating the gastrointestinal symtoms of patients whose gallbladders have been removed; for locating stones within the bile ducts; and in the diagnosis of cancer involving the biliary system.

The patient, fasting and well sedated, lies prone on the x-ray table. The injection site, usually in the mid-clavicular line immediately beneath the right costal margin, is disinfected and anesthetized with Xylocaine. Through a small incision at this point is passed an 18-gauge spinal puncture needle, directed cephalad, posteriorly at a 45 degree angle and parallel to the midline. When the needle has penetrated to a depth of approximately 4 inches, the stylet is removed and replaced by a plastic connector tube with 50-ml. syringe attached. While gently applying suction, the operator slowly withdraws the needle until bile appears in the syringe. Further withdrawal is halted, as much bile as possible is withdrawn, a radiopaque dye is injected (e.g., 20 ml. of 70 per cent Urokon Sodium) and an x-ray picture taken. Before removing the needle, the operator aspirates as much dye and bile as possible in order to forestall subsequent leakage via the needle tract into the peritoneal cavity and avoid the possibility of bile peritonitis.

Roentgenography of the Upper Gastrointestinal Tract

The entire gastrointestinal tract can be delineated by x-rays following the introduction of barium sulfate as the contrast medium. This material, a tasteless, odorless, nongranular and completely insoluble (hence, not absorbable) powder, is ingested in the form of a thick or thin aqueous suspension for purposes of upper gastrointestinal tract study ("upper G.I. series") and is instilled rectally for visualization of the colon ("barium enema"). For purposes of examining the upper gastrointestinal tract, the fasting patient is required to swallow barium under direct fluoroscopic examination. As the contrast medium descends into the stomach, the position, patency and caliber of the esophagus are visualized, enabling the examiner to detect or exclude any anatomic or functional derangement of that organ. He is able to make an important observation relating to the heart, namely, the presence or the absence of right atrial involvement. An enlarged right atrium invariably impinges on the esophagus, revealed by the resulting pressure defect in the esophagus.

The roentgenographic appearance of the lower esophagus after a swallow of thick barium suspension enables detection of esophageal varices, a manifestation of liver cirrhosis. Fluoroscopic examination is extended next to the stomach, as its lumen fills with barium. The motility and the thickness of the gastric wall and the mucosal pattern are observed for evidence of spasms, ulcerations, malignant infiltrates and other anatomic abnormalities, including pressure defects from without. The patency of the pyloric valve and the anatomy of the duodenum are also observed under the fluoroscope, with particular reference to possible ulceration of the mucosa, spasm of the wall or displacement of the structure as a whole by a tumor in the adjacent area.

During the fluoroscopic examination, roentgenograms are exposed, in order to obtain a permanent record of the findings. Additional roentgenograms are taken at intervals, for as long as 24 hours thereafter, as a means of estimating the rate of gastric emptying and the degree of small bowel motility. A truly detailed study of the small intestine involves the continuous infusion, via a duodenal tube, of from 500 to 1,000 ml. of a thin barium sulfate suspension. This is carried out as a separate procedure. The barium column fills the intestinal loops and is observed continuously by fluoroscope and filmed at frequent intervals as it progresses through the jejunum and the ilium.

The following are the nursing specifications that are applicable in connection with the G.I. series:

1. The patient is to receive nothing by mouth after 12 o'clock midnight prior to the test.

2. During this interim, the patient is to receive no purgative, however mild, and no other medication, unless specifically ordered.

3. Breakfast and the noonday meal are to be omitted on the day of the test.

4. The evening meal may be offered and nourishment provided until midnight.

5. After midnight the patient is to resume fasting. Nothing is permitted by mouth after midnight on the second day of the test until the final roentgenogram is taken.

6. Breakfast is again held on the second day of the test and the fasting continued until the last roentgenogram is taken.

Roentgenography of the Large Bowel (Barium Enema)

As the first step in an x-ray study of the colon, the fasting patient receives a rectal instillation of a barium sulfate suspension, which is viewed in the fluoroscope and then filmed. If the patient has been prepared satisfactorily, with the colonic contents having been evacuated completely by enemas, the contour of the entire colon, including cecum and appendix (if patent), is clearly visible and the motility of each portion readily observed.

The following orders may be specified for the patient who is to be prepared for barium enema:

1. A saline enema is administered early in the preceding evening.

2. Saline enemas are repeated until returns are clear.

3. The patient is to receive nothing by mouth after midnight.

4. Two hours after completion of the x-ray study, the patient is to receive an oil retention enema.

5. This is followed 2 hours later by saline clearing enemas.

6. On the following day, the oil retention enemas are again administered to assure adequate evacuation of the barium suspension.

Barium Double Contrast Enema

Examination of the colonic mucosa for detailed inspection of small lesions may be carried out by insufflating the lower gastrointestinal tract with air immediately following spontaneous evacuation of the barium enema.

Retrograde and Intravenous Pyelography

The position, the shape and the dimensions of the kidneys, the contour of the renal pelvis, the position and the caliber of the urethral lumina and the contours of the bladder may be visualized by roentgenography following the direct instillation of a contrast medium via the cystoscope (retrograde pyelogram), or following the intravenous administration of a contrast medium into the venous system whence it is cleared by the kidneys (intravenous pyelogram). The contrast medium for both examinations is an iodide salt, such as Skiodan (methiodal sodium), 100 ml. in a 10 or 20 per cent solution being infused for the retrograde pyelogram, and 20 to 40 Gm. in 100 ml. of sterile distilled water being given intravenously for the intravenous pyelogram. The patient is prepared for the intravenous pyelogram as follows:

1. A saline enema is adminstered in the evening prior to the test.

2. Nothing is to be received by mouth after 12 o'clock midnight.

3. Saline enema is repeated early in the morning of the test.

4. All nourishment, including breakfast, on the day of the test is withheld until the procedure is concluded.

Prior to either test, it must be ascertained that the patient is not allergic to the contrast medium. Skiodan sensitivity is excluded as follows:

1. Two ml. of Skiodan are diluted with 8 ml. of water.

2. The patient is required to hold this solution in his mouth for 15 minutes.

3. During this period he is carefully observed for evidence of numbness of the face or the lips, swelling of the tongue, burning sensations in any cutaneous area of flushing of the face and the neck.

4. If none of these phenomena has appeared, the patient is instructed to swallow the solution.

5. Throughout the ensuing hour, the nurse is to check the patient for possible

flushing of the skin, symptoms of nausea or abdominal cramps.

6. If a reaction is suspected on any basis, the nurse is to notify the doctor at once and prepare a hypodermic dose of epinephrine (0.5 to 1.0 ml. of a 1:1,000 solution) which is to be kept in readiness for immediate administration.

Roentgenography of the Central Nervous System

An extremely useful technic for the detection and the localization of spinal cord tumors and ruptured intravertebral disks that encroach on the spinal canal involves the withdrawal of a few ml. of spinal fluid, followed by the injection of air or of a contrast iodide solution. X-ray examination of the spinal canal following an air injection is referred to as an "air myelogram." Those myelograms in which spinal fluid is replaced by a radiopaque fluid are designated in accordance with the chemical used, for example, "Skiodan myelogram" or "Pantopaqe myelogram," etc. Injections of air in 25-ml. or larger volumes permit the x-ray visualization of the cerebral ventricles; this type of study is referred to as an "air encephalogram." Skull roentgenograms taken after direct aspiration of the cerebrospinal fluid in a cerebral ventricle and its replacement by air via a needle which has been inserted through the cranium and the intervening brain substance are termed "ventriculograms."

Preparation of the patient who is to receive an iodide solution as a contrast medium must include a sensitivity test, which is carried out according to the specifications outlined in connection with the preparations for pyelography. Other details of the patient's preparation will vary, depending on the nature of the test contemplated. In most instances this will include the administration of analgesic and hypnotic medicines prior to the procedure and the immobilization of the patient in a horizontal position for 24 hours or longer following the test.

Lymphangiography

Radiologic visualization of the lymphatic system is possible after the direct injection of contrast medium directly into lymphatic vessels in the hands and the feet. This technic affords a means of detecting lymph-node involvement by metastatic carcinoma, lymphoma or infection in sites that are otherwise inaccessible to the examiner except by the direct surgical approach—for example, in the pelvis, the retroperitoneum and deep in the axillae.

The first step in this procedure is the location of a lymphatic vessel in each foot (or hand) by injecting Evans blue dye intradermally between the first and the second digits and then, 15 to 20 minutes later, incising the skin proximal to the injection site. A blue lymphatic is identified, isolated, cannulated with a 25 to 30 gauge needle and infused very slowly with a contrast medium containing iodine and oil (Ethiodol). Approximately 10 ml. of this material is injected into the foot (or 5 ml. into the hand) at a rate not exceeding 7 ml. per hour. Appropriate x-ray pictures are taken at the conclusion of the injection, 24 hours later and periodically thereafter, as indicated. Injection of the feet delineates, for about an hour, the lymphatic channels in the legs and the thoracic duct and, for many weeks, the inguinal, abdominal and supraclavicular lymph nodes. Similar delineation of lymphatic vessels in the upper extremity, and of the axillary and the supraclavicular nodes, follows injection of the hand.

Apart from its diagnostic value in cases of unsuspected lymph-node disease, lymphangiography offers a means of evaluating the presence and the extent of metastases in patients who are known to have cancer. Moreover, since lymphomatous lymph nodes retain the contrast medium for 4 to 6 weeks after the injection, any change in their size that may occur in response to irradiation or chemotherapy can be measured and used as a criterion of therapeutic effect.

RADIOISOTOPE TESTS

Recent increases in the availability of isotope-tracer materials and improved methods of measuring radioactivity have opened entirely new approaches to the evaluation of the patient. Based on a variety of tracer technics, several ingenious tests of organ function have been devised. The localization of certain malignant tumors has become

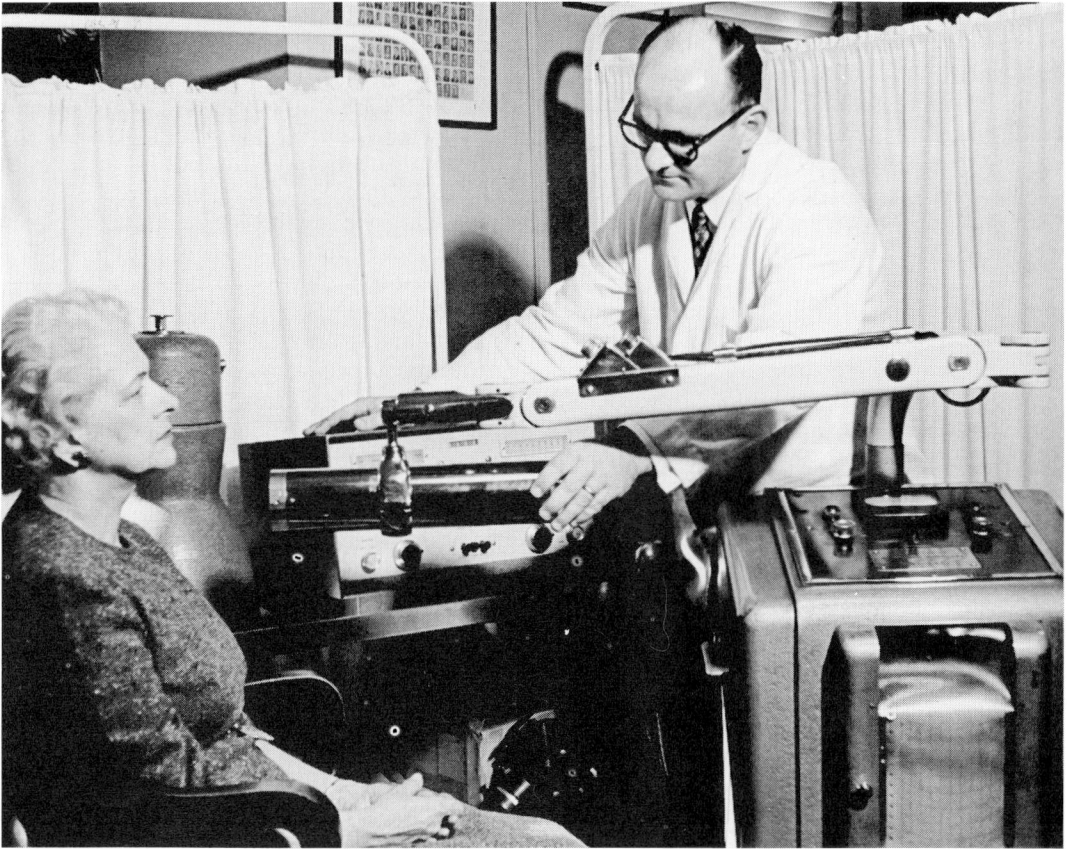

FIG. 24. Performance of 24-hour iodine uptake test. The physician has centered the scintillation probe and is measuring the energy transmitted from the gamma emissions by means of a pulse-height analyzer. (Photo by Caroline Bailey)

possible, and, in some instances, methods are now available for observing and measuring biologic processes which hitherto have not been susceptible to direct demonstration. Representative tests, now in wide use and certain of general acceptance, are summarized below.

Thyroid Tests with Radioiodine (I^{131})

The rate of I^{131} uptake by the thyroid gland, the plasma clearance of I^{131} and the urinary excretion of this isotope furnish reliable criteria of thyroid activity. Moreover, the distribution of radioactivity in the thyroid and elsewhere in the body after the administration of radioiodine affords a means of distinguishing malignant from benign thyroid nodules and a method for the detection of metastatic thyroid cancer.

I^{131} Uptake. The usual procedure is to administer orally to the fasting patient a solution of sodium iodide^{131} (or a capsule which has been prepared with an internal coating of I^{131}) in a dose of from 5 to 50 microcuries. After a standard time interval, e.g., 24 and 48 hours, the I^{131} that has been assimilated by the thyroid gland is measured on the basis of the radioactive counts per minute that are detected at a point above the isthmus of the thyroid gland. Hyperthyroid individuals accumulate a high proportion of the I^{131}, in some cases approximately 90 per cent, whereas hypothyroid individuals exhibit a very low uptake.

Thyroidal Iodide Clearance. The I^{131} clearance test measures the quantity of circulating blood that is cleared completely of iodide per unit time. After the intravenous injection of radioiodine, the radioactivity over the thyroid gland is measured continuously for 30 to 60 minutes, and the total amount of I^{131} accumulated by the gland per minute is computed. In addition, the plasma I^{131} content is measured in samples of blood collected 45 and 70 minutes after injection; these values are averaged. Thyroid I^{131}, divided by the mean plasma I^{131}, equals thyroid clearance (ml. of plasma cleared of iodide per minute). The mean clearance value for normal (euthyroid) individuals is 25 ml. per minute; for hyperthyroid patients, 250 ml. per minute; and hypothyroid patients, 1.6 ml. per minute.

I^{131} Excretion. Another test of thyroid activity using radioiodine involves measuring the urinary output of this isotope during the 24- to 48-hour period after its ingestion. A subject whose thyroid activity is normal (i.e., euthyroid individual) excretes from 40 to 80 per cent of the ingested iodine in 24 hours. Hyperthyroid individuals almost invariably excrete less than 40, and patients with hypothyroidism excrete more than 80 per cent of the tracer dose.

In addition to quantitative measurement of iodine uptake by the thyroid gland, the latter may be subjected to external scanning by means of a handheld scintillation counter or by a mechanical scanning device for evidence of irregularity in the deposition of radioactive iodine. The scintillation crystal is electromechanically linked to a recording device which automatically maps the activity in the scanned area, producing a so-called "scintogram," "scanogram" or "gammagram." Discovery of decreased I^{131} uptake in a localized area of the thyroid is construed as evidence of a malignancy. Scanning of the entire body to obtain the total body profile may be carried out in a search for a metastatic functioning of a thyroid metastasis.

Role of the Nurse in I^{131} Thyroid Tests

Although the nurse may not be involved directly in the performance of these tests, their validity may depend on her participation. But for nursing vigilance throughout the 24-hour observation period, the iodine excretion test proves worthless in a high proportion of cases. Valid results require the salvaging and pooling of every specimen voided during that interval. Experience has demonstrated that one specimen at least is unintentionally discarded and lost in 25 per cent of tests in the face of clear-cut and forceful admonitions given in advance by the physician and despite the desire of the patient to cooperate. Another source of error which may vitiate the iodine uptake, clearance and excretion tests is prior exposure of the patient to iodine. Such exposure, whether acquired in the form of a prescribed medication containing an iodide salt or as the result of the injection of an iodine-containing contrast medium in a bronchogram, venogram, pyelogram or gallbladder study, or an application of iodine to the skin, reduces the uptake of I^{131} and invalidates these tests. Thus, as soon as the physician is informed that a radioiodine excretion test or uptake test is in prospect, he should systematically eliminate any chance of such contact in the interim.

Radioactive Chromium (Cr^{51}) in Measurements of Blood Volume, Red Cell Longevity and Red Cell Sequestration in the Spleen

When sodium chromate[51] is added to samples of blood, the radioactive salt penetrates the red cell membranes, enters the erythrocytes and there becomes bound. These cells, for the remainder of their lifespan, are tagged with a radioactive label. Otherwise unaltered by the labeling process, the tagged cells can be used for a variety of in vivo tests, including measurements of the circulating red cell mass and red cell survival and for evaluating the role of the spleen in blood destruction. The preliminary step in all of these tests is the collection of from 10 to 50 ml. of venous blood into a sterile solution, to which is added sodium chromate[51]. A red cell suspension is prepared and reinjected into the patient, an aliquot sample of the suspension being tested for "specific red cell activity," i.e., number of radioactive counts per ml. of red cells per minute. After a minimum of 1 hour following the injection of tagged red cells, a venous sample is obtained and likewise tested for specific red cell activity. The ratio of these values is inversely proportional to the volume of circulating red cells and the volume of red cells in the injected sample. The normal red cell volume ranges from 25 to 35 ml. per kilogram of body weight. The circulating plasma volume is calculated from the circulating red cell volume and the venous hematocrit, determined as described above. The plasma volume in normal individuals ranges from 40 to 50 ml. per Kg. of body weight.

The rate at which labeled red cells are eliminated from the circulation, based on successive changes in red cell radioactivity during the ensuing weeks, reflects the longevity of the mean red cell population. The normal lifespan may range from 110 to 130 days. In cases of hemolytic anemia, the life span of the red cells is relatively brief, e.g., 10 days or less, in the most severe cases. The degree to which the spleen is responsible for the destruction of red cells is often an important consideration in patients with hemolytic disease, for if there is evidence of excessive trapping of erythrocytes in that organ, its removal may be undertaken in the expectation of lessening hemolysis and correcting the anemia. Such evidence can be obtained by "external monitoring" over the splenic area and over a corresponding area on the opposite side (i.e., over the liver) after the patient has received an injection of chromium^{51}-labeled red cells. The ratio of radioactive counts obtained simultaneously over these areas reflect the degree of red cell sequestration, hence, hemolysis in the spleen. If the splenic radioactivity exceeds liver radioactivity by a factor of more than two, splenectomy may be advised.

Radioactive (Cobalt^{57}-Labeled) Vitamin B$_{12}$, Absorption Test

Patients with pernicious anemia are constitutionally incapable of absorbing vitamin B$_{12}$, a characteristic that is unique. A radioactive tag (cobalt^{57}) in the B$_{12}$ molecule furnishes a simple means of detecting or excluding this absorption defect. The fasting patient receives a 1-microcurie oral dose of Co^{57}-labeled B$_{12}$ and the collection of urine is started. One to three hours later, a large quantity (1 mg., i.e., 1,000 micrograms) of nonradioactive B$_{12}$ is injected intramuscularly for the purpose of saturating the tissues with B$_{12}$ and thereby reducing the likelihood that any labeled B$_{12}$ that may be absorbed from the intestine might be removed by the liver or stored elsewhere in the body. After this "loading dose" of unlabeled vitamin, whatever B$_{12}$ may be contained in or enter the blood, including B$_{12}$ absorbed from the gut, is excreted in toto into the urine. Therefore, the proportion of the oral dose of cobalt^{57}-labeled B$_{12}$ that is absorbed in the blood of the patient can be calculated from the radioactivity of the urine that he excretes. This measurement is made 24 hours after the test dose.

As in the case of the I^{131} excretion test of thyroid function, the measurement is valueless unless the 24-hour sample includes all the urine that has been voided during the test period. A second measurement may be made at the end of 48 hours, in which case a second loading dose of unlabeled B$_{12}$ is injected intramuscularly at the beginning of the second day. Normal individuals excrete more than 10 to 20 per cent of the oral dose in 24 hours. The urinary excretion of less than 10 per cent is indicative of a malabsorption defect of some type, including pernicious anemia; the excretion of less than 3 per cent is presumptive evidence of pernicious anemia. Proof of this diagnosis may be secured by repeating the entire test, this time administering a preparation containing intrinsic factor along with the oral dose of Co^{57}-labeled B$_{12}$. Under these conditions, the patient with pernicious anemia will absorb the labeled vitamin normally, and it will be detected in the urine in normal quantities. In patients with absorptive defects due to gastrointestinal disease, the absorption of B$_{12}$, hence its urinary excretion, will not be increased by feeding intrinsic factor.

Radioisotope Studies of the Urinary Tract

Evaluation of Renal Blood Flow and Tubular Function. Certain iodine containing compounds, i.e., those employed in intravenous pyelography (see page 105) are selectively concentrated in the kidneys after intravenous injection. After the administration of such compounds labeled with radioiodine, the kidneys transiently become radioactive, and the degree of radioactivity, determined by external counters, provides a

The Clinical Study of the Patient

TABLE 3. SAMPLE SPECIFICATIONS AND NORMAL VALUES FOR INDIVIDUAL LABORATORY TESTS

Test	Samples	Containers*	Normal Values
Albumin, serum	Venous, 6 ml.	T	4.0–5.0 Gm. per 100 ml.
Amylase, serum	Venous, 6 ml.	T	Less than 150 units (Sumogyi)
Ascorbic acid	(See Vitamin C)		
Bilirubin, serum: total	Venous, 5 ml. (a); or capillary, 0.2 ml. (b)	T, K. Ox. or B. Ox. (a), Capillary (b)	Less than 0.8 mg. per 100 ml.
conjugated ("direct")	Venous, 6 ml.	T, K. Ox. or B. Ox.	Less than 0.4 mg. per 100 ml.
Bilirubin tolerance	Venous, 5 ml., before 5 min. and 4 hr. after test injection	T (3)	Less than 5% retention of test dose in 4 hr.
Bleeding time	——	——	2 to 5 min. (Duke)
Blood volume, total	Special sampling procedure and equipment		65–85 ml. per Kg. of body weight
Bromsulphalein retention (B.S.P.)	Venous, 5 ml., 45 min. after test injection	T	Less than 5% retained in 45 min.
Calcium, serum	Venous, 6 ml.	T	4.5–5.5 mEq. per liter (9–11 mg. %)
Carbon dioxide content, serum	Venous, 5 ml.	T with oil	25–32 mEq. per liter
Catecholamines, urine	24-hr. collection	Refrig. bottle (with 5 ml. conc. HCl)	Less than 200 micrograms per 24 hrs.
Cephalin-cholesterol flocculation	Venous, 3 ml.	T	Up to 2+ flocculation in 24 hrs.
Chlorides, serum	Venous, 5 ml.	T with oil	100–106 mEq. per liter
Cholesterol, serum (total)	Venous, 5 ml.	T	150–270 mg. per 100 ml.
Cholesterol esters, serum	Venous, 5 ml.	T	68–78% of total cholesterol
Clotting time, venous, in glass	Venous, 4 ml.	T (4)	6–12 min. (Lee-White)
Congo red retention	Venous, 6 ml., 5 and 65 min. after injection	T (2)	Less than 30% decrease in dye concentration in 1 hr.
Creatine, urine	24-hr. collection	Refrig. bottle	Up to 100 mg. per 24 hrs.
Creatinine, serum	Venous, 10 ml.	T	0.3–1.0 mg. per 100 ml.
Creatinine, urine	24-hr. collection	Bottle refrigerated in freezer	1.0–1.8 Gm. per 24 hrs.
Creatinine clearance	Venous, 10 ml. (a); two successive 30–60 min. urine collections (b)	(a) T (b) refrig. bottle	100–130 ml. cleared per min.
Fibrinogen, plasma	Venous, 2 ml.	K. Ox. or B. Ox.	200–330 mg. per 100 ml.
Galactose tolerance	Venous, 1 ml., taken before and 75 min. after intravenous test dose	K. Ox. (2)	No galactose present in 75-min. sample.
Globulins, serum			
Alpha 1	Venous, 3 ml.	T	0.2–0.4 Gm. per 100 ml.
Alpha 2	Venous, 3 ml.	T	0.5–0.9 Gm. per 100 ml.
Beta	Venous, 3 ml.	T	0.6–1.1 Gm. per 100 ml.
Gamma	Venous, 3 ml.	T	0.7–1.7 Gm. per 100 ml.
Glucose, blood	Venous, fasting, 3 ml.	K. Ox.	65–90 mg. per 100 ml. blood; 75–100 mg. per 100 ml. plasma
Glucose tolerance	Venous, 3 ml., before, and 30, 60, 120 and 180 min. after oral test dose (a); urine samples collected concomitantly (b)	(a) K. Ox. (5) (b) Bottles (5)	Peak concentration less than 150 mg. per 100 ml. plasma. Fasting level restored within 2 hrs.

TABLE 3. SAMPLE SPECIFICATIONS AND NORMAL VALUES FOR
INDIVIDUAL LABORATORY TESTS—(Continued)

Test	Samples	Containers*	Normal Values
Hematocrit reading	Venous, 3 ml. (a); or capillary, 0.2 ml. (b)	(a) B. Ox. (b) Cap.	Males: 42–52%; females: 38–48%
Hemoglobin, blood	Venous, 3 ml. (a); or capillary, 0.2 ml. (b)	(a) B. Ox. (b) MP	Males: 15.0–16.5 Gm. per 100 ml. Females: 14.0–15.5 Gm. per 100 ml.
Hippuric acid excretion	4-hr. urine collection following oral, or 1-hr. collection after intravenous, test dose	Empty bottle	Equivalent of at least 2.5 Gm. sodium benzoate excreted in oral test, and at least 0.7 Gm. in intravenous test
Icterus index	Venous, 3 ml.	B. Ox.	4–6 units
Iodine, protein-bound, serum (PBI)	Venous, 10 ml.	T	4–8 micrograms per 100 ml.
Iodine[131] excretion	24- or 48-hr. collection	Bottle	40–80% of ingested I[131] excreted in 24 hrs.
Iodine[131] uptake	——	——	14–45% of ingested radioactivity concentrated in thyroid gland in 24 hrs.
Iron, serum	Venous, 5 ml.	T (iron-free)	75–150 micrograms per 100 ml.
Lactic dehydrogenase (LDH), serum	Venous, 3 ml.	T	Less than 180 units
Leucine aminopeptidase (LAP), serum	Venous, 3 ml.	T	Less than 200 units
Lipase	Venous, 5 ml.	T	Less than 1.5 units
Nonprotein nitrogen (NPN)	Venous, 4 ml.	K. Ox.	25–40 mg. per 100 ml. whole blood; 20–30 mg. per 100 ml. plasma or serum
Osmotic fragility, red cell	Venous, 5 ml.	B. Ox.	1% hemolysis in .45–.50, 50% hemolysis in .35–40 and 90% hemolysis in .25–.30 Gm. % NaCl solution
Oxygen saturation, arterial	Arterial, 3 ml.	K. Ox. or heparin with oil	94–96%
pH, whole blood or serum	Venous, 1 ml.	T or heparin with oil	7.40–7.45 units
Phenolsulfonphthalein excretion (PSP)	Urine, 15-min., 30 min. and 2-hr. collections	Bottle (3)	20–40% of dye excreted in 15 min.; 60–90% in 2 hrs.
Phosphatase, acid, serum	Venous, 6 ml.	T	Less than 4 Gutman units per 100 ml.
Phosphatase, alkaline, serum	Venous, 6 ml.	T	Less than 4 Bodansky units per 100 ml.
Phosphorus, inorganic, serum	Venous, 5 ml.	T	3.0–4.5 mg. per 100 ml.
Plasma volume, total	Special sampling procedure and equipment		40–50 ml. per Kg. of body weight
Platelet count	Capillary, 0.05 ml.	MP or coverslips	250,000–400,000 per cu. mm.
Potassium, serum	Venous, 5 ml.	T	3.5–5.5 mEq. per liter
Proteins, serum (total)	Venous, 5 ml.	T or K. Ox.	6.5–8.0 Gm. per 100 ml.
Red cell count	Venous, 5 ml. (a); or capillary, 0.05 ml. (b)	(a) B. Ox. (b) MP	4.5–5.5 million per cu. mm.
Red cell indices	Venous, 5 ml.	B. Ox.	
Mean corpuscular volume (MCV)			80–92 cubic micra
Mean corpuscular hemoglobin (MCH)			27–31 micromicrograms
Mean corpuscular hemoglobin concentration (MCHC)			32–36%

TABLE 3. SAMPLE SPECIFICATIONS AND NORMAL VALUES FOR INDIVIDUAL LABORATORY TESTS—(Continued)

Test	Samples	Containers*	Normal Values
Red cell volume, total	Special sampling procedure and equipment		25–35 ml. per Kg. body weight
Reticulocyte count	Venous, 5 ml. (a); or capillary, 0.1 ml. (b)	(a) B. Ox. or (b) tube tube with stain	0.5–1.0% of normal red cell count (25,000–60,000 per cu. mm.)
Sedimentation rate, red cell (Wintrobe-Landsberg)	Venous, 5 ml.	B. Ox.	Less than 10 mm. in 1 hr.
17-ketosteroids	24-hr. collection		Males: 8–20 mg. Females: 5–15 mg.
Sodium, serum	Venous, 5 ml.	T	136–145 mEq. per liter
Sugar, blood	(See Glucose)		
Thymol turbidity	Venous, 3 ml.	T	Up to 4 Maclagan units
Transaminase, glutamic-oxalacetic, serum (SGO-T)	Venous, 3 ml.	T	Less than 40 units
Transaminase, glutamic-pyruvic, serum (SGP-T)	Venous, 3 ml.	T	Males: less than 50 units Females: less than 40 units
Urea-nitrogen, blood (BUN)	Venous, 3 ml.	K. Ox.	10–20 mg. per 100 ml.
Urea clearance	Venous, 3 ml. (a); Urine, 2 successive 30–60 min. collections (b)	(a) K. Ox. (b) bottles (2)	50–100 ml. of blood cleared per min.
Uric acid, serum	Venous, 6 ml.	T	2–5 mg. per 100 ml.
Urobilinogen, urine	Single sample (a); or 24-hr. collection (b)	Refrig. bottles	(a) Detectable in urine diluted 1:8–1:32; (b) 0–3.5 mg. per 24 hrs.
Vitamin A, serum	Venous, 5 ml.	T	40–100 international units per 100 ml.
Vitamin A tolerance	Venous, 5 ml., before, and 1 hr. and 2 hrs. after test meal	T (3)	200–300 micrograms per 100 ml. serum in postprandial specimens (or 5 times the fasting level)
Vitamin B_{12} absorption	24-hr. collection	Bottle	More than 10% of labeled B_{12} excreted in 24 hrs. (Schilling)
Vitamin C (ascorbic acid), plasma	Venous, 6 ml.	K. Ox.	0.7–1.4 mg. per 100 ml.
Vitamin C tolerance	24-hr. collection	Brown bottle, refrigerated	300 mg. (30% of intravenous dose excreted in 24 hrs.)
White cell count	Venous, 5 ml. (a); capillary, 0.05 ml. (b)	(a) B. Ox. (b) MP	5,000–10,000 per cu. mm.
White cell differential count	Capillary, 0.05 ml.	Coverslips	Segmented neutrophils 55–70% Band forms 2–5% Eosinophils 1–2% Basophils 0.5–1.0% Lymphocytes 20–30% Monocytes 3–5%
Xylose (d-xylose) tolerance	5 hr. collection following test meal	Bottle	More than 5 Gm. d-xylose excreted

*T = clean, dry test tube; K. Ox. = test tube or bottle containing potassium oxalate; B. Ox. = test tube or bottle containing balanced mixture of ammonium and potassium oxalate; Cap. = glass capillary containing dry heparin; MP = micropipette.

measure of renal function. Among the compounds that have been employed for this purpose are I^{131} Diodrast, I^{131} Hypaque and I^{131} Hippuran.

Having received an intravenous injection of the compound labeled with approximately 20 microcuries of I^{131}, the patient is placed in the sitting position before a pair of radiation counters, one directed toward the right and the other toward the left kidney. Both sites are counted simultaneously and continuously for 15 to 20 minutes by recording rate meters, to permit direct comparison of the two kidneys. A peak of radioactivity appearing within a few seconds reflects the renal blood flow; a second peak, approximately 5 minutes later, coincides with active tubular transport of the dye and filling of the renal tubules with concentrated dye. In patients with unilateral renal disease, differences between the two kidneys with respect to blood flow, tubular function, or both, are clearly demonstrable by this technic.

Isotopic Localization of Renal Tumor. Neohydrin is a diuretic compound that concentrates in the kidney tubules, but does not become concentrated in tumor tissue. After intravenous injection of Neohydrin labeled with radioactive mercury (Hg^{203}), it is possible to visualize the kidneys clearly by external scanning. If a space-occupying lesion is contained within the kidney, it is readily detected because of the absence of radioactivity in the involved area and the resultant defect in the scanogram.

Isotopic Measurement of Residual Urine. Residual urine in the bladder of a patient with urethral obstruction may be measured by injecting I^{131} Diodrast intravenously then, 1 to 3 hours later, measuring the radioactivity over the bladder before and after voiding. The difference between the pre- and the post-voiding counts, (after correcting for background activity not due to bladder urine) represents the counts voided. The residual urine volume equals the volume of *urine voided* divided by the *counted voided* times the residual counts over the bladder.

BIBLIOGRAPHY AND SELECTED READING

Books

French, R. M.: Nurse's Guide to Diagnostic Procedures, New York, McGraw-Hill, 1962.

Garb, Solomon: Laboratory Tests in Common Use, New York, Springer, 1959.

Ham, T. H.: A Syllabus of Laboratory Examinations in Clinical Diagnosis, Cambridge, Mass., Harvard, 1950.

Articles

Cassidy, C. E., and Vander Laan, W. P.: Laboratory aids to diagnosis in thyroid disease, New England J. Med. **258**:828-832, 1952.

Clinical Staff Conference, National Institutes of Health: Factitious diseases, Ann. Int. Med. **48**:1328-1340, 1958.

Cotran, R. S., and Kass, E. H.: Determination of the volume of residual urine in the bladder without catheterization, New England J. Med. **259**:337-339, 1958.

Emerick, R. W., *et al.*: Diagnostic use of radioisotopes in a general hospital, J.A.M.A. **154**:493-495, 1954.

Evans, F.: The basal metabolic rate determination, Am. J. Nursing **53**:1322, 1953.

Farrar, J. T., Zworykin, V. K., and Baum, J.: Pressure-sensitive telemetering capsule for study of gastro-intestinal motility, Science **126**:975-976, 1957.

Frank, N. R., and Shedyak, A. M.: Laboratory analysis of pulmonary functions, Am. J. Nursing **56**:875-879, 1956.

Geist, D. I.: Round-the-clock specimens, Am. J. Nursing **60**:1300-1302, 1960.

Goldring, W.: Clinical application of current tests of renal function, J.A.M.A. **153**:1245-1249, 1953.

Hart, E. L., and Magee, M. J.: Collecting urine specimens, Am. J. Nursing **57**:1323-1324, 1957.

LaDue, J. S.: Laboratory aids in diagnosis of myocardial infarction, J.A.M.A. **165**:1776-1780, 1957.

Petersdorf, R. G., and Bennett, I. L., Jr.: Factitious fever, Ann. Int. Med. **46**:1039-1060, 1957.

Phillips, E. T.: Fever—its causes and effects, Am. J. Nursing **56**:319-321, 1956.

Reagan, J. W.: Cytological studies, Am. J. Nursing **58**:1693-1695, 1958.

Roswit, B., *et al.*: Evaluation of diagnostic methods in diseases of thyroid function, with particular reference to radioiodine tracer tests, Am. J. Med. Sc. **223:**229-238, 1953.

Scoggins, M. L.: Preparing patients for x-ray examinations, Am. J. Nursing **57:**76-79, 1957.

Walters, M. E.: Surgical procedures in the x-ray department, Am. J. Nursing **57:**623-624, 1957.

Weber, R. W., and Elliott, J.: Needle biopsy of the liver, Am. J. Nursing **56:**190-191, 1956.

Wright, S. W.: Phenylketonuria, J.A.M.A. **165:**2079-2083, 1957.

7

Promotion of Comfort and Relief of Symptoms

RELIEF OF PAIN AND DISCOMFORT

The treatment of pain and discomfort is of two principal types: one employing physical, and the other using pharmacologic, methods. The two methods are often used simultaneously. Included in the first category are measures for the immobilization and the positioning of the patient or a portion of his anatomy, procedures involving hot and cold applications and the provision of protective dressings. Pharmacologic methods involve the use of non-narcotic analgesic agents, which reduce the intensity of pain and discomfort; narcotics, which not only relieve pain but also induce stupor; antispasmodics, which lessen the intensity of painful smooth muscle contractions; antitussives, which tend to control cough; and antiemetics, which have the effect of relieving nausea and vomiting.

Physical Measures

Immobilization

This is important, not only as a symptomatic but also as a specific form of therapy, in patients with inflammatory lesions and those suffering pain due to an interruption of the blood supply to some local region of the body. In the latter instance, the value of immobilization is its effect in lessening the oxygen requirement of the tissue deprived of its arterial blood supply and in decreasing the production of metabolic wastes which can no longer be cleared from the area at a normal rate, due to the circulatory interference. The immobilization of

regions in which there is inflammatory disease avoids such pain-provoking stimuli as mechanical friction and local pressure. Depending on the therapeutic requirements of a particular patient, adequate immobilization may be achieved by confining the movements of a single region or it may necessitate complete bed rest.

Position

The location of a painful region in relation to the rest of the patient's body has an important bearing on the degree of discomfort. Pain originating in areas of inflammation is partially attributable to the stimulus of local pressure which, in turn, is caused by an accumulation of tissue fluid, and any increase in tissue fluid aggravates the intensity of the pain. Relief of discomfort may be brought about by placing the affected region in an elevated position, which not only facilitates the drainage of fluid via the lymph channels but also reduces its production in the inflamed area. Pain associated with acute sinusitis, tonsillitis and cervical lymphadenitis is alleviated to an appreciable degree by the adoption of the sitting rather than a horizontal position, and an infected or traumatized extremity is most comfortable when supported in a position of elevation. Position is also an important consideration in the treatment of painful joint lesions, in which the factor of local pressure (i.e., within the joint cavity) is important in relation to the severity of symptoms. Thus, the pressure of synovial fluid in an arthritic joint is minimal, and the pain is least severe in a position of semi-flexion, when the capacity of the joint cavity is greatest.

Local Heat and Cold

Hot and cold applications often contribute greatly to the relief of pain. Their effects are exerted in one of three ways: through alterations of the volume and the rate of regional blood flow; through the relief of muscle spasm; and through a decrease in pain sensitivity.

Hot applications cause a local dilatation of the superficial capillaries, arterioles and venules. As a result, the rate of blood flow in the skin and the subjacent tissues is increased greatly, often more than doubled. Capillary pressure also is increased, and there is more transudation of fluid through the capillary walls, so that more lymph is formed, and the flow of lymph in this region is accelerated. Therefore, local inflammatory swellings are prone to subside more rapidly, tissue pressure tends to become reduced, and consequently pain is alleviated in response to heat. Moreover, there is a relaxation of the painful muscle spasm which almost invariably is associated with inflammatory processes. Heating of the abdominal wall stimulates intestinal peristalsis and therefore is indicated in the treatment of patients with painful abdominal distention due to paralytic ileus (see p. 633).

Cold applications stimulate the local arterioles to constrict, thereby reducing the rate of blood flow and lymph formation in the chilled area. This may be followed by a temporary reduction of inflammatory swelling, with corresponding relief of pain. Moreover, pain sensitivity may be reduced as a result of its effect on nerve function, in which respect marked chilling acts as a local anesthetic. As a matter of fact, gentle warmth, as well as cold, if applied for prolonged periods, may also diminish pain perception. Cooling of the abdominal wall decreases peristaltic movement and is therefore an important aspect of treatment in inflammatory conditions in the peritoneal cavity which are helped by intestinal immobilization.

Hot and cold applications alike are administered most efficiently in the form of wet compresses, depending on the location and the extent of the area to be treated and the degree and the speed of temperature alteration desired. However, there are many situations in which dry heat is preferable; this is administered by an electric warming device or by heliotherapy.

Nursing Precautions. It is essential that the nurse be thoroughly familiar not only with the details of their application but also with the risks entailed and the precautions indicated in connection with each method. The danger of thermal burns from injudicious heat therapy is well known, but the risks of introducing and spreading bacterial infection by contaminated wrappings and the destructive effects of heat on ischemic tissues are equally impressive and deserve similar emphasis.

Diathermy

Surface heat, i.e., warmth applied to the skin, does not raise the internal temperature significantly beyond a depth of 1 to 2 cm., barred from further penetration by an insulating layer of subcutaneous fat, and distributed elsewhere by the circulating blood. Effective heating of deeper tissues requires the application of physical energy of a type that is capable of deep penetration and yet can be absorbed by various tissues and thereby converted into heat energy. This method of tissue heating is termed "diathermy." Two types of diathermy apparatus are now applied in physical medicine: one produces ultrasonic waves—mechanical vibrations occurring at a rate of approximately 1 megacycle per second (approximately 50 times the frequency of audible sonic waves); the other radiates ultra-high-frequency electromagnetic waves (i.e., "microwaves"). Both instruments produce heat in tissues situated 5 to 10 cm. beneath the skin surface. Owing to certain problems in the mechanics of applying diathermy, in predicting the depth and the degree of heat that it produces and in evaluating the biological effects of deep heat, its clinical use has been confined thus far to specialists in physical medicine.

Analgesics

The Salicylates

Analgesic drugs most commonly used are the salicylates, particularly acetylsalicylic acid (aspirin), administered orally in doses averaging from 0.3 to 0.6 Gm. at intervals of from 2 to 6 hours, as required. The salicylates act on the central nervous system but do not affect consciousness. These drugs are particularly useful in the treatment of pain originating in muscles, joints and other integumental structures. The effectiveness of acetylsalicylic acid in controlling the pain of traumatic injury compares favorably with that of narcotic analgesics given in moderate dosage. The degree of analgesia that is obtained and the speed with which the joints improve in patients with acute rheumatic fever receiving salicylates are truly dramatic. Indeed the anti-inflammatory effect of the salicylates is such as to suggest a specific action, or an activity comparable with that of the steroid hormones. Apart from their analgesic properties, these drugs exhibit a potent antipyretic action in many infectious illnesses and are therefore unusually efficacious in the treatment of the generalized malaise, headache and muscle and joint pain associated with fever. On the other hand, their effectiveness in controlling visceral pain is relatively slight.

Complications attending salicylate therapy are few and relatively unimportant. Excessive sweating in febrile patients may be induced to the point of discomfort equal to that of the original malaise. Dyspepsia, consisting of acid eructations and a gnawing, burning pain in the epigastrium in patients receiving aspirin, can often be related to the irritating effect of salicylates on the gastric mucosa; occasionally this irritation is sufficient to produce a severe hemorrhagic gastritis and massive hematemesis. In order to avoid gastrointestinal disturbances, these drugs should be administered after, rather than before, meals or given in combination with a buffer. Salicylates in toxic doses stimulate the respiratory center, markedly increasing the rate and the depth of respiration and producing respiratory alkalosis (see p. 400).

Acetophenetidin (Phenacetin) is an analgesic, antipyretic and antipruritic drug with an action similar to that of aspirin, and it can be substituted for the latter without difficulty in the event that a patient develops salicylate sensitivity. Definite psychological benefits are obtained with phenacetin since it produces greater relaxation in the patient and controls his restlessness more effectively than aspirin. Phenacetin, in contrast to aspirin, exerts a cumulative action and may be responsible for toxic effects after prolonged usage. One of its toxic manifestations is the reproduction and the perpetuation of the very headache for which the drug was originally taken, providing the background for the establishment of a vicious cycle.

Another non-narcotic analgesic agent contained in many proprietary remedies is *acetanilid,* a drug which is similar to phenacetin, only more toxic and without any unique merit. *Antipyrine* (phenazone), *aminopyrine* (Pyramidon) and *phenylbutazone* (Butazolidin) are structurally related compounds which produce excellent antipyretic and analgesic effects. Antipyrine and aspirin given in the same dosage are equally effective and may be substituted one for the other. Edema and eruptions occasionally develop around the nose, the mouth and the genitals as the only common complication of antipyrine therapy. Aminopyrine, although an excellent analgesic, no longer is used to any great extent, owing to its association with fatal agranulocytosis which has occurred in a small proportion of individuals receiving this drug. Phenylbutazone produces striking benefit in acute rheumatic fever, rheumatoid arthritis, spondylitis and gout, both acute and chronic. Its efficacy, however, appears to be outweighed by its potential toxicity, renal, hepatic and bone marrow damage having been attributed to this drug in an appreciable number of patients.

Opium Alkaloids and Synthetic Opiates

The group of pharmacologic agents now to be considered possess, in varying degree, analgesic, sedative and hypnotic properties. Their pain-relieving qualities are explainable almost entirely on the basis of central nervous system response, the effect of which is to inhibit not only pain perception but also other cerebral cortical functions as well, accounting for the euphoria, the excitement, the stupor and the other phenomena attending their use. All the members of this pharmacologic group are capable of causing drug habituation, an extremely serious disadvantage. On the other hand, they have provided the most efficient and reliable means known to man for the relief of pain which otherwise would be intolerable, and through their use, incalculable physical suffering has been spared.

The opium alkaloids and the derivatives of opium that are most useful as analgesics include morphine, codeine, papaveretum (Pantopon), dihydromorphinone (Dilaudid), methyldihydromorphinone (Metopon), dihydrocodeinone (Hycodan), dihydrocodeine (Rapacodin) and papaverine. Nalorphine (Nalline), another synthetic derivative of opium, is not an effective analgesic but, instead, a potent antagonist of morphine and, as such, is useful in the treatment of morphine poisoning. With this exception, all drugs in this class are alike as regards their capacity to relieve pain, the most satisfactory relief being obtained in patients with pain of a dull, sustained type, in contrast to the spasmodic, colicky variety. They share other properties as well, some of which are therapeutically advantageous; others are extremely hazardous for the patient.

The important limiting factors in their use are the production of euphoria, their addicting properties, the tolerance to their action that develops in their recipients and their depressant effect on the respiratory center which is particularly dangerous in elderly individuals, in patients with exhausting respiratory diseases and in persons who are susceptible to vascular collapse. All of these drugs tend to reduce gastric and intestinal motility; therefore, they cause anorexia and constipation. All fail to relieve smooth muscle spasm; indeed, they may promote spastic contractions in the gallbladder and the biliary ducts, an undesirable effect in biliary tract disease which is eliminated partially by the simultaneous administration of amyl nitrite or nitroglycerin. A similar effect is exerted on the renal tract musculature; in view of this, atropine or one of the belladonna substitutes is indicated as an adjunct to morphine when the latter is employed for the treatment of renal colic. The tendency of the opium alkaloids to cause addiction to their habitual use, by far the most serious defect of narcotic therapy, is discussed later in this chapter.

Morphine sulfate, or morphine hydrochloride, in adults is administered in doses ranging from 2.5 to 15 mg., depending on the route of injection, as follows: 8 to 15 mg. subcutaneously or 2.5 to 15 mg. intravenously. These doses are repeated, if required, after a minimum of 1 hour in the case of a subcutaneous injection and after no less than 20 minutes following an intravenous injection. The dosage of morphine or of any narcotic drug should be reduced below the customary therapeutic range when treating elderly, young and small patients or cases complicated by debility, exhaustion, vascular collapse, respiratory depression, cyanosis, respiratory obstruction or pulmonary edema. On the other hand, the dosage requirements are increased in patients addicted to the use of these drugs and in persons suffering intense pain.

Codeine (methylmorphine) is administered as the sulfate or the phosphate salt in doses of 16 to 60 mg., given orally or subcutaneously. The analgesic potency of codeine is less than one sixth that of morphine, and its depressant effect is less with respect to the respiratory center and other cortical functions. It is more prone than morphine to produce nausea and, instead of a sedative effect productive of stupor or coma, it may cause restlessness and mental excitement.

Pantopon, a mixture of purified opium alkaloids, contains morphine in a concentration of approximately 50 per cent and is correspondingly as effective as an analgesic. It is administered orally or hypodermically in doses averaging 20 mg.

Dilaudid (dihydromorphinone hydrochloride) is 10 times as analgesic but only 4 times as soporific as morphine. It is supplied in 2- to 4-mg. doses which may be administered orally or, when slow absorption is desired, in the form of suppositories.

Metopon (methyldihydromorphinone), usually administered orally in 6- to 9-mg. doses, is regarded as being one of the most useful of the narcotic analgesics because of its relative effectiveness when given by mouth; its unusually prolonged action, which may persist for 10 hours; the degree of analgesia it produces, which is double that of morphine; its freedom from unpleasant side-effects; and its lesser tendency to establish addiction in its users.

Hycodan, administered orally in average doses of 5 to 10 mg. per 8 hours, is prescribed most frequently as a cough suppressor. It is more effective than codeine in this regard, but is more addicting.

Synthetic Narcotics

Agents resembling morphine in chemical structure, analgesic properties and, unfortunately, in addicting tendencies, include Demerol (meperidine), Levo-Dromoran (levorphan), Dolophine (methadone) and Nisentil (alphaprodine).

Demerol hydrochloride (meperidine hydrochloride) is a synthetic drug which not only exerts analgesic and sedative properties comparable with those of morphine but also has antispasmodic activity. The latter effect is obtained in part through depression of the parasympathetic nerve endings, as in the case of the belladonna alkaloids, and partly through a direct action on the smooth muscle fibers similar to that exhibited by the synthetic substitutes of belladonna. Demerol is peculiarly effective, therefore, in treating pain associated with smooth muscle spasm. This atropinelike effect is responsible for tachycardia, as well as other unpleasant side-effects, such as dizziness, sweating, nausea and vomiting, dryness of the mouth, and, in larger doses, cardiac arrhythmias, muscular in-coordination and convulsions. Because of these complications, Demerol can be given only in relatively small, and of necessity, relatively frequent doses. Repeated administration of a narcotic predisposes to the development of tolerance, with progessive lessening of therapeutic effectiveness and increasing dosage requirements. Complications of toxicity eventually appear, forcing the abandonment of Demerol and the substitution of morphine. The most useful application of Demerol is for the relief of intermittent, severe pain caused by smooth muscle spasm, as in patients with gastrointestinal, biliary or renal colic.

Other synthetic opiates, although varying to some extent in their analgesic effect and their tendencies to produce complications, are basically alike, the pharmacologic activity of these agents, as a group, resembling that of opium and its derivatives. With the possible exception of Demerol, which appears to have certain advantages in restricted situations, none has been demonstrated to be superior in any way to the opium alkaloids.

The analgesic action of the opium alkaloids and the synthetic opiates appears to be enhanced and prolonged when these drugs are supplemented by one of the tranquilizing agents described on page 135. The principal virtue of this combination is that patients, so treated, require less medication for the relief of pain, require it less often, and therefore are less vulnerable to narcotic addiction.

Antispasmodics

Certain drugs are useful in symptomatic therapy because they reduce the amplitude and the frequency of painful spasmodic contractions of smooth muscle, in particular the muscles of the gastrointestinal, the biliary and the genitourinary tracts. These drugs include *belladonna* and its chief alkaloid, *atropine,* and synthetics *Banthine* and *Pro-Banthine,* which block the parasympathetic stimulation of smooth muscle, and the synthetic belladonna substitutes, *Novatropine, Syntropan and Trasentine,* which act predominantly on the muscle fibers themselves, inhibiting their response to nervous stimuli. These agents are effective to a variable degree as analgesics in the treatment of ureteral, biliary and gastrointestinal colic and in the treatment of dysuria due to spastic contractions of the urinary bladder. Their side-effects are less pronounced than those of the belladonna alkaloids.

Unpleasant side-effects associated with belladonna and atropine therapy include alterations of the cardiac rate. A low dosage causes bradycardia. Larger doses cause tachycardia; mydriasis, or dilatation of the pupils, with resultant photophobia; and cycloplegia, or paralysis of the ocular muscles of accommodation. Moreover, they inhibit glandular secretion, with the result that sweating and salivation are decreased or halted; their use, therefore, may be attended by dryness of the mouth and an uncomfortable sense of warmth or, in some instances, actual fever.

These antispasmodic drugs are employed as follows: *belladonna tincture* is administered as 0.3 to 0.6 ml. (5 to 10 minims), one half hour before each meal, the dose being increased progressively until an optimum therapeutic response has been obtained. *Atropine sulfate* is given orally, subcutaneously or intravenously in 0.3- to 1.0-mg. doses, 2 to 4 times daily, as indicated. *Novatropine,* 2.5 mg. orally, *Syntropan,* 50 mg. orally (or 10 mg. subcutaneously), and *Trasentine,* 75 to 150 mg. orally (or 50 to 75 mg. subcutaneously), 2 or 3 times daily, represent the usual dosage schedules for 3 of the principal synthetic substitutes of belladonna.

Antitussives

Persistent or painful cough is usually the most distressing feature of an acute pulmonary infection. Not only does it promote fatigue, through the expenditure of muscular effort, but it also interferes with recuperative rest, to the end that a debilitated patient can become dangerously exhausted. Moreover, paroxysmal coughing can cause permanent damage to lung tissue, manifested in the form of chronic bronchiectasis or pulmonary fibrosis. Measures for the control of this symptom are decidedly justified on grounds of health, therefore, as well as comfort.

Agents of many sorts have been used to suppress a cough or to modify its severity. First of the effective suppressors was opium; the usefulness of this agent, however, is limited by its addiction liability. Of the antitussives available today, the most effective still are opium derivatives, the addicting potency of which, relative to therapeutic potency, is considerably less than that of the parent drug. Codeine has been used for this purpose and to a far greater extent than any other drug. Its merits, however, are surpassed by Hycodan, for, in contrast with codeine, this drug does not suppress coughing entirely or inhibit coughing to the extent that bronchial exudates are permitted to accumulate excessively. Hycodan, 5 mg., given in the form of a sustained release complex, i.e., linked to an ion-exchange resin in combination with an antihistaminic drug (phenlytoloxamine), suppresses coughing effectively for as long as 8 to 12 hours. To secure comparable relief from codeine, the latter generally would be required in a dose of 15 mg. given every 4 to 6 hours. At this dosage level, a number of codeine side-effects are inevitable, including nausea and constipation. Although Hycodan is relatively free of symptomatic complications, it is by no means free of addiction liability, its potency, in this respect, exceeding that of codeine to a degree that corresponds to its relative superiority as a cough suppressor.

Non-narcotic cough suppressors have long been sought. One of the most promising of these agents is Toryn (caramiphen ethanedisulfonate), which is administered at 4- to 6-hour intervals in 10- to 20-mg. doses. The action of this agent is considered to be peripheral rather than central, i.e., its effect may be to reduce the tone and diminish the reactivity of skeletal muscle in response to stretch stimuli.

With the expectation of increasing the volume of, or "loosening," the bronchial secretions and thereby alleviating a "dry" cough, certain medications are often prescribed which are described as "expectorants." Such drugs include ipecac, iodide salts and ammonium chloride. Whether or not bronchial secretions are, in fact, increased or loosened by such medication is not entirely clear. *In any case, this effect, if desired, can be accomplished readily, beneficially and without side-effects by drinking a sufficient volume of fluids.* Another form of antitussic therapy consists of steam inhalations, with or without the inclusion of a medicinal agent in the boiling water. Humid air, passing over an inflamed pharyngeal mucosa, is bound to be less irritating and therefore less likely to stimulate coughing than is dry air. Finally, it should be re-emphasized that the most effective antitussics, and the ones used most widely, are narcotic agents, any of which is capable of establishing a drug addiction if its use is sufficiently prolonged. From this it follows that such an agent should be reserved for patients with acute respiratory illnesses, whose prospects for an early recovery are good, and whose therapy is intended to be of short duration.

Antiemetics

The discomfort of pain is often equaled in severity by the distress associated with nausea and vomiting. These symptoms arise from a variety of causes, and the frequency of their occurrence classifies them as among the commonest. Vomiting is produced as a result of violent, rhythmic contractions of the stomach and the intestine which have the characteristics of peristaltic waves (described on p. 569) except for their direction, which is reversed, their effect being to propel the gastrointestinal contents toward the mouth instead of toward the rectum. Sensations of nausea, whether or not accompanied by vomiting, are also stimulated by, and coincide with, reverse peristalsis. The mechanism of this reversal is directed and controlled by nerve impulses which arise in the midbrain, from the "emetic center." This center, in turn, is activated by nerve impulses from "chemoreceptors" in the brain, i.e., nerve centers which are sensitive to the presence of abnormal constituents in the circulating blood, thereby explaining the production of nausea and vomiting by emetic drugs. The emetic center also responds to stimuli from nerve centers controlling balance, which explains motion sickness.

Control of motion sickness is aided by the administration of certain drugs which act both as sedatives and histamine antagonists, for example, Benadryl (diphenhydramine), Marezine (cyclizine) and Bonamine (meclizine). Other compounds control more effectively the nausea and vomiting that is induced by such emetics as disulfiram (Antabuse) in conjunction with ethyl alcohol; drugs used in the treatment of leukemia (see p. 323); the opium alkaloids, particularly apomorphine; methadone and meperidine; chlortetracycline (Aureomycin) and oxytetracycline (Terramycin). Torecan (Thiethylperazine) has been found especially effective in postoperative nausea. Nausea and vomiting occur spontaneously in response to inflammatory lesions involving the peritoneum or the intestinal wall, lesions that obstruct the gut or interfere with the passage of its contents, emotional stress, uremia and pregnancy.

Antiemetic activity, which tends to counteract these and other nausea-provoking stimuli, is provided by "tranquilizing" drugs of the phenothiazine series. The latter, which may be administered by mouth, by injection or in the form of an anal suppository, include Thorazine (chlorpromazine) and Sparine (promazine), both prescribed in doses of 30 to 300 mg. daily. Compazine (prochlorperazine), 40 to 60 mg. daily, and Trilafon (perphenazine), 4 to 16 mg. per day, serve as powerful and versatile antiemetics, effectively controlling nausea of every variety. Unhappily, all of these agents have demonstrated a capacity to produce dangerous complications in susceptible individuals, including bone marrow depression and hepatitis; therefore, none is dispensed unless the symptomatic relief that is anticipated is deemed sufficiently important to justify the risk.

Drug Addiction

There are several drugs other than narcotics, some with predominantly sedative effect and others which provoke emotional excitement or euphoria, that are habitually self-administered by maladjusted individuals. For these individuals the drugs serve no useful purpose excepting as a means of supporting the morale, elevating the mood and generating satisfying but unrealistic fantasies, or simply as a method of relieving unpleasant emotional tension. Excepting in the case of the narcotics, discontinuance of these drugs is not followed by the development of signs or symptoms suggesting a serious physiologic disturbance, nor does their habitual use lead to a significant increase in drug tolerance on the part of the patient.

The situation in narcotic addiction is far more serious. True addiction implies not only the continuous extratherapeutic use of a drug and a psychological dependence on the drug but also a conditioning of its recipient in a manner involving organic as well as psychological functions. Proof that such conditioning has occurred is supplied by the fact that withdrawal of the drug is followed at once by a characteristic train of symptoms and signs indicating a severe derangement of the autonomic nervous system. Indeed, it is the fear of these withdrawal symptoms rather than the pleasure afforded by the narcotics that is largely responsible for the slavery of drug addiction. Moreover, addiction implies the development of tolerance. A constantly increasing dosage must be employed in order to secure comparable degrees of euphoria, emotional release and protection against abstinence symptoms. The financial burden which the addict must assume is correspondingly greater.

The narcotic drugs chiefly used by addicts in the United States are heroin, morphine and cocaine. Heroin is the most habit-forming, not only because of the unusual degree of euphoria it affords but also because of its effectiveness in relatively small dosage and the consequent ease of illicit marketing. Of all the narcotic agents, codeine, with slight euphoric effect, is the least apt to cause addiction, and most codeine addicts, of whom there are relatively few, are individuals who originally received the drug for medicinal purposes, which is in complete contrast to other types of addiction.

Narcotic addiction in the vast majority of cases is a manifestation of a serious personality defect. This is equally true, of course, as regards addiction to alcohol and other nervous system depressants, irrespective of their individual pharmacologic properties. However, because of the social, the economic, the psychological and the physiologic incapacity associated with narcotic addiction, this latter poses a problem that is incomparably more serious, from the standpoints of both therapy and prevention, than those problems which relate to other types of drug habituation. Indeed, the responsibility for the prevention of addiction to narcotics is one of the most serious that is imposed on the medical profession; for, even granting the premise that addiction is invariably founded on a psychiatric defect, the precipitating factor in its development and the initial opportunity for its active expression may be the administration of a narcotic for the relief of pain. Therefore, it must be considered a potential complication of symptomatic therapy, ever to be dreaded and guarded against with unrelenting care.

Diagnosis

Drug addiction must be suspected if a patient fails to respond in characteristic fashion to narcotic therapy when the drug is administered in its customary dosage. Dependable confirmation may be supplied if numerous scars representing multiple hypodermic puncture wounds are found. The final and conclusive demonstration of current addiction, however, is contained in the characteristic symptomatology that develops within 12 to 24 hours following the withdrawal of the drug. The sequence of events is described as follows.

Initially the patient yawns, lacrimates, sweats and exhibits rhinorrhea. His appetite then fails. Goose-flesh and muscle tremors appear. Subsequently, in severe cases, the patient becomes increasingly restless, dyspneic, febrile, loses weight, goes into vascular collapse and, unless adequate measures are taken, may die. These symptoms can be relieved effectively and promptly by a resumption of the drug, in the dosage to which the addict has become habituated; this step should be avoided wherever possible, but it may be required as a life-saving measure, particularly in the event of an intercurrent acute illness. Resumption is unquestionably the wisest expedient when the syndrome is encountered elsewhere than in a hospital provided with trained personnel and the equipment necessary to meet the problems of abstinence in narcotic addiction cases.

Treatment

The cure of drug addiction is one of the most difficult of all therapeutic accomplishments, its most complicated aspect being the psychiatric rehabilitation of the patient. Hospitalization in institutions equipped with special facilities and staffed with qualified physicians, nurses and attendants is absolutely necessary. With regard to details of procedure, there is no precise uniformity of treatment. Some therapists adhere to the practice of gradual withdrawal of the drug, while others cease its administration abruptly. Some regimens entail the temporary substitution of a narcotic with less addicting potency; others employ no substitution therapy. The routine practiced most commonly consists of abrupt and complete withdrawal of all narcotics, the ensuing abstinence syndrome being treated vigorously on a symptomatic basis. Sedation is provided by means of barbiturates, chloral hydrate, paraldehyde and warm baths. Nitrites may be administered for the relief of muscle cramps, which may be intensely severe, and parenteral fluids may be given for hydration. Exercise is encouraged to the limits of tolerance and safety. In severe cases, the advent of vascular collapse may require the temporary administration of morphine, but this device is usually unnecessary, and within 3 or 4 days subsidence of the acute manifestations may be anticipated. With recovery of his appetite, weight and strength, the patient becomes primarily a problem of psychiatric rehabilitation, for the achievement of which the basis of his psychological defect must be discovered and methods devised for its healthy compensation.*

Prevention

Narcotic drugs, if administered repeatedly over a period of 2 weeks or longer, may produce addiction in any patient, no matter how stable his personality. Patients with personality defects and emotional tensions, ambitious yet lacking in confidence, torn with irreconcilable conflicts or tortured with an inescapable sense of guilt, may find solace so complete, and the sensuous patient such euphoric pleasure in narcosis, that only a few doses of the more potent agents may suffice to induce addiction. Such individuals may become addicted to drugs endowed with relatively little addicting potency, such as codeine, or may become habituated to the use of soporific agents of any type, however innocuous. Moreover, having once enjoyed this accessible and pleasant mode of escape, they may graduate to the use of a potent narcotic and at once become enslaved.

The above facts lead to certain obvious conclusions regarding the use of narcotic drugs in symptomatic therapy. First, narcotic agents never should be prescribed except when the need is specific and compelling and it is clear that no safer substitute will suffice. Moreover, under no circumstances should their administration be continued unnecessarily, regardless of the original indications for their use. In the treatment of chronic or recurrent illnesses, such as migraine, chronic arthritis, bronchial asthma,

* Attention is called to the United States Public Health Service's addiction treatment centers at Lexington, Ky., and elsewhere.

peptic ulcer and chronic ulcerative colitis, narcotic therapy is hazardous and rarely warranted. It is unwise, under any conditions, to inform a patient concerning the specific identity, or even the character, of any drug that is prescribed, whether it is a narcotic with limited or strong potentialities for addiction or merely a benign soporific. Finally, on concluding a course of narcotic therapy which has lasted 10 days or more, the patient should be observed carefully for the symptoms and the signs of the abstinence syndrome indicative of drug addiction.

THERAPEUTIC REST

Rest, varying in degree from the mere avoidance of strenuous exertion to complete bed confinement, is one of the most important and generally applicable of all therapeutic measures. Its therapeutic virtues have long been emphasized, and it is universally prescribed as a therapeutic mainstay in symptomatic conditions of almost every type.

Therapeutic Indications. Rest may be imposed as an obvious necessity in disabling illness. In other situations, its desirability may be evident to physician and patient alike because of an obvious relationship between physical exercise and the immediate appearance of symptoms, such as fatigue and malaise in the patient with fever, or chest pain in a case of coronary artery disease. However, there are many conditions in which the virtues of rest are less obvious; in arterial hypertension, for example, symptoms may be altogether lacking, or, if present, they may appear to be completely unrelated to exertion. If this is the case, adequate restriction of activity may require powerful persuasion on the part of the attending physician, his professional assistants and the patient's family. In most patients of this type treated at home, the prescription of complete bed rest is quite unrealistic, for the importance of complete inactivity always is overshadowed in the patient's mind by the urgency of domestic situations, and it may be a practical impossibility. Under these circumstances, regardless of other therapeutic indications, hospitalization may be required for the sole purpose of securing complete and continuous physical rest.

Rest, although frequently unavoidable,

should be imposed only when its necessity is clear, for prolonged rest, irrespective of the rationale behind it, is far from benign, its potential complications corresponding to the degree and the duration of inactivity imposed.

Partial curtailment of activity, as will become evident from later discussions, is indicated in a host of conditions; with judicious planning and careful supervision, unfavorable results ascribable to rest, per se, need hardly arise. Complete bed rest, on the other hand, poses a number of very difficult problems in medical and nursing care, and associated with it are certain definite risks.

Sleep and Sedation

The most effective form of rest is sleep, indispensable for the maintenance of good health and for its restoration when impaired. The rest that is secured during the hours of sleep is incomparably more effective than that afforded by wakeful repose, however peaceful. During slumber, all bodily activity and energy expenditure are at a minimum; metabolic processes of all types are able to operate at an abated speed and with maximum economy. There is a reduction of muscular tone throughout the body; the cardiac rate and output are diminished, and peripheral resistance to blood flow decreased, so that the arterial pressure is lowered and the work of the heart materially lessened. The cells of the central nervous system also share in this respite, as demonstrated by the electroencephalogram.

Throughout the waking hours most of the metabolic processes are in active operation, even if the body is still and recumbent. It is readily understandable, therefore, why any appreciable sleep deficit must lead inevitably to a state of fatigue, muscular inefficiency and a variety of organ dysfunctions, all completely reversible, perhaps, but corrected only by sleep. It is equally obvious that sufficient sleep must be a key provision in the program of therapeutic rest, as well as one of the most important requirements of hygienic living.

Insomnia is attributable to excessive activity on the part of the cerebral cortex. Cortical stimulation sufficient to cause persistent wakefulness may originate in painful or uncomfortable sensations due, for example, to unusual cold or warmth, excessive muscle tension resulting from the adoption of an unaccustomed posture obligated, perhaps, by a mattress of faulty design, or hypermotility of the gastrointestinal tract in response to the most recent meal. Fortunately, fatigue confers a very effective immunity against all types of sensory stimuli, whether tactile, ocular, auditory or olfactory, unless other factors directly affecting the central nervous system are also operative. Those reducing the threshold of sensory perception, causing wakefulness despite profound fatigue, include anxiety, pharmacologic stimulants such as caffeine, ephedrine, codeine and the amphetamines, and organic disease of the brain, particularly cerebral arteriosclerosis.

A complaint of "insomnia" is frequent among hospital patients; no satisfactory explanation for this insomnia may be readily available in terms of physical discomfort or of anxiety. One possibility to be considered in such instances is that the patient may have been obtaining the requisite amount of sleep regularly but intermittently during each 24-hour period. Being quite rested, he is disturbed easily and therefore is unduly alert to unfamiliar sights and sounds, cerebrates actively, perhaps apprehensively, and fails to sleep. In other cases, although the total duration of each night's sleep is adequate, it is the patient's impression that he has scarcely slept because of frequent awakening through the night.

Hypnotics

In illness, drugged sleep is preferable to no sleep, inasmuch as it provides far more effective rest than does sleepless repose. A number of soporific drugs are highly effective and, at the same time, relatively innocuous; drug sedation, therefore, has become the prevailing means of combating nocturnal sleeplessness. Often the routine administration of a soporific agent is practiced advantageously to ensure restful sleep during the first few nights of hospitalization, to combat the anxiety almost invariably aroused by this unfamiliar situation or to improve the effectiveness of other symptomatic measures. Too often, however, soporifics are supplied almost as a prophylactic routine throughout the entire period of hospitalization, irrespective of the patient's actual needs. It must be recalled that drug habituation is an unpredictable risk attending the prolonged use of any sedative or soporific agent and that certain identification of those who are susceptible is impossible.

Soporific and sedatives should not be supplied automatically or indefinitely because of unconfirmed complaints of persistent insomnia. Moreover, even if there is good evidence of wakefulness despite their use, every effort should be made to correct the situation by safer and more logical methods, and their administration should be discontinued as soon as possible. A routine order by the physician, specifying that a sedative is to be given "nightly, if necessary," expresses his confidence in the judgment that will be exercised by the nurse who must decide what is, and is not, necessary. The patient's physical comfort and emotional tranquillity should be assured. Elective procedures rarely take precedence over sleep.

Disturbing noises at night should be eliminated insofar as is possible and practicable. The temperature of the room should be reduced below the daytime level. Attempts to secure muscular relaxation should be made by means of any allowable device in the armamentarium of nursing care, including a trial of the warm immersion bath, cold applications on the forehead or a back massage, adjustment of the bed frame and clothing for maximum comfort and, most important, quiet.

Soporific Drugs

The barbituric acid derivatives are by far the most commonly employed of the sedative and soporific drugs presently available. Included in this group are phenobarbital (phenylethylbarbituric acid) (Luminal), the average adult dose being 30 to 60 mg.; *Nembutal* (pentabarbital sodium), 0.1 Gm.; *Amytal,* 0.1 to 0.3 Gm.; and *Seconal,* 0.1 Gm. Phenobarbital, because of its action in depressing excess motor excitability, is also prescribed in small doses (e.g., 30 mg. 3 times daily) for the purpose of obtaining a prolonged mild sedative effect in certain types of cases. Except for habituation, which has been discussed, and the rare occurrence of drug allergy, manifested by the appearance of a morbilliform skin rash, barbiturate therapy is practically devoid of complications.

Chloral hydrate is likewise an efficient soporific. It is administered orally in aqueous solution, highly diluted because of its irritant effects on the gastric mucosa, the adult hypnotic dose being 0.5 to 1.0 Gm.

Paraldehyde, a central nervous system depressant with pharmacologic properties quite similar to those of chloral hydrate, is one of the most valuable of the soporifics because of its low toxicity and the promptness of its action. Thus, in the usual adult dosage of 4 to 8 ml., it is capable of inducing sleep within 10 to 15 minutes without preliminary excitement and without residual side-effects. Although customarily given by mouth, this drug is suitable for intramuscular injection and is employed in doses as high as 20 or 30 ml. for the parenteral sedation of patients who are maniacal or experiencing acute toxic delirium. Its prinicpal disadvantage is its pungent persistent odor and its burning disagreeable taste.

THE PATIENT IN PAIN
Principles of Nursing Management

1. Evaluate the quality, intensity and duration of the pain.
   A. Determine the time sequence of the pain.
   B. Ascertain if the pain is related to an activity (eating, moving, etc.).
   C. Ask the patient to localize the site of pain.
2. Note the patient's behavior and reaction to pain.
   A. Observe for evidences of disparity between pain intensity and patient's physical appearance.
   B. Note the circumstances under which pain occurs.
   C. Listen and record the patient's descriptions of his pain sensations.
3. Attempt to determine what the pain signifies to the patient.
   A. Accept the behavior of the patient.

B. Observe and listen for evidences of fear and anxiety.

C. Listen with empathy and patience to complaints.

D. Develop a therapeutic relationship with the patient.

4. Prevent the occurrence of pain.

A. Relieve any evidences of pressure.

B. Ascertain if the patient has a full bladder.

C. Use measures to relieve intestinal distention.

D. Encourage the patient to turn and move frequently.

E. Maintain the patient in correct physiological positions.

5. Promote the general comfort of the patient.

A. Handle the patient carefully and gently.

B. Ensure general body warmth and relaxation.

C. Relieve hunger and thirst.

D. Relieve sensations of itching and burning.

E. Promote a therapeutic environment (temperature, ventilation, visitors).

F. Massage the patient's back.

G. Offer diversional activities.

6. Support the patient during painful diagnostic procedures and treatment.

A. Give a clear and adequate explanation to the patient.

B. Enlist the patient's cooperation during the procedure.

C. Teach the patient how to cope with his pain (deep breathe, immobilize parts).

D. Observe for untoward physical reactions.

E. Keep the patient informed of the progress of the examination or procedure.

F. Praise the patient for his participation.

G. Make the patient comfortable after a painful ordeal.

7. Relieve localized pain.

A. Elevate edematous or painful extremities.

B. Handle painful parts with care.

C. Apply heat, cold and counterirritants as indicated.

D. Encourage patient to participate in prescribed exercise program.

8. Administer agents to relieve pain when indicated.

A. Use specific drugs for the relief of nausea and vomiting.

B. Give ataractic agents to relieve anxiety.

C. Apply local anesthetics as indicated.

D. Give soporifics to induce sleep.

E. Administer muscle-relaxant drugs and antispasmodics.

F. Give analgesic drugs for more intense pain.

G. Evaluate patient for signs of hypersensitivity, respiratory depression and toxic effects.

BIBLIOGRAPHY AND SUGGESTED READING

Books

Crowley, D. M., *et al.:* Pain and Its Alleviation, U.C.L.A. (School of Nursing), 1962.

Nordmark, M. T., and Rohweder, A. W.: Science Principles Applied to Nursing, pp. 171-180, Philadelphia, Lippincott, 1959.

Articles

Beckman, H.: Expectorants, J.A.M.A. **167:** 1638-1639, 1958.

Conference on Therapy: Treatment of cough, Am. J. Med. **14:**87-98, 1953.

Editorial: On muscular cramps, J. Chron. Dis. **1:**100-102, 1955.

Fraser, H. F., and Grider, J. A.: Treatment of drug addiction, Am. J. Med. **14:**571-577, 1953.

Hunter, J.: The mark of pain, Am. J. Nursing **61:**96-99, Oct., 1961.

Isbell, H., and White, W. M.: Clinical characteristics of addictions, Am. J. Med. **14:**558-565, 1953.

Knapp, P. H.: Drugs and the doctor; some aspects of addiction in general medicine, Boston M. Quart. **3:**110-115, 1952.

Knudson, A. B. C.: Physical medicine and rehabilitation: effectiveness and progress in restoration of the chronically ill and aging, Ann. Intern. Med. **48:**139-145, 1958.

Newberry, W. B., Jr.: Sedatives have their place, but . . . , Am. J. Nursing **57:**1285-1286, 1957.

Report to the Council: Precautions regarding salicylates, including aspirin, J.A.M.A. **158:** 831, 1955.

Schwan, H. P.: The biophysical basis of physical medicine, J.A.M.A. **160:**191-197, 1956.

Solomon, P.: Insomnia, New England J. Med. **255:**755-760, 1956.

Townsend, E. H., Jr.: Prolonged cough suppression, New England J. Med. **258:**63-67, 1958.

Vaisrub, S.: Nocturnal disorders of medical interest, Ann. Intern. Med. **35:**323-330, 1951.

Wikler, A., and Rasor, R. W.: Psychiatric aspects of drug addiction, Am. J. Med. **14:** 566-570, 1953.

8

Psychological Considerations

Portions of this chapter were contributed by
RACHEL BLISS, R.N., M.A.
Assistant Professor of Nursing,
University of Illinois, College of Nursing

EFFECTIVE NURSE-PATIENT INTERACTION

Most students enter nursing at least in part because of a sincere feeling of kindliness toward people and a real desire to help them when they are sick. This kindliness usually is carried into the clinical situation, and an attempt is made to apply it to patient care. Sometimes students are confused because their efforts to help patients do not seem to bring forth the results that they anticipate or may even precipitate undesirable reactions.

Although kindness is a necessary quality, it alone cannot always assure the nurse the result that she seeks. To be an effective tool, kindness must be reinforced with knowledge. It must have direction based on scientific principles.

For instance, the nurse who succumbs to the patient's request to bathe him, when the physician's order permits him to bathe himself, may be doing him an actual disservice. The exercise utilized for this activity may be an essential therapeutic requirement for this patient's recovery from his illness.

A common misconception among nurses (and students) is that meeting the emotional needs of patients is always time-consuming and frequently difficult to accept as an added responsibility to an overloaded patient assignment.

Actually, well-directed attention to the psychological needs of the patient can be time and energy saving for both patient and nurse. It can result in better cooperation on the part of the patient in therapeutic procedures; it can relieve tension and anxiety in the patient, promoting his recovery or adding to his comfort. It can free the nurse of the anxiety created by feelings of frustration and inadequacy caused by negative responses from patients and permit her the confidence necessary for effective nursing.

How much and what kind of knowledge regarding the patient's psychology (and her own) does the nurse need in order to give care to the ill patient? This question can probably best be answered by defining a psychological component of good nursing: effective nurse-patient interaction.

From a psychological point of view, there must be, in good nursing, the kind of nurse-patient interaction that will be conducive to an environment in which the patient is most likely to respond to the therapeutic program of the physician and that will most effectively help the patient get well (or feel better) mentally and/or physically.

This kind of nurse-patient interaction, the kind in which nurses meet the emotional as well as the physical needs of patients, does occur without benefit of specific psychological or psychiatric training. However, skill in such interaction usually occurs more rapidly and more consistently with the identification and the study of the prinicples involved. Marion Kalkman says:

A child who plays with a box of paints splashes color haphazardly, but a student of art learns the value of each color and chooses them purposefully in order to create something beautiful. So the nurse will learn to use purposefully those techniques which are most effective and beneficial to her patient. Too long have nurses muddled through their personal contacts with their patients without really knowing how to manage the psychological problems that arise. This lack of knowledge has earned nurses the undeserved reputation of being hard or unsympathetic toward their patients.*

Miss Kalkman made these statements with reference to psychiatric nursing, but they apply equally to all other clinical areas. Any time a nurse meets an emotional need of a patient she is, in essence, doing psychiatric (or psychological) nursing.

The nurse who is asked to give an enema to a patient surely would not merely collect her equipment, carry it to the bedside and perform the procedure. She would first tell her patient what she was going to do and why she was going to do it. We would also expect her to screen her patient or take whatever measures were necessary to ensure his privacy. Then she would likely talk to him while performing the procedure, checking on his comfort or giving him reassurance about his illness, as indicated. All of these measures constitute psychological aspects of nursing care.

Appreciation of Behavioral Motivation

The nurse must understand the *fundamental dynamics of behavior* in order to understand *motivations* for her patient's behavior. Understanding *why* the patient behaves as he does is frequently necessary in order for the nurse to accept the patient's behavior with a nonjudging attitude; it always adds to the degree of accuracy with which she can evaluate her patient's needs.

For the person untrained in the skills of human relations, there is sometimes a tendency to think of "needs" in purely physical terms, that is, in terms of the need for food, clothing, shelter and the like. Study of the total person quickly reveals the inadequacy of this procedure. It is common knowledge that if two patients are provided with identical care, they will respond differently to it.

* Kalkman, M. E.: Introduction to Psychiatric Nursing, New York, McGraw-Hill, 1950.

In order to understand this phenomenon, it is necessary to have a basic familiarity with the derivation of individual human behavior patterns.

It is assumed that by the time the student begins her first clinical nursing experience she will have had at least one course with content concerning human growth and development. From this experience she will know that the human infant enters this world with a biologic endowment unique to him. She will also know that in the maturation process physical, sociocultural and psychological influences interact to determine the possible development of his potential and to shape his personality. The newborn infant is quite a helpless creature. Both his physical and emotional needs are many for actual survival. The growth process follows a more or less orderly pattern. For convenience of study, it is usually divided into stages of development which, to a degree, correspond to chronologic age ranges. During each stage the child is confronted with specific developmental problems which require some kind of resolution. The quality of this resolution has an effect, either positive or negative, on character structure. It is felt to be determined by the interaction of the previously mentioned influences and their action on his biologic endowment. If, for instance, early dependency needs are not adequately met, the child will not develop an immunity to such needs. Unless corrective experiences occur, he will enter each subsequent stage of development with a deficiency that snowballs, producing an adult whose dependency needs are literally insatiable. Strengths and weaknesses in his capacity to adapt to the stress of illness will reflect his life experiences and his consequent pattern of adaptation.

Much has been written in psychiatric nursing literature defining a therapeutic environment for the mentally ill. Such an environment is usually described as one which endeavors to fulfill basic human needs: the need for acceptance, respect, recognition, security and the like; the need for a comfortable degree of self-esteem. The physically ill patient will respond no less beneficially to such an environment. Regardless of adaptive capacity, all patients—the most flexible patients—will manifest these needs to the observing nurse.

An individual, in the process of daily living, has the ever-present job of integrating the demands of his instinctive desires, his self-controlling force (conscience) and the world of reality to which he is exposed. Inherently, he strives for comfort (physical and emotional) and attempts to ward off discomfort. In his efforts toward this end he uses psychological technics which seem to fall into patterns of behavior called mental mechanisms. These mechanisms are employed by the mentally healthy as well as by the mentally sick. They reduce the tension of internal conflict and save psychic energy. For instance, a student may say (and feel) that a low grade that she received on an examination was the result of a headache which she had at the time she took the examination, which reduced her efficiency. Her explanation of the low grade may be completely accurate. Another equally accurate explanation for her performance may be that she did not study adequately for the examination. There may have been other relevant factors involved. The student selected the one of several causative factors which she could tolerate without undue anxiety. The mechanism is called *rationalization*. It is usually used unconsciously and is usually harmless to the psychological functioning of the individual.

Mechanisms employed vary in both degree and kind and, dependent on such use, may be normal or pathologic. The determining factor is whether or not the particular pattern of behavior is a realistic effort toward problem solving or one that denies and distorts reality. The patient who refuses the medication which the doctor has ordered for him because he feels that he does not need it may be using the mechanism of *denial*. It can be pathologic and destructive to him. It may offer him temporary relief from the anxiety created by the need to accept his illness, but it can interfere with his capacity to cooperate in the therapeutic plan formulated for him and with the ultimate success of treatment.

Interpretation of Aberrant Behavior

The nurse must develop *skills of observation* in order to see, hear and even "feel" patient's needs which may not be expressed overtly (or may be camouflaged). She must be able to coordinate her impressions about the patient derived from these sources and note consistencies or inconsistencies in her patient's behavior. She must know that behavior involves more than merely action, that it also involves a person's thoughts and emotions.

Mr. Brown's irritability surprised Miss Smith, the sophomore nursing student assigned to give him morning care. She had been assigned this patient on previous days, and he had been pleasant and friendly. She thought that her approach had been the same this morning, but he responded to her "Good morning" with, "Don't bother me! I don't want a bath! Can't people ever leave you alone around here? I need some sleep!" This change frightened Miss Smith. As she continued to collect the equipment necessary for his bath, she noticed that her patient looked more tired than he had when she had seen him on previous days. His face looked drawn and tense. His eyes lacked their usual luster. She said, "You look tired this morning, Mr. Brown. Didn't you sleep well last night?" He replied, "How well do you think you would sleep if the doctor told you that you'd have to stay in bed for six more weeks? I've got a wife and three kids to support. My oldest girl is in college. What are they supposed to do for money while I'm lying here? I don't have that much sick-time coming on my job." Miss Smith asked, "When did Dr. Jones tell you about this, Mr. Brown?" He said, "He came in about 7:30 last night; he told me then."

It is important that the nurse learn to realize what illness means to the patient. She can increase her understanding of the patient's problem by observing him carefully and then by interpreting her observations in the light of her knowledge of human behavior.

The Nurse's Emotional Responses

The nurse must *understand her own reactions and how they affect her patients*. Up to this point an attempt has been made to give a brief overview of the development and the dynamics of behavior. Human nature is kind and protective of us. It permits us to view the behavior of other people analytically and critically, with generally little personal anxiety. To look at our own reactions objectively is less easy for us. However, it is a necessity for effective nursing.

As we learn about human development and the dynamics of behavior, we become more aware of our own needs and those of others. When this occurs, we learn to differentiate between the two, to evaluate each more objectively and to handle each more effectively. Without this differentiation, it is impossible to appraise accurately the needs of another person because they are then seen through the eyes of our own experiences and attitudes. The appraisal *must* be based on the facts of the other person's experiences, from which his needs are derived.

The concept of objectivity in evaluation of patient needs is not too difficult to understand. The philosophy of patient care on which the concept is based is readily acceptable to most students. However, performance in nursing based on the concept will be exceedingly difficult if the acceptance is intellectual only. It must also become a part of the emotional make-up of the student.

Miss White, a nursing student, tried to get her patient to accept his morning bath. His refusal, on the grounds that he had had one on the previous day and did not feel in need of another, did not discourage his nurse. She tried repeatedly to convince him that the bath would make him feel better. The patient's resistance confused Miss White no less than her insistence irritated him. After all, a daily bath does make one feel better. She knew this from personal experience. But was this also his experience? Had he not for fifty-odd years been comfortable with taking a weekly bath, making the more frequent ones seem a nuisance to him? Was the student's plea for cleanliness on the basis of comfort consistent with his experience? Might the student, consciously or unconsciously, have been guided by a desire to please her superior with a completed assignment, as well as by a consideration of her patient's welfare?

Miss Jones was a conscientious, capable student. Past performance had given repeated evidence of these characteristics. She always completed her assignment and frequently found time to offer help to fellow students. This morning she had less than usual to do because one of her patients was off the ward having some special tests in another department of the hospital. Somehow, in spite of these circumstances, Miss Jones "just didn't get to" Mr. Green, the last patient on her assignment. In fact, she was not quite sure why she had decided to give him his care last. Her other patients were less ill than he, and she was in the habit of caring for her sicker patients first. Mr. Green had cirrhosis of the liver. Miss Jones was present when he was admitted to the hospital. He was emaciated, dirty and in a state of confusion. Miss Jones was told that the latter condition was due to delirium tremens and caused by excessive drinking of alcohol. She had an uncle who was an alcoholic. She had heard her mother say that he sometimes had "DT's," and she knew it would someday be the end of him. Her mother was always irritable when this uncle came to visit.

Patient behavior that conflicts with the student's moral code or cultural values is frequently very difficult for her to handle. Acceptance of it is allied with condoning or commending the behavior. Only knowledge that it is the result of his life experiences, and currently necessary to him, can help the student to view it objectively.

The "Difficult" Patient

Occasionally the student will encounter a patient who seems to defy all her efforts to please him. She may notice that his pillow has slipped, so that his chin is resting on his chest, and will fluff and replace it in an obviously more comfortable position, only to hear him say, "When are you going to get out of here?" She may give him an injection of a medication for relief of pain and say, "I hope you will soon be feeling better," only to hear him grunt and mutter something about the doctors and the nurses liking to see him suffer. Such responses from patients will be only too familiar to the experienced nurse. In spite of the fact that such patient reactions are greatly in the minority, when they do occur they can be quite devastating to the student (or to the experienced nurse).

Obviously, all patients (and all people) do not always feel like being pleasant. Consistent ill-humor is another matter. It is important that the student learn to distinguish between the two. It is important that she evaluate carefully negative (as well as positive) responses from patients. A negative response may be the result of a deficiency on the part of the nurse in evaluating, and consequently meeting, the patient's needs; it may be the result of a momentary low point (for any reason) in the patient's ability to be pleasant; it may be due to the characteristic disposition of the patient, which is most accurately described as "ornery."

The previous discussion of behavior development should suffice to imply that it is unlikely that any person is born with an unpleasant disposition, even though constitutional differences are evident at birth. It seems unnecessary to doubt that life experiences are influential in shaping one's characteristic pattern of behavior. If we can assume that this is true, and a particular patient with whom we come in contact has been so unfortunate as to have had experiences resulting in the formation of such a personality pattern, and this pattern of behavior has developed over a period of whatever number of years he may have lived, is it not then unrealistic to assume that we should be able to change his characteristic responses in a matter of a few minutes, hours or days?

The above behavior has been described not to remove from the student any responsibility for dealing with such situations in a positive fashion, or to condone unkind treatment of her patient, but in an attempt to help her construct a therapeutically effective approach to such a problem.

This kind of situation tends to create a vicious cycle. The patient responds negatively; the conscientious student feels that she must be inadequate as a nurse or she should somehow be able to please him; feeling inadequate lowers her self-esteem and makes her uncomfortable; she dislikes being uncomfortable and, in retaliation, attacks the patient (the source of her discomfort) by consciously or unconsciously rejecting him.

It is probably a valid generalization to say that unpleasant people are unhappy, lonely people. For all people illness is a time of stress. Stress from any cause is anxiety provoking. The stress of illness is sometimes extreme, bringing on fears of loss of economic security, disability, body mutilation, death or numerous other individualized fears.

Fear and anxiety provoked by illness are difficult enough for the person who has previously received much gratification from living. For the person for whom life, prior to his illness, has been a more or less unhappy experience, the added stress and associated fears of illness can be overwhelming.

It can provoke in the person a state of near panic, which, in turn, can manifest itself in behavior that is an exaggeration of the patient's usual more or less unpleasant behavior. No patient so desperately needs understanding acceptance as does such a patient; no patient is less able to show appreciation for kindness received.

The student who has learned to recognize her patient's behavioral capacity, and can accept her role in the situation without demanding immediate gratification for her efforts, will show evidence of much professional growth.

Patient Dependency

Sometimes the student who has handled the situation with judgment and skill encounters yet another problem if contact with her patient has been a fairly long or consistent one. Her very skill in caring for him may bring him the gratification so sadly lacking in his experience. As a result of this more pleasant experience, he may be reluctant to break this relationship when the student must leave him for another assignment. Two important questions arise. First, has the student erred (in spite of her good intentions) by permitting such a relationship to develop? Second, might she have permitted her patient the benefits of the relationship and at the same time avoided (or lessened) for him the trauma of separation?

In answer to the first question, one might paraphrase a familiar quotation and say: " 'Tis better (for this patient) to have had loving nursing care and lost it than never to have had it at all." The nurse who has been able to promote in such a patient a relationship of mutual respect and confidence may have provided him with as essential an ingredient for his recovery as any medication his doctor might prescribe.

So often meaningful, therapeutic relationships with patients are discouraged on the grounds that the patient will become too emotionally dependent on the student. She is advised against getting "emotionally involved" with her patients. Undeniably, there are hazards in such relationships. Chief of the hazards is that the involvement may become uncontrolled and consequently destructive to both student and patient.

It is a first consideration, and of utmost importance, that the student understand that the relationship is a therapeutic tool and as such must be used with purpose and direction. It can then be an invaluable tool.

The problem of dependency is a highly complex one. Unfortunately, there is a connotation of pathology in the very use of the word. Inherently, we all have dependent, as well as independent, strivings. Imbalance in the relationship of the two can be pathologic and, if so, may then need to be handled under the guidance of the specially trained therapist.

In such situations as the above, the problem of healthful human interaction is frequently one of greater *immediate* concern than that of dependency. As previously stated, a characteristic pattern of unpleasant behavior on the part of a patient tends to provoke rejection of him and thus reinforce his previous experience. He needs a positive interpersonal relationship in order to lessen feelings of loneliness and despair. In order to be motivated to get well, he needs to feel that someone really cares whether or not he gets well; that the world is not such a bad place after all; that if he can have one satisfying relationship, perhaps he can have more. He needs to have rekindled the fire of interpersonal response.

The student can usually give her patient the benefits of such a relationship with minimal or no negative effects if she is guided in her approach by two important principles: (1) The limitations of her contacts with him must be defined early in the relationship, and he must be reminded of them at intervals; and (2) other persons must be introduced into the situation gradually so that the termination of services by the student will leave no major gap in his experience.

If the situation permits, the student should tell her patient on her first contact with him how often and for what period of time she will be giving him nursing care. Such information tells the patient the amount of care that he may anticipate from her. If her assignment should be changed before the expected termination, or if she should need to be absent for any reason during the period of assignment, the patient should be informed as well in advance as possible. Honesty and consistency in the relationship promote trust.

If the patient obtains satisfaction from the care he receives, he may have difficulty remembering that it must end on a given date, even though he has been told. The student should occasionally take the opportunity to remind him tactfully of this fact.

If a student has been so skillful as to develop in her patient a degree of trust in her, he will be more inclined than previously to respond to others. This will be particularly true if the student conveys to him her trust in the third person. Obviously, the same criteria for success in a relationship with the patient will hold true for all who attempt it. However, it is important that the patient be encouraged to develop a rapport with as many other people as he can tolerate, so that the removal of any one person will not destroy the consistency of his experience.

Here, again, the student will need to look critically at her own reaction in the situation. Success with the patient will bring her justifiable gratification and pleasure. She should enjoy the experience, recognizing that her own need for gratification is normal, but that it must not interfere with her efforts to help her patient transfer the confidence he has gained from her to other people. If she is able to perform in this manner, she will promote growth in both her patient and herself.

Nursing Support

The student must communicate *warmth, interest in her patient and confidence in herself as a nurse and as a person.* Although some special problems have been highlighted because they tend to be particularly difficult, by far the great majority of patients will be receptive to the student's efforts if the nursing care that she offers them is thoughtful and sincere.

For the average patient, hospitalization is a relatively infrequent and therefore strange experience. It usually involves many unknowns, including those of the environment, the personnel and the illness. The patient enters the situation from one in which he felt the security of familiar surroundings and familiar people. Prior to the onset of the illness which brought him to the hospital, he may have had no physical symptoms to cause him concern. Reinforcing his apprehension is his feeling that the situation is all out of his control, rendering him at the mercy of the medical and nursing staffs. He is dependent on them, and he knows it. Generally, he is somewhat weary from the strain of illness and is glad to relinquish control if he has confidence in those who are responsible for his care. He hopes that they will give him competent care, that they will not make too many demands on him and that they will be tolerant of his weaknesses.

How can the student let the patient know that she is interested in him and wants to help him? The ways are many and will need to vary according to the student's personality and that of her patient. The pat on the hand that will be welcomed by one patient and indicate acceptance and reassurance to him may be quite upsetting to another. The latter patient might interpret the gesture as "babying" him, implying that he is not the man he would like to think himself to be. Patting a patient on the hand may come as a spontaneous expression of warmth and empathy from one student; it might make another feel very self-conscious and awkward. The patient will know the difference, and he will feel uncomfortable in the latter situation. Generally, it may be preferable to avoid touching the patient, as unnecessary bodily contact is sometimes anxiety provoking, stimulating sexual or dependency feelings. The many other methods of expressing warmth and interest include such gestures as giving the patient an understanding glance or a kind word, adjusting a lamp or a window shade so that light will not shine in his eyes, getting him fresh drinking water, etc. Interest is communicated by skillfully evaluating and meeting the patient's needs. The student who reads to her patient while he has pain that might be within her control to lessen or eliminate will make the patient feel that she neither understands his needs nor cares about him.

Interest in a patient is communicated by undivided attention, perhaps for a moment, perhaps for an hour or more—but undivided. Physical proximity helps little if the face is turned toward the patient while the eyes wander and the ears are closed.

Sometimes students contribute considerably more to the patient's emotional comfort than they can recognize.

Miss Gray, a nursing student, spoke to her instructor about her feeling of inadequacy while caring for Mrs. Green, a terminally ill cancer patient: "I just felt terrible. She kept wanting to know if I thought she was going to die. I didn't know what to say. Actually, I didn't say much of anything; I pulled a chair up to her bed and sat down and let her talk. I knew that I had to get my other patients finished, and the phone kept ringing, but I didn't let her know. I just stayed with her. She talked for quite a while and then she fell asleep. I guess that was good, because she's had trouble sleeping."

It is possible that a narcotic might have been less effective in producing sleep for this patient. The student's undivided attention may have given the patient not only the opportunity to express her fears but also may have relieved somewhat the feeling of loneliness that often is a part of the great anxiety of severe illness. The student may have afforded the patient the relief of tension and consequent relaxation necessary for sleep.

PSYCHOPHARMACOLOGY

The administration of a drug with the specific intention and reasonable expectation of normalizing the mood of an anxious, hostile or depressed patient reflects an important advance in the field of pharmacology and constitutes a new departure in psychotherapy. Prior to 1940, chemotherapy in psychiatry was limited almost entirely to the use of sedatives and soporifics (p. 124) to suppress anxiety, limit overactivity and induce sleep. Subsequently, a number of agents have been developed which have their predominant effects on the central nervous system, modifying emotional reactions and coloring mood without inducing sleep or otherwise interfering with cerebral function. Several of these agents have since been marketed and prescribed on a stupendous scale, some for their excitatory, others for their mollifying, action. Drugs in the first category are the so-called "psychic energizers" employed extensively in treating depressive states, fortifying abstinence in alcoholism and curbing the appetite of the obese. The second group, representing the "tranquilizers," comprises a large assortment of drugs which are designed to quell emotional turbulence and to alleviate anxiety. Men of ancient Greece called their tranquilizers (wine, women and song) "ataractics," from *atarax,* meaning "peace of mind." Our tranquilizers, in modern medical parlance, are the "ataractic" drugs. More than 50,000,000 prescriptions for peace pills have been issued in a single year.

Tranquilizing Agents

Ataractic therapy aims to restore emotional balance to the distraught patient without putting him to sleep, reducing his energy, or impairing his mental faculties, his judgment or his motor coordination, and without introducing organic complications or risking drug addiction. Of the many ataractics now available, none achieves this objective in its entirety. Side-effects which occur most frequently, and of which the nurse should be aware, include anorexia, gastrointestinal dysfunction, chronic fatigue, visual disturbances, drowsiness, muscular in-coordination, tremors, dermatitis and menstrual irregularity. Drug tolerance, evidenced by declining effectiveness and rising dosage requirements, is acquired by many patients, a fact which carries the disturbing implication that drug habituation may constitute a risk that is inherent in this type of chemotherapy. Bone marrow function may be disturbed and resistance to infection impaired as the price of tranquility.

Ataractic drugs which are known to be efficacious and comprise the vast majority of tranquilizers in current use belong to 1 of 4 categories: (1) rauwolfia (Raudixin) and the rauwolfia alkaloids, including reserpine (Serpasil, Reserpoid, Sandril or Serpiloid), rescinnamine (Moderil) and deserpidine (Recanescine, Raunormine and Harmonyl); (2) the phenothiazine compounds, including chlorpromazine (Thorazine), promazine (Sparine), prochlorperazine (Compazine), perphenazine (Trilafon), thiopropazate (Dartal), mepazine (Pacatal), fluphenazine (Permitil; Prolixin), trifluoperazine (Stelazine) and thioridazine (Mellaril); (3) the benzhydrol compounds, pipradrol (Meratran), azacyclonol (Frenquel), benactyzine (Suavitil) and hydroxyzine (Atarax); and (4) the Propanal derivatives, mephenesin (Tolserol) and meprobamate (Miltown or Equanil).

Ataractic drugs have been used with varying reports of success in the management of all varieties and gradations of psychic overactivity and psychoneurosis, from simple emotional grief, neuromuscular tension states and psychosomatic disturbances, at one end of the spectrum, to frank manifestations of severe psychoses, at the other. The relative merits of the individual drugs in treatment of specific disorders are not yet fully established. In general, considering the group as a whole, the most satisfactory results have been experienced by anxious patients with tension headaches and backaches, who are restless, irritable, fatigued and unable to sleep. The ataractics have been used with notable success in the "normalizing" of patients who are anxious for no apparent cause, whose anxiety is mounting in severity and who appear to be approaching a psychotic break. Regardless of the nature of the therapeutic indications, none of these agents should be employed excepting under close clinical observation. None is completely devoid of risk, and self-medication with any one of these invites serious trouble.

Among the complications that have attended the use of the Rauwolfia alkaloids have been mental depression, convulsive seizures and various autonomic disturbances, such as bradycardia, flushing, nasal congestion, salivation, vomiting, diarrhea and hypotension with syncope. Undesirable side-effects of the phenothiazine compounds include tachycardia, dryness of the mouth and vivid dreams. More dramatic complications are transient extrapyramidal disorders characteristic of parkinsonism (page 949), jaundice (page 649) and convulsive seizures. One drug in this group (thioridazine) has been responsible for pigmentary retinopathy, accompanied by temporary visual impairment and brownish coloring of vision. Most serious of all are certain blood dyscrasias, notably leukopenia (page 470), thrombocytopenia (page 476) and anemia, which may be produced by any of the ataractic drugs in current use.

One important fact relating to the use of tranquilizers must be realized by the nurse: Ataractic chemotherapy provides temporary relief from certain unpleasant emotional disturbances, but its action is not curative, and as a symptomatic device it is no more than a temporary expedient. The patient's real problem, of which the symptoms are merely an expression, is not resolved or even simplified by their amelioration. If these symptoms are of such severity as to render the patient helpless, confused or incapable of attacking the basic problem constructively, symptomatic relief is a worthwhile objective, not only because of the comfort which it affords, but also because of the opportunity which it may provide for investigation and correction of the underlying disturbance. Tranquilizer therapy, administered solely as a comfort measure, without regard for the underlying situation, is not truly helpful, may be harmful and is usually unwarranted.

Awareness of tension, sensations of anxiety and reactions of grief are natural phenomena experienced by all normal individuals. When reactions such as these occur without apparent justification or with inexplicable intensity, some psychological aberration should indeed be suspected. Barring the exceptional case, however, these experiences, though painful, are to be construed as being normal, not pathologic, manifestations, which are of value, not detrimental, to the sufferer. Relief from emotional tension is the goal that motivates the individual in most of his activities and compels the solution of problems which, but for tensions and stress, would remain unsolved. Relief of tension, supplied with no effort and no accomplishment, but with pills, produces a cheap brand of tranquility, a type that is worthless to the normal individual and a threat to his welfare.

Psychic Energizers

Another form of psychochemotherapy is exemplified by Dexedrine (d-amphetamine) and Marsilid (iproniazid). These drugs exert a stimulating effect on cerebral function, their excitatory action being used to advantage in treating depressive states, controlling petit mal attacks (Chap. 41) and combating withdrawal symptoms in drug addicts. Their many other applications will be considered elsewhere in the text rather than in this section.

Depending on the dose ingested, and the tolerance of the individual who ingests this drug, all degrees of nervous excitation may be produced by Dexedrine. A small dose, e.g., 2.5 mg., causes barely detectable elevation of mood, a sense of alertness and increased energy and an improved ability to concentrate. A 5- to 15-mg. dose may induce definite euphoria (disproportionate sense of well-being); insomnia for several hours, regardless of fatigue; manifestations of increased tension and overactivity; and loss of appetite. Given in doses exceeding the therapeutic range, Dexedrine induces manifestations of severe anxiety and confusion, exaggerates abnormal patterns of behavior and may precipitate hallucinations or even convulsions.

The excitatory, energizing effects of Dexedrine or Marsilid are the antitheses of those produced by the tranquilizers, yet both types of agent serve as psychological restoratives. The therapeutic value of the tranquilizers resides in their capacity to relax tension, eliminate panic and resolve confusion, thereby favoring concentrated, orderly and constructive thought processes. Dexedrine and Marsilid, used in their proper role, combat depression effectively by quickening and diversifying thought processes which have become obsessive or repetitive.

Used in the absence of proper indications, or without benefit of close supervision, tranquilizers and energizers alike are a distinct hazard to mental health. The artificial creation of moods that are divorced from reality, by means that are independent of the normal psychological mechanisms, too often serves as a pleasant diversion, indulgence in which can lead to drug dependency and eventual disintegration of the personality.

PATIENTS WITH MENTAL AND EMOTIONAL PROBLEMS

The nurse will encounter patients with all degrees of emotional health or illness in the nursing siuation. Neurosis provides the person with no immunity to physical ills, nor does psychosis. No attempt will be made to speculate on percentages of patients whose emotional state would place them in the category of mentally healthy or neurotic. Perhaps each of us manifests some neurotic symptomatology at some time.

The far greater percentage of patients will vary from the very stable personality (in terms of rather abstract norms) to patients with varying degrees of behavior deviations.

While recognizing that some exaggeration of behavior patterns is normal for all people under the stress of illness, it is necessary that the student be alert to rapid or unusual changes in the behavior of her patient. Such changes may be indicative of an alteration in the mental or physical condition of the patient which may require some change in therapy and should be reported immediately to the nurse in charge or to the doctor.

The Patient with Acute Anxiety

The problems involved in the care of the acutely apprehensive patient can be as complex as any that confront the professional nurse. When an anxiety state develops in the course of an organic disease, the symptoms of the latter may be grossly distorted, compounding the difficulty of diagnosis and treatment; the confidence and the morale of a patient are undermined, and his cooperation may be lost. Vital physiologic processes, too, are affected, anorexia often interfering with nutrition, and insomnia with rest.

Diagnosis

An anxiety state may be suspected and its severity evaluated on the basis of certain observations which are familiar to those in constant association with ill patients. The correct interpretation of these manifestations is obviously very important, for very often it determines the success or the failure of treatment.

The emotional reactions of the patient suffering from acute anxiety often suggest a reversion toward immaturity, corresponding in degree to the level of apprehension and the basic character of the personality. Evidences of this trend may include signs of decreased emotional stability, a lessening of educated inhibitions and the willing adoption of a dependent role. Depending on the personality pattern, however, there may be a predominant display of aggressiveness or an attitude of hostility. In many patients the only indication of anxiety is an obvious exaggeration of suffering, the symptoms, as described by the patient, being dispropor-

tionately severe, numerous and variable. Physical signs of diagnostic value may include the presence of muscular tremors involving the extremities and an increase in the general muscular tone, as evidenced by involuntary resistance to passive muscular movement and hyperactivity of the deep tendon reflexes. The pupils may be dilated and the eyes excessively moist, as though the patient were constantly on the verge of tears.

Treatment and Nursing Care

Reactions of the type that occur when apprehension is unconcealed and is clearly justified on the basis of an obvious problem or a difficult situation usually respond to simple reassurance, guided by sound experience, common sense and, above all, friendly interest in the patient's personal problems.

It is important that the patient be informed adequately regarding his medical problems; that such information, although not necessarily complete, be wholly reliable; and that he understand correctly all statements of professional import. He need not be bombarded by a wealth of medical data, which may be confusing to a layman and only serve to aggravate his anxiety, but he should be told enough to ensure his cooperation in the therapeutic program and to confirm his confidence in his medical advisors. Statements which imply that his symptoms are the product of his imagination or invention, inconsequential and without foundation, are highly disturbing to the patient, add to his sense of insecurity, arouse his resentment and seriously aggravate the existing tension. Obviously, precisely the opposite effects are to be desired. The first objective of psychotherapy is the relaxation of emotional tension, and, to this end, every effort must be made to avoid uncertainty and confusion in the mind of the anxious patient, to establish and support his confidence and to reinforce his optimism, not through false or misleading representations and predictions, but by constantly stressing the more hopeful elements of the truth.

Diverting activity is an important aspect of psychotherapy, the objective being to disengage the patient's interest from his personal problems. Every patient, of course, should be encouraged to do as much for himself as possible, commensurate with health and strength. Occupational therapy of a creative type is useful for patients of all ages. Participation in ward activities and assistance in the performance of nursing or household duties always are to be encouraged. The occupational therapy staff can supply a variety of materials and useful suggestions for the cultivation of new interests and hobbies. Finally, if domestic or economic problems are disturbing to a patient, the social service department may be consulted for advice and assistance.

The Delirious Patient

The student occasionally may be astonished to find a patient with whom she had only a short time before enjoyed a fine conversation now in a state of complete confusion and disorientation. The patient may be having a *delirious reaction* due to a toxic condition causing temporary brain dysfunction. In addition to confusion and disorientation, such patients frequently have vivid hallucinations. These symptoms tend to make them very fearful and excitable.

Delirious states present a nursing problem of great challenge. The patient is frequently quite ill and requires skilled physical care. In addition, the psychological problems are many. The confused state of the patient makes him subject to many hazards. Such patients frequently harm themselves seriously or even commit suicide, not out of intent but as a result of their confusion or response to their hallucinations. They drink poisonous solutions if such are left unguarded within their reach; they walk out of windows, mistaking them for doors; they strangle themselves with their bedclothing, due to their extreme restlessness and thrashing about in bed; they fall out of bed while reaching for hallucinatory objects. The list of possible hazards is almost limitless.

Such patients need to be watched carefully to protect them from harm. Mechanical restraints are especially contraindicated, as they tend to add to the patient's confusion and increase his apprehension. They can also be an instrument in which the patient may accidentally become entangled and strangle himself. Only careful watching of

the patient can effectively ensure him against harm.

The student's attentions can offer the patient two other major psychological benefits, one during his state of extreme confusion and excitement, and the other during his period of convalescence. If the nurse's approach to the patient is a direct, simple, secure one, her calm can have a stabilizing effect on the patient and can make him less fearful. During the patient's period of convalescence he may remember with some vagueness and much anxiety his frightening confusion and hallucinations. The nurse's explanation of the experience, and the fact that he may expect no recurrence, can be very reassuring to him.

Although caring for a patient with a delirious reaction can be very trying, there is probably no nursing situation in which the rewards are greater. Just as the symptoms occurred so abruptly, so they usually disappear. As the patient improves physically, so does the mental state. The student once more may be surprised, but this time pleasantly, to hear the patient whose confusion was still quite apparent when she left him the day before greet her in completely lucid fashion when she approaches him the next day.

The Psychoneurotic Patient

There are other stress situations which are likewise threatening to the individual and provoke severe anxiety reactions; the source of these, however, is of an entirely different sort, namely, some irreconcilable conflict between strong opposing forces in the primitive emotions. The nature of this conflict is often such that it would be condemned as unworthy or socially unacceptable were it openly recognized, but its character and, for that matter, its existence are unknown even to the patient himself, being concealed in his subconscious mind. This concealment does not eliminate its existence, however, or in any sense resolve the opposing forces. Nor does it cause the emotional reactions to lose any of their intensity; these find their open expression when they appear, energetic but in disguise, in the form of organic signs and symptoms, manifestations which are referred to as "psychoneurotic reactions."

The patient apparently seeks relief from

his emotional stress by directing his attention to sensations arising from the activity of some organ, particularly one of an involuntary type, such as the beating of the heart, the peristaltic movements of the gastrointestinal tract or the movements of respiration. Consequently, he experiences symptoms of cardiac palpitation, dyspepsia or breathlessness—symptoms, however, which are merely exaggerated perceptions of normal physiologic activity—uncomfortable, to be sure, but more tolerable than contemplation of his basic problem. These symptoms, to his conscious mind, imply the presence of organic disease, which becomes not only a logical but a wholly acceptable basis on which to explain the physical responses to his emotional strife. An individual may be greatly disturbed, for example, because of some social, domestic or economic situation which is humiliating, dangerous to his security and prestige and of which he is not proud. By way of an alibi reaction he may proceed to focus his emotional interest on his heart. He may become increasingly aware of the sensations stimulated by its contractions until they become distinctly uncomfortable and he has persuaded himself that he has a heart disease. He then protects himself socially behind that diagnosis, which for the benefit of his family and friends he describes in the most dramatic terms possible. A similar mechanism operates occasionally, and only on a temporary basis, in many normal individuals at some time or other in their lives when subjected to intolerable stress, attributable perhaps to an obligation to risk grave personal danger, fear of humiliation or a sense of guilt.

Psychoneurotic symptoms are of all varieties and all grades of severity. As will become evident in the course of subsequent discussions concerning the clinical features of disease, there is hardly an organic symptom that cannot be, and is not, duplicated by a psychoneurotic reaction. These reactions are not built up in the consciousness, nor is the patient responsible for the precise details of their operation. They are compensatory phenomena, and their role is a guardian one, the object of their protection being self and self-esteem. They arise instinctively, and their development is possible in anyone, depending on the character of the emotional conflict, the degree of resulting stress, the quality of the innate personality and a host of environmental factors, all of which are responsible for individual differences in susceptibility.

Treatment and Nursing Care

The treatment of patients exhibiting psychoneurotic symptoms, whether partially or wholly psychogenic in origin, is designed to alleviate anxiety through a direct attack on the stress-promoting factors and to effect a more suitable adjustment on the part of the individual to whatever problems must be faced. First, it must be determined by careful physical and laboratory examinations to what extent his symptoms may be referable to organic disease. Then attempts are made, by means of appropriate psychiatric study, to identify his personality pattern and to unmask the psychoneurotic reactions which are contributing to his illness.

Treatment may require an initial period of rest, isolation from personal problems and relief from responsibility. In the majority of cases, however, therapy may be initiated at once, with the integration of the patient into a well-organized program and a full schedule of planned activity, physical and intellectual, and planned rest.

At the outset, the patient's activities should be scheduled as closely as possible in accordance with a definite daily routine. This procedure has two principal merits. It promotes the formation of good hygienic habits relative to diet, rest and exercise, a good method of establishing order in a disturbed emotional life being the proper organization of all activities. Secondly, through self-discipline and the repeated necessity for actively integrating all phases and functions of his personality as he carries out such a program, the patient is empowered to overcome the disintegrating forces which stem from his basic conflicts. He should not have assistance in the conduct of his scheduled routine; he himself must have it in mind, plan his actions accordingly and act of his own volition in each situation.

The basis of psychotherapy in the treatment of the psychoneurotic patient is reassurance. Early in the treatment the physician should discuss the therapy that is proposed, clearly and in simple terms, but without unnecessary reference to the symptoms, much as the patient would like to have these discussed, for too keen an interest in these sensations has been a prominent factor in the causation of his disability. What should be emphasized, rather, and in as optimistic terms as are justified, is the goal that the patient should attain, particularly the part he himself is to take in its attainment. The origin of the anxiety reaction should be clarified to the patient as soon as it is discovered, and the mechanism of his symptomatology then should be explained in full. The patient should be convinced of the fact that the existence of many of his physical symptoms, and the severity of all of them, are the result rather than the cause of his anxiety and that treatment, to be effective, must be conducted on that basis.

A prerequisite to complete therapeutic success in the treatment of psychoneurosis, however, is the ability to convey to the patient an adequate interpretation of his disabilities, including their pathogenesis, an awareness that a basic conflict exists and an appreciation of its significance. A more effective and healthful method of solving his fundamental difficulties must be offered as an alternative to the one adopted. Recognition of his problem may be so nearly within the conscious sphere that as soon as the proper explanations are suggested their validity may be apparent at once to the patient; he then may seek and perhaps find his own solution; in other words, he auto-analyzes himself and "sees his way out." Unfortunately, however, psychoneurosis is more often a reflection of a long-standing, deep-seated psychological mechanism, one that is completely resistant to superficial psychotherapy and not altogether amenable to any form of treatment, however intensive and skilled. The psychiatric problems that are involved in attempting to identify and resolve the basic emotional conflicts harassing these patients are complex in the extreme and far removed from the scope of the present text.

The Psychotic Patient

This patient will be encountered relatively rarely for two reasons: (1) because psychotics make up a very small percentage of the emotionally ill, and (2) because only in special situations are known psychotic patients cared for on a medical or surgical unit. Such situations involve conditions which require equipment, procedures and medical and nursing care not ordinarily available in a psychiatric unit. It is hoped that the student will not be assigned the care of a patient known to be psychotic if she has not yet had psychiatric nursing theory and practice. It is in this experience that the special knowledge and skills necessary for the care of such a patient are usually taught.

THE NURSE AND THE DISTURBED PATIENT

The nurse can be of invaluable assistance in allaying the anxieties of the disturbed patient and in helping him to adjust to the new and threatening situations that develop in the course of his illness. Her efforts and those of his physician should be coordinated very closely lest the patient be confused and disturbed as a result of inconsistencies in their discussions, or his confidence weakened by apparent indecision or by what seems to be evasive tactics on their part. All discussions and explanatory comments offered by the nurse should be modeled closely after those of the physician or directed according to his specific instructions and dictated invariably by common sense.

The extent to which the nurse wins and holds the confidence of her patient may determine the shape of his morale, the freedom with which he communicates his problems and the manner in which he cooperates in their solution. Unfortunately, those cases which demand the closest kind of rapport, namely, patients with psychological disturbances, are the very ones in which proper rapport may never be achieved or may be lost as a result of a misconception on the part of the nurse regarding her role in the nurse-patient relationship. This relationship usually is discussed in terms of the patient's response to various factors in his environment and the responsibilities of the nurse in relation to these. The nurse originates or selects and transmits appropriate stimuli; the patient receives these and reacts accordingly. The situation in actual practice is not always as pictured, however, for from time to time the nurse discovers that her patient has contrived to exchange roles with her. It is he who is sending; she is receiving. The signals are his; she is reacting. If such a predicament is to be avoided, the nurse must become familiar with certain abnormal behavior patterns, learn what these mean in terms of nursing needs and be cognizant of the problems that they create in the provision of good nursing care.

Development of an effective nurse-patient relationship may be thwarted by a reaction of hostility toward the patient, which has been engendered by the patient with subconscious motivation and purposeful intent. Depending on his maturity level, he may accomplish this by adopting an arrogant pose, making excessive demands, flaunting regulations and being generally obnoxious. More sophisticated, but equally provocative, are the tactics of the patient whose incessant complaints, disparaging attitude and vocal criticism are calculated to force the nurse into a defensive position and an exchange of hostilities, as a result of which he has both justified and relieved his aggressive tension and has alienated the nurse, thereby improving his defenses and protecting his anxious secrets. Another troubled patient, by skillful dramatics and fabrication, succeeds in appropriating the attention of the unwary nurse and a share of her emotions as well—substance for the imaginary foundations of his own. A serious impediment to good nursing care is the hostile reaction that often follows the discovery of a patient's deception and artifact, as has been discussed in relation to factitious fever (p. 56). Contempt for the malingerer (plus resentment, if he is suing for compensation) blinds the nurse and the physician to a fact that should have been self-evident, namely, that the act of malingering, per se, is proof of serious mental illness, one that has reduced the patient to a state of pathologic dependency.

Finally, the nurse must be alert to quell any unfavorable reactions that might be aroused by patients with symptoms and signs of organic disease which do not correspond in severity, who appear to be stubbornly reluctant to abandon their symptoms in response to vigorous therapy. Failure of a patient to improve as expected carries, of course, the unpleasant implication that the treatment has been wrong. An alternative and more attractive hypothesis places the blame on the patient, so professional concern gives way to unprofessional annoyance and the patient thenceforth is a "chronic complainer." The psychoneurotic individual with organic disease poses a real challenge for the nurse, and if the nursing care is of a high order of excellence, the achievement is a tribute to her mature personality and superior emotional discipline, as well as her technical competence.

The problems that have just been discussed illustrate some of the pitfalls that must be foreseen and circumvented by the nurse if she is to perform her role capably. Whether or not they prove to be stumbling blocks and barriers to good nursing care is up to the nurse, for any obstruction that may materialize is the product of her own emotions. The nurse who is truly expert is one who can be close and attentive to her patients, observe and hear them without prejudice and appreciate their problems fully without allowing her own emotions to become engaged in the process. The quality that enables her to function so admirably while retaining, and because she retains, her own identity is known as *empathy,* as distinguished from *sympathy*.

Sympathy, implying a sense of compassion and emotional participation in the patient's problems, is no asset but an impediment in the conduct of nursing care. A show of sympathy does not win the patient's confidence; on the contrary, it may prove to him that she has been misled. A show of annoyance in response to a patient's provocations notifies him that he is accepted at face value, i.e., that his camouflage is effective. A malingerer would prefer sympathy to censure and condemnation, but neither approach will deter him from malingering, and he is prepared to go to considerable lengths to ensure protective care. The "chronic complainer" is in need of meticulous, objective appraisal rather than the sympathy which was withdrawn.

Sympathy involves emotions and moods; it refers to an attitude which may or may not be adopted, or one that can change. The nurse who permits herself to be sympathetic can also become unsympathetic. With her patients' welfare at stake, she cannot afford to indulge in emotional attitudes which destroy objectivity and obliterate logic. The role of the nurse is to make decisions and to act without emotional encumbrances, to make observations undistorted by emotion and to appreciate the problems of her patients without emotional entanglement. Hers is an empathic role.

BIBLIOGRAPHY AND SUGGESTED READING

Books

Bird, B.: Talking with Patients, Philadelphia, Lippincott, 1955.

Nordmark, M. T., and Rohweder, A. W.: Science Principles Applied to Nursing — A Reference for Nurse Educators, pp. 220-276, Philadelphia, Lippincott, 1959.

Peplau, H. E.: Interpersonal Relations in Nursing, New York, Putnam, 1952.

Articles

Aring, C. D.: Sympathy and empathy, J.A.M.A. **167**:448-452, 1958.

Brill, N. Q.: Understanding yourself, Am. J. Nursing **57**:1325-1326, 1957.

Ebaugh, F. G.: The old-fashioned tranquilizer, J.A.M.A. **166**:1610-1612, 1958.

Gregg, D.: Reassurance, Am. J. Nursing **55**: 171-174, Feb., 1955.

————: Anxiety—a factor in nursing care, Am. J. Nursing **52**:1363-1365, 1952.

Hart, B., and Rohweder, A. W.: Support in nursing, Am. J. Nursing **59**:1398-1401, 1959.

Jourard, S. M.: How well do you know your patients? Am. J. Nursing **59**:1568-1571, 1959.

Knowles, L. N.: How can we reassure patients? Am. J. Nursing **59**:834-835, 1959.

Norris, C.: The nurse and the crying patient, Am. J. Nursing **57**:323-327, 1957.

Stevens, L. F.: Understanding ourselves, Am. J. Nursing **57**:1022-1023, 1957.

Ziskind, E.: Isolation stress in medical and mental illness, J.A.M.A. **168**:1427-1431, 1958.

Pamphlet

Milt, H.: How to Deal with Mental Problems, a 13-page pamphlet available from the National Association for Mental Health, 10 Columbus Circle, New York 19, N. Y.

Unit IV

9

Nutritional Needs and Problems

By ELEANOR DAWBER, B.S.
Instructor, Food and Nutrition,
Simmons College, Boston, and
Instructor, Nutrition and Diet Therapy,
Newton-Wellesley Hospital, Newton, Mass.

A healthy nutritional state is maintained by eating regularly a diet which is properly balanced and which supplies all of the essential nutrients in adequate amounts. The specific quantity of each nutrient that should be included each day is specified in Table 4, representing the dietary allowances that are currently recommended by the Food and Nutrition Board of the National Research Council. All of these nutrients are amply provided by a diet that is comprised solely of the common, readily available food items. Many of the commonest foods are enriched artificially with vitamin and mineral supplements, a practice that has become widespread and has simplified greatly the problem of food selection.

FOOD GUIDE ("THE BASIC FOUR")

As a practical aid to diet planning, the Institute of Home Economics has published a "Daily Food Guide," which divides the common foods into four groups, based on their nutrient properties, and indicates the minimum extent to which each group should be represented in the daily diet, as follows:

Milk Group

Adults, 2 or more cups; children, 3 or 4 cups; adolescents and pregnant women, 4 or more cups; and nursing mothers, 6 or more cups

Meat Group

2 or more servings daily, each of the following counting as 1 serving:

2 to 3 ounces lean, cooked beef, veal, pork, lamb, poultry or boned fish
2 eggs
1 cup cooked dry beans, dry peas or lentils
4 tablespoons peanut butter

Vegetable-Fruit Group

4 or more servings daily, including:
1 serving of citrus fruit, noncitrus fruit or a vegetable, if a good source (or 2 servings if only a fair source) of vitamin C
1 serving of a dark green or deep yellow vegetable (every other day, at least) as a source of vitamin A
2 or more servings of another vegetable (including potato) or fruit

Bread-Cereal Group

4 or more servings daily, each of the following representing 1 serving:
1 slice of bread (whole grain, enriched or restored)
1 ounce ready-to-eat cereal
½ to ¾ cup cooked cereal, corn meal, grits, macaroni, noodles, rice or spaghetti
If food from each group is ingested daily in the amounts recommended, all of the nutrients which are known to be essential will be supplied in adequate quantities.

THE MAJOR FOOD COMPONENTS

The nutritive value of any particular food depends on its content of specific nutrients, such as proteins, carbohydrates, fats, vitamins and minerals, and on its caloric value, i.e., the amount of heat it is capable of generating when metabolized in the body.

143

TABLE 4:
Food and Nutrition Board, National Research Council
Recommended Daily Dietary Allowances[1], Revised 1958

DESIGNED FOR THE MAINTENANCE OF GOOD NUTRITION OF HEALTHY PERSONS IN THE U.S.A.

(Allowances are intended for persons normally active in a temperate climate)

	Age Years	Weight kg. (lb.)	Height cm. (in.)	Calories	Protein gm.	Calcium gm.	Iron mg.	Vitamin A I.U.	Thiam. mg.	Ribo. mg.	Niacin[2] mg. equiv.	Asc. Acid mg.	Vitamin D I.U.
Men..............	25	70 (154)	175 (69)	3200[3]	70	0.8	10	5000	1.6	1.8	21	75	
	45	70 (154)	175 (69)	3000	70	0.8	10	5000	1.5	1.8	20	75	
	65	70 (154)	175 (69)	2550	70	0.8	10	5000	1.3	1.8	18	75	
Women..............	25	58 (128)	163 (64)	2300	58	0.8	12	5000	1.2	1.5	17	70	
	45	58 (128)	163 (64)	2200	58	0.8	12	5000	1.1	1.5	17	70	
	65	58 (128)	163 (64)	1800	58	0.8	12	5000	1.0	1.5	17	70	
	Pregnant (second half)			+300	+20	1.5	15	6000	1.3	2.0	+3	100	400
	Lactating (850 ml. daily)			+1000	+40	2.0	15	8000	1.7	2.5	+2	150	400
Infants[4]..............	0-1/12[4]				See Footnote 4								
	2/12-6/12	6 (13)	60 (24)	kg. x 120		0.6	5	1500	0.4	0.5	6	30	400
	7/12-12/12	9 (20)	70 (28)	kg. x 100		0.8	7	1500	0.5	0.8	7	30	400
Children..............	1-3	12 (27)	87 (34)	1300	40	1.0	7	2000	0.7	1.0	8	35	400
	4-6	18 (40)	109 (43)	1700	50	1.0	8	2500	0.9	1.3	11	50	400
	7-9	27 (60)	129 (51)	2100	60	1.0	10	3500	1.1	1.5	14	60	400
	10-12	36 (79)	144 (57)	2500	70	1.2	12	4500	1.3	1.8	17	75	400
Boys..............	13-15	49 (108)	163 (64)	3100	85	1.4	15	5000	1.6	2.1	21	90	400
	16-19	63 (139)	175 (69)	3600	100	1.4	15	5000	1.8	2.5	25	100	400
Girls..............	13-15	49 (108)	160 (63)	2600	80	1.3	15	5000	1.3	2.0	17	80	400
	16-19	54 (120)	162 (64)	2400	75	1.3	15	5000	1.2	1.9	16	80	400

[1] The allowance levels are intended to cover individual variations among most normal persons as they live in the United States under usual environmental stresses. The recommended allowances can be attained with a variety of common foods, providing other nutrients for which human requirements have been less well defined. See text for more detailed discussion of allowances and of nutrients not tabulated.

[2] Niacin equivalents include dietary sources of the preformed vitamin and the precursor, tryptophan. 60 milligrams tryptophan equals 1 milligram niacin.

[3] Calorie allowances apply to individuals usually engaged in moderate physical activity (page 2). For office workers or others in sedentary occupations they are excessive. Adjustments must be made for variations in body size, age, physical activity, and environmental temperature.

[4] See text for discussion of infant allowances. The Board recognizes that human milk is the natural food for infants and feels that breast feeding is the best and desired procedure for meeting nutrient requirements in the first months of life. No allowances are stated for the first month of life. Breast feeding is particularly indicated during the first month when infants show handicaps in homeostasis due to different rates of maturation of digestive, excretory, and endocrine functions. Recommendations as listed pertain to nutrient intake as afforded by cow's milk formulas and supplementary foods given the infant when breast feeding is terminated. Allowances are not given for protein during infancy.

Distributed as a public service to workers in the field of Nutrition by:
J. B. ROERIG AND COMPANY
800 Second Avenue
New York 17, N. Y.

Reprinted by permission of:
National Academy of Sciences
National Research Council (Publication 589)
Recommended Dietary Allowances
Revised, 1958

Carbohydrate

Carbohydrates include starches and sugars. These foods become oxidized in the body, forming carbon dioxide and water and releasing energy. Among the principal dietary sources of carbohydrate are grains, fruits, vegetables, syrups and sugars. Carbohydrates account for the production of nearly half of all the calories that are supplied by the average American diet. Wide variations in carbohydrate intake are perfectly compatible with normal health.

Carbohydrate functions primarily as a source of energy, the metabolism of 1 gram yielding 4 calories. If carbohydrates were not available, proteins would be utilized as fuel; adequate carbohydrates make this substitution unnecessary, so that the proteins continue to be available to carry out their unique function, namely, the building of tissue. Moreover, carbohydrates provide the starting material for the synthesis of certain amino acids in the body. The presence of carbohydrate in the diet insures that dietary (or body) fat will not be oxidized excessively. Thus, under conditions of severe carbohydrate restriction, fats proceed to become oxidized and the intermediate products of fat metabolism accumulate in the blood, producing ketosis (see page 832). This complication develops most often in association with diabetes mellitus, in patients whose diabetes is severe and poorly controlled. It may be observed also as a consequence of improperly planned reduction diets, which provide insufficient carbohydrate. When dietary carbohydrate is excessive in relation to the patient's caloric needs, it is converted to fat and stored as adipose tissue throughout the body.

All carbohydrates are reduced to simple sugars by digestion. After absorption, these sugars are converted to glycogen, which is stored in the liver. Liver glycogen provides a ready source of glucose, capable of maintaining an adequate concentration of blood sugar during extended periods of fasting. (Muscle glycogen is a complex glycogen-phosphorus compound that is decomposed with extraordinary rapidity, supplying energy for muscular activity almost instantaneously on demand.)

Fat

Fats, yielding 9 calories per gram when metabolized, represent a concentrated source of energy. Forty per cent of all food calories in America are derived from ingested fat. Dietary fats are derived principally from meat, dairy products and cooking fats. Some food fat is grossly visible, as in the case of butter, oils and meat. However, even if all visible fat were removed from the diet, a considerable quantity of invisible fat would still be left—as much as one half of the entire fat intake. Whole milk, egg yolk and lean meat are examples of foods high in invisible fat content. Certain cooking practices, such as frying in deep fat, enhance greatly the amount of fat already present in the food. On the other hand, broiling and roasting tend to reduce the total dietary fat.

After their ingestion, food fats are emulsified and hydrolized in the intestine. Eventually, they are absorbed, largely in the form of fatty acids. They may recombine thereafter to form neutral fat once more, or they may be transported to fat depots and stored. On the other hand, they may be oxidized to produce carbon dioxide and water, depending on the body's need for energy. When the demands for such energy become excessive, as in starvation or in uncontrolled diabetes mellitus, increased breakdown of body fat occurs. This breakdown is attended by a corresponding increase in the intermediate products of fat metabolism. These substances are acidic, and when they accumulate they produce a state of acidosis, a constant feature of uncontrolled diabetes mellitus (see page 827).

Saturated and Unsaturated Fats

True fats are combinations of glycerol and fatty acids. The latter can be divided roughly into 2 groups: saturated and unsaturated, depending on the number of carbon atoms joined by double bonds: the greater the number, the less saturated the fat. As a general rule, animal fats are relatively saturated, and they are solid at room temperature. On the other hand, vegetable fats and fish oils are relatively unsaturated and are usually liquid at room temperature. The addition of hydrogen to unsaturated oils in the course of commercial processing renders them less saturated and more solid.

The current interest in the relationship of dietary fat to the pathogenesis of coronary heart disease has stimulated a vast amount of research in connection with the effect of various diets on the lipids of the blood, and on the incidence or the progression of atherosclerosis. Whereas it has been demonstrated quite clearly that both a reduction in total fat intake and a shift from saturated to unsaturated fatty acids in the diet can lower the concentration of cholesterol and other lipids in the blood, the merits and the ultimate value of these changes remain to be established.

The palatability of food and the satiating effects of a meal are increased by the inclusion of fat in the diet. One reason for the latter is that fat tends to delay gastric emptying: the emptying time of the stomach is prolonged following the ingestion of fat, an important consideration for the dietary management of peptic ulcer (see page 596). As for palatability, low-fat diets are far from tasty and are likely to discourage eating. This effect may be the antithesis of the one desired, as in the case of the patient with liver disease who is anorexic, eats reluctantly and with difficulty, but whose principal therapeutic need is food and for whom the restriction of dietary fat therefore is not indicated.

Protein

Proteins are complex organic compounds containing nitrogen. They supply 10 to 15 per cent of the calories in the average American diet. Important food sources of proteins are meat, fish, poultry, eggs and milk. Proteins are built up from amino acids. Conversely, in the process of digestion dietary proteins are broken down into their constituent amino acids, and as such are absorbed. Tissue proteins and proteins in tissue fluids are synthesized from proper combinations of amino acids. If the synthesis of a particular protein is to occur, all of the amino acids required in its structure must be available at the same time.

Amino acids are designated as *essential* or *non-essential*. Essential amino acids are those that must be supplied in the diet, since the body is incapable of manufacturing them. The food proteins that supply all of the essential amino acids are referred to as *complete* proteins, and are said to be of "high biologic value," since a given amount of such a protein will support the maximum synthesis of tissue protein. Foods supplying proteins of "high biologic value" include milk, eggs, meat and fish.

Incomplete proteins are proteins that lack one or more of the essential amino acids. Appropriate combinations of incomplete proteins may supply adequately all of the essential amino acids by supplementing each other.

Amino acids that are not utilized for protein synthesis are metabolized, i.e., consumed for energy, and the excess nitrogen liberated therefrom is excreted for the most part as urea by the kidneys.

Since there are no storage depots for protein in the body—comparable, for example, to the glycogen stores of carbohydrate, or to adipose tissue, where fat is stored—it is important that the body have uninterrupted access to, and ample supplies of, dietary protein.

In order to support the manufacture of new tissue, which is constantly in progress, the body must be supplied with nitrogen in quantities that are sufficient at least to compensate for the amounts lost in urine and feces. The body is said to be "in positive nitrogen balance" when nitrogen intake exceeds nitrogen output. The existence of a positive nitrogen balance signifies that at this time tissue formation is surpassing tissue breakdown. A negative nitrogen balance signifies the reverse.

Calories

The term *calorie*, employed in relation to nutrition, is an abbreviated form of *kilogram-calorie*, the correct designation; i.e., 1 calorie (dietetic) represents the quantity of heat required to raise the temperature of 1 kilogram (2.2 pounds) of water 1° C. The heat produced as a result of food metabolism amounts to 4 calories per gram of carbohydrate, 4 calories per gram of protein and 9 calories per gram of fat. The energy requirements of the normal human adult under resting, basal conditions are estimated to be about 1 calorie per kilogram of body weight per hour. Moderate activity increases the caloric needs by a factor of about 50 per cent. If the caloric requirements fail to be met by the ingestion of sufficient food, the carbohydrate, fat and protein of the body tissues or in the body stores must serve as fuel.

Vitamins

Vitamins are organic food compounds that function primarily in enzyme systems and facilitate the metabolism of amino acids, fats and carbohydrates. Each vitamin plays a distinctive and highly specific role in the metabolic processes. The use of vitamin supplements may be recommended to correct dietary deficiencies, but these should not substitute for efforts to secure an adequate daily vitamin intake from a well-rounded selection of foods.

Vitamins are designated by the letters A, B, C, D, E, and K. In addition, a number of vitamin B subgroups have been discovered; these bear the additional designation of a number, e.g., B_{12}. In instances where chemical identification has been accomplished, the chemical name is preferred, e.g., *ascorbic acid.*

Fat-Soluble Vitamins

Vitamins are often classified on the basis of their solubility in fat or water. The fat-soluble vitamins are A, D, E and K. By virtue of their solubility in fat, they are capable of being stored in the body.

Vitamin A. This vitamin is required for the formation of visual purple, a substance in the retina that permits sight in semidarkness. It is needed also for the normal growth and for the integrity of epithelial structures, including the surface of the skin and the eyes, and the linings of the genitourinary, the respiratory and gastrointestinal tracts. This vitamin is probably synthesized in the intestinal wall. Its precursor in the diet is a hydrocarbon pigment, *carotene*. Yellow and dark green vegetables are particularly rich sources of carotene. Vitamin A is supplied most efficiently in the form of fish liver oil; but egg yolk, butter, cream and animal livers are also good sources. The principal depot of vitamin A in the body is the liver.

Vitamin D. This vitamin plays an important role in mineral metabolism. The principle function ascribed to vitamin D is related to the absorption of calcium and phosphorus from the gastrointestinal tract. The richest sources of vitamin D include fish liver oils, irradiated foods and viosterol. Fresh milk and most of the commercially prepared evaporated milks are fortified with 400 international units of vitamin D per quart, the amount recommended as the daily dietary allowance for infants, children and women who are pregnant or dieting. Most margarines contain 15,000 international units per pound. There are no reliable natural food sources. Exposure to sunlight of cholesterol derivatives present in the natural secretions of the skin endow these compounds with the properties of vitamin D. Excessive intake of vitamin D produces a toxic state, with derangement of the calcium balance, elevation of the serum calcium to excessively high levels and metastatic calcification in the soft tissues.

Vitamin E. The role of vitamin E in human physiology and nutrition remains to to be determined.

Vitamin K is essential for the synthesis of prothrombin, which is necessary for the clotting of blood. Ample amounts of this vitamin are formed continuously under normal conditions by bacterial flora of the human intestinal tract. Because of vitamin K's wide distribution in nature, and its endogenous production within the gut, no definite dietary requirements have been specified.

Water-soluble Vitamins

The water-soluble vitamins include all elements of the B complex and vitamin C (ascorbic acid).

The B-complex Vitamins. The B complex comprises at least a dozen separate members. Although their complete role is not entirely clear in every instance, it is certain that all are essential for the metabolic reactions that take place constantly in all living cells, and that all are involved in the oxidation of food to produce energy.

In the planning of normal and therapeutic diets, an effort is made to include adequate sources of three of the B complex: namely, thiamine, riboflavin and niacin. Other members of the B complex are just as necessary to human nutrition but in all probability will be supplied in adequate quantities if these three are supplied.

Good food sources of thiamine, riboflavin and niacin are whole-grain or enriched cereal products, meat and liver. Milk contains riboflavin in relatively large amounts.

The water-soluble vitamins are not stored by the body for any appreciable length of time; therefore, it is necessary to include an adequate source in the daily diet.

THIAMINE. This component of the enzyme cocarboxylase functions in the release of energy from the metabolism of carbohydrate. The daily requirement of thiamine is related to the amounts of carbohydrate being metabolized. Specific values are cited in Table 4.

RIBOFLAVIN. This vitamin (B_2) functions in many important enzyme systems. It is essential in the metabolism of amino acids, fatty acids and carbohydrate.

NIACIN (NICOTINIC ACID). This vitamin is a component of two coenzymes that effect the release of energy from food in the body. The amino acid tryptophane can be converted to niacin, and when planning the diet, this amino acid should be taken into account as a potential source of niacin.

FOLIC ACID (PTEROYLGLUTAMIC ACID). Required for normal tissue growth, including the normal production of red and white blood cells by bone marrow, folic acid plays a key role in purine metabolism. Folic acid occurs in green vegetables, cauliflower, liver, kidney, muscle meat, wheat and cereals. Also, it is produced by bacteria in the intestine.

VITAMIN B_6 (PYRIDOXINE, PYRIDOXAL AND PYRIDOXAMINE). This vitamin is concerned with the metabolism of tryptophane, one of the essential amino acids, and with the synthesis of unsaturated fatty acids. The daily requirement is estimated to be 1 to 2 mg.

VITAMIN B_{12} (CYANOCOBALAMIN). Formed as a metabolite by the bacterial intestinal flora and supplied in the diet by liver and eggs, this material is necessary for normal growth in childhood and is essential throughout life for the normal structure and function of the bone marrow, the gastrointestinal tract, the nervous system and various other tissues. Minute quantities of B_{12} (0.5 to 2.0 micrograms) suffice to meet the daily requirements of a normal individual. On the other hand, patients with gastrointestinal abnormalities which impair absorption may require far larger quantities of the vitamin if they are to avoid the complications of B_{12} deficiency, i.e., macrocytic anemia, atrophy of the gastrointestinal epithelium and degenerative lesions in the central nervous system of the type that are characteristic of primary pernicious anemia.

Vitamin C. Ascorbic acid is required for the normal formation and the maintenance of the intracellular cementlike substance. Rich food sources of vitamin C are citrus fruit and citrus juices, tomatoes and green peppers. Potatoes and cabbage are also important sources. Vitamin C is destroyed easily by heat and oxidation. To preserve the vitamin C content, fruit and vegetables should be refrigerated. For the same reason, vegetables should be cooked for the shortest possible time, using a minimum amount of water. The recommended amount of vitamin C for an average adult is 70 mg. daily. This is supplied by 6 oz. orange juice or by 1 grapefruit.

Minerals

Calcium and Phosphorus

These minerals are required for skeletal calcification and normal dentition.

The calcium in the blood serves several major functions. Some of the most important of these have to do with the normal clotting of blood, normal functioning of nerve tissue and the contraction of muscle fibers. The recommended daily intake for the average adult is 0.8 Gm. However, it has been shown that in the absence of stress an adult can adjust favorably to widely varying levels of intake. The need for calcium is increased during childhood, pregnancy and lactation. In the United States, milk and cheese are the principal sources of dietary calcium. Good amounts of calcium are available also in canned sardines, canned salmon with bones, and turnip and mustard greens.

Phosphorus plays many roles in relation to basic metabolic activities. It is widely distributed in nature, being present in large amounts in fish, meat, cereals, milk and milk products. The daily requirement of phosphorus, i.e., 1.5 Gm., is met readily by these dietary sources, and a deficiency of this mineral is unlikely solely on the basis of an inadequate diet.

Iron

This mineral is required for hemoglobin production, as discussed on page 460. Approximately 10 per cent of the iron ingested in food is absorbed from the gastrointestinal tract. The normal adult male requires little dietary iron, i.e., 1 to 2 mg. daily. The adult menstruating female's requirement of iron is 15 to 20 mg. daily. Iron requirements are increased during pregnancy and periods of active growth. Lean meat, liver, shellfish and egg yolk are good sources, and apricots, prunes and raisins, relatively good sources of iron. The widespread enrichment of cereals and flours has been a decided factor in the improvement of iron intake.

Sodium

This mineral is concerned with the regulation of the osmotic pressure, the acidity and the volume distribution of the extracellular body fluids. Most of the sodium that is ingested is excreted in the urine, and lesser amounts are lost in the feces and in sweat. The total excretion of sodium is determined by its intake, which usually amounts to 2 to 6 grams daily. This amount is considerably in excess of that needed by the body, and for the most part represents sodium which has been added in the form of salt for purposes of cooking, processing and flavoring food. When the sodium intake is greatly reduced, its excretion decreases likewise, and only rarely does the amount of sodium in the body drop to levels sufficiently low to produce symptoms of hyponatremia, i.e., weakness, prostration or shock. Restriction of sodium intake to prevent or decrease edema in cardiac, renal and hepatic diseases, and to lower blood pressure in hypertension is a therapeutic procedure of major medical importance.

Potassium

Just as sodium is the principal cation of the extracellular fluid, potassium performs the same role in the intracellular fluid. Potassium also is necessary for normal carbohydrate and protein metabolism and plays an important role in the transmission of nerve impulses. The administration of some diuretic agents designed to produce increased excretion of sodium may remove also considerable potassium from the body and produce potassium deficiency (hypokalemia). This deficiency may occur in diarrheal diseases and diabetic coma treated with insulin. Potassium deficiency gives rise to extreme muscular weakness. An excess of potassium in the blood (hyperkalemia) occurs spontaneously in cases of adrenal insufficiency (Addison's disease) and as a complication of renal failure; if marked, it poses a serious risk from the standpoint of cardiac arrythmia. The minimum requirement is 2 to 4 grams a day; the supply is ample in almost every sort of diet. The richest sources are cereals, green vegetables, meat and certain fruits.

Iodine

This mineral is the key constituent of the thyroid hormone. The daily requirement is believed to be 150 to 300 mcg. This amount is readily obtained in coastal areas of the United States from salt-water fish and locally raised produce. The Great Lakes region and the Pacific Northwest are areas in which the indigenous crops are relatively deficient in iodine and where the daily requirement may not be provided in the diet. Table salt fortified with iodine is the method of choice for supplying sufficient iodine in these areas. A patient on a restricted sodium diet may require an iodine supplement from another source.

Fluorine

Fluorine is a normal constituent of the body, found primarily in the bones and the teeth. As little as 1 part fluorine per million in drinking water brings about a striking decrease in tooth decay in children. The fluoridation of water is now an accepted public health measure in almost 4,000 communities throughout the country. The amount used in water and obtained from dietary sources is not enough to produce toxic manifestations.

TABLE 5.

Effect of Dietary Modifications on the Major Food Groups by Two Therapeutic Diets

Food Group	Normal Adult Diet	Bland Diet	Restricted Sodium Diet 500 mg.
Milk	2 cups or more	2 cups or more	2 cups only
Vegetables	2 or more and potato	2 or more cooked without skins or seeds. No gas producing vegetables	Unrestricted fresh or canned without salt *except* celery, beets, beet greens, spinach, kale, sauerkraut, chard, dandelions, frozen peas
Fruits	2 or more 1 citrus	Orange juice. Any cooked or canned fruit without seeds or skin.	Unrestricted
Bread and Cereal	4 or more enriched	4 or more; white refined & enriched; White crackers; Macaroni; Rice	Unrestricted "salt free bread"; unrestricted regular cooked cereal, puffed wheat, rice, shredded wheat
Meat, fish, poultry, Cheese-eggs	4 oz. or more 1 egg or more	4 oz. or more tender meat, poultry or fish; no spicy "prepared meat"; Mild American, cottage cheese; 1 egg or more	Not more than 5 oz. fresh meat, fish, poultry. *Avoid* all processed or canned meat or fish. Salt free cheese only; 1 egg a day
Fat	As tolerated for sufficient calories	As tolerated Do not fry food	Unrestricted salt free butter and margarine or cooking oil.
Other	Sugar	No coffee, tea, broth or excessively spicy foods	No *salt* in cooking or at the table; use pepper & herbs; Sugar

Any combinations of the above foods allowed to make casserole dishes or desserts.

Trace Elements

A number of trace elements are essential for the functioning of numerous enzyme systems. Among these elements are magnesium, zinc, cobalt, sulfur and copper. They are needed in such small amounts and are so ubiquitous, in foods of all categories, that problems of deprivation rarely occur.

THERAPEUTIC DIETS

The normal diet, with relatively minor revisions, may serve as the basis for the therapeutic diet. The need for revision or modification may involve primarily total food intake to alter body weight. It may involve a change in food consistency to compensate for mechanical defects in the oropharynx, the esophagus or the gastrointestinal tract, or to aid the intestinal tract to tolerate and digest food better. Diets so modified are known as *bland, liquid, soft* and *low roughage.* Another type of modification entails increasing the amount of a particular nutrient for which a specific demand exists in the body. Metabolic abnormalities and inability of the body to handle certain nutrients also require modification of the diet. Examples of these are the restriction of sodium in congestive heart failure, the restriction of carbohydrate in diabetes, the omission of protein containing the amino acid phenylalanine in phenylketonuria, and the omission of lactose in galactosemia. Allergic reactions to a particular food may require the omission of the offending item.

To be acceptable to the patient the diet must be of a type that is practicable to prepare. Every effort must be made to tailor the diet in accordance with the food pattern to which the patient is accustomed, while keeping within the diet prescription. Instructions to the patient should stress the advantages of selecting foods which are common, readily obtained and easy to prepare in the home.

How therapeutic diets are constructed, namely through simple modifications of the basic normal pattern, is exemplified by the "bland" and the "restricted sodium" diet, illustrated in Table 5.

PATIENTS WITH NUTRITIONAL PROBLEMS

Deficiency States

Generalized nutritional deficiency or starvation results if most or all of the necessary food elements are lacking in the diet. Specific deficiency states, on the other hand, are caused by a diet which is defective with respect to one nutrient element or a single group of nutrients. Certain clinical features of starvation may suggest a specific deficiency disease, but this is by no means a constant observation. Quite the contrary, the need for specific nutrients is lessened progressively in the case of generalized malnutrition. Thus, an individual on a low carbohydrate intake requires less thiamine than one whose diet has an average or an increased carbohydrate content. The converse, likewise, is true, namely, the development of a specific nutritional disease does not imply the existence of generalized malnutrition. One would hardly describe as "starved" the average patient with anemia due to iron deficiency, night blindness due to vitamin A deficiency or pernicious anemia due to a lack of vitamin B_{12}. Classical scurvy may develop in an individual whose outward appearance would seem to indicate an excellent state of nutrition, and many alcoholic patients with beriberi are actually obese.

Deficiency diseases are not always attributable to dietary defects; some result from impairment of gastrointestinal absorption, others from the defective utilization of particular food elements after their absorption. Failure of absorption is a common complication of chronic diarrhea. The inadequate production of bile or a blockage of the bile duct may impair the absorption of fats and fat-soluble vitamins. If the volume of pancreatic juice is too small, or if its entry into the gastrointestinal tract is obstructed, the enzymatic hydrolysis of proteins, fats and carbohydrates is reduced, and the absorption of these materials is prevented. Gastric achylia curtails the efficiency of protein hydrolysis; it also interferes with the extraction of iron from the food and the dissolving of this mineral preparatory to its absorption through the intestinal wall. The metabolism of absorbed nutrients is disturbed in a number of conditions, notably liver disease, generalized infections and certain endocrine disorders, including Simmonds' disease and Addison's disease.

Finally, deficiency disorders may occur as the result of still another factor, namely, an increase in the nutritional requirements of an individual due to an increase in his body metabolism which is not compensated for by a corresponding increase in his diet. This situation commonly is associated with hyperthyroidism and with prolonged febrile illnesses, but most important is its occurrence in normal pregnant women and rapidly growing children whose dietary intake is less than optimal.

Avitaminoses

Vitamins are specific organic nutrients needed by the body for its normal growth and metabolism. If the diet is deficient in vitamins or in the substances from which they can be derived (termed *vitamin precursors*), if the absorption of these from the gastrointestinal tract is inadequate or if they are not utilized properly in the body, the inevitable result is a vitamin-deficiency disease (an avitaminosis) which is curable only by the administration of the vitamin in question, or, if absorbable and utilizable, its precursor.

Vitamin A Deficiency. This causes night blindness, and the degree of visual adaptability in darkness is used as a clinical test to determine this deficiency. Xerophthalmia (inflammation of the cornea) and abnormal vascularization of the cornea are also caused by its lack. Certain skin disorders are attributable to vitamin A deficiency, but inasmuch as many avitaminoses may be associated with similar lesions, the relationship is not established. Moderate degrees of vitamin A deficiency, from studies of visual dark-adaptation, are not uncommon among the general population. Medically this vitamin can be provided in most concentrated forms in fish-liver oils.

Vitamin B Deficiencies. These are responsible for a variety of symptoms and signs which occur in all manner of combinations. Rarely are these nutritional disorders attributable to the lack of one single vitamin; moreover, a deficiency of any one of the group, by affecting the absorption and the utilization of the others, produces in effect a multiple deficiency state, and the relative importance of any individual member of the B complex is often difficult to determine. It is a sound therapeutic principle to regard all deficiency states, the "B" deficiencies included, as compound, rather than simple, defects.

The clinical manifestations of vitamin B deficiency include the following: nerve dysfunction, evidenced by muscle pain, tenderness and weakness on exertion, cured promptly by thiamine (which nerve tissue requires for glucose utilization); anatomic peripheral polyneuritis, as it occurs in beriberi, pellagra, diabetes, hyperthyroidism and pregnancy, characterized by constant muscle weakness, sensory impairment and loss of tendon reflexes in the extremities. Also included are angular mouth lesions (perlèche), occasionally but not always curable with riboflavin alone; pellagrous dermatitis, due mainly to nicotinic acid deficiency and marked by pigmentation and desquamation in skin areas where there is exposure to irritation of any sort (trauma, infection, sunlight, etc.); diarrhea, as it occurs in pellagra, and some cases of glossitis, cured by nicotinic acid; the psychosis of pellagra and beriberi, which, if acute, responds rapidly to nicotinic acid. Cardiovascular disease, characterized by persistent peripheral arteriolar vasodilatation, resulting in edema, tachycardia and cardiac dilation, and exemplified by beriberi heart disease, may be cured by thiamine (if uncomplicated by hypoproteinemia). Degenerative spinal cord changes (combined system disease) and the anemia of certain deficiency states are attributable to a deficiency of vitamin B_{12}.

Pellagra (Rough Skin). This is a deficiency disease affecting the skin, the gastrointestinal canal and the nervous system. It is due to a lack, in the diet, of niacin.

The severity of pellagra's manifestations periodically waxes and wanes, exacerbations usually beginning in the spring and subsiding gradually, each attack leaving the patient in worse condition. This disease is seen particularly among the poorer classes, the inmates of institutions and occasionally among members of well-to-do families who are on faulty diets. Precipitating factors include enteric infections, systemic infections of any type, gastric achylia and alcoholism.

The initial symptoms of pellagra may consist solely of soreness of the tongue, which becomes red and raw; nausea; vomiting and diarrhea. Skin lesions which are symmetrical and sharply defined appear early; the back of both hands, from the wrist to the last finger joint, and later the forehead and the feet, become "sun-burned." Then the skin peels and becomes more and more pigmented. It becomes progressively dryer, thicker and rougher, but finally thin and atrophic. After several attacks the nervous symptoms begin: headaches, insomnia and depression, in time complicated by paralysis and eventually dementia. Some patients have many attacks. Without benefit of specific treatment, a large percentage of cases terminate fatally.

Most of the signs and symptoms clear up on administration of nicotinic acid, but whole yeast and liver are more satisfactory therapeutic agents, containing, as they do, not only this vitamin, but all those in the B group.

VITAMIN B_{12} AND FOLIC ACID DEFICIENCIES. The macrocytic anemias associated with pernicious anemia, diarrheal disorders, sprue, pellagra, pregnancy and starvation are discussed in Chapter 25. It will be recalled that pernicious anemia is a complicated deficiency state, due to a defect involving the gastric mucosa and interfering with the absorption of vitamin B_{12}; vitamin B_{12} deficiency is responsible for the gastrointestinal, neurologic and hematologic manifestations of this disease. Restoration and maintenance of good health in these patients requires the periodic administration of B_{12} by intramuscular injections for the duration of their lives.

The so-called "nutritional macrocytic anemia" that occurs as a rare complication of pregnancy, liver disease and various malabsorptive states is indistinguishable from pernicious anemia from the hematologic standpoint. However, it is based on a deficiency, not of vitamin B_{12}, but of folic acid. This nutrient is administered by mouth with the expectation of achieving marked improvement, if not permanent cure, in the majority of the patients, depending on the nature and the severity of their underlying disorder.

Vitamin C Deficiency. Severe vitamin C

deficiency results in *scurvy*. This disease is marked by the occurrence throughout the body of blood leakage from capillaries which are too fragile because the cells of their walls are not solidly cemented together. Hemorrhages take place from the nose; in the gastrointestinal and the genitourinary tracts; into the joints—causing painful, bloody, joint effusions; about the hair follicles, causing petechial spots; into the subcutaneous tissue spaces, giving rise to large ecchymoses; into the bone epiphyses; and under the periosteum (in children giving rise to specific signs at x-ray examination). In fact, wherever there are capillaries to rupture, hemorrhage may occur.

The child with scurvy is pale, restless and irritable. He may develop localized swellings of the limbs due to hemorrhages under the periosteum of the bones or under the skin. The adult becomes sallow, weak and short of breath and may complain of rheumatic pains in the legs. The disease is diagnosed clinically when there are spongy, bleeding gums and hemorrhagic tendencies, when there is an increased susceptibility of the skin capillaries to rupture and when there is a low ascorbic acid level in the blood. A patient should be treated at once with fresh fruit juice, either orange or lemon, or, better, crystalline ascorbic acid (which these foods contain), and afterward put on a diet rich in fresh fruits. The cure is astonishingly rapid; all traces of the disease often disappear in less than a week.

Vitamin D Deficiency. Severe vitamin D deficiency in infants and young children results in *rickets*. This disease is brought about through faulty absorption from the gastrointestinal tract of calcium or phosphorus needed for bone structure; this abnormality is corrected by the administration of vitamin D. Faulty bone formation in growing children leads to deformity involving practically the entire skeleton, hence rickets is an exceedingly important disease in children, whose bones, if too soft at that period, become permanently distorted. In adults, under the same conditions of calcium lack, there also occurs bone softening (osteomalacia), but the consequences usually are less serious.

Any condition causing prolonged calcium deficiency will cause bone changes analogous to those seen in rickets and osteomalacia. Thus, it occurs in pancreatic infantilism, renal rickets, in pregnant women on a low-calcium diet, in fatty diarrheas of children, etc. Also, rickets can result from phosphorus deficiency, since the bone requires both elements in its structure. Failure of calcium to be absorbed from the gastrointestinal tract for any reason—for example, in vitamin D deficiency—impedes the intestinal absorption of phosphorus, possibly due to the excretion of calcium and phosphorus together as an insoluble salt in the stools.

Vitamin K Deficiency

Vitamin K deficiency is responsible for hemorrhagic disease of the newborn, the prevention of which defect is ensured by the routine administration of one of the synthetic analogues of this vitamin (e.g., Hykinone, Synkamin or Menadione), given orally to the mother in dosages of 50 to 100 mg. immediately preceding delivery. Vitamin K deficiency also accounts for the hemorrhagic tendency associated with certain types of liver disease. It is observed also in patients with obstructive jaundice, absorption of the vitamin being impaired in these patients because of the absence of bile in the gastrointestinal tract. Hypoprothrombinemia, occurring on this basis, is corrected by the parenteral administration of any of the synthetic vitamin K preparations. If, however, the defect is attributable to liver disease and to a failure of vitamin K utilization, rather than to failure of its absorption, treatment with these drugs may be disappointing, correction of the defect requiring the transfusion of whole blood or plasma or the parenteral injection of K_1 oxide emulsion. Further details regarding the character and the treatment of hypoprothrombinemia are discussed on page 478.

Mineral Deficiencies

Inorganic elements often are implicated in deficiency syndromes, including those of extrinsic and of intrinsic origin. Iron, calcium, phosphorus, iodine, the cations (basic) and the anions (acidic) of the serum are most important in this respect. By an extrinsic deficiency is meant that type of deficiency which is due to insufficient ingestion of the substance in question; by deficiency of intrinsic origin we refer to depletion of the substance due to one or another pathologic process, as, for example, vomiting or hemorrhage.

Iron Deficiency. This gives rise to hypochromic anemia, inasmuch as iron is necessary for hemoglobin formation. It is most apt to occur as a result of acute or chronic hemorrhage, when there is inadequate replacement of the lost iron through the ingestion of iron salts or iron-containing foods (best represented by dried fruits, beans, peas, meats and whole-wheat products). It is also associated with pregnancy, in the course of which there is an increased demand on the mother (by the fetus) for iron.

Calcium and Phosphorus Deficiencies. These deficiencies, causing rickets in children and osteomalacia in adults, may result from insufficient ingestion of these substances in the diet (their concentration being highest in milk, whole-grain breads and cereals, vegetables, cheese and eggs) or from vitamin D deficiency, impeding their proper absorption from the gastrointestinal tract. A lowering of the plasma-calcium level may arise due to circumstances causing an increase in the plasma phosphorus, such as chronic renal disease or hypoparathyroidism, with tetany the result. In hyperparathyroidism, the bones are depleted of calcium and phosphorus, possibly through abnormal stimulation of their urinary excretion (Von Recklinghausen's disease).

Iodine Deficiency. This is responsible for colloid goiter when the deficiency arises in adult life, and cretinism when the supply is diminished during the stage of fetal development, provided the mother fails to furnish sufficient thyroid hormone.

The Anorexic Patient

The nutritional state of an individual with normal digestive and metabolic function is determined by the quality and the quantity of the food he eats, and, assuming that an adequate diet is accessible, his food intake is controlled principally by his appetite. The magnitude and the satiability of the appetite are subject to a variety of influences, emotional as well as physiologic. Basically, it reflects the intensity of hunger sensations

and the frequency with which these occur, but the interpretation of his sensations by each individual and the responses which they evoke are conditioned from the time of infancy by a great many factors. In healthy and emotionally adjusted persons it corresponds fairly closely to the nutritional requirements of the body; otherwise, there is no such correspondence, and, as a result, the food intake may be inadequate, excessive or irregular and the food selection poor.

Hunger sensations originate in the stomach wall, stimulated by the slow, powerful muscular contractions of that organ which start as soon as it is empty of its contents and continue intermittently until more food is introduced at the next meal. These contractions are inhibited, and the appetite correspondingly diminished, in the course of most illnesses, particularly during the active stages of infections and in almost all disorders which involve the digestive organs. Moreover, there are inhibitory influences which are entirely independent of the presence or the absence of organic disease, including unfavorable psychological responses, emotional disturbances, such as fear and anxiety, and all types of physical discomfort. Abnormal stimulation of the appetite, on the other hand, may be caused by irritation of the gastric mucosa, as by alcoholic beverages or salicylates. Commonly, it is associated with diabetes mellitus and is a persistent phenomenon in some individuals whose excessive hunger, or "bulimia," reflects a state of chronic anxiety and frustration, release of their emotional tension being afforded, via some psychological reflex mechanism, by the ingestion of food. The difficult problems arising in the prevention and treatment of obesity, the result of meals which are too large and too frequent, are discussed in a later section of this text.

The Role of the Nurse. The nourishment of the ill patient is one of the most important problems of nursing care. By helping to create a pleasant physical and psychological environment and by encouraging the patient, as well as by providing physical aid in the eating process, the nurse may play a major role in developing and maintaining an optimum nutritional state. If for any reason the patient is forced to go without food for varying periods, he should be reassured of the harmlessness of fasting, even if prolonged.

Ingestion of food in the usual manner is the most desirable way in which to achieve a good nutritional state. If because of inability or unwillingness to eat it becomes necessary to feed the patient artificially, the gastro-intestinal route is still by far the best. Nutritious foods can be prepared in a fluid state, capable of passing through a tube inserted into the stomach, which will supply the patient with an adequate, balanced diet. Very satisfactory preparations for tube feeding can be made from milk and eggs, fruit juices and strained and pureed foods. Commercial preparations with comparable nutrient properties are readily available. However, assuming that the oral route is available, the patient should be fed, receiving whatever assistance he needs. In consideration of the psychological factors involved, the meals should be served as attractively as possible and with full attention to the following details:

Select the menu with due regard for the patient's preferences and prejudices, which will have been explored in the course of a detailed nutritional history.

Prepare food combinations which are colorful and appetizing in appearance.

Eliminate all concentrated fats except butter; remove all visible fat from meat and fatty surface layers from soups.

Ensure that the food is palatably seasoned and is served at the proper temperature.

Do not present the entire meal all at once, but serve food courses individually.

Offer small, rather than large, portions.

The service should be neat and conducted with meticulous regard to cleanliness.

Eliminate all unpleasant odors in the patient's room.

Screen all unappetizing spectacles from the patient's view.

Present a cheerful demeanor and take pains to avoid antagonism. Lend all possible encouragement, reassurance and assistance. If necessary, cajole the patient into accepting nourishment, but never scold or threaten.

Notify dietitian of patients who present feeding problems.

Obesity

Obesity, or the presence of abnormal amounts of fat stored in the fat depots of the body, is due to excessive food ingestion in proportion to the caloric requirements of the individual. Some persons must forever watch their diet lest they gain weight. Others eat all they wish and remain thin.

There are two fundamental differences between these two groups: (1) the obese individual eats more, and, (2) his energy output is less, relative to his intake, than that of the slender individual. Obese individuals, all their protestations to the contrary, ingest more calories and spare themselves physically more than slender individuals. They are excessively fond of foods with high fat and carbohydrate content, and their appetite is unduly great. Hunger returns too promptly following a meal; this is appeased too often by a between-meal snack. They also are prone to relax easily, move slowly and exercise little.

The dangers of obesity, which are not inconsiderable, are related chiefly to the unavoidable strain which it imposes on the heart, the kidneys and the pancreas. It tends to aggravate hypertension and precipitates diabetes mellitus in individuals so predisposed.

Treatment. The treatment is to lessen the food intake and, in some cases, to increase the muscular activity. An obesity diet is ordered which satisfies the basal requirements and no more. Such a diet, for sedentary workers, provides approximately 1,200 calories daily, the proportion of fatty constituents being absolutely minimal. Multiple small feedings are preferable to one or two comparatively large meals each day, the object being to forestall the development of those acute hunger sensations so devastating to the morale. The patient must be impressed by the importance of eating his meals slowly, with great deliberation, and cautioned not to bolt his food voraciously. Bulky, low-caloric foodstuffs, such as green vegetables, should replace the high-caloric fried, fatty meats, pastries and sweets. Coffee or tea (without cream) between meals is a very useful device for curbing the appetite at mealtime.

TABLE 6—Desirable Weights for Men and Women
According to Height and Frame. Ages 25 and Over

Height (In Shoes)*	Weight in Pounds (In Indoor Clothing)		
	Small Frame	Medium Frame	Large Frame
	Men		
5' 2"	112–120	118–129	126–141
3"	115–123	121–133	129–144
4"	118–126	124–136	132–148
5"	121–129	127–139	135–152
6"	124–133	130–143	138–156
7"	128–137	134–147	142–161
8"	132–141	138–152	147–166
9"	136–145	142–156	151–170
10"	140–150	146–160	155–174
11"	144–154	150–165	159–179
6' 0"	148–158	154–170	164–184
1"	152–162	158–175	168–189
2"	156–167	162–180	173–194
3"	160–171	167–185	178–199
4"	164–175	172–190	182–204
	Women		
4' 10"	92– 98	96–107	104–119
11"	94–101	98–110	106–122
5' 0"	96–104	101–113	109–125
1"	99–107	104–116	112–128
2"	102–110	107–119	115–131
3"	105–113	110–122	118–134
4"	108–116	113–126	121–138
5"	111–119	116–130	125–142
6"	114–123	120–135	129–146
7"	118–127	124–139	133–150
8"	122–131	128–143	137–154
9"	126–135	132–147	141–158
10"	130–140	136–151	145–163
11"	134–144	140–155	149–168
6' 0"	138–148	144–159	153–173

* 1-inch heels for men and 2-inch heels for women.
Note: Prepared by the Metropolitan Life Insurance Company. Derived primarily from data of the Build and Blood Pressure Study, 1959, Society of Actuaries.

Therapeutic exercise is to be recommended only for the young and those accustomed to it, among whom the average obese individual is not included. Such treatment can stimulate the appetite remarkably, an unfortunate effect, and, unless the cardiovascular system is in excellent repair, may actually be dangerous. Thyroid preparations, unless there is good evidence that the metabolic rate is abnormally low, have no more place in the treatment of obesity than has overexercise, and for reasons which are quite analogous.

The amphetamine drugs, including Benzedrine and Dexedrine, reduce the appetite effectively and are very helpful, for a time, in curtailing the diet. But these agents, too, have their limitations; drug tolerance develops in many cases, resulting in the need for progressively larger doses, which eventually may interfere with normal sleep.

A novel approach to the dietetic management of obesity has been the imposition of total fasting for an initial period of 4 to 14 days while the patient is hospitalized, and for briefer periods thereafter on an ambulatory basis. Although seemingly drastic, this regimen is tolerated well, is attended by surprisingly little discomfort, has produced no obvious complications and has proven effective in many "intractable" cases, weight loss averaging 2.5 pounds per day of fast. Obviously, the lost weight will be regained and this therapeutic accomplishment nullified if the earlier eating habits are resumed. These habits must be revised permanently, according to the principles outlined above, and medical supervision should be continued until a satisfactory program appears to be established.

PROBLEM SOLVING ACTIVITY

Iron, cobalt, vitamin B_{12} and protein all have a function in blood formation.

1. What is the function (relating to blood) of each of these nutrients?

2. What is the deficiency disease resulting from an inadequate intake of iron?

3. What disease results from an inadequate absorption of Vitamin B_{12}?

4. What foods would you encourage for a patient who has just lost a large amount of blood?

5. In what clinical conditions is Vitamin K given?

SOURCES FOR NUTRITION EDUCATION

American Can Company
100 Park Avenue
New York 17, N. Y.

American Dietetic Association
620 N. Michigan Avenue
Chicago 11, Illinois

American Institute of Baking
400 East Ontario Street
Chicago 11, Illinois

American Meat Institute
59 East Van Buren Street
Chicago 5, Illinois

Cereal Institute
135 South LaSalle Street
Chicago 3, Illinois

Corn Industries
Research Foundation, Inc.
3 East 45th Street
New York 17, N. Y.

Evaporated Milk Association
228 North LaSalle Street
Chicago, Illinois

General Mills, Inc.
Minneapolis, Minnesota

H. J. Heinz Company
Pittsburg 30, Pennsylvania

National Dairy Council
111 North Canal Street
Chicago 6, Illinois

The Nutrition Foundation, Inc.
99 Park Avenue
New York 16, N. Y.

Official Agencies

United States Department of Agriculture
Agriculture Research Service
Washington, D. C.

World Organizations

Food and Agriculture Organization
of the United Nations
North American Regional Office
1325 C Street, S.W.
Washington, D. C.

BIBLIOGRAPHY AND SUGGESTED READING

Books

Cooper, L. F., Barber, E. M., Mitchell, H. S., and Rynbergen, H. J.: Nutrition in Health and Disease, ed. 14, Philadelphia, Lippincott, 1963.

Krause, M. V.: Food, Nutrition and Diet Therapy, Philadelphia, Saunders, 1961.

Mowry, L.: Basic Nutrition and Diet Therapy for Nurses, St. Louis, Mosby, 1962.

Proudfit, F. T., and Robinson, C.: Normal and Therapeutic Nutrition, New York, Macmillan, 1961.

Sense, E.: Clinical Studies in Nutrition, Philadelphia, Lippincott, 1960.

Turner, D.: Handbook of Diet Therapy, Chicago, University of Chicago Press, 1959.

U. S. Department of Agriculture: Food—The Yearbook of Agriculture, Washington, D. C., U. S. Government Printing Office, 1959.

Articles

Conference on Therapy: Treatment of obesity, Am. J. Med. **13:**478-487, 1952.

Darby, W. S.: Nutritional deficiency diseases today, J. Am. Dietet. Ass. **57:**17-21, 1957.

Feinstein, A. R., Dole, V. P., and Schwartz, I. L.: The use of a formula diet for weight reduction of obese outpatients, Ann. Intern. Med. **48:**330-342, 1958.

Griffith, W. H.: The physiologic role of vitamins, Am. J. Med. **25:**666-679, 1958.

Lorincz, A. L.: Nutrition in relation to dermatology, J.A.M.A. **166:**1862-1867, 1958.

McConnell, J. F.: The deposed one, Am. J. Nursing **61:**78-81, Aug., 1961.

Newton, M. E.: What every nurse needs to know about nutrition, Nursing Outlook **8:** 316-317, 1960.

Pennington, A. W., *et al.*: Symposium on obesity, New England J. Med. **248:**959-975, 1953.

Sailor, N. M.: Nutrition knowledge applied to everyday living, Nursing Outlook **9:**756-759, 1961.

Spies, T. D.: Some recent advances in nutrition, J.A.M.A. **167:**675-690, 1958.

Stare, F. J.: Nutritional challenges for physicians, J.A.M.A. **178:**924-927, 1961.

Symposium on overnutrition: Am. J. Clin. Nutr. **9:** 1961.

10

Parenteral Therapy

An increasing knowledge of the chemical composition of body fluids in recent years has brought with it a greater awareness of the importance of restoring normal water and electrolyte balance in the bodies of patients who have a disease or are subjected to surgery. To attain this end, parenteral fluid therpay, whether for nutrition, maintenance or replacement, is planned and adapted to meet the particular need. The only way a physician can meet adequately the fluid needs of a patient is by knowing his intake and fluid losses. In nursing, it is as imperative to keep accurate intake and output records as it is to administer medications, oxygen and so forth.

In this chapter, an attempt will be made to clarify some of the physiologic, the chemical and the nutritional changes which take place in the normal adult and in individuals who are sick.

Although the whole subject of fluid balance is a complex one, the nurse ought to have an understanding of the problem. As a result, she will be of greater assistance to the physician and be better able to administer more intelligent nursing care to her patient.

BODY WATER

The total body water is divided into two main divisions: extracellular and intracellular fluid. Extracellular fluid includes plasma (about 5 per cent of body weight) and interstitial fluid (about 15 per cent of body weight). Intracellular fluid is equal to about 50 per cent of body weight. Hence, 70 per cent of body weight is water (Fig. 25).

Fluid exchange occurs in a definite way. For instance, the skin can lose fluid only, the gastrointestinal tract can absorb or lose fluid, the lungs lose fluid by evaporation, and the kidneys lose fluid and many other substances. Ordinarily, fluid is taken through the gastrointestinal tract and is excreted in the urine, the feces and the perspiration and through losses from the lungs (Fig. 26). Abnormally, fluid is lost by vomiting, diarrhea, fistula, perspiration, hemorrhage and exudation. It is estimated that daily water loss by evaporation is about 2,000 ml.; water loss in the urine averages about 1,500 ml. To this total daily loss of 3,500 ml. must be added the approximate amount of fluid loss in vomiting, drainage, diarrhea or any other abnormal or unusual loss. These losses are corrected by oral intake of food and fluid and/or parenteral injection.

Specific Body Water Needs

Fluid Balance

Water is second only to oxygen as a vital physiologic necessity. Man can be starved, can lose almost all of his glycogen and fat, half of his body protein, 40 per cent of his body weight and still live. However, a loss of 10 per cent of his water content is serious, and a loss of 20 per cent is fatal.

According to Bowen (Fig. 27), the amount of fluid secreted by the gastrointestinal tract in 24 hours is close to 8,200 ml., an amount equal to the total blood volume. Consequently, vomiting, diarrhea and draining intestinal fistulae can and do result in the loss of considerable amounts of water and electrolytes.

The water loss sustained during surgical procedures by evaporation and perspiration is about 1,000 to 1,500 ml. In addition, fluid losses due to hemorrhage may vary from 1,000 to 3,000 ml. Furthermore, due to anesthesia and the operative procedure, it is usually impossible to give fluids by mouth for 1 or 2 days and even longer. Therefore, in order to maintain a *fluid balance* (fluid intake equal to fluid loss) fluid must be given parenterally. In addition to the loss of fluid at operation, many patients may lose fluid by vomiting or from drainage due to intestinal, biliary, pancreatic or other fistulae. In these patients also, the fluid balance is disturbed. In some instances, especially those in which there has been an inability to take fluids, as in carcinoma of the esophagus, or in those in which there has been prolonged fluid loss by vomiting, as in pyloric or intestinal obstruction, the fluid deficit may be present even before operation. Patients in whom there is a marked and prolonged fluid deficit are said to be *dehydrated* (Fig. 26). Accompanying symptoms are hot, dry skin, thirst, dry tongue, sunken eyes, temperature elevation and scanty urine. Fluid replacement is given preferably by mouth, but in those situations in which fluids cannot be given orally they must be administered parenterally, usually intravenously.

A fairly accurate clinical estimate of the fluid loss may be obtained by the amount of the urinary output; hence, it is extremely important to measure the urine. In most cases an output varying between 1,000 and 1,500 ml. is considered to be adequate.

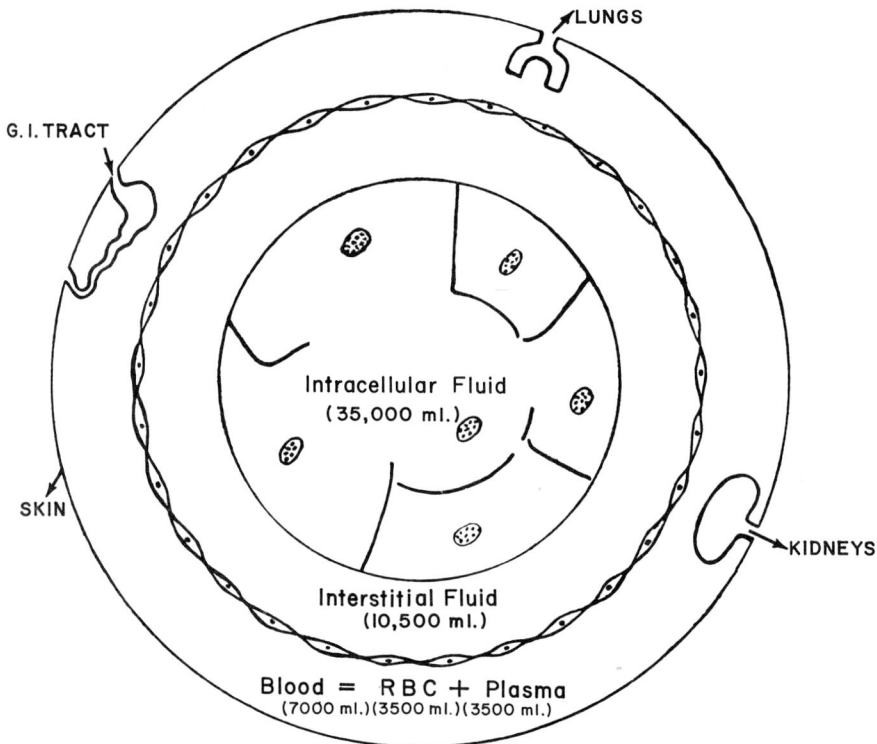

Fig. 25. A diagram illustrating the 3 main compartments of the body separated from each other by definite anatomic barriers, i.e., the capillary and the cell walls. The inner sphere is the intracellular space containing the fluid inside the cells of muscles, liver, etc., separated from the rest of the body by cell membrane. The outer space represents circulating blood. In the space between is the interstitial (or intercellular) fluid. The barrier between the blood and the interstitial fluid is the wall of the blood capillary membrane. (Adapted from Elman, Robert: Fluid balance from the nurse's point of view, Am. J. Nurs. **49**:222)

Electrolytes

Body fluids contain many chemical compounds. Some of them are present as intact molecules; others are split into separate electrically charged components known as *ions*. Compounds that break up into ions are called *electrolytes*. Ions may carry positive charges (*cations*) or negative charges (*anions*). Examples include sodium (Na^+), potassium (K^+), calcium (Ca^{++}), magnesium (Mg^{++}), bicarbonate (HCO_3^-), chloride (Cl^-), phosphate ($PO_4^=$) and sulfate ($SO_4^=$) ions.

Electrolyte concentrations can be expressed in terms of milligrams per 100 ml. or, preferably, as milliequivalents per liter (mEq./L.), a value that indicates the combining power of the ion and hence is more meaningful. One *equivalent* equals the molecular weight, expressed in grams, of an anion or a cation, divided by its chemical valence (1 in the case of Na^+, K^+, HCO_3^- and Cl^-; 2 in the case of Mg^{++}, $PO_4^=$, and $SO_4^=$). A *milliequivalent* represents the molecular weight in milligrams, instead of grams, i.e., it is one one-thousandth of an equivalent. One milliequivalent of any anion will combine with precisely one milliequivalent of any cation. For example, the atomic weight of sodium is 23, and one milliequivalent of sodium therefore is 23 milligrams; the molecular weight of the bicarbonate ion is 61 and one milliequivalent, 61 mg.; and the relative weights of these two ions in sodium bicarbonate are 23 and 61, respectively. The atomic weight of calcium is 40; therefore, one milliequivalent of calcium ion (Ca^{++}) is 20 mg., and if the concentration of calcium in the serum is 10 mg. per 100 ml., there are 5 milliequivalents per 1,000 ml. (5 mEq./L.).

Ordinarily, the body maintains a constant internal environment through mechanisms of homeostasis. However, in many medical and surgical patients, fluid and electrolyte balance becomes disturbed. When fluids are lost from the body, there is likewise a loss of the body electrolytes; thus, in vomiting, diarrhea or intestinal or biliary fistulae, electrolytes as

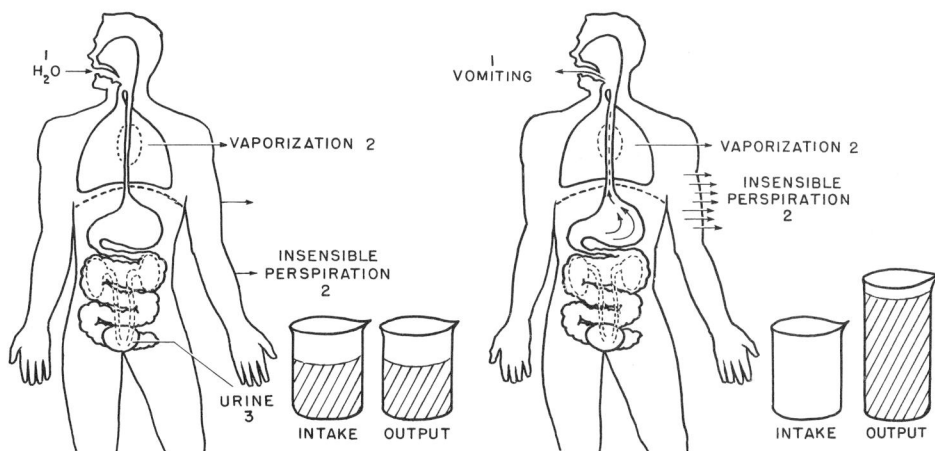

FIG. 26. Fluid balance and imbalance in an individual. (*Left*) Normal fluid balance. (1) Water taken in as such. (2) Water lost by vaporization from the lungs and the skin (insensible loss). (3) Water lost in urine. The small amount normally lost in the feces is not indicated. The amount lost as sensible perspiration is highly variable and is not indicated. Daily intake and output are equal. (*Right*) Output exceeds intake. (1) Water lost by vomiting. None is taken in either as such or in food. The only source is the water of oxidation produced in the cells as the body tissues are consumed. (2) Water lost by vaporization. The insensible loss from the skin is increased, due to the elevation of the body temperature or to hot weather. Little or no urine is formed. The variable loss by sensible perspiration is not shown.

well as fluids are lost. Because of the fact that these fluids vary in their electrolyte composition, there is a difference in the electrolyte loss by these various means. Thus, in vomiting, the loss is mostly the hydrochloric acid of the stomach, and the ion loss is chloride; the basic ion, sodium, is retained. On the other hand, the loss from intestinal fistulae contains more of the basic ions— calcium, sodium and potassium. Under normal conditions, the acid-base balance is maintained by the kidneys and the lungs; but under certain conditions, such as immediately after operation, sodium excretion may be less than normal, and potassium excretion may be increased. These variations produce disturbances in acid-base balance and must be taken into account in administering postoperative electrolyte solutions.

Abnormal Electrolyte Patterns. Described below are several common electrolyte patterns that are of paramount concern to the nurse.

Dehydration hypertonicity is a problem that frequently confronts the nurse in patients who have pulmonary congestion or infection. This phenomenon results from loss of body water predominantly or exclusively (little or no electrolyte loss being entailed). The loss occurs through evaporation of moisture in the expired air of patients who are dyspneic, or hyperventilating, and breathing through their mouths. Evaporation is enhanced and the water loss increased by fever. The problem is aggravated severely by tracheotomy, which favors rapid drying of the moisture-laden tidal air in the trachea. An extreme example of the situation is found in sunstroke, excessive exposure to the hot sun and dry air leading to hyperventilation, hyperthermia and eventual desiccation. Dehydration hypertonicity is characterized by a rising hematocrit and by increasing concentrations of sodium and chloride ions in the plasma, hyperproteinemia and azotemia. Patients who are mildly affected may exhibit no more than fever, oliguria and delirium, the severest cases progressing to coma, convulsions and death. Treatment consists in correction of the water deficit by the parenteral administration of a 5 per cent aqueous solution of dextrose. More important is pre-

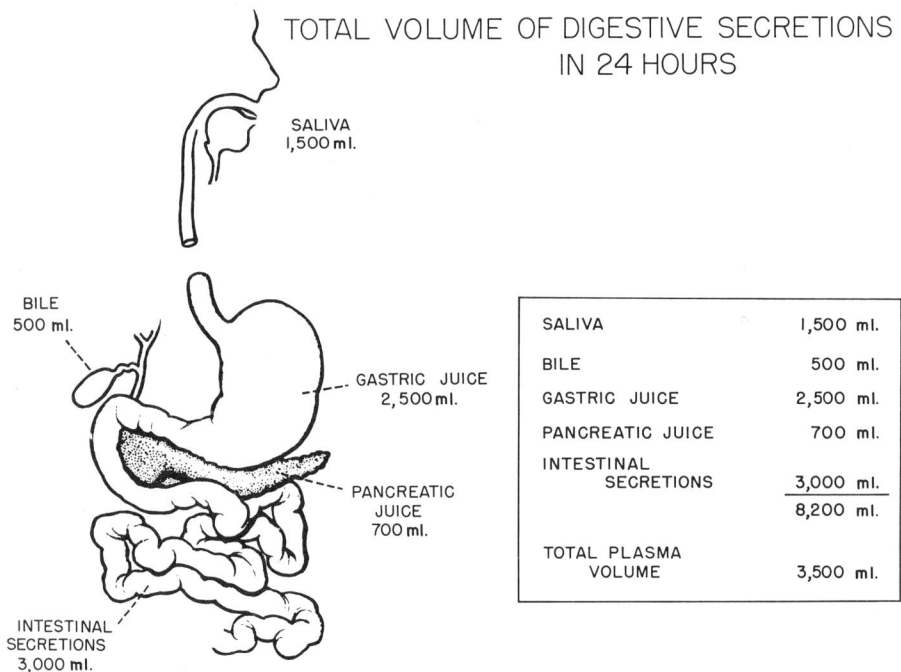

TOTAL VOLUME OF DIGESTIVE SECRETIONS IN 24 HOURS

SALIVA
1,500 ml.

BILE
500 ml.

GASTRIC JUICE
2,500 ml.

PANCREATIC JUICE
700 ml.

INTESTINAL SECRETIONS
3,000 ml.

SALIVA	1,500 ml.
BILE	500 ml.
GASTRIC JUICE	2,500 ml.
PANCREATIC JUICE	700 ml.
INTESTINAL SECRETIONS	3,000 ml.
	8,200 ml.
TOTAL PLASMA VOLUME	3,500 ml.

Fig. 27. Total volume of digestive secretions produced in 24 hours. (Adapted from Bowen, Arthur: Intravenous alimentation in surgical patients, Mod. Med.)

vention, which can be achieved by supplying fluids at rates that are commensurate with losses.

Water intoxication, or "dilutional hypotonicity," is the converse of the situation described above. This results from the ingestion (or therapeutic administration) of water in volumes that are excessive in relation to the fluid output; it occurs most often in patients with reduced renal function who have received liberal quantities of dextrose solution by parenteral injection. Patients with cardiac, renal and liver disease are especially vulnerable. A parallel decline in the hematocrit reading and in the concentrations of sodium, chloride and protein in the plasma is characteristic, and diagnostic, of water intoxication. Assuming that diuresis has been established, and is active, and provided that no cerebral symptoms are apparent, no therapy is indicated other than the halting of fluids. On the other hand, if mental aberrations are detected, loss of alertness is observed or symptoms of headache, nausea or vomiting develop, the patient may receive hypertonic sodium. The latter is given intravenously in the form of 3 per cent sodium chloride solution, starting with a test dose of 300 ml. Treatment then proceeds in accord-

PERTINENT DEFINITIONS:

Azotemia — excessive accumulation of nitrogenous bodies in the blood

Proteinemia — protein in the blood plasma

Natremia—sodium in the blood plasma

Kalemia — potassium in the blood plasma

	Female	Male
Normal hematocrit % vol. of packed RBC/100ml.	39-47	44-52

ance with the changing electrolyte pattern and the condition of the patient.

Congestive heart failure is responsible for another variety of dilutional hypotonicity which is brought about by excessive retention of water. Sodium is also retained, even to the extent that the exchangeable body sodium may be doubled; nevertheless, no matter how marked the sodium retention may be, the latter invariably is exceeded by the retention of water in these cases, with the result that the body fluids are not only expanded in volume but also are hypotonic. The typical pattern is marked by hyponatremia,

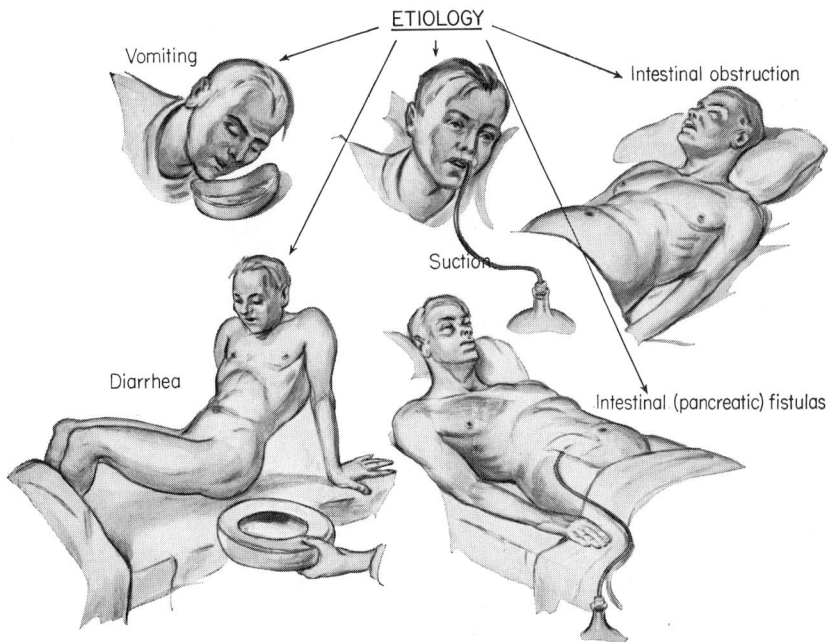

FIG. 28. The more common causes of primary salt depletion. (Thorek, P.: Illustrated Preoperative and Postoperative Care, Philadelphia, Lippincott)

ACID-BASE BALANCE (NORMAL)

I LITER EXTRACELLULAR FLUID

pH normal

7.35–7.45

Acid

Alkaline

I Part

20 Parts

6.

8.

CARBONIC ACID

BASE BICARBONATE

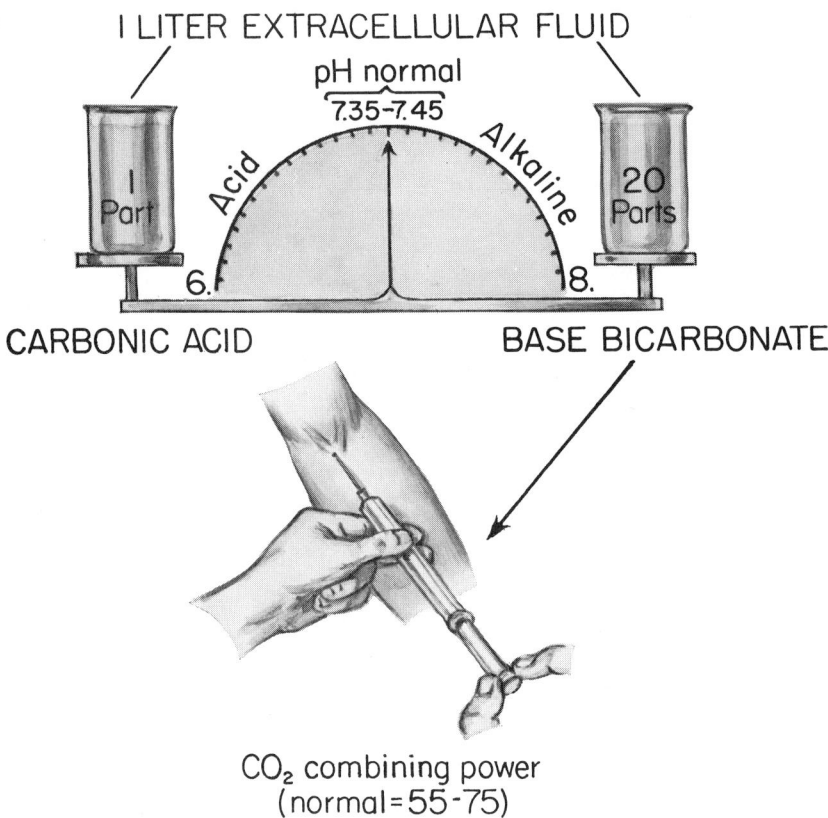

CO_2 combining power
(normal = 55–75)

Fig. 29. Normal acid-base balance is in a pH range between 7.35 and 7.45. If the pH drops below 7.35 acidosis (acidemia) results; if the pH is above 7.45, alkalosis (alkalemia) is present. In each liter of extracellular fluid there is approximately 1 part of carbonic acid to 20 parts of base bicarbonate. (Thorek, P.: Illustrated Preoperative and Postoperative Care, Philadelphia, Lippincott)

hypoproteinemia, hyperkalemia and slight azotemia. Treatment must provide for ample caloric nutrition, restriction of sodium and water intake, the administration of diuretics and a course of digitalis (see p. 542).

Starvation may result in similar changes in the electrolyte pattern, including hyponatremia, hypoproteinemia, moderate hyperkalemia and considerable expansion of the extracellular fluid volume. These patients require ample caloric nutrition. This may be fortified by infusions of concentrated glucose and insulin and supplemented by transfusions of red cells, as required.

Hypertonicity from "solute-loading," rather than water loss, is brought about by the spontaneous accumulation (or therapeutic administration) of osmotically active substances to a degree that is excessive in relation to the volume of water that is re-tained. This situation develops occasionally as a result of incautious tube feeding of an unconscious patient, incapable of registering thirst, who receives nothing but concentrated solutions of glucose and amino acids. It is encountered occasionally in an infant who has been fed cow's milk without sufficient water supplement. The problem is particularly apt to arise in instances of bleeding peptic ulcer, the patient having received liberal quantities of milk and cream, but insufficient water, and is absorbing from his gut an additional solute load in the form of digested blood. Moreover, it is likely to be aggravated further through wastage of water by kidneys which recently have sustained tubular damage in the course of oligemic shock and temporarily are incapable of concentrating urine and conserving water. Laboratory findings include marked hypernatremia, moderate elevation of the hematocrit reading and azotemia. Treatment consists in providing water until the excess solute has been unloaded.

Desalting and dehydration may occur acutely as a result of very rapid and substantial loss of fluid and electrolytes from the gastrointestinal tract in patients who have gastric or small bowel obstruction, ulcerative colitis, cholera, dysentery or infantile diarrhea. The patient becomes febrile and apathetic; the pulse mounts; the hematocrit rises; urine volume diminishes to the point

of anuria; hypotension progresses into shock and, barring vigorous treatment, death may ensue. Treatment at this stage involves the administration of sodium chloride in large quantities, supplemented by infusions of potassium as soon as the patient begins to void urine. If the arterial pressure is significantly depressed, the administration of plasma, or concentrated serum albumin, is indicated in amounts that may be predicted from the degree of hematocrit elevation. This phase, if survived, is followed by one marked by general electrolyte depletion, anemia, hy-

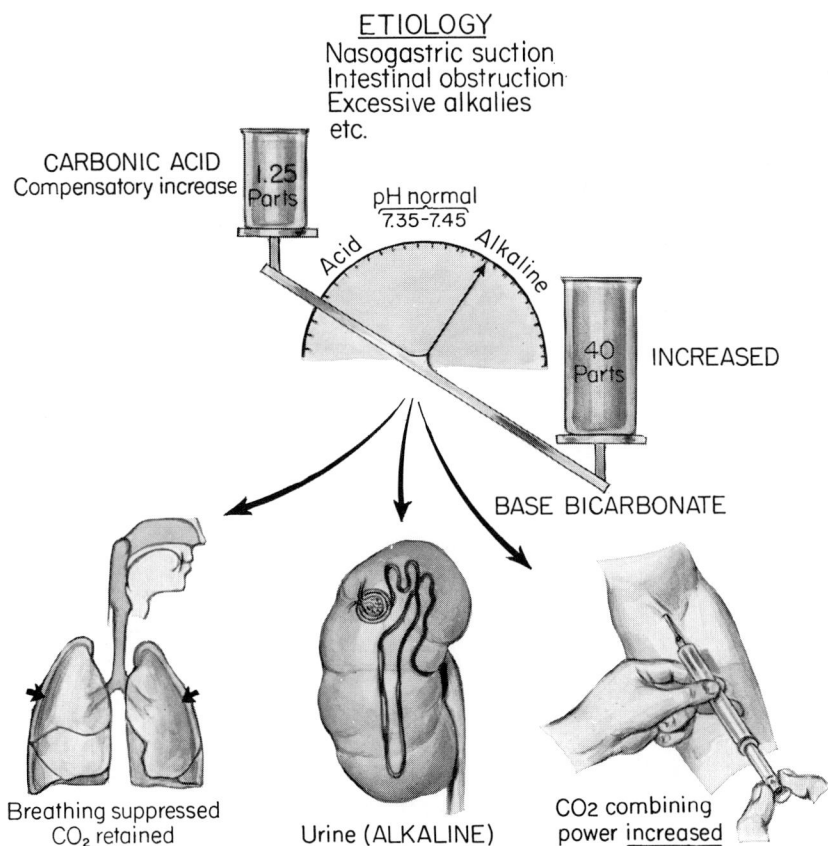

ETIOLOGY
Nasogastric suction
Intestinal obstruction
Excessive alkalies
etc.

CARBONIC ACID
Compensatory increase

1.25 Parts

pH normal
7.35-7.45

Acid   Alkaline

40 Parts   INCREASED

BASE BICARBONATE

Breathing suppressed
CO_2 retained

Urine (ALKALINE)

CO_2 combining
power increased

FIG. 30. Metabolic alkalosis (base bicarbonate excess). In this condition the base bicarbonates are increased, and the pH is increased. The normal acid-base ratio of 1 to 20 is now changed to 1.25 to 40. The lungs attempt to compensate by withholding carbonic acid (CO_2); hence the breathing is suppressed. A compensatory increase in carbonic acid may result. The kidneys attempt to compensate by retaining hydrogen ions and excreting bicarbonate ions; the urine becomes alkaline. The CO_2 combining power is increased. (Thorek, P.: Illustrated Preoperative and Postoperative Care, Philadelphia, Lippincott)

poproteinemia and either metabolic alkalosis or acidosis, depending on the character of fluid that was lost, i.e., whether it was acid or alkaline. In either case, restoration of the normal metabolic status requires re-expansion of the plasma volume with plasma, serum albumin or whole blood and the parenteral administration of sodium chloride, potassium and bicarbonate solutions.

Venous hemorrhage and thermal burns result in losses not only of water and electrolytes but also the proteins of the plasma and intracellular proteins.

ACIDOSIS AND ALKALOSIS. Whether a fluid is acid or alkaline, and to what degree, depends on the concentration of hydrogen ions in the solution, a value that is expressed in terms of *pH*. (pH units express logarithmically the hydrogen ion concentration in equivalents of H^+ per liter of solution.) A neutral solution has a pH of 7: it contains $1/10^7$ equivalents (0.0000001 grams) of H^+ per liter. The pH of an acid solution is less than 7; the lower the pH, the greater the acidity. Conversely, pH values above 7 denote alkalinity. The most acid of all the body fluids is the juice that is secreted by the normal stomach in response to a meal. The pH of

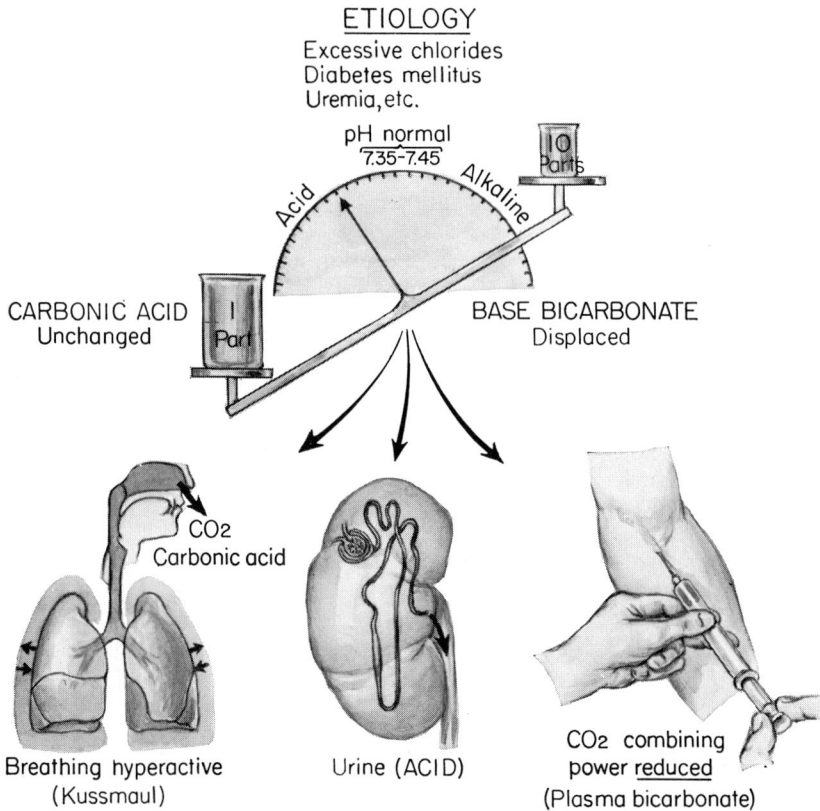

FIG. 31. Metabolic acidosis (base bicarbonate deficit). In this condition chlorides, organic acids and ketone bodies *displace* the base bicarbonate, and the pH of the extracellular fluid drops below 7.35. The lungs attempt to compensate by hyperactive breathing, thus blowing off excess carbonic acid (CO_2). The kidneys attempt to compensate by excreting hydrogen ions (acid) and conserving base bicarbonate. The CO_2 combining power is reduced. Although this illustration shows the carbonic acid unchanged, it may actually be lowered by hyperactive breathing. (Thorek, P.: Illustrated Preoperative and Postoperative Care, Philadelphia, Lippincott)

such juice may be as low as 2, in which case it contains $1/10^2$ equivalents (0.01 equivalents or grams) of hydrogen ions per liter. Most of the body fluids are slightly alkaline (pH 7.35 to 7.45). The acid-base balance is maintained by a system of buffer substances that take up or release hydrogen ions as the situation requires. The most important of the buffer teams in the extracellular fluid is comprised of carbonic acid (H_2CO_3) and bicarbonate (HCO_3^-). The bicarbonate ion usually is measured as the carbon dioxide content of venous plasma, normally 25 to 30 mEq. per liter.

Acute alkalosis and hypokalemia represent a pattern that is characteristic of patients who have vomited severely and lost large volumes of gastric HCl. The plasma carbon dioxide content becomes markedly elevated; the hematocrit reading, plasma sodium concentration and blood urea nitrogen likewise are increased, while the potassium and the chloride levels decline. These patients become distended, apathetic and weak. In order to restore the potassium deficit, potassium chloride is supplied in large excess over sodium salts or protein.

Diabetic acidosis presents an unusually complicated situation in which both intracellular and extracellular water is lost. Sodium, combined with organic acids, is lost, together with water, in the urine. Potassium migrates, with intracellular water, through the cell membranes into the plasma and thence into the urine. The electrolyte pattern is characterized by signs of dehydration, acidosis, hyponatremia and hypokalemia. As soon as insulin therapy is commenced and parenteral fluids are administered, potassium proceeds to leave the plasma and re-enter the cells, as a result of which the potassium concentration falls to a hazardous level very rapidly, unless potassium has been included among the injected materials.

The electrolyte disturbances and water shifts that are associated with diabetes insipidus, adrenal insufficiency and various types of renal failure are described elsewhere in the text, in conjunction with other manifestations of the underlying diseases.

Restitution of Normal Pattern. Serious electrolyte disturbances which endanger the patient and require vigorous, complicated treatment often can be forestalled by relatively simple measures, provided that these situations are recognized and appropriate measures are applied at a sufficiently early stage in their development. (Some disorders, such as hypotonicity due to overdilution, or hypertonicity from solute-loading, representing complications of therapy rather than disease, of course, should have been foreseen and avoided altogether.) For the administration of corrective fluids, the oral route should be utilized to whatever extent this is possible. Electrolyte solutions may be tolerated when food is not. The solution shown below, given by mouth in amounts sufficient to balance fluid losses, effectively prevents and relieves metabolic acidosis and alkalosis alike.

The majority of patients with serious dehydration and electrolyte derangements are unable to ingest or absorb the necessary fluids in adequate amounts and with sufficient rapidity when supplied by mouth or by tubal feedings. Under these circumstances, nutrition and hydration must be accomplished by means of parenteral therapy, the technical aspects of which are now to be considered.

Electrolyte and Nutrient Solutions

The principle on which all electrolyte therapy is based, whether prophylactic or corrective, oral or parenteral, postulates that, for every 100 calories metabolized, a patient requires 3 millimoles (0.06 Gm.) of

ELECTROLYTE REPAIR SOLUTION FOR ORAL ADMINISTRATION

Ingredients		Ionic Concentration (mEq./L.)	
Sodium chloride:	1.0 Gm.	Sodium:	30
Sodium bicarbonate:	1.0 Gm.	Potassium:	13
Potassium chloride:	1.0 Gm.	Chloride:	30
Dextrose:	5.0 Gm.	Bicarbonate:	12
Distilled water:	q.s. ad 1,000 ml.		

sodium chloride, 2 mEq. of potassium ion and 150 ml. of water. Available to meet these requirements, and to correct abnormalities in the electrolyte pattern, are several solutions which are suitable for parenteral injection. Of these, the most widely used are isotonic saline, solutions containing the sodium and chloride ions in the proportion in which they are found in the body and solutions in which the potassium ion is the principal ingredient.

Sodium and Chloride Ions

Solutions which are employed specifically for the restoration of body water, sodium ion and chloride ion include isotonic saline solution, in which these ions are present in equimolar concentrations, and a solution in which sodium and chloride ions are contained in the proportion in which they are found in the body (i.e., in a ratio of about 1.5 to 1), 40 per cent of the chloride having been replaced by lactate, or bicarbonate, which is promptly metabolized in the body. The composition of these solutions is indicated below.

Isotonic saline is entirely effective in the treatment of most cases with dehydration, even when complicated by acidosis or alkalosis, provided that the kidneys are capable of excreting the excess chloride that is supplied by this solution. However, if the renal function is impaired and chlorides are not excreted efficiently, the electrolyte imbalance may be increased as a result of saline infusions. In most cases with dehydration and acidosis, a mixture of sodium chloride and sodium lactate (or sodium bicarbonate) is preferable to sodium chloride solution. This is true because it supplies sodium and chloride in the same ratio that normally exists in the plasma and can be administered without the risk of causing a preponderant accumulation of either ion, despite renal impairment.

Patients whose electrolyte pattern indicates hyponatremia and hypotonicity of the body fluids (see p. 163) are treated most effectively with hypertonic sodium solution. This is usually administered in the form of 3 per cent saline (NaCl, 3 Gm./100 ml.).

Potassium

After repeated or prolonged bouts of diarrhea, and following a prolonged course of parenteral therapy which has not included the administration of this element, potassium deficiency is inevitable. Hypokalemia, in addition to other electrolyte disturbances, also is an important consideration in cases of severe acidosis or alkalosis. Alkalosis is particularly prone to produce K deficiency, the "alkalotic kidney" permitting this element to be wasted in the urine. Furthermore, K deficiency itself favors alkalosis by producing kidney damage ("clear cell nephrosis") of a type which promotes sodium retention, therefore, alkalosis.

Potassium replacement should be carried out at a rate of 3 mEq. per kilogram of body

ISOTONIC SODIUM CHLORIDE SOLUTION (PHYSIOLOGIC SALINE)

Ingredients	Ionic Concentration (mEq./L.)
Sodium chloride: 8.5 Gm.	Sodium: 145
Distilled water: q.s. ad 1,000 ml.	Chloride: 145

SODIUM CHLORIDE—SODIUM LACTATE SOLUTION

Ingredients	Ionic Concentration (mEq./L.)
Sodium chloride: 6.4 Gm.	Sodium: 150
Sodium lactate: 5.6 Gm.	Chloride: 108
Distilled water: q.s. ad 1,000 ml.	Lactate: 42
or	
Isotonic saline solution: 750 ml.	
Sixth-molar sodium lactate solution: 250 ml.	

weight per 24 hours. Patients who are maintained on parenteral nutrients exclusively should receive 1 to 3 mEq. of potassium per 100 calories administered in order to avoid potassium depletion. The concentration of potassium in an intravenous solution should not exceed 40 mEq. per liter, and each day's ration of potassium should be injected over a period of not less than 4 hours.

Two solutions capable of restoring and preventing potassium deficiency are specified below. The second of these, containing NaCl and KCl, is designed primarily for electrolyte maintenance in patients on constant gastric suction. The inclusion of dextrose in these solutions not only supplies calories but also ensures hypotonicity, the concentration of inorganic ions being so low that, except for this addition, hemolysis might result from their injection.

Nutrient Solutions

Conditions occasionally arise in which both oral and tube feedings become impossible or are contraindicated, and in which recourse must be had to parenteral nutrition. The parenteral nutrient used most frequently is 5 per cent dextrose, i.e., a solution containing 50 Gm. of dextrose per 1,000 ml. water or isotonic saline, and providing therefore 200 calories per liter.

Higher concentrations are employed in the treatment of patients with oliguria whose total fluid intake must be reduced to a minimum, a suitable regimen in such cases being the daily intravenous injection of 300 to 500 ml. of a solution containing 15 to 20 Gm. of dextrose per 100 ml. of distilled water, other fluids being withheld pending the resumption of urine excretion. Concentrated solutions of this type should be administered with caution, for hypertonic fluids exert a dehydrating and irritant effect on exposed tissues. Their injection, if unduly rapid or continued without interruption for prolonged periods of time, causes intravascular thrombosis and obliteration of the veins at the sites of injection.

Parenteral solutions containing amino acids and fat emulsions likewise are available for intravenous administration. The need for either is extremely limited.

METHODS OF ADMINISTERING PARENTERAL FLUIDS

Four routes are available for the parenteral injection of fluids, namely, the intravenous, the intramuscular, the subcutaneous and the intramedullary. Their relative advantages and inherent limitations determine the method of injection to be selected in individual cases.

Intravenous Infusions

The venous route is preferred above all others for the administration of parenteral fluids (Fig. 32). The rate of absorption by this method can be controlled with greater precision, greater flexibility is possible with respect to the character of material infused, and there is less discomfort associated with this procedure than with any other method.

POTASSIUM CHLORIDE—DEXTROSE SOLUTION

Ingredients		Ionic Concentration (mEq./L.)	
Potassium chloride:	2.25 Gm.	Potassium:	30
Glucose:	50 Gm.	Chloride:	30
Distilled water:	q.s. ad 1,000 ml.		

POTASSIUM-SODIUM-CHLORIDE-DEXTROSE

Ingredients		Ionic Concentration (mEq./L.)	
Potassium chloride:	3.0 Gm.	Potassium:	40
Sodium chloride:	4.5 Gm.	Sodium:	80
Dextrose:	25.0 Gm.		
Distilled water:	q.s. ad 1,000 ml.		

Fluids injected intravenously are absorbed and distributed throughout the body at a rate that corresponds exactly with the speed of injection. Thus, the intravenous method offers a measure of safety, as regards the production of pulmonary edema, that alternate procedures lack. The type of patient in whom the risk of overhydration is especially important to consider is one whose plasma proteins are deficient, serum sodium concentration is low and body water is increased, exemplified by certain patients with congestive heart failure and others with chronic renal disease.

The solution in the reservoir usually should be at room temperature. The solution is given at a rate of about 60 to 80 drops a minute or as ordered by the physician.* The amount and the type of solution

* It may be necessary to check the type of equipment being used in order to determine the speed of injection, since the size of a drop may vary or be changed by a drop meter. See "Speed of Infusion" on page 172.
The flow rate ideally should be specified (and measured) in terms of ml. per minute.

are indicated in the doctor's orders. Drugs may be introduced into the tubing with a syringe and a needle using sterile precautions.

If the circulation is good, the fluid is lost rapidly through the kidneys and other excretory organs or by absorption into the tissues, so that the procedure must be repeated frequently. For this reason, intravenous infusion should be considered as having only a temporary effect in increasing the volume of circulating fluids. More lasting effects are obtained by a transfusion of blood or plasma.

Intravenous needles cannot be left *in situ* for periods longer than 24 to 48 hours without producing an inflammatory reaction locally. There follows a painful thrombophlebitis, and the vein, occluded by clot, is thenceforth eliminated as an infusion route. Patients who require continuous or intermittent intravenous therapy therefore pose a knotty technical problem, for which there are three possible solutions: (1) the needle may be withdrawn at 12- to 24-hour intervals and replaced in another vein; (2) the vein may

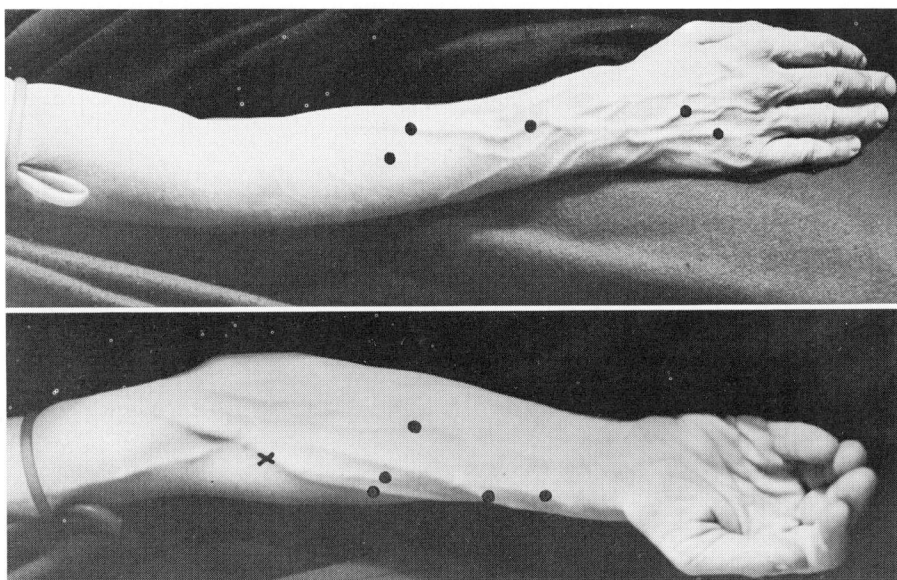

Fig. 32. Sites of election for the insertion of intravenous needles for the parenteral administration of fluids or blood transfusion. Preferably, injections are made into the distal portion of the extremity, at the points indicated by dots, rather than in the anterior cubital fossa (e.g., at point x), to avoid the necessity for immobilizing the elbow and the risk of the needle's becoming dislodged during the injection.

be incised, its lumen cannulated and the cannula sutured in place; (3) the vein may be catheterized with a small polyethylene tube. This catheter is threaded into a vein through the lumen of a hypodermic needle. The needle is then withdrawn, leaving the tube in place. Its proximal end may serve to accommodate an intravenous needle. Such plastic catheters can be left undisturbed and remain patent for as long as 6 weeks. However, research continues in an effort to find an indwelling catheter that will not evoke a foreign body reaction.

For the details involved in intravenous therapy administration, the student is referred to her textbook on fundamentals of nursing.

Intramedullary Injections

Although rarely utilized in parenteral therapy, the bone marrow cavity offers ready access to the circulating blood and is one injection site that is almost always available. The bone marrow communicates directly with the venous circulation, and, therefore, injected materials arrive in the blood stream as rapidly as they enter the body. The majority of crystalloid solutions, including amino acid preparations, as well as those containing protein, such as plasma, and even whole blood, can be administered successfully by this route. The site of preference for intramedullary infusion in an adult is the iliac crest; in a child, the tibia. An excellent needle for this purpose is one of the 14-gauge caliber which is equipped with a sharp tip of hard steel, but the shaft of which is composed of a malleable metal. After penetrating the bony cortex, its rigidity reinforced by a rigid stylet, and its tip solidly within the marrow cavity, the stylet is removed and the shaft bent at right angles before the infusion set is connected. Its projection now relatively slight, the needle is not likely to be dislodged by lateral pressure, and it is incapable of deep penetration as a result of a direct blow, so that no protective or supporting device is needed to maintain its position during the infusion. It may be allowed to remain in place for as long as 72 hours without risk, technical difficulty or discomfort to the patient. Maximum infusion rates achieved via the bone marrow are between 2,500 and 3,000 ml. per 24 hours.

PYROGENIC REACTIONS TO FLUID THERAPY

The most common and troublesome of all complications associated with parenteral fluid therapy is the so-called "pyrogenic reaction." The appearance of chills and fever in patients receiving intravenous material is almost always attributable to the injection of organisms, living or dead, into the blood stream of the recipient.

The febrile reaction characteristically begins between 30 and 60 minutes following the entry of the bacterial contaminant into the blood of the recipient. The development of fever is generally abrupt and is accompanied by a shaking chill. The body temperature at its peak ranges from 100° to 106°, its duration lasting from less than 1 hour to as long as 12 or even 24 hours. Associated with the reaction are headache, backache, generalized malaise, anorexia, nausea and occasional vomiting. In very severe reactions a state of vascular collapse may supervene; this is marked by an abrupt drop in arterial blood pressure—an ominous development in seriously ill patients. The problems that are created by reactions of this type in transfusion recipients and their differentiation from hemolytic reactions due to incompatible blood are discussed in Chapter 11.

Treatment and Prevention

No measures of specific therapeutic value are available with which to halt or control the course of the pyrogenic reaction. Antipyretic agents such as aspirin and acetophenetidin may reduce the height of the fever, but they may or may not alleviate the patient's discomfort, for profuse sweating, nausea and vomiting occasionally provoked by these drugs may overshadow in unpleasantness the symptoms attributable to the fever per se. The administration of antihistaminic drugs or antipyretics prior to, or immediately following, a parenteral injection is prescribed occasionally in the hope of preventing this complication, but there is no logical basis for this expectation. Therapeutic measures which improve the patient's comfort while chilling is in progress include the application of extra blankets and the provision of warm drinks, if these are tolerated and acceptable, and the use of sedatives and analgesic drugs, such as salicylates, codeine or Demerol.

The essence of therapy, of course, is prevention, and reactions of this type are very definitely preventable. The most dependable insurance against their development is the exclusive use of commercially prepared, disposable materials for parenteral therapy, all solutions and all equipment being discarded after use. Under these circumstances the only important precaution that must be observed is the prevention of bacterial contamination through incautious exposure of the solution to the air or the addition of materials not contained in the original equipment before or during the injection.

A contaminated needle as the source of a pyrogenic reaction is commonly overlooked in the investigation. Any hypodermic needle which is to be reused must be properly cleaned and sterilized. The only safe alternative is to use new disposable needles exclusively.

NURSING SUPERVISION OF PARENTERAL THERAPY

All recipients of parenteral fluids should be observed repeatedly during the procedure in order to detect at the earliest possible moment any signs indicative of an unfavorable response. Particular attention should be paid to the appearance of the injection site; the flow rate, as observed in the drip counter; the character of the respiration; the occurrence of coughing; and the color of the mucous membranes. An increase in the respiratory rate, the onset or increase of coughing or development of cyanosis suggests an overloading of the patient's circulation with transudation of fluid from the blood into the alveoli of the lungs. Immediately upon discovery of these signs the injection should be halted and the responsible physician should be informed regarding the sequence of events and the condition of the patient.

Sequence and Speed of Infusion

Intravenous infusions that are prescribed for nutritional and electrolyte maintenance are scheduled on a day-to-day basis, the nurse verifying the order in which particular solutions are given and regulating the rates of injection. Her decisions in these matters are guided by certain basic considerations, as follows.

Parenteral nutrition should be as nearly free of interruption as can be arranged from a practical standpoint. Interruptions for periods longer than 12 hours are undesirable and should be avoided.

Parenteral dextrose can be metabolized no more rapidly than 1 Gm. per kilogram (4.5 Gm. per 10 pounds) of body weight per hour. Consequently, a patient weighing 120 pounds should receive in 1 hour no more than 55 Gm. of intravenous dextrose, that is, less than 1,100 ml. of a 5 per cent, or 550 ml. of a 10 per cent, solution.

Hypertonic solutions, i.e., those having greater osmotic activity than the body fluids, should be injected no more rapidly than 3 to 4 ml. per minute, or approximately 1 drop per second, if the recipient vein is to escape damage and thrombophlebitis is to be avoided. (Sodium chloride, 0.85 Gm. per 100 ml., is an isotonic, or "normal," solution, approximately; thus, 0.85 per cent saline containing dextrose, 5 Gm. per 100 ml., is decidedly hypertonic. Dextrose, 7 Gm. per 100 ml. water, is approximately isotonic; accordingly, 10 per cent dextrose in water is hypertonic and 10 per cent dextrose in normal saline is exceedingly hypertonic.)

Potassium must be administered slowly in order to minimize the risk of cardiac arrest, which is especially hazardous in cases of renal failure. The concentration of potassium in intravenous solutions should not exceed 40 mEq. per liter, and a 30-mEq. solution is preferred. If the nurse is instructed to prepare a solution for intravenous injection by diluting a concentrated stock solution of a potassium salt, she has been assigned a grave responsibility. She must be fully aware of this and follow her instructions precisely and most attentively, for a dilution error could be fatal. A solution containing either dextrose, sodium chloride, or both, is suitable as a diluent for such a stock concentrate, as long as the combined concentration of sodium and potassium does not exceed 150 mEq. per liter. The daily quota of potassium should be administered over a period of no less than 4 hours. If the prescribed amount is contained in 1 liter of fluid, the rate of injection should be adjusted to approximately 60 drops per minute.

Amino acid injections should be instituted slowly, i.e., at a rate not exceeding 2 ml. per minute, or 1 drop every 2 seconds. After a period of 10 minutes, if the injection is well tolerated, the injection rate may be increased to 120 drops or more per minute. (Fat emulsions must be given precisely in accordance with the distributor's instructions.)

The addition of one or more injectable vitamins to an intravenous dextrose or electrolyte solution may be prescribed. The procedure must be accomplished with meticulous sterile technic, the solution so treated should be labeled appropriately and the mixture discarded if not used within the ensuing 4 hours.

The precise sequence in which parenteral solutions are infused is relatively unimportant except from the standpoint of the distribution, in time, of caloric nutrition and potassium therapy, as specified above.

Intravenous Teams

Intravenous therapy is so generally used in hospitals today that it often is turned over to intravenous teams. These teams, composed of technicians or nurses highly trained in giving intravenous injections, serve the entire hospital. Thus, the patients are not delayed in receiving their intravenous therapy by the fact that internes or residents may be in the operating room or elsewhere and unable to introduce the needles into the vein.

BIBLIOGRAPHY AND SUGGESTED READING
Books

Of Water, Salt and Life—An Atlas of Fluid and Electrolytic Balance in Health and Disease, Milwaukee, Lakeside Laboratories, 1956.

Parenteral Administration, North Chicago, Illinois, Abbott Laboratories, 1959.

Snively, William D.: Sea Within, Philadelphia, Lippincott, 1960.

Articles

Adriani, J.: Venipuncture, Am. J. Nursing **62:** 66-70, March, 1962.

Chow, R.: Innovations in I.V. equipment, Am. J. Nursing **62:**80-81, March, 1962.

Dunning, M. F. and Plun, F.: Potassium depletion by enemas, Am. J. Med. **20:**789-792, 1956.

Farr, H. W.: Fluid and electrolyte balance—with special reference to the gastro-intestinal tract, Am. J. Nursing **54:**826-831, 1954.

Imperiale, M., and Krebs, T.: The intravenous therapy nurses, Am. J. Nursing **61:**53-54, May, 1961.

Jorgensen, H. E.: Studies in metabolism of trauma — postoperative sodium retention, Surg., Gynec., & Obstet. **108:**339-342, 1959.

Lowe, C. U.: Principles of parenteral fluid therapy, Am. J. Nursing **53:**963-965, 1953.

Moore, F. D.: Common patterns of water and electrolyte change in injury, surgery, and disease, New England J. Med. **258:**277-286, 325-333, 377-384, 427-432, 1958.

Neyzi, O., Bailey, R. N., and Talbot, N. B.: Effects of varying infusion time in maintenance of fluid therapy, New England J. Med. **258:** 1239-1244, 1958.

Rademaker, L.: Reactions to intravenous administration of solutions, J.A.M.A. **135:**1140-1141, 1947.

Snively, W. D., and Brown, B. J.: In the balance, Am. J. Nursing **58:**55-57, Jan., 1958.

The dangers of intravenous therapy, Am. J. Nursing **59:**369, 1959.

Van Pelt, V. M.: A new fluid intake and output record, Am. J. Nursing **61:**80-82, Oct., 1961.

Wempe, B. M.: The new and the old intramuscular injection sites, Am. J. Nursing **61:**56-57, Sept., 1961.

Wolf, E. S.: The nurse and fluid therapy, Am. J. Nursing **54:**831-833, 1954.

11

Blood Transfusion

THE NURSE IN THE DONOR CLINIC

With the passage of time, nurses have been required to undertake an ever-increasing measure of responsibility in connection with transfusion therapy, including the taking of blood from donors and the conduct of donor clinics. The problems relative to blood procurement, which are of most immediate concern, are the selection and care of donors, the technical aspects of venesection and the possible complications of this procedure. Nursing responsibilities include the screening of potential donors on the basis of medical history and physical qualifications; the maintenance of sterile supplies and all other equipment and materials used in conjunction with donor phlebotomy; the training and the supervision of auxiliary workers assigned to the donor clinic; the performance of phlebotomy; the precise, unequivocal identification of donor blood and pilot samples; and the appropriate disposition of these donor units and test samples. The nurse is a key figure in public relations, the competence with which she performs her tasks in the donor clinic coloring the reputation not only of this unit but also of the entire hospital.

Donor Screening

Every prospective donor must be seen, questioned and examined before he donates blood, both for his own protection and that of the patient destined to receive his blood.

Measurements are made of the body weight, which must exceed 110 pounds; the arterial pressure, the acceptable limits of systolic pressure ordinarily being regarded as between 100 and 160 mm. Hg; the pulse rate, which should be between 60 and 110 beats per minute; and the body temperature, which, of course, must be normal.

Small individuals, whose body weight is less than 110 pounds, are considered unsuitable because the volume of their circulating blood is generally inadequate to support comfortably a loss of 450 ml. Candidates with arterial hypertension are disqualified, unless the procedure is requested specifically by their personal physicians, since they are unusually vulnerable to the risk of coronary thrombosis in the event of vascular collapse and sudden hypotension following the procedure; or, conversely, they may sustain a profound rise in pressure, preceding, during or following venesection, which conceivably could be responsible for a cerebral hemorrhage or an arterial rupture elsewhere in the body. Patients with marked hypotension are often regarded as prone to vascular collapse. Bradycardia may indicate the presence of complete heart block, and tachycardia may be a sign of vasomotor instability, with an increased tendency to fainting, of an infection or of hyperthyroidism. Women who are pregnant or have delivered within the preceding 9 months are not accepted because of the huge nutritional drain which is imposed by pregnancy.

Prospective donors are disqualified if evidence of any of the following conditions is obtained on the basis of medical history, signs or symptoms: acute or chronic alcoholism; an acute or chronic respiratory infection; malarial infection, past or present, including those patients who have resided in a malarial area and are meanwhile receiving suppressive antimalarial therapy; any other type of transmissible parasitic disease, such

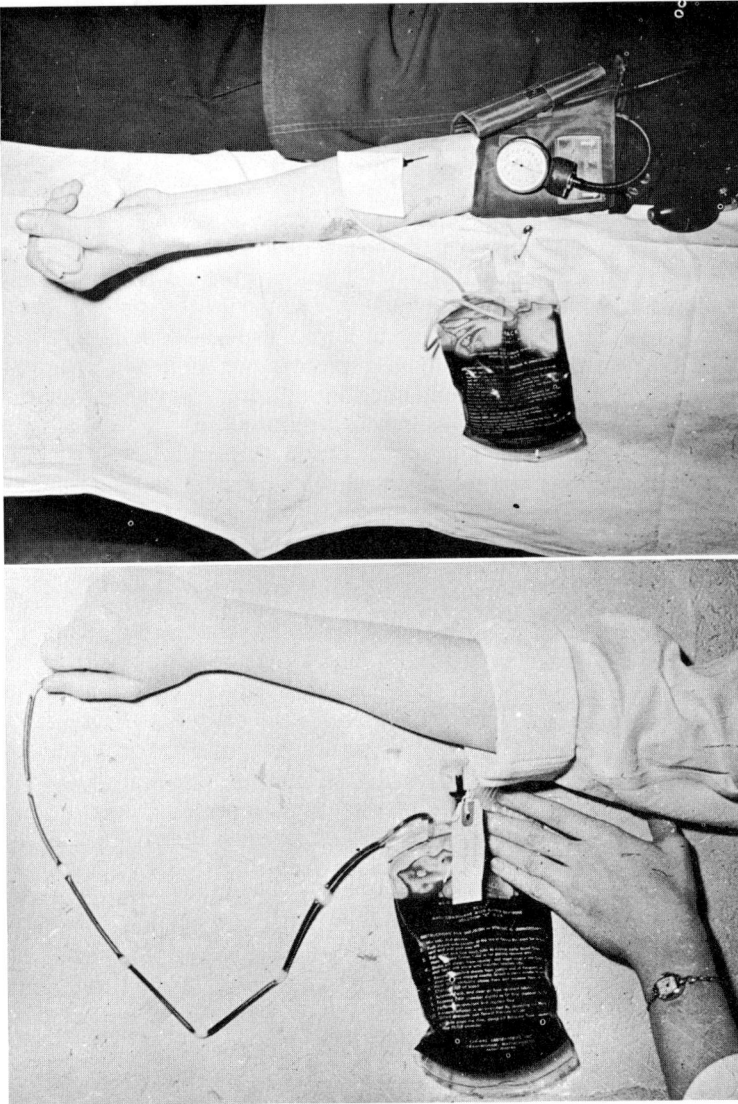

FIG. 33. (*Top*) Donor phlebotomy (plastic bag technic). Venous blood is flowing into a flexible polyvinyl bag that contains 75 ml. of acid-citrate-dextrose (ACD) solution as an anticoagulant and red cell preservative. (*Bottom*) The bag, containing approximately 450 ml. of donor blood, has been sealed off by fusing the donor tube at several points with a dielectric sealer. Each pair of seals encloses a small volume of blood which, thereafter, is available for testing without the necessity of entering the bag itself for a sample. (William Richardson-Jones, M.D., Miami)

as relapsing fever and Weil's disease; severe allergy of any type; any major illness within a 2-month period; a history of jaundice occurring at any time in the past, or a history of having resided in a common domicile with an individual who has a history of jaundice occurring within a 12-month period.

Phlebotomy

The technic of venesection may be described briefly as follows. The donor, having just received a full glass of water to assist the rapid restoration of his blood volume, is placed in a comfortable position, head resting on the same horizontal plane as the trunk. A blood pressure cuff is applied to the upper arm and inflated to a level between the diastolic and systolic pressure, e.g., approximately 100 mm. Hg, in order to distend and locate the antecubital vessels. After a vein has been selected the cuff is deflated and the skin overlying the puncture site is cleansed. Before venesection, the labeling of the donor-blood bottle and the tubes that are to receive the lab specimens is completed. Even if these labels have already been subjected to a routine check, they should be scrutinized once more with the utmost care, for it is quite clear that clerical errors, particularly those involving the placement of labels, are the most frequent cause of serious transfusion accidents, numerous fatalities having been attributable to misdirection or faulty identification of donor blood.

Following reinflation of the cuff to the original pressure, venipuncture is performed, and the blood is allowed to flow until the volume of blood collected is sufficient (Fig. 33). The volume of blood drawn from the donor should not exceed 450 ml. The blood pressure cuff is deflated, and the needle is released. The venesection may be considered complete after the blood bottle has been capped securely and sealed and specimen or "pilot" tubes have been filled.

The donor should be required to rest for a minimum period of 5 minutes and then adjust himself to the sitting posture. After the wound has been examined carefully for residual bleeding, a pressure dressing is applied to the arm, and the donor is permitted to regain his feet unless there is evidence of unusual weakness or faintness, in which event a longer rest is prescribed. Whatever his appearance, it is important that the donor remain in the near vicinity and under observation for a period of at least 20 minutes after leaving the table. During this interval he should drink a glass of liquid refreshment, one that is neither very hot nor very cold; permission to smoke, however, should be refused until he is considered for release.

Complications of Blood Donation

Local damage at the site of venipuncture occasionally occurs in blood donors. This may produce subcutaneous bleeding or inflammatory lesions, the former developing while the patient is still under observation and the latter many hours afterward. Continuous bleeding, although conceivably due to a blood disorder accompanied by a failure of the normal clotting mechanism, actually is rarely attributable to this cause but usually is due to laceration of the vein owing to some technical difficulty associated with the venipuncture or the withdrawal of the needle. Excessive probing within the subcutaneous tissue while searching for the

lumen of the vein or through-and-through perforations of the vein often are responsible for damage adequate to explain the occurrence of both external and subcutaneous hemorrhage with subsequent hematoma production. A technical error which invariably results in bleeding of this type is failure to release the cuff pressure prior to the withdrawal of the needle. However, if the venipuncture has been performed carefully and correctly and a pressure dressing has been applied securely no earlier than 5 minutes following the bleeding, and if the arm has been extended in an upright position, hemorrhage is rarely encountered.

Fainting in blood donors is a fairly common occurrence for which there are many possible causes. Emotional factors play a decided role in the genesis of this phenomenon, as is evident from the contagious element apparent when several donors are bled in a common room; the observing of such an attack by individuals who are about to be, or just have been, bled often precipitates a similar response in other donors. The fasting state, if prolonged, is likewise a predisposing factor in the production of faints. Because of this correlation, most blood bank regulations which formerly forbade the ingestion of food within 6 or 8 hours now have been revised in the opposite direction; donors are requested to have a light meal within 4 or 6 hours prior to venesection, and at all events to drink a full tumbler of some fluid, e.g., water, milk or fruit juice, immediately before giving blood.

Attacks of fainting usually occur at the conclusion of the procedure, immediately after resumption of the upright posture or shortly thereafter, for this position aggravates the severity of hypotension that reflects the loss of blood volume. The warning signal which should be looked for in all donors during the bleeding and afterward is the development of pallor. On the appearance of this sign, the donor should be obliged to lie down, or, if this cannot be arranged at once, he should sit with his head lowered between and below the level of the knees. This posture, and the reclining position with the feet on the bed and the knees flexed, improves the cerebral arterial circulation and tends to forestall fainting as well as to revive persons who have fainted. A donor who has fainted or feels faint should be kept under observation for a period of at least 30 minutes lest the phenomenon recur under less favorable circumstances.

Anginal pain, that is, pain located in the anterior chest in the region of the sternum or over the heart, is precipitated occasionally in donors who are afflicted with unsuspected coronary heart disease. The development of any symptom of this sort is always an occasion for serious concern because of its implication relative to the possibility of a recent acute coronary thrombosis. Convulsions, the most dramatic sequel to venesection, may be precipitated in epileptic individuals, including those with a latent susceptibility to seizures. Angina pectoris and epilepsy are discussed elsewhere in this text (Chaps. 27 and 41).

Inflammation of the tissues in the area of venipuncture may result from the introduction of bacteria into the soft tissues owing to faulty technic in cleansing and sterilizing of the skin or in protecting the needle from contamination prior to its use. Sterile inflammatory processes which develop within a few hours following the procedure usually are due to procaine sensitivity.

BLOOD GROUPS AND BLOOD GROUP COMPATIBILITY

There are distinctive differences in the immunologic properties of blood, as a result of which the blood of one individual may be incompatible with another's on the basis of "blood group." Human blood is classified into four "major" blood groups, designated as group A, group B, group AB and group O. The relative incidence of these, among Caucasians, is approximately as follows:

GROUP	INCIDENCE %
A	40
B	15
AB	5
O	40

The above letters refer to an inherited property of an individual's red cells, i.e., whether, of two proteins labeled "A" and "B," one, both or neither is incorporated in the red cell, group O indicating the absence of both. A second characteristic which distinguishes bloods of different groups is the presence or the absence of certain proteins in their plasma, called anti-A and anti-B, which react immediately and specifically on contact with the proteins A and B of the red cells and cause the latter, if "incompatible," to clump, or "agglutinate." Because of this agglutination reaction, the substances "A" and "B" of the red cells are referred to as "agglutinogens," whereas the plasma proteins which react with these are referred to as "agglutinins." The plasma agglutinins which are present in the blood of each group are indicated as follows:

ABO GROUP (RED CELL AGGLUTINOGEN)	PLASMA AGGLUTININ
A	Anti-B
B	Anti-A
AB	None
O	Anti-A and Anti-B

There is no group, it will be noted, in which plasma agglutinins are capable of reacting with cells of the same group, for, if this were the case, these red cells would be agglutinated constantly by antibodies in their own plasma, a situation obviously incompatible with life. Thus, group-A blood contains anti-B, but no anti-A, agglutinins; in group B, the reverse situation is encountered; group-O blood contains both anti-A and anti-B agglutinins, whereas in group AB neither anti-A nor anti-B agglutinins are present.

So far as the ABO blood groups are concerned, the essential precaution to consider in planning a blood transfusion is to exclude the possibility that agglutinins that are capable of reacting with agglutinogens of the donor red cells (agglutinating the latter) are contained in the recipient's plasma. This reaction, if it occurs in the recipient's blood stream, usually results in the prompt destruction of the donor cells, the most dangerous consequence of which is in the liberation of large amounts of hemoglobin. The hemoglobin, filtering through the kidney glomeruli, becomes concentrated in the kidney tubules to such a degree that precipitation of a pigment occurs, impairing or halting altogether the excretion of urine. Moreover, restoration of renal function may not be regained for several days, before which death may supervene.

Compatible and Incompatible Blood Group Combinations

Group-O patients, since they possess both anti-A and anti-B agglutinins, cannot receive donor blood belonging to groups A, B or AB, only group-O donors being acceptable. Group-A patients must not receive group-B blood in view of the anti-B antibodies contained in their plasma, and group-A donors are similarly unacceptable for group-B recipients.

Group-O red cells are not agglutinated by either anti-A or anti-B agglutinins and therefore may be transfused not only into patients belonging to group O but also into group-A and group-B patients as well. Incompatible anti-A and anti-B agglutinins in donor blood, unless present in high concentration, cause relatively little red-cell damage in group-A, group-B or group-AB recipients. On this basis, group-O individuals whose agglutinins have been measured and found to be in low titer may serve as "universal donors" for the transfusion of patients belonging to any ABO group (assuming no blood-group incompatibility exists on some other basis).

Just as group-O blood may be used for transfusion into patients belonging to all major blood groups, those patients belonging to group AB, since they possess neither agglutinin, may receive without danger donor blood of any ABO group, and therefore are referred to as "universal recipients." With these two exceptions, however, the selection of every donor must be such that his ABO group corresponds exactly to that of the recipient, and prior to every transfusion a "compatibility test" must be performed.

Rh Types

Bloods of different individuals are distinguishable not only by differences in ABO grouping but also according to their "Rh type."* In contrast with the 4 ABO groups,

* The term "Rh" has its origin in the fact that the existence of this red cell factor was first recognized through its similarity to one previously discovered in the Rhesus monkey.

the Rh types are relatively numerous; moreover, there are no naturally occurring anti-Rh agglutinins in normal human plasma which correspond to the anti-A and anti-B agglutinins. However, and herein lies the practical importance of the Rh types, anti-Rh agglutinins may appear in the plasma of an individual lacking particular Rh factors in the red cells. For example, an anti-Rh agglutinin may appear in an "Rh-negative" person following transfusions of "Rh-positive" blood which contain the Rh factor, or, in an Rh-negative woman, following a pregnancy with an Rh-positive fetus, the Rh factor in the fetus having been inherited from its father. By whatever mechanism the production of anti-Rh antibodies is stimulated in susceptible individuals, whether through repeated transfusions of Rh-positive blood or by the harboring of an Rh-positive fetus, the agglutinating action of these agglutinins on Rh-positive red cells is similar to that of anti-A and anti-B agglutinins on cells belonging to groups A and B, respectively. Moreover, the use of Rh-positive donor blood in Rh-negative recipients who have been "sensitized" previously, i.e., stimulated to produce anti-Rh antibodies by earlier transfusions or pregnancies, may result in an accident similar to the type which has been described.

Approximately 85 per cent of Caucasians and 92 per cent of Negroes are classed as being "Rh-positive," since they possess the most important of the many Rh agglutinogens, the one most apt to stimulate the production of anti-Rh antibodies in those who lack it. Inasmuch as sensitization by other Rh agglutinogens is relatively uncommon, the majority of individuals are quite unlikely to experience complications as a result of Rh-incompatible transfusions or pregnancies. On the other hand, the remaining 15 per cent of Caucasians and 8 per cent of Negroes who lack this agglutinogen are susceptible to sensitization by this, the most potent of the Rh factors, producing antibodies which agglutinate cells of this type after multiple transfusions, unless Rh-positive donors are specifically excluded. In the case of Rh-negative girls and women, until they have passed the child-bearing age, this exclusion is extremely important, for the odds that their husbands will be Rh-positive are about six to one, and the odds that their future offspring, if any, will also be Rh-positive are of approximately the same order of magnitude.* The danger of an Rh-negative woman becoming sensitized as a result of bearing an Rh-positive child is fortunately not great. In less than 5 per cent of matings in which the woman is Rh-negative and the husband Rh-positive are there complications attributable to Rh differences—*unless the woman, at some earlier time in her life, has been transfused with Rh-positive blood, in which event the risk is increased about tenfold.* Thus, if her infant is Rh-positive, there is at least a 50 per cent chance that its red cells will be damaged by agglutinins produced by its mother before the time of delivery. The resulting disease, called "erythroblastosis fetalis" or "hemolytic anemia of the newborn," is described in Chapter 25.

TRANSFUSION THERAPY
Clinical Use of Blood and Blood Components

The intravenous injection of whole blood, whole plasma or plasma albumin is the most effective method of correcting a blood volume deficiency, or "oligemia," whether it be due to the loss of whole blood or to a predominant loss of plasma. A blood volume deficit which occurs rapidly enough and is of sufficient severity to cause circulatory failure ("shock") may result from acute hemorrhage with loss both of red cells and plasma, or from leakage of plasma in burned tissues. The type of restorative treatment that is offered, i.e., whether by means of whole blood transfusion or injections of plasma or plasma albumin, depends on the nature of the resultant deficiency. Optimum replacement in the case of hemorrhage ordinarily is accomplished by means of whole blood, for plasma transfusions under these circumstances, although effectively expanding the blood volume, make no provision for

the restoration of red cells, and the resultant anemia may be sufficiently severe to prevent recovery of the patient. Whole blood transfusions or injections of red cell concentrates (whole blood from which most of the plasma has been removed prior to injection) also are indicated in the treatment of several types of anemia, depending on their severity and responsiveness to other forms of treatment.

Fresh whole blood is given to maintain the platelet level in patients undergoing extensive surgery who require massive blood replacement. Similar transfusions are employed to elevate the platelet count in patients with thrombocytopenic purpura; most effective for this purpose is blood from individuals with polycythemia vera, whose platelet counts may exceed one or two million. Fresh whole blood or freshly frozen plasma† may be used also as a source of two other blood components which likewise deteriorate rapidly in storage, i.e., the antihemophilic factor and the labile Factor V, which accelerates prothrombin conversion (see p. 478). Plasma fractions containing specific components in high concentration provide the most efficient method of replacement therapy in cases of fibrinogen deficiency and hemophilia. Albumin, relatively free of admixture with other proteins, is available in the form of a 25 per cent solution; this material, in contrast with whole plasma, is capable of being sterilized by pasteurization and therefore can be used without fear of viral infectivity, which is a tremendous advantage. Concentrated plasma albumin (or whole plasma) may be used to expand the blood volume of patients with oligemic shock and to elevate the plasma protein concentration in cases of hypoproteinemia due to nephrosis or cirrhosis.

Transfusion Technic

Methods of injecting blood are similar in most respects to those employed in other types of parenteral therapy. However, there are certain technical considerations of importance which apply specifically to blood

---

* If the husband is heterozygous with respect to the Rh factor, i.e., if the Rh-positive character is inherited from only one of his parents, only one-half of their children will be Rh-positive.

† The term "freshly frozen" applies to plasma which has been separated and frozen immediately after collection of the donor blood and stored continuously in the frozen state.

transfusion and relate in part to the handling of the material before its injection. For example, blood never should be allowed to remain uncooled for any appreciable length of time (more than 2 hours) following its collection from the donor or its removal from the storage refrigerator, if rapid deterioration of the red cells is to be avoided.

Blood should be administered by a closed-system technic, using a glass transfusion bottle which is vented through a protected airway tube or a plastic system such as is shown in Figure 33, composed of a collapsible bag with attachments for phlebotomy and transfusion.

When blood is administered from the bottle or bag in which it was collected, a filter must be introduced into the connecting tubing to remove small clots before the blood enters the vein. The same precautions as for the giving of fluid by intravenous infusion must be observed. The nurse should observe and record the time at which the blood is given and the amount, any rise in temperature, rise in pulse, difficulty in respiration, nausea and vomiting.

Role of the Nurse

The first step in the performance of every transfusion is to check the labels identifying the donor blood and to confirm the identity of the patient who is to receive it!

The insertion of the intravenous needle and the arrangement of the recipient set, although classically the responsibility of the attending physician, is also quite properly and often necessarily within the capacity of the professional nurse. Judgment in the selection of a suitable vein and skill in the use of intravenous needles are usually acquired very readily, provided that the original technical instruction was correct and opportunities for practical experience have been sufficiently frequent. The importance of these technics, formerly considered entirely outside the province of nursing care, stems from the fact that parenteral therapy has increased in usage to such an astounding degree that most hospitals, unless staffed with resident physicians, would find it impossible to conduct treatment of this sort on an adequate scale without the participation of competent nursing personnel. Moreover, even when professional medical assistance is amply available, there is often a tendency to schedule parenteral injections, including transfusion therapy, in a manner that is something less than ideal, large infusions being administered at infrequent intervals, whereas smaller injections, given regularly and more frequently, might be preferred on physiologic grounds. Finally, assuming that all such treatments could be performed by the attending physicians and scheduled in a manner that is always optimal from the patient's standpoint, the necessity for readjustment of the injection set is still an unavoidable problem. This function can be fulfilled best by a competent nurse who is close at hand in a position to recognize and remedy the situation at once.

Patients receiving whole blood or red cell transfusions should be attended closely for at least 10 minutes after the start of the infusion, and the rate of injection during this period should not exceed 20 drops per minute. Thereafter, if no untoward reaction is apparent, and unless rapidity of injection is undesirable for other reasons, the rate may be increased. It is important that the flow be continuous. If it ceases, corrective measures should be undertaken by the nurse, if able to do so; otherwise, the physician must be notified immediately. Most important, she must be prompt to note the appearance of any unfavorable response on the part of the recipient which might signify the development of a transfusion complication.

TRANSFUSION COMPLICATIONS

Transfusion therapy, whether conducted with whole blood, red cells or plasma, entails a number of calculated risks, for certain of its potential complications cannot be prevented with absolute certainty, and some are sufficiently dangerous to merit serious consideration whenever treatment of this type is contemplated.

Circulatory Overloading

Pulmonary congestion may occur, whatever the nature of the transfusate, if the volume of injected material is excessive in relation to the patient's cardiac reserve. This is an unusual complication in recipients who have sustained a blood loss sufficient to precipitate shock, unless therapy is conducted very carelessly, but is far from uncommon in individuals whose blood volume is normal or excessive at the start. Precautions for the prevention of pulmonary edema are particularly important in elderly patients, especially those suffering from cardiovascular disease. Pulmonary congestion is suggested by the development of cyanosis and dyspnea. Later, if the injection is continued, pulmonary edema is precipitated, heralded by stertorous breathing, persistent coughing and the production of frothy sputum.

Treatment demands that the transfusion be stopped immediately. The patient is placed in an orthopneic position, tourniquets are applied on the extremities in rotation, and, unless there is obvious and prompt improvement, venesection is employed without delay as the surest method of relieving this dangerous situation.

Transmission of Infection

Infections of many types can be transmitted from a blood donor to a transfusion recipient if there are bacteria, viruses or parasites in the donor blood at the time of the venesection. Of these, the most important to consider are syphilis, hepatitis and malaria. Syphilitic infection by transfusion is a relatively uncommon accident because of the precautions usually enforced in the screening of prospective donors and the serologic tests that are required before donor blood is released for transfusion. Malaria is a more frequent complication, since exclusion of this disease in donors, particularly of those types of malaria characterized by prolonged symptom-free intervals, is very difficult.

Virus hepatitis, of all transfusion risks, at present is recognized to be one of the most important. There are two distinct varieties of hepatitis, one called "epidemic hepatitis" and the other, "homologous serum jaundice." The incubation period characteristic of the epidemic type is from 3 to 4 weeks; of homologous serum jaundice, from 2 to 6 months. The risk is multiplied with successive transfusions on the basis of statistical probabilities, for it is estimated that one or the other of these viruses is present in the circulating blood of one out of every 300 to 600 individuals. The highest incidence of these diseases is in recipients of plasma prepared from large pools of donor blood.

Allergic and Pyrogenic Reactions

Allergic reactions in the form of urticaria (hives) or, far less commonly, asthmatic breathing may appear in the course of transfusion. In an effort to avoid this type of complication, allergic individuals generally are disqualified as blood donors, owing to the possibility that their blood may contain antibodies capable of reacting with protein materials (allergens) in the recipient's circulating blood. Nevertheless, hives may be anticipated in approximately 3 per cent of the cases. Allergic manifestations are most successfully treated by means of epinephrine, 0.5 ml. of a 1:1,000 solution being injected subcutaneously or, if respiratory difficulty is severe, 0.25 to 0.5 ml. intravenously. The oral administration of one of the antihistaminic agents, such as Benadryl or Pyribenzamine, is usually quite as effective, although relief may not follow for a period of from 10 to 20 minutes.

Pyrogenic reactions due to bacterial contaminants are quite as common, if not more so, in transfusion recipients as in patients receiving fluids of the crystalloid type. These reactions are characterized by the sudden onset of chills and fever 40 to 60 minutes following the start of a pyrogenic infusion or, in this case, transfusion. Headache, nausea and vomiting may accompany the fever at its height. The total duration of the reaction may be as brief as 20 minutes or as prolonged as 8 hours. Treatment consists in supplying extra blankets, as needed, and reducing discomfort by administering analgesics. The salicylates usually are effective in such cases; intramuscular Demerol (25 to 50 mg.) may be indicated in some instances, when symptoms are severe and oral medication is not tolerated.

Some of these febrile, nonhemolytic transfusion reactions have been attributed to the presence of "leuko-agglutinins" (white blood cell antibodies) in the blood of the recipient, implying the development of an immunity against foreign leukocyte antigens introduced in the course of earlier transfusions. Preliminary processing of the donor blood by removal of the buffy coat after centrifuging has been recommended as a means of rendering it nonpyrogenic for such individuals. The usual explanation, however, implicates the familiar airborne bacterial contaminants that likewise are responsible for the "intravenous chills" described on page 171. The pyrogenic reactions that result from the use of improperly prepared transfusion sets are not always brief and harmless; at best they are unpleasant in the extreme; for very ill patients they can be fatal. From this standpoint, commercial disposable transfusion sets are incomparably superior to reusable equipment of any type yet devised, and their exclusive use is highly recommended.

Incompatible Transfusions

Most dangerous of all transfusion complications is the hemolytic reaction which follows the injection of red cells which are agglutinated by the plasma of the recipient. Transfusions which cause this complication are those in which donor blood contains the A or B antigen, when this particular antigen is lacking in the recipient. This type of reaction may also follow the injection of a red cell antigen other than A or B, provided the recipient lacks it and has been sensitized to it as a result of previous transfusion or pregnancy.*

An example of an ABO incompatibility would be the use of a group-A donor for a group-O recipient. The second type of situation would be exemplified by the use of an Rh-positive donor for an Rh-negative recipient.

An incompatibility which involves one of the major (ABO) blood groups almost always precipitates an immediate reaction in an unanesthetized patient, symptoms usually developing before the injection has been in progress for 10 minutes. The recipient may complain first of chilliness, headache and backache or abdominal distress and then exhibits a shaking chill followed by a high fever. There may be a precipitous fall in arterial blood pressure, accompanied by

* Such antigens are numerous and include, among others, those belonging to the Rh, the Kell, Kidd, Duffy and MNS blood group systems.

clinical evidences of profound vascular collapse.

When symptoms of this sort appear, or, indeed, if there is any untoward manifestation in the course of a transfusion, this is the signal for halting the procedure immediately, recognizing that, whereas incompatible blood given in amounts of less than 100 ml. rarely causes death, such blood in amounts exceeding 300 or 400 ml. is lethal in a substantial proportion of patients. The promptness with which symptoms of incompatibility usually develop, namely, within 10 minutes, regardless of the precise volume of material injected, is the basis for insisting on the constant attendance of transfused patients for the first 10 minutes at least and on slowness of injection during the initial period. Patients receiving incompatible blood while under general anesthesia unfortunately may provide no overt evidence of incompatibility, except perhaps an inexplicable drop in arterial blood pressure, and the risk of blood transfusion under these circumstances, without an effective alarm system, is multipled greatly.

The sequence of events which follow the initial clinical response in patients receiving large volumes of incompatible blood is usually as follows: the patient may void a small volume of urine, dark-red or wine-red in color, and thereafter excrete little or no urine for several days. During this period he may look and feel quite well, but if, by the end of the second week, there has been no spontaneous diuresis, the manifestations of uremia supervene. The patient becomes obviously ill, progressively more so each day, complaining of nausea, vomiting, general malaise, weakness, abdominal pain and diarrhea. Finally, after a few days of increasing lethargy and deepening stupor, death may be anticipated. A fatal outcome is by no means the rule, however, for in a considerable proportion of cases, after a period of oliguria lasting 2 weeks or more, there develops a brisk diuresis followed by rapid and complete recovery. In the mildest cases the only obvious indication of a transfusion accident may be transient hemoglobinuria unaccompanied by untoward symptoms of any sort, the subsequent clinical course being completely uneventful. Transfusion reactions attributable to an Rh incompatibility are generally of the milder variety, chills, fever and transient hemoglobinuria perhaps comprising the entire symptomatology, but with each succeeding transfusion of Rh-incompatible blood the severity of these reactions increases until they are entirely those characteristic of a major blood group incompatibility.

Hemolytic transfusion reactions which are entirely asymptomatic occasionally are observed following transfusions of "universal donor" blood; the donor red cells are completely unaffected, but the red cells of the patient sustain damage caused by the incompatible agglutinins contained in the donor plasma. This is particularly apt to occur when patients belonging to groups A, B or AB receive group-O blood containing anti-A and anti-B agglutinins in high concentration. Hemoglobinemia and hemoglobinuria do not often occur as complications of such transfusions, or, if they do develop, they are of very brief duration and completely without residual impairment of kidney function. Patients belonging to groups A, B or AB who repeatedly receive large volumes of incompatible plasma over a period of several days may exhibit a mild degree of icterus because of the excessive destruction of their own red cells, but other than the appearance of jaundice and signs of progressive anemia, there is little evidence to indicate a hemolytic reaction. Such hemolysis is nonetheless undesirable, obviously, and can be avoided by neutralizing the incompatible agglutinins before they are injected into the patient. This is accomplished by adding purified blood group A and B substances to the plasma or group-O blood prior to transfusion.

Responsibilities of the Nurse

If the nurse suspects that a transfusion reaction may be developing, the injection of blood must be stopped abruptly, and the physician responsible for the patient should be summoned immediately. During the interim the nurse prepares to carry out certain procedures indicated in all cases in which an obvious or suspected reaction has occurred or is in progress.

1. The transfusion set is disconnected, and the needle either is withdrawn or is connected to an intravenous set for the slow administration of sodium chloride or another crystalloid solution, if it is desirable to keep this particular needle in place and patent for the purpose of securing blood specimens or for continued therapy.

2. *Do not empty the contents of the blood bottle or set!* This equipment should be sent at once, intact and with all labels attached, together with an explanatory note, to the laboratory responsible for the blood grouping and compatibility tests for an immediate repetition of these tests.

3. Secure a test tube containing about 0.5 ml. of sodium citrate solution (approx. 3 per cent concentration) for the collection of a blood sample required for the exclusion of hemoglobinemia (the presence of free hemoglobin in the plasma is indicative of a hemolytic reaction).

4. Arrange that this collection be made as soon as possible. Use a 5-ml. or 10-ml. syringe rinsed with sterile sodium chloride or sodium citrate solution; this sample should be obtained with the utmost care and should be sent at once to a laboratory for immediate separation of the plasma and inspection of the latter for the presence or absence of free hemoglobin.

5. Arrangements are made in detail for a sampling of the next voided specimen of urine; this, as soon as it is secured, is likewise sent to the laboratory for hemoglobin tests.

If a hemolytic reaction is diagnosed on the basis of these examinations, an intravenous infusion of mannitol is given (approximately 100 Gm. in 20 per cent concentration). After 1 liter of fluid is received, however, unless the patient is also suffering from dehydration or blood loss, no further parenteral treatment is indicated until the renal function can be estimated. Thus, one must foresee the possibility that practically no urine may be secreted for many days, and, during this period, if death occurs, it is far more likely to result from excessive fluid therapy than from kidney failure alone. If complete anuria or severe oliguria does develop, oral feeding is halted; all nutrient and

SUMMARY OF THE PROBLEMS OF THE TRANSFUSION RECIPIENT

Transfusion Complications	Nursing Implications

1. *Circulatory Overloading*
If the volume of the blood exceeds the cardiac output, the following symptoms of pulmonary congestion may occur:
   a. dyspnea
   b. cough
   c. frothy sputum
	Stop the transfusion immediately.
	Known cardiac patients and elderly patients should receive blood at a slower rate.
	Place the patient upright with his feet and legs in a dependent position.
	Apply rotating tourniquets if indicated.

2. *Transmission of Disease* The virus of hepatitis and malarial parasites may be transmitted from donor to recipient via infected blood. There is no known laboratory test to exclude these diseases in the donor.	A careful history should be taken of every donor.

3. *Febrile (Pyrogenic) Reactions*
These may be due to bacterial proteins in needles, blood, bottles, etc., or possibly to the presence of leuko-agglutinins in the recipient's blood.
Symptoms: (may occur after blood is discontinued)
   a. sudden chilling and fever
   b. headache
   c. nausea and vomiting
	Stop the transfusion immediately.
	Take the temperature one-half hour after the chill and as indicated thereafter.

4. *Bacterial Contamination*
Bacteria may gain access to the blood and multiply.
Symptoms:
   a. severe fever and chills
   b. nausea and vomiting
   c. persistant shock-like state
	Stop the blood immediately. Send the remainder of the blood to the laboratory.
	Call the physician immediately.
	Use rigid asepsis with transfusion equipment.

5. *Allergic Reactions*
Allergic individuals should not donate blood, for their blood may contain antibodies capable of reacting with allergens in the recipient's blood.
Symptoms:
   a. hives
   b. laryngeal edema
   c. asthmatic wheezing
	Stop the transfusion.
	The individual who has had a previous allergic reaction to blood may be given an antihistamine before subsequent transfusions.
	Prepare epinephrine if respiratory distress is severe.
	Watch for indications of laryngeal edema.
	Antihistamine drugs may be given orally.

6. *Hemolytic Reactions*
Hemolysis follows when incompatible red cells are injected into the patient's circulating blood.
Symptoms:
   a. chilliness
   b. feeling of head fullness
   c. oppressive feeling in the chest
	Positively identify patient and blood before transfusion is started.
	Stay with the patient during the first 10 minutes that he is receiving the transfusion.
	Administer blood at 20 drops per min. during this period.
	Stop the transfusion immediately if the symptoms occur.
	Call the physician at once.

Transfusion Complications (Continued)	**Nursing Implications (Continued)**
d. sharp pain in lumbar area	Give mannitol as indicated.
e. flushing of face	Encourage fluid intake for next few hours.
f. distention of neck veins	Measure and save all urine voided. Keep accurate intake and output record.
g. fall of blood pressure	Send blood and transfusion equipment to the laboratory for immediate repetition of typing and cross-matching.
h. vascular depression	

hydration therapy is supplied in the form of intravenous solutions, the selection of which must depend on the particular requirements of the individual patient. On no account must the total volume each day be allowed to exceed by a margin of more than 1 liter the amount of urine secreted within the preceding 24-hour period in extremely hot weather or 500 ml. when the room temperature is moderate and perspiration is minimal.

The nursing staff must be fully aware of its responsibilities in relation to the measurements of fluid volumes received and excreted and of the necessity for complete and accurate recording of this information, vitally required for the control of water balance and the conduct of parenteral therapy in these patients. Precision in this regard is an absolute necessity, for as long as anuria persists the patient's life is balanced perilously between two threats: dehydration and gross electrolyte imbalance on the one hand and, on the other, overhydration resulting in pulmonary edema—in other words, therapeutic drowning. Either of these disasters may easily destroy life while there may yet be time for the spontaneous recovery of kidney function and the patient's own salvation.

BIBLIOGRAPHY AND SUGGESTED READING

Allen, F. H., Jr., Emerson, C. P., and Soutter, L.: Blood grouping, blood banking, and blood transfusion, New England J. Med. **245:**367-375, 410-424, 456-464, 1951.

Crouch, M. L. and Gibson, S. T.: Blood therapy, Am. J. Nursing **62:**71-76, March, 1962.

Donohue, D., Gabrio, B., and Finch, C.: Preservation and transfusion of blood, J.A.M.A. **161:**784-788, 1956.

Rath, C. E.: The prevention and management of blood transfusion hazards, Am. J. Nursing **55:**323-326, 1955.

Scott, C. S.: Blood bank operation, Nursing Outlook **5:**204-206, 1957.

Unger, L. J.: Human blood plasma and plasma substances, Am. J. Nursing **54:**50-52, 1954.

12

Oxygen Inhalation Therapy

Oxygen is required for life. *Anoxia* or, more precisely, *hypoxia,* refers to a deficiency of oxygen, and *hypoxemia* indicates an insufficient oxygenation of the blood. *Cyanosis* is the slightly bluish or grayish discoloration of the skin that results from a deficiency of oxygen and an excess of carbon dioxide in the blood. (Normal air contains 20.93 per cent oxygen, 79.04 per cent nitrogen and 0.03 per cent carbon dioxide.)

The purpose of oxygen therapy is to provide and maintain a normal supply of oxygen for blood and tissues and to correct deficiencies that may exist in the removal of carbon dioxide. Oxygen is supplied in concentrations above that found in normal air, thus raising the oxygen tension in the inspired air. As a result, a more complete respiratory exchange in the lungs becomes possible, the hemoglobin leaving the lungs with a higher percentage of oxygen than is possible when ordinary air is inspired and the deficiency of oxygen in the tissues is overcome. A concentration of 45 per cent oxygen usually is required to relieve cyanosis.

INDICATIONS FOR USE

Any condition (such as pulmonary congestion, bronchial asthma, pneumonia, acute myocardial infarction due to coronary thrombosis, chest trauma) that reduces the oxygen-carbon dioxide exchange, which in turn reduces the oxygen supply to the blood, warrants the use of oxygen therapy.

In surgery, oxygen may be given as a prophylactic measure both during and after operation. Oxygen therapy also is indicated in the treatment of patients who have some temporary partial obstruction in the air passages (as after thyroidectomy), and in those who have a deficient respiration due to pain in an upper abdominal wound. Inhalations of oxygen have been found to aid in the treatment of ileus when it is of the reflex or paralytic type.

Regardless of the indication for oxygen, if the patient is conscious and would benefit by an explanation of the apparatus to be used, the nurse should do so.

PRECAUTIONS TO OBSERVE IN HANDLING OXYGEN

Because oxygen supports combustion, sparks and open flames must be kept away from the area where this gas is used. The patient and his visitors must be given emphatic instructions in this regard, and "No Smoking" signs should be displayed.

No electrical appliances should be used by a patient in an oxygen tent; this includes radios, heating pads, electric razors and call buttons. Where electrical equipment is called for in the treatment of a patient in an oxygen tent, the oxygen therapy must be discontinued while such equipment is in operation.

Wool, nylon and any fabric that is capable of producing static electricity and sparks are not to be used in areas where the concentration of oxygen is higher than that found in the atmosphere.

Piped oxygen has many advantages over oxygen obtainable in cylinders. It is readily available, and it is safer. When oxygen from cylinders is used, the dangers must be recognized. The standard, large steel tank holds 244 cubic feet of 99.5 per cent pure oxygen at a pressure of 2,200 pounds per square inch.* A full tank of oxygen has a dome-

---

*When delivering oxygen at a rate of 7 to 15 L./min., this tank will last approximately 18 hours.

shaped steel cap screwed on top to protect the cylinder outlet. When oxygen is required, the cap is removed, and the cylinder valve must be loosened slightly ("cracked") to allow the gas to blow dust particles from the outlet. This is done slowly because of the high pressure involved; if the valve is turned too rapidly, the hissing noise and pressure is great. Should "cracking" have to be done in the hearing distance of the patient, it is well to let him know what to expect before the valve is turned.

At this time a reducing device or regulator is attached. The purpose of the oxygen regulator is twofold: (1) to indicate the amount of oxygen in the tank; and (2) to "step-down" the force of the oxygen that is under pressure to a usable and regulated level. Consequently, a regulator has two gauges that indicate both. When the tank is in position at the bedside, it should be strapped to the bed or chained to the carrier, so that it will not be accidentally knocked over. (It is necessary to check the cylinder gauge periodically at specific intervals to assure the patient of an adequate supply of oxygen. When the gauge registers 1/4 full or 55 cubic feet, it is time to order another tank of oxygen.)

It is advisable to humidify the gas by bubbling it through water, since the prolonged use of dry gas will dehydrate the patient's respiratory mucous membrane.

The supply of oxygen is now ready to be connected to the method of choice.

METHODS OF OXYGEN ADMINISTRATION

Oxygen may be administered by means of an oropharyngeal (nasal) catheter, a mask or some form of tent.

Oropharyngeal (Nasal) Catheter

An oropharyngeal catheter is one of the simplest and most convenient methods of administering oxygen. Oxygen is bubbled through water to humidify it before it enters the catheter, in order to lessen the drying

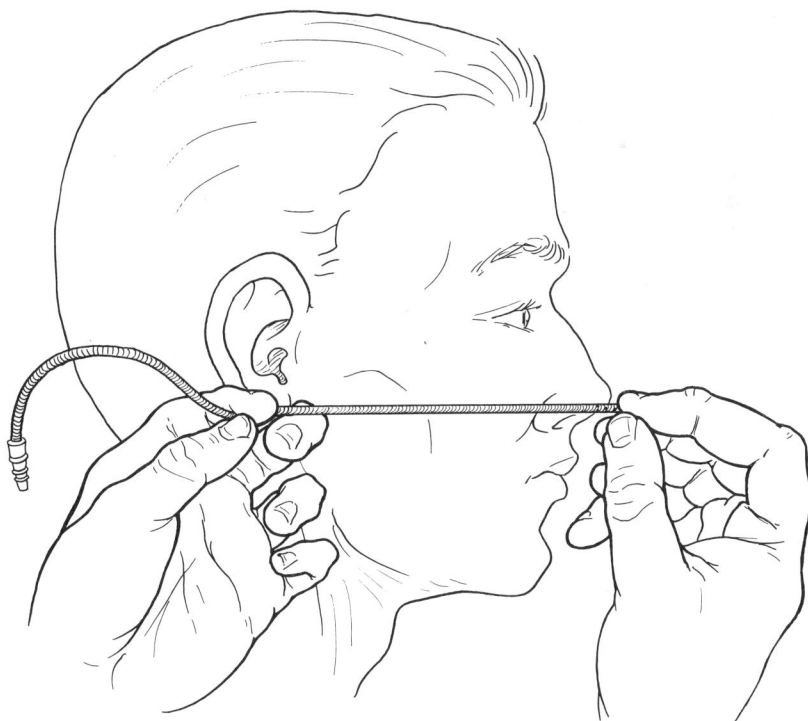

Fig. 34. Illustrates the method of approximating the distance that the oropharyngeal catheter should be inserted in the nose by measuring the length from the external nares to the tragus or ear lobe.

and consequent irritating effect on the mucous membrane that is the chief disadvantage of this method. Curved metal tubes are available that fit into the nostrils and are strapped to the forehead. However, more commonly, the plastic or rubber catheter (No. 10 F.) is used. If the catheter has many pinhead holes for a distance of about 2 to 3 cm. from the tip, oxygen is introduced more diffusely rather than being concentrated at one outlet. The distance a catheter is to be passed is determined by measuring the distance from the tip of the patient's nose to the tip of his ear (Fig. 34). This length is marked on the catheter, a piece of adhesive tape being used for the purpose. Then, with the oxygen flowing through the catheter, moisten the catheter with water and pass it through the nostril up to the adhesive marking.

To ensure correct position of the catheter, the nurse may depress the tongue carefully and note whether the tip of the catheter is visible behind the uvula. Adjust the catheter, if necessary, before securing the catheter to

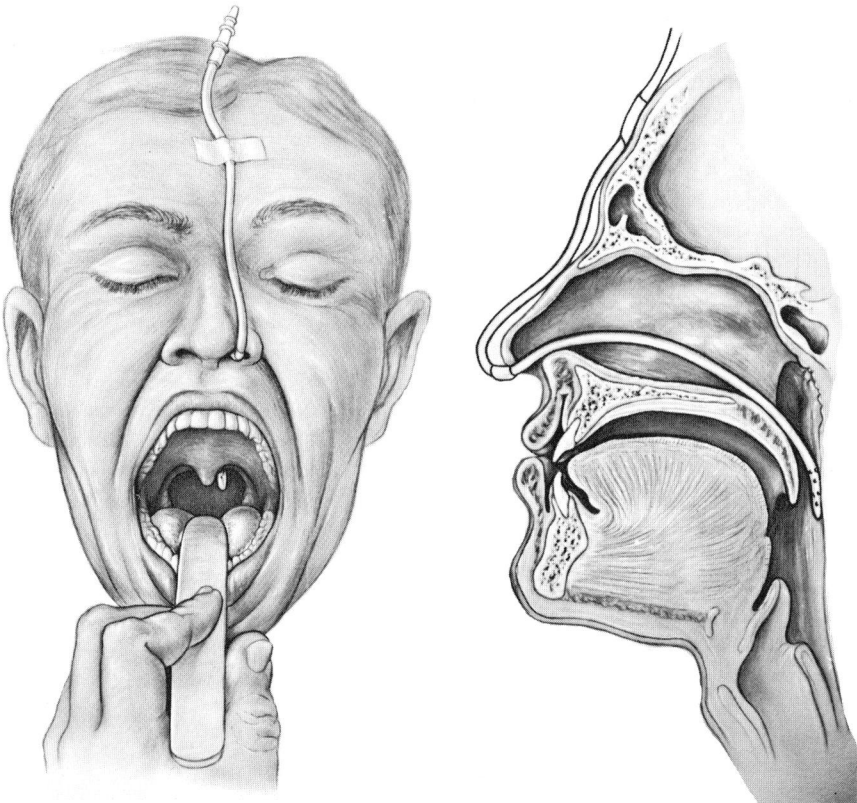

Fig. 34 (*Continued*). (*Left*) The full-face view shows the only certain method of checking the location of the tip of the nasal catheter in the unconscious patient. If the catheter tip is too high, a lower oxygen concentration than desirable will be delivered. If the catheter tip is too low, oxygen will pass down the esophagus and distend the stomach. This figure also illustrates the adhesive marker placed on the catheter at the external nares to fix the proper distance that the catheter is reinserted after cleaning. To ensure stability the catheter may be taped to the forehead. (*Right*) The sagittal view shows the nasal catheter in place and shows the numerous holes made in the tip so that a stream of oxygen will not be directed against any one region of the pharynx. (Beal, J.M.: Manual of Recovery Room Care, p. 19, New York, Macmillan)

the side of the patient's face. Such a catheter should be removed by the nurse every 8 hours. A clean catheter should be available to reinsert immediately. This technic will prevent undue crusting of secretions on the catheter and possible blocking of the oxygen outlet. Changing from one nostril to the other may be more comfortable for the patient. Catheters should not be forced into the nostril. The rate of oxygen flow should be adjusted according to the desired concentration; 6 to 8 liters per minute seems to provide a maximum of efficiency with a minimum of discomfort to the patient. This method will provide approximately 35 to 40 per cent concentration in the alveolar air; somewhat less is absorbed if the patient breathes through his mouth. (See Fig. 34, *Cont.*)

Oxygen Mask

Various types of face masks have been designed for efficient and economical administration of oxygen in high concentrations. The efficiency of masks which permit the mouth to remain unenclosed depends entirely on the patency of the patient's nostrils; thus, if oxygen concentrations approaching 100 per cent are to be secured, the mouth must be kept tightly closed, the patient breathing exclusively through the nose. The same requirement does not apply in the case of the oral-nasal mask which encloses both nose and mouth.

The principal drawback associated with the use of facial masks is the necessity for close contact at every point between their edges and the skin of the face, a perfect adjustment sometimes being extraordinarily difficult to accomplish. Another and more important disadvantage, and one which seriously detracts from their usefulness, is the fact that devices of this type are tolerated poorly by the majority of dyspneic and anxious patients. Indeed, it would appear that those individuals whose need for supplemental oxygen is greatest, who could benefit most from the high oxygen concentrations delivered by this technic, are the very ones who are most prone to resist the application of an oxygen mask. Their unfortunate hostility toward the oxygen mask may be attributable to a sense of suffocation and confinement which follows to some extent

the application of any mask, even those which enclose only the nose. In a situation of this sort, the nurse must exercise the most persuasive reassurance at her command, and this, together with the judicious use of hypnotic and sedative agents, may permit the satisfactory application of a mask, by all odds the most efficient device available for the prolonged administration of oxygen in high concentration.

When applying the mask, care should be taken to see that the facial strap is optimally placed and adjusted to a comfortable degree of tension. If the mask is in proper position, the breathing bag will deflate and inflate alternately, coincident with inspiration and expiration, respectively. The flow should be so regulated that the breathing bag is not completely collapsed during inspiration. These movements should be checked frequently and the mask readjusted accordingly. At intervals of 2 or 3 hours, or oftener, it is removed altogether and the face cleansed.

Oxygen Tent

An oxygen tent may be employed whenever the other means are not feasible.

The oxygen tent is essentially an air-conditioning unit supplied with oxygen which is refrigerated and delivered under forced draft. There are many varieties of tents capable of providing a properly humid atmosphere, the temperature of which is adjustable within a suitable range (from 68° to 72° F.) and the oxygen content of which can be maintained at a desirable level (60 per cent in the drape tent and close to 95 per cent in the open-top variety).* The drape tent permits maximum mobility on the part of the patient and is least restrictive as regards posture and visibility. It has an external cooling system which eliminates the possibility of water leakage within the tent or wetting of the patient with water of condensation. The amount of oxygen required for its operation is relatively great, due to the unavoidable leakage of the gas through the bedclothes and its escape beneath the margins of the

* The open-top tent is used especially in giving oxygen to children or to patients who need extra humidification.

drape, unless the drape is arranged and protected carefully.

Plastic or similar type mattress covers will prevent oxygen from being diffused through the mattress. The sides of the tent are tucked securely under the mattress and a draw sheet is placed over the free front edge. In giving nursing care through the openings, the nurse should see to it that the tent is kept close round her arm.

Before the patient is placed in the tent he should receive a detailed explanation of the device and its purpose, as the most effective method of reassurance. The rate of oxygen delivery will be specified, in liters per minute, by the physician, and the nurse will adjust the flow gauge accordingly, after a preliminary flooding of the tent (15 liters per minute for 2 minutes) with oxygen. Frequently she must check the concentration of oxygen in the tent, the flow gauge, indicating the delivery rate, and the pressure gauge (which registers the amount of oxygen remaining in the tank).

Temperature readings should be made at frequent intervals. Comfort in an oxygen tent requires adequate protection against chilling by the provision of appropriate bed garments and the draping of a lightweight cotton blanket like a shawl about the neck and the shoulders. The patient's posture should be adjusted for comfort and to assure maximum ease of respiration.

The patient is fed and cared for through the sleeves of the tent. These are opened no oftener and no longer than necessary. When nursing care requires more complete access to the patient than the sleeves afford, the nurse can tuck the drapes under the pillow and proceed with her mission. Thus, the patient can be bathed and his bed made while oxygen inhalation continues. He should be provided with a tap bell so that he may call the nurse when necessary.

A word of caution: The patient in a tent may appear to be partitioned away from his surroundings. However, he can see and hear perfectly well what goes on about him, and individuals in his vicinity must be no less discreet in their discussions than they would be at the bedside of a patient who is not in a tent.

COMPLICATIONS AND HAZARDS

In addition to the dangers inherent in the use of oxygen with regard to combustibility and explosiveness, discussed above, the patient must be guarded against asphyxiation and narcosis.

Asphyxia

Patients receiving oxygen inhalations by means of oral-nasal masks or closed tents must be protected from the danger of asphyxia resulting from unexpected and unobserved depletion of the oxygen tank. This tragic accident is entirely avoidable through scheduled inspection of the pressure gauge and flowmeter during the procedure. These inspections should include the careful observation of the patient, noting in particular the nature of the pulse and respiration; the occurrence of coughing and type of sputum produced, if any; the color of his skin, lips and nail beds, with respect to the presence or degree of cyanosis; and his mental status. Oxygen pressures, flow rates and vital signs should be recorded accurately and according to schedule. Any change that is observed in the patient's condition should be described in detail and, if it is the least bit ominous, communicated to the physician at once.

Carbon Dioxide Narcosis

This complication presents a serious problem in the treatment of patients with chronic emphysema and generalized pulmonary fibrosis. The only serious complication related to oxygen inhalation per se is one with which the nurse should become thoroughly acquainted, for upon her may rest the major responsibility for its prompt recognition and for the action that must follow immediately if certain patients are to survive. These are patients with lung disease of a type which has resulted in generalized scarring of pulmonary tissue throughout both lungs and serious loss of respiratory efficiency. Prompt equilibrium between atmospheric air and the circulating blood is no longer established; the amount of oxygen absorbed during inspiration and the amount of carbon dioxide excreted during expiration are far less than normal. Therefore, these patients are oxygen deficient and, moreover, retain excessive

FIG. 35. Plastic type of oxygen tent with zipper front. In this type of transparent tent the patient does not feel enclosed. In addition, the nurse is able to communicate with the patient without opening the tent or disturbing its oxygen content. (Southern Oxygen Company)

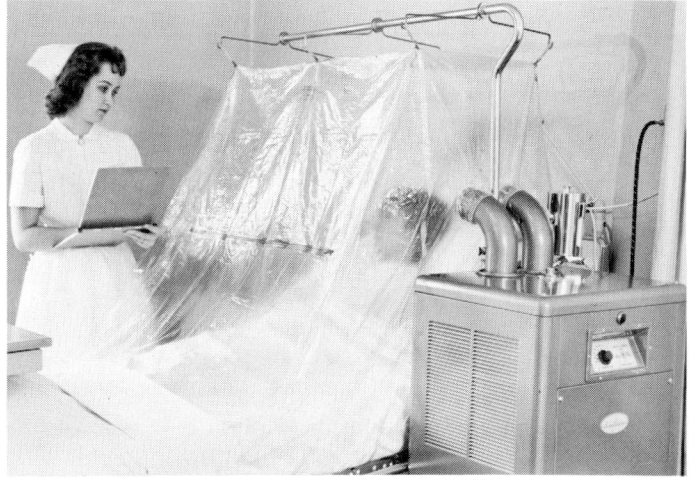

amounts of carbon dioxide in their blood. Herein lies the root of the problem.

Whereas the most potent stimulus responsible for increasing the rate and the depth of respiration normally is provided by a rise in the concentration of carbon dioxide in the blood, the respiratory center in these patients, long accustomed to a high carbon dioxide level, no longer responds to that stimulus, depending, instead, on a decreased blood oxygen—a stimulus only when it is very low. If a severely hypoxemic patient of this type inhales oxygen, the oxygen level in the blood rises, with the result that the only respiratory stimulus that remains effective now ceases to function. Respiration becomes progressively slower and more shallow, no faster or deeper than just sufficient to maintain the lowest oxygen level to which the patient has been accustomed and much less rapid and deep than had been customary. The most dangerous aspect of this situation is the increasing accumulation of carbon dioxide in the blood, the concentration of which soon reaches toxic levels. The patient becomes drowsy, then loses consciousness completely. Death is inevitable unless the respiratory function can be restored promptly.

Once the nurse becomes aware of any change in the patient's mental clarity or level of consciousness which suggests the possibility of carbon dioxide narcosis, oxygen inhalation should be interrupted at once and a physician notified of the emergency. If the oxygen is withdrawn in time, these symptoms should improve within the space of a few minutes. If consciousness has been lost, it may not return for many hours after the withdrawal of oxygen, and it may never be regained. The chances of survival decrease in proportion to the time elapsing between the loss of consciousness and the cessation of oxygen therapy. The chances of recovery are improved if artificial respiration is applied immediately, preferably in a mechanical respirator.

BIBLIOGRAPHY AND SUGGESTED READING

Book

Nordmark, M. T., and Rohweder, A. W.: Science Principles Applied to Nursing—A Reference for Nurse Educators, pp. 59-70, Philadelphia, Lippincott, 1959.

Articles

Burch, G. D., *et al.*: Influence of temperature and oxygen concentrations in oxygen tents, J.A.M.A. **176**:1017-1025, 1961.

House, J. A.: Safe practice in oxygen therapy, Hosp. Man. **81**:106-108, 1956.

Livingstone, H. M.: Nursing care in oxygen therapy, Am. J. Nursing **57**:65-68, 1957.

Macpherson, C. R.: Oxygen therapy—an unsuspected source of hospital infections? J.A.M.A. **167**:1083-1086, 1956.

McQuillan, F. L.: Safety in the administration of oxygen therapy, Nursing World, **130**:10-15, 1956.

Pons, E. R., Jr.: Ambulatory use of oxygen, Am. J. Nursing **60**:1775-1776, 1960.

13

Antimicrobial Chemotherapy

Exposure of tissue cells to the "foreign" proteins and chemicals produced by certain micro-organisms leads to a disruption of cellular metabolism and eventual dissolution of those cells. As a result of bacterial enzyme activity, capillary blood may be clotted and tissues thereby deprived of oxygen and nutrients. Carbohydrates from lysed tissue cells may be fermented, and intracellular protein degraded and liquefied, with liberation of toxic materials which have widespread systemic effects. Destructive activities such as these, together with certain defense reactions on the part of the individual harboring these pathogenic organisms, are manifested by a sequence of symptoms and signs which we recognize as being characteristic of infection: malaise, anorexia, fever, toxemia, anemia and, at the site of a localized infection, pain, hyperemia and edema, gangrenous necrosis and possibly gaseous crepitation. The clinical picture of infection depends on the nature of the pathogen, its virulence, portal of entry and the number of micro-organisms involved. It is equally dependent on the resistance of the host and the extent to which this may receive therapeutic support. The present chapter is concerned with antimicrobial chemotherapy in the treatment of infections. This type of therapy creates problems of nursing care which certainly are complex and unique, and which therefore deserve separate and early consideration.

ANTIBIOTICS

During recent years a number of compounds have been discovered which exert an extraordinary degree of antimicrobial activity in proportion to human toxicity and therefore are admirably adaptable for use in the chemotherapy of infection. Many are biosynthetic products, that is, manufactured by living cells, especially yeasts and fungi, in the process of their metabolism. In recognition of their origin and their capacity to inhibit the metabolism and the growth of other micro-organisms, these agents have been labeled "antibiotics." The therapeutic effectiveness of the antibiotic drugs, based on the reduction of mortality and morbidity that they have accomplished, has seen no parallel in materia medica. Whereas the anti-infectious activity of most antibiotics is limited to but a few types of infection, the number of agents with differing specificity is large and is expanding constantly. Moreover, the medical armamentarium includes a few "broad-spectrum" antibiotics which are effective against a wide variety of infectious agents. There are also some useful compounds other than the antibiotics so that most categories of infectious disease are now susceptible, to some extent at least, to one or another type of antimicrobial chemotherapy.

Individual antibiotic drugs, the clinical use of which is currently prevalent or increasing, are the following.

Penicillins

Penicillin, produced by the Penicillium mold and now synthesized in pure crystalline form, is by far the most extensively used of all chemotherapeutic agents, being almost completely devoid of toxicity and highly effective in a wide variety of infections. Almost all cocci are susceptible to the drug. These include gram-positive cocci, such as the pneumococcus, the streptococcus and the staphylococcus, and gram-negative cocci, such as the meningococcus and the gonococcus. It is likewise effective against gram-positive bacilli, including those causing anthrax, tetanus and gas gangrene. Its activity extends also to a few gram-negative bacilli, including *Hemophilus influenzae.* Moreover, penicillin destroys most spirochetes, including those responsible for syphilis, yaws, Weil's disease and rat-bite fever.

Oral penicillin is effective in doses of 200,000 to 500,000 units, given 4 or 6 times daily. Among the many dosage forms in which the drug is available for oral administration are the following: buffered potassium penicillin G, which is used most commonly; benzathine penicillin G, the most palatable variety; pencillin G with probenecid, the effect of the latter being to inhibit the urinary excretion of penicillin and therefore raise its concentration in the blood; and penicillin V, in which form the drug is not released for absorption until it has passed into the alkaline environment of the small intestine, having escaped the destructive action of the acid gastric juice. Sodium and potassium salts of penicillin often are given intramuscularly, and may be administered intravenously, in doses of 50,000 to 100,000 units every 4 to 6 hours. Slowly absorbed compounds of pencillin, or "depot penicillin," i.e., procaine penicillin or benzathine penicillin, must be given by intramuscular injection—never intravenously—the usual dose being 300,000 to 600,000 units once or twice daily.

Toxic complications associated with penicillin therapy are relatively infrequent and rarely serious. Sensitivity phenomena are encountered in about 1 patient in 200, occurring most frequently following topical applications of penicillin, least frequently following its oral administration. Delayed sensitivity develops occasionally, producing symptoms and signs which are comparable in all respects to those encountered in serum sickness, including edema of the face, hands and feet, pains in the small joints, fever and urticaria. These phenomena, indicating penicillin sensitivity, usually have their onset 7 to 10 days following the initial dose of the drug (on first exposure), occasionally not before 2 to 3 weeks have elapsed. The reaction usually clears completely within a period of 2 weeks after the cessation of penicillin therapy. Acute anaphylactoid reactions have been described, especially in association with the administration of depot penicillin, and

have been responsible for a few fatalities. On the other hand, oral penicillin therapy has been virtually free of serious complications.

Methicillin (Staphcillin) and oxacillin (Prostaphlin) are two synthetic penicillins which are particularly effective against the staphylococcus, an organism exceedingly prone to become resistant to the action of penicillins G and V, as well as to other antibiotics. Methicillin is not absorbed after peroral administration; therefore, it must be supplied by injection. For adults, the average dose is 1 Gm. intramuscularly every 4 hours, or 6 to 8 Gm. daily by continuous intravenous infusion; for infants, these amounts usually are halved. Oxacillin is effective by mouth, given every 4 hours in doses of 10 to 20 mg. per Kg. of body weight, no dose being administered less than 1 hour before, or 2 hours after, a meal. Complications attending the use of methicillin and oxacillin include: (1) pain at the site of injection; (2) gastrointestinal disturbances; and (3) skin rashes. Granulocytopenia (p. 469) has been encountered as a rare but hazardous complication of methicillin therapy.

Tetracyclines

This group of antibiotics includes chlortetracycline (Aureomycin), oxytetracycline (Terramycin), tetracycline (Achromycin) and demethylchlortetracycline (Declomycin). Very similar as regards their chemical structure, antimicrobial activity and method of administration, and all exhibiting an unusually wide range of effectiveness, these agents are classed as "broad-spectrum" antibiotics. Both gram-positive and gram-negative bacteria are susceptible to their bacteriostatic action, as well as certain of the larger viruses and the rickettsiae. Their numerous therapeutic applications include the treatment of infections due to the pneumococcus, the streptococcus, the staphylococcus, the meningococcus and the gonococcus; treponemal infections, including syphilis, yaws and Vincent's angina; surgical infections due to *E. coli* and *Aerobacter aerogenes;* urinary tract infections due to susceptible organisms; shigella infections of the gastrointestinal tract; *H. influenzae* infections; pertussis;

brucellosis; intestinal amebiasis; many viral and rickettsial infections; occasional cases of plague and tularemia.

These drugs are administered orally whenever possible, or intravenously if the oral route is not available. Intramuscular injections of tetracycline are undesirable, because of their painful character, but feasible, and are employed if there is no alternative. The average adult dose is 1 to 2 Gm. daily, given in divided doses, preferably with milk. Demethylchlortetracycline, which is cleared through the kidneys much more slowly and persists considerably longer in the blood stream than other tetracyclines, may be given in smaller doses. With respect to toxic complications of tetracycline therapy, it may be pointed out that symptoms of gastrointestinal irritation are common, especially in association with oxytetracycline and chlortetracycline. Prolonged administration of these broad-spectrum antimicrobials inevitably promotes an overgrowth of nonsusceptible organisms, of which the most feared is the staphylococcus. A debilitated patient is not likely to survive a complicating staphylococcus enterocolitis, which carries an over-all mortality rate of 40 per cent.

Chloramphenicol

Chloramphenicol (Chloromycetin) exhibits the same range of antimicrobial activity as do the tetracyclines and similarly qualifies as a broad-spectrum antibiotic. It likewise is absorbed from the gastrointestinal tract and is effective therapeutically when given by mouth, the usual oral dose being 1 to 2 Gm. daily. The drug is available also in forms which are suitable for intramuscular or intravenous administration. Its principal use has been in cases of salmonella and shigella infections. It is regarded as being the treatment of choice for typhoid fever. Chloramphenicol has been implicated as the cause of bone marrow failure in a small percentage of recipients. Most susceptible to this complication have been white children under the age of 10 years, females outnumbering males in this group 2 or 3 to 1.

Erythromycin and Erythromycinlike Drugs (Carbomycin, Oleandomycin and Spiramycin)

This group, of which erythromycin is the most active and useful, resembles penicillin in antimicrobial properties. Erythromycin, in particular, constitutes an excellent alternative to penicillin therapy in the treatment of infections caused by penicillin-resistant organisms, having proved to be most valuable in cases of pneumococcal meningitis, *H. influenzae* and staphylococcal infections. Whereas approximately 70 per cent of staphylococcus infections in hospitalized patients prove to be resistant to penicillin, and approximately 40 to 60 per cent to chlortetracycline and its analogues, less than 10 per cent are resistant to erythromycin. This drug is given orally in doses ranging from 100 to 600 mg. every 4 to 8 hours. Equivalent effects are obtained with 250 mg. of erythromycin administered by intravenous injection at 8-hour intervals. Toxic complications have been relatively few and mild, consisting mainly of abdominal cramps and diarrhea in a small percentage of recipients.

Streptomycin and Dihydrostreptomycin

These drugs are active against gram-negative and gram-positive bacteria, certain mycobacteria and some rickettsiae. Their principal use is in the treatment of tuberculosis, as described in Chapter 43, their other important uses being in the control of gram-negative bacterial infections and cases of Friedlander's pneumonia and tularemia. Patients with Friedlander's pneumonia generally receive 1 Gm. of streptomycin and 1 Gm. of dihydrostreptomycin each day by intramuscular injection, together with chloramphenicol. Patients with a streptococcus viridans infection may receive a combination of streptomycin, dihydrostreptomycin and pencillin. As in the case of penicillin, streptomycin produces sensitization phenomena in an appreciable number of patients, with manifestations of fever and the appearance of skin eruptions. A more serious complication is 8th nerve toxicity, vestibular disturbances being associated more often with streptomycin, and deafness occurring more commonly in patients who have received dihydrostreptomycin. Transient renal dysfunction, with proteinuria and moderate nitrogen retention, is not uncommon after prolonged therapy.

Neomycin

This agent is distinguished by the broadest spectrum of antimicrobial activity of any antibiotic known. It is particularly valuable in the treatment of proteus, pseudomonas and pyocyaneus infections. Administered by aerosol, it is efficacious in the treatment of infectious asthma, chronic bronchitis, bronchiectasis and in patients with lung abscess prior to surgery. A common type of neomycin aerosol is prepared by dissolving 0.5 Gm. of the drug in 2 ml. of water; to 1 ml. of this solution are added 2 ml. of superinone (Alevaire) or isopropylarterenol (Isuprel). Such an aerosol is usually administered twice daily for approximately 5 days. Intravenous neomycin is indicated in cases of overwhelming staphylococcus, proteus or aerogenes infections, especially staphylococcal pneumonia, enteritis endocarditis and meningitis. For intravenous use, 0.5 Gm. of the drug are dissolved in 500 ml. of saline solution; this is administered twice daily. Approximately 20 percent of patients receiving intravenous neomycin experience progressive and irreversible deafness. Neomycin in 5-mg. doses may be infused intrathecally and in 500-mg. amounts injected into the pleural, peritoneal or joint cavities. Neomycin is given orally, either alone or in conjunction with phthalylsulfathiazole (Sulfathalidine), with the object of preparing the bowel for surgery, treating bacterial diarrheas and decontaminating salmonella carriers. The dosage schedule usually employed for this purpose involves the ingestion of 1.0 Gm. 2 or 4 times daily.

Polymyxin B

Polymyxin B is active against gram-negative bacteria other than proteus and is useful particularly in the treatment of *Pseudomonas aeruginosa* (pyocyaneus). The drug is applied topically in a concentration of 0.5 mg. per ml., often mixed with neomycin, 1 mg. per ml. Pyocyaneus meningitis, an occasional complication of spinal anesthesia, is treated by combined intramuscular and intrathecal polymyxin B, 50 mg. of the drug injected intramuscularly every 6 hours and from 5 to 10 mg. given intrathecally once daily for 3 weeks. A combination of polymixin B, 50 mg. injected intramuscularly 3 times a day, and Aureomycin, 0.5 Gm. 4 times daily by mouth for a total of 4 to 6 days, is an effective regimen for the control of pyocyaneus infections of the urinary tract. Polymyxin B occasionally is given by mouth in 15- to 20-mg. doses in cases of shigella and pyocyaneus diarrhea in children. One of the complications of polymixin B therapy is the production of pain at sites of injection, which may force abandonment of the intramuscular route. Under these circumstances the drug may be given intravenously in the form of a solution containing 200 mg. of polymyxin B per 2,000 ml. of fluid. Patients who receive polymyxin B in excess of 200 mg. per day may exhibit transient signs of renal toxicity. A relatively minor side-effect is a transient "prickly" sensation in the vicinity of the mouth and the tongue, described by approximately 30 per cent of recipients.

Kanamycin (Kantrex)

This is used effectively in the treatment of infections due to staphylococci that are resistant to other antibiotics. It is also active against most gram-negative bacilli, *Aeorbacter aerogenes,* tubercle bacilli and some pseudomonas. It is not absorbed from the gastrointestinal tract and therefore must be given by intramuscular injection, 3 or 4 0.5-Gm. doses being administered daily in most cases. Patients who have received Kanamycin for prolonged periods of time are apt to exhibit proteinuria and may experience symptoms of 8th nerve toxicity, comparable with those produced by streptomycin.

Bacitracin

Bacitracin is effective exclusively against gram-positive organisms, and its clinical value is limited almost entirely to patients with staphylococcal infection. It is employed principally in the form of topical applications, compounded with neomycin, in patients with skin sepsis and infections involving body cavities.

Amphotericin B

An actively fungicidal and fungistatic antibiotic, this is effective in the treatment of certain systemic mycotic infections, notably coccidioidomycosis. A common routine involves the intravenous injection, on alternate days, of from 1.0 to 1.6 mg. of the drug per kilogram of body weight, dissolved in 5 per cent dextrose and injected over periods extending for at least 6 hours. Amphotericin B, in doses of 25 mg., may be infused into joint cavities; 0.5 to 0.7 mg. may be injected intrathecally. Dosages exceeding the levels indicated above are toxic, producing chills, fever and azotemia, indicating renal dysfunction.

Griseofulvin

Griseofulvin (Fulvicin, Grifulvin) is a fungistatic antibiotic used for the systemic treatment of superficial fungus diseases of the skin. Effective against species of *Microsporum, Trichophyton* and *Epidermophyton,* this agent is of particular value in treating children with ringworm of the scalp and patients of all ages with fungous infections of the glabrous (hairless) skin, feet or nails. It is supplied by mouth in daily doses of 1 to 2 Gm. for several weeks. Minor complications of griseofulvin therapy include headache and transient mental confusion. Skin eruptions of various types, and a clinical picture resembling serum sickness, have been reported. The most serious development has been the appearance of leukopenia in an occasional griseofulvin recipient. Rarely this has progressed to a dangerous granulocytopenia. On this account, blood cell counts should be carried out periodically as an integral part of griseofulvin therapy.

Nystatin

Nystatin (Mycostatin), an antifungal antibiotic, effective on surface application, is useful in the treatment of monilial infections of the vagina and the mouth. Tablets or suppositories containing 10,000 to 100,000 units of the drug are applied locally in the treatment of vaginitis. Solutions of nystatin are used on intertriginous areas of infected skin, and troches compounded of the drug are employed in the treatment of oral moniliasis.

SULFONAMIDES

An exceedingly important group of antimicrobials are the sulfonamide drugs, which exhibit a broad spectrum of bacteriostatic and bacteriocidal activity and have demonstrated their usefulness in a wide variety of clinical infections. Highly susceptible organisms include the hemolytic streptococcus, staphylococcus, pneumococcus, meningococcus, gonococcus, *Cl. welchi, B. anthracis, C. diphtheriae, H. influenzae, K. pneumoniae, H. ducreyi,* Brucella, V. *cholerae,* Shigella, *P. pestis,* Actinomyces and *D. granulomatis,* as well as the viruses of trachoma, lymphogranuloma inguinale, psittacosis, ornithosis, molluscum contagiosum and follicular conjunctivitis. *E. coli,* Proteus, *A. aerogenes* and *Ps. aeruginosa,* although somewhat less susceptible, nevertheless are destroyed by these drugs in higher concentrations, such as are attained in the urine of recipients. The sulfonamides that are absorbed from the gastrointestinal tract after ingestion and, therefore, are effective in the treatment of systemic infections, especially urinary tract infections, include the following: sulfadiazine, sulfamerazine, sulfamethazine, sulfisoxazole (Gantrisin), sulfacetamide (Sulamyd), sulfadimetine (Elkosin, Sulfisomidine) and sulfamethoxypyridazine (Kynex, Midicel). The average dosage in which most of these drugs are administered is 1 or 2 Gm. every 6 to 8 hours by mouth, a double quantity being supplied on the first day as the "loading" dose. Sulfamethoxypyridazine, of which less is excreted in the urine than other sulfonamides, is effective in corresponding lower doses, for example, 0.5 Gm. daily or every other day. The sodium salts of sulfadiazine and sulfamerazine and the diethanolamine salt of sulfamethoxypyridazine may be given by intramuscular or intravenous injection. Almost all of these agents are available in the form of solutions and creams designed for topical applications.

In contrast with the drugs listed above, which are absorbed readily from the intestine, certain other sulfonamides are absorbed very little, which renders them suitable for the treatment of intestinal infections and for preoperative sterilization of the bowel. This group includes the following: succinyl-sulfathiazole (Sulfasuxidine), given in a dose of 0.5 Gm. per Kg. of body weight the first day, followed by 0.25 Gm. per Kg. on 5 successive days, the daily dosage being divided into 6 equal quantities and ingested at evenly spaced intervals throughout the 24 hours; phthalylsulfathiazole (Sulfathalidine), administered in one quarter to one half the doses specified above for Sulfasuxidine; phthalylsulfacetamide (Thalamyd), given by mouth in doses of 0.2 Gm. per Kg. per day, in divided doses, for 3 to 5 days, and for 2 days postoperatively, or, for dysentery, 1.0 Gm. 3 times daily after meals for 5 to 10 days; paranitrosulfathiazole (Nisulfazole), given by rectal instillation in doses of from 10 to 60 ml. of a 10 per cent solution 3 times each day and at bedtime; and salicylazosulfapyridine (Azulfidine), the average dose being 1.0 Gm. by mouth 4 to 6 times each day for the first few days, and later, one half this amount.

The principal disadvantage attending the use of the sulfonamide drugs is the frequent occurrence of clinical complications. These include the production of skin eruptions and drug fever in susceptible individuals, and renal disturbances, due to the precipitation of insoluble sulfonamide derivatives in the renal tubules. The latter phenomenon may result in hematuria or, if extensive, complete mechanical obstruction and renal failure. This complication can be forestalled by ensuring adequate hydration and supplying, as an adjunct, some alkalinizing salt, e.g., sodium citrate solution, in an amount sufficient to elevate the urine pH above 6 or 7 units. Bone marrow disturbances, manifested by granulopenia, thrombocytopenia or anemia, may develop in any patient receiving a sulfonamide. In view of this possibility, hemoglobin measurements, leukocyte counts and examinations of the blood smear should be carried out periodically as a routine precaution in all patients receiving this form of antimicrobial therapy.

FURAN DERIVATIVES

Nitrofurantoin (Furadantin) is a useful urinary antimicrobial with a broad antibacterial spectrum which encompasses both gram-positive and gram-negative organisms. In concentrations that are achieved after oral ingestion, the drug is bacteriocidal for *E. coli, Staphylococcus albus* and *aureus, S. pyogenes* and *A. aerogenes,* as well as for certain species of proteus, *Ps. aeruginos* and *A. fecalis.* Its principal application is in the treatment of urinary tract infections which have proved to be refractory to other antimicrobials. The average dose of Furadantin is 7.5 mg. per Kg. per day, this amount being divided into 4 portions that are ingested at meals and at bedtime. A maximum of 14 days on this regimen constitutes a course of therapy. A similar course should not be repeated within 4 weeks. Lower doses, e.g., 2 to 4 mg. per Kg. per day, are tolerated well and may be given without interruption for many weeks, or even **months.**

Except for nausea and vomiting in a small percentage of recipients and rare instances of hemolytic anemia in "primaquine-sensitive" individuals (see p. 199), no untoward reactions of significance have been reported.

Nitrofurazone (Furacin) is a potent bacteriostatic and bacteriocidal agent which is active against a wide variety of gram-positive and gram-negative organisms. Its clinical use is mainly in the form of a soluble dressing (1:500 concentration in a polyethylene glycol base) for topical application. Such dressings are used with favorable effects in the treatment of mixed wound infections and infected skin lesions.

Approximately 5 per cent of patients become sensitized to the drug, many within the first few days of treatment, as indicated by the appearance of a pruritic, erythematous eruption at the site of application.

ISONIAZID AND PARA-AMINOSALICYLIC ACID

Isoniazid (Nydrazid, Pyrizidin, Tyvid) is actively bacteriostatic and bacteriocidal against the tubercle bacillus and is the most effective drug that has become available thus far for the chemotherapy of tuberculosis. The drug is given by mouth in daily doses of from 3 to 5 mg. per Kg. of body weight per day, this amount being divided into 2 equal portions which are taken at 12-hour intervals.

Toxic side-effects of isoniazid therapy may include the development of peripheral neuritis and/or manifestations of central nervous system dysfunction, such as restlessness, insomnia, muscular twitching and paresthesias. Peripheral neuritis can be prevented, even when giving much larger than normal doses of the drug, (e.g., 20 mg. per Kg.) by administering pyridoxine hydrochloride, 50 mg. daily, as an adjunct. (Other complications of isoniazid may continue to occur, however, despite pyridoxine.) Since isoniazid lowers the threshold for convulsions, individuals with epilepsy or convulsive disorders of any type should be treated with caution and observed closely during isoniazid therapy. Side-effects have been infrequent and mild, consisting mainly of dryness of the mouth and disturbances in micturition. Purpura, jaundice and agranulocytosis have been reported, but such instances have been remarkably rare.

Para-aminosalicylic Acid (PAS) has bacteriostatic activity which is limited strictly to *M. tuberculosis.* The clinical action of PAS and of streptomycin are synergistic (i.e., mutually reinforced); moreover, the opportunity for the development of resistant strains of tubercle bacilli is reduced when both drugs are administered simultaneously. (This applies to combinations of streptomycin and isoniazid.) PAS is administered orally in doses of from 8 to 16 Gm. daily, each dose being divided into 4 or more equal portions.

A certain number of patients receiving PAS experience anorexia, nausea, vomiting and diarrhea; these symptoms are often relieved by the administration of aluminum hydroxide gel with each dose. An occasional hypersensitivity reaction may be encountered, mainfested by a pruritic dermatitis and fever. Leukopenia and signs of renal irritation likewise may occur. Children receiving large doses of PAS, which is an organic acid, should receive the drug in the form of its sodium salt to avoid acidosis.

SULFONES

The sulfones comprise a group of drugs derived from a parent compound, DDS (4,-4'diaminophenylsulfone), which has bacteriostatic activity against *M. tuberculosis* and far more useful activity against the organism of leprosy. The drugs in current use for the treatment of leprosy include **sulfoxone sodium (Diasone),** given in a dose of 0.3 Gm. daily, which is increased to 0.5 Gm. for 2 weeks of every month, and **Promizole,** the recommended dosage of which, for the first few weeks, is 0.5 Gm. 3 times daily; this is increased gradually until a total of 6 to 8 Gm. is received each day. Promizole is also used in conjunction with streptomycin in the treatment of tuberculous meningitis and miliary tuberculosis in childhood. DDS itself is gradually superseding its derivatives, Diasone and Promizole, in the treatment of leprosy. This drug is administered, either orally or by deep cutaneous injection, in doses of 500 mg. This amount is suspended in a coconut oil and injected twice weekly.

Untoward reactions to DDS may include anorexia, nausea and vomiting, headache, nervousness, blurring of vision and paresthesias. Far more serious is methemoglobinemia and an acute hemolytic anemia, which develops to some extent in almost all recipients of this drug and is the basis for the routine interruption of therapy at two-week intervals. All toxic complications of the drug disappear upon its withdrawal.

QUINOLINES, EMETINE AND STILBAMIDINE

Chloroquine (Aralen, Resochin) is an extremely effective antimalarial drug and is active against amebae as well. Its most valuable property is its action against the erythrocytic forms of the malarial parasites, *P. vivax* and *P. falciparum,* as a result of which the parasitemia of acute malarial attacks can be controlled rigidly. Falciparum malaria, as a rule, is cured completely; relapses in vivax malaria are deferred, but not necessarily prevented, by the initial therapy. Acute attacks of vivax or falciparum malaria are treated with an initial loading dose of 1.0 Gm. by mouth, followed after 6 to 8 hours by an additional 0.5 Gm., and a single 0.5-Gm.

dose ingested on each of 3 successive days. Cases of vivax malaria receive 0.5 Gm. weekly thereafter to assure freedom from relapses.

Chloroquine, in addition to its antimalarial properties, has unique amebicidal activity and is most efficacious in the treatment of extra-intestinal amebiasis, including the hepatic and pulmonary varieties. Intestinal amebiasis is not improved by this agent, however. Chloroquine is usually administered in daily doses of 1.0 Gm. for 2 days, followed by 0.5 Gm. daily for 2 or 3 weeks. In addition to extra-intestinal amebiasis, chloroquine is reportedly effective in giardiasis, clonorchiasis, taeniasis and leishmaniasis and possibly is of benefit both in discoid and in disseminated lupus erythematosus.

Chloroquine, in the recommended dosage range, does not produce dangerous toxicity; mild, transient headache, visual disturbances, gastrointestinal complaints and pruritis are approximately the extent of the complications.

Primaquine is the most valuable antimalarial agent that has become available to date, the only one capable of curing vivax malaria. The recommended dose for accomplishing a cure in relapsing vivax malaria, temperate zone variety, is from 10 to 15 mg. of primaquine base daily for 14 days; for the Southwest Pacific variety, the dose is from 30 to 45 mg. of base daily for 14 days.

The toxic properties of primaquine, administered in therapeutic doses, are significant only in relation to one specific segment of the population, which comprises about 10 per cent of Negroes, individuals who appear to lack normal quantities of a red cell enzyme (glucose-6-phosphate dehydrogenase). These "primaquine-sensitive" patients exhibit methemoglobinemia, signs of intravascular hemolysis and hemolytic anemia in response to the drug. The severity of this reaction is proportional to the degree of exposure to the toxic agent. Primaquine therapy in susceptible individuals is not precluded, provided that its dosage is limited to 15 mg. per day.

Diiodohydroxyquin (Diodoquin, Yodoxin) is directly amebicidal, exhibiting powerful activity against both motile and encysted forms of the parasite. Therapeutically, it is active only against those organisms that are located within the enteric canal; accordingly, it is ineffective in cases of amebic hepatitis or amebic abscess of the liver. Its chief clinical value is in cases of intestinal amebiasis; it is effective also in balantidial enteritides, in lambliasis, *Trichomonas vaginalis* vaginitis (in the form of topical applications) and in the treatment of certain pyogenic and fungal infections of the skin. For intestinal amebiasis the total daily dose is 0.2 Gm. per 15 pounds of body weight for 15 to 20 days; a dose of 0.65 Gm. daily is adequate for asymptomatic carriers of amebae.

Emetine exerts a direct lethal effect on *Entamoeba histolytica* and is of great therapeutic value in severe cases of amebic diarrhea and acute amebic dysentery. Its most important role is in the treatment of amebic abscesses and amebic hepatitis, its therapeutic efficacy in such cases being equaled only by chloroquine. The optimum route of administration is by deep subcutaneous injection. A course of emetine therapy consists of 2 injections daily of a dose totaling no more than 60 mg. for no longer than 10 days (or up to 1 mg. per Kg. per day to a total dose of no more than 10 mg. per Kg. per course). Emetine therapy should not be repeated in less than 6 weeks.

Toxic symptoms relate principally to the cardiovascular system. They may consist of hypotension, precordial pain, tachycardia and EKG abnormalities which reflect toxic myocarditis. In view of the risk of toxicity, the recipient should be at bed rest and under close scrutiny during emetine therapy and for several days thereafter. Patients with organic heart disease should receive this drug only if the indications are truly compelling, for example, in the event that active amebic hepatitis or amebic abscess is not controlled by chloroquine.

Stilbamidine (Hydroxystilbamidine, Isethionate) is of value in the chemotherapy of various protozoan infections, particularly trypanosomiasis and leishmaniasis. It is effective also in systemic fungal infections, notably systemic blastomycosis. This drug is administered by slow (2-hour) intravenous drip, each dose dissolved in 250 ml. of 5 per cent dextrose or isotonic salt. The usual course involves the administration of 50 mg. on the first day, 100 mg. on the third and 150 mg. on alternate days thereafter, for a total of 15 injections. A course of stilbamidine should not be repeated within 60 days.

Toxic effects of stilbamidine include immediate reactions following injections that are completed too rapidly, marked by hypotension, flushing, salivation, headache, nausea and vomiting, symptoms that are explainable on the basis of histamine release. The most serious of the toxic complications of stilbamidine therapy is a neuropathy that may first become evident 2 to 5 months after therapy is ended, characterized by paresthesia, anesthesia and hypalgesia in the distribution of the trigeminal nerve, or, less commonly, in areas about the neck or the waist. Recovery is the rule, but in some patients symptoms appear to persist indefinitely.

BIBLIOGRAPHY AND SUGGESTED READING

Cohen, L. S., and Cluff, L. E.: The sulfonamides, Am. J. Nursing, 61:54-58, June, 1961.

Dameshek, W.: Chloramphenicol—a new warning, J.A.M.A. 174:1853-1854, 1960.

Feinberg, S. M., and Feinberg, A. R.: Allergy and penicillin, J.A.M.A. 160:778-779, 1956.

Finland, M.: Treatment of pneumonia and other serious infections, New England J. Med. 263: 207-221, August, 1960.

Frenay, M. C. A.: Drugs in tuberculosis control, Am. J. Nursing 61:82-85, April, 1961.

Hall, J. W.: Drug therapy in infectious diseases, Am. J. Nursing 61:56-60, February, 1961.

Randall, M. G.: Anaphylactic reactions to penicillin, Nursing Outlook 4:617-619, November, 1956.

Romansky, M. J.: Steroid therapy in systemic infections, J.A.M.A. 170:1179-1183, 1959.

Rothstein, E.: The 19th Veterans Administration-Armed Forces Conference on the chemotherapy of tuberculosis, New England J. Med. 263:585-591, 1960.

Staphcillin (Bristol Laboratories): Am. J. Nursing 61:58-59, March, 1961.

Weinstein, L., Madoff, M. A., and Samet, C. M.: The sulfonamides, New England J. Med. 263: 793-800, October 20, 1960; 842-849, October 27, 1960; 900-905, November 3, 1960; 952-957, November 10, 1960.

Weiss, M.: Chemotherapy and tuberculosis, Am. J. Nursing 59:1711-1714, December, 1959.

Witten, V. H., Sulzberger, M. B., and Krasner, F.: Blood counts and long-term antibiotic therapy, J.A.M.A. 173:1458-1461, 1960.

14

The Preoperative Patient

SURGERY IN THE PAST

Surgery was performed long before the dawn of civilization with the aid of a sharpened flint. Neolithic skulls with trephined holes show evidence of bony repair and prove that patients did survive major operations. Surgery developed remarkably in ancient India; a clear-cut and logical classification of surgical operations is given in the famous writing, the Samhita. It is recorded also that women who helped with the sick had to have clean hands and nails cut short. In Greece (400 B.C.) Hippocrates knew and described surgical conditions varying from a clubfoot to a fracture of the vertebra. Prostheses, such as false limbs and dentures, were made for patients. Plastic operations were performed, and bladder stones were removed. Surgery advanced more rapidly than medicine, probably because its results were more dramatic. Surgical nursing as such is not mentioned in these early histories, but it must have existed.

One of the many stories in the Bible at the beginning of the Christian era is:

And he went to him, and bound up his wounds, pouring in oil and wine, and set him on his own beast, and brought him to an inn, and took care of him.　　　　　LUKE 10:34

The good Samaritan gave nursing care. He found a man who had been beaten cruelly by thieves. After he had cared for his wounds, the Samaritan took his patient to an inn and continued to care for him. One realizes that the emphasis of his care was on the person with the wound and not the wound alone.

There were no remarkable developments in surgery or in nursing for many centuries after the beginning of the Christian era. Through these years there is reference to two

groups of nurses: those associated with some religious group and those of the Sairey Gamp type who nursed for hire. Little mention is made of nurses who cared specifically for surgical patients. At the time of Lister's introduction of carbolic acid as an antiseptic in the 19th century, one is made aware that nurses assisted in the operating room. About this time the seeds of present-day nursing were planted by Florence Nightingale as she cared for the wounded soldiers in the Crimean War. In particular, she emphasized the significance of good hygiene, and she was a strong advocate of planned instruction for nurses.

Up to the 19th century tradition had a strong influence and a restricting effect on progress. The general practitioner treated all ills. There were few who limited their practice to surgery and almost none who limited their field to specialized types of surgery. However, following the industrial revolution, tradition relaxed, and the more highly skilled tasks necessary to operate machinery introduced specialization. A parallel in the medical field was the rise of the specialist. If a person had difficulty with his ear, he went to an ear specialist. Now we are living in an age in which we are seeing a return in the professions to the more desirable middle course. Our emphasis today is not on the ear as such but on the person who has an ear problem. And so, in surgical nursing, our concern is not the appendectomy but the patient who has undergone surgery for appendicitis.

SURGERY AT PRESENT

The greatest progress in the care of the surgical patient has taken place since the beginning of the present century. An increasing knowledge of disease as a result of research has permitted the development of many diagnostic aids. Some of these depend upon roentgenograms and others upon various laboratory procedures: chemical, bacteriologic, pathologic and so forth. The result is that the diagnosis of disease is made with more exactness and certainty than was possible from the simple clinical examinations of previous days. It became apparent that the nutritional condition of the patient was an important factor in the outcome of a surgical procedure. The surgeon recognized the value to the patient of a normal fluid and electrolyte balance. In addition, he realized that good nutrition depended upon the maintenance of normal vitamin intake and a replacement of vitamins if there had been a loss of them. The significance of protein in the body nutrition has led to increasing at-

tention to its intake in the surgical patient, both before and after operation. When this food element cannot be taken by mouth, water-soluble protein may be given intravenously. In addition, replacement of protein and hemoglobin now is achieved commonly by plasma and blood transfusions. Blood also is used extensively during and after operation to replace blood loss and to prevent shock.

In the operating room the surgeon has been aided by progressive improvement in instruments, equipment and conveniences in construction. Improvement in the understanding and the practice of asepsis and various technical procedures enables surgeons to perform operations that would not have been possible before. Not the least of these improvements has been the development of the anesthesiologist, and with him have come

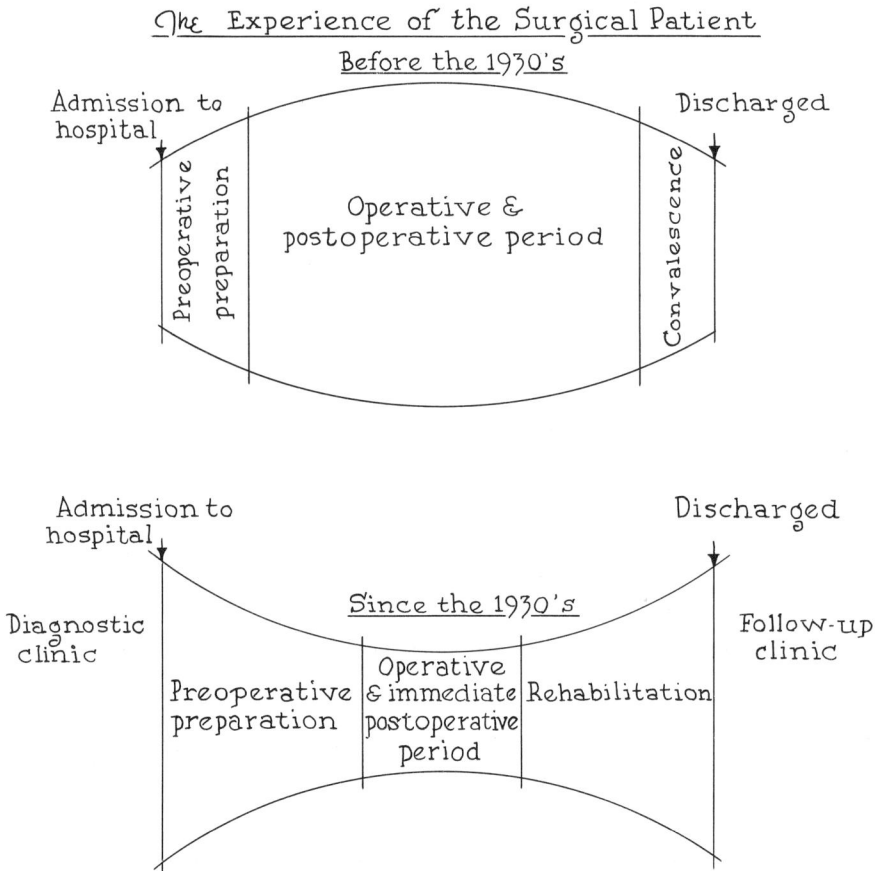

FIGURE 36

many advances in the technic of the administration of anesthesia. These advances have made it possible to deal surgically with lesions in the chest, the brain, the heart and the great vessels and with extensive malignancies in many parts of the body—something unheard of before.

One of the most striking developments has been the result of research in the control of infection. The discovery of the sulfona-

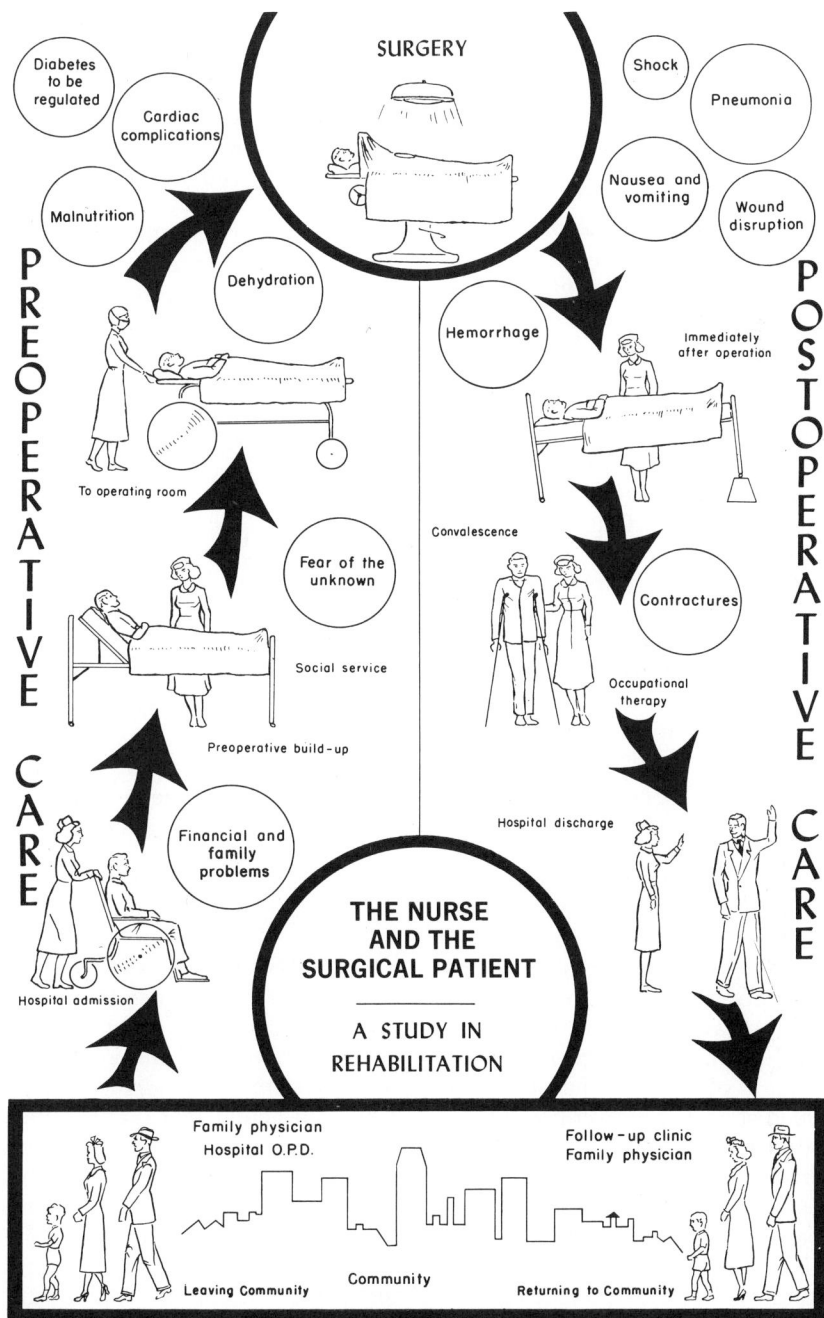

FIGURE 37

mides and the production of more effective and less toxic drugs were followed by the advent of the antibiotics, so that many infections which led previously to surgery now can be treated conservatively. These drugs may be used to prevent infections after operations and, should they arise, to treat them, and this has reduced greatly the operative hazard.

Many new fields of therapy have opened for the surgical patient. To mention them all would be impossible, but the therapeutic use of radiant energy, such as radium, x-rays and radioactive materials, may be used as an example.

A final advance in the care of the surgical patient is the change in attitude of all those who have a part in his care. It is recognized that the care of the surgical lesion is only a part of the care of the patient as a person: the important thing is to rehabilitate the patient and to return him to his home a healthy, happy, contributing member of society. This concept has many aspects. It may be concerned with the psychosomatic cause of the surgical disease, such as the influence of mental stress and overfatigue upon the production of peptic ulcer, or it may deal with the development of a mental attitude toward the acceptance of a colostomy or an amputation. In this rehabilitation, the patient and even his family frequently require training and instruction. Realizing that the best rehabilitation is a return to normal activities at an early date, there has been a gradual trend toward getting the patient out of bed as soon as possible after operation. Experience has proved that wounds heal well, that complications are decreased and that the general metabolism and the morale of the patient are improved by early ambulation. Prosthetic appliances that permit a more normal life for patients who have deformities have helped a great deal. Along with these important contributions to the rehabilitation of patients has come an increasing interest in the prevention of disease. Periodic health examinations, cancer detection clinics and industrial and public health education are playing an increasingly important part in the prevention of disease and the early detection of what would lead to serious surgical lesions if neglected.

THE NURSE AND THE SURGICAL PATIENT

With this improvement in the care of the surgical patient has come a change in the attitude, the functions and the responsibilities of the nurse. Although she still is expected to understand and carry out bedside nursing required in the care of the surgical patient, she also is expected to understand and take an important part in all phases of the patient's care.

The nurse, from her daily contact with the patient and the opportunity it affords her to observe him, can begin the rehabilitation of the patient even before operation. She must be able to carry out the immediate details of treatment while maintaining the over-all purpose of surgical care as related to the patient as a whole. This demands increasing knowledge and, therefore, increasing study. But it is important that with this increasing knowledge and responsibility she should not lose the human attribute that the connotation of the word "nurse" implies. The highly educated nurse with a scientific knowledge does not help the patient unless this knowledge is directed toward making the patient a more comfortable, healthy and contented individual. In present-day practice, less highly trained individuals may be given responsibility for certain types of care that do not demand extensive preparation. Thus nurses' aides, practical nurses and surgical technicians are being employed more widely to take over some of the less responsible duties. However, the professional nurse must realize that her responsibility to her patient entails careful supervision of auxiliary personnel who have less training.

PREOPERATIVE CARE

When a patient goes to a hospital for an operation, he enters an environment that not only is strange and different but often is associated with much anxiety, many misgivings and even actual fear. This applies not only to the patient but often even more so to the members of his family who accompany him. The nurse, who is in most intimate contact with the patient during his stay in the hospital, must realize the large part she plays in the psychological, as well as the physical, care of the patient. Able to predict the emotional responses of a patient in the hospital, she can reassure him by her attention and aid. A sympathetic understanding and an optimistic manner add to the patient's mental and physical comfort.

Admission of the Surgical Patient

When the admission requirements are completed, it is wise to obtain the name, the address and the telephone number of the nearest relative or friend. These particulars can be kept in a convenient place on the chart.

The assignment of a patient to his bed or to his room should be done with his condition and individual preferences in mind. If he is assigned to a ward, psychologically it is better for him to be placed near someone who is cheerful and convalescing from surgery rather than near one who is acutely ill or one who is bitter and pessimistic. Patients not only have been frightened out of the hospital; they have been frightened to death. Such cases are on record.

After the temperature, the pulse and the respiration are taken and recorded, the time may be opportune to weigh the patient and to secure a urine specimen. Hospital apparel usually consists of a short cotton gown tied in the back. A dressing gown or a house coat and bedroom slippers are a necessity. Every patient should have a toothbrush and a washcloth. His clothing and valuables are given to his family, or they are kept in the hospital, according to the policies of the institution.

The physician is notified of the admission of the patient. If he presents an emergency problem, medical attention takes precedence over the admission routine just outlined. A written permission for operation is obtained as soon as this method of treatment is decided upon.

Operative Permit. A patient may sign his own permit for operation if he is of age and in his right mind. Before he gives his permission, he has a right to know the nature of the operation and what to expect after it. This is the responsibility of the surgeon. If the patient is a minor, unconscious or irresponsible, permission must be obtained from a relative. For this reason, it is wise to retain a member of the family at the time of admission until this point is decided. Also, this person may contribute greatly to the history of the patient's illness.

Psychological Preparation

The student who is studying and practicing surgical nursing learns that essentially she is caring for a person with a surgical condition. She becomes aware that mind, body and soul should be in a healthy condition. One knows that any kind of surgical procedure always is preceded by some type of emotional reaction in a patient, whether it is obvious or not.* From the psychological point of view, she will learn that a mind that is not at peace influences directly the proper functioning of the body. Fear of the unknown, of death, of anesthesia or of cancer may or may not be apparent immediately, but other fears may be more intangible and overt; those, for example, regarding the possible loss of a job, the need to support a family or the possibility of permanent incapacity. Not infrequently one sees a sick body that has resulted wholly from emotional insecurity, such as is evident many times in patients with a stomach ulcer or an inflamed, ulcerating colon. Emotional upsets are more apparent in illness. Consequently, the nurse who learns this early in her career will be more tolerant and understanding. Unfortunately, all adults are not mature persons. They may be adult physically but not emotionally.

An essential part of the preoperative phase of patient care is the diagnostic study. The nurse should understand the purpose of each test and help to keep the patient informed. Too many times, a patient feels that he is a guinea pig. There need be no such reaction if the nurse assumes her full role.

* Recently, a team of physicians and psychologists made a study of the reasons for delay in surgical patients seeking medical and surgical care. It was concluded that 42 per cent of the 200 patients studied who did delay, did so because of psychological, psychodynamic and emotional factors operating before, during and after the individual's recognition of a sign or symptom of illness. Titchener, J. L., et al.: Problem of delay in seeking surgical care, J.A.M.A. **160**:1187, 1956.

The summation of diagnostic tests serves as a road map for the physician in directing him to his goal—the cure of illness.

Bird* acknowledges the psychological contribution of comfort and reassurance but emphasizes that even more important is the need to

keep open the patient's lines of communication to see that he is properly informed of everything he should know, that he does not receive misinformation, and that he himself can communicate freely with his surgeon and his relatives, thus allowing him to make his own requests and to ask his own questions. Other lines to be kept open are those between the relatives and the surgeon, between the nurse and the surgeon, and between all other working personnel.

Communication lines break down because of the number of persons who come in contact with the patient, the strangeness of the surgical floor (strange apparatus, a seemingly new language, increased tempo of activity) and the patient's own fears and anxieties. Such breakdowns in satisfactory interrelations leave the patient upset, bewildered and even unable to follow simple directions. Often in the course of conversation, something which was mentioned by a nurse or a physician becomes exaggerated out of all proportion to its importance. For example, because of a filled schedule, an operation had to be postponed. The patient was told that "something had come up." As he thought about this remark, the patient began to worry that something concerning himself was unsatisfactory; therefore, his condition must be deteriorating.

Let us examine the causes of fear which a preoperative patient may experience.

Fear of anesthesia was justified years ago, when little was known of the control and the effect of anesthetic agents. But with refined methods, tested drugs and skilled anesthetists, the hazards are minimized. The ease with which a patient accepts an anesthetic today is attributed to the adequate physical and mental preparation that he receives. The price of poor preparation is a difficult period of induction, followed by an unpleasant emergence from the anesthetic agent. The

* Bird, Brian: Psychological aspects of preoperative and postoperative care, Am. J. Nursing 55:685, 1955.

nurse in her daily association with her patient can do much to dispel false conceptions and misinformation. In instances in which the anesthetist visits the patient the day before surgery, real confidence is established, and the patient accepts the anesthetic more gracefully.

Often the fear of the anesthetic is secondary to the *fear of pain or of death.* Will I feel the knife? What if the anesthesia wears off? The patient needs reassurance that the anesthetist will be in constant attendance to take care of these problems. Some surgeons will not operate on a patient who is convinced that he will die. This is a real fear, and it cannot be dismissed lightly. Good rapport between patient and nurse, together with tact on the nurse's part, may bring him to a realization that his fear is magnified. It will help him greatly if those responsible for his care build up his confidence.

The *fear of the unknown* is the worst of all. Therefore, the more understanding one has of the probabilities for the future, the better is the adjustment. The nurse can do much to allay the anxieties of her patient and induce a certain peace of mind. A patient frequently will express fears and misgivings to the nurse but hide them from the surgeon. In such circumstances the nurse should communicate these evidences of anxiety privately to the surgeon.

When some of these fears have been expressed, brought to light and examined in their proper perspective, it is possible and even essential to get the patient to reveal what the operation means to him. Have him express his thoughts with regard to the importance and the meaning of this surgery for the immediate future and the more distant future. This is usually done by the surgeon, but, in the event that questions remain, the nurse may be in a position to elicit these from the patient. The importance of adequate lines of communication between surgeon and nurse must be emphasized here as they work together to prepare their patient for surgery.

The average person has many *worries* when he is well, but he has more when he is ill. He may have financial problems, family responsibilities and employment obligations; in addition to these, he may fear a poor prognosis or the probability of a handicap in the future. These problems can be investigated by the nurse. If the difficulty is of such a nature that a medical social worker can give assistance, the aid of such a person should be enlisted. If the worry stems from fear of what the prognosis is likely to be, the physician should be informed.

The significance of *spiritual therapy* must not be forgotten. Regardless of the religious affiliation of the patient, the nurse must rec-

PSYCHOLOGICAL PREOPERATIVE PREPARATION
OF THE PATIENT

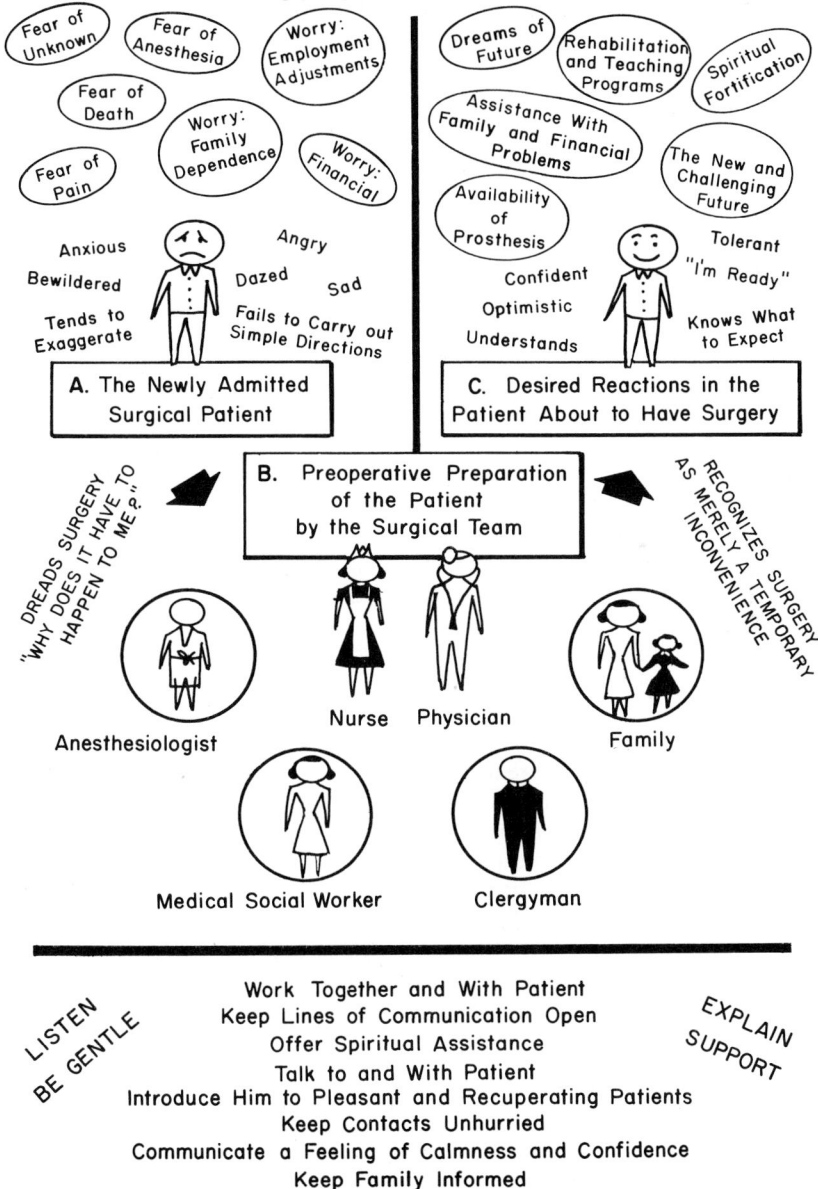

FIGURE 38

ognize that faith in a Higher Power can be as therapeutic as medication. Every attempt must be made to help the patient achieve the fullest spiritual help that he requests. This may be accomplished by participating in prayer, by reading passages from the Scriptures or by calling a clergyman. Such ministration by the nurse implies that she be informed about different religious beliefs. Faith has great sustaining power; the beliefs of each individual patient should be respected and supported.

The interval of time preparatory to surgery may become very extended. *Recreational and diversional activities,* such as reading, listening to the radio, watching television, handcrafts, games and so forth, are useful. The nurse can arrange for individuals with similar interests to meet. Many times patients can help one another.

In her association with her patient, the nurse must be cautious and tactful. A detailed discussion of the medical problems of her patients does not come within her sphere. It is the physician's place to discuss surgical procedures, prognosis and future treatment. Much trouble can be avoided if the nurse knows her limitations, as well as her strong points, in her relationship to her patient.

Perhaps the most valuable facility at the disposal of the nurse is her ability to *listen* to the patient. By engaging in conversation and using the principles of tactful interviewing, the nurse can acquire invaluable bits of information. An unhurried, understanding and kind nurse invites confidence on the part of her patient.

Lastly, every patient should be treated as an individual who has fears and hopes quite apart from the fears and hopes of the next person. To understand and help one patient may require a completely different approach from that used on another.* (See Fig. 38.)

Early Physical Preparation

Before treatment is initiated, the patient will be given a physical examination. The

---

* A recent development in nursing, which is of inestimable value to the preoperative patient who has problems, is the nursing conference in which members of the nursing team and members of associated disciplines participate. On occasion the patient may be a member of the conference and receive guidance and assistance.

---

physician and the nurse must respect his feelings and his sense of modesty. In bathing the patient, the nurse may note significant physical findings, such as a rash, decubitus ulcer and so forth, that may be contributory.

Diagnostic Tests. There may be many diagnostic tests, such as blood counts, roentgenographic studies, gastric analyses, tissue biopsies and stool and urine examinations. In all these tests the nurse plays an important part. She is in a position to help her patient to understand the need for diagnostic studies. She is aware that it is important to collect specimens and to describe them accurately in her charting. She must arrange for their safe transportation to the laboratory. The nurse knows that blood pressure, temperature, pulse and respiration are important indices of the condition of the patient and, therefore, must be charted correctly.

Preoperative Condition. Common conditions that affect a surgical risk may be dehydration and malnutrition. Perhaps the patient has been vomiting and, as a result, there is a disturbed fluid and electrolyte balance. To remedy this condition, the physician may order parenteral fluids of various types. In such a situation it is important to keep a good record of total intake and output. Malnutrition may be alleviated by high caloric diets with adequate vitamins and proteins. This is important, because vitamin C and protein are significant in tissue repair. Dental caries and poor mouth hygiene should be taken care of by the frequent use of a toothbrush and a mouthwash.

Patients with associated cardiac, diabetic or respiratory complications may require appropriate treatment before operation. Obesity increases the seriousness of these complications to a great extent. Their fatty tissues are not highly resistant to infection; therefore, dehiscence and wound infections are more common. They are difficult to nurse because of their weight, they breathe poorly when lying on their side and so are subject to hypoventilation and postoperative pulmonary complications, distention and phlebitis.

It is important for the nurse to remember the effect of old age or senescence. Reactions to injury are less pronounced and slower in appearing. The aged do not stand dehydration at all well. Their long established diabetes, anemia, obesity, hypoproteinemia and so forth must be considered. Certain drugs are dangerous because they are poorly tolerated. Scopolamine, morphia and the barbiturates are likely to cause confusion and disorientation, even excitement and apprehension. Some drugs have a cumulative effect. Sleeping and eating habits and the use of alcohol and laxatives, as well as the nightly "sleeping" medicine, must not be dismissed as unimportant. (See pp. 340-341.)

To summarize, the preparation and the care of the patient before operation are guided by an understanding of him as a unique, multifaceted individual. *Our objective is known; that is, to get the patient into the best possible condition for surgery. The means of achieving that goal are determined by the needs of the individual patient.*

General Preoperative Nursing Care

Surgeons and hospitals differ greatly in the detail of preparation for operation, but the general principle remains the same: to make the patient as clean as possible, externally and internally, and to cause the least possible amount of physical and mental exhaustion in doing so. The reasons for preoperative procedures are obvious. All sources of infection must be eliminated, hence the scrupulous cleanliness of the operative site. The intestines and the bladder must be empty to prevent their contents from being discharged involuntarily while the patient is under the influence of the anesthetic and to preclude an accidental incision in them, as sometimes occurs in an abdominal operation when these organs are distended. This is true particularly of the bladder and is the chief reason why it must be empty before a patient is sent to the operating room for a laparotomy.

Any preparation of the patient before operation should be carried out in the most efficient and capable way. Never approach a patient with an air of indecision: to do so causes him to lose confidence at once, and lost confidence is not regained easily. Determine exactly what procedures are to be performed and proceed with them in a systematic manner. If the treatment seems to be at all alarming to the patient, explain to him what you are about to do. Always work quietly, thoroughly and neatly; bustle, confusion and noise harass the patient.

During this period of preparation, from the time of admission to the actual operation, one of the most important responsibilities of the nurse is very close observation of the patient. Any sneezing, sniffling and coughing must be reported to the attending surgeon at once. Failure to do so may lead to postoperative pulmonary complications in the patient.

It should be the aim of every nurse to send her patient to the operating room in the best condition possible, so that convalescence will not be impaired. To this end she must remember that there is a great difference in the complaints of patients, and that any technic may have to be altered to suit individual needs. She must use her judgment and, when in doubt as to the advisability of a certain procedure, ask for instructions.

Bath. The patient should have a warm bath the night before operation.

Hair. A shampoo several days before operation is advisable, unless the condition of the patient does not warrant it.

Mouth and Teeth. The teeth should be brushed thoroughly twice a day and the mouth rinsed with a mild antiseptic solution at least 3 times a day.

Diet. When the operation is scheduled for the morning, the meal the evening before may be an ordinary light diet. Water may, and should be, given freely up to 4 hours before operation. In dehydrated patients, and especially in older ones, fluids often are encouraged by mouth before operation. In addition, and especially in patients to whom fluids cannot be given by mouth, they are administered by vein. If the operation is scheduled to take place after noon and is not to be upon any part of the gastrointestinal tract, the patient may be given a soft diet for breakfast.

Starvation, exhaustion, prolonged loss of fluids from fistulous tracts or vomiting results in loss of calories, vitamins and proteins (hypoproteinemia). The preparation of such patients for operation demands the use of

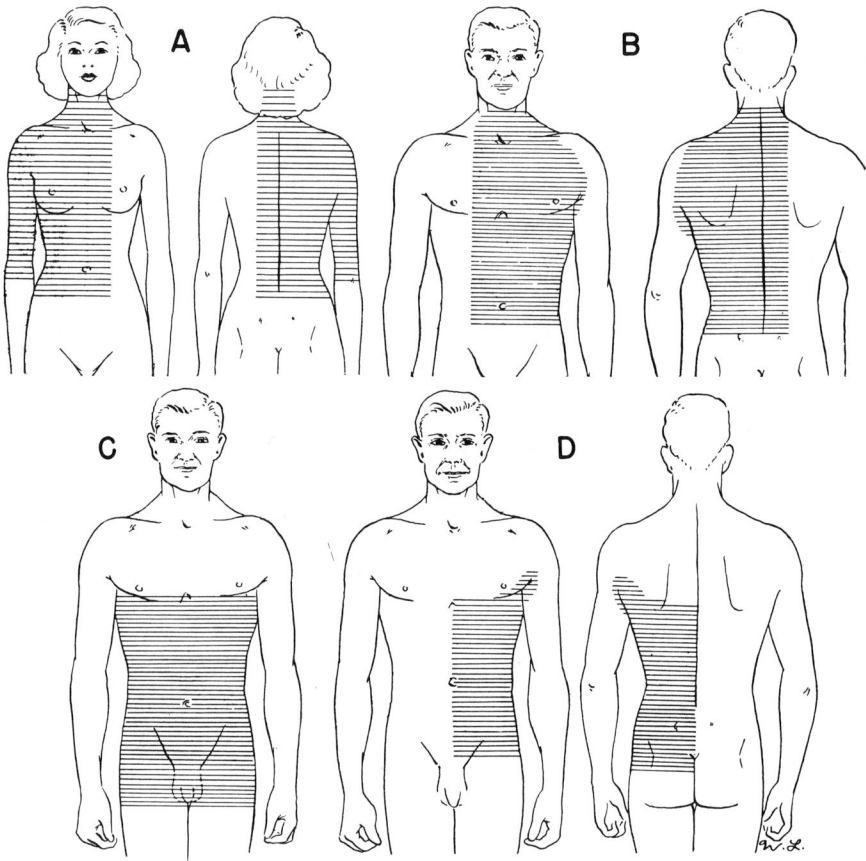

FIG. 39. Areas to be prepared for operation. The shaded areas are those to be shaved. (A) Preparation for amputation of breast. Note that the area to be prepared includes the front and the back of the trunk and extends from the neck to the umbilicus. The axilla and the upper portion of the arm also are included. (B) Area of preparation for operation on the thorax. (C) Area of preparation for operation upon the abdomen (laparotomy) and for hernia. The preparation should extend from the nipple line to well below the crest of the ilium. For herniorrhaphy the upper limit of preparation may be the area of the umbilicus. (D) Area to be prepared for nephrectomy. Note that the preparation should be on both the anterior and the posterior sides of the trunk. (E) Area to be prepared for operations on the perineum. These areas should be shaved completely for all gynecologic operations, operations around the anus and for such combined operations as an abdominoperineal resection of the rectum.

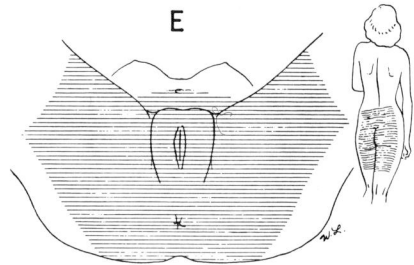

transfusions of blood, plasma or amino acid preparations. The particular vitamins needed may be added as indicated.

Enema. A warm soapsuds enema may be given the evening before operation, and may be repeated if ineffectual. Unless the condition of the patient presents some contraindication, the commode, and not the bedpan, should be used in evacuating the enema.

Preoperative Skin Preparation

The purpose of skin care preoperatively is to render the skin as clean and free of bacteria as possible without causing irritation or damage to the skin, without impairing its natural protective function, and without interfering with subsequent wound healing. [*]

When there is time, such as in surgery of a nonemergency nature, the physician may suggest that the patient use a soap containing hexachlorophene to cleanse the skin area for several days before surgery in order to help to reduce the number of skin organisms. After the bath, the area in the region of the operative field is cleansed particularly by the use of warm water and soap. Any adhesive or grease may be removed readily with a sponge moistened in benzene or ether, if the odor is not objectionable to the patient. All hair must be shaved from the part to be operated upon. Be very sure to have a sharp razor and to shave thoroughly a sufficiently wide area. (It is embarrassing to have a surgeon call for a razor after the patient is placed on the operating table.) Scratches should be avoided, and any skin eruptions must be reported because they are potential sites of infection.

Instructions as to special preparation will be found under the various operations.

Some surgeons require nothing further in the way of local preparation than thorough shaving and cleansing of the part until the patient reaches the operating room. Others prefer to have the operative area washed further with an antiseptic solution, such as 1:750 Zephiran Chloride, and the area covered with a dry, sterile dressing. If iodine is to be applied to the skin, the skin must be perfectly dry; washing and shaving should

be done at least 6 hours before. Also, because of the danger of blistering, great care must be taken not to apply too much iodine. It should not be used on the scalp, the face, the axilla, the perineum or the scrotum. In summer, iodine may blister a sweaty skin.

When using solutions on the abdomen, be careful to prevent any excess from trickling down into the groin, as this may cause severe burns of the scrotum or the labia.

The value of chemical depilatories is being studied.[†]

Operative Fields

Cranial Operations. Obtain specific instructions from the surgeon as to the extent of shaving that is necessary.

Thyroid and Neck Operations. Shave the anterior neck from under the chin to the nipple line. The area should be shaved back to the hair line and to meet the bed line when the patient is lying supine.

Operations upon the Chest. Shave the affected side from the spine posteriorly to beyond the mid-line anteriorly, and from the clavicle to the umbilicus.

Breast Amputation. Shave the axilla on the affected side. Skin preparation should extend from above the clavicle to the umbilicus, from beyond the mid-line anteriorly to beyond the mid-line posteriorly. Particular care should be taken in cleansing the folds underneath the breast.

Operations upon the Abdomen. Shave from the nipple line in males and from below the breast in females to, and including, the pubic area. Laterally, shaving should extend to the anterior axillary line. Particular care should be taken in cleansing the umbilicus and the inguinal creases.

Inguinal Hernia. Shave the lower abdomen from the umbilicus downward, including the suprapubic area and about 6 inches of the upper thigh on the affected side. Particular attention should be paid to cleansing the groin.

Operations on the Lower Bowel and the Rectum. Shave the entire abdomen as for any abdominal operation and prepare the perineum as for any anal operation.

---

[*] Knocke, F. J., and Knocke, L. S.: Orthopaedic Nursing, p. 279, Philadelphia, Davis, 1951.

[†] Prigot, A., *et al.:* Evaluation of a chemical depilatory for preoperative preparation of 515 surgical patients, Am. J. Surg. 104:900-906, Dec., 1962.

Anal Operations. Shave the area for a distance of about 10 inches from the anus. A suprapubic preparation is not necessary in male patients, but a partial perineal shave should be carried out in female patients.

Amputations. The area should be shaved and the skin cleansed for a distance of about 12 inches above and below the proposed site of amputation. It is important for the nurse to know where the amputation is to be performed. Thus, in gangrene of the foot, the amputation often is through the thigh, and it is necessary, therefore, to prepare the thigh.

Skin Grafts. Shave both anterior thighs or the area from which a graft is to be taken. Request instructions. In many hospitals the preparation of the operative field is done by aids or technicians from the operating room staff.

Operations upon the Spine. Shave and prepare the skin for an area of 12 inches above and below the site of operation. Ask the surgeon for instructions.

When the nurse is not sure about the area to be prepared, she always should ask for instructions.

Immediate Preoperative Preparation

The patient is summoned to the operating room about 20 minutes before the anesthesia is to be started. Previous to this the nurse clothes the patient in the regulation short gown, leaving it untied and open in the back. Occasionally, long leggings are added. Further, for a woman, long hair is plaited in two braids, all hairpins are removed, and the head and the hair are covered entirely with a cap. The mouth must be inspected and all dentures or plates, chewing gum and so forth removed. Jewelry should not be worn to the operating room; even wedding rings should be taken off. If a patient has any real objection to the removal of a ring, a narrow tape may be tied to the ring and then fastened securely around the patient's wrist. All articles of value, including dentures, should be labeled clearly with the patient's name and left in charge of the head nurse.

All patients (except urologic cases) should void immediately before being sent to the operating room. Unless the patient is in a weakened condition, the use of the commode or the bathroom rather than the bedpan should be urged. The bladder must be empty, but catheterization should not be resorted to except in an emergency. The amount of urine voided should be measured and recorded with the time of voiding on the preoperative check slip or the anesthesia chart.

Preanesthetic Medication

The administration of any anesthetic (general, spinal, regional or local) is facilitated greatly by the use of preanesthetic medication. Such medication is ordered to meet the needs of the particular patient. The drugs used most commonly are (1) the opiates— morphine and meperidine (Demerol), (2) the barbiturates—pentobarbital (Nembutal) and secobarbital (Seconal Sodium) and (3) the belladonna derivatives—atropine and scopolamine.*

Opiates and barbiturates tend to allay the anxiety and the apprehension of the patient. They also reduce the metabolic rate and, by so doing, permit the induction of surgical anesthesia with smaller quantities of anesthetic agents. The belladonna derivatives reduce the amount of secretions in the mouth and the respiratory tract and help thereby to maintain a clear airway. They tend also to obtund certain harmful reflexes that may occur during operation on the chest and the abdomen.

These drugs should be given from 45 to 75 minutes before anesthesia is begun. Therefore, it is most important that the nurse give this medication precisely at the time it is ordered, otherwise its effect will have worn off or—what happens more often—it will not have begun to act when anesthesia is started.

Very frequently operations are delayed or schedules changed, and it becomes impossible to order medication for a given time. In these situations the preoperative medication is ordered "on call from operating room." Although this is far from ideal and should be avoided whenever possible, the nurse can help by having the medication ready to give

* Fuerst, E. V., and Wolff, L.: Fundamentals of Nursing, ed. 2, Moving a patient from the bed to a stretcher, pp. 287-290, Philadelphia, Lippincott, 1959.

Patient ___JANE EVANS___ Ward ___THOMAS E-1___

	Remarks:	YES	NO
1. Operative area prepared		✓	
2. Operative area inspected by head nurse or supervisor		✓	
3. Jewelry		✓	
a. Removed			
b. Tied on			
4. False teeth removed	NONE		
5. Hair prepared - covered if necessary Hairpins removed		✓	
6. Voided or catheterized Amount:	350 cc		
Time:	8:40 A.M.		
7. Preanesthetic Medication Time:	8:30 A.M.	✓	
8. Side rails applied after giving preanesthetic Medication		✓	
9. Pulse and respiration taken Pulse:	78	✓	
30 minutes after preanesthetic Resp: Medication	18	✓	
10. Morning T P R charted		✓	
11. Operative permit signed and on chart		✓	
12. Blood report on chart		✓	
13. Urine report on chart		✓	
14. Doctor's order sheet on chart		✓	
15. Identification wristlet applied.		✓	
16. Colored nail polish removed (from at least 2 fingers)		✓	

Signature of Nurse: ___Janet Bender___

Date: ___July 9___

FIG. 40. Preoperative check list which is attached to the patient's chart and is checked immediately before the patient is taken to the operating room.

and by administering it as soon as the patient is called for. It usually takes from 15 to 20 minutes to get a patient ready for the operating room. If the nurse gives the medication before she attends to the other details of preparing the patient, she will have allowed the patient at least partial benefit of the preoperative medication and will have contributed to a smoother and more pleasant anesthetic and operative course. A last-minute check concludes the preparation (Fig. 40).

NAME_____
ROOM_____

You are about to join a very
Exclusive Club...

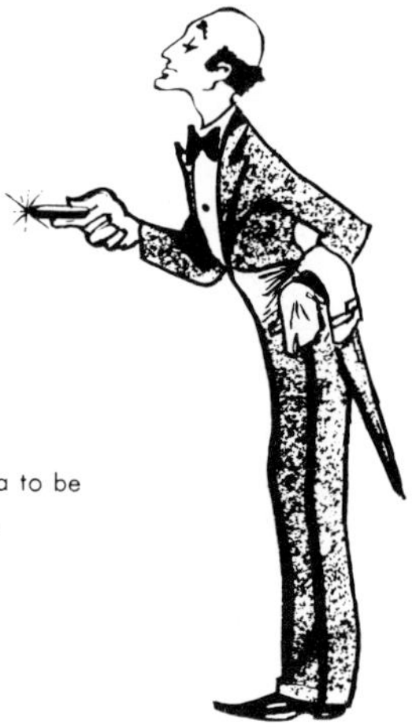

Your doctor wants you to be fully aware of how painless the "initiation ceremonies" will be for your membership in the

"Did I Tell You About My Operation Club"

1. You will receive dinner about 5 P.M. the night before your operation.

2. Enemas may be ordered following evening meal. Skin area around the area to be operated on will be shaved. This will be done the evening before surgery. However, in some cases it may be done in the morning before surgery.

3. A sleeping pill may be ordered for you in the evening if you need it.

4. You will not eat or take anything by mouth after 12:00 P.M. if you are scheduled for surgery the following morning.

5. Ladies! The nurse will ask you to remove your nail polish, jewelry, hair pins and makeup.

6. About one hour before surgery, you will receive a hypodermic, a hospital gown and a surgery "hairdo".

7. You will then be on the way to surgery.

8. After surgery, you will be taken to the "recovery room" where you will get special attention until you awake. Your family will be notified of your progress in the recovery room.

9. After you are awake, you will be returned to your freshly made bed.

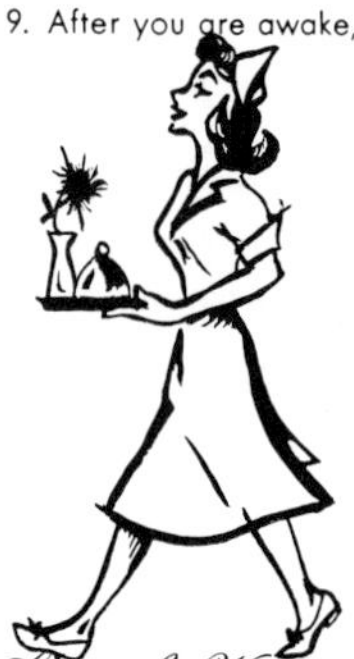

If you have any questions ask your nurse

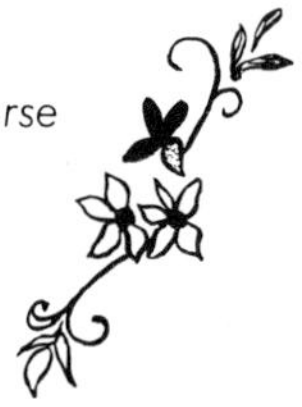

Louis A. Weiss MEMORIAL HOSPITAL • 4646 NORTH MARINE DRIVE • CHICAGO 40, ILLINOIS

FIG. 41. Patient instruction card. (Memorial Hospital, Chicago, Ill.)

Transportation to the Operating Room*

The patient then is transferred to the operating room in bed or on a previously prepared stretcher. This should be made as comfortable as possible and must be made up with a sufficient number of blankets to ensure against chilling from draughty corridors. A small pillow at the head usually is acceptable. The top covers of the stretcher should be long enough to tuck in at both the patient's feet and shoulders. The nurse always should remain with the patient until relieved by one of the anesthetists. The chart should be given to the anesthetist or a nurse; it never should be left with the patient.

THE PATIENT'S FAMILY

Many hospitals now are providing a special waiting-room for the family of the patient who is having surgery. This room may be equipped with comfortable chairs, television, telephone and facilities for light refreshment. Volunteers may remain with the family, serve them coffee, boost their morale, and even keep them informed of the patient's progress. After surgery, the surgeon may meet the family here, join them for coffee and report his findings.

The family never should judge the seriousness of an operation by the length of time the patient is in the operating room. He may be in surgery much longer than the actual operating time for several reasons:

1. It is customary to send for the patient some time in advance of the actual operating time.

2. Anesthetists often make additional preparation that may take from ½ to 1 hour.

3. Occasionally, the surgeon takes longer than he expected with the preceding case, hence delaying the time of beginning the next operation.

4. After surgery, the patient may be kept on the operating floor or recovery room to ensure satisfactory emergence from the anesthetic.

Those waiting for the postoperative patient

should be told what to expect when the patient arrives, such as a blood transfusion, suction bottles, nasal tube, airway, oxygen tent, tracheostomy tube and so forth. A point needing emphasis is the situation in which it appears that the prognosis of the patient is more negative than positive. Even when the odds appear against the patient, it is not within the prerogative of the nurse to relay this information to the family.

BIBLIOGRAPHY AND SUGGESTED READING

Articles

Bird, B.: Psychological aspects of preoperative and postoperative care, Am. J. Nursing **55**: 685-687, 1955.

Connolly, M. G.: What acceptance means to patients, Am. J. Nursing **60**:1754-1757, Dec. 1960.

Dumas, R. D.: Psychological preparation for surgery, Am. J. Nurs. **63**:52-55, Aug., 1963.

Gregg, D. E.: Reassurance, Am. J. Nursing **55**:171-174, 1955.

Hart, E. L., and Magee, M. J.: Collecting urine specimens, Am. J. Nursing **57**:1323-1324, 1957.

Hershey, N.: Whose consent is necessary? Am. J. Nursing **62**:94-95, Oct., 1962.

Hulse, W. C., and Lowinger, L.: The psychological management of the pre- and postoperative patient—the preoperative period, Am. Pract. **7**:927-933, 1956.

Isserman, F. M.: Spiritual preparation of the surgical patient, Hosp. Topics **33**:24-27, May, 1955.

McCaskill, C. L.: Transporting patients to the operating room, Nurs. Outlook **4**:562-564, 1956.

Preoperative and postoperative care, a symposium, Modern Medicine **25**:118, Aug. 15, 1957.

Van Schoick, M. R.: Emotional factors in surgical nursing, Am. J. Nursing **46**:451-453, 1946.

Via, S. C.: A presurgical conference, Am. J. Nursing **60**:1646, Nov., 1960.

Walter, C. W.: Preoperative skin preparation, Hosp. Topics **33**:65-68, Sept., 1955.

What is the nurse's responsibility in securing consent forms for treatment? If You Ask Me, Am. J. Nursing **62**:42-43, Aug., 1962.

* Film: Transporting the Patient for Surgery (16 mm. color, sound, 18 min.) available from ANA-NLN Film Library, 13 E. 37th St., New York, N.Y.

Williams, R. D., and Zallonger, R. M.: Principles of surgical nutrition, Am. J. Clin. Nutr. **3**:449-455, 1955.

Books

Bird, B.: Talking With Patients, Philadelphia, Lippincott, 1955.

Dripps, R. D., Eckenhoff, J. E., and Vandam, L. D.: Introduction to Anesthesia, ed. 2, Chap. 4, Philadelphia, Saunders, 1961.

Leibman, S.: Stress Situations, Chap. 2, Emotional Reactions to Acute Illnesses, Philadelphia, Lippincott, 1955.

Richardson, H. B.: Patients Have Families, New York, Commonwealth Fund, 1945.

Rosenbaum, M., and Cohen, Y.: Psychological preparation of the individual for medical and surgical care *in* Leibmann, S. (ed.): Understanding Your Patient, Chap. 2, Philadelphia, Lippincott, 1957.

PATIENT TEACHING AIDS

For Children

Dudley, N.: Linda Goes to the Hospital, Coward, 1953. (Preparation for an operation)

Radler, H. B.: All About an Operation, Society of Memorial Center, 444 East 68th St., New York 21, N. Y., 1956.

A Sea Captain's Voyage, a 12-page mimeographed and illustrated brochure depicting pre- and postoperative care. Attractive for children of reading age. Mimeographed by Baptist Memorial Hospital, Memphis, Tenn.

For Adults

Cunningham, R. M.: Your Operation, Public Affairs Pamphlet No. 267, New York, Public Affairs Committee, Inc., 1958.

Reiter, B.: You and Your Operation, New York, Macmillan, 1957.

15

The Patient in the Operating Room: Anesthesia

RECEPTION AND GREETING OF THE PATIENT

It is important that someone be with the preoperative patient at all times. Even though he has had preoperative medication, appears to be dozing and seems to be secure on the stretcher with a strap in place, he should not be left alone. It is desirable to have the patient brought directly to the anesthesia room, where he is greeted by name and made to feel that he is in safe hands. If no other waiting area is available, often he has to wait a few minutes in the corridor. Wherever he must wait before preparations for the administration of anesthesia are made, certain conditions should prevail. The area must be quiet for maximum effectiveness of the preoperative medication. He should not have to hear undesirable sounds from other patients or conversations which might be misinterpreted, exaggerated or out of range for accurate perception.

Patients occasionally assume an attitude of disinterest toward the equipment in an operating room; however, most people exhibit considerable curiosity. Some operating rooms are equipped with soft-playing piped music which is conducive to quiet relaxation.

It is assumed that preoperative preparation has covered quite a span of time before the patient comes to the operating room. However, many times the waiting patient with his eyes closed is reviewing some personal thoughts; then, a question or concern about some one thing may occur to him. Its value may even become overly exaggerated. Someone in attendance should be available to answer or attempt to find the answer to his query.

Skill in communication is accomplished not only verbally but also by facial expression, manner and a reassuring touch or warm grasp of the hand. Without a doubt it is important for the patient to have the security of someone nearby who is familiar, such as the nurse who helped to prepare him before coming to the operating floor, the nurse who greeted him in surgery and told him she would stay with him during his operation and be with him in the recovery room or the anesthesiologist who visited with him the day before and discussed his anesthetic agent and its induction.

Attention to physical needs will add greatly to his comfort. Keep the patient out of drafts, add a blanket if he is cold or remove a cover if he is too warm. Respect his modesty at all times and avoid unnecessary exposure. Knee straps should be applied loosely to prevent circulatory impairment. If there is any need to discuss something which the patient should not hear, this should be done well out of hearing range of the patient; even if he appears to be asleep, he may be acutely aware of all sounds.

THE ANESTHETIST AND THE PATIENT

The surgical patient usually is interested in and even concerned about the types of anesthesia that he is to receive. He has heard friends or relatives discuss the subject on the basis of personal experience or hearsay, and not infrequently he has formed definite opinions as to the merits or the demerits of the various methods in vogue. Therefore, it is helpful for the anesthetist to visit the patient in his own room before

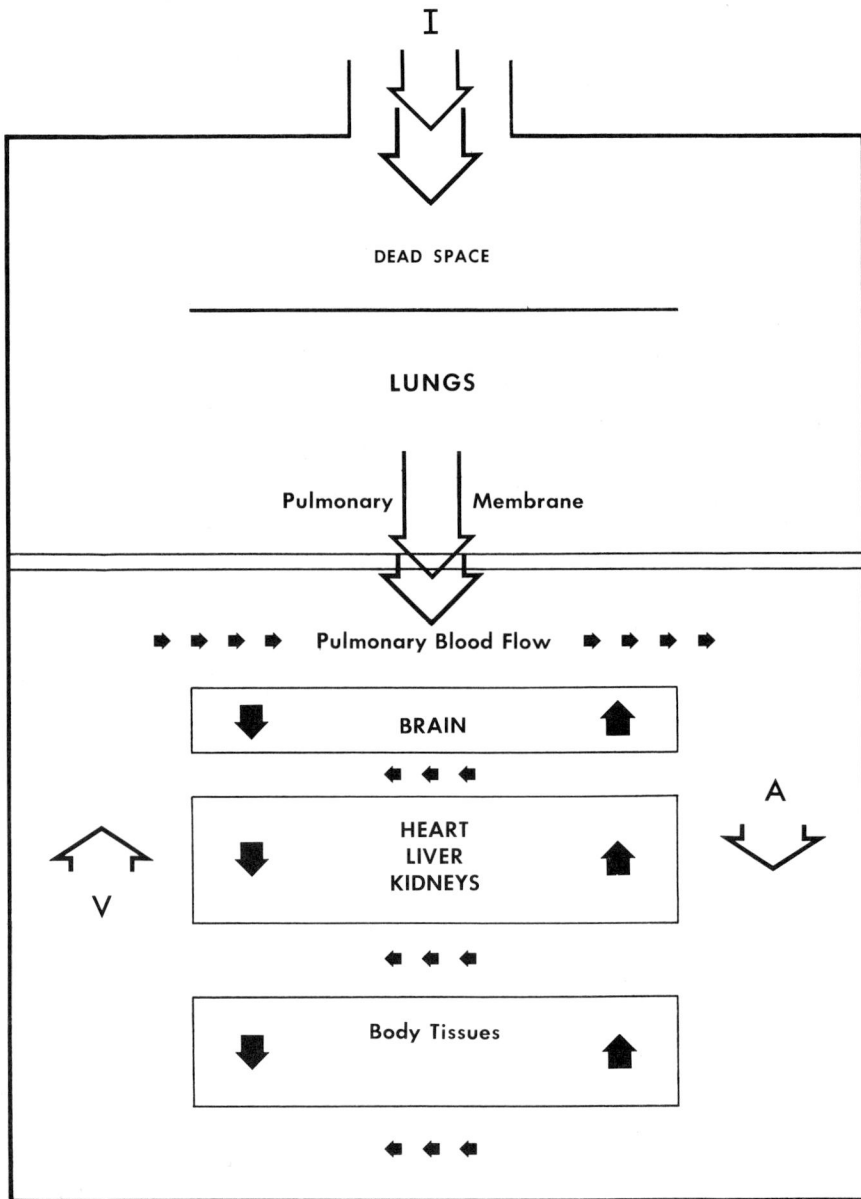

FIG. 42. Diagram illustrating some of the physiologic and physical factors underlying the uptake of inhalational anesthetics by the body. An anesthetic gas is given by mask at the mouth which, when carried to the brain by the circulating blood, will give rise to anesthesia. First, the anesthetic is breathed and mixed with the functional residual air of the lungs. Failure of the anesthetic in the tracheobronchial passages to come into contact with the pulmonary membrane is shown by the dead space area. The arrow pointing across the pulmonary membrane represents diffusion of the anesthetic gas across the membrane and solution of the anesthetic in the circulating pulmonary blood. The subsequent distribution of the anesthetic in the blood to the body is shown by the directional arrows. On the arterial side of the circulation, the tension of the anesthetic reaching the organs and the tissues is the same for all. The mass of the brain is pictured as being smallest, yet the volume of the blood flow to it is large. The body tissues, with the greatest mass, have the least blood flow.

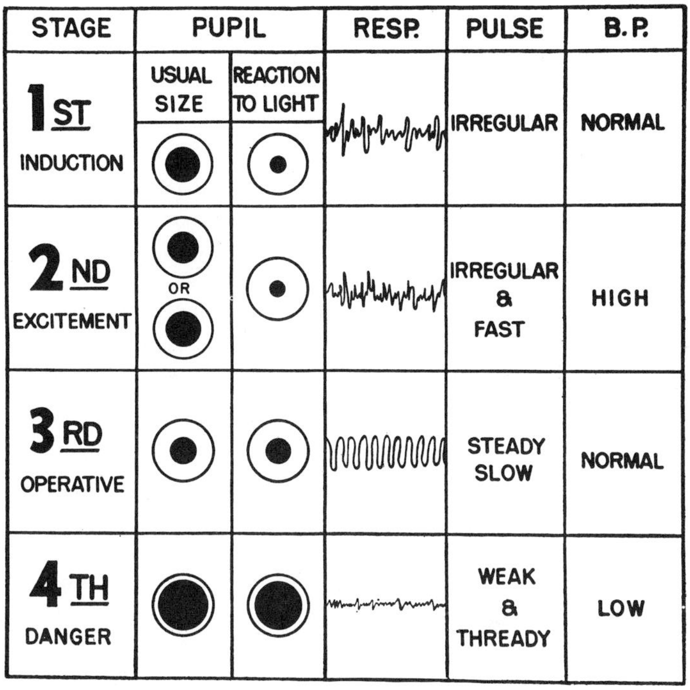

FIG. 43. Stages of anesthesia. (U. S. Army Manual, TM 8-230, Medical and Surgical Technicians)

STAGE	PUPIL		RESP.	PULSE	B.P.
	USUAL SIZE	REACTION TO LIGHT			
1ST INDUCTION	●	●	(tracing) IRREGULAR	IRREGULAR	NORMAL
2ND EXCITEMENT	● OR ●	●	(tracing)	IRREGULAR & FAST	HIGH
3RD OPERATIVE	●	●	(tracing)	STEADY SLOW	NORMAL
4TH DANGER	●	●	(tracing)	WEAK & THREADY	LOW

operation, introduce himself and point out that he has come for the purpose of allaying the fears that he knows exist in the minds of so many people. This preoperative contact builds up confidence and enables the patient to recognize a familiar face as he is being wheeled onto the operating floor. Uncertainty and anxiety are relieved, in part at least, and a much smoother course can be anticipated.

Today, with the increasing technical demands placed on the surgeon through bolder intervention in the abdomen, the chest and the brain, it is of the utmost importance that he be freed of the responsibility of watching the patient's anesthetic progress while he is operating. Consequently, the physician-anesthetist, especially trained in the art and the science of anesthesiology, has come into existence. To him, after consultation with the surgeon, can be delegated the choice of anesthesia, the technical problems relating to the administration of the anesthetic agent and the supervision of the patient's condition during the operation. This enables the surgeon to devote his entire energy to the surgery itself. Such a "sharing" of responsibility obviously benefits the patient.

Such supervision and observation today include not only attention to the blood pressure, the pulse and respiration but also, in many instances, the permanent recording of the patient's electrocardiogram, electroencephalogram, tidal volume, blood oxygen saturation, blood pH, pulmonary gas concentrations and body temperature. By meticulous attention to the cause-and-effect relationship of vital changes during operation, the anesthesiologist has contributed greatly to the development of devices with which to ventilate the patient's lungs or to circulate and aerate his blood, should his physiologic mechanisms, through the exigencies of surgery, become incapable of performing these functions.

Diffusion of the anesthetic gas into and out of the organs and tissues according to the prevailing pressure gradient is shown by arrows. Finally, recirculation of the anesthetic to the lungs is shown on the venous side of the circulation. On the venous side, the tension of anesthetic gas is an average of the tensions of the anesthetic returned from the organs and the tissues. (Modified after Haggard, Journal of Biochemistry) (Dripps, R. D., Eckenhoff, J. E., and Vandam, L. D.: Introduction to Anesthesia, ed. 2, p. 60, Philadelphia, Saunders)

In the event that physicians so qualified are not available, the skill of nurses trained especially in anesthesia, preferably by a physician, must be called upon.

In the anesthetizing room the patient is transferred to the operating table, and a last-minute check of his condition is made, blood pressure, pulse and respiratory rates in particular being noted. Then the anesthetic previously selected is administered. When all is in readiness for the beginning of the operation, the patient is wheeled into the operating room.

TYPES OF ANESTHESIA

Anesthetics have been divided into two classes according to whether they suspend the sensations (1) of the whole body (general anesthetics) or (2) of parts of the body (local, regional or spinal anesthetics). General anesthesia can be obtained by inhalation, intravenous or rectal technics.

Inhalation Anesthesia

Liquids producing anesthesia by inhalation of their vapor: ethyl ether, halothane, divinyl ether, trichlorethylene, ethyl chloride, chloroform.

Gases also administered by inhalation, usually in combination with oxygen: nitrous oxide, ethylene and cyclopropane.

These substances, when inhaled, enter the blood through the pulmonary capillaries and, when in sufficient concentration, act on the cerebral centers in such a manner as to produce loss of consciousness and of sensation. When the administration of the anesthetic has been discontinued, the vapor or gas is eliminated via the lungs in respiration.

Physiologic and Physical Factors. General anesthetics produce anesthesia because they are delivered to the brain at high partial pressure. Relatively high amounts of anesthetic must be given during induction and the early maintenance phases because of recirculation of the anesthetic and its deposition in body tissues. As these depots become saturated, smaller amounts of the anesthetic agent are required to maintain anesthesia, since equilibrium or near equilibrium has been achieved between the brain, the blood and the other tissues. The relationship between the various parts of the body as it influences the course of anesthesia may be seen in Fig. 42. On viewing this diagram, it becomes apparent that anything that influences peripheral blood flow, such as lean tissues or a condition of shock, may cause only small amounts of anesthetic to be required. Conversely, when peripheral blood flow is unusually high, as it is in the muscularly active or the apprehensive patient, the brain receives a smaller quantity of anesthetic which, in turn, means that induction is slower and that larger than usual quantities of anesthetic will be required.

Stages of Anesthesia

Anesthesia generally is described as having 4 stages, each of which presents a definite group of symptoms (Fig. 43).

Stage of Beginning Anesthesia. As the patient breathes in the anesthetic vapor, a feeling of warmth steals over his body, dizziness is experienced, and he seems to be detached from the world. He experiences a ringing, roaring or buzzing in his ears, and then, though still conscious, he is aware that he is unable to move his limbs voluntarily. During this stage noises are greatly exaggerated; even low voices or minor sounds appear distressingly loud and unreal. For this reason, unnecessary noise or motion must be prevented at all costs while anesthesia is being started.

Stage of Excitement. This stage—characterized variously by struggling, shouting, talking, singing, laughing or even crying—frequently may be avoided by judicious suggestion before anesthesia is begun and by its even and slow administration. The pupils of the eyes are dilated but contract if exposed to light, the pulse rate is rapid, and respiration is irregular.

Because of the uncontrolled movements of the patient during this stage, the anesthetist always should be attended by a nurse and an attendant, who should be ready to apply restraining straps if occasion demands. The patient should not be touched except for purposes of restraint, and in no circumstances should there be any palpation of the operative site.

Stage of Surgical Anesthesia. The stage of surgical anesthesia is reached by continued administration of the vapor or gas.

The patient is then entirely unconscious, lying quietly on the table. The pupils are small, but they retain their contractile power on exposure to light. Respiration is regular, the pulse rate is about normal and of good volume, and the skin is pink or slightly flushed. By proper administration of the anesthetic this stage may be maintained for hours.

Stage of Danger. This stage is reached when too much anesthesia has been given and when the patient has not been observed carefully. The respiration becomes shallow, the pulse weak and thready; the pupils become widely dilated and no longer contract when exposed to light. Cyanosis develops gradually, and, unless prompt action is taken, death follows rapidly. If this stage should develop, the anesthetic is discontinued immediately, and artificial respiration is given. Stimulants may be administered.

During the administration of an anesthetic, there is, of course, no sharp division between the various stages. The patient passes gradually from one stage to another, and it is only by close observation of the signs exhibited by the patient that an anesthetist can have complete control of the situation. The condition of the pupils, the blood pressure and the respiratory and the cardiac rates are probably the most reliable guides to the patient's condition. The anesthetist should focus his attention entirely on the patient and not be diverted by an interest in the details of the operation or by other activities of the room.

The administration of an anesthetic is attended by other physiologic activities that have not been mentioned. Some anesthetics, especially ether, produce a hypersecretion of mucus and saliva. This may be eliminated largely by the preoperative administration of atropine. Vomiting occurs not infrequently, especially when the patient comes to the operating room with a full stomach. The head should be turned sharply to the side, if gagging occurs, and a basin provided to collect the vomitus. The head of the table should be lowered to permit material to flow out of the mouth by gravity. Suction apparatus always should be available.

During the anesthesia, the temperature may fall. Because of this, every precaution should be taken against chilling the patient. A warm bed and blankets always should be provided. Sugar metabolism is much reduced, with the result that acidosis may develop.

In addition to the dangers of the anesthetic itself, the anesthetist must guard against asphyxia. This may be due to foreign bodies in the mouth, spasm of the vocal cords, falling back of the tongue or aspiration of vomitus, saliva or blood.

Methods of Administration

Open-Drop Method. Sometimes this method is used for the anesthetics that are

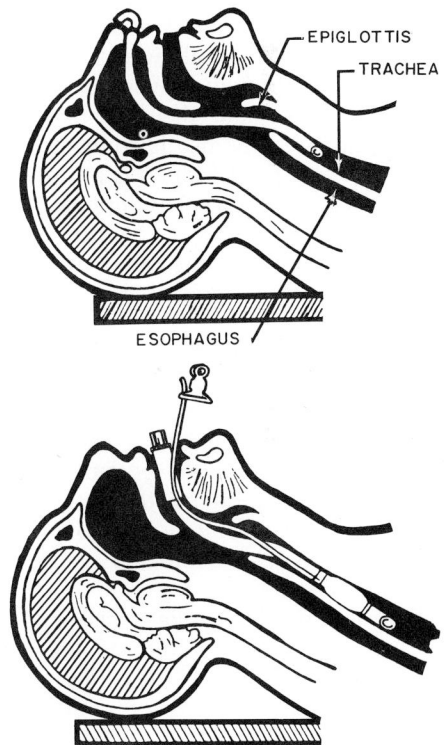

FIG. 44. Endotracheal anesthesia. (*Top*) Magill tube in proper position, intranasal intubation being used. Note metal elbow at proximal end of tube. This adaptor is used to keep the tube from entering the nose beyond reach of extubation. It can be used also to attach to anesthetic equipment. (*Bottom*) Oral intubation. The tube in position with the cuff inflated. (Surgical Equipment)

liquid. The fluid is dropped slowly on 8 layers of gauze held over the patient's nose and mouth. The patient inhales the vapor that evaporates from the gauze. Care must be taken to prevent a drop of the anesthetic from entering the eye. If this occurs, the eye should be irrigated immediately with saline solution and followed by a drop of sterile liquid petroleum.

Vapor or Gas Administration with Mask. Liquid anesthetics may also be given by causing the patient to breathe air or oxygen containing the vapor arising from the liquid. Ether, especially, is used in this manner, frequently in combination with the gas anesthetics. The vapor is conducted to the patient by a tube and a mask.

The gases (nitrous oxide, ethylene, cyclopropane and oxygen) are contained in tanks under pressure and are allowed to escape at the proper rate through valves opening into a mixing chamber and then usually into a large rubber bag. The bag is connected by a flexible tube to a mask, which is put over the patient's face. A reservoir containing ether often is attached to the mechanism so that, by turning a valve, a regulated amount of ether vapor may be given with the gas if this is desired.

Intrapharyngeal Anesthesia. Many operations upon the mouth and the lower part of the face will not permit the use of the ordinary inhaler. After anesthesia has been induced in these cases, it is possible to continue its adminstration by the introduction of ether by the vapor method, through small rubber tubes that lead into the pharynx by way of the nostrils.

Endotracheal Anesthesia. The endotracheal technic consists of introducing a soft rubber or other variety of tube directly into the trachea, either by exposing the larynx with a laryngoscope or by passing it "blindly." It may be inserted either through the nose or the mouth.

This technic has many advantages, but the most important is the most obvious—the patient has a clear airway. There is no danger of respiratory obstruction, either from the falling back of the tongue against the posterior pharyngeal wall (swallowing the tongue) or from spasm of the vocal cords. The endotracheal method has its greatest use in chest surgery, in which the thorax is open and the patient must depend upon the anesthetist to assist him in breathing or take over breathing for him completely by rhythmic compression of the breathing bag. But many other types of operation have been made possible or made safer by this technic: for example, neurosurgical, dental, plastic and nose and throat procedures, in which the anesthetist does not have immediate access to the patient's face or any procedure on a patient in whom, because of obesity or anatomic abnormality, the airway may become compromised.

Another important advantage of endotracheal intubation is that it provides a convenient method of aspirating secretions, blood or other foreign material from the trachea and the bronchi. This is not only important in anesthesia, but it is invaluable in the nursing care of very ill patients.

Often the advantages overshadow some disadvantages. Care must be taken in inserting the tube to prevent injury to the lips, the tongue and the teeth. Other complications must be prevented, during intubation, such as increased resistance to breathing, obstruction or dislodgment of the tube, and coughing by the patient. Other complications may develop after removal of the tracheal tube: (1) laryngospasm, which may occur in the lightly anesthetized patient and can be treated by the administration of 100 per cent oxygen; (2) tracheal collapse; (3) edema or infection of the larynx or the trachea; (4) hoarseness; and (5) sore throat.

Drugs Used for General Anesthesia
Inhalation Volatile Liquid Anesthetics

Ethyl Ether generally is considered the best and the safest of the general anesthetics. It is a clear, volatile, inflammable fluid. It may be given by any of the methods mentioned.

ADVANTAGES. It produces anesthesia with relaxation admirably suited for surgical operations.

It is not highly toxic, and it has a wide margin of safety between the dosage required for anesthesia and the toxic dose. The signs of a toxic dosage usually appear in sufficient time to allow for resuscitation of the patient and avoid a fatal outcome.

No accurate statistics are available, but various authors give mortality figures at from 1 death in 16,000 to 1 in 30,000.

In emergencies, ether may be given by unskilled persons under the guidance of the surgeon.

DISADVANTAGES. Ether vapor, especially in high concentration, irritates the respiratory mucous membrane. Its administration may be followed by increased secretions of the respiratory tract and by nausea and vomiting in the postoperative period. In the presence of respiratory diseases it is advisable to avoid ether whenever possible. The period of induction and of "coming out" is longer than for most of the other anesthetics.

Halothane (Fluothane); methoxyflurane (Penthrane). In recent years, great emphasis has been directed toward obtaining a non-explosive, potent general anesthetic which did not possess the toxicity of a drug such as chloroform. Two such drugs are now available—halothane and methoxyflurane. Both are clear, sweet-smelling liquids. Anesthesia is produced by inhalation of the vapor. They are both less volatile than ether and many times more potent. Evidence indicates they are even more potent than chloroform. Their main advantage is that they are neither explosive nor inflammable in therapeutic ranges even when mixed with oxygen. Induction with halothane is extremely rapid; with methoxyflurane considerably slower. Muscular relaxation is excellent with methoxyflurane, fair with halothane. To obtain good muscular relaxation with halothane, concentrations must be used which may severely depress circulation and/or respiration. Overdosage with these drugs is quite easy. They should be administered by special vaporizers which permit careful regulation of the inspired vapor concentration. In inexperienced hands, these drugs may be extremely dangerous. They do not possess the same margin of safety as ethyl ether.

Divinyl ether (Vinethene) is a clear, colorless volatile liquid. When given by the slow-drop method on gauze over the nostrils, it produces a rapid and a not unpleasant anesthesia from which the patient recovers rapidly with little or no nausea or vomiting. It is useful for short anesthesia. Kidney damage and liver damage may follow its use, particularly if it is given for operations of long duration.

Trichlorethylene (Trilene) is a weak anesthetic agent. It is useful to supplement nitrous oxide anesthesia and to provide pain relief without unconsciousness in obstetrics, urology and dentistry.

DISADVANTAGES. It may produce very rapid respiratory rates. It cannot be administered from the more common types of anesthetic machines.

Ethyl chloride at ordinary room temperature is a gas. Usually it is dispensed under compression from a glass tube with a tiny hole in one end. The spray tends to freeze tissues and render them less sensitive to a surgical incision.

As a general anesthetic it is rapid in its action and is administered by inhalation. It is used occasionally for short anesthesia and as a preliminary to ether. The rapid action of the drug makes it very dangerous for general use.

*Inhalation Gaseous Anesthetics**

Nitrous Oxide. This general anesthetic causes the least disturbance of bodily function if it is given with a concentration of oxygen not less than that of air (21%).

ADVANTAGES. The onset and the emergence from anesthesia are rapid and usually uneventful. Therefore, it is useful for short procedures on outpatients. It has a fairly pleasant smell. It is non-explosive and can be used with the electrocautery.

DISADVANTAGES. Nitrous oxide is a weak anesthetic. Its lack of potency can be overcome by adequate preanesthetic medication or by supplementation with an anesthetic vapor, such as ether, or an intravenous barbiturate or narcotic. Without these, if

* The Division of Simplified Practices of the National Bureau of Standards, Washington, D.C. has recommended the following color markings for the tanks containing these particular gases:

Oxygen .... green
Carbon dioxide .... gray
Nitrous oxide .... light blue
Cyclopropane .... orange
Helium .... brown
Ethylene .... red
Carbon dioxide & oxygen....... gray and green
Helium & oxygen .... brown and green

Anesthetics (General and Basal) and Adjuncts to Anesthesia†

Classification*	Official, Generic, or Chemical Name	Commercial Names or Synonyms
1. *Volatile (Inhalation) Anesthetics* (a) *Liquids* with Volatile Vapors	1. Ether U.S.P. (Diethyl Oxide) 2. Vinyl Ether U.S.P. (Divinyl Oxide) 3. Chloroform U.S.P. (Trichlormethane) 4. Ethyl Chloride U.S.P. (Monochlorethane) 5. Trichlorethylene U.S.P. (Trichlorethene) 6. Fluroxene (Trifluroethyl vinyl ether) 7. Halothane N.N.D. 8. Methoxyflurane	Diethyl Ether; Ethyl Ether; Sulfuric Ether Vinethene; Divinyl Ether Kelene; Anodynon; Narcotile Trilene; Trethylene Fluomar Fluothane Penthrane
(b) *Gaseous Anesthetics*	1. Nitrous Oxide U.S.P. (Nitrogen Monoxide) 2. Ethylene U.S.P. 3. Cyclopropane U.S.P. (Trimethylene)	Laughing Gas Ethene; Olefiant Gas

2. *Basal Anesthetics* (Nonvolatile; Administered intravenously or rectally, usually in doses adequate for rapid induction but not for deep surgical planes of anesthesia)	1. Tribromoethanol Solution U.S.P.
	 2. Ultra-short Acting Barbiturates
	   a. Thiopental Sodium U.S.P.
	     (Thiopentone)
	   b. Hexobarbital Sodium N.F.
	     (Hexobarbitone)
	   c. Thiamylal Sodium
	   d. Thialbarbitone Sodium
	   e. Methitural Sodium
	 3. Steroid Anesthetic: Hydroxydione
	 4. Methohexital Sodium N.N.D.
		Avertin with Amylene Hydrate
		
		 Pentothal Sodium
		
		 Evipal Sodium
		
		 Surital Sodium
		 Kemithal Sodium
		 Neraval Sodium
		 Viadril
		 Brevital Sodium

3. *Adjuncts to Anesthesia*
 (a) *Preanesthetic Medication* (Some used also postoperatively)
 	
 (b) *Skeletal Muscle Relaxants*
 	
 (c) *Non-anesthetic Gases*
	Depressants;
	 Morphine salts U.S.P.
	 Meperidine Hydrochloride U.S.P.
	 Barbiturates
	   ex: Pentobarbital Sodium U.S.P.
	   ex: Amobarbital Sodium U.S.P.
	   ex: Secobarbital Sodium U.S.P.
	 Anticholinergics
	 Atropine Sulfate U.S.P.
	 Scopolamine Hydrobromide U.S.P.
	 Miscellaneous
	 Chlorpromazine Hydrochloride U.S.P.
	 Promethazine Hydrochloride N.F.
	 Combinations of all the above
	 Tubocurarine Chloride U.S.P.
	 (d-Tubo.) and other Curare Derivatives
	 Gallamine Triethiodide N.N.D.
	 Succinylcholine Chloride U.S.P.
	 Decamethonium Bromide
	 Benzoquinonium Chloride
	
	 Hexafluorenium Bromide
	 Oxygen, Carbon Dioxide, Helium
		
		 Demerol, Pethidine; Dolantin
		
		 Nembutal; Pental; Embutal
		 Amytal Sodium
		 Seconal Sodium
		
		 Hyoscine Hydrobromide
		
		 Thorazine Hcl
		 Phenergan Hcl; Lergigan
		
		 Tubadil, Tubarine
		
		 Flaxedil Triethiodide
		 Anectine; Quelicin, Sucostrin
		 Syncurine; C-10
		 Mytolon Chloride
		 Mylaxen

* According to method of administration; physical, chemical and pharmacological properties.
† Morton J. Rodman, Ph.D., Prof. of Pharmacology, Rutgers University, Newark, New Jersey. Adapted from R.N., A Journal of Nursing, April, 1957 and revised by Dr. Morton Rodman, 1962.

nitrous oxide alone is being used for induction, it may be necessary to reduce the oxygen to 10 per cent or less. This is dangerous in certain individuals, such as those suffering from heart disease or anemia.

Ethylene is a colorless, highly inflammable gas possessing a characteristic sweetish odor that reminds one somewhat of burnt matches. It is like nitrous oxide but has a more unpleasant odor and is explosive.

ADVANTAGES. Rapid induction of anesthesia and rapid recovery.

No irritation of the respiratory mucous membrane.

DISADVANTAGES. It has an odor that is offensive to some.

Oozing from wounds seems to be increased, and the clotting time is prolonged.

Cyclopropane is much more potent than nitrous oxide or ethylene and can produce anesthesia in concentrations of from 15 to 20 per cent. The remainder of the anesthetic mixture can consist of oxygen; therefore, the patient has a more than adequate supply at all times. Cyclopropane is relatively nonirritating. It is a powerful depressant to breathing and for this reason should be administered only by an expert. Occasionally, marked disorders of the heart rate and rhythm occur during cyclopropane anesthesia. These increase with respiratory depression and deepening of anesthesia.

Explosibility

All the inhalation anesthetics discussed, with the exception of nitrous oxide, halothane and methoxyflurane, form explosive mixtures with air or oxygen. Therefore, they should be avoided if possible when the electric cautery and the electric desiccator are to be used. In addition, the spark of static electricity may set off an explosion. For this reason woolen blankets should not be used to cover the patient on the operating table. Nor should sharkskin or silk uniforms be permitted near the gas machine or the anesthetized patient. Finally, no one should touch the patient in the vicinity of the breathing mask lest a spark be generated and cause an explosion. The hazard of explosion is present always, but such unfortunate accidents will be extremely rare if common sense is exercised.

Muscle Relaxants

Using muscle relaxants, it is possible to give a lighter degree of anesthesia by using a less potent anesthetic agent at a reduced dosage. Purified curare was the first widely used muscle relaxant; tubocurarine was isolated as the active principle. Since then, synthetic muscle relaxants have been introduced that have supplanted the original drugs. They act more rapidly than curare. The full effect of a dose occurs in from 60 to 90 seconds after administration and persists for from 1 to 2 minutes. The return to normal occurs in about 3 to 5 minutes. Because of its fast action and rapid elimination, the drug is repeated each time that relaxation is needed. Serious depression of respiration may occur if the dose that is given is too great; therefore, careful observation of the volume of breathing is of particular importance.

Intravenous Barbiturate Anesthesia

General anesthesia also can be produced by the intravenous injection of various substances. An extremely short-acting barbiturate, thiopental (pentothal sodium) is the anesthetic in most common use today for this purpose. This substance leads to unconsciousness within 30 seconds. The onset of anesthesia is pleasant; there is none of the buzzing, the roaring or the dizziness known to follow the administration of an inhalation anesthetic. For this reason induction of anesthesia with an intravenous agent is the favorite of patients who have experienced various methods. The duration of action is brief, and the patient awakens with little nausea or vomiting. Thiopental frequently is given in addition to other anesthetic agents. It is especially useful to relieve the anxiety of the patient with spinal anesthesia.

Thiopental is a powerful depressant of breathing, and its chief danger lies in this characteristic. It should be administered only by skilled anesthetists and only when some method of giving oxygen is available immediately should trouble arise. Sneezing, coughing and choking sometimes are noted.

Intravenous anesthesia has the advantage of being nonexplosive, of requiring little equipment and of being so easy to take. The low incidence of postoperative nausea and vomiting makes the method useful in eye surgery, in which retching endangers vision in the operated eye. It is useful for short procedures, but is used less often for abdominal surgery. It is not indicated for children, who have small veins and who are more susceptible to respiratory obstruction. The reasons in both instances are apparent.

Spinal Anesthesia

It must never be forgotten that the patient under spinal, regional or local anesthesia is awake and aware of his surroundings. Careless conversation, unnecessary noise, unpleasant odors—all are noticed by the patient on the operating table and reflect discredit on the operating room staff. Quiet must be insisted upon. The diagnosis must not be made aloud if the patient is not to be made aware of it at once.

Anesthesia of the lower extremities, the abdomen and even of the chest may be induced by the introduction of anesthetic drugs into the subarachnoid space (Figs. 45 and 46). A spinal puncture is made with sterile precautions, and the drug is injected in solution through the needle. As soon as the injection has been made, the patient is placed on his back. As a rule, the head and the shoulders are lowered, depending on the height of anesthesia desired. In a few minutes anesthesia and paralysis appear, first of the toes and the perineum and then gradually of the legs and the abdomen. The drugs generally used are procaine, Pontocaine and Nupercaine.

ADVANTAGES. It is administered easily, is inexpensive, and requires a minimum of equipment. The anesthesia produced usually is rapid in onset, and there is excellent muscular relaxation. The patient may remain awake, if that is desirable. It is a relatively safe anesthesia in experienced hands. Mortality figures compare favorably with those of the safer general anesthetics.

DISADVANTAGES. Soon after the administration of the drug there may be a marked fall in blood pressure, caused by a paralysis of the vasomotor nerves. This phenomenon is noted most often when the anesthesia ascends to the upper abdomen and the chest. The preoperative administration of drugs such as ephedrine or methoxamine may be used to prevent the marked decrease in blood pressure. The inhalation of oxygen,

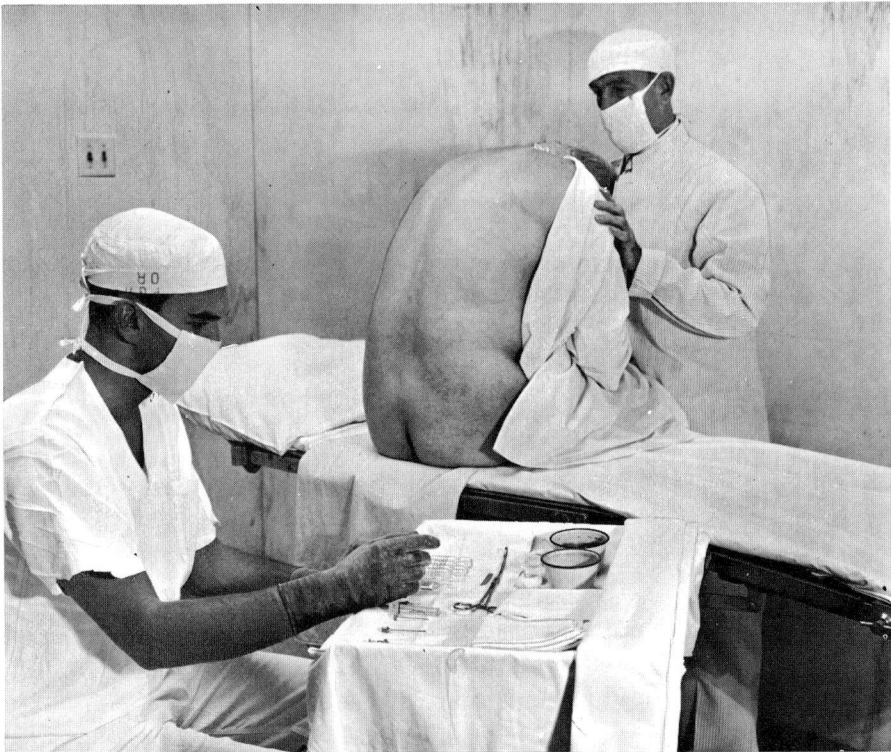

FIG. 45. Sitting position for spinal puncture.

the intravenous administration of blood, plasma or saline and the injection of stimulant drugs such as ephedrine, methoxamine, or phenylephrine, are measures of value once the blood pressure has fallen. Nausea, vomiting and pain not infrequently occur during surgery under spinal anesthesia. As a rule, this is due to traction on various structures, particularly those within the abdominal cavity. These reactions may be avoided by the simultaneous intravenous administration of a weak solution of Pentothal.

When the anesthetic drug reaches the upper thoracic and cervical cord in high concentration, a temporary, partial or complete respiratory paralysis may occur. This complication is treated by maintaining artificial respiration until the effects of the drug on the respiratory nerves have worn off.

Such postoperative complications as headaches, paralysis or meningitis may occur.

Several factors are involved: the size of the spinal needle used, the leakage of fluid from the subarachnoid space through the puncture site, the activity of the patient and the degree of the patient's hydration. Any measure which can increase the cerebrospinal pressure is helpful in relieving headache. These include keeping the patient flat and quiet, applying a tight abdominal binder and injecting fluid into the subarachnoid space.

"Serial" Spinal. A malleable needle or the tip of a plastic catheter may be left in the subarachnoid space during operation. Thus, more anesthetic may be injected as needed. Greater controllability of dosage is afforded by this technic; however, there is greater potential for postanesthetic sequelae.

Epidural or Peridural Anesthesia. This anesthesia is obtained by the injection of a local anesthetic into the spinal canal in the space surrounding the dura mater. Interest in this approach has increased probably be-

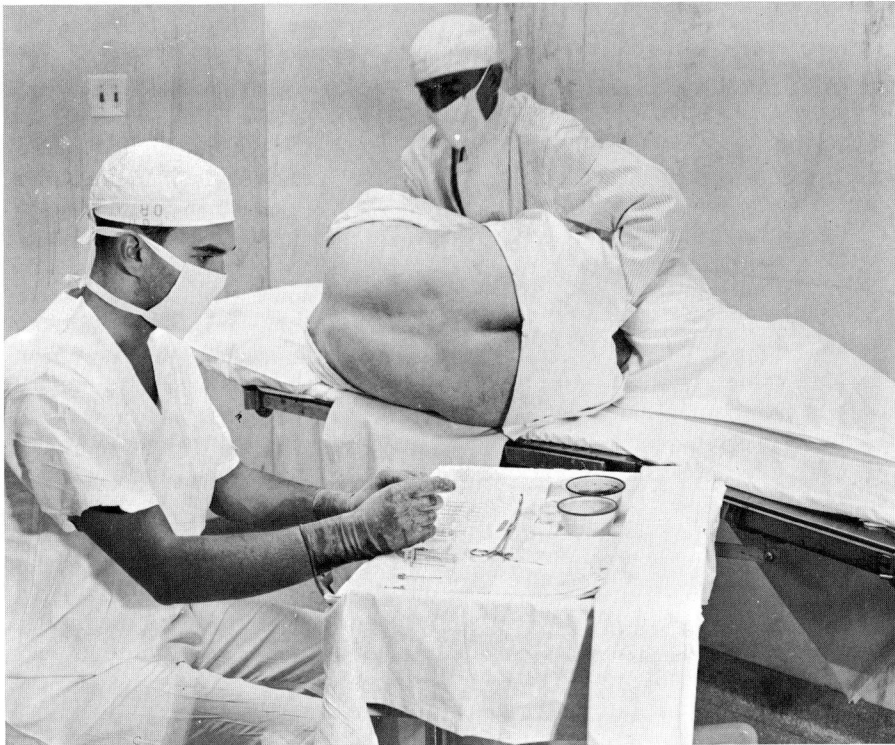

FIG. 46. Spinal anesthesia being given in lateral position. Note position of assistant, one arm behind the patient's knees and the other behind patient's neck in order to arch the back.

cause of a desire to find a method of spinal anesthesia without the undesirable neurologic sequelae, notably headache, which occasionally result from the subarachnoid injection.

The advantages of epidural anesthesia appear to be the absence of neurologic complications and less disturbance of blood pressure. One disadvantage lies in the greater technical problem of introducing the anesthetic into the epidural rather than the subarachnoid space. Another is that the level of anesthesia is less controllable.

Nursing Care After Spinal Anesthesia

In addition to taking the blood pressure, the nurse should observe these patients closely and make notes as to the time of return of motion and sensation in the legs and the toes. When there is complete return of sensation in the toes (appreciation of pinprick) the patient may be considered to have recovered from the effects of the spinal drug.

Regional Anesthesia

Regional anesthesia is that branch of local anesthesia in which, by an injection into or around the nerves, the area supplied by these nerve trunks is anesthetized. Motor fibers are the largest and have the thickest myelin sheath. Sympathetic fibers are the smallest and have a minimal covering. Sensory fibers are intermediary. Thus a local anesthetic blocks the motor nerves least readily and the sympathetic nerves most readily. An anesthetic cannot be regarded as having "worn off" until after all 3 systems (motor, sensory and autonomic) are no longer affected by the anesthetic. There are many types of this anesthesia, depending upon the various nerve groups that are injected.

Brachial Plexus Block. This produces anesthesia of the arm.

Paravertebral Anesthesia. This produces anesthesia of the spinal nerves supplying the abdominal wall and the viscera.

Transsacral (Caudal) Block. This produces anesthesia of the perineum and, occasionally, the lower abdomen.

An addition to obstetric anesthesia has been an adaptation of caudal block analogous to the change from a single-injection spinal to serial spinal. This adaptation is called *continuous* or *serial caudal*. A malleable needle or a nylon ureteral catheter is inserted into the caudal canal. This is allowed to remain in place and is attached by a rubber tube to a reservoir of anesthetic solution. When the woman in labor complains of pain, an injection is made, and subsequent injections are given as indicated. These may be continued for from 20 to 30 hours. The patient is conscious during the entire labor, and the fetus is spared the depression caused by drugs given to relieve maternal distress. The mechanism of labor is changed somewhat by this method. The second stage is longer, and operative deliveries are more frequent.

The method is not entirely without harm. Infections have occurred at the site of the injection. The level of anesthesia may become too high, and respiratory and circulatory difficulties may follow. With a drop in blood pressure the fetus may be endangered. Convulsions can occur, and the nurse should report at once any marked restlessness, anxiety, tremor or twitching.

Local Infiltration Anesthesia

Infiltration anesthesia is the injection of a solution containing the local anesthesia into the tissues through which the incision is to pass. Often it is combined with a local regional block by injection of the nerves immediately supplying that area. Local anesthesia is popular for several reasons:

1. It is simple to use, economical and nonexplosive. The amount of required equipment is minimal. Postoperative care is lessened.

2. Undesirable effects of general anesthesia are avoided.

3. It is ideal for use in short and superficial operations.

In operations upon the abdominal viscera, complete anesthesia is not obtained by infiltration or local block of the anterior abdominal wall, because the viscera are supplied by nerves that have not been affected by the anesthetic. For this reason, a separate injection must be made into the region of the splanchnic nerves, which supply the abdominal organs, except those of the pelvis. This injection may be made from the back (posterior-splanchnic anesthesia), or anteriorly, after opening the abdomen.

Local anesthesia is administered often in combination with epinephrine (5 to 10 minims to the ounce). Epinephrine has the property of causing a local constriction of the blood vessels, which in turn prevents rapid absorption of the anesthetic drug and so prolongs its local action.

Contraindications for Local Anesthesia

Local anesthesia is the anesthesia of choice in every operation in which it can be used. However, it is contraindicated in surgical operations upon highly nervous, apprehensive patients. The emotional trauma experienced by these individuals under local anesthesia may be more harmful than that following a general anesthetic. A patient who begs to be put to sleep rarely does well under local anesthesia.

For some kinds of operations, local anesthesia is impractical because of the number of injections and the amount of anesthetic required, as for example, a radical mastectomy.

Technic of Local Anesthesia

The technic for the introduction of local infiltration requires few extraordinary materials. For the ordinary case the following are all that are needed:

1. Flask of sterile ½ per cent procaine solution.
2. Sterile beaker or medicine glass.
3. Sterile syringes and needles to fit. If the syringe and the needles are kept in alcohol, they should be rinsed thoroughly in sterile water before being used.
4. Sterile sponges.

The skin is prepared as for an operation and, with a small-gauge needle, a little of the anesthetic is injected into the skin layers. This produces a blanching or wheal. The anesthetic then is carried ahead of the needle in the skin until an area as long as the proposed incision is anesthetized. A larger, longer needle then is used to infiltrate the deeper tissues with the anesthetic. The action of the drug is almost immediate, so that the operation may begin as soon as the injection is finished. The anesthesia lasts from ½ hour to 1 hour.

Drugs Used for Local Anesthesia

Cocaine

Cocaine is a white crystalline powder that is soluble readily in water.

USES. In from 1 to 4 per cent for anesthesia of the eye or of the mucous surface of the nose, the mouth and the urethra.

In from 0.1 to 1 per cent solutions for anesthetizing the skin.

In crystalline form for application to mucous surfaces.

DISADVANTAGES. It is highly poisonous, 1 gr. being regarded as the maximum dose for subcutaneous injections. Even this dose may produce acute toxic symptoms if rapidly absorbed or injected into a vein. The cause of the poisoning is the action of the drug on the centers of the medulla, causing respiratory failure and cardiac depression. The first symptom is a feeling of faintness. Nausea and vomiting occur, the pulse rate increases, and respiratory failure follows. In the event of cocaine poisoning with respiratory paralysis, life may be saved if artificial respiration is practiced until the effect of the drug wears off.

Prolonged sterilization by heat decomposes the drug.

Procaine (Novocaine)

Procaine is the least toxic of the local anesthetics. It is used in ½ and 1 per cent solutions, and as much as 2 Gm. may be injected without toxic effects. It has supplanted cocaine for general use. Although its effects as an anesthetic are not quite as marked as those of cocaine, its lack of toxicity recommends its use.

ADVANTAGES. It may be sterilized by heat.

It is very slightly toxic.

Its anesthetic effects are sufficiently potent for all ordinary requirements.

Tetracaine (Pontocaine)

This local anesthetic agent has a toxicity from 3 to 5 times that of cocaine; however, it is used in much smaller doses. The chief use of tetracaine is for spinal anesthesia; the advantage is that it can give up to 2 hours of anesthesia.

Lidocaine (Xylocaine)

Lidocaine has achieved wide usage because of the rapid onset of action, the freedom from local irritative effect, and the longer duration of action as compared with procaine. Apparently, it has a tendency to spread from the site of injection.

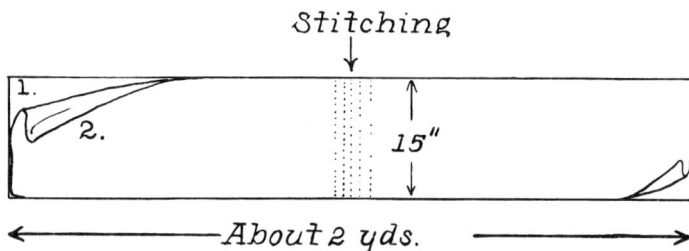

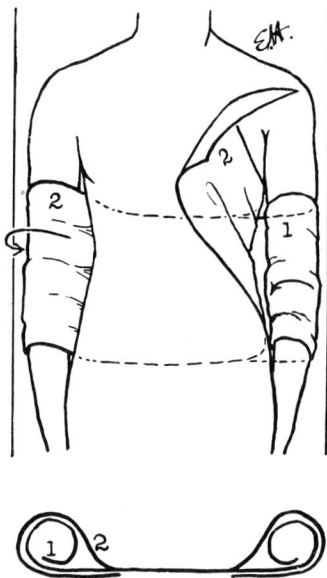

FIG. 47. Combination arm holder and body lift for use on operating table.

Mepivacaine (Carbocaine)

Mepivacaine is most similar to lidocaine. It is found to act equally quickly but to increase the duration of anesthesia by approximately 20 per cent. Tissue irritation appears to be minimal.

Induced Hypothermia

Deliberate cooling of the body (hypothermia) can be used as an adjunct to anesthesia in cardiac and neurosurgical operations, in which the reduction of tissue metabolism by cooling exerts a protective effect.

Induced hypothermia is a technic that is used to reduce the body temperature of the patient to below the normal (about 28° to 30° C. or 82° to 86° F.) in order to de-

crease the rate of metabolism. An individual who has been severely injured and is receiving an insufficient amount of blood flow to the tissues has a better chance of survival with the use of hypothermia because the body tissues and organs require less blood when the body temperature is kept at a subnormal level. That is, the oxygen uptake is reduced in linear fashion by the lowering of the body temperature.

Induction

The simplest way of reducing the body temperature is by the application of partially-filled ice bags* molded over the body and the extremities; however, specially devised blankets with coils for either heating or cooling by means of circulating water may be used. When the desired temperature is reached, some of the bags may be removed. A flexible electric thermometer provides an available temperature reading.

The nurse has special responsibilities when hypothermia is used for therapeutic purposes. These include: acute awareness of slight changes in the patient's blood pressure, pulse, respiration and level of consciousness which should be checked and recorded every 15 minutes. Thus, cardiac irregularities or respiratory difficulties can be detected early and treated. Shivering is a serious problem that can result in a multitude of difficulties if left uncorrected. Other dangers of prolonged hypothermia are: cardiac arrest; edema; disturbance of fluid balance; and fat necrosis. During hypothermia, an indwelling catheter is usually in place in

---

* Graves notes that 2 sizes of bags are most desirable. One that measures 36 x 12 inches is ideal for molding over the arms and the legs. The other measuring 12 x 12 inches is used to cover the chest and the abdomen.

the bladder and a venesection is performed. An accurate recording of both the intake and the output is necessary.

Induced hypothermia may be used for the duration of an operation or it may be prolonged for from 3 to 5 days depending on the objective. For prolonged treatment, care of the eyes, the mouth and the skin are important. Maintenance of proper body alignment is essential and the patient should be turned to alternate sides every 2 hours.

Rewarming

Ice bags are removed and the patient is allowed to rewarm at his own rate. At this time, hot water bottles are contraindicated because of the danger of burning the skin. Following the return to a normal body temperature, the patient continues to have his vital signs checked periodically and a gradual return to a normal diet is planned. Problems that require special observation may include: an increased bleeding tendency; gastric distention; skin changes resulting from exposure to cold.

Artificial Hypotension During Operation

Another new development is that of producing *deliberate hypotension*. This is accomplished by spinal or intravenous injection of drugs which affect the sympathetic ganglia. The resultant hypotension reduces bleeding at the operative site, thereby allowing for more rapid surgery. Such a technic has been successful in brain surgery, radical neck dissection and radical pelvic surgery.

POSITION ON OPERATING TABLE

The position in which the patient is placed on the operating table depends upon the operation to be performed as well as the physical condition of the patient. Factors to consider:

(1) The patient should be in as comfortable a position as possible, whether asleep or awake.

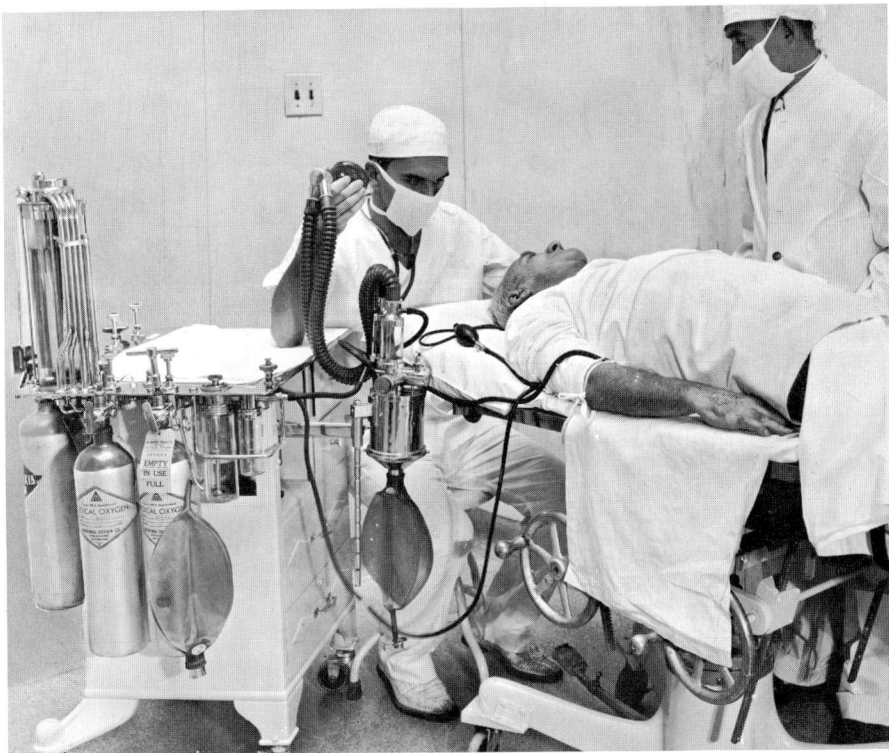

FIG. 48. Patient on operating table ready for anesthesia, with blood pressure cuff applied. Note presence of orderly. Arm holder-lift ready for use.

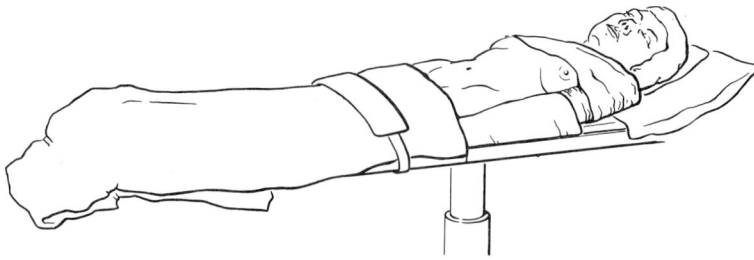

(A) Patient in position on the operating table as prepared for a laparotomy. Note the strap above the knees and the arm holder in use.

(B) Patient in Trendelenburg position on operating table. Note padded shoulder braces in place.

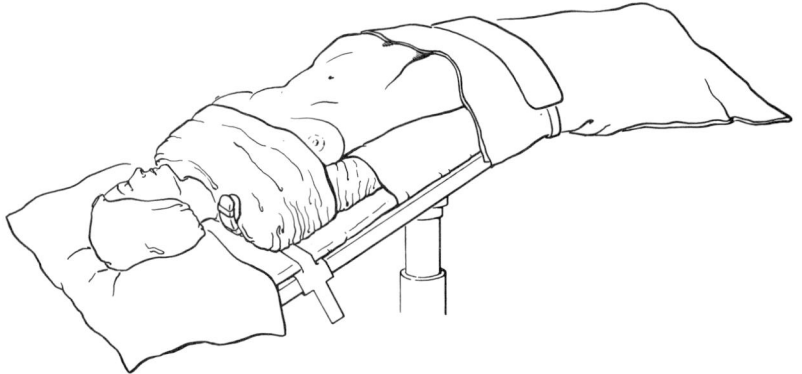

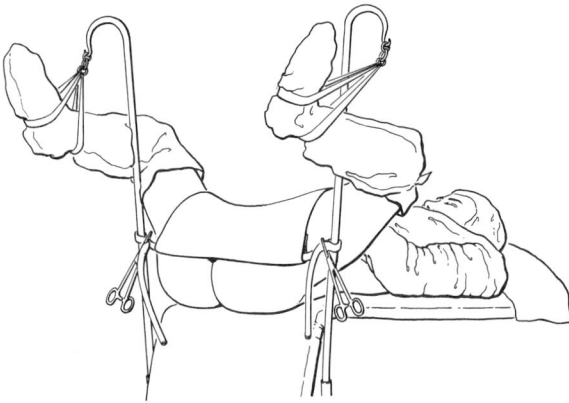

(C) Patient in lithotomy position. Note that the hips extend over the edge of the table.

(D) Patient on operating table for kidney operation, lying on his well side. Table is broken to spread apart space between the lower ribs and the pelvis. The upper leg is extended; the lower leg is flexed at the knee and the hip joints; a pillow is placed between the legs. Note the sandbag, which helps to support patient's chest.

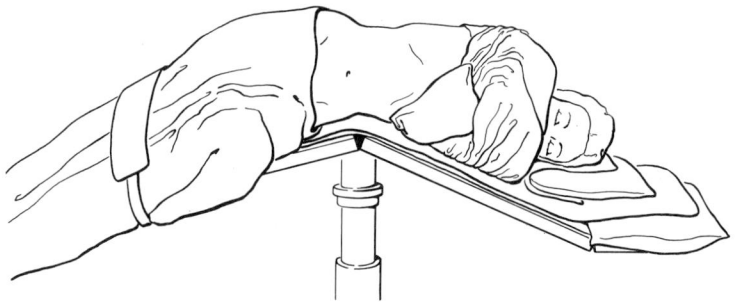

FIGURE 49

(2) The operative area must be adequately exposed.

(3) Circulation should not be obstructed by an awkward position or undue pressure on a part (Fig. 47).

(4) There should be no interference with the patient's respiration as a result of pressure of the arms on the chest or from constriction of a gown about the neck or the chest.

(5) Nerves must be protected from undue pressure. Improper positions of arms, hand, legs or feet may cause serious injury or paralysis. Shoulder braces must be well padded to prevent irreparable nerve injury, especially when the Trendelenburg position is necessary.

(6) Concern for the patient as an individual must be practiced, particularly with the very thin, the elderly or the obese.

Dorsal Recumbent Position. The usual position is flat on the back, with the arms at the side on the table, palms down (Fig. 48). This position is used for most abdominal operations, except for those upon the gallbladder and the pelvis, and for other operations as described below (Fig. 49A).

Trendelenburg Position. This position usually is employed for operations on the lower abdomen and the pelvis to obtain good exposure by displacing the intestines into the upper abdomen. In this position the head and the body are lowered, so that the plane of the body meets the horizontal at an angle. The knees are flexed by "breaking" the table, and the patient is held in position by padded shoulder braces (Fig. 49B).

Lithotomy Position. This is the position in which, with the patient on his back and under the influence of an anesthetic, the legs and the thighs are flexed to right angles. The position is maintained by placing the feet in stirrups. Nearly all perineal, rectal and vaginal operations require this posture (Fig. 49 C).

For kidney operations, the patient is placed on his well side in Sims's position with an air pillow 5 or 6 inches thick under the loin, or he is placed on a table with a kidney or back lift (Fig. 49 D).

For chest and abdominothoracic operations, the position varies with the operation to be performed. The surgeon and the anesthetist place the patient on the operating table in the proper position.

Operations on the neck, as for goiter, are performed with the patient on his back, the neck extended somewhat by a pillow beneath the shoulders.

Operations on the skull and the brain demand special positions and apparatus, these usually are adjusted by the surgeon in charge. Restraining straps are applied after the anesthetic is begun.

BIBLIOGRAPHY AND SUGGESTED READING

Adriani, J.: Local anesthetics, Am. J. Nursing **59**:86-88, Jan., 1959.

Breckenridge, F. J., and Bruno, P.: Nursing care of the anesthetized patient, Am. J. Nursing, **62**:74-78, July, 1962.

Catenacci, A. J., Anderson, J. D., and Boersma, D.: Anesthetic hazards of obesity, J.A.M.A. **175**:657-665, Feb. 25, 1961.

Dripps, R. D., Eckenhoff, J. E., and Vandam, L. D.: Introduction to Anesthesia, ed. 2, Philadelphia, Saunders, 1961.

Genereux, T. B.: Positioning patients in the operating room, Am. J. Nursing **59**:1572-1574, Nov., 1959.

Goodman, L. S., and Gilman, A.: The Pharmacological Basis of Therapeutics, ed. 2, Central Nervous System Depressants, pp. 20-323, New York, Macmillan, 1955.

Greisheimer, E. M.: The physiological effects of anesthesia, Am. J. Nursing **49**:337-343, 1949.

Hale, D. E. (ed.): Anesthesiology, by Forty American Authors, Philadelphia, Davis, 1955.

Hingson, R., Ross, E. F., and Costley, E. C.: A current analysis of the cost of anesthetic agents, Hosp. Topics **36**:104-107, Feb., 1958.

Jenkins, M. T., and Crasilneck, H. B.: Hypnoanesthesia, Am. J. Nursing **59**:958-961, July, 1959.

Murphree, H. B.: The use of potent analgesics, Am. J. Nurs. **63**:104-109, Sept., 1963.

Niazi, S. A., and Lewis, J. F.: Profound hypothermia in man, Ann. Surg. **147**:264-266, 1958.

Patient monitoring is more than just a dream, Am. J. Nursing **61**:60-61, Nov., 1961.

16

Operating Room Nursing

The student of nursing will enjoy her experience in the operating room because she will find the answers to many of the problems she has encountered in her care of surgical patients on the divisions. Only by observing, assisting with and understanding the experiences of the operative patient can the nurse interpret intelligently her own function in relation to each individual surgical patient. For the experience to be a satisfying one, the student must learn the principles involved in surgical asepsis as well as those related to the psychological and physical experiences of the patient.

Alexander* has expressed the significance of patient-centered care in the operating room as follows:

We would all agree that persons who enter our operating rooms as patients are very important people. We would agree that the people who care for patients are important. We know that good nursing care is given when all personnel carry out their prescribed tasks correctly, completely, and safely. We also know that optimum care requires expert assistance from the personnel in other departments in the hospital—the bacteriologist, the pathologist, the engineer, the nursing teams stationed in the units, the supply room, and the recovery room, as well as the educational leaders, the medical staff, and the administrators.

The gowned, masked personnel who hurry down the halls as they pass the worried patients, the many instruments lined row upon row on the numerous draped tables, the odor of disinfectants, the searching lamps, the buzzing saw, the placing of a patient on the operating table as if he were a contortionist—all are necessary in our operating room, but they should not push away the personal, gentle touch in caring for each patient. How the personnel accept their duties and work together influence and often determine how the patients accept their problems.

The nurse consciously uses her voice, her hands and her movements with gentleness because she knows that it is a manifestation of good nursing. She is aware that all activity in the operating room is carried out primarily and solely for the patient. *Whether he is conscious or anesthetized, the patient must be respected, protected and cared for as carefully as we would want those dearest to us to be treated.*

Other important objectives are:

To see and appreciate surgical problems as they affect the patient; to observe the skill necessary to correct these problems.

To understand and apply the principles of surgical asepsis in the clinical area where such technic is practiced in its fullest sense.

To learn to work effectively on a team in which every member is necessary and important, and the element of time is a precious one.

To recognize the value of emotional stability and mental alertness, particularly in a tense or emergency situation.

To appreciate the responsibility of the professional nurse in maintaining a well-organized unit and in practicing satisfactory interpersonal relations.

To appreciate the underlying safety measures which dictate the specific way in which technic is practiced, thus providing the safest possible care for the patient.

The development of the technical skill of operating room nursing is dependent upon much more than the perfect mechanical accomplish-

* Alexander, E.: Patient-centered care, Hospital Topics 33:75-76, Dec., 1955.

ment of certain actions. It is based on logical thought, evaluation of previous trials, and anticipatory thinking. It is rooted in a motivation of service, a keen desire to be helpful to patients in need of special surgical service, of which nursing is a part. The satisfaction which comes from giving good assistance through technical excellence may be compared to that gained from any nursing service. It will be increased or decreased in proportion to our appreciation of our fellow-man and his need for the services which we can give.*

TEAMWORK IN THE OPERATING ROOM

When a patient arrives in the operating room, essentially 4 different groups are preparing for their roles in his care. The first group is the anesthesiologist and his assistants who greet the patient, administer the anesthetic agent and place him in the proper position on the operating table. The second team is the nurses who prepare the operating room for the reception of the patient and assist throughout the operation. Such a nurse does not scrub but remains unsterile and often is referred to as the circulating nurse (unsterile nurse). The third group is the nurses who scrub, set up the sterile tables to include all the instruments, sponges, sutures, etc., that will be necessary for the particular operation, and this nurse is referred to as a "scrub" nurse (sterile nurse). The fourth group is the surgeon and his assistants who scrub and perform the operation. Auxiliary personnel, such as surgical technicians and licensed practical nurses, are being trained to take over some of the less exacting functions of the nursing group.

Regardless of the particular responsibilities of each worker, the concept of team work should be practiced. Every member of an operating room group must work together so that the corps of workers may function, not as individuals but as one unit, having one common interest—the welfare of the patient.

The responsibilities of everyone associated with the operating room should be outlined clearly. This avoids many errors and fixes

* Redmond, M.: Psychological Aspects of Operating Room Nursing, Workshop on Military Operating Room Nursing, 1956.

responsibility at all times. If lists enumerating the duties of each person are placed where all may see and read them, endless difficulties will be avoided. More work will be accomplished in a shorter length of time, one person will not wait for another to do some task if she knows it to be part of her own particular duties, and, if something has not been done or has been done improperly, the head nurse will be in a better position to handle the situation.

MAINTENANCE OF SURGICAL ASEPSIS

Principles Regarding Health and Operating Room Attire

Good health is essential for any professional person in the operating room. Colds, sore throats and infected fingers are a distinct menace and must be reported at once to the nurse in charge. A series of wound infections in postoperative patients was traced in one instance to a mild throat infection among operating room nurses. Therefore, it can be understood readily how very important it is for nurses to report any seemingly slight ailment without delay.

Wearing apparel must be clean. All clothing, including the headgear, should be changed daily. A mask requires changing much more frequently, certainly between operations, and oftener if necessary. Operating room dress should be worn on the operating floor only. Shoes used in the operating room should not be worn on the street.

The style of the clothing and the shoes should be plain. This will facilitate cleaning, allow ease in dressing and ensure the comfort of the wearer. For example, a turban or a headpiece which requires skill and practice to put on properly may be applied poorly by the novice, and the purpose for which it is intended is lost.

Garments and shoes must be safe.

1. *Headgear* should completely cover the hair so that single strands of hair or particles of dandruff or dust do not fall on sterile fields.

2. *Mask.* This is worn to minimize airborne contamination. The mask must do this effectively; in addition, it should leak no air, not interfere with breathing, be compact, comfortable, and not hinder speech or

vision. A disposable plastic mask is now available which has a filter that is held away from the nose and the mouth. Tests prove its superiority over gauze masks. Forced expiration, such as that produced by talking, laughing, sneezing and coughing, should be avoided, since it deposits organisms on the masks.* To increase filtering efficiency, gauze masks should be laundered before use.

3. *Conductive Shoes.* Shoes with rubber soles are nonconductors of electricity, and there is danger of generation of static electricity under such conditions. Static electricity may ignite anesthetic gases to produce explosions in the operating room. Shoes with conductive soles or conductive slip-ons produce a grounding of the wearer which avoids the generation of static electricity and so removes the danger from this source. Soles must be conductive and should be cleaned after each wearing to remove bacteria lodged in blood stains and dirt, which tend to insulate the bottom of the shoe. Shoes can be tested for conductivity by using an insulation tester. In the absence of conductive shoes, conductive slip-ons or booties may be worn.

4. *Clothing.* Cotton clothing must be worn in the operating room. Wool, nylon, rayon, sharkskin, Orlon, Dacron, celanese and cellulose acetate are potential sources of hazard because the rate of static build-up is so rapid with these materials that sparking is hard to control with certainty. It is acceptable to wear nylon or other synthetic undergarments if the whole garment is in contact with the skin. A nylon slip is not acceptable; the bodice of the slip qualifies, but the free-hanging skirt is dangerous.

Principles of Surgical Asepsis

Ways and means of making an article sterile have been discussed in Chapter 4, "Antisepsis and Asepsis." Following the sterilization process, the responsibility of the operating room personnel is to maintain asepsis by practicing a well-defined technic or procedure based on sound principles.

---

* "Silence is more valuable than masking in reducing wound contamination during surgical procedures, according to a study made on the sources of wound infection in the Boston City Hospital. 'The tongue is only three inches long, but it can kill a man six feet tall.'" From Byrne, J. J., and Okeke, N. E.: Silence: a valuable control for surgical wound infection, Am. J. Surg. 94:398, 1957.

Conscientiousness, alertness and honesty are personal qualifications necessary to execute these principles. The facing outline will serve to emphasize the principle involved, what is implied and how the nurse can apply the principle concerned.

TECHNIC OF SCRUBBING, PUTTING ON GOWN AND GLOVES

Scrubbing

Preoperative skin disinfection is done to remove from the hands and the arms as much dirt, fats, transient and resident bacterial flora as is possible. During an operation, should a glove become torn, the possibility of introducing organisms into the wound is lessened provided that a satisfactory preoperative scrub has been done. The normal bacteria on a person's skin vary in different parts of the body. On smooth surfaces, they may be few, whereas, in protected areas, such as creases, there may be many.

Immediately before scrubbing, the headgear can be adjusted and the mask tied so that the nose and the mouth are completely covered. For those who wear glasses, an effective method of preventing foggy glasses ("steaming up") is to rub them with a piece of soap and then wipe them clean. At the scrub sink, the water is adjusted to the proper temperature and flow.

The kind of surgical scrub (which consists of mechanical cleansing of the hands and the arms that may be followed by immersion in a chemical disinfectant) depends on the needs of the individual scrubbing. Naturally, one who contacts soil more frequently, such as an individual with an avocation of gardening, needs a longer period for scrubbing. Likewise, one who scrubs less frequently, such as once every 3 or 4 days, will need a longer scrub than the person who scrubs daily. Whatever the procedure, and there are several, certain principles must be observed:

1. The nails should be kept short; special attention must be given to the subungual space with a sterile stainless steel nail file early in the scrub.

2. Use a soft but firm bristled brush. Nylon brushes for scrubbing are most durable. After each person's use, they are terminally sterilized by autoclaving for 30 minutes at 250° F.

OUTLINE OF PRINCIPLES AND APPLICATIONS

Principle	Implication	Guides to Action
An article which is sterile remains so until it is contaminated.	A package of sterile dressings on a shelf will remain sterile unless organisms are introduced.	Keep closets clean and free from vermin, dust and so forth.
A sterile area or field can become contaminated:		
1. By becoming wet if the underlying area is unsterile.	A sterile drape on a table can become wet from splashing water or fluid dropped from a container of surgical gut.	Place a sterile drape of moisture-proof polyvinyl over the table or the operative field before placing sterile drapes. Drop articles wet with a germicide (such as ampules, cystoscope) onto a sterile metal tray in which a sterile towel is placed to absorb moisture. Dry thoroughly all wrapped packages after sterilization to prevent moisture from condensation when the packages come in contact with a cold surface.
2. By dropping anything unsterile onto a sterile field.	Powder falling from surgically clean hands prior to donning sterile gloves. An unsterile arm reaching over a sterile field.	Avoid powdering hands over a sterile field. Avoid reaching over a sterile field (1) to drop a sterile object or (2) to reposition the overhead light.
3. By infectious or soiled materials from a wound.	*B. coli* and other organisms are present in the gastrointestinal tract. Pathogenic organisms are present in an abscess.	Limit the contaminated field to as small an area as is practical. As soon as surgery has been completed in this area, remove all contaminated linens, dressings, instruments and gloves. Reestablish a sterile area with sterile replacements.
4. From airborne sources, since air currents are capable of transporting contaminants.	Dust, human expirations from the nose and the throat, and thrown soiled sponges are possible sources.	Anyone with a respiratory infection should not be near a sterile field. The nose and the mouth must be covered with an effective mask; clearing the throat, unnecessary speaking, etc., should be at a minimum. Excessive traffic should be forbidden. Floors must be damp mopped with an effective detergent-germicide. Clean garments and shoes should be worn by all O.R. personnel.
A sterile area (field) remains sterile even when sterile articles are added to it.	A sterile article may be moved to another sterile area by 1. The use of a sterile gloved hand 2. The use of sterile-tipped transfer forceps 3. Being dropped onto it, such as dressings or a knife blade.	Sterile gloved hands must remain within constant view of their owner; hence it is desirable to keep hands at or above the waistline. See p. 246. Handling of sterile transfer forceps. See pp. 245 and 247. Opening a sterile pack or package.

Over and above these principles, many policies or procedures need to be reviewed to emphasize the many activities that are related to the successful practice of aseptic technic. The most important of these procedures are the following:

Keep sterile areas in view to prevent accidental contamination.

APPLICATION

STERILE AREAS	UNSTERILE AREAS
Top of a sterile drape	Sides and back of a sterile draped table (A suture or a ligature hanging over the edge of a table is considered unsterile.)
Above the anterior waist and anterior aspect of sleeves of a sterile gown	Back of sleeves of sterile gown Below waist of sterile gown Under arm of sterile gown Collar area and back of sterile gown
Sterile gloved hands resting on a sterile drape or kept within the individual's view, always above the waist	Sterile gloved hands on the waist at the side or below the waist
A table, draped from front to back, which permits full view of the sterile area	Draping a table from back to front is awkward, and all parts of the top side of the drape may not be visible.
Innermost side of a wrapper or cap that encloses a sterile article	Edge of wrapper on a sterile package or edge of cap on a sterile flask or tube

"Scrubbed" persons keep away from unsterile areas; circulating personnel keep away from sterile areas.

APPLICATION

"SCRUBBED" PERSONS	CIRCULATING PERSONS
1. Stand a safe distance from operating table while patient is being draped.	1. Face sterile areas or scrubbed persons to prevent accidental contact.
2. Face sterile areas when passing them.	
3. Turn back toward circulating persons or unsterile areas.	
4. Keep hand dips and sterile table at a safe distance from operating area so that one's back will not touch them.	
5. Never squeeze through a narrow space; rather, ask the "unsterile" person to move, or ask someone to move unsterile equipment.	

3. Use an antiseptic detergent for scrubbing such as pHisoderm containing hexachlorophene.* This has been proved to provide greater cleansing power, and it remains persistently bacteriostatic for hours and even days.

* pHisoderm is a sudsing emollient skin detergent which cleans rapidly and thoroughly. When 3% hexachlorophene, G-11 (a phenol derivative) is combined with pHisoderm, a powerful antiseptic is formed ("pHisoHex" Winthrop-Stearns). By adsorption and retention, a film encases the hands and the arms, thereby resisting bacteria. Experiments have shown that the film remains for some time, exerting prolonged antibacterial activity. Only a

4. Lather well and rinse frequently. No chemical agent can be relied upon as a substitute for conscientious mechanical cleansing of the skin.

5. The duration of the scrub may be determined by a time limit set on the conscientious scrubbing of one part after another in a prescribed manner, or it may be determined by a certain number of strokes per part. A practical, reliable and intelligent

small amount is necessary for a scrub. It is nonirritating and nontoxic, since it has the same pH as skin; it is hypoallergenic and can be used on mucous membranes.

procedure should be followed. A common practice is to scrub for 10 minutes at the beginning of the operating day and 3 minutes between operations. This is usually set up in each hospital by a committee on aseptic procedure.

Aids in determining the "kind" of scrub procedure to follow are these: (A) Take the scrubbing test in which 10 per cent lampblack mixed with salad oil is rubbed into the hands and the forearms. The student is blindfolded, provided with soap, brush and running water and is instructed to scrub until he thinks his hands are clean. The results can serve as a guide.* (B) Review pertinent literature.†

6. Following the scrub, rinse hands and arms thoroughly, discard soap, and turn off water, using the elbow or knee.

7. Immerse hands and arms for 1 minute in 1:1,000 aqueous Zephiran or in 70 per cent isopropyl alcohol containing hexachlorophene. (Many surgeons prefer to omit the rinsing of hands and arms with an antiseptic solution. Instead, they advocate that on completion of the scrub, simply dry the hands and the arms with a sterile towel, leaving a film of antiseptic detergent in order that it continue its effective action.)

Gowning and Gloving

After scrubbing and disinfecting the hands and the arms, a sterile gown and gloves are put on. These are worn to allow the wearer to participate in the surgical operation while maintaining a state of asepsis in as practical a way as is possible. The sterile gown may be obtained from an open pack, or it may be handed by someone already scrubbed. Since gowns are folded inside out to facilitate donning without touching the outside, the scrubbed person will hold the neckband and

gently let the gown unfold from his extended hands. As the gown unfolds, the armholes should face the wearer. Slip the hands into the armholes and hold the hands upward.

The circulating nurse can assist by reaching inside the gown and pulling the sleeves over the hands on the scrubbed person (Fig. 50). Tapes at the back are tied. If the gown has tapes at the waist, the circulating nurse reaches for the ends of them without touching the gown, draws them back and ties them. Surgeons usually prefer to have their gowns tied loosely, whereas nurses often want the gown tied more snugly.

NOTE: A gown is sterile only as long as it is dry. If it is wet from perspiration or in any other way, it must be considered as being contaminated.

A surgeon was dressed in a sterile manner, wearing the usual operating room suit, cap, mask, gown and gloves. A culture was taken by a moist swab from the front of his gown. The surgeon then washed his hands in the usual basin of sterile saline, splashing his gown in so doing. Another culture was taken in a similar manner from the moist area of his gown within a matter of a few seconds. The first culture was sterile while the second was replete with bacteria.‡

In the entire procedure of putting on sterile gloves, one principle must be followed; the surgically clean hand may touch the inside of the glove only; should it touch the outside, the glove must be considered as being contaminated and must be discarded. Glove lubricant that is available in individual containers minimizes the spread of dust particles. Its purpose is to lubricate the hands so that they will glide more easily into the gloves.

It has been proved that talcum powder in a wound may cause adhesions and granulomas which result from both a chemical irritation and a foreign body reaction. Therefore, talcum has largely been replaced by starch. However, powder contamination of the operative field must still be minimized, since any powder is a foreign body. This can be done by: (1) keeping air contamination to a minimum and (2) thorough wash-

* See Lilienthal, H., and Ziegler, J.: A study in the disinfection of hands, Ann. Surg. 83:831-836, 1926.

† Caswell, H. T., et al.: Bacteriologic and clinical experiences and the methods of control of hospital infections due to antibiotic resistant staphylococci, Surg., Gynec. & Obst. 106:1-10, 1958.
Walter, C. W.: Scrubbing for surgery, Am. J. Nursing 52:188-189, 1952.
Walter, C. W.: Preoperative skin preparation, Hosp. Topics 55:74-79, Sept., 1955.

‡ Beck, W. C., and Collette, T. S.: False faith in the surgeon's gown and surgical drape, Am. J. Surg. 83:125, 1952.

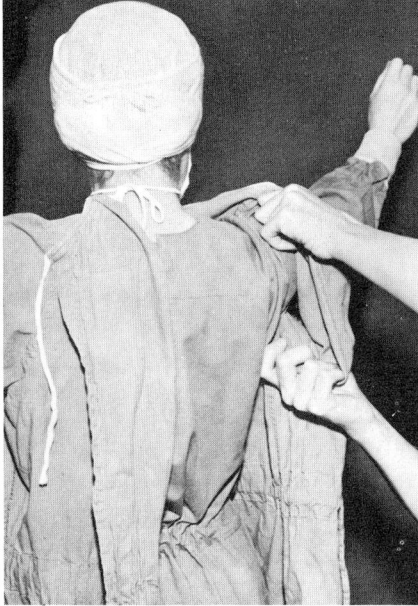

FIG. 50. Method of putting on sterile gown. The unsterile nurse at the back of the scrub nurse or doctor grasps the axillary seam from within the gown. By pulling on this seam toward the chest wall, the sleeve is drawn easily over the damp hand to its proper position.

ing of the gloves to make them as free of powder as possible.

Corn starch, with a dispersal agent such as 2 per cent magnesium oxide or 3 per cent magnesium carbonate, appears to be the best glove lubricant at present.*

Bio-Sorb Cream (Johnson and Johnson) is satisfactory for lubricating the hands.

* For more detailed investigation, read (1) Lee, C. M., Jr., Collins, W. T., and Largen, T. L.: A reappraisal of absorbable glove powder, Surg. Gynec. & Obst. 95:725-737, 1952 and (2) Karlin, S.: Unnecessary contamination from glove powder, Hosp. Topics 35:100-101, 1957.

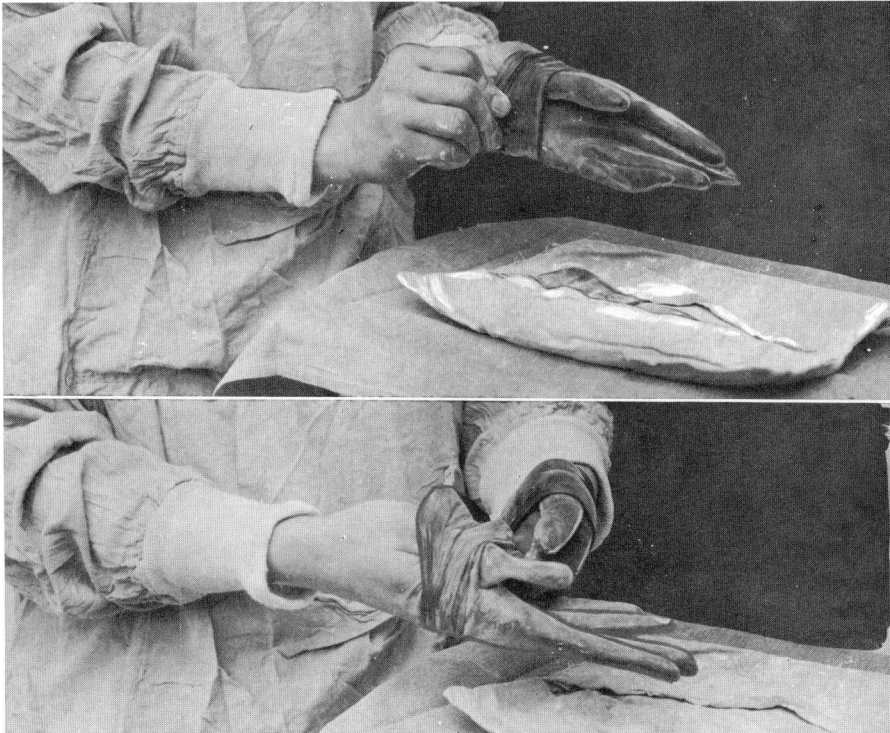

FIG. 51. (*Top*) Pulling on left glove without touching outside. (*Bottom*) Pulling on right glove by inserting gloved fingers into cuff.

Steps in Putting on Sterile Gloves

1. The turned-back cuff of the left glove should be grasped with the right hand in putting on the left glove.

2. The gloved fingers of the left hand should then be placed inside the turned-back cuff of the right glove; slip the right hand into the glove.

3. When both hands are gloved, the gown cuff should be folded snugly at the wrist and the glove cuff pulled up over it.

Getting sterile gloves on over hands and gown cuff without contaminating them has never been accepted as completely foolproof. The area of hazard is the inner cuff, which makes contact with skin surfaces. If the glove is donned carefully and the cuff does not roll down or the gown sleeve pull out because of excessive reaching, the conventional procedure is acceptable. However, Brooks and Rockwell* have presented a

* Brooks, H. L., and Rockwell, V. T.: Simple procedures for processing, donning surgical rubber gloves, OR Nursing 2:41-54, July-Aug., 1961.

"closed gloving method," which attempts to eliminate the hazard explained above. They describe the putting on of sterile gown and gloves as follows:

Slide hands in sleeves only as far as the sleeve-cuff seam. Grasp the inside of sleeve-cuff seam with thumb and index finger. After the gown is tied and pulled down by the unsterile circulating nurse, pick up a glove with one sleeve-covered hand and place it, thumb down, on the palm side of the other arm with glove fingers pointing toward the shoulder (Fig. 53, *top, left*).

Grasp the wrist edge of the glove that is against the sleeve with the fingers that hold the seam, and grasp the uppermost glove wrist edge with the sleeve-covered fingers of the other hand (Fig. 53, *top, right*).

Pull the glove wrist over the gown cuff, using care not to fold the gown cuff back or to expose the fingers inside it (Fig. 53, *bottom, left*).

With the other sleeve-covered hand, grasp both glove and gown cuffs and pull glove on (Fig. 53, *bottom, right*). Put the second

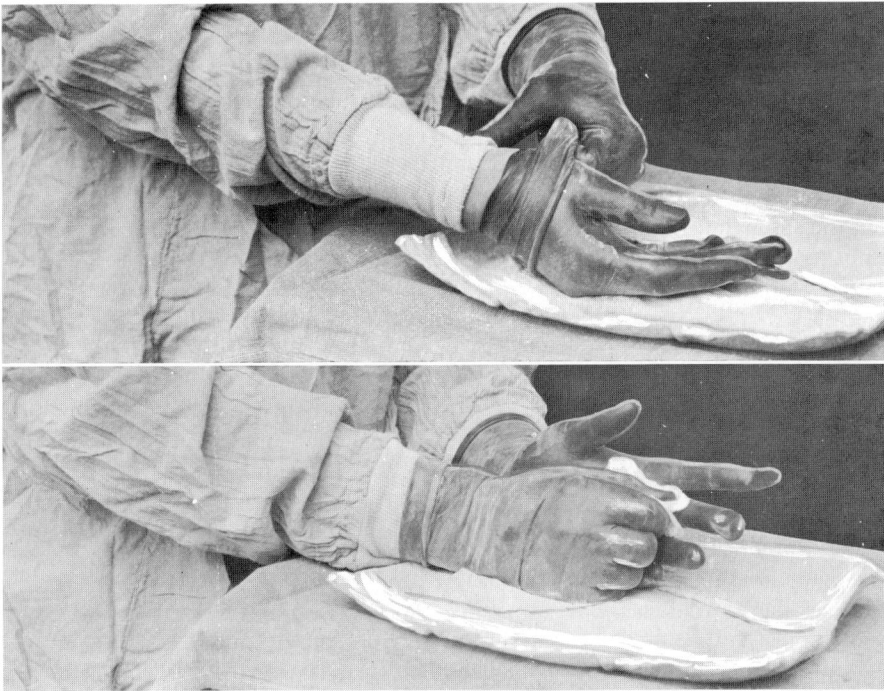

Fig. 52. (*Top*) Folding glove cuff over gown cuff. (*Bottom*) Working on glove fingers with sterile gauze.

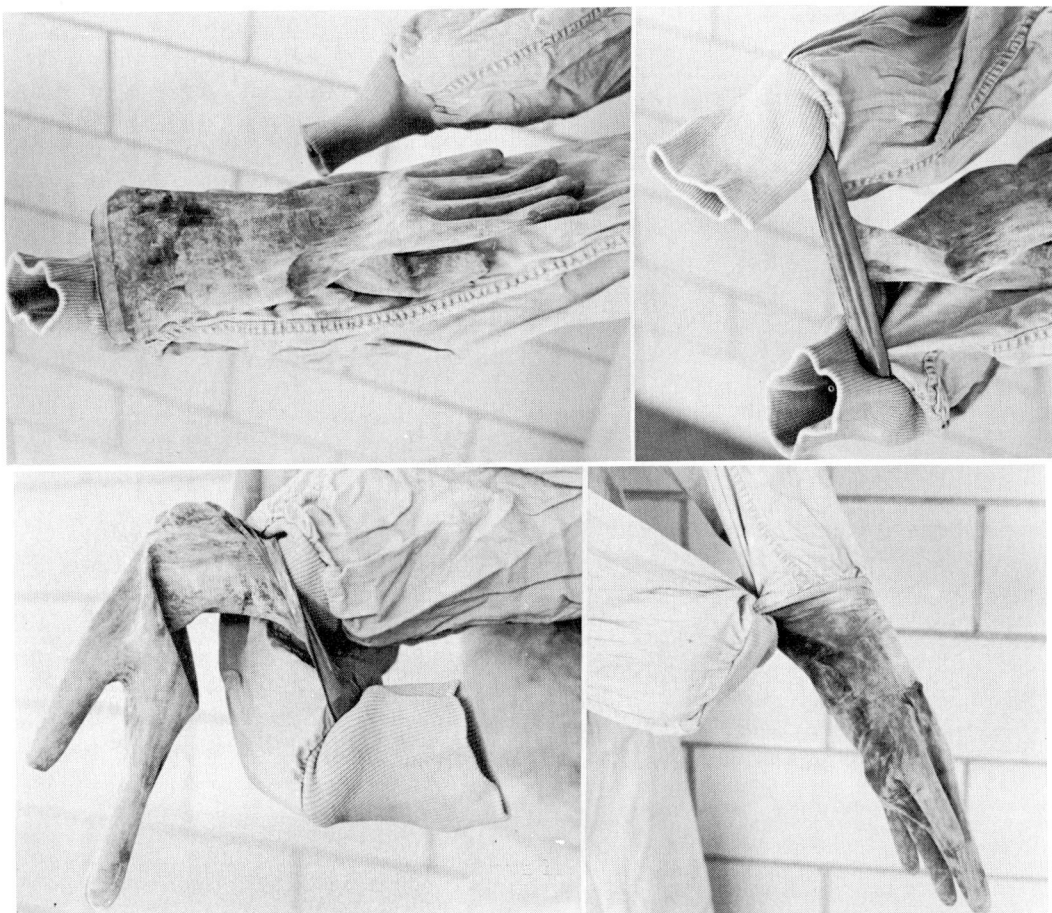

FIGURE 53. (From Hospital Topics)

glove on in the same manner, using the newly gloved hand to hold the glove.

Offering the Gown and the Gloves to the Surgeon

Many hospitals follow the procedure whereby the scrub nurse holds the sterile gown and gloves for the surgeon in such a way that he is able to get into them easily. In this procedure, the following steps are followed:

1. The scrub nurse shakes out the gown at arm's length, holding it at the neckband. The outside of the gown faces her.

2. By making a cuff, using the neck area of the gown, the scrub nurse can protect her gloved hands underneath this cuff.

3. She offers the inside of the gown to the surgeon. (The circulating nurse pulls the gown on and ties it.)

4. Pour lubricant into his hands.

5. Hold the right glove with fingers on the inside of turned-back cuff (Fig. 54). Hold the palm of the glove toward the surgeon. Stretch the cuff to allow him to introduce his hand. Keep thumbs outward to avoid touching his hand.

6. The surgeon makes a fold on the cuff of his gown and keeps it in position as he inserts his hand into the glove.

7. The nurse unfolds the turned-back cuff of the glove to cover the gown cuff.

SURGICAL DRAPING

Surgical draping is a procedure whereby an unsterile field is covered with a sheet (or sheets) made of linen*, plastic or specially prepared waterproof paper. The areas to be

* The term "linen" is used broadly to indicate a woven cloth.

FIG. 54. (*Top*) Method of holding gloves for surgeon. Fingers of both hands are placed on inside of turned-back cuff (the outside of the glove), thumb up. Cuff then is stretched slightly to allow surgeon's hand to slip in freely. (*Bottom*) Holding gloves for surgeon. Surgeon has inserted hand into glove with quick thrust, nurse is pulling cuff of glove over surgeon's sleeve.

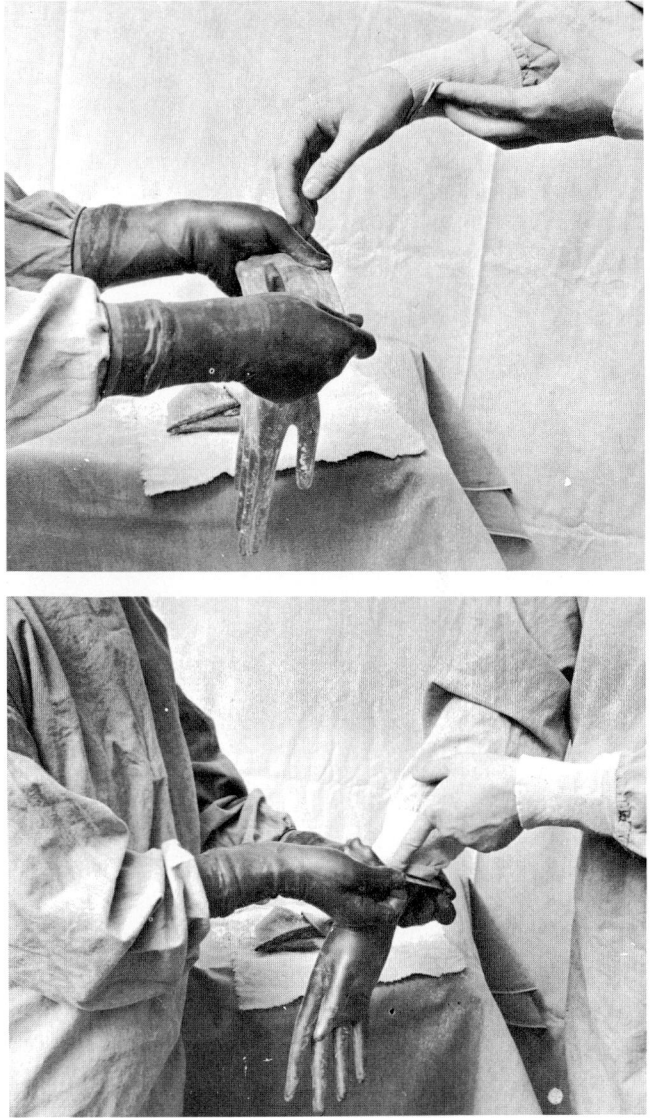

draped are the patient, the instrument tables and the hand-dip stands.

Regardless of the kind of material from which the drape is made, the principles of sterilization and handling remain the same.

Folding of Drapes or Sheets

The manner in which sheets or drapes are folded before sterilization is determined by

1. Its use following sterilization

Every sterile drape is used to provide a sterile area. The underside is not kept sterile, since it comes in contact with an unsterile surface. To facilitate handling and the keeping of one side sterile, the use of a cuff, a turned down corner, fanfolding or rolling is advisable in the folding process. With these kinds of folds, the draper can safely grasp the drape and protect her sterile gloved hands and the upper outer surface of the sheet from contamination.

2. The ease with which steam can penetrate the layers during the process of sterilization

Imagine a sheet of polyvinyl plastic material which is folded like a man's handkerchief; it is obvious that steam would not enter the innermost parts of the sheet.

After preparation of the patient and application of sterile drapes, a waterproof cover

Guide for Handling of Drapes

ACTIVITY	PRINCIPLE
1. Handle drapes as little as possible. Avoid shaking and flourishing of linens.	Air currents are capable of carrying contaminants.
2. Making a cuff or turning the corners of the drape over the gloved hand will afford protection as the sterile person places the drape in position.	Contact with an unsterile surface contaminates a sterile object.
3. A scrubbed person places drapes on a table or a patient in such a way that the side closest to her is covered first.	Contact with an unsterile surface contaminates a sterile object.
4. That part of the drape which falls below the top level of the table is considered unsafe as a sterile area.	When a question exists regarding sterility, the object (or field) is considered as being unsterile.
5. Drapes that have holes, tears or worn spots should not be used.	A portal of entry which allows contact with an unsterile surface immediately renders an otherwise sterile field contaminated.
6. Drapes should not be held so high that they touch the lights or so low that they touch the floor.	Contact with an unsterile surface contaminates a sterile object.

of plastic material may be used to cover the lower part of the patient. The purpose of this is to prevent contamination by dampness from penetrating the sterile covers to the unsterile area below. Many surgeons prefer to cover the waterproof material with a wet towel. This prevents instruments from slipping, even where the area is not flat. This towel can be changed if it becomes soiled. Waterproof plastic surgical drapes are available commercially.* They are sterile, with an aperture covered with adhesive which seals off and demarcates the operative site. Such a drape remains in position without slipping.

HANDLING OF STERILE EQUIPMENT BY THE CIRCULATING NURSE

To supply the sterile nurse with the necessary articles for an operation, the circulating nurse must know how to handle sterile materials safely. The most common activities are:

1. To use a sterile transfer forceps
2. To open a sterile package
3. To remove a lid from a sterile jar or container
4. To pour sterile solutions

The use of a transfer forceps and the

* Scotch Surgical Drapes are made by Minnesota Mining and Manufacturing Co., St. Paul, Minnesota.

removal of a lid from a sterile container imply that stock materials are used on individual setups. It is preferred that all materials for use on a particular patient be packaged individually, thereby eliminating a stock source of supplies and the transfer forceps. The chief reason for this procedure is to eliminate potential sources of contamination through faulty handling.

Each of the above activities will be described in detail.

Use of Transfer or Pick-Up Forceps

One of the most common methods of transferring a sterile object from one place to another is by means of a sterile transfer forceps. Such a forceps and its container are first sterilized (a single forceps for each container); then a germicide is added to the container, and the forceps is placed so that the prongs or the legs are immersed. Thereafter, only that end of the forceps which is in the germicide is considered as being sterile. The activities and the principles involved in the safe handling of these forceps are as shown on page 246.

Caution: Do not use transfer forceps to pick up anything with an adhering base, such as petroleum gauze. Should this occur, clean and resterilize the forceps; otherwise, anything picked up by the forceps will adhere to it.

The forceps illustrated in Figure 55 automatically eliminates many of the possible sources of contamination and is highly recommended. The pistol-like grip permits comfortable handling; the bend in the instrument eliminates the need for consciously keeping the prongs pointed downward; and the type of prong permits the grasping of circular objects as well as fine surgical needles. The collar serves as a cap for the germicide container, thereby controlling unnecessary evaporation. A springlike guard within the container eliminates the problem of having the forceps touch the side above the solution level.

Opening a Sterile Package

This may be done by placing the package on a table and undoing the wrapper in such a way that only the outside cover is touched by the circulating nurse. Or she may hold the package in her left hand and unwrap with the right hand (Figs. 56 and 57).

The scrub nurse may take the offered package, or it may be dropped safely on a sterile field. The loose ends of the wrapper must be drawn back and away from the inner sterile package and the sterile field. The arm and the hand of the circulating nurse must not reach over the sterile field.

Handling a Sterile Covered Container

The hazards of using sterile covered containers must be understood. Each time the lid is removed there is a possibility of airborne contamination; hence, unnecessary or prolonged removal of the lid should be avoided. When several persons use a common container, the risk of contamination exists. To minimize these problems, each person using such a container must be thoroughly familiar with the handling of it. (See Guide, p. 246.)

Pouring Sterile Solutions

Sterile flasks or pitchers are covered with a top which fits over the outer edge of the flask or bottle. To remove the cap, touch

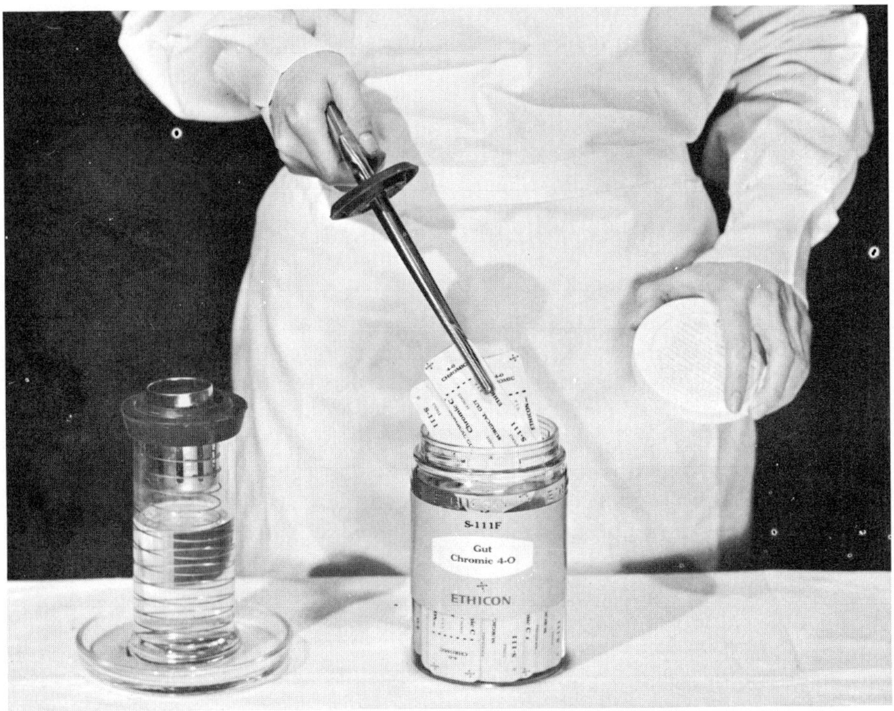

FIG. 55. By using a safe transfer forceps, the operating room nurse is able to remove several foil packets of surgical gut at one time. (Ethicon, Inc., Somerville, N. J.)

Guide for Handling of Forceps

ACTIVITY	PRINCIPLE
When withdrawing the forceps from the germicide container, do not allow the forceps to touch the side or the top of the container.	A sterile object becomes contaminated when it touches an unsterile area. (The area not covered with germicide solution cannot be considered sterile.)
Keep the forceps blades pointed downward at all times. If this is not done, germicide solution will flow toward the unsterile handle. When the forceps are returned to the correct position, the blades become contaminated.	Gravity pulls liquids downward.
When using the forceps, keep them within view at the level of the waistline or above it.	A sterile object or area remains sterile unless it is contaminated. (A possibility of contamination exists when a sterile object is out of view.)
Drop the sterile article gently on the sterile field; the forceps must not touch the field.	After an operation has begun, the sterile set-up is sterile for that patient alone; should a sterile transfer forceps touch such a field, it is no longer sterile for any other field.

Guide for Handling of Sterile Covered Container

ACTIVITY	PRINCIPLE
Remove the lid only when necessary and replace it as soon as possible.	The possibility of airborne contamination exists.
In removing the lid, hold it in such a way that the sterile undersurface faces downward.	Because of gravity, dust particles, etc., fall downward.
If it is necessary to set the lid down, the sterile undersurface faces upward.	Contact with an unsterile surface contaminates a sterile object.
The rims of the lids and the container are considered as being unsterile.	(Proximity to unsterile surfaces makes the rim of the lid and container a doubtful area.) When sterility is doubted, consider the object (or field) as being contaminated.
Unused sterile objects are not to be returned to the sterile container.	Air currents are capable of carrying contaminants.

---

only the top outer surface and avoid touching the edge. If the flask or the bottle has a pouring lip, such as the "Pour-o-vac," sterile fluids can be dispensed safely.

They can be resealed and opened repeatedly without danger of contamination. When used carefully, the paper flask hood also provides a safe means of transferring sterile fluid to the operative field. The traditional technic of pouring a quantity of fluid over the lip is sloppy and bacteriologically ineffectual.*

When pouring solutions, the flask or the

pitcher must be held high enough so that the unsterile outside of the container or the hand of the pourer will not touch the receiving sterile basin. On the other hand, it should not be held so high that the solution will splash. When the flask is too warm to handle, special tongs are available to grasp the flask safely.

PREPARATION OF TABLES FOR THE OPERATION

At this point the circulating nurse and the scrub nurse work together as a team to set up the various tables needed for a particular operation.

* Walter, C.: Aseptic Treatment of Wounds, p. 219, New York, Macmillan, 1948.

Laparotomy Pack. The circulating nurse unwraps the outer cover of the laparotomy pack. This contains gowns, hand towels and drapes for the doctor's instrument table, the Mayo stand and the patient—plus extra towels. What is included is a matter of preference; however, the significant points to remember are (1) to keep the size consistent with proper sterilization qualifications, (2) to arrange materials in the order of their use,

(3) to place the pack in a certain position on the table so that when the pack is opened the articles will not need to be moved but can be used where they are and (4) to use the double thickness covers as drapes for the nurse's table.

Basin Set. This usually contains the hand-dip basins, a basin for saline for sponges, a basin for the specimen, one for discarded sponges, a container with a towel

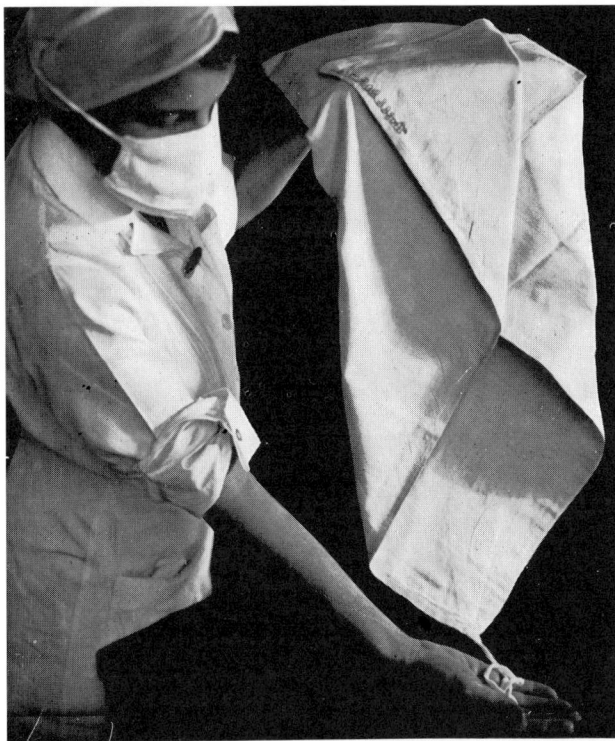

Fig. 56. (*Top*) The first step is unwrapping the package.

Fig. 57. (*Bottom*) The package completely unwrapped and ready to hand to a sterile nurse or to place on a sterile table.

(The Surgical Supervisor, American Sterilizer Co., Erie, Pa.)

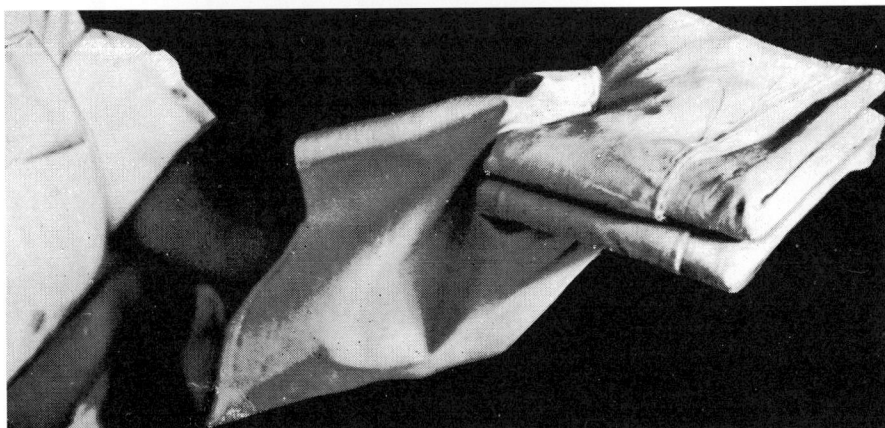

in which to break suture tubes if glass tubes are used and containers and sponges for the skin preparation of the patient (unless this is set up as a special unit).

Gowns and Gloves. This consists of a package of sterile gowns and a package of sterile gloves for the surgeon and his assistants.

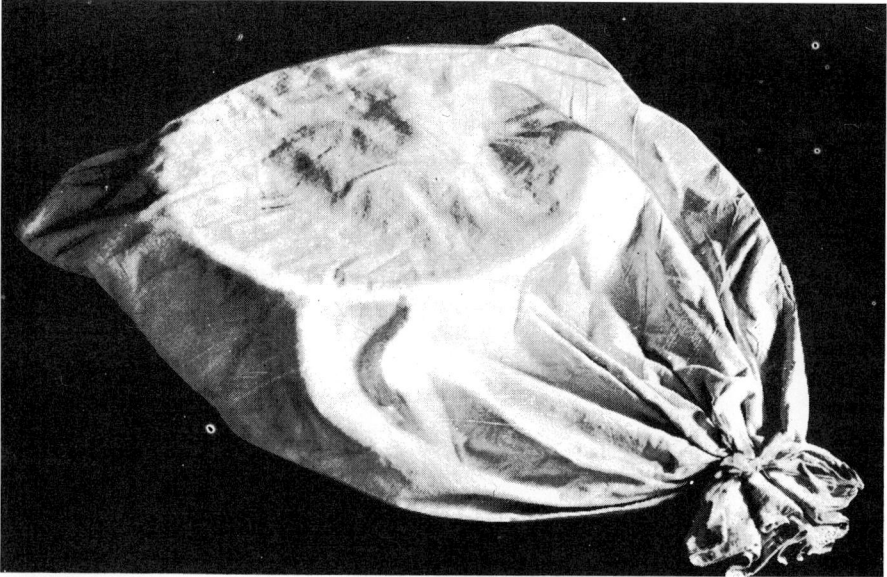

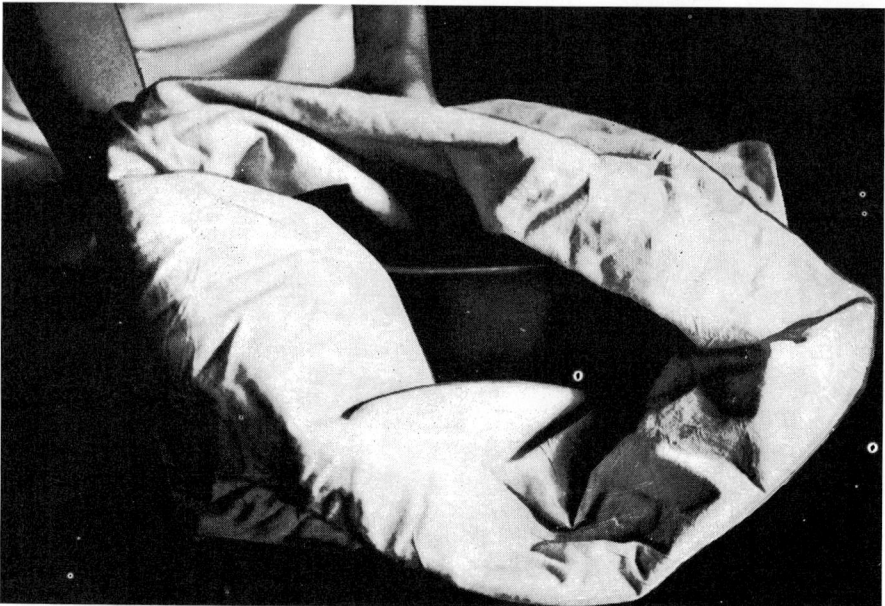

FIG. 58. (*Top*) A basin set enclosed in a bag.
FIG. 59. (*Bottom*) Suggesting the first step in removing the bag in the surgery. The open edge is held away from the individual. A cuff is turned back along the entire surface of the bag. The left hand holds the set while the right hand peels the bag away from the set over the left arm. (The Surgical Supervisor, American Sterilizer Co., Erie, Pa.)

After the tables are draped, the circulating nurse provides the following additional supplies: Knife blades (Figs. 61-63), suture materials (Figs. 64-67), instruments, solutions, and any additional supplies.

LIGATURES AND SUTURES

After the instruments are placed (according to the prescribed pattern in the local hospital), the "scrubbed" nurse will select and prepare ligatures and sutures according to the needs of the operation and the preference of the surgeon.*

Generally, a *ligature* (a tie) is a free piece of suture material, not threaded on a needle, and of considerable length (10 to 18 in.) or on a spool, for the purpose of tying blood vessels that have previously been clamped with an artery forceps. Spiral-wound suture

* Types of suture materials are discussed on pages 263-267.

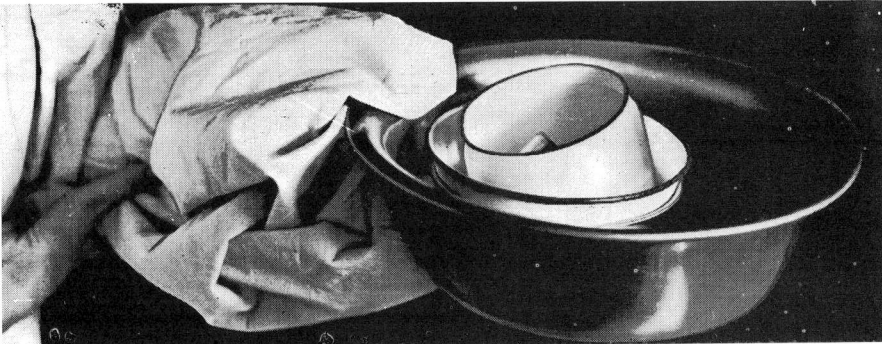

FIG. 60. The basin set is ready to hand to the sterile nurse or to place on a sterile table. (The Surgical Supervisor, American Sterilizer Co., Erie, Pa.)

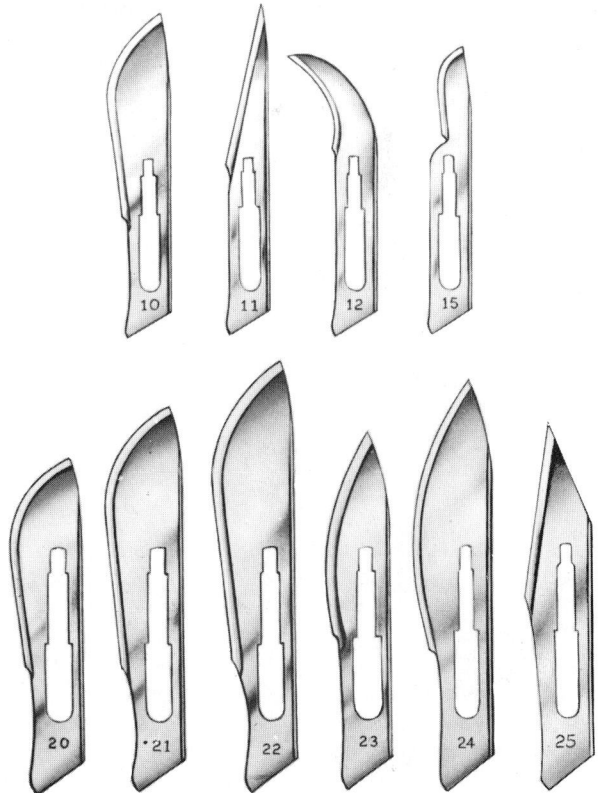

FIG. 61. The most common kinds of knife blades. (Bard-Parker Co., Danbury, Conn.)

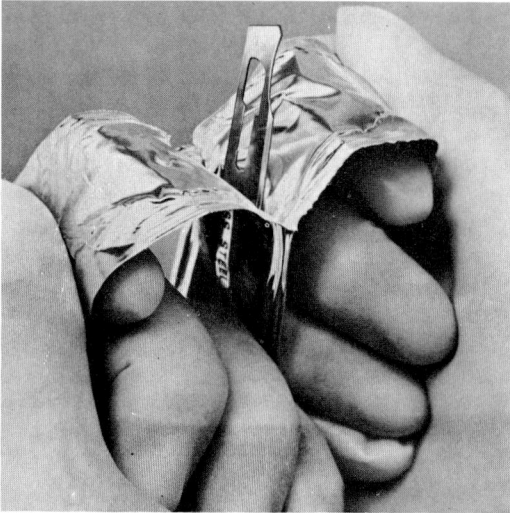

FIG. 62. Unopened packets of individually wrapped knife blades are put in the instrument pack and autoclaved with them. The scrub nurse opens the packet by pulling two tabs which expose the sterile blade for use. (A-S-R Products Corporation)

tissue, for checking the flow of blood, fastening drainage tubes in position, etc. Sutures are either *interrupted,* each stitch tied separately, or *continuous,* the thread running in a series of stitches, only the first and last of which are tied. The length of sutures naturally varies considerably. Each depends on the character of the work and the nature of the operation. Deep work, in the pelvis for instance, requires a much longer suture than would be necessary in suturing in an area closer to the surface of a wound. Experience and judgment, along with the desire of the surgeon, must be the determining factors in details of sutures and ligatures.

Testing of suture material is usually unnecessary if it is purchased from reliable firms who gauge and test for tensile strength. However, if testing is undertaken, it must be done carefully. A length of suture material is tested by holding the ends in each hand and exerting a firm, steady pull. Any jerking will weaken it considerably (Fig. 65). It is injurious to handle suture material any more than is absolutely necessary, such as constantly drawing it through the fingers, etc. Catgut sutures which have been folded in glass tubes are kinked and inconvenient to use. By a brief dip in sterile saline and gentle stretching, these kinks are easily removed by the suture nurse before the suture is handed to the surgeon. This is especially important in

material is available and is more convenient to use than a suture wound on a reel.

A *suture,* on the other hand, is a catgut, silk, cotton or metal thread, 18 or more inches long threaded on a needle and is used for sewing or suturing together the edges and the surfaces of

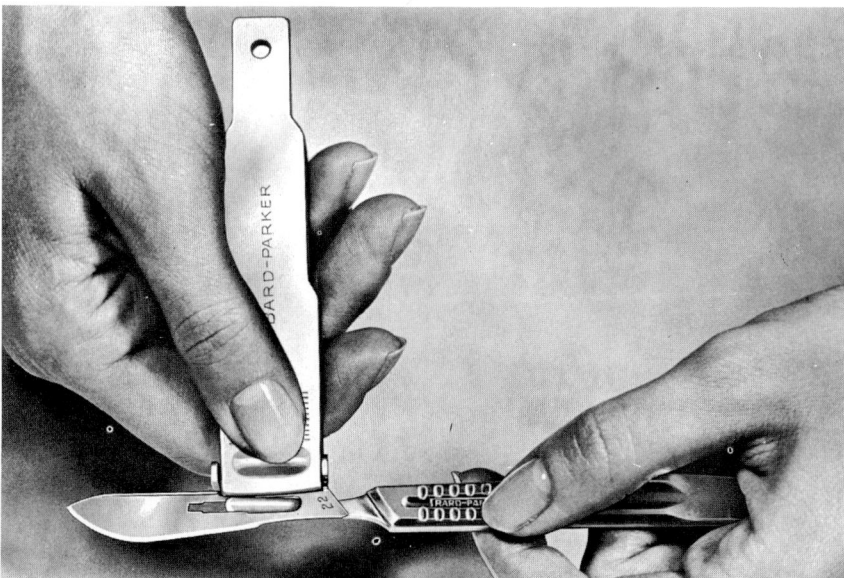

FIG. 63. Attaching or removing a knife blade can be done safely by using an instrument especially designed for this task. Under aseptic conditions sterile rubber gloves would be worn. (Bard-Parker Co., Danbury, Conn.)

heavier types of surgical gut sutures. Prolonged soaking should be avoided because it makes the gut rubbery and reduces its tensile strength. Surgical gut tubes should not be broken until the "scrubbed" nurse is ready to prepare her sutures. When breaking glass suture tubes, a sterile cover is wrapped around the filled tube and broken in a prescribed manner (Fig. 64). The foil packet is notched for easy tearing.

When a suture is being used (Figs. 66-68), a duplicate should be kept in reserve. The end of a suture never should be wrapped around a needle holder nor should it be dragged over the instruments or drapings. A needle which has been used should be replaced in the holder as soon as the surgeon lays it down. Constant checking to see that all needles are accounted for is necessary. Suture material which is cut on the bias facilitates threading. Gloves which are clean and wet make the handling of instruments and sutures much easier than dry, sticky gloves.

IMMEDIATELY BEFORE THE OPERATION

Immediately before the patient is wheeled into the operating room, the nurse should see to it that each sterile table is covered with a sterile drape. The overhead light is turned on, and the circulating nurse assists the anesthetist and the technician or orderly in moving the patient and the anesthesia equipment into the room. At this time, lights are adjusted, covers on the sterile tables are removed, footstools are placed where necessary, and the field of operation is ready to be prepared. The sheet covering the patient is withdrawn to expose the area. Consideration for the patient is observed at all times. The preparation of the skin is done by the surgeon or one of his assistants.

The drapes are placed in such a way that the patient is completely covered except for the site of incision. A screen over the head of the patient holds the drapes away from his face and affords working space for the anesthetist. Metal towel clips hold sterile drapes in place.

Responsibilities of the "Scrub" Nurse:
1. Arrange the instruments so that they are readily accessible.

2. Place knife blades on handles (Fig. 63).
3. Count sponges with the circulating nurse.
4. Arrange suture materials, and prepare the ligatures and sutures which will be used first.
5. Since it is imperative that every piece of equipment be in good working order, it is essential that it be checked immediately before use. This includes suction tubing and tips, needles, instruments and sutures.
6. Cover the table with sterile drapes until the patient is in the operating room and the surgeon is ready to drape the operative field.

DURING THE OPERATION
Principles of Operative Procedure
Surgery may be done for a variety of reasons: to remove foreign bodies, to remove diseased parts, to repair poorly functioning parts, to diagnose or for exploratory purposes. Whatever the reason, all precautions are taken to handle tissue gently and carefully. The incision will heal best when a clean smooth cut is made; the scalpel blade must not produce a jagged tear. For adequate exposure and a minimum of trauma from retractors, the incision should be adequate.

Hemostasis is the process of controlling hemorrhage and is of importance for these reasons: (1) it prevents blood loss and shock; (2) the likelihood of postoperative

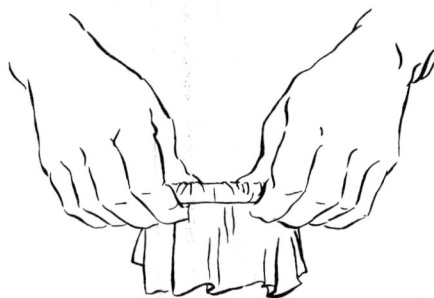

FIG. 64. When breaking glass suture tubes, a sterile towel or gauze is wrapped around tube to protect gloves and hands. By grasping tube by the ends and pulling against the thumbs, the tube is broken easily. (Davis & Geck, Inc., from Manual of Sutures and Ligatures)

hematoma is lessened; (3) the surgeon is able to dissect more accurately in a bloodless field.

Naturally, blood vessels will be severed. In order to make the operative field dry and visible, it is necessary to minimize bleeding by *sponging* as well as using other means of control. When an assistant uses a sponge in a wound, it must be used to blot by gentle pressure; rubbing or using force injures delicate tissues. It is much better to conserve the patient's own blood by carefully controlling all blood vessels and bleeding areas before significant amounts of blood are lost than to replace lost blood.

Next to the scalpel, the *hemostat* probably is the most common of all surgical instru-

ments. It is of simple design with a screw lock having slender jaws for grasping and compressing a blood vessel. Hemostats may have straight or curved tips, and are of various sized blades according to the needs of the operative procedure and the preference of the surgeon. Sometimes the pressure of the instrument on the vessel is sufficient to constrict and seal it; however, the surgeon usually slips a *ligature* (a thread or a tie) around the captured vessel. After tying it securely, the hemostat is released, the excess thread is cut, and the vessel is sealed.

In neurosurgery, two common methods of controlling hemorrhage are the use of *bone wax* and *silver clips*. Bone wax, composed mainly of beeswax, is used to seal bleeders in bone. Silver clips are small thin pieces of wire which are applied with a special forceps to the end of a vessel and pinched to occlude the lumen and stop the bleeding.

Oxidized cellulose (Oxycel, Surgicel) is a hemostatic absorbable substance made of especially treated gauze or cotton which when applied directly to a bleeding area checks capillary oozing. It absorbs fluids, and it swells and becomes sticky, forming a jellylike mass or coagulum. It is available in gauze-type pads, pledgets or strips.

Gelatin sponge (Gelfoam, Gelfoam Powder, Gelfilm) is an absorbable substance made from gelatin which has been beaten to a foamy consistency, dried and heat sterilized. It can be cut to any size or shape; when placed in an area of capillary bleeding, fibrin is deposited within its spaces, the sponge swells, and an effective clot is formed.

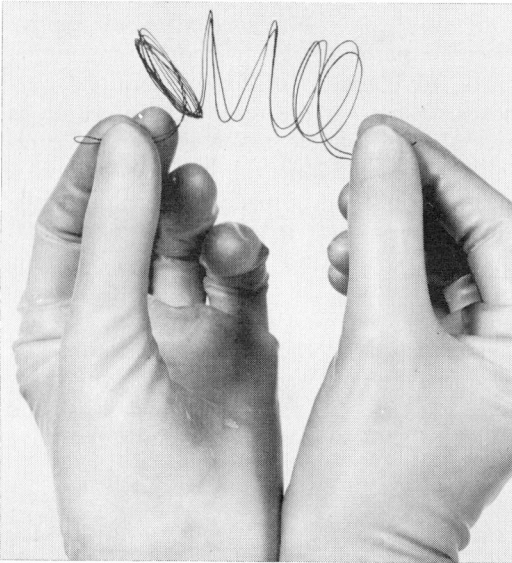

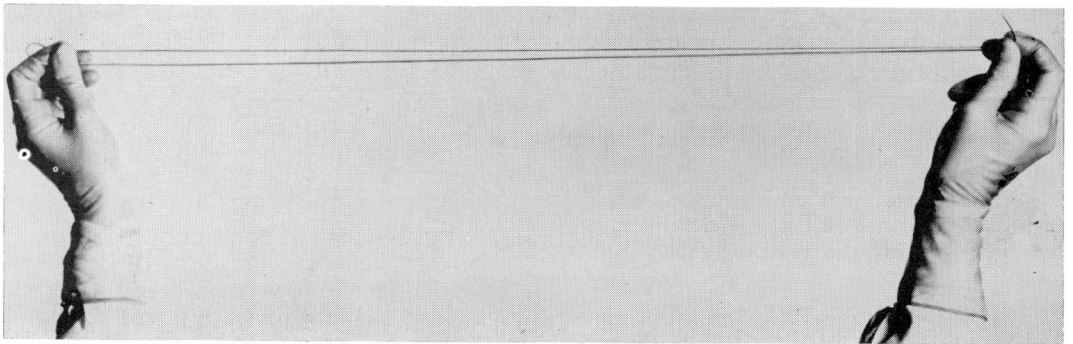

Fig. 65. Unwinding surgical gut sutures. Strand is gently pulled out straight with an even pull to remove kinks. (Davis & Geck, Division of American Cyanamid Company)

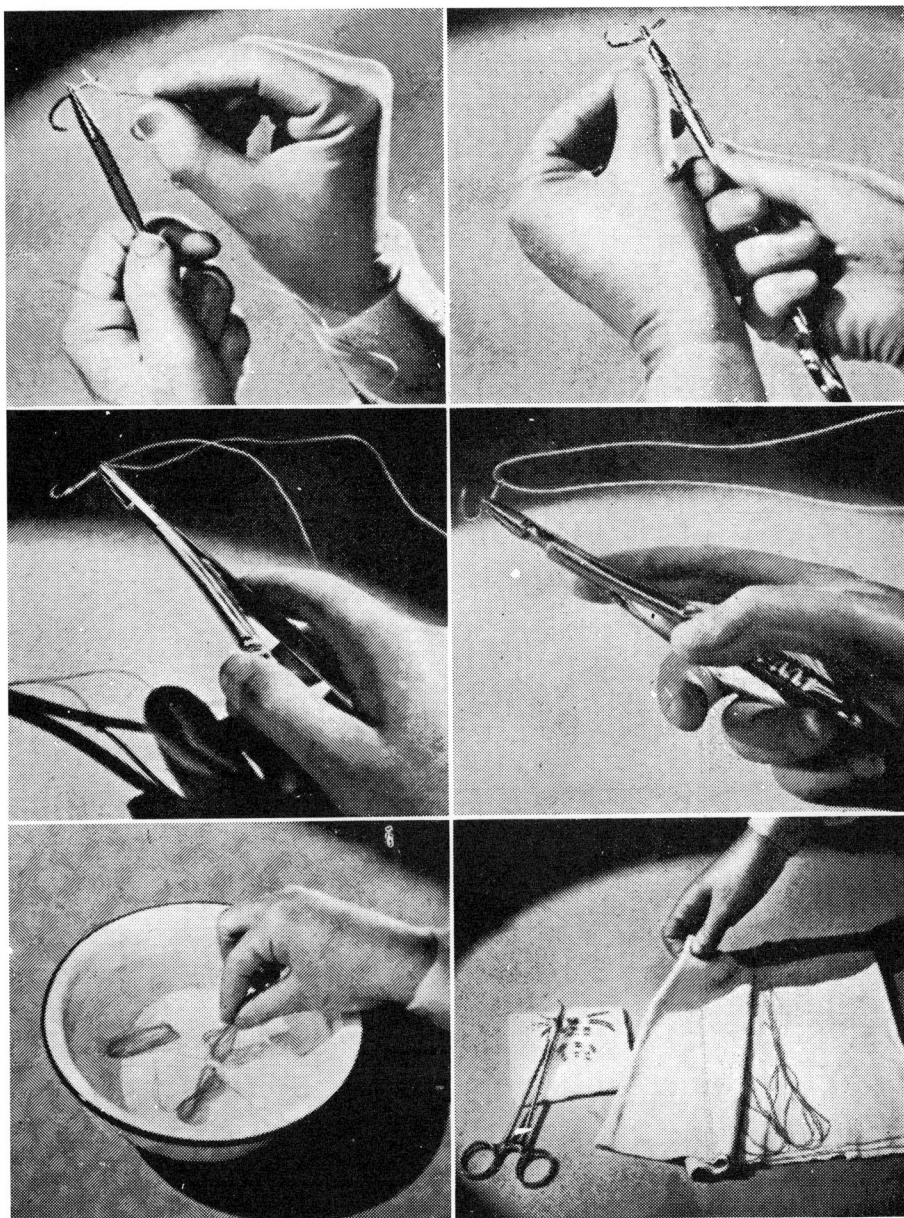

FIG. 66. Hints on handling sutures. (*Top*) Needle should be threaded from inside the curve, it is less easily unthreaded. (*Center*) Needle holder should not grasp needle close to eye but about one third the distance down the shaft. This prevents breaking of needle when in use. (*Bottom*) Sutures should not be soaked in water or saline but dipped and placed between the layers of a sterile towel. (Ethicon, Inc., Somerville, N. J.)

Responsibilities of the Circulating Nurse

The circulating nurse has many functions during an operation. Stated simply, she is responsible for maintaining a neat, quiet, well-organized operating room and must be able to anticipate and meet the needs of the "scrub" nurse, the surgeon, the anesthetist and the patient. Above all, she is as much responsible for the safety and the comfort of the patient as any other person. Some of her activities include the following:

1. Observe technic at all times to see that it is maintained properly. If there is a break, it must be remedied.

2. Assume responsibility with the other members of the team for the comfort and the safety of the patient.

3. Keep the "scrub" nurse supplied with dressings, suture materials, etc.

4. Attach the suction apparatus and check to see that it is functioning properly.

5. Place buckets strategically to receive discarded sponges.

6. Retrieve instruments, etc., which accidentally fall from the table.

7. Replace saline or water in basins as necessary.

8. Regulate temperature of the room as necessary.

9. Count, with the "scrub" nurse, all sponges opened for use, and permit no gauze of any kind to be carried from the operating room during an abdominal operation.

10. Take care of specimens.

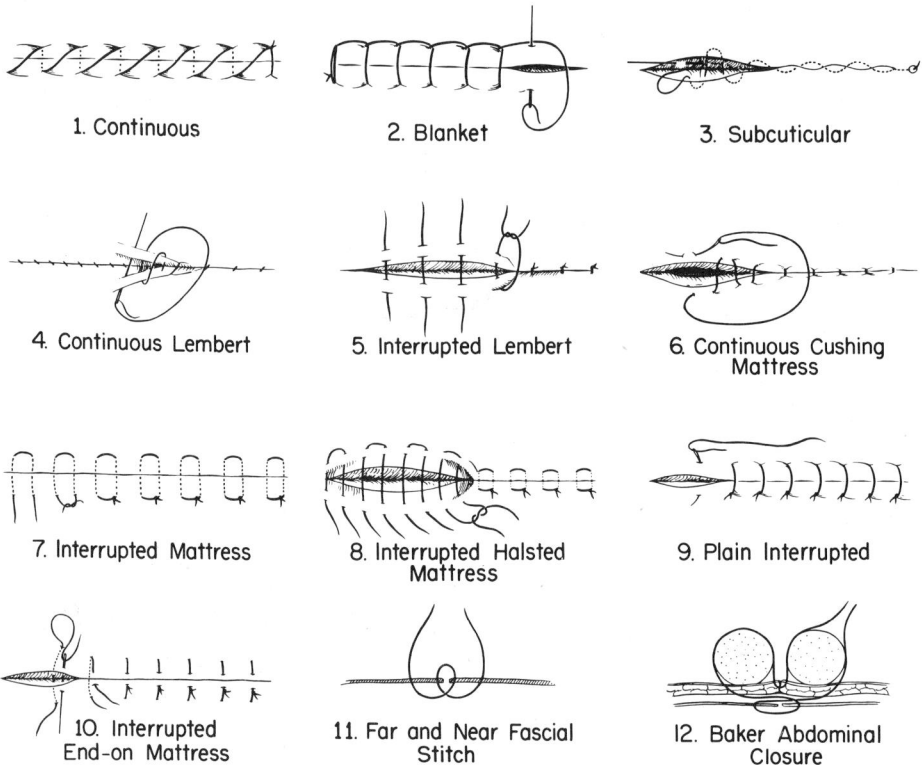

Fig. 67. Types of sutures commonly used. Types 4, 5 and 8 are utilized on the intestine, Types 3 and 10 on the skin, Type 11 on the fascia and Type 12 on the entire thickness of the abdominal wall (or thoracic wall). The other sutures depicted have more general applications. (Allen, J. G., *et al.*: Surgery: Principles and Practices, p. 19, Philadelphia, Lippincott)

11. Prepare dressing materials to be used following wound closure.

12. Direct the cleaning and the preparation of the room for the next patient.

From the responsibilities listed, it is evident that the circulating nurse must be prepared for her position. Essential attributes which she should possess are these: (1) ability to organize activities and direct personnel, with due understanding of interpersonal relations; (2) ability to anticipate needs; (3) ability to differentiate between situations which demand immediate attention and those of lesser import; (4) ability to maintain a quiet, neat and well-equipped unit; (5) understand thoroughly the principles of asepsis and (6) ability to teach actively and by the example she sets.

Responsibilities of the "Scrub" Nurse

Individual surgeons have individual preferences in their effort to standardize operative procedures. The "scrubbed" assistants learn how best to work with him as a smooth-working team. Some general suggestions are offered to help the "scrub" nurse in her important role.

To begin with, she is guided and directed constantly by what the surgeon is doing. This means almost constant attention to the

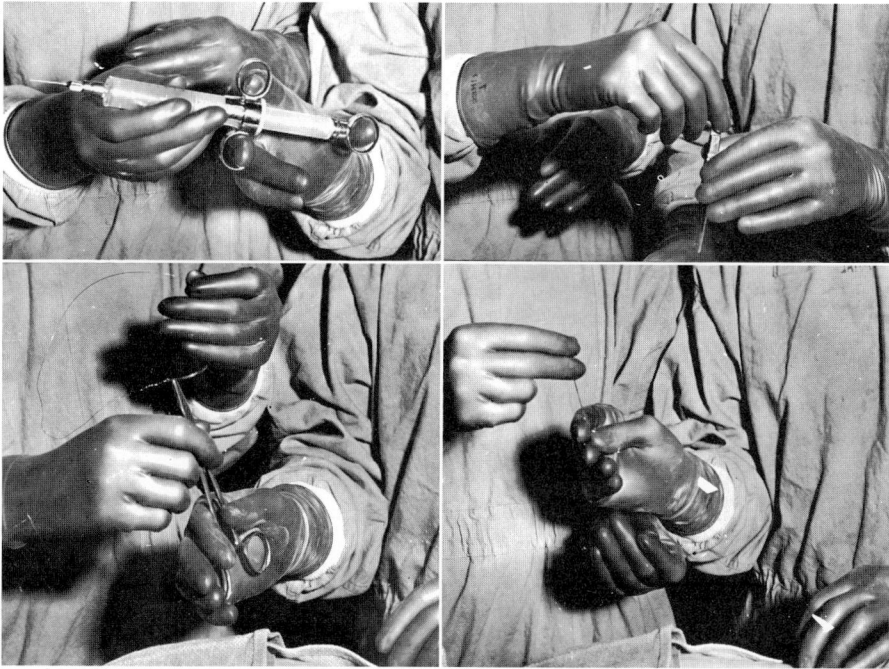

Fig. 68. The "scrub" nurse—technic of passing sutures and instruments.

(*Top, left*) Passing the syringe. The ring type of syringe should be passed so that the rings may be grasped easily by the surgeon in the fingers of the right hand.

(*Top, right*) Forceps to be passed by grasping the end in the fingers, the open part of the forceps down. As most surgeons are right-handed, the forceps usually are passed to the surgeon's left hand.

(*Bottom, left*) Method of passing a needle holder. Handle portion of the needle holder should be placed firmly in the right hand of the surgeon. The nurse should pass the needle holder, holding it in such a way that the surgeon may grasp it without looking. The nurse should be careful that she is not caught by the needle.

(*Bottom, right*) Passing a straight needle to the surgeon. The tip of the needle is held between the fingers and the thumb of the nurse's right hand. The eye end of the needle then is placed in the fingers of the surgeon's right hand.

SPONGE COUNT

Doctor *RANDOLPH*   Operation *CHOLECYSTECTOMY* Date *MAY 15.19.*

	Raytec 4x8	Large Laps	Small Laps	Pushers
Operation started with	12	6	4	12
Sponges added	12	—	4	12 + 12 + 12
Sponges added				
TOTAL SPONGES TO SCRUB NURSE	24	6	8	48
At counting time: Circulating nurse	21	5	8	46
Scrub nurse	1	1	0	0
TOTAL AT PRELIMINARY SPONGE COUNT	22	6	8	46
Sponges needed:	2	0	0	2
Surgeon	2			2
TOTAL AT FINAL SPONGE COUNT	24	6	8	48

Signature *Sue Randall*

FIG. 69. A sample of a sponge count record. This is kept by the circulating nurse in the operating room. The number of sponges at the beginning of the operation are recorded. As more sponges are required, they are charted. The record indicates the number of sponges accounted for during the preliminary and final sponge counts.

wound. The scalpel is discarded, after the skin incision is made, and replaced with a fresh one. Since the skin cannot be sterilized, the blade used on the skin is considered as being contaminated.

The next step is to provide ligatures for tying the vessels which are clamped. If the nurse holds each end of a surgical gut "tie," the surgeon is able to grasp the suture in the middle. When cotton, nylon or silk ligatures are used, the surgeon often ties from a reel or a bobbin of ligature material. In such case the bobbin should be handed to the surgeon, with a 6" or 8" length of ligature material hanging free. All ligatures must have excess threads cut after the tie is completed; therefore, an assistant must be provided with scissors.

By knowing these basic steps, a nurse is soon able to anticipate the needs of the surgeon and his assistants without being told. Some surgeons use a sign language, so that the nurse knows by a gesture what he would like next. The simple routine of scalpel, sponges, hemostat, ligature and scissors is fairly consistent. Common sense has to be practiced too. For example, suppose that after a ligature has been passed to the surgeon, he ties the bleeding vessel, and his assistant releases the hemostat. In the usual order, the scissors would be passed next. However, suppose that at that instant, a vessel begins to bleed profusely. The wisdom of passing a scissors or a hemostat can be readily determined.

The "scrub" nurse learns to anticipate intelligently the needs of the surgeon. This can be done only by watching the field of operation carefully. There may be instances in which the view of the nurse is obstructed, but she should make every effort to see and understand the progress of the operation. She is responsible for keeping the field neat and uncluttered—this includes removal of loose ends of suture or ligature material. She should ask quietly for new supplies, work rapidly and efficiently. This implies that her tables should be arranged in such a way (and she should know the arrangement) that she can reach any article without having to turn her head to look for it. Obviously, this can come only with practice. The surgeon should not expect a new nurse to have this skill, nor should a new nurse be placed in a situation for which she is not properly prepared and supervised.

Passing Instruments. In passing an instrument, place it in the surgeon's hand in the position in which he is going to use it. Pass a needle in a needle holder the same way; support the suture so that it does not drag, and have the needle pointing in the direction in which the surgeon will use it (Fig. 68).

A basin should be provided to receive any specimen. Care must be taken that cultures or other specimens are cared for properly.

Sponge Count. This is necessary in all large wounds and when body cavities (abdominal and chest) are entered during operation. To ensure the patient's safety in the operating room, it is strongly recommended that sponges containing radiopaque materials be used. Four sponge counts are taken routinely in most hospitals:

1. Unsterile sponges are counted at the make-up of the unsterile pack.
2. Sterile sponges are counted by the "scrub" or circulating nurse, or both, immediately before surgery starts.
3. A sponge count is instituted by "scrub" and circulating nurses when the surgeon begins to close the peritoneum.
4. After closure of peritoneum or chest a fourth count is taken to ensure that all sponges are accounted for (Fig. 69).

After the skin is closed and dressings have been applied, the "scrub" nurse collects all drapes and removes all tables from the operating room. She is personally responsible for taking care of any specimens and seeing that they are labeled properly and transported to the laboratory. She also should remove needles from holders, knife blades from knife handles, etc., so that whoever is responsible for instrument cleaning is not cut accidentally. Dressings and linens which were not used do not have to be discarded. They can be repackaged later and autoclaved.

Drainage Materials

Drainage is required to permit easy escape of pus, blood, or such fluids as otherwise might collect in wounds and delay their healing. The most common materials used for this purpose are gauze, rubber tissue, rubber tubes, and catheters.

Gauze, folded in some manner to exclude any cut edges coming in contact with raw surfaces, is used where capillary drainage is desired. Bandage gauze should not be used because the sizing (starch) and the close mesh employed in its manufacture make a stiffer material and one that has less capillarity. Gauze folded in various widths may be used as packing for the control of capillary or venous hemorrhage. Gauze drains become clogged within 24 hours and are not useful after that time. When drains are required for a longer period, rubber in some form is the material of choice. Rubber tissue may be used alone or in combination with gauze. The latter is known as a "cigarette" drain. The ends of the gauze should project beyond the rubber casing to get the best results. It must be borne in mind that gauze sterilized in rubber becomes friable. Hence, the nurse should test the gauze each time before it is used, or better, the cigarette drains may be freshly prepared each time, using gauze packing and Penrose tubing which have been sterilized separately. This drain has the advantage of capillarity and at the same time does not clog or adhere to the edges of the wound. Cigarette drains are used in many instances, especially in abdominal wounds. When drainage is necessary in a small wound, rubber tissue is used.

Rubber tubes of varying size and thickness make excellent material for drainage. They should have sufficient lumen to carry secretions and should be of adequate thickness to prevent their collapse. Tubes may be split lengthwise or "fenestrated" (perforated with small holes) to permit easy flow of the fluids to be drained through the tube to the exterior. If a small gauze wick is placed within the lumen of the tube, the advantage

of capillarity is added. Some of the varieties are shown in Figure 70.

Another drain is the sump drain which is a perforated glass or metal tube into which a rubber tube is inserted. This permits continuous suction removal of materials and has the advantage of not clogging.

BETWEEN OPERATIONS

Every possible precaution should be taken to avoid undue haste; at the same time, as little time as possible should be lost in going from one operation to another. Sufficient time must be allowed for the proper cleaning of the room and the floor. Nothing—instruments, supplies, suture material, etc.—that has been used for one case should be used for another without resterilization. Gowns, masks and gloves must be changed between patients.

Procedure After a Contaminated Case

A contaminated or "dirty" case is an operation in which pus or gangrene is found associated with frank infection. The care of all materials which have been used on a contaminated case differs very little from that given so-called "clean" cases. The basic principle is that all contaminated articles, gowns, gloves, instruments, sponges, drapes, must be handled as little as possible as they are prepared and transported to the sterilizer or place of disposition; they should be disposed of imme-

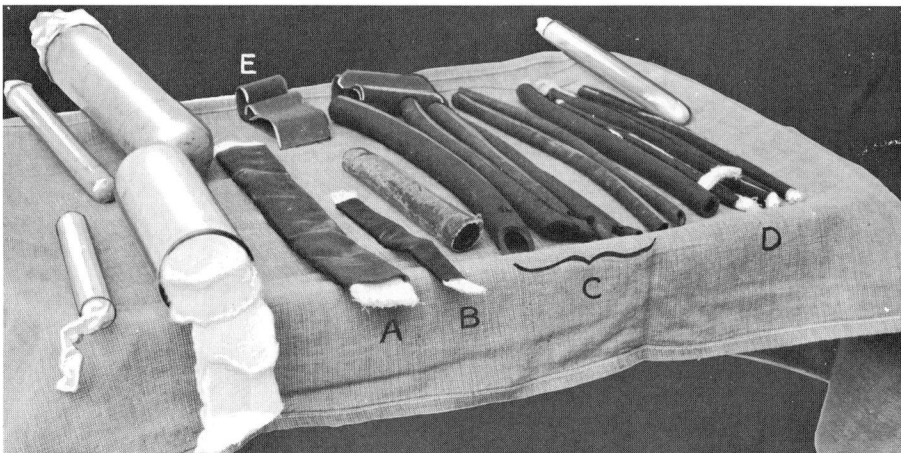

FIG. 70. Drainage materials. Gauze packed in glass tubes. (A) Cigarette drain, large size. (B) Cigarette drain, small size. (C) Fenestrated rubber tubes. (D) Split rubber tube drains with gauze wicks. (E) Rubber dam or tissue.

diately. One person, usually the "scrub" nurse, remains contaminated to receive all soiled linens in a special bag marked "contaminated" and all gloves which members of the operating team have washed in a glove basin before removing. All contaminated rubber goods will be sterilized together in the washer sterilizer. Instruments should be opened before sterilizing. Needles can be collected in a metal needle box and autoclaved; glass suture tubes are immersed in a germicide. Unused sponges, dressings and linens are received in a dry linen bag and autoclaved. Soiled sponges and other discarded items are collected in a paper bag before being transported to the incinerator. Solutions and suction bottle contents are all collected in a kick bucket and emptied into the hopper. Instrument tables, operating tables, buckets and other utensils are scrubbed thoroughly with a germicide.

If the septic areas and articles are cleansed thoroughly, sterilized or disposed of, the room may be prepared for the next case. It is not necessary to quarantine the room. For spots of blood and pus on the floor, Walter recommends disinfecting the area with lime paste and washing the floor with sodium hypochlorite or any other suitable germicide. When a patient who has tuberculosis comes to the operating room, he should wear a mask. Intubation tubes and anesthesia face masks following their use on a patient with tuberculosis should be scrubbed inside and out and immersed in an appropriate chemical disinfectant.

During gastrointestinal surgery, instruments and sponges can be kept isolated on the patient by first covering the "clean" drapes with sterile plastic material such as polyvinyl chloride films or waterproof cellophane. On top of this a sterile drape is placed, and all articles placed on this drape are then considered contaminated. When the gastrointestinal tract is closed, all "dirty" materials must be removed, including contaminated gowns and gloves.

Care of Specimens

A *specimen* is any tissue removed from a patient during an operation. Most specimens are sent to the pathology laboratory for examination, whereas cultures, spinal fluid,

urine and smears are sent to the bacteriology laboratory. The nurse's responsibility is twofold: (1) the specimen must be labeled properly, and (2) it must be sent to the proper laboratory.

Each specimen should be handled carefully so as not to destroy any natural landmarks or characteristics which aid in the diagnosis. Each specimen should be placed in a container of adequate size and covered with the solution recommended by the local laboratory. Allowing a specimen to dry produces autolysis, and the specimen becomes useless for study. There are several exceptions to this general rule, and the nurse should familiarize herself with the policies of the local laboratory. For example, specimens for frozen section are taken to the laboratory immediately after they are obtained. For D & C specimens, some surgeons prefer to have the specimen rinsed of excess blood, with citrate, before placing in formalin. Smears may be placed in equal parts of 95 per cent alcohol and ether.

Early in the nurse's orientation to the operating room, she should become familiar with the correct procedure to follow in the local hospital. When it is realized that the future of many patients depends on a small specimen of tissue and its laboratory studies, the nurse's responsibility for safeguarding and caring for it is a real and great one.

AT THE END OF THE OPERATIVE SCHEDULE

After the day's operations, the entire operating suite must receive a thorough cleaning, with particular attention to the operating room proper. Soiled linen must be sorted carefully to prevent valuable instruments being sent to the laundry.

Floors should be cleaned and disinfected daily with a detergent germicide; the iodophorms and the phenolics combine these actions. All tables, stools, basin racks, etc., must be well washed to remove blood stains and any other foreign material. The operating table and pad should be cleaned thoroughly with a detergent germicide.

The care of instruments, needles, gloves, etc., after use is taken up in detail on pages 261-269.

All unused sterile supplies, including packages that have been opened, must be resterilized, even though the contents apparently have not been touched. When in doubt, resterilize.

Utensils and special apparatus must be cleansed and sterilized or put away, as the case may demand. Everything that has been used during the course of the day's operations should be returned to its rightful place in condition to be used again at a moment's notice. The operating room must always be in a state of preparedness.

SAFETY PRACTICES IN THE OPERATING ROOM

Throughout the chapter devoted to operating room nursing, safety measures have been emphasized. However, inasmuch as safety practices never can be overemphasized, this section will explore further the conditions and the activities which are potentially hazardous and what might be done to eliminate them.

The operating room nurse has a responsibility for the safety of every patient who comes to her department. Emergency equipment always should be available and in usable condition. This includes suction apparatus, airways, drugs, etc. No excuse is acceptable when a patient's life is lost due to negligence.

All solutions which are used in the operating room should be labeled plainly. In order that mistakes may be averted, the policy of tinting solutions is helpful. There is no justification for a patient's receiving an injection of ether when the surgeon assumed that he was using procaine.

Although it is not the direct responsibility of the nurse to check anesthesia equipment, she must be aware of the importance of maintaining proper connections of tubing leading to gas machines, suction outlets, air under pressure, etc. For example, a wrong connection made by a well-intentioned nurse or auxiliary worker may result in a patient's receiving carbon dioxide when his precarious condition demands oxygen.

Occasionally, a needle breaks and is lost in the tissues of the patient. This may be a hollow needle which can break at the hub during an injection or it may be a suture needle. It is extremely important that such

an accident be reported to the surgeon, who will initiate steps to localize and remove the foreign object.

The recovery of all instruments and sponges used during an operation is imperative. Even though the surgeon assumes the responsibility for a correct count, the nurse is in a unique position to verify such an accounting.

Explosive Hazards and Safety Precautions

Walter* describes 4 factors which operate simultaneously to produce explosive combustion of anesthetic gases in the operating room: (1) a flammable gas, (2) the presence of oxygen, (3) a source of ignition and (4) carelessness. To control the first 2 factors, a closed technic of administering the gas is recommended. All personnel should keep away from the anesthesia area, at least 2 feet away from anesthesia equipment and the patient securing the anesthetic agent. A source of ignition may be from:

1. Flames, such as cigarettes, alcohol lamps;

2. Electrical equipment, such as motors, heaters, hot plates, x-ray equipment, cauteries, switches, lamps, endoscopes;

3. Static electricity, such as friction from rubber goods, clothing, tearing of adhesive, shuffling of feet or personnel moving about the room; and

4. Clicking together of metal parts, such

Anesthesia Drugs which are Flammable

Ether	Ethylene
Vinethene	Cyclopropane
Ethyl Chloride	Divinyl Ether

Any of these in a gaseous vapor form, mixed with nitrous oxide, air or oxygen, form explosive mixtures.

Anesthesia Drugs which are not Flammable

Nitrogen	Chloroform
Carbon Dioxide	Nitrous Oxide
Helium	Trichlorethylene
Oxygen	Fluothane

---

* Walter, C.: Electrostatics in the Operating Room, Hosp. Topics **31**: Sept., 1953.

as slip joints, and dropping of instruments.

All electric equipment should be Underwriters'-approved. Cords of portable lamps and electrical appliances should be flexible, continuous and without connections or switches. They should be equipped with explosion-proof plugs.

Another essential safety factor in the operating room is to maintain conductive pathways so that electrical contact is provided. Conductive parts of tables or equipment which are worn should be replaced. Suture ends, dirt, blood or pus must not be allowed to accumulate on castors of tables which tend to insulate them from the floor. Wax which is nonconductive should not be applied to the floor. A system of checking or testing the safety of equipment is essential to the safety of the surgical patient and should be enforced rigorously.

Wool blankets and plastic sheets should not be used around anesthetic-gas equipment or patients anesthetized with combustible-gas mixtures. Cotton blankets are preferred; however, these blankets must be free of synthetic fibers such as nylon, dacron, etc. It is preferable not to warm cotton blankets, since this removes moisture which if present cuts down on the possibility of static sparks. (Physiologically, a superwarmed blanket may be more harmful to the anesthetized patient than one at room temperature.) Conductive rubber mattresses, pads and pillows, breathing tubes, bags and masks should be used. Operating tables should be fitted with conductive straps for connecting the bare skin of the patient with the conductive system. Receptacles and plugs that cannot be pulled apart accidentally should be installed where needed. Unless they are of the explosion-proof type, they should not be placed lower than 5 feet above the floor.

Personnel contribute to the fourth factor mentioned above, namely carelessness. Proper wearing apparel has been described on page 235. The nurse is in a position to be informed and to pass this information on to others not so informed. This responsibility for teaching, particularly in the operating room, is one major area of difference between professional and nonprofessional personnel. Only by accepting fully her obligations to her patient and to her profession will the nurse justify assuming a key position in the operating room.

STERILIZATION AND CARE OF VARIOUS ARTICLES
Instruments

The care, the handling and the use of surgical instruments holds a high priority position in the care of the surgical patient. Because of their real value to the skillful performance of the surgeon, it is imperative that surgical instruments be kept in excellent working order.

The nurse needs to know the proper care of instruments whether she is responsible for them herself or delegates their care to auxiliary workers. It is in the cleaning that an instrument is subjected to most abuse. Too often, unskilled or unsupervised personnel are entrusted with this important responsibility.

After use, all instruments should be cleaned thoroughly. They may be cleaned in the washing sterilizer or by ultrasonic means.* If they are cleaned manually, instruments should be scrubbed with a detergent; abrasives must be avoided. For inaccessible soil which collects on serrations of the jaw and the locks and the catches, instruments can be soaked in a detergent. The cleaning agent chosen should be corrosion-inhibited and should not leave a residual film on the instrument. Corrosion will occur if moist instruments are allowed to stand exposed to air. This will interfere not only with sterilization but also with the smooth working of an instrument.

To ensure thorough drying, instruments can be placed on trays and exposed to the hot air oven, a steam radiator or a steam sterilizer. Another effective way is to place the tray in the chamber of the dressing autoclave, which has the heat turned on in the jacket. In damp climates, instrument closets can be equipped with a "damp chaser" similar to that used in pianos. These dehumidifiers are heating elements run on ordinary current to keep the cabinet dry.

* An ultrasonic cleaner removes soil most effectively by means of high frequency sound waves; 100 instruments can be completely processed every 3 minutes. (American Sterilizer Co., Erie, Pa.)

The question of oiling instruments remains a controversial one. Walter states that with proper cleaning, sterilization and storage, instruments need no oiling. Oiling introduces a hazard in that the oil film protects bacteria trapped beneath it from contact with steam in the sterilizer. Oiled instruments are sterilized adequately only in an instrument-washer sterilizer, which removes the film of oil and exposes all surfaces of the instrument to moist heat.*

Ahearn† compromises by saying that if the proper oil is used, many of the original objections to oiling instruments are overcome. A highly volatile oil which is sufficiently light to penetrate the grain of the steel and not form a film that will harbor dangerous bacteria should be used. A volatile oil is chosen so that the excess will vaporize quickly when exposed to the heat of the sterilizer. The oil should be applied sparingly with a metal "pin" and only on the inside of the box or screwlock and on the screw heads of scissors. Conscientious cleaning of the locks of instruments will obviate much of the need for oiling, inasmuch as ordinary dirt and baked-on blood are often responsible for imperfect function.

The following suggestions will help in minimizing unnecessary wear‡:

1. Do not handle instruments unnecessarily. The habit of idly opening and closing a hemostat merely to feel it click causes more wear than ordinary surgical use.

2. Be cautious in loading the sterilizer, and do not stack heavy instruments on top of delicate, finely tooled instruments.

3. When disassembling instruments, such as tonsil snares, for cleaning, be sure that original parts are reassembled as they were originally.

4. Keep a supply of tools at hand to prevent the use of surgical instruments for jobs for which they were never intended.

5. Avoid use of the normal saline solution to "soak" instruments during the operation. Salt has an extremely high corrosive action on all steel.

* Walter, C.: O R question box, Hosp. Topics **34:** Oct., 1956.
† Ahearn, G.: Care of surgical instruments, Hosp. Topics **35:**106, Apr., 1957.
‡ *Ibid.*, p. 106.

Let the surgeon who uses the instrument be the judge of its performance. If he determines that an instrument is useless, mark it for repair immediately and do not return it to use until its performance is perfect.

Sterilization. Instruments should be unlocked before sterilization; this allows for proper sterilization of all surfaces. The preferred method of sterilizing instruments preoperatively is steam under pressure, 250° F. (120° C.) for 15 minutes, with 15 to 17 lbs. of pressure. Instruments may also be sterilized in a hot oven for 1 hour at 320° F. The disadvantage here is the length of time.

For routine washing and sterilizing of soiled or contaminated instruments, the instrument-washer-sterilizer is recommended. The cleansing process is accomplished chiefly by exposing the instruments to an effective detergent solution in the washer; ultimately, sterilization takes place when the temperature reaches 270° F.

For emergency sterilization, 270° F. at 27 lbs. for 3 minutes is perfectly safe.

Boiling water for 30 minutes may be used; it is recognized that some spores can withstand this method. When an alkali has been added to the water, the time of boiling may be reduced to 15 minutes.

Chemical disinfection is discussed on p. 45.

Cutting Instruments

Knives, scissors, chisels and other sharp instruments depend on the sharpness of their edges for proper performance. Every effort must be exerted to protect the blades from injury. This is accomplished by cleaning them carefully, avoiding abrasives and preventing them from coming in contact with hard surfaces. They must be sterilized in the least injurious and safest way.

Knives may have the blade permanently attached, or it may be detached. One of the safest methods of attaching or removing a detachable blade is by using a special forceps (Fig. 63).

Scissors are made in a variety of types for various uses; on the whole, they are delicate and should not be used for purposes other than the use specifically intended. They are easily sprung, and the fine adjustments can be damaged with very little effort.

Sterilization. Cutting-edge instruments and those so delicate that moist heat destroys them should be sterilized by dry heat at 320° F. (160° C.) for 1 hour. Scissors and instruments of stainless steel which are made properly are not injured by heat and can be sterilized safely by autoclaving at 250° F. for 15 minutes. Sharp instruments should not be piled on top of one another, because of the possibility of injuring the cutting edges. Knife blades can be purchased individually wrapped and sterile, and that is the safest method. Blades can be disinfected in a germicide; however, the hazards involved in germicidal disinfection must be recognized. When germicides are used, the blade must be washed carefully before use. The germicide is so powerful that if it comes in contact with tissue, it produces an immediate death of tissues, with consequent complications in wound healing.

Instrument Setups

After the instruments have been sterilized, the nurse arranges them for the next operation. For a simple operation such as a biopsy of lymph node, suturing of a laceration, etc., the instruments, suture materials, drapes and dressings can be conveniently placed on one table. Basic instruments for a simple setup are as follows:

Sponge forceps and towel clips
Scalpel
Scissors (dissecting and nurse's)
Forceps, plain and toothed
Hemostats, straight and curved
Allis forceps
Retractors
Suture needles and needles
Grooved director and/or probe

Modifications of this setup are made in terms of the type of operation and the preference of the surgeon. If the arrangement of this table is standardized, it becomes a simple matter to make minor additions for such operations as hemorrhoidectomy, minor amputations, minor plastic operations, tonsillectomy, etc. For an incision and drainage of an abscess, a culture tube and drainage material should be added.

For a simple abdominal procedure, such as an appendectomy or herniorrhapy, or a larger dissecting operation such as a mastec-tomy or radical neck dissection, a Mayo instrument stand plus an instrument table is usually used. The Mayo stand ordinarily contains the basic instruments found in the simple setup described above. The instrument table is convenient for the specialty instruments as well as drains, suture material, dressings, etc. From such a setup as the basic Mayo stand and appendectomy instrument table, the more major procedure setups can be developed.

Suture Materials

Sutures and ligatures are of two main types: those which are absorbed by the body and those which are not. Surgical gut (catgut), Cargile membrane, kangaroo tendon and fascia lata are of the *absorbable* type, while silk, linen, cotton, nylon, Dacron (e.g., Mersilene polyester fiber), surgical steel and tantalum wire, silk-worm gut and so forth comprise the *nonabsorbable* group. For the most part, absorbable sutures are used under the skin, while the nonabsorbable kind may be used almost anywhere. The criteria of the surgeon is to select a suture material which is strong enough to hold tissues in approximation, cause minimal interference with healing, incite minimal foreign body reaction and is easy to handle and inexpensive.

Absorbable Sutures

Surgical Gut (catgut) is made from the submucous layer of sheep's intestine, which is cleaned, dried, twisted into threads of various sizes and prepared for use by special processes which include innumerable inspections of gauge and tensile strength and scrupulous sterilization.

Standard lengths of surgical gut are between 54 and 60 inches. Shorter strands, usually packaged 2 or 3 strands in a glass tube, are available. Sutures are either wound on a reel or coiled, depending on the type of package containing them. Surgical gut sutures usually are in a fluid consisting of alcohol and water, not for purposes of sterility but to maintain the gut in finest ready-to-use condition as it is removed from its hermetically sealed container. (This fluid must not be confused with *sterilizing* solution that protects the *exterior* of the suture tubes or packets. This will be discussed in more detail

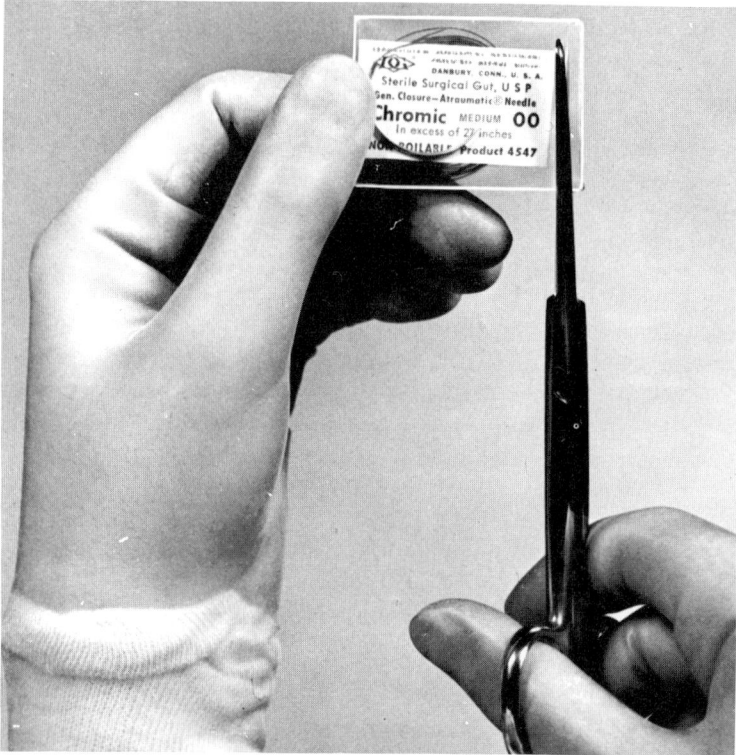

Fig. 71. The plastic envelope must be cut before removing the surgical gut. (Davis & Geck, division of American Cyanamid Co.)

later.) Surgical gut is processed either *boilable* or *nonboilable,* which means that the former must be autoclaved or boiled, whereas the latter type must be sterilized by immersion in an antiseptic for at least 18 hours if the sutures are not already provided in a sterile-pack container rendering them ready for use as they are removed from the sterilizing solution. The suture label indicates whether the suture is boilable or nonboilable. If nonboilable, it must not be autoclaved or boiled, as this will literally cook the gut. Nearly all surgical gut used now is the nonboilable type and is available in plastic and foil packets.* The plastic or foil packet (Fig. 71) is cut, pulled apart or notched for easy tearing to expose a sterile sealed inner envelope containing the suture material.

Surgical gut is made in different sizes. The strands are graded according to their caliber and range from 7/0, the finest size, to the very coarse size 5. The sizes in most com-

mon use are 000, 00, 0 and 1 (Fig. 72). The length of time for complete absorption of surgical gut in a wound is reckoned by the action of certain hardening agents. Therefore, "Type A, Plain Surgical Gut," has not been treated to alter its digestion rate. Such untreated gut is absorbed in 5 to 10 days. Chromic gut refers to gut which has been treated by a tanning process with chromic salts; this prolongs the absorption time. Type B, Mild Chromic, Type C, Medium Chromic and Type D, Extra Chromic indicate that such gut resists digestion for varying periods of time, usually 10 to 40 or more days.

Surgical gut is the most popular suture material. The advantages are: (1) it is absorbed eventually, (2) it is easy to handle, (3) standardized sizes are available for different uses, and (4) it can be used in a variety of tissues beneath the skin. The disadvantages are: (1) it produces some tissue reaction,† (2) it is expensive, and (3) it cannot be used on the skin.

* If they are not sterile, packets and tubes must be washed thoroughly with a detergent and dried before they are placed in a recommended disinfecting solution for 18 hours.

† Tissue reaction is the response of tissue to injury; a repair process is set up immediately.

Fascia lata is prepared after it is obtained from the fibrous tissue in the thigh of an ox. It comes in strips or sheets and is used in reconstructive orthopedic surgery as well as for the repair of hernia in operations where an especially strong absorbable suture is required.

Nonabsorbable Sutures

Surgical silk is obtained from the silkworm and goes through many processes before it can be used for surgical suturing. Silk may be black, colored or white; however, black is seen more easily in tissues and is preferred. It may be twisted or braided, and it comes in sizes comparable with surgical gut. Size range is from very fine to very coarse: A-B-C-1 to 8. It is available in sterile tubes and envelopes and can be purchased on unsterile spools which can be rewound in smaller amounts and sterilized. Metal or glass spools, rubber tubing and flat sheets of metal have been used with success in the rewinding process. Care must be taken to wind silk loosely and evenly. If wound tightly on something which expands during the sterilization process, the tensile strength of the silk will be reduced, since silk contracts with heat. Suture manufacturers offer silk and cotton suture materials in ready-to-use packages in addition to spools of the same materials. For example, these include 17 strands, 18 inches long, within a sealed envelope, which may be autoclaved as an entire unit. Also, 17 strands, 18 inches long, are available in glass tubes and foil packets, sterile and ready-to-use from their containers. These package improvements offer the advantage of timesavings and simplified procedures in the operating room.

Untreated silk has a capillary action; by this process, fluids may pass along the strand, thus permitting infection to be drawn into the wound. By treating it to render it *serum proof*, silk can withstand the action of body fluids and moisture.

The advantages of silk are: (1) it has high tensile strength, (2) it is relatively inexpensive, and (3) there is less tissue reaction than with surgical gut. Disadvantage is that the necessary meticulous technic prolongs operating time.

Silk should be sterilized by autoclaving at 250° F. for 15 minutes. However, for maximum tensile strength, silk should be used *dry,* not dipped in solution. Spooled silk should be removed from the spool before autoclaving.

Surgical Cotton differs from ordinary sewing cotton in that it is boiled in soda to remove the cotton fiber wax, and it is colored with certified dyes. It comes in the same sizes as silk and is sterilized in the same manner. Cotton shrinks during the sterilization process; therefore, it should never be autoclaved on a glass or metal spool. Contrary to usage of silk *dry,* cotton should always be used *wet* for maximum tensile strength. The choice of surgical silk or surgical cotton depends entirely upon individual surgeons' preference for a given application.

Surgical Nylon is a synthetic polyamide available in two forms: monofilament and multifilament (braided). Monofilament is used primarily for skin closure, tension sutures and plastic surgery. The chief disadvantage is that a triple knot must be tied in the small sizes and a double square knot in the larger sizes. Braided nylon has the same

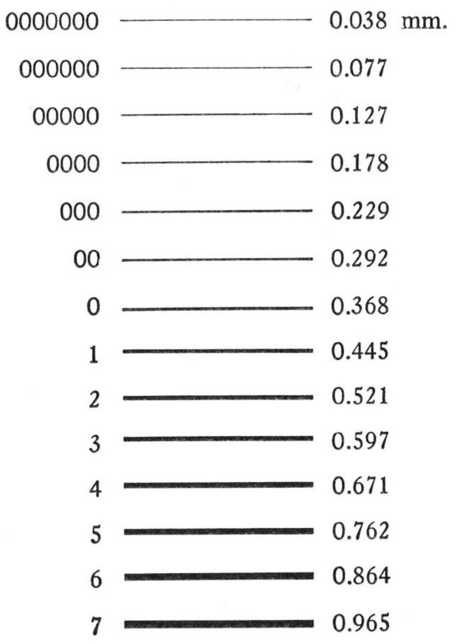

0000000	0.038 mm.
000000	0.077
00000	0.127
0000	0.178
000	0.229
00	0.292
0	0.368
1	0.445
2	0.521
3	0.597
4	0.671
5	0.762
6	0.864
7	0.965

FIG. 72. U.S. Pharmacopoeia suture gauges. (Ziegler, P. F.: Text Book of Sutures, Bauer & Black, Chicago, Ill.)

uses as cotton and silk. It is strong and relatively inert, causing little tissue reaction when imbedded in tissues.

Surgical Wire of silver, bronze and copper has been used in surgery for a long time. Stainless steel and tantalum are the most popular today. Wire comes in various gauges and has the advantage of being strong and permanent and of causing little or no local reaction in the tissue in which it is placed. It is frequently used not only for skin closure but also as a buried suture in the fascial layers of a wound. Steel alloy wire is relatively cheap, and it may be tied in knots almost as easily as silk and surgical gut. Meticulous technic is necessary so that kinks are not produced, thereby weakening the suture material. All ends must be cut close to the knot to prevent irritation except when the wire is used for skin closure. Tantalum is expensive, which seems to be its only disadvantage. Wire is sterilized by autoclaving at 250° F. for 15 minutes.

Silver Wire Clips are made for use in controlling bleeding from vessels in brain, stomach and nerve surgery. A dispenser is available in which clips are harbored and dispensed, Michel clips are metal-toothed clips applied to hold skin edges in approximation. They require a special forceps for both appli-

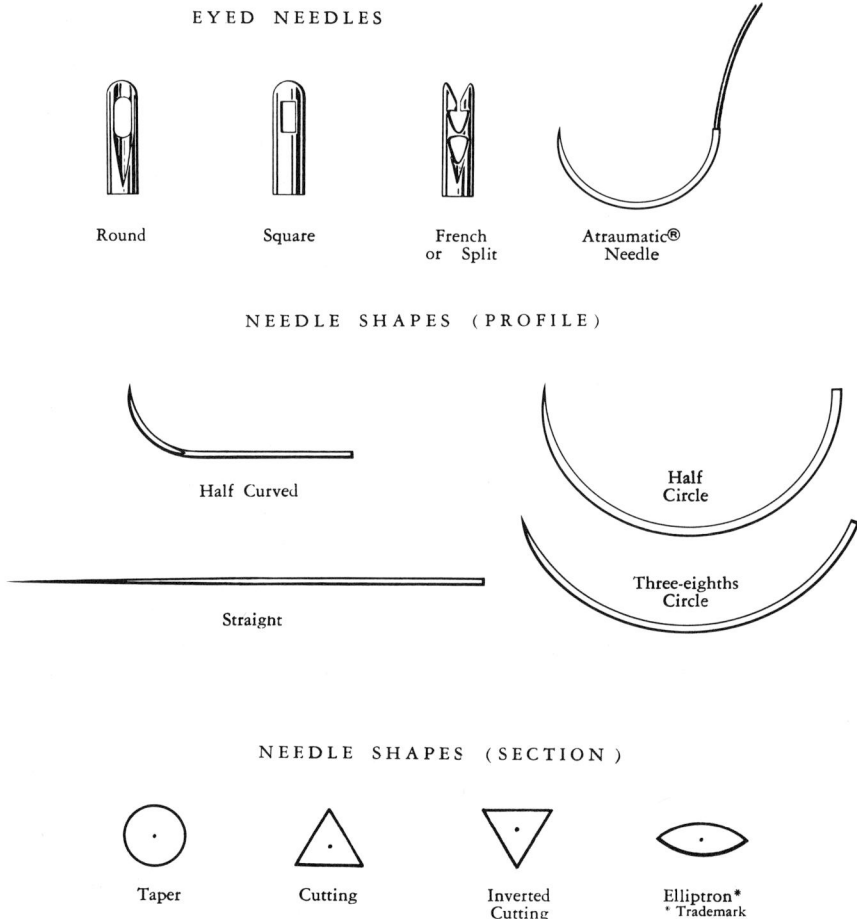

EYED NEEDLES

| Round | Square | French or Split | Atraumatic® Needle |

NEEDLE SHAPES (PROFILE)

Half Curved

Half Circle

Three-eighths Circle

Straight

NEEDLE SHAPES (SECTION)

| Taper | Cutting | Inverted Cutting | Elliptron* * Trademark |

FIG. 73. Basic needle chart. (American Cyanamid Co., Surgical Products Div., Danbury, Conn.)

cation and removal. Clips and forceps may be sterilized by autoclaving with the instruments.

Silkworm Gut is a strong, smooth material used for tension sutures, especially in the closure of abdominal wounds, or those in which there is particular strain. The strands come 10 to 12 inches in length and vary considerably in thickness. The size is identified by the terms fine, medium and heavy. Because the strands are of unequal length and of uneven diameters, this suture material is being replaced by wire, nylon and heavy silk. It can be sterilized by autoclaving. After sterilization, the gut may be stored in 70 per cent alcohol until used. Silkworm gut is exceedingly stiff and unpliable and must be soaked in hot sterile water for at least 10 minutes before use.

Stainless steel mesh may be used in herniated areas to reinforce tissue and is used to a limited extent in plastic surgery. After the size of the piece of mesh to be implanted is determined, allow an extra 3/16 to ½ inch all around. This extra margin is folded over to provide a double thickness through which sutures are placed; this procedure also eliminates sharp edges. Wire scissors are used to cut it. Stainless steel has replaced tantalum for this use, thereby making the implant less expensive. Good results have been reported.

Suture Needles

The surgeon's needle must be sharp and made of properly tempered steel so that it is sufficiently malleable not to break easily. Classification of needles may be done in several ways. They may be grouped *according to shape,* such as straight, curved or half-curved (Fig. 73).

Another classification is *according to the tip* of the needle: cutting-point or taper-point. Cutting needles may be the conventional 3-edged triangular style, reversed cutting edge (an improved design) and trocar (not widely used). These needles may cut into tissue to allow for the easier passage of the suture. This is necessary in suturing dense tissue such as skin, cervix of the uterus and tendon. The taper needle is used for the suturing of such delicate structures as the intestine, brain, mucous membranes and nerves.

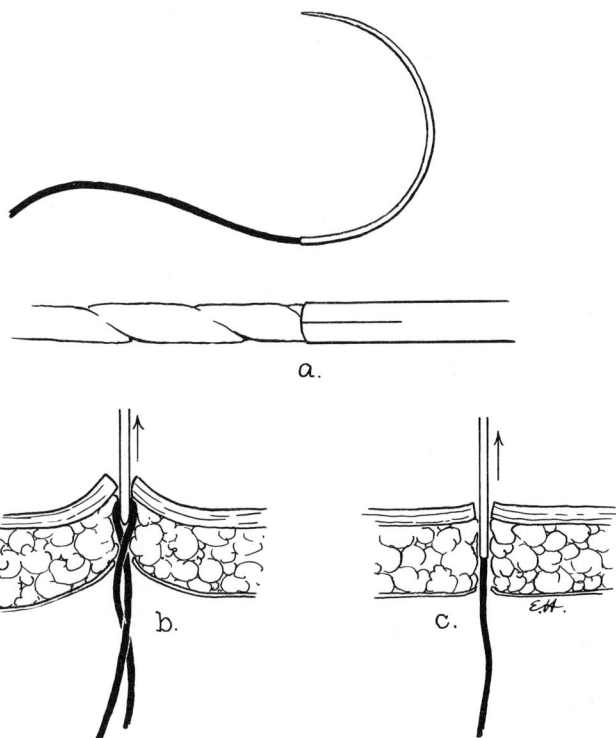

Fig. 74. Atraumatic needle and suture for intestinal sutures. Needle and suture are of same size, and, when pulled through tissue, suture fills needle hole (c). Ordinary suture and needle (b) for comparison.

A third classification may be *according to the eye* of the needle: ordinary eye, French or split eye and atraumatic or swaged-on needle. The French eye has a slit from the end of the needle to the eye, through which the suture is drawn to thread it. This kind of needle can be threaded more quickly than the ordinary eye needle (Fig. 74). The atraumatic or swaged-on needle is really an eyeless needle. In the manufacturing process the suture is inserted within the metal of the needle so that the diameter of the suture is not greater than the needle.

Eyeless needles are popular for several reasons: (1) they do not have to be threaded, (2) they produce a minimum of tissue trauma, and (3) there is less damage to the suture strand (Fig. 74).

Needles also come in various sizes. Different surgeons, with their individual technics, use different needles. Experience and the wish of the surgeon are the only real guides as to the various uses of needles, although good judgment on the nurse's part is always a valuable asset. Straight needles are generally used without a needle holder, while all curved needles are used with a holder. The jaws of the needle holder should be placed so as to grasp the needle about ⅔ of the distance from the needle tip to the eye end. The clamps of the holder never should come together directly on the eye of the needle. Almost invariably the needle will break if this is done.

Sterilization. Suture needles are arranged in some definite order on a towel or an anchor-spring needle holder. After use, they are placed in a perforated stainless steel box and washed with the instruments in the instrument-washer-sterilizer. They may be scoured or run through emery powder, washed, rinsed thoroughly and dried. "The disinfection of suture needles by immersion in germicide is an obsolete, unsafe technic."*

Articles of Rubber

Rubber is found in a number of articles such as tubing, drainage tubes, bulbs, rubber dam and gloves. Unfortunately, rubber can be damaged easily; therefore, it is important to know how to care for and sterilize it properly. This is necessary not only for economical reasons but also for the proper functioning of the article, as well as the safety of the patient and the personnel.

Rubber soiled with any of these should be cleansed as soon as possible.†

1. Petroleum by-products and hydrocarbon solvents
    A. Petrolatum
    B. Mineral oil
    C. Cleaning fluid
    D. Benzene
    E. Acetone
2. Vegetable oils: eucalyptus, wintergreen, pine, etc.
3. Glycerin
4. Ether
5. Esters which are most commonly found in medications but are also in white wax, yellow wax (beeswax), benzyl benzoate USP, methyl and ethyl salicylate common in liniments.
6. Oxidizing acids: sulfuric, hydrochloric, etc.
7. Copper and manganese, indigenous to most sterilizer fabrication
8. Phenols and cresols
9. Ozone which is generated by fluorescent light, electric motors and diathermy machines.
10. Excessive heat and sunlight.

Rubber Gloves

Rubber gloves protect the wearer and the patient; they are used in all situations where blood and body fluids are contacted. Gloves are expensive, and their lives are relatively short. Therefore, it is good sense to care for them meticulously.

Before gloves are removed, the user should carefully wash off all soil in cold running water. This prevents drying and caking of blood and pus, which makes it very difficult to remove later. Then gloves are washed in a washing machine or a laundromat in which an alkaline detergent, such as trisodium phosphate, renders soluble any remaining soil.

After removing gloves from the washing machine, they are ready for drying, powdering, testing, sorting and packaging.

---

* Walter, *op. cit.*, p. 16.

† Errera, D. W., and Walter, C. W.: The care and sterilization of catheters, drains and tubes, Hosp. Topics 34:93, Aug., 1956.

Sterilization. Packages of gloves are placed in the autoclave in such a way that each glove is standing on edge with the thumb uppermost. In this position steam may enter all the fingers, and the presence of air pockets is eliminated. Place glove trays in the upper half of the sterilizer. Gloves should be sterilized alone and removed from the sterilizer at the end of the sterilizing period, which is 10 minutes at 250° F. (121° C.). After sterilization, gloves should dry thoroughly; therefore, it is recommended that at least 24 to 48 hours elapse before they are used.*

Disposable Gloves. Many hospitals now use disposable rubber gloves which are delivered packaged and sterile in paper wrappers. They have the distinct advantage of requiring no care in powdering, washing and sterilizing, and the wearer has the advantage of always having new gloves without patches. Available also are synthetic gloves for personnel who are allergic to rubber.

Cystoscopes

Cystoscopes, urethroscopes, proctoscopes and other such instruments containing delicate lenses cannot be sterilized by heat, owing to the unequal expansion of glass and metal. They should not be subjected to contact with alcohol, which will loosen the cement with which the lenses are fixed. In urology and proctology, the organisms encountered most frequently are of the vegetative type. Because of this, the disinfection of scopes can be accomplished safely by immersing them in a solution of Zephiran 1:1,000 for a half hour. Scopes should be rinsed thoroughly in sterile cold water before use.† If the scope has the lens held in place by a heat-resistant plastic compound, such an instrument can be autoclaved.

Ureteral and Radio-opaque Catheters

Ureteral and radio-opaque catheters made of nylon can be sterilized by autoclaving for 30 minutes at 250° F. For catheters which are not stable in high temperatures, submerge in aqueous solution of quaternary ammonium compound for the recommended time. It is important to flush the catheter with the disinfectant in order to remove any air bubbles which would hinder the sterilizing process. Before use, the catheter should be washed on the inside and the outside with sterile water or saline. Many catheters are plastic and disposable, thereby eliminating the need for cleaning and sterilizing.

Radium Tubes

Tubes containing radium are disinfected when necessary by soaking in a chemical disinfectant. Tubes should be rinsed in sterile water before use. Radium in any shape or form always must be handled with forceps, never with the hands, even though gloved. Unprotected undue exposure of any part of the body may result in a burn.

Operating Motors

Motors for bone surgery are contained in removable outer shells that can be sterilized by autoclaving. The chuck, all drills, doweling apparatus, saws, etc., can be autoclaved. The motor must not get wet. No attempt is made to sterilize it. Oil should be applied as directed. Motors that can be autoclaved in toto are most generally used.

BIBLIOGRAPHY AND SELECTED READING
Books

Alexander, E. L.: Care of the Patient in Surgery (including techniques), ed. 3, St. Louis, Mosby, 1958.

Cutler, E. C., and Zollinger, R.: Atlas of Surgical Operations, ed. 2, New York, Macmillan, 1949.

Davis and Geck Suture Manual, Danbury, Conn., Amer. Cyanamid Co., 1963.

Ethicon Suture Handbook, Somerville, N. J., Ethicon, Inc., 1958.

Guest, P. G., Sikora, V. W., and Lewis, B.: Static Electricity in Hospital Operating Suites, Bulletin 520, Bureau of Mines, U. S. Government Printing Office, 1953.

Hall, E. D.: Surgical Instrument Guide for Nurses, New York, Weck, 1954.

Madden, J. L.: Atlas of Technics in Surgery, New York, Appleton, 1958.

Manual of Operative Procedure, ed. 11, Somerville, N. J., Ethicon, Inc., 1958.

---

* For more detailed information, see Walter, C., and Errera, D. W.: Care and Sterilization of Rubber Gloves, Hosp. Topics 35:101, Aug., 1957.

† Note: For the disinfection of scopes and catheters when tubercle bacillus or spores are present, see Spaulding, E. H., and Emmons, E. K.: Chemical disinfection, Am. J. Nursing 58:1241, 1958.

Perkins, J. J.: Principles and Methods of Sterilization, Springfield, Ill., Thomas, 1956.

Recommended Safe Practice for Hospital Operating Rooms, NFPA, No. 56, ed. 7, Boston, National Fire Protection Assn., 1956.

Walter, C. W.: Aseptic Treatment of Wounds, New York, Macmillan, 1948.

Articles

Adams, R., and Fraser, R.: Plastic skin drapes, Am. J. Nursing, **59:**845-847, June, 1959.

Barrett, R. H.: Explosion hazards in the operatting room, Hosp. Topics **33:** 86-88, Oct., 1955.

Barton, J.: What would you do in case of operating room explosion? Modern Hospital **86:** 51-53, 1956.

Beck, W. C.: Justified faith in surgical drapes (waterproof paper drapes), Am. J. Surg. **105:**560-562, Apr., 1963.

Creber, I.: Safety measures in the operating room, Nursing Outlook **6:**528-531, Sept., 1958.

Fire in the operating room, Nursing Outlook, **5:** 412-413, 1957.

Gale, D., and others: Re-evaluation of scrub technic for preoperative disinfection of the surgeon's hands, Ann. Surg. **155:**107-118, 1962.

Griffin, N. L.: Preventing fires and explosions in the operating room, Am. J. Nursing **53:**809-812, 1953.

Prioleau, W. H.: Uncovered scalp hair as a source of contamination, Hosp. Topics **36:** 107, Feb., 1958.

Riley, R. L.: Protective measures—reasonable or ritualistic? Nursing Outlook **7:**38-39, Jan., 1959.

Rockwell, V. T.: Surgical hand scrubbing, Am. J. Nurs. **63:**75-81, June, 1963.

Shaw, W. M.: Simple method of electrically grounding personnel in the operating rooms, Anesthesiology **17:**621-623, 1956.

Walter, C.: Patient safety in the operating room, Hosp. Topics **29:**50-54, July, 1951.

Wiltrakis, G. A.: Safety in the operating room, Hosp. Topics **31:**64, Jan., 1953.

Wolff, E. L.: Developing procedures for draping patients, Am. J. Nursing **56:**590-593, 1956.

17

The Postoperative Patient

The prime objective of postoperative nursing care is to assist the patient in his return to normal function as quickly, safely and comfortably as possible.

Considerable effort should be expended on *anticipation* and *prevention,* if possible, of difficulties in the postoperative period. The nursing care of the patient after operation is second in importance only to the operation itself. The knowledge, the skill and the ability required by the nurse make this type of nursing one of the most satisfying. She is a most valuable person to the patient, to his family and to the surgeon.

RECOVERY ROOM

The recovery room is a unit on the same floor as or near the operating rooms, where there is a concentration of (1) nurses who are especially prepared in caring for the immediate postoperative patient; (2) anesthesiologists and surgeons; (3) special eqiupment, medications and replacement fluids and (4) patients who are under anesthesia or are recovering from it. With this setting, the newly operated patient is given the best care available by those best qualified to give it.

The room should be quiet, neat and clean; unnecessary equipment should be removed. Many units are equipped with shelf space running the length of the wall, thus eliminating the use of small mobile tables which often are where they are least needed. Other features of this room might be: (1) walls and ceilings painted in soft pleasing colors, (2) indirect lighting, (3) soundproof ceiling and (4) equipment which controls or eliminates noise, e.g., synthetic emesis basins, rubber bumpers on beds and tables and so forth, as well as isolated quarters (glass encased) for noisy patients. These seemingly luxurious features may be added at little extra cost, yet psychologically they are of real value to the patient.

Equipment will include every type of breathing aid: oxygen, laryngoscopes, tracheotomy sets, bronchial instruments, catheters, mechanical ventilators and suction equipment; another necessity is equipment for meeting circulatory needs, such as blood pressure apparatus, parenteral equipment, universal donor blood, plasma expanders, intravenous trays and cut-down trays, cardiac arrest equipment, defibrillator, venous catheters and tourniquets. Surgical dressing materials, narcotics and emergency drugs should be available also.

The recovery bed should be one which affords easy access to the patient, is safe, easily movable, can assume Trendelenburg and reverse Trendelenburg position easily and which possesses features which facilitate care, such as available receptacles for intravenous poles, side guards, wheel brakes and chart storage rack (Fig. 75).

The temperature of the room should be about 68° F. to 70° F. during the day and about 60° F. at night. There should be an abundance of fresh air but no draughts.

A patient remains in this unit until he has reacted from the anesthetic agent, that is, has a stable blood pressure, good air passage and a reasonable degree of consciousness.

Some hospitals have set up an "Intensive Care Unit" to which are admitted all patients requiring special care. These include those who have recovered from anesthesia but who demand intensive care, patients from other areas of the hospital who require special care, e.g., those with cardiac problems, hemiplegia, gastrointestinal bleeding and burns, and others in critical condition. The equipment is similiar to that described for the Recovery Room, and the nursing staff is specially trained to the care of critically ill patients.

271

REMOVING PATIENT FROM OPERATING TABLE

The removal of the patient from the operating table to the bed or the stretcher should be done with the least possible delay and exposure. Exposure of the perspiring patient predisposes to pulmonary complications and postoperative shock. The site of the operation should be kept in mind every time a newly operated patient is moved. Many wounds are closed under considerable tension, and every effort should be made not to place any further strain on the sutures. Thus, in patients in whom a thyroidectomy has been performed, the head should not be allowed to hyperextend; in breast amputations, the arm of the operated side should be held close to the body; in nephrectomy, the patient should not be allowed to lie on the affected side; and so on.

Attention has been called to the problem of serious arterial hypotension which may occur when a patient is moved from a lithotomy position to a horizontal position, from lateral to supine, from prone to supine and even from movement of the anesthetized patient to the stretcher; it must be done slowly and carefully.

As soon as the patient is placed on the stretcher or bed, he is covered with lightweight blankets that have been arranged previously on the stretcher. The wet and soiled gown and socks should be removed, a dry gown applied, and the bedding tucked in along the sides as well as at the bottom. On the stretcher the patient is held with straps above the knees and the elbows. The straps serve the double purpose of securing the blankets and of restraining the patient should he pass through a stage of excitement as he recovers from the anesthetic. Siderails should be raised to the position affording protection.

PRINCIPLES OF IMMEDIATE POSTOPERATIVE NURSING CARE

Transfer of the postoperative patient from surgery to the recovery room is the responsibility of the anesthesiologist, with some member of the special care unit in attendance. If a nurse has been assigned to a par-

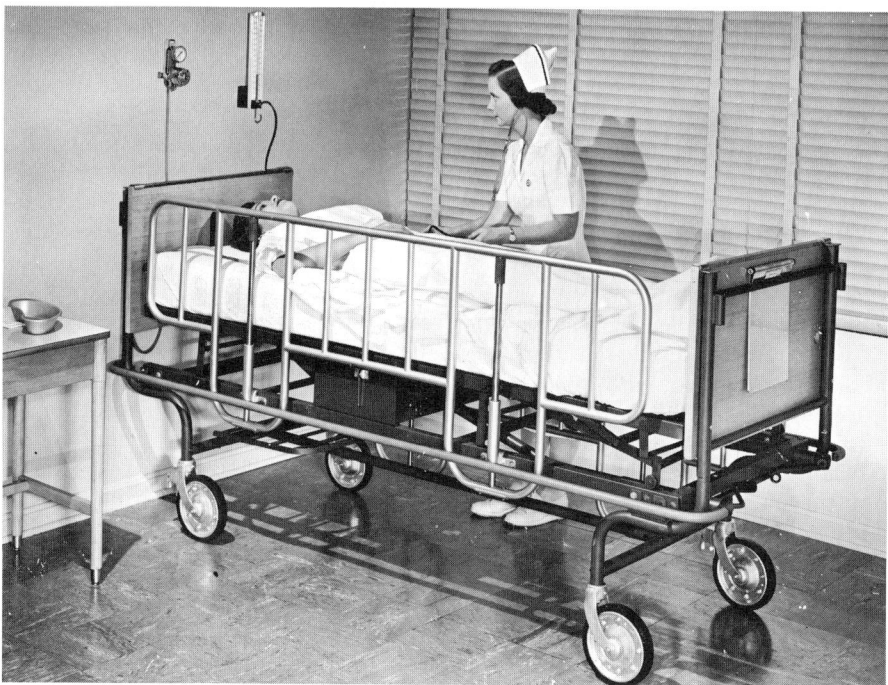

FIG. 75. Recovery bed in position for use with vital postoperative equipment. (Hill-Rom Co., Batesville, Ind.)

ticular patient, she would assist also. The nurse needs to know what operation was performed, any untoward problem which has occurred in the operating room that may have a bearing on postoperative care, and what pathology was encountered (if a malignancy, whether the patient or his family know). She needs to know the patient's present condition, complications that might develop and special symptoms to watch for. She should be provided with immediate postoperative orders in writing. In most hospitals a physician remains in the unit while the nurse checks (1) the patient's blood pressure, pulse and respirations and (2) his airway, tubing, drains, catheters, infusions and other supportive aids as may have been instituted in the operating room.

The chief immediate postoperative hazards are those of shock and anoxemia due to respiratory difficulties. Shock can be avoided largely by the timely administration of intravenous fluids and blood and by appropriate drugs. The *respiratory difficulties* may be treated as they arise, or better, the patient can be treated so that they do not arise. These disturbances are confined almost entirely to those patients who are under prolonged or deep anesthesia. Patients given local anesthesia, nitrous oxide or ethylene usually are "awake" a few minutes after leaving the operating room. However, those patients having prolonged anesthesia usually are completely unconscious, with all muscles relaxed. This relaxation extends to the muscles of the pharynx; therefore, when the patient lies on his back the lower jaw and the tongue fall backward, and the air passages close more or less completely (Fig. 77). The patient gives evidence of this difficulty in breathing by choking, noisy and irregular respirations, and in a short time a blue duskiness (cyanosis) of the skin appears. The treatment of this complication is to push forward on the angle of the lower jaw as if to push the lower teeth in front of the upper

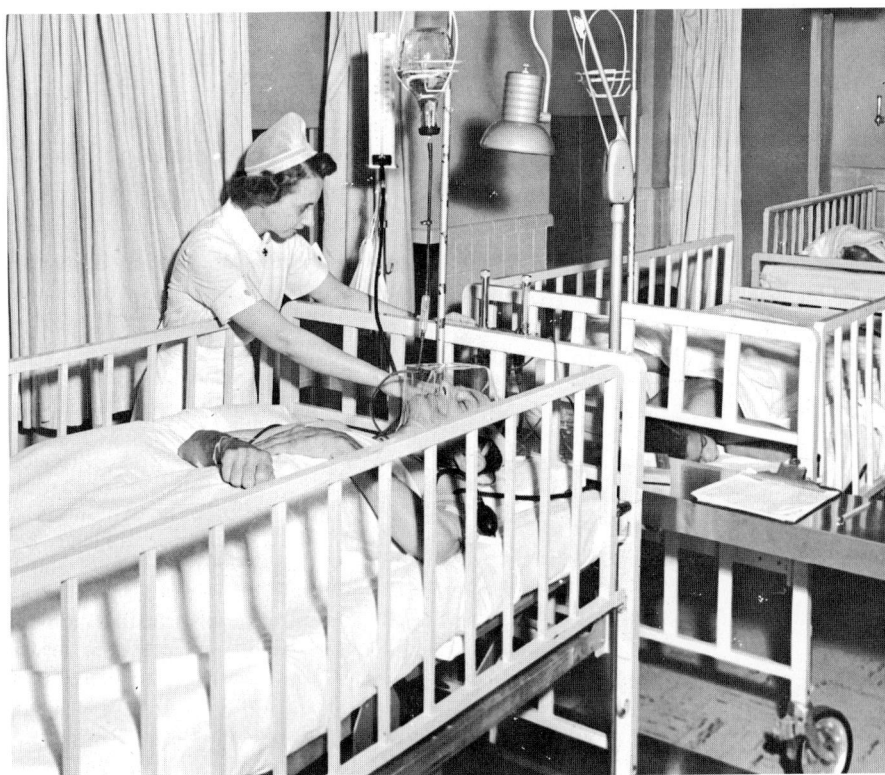

Fig. 76. Recovery room.

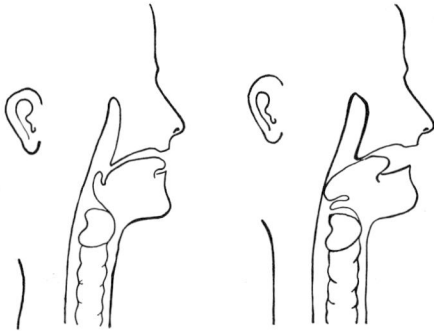

FIG. 77. Respiratory obstruction. (*Left*) With the tone of muscles normal, the tongue is in its usual position. (*Right*) With the muscles relaxed, the chin drops back, and the tongue comes in contact with the posterior wall of the pharynx, thereby shutting off the respiratory passages. (Greisheimer, Esther: The physiological effects of anesthesia, Am. J. Nursing *49*:338)

(Fig. 78). This maneuver pulls the tongue forward and opens the air passages. At times it may be necessary to grasp the tongue between gauze and pull it forward for a time. This prevents the respiratory obstruction, and the maneuver should be continued when necessary until the patient has regained reflex functions sufficiently to carry on normal respiration.

Often the anesthesiologist leaves a hard rubber or plastic "airway" in the mouth or a rubber nasal catheter in the nose. By both devices a patent airway is maintained. Such a device should not be removed until the patient expresses a desire to have it removed (Figs. 79 and 80).

Not infrequently the respiratory difficulty is produced by an excessive secretion of mucus. Turning the head to the side will allow the collected fluid to escape from the side of the mouth. If vomiting occurs, the head should be turned sharply to the side and the vomitus collected in the emesis basin. The face should be wiped with gauze or paper wipes.

A very important point for the nurse to remember is that the only sure way of knowing whether a patient is breathing or not is to place the palm of her hand over the nose and the mouth of the patient in order to feel the exhaled breath. Movements of the thorax and the diaphragm do not necessarily mean that a patient is breathing. Mucus or vomitus obstructing the pharynx or the trachea should be aspirated with a nasal catheter introduced into the nasopharynx or the oropharynx. In most recovery rooms, wall suction or suction machines are available for this purpose. The introduction of the catheter into the nasopharynx or the oropharynx is not dangerous, and the catheter can be introduced safely a distance of 6 to 8 inches if secretions are obtained at this level. Oxygen may be given by mask, tent or intranasally.

Nursing Principles During Recovery from Anesthesia

A nurse should be in constant attendance while the patient is recovering from anes-

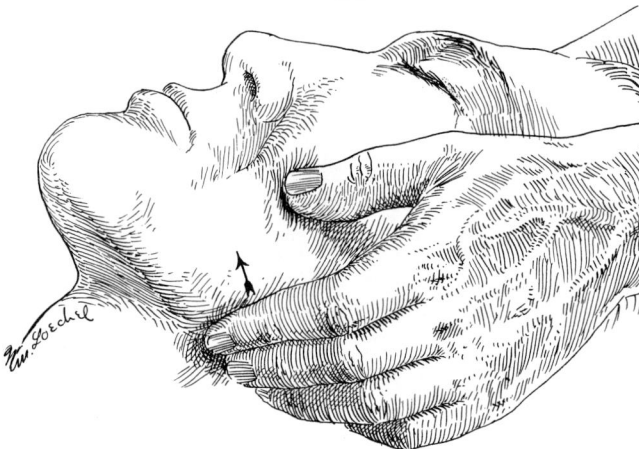

FIG. 78. Position of hand to hold the jaw forward after inhalation of anesthesia. Note that the fingers are placed behind the angle of the jaw, and the direction of the arrow shows the direction of pressure being exerted on the jaw. As the jaw is pushed forward the tongue is brought forward so as to keep an open airway. This is important, especially after operation under general anesthesia in children, for instance, in tonsillectomy.

FIG. 79. Diagrammatic view to show methods by which an airway prevents respiratory difficulty after anesthesia. The airway passes over the base of the tongue and delivers air into the pharynx in the region of the epiglottis. Patients are often brought from the operating room with an airway in place. This should remain in place until the patient recovers sufficiently to breathe normally. Usually, as the patient regains consciousness, the airway causes irritation; then it should be removed.

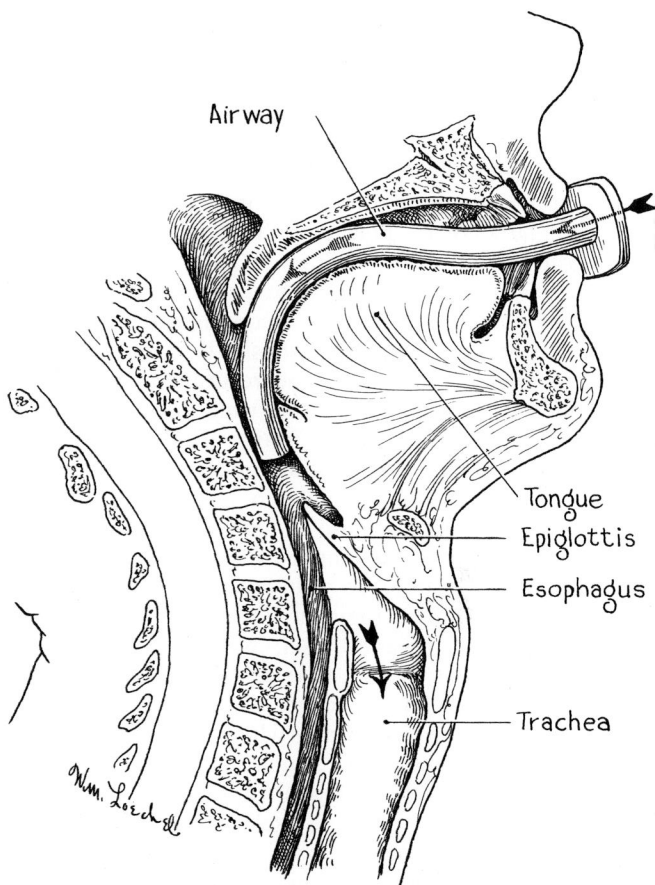

thesia. *Never leave a patient alone, even for an instant.* The following are her chief responsibilities:

1. Maintain a patent airway (discussed in section immediately preceding this).

2. Carry out any "stat" orders immediately. This usually refers to drug or oxygen therapy.

3. Turn the patient's head to the side when he vomits. Wipe the lips and the mouth with paper wipes or gauze. Note the amount and the nature of the vomitus and record them. Frequent aspiration of the nasopharynx and the oropharynx may be indicated. A clean rubber or plastic catheter is essential for this, and a basin of water for cleansing the suction tip. Caution is necessary in suctioning the throats of patients who have had tonsillectomies, since irritation of the operative area may cause bleeding or

added discomfort. Moisten the lips to relieve thirst.

4. Observe the patient for signs of respiratory obstruction, shock and hemorrhage. The chief guides are the appearance of the patient, the pulse, the respiration and the temperature. The pulse and the respiration should be counted at frequent intervals for the first 2 hours, and every half hour for the next 2 hours. Thereafter they may be taken less frequently if they remain stable. The blood pressure is taken as often as ordered. A temperature of over 100° or under 97° F., respirations of over 30 or under 16 and a systolic blood pressure of under 90 are usually considered reportable at once. Make notes on the general condition of the patient —for example, his color, good or cyanotic; skin, cold and clammy, warm and moist; excessive mucus in the throat and in the nostrils.

5. Position. Until the patient regains consciousness, the bed is kept flat. Unless contraindicated, the unconscious patient is positioned on his side with a pillow at his back and with his chin extended to minimize aspiratory danger. His knees are flexed to reduce strain on the abdominal sutures. If indicated, he may be placed in Trendelenburg position to prevent or treat shock.

6. Keep the patient as quiet and as comfortable as possible. When he is coming out of the anesthesia he may be restless. If it is at all possible, he should not be restrained, but he must be protected from injuring himself. Usually an infusion is running. If the arm is splinted, the needle will not be dislodged. However, the patient can pull the needle out with his free hand. Patients who have had hyoscine (scopolamine) or Amytal before operation should be watched closely for several hours after they have recovered from the effects of the anesthesia. Not infrequently, these drugs cause a type of delirium. Patients have been known to get out of bed and do other injurious things while under their influence. When the patient is fully conscious, deep breathing and turning every hour are necessary to prevent atelectasis or other pulmonary complications.

7. Attach any drainage apparatus when drainage is to be collected in a bottle—for example, from cholecystostomy or choledochostomy tubes, catheters, enterostomy drains

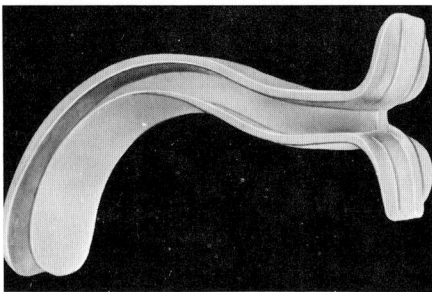

Fig. 80. The Berman Disposable Oral Airway is made of polyethylene and features a central partition which leaves either side free for easy insertion of catheters and easy cleaning. It is inexpensive enough to permit the use of a fresh, uncontaminated airway for each patient.

and chest tubes. In case of underwater drainage tubes, such as those used after thoracotomy, clamps should be available to clamp the tube in order to prevent air from entering the chest if the bottle is accidentally broken or the apparatus disconnected.

8. Begin postoperative treatment as ordered—for example, attach nasogastric tube to suction-drainage apparatus.

9. Inspect dressings from time to time to detect signs of undue hemorrhage or abnormal drainage. Reinforce dressings, if necessary, making note of time of application, on nurse's record.

10. Report any alarming or peculiar symptoms to the surgeon at once. This includes any mental phenomena or uneasiness on the part of the patient. A patient's statements concerning his condition never should be disregarded entirely.

11. Keep an intelligent and accurate record. The volume and the character of the intake and the output must be charted conscientiously. (See Fig. 90.)

The Patient's Postoperative Symptoms

Often the inexperienced nurse will be at a loss to differentiate between important and unimportant symptoms; and, in fact, the experienced nurse sometimes may be puzzled as to whether or not to notify the surgeon of a certain change in condition. The safest plan always is to call for advice when in doubt. However, in order to be able to decide intelligently, there are a few general rules that may be of some assistance. Of course, any severe symptom always is important. Any apparently slight symptom that tends to recur repeatedly or to increase in severity should be regarded as significant—for example, hiccough may or may not be of importance, depending on the duration. A symptom seemingly may be of no consequence in itself but when associated with other definite changes may foretell danger; for example, a repeated sigh means nothing, but, when accompanied by great restlessness, increasing pallor, rising pulse rate and so forth, it becomes one of the clinical signs of dangerous hemorrhage. Any progressive and steady change for the worse in the general condition of the patient, even with no outstanding symptoms evident, is of the gravest

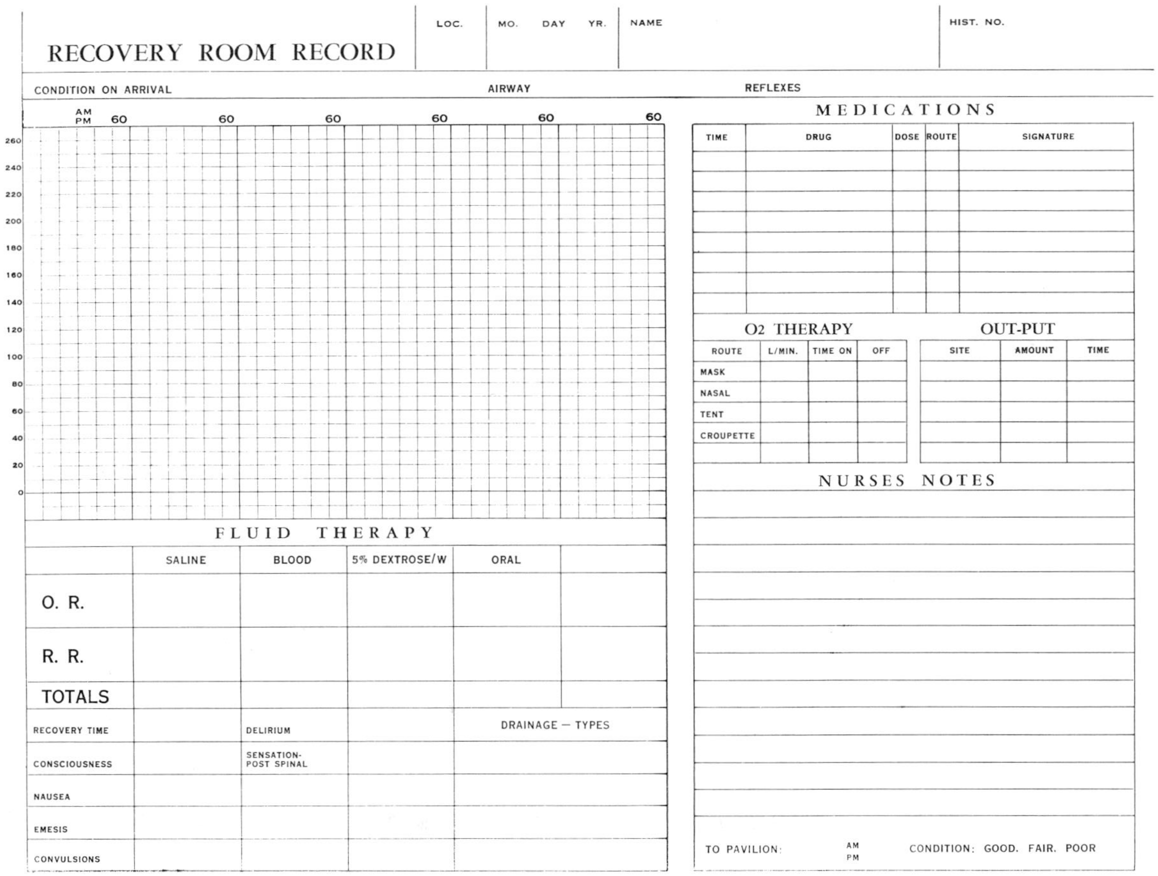

Fig. 81. A rapid visual appraisal of the patient's immediate postoperative condition is available from this concise chart. (The New York Hospital, New York, N. Y.)

importance. And, as has been mentioned already, the patient's complaints and statements never should be passed over without investigation.

If the physician in charge of the patient is to be notified for any reason, be sure to have all necessary information literally at your fingertips before going to the telephone. Know the latest temperature, the pulse and the respiration figures, and always take the patient's chart and the nurse's record with you to the telephone, in order to refer to them should occasion arise. Learn to state the patient's condition concisely and accurately, and be prepared to answer all questions intelligently.

NEEDS OF THE PATIENT RETURNING TO COMPLETE CONSCIOUSNESS

As the patient returns to consciousness, he usually expresses concern about the outcome of the operation, his family, and his awareness of discomfort. Brief but appropriate information can be given to him. When his condition permits, a close member of his family may see him for a few moments. Thus, the family is reassured, and the patient feels more secure.

Hypodermic injections of morphine, Dilaudid, Demerol or Methadon often are ordered for pain and restlessness. Such an order usually is written "p.r.n." (Latin for "pro re nata"—as required by circumstances) for a certain number of doses. The time of administration frequently is left to the judgment of the nurse, but she should realize that pain in the first 24 hours after an operation requires relief by narcotics, and these drugs should not be withdrawn when the patient is in pain. There is seldom any method of relieving pain in the operative region, but the following suggestions may be useful in assuaging general discomfort temporarily and rendering the hypodermic medication more effectual when finally it is given:

1. **Change position.** Give added support with pillows. A small pillow in the hollow of the back is comforting.

2. **Encourage deep breathing.** A most important point in the care of the patient after the anesthesia is to prevent pulmonary complications. This is another significant reason why the *radical alteration in the position* of the patient is important. He is able to expand his lungs better when this is done. Patients are *encouraged to cough* in an effort to clear the respiratory passages of secretions. A third method of causing gas exchange in the lung is to encourage the patient to *take deep breaths*. This may be done by the use of a blow bottle. This is merely a gallon bottle half filled with water. A length of rubber tubing with a mouthpiece is attached to the bottle and the patient is asked to "blow bubbles" for 5 minutes in every hour. Unless the patient is told why it is important for him to do this simple procedure, the nurse may not get his cooperation. Another method of stimulating deep respirations is by the use of carbon dioxide inhalations. This may be carried out by using a face mask attached to a gas tank or simply by instructing the patient to blow in and out of a paper bag. In a fourth method the patient should be shown how to take a deep breath, hold it a second and then give a hard cough as he starts to expel the air. On the second or the third exercise of this kind, he will often expectorate suddenly a viscid mass of mucus and clear his lung.

3. **Wash the face and the hands.** Cold cloths applied to the forehead often are soothing.

4. **Give a mouthwash.** At the same time wipe the lips with a cool gauze sponge when water by mouth is not permitted.

5. **Rub the back with lotion or alcohol.** The extremities may be stroked very lightly with alcohol. *They never should be rubbed vigorously*. To do so may dislodge a thrombus and result in embolism and death.

6. **If permissible give water in small quantities when nausea ceases.** If small amounts are retained by the patient, the quantity given at one time may be increased gradually. Water is best either hot or cold; otherwise, it is likely to cause nausea. There are times when a large glass of water will do a patient no harm, even when he is nauseated, but this never should be given without the proper authority. Patients usually ask for cracked ice, and usually it does no harm in small amounts. If orders are that the patient is to have nothing by mouth,

FIG. 82. Position for immediate postoperative patient which permits drainage of mucus from the mouth and general relaxation. (Winters, M. C.: Protective Body Mechanics in Daily Life and in Nursing, Philadelphia, Saunders)

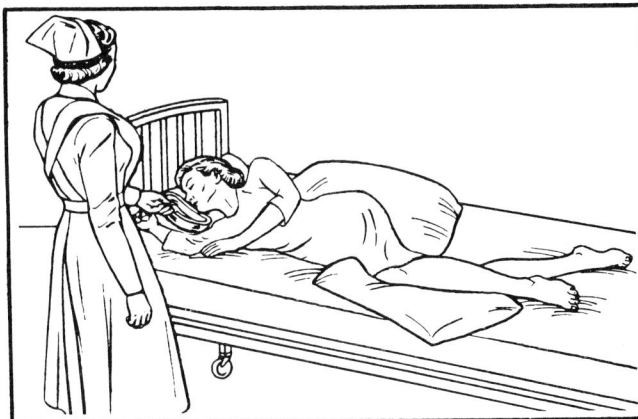

cracked ice wrapped in a piece of gauze is refreshing and soothing to the lips.

7. Remove blankets. If the patient has been put between blankets, they should be removed on complete recovery from the anesthesia—when the temperature, the pulse and the respirations are within normal limits; or they may be removed promptly but carefully when they are the cause of excessive perspiration. Recovery beds should be made in such a manner that the patient is left between sheets when these extra blankets are withdrawn. Cool sheets usually are a most gratifying change and often very soothing. However, care must be taken that the change is not too abrupt: if the patient complains of excessive heat, remove the under blanket first and the upper blanket a little later. In warm weather too many blankets will cause marked perspiration and the consequent loss of a large amount of fluid. Therefore, it is advisable as a rule not to use blankets on the recovery bed during warm periods in the summer months. Remember that patients who have been anesthetized are susceptible to chills and draughts. Remember, also, that the obese patient perspires profusely and so loses fluid and salt much more rapidly than the patient who is of normal weight.

8. Elimination. URINATION. The length of time a patient may be permitted to go without voiding after operation varies considerably with the type of operation performed. Following gynecologic and abdominal operations patient catheterization may be required at the end of 8 or 10 hours (sometimes sooner), and in others it may be put off for from 16 to 18 hours. Generally speaking, every effort must be made to avoid the use of the catheter. Exhaust all known methods to aid the patient in voiding—let water run, apply heat and so forth. Never give a patient a cold bedpan. When a patient complains of not being able to use the bedpan, some surgeons permit the use of the commode rather than resort to catheterization. Of course, this applies only to suitable cases. Male patients sometimes are permitted to sit up or stand beside the bed, but this should not be allowed unless an orderly is in attendance to prevent any accidents from falling or fainting. All urine, whether voided or catheterized, must be measured and the amount noted on the nurse's record. A separate intake and output chart (p. 288) should be kept on all aged and all very ill patients. (See also p. 304, Urinary Retention.)

DEFECATION. Each defecation should be recorded. If the bowels do not move spontaneously every other day, a cleansing enema usually is given. As a rule, cathartics are not given to postoperative patients, especially if the operation has been on the abdomen.

9. Psychological Support. Almost all postoperative surgical patients have need for psychological support during the immediate postoperative period. The questions posed by an awakening patient often indicate his deep feelings and thoughts. Perhaps he shows concern about the operation and the findings or about his future—whatever his expression, the nurse should be in a position to answer his query reassuringly without going into a discussion of details. The immediate postoperative period is not the time for dis-

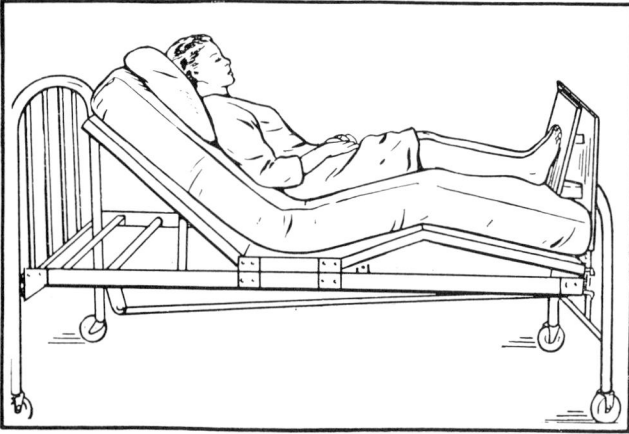

FIG. 83. In Fowler's position the patient's position is arranged so that flexion of hips and knees correspond to the bend in the mattress provided by the gatch. The trunk is in good alignment. Foot support adds to comfort and helps prevent patient from sliding down in bed. This position is contraindicated in the immediate postoperative period and in certain cardiovascular conditions. (Winters, M. C.: Protective Body Mechanics in Daily Life and in Nursing, Philadelphia, Saunders)

cussion of operative findings or prognosis. On the other hand, these questions ought not to be dismissed lightly, for they may offer clues which suggest the method to select in directing future treatment and rehabilitation. The function of the recovery room nurse cannot be limited to bedside procedures, safety measures and the relief of pain; an understanding regarding the significance of psychological support is also important. If the nurse has never seen the patient before, a definite handicap is immediately presented. The nurse who knows the patient and accompanies him through the immediate preoperative and operative experiences is in a unique position to offer valuable support. In the absence of such continuous care by one nurse, pertinent nurses' notes on the chart will help the recovery room nurse to recognize the particular needs of each individual patient.

BODY ALIGNMENT AND GOOD BODY MECHANICS

(Also see: Rehabilitation, Chapter 21, p. 361.) Poor posture for the surgical patient can result in the development of complications with subsequent delay in convalescence. These include pulmonary complications which result from inadequate chest expansion, improper drainage from body cavities, contractures, decubiti, circulatory impairment and urinary and gastrointestinal difficulties.

The principles of proper body alignment and good body mechanics are an essential part of good surgical nursing. These apply to the nurse as well as to her patient.

Dorsal Position

The patient lies on his back without elevation of the head. In most cases this is the position in which the patient is placed immediately after operation. The head usually is turned to one side to facilitate easy evacuation of vomitus and to prevent its aspiration into the lungs. Bed covers should not restrict the movement of the toes and the feet of the patient.

This position is maintained until the patient has recovered from the effects of the anesthetic and has regained sufficient reflex activity to swallow, cough and so forth. This position may be employed to advantage many times when the necessity for drainage does not demand the Fowler position. It is believed that when the patient is flat in bed, respiration often is more free and turning is easier, advantages that are important in the prevention of respiratory complications.

Head Low Dorsal (Trendelenburg) Position

The patient lies on his back with or without a pillow under his head, and the foot of the bed is raised from 1 foot to 3 feet. This position increases the blood flow to the cerebral centers. It is indicated in the treatment of shock and hemorrhage, both before and after operation.

Sims or Lateral Position

The patient lies on either side with the upper arm forward. The under leg lies slightly flexed, the upper leg is flexed at the thigh and the knee. The head is supported on a pillow, and a second pillow is placed longitudinally under the flexed knee. This position is used when it is desirable to have the patient change position frequently, to aid in the drainage of cavities, as of the chest, the abdomen and so forth, and to prevent postoperative pulmonary, respiratory and circulatory complications. (See Fig. 82.)

Fowler Position

Of all the positions ordered for a patient, perhaps the most common, as well as the most difficult to maintain, is the Fowler. The difficulty in most instances lies in trying to make the patient fit the bed rather than having the bed conform to the needs of the patient. The patient's trunk is raised to form an angle of from 60° to 70° with the horizontal (Fig. 83). This is a comfortable sitting position. Patients with abdominal drainage usually are put in Fowler position as soon as they have recovered consciousness, but great caution must be observed in raising the bed. It is not an unusual occurrence for a patient to feel faint after the raising of the head of the bed, and for this reason a close watch must be kept on the pulse rate and the color. If the patient complains of any dizziness, the bed must be lowered at once. However, if the condition of the patient is good, the head of the bed may be raised within 1 or 2 hours. There is less slipping of the patient when the knee area is elevated before the head is raised.

The nurse must determine whether or not the patient is in correct position and comfortable. Often very short people are most uncomfortable in the ordinary hospital bed and must be supported by pillows. It is advisable to place a support against the feet to prevent slipping down in bed, to prevent footdrop and to make the patient feel more secure.

When the Fowler position is ordered for a patient, it is the nurse's responsibility to see that this position is maintained at all times. It is not sufficient to arrange the patient in a faultless manner: he must remain so. No matter how correctly placed or how well supported by pillows the patient is, he will slip down in the course of time and frequent lifting up in bed and readjustment of the pillows will be necessary. Another

significant reason for maintaining good body posture is that it affords better functioning of all organs, including those of respiration.

Jackknife or Semi-Fowler Position

This position is one used to relieve tension following the repair of inguinal or abdominal hernia. It is produced by raising the head of the patient from 10 to 12 inches and flexing the knees.

The Patient's Comfort and Changes of Position

Hampered by dressings, splints or drainage apparatus, the patient very frequently is quite unable to shift his position. Lying constantly in the same position may be the cause of pressure sores or hypostatic pneumonia, to mention only two of the more serious resulting complications. Turning a pillow from one side to another presents a cooler side as it touches the patient. Proper support for the arms and the hands offers a measure of comfort. A foot support encourages the patient to stretch his foot muscles and spread his toes, which is a relaxing maneuver. The helpless patient must be turned from side to side at least every 2 hours, and he should have his position changed as soon as he becomes uncomfortable.

When a patient is unable to turn himself, it may be necessary for the nurse to have one or two assistants. The number of persons needed depends on whether the patient must be moved in one unit or not and on his height and weight. At all times, the nurse should practice good body mechanics herself. Often back strain can be prevented if, instead of bending at the waist, the nurse can lift her patient with her back erect, bending at the knees and the hips.

EARLY POSTOPERATIVE AMBULATION

Almost all types of surgical patients are allowed and encouraged to be out of bed within 24 to 48 hours after operation. The advantages of early ambulation are seen in a reduction of postoperative complications. Atelectasis and hypostatic pneumonia are relatively infrequent when the patient is ambulatory. Ambulation increases respiratory exchange and aids in preventing stasis of bronchial secretions within the lung. Postoperative distention is almost absent, due to the increased tone of the gastrointestinal tract and the abdominal wall. Therefore, frequent enemata are unnecessary. Thrombophlebitis or phlebothrombosis are less frequent because ambulation increases the rate of circulation in the extremities, thereby preventing stasis of venous blood. Clinical as well as experimental evidence shows that the rate of healing in abdominal wounds is more rapid by early ambulation, and the occurrence of postoperative evisceration has been no greater than formerly: in some series of cases actually it has been less when the patient was allowed to be out of bed soon after operation. Statistics indicate that pain is decreased, as shown by the number of hypodermics required. Comparative records also indicate that the pulse rate and the temperature return to normal sooner when the patient attempts to regain his normal preoperative activity as quickly as possible.

Re-establishing a normal physiology includes a resumption of a full diet. Normal intestinal function returns in 2 or 3 days. This is indicated by the appearance of peristaltic sounds and the passage of gas. After this time the diet may be increased rapidly. In a few instances, a more adequate diet may be given earlier (usually, patients with operations on the extremities, following thyroidectomy, etc.). Finally, there are the further advantages to the patient of a shorter stay in the hospital, with the consequent lower expense.

Early ambulation should not be overdone. The condition of the patient must be the deciding factor. The very ill and feeble aged patient must be given every consideration. First of all, he must be placed almost upright in bed until all suggestion of dizziness has passed. This position can be obtained by raising the head of the bed. Then, he may be placed completely upright and turned so that his legs hang over the edge of the bed. After this preparation, he may be helped to stand beside his bed. When he has become accommodated to the upright position, he may take a few steps to a chair or around the bed. The nurse should be at his side to give support, both physical and moral. Care must be taken not to tire the patient, and the extent of the first few periods of ambulation should vary with the type of operation and the physical condition and the age of the patient.

Convalescent Bed Exercises

When early ambulation is not feasible due to circumstances already mentioned, *convalescent bed exercises* may accomplish to some extent the same desirable results. General exercises should begin as soon after operation as possible—preferably within the first 24 hours—and they should be done under supervision to ensure their adequacy. These exercises are done to prevent the development of contractures and other deformities as well as to permit the patient the fullest return of his functions:

1. Deep breathing exercises for complete lung expansion

2. Arm exercises through full range of motion, with specific attention to abduction and external rotation of shoulder

3. Hand and finger exercises

4. Foot exercises to prevent foot drop and toe deformities and to aid in maintaining good circulation

5. Exercises to prepare the patient for ambulation activities.

6. Abdominal and gluteal contraction exercises

POSTOPERATIVE DIET

Patients have nutritional and fluid needs even more after operation than before it. Although these requirements may be supplied fairly well by the intravenous administration of amino acids, glucose, saline and blood (see pp. 169-171), this method of feeding a patient is much less efficient than giving food by mouth.

In many instances, even though a major operation has been performed, there is no reason why a normal diet cannot be given. Thus, after a thyroidectomy, a breast amputation, a lung resection or a herniorrhaphy, the patient may receive a full diet if he desires it. The patient should be encouraged to eat normally, because many patients are afraid to eat. By eating a normal diet, many of the unpleasant "gas pains" and enemas can be avoided. However, food should not be forced on the unwilling patient. The desire of the patient for food is one of the best indications of a normal recovery.

Usually liquids are desired first by the patient after operation. They also are tolerated by him. Water, fruit juices and tea with lemon and sugar may be given in increasing amounts if vomiting does not occur. Fluids administered should be cool, not ice cold or tepid. The fluids supply relatively few calories. If fluids are tolerated well, gelatin, junket, custard and cornstarch pudding may be added gradually; even buttered toast, milk and creamed soups. As soon as the patient tolerates liquids well, solid food may be given.

CARE OF THE WOUND

Rigid Asepsis

The most important requisite for the successful care of wounds is rigid asepsis. Bacteria are excluded from wounds during the period of operation to the full extent of the facilities for sterility in the operating room. Organisms that enter the wound usually are destroyed by the natural powers of resistance of the body. Accidental wounds are potentially infected wounds. Therefore, the surgeon is concerned with the removal of as much of the infection as possible and with the protection of the wound from further invasion by bacteria.

Wound Classification

Wounds are classified as (1) incised, (2) contused, (3) lacerated or (4) puncture, according to the manner in which they were made.

Incised wounds are those made by a clean cut with a sharp instrument. They are made by the surgeon in every operation.

Contused wounds are made by blunt force and are characterized by considerable injury of the soft parts, hemorrhage and swelling.

Lacerated wounds are those with jagged, irregular edges, such as would be made by glass, barbed wire and so forth.

Puncture wounds have small openings in the skin, such as those made by a bullet, a knifestab and the like.

Clean wounds (those made aseptically) usually are closed by sutures after all bleeding points have been ligated carefully. All other wounds are potentially infected and cannot be closed until every effort has been made to remove all devitalized tissue and infection. Therefore, a formal operation is performed for the purpose of cutting out the infected and devitalized tissue. This operation is called *débridement*. Often it is well to insert a small drain before suturing the wound to prevent the collection of blood and lymph, which would retard healing if it were allowed to remain. (See p. 23, Reparative Process.)

The Purpose of Dressings

There is a trend* toward the elimination of dressings, either shortly after surgery or within the immediate postoperative period, wherever possible or feasible. On clean, dry incisions, it is noted that when the initial dressing (applied in the operating room) is removed, usually it is not replaced. Generally, initial dressings on clean, dry incisions are left in place until the sutures are removed, and if a dressing is replaced at all, its purpose is more an esthetic than a necessary one.

In the absence of dressings, a wound heals with fibrin. The apparent advantages of no dressings are that it: (1) eliminates the conditions necessary for growth of organisms (warmth, moisture and darkness), (2) allows for better observation and early detection of wound difficulties, (3) facilitates bathing, (4) tends to minimize the operative procedure, (5) avoids adhesive tape reaction, (6) appears to be more comfortable for the patient and facilitates his activity and (7) is economical.

A dressing is applied to a wound for one

* Adapted from Postoperative Wound Care Study Report, Department of Nursing, University of Chicago Clinics.

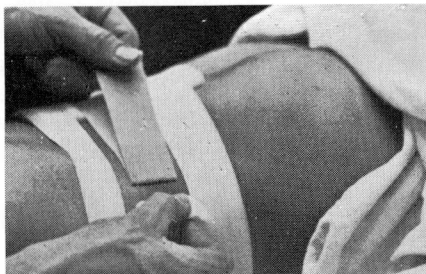

FIG. 84. Removing adhesive strips.

or more reasons: (1) to absorb drainage, (2) to prevent contamination from feces, vomitus and urine, (3) for splinting or immobilization of the wound, (4) to protect the wound from mechanical injury, (5) to promote hemostasis, as in a pressure dressing and (6) for the mental and physical comfort of the patient. Substitute materials, such as sprayed plastic dressings, are being tested, and the few observed seem to be providing satisfactory service for clean and dry incisions. Then, on clean, dry wounds it seems superfluous to be concerned with the ability of the dressing to absorb secretions, since there are practically no secretions to be absorbed. Texture, comfort and perhaps screening ability against micro-organisms (although this latter is a doubtful prerequisite) can be given more emphasis than power of absorption in such dressings. In spite of the advantages and the disadvantages mentioned above, most surgeons prefer to apply a dressing at the time of operation and a second dressing between 4 and 5 days later, after the removal of sutures. These dressings are purely protective from a mechanical point of view, and they give the patient a sense of security which is not present if wounds are treated without dressings.

Surgical Dressing Technic

The prerequisite to flawless surgical dressing technic is for surgeons and nurses to agree on a standard. Thereafter, it becomes a matter of repeated teaching and supervision to ensure that such handling of dressings actually is carried out.

Because of the dangers of contamination and spread of infection, the surgical dressing carriage as it has been used in the average hospital is not recommended as a safe adjunct in the changing of surgical dressings. In situations where such a cart is used by one nurse only, control over cross contamination may be minimized.* A more desirable and safe technic is to use a sterile dressing pack for each patient.† With this technic, a surgical dressing cart may be used as a stock

* Garrett, E. G.: The dressing nurse, Am. J. Nursing **61**:57, January, 1961.

† Suddarth, D. S.: Individual dressing packs, Am. J. Nursing **60**:991-992, July, 1960.

table to hold the individually wrapped sterile supplies, including individual flasks of antiseptic solution.

Nursing Responsibility

The surgical nurse should be available to assist the physician in the changing of dressings for several reasons:

1. The "team" working together assures the patient of expert care.

2. The nurse, as a witness to the dressing, is better informed concerning her patient and therefore can give him more intelligent care.

3. The nurse can obtain additional sterile materials as needed and can insure proper disposal of contaminated articles.

4. While all initial postoperative dressings are done properly only by the surgeon, subsequent applications may be done by the nurse.

5. The condition of surgical dressings should be noted on the patient's chart as carefully as any medication or treatment, and pertinent observations should be recorded by the nurse.

Dressing Procedure

Preparation of the Patient. The patient should be told that the surgeon is going to change the dressing, and that it is a simple procedure associated with little discomfort. *Dressings should not be done at mealtime.* If the patient is in an open unit, the curtains should be drawn to ensure his privacy. When the dressing has a foul odor or the patient is unusually squeamish, it is better to wheel his bed to the treatment room, away from other patients. He should not be exposed unduly; his sense of modesty should be respected.

Stitches or clips used to approximate the skin edges are of no value after the 5th, the 6th or the 7th day. The nurse should be prepared for the first dressing at that time.

Removal of Adhesive. The adhesive should be removed by pulling it parallel with the skin surface and not at right angles. (Fig. 84.) Nonirritating solvents are available which come in aerosol containers and aid in removing adhesive tapes painlessly and quickly. The nurse removes the old dressing by means of an unsterile forceps and places

FIG. 85. Nonallergic tape used to hold abdominal dressings. (Larson, P. N., M.D., Minneapolis, Minn.) (Minnesota, Mining and Manufacturing Co.)

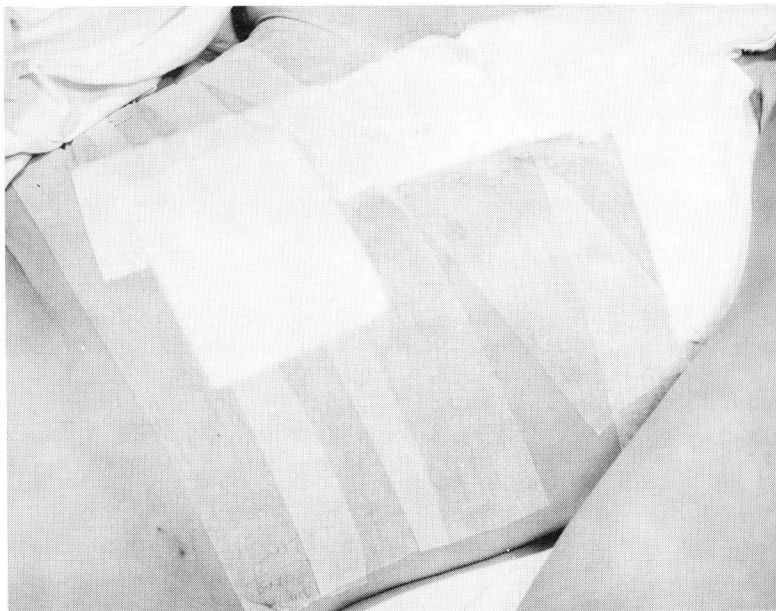

this dressing in a paper bag for easy disposal. She then hands the surgeon a sterile cover which becomes the sterile field.

A Routine Dressing. To carry out aseptic technic, the nurse must know how to handle the transfer forceps correctly. (See p. 244.) For the routine dressing, an individual pack usually contains scissors, forceps, hemostat and grooved director that has been sterilized in an envelope cover of muslin. When the tray has been properly opened, the nurse drops 2 or 3 sterile cotton balls on the sterile field if they are not already on the tray. Using a forceps, the surgeon grasps a cotton ball and holds it over the emesis basin as the nurse pours a small quantity of the desired antiseptic. After cleansing the wound and the surrounding skin with an antiseptic, the stitches are removed, and the nurse provides sterile gauze compresses and adhesive strips for the new dressing. A surgical tape is available which is useful for patients who are allergic to the rubber base in the usual adhesive tape. This 3M brand Micropore surgical tape is porous in structure and permits ventilation and prevents maceration. (Fig. 85.) Tension sutures are allowed to remain in place for a longer period of time in some instances.

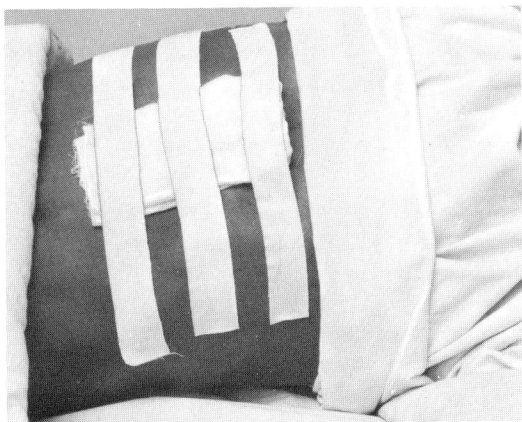

FIG. 86. Adhesive strips applied to abdominal wound. Note that sufficient gauze is exposed between adhesive to allow for inspection and ventilation.

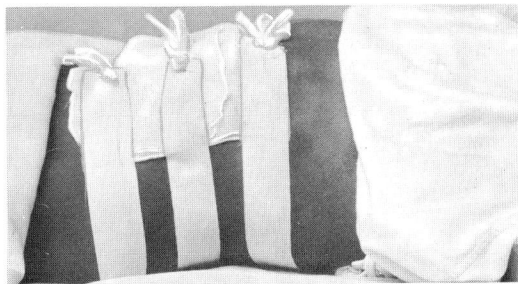

FIG. 87. Montgomery tape dressing, for use when dressings have to be changed frequently.

If there is any doubt concerning the sterility of an instrument or a dressing, it should be considered to be unsterile. In no circumstance should the nurse touch soiled dressings with her hands.

The Dressing of Draining Wounds. It may be necessary to dress draining wounds as soon as 24 hours after operation. Nothing causes a patient more unnecessary discomfort than a dressing saturated with drainage fluids. It dries on the edges and becomes stiff and scratchy, and the odor frequently is very offensive if not actually nauseating. The nurse may relieve such a situation by changing the outer layers of the dressing at frequent intervals between dressings.

When it is necessary to dress the wound daily, either adhesive with tapes or a laced dressing is more convenient than simple adhesive strips. (Figs. 86-88) These should not be applied so tightly that the dressings beneath are unable to retain drainage.

A scultetus binder also makes an effective, convenient dressing. (Fig. 89)

When the edges of the wound gape and the gauze has become adherent to the tissues, the patient may be spared considerable pain by moistening the dressings with peroxide of

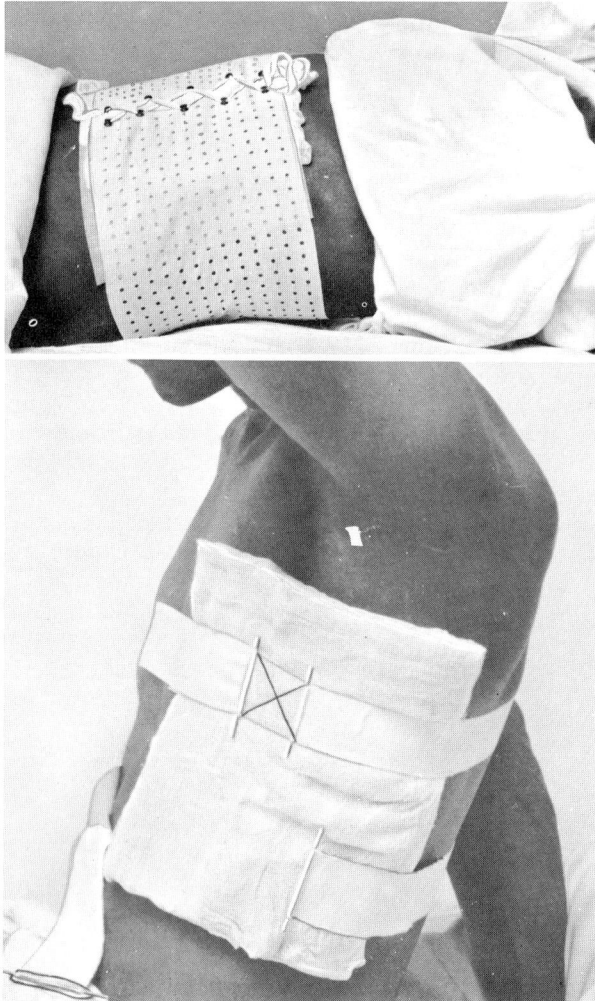

FIG. 88. (*Top*) Laced dressing. (*Bottom*) Adhesive matchstick dressing with rubber bands. For use when dressings have to be changed frequently.

Fig. 89. Scultetus binder. Dimensions of binder and method of sewing are shown, also the method of application of binder. The tails should overlap from below upward, and the binder should fit snugly.

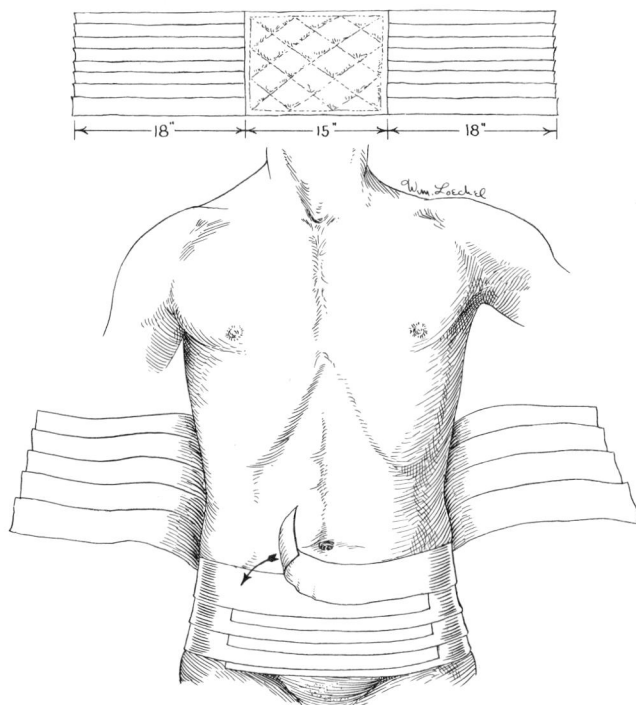

hydrogen. For this purpose a syringe and a basin containing the solution must be provided. As the surgeon applies the peroxide, the nurse should hold a waste pan to prevent the solution from soiling the bed.

When *drainage tubes* are being shortened, the nurse should have a sterile safety pin ready to insert in the new tube end. If the tubes are removed, the surgeon frequently inserts a piece of rubber tissue or packing to prevent too early a closing of the drainage tract. These materials should be at hand and ready for use.

The drainage from an infected wound frequently proves to be irritating to the surrounding skin. Often this situation may be avoided by the use of a protecting ointment or dressing. Petrolatum gauze and zinc oxide ointments are favorite preparations. When the discharge from the wound contains the digestive enzymes, as in pancreatic or intestinal fistulae, ileostomy and cecostomy wounds, more active measures to protect the skin must be taken. In some cases, the enzyme-containing secretion may be aspirated by constant suction. In others, the skin surrounding the wound may be protected by such adhering ointments as zinc oxide oint-

ment containing aluminum filings or by a creamy paste mixture of aluminum hydroxide gel and kaolin (Protogel, Wyeth) which is both soothing to the skin and a neutralizer of the enzymes in the secretions. These must be applied to an absolutely dry skin surface.

When a drainage tube is attached to drainage tubing and a bottle, it is necessary to check the tubing frequently for kinking, coiling and looping which would restrict the flow of drainage.

The Completion of a Dressing

Dressings are held in place by adhesive or Scotch tape. There are available many types and widths of adhesive tapes. The usual white adhesive tape is most frequently used in locations on the extremities or when seepage of secretions is a factor; waterproofed adhesive is available. A transparent adhesive without cloth backing also is available. Some patients who are sentitive to the adhesive material may be better treated by the use of Scotch tape which in many cases proves nonirritating.

Elastoplast (elastic adhesive bandage) is preferable for holding dressings in place over mobile areas, such as the neck or the extremities, or where pressure is required. When the dressing is completed, the soiled dressings are wrapped in the bag and deposited in the large covered utility can to await its removal to the incinerator.

CHARTS AND NURSES' RECORDS

To keep a record of all observations and treatments bearing on patient care is an essential function of the nurse (Fig. 90). Accuracy and neatness in the matter of charts and records usually bespeak thorough nursing with keen observation and attention to detail. For this reason, the record should be kept up to date. Such a nurse's report is worth more than one in which the whole record for the day is written in 5 minutes before the nurse reports to her successor.

In general, printing rather than script is

FORM M-241 3M 2-58

RHODE ISLAND HOSPITAL

FLUID BALANCE AND BURN CHART

Feb. 7, 19..

	INTAKE			OUTPUT				Urine SG and/or Chloride	Urine PH	Hmt.	Hemoglobin	OTHER
	P.O. Tube	I.V.	Other	Urine	Int. Tube	Vomitus	Other					
A.M. 8	30											
9												124/68 P-82
10	30									11.2	35%	
11		1000		400				1.010				
12	30											120/70 P-74
P.M. 1		1000										
2	30											
3		500		200								118/68 P-76
4	30				300		200					
8 hr. Total	150	2500		600	300		200					
5												
6	30											130/74 P-78
7												
8	30	1000		400				1.008				
9												130/74 P-76
10	30			200								
11												
12					250		150					128/72 P-70
16 hr. Total	240	3500		1200	550		350					
A.M. 1												
2												
3												122/70 P-72
4												
5												
6	30											120/68 P-74
7				600	275		100	1.012				
24 hr. Total	270	3500		1800	825		450					

Total Intake 3770 cc   Total Output 3075 cc

Weight (Kgm) (A.M.)   72 Kgm.

Balance   +695 cc

FIG. 90. Front and back of the chart used in the Intensive Care Unit—Rhode Island Hospital, Providence, R. I.

preferable since usually it is more legible. Statements should be concise, pertinent and brief. The recording of the reactions of a patient to a treatment may be more important for his future therapy than the treatment itself. Hence, significant conversation, facial expressions, and general behavior of an individual ought to be charted when such activities seem to be worthy of attention. Cultural practices of the patient which reflect past experiences and indicate future tendencies may affect future treatment; therefore, these should be recorded by the nurse. This will be of value not only to the physician but also to the next nurse coming to care for this patient.

RHODE ISLAND HOSPITAL
TREATMENT AND NURSING NOTES

Date and Hour	Medications and Special Orders	Description of Excreta Condition of Patient, Effect of Medication
9 A.M.	DICRYSTICIN TAMP. I.M. B.I.D. (H. Olsen) #18 CHAFFIN TUBE	UP OUT OF BED THIS A.M. WALKING CECOSTOMY DRESSING DONE BY DR. BROWN DRAINAGE DARK BROWN FECAL MATTER. INSERTED IN CECOSTOMY (BY DR. BROWN) AND PLACED ON GRAVITY DRAINAGE.
9+12+3	IRR. LEVIN TUBE + CECOSTOMY TUBE	DARK GREEN BROWN DRAINAGE DARK BROWN FECAL MATTER
9 30	1000 INVERT SUGAR 10% IN WATER c̄ 3 AMP. VIT. B. AND 3 AMP. VIT. C 40 mg. KCL I.V. (H. Olsen)	ABDOMEN DISTENDED — RECTAL TUBE INSERTED WITH FAIR FLATUS RESULTS. BEING REMINDED TO TAKE DEEP BREATHS EVERY HOUR. PARTICIPATING IN
12 NOON	ACHROMYCIN 100 MGM. I.M. q. 6° (H. Olsen)	QUADRICEPS — SETTING EXERCISES
1 P.M.	500 INVERT SUGAR 10% IN WATER c̄ 3 AMP. VIT. B. AND 3 AMP. VIT. C. (J. Baer)	UP AND OUT OF BED WALKING TWICE THIS P.M. (Helen Olsen)
3 P.M.	GLYCERINE AND WATER ENEMA	FAIR FECAL AND EXCELLENT FLATUS RESULTS. ABDOMEN LESS DISTENDED.
6 P.M.	ACHROMYCIN 100 MGM. I.M. q. 6°	LEVIN TUBE AND CECOSTOMY TUBE DRAINING WELL AND IRRIGATING WELL
6 30	1000 5% DEXTROSE IN WATER I.V. (J. Baer)	
9 P.M.	DICRYSTICIN ½ AMP. I.M. B.I.D.	SLEEPING MEDICATION REFUSED (Jane Baer)
12 M.	ACHROMYCIN 10 MGM. I.M. q6°	
	FEBRUARY 8, 19	
		COMFORTABLE - SLEEPING ALL NIGHT
6 A.M.	ACHROMYCIN 100 MGM. I.M. q.6° (B. Calvin)	LEVIN TUBE AND CECOSTOMY TUBES DRAINING WELL

FIGURE 90 (*Continued*)

The nurse prepares the important temperature chart that shows fluctuations in the vital signs of the patient. All medications and treatments should be recorded with the time of administration. The effects produced and/or the results noted must be recorded. For example, in recording the results of an enema, the kind, the amount of solution given and the effectiveness are desired. Merely to chart "Eff." or "Not eff." is not sufficient. By effectiveness is meant, what type of return (color and consistency as well as amount)? Was there much flatus? How did the patient feel during and after the enema?

At the end of each period of 8 or 12 hours, a brief summary is charted, depending on the desires of the surgeon. This may be merely fluid intake and output or it may be more extensive. A 24-hour résumé is more nearly complete and should include the condition of the patient, the medications and the treatments given during that time, the intake and the output and so forth.

Complete fluid intake and output charts are essential on some patients. The nurse must remember that the fluid intake includes all fluids given to the patient by any method during the 24-hour period. This includes liquid foods as well as water taken by mouth and all fluids given parenterally as well as fluids used for irrigating gastrointestinal suction tubes. Fluid output consists of all measurable fluids given off by the patient in 24 hours. This includes urine voided, vomitus and drainage. These fluids are recorded in milliliters and are totaled at periods of 12 and 24 hours.

In many hospitals it is required that each nurse sign or initial that portion of the nurse's record which represents the time she was responsible for the patient's care. When the patient is discharged, the nurse is responsible for seeing that the complete chart is in order and is sent to the record room. This completes her responsibility.

BIBLIOGRAPHY AND SUGGESTED READING

Books

Beal, J. M.: Manual of Recovery Room Care, ed. 2, New York, Macmillan, 1962.
Dressing Procedure Guide—Wound Classification and Dressing Requirements, 4-page brochure: Johnson & Johnson, New Brunswick, N. J.
Sadove, M. S., and Cross, J. S.: The Recovery Room, Philadelphia, Saunders, 1956.

Articles

Barbie, G. C.: More about bedrails and the nurse, Am. J. Nursing 57:1441-1442, 1957.
Bean, H.: What a patient thinks about early ambulation, Am. J. Nursing 54:169-171, 1954.
Bearsley, J. M., and Carvisiglia, F. F.: A special care ward for surgical patients, Nursing World 131:11-13, March, 1957.
Bird, B.: Psychological aspects of preoperative and postoperative care, Am. J. Nursing 55:685, 1955.
Clarke, A. R.: Progress report on recovery rooms, R.N.—A Journal for Nurses 20:36-45, April, 1957.
Collins, J. B.: A revised charting procedure, Am. J. Nursing 56:1140-1141, 1956.
Coppolino, C. A., and Wallace, G.: Trimethobenzamide antiemetic in immediate postoperative period, J.A.M.A. 180:326-328, 1962.
Dripps, R. D., and Waters, R. M.: Nursing care of surgical patients—the "stir-up," Am. J. Nursing 41:530-534, May, 1941.
Eastwood, D. W., and Mabrey, J. K.: Suction and the maintenance of an airway, Am. J. Nursing 53:552-553, 1963.
Garrett, E. G.: The dressing nurse, Am. J. Nursing 61:57, Jan., 1961.
Hayes, M. A.: Postoperative diet therapy, J. Am. Dietetic Assn. 35:17-18, Jan., 1959.
Heifetz, C. J., Lawrence, M. S. and Richards, F. O.: Comparison of wound healing with and without dressings, Arch. Surg. 65:746-751, 1952.
Jensen, F. T.: Recovery service without a recovery room, Am. J. Nursing 59:988, July, 1959.
Ludlam, J. E.: Bedrails—up or down? Am. J. Nursing 57:1439-1440, 1957.
McMahon, J., and Fife, G.: Nursing problems in recovery from anesthesia, Am. J. Nursing 45:618-622, 1945.
Modell, W.: The search for a morphine substitute, Am. J. Nursing 57:1565-1567, 1957.
Poppe, J. K., and James, R. B.: Intratracheal suctioning, Am. J. Nursing 45:538-540, 1945.
Rosenfeld, E. D.: Planning and managing the recovery room, Hosp. Topics 34:106-111, Oct. 1956.
Rourke, H.: The family lounge, Nursing Outlook 6:466-467, 1958.
Suddarth, D. S.: Individual dressing packs, Am. J Nursing 60:991-992, July, 1960.

18

Postoperative Discomforts, Complaints and Complications

POSTOPERATIVE DISCOMFORTS AND COMPLAINTS

By knowing that the patient may experience some discomforts postoperatively, the nurse will be alerted to recognize their early manifestations and then proceed to alleviate them as best she can. This chapter should help the nurse to achieve these objectives.

Pain

Pain is among the earliest postoperative symptoms. It can be expected as soon as the patient returns to consciousness. During the first 24 hours the pain is considered to be due to the cutting, the retracting and the suturing incidental to the operation, and for this discomfort morphine or a similar narcotic should be given as ordered. If the patient still complains, the surgeon should be notified.

The pain in abdominal operations is aggravated continually by vomiting, coughing and respiratory movements, and often in these cases it is wise to administer the morphine before the patient has recovered entirely from the anesthetic, so that he will pass several additional hours in quiet sleep. When hyoscine has been given before operation or when a basal anesthetic (page 225) such as thiopental has been used, often recovery from anesthesia is long. In such patients, morphine may be withheld until the necessity for its use arises.

Although pain in the first 24 hours usually is due to the operative procedures, the nurse never should omit a thorough inspection of the wound and the dressings for causes of discomfort. Pins from dressings or drainage tubes may be sticking into the patient, or the bandage may be too tight. Pain occurring after operations on bones or joints in which splints or a cast has been applied demands immediate attention. Pressure points occur very frequently because of insufficient padding or because the bandages have been applied too firmly. These difficulties may be overcome easily if they are found early, but if the danger sign, pain, is disregarded, the patient may go without treatment until pressure causes necrosis of skin or tendons or paralysis of nerves. The pain in these patients may be very short-lived, but it never should be neglected for a single moment.

Pain is a symptom that differs markedly in acuity in various patients. A neurotic patient with a small wound may complain much more than a phlegmatic individual after an extensive operation. Not only does the mental state of the patient affect the amount of pain he experiences, but there seems to be an actual difference in the amount of pain experienced by individuals of the same type. Some races—the Negro, the Chinese and the Germanic types—seem to bear pain well, while the Jewish, the Italian and other Latin races do not. Pain seems to be experienced less keenly in old age than in youth and middle age. Pain is the result of two factors, the lesion and the patient, and in order to arrive at an intelligent appreciation of its true significance, both must be thoroughly understood. When the patient complains of pain, the nurse should find its location, whether it is intermittent or constant, and whether it is dull, sharp or colicky in character. She should ascertain whether there is any constant radiation of the pain— whether it is down the legs; whether it is in the back; whether it occurs on taking a breath; or whether it is worse at night than during the day. These facts should be noted on the nurse's record and communicated to the surgeon, because with this information he may be able to diagnose the cause more accurately and prescribe for its relief.

Headache after spinal anesthesia may occur for a few days. By keeping the patient flat and quiet and administering aspirin, the headache may be controlled. (See p. 227.)

Treatment

The treatment of postoperative pain depends on its cause. After making sure that there is no removable cause for discomfort in the wound or the dressings, other reasons for discomfort should be investigated, and proper specific treatment instituted. As a general rule, pain that occurs after 24 hours usually is due to causes other than the operation.

Abdominal distention is a common cause, and often relief may be given by the insertion of a rectal tube or, better, by the use of a small enema. The sharp pains of a postoperative pleurisy may be relieved almost completely by tight adhesive strapping.

Drugs should be used in conjunction with other forms of treatment rather than instead of them. Morphine or Demerol are the most effective, and should not be withheld if the indications for their use arise. The morphine habit rarely develops in a patient to whom it is given for actual pain. However, as soon as possible it may be replaced by codeine and the coal-tar group, such as aspirin and phenacetin. In patients who exhibit an idiosyncrasy to morphine, Demerol often is substituted with good results.

Certain patients come to depend on their "hypodermic," especially at night, and complain of pain and discomfort that obviously are not as severe as they represent them to be. In such cases a hypodermic of sterile saline solution may act as a placebo. This procedure never should be resorted to without the knowledge and the written consent of the surgeon.

Vomiting

Vomiting is a frequent postoperative symptom. The nurse should have a basin at hand for vomitus and should turn the patient's head to one side. Also, she should keep the patient and the bed clean. In case of an abdominal operation, the patient will appreciate it if she will support the wound with her hand during the retching. The nurse should provide a mouth wash after the patient has vomited.

There are three types of postoperative vomiting, according to its duration: (1) vomiting when coming out of the anesthetic, (2) vomiting that is continuous through the first day and night and (3) vomiting that is excessive or prolonged.

When Coming Out of the Anesthetic

The vomiting that occurs as the patient is coming out of the anesthetic relieves the stomach merely of mucus and saliva swallowed during the anesthetic period. This type of vomiting also may occur occasionally after operations done under local anesthesia. Its duration is short (from 2 to 8 hours at most), and it requires no special treatment beyond the washing out of the mouth and the withholding of fluids for a few hours.

When Continuous Through the First Day and Night

Vomiting that continues for the first day and night may be due to one of several causes:

Effects of the Anesthesia. These may persist so that some patients may be nauseated and vomit long after they have regained consciousness. This occurs especially in patients who have had ether. If such patients are given a large glass of warm water with a half teaspoonful of sodium bicarbonate dissolved in it, they usually will vomit immediately, bringing up with the fluid considerable amounts of ether-laden mucus. After one or two such spontaneous gastric lavages, the patient usually will be relieved, and, after an hour or two, fluids may be given by mouth. Ginger ale and other effervescent drinks are often tolerated better than other fluids. Very frequently a hypodermic of morphine may give the patient several hours' rest, at the end of which time the nausea and the vomiting will have ceased.

Paralysis of Intestinal Activity. Frequently, there is considerable injury to the abdominal organs during an operation, with resultant paralysis of intestinal activity for a period longer than usual. Such patients have what in effect is a sterile peritonitis: fluids from the upper intestinal canal do not move onward; they dam back and are vomited. Nasal catheter drainage of the stomach for a time is the most effective treatment.

Idiosyncrasy to Morphine. The patient may be affected in an unusual way by morphine or other medication. Usually he vomits soon after the administration of the drug. An experienced nurse will recognize this idiosyncrasy and will report her suspicions to the surgeon and ask for instructions.

When Excessive and Prolonged

The causes of vomiting that continues without much remission for from 3 to 7 days, retarding the patient's recovery or even threatening his life, usually are serious and will be discussed separately. Such conditions may be enumerated as follows:

1. Intestinal obstruction
2. Acute dilatation of stomach
3. Uremia or kidney insufficiency
4. Hemorrhage in operations upon stomach
5. Peritonitis

At times, even without any apparent marked organic cause, vomiting will continue longer than usual. Such patients usually are highly nervous, apprehensive individuals, and it frequently taxes the ingenuity of both doctor and nurse to the utmost to keep anything in their stomachs. In these patients, charged water, ginger ale or other effervescent drinks may be tried after evacuation of the stomach through a nasal catheter. Antiemetic and antinauseant drugs such as Compazine, Tigan, Vesprin, Vistaril and Bonadoxin may be used intramuscularly or by mouth to give prompt relief.

Restlessness

Discomfort. Restlessness is a postoperative symptom that should not be passed over lightly. The most common cause probably is the general discomfort following an operation, especially pain in the back, headache and thirst. This discomfort may be relieved largely by a gentle massage with lotion or alcohol, followed by a dose of aspirin (which may be repeated if necessary).

Tight Drainage-soaked Bandages. Often these cause enough discomfort to make a patient restless and ill at ease. Fresh dressings usually improve the patient's spirits and make him more comfortable. Severe pain should not be permitted to be the cause of restlessness. Morphine or other narcotics should be given until relief is obtained. They should not be given for restlessness or sleeplessness. Milder somnifacients should be used.

Retention of Urine. This occurs not infrequently after operation and may be the sole cause for restlessness.

Severe Toxemia. This condition frequently produces a very restless patient. For such a patient little can be done until the toxins have been eliminated from the blood. He is quieted best by adequate doses of morphine.

Flatulence and Hiccup. Flatulence and hiccup may be causes of restlessness. Their recognition and their treatment will be discussed later (pp. 294 and 302).

Hemorrhage. Probably the most serious cause of restlessness is hemorrhage. This is discussed on page 298.

Sleeplessness

Frequently, sleeplessness is associated with restlessness in patients after operation. However, there are many patients who simply cannot sleep. When this situation continues for 2 or 3 days, it is the cause of considerable anxiety to the surgeon. It is in such a situation that a competent nurse is most valuable. She must recognize that a patient taken suddenly from an active life and put to bed in strange surroundings may have cause for inability to sleep. The prolonged rest and periods of sleep secured during the daytime leave him wide awake at a time when in ordinary circumstances he would be asleep. Often, hospital noises prevent a patient from sleeping.

Treatment

The nurse should help to reduce noise to a minimum, provide diversion for her patient and cut the daytime naps short, so that at night he is ready to welcome a "good sound sleep." At bedtime she may give a gentle massage, particularly of the back and the neck, ventilate the room thoroughly and dim the lights. If these ordinary measures do not promote sleep, further causes of insomnia must be looked for. Many patients are used to some form of food before going to bed. Frequently these patients will go to sleep after they have been given (their condition permitting) a cup of warm milk or cocoa and crackers or other food that is easily assimilated.

Worry and anxiety keep many patients awake. If it is possible to ascertain the cause of their worry, attempts can be made to relieve it. Perhaps it concerns their surgery, length of convalescence, readjustment to a new way of life—whatever it may be and however deep the worry, there is always a bright side of the picture. An understanding nurse can help such an individual. Spiritual comfort can provide an inner peace.

Medications. To this type of patient, bromides or barbiturates may be given with benefit. They should be given cautiously and in doses just sufficient to produce the desired effect. Demerol is a useful analgesic.

Thirst

Thirst is a troublesome symptom after many general anesthetics, and even after some cases of local anesthesia. It is due in large measure to the dryness of the mouth and the pharynx, caused by the inhibition of mucous secretion after the usual preoperative injection of atropine. Many patients operated on under local anesthesia will complain of thirst during the operation. In addition, there is a considerable loss of body fluids due to perspiration, increased mucous secretion in the lungs and more or less loss of blood, so that the factor of dehydration also enters into the cause. To combat the loss of fluids, solutions are given into the vein for the first few hours after operation. Even though an adequate amount of fluid is taken by these methods, often it does not relieve the thirst.

The sticky, dry mouth demands fluids, and fluids may be given to most patients as soon as the postoperative nausea and vomiting have passed. Sips of water or hot tea with lemon juice serve to dissolve the mucus

better than cold water. Small pieces of ice given to the patient may be very much enjoyed, and the amount of fluid given by this method is so small relatively that it is permitted even in patients in whom fluids are withheld by mouth. As soon as the patient can take water by mouth in sufficient quantities, the parenteral administration should be discontinued.

When operations have been performed on the mouth, the esophagus and the stomach, and about the duodenum, water usually is withheld for about 24 hours—often longer. Mouthwashes containing some weak alkali to dissolve the mucus are the best. A solution of equal parts of boric acid 4 per cent and glycerin also may be used. It seems to leave the mouth "wet" and allays thirst somewhat. A damp gauze cloth laid over the mouth will tend to moisten the air breathed and will be gratifying to many patients. Hard candies, chewing gum, even paraffin wax, may be chewed. This stimulates the flow of saliva and tends to keep the mouth moist.

Abdominal Distention

Distention of the abdomen after operation is very common. The trauma to the abdominal contents by operation produces a loss of normal peristalsis for 24 to 48 hours, depending on the type and the extent of the operation. Even though nothing is given by mouth, swallowed air and gastrointestinal secretions enter the stomach and the intestines and if not propelled by peristaltic activity, they collect in the intestinal coils to produce distention. Most often the gas collects in the colon; hence, a rectal tube or a small enema may be expected to give relief. After major abdominal surgery, distention may be avoided by frequent turning and movement by the patient and by the prophylactic use of a gastric or an intestinal tube. By this means the air which is swallowed (swallowed air provides most of the gas that produces distention) may be aspirated from the stomach and the upper intestine.

Certain patients swallow air as a part of anxiety reaction. If these characteristics can be recognized, the gastric suction tube may be used for a longer time than usual, until full peristaltic activity (passage of flatus) is resumed.

Distended Bladder. A distended bladder

frequently is the cause of a distention of the lower abdomen. This is discussed on page 304.

Constipation and Diarrhea

The care of the bowels after operation is a responsibility shared alike by surgeon and nurse. The nurse, who is with the patient constantly, must be prepared to give accurate reports as to the number and the character of the stools, the effectiveness of enemas and so forth.

Constipation

The causes of constipation after operation may be innocent or serious. The irritation and the trauma to the bowel at the time of the operation may inhibit intestinal movement for several days, but usually peristaltic function returns after the third day, following early ambulation, perhaps a simple enema and an increase in diet. Local inflammation, peritonitis or abscess may cause constipation, but the treatment of the causal condition is indicated. Constipation has been mentioned as being a constant symptom of intestinal obstruction.

Fecal Impaction. An avoidable cause of postoperative constipation is fecal impaction. This complication is a result of neglect and never should be permitted to occur. Early ambulation and regard for proper fluids and diet can prevent this problem in the majority of patients. Those affected usually are individuals past middle age, weakened somewhat by operation, whose bowel movements have been small in amount for several days. Enemas appear to be fairly effective, but distention usually will continue and the patient will have both general abdominal and local discomfort. He often states that he feels that the bowel wants to move but that movement gives no relief. Diarrhea may occur and persist, due to irritation of the upper rectum and the sigmoid by dammed-up fecal material. The diagnosis is made easily by inserting the gloved finger into the rectum. A hard fecal mass that fills the rectum will be palpated.

TREATMENT. The treatment of the condition is to remove the impaction. Enemas of 6 ounces of liquid petrolatum (oil enema) often are effective in softening the mass and helping its discharge. The harder masses may not be moved by this treatment. In these cases, the impaction may be broken up with the gloved finger, or by injecting from 1 to 2 ounces of hydrogen peroxide into the rectum. The foaming action of the drug tends to break up the fecal masses, which then may be evacuated.

It must be borne in mind also, in this connection, that many people, especially thin females and older people, are constipated habitually, and often give a history of having taken some form of laxative drug every day for years. These patients should be allowed to return to their former bowel habits as soon as possible after operation—at least until they have recovered from their operation. As a general rule it is best not to give cathartic drugs for at least a week after an abdominal operation, and for a much longer time when drains have been inserted. Enemas usually are effective in evacuating the lower bowel, and cathartic drugs never should be given except on the physician's orders. An exception to this rule may be made in the case of liquid petrolatum (paraffin oil). This substance causes no irritation to the bowel and may be used without danger in doses of 1 ounce once or twice daily (by order of the physician).

Diarrhea

After operations diarrhea is rare. The patient may have from 5 to 10 liquid stools of small amount a day. This should be reported at once. Fecal impaction has been mentioned as the most frequent cause of this complication in the aged.

Local irritation, such as a pelvic abscess, is the most frequent cause of diarrhea after operations in which a peritonitis was found. The gloved finger will find a tender mass bulging into the rectum. Surgical drainage usually is required, although at times these abscesses will rupture spontaneously and drain into the rectum. Diarrhea due to a pelvic abscess is usually "spurious" in type —that is, not a true diarrhea but simply the expulsion of small amounts of liquid from the rectum. It is associated often with *tenesmus* (straining). The patient also may have painful urination.

POSTOPERATIVE COMPLICATIONS

The danger from a surgical problem is not only the risk of the operative procedure; there is also the very definite hazard of postoperative complications that may prolong the convalescence or even be an important contributing cause in an unsuccessful operative result. The nurse plays an important part in the prevention of these complications and in their early treatment should they arise. The signs and symptoms of the more common postoperative complications are discussed below. In each instance the most improved methods of prevention and the usual treatment are emphasized.

It should be borne in mind constantly that attention must be paid to the patient as an individual as well as to his particular surgical condition.

Shock

One of the most serious postoperative complications is shock. It was, for a time, the cause of many operative fatalities. However, adequate attention in recent years to preoperative fluid balance and surgical preparation, together with the intelligent use of whole blood and blood substitutes during and after operation, has prevented this complication to a large extent.

Shock, for practical purposes, may be defined as a disproportion between the circulating blood volume and cardiovascular tree. It may be due either to an inadequate amount of blood in the circulation or, if a normal amount of blood is present, to a relative insufficiency due to dilatation of the vascular tree.

There are many causes of shock, and in almost all instances it is due to a combination of two or more factors. These factors may be of three main types. The first is *neurogenic,* sometimes called *primary* shock. It may result from anesthetics, especially spinal anesthesia, or neurogenic factors such as fear of operation, the sight of blood or the hustle and bustle in the strange atmosphere of the operating room. Under this heading might also be placed the trauma of an extensive or prolonged operative procedure, especially in a debilitated patient. The second type is that due to blood loss or *hematogenic* shock. Often there is more blood loss at operation than the surgeon realizes. The handling of body tissues may cause local trauma and loss of blood and plasma from the circulation, thereby creating a decrease in the circulating blood volume.

The third type is *toxic* shock. This is rather ill-defined and is not well understood. It is characterized by a change in the capillary endothelium that permits loss of blood and plasma through the capillary walls into the surrounding tissues. This is thought to be caused by a toxic factor that enters the blood stream from infection.

Symptoms of Shock. No matter what the cause, the symptoms of shock are due to a breakdown of the vascular system and an insufficiency of the circulation. The result then is an apathetic patient in whom all sensations are markedly dulled. The skin is cold and moist, the lips are somewhat cyanotic, the pulse is rapid and thready, the respiration is rapid and shallow, and the temperature is subnormal. The blood pressure begins to fall.

Effects of Shock. Continued shock and its associated low blood pressure result in undesirable body changes. One of these is anoxia. *Anoxia,* a lack of oxygen in the body tissues, may be the result of *anoxemia,* decreased oxygen content in the blood. Oxygen, which combines with hemoglobin for transportation throughout the body, may be insufficient to provide the tissues with their normal requirements. Some of the more specialized tissues—the brain, the spinal cord and the kidneys—undergo degenerative changes rapidly when they are not supplied with adequate oxygen. These changes in the brain may be manifested by a permanent lack of nervous control of the vascular system and vascular collapse, paralysis of one or more parts of the body, or by *hyperpyrexia.* The last is an excessive fever, sometimes as high as 108° or 109°F., that presages usually a fatal outcome and is the result of changes in the hypothalamic area. Later symptoms may include loss of memory and psychogenic alterations. When the kidney is deprived of oxygen for a sufficient period of time, kidney depression or failure may occur. Kidney depression, *oliguria,* is manifested by a decreased kidney secretion and urinary output. Kidney failure or *anuria* is evidenced by a lack of urinary secretion. Thrombosis with subsequent emboli also may occur throughout the body due to stasis of blood resulting from decreased circulation (see p. 302).

Principles of Treatment. The best treatment for shock is prophylaxis. This consists of adequate preparation of the patient, mental as well as physical, and anticipation of any complication that may arise during or after operation. The proper type of anesthesia should be chosen after careful consideration of the patient and his disease. Blood and plasma should be available if indicated. Operative trauma should be kept at a minimum. After operation, factors that may promote shock are to be prevented. Pain is controlled by making the patient as comfortable as possible and by using narcotics judiciously. Exposure should be avoided. In the recovery room the patient can be watched and cared for by nurses trained especially in the recovery of patients from anesthesia. In addition, a quiet room is advantageous in the immediate postoperative period in reducing mental trauma.

1. RESTORATION OF BLOOD VOLUME. This, of course, is the most important goal to be achieved in the treatment of shock. However, if the depressed circulation cannot be restored immediately, one must protect the vital centers of the brain. Irreversible changes may take place in a short period of time if the volume of the circulating blood is inadequate. The foot of the bed should be elevated and the head lowered, so that the heart can maintain the circulation more easily to these vital centers. In addition, some surgeons apply elastic bandages to the extremities, bandaging toward the trunk. By this procedure the available blood may be kept in a smaller circulating area, thus raising the blood pressure.

The quickest method of supplying an adequate amount of circulating blood is by transfusion. When blood is not available, a blood substitute, such as plasma or plasma volume expanders (Dextran), should be employed. Solutions of the electrolytes, glucose and saline solutions, should be used only when blood or plasma is not available, and then only until one or the other can be obtained.

2. RELIEF OF PAIN. Pain should be relieved as far as possible by the intelligent use of narcotics. However, when the circulation is depressed, as it is in shock, the effect of morphine or other narcotics will be delayed. Therefore, one must avoid overloading the patient with drugs that may accumulate during shock and become overwhelming when the circulation has been restored to normal. Other measures are used sometimes to alleviate pain. One of the most useful is procaine block of the peripheral nerves. This is satisfactory especially after operations on the chest, where relief can be obtained by intercostal nerve blocks.

3. BODY HEAT. Present opinion is that body heat should be maintained by dry blankets at only slightly higher than normal body temperature. If temperatures above body heat are employed, further dilation of blood vessels throughout the body may occur. This creates an even greater disproportion between the circulating blood volume and the cardiovascular tree. Warm drinks, such as hot tea or coffee, may be given by mouth unless they are contraindicated.

4. OXYGEN. As patients in shock have some anoxemia, to increase the available oxygen to the blood may be beneficial. Done to improve oxygenation of vital organs and tissues, thereby decreasing the work of the heart, this treatment works most easily by mask or intranasal catheter. An oxygen tent is bulky and cumbersome, and it takes too long to assemble it. However, if one is immediately available, it will achieve the same purpose.

5. DRUGS. Certain drugs may cause a temporary rise in blood pressure. These drugs act by constricting the vessels in the peripheral circulation or by stimulating the brain centers, but they have a transient effect, and sometimes the effects are more harmful than beneficial. All vasopressor drugs must be withdrawn gradually, for an abrupt discontinuance can produce a sudden hypotensive effect. They should be used with caution, and only on the surgeon's orders. These drugs include Levophed or an extract of the adrenal cortex known as desoxycorticosterone, Pituitrin, ephedrine and caffeine-sodium benzoate.

The Nurse's Responsibility. From a glance at the above outline, the nurse's responsibility should shock develop is (1) to keep the patient on his back and elevate the foot of the bed, (2) to apply dry, gently warmed blankets, (3) to call the surgeon, (4) to obtain a tank of oxygen and a mask or an intranasal catheter with tubing and attachments and (5) to have the following articles ready for immediate use: a sphygmomanometer and a stethoscope; an intravenous tray, preferably with plasma or glucose and salt solution; a hypodermic syringe in case the surgeon decides to use some drug mentioned above.

Hemorrhage

Classification. Hemorrhage is classified as (1) *primary,* when it occurs at the time of the operation; (2) *intermediary,* when it occurs within the first few hours after an operation, due to a return of blood pressure to its normal level and a consequent washing out of the insecure clots from untied vessels; and (3) *secondary,* when it occurs some time after the operation, due to the slipping of a ligature because of infection, insecure tying or erosion of a vessel by a drainage tube.

A further classification frequently is made according to the kind of vessel that is bleeding. *Capillary* hemorrhage is characterized by a slow general ooze; *venous* hemorrhage bubbles out quickly and is dark in color; *arterial* hemorrhage is bright in color and appears in spurts with each heartbeat.

When the hemorrhage is on the surface and can be seen, it is spoken of as *evident;* when it cannot be seen, as in the peritoneal cavity, it is spoken of as *concealed.*

Symptoms. Hemorrhage presents a more or less well-defined syndrome, depending on the amount of blood lost and the rapidity of its escape. The patient is apprehensive, restless and moves continually; he is thirsty; and the skin is cold, moist and pale. The pulse rate increases, the temperature falls, respirations are rapid and deep, often of the gasping type spoken of as "air hunger." As the hemorrhage progresses, the blood pressure and the hemoglobin of the blood fall rapidly, the lips and the conjunctiva become pallid, spots appear before the eyes, a ringing is heard in the ears, and the patient grows weaker but remains conscious until near death. The nurse must notify the surgeon immediately and carry out emergency measures until he arrives.

Treatment. Often the effects of hemorrhage after an operation are masked by those due to the anesthetic and to shock; therefore,

the treatment of the patient is in a general way almost identical to that described for shock, viz., (1) keep the head low and (2) administer morphine to keep the patient quiet. The wound always should be inspected to find out, if possible, the site of the bleeding. A sterile gauze pad and a snug bandage with elevation of the part, arm or leg, are indicated.

A transfusion of blood is the most logical therapeutic measure, and in the case of serious operation, the blood of the patient is typed and blood is secured beforehand. If blood is not available when needed, saline solution, plasma or a plasma volume expander (Dextran) may be given intravenously to tide the patient over temporarily until the blood can be secured (see pp. 169 to 185).

In giving fluids by vein in cases of hemorrhage, remember that too large a quantity or too rapid administration may raise the blood pressure enough to start the bleeding again, unless the hemorrhage has been well controlled.

Pulmonary Complications

Respiratory complications are among the most frequent and serious with which the surgical team has to deal. Experience has shown that they may be avoided in large measure by careful preoperative observation and by taking every precaution during and after the operation. It is well known that those patients who have some respiratory disease before operation are more prone to develop serious complications after operation. Therefore, the careful surgeon will perform only emergency operations when acute disease of the respiratory tract exists. The nurse may aid by reporting any symptom, such as cough, sneezing, injected conjunctiva and nasal discharge, to the surgeon before the operation.

During and immediately after the operation, every effort should be made to prevent chilling and to keep the patient warm. Aspiration of the nasopharynx in the immediate postoperative period in the recovery room removes secretions which would otherwise embarrass respirations in the postoperative period. Occasionally, when secretions form which cannot be coughed up by the patient, aspiration through the bronchoscope may be practiced, and, in very debilitated patients where retained secretions are a complicating factor, a tracheotomy may be performed which permits the nurse to aspirate the trachea directly through the tube as necessary.

The predisposing and exciting causes of pulmonary complications may be any of the following:

1. Infections in the mouth, the nose and the throat.

2. The irritating effect of the anesthetic, especially ether, on the respiratory mucous membranes, with a resultant increase in mucous secretion.

3. The aspiration of vomitus.

4. Shallow respiration after operations, especially those on the upper abdomen, because of the pain in the wound that deep respiration will cause.

It seems probable then that in many cases the cause is largely a lack of complete aeration of the lungs. The mucous formed is not coughed up, bacterial action comes into play and, when the affection is limited to the larger air passages, a *bronchitis* results. If the process involves the pulmonary alveoli, a *bronchopneumonia* occurs. Penicillin and the sulfa drugs frequently are used both in the prophylactic and the active treatment of respiratory complications.

The increased metabolism, more complete pulmonary aeration and the general improvement of all body functions incidental to getting the patient up out of bed have led many surgeons to regard getting him up as one of the best prophylactic measures against pulmonary complications. When the patient's wound or condition otherwise permits, it is not unusual to allow him to get up on the second or the third day after operation, and even on the first day. This practice is especially valuable in preventing pulmonary complications in older patients.

Atelectasis

When the mucous plug closes one of the bronchi entirely, there is a collapse of the pulmonary tissue beyond, and a massive *atelectasis* is said to result (Fig. 91). The prophylactic treatment of these conditions then would seem to include measures to promote full aeration of the lungs. The nurse should instruct her patient to take at least 10 deep inhalations every hour. Frequently, some surgeons recommend some apparatus (a spirometer, blow-bottles or ordinary paper bags) into which the patient blows in an effort to expand the lungs fully. Turning

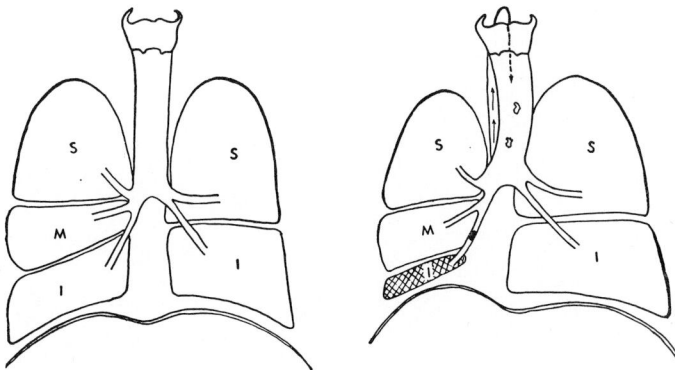

Fig. 91. Atelectasis. (*Left*) Normal expansion of all lobes of lungs. (*Right*) Plug of mucus or vomitus in bronchus leading to inferior lobe of right lung, with atelectasis of lobe. Arrows indicate the path followed by vomitus from the esophagus into the trachea before protective reflexes have returned following anesthesia. (Greisheimer, E. M.: The physiological effects of anesthesia, Am. J. Nursing *49*:339)

the patient from side to side results occasionally in coughing, with expulsion of the mucous plug, and recovery. At times the mucous plug may be removed by aspiration through a bronchoscope.

Bronchitis

This pulmonary complication may appear at any time after operation, usually within the first 5 or 6 days. The symptoms vary according to the disease. A simple bronchitis is characterized by cough productive of considerable mucopus, but without marked temperature or pulse elevation.

Treatment. A most effective method of treatment of bronchitis is the inhalation of steam, which may be administered by electric vaporizers. In using these the nurse must be careful to see that they are kept filled with water and are so placed that burning of the patient would be impossible. Figure 92 shows a vaporizer that stands on the floor. Smaller types for table use are more apt to be spilled. (See Chap. 23, p. 419.)

Bronchopneumonia

Bronchopneumonia is perhaps the second most frequent pulmonary complication. Besides a productive cough, there may be considerable temperature elevation, with an increase in the pulse and the respiratory rates.

Treatment. The patient is encouraged to take fluids, and expectorant and supportive

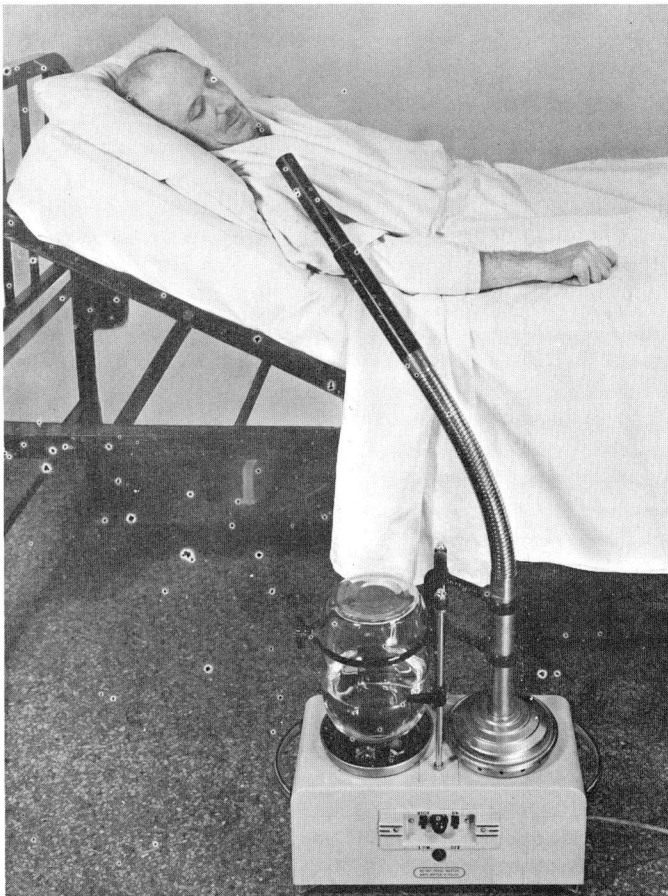

FIG. 92. Patient receiving inhalation from Colson vaporizer. The tube also may be inserted under a croup tent to supply steam and medication.

drugs are given him. Distention should be watched for and prevented, if possible, so as to avoid added respiratory or cardiac embarrassment. Most of these patients are effectively treated by the use of antibiotics.

Pleurisy

Pleurisy is not an uncommon occurrence after operation. Its chief symptom is an acute, knifelike pain in the chest on the affected side that is particularly excruciating when the patient takes a deep breath. Also, there usually is some slight temperature and pulse rise, and respirations are rapid and more shallow than normal.

Treatment. A tight adhesive strapping, applied during full expiration, will relieve the pain almost at once. Aspirin, 0.6 Gm. (gr. x), may be given if it is needed.

Pleurisy with effusion may result secondary to a primary pleurisy. In these cases aspiration of the chest frequently becomes necessary.

Lobar Pneumonia

Lobar pneumonia is a less frequent complication after operation. Usually it begins with a chill, followed by high temperature, pulse and respiration. There may be little or no cough, but the respiratory embarrassment, the flushed cheeks and the evident illness of the patient make a combination of clinical signs that are distinctive. The disease runs its usual course with the added complication of the operative wound.

Treatment. The treatment is as for bronchopneumonia, with liberal use of the antibiotics and the sulfonamides. (See Chap. 23.)

Hypostatic Pulmonary Congestion

Hypostatic pulmonary congestion is a condition that develops too often in old or in very weak patients. Its cause is a weakened heart and vascular system that permit a stagnation of blood at the bases of both lungs. It occurs most frequently, perhaps, in elderly patients who have sustained a fractured femur and are not mobilized effectively. The symptoms frequently are not marked for a time—perhaps a slight elevation of temperature and pulse and respiratory rate, also a slight cough. But physical examination will reveal dullness and rales at the bases of the lungs. If the condition goes untreated, the outcome may be fatal.

Treatment. Prophylaxis is the important thing. When the surgical condition permits, such a patient should be turned from side to side frequently and given cardiac stimulants. Also, he should be allowed out of bed as soon as possible. Many times this pulmonary complication becomes more serious than the original surgical condition, in which case the surgical condition may be disregarded in measure to permit proper treatment of the hypostatic pneumonia.

Because of reduced aeration in many of the pulmonary complications, which means that less oxygen reaches the blood, many clinics are employing an oxygen tent in treatment. This apparatus, which consists of a large hood that encloses the patient's head and shoulders, delivers oxygen in high concentration combined with a small amount of carbon dioxide. By this means the patient receives more oxygen with each respiration, cyanosis is lessened, and the general condition is improved. The nurse is required to see that the tent fits closely about the shoulders of the patient. (See p. 189.)

Pulmonary Embolism

An *embolus* is defined as a foreign body in the blood stream. In most cases it is formed by a blood clot that becomes dislodged from its original site and is carried along in the blood. When the clot is carried to the heart, it is forced by the blood into the pulmonary artery, where it plugs the main artery or one of its branches. The symptoms produced are among the most sudden and startling in surgical practice. A patient passing an apparently normal convalescence suddenly cries out with sharp, stabbing pains in the chest and becomes breathless, cyanotic and anxious. The pupils dilate, cold sweat pours out, the pulse becomes rapid and irregular, then imperceptible, and death usually results. If death does not occur within 30 minutes, there is a chance of recovery.

This complication may arise at any time after operation. It is probable that movements of the patient dislodge the clot, because pulmonary embolism seems to occur most frequently immediately after the patient has been taken out of bed or put to bed again for the first time after operation.

Treatment. If death does not occur at once, oxygen or fresh air should be given in abundance, with the patient in the sitting position to help respiration. Attempts should be made to quiet and reassure the patient, and drugs (morphine) should be given to prevent the panic that rapidly will wear out the overworked, dilating heart.

Femoral Phlebitis or Thrombosis

This complication occurs most frequently after operations upon the lower abdomen or in the course of severe septic diseases, such as peritonitis and ruptured ulcer. An inflammation of the vein occurs associated with a clotting of blood; this may be mild or severe. The cause of the complication may be injury to the vein by tight straps or leg-holders at the time of operation, concentration of blood by loss of fluid or dehydration, or, more commonly, probably the slowing of the blood flow in the extremity due to a lowered metabolism and depression of the circulation after operation. It is probable that several of these factors may act together to produce the thrombosis commonly seen. The left leg is affected more frequently. The first symptom may be a pain or a cramp in the calf. Pressure here gives pain, and a day or so later a painful swelling of the entire leg occurs, often associated with a slight fever and sometimes with chills and sweats. The swelling is due to a soft edema that pits easily on pressure. There is marked tenderness over the anteromedial surface of the thigh, and frequently the vein itself may be palpated as a firm pencil-like mass that may be rolled under the fingers.

A milder form of the same disease is termed *phlebothrombosis,* to indicate intravascular clotting without marked inflammation of the vein. The clotting occurs usually in the veins of the calf, often with few symptoms except slight soreness of the calf. The danger from this type of thrombosis is that the clot may be dislodged and produce an embolus. It is believed that most pulmonary emboli (p. 301) arise from this source.

Treatment

The treatment of thrombophlebitis or phlebothrombosis may be considered as (1) prophylactic and (2) active.

Prophylactic Treatment. Efforts are directed toward preventing the formation of a thrombus and include such measures as adequate administration of fluids after operation to prevent blood concentration, leg exercises, bandaging of the legs and getting the patient out of bed early to prevent stagnation of the blood in the veins of the lower extremity.

Active Treatment. Some surgeons believe that ligation of the femoral veins is an important therapeutic method. The rationale behind this method of therapy is to prevent pulmonary embolism from the breaking off of thrombi.

Anticoagulant therapy has taken a prominent place in the prophylaxis and the treatment of phlebitis and phlebothrombosis. Heparin, given intravenously by the drip method or intramuscularly in an oily menstruum, reduces the coagulability of the blood rapidly and is used most often when an immediate effect is desired. Repeated checks of the coagulation time of the blood are necessary to control its administration. Dicumarol or similar acting drugs are used for the same purpose. It is given by mouth and does not become effective for about 24 hours. Its daily dosage is controlled by daily estimations of the prothrombin time of the blood.

Both as a prophylactic and an active treatment of phlebitis and thrombosis, wrapping the legs from toes to groin with snug elastic adhesive bandages, or wearing elastic stockings, has much virtue. These bandages prevent swelling and stagnation of venous blood in the legs and do much to relieve pain in the phlebitic extremity.

Hiccup (Singultus)

Hiccup occurs not infrequently after abdominal operations. Often it occurs in mild transitory attacks that cease spontaneously or with very simple treatment. When hiccups persist they may produce considerable distress and serious effects such as vomiting, acidbase and fluid imbalance, malnutrition, exhaustion and possibly wound dehiscence.

Hiccup is produced by intermittent spasms of the diaphragm. It is associated with a coarse sound, a result of the vibration of the closed vocal cords as the air rushes suddenly into the lungs. The cause of the diaphragmatic spasm may be any irritation of the phrenic nerve from its center in the spinal cord to its terminal ramifications on the undersurface of the diaphragm. This irritation may be direct—such as a stimulation of the nerve itself by a distended stomach, peritonitis or subdiaphragmatic abscess, abdominal distention, pleurisy or tumors in the chest pressing on the nerves; or indirect—such as toxemia, uremia and so forth that stimulate the center; or reflex—such as irritations from a drainage tube, exposure to cold, drinking very hot or very cold fluids or obstruction of the intestines.

Treatment. The multitude of remedies suggested for the relief of this condition is proof that no one treatment is effective in every case. The best remedy, of course, is removal of the cause, which in some cases is easy—for example, gastric lavage for gastric distention, shortening or removal of drainage tubes causing irritation, or adhesive strapping in pleurisy. At other times the removal of the cause is almost impossible; then attention must be directed toward the treatment of the hiccup itself. Many simple remedies —such as drinking a half glass of water in which a teaspoonful of sodium bicarbonate has been dissolved, swallowing ice, stopping the patient from talking, sucking a lemon, taking a little vinegar, salt or sugar—have been used and often with success. Probably the most efficient of the older and simpler remedies is to hold the breath while taking large swallows of cold water.

After studying the problem recently, a group of anesthesiologists recommend treatment ranging from the simplest to the most drastic until relief is obtained. Their suggestions, in order, are:

1. Finger pressure on the eyeballs through closed lids for several minutes

2. Induced vomiting

3. Gastric lavage

4. Intravenous injection of atropine

5. Inhalation of carbon dioxide (breathing in and out of a paper bag or more technical administration)

6. Should these fail, a phrenic nerve block

7. As a final resort, a phrenic nerve crush*

Intestinal Obstruction

Intestinal obstruction is a complication that may follow abdominal operations. It occurs most often after operations on the lower abdomen and the pelvis, and especially after those in which drainage has been necessary. The symptoms usually appear between the third and the fifth days. The cause is some obstruction of the intestinal current—frequently a loop of intestine that has become kinked from inflammatory adhesions or that has become involved in the drainage tract. A typical situation is that of a patient with a ruptured appendix, having pelvic drainage. He had his enema on the third day, and it was reported to be effective. He was fed a soft diet and, after a day or two, he complained of sharp, colicky, abdominal pains with a pain-free interval between. Usually there is no temperature or pulse elevation. At first the pains are localized, and this point should be noted by the nurse, because the localization of the early pains represents in a general way the loop of intestine that is just above the obstruction.

Usually, the patient will continue to have abdominal pains, with shorter and shorter intervals between. If the ear or a stethoscope is placed on the abdomen, sounds may be heard that give evidence of extremely active intestinal movements, especially during an attack of pain. The intestinal contents, being unable to move forward, distend the intestinal coils, are carried backward to the stomach and are vomited. Thus, vomiting and increasing distention gradually become more prominent symptoms. Hiccup often precedes the vomiting in many cases. The bowels do not move, and enemas return nearly clear, showing that very little of the intestinal contents has reached the large bowel since the enema on the third day. Unless the obstruction is relieved the patient

* Friedgood and Ripstein report that chlorpromazine was effective in the treatment of severe hiccups in 46 patients out of 50. It is effective when given orally or parenterally but acts more rapidly if injected intravenously. See Friedgood, C. E., and Ripstein, C. B.: Chlorpromazine (thorazine) in the treatment of intractable hiccups, J.A.M.A. **157**:309, 1955.

continues to vomit, distention becomes more pronounced, the pulse becomes rapid, and the end is a toxic death.

Treatment. Sometimes the distention of the intestine above the obstruction can be prevented by the use of the constant-suction drainage with the Miller-Abbott, Harris or Cantor tubes, in which case the inflammatory reaction of the bowel at the site of the obstruction may subside and the obstruction is relieved. (See Fig. 93.) However, at times it is necessary to relieve the obstructed intestine by operation. In addition, intravenous infusions of saline usually are given. (See the section on intestinal obstruction for a more complete discussion of the treatment and the postoperative care, p. 632.)

Urinary Retention

Urinary retention may follow any operation, but it occurs most frequently after operations on the rectum, the anus and the vagina, and after herniorrhaphies and opera-

tions on the lower abdomen. The cause is thought to be a spasm of the bladder sphincter.

Not infrequently patients are unable to void in bed but, when allowed to sit or stand up, do so without difficulty. When standing does not interfere with the operative result, male patients may be allowed to stand by the side of the bed or female patients to sit on the edge of the bed with their feet on a chair or a stool. However, many patients cannot be permitted this liberty and other means of encouraging urination must be tried. Some people cannot void with another person in the room. These patients should be left alone for a time after being provided with a warm bedpan or urinal.

Frequently the sound or the sight of running water may relax reflexly the spasm of the bladder sphincter. A bedpan containing warm water or an irrigation of the perineum with warm water frequently will initiate urination for female patients. A small warm

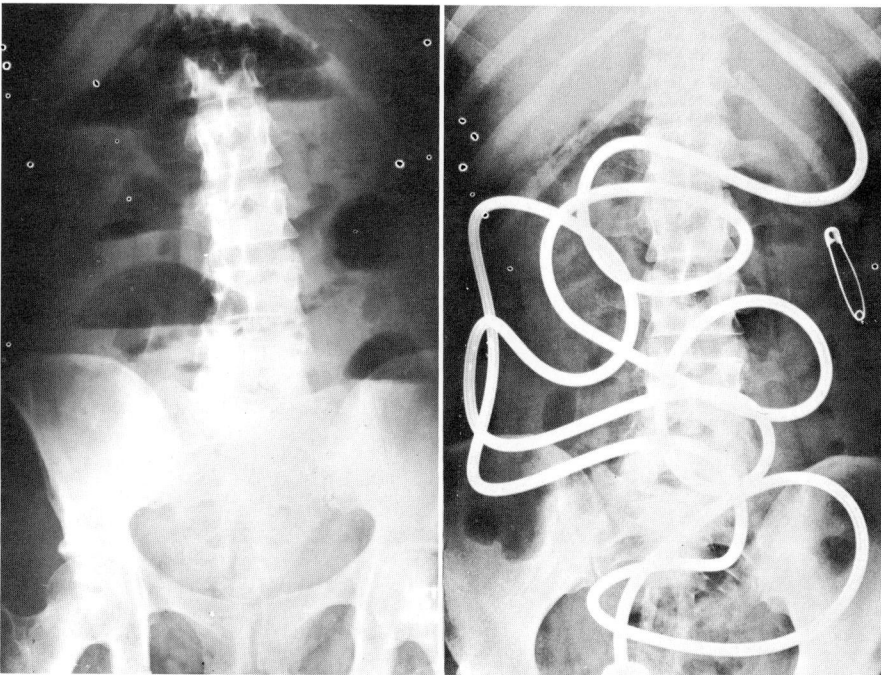

FIG. 93. (*Left*) Marked intestinal distention 4 days after exploratory operation. (*Right*) Twenty-four hours later, after Miller-Abbott tube had decompressed the intestines by constant suction. The tube may be seen following the coils of the intestines.

enema often is of value in such a situation. If the retention of urine continues for some hours, the patient will complain of considerable pain in the lower abdomen, and the bladder frequently can be palpated and seen in outline distending the lower anterior abdominal wall.

When all conservative measures have failed, catheterization must be practiced. If the patient has voided just before operation, this procedure may be delayed in most cases for 12 to 18 hours. There are two reasons for wishing to avoid catheterization: (1) there is the possibility of infecting the bladder and producing a cystitis, and (2) experience has shown that once a patient has been catheterized, frequently he needs subsequent catheterizations.

Many patients may exhibit a palpable bladder, with lower abdominal discomfort, and still void small amounts of urine at frequent intervals. The keen nurse will not mistake this for normal functioning of the bladder. This voiding of from 1 to 2 ounces of urine at intervals of from 15 to 30 minutes is, rather, a sign of an overdistended bladder, the very distention being sufficient to allow the escape of small amounts of urine at intervals. The condition usually is spoken of as the "overflow of retention." A catheter usually will relieve the patient by draining from 20 to 30 ounces of urine from the bladder. "Incontinence of retention" may be evidenced by a constant dribble of urine, yet the bladder remains overdistended. Overdistention injures the bladder; catheterization is indicated. There often is a definite psychic element in urinary retention.

Urinary Incontinence

Incontinence of urine is a frequent complication in the aged, either after operation or after shocking injuries. It is due probably to weakness with loss of tone of the bladder sphincter. This symptom frequently disappears as the patient gains in strength and normal muscular tone is regained.

Treatment. Treatment of urinary incontinence is difficult. In many patients, an indwelling catheter may be inserted. In some individuals the giving of a bedpan hourly may keep the bed dry. (See p. 971 for management of neurogenic bladder.) It is well to place a large pad under the patient to absorb the urine. Special pants for incontinent patients are available. The incontinent patient must be watched carefully to prevent the development of bedsores.

Delirium

Postoperative delirium occurs occasionally in several groups of patients. The most common types are:

Toxic

Toxic delirium occurs in conjunction with the signs and the symptoms of a general toxemia. These patients are very ill, usually with a high temperature and pulse rate. The face is flushed, and the eyes are bright and roving. These patients move incessantly, often attempting to get out of bed and disarranging the bedclothes continually. They present a marked degree of mental confusion. These states are seen in surgical conditions, most often in patients with general peritonitis or other septic conditions.

In such patients elimination is promoted by encouraging the intake of fluids, and the causative condition is treated by antimicrobial therapy. At times, however, the outcome is fatal.

Traumatic

Traumatic delirium is a mental state resulting from sudden trauma of any sort, especially in highly nervous people. The malady may take the form of wild maniacal excitement, of simple confusion with hallucinations and delusions or of melancholic depression. Sedative drugs—chloral hydrate, paraldehyde and morphine—are used in treatment. Usually the state begins and ends suddenly.

Delirium Tremens

Individuals who have used alcohol habitually over a long period of time are very poor surgical risks. The alcohol has damaged practically every organ and in the event of accidents or serious surgical procedures their resistance is much below that of the average person. These patients always take anesthesia poorly.

After operation the patient may do well for a few days, but the prolonged abstinence from alcohol causes him to become restless, nervous and irritated easily by little things. The facial expression changes entirely. He sleeps poorly and often is disturbed by unreal dreams. When approached by the doctor or the nurse he appears to awake suddenly, asks "Who are you?" and, when he is told where he is, he will appear to be fairly normal for a short time. These symptoms should be watched for in patients who have been alcoholics, because by active treatment at this stage the more violent delirium may be avoided.

Active delirium tremens may come on suddenly or gradually. After a period of restless, nervous, semidelirium, the patient finally loses entire control of his mental functions and "horrors reign supreme." "His mind is a chaos of everchanging ideas." He talks incessantly, tries to get out of bed to get away from the hallucinations of fear and persecution that torment him continually. If attempts are made to restrain him, he may fight maniacally and often will injure himself and others. "In this stage the patient is obviously sick." He is sleepless, he perspires freely and the limbs display a marked tremor.

Finally, after many hours of torture, the patient becomes stuporous.

Treatment. When possible, the treatment of these patients should begin 2 or 3 days before operation by most thorough elimination from the kidneys, the bowels and the skin. These measures should be continued after operation, especially if any of the early signs of the condition develop. Sedative drugs — and/or tranquilizers — should be given in quantities to keep the patient quiet. Stimulation often is required, especially in the older alcoholics, in the form of whisky, strychnine and caffeine. The chief cause of the symptoms in chronic alcoholics has been shown to be a depletion of the carbohydrate stores of the body and an inadequate ingestion of vitamins. Therefore, glucose is given intravenously, and vitamins are administered in concentrated form by mouth and by injection.

RESTRAINT. In the postoperative care of patients, it is wise for the nurse to explain the necessity for the patient's remaining in bed until the surgeon permits him to get up. Often patients prefer to get out of bed to void or get a drink of water rather than

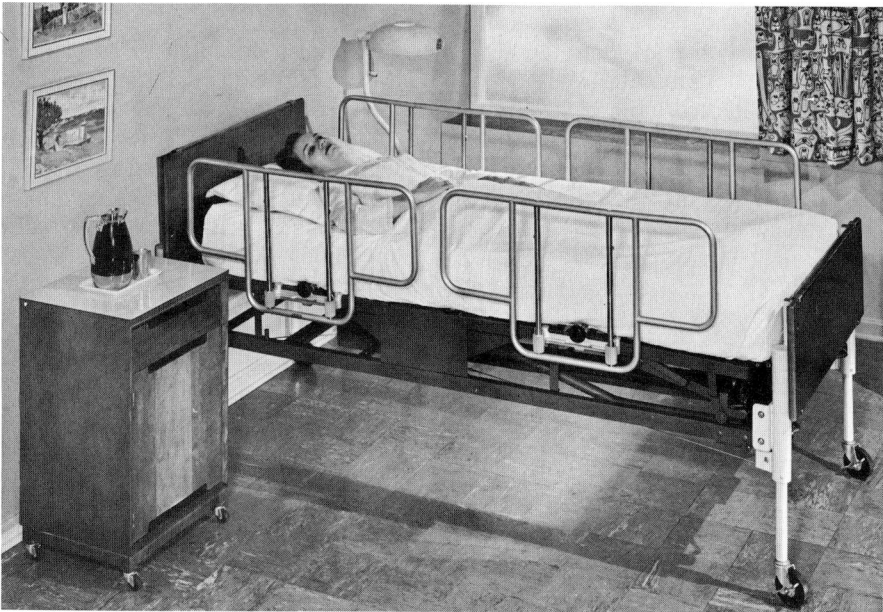

FIG. 94. Metal side attachment for hospital beds used when patients are restless and likely to get out of bed. (Hill-Rom Co. Inc., Batesville, Ind.)

bother the nurse. This may lead to serious complications that a word or two of explanation can prevent. However, in some cases it may be impossible for the patient to grasp this. This is true of patients who are disoriented, and especially of older individuals. In such patients, the simplest form of restraint is the use of a bed with siderails or side protection. This permits the patient to move about in bed but prevents him from getting out of bed easily and injuring himself.

To protect both patient and nurse, often it becomes necessary to apply some form of restraint in cases of delirium. In the milder forms, a restraining sheet may be used: an ordinary sheet folded lengthwise to be from about 12 to 15 inches wide, applied firmly over the thighs and held by wrapping each end round the bed frame.

Restraint of the upper extremities may be obtained by applying straight splints to hold the elbow joint in extension or by bandaging the fingers over a roller bandage held in the palm.

Nursing Care. The psychological effect of being restrained can be severe; therefore, any form of restraint should be applied *only as a last resort.* All other means of making the patient quiet should be tried first. If possible, he should be isolated from other patients. Any article in his vicinity which could be used harmfully should be removed.

When restraints are used, the patient should be in a comfortable and natural position and care should be taken that the part is not so constricted as to interfere with the circulation. Restraint to the chest should be avoided, if possible. The appearance of cyanosis in hand or foot indicates that the appliance is too tight. The appliances should be padded carefully and so used as to prevent chafing or pressure sores. The skin underneath them should be inspected frequently, bathed carefully and massaged at least every 2 or 3 hours. Even though restraints are applied, the patient never should be left unwatched. Any patient needing restraint should have constant and careful nursing attention.

Wound Complications

Infection

In the field of postoperative sepsis, staph-ylococcal infections appear to be an increasing problem; many of these infections are caused by antibiotic-resistant organisms.* Other infections may result from colon bacillus, streptococcus and, occasionally, infections by other organisms. The most important area of prevention lies in meticulous wound management and surgical technic. In addition, housekeeping cleanliness and environmental disinfection are important. When the inflammatory process occurs, it usually begins to show symptoms in from 36 to 48 hours. The patient's pulse rate and temperature increase, and the wound usually becomes somewhat tender, swollen and warm. At times, when the infection is deep, there may be no local signs. When the surgeon makes a diagnosis of wound infection, usually he removes one stitch or more and, under aseptic precautions, separates the wound edges with a pair of blunt scissors or a hemostat. The infection opened, he will call for a drain of rubber or gauze, which an alert nurse will have ready for him. In addition, many surgeons will require some form of warm antiseptic solution with which to flush the wound.

Hematoma (Hemorrhage)

The nurse should know the location of the patient's incision so that she may inspect the dressings for hemorrhage at intervals during the first 24 hours after operation. Any undue amount of bleeding should be reported to the surgeon. At times concealed bleeding occurs in the wound but beneath the skin. This hemorrhage usually stops spontaneously but results in clot formation within the wound. If the clot is small, it will be absorbed and need not be treated. When the clot is large, the wound usually bulges somewhat, and healing will be delayed unless it is removed. After the removal of several stitches, the clot is evacuated, after which the wound is packed lightly with gauze. Healing occurs usually by granulation, or a secondary closure may be performed.

---

* Howe, C. W.: The problem of postoperative wound infections caused by *Staphylococcus aureus,* Ann. Surg. 146:3, 1957.

Rupture (Disruption, Evisceration or Dehiscence)

This complication is especially serious in the case of abdominal wounds. It results from the giving way of sutures and from infection; also, more frequently, after marked distention or cough. The rupture of the wound may occur suddenly, with the escape of coils of intestine onto the abdominal wall. Such a catastrophe causes considerable pain and often is associated with vomiting. Frequently the patient says that something gave way. When the wound edges part slowly, the intestines may escape gradually or not at all, and the presenting symptom may be the sudden drainage of a large amount of peritoneal fluid into the dressings.

When rupture of a wound occurs, the attending surgeon should be notified at once. The protruding coils of intestine should be covered with sterile gauze.

A scultetus binder, properly applied, is an excellent prophylactic measure against an accident of this kind, and often it is used in the primary dressing, especially for operations on individuals with weak or pendulous abdominal walls. (Fig. 89.) It is used often also as a firm binder when rupture of a wound has occurred. Vitamin deficiency or lowered serum protein or chloride may require correction.

Keloid

Not infrequently in an otherwise normal wound the scar develops a tendency to excessive growth. Sometimes the entire scar is affected; at other times the condition is segmented. This keloid tendency is unexplainable, unpredictable and unavoidable in some individuals. (See p. 769 and Fig. 301.)

Much investigation has been done along the lines of prevention and cure. Careful closure of the wound, complete hemostasis, pressure support without undue tension on the suture lines—all are reputed to combat this distressing wound complication.

BIBLIOGRAPHY AND SUGGESTED READING

Books

Harkins, H. N., *et. al.*: Surgery: Principles and Practice, ed. 2., Postoperative Pain, Chap. 14, Section 3, pp. 236-244, and Postoperative Urinary Retention and Oliguria, Section 5, pp. 246-249, Philadelphia, Lippincott, 1961.

Sadove, M. S., and Cross, J. H.: The Recovery Room, Chap. 2, Principles of Recovery Room Management, Philadelphia, Saunders, 1956.

MacBryde, C. M.: Signs and Symptoms, ed. 3, Chap. 3, Pain, pp. 49-64, Philadelphia, Lippincott, 1957.

Articles

Calabro, J. J.: Hiccups, Am. J. Nursing **55**:1365-1366, 1955.

Haggerty, R. J.: Levarterenol for shock, Am. J. Nursing **58**:1243-1244, 1958.

Hunter, J.: The mark of pain, Am. J. Nursing, **61**:96-99, Oct., 1961.

Kaufman, M. A., and Brown, D. E.: Pain wears many faces, Am. J. Nursing **61**:48-51, Jan., 1961.

Klutsch, W. P., and Douglas, D. W.: Postoperative wound disruption, Am. J. Surg. **84**:678-683, 1952.

Maddock, W. G.: Gastrointestinal distention, Am. J. Nursing **56**:893-895, 1956.

Prout, H. C.: The modern concept of surgical shock, Am. J. Nursing **58**:78-79, 1958.

Reams, G. B., and Powell, E. J.: Postoperative catheterization—yes or no? Am. J. Nursing **60**:371, 1960.

Simard, O. M.: Nursing during levarterenol therapy, Am. J. Nursing **58**:1244-1245, 1958.

Stanton, J. R.: Venous thrombosis and pulmonary embolism, Am. J. Nursing **55**:709-711, 1955.

19

Cancer Nursing

The nurse is a very important member of any team fighting cancer. In the hospital her skill is a necessary adjunct to that of the surgeon, the radiologist and the internist. Within the community as a public health nurse, she regularly calls on the patient with cancer who is being treated at home. In industry, she not only must contend with illness of employees themselves but often worries about the health of their families as well. Directly or indirectly, her knowledge and influence supplement the doctor's plan of action for the diagnosis, the treatment, the rehabilitation or the terminal care of those who are cancer victims. (American Cancer Society, Inc.)

INTRODUCTION

Each cell in the human body is thought to have a definite function that it performs in conjunction with the other cells to form a useful machine. Thus, the skin cells protect the body surface; the cells of the breast secrete milk; the muscle cells contract, giving us movements. All these various groups of cells are held together by connective tissue. However, at times certain cells take on a new form of growth that is not useful. They cease to cooperate with their fellows of like nature to form a useful machine. They grow independently, often rapidly, taking nourishment from the body and giving nothing in return. Such a group of cells, similar in form to the normal cells but serving no useful purpose, is called a *neoplasm* or *tumor.*

The question, "What makes apparently normal cells adopt these strange forms of growth?" long has been asked, but a satisfactory answer has not been found as yet.

Extensive studies seem to show that there may be certain hereditary tendencies toward tumor formation, and that irritation of long standing from any cause may excite cells to this abnormal development. The role of viruses, parasites and chemicals as potential causative agents also has been studied. These factors may play a part, but the real exciting cause has not been discovered as yet. Infection, as we generally speak of it, does not seem to play a role in tumor causation.

CLASSIFICATION OF CYSTS AND TUMORS

Cysts

A *cyst* is an abnormal collection of fluid within a definite sac or wall. Cysts may form in several different ways. When the outlet to a gland becomes blocked and the gland continues to secrete, a *retention cyst* is formed. The common sebaceous cyst or wen is an example. Remnants of fetal organs may secrete a fluid, often forming a cyst of considerable size especially when springing from the pelvic organs of the female. This is called an epidermoid cyst. An extravasation of blood in the tissues may become surrounded by a definite wall and form an *extravasation cyst.*

Cysts may be formed by parasites, especially the *Taenia echinococcus (Echinococcus granulosus)* or dog tapeworm. These cysts, spoken of as *hydatid cysts,* often are of considerable size and usually are found in the liver.

Treatment. Cysts should be removed when possible because occasionally they change into malignant growths. They often may become infected; then incision and drainage are necessary.

Benign or Nonmalignant Tumors

Some tumors are surrounded by a definite capsule, remain localized in the tissue from which they spring, and disturb their host only by pressure on the surrounding structures and by robbing the normal tissues of their blood supply. These tumors usually grow rather slowly, and once removed they do not tend to recur. Such tumors are spoken of as *benign* or *nonmalignant*.

Malignant Tumors

Other neoplasms are not surrounded by a capsule, but grow by invasion into the tissues surrounding them. They invade the blood vessels or the lymphatics and extend rapidly along these open channels. Often the tumor cells are broken off and carried by the blood and the lymph to other parts of the body, where they set up a secondary growth. Secondary growths are looked for at the nearest lymph filter, the lymph nodes. Here cells are caught and begin to form an independent tumor like the parent or primary growth. Thus, in every case of cancer of the breast, the axilla is examined carefully for enlarged lymph nodes, because it is known that the lymph flow from the breast is through the axillary lymph nodes. Tumor cells invading the blood vessels are carried to organs where the venous blood passes through a capillary bed; thus we see secondary tumor appearing in the lung from a cancer of the breast or in the liver when the cells are carried by the portal venous system from a tumor in the abdomen. This property of these tumors is called *metastasis,* and the new or secondary growth is called a *metastatic growth*. The cells of these tumors grow rapidly and under the microscope resemble the rapidly growing cells found in the embryo. They invade the surrounding tissues in such a manner that it is nearly impossible to remove all the tumor cells and, therefore, they tend to recur after the main body of the tumor has been removed.

The rapid growth of the tumor and its secondary growths sap the vitality of its host, with the result that there is a rapid loss of weight and strength. These tumors bleed easily, producing a loss of the red cells in the blood—an anemia. The patient finally becomes thin, pale and weak, a shadow of his former self. This condition is spoken of as *cachexia*. The course of the disease ends in death. These tumors are called *malignant*.

At times a tumor that was at first benign may take on malignant characteristics. For this reason it is well to remove all tumors as soon as they are discovered in most instances.

The characteristics of these two classes of tumors are summarized in the columns below.

Subdivisions on Basis of Tissue

Neoplasms are subdivided further according to the kind of tissue of which they are formed. In embryonic life there are

TABLE 7. Classification of Tumor Cells

Type of Cell	Benign	Malignant
Epithelium	*Papilloma*	Cancer—Carcinoma
Skin Epithelium	Wart (Verrucae)	Epithelioma
		Melanoma
Gland Epithelium	Adenoma	Adenocarcinoma
Connective Tissue:	Fibroma	Fibrosarcoma
Fatty Tissue	Lipoma	Liposarcoma
Bone	Osteoma	Osteosarcoma
Cartilage	Chondroma	Chondrosarcoma
Muscle Tissue:	Myoma	Myosarcoma
Endothelial Tissue:		Endothelioma
Blood Vessels	Hemangioma	Hemangiosarcoma
Lymph Vessels	Lymphangioma	Lymphangiosarcoma
Nevus Cell (Pigmented)	Nevus—mole	Melanoma

Benign	*Malignant*
Adult type of cell	Young type of cell
Slow growth	Rapid growth
Often encapsulated	Never encapsulated
Never grow into surrounding tissues	Invade surrounding tissues widely
Always remain localized at original site	Form secondary growths by metastasis
Do not tend to recur when removed	through both the lymph and the blood stream
Harm the host only by pressure of growth on surrounding structures	Tend to recur when removed
	Cause loss of weight and strength, anemia, cachexia and, eventually, death

three divisions of tissue from which all others are formed. These tissues are called (1) endoderm, (2) mesoderm and (3) ectoderm.

Endoderm is the tissue from which the lining membranes (mucosa) of the respiratory tract, the gastrointestinal tract and the genitourinary tract are formed.

Mesoderm is the tissue from which muscles, bones, fascia and connective tissue are formed.

Ectoderm is the tissue from which come the skin cells and the cells composing its hair follicles, sweat glands and the entire nervous system.

FORECAST OF CANCER DEATHS
(IF PRESENT RATES CONTINUE)

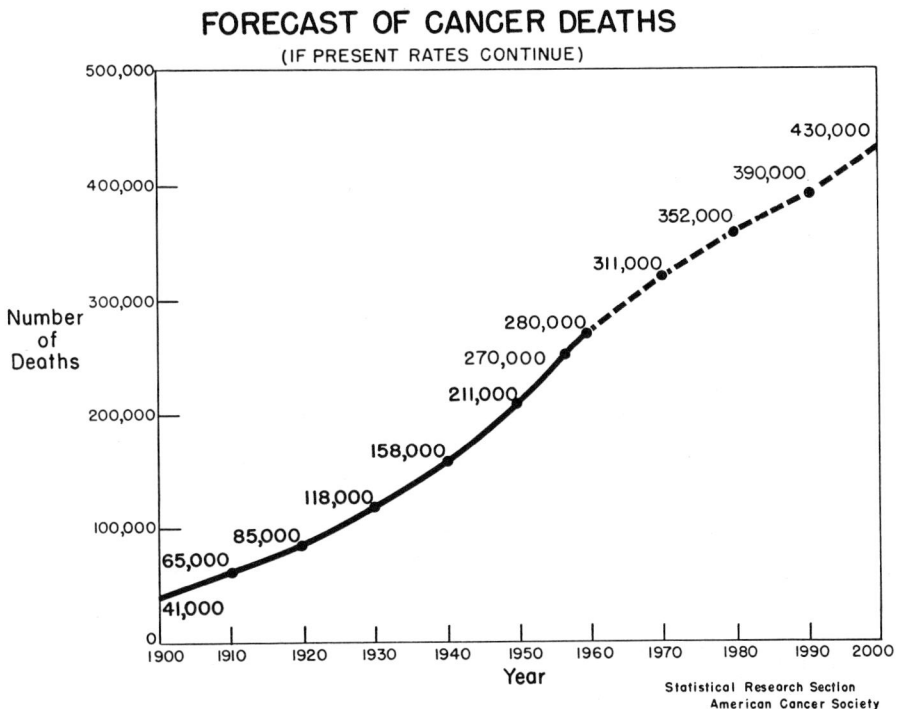

Statistical Research Section
American Cancer Society

FIG. 95. Forecast of Cancer Deaths. Note that the solid line through 1961 tells the actual number of deaths from cancer, while the dotted line is a statistician's prediction for the years to come—if present rates continue. It is hoped that some more effective means will be found to prevent deaths from cancer. (Cancer and the Nursing Profession, American Cancer Society, 1958; revised according to 1963 Cancer Facts and Figures, American Cancer Society)

TABLE 8.   Relation of Cancer to Leading Causes of Death in the United States

	Number of Deaths	Per Cent of Total Deaths		Number of Deaths	Per Cent of Total Deaths
All Causes	1,702,000	100.0			
1. Heart disease	668,170	39.3	8. Diabetes mellitus	28,850	1.7
2. Cancer	269,820	15.9	9. Congenital malformations	21,030	1.2
3. Cerebral hemorrhage	192,350	11.3	10. Cirrhosis of liver	20,570	1.2
4. Accidents	92,760	5.5	11. Suicide	19,170	1.1
A. Motor vehicle accidents	37,520	2.3	12. Nephritis	13,320	0.8
B. Other accidents	55,240	3.2	13. Hypertension without heart mention	12,490	0.7
5. Diseases of early infancy	66,890	3.9	14. Ulcer of stomach and duodenum	11,080	0.7
6. Pneumonia and influenza	54,510	3.2	15. Tuberculosis	10,470	0.6
7. General arteriosclerosis	34,840	2.0	Other and ill defined	185,680	10.9

Note: These are preliminary estimates by U. S. National Office of Vital Statistics based on 10 per cent sample of death certificates in 1961.
(1963 Cancer Facts and Figures, American Cancer Society)

TABLE 9. Cancer Status Chart Showing Leading Sites of Involvement

Site	Estimated New Cases 1963	Estimated Deaths 1963	Danger Signal (When lasting longer than two weeks see your doctor)	Safeguards	Comment
Breast	64,000	25,000	Lump or thickening in the breast.	Annual checkup. Monthly breast self-examination.	The leading cause of cancer death in women.
Colon and Rectum	73,000	41,000	Change in bowel habits; bleeding.	Annual checkup, including proctoscopy.	Considered a highly curable disease when digital and proctoscopic examinations are included in routine checkups.
Kidney and Bladder	28,000	14,000	Urinary difficulty. Bleeding—in which case consult your doctor at once.	Annual checkup with urinalysis.	Protective measures for workers in high-risk industries are helping to eliminate one of the important causes of these cancers.
Lung	47,000	41,000	Persistent cough, or lingering respiratory ailment.	Prevention: learn facts about smoking. Annual checkup. Chest x-ray.	The leading cause of cancer death among men, this form of cancer is largely preventable.
Mouth, Larynx and Pharynx	19,000	9,000	Sore that does not heal. Difficulty in swallowing. Hoarseness.	Annual checkup, including larynx.	Many more lives should be saved because the mouth is easily accessible to visual examination by physicians and dentists.
Prostate	32,000	16,000	Urinary difficulty.	Annual checkup, including palpation.	Occurs mainly in men over 60. The disease can be detected by palpation and urinalysis at annual checkup.
Skin	68,000	4,000	Sore that does not heal, or change in wart or mole.	Annual checkup. Avoidance of overexposure to sun.	Skin cancer is readily detected by observation, and diagnosed by simple biopsy.
Stomach	25,000	19,000	Indigestion.	Annual checkup.	A 40% decline in mortality in 20 years, for reasons yet unknown.
Uterus	40,000	14,000	Unusual bleeding or discharge	Annual checkup including pelvic examination and papanicolaou smear.	Uterine cancer mortality has declined 50% during the last 25 years. With wider application of the "pap" smear, many thousand more lives can be saved.
Leukemia	16,000	14,000	Leukemia is a cancer of blood-forming tissues and is characterized by the abnormal production of immature white blood cells. Acute leukemia strikes mainly children and is treated by drugs which have extended life from a few months to as much as three years. Chronic leukemia strikes usually after age 25 and progresses less rapidly.		Cancer experts believe that if drugs or vaccines are found which can cure or prevent any cancers they will be successful first for leukemia and the lymphomas.
Lymphomas	19,000	15,000	These diseases arise in the lymph system and include Hodgkin's and lymphosarcoma. Some patients with lymphatic cancers can lead normal lives for many years.		

(1963 Cancer Facts and Figures, American Cancer Society).

Total Male	Incidence 223,000 % of total	Mortality 131,500 % of total
Head & Neck	7%	6%
Lung	14%	19%
Breast	1%	1%
Stomach	7%	11%
Urinary Tract	6%	6%
Rectum & Colon	13%	14%
Genitalia	11%	11%
Skin	16%	2%
Leukemia & Lymphoma	8%	10%
Others	19%	22%

Total Female	Incidence 227,000 % of total	Mortality 118,500 % of total
Head & Neck	2%	2%
Lung	2%	2%
Breast	21%	19%
Stomach	4%	7%
Urinary Tract	3%	3%
Rectum & Colon	14%	16%
Uterus	18%	13%
Skin	11%	1%
Leukemia & Lymphoma	6%	8%
Others	19%	27%

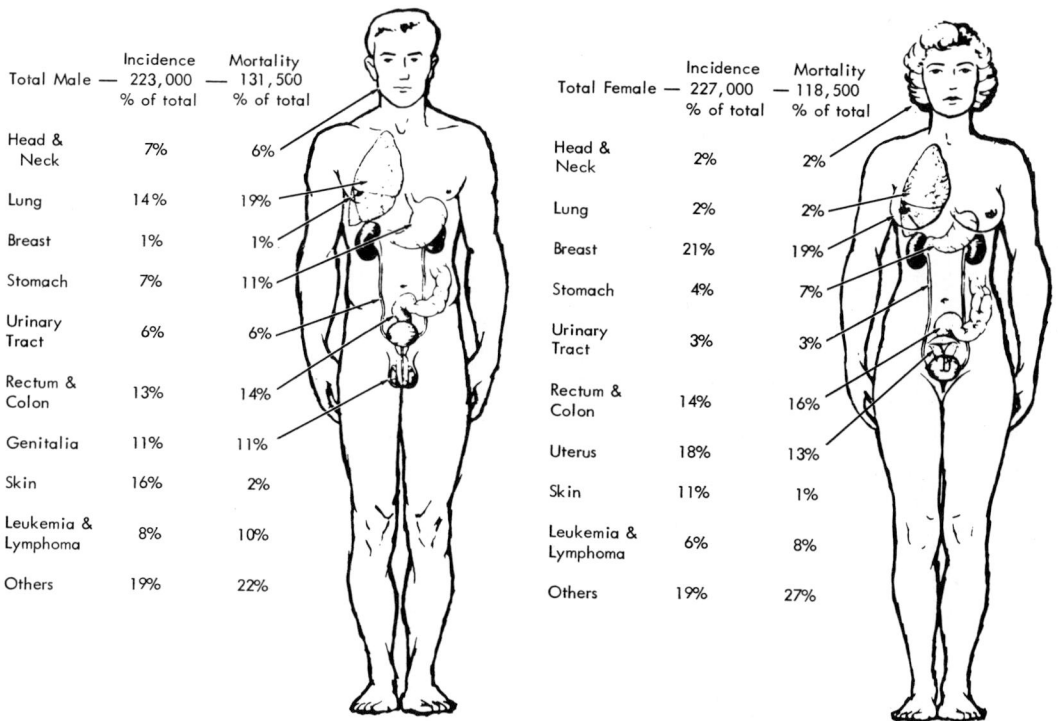

FIG. 96. Incidence and mortality by major site. (Cancer Detection, American Cancer Society, 1958)

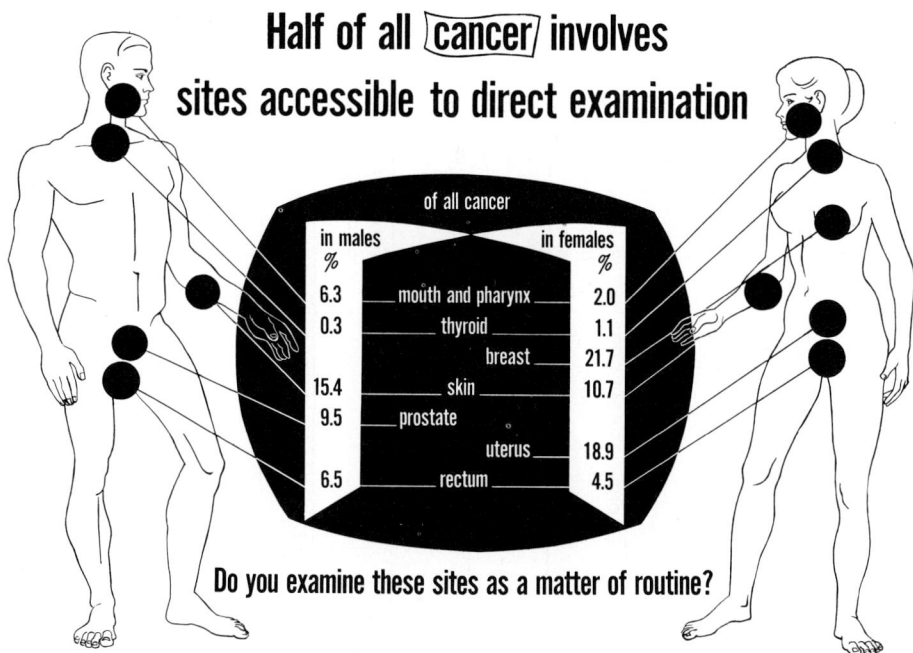

Half of all cancer involves sites accessible to direct examination

of all cancer

in males %		in females %
6.3	mouth and pharynx	2.0
0.3	thyroid	1.1
	breast	21.7
15.4	skin	10.7
9.5	prostate	
	uterus	18.9
6.5	rectum	4.5

Do you examine these sites as a matter of routine?

FIG. 97. Nearly 60 per cent of cancer in women occurs in sites that are accessible to direct examination; just under 40 per cent of cancer that occurs in men is accessible to direct examination. (Chart: National Cancer Institute)

Complex Tissues

Some tumors, thought to arise from embryologic maldevelopment, contain more than one of the embryonal tissues. Those which contain two of the tissues, called *teratomas* or *dermoids,* are not infrequently seen in operations on the ovary or the testicle. They may contain bone, teeth, muscle—all of which arise from the mesoderm—and hair, skin and sebaceous glands, which develop from the ectoderm.

New growths often are composed of more than one tissue and are named accordingly —fibroadenoma, fibrolipoma, osteosarcoma and so forth.

INCIDENCE OF VARIOUS MALIGNANCIES

The importance of malignant growth to the nursing and the medical professions can be understood if some of the facts concerning its incidence are reviewed. It is estimated that in the United States malignancy annually exacts a toll of at least 270,000 lives, ranking second as the principal cause of death, being exceeded only by heart disease. More than 1 out of 6 deaths that occur in adults is caused by malignancy. It is estimated that more than 88,000 cancer patients might have been saved in 1963, for example, had they recognized early symptoms and sought prompt treatment. Cancer affects men and women of all ages and of all races. No organ of the body is exempt.

THE NURSE AND THE CANCER PATIENT

The hope of cure in malignant disease depends on treatment of the malignancy before it is spread beyond the possibility of removal. This means that treatment should be given as soon as possible after the malignancy is recognized, but it must also be understood that in some patients even by that time there may have been a spread of tumor, which would make it impossible to cure by our present methods of therapy. Rapid progress is being made in the education of the public as to the dangerous consequences of untreated tumors. The intelligent nurse is one of the most effective agents in the dissemination of such information. Not infrequently her patients or their friends will question her concerning "a lump that has formed" or a rapid loss of weight with increasing "indigestion."

In order to answer such questions she should remember that these symptoms and signs suggest malignant disease: *a swelling, usually painless, growing progressively larger; the abnormal appearance of blood from the stomach, the bowel or the pelvic organs; loss of weight; slowly increasing "indigestion"; or an ulcer that refuses to heal.* If these symptoms occur in a person past middle age, they are especially suggestive, because cancer occurs most frequently at that time of life.

Knowing that only early treatment can cure, the nurse should urge an immediate examination by a physician. The diagnosis is confirmed by the use of biopsy, cytologic test, endoscopy, roentgenogram, or blood tests.

The responsibility of the nurse begins in the early stages of cancer detection and progresses through the following roles: (1) supporting the patient undergoing diagnostic procedures, (2) meeting the fluid and nutritional needs of the patient, (3) assisting in carrying out treatments of the malignancy itself, (4) recognizing the psychological and spiritual needs of the patient, (5) assisting in the rehabilitation and convalescence of the patient, (6) assisting in the follow-up of all treated patients, (7) aiding in the collection of data for research and (8) assisting in planning for the care of individuals whose disease has not been terminated.*

In caring for patients with a malignant tumor, the nurse finds that the team of which she is a member never is limited to

* Principal agencies supplying information on Cancer:

American Cancer Society, 521 W. 57th St., New York 19, N.Y., with divisions located in each state and principal cities in the United States.

National Cancer Institute of the U. S. Dept. of Health, Education, and Welfare, Public Health Service, Bethesda, Md.

State Departments of Health.

Also see *Cancer and the Nursing Profession,* a brochure describing the importance of the nurse in cancer control, management and treatment, American Cancer Society, 1957.

the surgeon, the patient and the nurse, but includes often the medical social worker, the nutritionist, the occupational and physical therapists, the psychiatrist and the clergyman. Over and above this, one cannot overlook the fact that the patient's family plays a significant role.

TREATMENT OF NEOPLASMS

It has been learned that malignant neoplasms usually lead to certain death if untreated, and that benign tumors frequently become malignant without warning. Therefore, it must be realized that the patient who is the host to a tumor of any kind is the potential victim of a fatal disease. At present, three methods have proved their value in the treatment of cancer: surgery, radiation and chemotherapy.

Surgery of Cancer

Actually, surgery plays a part in the management of every growth that is suspected of being a cancer. When a piece of tissue is taken from a suspicious growth for examination under the microscope (*biopsy*), this procedure is a surgical one. Proof of malignancy can be definitely established by such a study. When the diagnosis is established, the surgeon removes the original growth, and in addition he removes the lymphatics that drain the area in which the growth is situated. Therefore, in operations for carcinoma of the breast, the overlying skin and the underlying muscles are removed with the breast, and the lymphatic channels of the axilla are dissected out carefully, along with any metastatic nodes that can be discovered.

Another type of cancer surgery may be called *preventive* or *prophylactic surgery,* which is of utmost importance in the control of cancer. This involves the removal of those lesions which, as known from past experience and study, are apt to develop into cancer if they are left in the body. An example would be the removal of small tumors (polyps) that often grow in the colon. These may be detected by roentgenograms or sigmoidoscopy.

Surgical removal of the entire cancer is regarded as the best method of cancer treatment. This often requires rather extensive operations and is only curative if the operation can be performed before the tumor has spread to areas that cannot be removed.

There is another field in which surgery aids in the control of cancer. This involves the removal of, or operations on, the different glands of the body which produce hormones that are known to affect the natural course of development of certain cancers. An example of this type of surgery is the removal of the ovaries in women who have had cancer of the breast and have not yet reached the menopause. The physician will do this if he thinks that by so doing he can increase his patient's chance of cure or reduce the rate of growth of the tumor.

Palliation of cancer is an attempt to relieve the complications of cancer; such complications may be ulcerations, obstruction of the gastrointestinal tract, pain produced by extension of the tumor to surrounding nerves, and bleeding and nutritional loss from the extensive tumor growth. Therefore, palliative surgery implies many sorts of operative procedures, depending on the complication which presents. Such operations are performed by the surgeon with the knowledge that he cannot produce a cure but with the hope that he can give the patient improved health and comfort for a longer period of time than would otherwise be the case. Thus, in bleeding or obstructing tumors of the stomach or the bowel, usually the tumor is resected in spite of the fact that the patient may have metastatic extension to the liver and with the knowledge that the operation is only a palliative rather than a curative one.

In addition to these attempts to remove the complications of tumors, sometimes other measures are employed, especially in an attempt to relieve pain. These include radiation therapy with x-rays or radium and operations on nerves, the spinal cord or the brain to divide the pathways which carry pain sensation; the use of hormones in the case of tumors which are affected by hormone stimulation, such as those in the breast or the testes, and the removal of hormone-producing glands such as the pituitary, the adrenal, the ovary and the testis. None of these procedures can produce a cure for the cancer, but they may relieve pain and in some patients may produce a regression of the tumor for a time.

Radiation of Cancer

Radiation and Nursing*

Basic Physical Description. Everything in our universe, including man, has been subjected to radiation since the universe was formed. This ever-present radiation, called natural background, is a normal part of nature's balance and presents no hazard to ordinary living. However, about 1895, man discovered ways of creating artificially almost all of nature's natural forms of radiation and then went on to create new forms in infinite number, power and variety.

While the number of radiation sources available to man today is very large, there are only two different basic types or kinds which are important in nursing. However, either of these may arise from a variety of different sources.

X-ray is a good example of electromagnetic radiation, one of the basic types. It is made up of rays or waves of very high electric energy traveling at very high speeds. When electromagnetic radiation arises from natural or artificially created radioactive isotopes, instead of an x-ray machine, it is called *gamma radiation*.

The other basic radiation type is represented by *alpha* and *beta* particles which are actual parts of radioactive atoms; these break away and travel at high speeds and with great energies to produce the same effects in man as x-rays or gamma rays but each in differing amounts.

All four of these act on living tissue in the same way, by ionization or, in other words, alteration of atoms in the chemical systems of the cell. If the level of radiation and its resulting intracellular ionization is low enough, no irreversible damage will be done to the cell or organism as a whole. However, if the level is high enough, the cell may be altered or even destroyed. When such ionization occurs in the cells of the gonads, genetic mutations may result. Radiation effect is cumulative; the ionization that occurs in cells is not reversible.

* In collaboration with Sandra L. Betz, R.N., Isotope Nurse-Technician, Radiology Dept., Hospital of the University of Pennsylvania.

Radiation Detection and Control. While these radiations are very powerful, they cannot be directly seen, heard, smelled, tasted, felt or in any other way detected by ordinary human senses. So their characteristic ability to ionize matter through which they pass is utilized in designing instruments to detect and measure them. Simply, such instruments record the number of rays or particles of radiation which pass through the detecting unit in a given period of time. These instruments, such as Geiger counters, will detect radioactivity and measure its general strength.

Radiation has an additional ability to affect the emulsion of photographic film as light does in a camera. Film badges can be worn while working with or near radiation. After development of the film from the badge, extent of exposure can be determined. This knowledge of total radiation exposure is very important. Within certain limits, cells live quite well while being constantly exposed—there is always a low continuous radiation background. At the other extreme, too much radiation exposure can cause physical damage and death.

In this country, and in much of the world, laws require that radiation sources and devices may be used only by persons trained in their theory and operation, who agree to abide by the specified standards and limits. Properly observed, they should enable anyone to work with or near radiation throughout his life without noticeable physical damage, shortening of life expectancy or genetic harm to future generations. Detailed specific dosage and exposure limits need not concern the average nurse, who is not working directly in a radiology department, so long as she does observe carefully the precautions outlined by the hospital radiologist for any particular case involving radiation. Her exposure ordinarily will be only occasional and, assuming proper precautions, very slight.

X-ray in Diagnosis and Therapy. Generally, radiation is used in medicine in three ways—for diagnosis, therapy or research. For any of these, the available radiation sources can be listed simply as roentgenographic and fluoroscopic machines (x-rays), natural and artificial radioactive isotopes and the high energy particle machines. The uses of roentgenograms and fluoroscopy are familiar to all of us. Probably the only comment needed here is a reminder again that while radiation exposure is cumulative, the probable advantages of its use outweigh any possible hazards. Of course, the radiologist takes care to see that this slight calculated risk is always minimized and that no patient is ever exposed unwisely.

X-ray Therapy

Ionizing irradiation is the traditional alternative to surgery as a therapeutic approach to malignant diseases and remains the therapy of choice for most nonresectable tumors. Depending on the type of tumor to be treated, x-ray or isotope radiotherapy may be preferred. If the patient is to receive x-ray irradiation, the radiologist devises a program involving repeated exposures to fractional doses, directed in such a manner as to produce effective ionization within the tumor while avoiding unnecessary irradiation of normal structures. Low-voltage, high-voltage or supervoltage equipment is available for generating x-rays with energies that are appropriate for tumors of all sizes and in all locations. The lesions which are most likely to respond to x-radiation are those originating from the reticuloendothelial tissues, i.e., leukemias and lymphomas, and from embryonal-type tissue, such as teratomas, for example. The least radio-sensitive are tumors of nerve tissue, bone and muscle. X-ray therapy is notably successful in carcinoma of the larynx, the nasopharynx, the tongue, the lip and the skin. Some regression is to be expected in most types of tumor so treated, especially if irradiated during phases or rapid growth. Postoperative irradiation of a tumor site is practiced commonly and is indicated, especially if the excised tumor is small and its histology is indicative of high-grade malignancy.

Radiation Hazards. Radiation damage will never be wholly eliminated as a complication of radiation therapy. Radiation damage may be discussed in two categories: (1) in terms of complications, both immediate and late, that affect the exposed individual directly, and (2) in terms of gonadal injury and gene mutations which threaten his progeny. So far as mutations are concerned, the effects of radiation on human germ plasm may be reflected in an increased incidence of stillbirths and congenital defects among the offspring of exposed individuals, similar abnormalities affecting their progeny and generations to follow, *ad infinitum*.

The early complications that involve the individual himself are related to the relatively high susceptibility of rapidly growing tissue to the effects of ionization and stem from the diffuse quality of the destruction which it causes. The fact that the injury extends to all components of the exposed tissue and affects most severely the cells that are growing fastest, i.e., those engaged in tissue regeneration and repair, accounts for the slow healing and extensive scarring that are characteristic of radiation damage.

The skin is especially vulnerable to radiation injury by virtue of its exposed location. Healing is likely to be protracted and permanent changes are unusually extensive.

Bone marrow is one of the most radiosensitive of normal tissues, and damage to the marrow is potentially the most lethal of the complications of excessive irradiation. Interruption of marrow function results promptly in a fall in circulating platelets to thrombocytopenic levels, giving rise to a hemorrhagic diathesis for which there is, as yet, no adequate replacement therapy. Agranulocytosis develops concomitantly, causing a heightened susceptibility to bacterial infection which may prove to be as hazardous as thrombocytopenia. Fortunately, antibiotic therapy affords adequate protection against sepsis in the majority of patients. Radiation cataracts have been described from excessive exposure of the eyes to neutron or x-radiation, and diffuse, incapacitating fibrosis of the lungs may follow injudicious irradiation of the thorax. Damage to the fetus in utero, with production of congenital malformations, is apt to occur as a result of irradiation during the period from the second to the sixth week of gestation.

Among the most serious of the late consequences of irradiation damage is the increased susceptibility to malignant metaplasia and the development of cancer at sites of earlier irradiation. Evidence cited in support of this relationship refers to the increased incidence of carcinoma of skin, bone and lung after latent periods of 20 years and longer following irradiation of those sites. Further support has been adduced from the relatively high incidence of carcinoma of the thyroid 7 years and longer following low-dosage irradiation of the thymus in childhood, and from the increased incidence of leukemia following total body irradiation at any age. Evidence for long-range damage from irradiation in the form of gene mutations in exposed germ plasm is derived almost entirely from observations on insects and small animals and is based on analogy. Statistical arguments and analogies aside, the potential capacity of radiation to produce gene mutations can scarcely be discounted; the existence of the threat cannot be denied. Accordingly, precautions against unnecessary or excessive exposure to radiation are appropriate, and every available safeguard against radiation damage is definitely indicated.

Improvements in equipment for diagnostic radiology are clearly desirable and are constantly in progress. Policies have been recommended, more rigid than those of the past, regarding the extent to which diagnostic x-ray examinations should be carried out and the frequency with which they should be repeated. Prophylactic examinations for possible pregnancy or for purposes of pelvimetry, for example, are discouraged, as are all x-ray studies that are undertaken in the absence of disease. Perhaps the most important aspect of any program that might be designed for the prevention of radiation damage concerns the education of practitioners who are equipped with radiologic apparatus but are untrained in radiology.

Finally, it needs to be emphasized that the benefits of radiation therapy should never be denied to a patient with a radiosensitive neoplasm because of considerations regarding long-range radiologic safety. As a result of intensive publicity regarding the dangers of radioactive fallout and the complications of radiation damage in general, anxiety over the potential complications of radiotherapy, including x-ray irradiation and the use of radioisotopes, is prevalent among the laity. The nurse is very likely to be in a position to allay such fears in the minds of many patients for whom irradiation has been recommended but who are inclined to refuse it on the grounds of its inherent risks.

Roentgenologic Precautions. The safety of the patient, the therapist, the nurse, the x-ray technician and any other personnel who might be present during radiography, fluoroscopy or radiotherapy demands strict observance of certain precautions, including the following:

1. No one should be in the room with the patient who is undergoing x-ray therapy or roentgenography.

2. The fluoroscopic equipment and technic should be such as to prevent the leakage of radiation.

3. Each individual in the fluoroscopic room should protect himself from scattered radiation by wearing a lead apron and, if indicated, lead-impregnated gloves.

4. Complete protection of the patient's gonads during radiography and x-ray therapy should be assured by means of appropriate lead shielding.

The nurse should be familiar with these stipulations and their purpose so that she may explain them to the patient.

When a patient is receiving x-ray therapy, he ought to know why he seems to be left alone when receiving treatment and that a technician is always nearby, who can see him through a window. Also, the patient should know that there is an intercommunication system which allows him to talk to the technician. It is well to remember that external radiation will never cause any patient to become radioactive himself. He cannot possibly present any radiation hazard to himself, other patients or the nurse.

Nursing Care. Radiation may have a marked systemic effect upon the patient and lead to nausea, vomiting, fever, loss of appetite and a feeling of extreme malaise. Although this postirradiation upset may be only temporary, lasting from a few days to a week or more, it is during this period that good nursing care is most essential. The giving of sedatives, the careful selection of fluids and foods that will not induce or aggravate nausea and the constant reassuring attitude of the nurse are extremely helpful. Liver extract and vitamins B and C are given in many cases, and the administration of intravenous glucose is helpful. Pyridoxine and dimenhydrate (Dramamine) given orally may be helpful in minimizing nausea and vomiting.

Skin reactions with reddening and blistering not infrequently occur following irradiation therapy; in such patients the area is kept dry. If vesication of the skin occurs, the area should be treated with bland ointments such as boric acid or vitamin A and D ointment. Even long after a course of radiation therapy, the treated skin will remain sensitive, and the patient should be cautioned against further irritation from friction, extremes in temperature and exposure to sunlight.

Radioisotope Therapy

Beta and Gamma Irradiation. The use of radioactive isotopes affords a method of delivering ionizing radiation that is extraordinarily versatile, one that is applicable to most types of cases, is convenient to administer and is relatively inexpensive for the patient.

TELETHERAPY. Radiation of a type similar to that delivered by supervoltage x-ray apparatus is obtained from radio-cobalt. Cobalt[60] emits 2 gamma rays with energies of 1.1 and 1.3 million electron volts. A weak beta emission from this isotope is screened out by means of interposing a thin metal filter between the source and the target. Assuming that the quantity of cobalt[60] is adequate, this and its protective casing (i.e., the "cobalt bomb") can be located at a considerable distance from the patient. The advantage of this arrangement is that the radiation dose absorbed by the skin and by the internal target become approximately equal, whereas if the source is in near proximity to the patient, his skin is exposed to relatively intense radiation.

EXTERNAL MOLDS. Cobalt[60] is employed also in external mold therapy, a method of irradiation in which the isotope, packaged and screened within an appropriate container, is applied directly to the skin surface. This method of application is of particular value in treating carcinomas of the lip, the ears, the scalp, the mouth, the larynx and the penis.

Another gamma emitter used in external molds is radioactive tantalum (Ta[182]).

Available in the form of flexible wire, this may be bent to conform to anatomic variations. For example, it may be applied in the form of a ring to the exterior surface of a retinoblastoma which involves the eyeball and the optic nerve. Radioactive strontium (Sr[90]) and yttrium (Y[90]), both pure beta emitters, are used in external molds for shallow irradiation of neoplasms in the eye. A most convenient method of applying beta radiation to superficial malignancies of the skin utilizes "plaques" consisting of bakelite, polyethylene plastic or blotting paper impregnated with radiophosphorus (P[32]). These are cut and molded to size and shape, then taped in place over the lesion.

INTRACAVITARY ISOTOPE THERAPY. Liquid radioisotopes—for example, solutions of radioactive colloidal gold (Au[198]), radioactive sodium (Na[24]) and bromine (Br[82]) —have been placed in balloons within the bladder for beta irradiation of the internal bladder wall to a depth of a few millimeters. Deeper penetration of the bladder is accomplished by gamma emission from a cobalt[60] source located in the center of a balloon which is distended within the center of the bladder. Capsules containing tantalum (Ta[182]) may be packed into the body of the uterus, the canal of the cervix or into a maxillary sinus.

INTERSTITIAL ISOTOPE THERAPY. Radioisotopes are available in the form of needles which can be implanted directly within the tumor tissue. Interstitial irradiation also may be applied by injecting a radioisotope solution directly into the substance of the tumor and the surrounding tissue. Colloidal solutions of radioactive colloidal gold (Au[198]) are especially suitable for this form of application. Radioactive colloidal gold also is injected into the pleural cavity, the colloid gradually precipitating onto the serosal surface which is thereafter exposed to a pure beta emission.

INTERNAL IRRADIATION. Other clinical applications of radioisotopes include the treatment of myelogenous leukemia and polycythemia vera by intravenous injections of sodium phosphate (P[32]). Solutions of radioiodine (I[131]) are administered orally in patients with hyperthyroidism. The effectiveness of these measures is attributable to the fact that, in each instance, the target tissue has an affinity for, and concentrates within its substance, the therapeutic agent, radioiodine becoming localized in the thyroid gland and metastatic thyroid tissue throughout the body, and radiophosphorus accumulating in the bones, where it is in close proximity to the proliferating marrow.

Protection of the Nurse. The receipt of a radioisotope in therapeutic dosage converts an individual temporarily into a radiation source, and the care of such an individual requires certain modifications if the nurse is to avoid the hazards of radiation exposure. Such considerations do not apply, of course, in relation to patients undergoing radioisotope tracer tests, because of the relatively minute quantities of radiation that these involve.

The amount of radioactivity that the nurse receives as she works near the patient depends on three factors: (1) her distance from the patient (doubling the distance from a radiation source will cut the intensity received to one fourth), (2) the amount of time spent in actual contact with him and (3) the degree of shielding provided. Such shielding usually is chosen according to the type of radiation in use, since alpha particles will be absorbed by even a sheet of tissue paper, while gamma rays, on the other hand, may penetrate many inches of solid lead. During the first 24 to 72 hour period, which is the time of greatest radioactivity, actual nursing care must be limited to essential care. The patient should know why he must stay in bed or within his room during his course of treatment and why the nurse may not remain in his room longer than it takes to perform her nursing tasks.

INTERNAL USE. The protective factors of time, distance and shielding help greatly with external radiation, but of these three, only time can be controlled when the radiation source has become internal through absorption, ingestion, injection, or other means.

All radioactive isotopes, by the very nature of their radioactivity, are destroying themselves at a rate which is constant but varies from one isotope to another. Each radiation particle or ray given off is the result of the destruction of one radioactive atom.

So in time, all of the radiation will disappear. Since this rate is constant, we can say that one half of the radioactivity will be dissipated in a given time. For each isotope, we call this time the *physical half-life*.

In the body, any chemical substance is disposed of sooner or later by normal metabolic processes, so we can determine for any isotope how long it will take for one half to disappear from the body on a purely chemical and biologic basis. This we call its *biologic half-life*. Since both of these factors are affecting any internal isotope, the result is an *effective half-life* which is a combination of the other two.

We cannot change distance or add shielding for internal isotopes, but by altering the metabolic uses and the body distribution of an isotope, we can change its effective half-life and thus vary time of exposure.

In considering problems of internal radiation sources, it is also extremely important to know the body's pattern of distribution, metabolism and excretion of each different isotope. It is apparent that an isotope which is completely dispersed throughout the body, or a major portion of it, is less hazardous to any one organ or tissue than another isotope which is concentrated by the body into a very localized organ or area.

For instance, such concentration occurs with radioactive iodine in the thyroid gland, where most of the body's iodine is found. Naturally, an isotope which is excreted rapidly is less hazardous than one which is bound in the body for long periods of time.

It is easiest to consider the nursing problems of radiation sources in two major groups—those resulting from sealed sources, which are physically implanted in the patient, and the different types of problems resulting from non-sealed sources, which may be introduced into a patient.

Sealed internal radiation, such as radium, radon, iridium or gold seeds, is controlled from the moment of application, in that the agent used is encased in a nonradioactive metallic covering so that it cannot directly contaminate any other object or tissue, even as it continues to radiate. The casing material will absorb all alpha radiation and most of the beta, so that the resulting hazard is one primarily of gamma radiation.

It is important that the nurse never fear such a patient. His internal radiation source cannot, in any way, be transferred to another person without actual contact. In addition, because the radiologist exercises safety controls, and as long as his orders and prescribed precautions are followed, the patient's internal radiation will not cause any other person to exceed normal exposure limits.

However, the radiation remains present, and, while giving the patient all the care that he needs and wants, the nurse should not linger with him unnecessarily.

In the unusual circumstance of a sealed source, such as a radium needle, becoming dislodged and perhaps falling on the bed or the floor, or being found in a dressing, it should be handled only with a long-handled forceps or tongs and reported immediately to the radiologist in charge of the case.

The nurse should never discard a dressing or a bandage from such a patient until she is sure that it does not contain a radioactive source, which would not only become a hazard to others, but especially in the case of radium, also would be an expensive loss.

The problems of *unsealed sources* are a bit more troublesome but when properly handled are no more dangerous. In these patients the radioactivity may be widely spread in the body, depending on a particular isotope's biologic distribution pattern. It may be localized or can appear in any body tissue or fluid.

Probably the most widely used unsealed radioactive source is radioactive iodine, valuable in diagnosis and treatment of diseases of the thyroid gland. Of all the isotopes, it is the one most likely to be encountered by the average nurse and is a good example for discussion of precautions to be followed with unsealed sources in general.

Except in unusual cases of large doses used for treatment, the radiation from a patient receiving iodine will be no important exposure hazard in ordinary nursing care; and even with the largest dose, common sense observation of time and distance factors can control this problem.

However, since radioactive iodine, like most isotopes, circulates in the blood stream and is excreted by the kidneys, both blood and urine of iodine patients will contain radioactivity. In addition, it can be secreted by the sweat glands and will be found in the vomitus of a patient who has recently taken an oral dose.

With iodine doses of the size used routinely for diagnostic purposes, the only major precaution is the careful handling and disposal of the patient's body fluids.

It is also wise to exercise extra care with bedpans as well as with any syringes and needles used, simply by seeing that all such contaminated objects are thoroughly washed before being returned to general use. It should be needless to add that the nurse's hands, especially, should be washed with extra care.

Wound dressings and bedclothes from patients who have received small tracer doses need only be wrapped well with paper or nonradioactive linens (so that no possible contamination is left exposed) and stored until safe for disposal.

In caring for patients who have received larger treatment doses, precautions must be somewhat more strict. In these cases items such as bedpans should be marked and used for that patient alone and never handled without rubber gloves. Dressings and bedclothes should also be handled with gloves during the first 2 or 3 days after administration of the dose, then treated as described above for tracer patients.

Since the radioactivity of iodine will decline to one half in 8 days, and since the iodine is constantly being removed by the kidneys as well, all of these precautions become less important after the first 3 days and can usually be relaxed in 1 week.

Another radioactive isotope in general use is radioactive phosphorus. Essentially the same precautions apply here except that elimination is primarily in the feces instead of the urine. Since radioactive phosphorus emits no gamma radiation, as iodine does, phosphorus patients constitute no hazard as an external source.

Few nurses will encounter patients who have been treated with radioactive colloidal gold. In most instances, the gold will be localized by injection into a single organ or body cavity. When administered intravenously the liver and the splenic tissue will

TABLE 10. Common Cytotoxic or Alkylating Agents

Agents	Route of Administration	Toxic Symptoms	Neoplastic Conditions Treated
Mechlorethamine HCl. (Mustargen, nitrogen mustard)	I.V.	Nausea and vomiting	Carcinoma of breast, ovary and lung; chronic leukemia; lymphoma
Triethylene Melamine (TEM) N,N',N''-Triethylene-thiophosphoramide (Thio-TEPA)	I.V. Oral I.V. Oral	Therapeutic doses depress peripheral blood-cell count; excessive doses cause severe bone marrow depression with leuko-penia, thrombocytopenia and bleeding.	Carcinoma of breast, ovary and lung; lymphoma
Chlorambucil (Leukeran)	Oral		Chronic leukemia; lymphoma

(Adapted from Karnofsky, D. A.: Cancer chemotherapeutic agents, CA 11:60–61, March–April, 1961)

remove essentially all of the radioactive material from the blood within a very few hours. While direct contamination is less of a problem here, more attention must be given to the time spent with, and the distance from, the patient.

It is important to remember always that while the use of radiation may create new nursing problems, it is justified by its value to the patient.

By understanding radiation and the problems of its use, regular nursing care can proceed safely, without worries of danger to the nurse and, most important, with no patient ever being neglected because of unreasonable fears or misunderstandings.

Chemotherapy of Cancer

Interest in the treatment of cancer by chemical agents (chemotherapy) has increased considerably since World War II. The hope for a cancer cure by this means depends on an understanding of the biochemical and metabolic differences between normal and neoplastic cells that will enable tumor cells to be destroyed while healthy tissue remains intact. *In general it can be said that as yet no drugs have been discovered to cure malignant tumors;* however, cancer chemotherapy may (or may not) offer some help to patients for whom surgery and irradiation are no longer beneficial. Some of the drugs produce a regression of the tumor or its metastases, and the use of chemotherapeutic agents at the time of surgery may reduce or slow up the appearance of secondary growths. In some patients, pain and other symptoms are relieved for a time.

Chemotherapeutic agents are especially useful in the treatment of lymphomas and leukemias, diffuse tumors usually not amenable to surgical therapy. In such patients, the use of chemotherapeutic agents may prolong life for many years, with a remission

TABLE 11. Common Antimetabolites

Agents	Route of Administration	Toxic Symptoms	Neoplastic Conditions Treated
Amethopterin (Methotrexate) Aminopterin sodium (4-amino folic acid)	Oral Oral	Oral and digestive tract ulcerations; bone marrow depression with leuko-penia, thrombocytopenia, and bleeding	Acute leukemia; uterine chorio-carcinoma; testicular tumors
6–Mercaptopurine (Purinethol)	Oral	Therapeutic doses usually well-tolerated; excessive doses cause bone marrow depression.	Acute leukemia; chronic myelocytic leukemia
5-Fluorouracil (5-FU)	I.V.	Stomatitis; nausea; gastro-intestinal injury; bone marrow depression	Carcinoma of colon and rectum

(Adapted from Karnofsky, D. A.: Cancer chemotherapeutic agents, CA 11:60–61, March–April, 1961)

TABLE 12. Steroid and ACTH Compounds

Agents	Route of Administration	Toxic Symptoms	Neoplastic Conditions Treated
Androgen (Testosterone propionate) (Fluoxymesterone, Halotestin)	I.M.	Fluid retention; masculinization	Carcinoma of breast
Estrogen (Diethylstilbestrol) (Stilbestrol)	Oral	Occasional nausea and vomiting; fluid retention; femininization; uterine bleeding	Carcinoma of breast and prostate
Progesterone (Delalutin)	I.M.		
Adrenal cortical compounds (Cortisone acetate) (Cortogen, Cortone)	Oral		
Hydrocortisone (Cortef, Cortril, Hycortole)	Oral	Fluid retention; hypertension; diabetes; increased susceptibility to infection	Acute leukemia; lymphomas; carcinoma of breast; chronic lymphocytic leukemia; and miscellaneous conditions
Prednisone (Deltra, Meticorten)	Oral		
Adrenocorticotropic Hormone (ACTH)	I.V. I.M.		

(Adapted from Karnofsky, D. A.: Cancer chemotherapeutic agents, CA **11**:60–61, March–April, 1961)

but never a cure. In solid tumors the mass may become smaller, and surface ulcerations may heal for a time. Cure is not to be expected.

In general, the chemotherapeutic agents may be divided into 4 different groups. (In each group some of the more common drugs are described.)

1. The poisons (or cytotoxic or alkylating agents), of which the nitrogen mustards and the polysaccharides are examples. These poisons destroy both normal and tumor cells. It is believed that cells in mitosis (rapidly growing tumor cells) are more sensitive to toxicity than normal adult cells, and that tumors of well-differentiated cells are less sensitive to toxicity than those of less well-differentiated cells in some tumors.

The chief disadvantage of most of these drugs is their destructive effect on bone marrow, one of the body's chief sources of new blood cells.

2. The mitosis inhibitors, colchicine and its derivatives. These drugs inhibit the normal nutritive sequence; unfortunately they are too toxic when given in effective doses.

3. The antimetabolites, folic acid and purine antagonists. These are synthetic substances similar to those that nourish the normal cell during its growth and development. However, they differ enough in their chemical composition so that, although the drugs are taken into the cell substance, they cannot be used by the cell. Thus, they deceive the cell, and act as a monkey wrench in the cellular machinery.

4. Steroid Compounds, ACTH, and Castration. Alteration of the endocrine environment is a major approach in the chemotherapy of certain types of neoplastic disease: namely, tumors arising in organs usually under hormonal influence, such as the prostate (castration) and the breast (androgen and estrogen therapy). Oophorectomy, adrenalectomy and pituitarectomy represent similar forms of therapy.

None of these measures cures malignancy. They are efforts to make the physiology of the host less favorable for the growth of cancer.

Methods of Administration

The cancer chemotherapeutic drugs may be given intravenously or by mouth, depending on the drug. In addition, efforts may be made to introduce the drug in high concentration into the tumor area by injection into its vascular supply. These efforts require complicated perfusion technics that usually are carried out in specialized clinics.

Perfusion. This technic allows the administration of large doses of extremely toxic drugs to an isolated extremity, organ, or region of the body. Such a dose could not be tolerated by the entire body.

The usual vessels perfused for a lesion in the lower extremity are iliac, femoral and popliteal arteries and veins. The axillary artery and vein are injected in upper extremity perfusion. The abdominal aorta and the vena cava are used in pelvic perfusion.

On admission and preoperatively the patient is weighed, since the amounts of chemotherapeutic drug and heparin given are calculated on the basis of kilograms of body weight. Blood, urine, and x-ray studies also are done. Preparation of the patient for surgery includes the answering of his many questions, since perfusion is a relatively new procedure.

In the operating room by means of a pump-oxygenator, the patient's blood is circulated in a closed system for the involved part of the body. The chemotherapeutic drug is injected in concentrated doses. The duration of the perfusion depends on the drug, and the extent and the location of the growth. During the procedure, efforts are made by tourniquets and/or ligatures to prevent seepage of the drug into the systemic circulation. Obviously, it is easier to prevent leakage into the systemic circulation when an extremity is involved but much more difficult when the torso is perfused.

Postoperatively, blood tests are done frequently to check on bone marrow depression. Tissue in the local area is observed frequently for any reaction such as erythema, mild edema, blistering and petechiae. Any noticeable change is charted with full description. Pain usually is not a problem but if it is present, it may indicate severe injury to normal tissue.

The patient who has had an aortic perfusion should be observed for signs of malaise, nausea, vomiting, rising temperature, blood pressure and pulse (note signs indicative of a hypotensive reaction). Fluids are given intravenously for the first 48 hours; all the patient's total intake and output are recorded accurately. The patient is turned frequently, because pressure areas develop easily. The principles of effective postoperative care are followed carefully, including the emotional support of the patient.

Nursing Care in Cancer Chemotherapy

The best of nursing care is required for patients receiving cancer chemotherapy. Many of these drugs are highly irritant. They produce local thrombophlebitis if the intravenous injections are given too rapidly, and they cause marked tissue reactions if the solution escapes into the tissues around a vein. Nausea and vomiting are common gastrointestinal symptoms that may persist for a considerable period (6 to 12 hours) after the administration of the drugs. Chills and fever appear after the administration of some of the drugs. In some instances, the toxic manifestations include ulceration of the gums and the buccal mucosa, abdominal cramps and marked anorexia.

Systemic effects of cancer chemotherapy are sometimes serious and may be fatal. Leukopenia and anemia, reflecting bone marrow destruction, are common complications that demand careful and repeated blood counts. Their appearance is an indication for reducing the drug dosage or substituting another drug.

The nurse must be constantly on the alert for the appearance of untoward reactions and symptoms. She must be prepared for even a fatality after the use of some of the chemotherapeutic agents in very ill patients.

It is of course important that the responsible relatives know about the possible effects of these drugs, and hope for improvement but never for cure may be held out to them.

PSYCHOLOGICAL ASPECTS OF NURSING THE CANCER PATIENT

The physician responsible for the patient and the patient's family make the decision as to whether the patient should or should not be told that he has cancer. Any questions that may arise are to be directed to the physician. It is up to the nurse to find out from the physician what information he has given the patient.

The manner in which a patient accepts the information that he has cancer often depends on his philosophy of life and his views of life and death. The greatest comfort may be spiritual consolation. The nurse should arrange to have those spiritual resources available that are most likely to meet his individual needs.

In modern cancer therapy it may happen frequently that extensive surgery and irradiation therapy may produce changes that are disfiguring or mutilating and not easily borne by the patient. The problems thus created may be almost overwhelming. They begin before operation, when the question is raised as to how much the patient should be told about the details of his disease and his operation; they must be handled differently in each patient. It is probably best that the nurse should not be called on to divulge the details of diagnosis and treatment.

The adaption that has to be made to the therapeutic measures for the malignancy must begin in the preoperative period. The patients are particularly in need of support and reassurance in order to establish confidence in the skill of the surgeon and the hospital environment. When the patient approaches surgery with a sense of hopefulness and expectation, excellent results can be anticipated from a psychological point of view. If, however, he approaches surgery with the conviction that the operation is going to be painful, disfiguring and mutilating, it is almost to be expected that he should show depression and a marked sense of weakness postoperatively. The postoperative symptoms of depression may be sleep disturbance, loss of appetite, and other manifestations that may persist for an indefinite period. In their depression, patients may think there is hostility on the part of nurses, doctors and attendants.

Even when the physician is not blamed directly, often he is looked on unconsciously as the injuring party; hence, resentment may appear particularly toward nurses in the immediate environment, social workers, and even members of the family. The symptoms often take more demanding attention. The nurse must recognize this attitude as a part of the normal process of repair and should work through the anger and the resentment to win the patient over to a more normal attitude.

In other instances, patients may assume feelings of dejection accompanied by a sense of helplessness. Such anxiety often makes the patient turn to other people for help, advice, consolation and reassurance. This state is often only temporary, and the nurse, who is closest to him, can be of invaluable aid during this period of rehabilitation. Kindness and warmth give the patient the security he needs.

The nurse, of all medical personnel, has the most sustained and intimate contact with the patient during his hospitalization. Therefore, she is the person to whom the patient will turn most often for kindness and support during the early postoperative period. If the nurse is able to meet these needs, not only will the pressure and the anxiety be alleviated, but also the patient's perception of his hospital experience will be modified.

In summary, the psychology of cancer patients is the psychology of a person who is facing a fundamental struggle with security and his self-value. Such problems can be met best by professional persons. The nurse is in a very advantageous position to aid the patient in his efforts to overcome depression and anxiety and to resume normal function after surgery.

TERMINAL NURSING CARE

Some authorities claim that the most important aspect in the care of the terminal patient is good nursing. Frequent changes of bed linen, cleanliness and keeping the patient warm are all comfort measures that can relieve a great deal of pain. During this care probably the most common emergency that the nurse should anticipate is hemorrhage, due to erosion of blood vessels by the malignancy itself, secondary necrosis or the sloughing of tissue following irradiation. In some instances, the nurse can control bleeding by digital pressure. In cases of hemorrhage that cannot be controlled by local measures, the patient should be kept quiet in the recumbent position, and the physician should be notified. The nurse should have the necessary equipment available for treating shock and hemorrhage (see pp. 296, 298).

Ambulation

The patient should be kept ambulatory as long as possible; however, the nurse must recognize when it is undesirable for him to get out of bed.

Nutrition and Hydration

The main limiting factor in attaining and maintaining a good nutritional level is anorexia. Specific food needs vary depending on the location of the tumor. For instance, the needs of a patient with cancer of the stomach may be quite different from those of a patient with cancer of the liver or the lungs. Small, frequent feedings are more likely to be accepted, together with protein supplementation and parenteral vitamin administration. Dehydration and electrolyte imbalance have to be prevented by correcting inadequate fluid intake and output.

Skin Care

Good skin care is imperative. Tissues do not repair so easily as in the normal individual; therefore, preventive measures may eliminate much discomfort. Back and body massages are helpful; in addition, they are conducive to relaxation and help to relieve pain.

Pain

The nurse must be able to judge whether her patient needs a soothing treatment, a sedative or a hypnotic. Usually, drugs can be given sparingly at first and then gradually increased in kind and amount. One must be cognizant of the effects of drugs on the debilitated and the older patient. These individuals have increased sensitivity and may have a chain-type reaction to narcotics. First, they are drowsy, take less food, become dehydrated, retain urine, and have gastrointestinal irritation, nausea and vomiting and ultimately develop a disturbed electrolyte and fluid balance. Of course, the treatment for such a condition would be to discontinue these medications or decrease their dosage.

Esthetic Factors

Facial tumors are often unsightly; the patient usually is very sensitive about his appearance. Such lesions should be covered if possible. Other features of the patient should be accented to detract attention from the tumor site. This can be done by careful grooming, attractive garments, etc. Bright lights in a room should be replaced by softer lights, inasmuch as shades of light and dark can tone down unsightly areas. The nurse should use her ingenuity in helping this individual to bear his burden more easily.

One of the most unpleasant features of cancer in exposed areas on the body is the foul odor that appears sooner or later. This is due to the sloughing of tissues. Every effort should be made to keep the patient and his room clean. Dressings should be changed frequently, removed quickly from the patient's room and deposited in a metal-covered container until they are sent to the incinerator. Bedclothes and the patient's clothing ought to be changed when soiled. The use of absorbent or oakum pads may help when drainage is present. The room should be ventilated properly. Deodorants may be necessary. Several of the essential oils, such as oil of geranium, oil of eucalyptus or oil of orange, will meet the situation. Neutroleum alpha is lasting and not unpleasant when one or two drops are applied to the dressing or to the bedclothing. Powdered charcoal in the dressing or potassium permanganate solution 1:2,000 as an irrigation often helps. Activated zinc peroxide is also effective in cleansing and deodorizing these wounds. Commercially prepared products are now available and can be disseminated from a bottle with a wick or by means of an electric deodorizer to absorb odors. These are quite successful.

The nurse should have a rational psychological approach toward death. She is often the person to whom the patient turns when he wants to talk about himself, his fears, his hopes, etc. To be able to listen and to offer encouragement are extremely important assets. Many times a patient demonstrates hostility and rebellion. In spite of this, the nurse must remain tolerant and show her patient that she stands by him in spite of his unpleasant actions. In this manner, eventually she will be able to discover the reason for his outbursts and then help him to resolve them. (See "Psychological Aspects of Cancer Patient Care," above.)

Occupational and Recreational Therapy

Statistics reveal that the home is best suited for the care of this patient for several reasons. He is in a familiar environment and can see his friends and family. Many times, he can perform some household duties and thereby feel that he is helping. The financial burden on the family is reduced. The family knows what is happening to him, which often is not the case when he is in an institution. The home is more conducive for him to pursue his hobbies, such as caring for tropical fish, developing a miniature garden, etc. Much of the responsibility for his care rests with the family. The nurse and the physician can help them greatly in making the adjustment an easier one. For patients who do not have a home, the next best available environment should be sought. The nurse with sympathetic understanding can help her patient in making contact with the proper agencies for the adjustment of his social and economic problems.

Nursing in Cancer of the Various Organs is discussed as each condition is studied in this text.

THE FOLLOW-THROUGH

Does every patient with a colostomy have a chance to learn how to keep himself clean and free from odors, without encumbering gadgets? Does every woman who has lost a breast get an understanding talk or two or more from her doctor (and nurse) directed toward readier acceptance of her deformity? And does she get pin-pointed, fact-full advice as to where she can obtain a falsie that will suit even her? Is every "laryngectomee" exposed to expert instruction on how to talk in spite of his lost chords?

Too often the answer to these and similar questions is "No."

The total treatment of cancer embraces detection, curative or palliative treatment and— depending on our success—rehabilitation. If we are to treat the patient and not only the disease, then rehabilitation — the follow-through—whether it takes the form of plastic surgery, prostheses, psychology, or whatever, must be recognized and practiced as an integral part of getting sick people well.*

BIBLIOGRAPHY AND SUGGESTED READING

Articles

Alston, F., Hilkemeyer, R., White, M., and Schmolke, H.: Perfusion, Am. J. Nursing **60:**1603-1607, Nov., 1960.

* CA: A Bulletin of Cancer Progress, Vol. 1, No. 5, July, 1951.

Barckley, V.: What can I say to the cancer patient? Nurs. Outlook **6:**316-318, June, 1958.

Barnett, C.: A defense of sweetness, Am. J. Nursing **61:**99-101, Feb., 1961.

Bocker, E. H., and Schultz, G. R.: Foundations of radiological health, Am. Assoc. Ind. Nurses J. **10:**11-15, Aug., 1962.

Brauer, P. H.: Should the patient be told the truth? Nurs. Outlook **8:**672-676, Dec., 1960.

Burnett, M. K.: The nurse in an industry with a radiation hazard, Am. Assoc. Ind. Nurses J. **10:**16-18, Aug., 1962.

Burns, P., and Parker, H.: When radioactive iodine or gold is used, Am. J. Nursing **56:**1404-1406, Nov., 1956.

Ellison, R. R.: Treating cancer with antimetabolites, Am. J. Nursing **62:**79-82, Nov., 1962.

Fitzpatrick, G. M., and Shotkin, J. M.: Pelvic perfusion, Am. J. Nursing **61:**79-81, June, 1961.

Golbey, R. B.: Chemotherapy of cancer, Am. J. Nursing **60:**521-525, April, 1960.

Kaplan, H. S.: New horizons in radiotherapy of malignant disease, J.A.M.A. **171:**133-138, 1959.

Karnofsky, D. A.: Cancer quackery: its causes, recognition and prevention, Am. J. Nursing **59:**496-500, April, 1959.

McGrath, M. J.: The care of the patient in terminal illness, Canad. Nurse **57:**566-568, June, 1961.

McIntyre, P. H.: Total body irradiation, Am. J. Nursing **61:**62-64, Sept., 1961.

Miller, I.: The patient's right to know the truth, Canad. Nurse **58:**25-29, Jan., 1962.

Mullan, J. F., and van Schoick, M. R.: Intractable pain, Am. J. Nursing **58:**228-230, 1958.

Oken, D.: What to tell cancer patients, J.A.M.A. **175:**1120-1128, 1961.

Pearson, O. H., et al.: Hypophysectomy in treatment of advanced cancer, J.A.M.A. **161:**17-21, 1956.

Proceedings of Staff Meetings of Mayo Clinic: What shall we tell the cancer patient? Am. Pract. **11:**915-917, 1960.

Ravdin, R. G., and Elkins, W. L.: Chemotherapy of solid tumors, Surg. Clin. N. Amer. **40:**1641-1656, 1960.

Stahlin, J. S., Jr.: Regional chemotherapy for cancer: experiences with 116 perfusions, Ann. Surg. **151:**605-619, 1960.

Sutherland, A. M.: Psychological impact of cancer and its therapy, Med. Clin. N. Amer. **40:**705-720, 1956.

Titchener, J., *et al.*: Problems of delay in seeking surgical care, J.A.M.A. **160:**1187-1192, 1956.

Zaino, C.: Eliminating the hazards from radiation, Am. J. Nursing **62:**60-61, April, 1962.

Pamphlets

Ogg, E.: When a family faces cancer, Pub. Affairs Pamphlet No. 286, New York, Public Affairs Committee, Inc., 1959.

Sinclair, Warren K.: Handbook of Rules for Administration of Radioactive Materials to Patients, New York, E. R. Squibb, 1962.

20

Problems Associated With Aging and Long-Term Illness

MODIFYING FACTORS

A medical problem almost never is found to be a simple product of a patient plus an illness. Other factors modify the character of the medical problem and frequently influence the conduct of both medical and nursing care. These aspects may have no direct relation to the disease itself but originate in the patient's environment or his general status. Situational elements in this category may include: the patient's age; the duration of his illness and its prognosis; his position in the family and community; his economic status and his financial responsibilities; the character of his family and its attitude toward him and his illness; stress-producing factors of all types; medico-legal complications, as in compensation cases; the climate and the weather.

There are many factors of comparable importance, but the significance of these is relatively restricted; they are discussed in conjunction with the disorders in which they are particularly influential. Of those cited above, three, with therapeutic implications of peculiar importance, are now to be examined: the age of the patient, the chronicity of disease and the gravity of prognosis.

The aging process begins with conception and ends with death. The treatment of very young and of elderly patients often is complicated by problems that relate strictly to age—problems warranting a degree of specialization of medical and nursing practice in the respective fields of pediatrics, ephebiatics and geriatrics. The sources of divergence between the problems of childhood and old age are multiple, principally related to differences in their susceptibilities, their responses to specific etiologic factors and their recuperative powers. Moreover, the psychological aspects of their individual situations are markedly different as regards both the psychogenic factors that are involved and the nature of the psychological responses characterizing their age group.

Pediatrics

This field of medicine and nursing is not included here, because this textbook is concerned primarily with the adult. The student is directed to pediatric textbooks and references.

Ephebiatrics

Adolescence marks a phase of rapid body growth, the stage of sexual maturation and a period of emotional turbulence. From the standpoint of nursing care, the most important feature distinguishing this age group is a psychological attribute, the effect of which is to impose a firm communication barrier between the adolescent and the adult. Neither child nor adult, the teenager is in an anomalous position. Vigorously rejecting the trappings of childhood, a status recently departed and now abhorred, he now strives in every way to establish himself as an adult, a tormenting aspiration with no prospect of mate-

330

TABLE 13. Increase of the Middle-Aged and Older Populations

Year	Middle-aged and Older People in the Population		
	Total Population	45–64 years	65 years and over
Both sexes			
1850	23,200,000	2,300,000	600,000
1900	76,000,000	10,400,000	3,100,000
1950	150,700,000	30,600,000	12,300,000
1975 (est.)	235,000,000	43,810,000	21,800,000

(Adapted from Tibbitts, C., and Donahue, W.: Aging in Today's Society, p. 13, Englewood Cliffs, N. J., Prentice-Hall,1960.)

rializing in the immediate future. Considerably inadequate in his own estimation and by his own standards of adulthood, he is constantly on guard against the likelihood of slight and humiliation at the hands of disparaging, patronizing adults who fail to identify him as another adult. Blanket protection against this threat is sought by adopting a defensive, i.e., hostile, attitude toward adults in general. There are all degrees of hostility and many ways in which it is reflected. Normally it expresses itself in the form of diffidence in the company of, and avoidance of close association with, older individuals. Exchanges of confidence are limited strictly to his contemporaries who, of course, share his basic attitudes and are "on his side."

This reluctance to confide in adults has a very definite influence on the doctor-nurse-patient relationship and therefore on the diagnosis, the treatment and the nursing care of the sick adolescent. Emotional disturbances are frequent and profound at this age, commonly overlying and distorting the clinical features of organic disease and occasionally engendering serious psychological aberrations. Problems of this type, demanding the closest rapport between patient, doctor and nurse for their solution, are especially difficult in this age group, owing to the natural obstacle in communications. Removal of the obstacle is a prerequisite to effective medical and nursing care. The patient will be induced to remove it, lower his guard and yield his confidence under one condition only, namely, that he be accepted by his seniors in the status of an adult. The nurse, principal observer and active therapist in immediate contact with the hospitalized adolescent, must not fail to take steps for the

achievement and the maintenance of good rapport with her young patient. By a convincing display of personal interest in matters of interest to the patient and personal respect for him as an adult, the goal is accomplished.

Some hospitals now admit teen-age patients to a "Teen-Age" floor which is apart from children and adult units. Snack bars, telephones, visiting hours and so forth are provided and geared to their interests.

Geriatrics

. . . Nobody grows old by merely living a number of years. People grow old only by deserting their ideals. . . . You are as young as your self-confidence, as old as your fear; as young as your hope, as old as your despair. In the central place of every heart, there is a recording chamber; so long as it receives messages of beauty, hope, cheer and courage, so long are you young. When the wires are all down and your heart is covered with the snows of pessimism and the ice of cynicism, then, and then only, are you grown old . . .

GENERAL DOUGLAS MACARTHUR
(*Time*, Vol. 63, Feb. 24, 1954)

Much attention is being focused on how to age gracefully and on how to be healthier, happier and more active in later years. The reason for increasing emphasis on this age group is that the number of persons 65 years old or more has almost quadrupled in the past half century (see Table 13).

SOCIOLOGIC AND HEALTH PROBLEMS OF THE AGING

As a result of the scientific and sociologic advances that have occurred during the past century, man's life expectancy has increased remarkably. Since there has been no commensurate increase in birth rates, the older age group now comprises a relatively substantial segment of the population. Moreover, it is expected that this segment will continue to expand at an accelerated pace for many decades to come. The impact of its

growth has been felt in many areas of our social and economic situation, including the fields of medicine and nursing. The importance of this segment from the standpoint of distribution of nursing requirements today and in the future is evident from the information given in Figures 97 and 98.

Geriatrics, i.e., care of the aged, has come to deserve specific emphasis in the nursing curriculum. This specialty has as its prime concern the health and the well-being of a large and an important segment of the patient population, and it deals with problems of therapy and rehabilitation that are inherently and uniquely complex.

Sociologic Factors

Current population trends, marked by an increasing accumulation of older members, must be followed by major adjustments in our socioeconomic planning. Individual attitude patterns must be reoriented on a similar scale. Youth must be educated to its inevitable responsibilities for the aged and educated to the concept of living cooperatively and effectively with one of the aged. The situations confronting the elderly individual in his life of retirement are often very complex, incapable of being resolved without the active participation of others. Modes of living must undergo radical revision in many cases if the old person is to remain at peace with himself and with others. His contemporary friends and relatives are departing from the scene or have already left; he feels increasingly isolated, helpless and anxious. He needs help but is not inclined to seek it. Nevertheless, help must be supplied and the young must supply it. Those assuming the responsibility for care of aged persons should recognize that the mental health of these persons depends on their opportunity to know security and to prove their usefulness in the conviction that they "belong."

An aged person, perhaps, has become aware that he has lost his status as the head of a family. He is now the dependent, rather than the head of the family. Evidences of deterioration have become increasingly obvious, such as forgetfulness, loss of the ability to concentrate and confusion. These are the characteristics of senility which, if pronounced, may require custodial care.

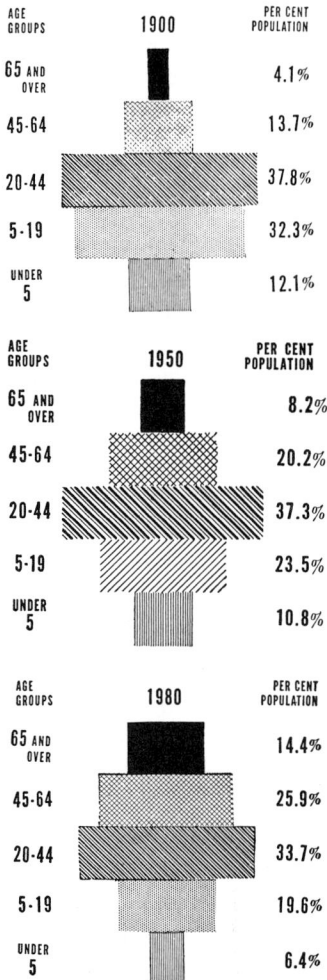

FIG. 98. Age distribution in the general population in 1900 and in 1950, and as predicted for 1980, illustrates the striking increase in the number of persons who are middle-aged and over. (Stieglitz, E. J.: The Second Forty Years, rev. ed., Philadelphia, Lippincott)

Fig. 99. This chart illustrates the relationship between age and the incidence of chronic illness. Beyond the age of 50, the incidence of invalidism increases rapidly as persons grow older. (Stieglitz, E. J.: Geriatric Medicine, ed. 3, Philadelphia, Lippincott)

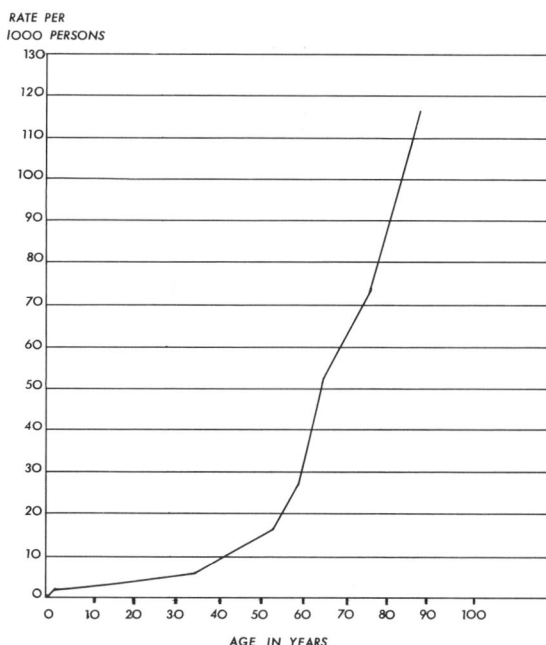

However, most old people retain their faculties. Some are acutely aware of their dependent status. They may acquire the impression that they are looked upon as a nuisance; they may feel something like a displaced person. It may be the responsibility of the nurse to advise this individual and help to correct such an attitude before it develops into one of resentment and hostility, which it is very apt to do. The nurse may need to instruct the family as follows:

Employment. With no job, the retired elderly person possesses much leisure time for morbid reflection. If possible, gainful employment should be sought for him in order that he may feel more effective and be reassured of his worth. Although the financial reward may not be great, usefulness will be felt.

Public Assistance. It is possible that the aged person needs to alter his concepts of public assistance in order to overcome his resentment over the necessity for accepting what he might regard as "charity."

Family Life. The discontinuance of solitary living in order to share another's household may seem to be undesirable from the standpoint of the elderly person, but he must be convinced of its necessity for the sake of healthful living. It may be necessary for younger members of the family to compel such a decision on the part of their older relative, obliging him to make the move without procrastination, willing or not, in order to protect his health and assure his well-being. The younger persons, although recognizing these needs and perfectly willing to discharge their responsibilities in the matter, may view with considerable misgivings the prospect of integrating the older member into their household. The nurse may be in a position to provide help with the reassuring prediction that the arrangement that is contemplated will prove to be even more rewarding for the young than for the old, whose contribution, in recompense for security, will be in terms of a companionship which promotes stability, aids perspective and achieves maturity.

Medical Aspects

Data issued by the U. S. Public Health Service indicate that approximately 5.5 million persons in this country are incapacitated each year by a chronic illness, i.e., by an illness lasting longer than 3 months. Almost one half of the chronically ill (45 per cent) is comprised of patients over 65 years of age, although this age group represents less than 8 per cent of the total population. The incidence of chronic disease in this group is approximately 17 per cent, as contrasted with an incidence of about 6 per cent in the age group between 45 and 64 and only 1.3 per cent in persons younger than 45.

Many of the disabilities that are particularly associated with old age develop as a result of degenerative vascular disease, namely, arteriosclerosis. Multiple occlusions of the arteries in the cerebral cortex are responsible for the mental deterioration of the "senile" patient; because of these occlusions he can no longer integrate his thoughts or observations, he loses the ability to recall recent events, becomes increasingly irritable and exhibits signs which in many respects seem to represent a childhood reversion. The individual caring for the patient of advanced years must take cognizance of this difficult complication, namely, mental disability due to cerebral degeneration, and the professional approach should be guided accordingly. Firmness in opposition to the expressed desires of the patient is often necessary; invariably, however, this should be accompanied by a display of reassurance and friendly understanding in order to preserve his sense of security. The elderly patient is always fearful of becoming incapacitated and dependent without protection far more than he is of acquiring disease; even the early prospect of death arouses less apprehension.

Apart from intellectual deterioration, disorders of motor and sensory function are common in elderly individuals; these are manifested in the form of muscular weakness, spasticity, tremors and various types of sensory disturbances. Loss of pain perception can be responsible for dangerous accidents—burn injuries, for example, through prolonged exposure to heat which is not perceived. In this regard, an extra blanket is safer than a hot-water bottle. Damaging falls may be caused by loss of position sense, related to a difficulty in maintaining equilibrium and to an uncertainty of gait, and it may be impossible to perform any act requiring precise muscular control. A cerebral hemorrhage, or the sudden occlusion of a large arteriosclerotic artery in the brain, if not immediately fatal, may seriously disable the patient, sometimes rendering him permanently unable to perform any serviceable motion of his extremities and completely incapable of caring for himself in any way. In other instances the degree of incapacity may be less, perhaps involving but one extremity and only to a partial degree.

However, regardless of the exact character of the neurologic disability, the medical management of these patients is a very serious

responsibility and, considering the details of protective care alone, may be an extraordinarily difficult problem.

Occlusive vascular disease involving the lower extremities, another complication of arteriosclerosis, is responsible for "intermittent claudication," that is, pain in the legs on walking, and may even provide the basis for gangrene, necessitating amputation of one or both extremities.

Arteriosclerosis is equally prone to involve the coronary arteries of the heart and those supplying the kidneys. Therefore, the elderly patient is unusually subject to cardiac disorders which may limit seriously his capacity for physical exertion, as well as to impairment of his kidney function with the ultimate prospect of chronic uremia. Gastrointestinal disturbances commonly occur in the older age groups because of a reduction of the blood supply to the gastrointestinal tract, arteriosclerotic changes or neoplastic disease involving that organ system. Gastrointestinal disturbances create problems in dietetic management and symptomatic therapy.

Softening of the bones due to their demineralization (senile osteoporosis) must be regarded as a possible hazard in any elderly individual, rendering him abnormally susceptible to major fractures. The joints are very often affected by degenerative ("hypertrophic") arthritis, causing pain and limiting the motion of the back and of the weight-bearing joints of the legs.

A variety of disorders occur with increasing frequency with advancing age including: malignant neoplasia; pulmonary emphysema with fibrosis and impairment of respiratory function; atrophic and ulcerative lesions affecting the skin and the mucous membranes; and, in the male, enlargement of the prostate gland with urinary obstruction. Descriptions of these and of other degenerative disorders are included in the appropriate sections of this text. By and large, they are not confined to the elderly and assume no unusual characteristics associated primarily with advanced age.

THE NURSE AND THE ELDERLY PATIENT

Is the nursing care which the older person should receive any different from that given to those of a younger age group? Essentially, it is not different but it has more depth; more is required of the nurse.

The nurse who cares for the elderly must possess and display an emotional maturity. On greeting the newly admitted patient the nurse should make him feel welcome and at home. If his condition permits, he should be introduced to nearby patients. At this early meeting, the nurse can observe any incapacities such as difficulty in hearing, tremor of an extremity, a stiff joint and so forth. In elderly patients more than in patients of the younger age group, a sudden change from accustomed surroundings to the bleak and impersonal routine of a hospital produces a feeling of insecurity and emotional disturbance. The understanding nurse can do much to help the patient over this hump of transition between home and institution. If he can be placed near another patient with whom he can talk it will help him to adjust to the hospital environment. The single and most constant symptom in elderly persons upon a sudden transfer from a familiar environment to strange hospital surroundings is that of disorientation, which is greatly intensified at night. Relatively simple measures such as illumination from a night light or the presence of a familiar person may prevent any evidence of disorientation.

By listening to her patient, a nurse may not only enhance his self-esteem but also may gain an over-all picture of his interests, beliefs and reactions. These can be helpful in diagnosis, prognosis and in planning for his total care. An illustration of this is a patient who had harbored false concepts about medicine which were accepted as sound medical practice in his youth. Until these ideas were expressed and corrected, they served as a hurdle to effective therapy.

The successful nurse early recognizes differences in older people. Some may be old and decrepit physically but are alert mentally and fresh in spirit. Very readily one may detect an inherent sense of humor, a philosophical frame of mind or a thwarted and depressed personality. Often the patient's temperament will direct his course of progress. Keen observation of these manifestations will present a challenge to the nurse as she develops a plan of care for her geriatric patient.

A fixed routine may provide a sense of security for some elderly persons. To know that a certain activity will take place at a certain time provides a schedule which allows him to anticipate and to do a certain amount of his own planning. The nurse can strengthen his further belief that he matters when she remembers his desires and idiosyncrasies even when they seem trivial. Having very little ice in the water pitcher may account for an adequate or an inadequate intake of fluids. These little things are significant aspects of individualized patient care.

During the period of diagnostic study or preoperative build-up, diversional aids such as visits, radio, television, newspapers, letters and gifts are significant. The older person has less tendency to live in the past if his present is filled with interesting activities.

Before procedures or examinations are done they should be described to the older patient in order to eliminate fears and tensions. Most of these individuals object to being hurried; therefore, sufficient time should be planned in preparation for a treatment. Every effort should be made to establish the confidence of the older patient in those individuals responsible for his care. If it is possible to learn of the socioeconomic background of the patient, a more tolerant understanding of his present condition and problems will result.

SIGNIFICANT CHARACTERISTICS OF THE OLDER PATIENT

Environmental and Physical Needs

One of the most disturbing *environmental factors* to the geriatric person is noise. Therefore, every attempt should be made to control unpleasant sounds such as dropping metal objects on a hard floor, handling dishes carelessly in the kitchen, banging elevator doors and so forth.

In general, the older patient does not like very much fresh air; therefore, indirect means of ventilation must be utilized. It is difficult to alter the *sleeping habits* of an individual; hence, any adjustment that can be made in the patient's behalf is desirable. Frequently, one has a patient who takes naps during the day and then complains of inability to sleep at night. In most instances, day napping should be discouraged in favor of a good night's sleep.

The nurse should employ whatever nursing measures that seem to be indicated to overcome insomnia, using every effort to make the patient comfortable, but reserving the use of soporific medications for such times as specific indications may exist, and then only as a final resort. Drugs pose a greater hazard to the elderly than to the younger patient, and their administration on a routine basis should be governed by an attitude of conservatism and circumspection on the part of the nurse.

The aging process and the inelasticity of the *skin* predispose to decubiti. The older patient is often content to lie in bed without moving. He must be encouraged to move and get out of bed as frequently as is permissible. Mineral oil, lanolin creams or baby oil can be used on dry skin; alcohol should not be used, since it causes drying of the cutaneous tissues. Some authorities say that bathing once or twice a week is sufficient, since frequent bathing removes the natural oil from the skin. It is exceedingly important that adequate attention be given to the removal of soapy water from the skin after each bath. The danger of residual soap and consequent lysis of the skin is greatest between the toes and the fingers and in areas where there are folds. The feet especially

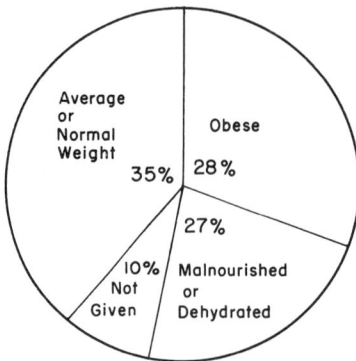

I. GENERAL CONDITION

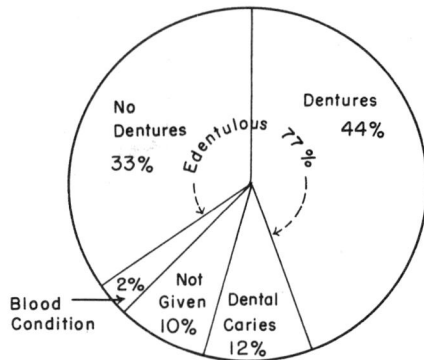

II. DENTAL CONDITION

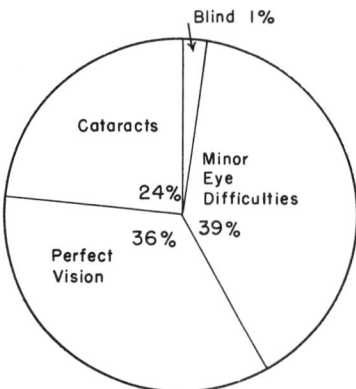

III. VISUAL ACUITY

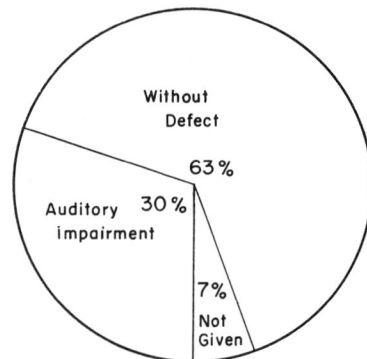

IV. AUDITORY ACUITY

Fig. 100. This chart shows the general physical conditions of an unselected group of surgical geriatric patients. (Sholtis, L. A.: Nursing the elderly surgical patient, Am. J. Nursing **51:** 727)

become dry. It is well to remember that before cutting nails, the feet should be soaked in warm water. Nails should be cleansed and trimmed with care in order to prevent infection as well as injury to the patient. Corns and calluses and tough toe nails may require the care of a podiatrist. Shower or bathtub bathing using water of moderate temperature is preferred to the bed bath. The hair and the scalp should be inspected regularly and given whatever attention the nurse may find necessary. The nurse should anticipate that the geriatric patient needs help to prevent accidents. Safety measures should be utilized. The patient often experiences stiffness and pain when he begins to move or change his position. Because neuromuscular control as well as sensory function may be impaired, the aged bone structures are injured easily.

Further, *visual impairment* may predispose the patient to accidents (Fig. 100). Side rails in the bathroom should be available, and all rooms should be well lighted. At the bedside there should be a footstool with a broad base and nonskid tips. The older patient's bed is equipped with side rails to remind him to remain in bed at night. They are useful to hold onto when raising oneself to the sitting position and when turning over in bed.

The nurse who takes care of the older patient should know of any *hearing impairment*. Perhaps only one ear is involved, or he may not hear certain ranges of sound; whatever the difficulty, simple gestures and signals by the nurse may be understood clearly. Most patients who have diminished hearing are reluctant to call attention to it; therefore, it is up to the nurse to take the initiative in discovering this or any other handicap.

Many of our older patients have lost a number of their own *teeth* or possess remnants of them. (Fig. 100.) Those who have dentures occasionally present difficulties with poorly fitting sets. This can be serious, inasmuch as constant irritation from a jagged tooth or an ill-fitting denture can lead to cancer of the mouth. Dentures should be cleaned at least twice daily; when they are not being worn a receptacle should be available for them. Frequently, the mouth is the most neglected part of the body. The nurse should encourage and help the patient in carrying out good mouth hygiene. By a careful evaluation of the condition of the mouth, the nurse is able to meet the patient's nutritional needs better, to request dental attention if necessary and to prevent postoperative pulmonary and systemic infections.

Nutritional Needs

Diet for the elderly patient demands consideration. Persons in this age group are especially prone to develop faulty dietary habits. Many depend to an undesirable extent on foods that are prepared with the least effort and which, in the individual's opinion, can be purchased most economically. Therefore, the proportions of carbohydrates in their diet may be excessively high, as in the "tea-toast" regimen, and their protein consumption far below the minimum requirements.

Interest in food may be very slight; social and environmental factors which usually operate to stimulate the appetite may be altogether lacking. Therefore, the selection of food items and the character of the environment are important to consider.

Merely because the patient is old, it does not necessarily follow that his food must be soft and bland. Reduced activity may have diminished the appetite, in which event it is especially important that the food be served attractively and be as palatable as possible (Fig. 101). Orders for special diets may be furnished by the physician, if indicated; otherwise, food should be selected for the elderly patient on the same basis as for any other patient. An adequate, well-balanced regimen should be planned and presented. The nurse should have checked the condition of the mouth and the teeth in advance to be certain that the patient can chew. If the patient is unable to feed himself, arrangements should be made for his feeding, which should be accomplished in a leisurely manner. Unfamiliar foods or methods of cooking should be avoided when feeding the elderly.

The foregoing discussion refers primarily to the problem of undernutrition in the aged. Less of a problem from the standpoint of numerical incidence but even more serious in individual cases, and equally deserving of consideration, is the problem of overnutrition. The majority of persons who have been constantly overnourished for many years retain with tenacity until death their habit of overeating and their obesity. An overweight patient with a disorder of locomotion due, for example, to hemiplegia, a fractured femur or arthritis affecting the weight-bearing joints, poses a vastly more difficult problem in treatment, rehabilitation or restoration, than does an individual who is not burdened with excess poundage. Standing may prove impossible, and a state of self-sufficiency unattainable, because of obesity complicating a disorder of locomotion which otherwise would not have been incapacitating. In a patient with an acute pulmonary infection or congestive heart failure the effect of obesity may be lethal.

Weight reduction, when it can be achieved, invariably accelerates the rehabilitation of such patients. Its accomplishment, however, is no more simple than in younger individuals. In a large proportion of cases the attempt is doomed to failure or is rewarded by no more than limited success. Efforts to revise an eating habit of several decades' standing are apt to provoke extreme emotional distress or to meet flat rebellion, and therefore should be undertaken with circumspection and a proper sense of values.

Elimination Problems

The problem of elimination is involved in

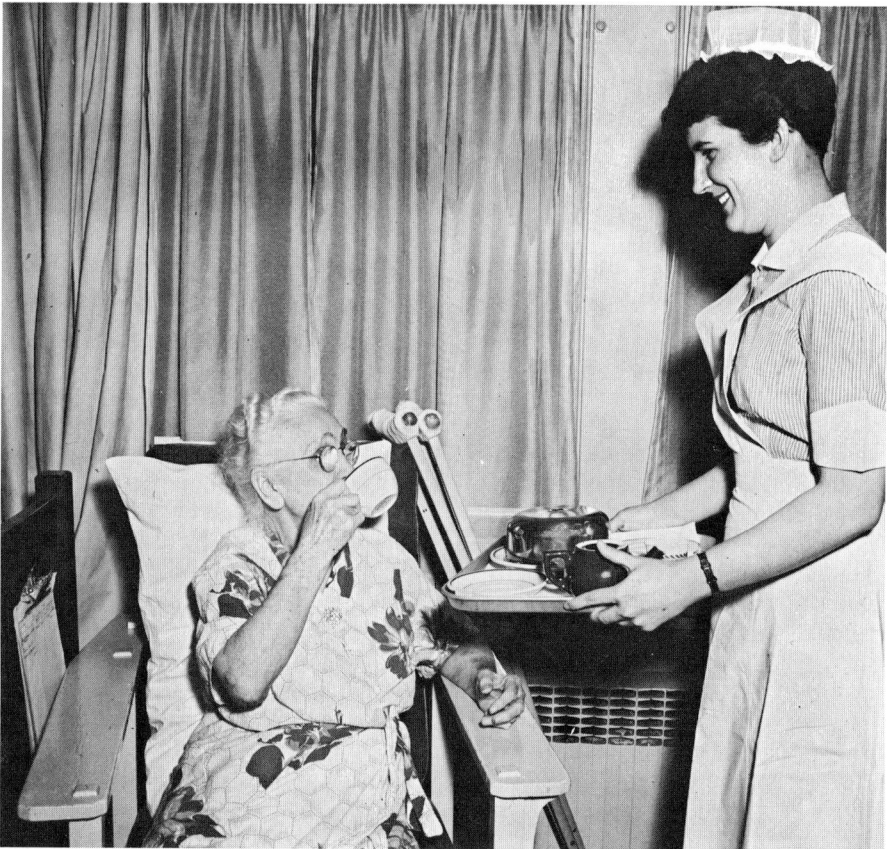

FIG. 101. Reduced activity may have diminished the appetite, in which event it is especially important that the food be served attractively and be as palatable as possible. The selection of food items and the character of the environment, therefore, are important to consider. (School of Nursing, Massachusetts Memorial Hospitals)

the nursing care of many elderly patients. If an indwelling catheter has been inserted or other technical maneuvers are required, these should be explained fully to the patient in order to alleviate his fears. Perineal care should be given regularly to males and females alike. The nurse must assure herself that the patient clearly understands the use of the bedpan and will request it without hesitation whenever or however often it is needed. Problems associated with incontinence and the wet or soiled bed are discussed on page 342.

Bowel elimination is often of prime concern to the aged, and care must be taken to see that it is accomplished properly. The nurse must keep the physician informed regarding the regularity of his patient's bowel function. The patient must be given an adequate opportunity to evacuate the bowels.

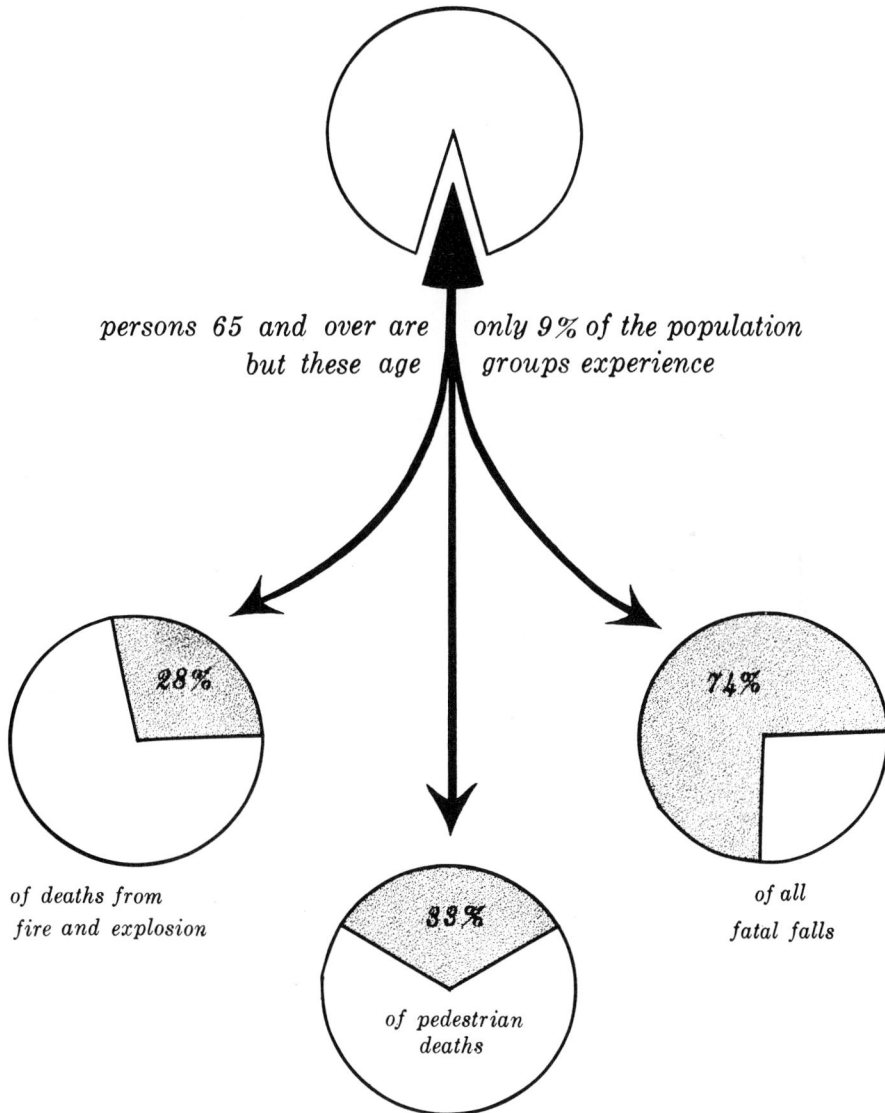

persons 65 and over are but these age   *only 9% of the population groups experience*

28%

74%

33%

of deaths from fire and explosion

of pedestrian deaths

of all fatal falls

Fig. 102. Older persons incur far too large a share of accidental death. (Accidental Injury Statistics, U.S. Dept. Health, Education and Welfare, May, 1961)

This function is very difficult for some aged persons to perform, particularly for those who are in the hospital for the first time. However, it will be the responsibility of the nurse to provide the necessary reassurance and to explain clearly the use of equipment in order to avoid unnecessary complications.

The Patient's Family

Another aspect of geriatric nursing involves the family of the elderly patient. It may be the responsibility of the nurse to educate and orient its members to various aspects of the social situation and to give instruction concerning responsibility or the immediate and follow-up care of the elderly relative. The family's cooperation should be enlisted as early as possible in the therapeutic planning in order to be assured that convalescent care will be satisfactory and that the patient will have maximum protection against possible complications and further recurrences of his disease.

The Elderly Person and Accidents

Accidents constitute a major, but insufficiently emphasized, cause of death and disability among the aged. Although persons of 65 and over comprise only about 9 per cent of our population, they experience a far greater share of fatal accidents (Fig. 102). Rusk* states that a study in 1957 showed that the average hospital stay for accidents of persons 65 years old and over was 24.1 days, as compared with 17 days for the total population and 4.8 days for children under 15. The most common disabilities that keep older persons in hospitals and nursing homes are strokes and fractured hips.

Mersdorf, National Safety Council specialist, stresses that persons above 65 usually are less able or less willing (1) to perceive danger—because of failing sensory abilities; (2) to organize and interpret warning signals rapidly — because of slowing mental abilities; (3) to move in a rapid and coordinated manner—because of muscular and skeletal impairment; and (4) to compensate for physical impairment—because they do not wish to burden others or even to admit that they are growing older.

* Rusk, H. A.: Aged and accidents, the ·New York Times, p. 68, March 12, 1961.

The home is where most of the accidents involving older persons take place; falling is the greatest single cause; and the staircase is the most dangerous place. Here are some suggestions to help older persons to avoid accidents: (1) all stairs should have handrails; (2) grab bars should be next to the bathtub, the shower and the toilet; (3) shoes should fit, and the laces must be tied securely; loose slippers are a hazard; (4) belongings and whatever an older person uses should be stored at a level that is between the hip and the eyes, in order to avoid climbing or bending; and (5) older pedestrians, who are prone to think that they have the right of way on streets and highways must be reminded to take precaution, since their hearing and vision often are impaired, and the conditions listed by Mersdorf above often are present.

(See also "Accidents" in the Emergency and Disaster Unit, p. 1166.)

SURGERY OF THE ELDERLY PATIENT

Preoperative Care

Because of improved technic, means to combat infection and good preoperative preparation and postoperative care, no individual need be denied the benefits of surgery because of age. For example, whereas about 2 decades ago prostatectomy after age 80 still had an operative mortality of 1 in 3, today at representative hospitals, the risk is only 0.5 per cent to 5 per cent.

Preparation for surgery demands a careful evaluation of the cardiovascular and the urinary systems as well as the nutritional status in the older patient. Although he may be admitted for a specific problem, it is usual for him to have several other difficulties. Ideally, all deficiencies should be eliminated before he goes to the operating room; practically, some compromises are necessary.

Psychological Aspects. Confidence will be strengthened if the geriatric patient fully realizes that the contemplated operation is less hazardous than the disease it is expected to remedy. Years of living have a tendency to broaden his ability to adjust to crises. He accepts adjustments more easily; this is particularly advantageous when he is given an anesthetic, for usually he has a smooth induction, maintenance and recovery. On the other hand, one must not assume that he is unconcerned. His attachment to life may be as real as the younger individual's, because in old age one is more conscious of the shortness of the remaining years.

Preoperative Medication. Drug sensitivity usually is increased in elderly individuals, so that dosages are generally smaller. Preoperative medication is given earlier in the aged because of delayed absorption. In those individuals who have cerebral arteriosclerosis, barbiturates and scopolamine may cause excitement; therefore, paraldehyde, chloral hydrate or tincture of opium may be preferable. Some physicians do not prescribe morphine for the older person. When it is given, the respiratory rate must be observed carefully. If sedatives are given, often one third to one half the usual adult amount is prescribed.

Enemas may be ordered the evening before rather than the morning of surgery because of the inclination of the rectum to retain fluid for several hours.

Position on Operating Table. In the operating room the older patient should be handled thoughtfully with no unnecessary exposure. One must have utmost patience in positioning him, since he cannot relax and allow others to move him as desired. Often his joints and muscles are painful when moved. His final position should be relaxed and as comfortable as possible. Extremes in positioning are to be avoided since they hinder circulation.

Anesthesia. Practically all the anesthetic agents used in the younger patient can be used in those past 65. Intravenous Pentothal Sodium has been used as a very satisfactory induction anesthetic. Complicated gas machines may be frightening; consequently, the prick of a needle may be more tolerable than a rubber face mask. Most experienced anesthesiologists prefer to give a mixture of cyclopropane and oxygen by the intratracheal method. This, combined with the curare drugs as needed for relaxation, has the advantage that there is complete control of the anesthesia at all times. The gas concentration can be varied as needed, and adequate oxygenation can be maintained at all times.

Spinal anesthesia also may be used for geriatric patients. It must be remembered that even though their blood vessels may be quite inelastic, they may have a profound drop in pressure. If the blood pressure drop is sudden and prolonged it may lead to circulatory insufficiency. This in turn may cause thrombosis, followed by embolism, infarction and anoxemia. To maintain blood pressure at a normal level is of utmost importance in these individuals.

Going to the other extreme, it is well to remember that sudden increases in blood pressure from excessive or over-rapid infusions may cause pulmonary edema.

Postoperative Care

The immediate postoperative care is the same as that for any patient. However, the older person can chill more easily, and the possibility of shock is greater. Keeping him warm and turning him from side to side after he regains consciousness are essential. His position should be changed frequently not only for his comfort, since he often complains of aches when lying in one position, but also to avoid pulmonary and circulatory complications.

Since lung expansion is decreased, the geriatric patient is more prone to develop pneumonia. Secretions in the upper respiratory tract usually are removed by the anesthesiologist with an endotracheal aspiration tube. Thereafter, in the recovery room the nurse should encourage the patient to cough and take deep breaths. If secretions continue to accumulate, it may be necessary to do a temporary tracheotomy to facilitate breathing and aspiration of secretions.

Hydration. Fluids should be encouraged for many known reasons. Occasionally, the older patient will not take liquids because the nurse has used too much ice, and he may not be used to that. One older man did not drink fluids because the nurse always filled his glass full; the prospect of drinking a glass full of water overwhelmed him. When another nurse poured a quarter of a glassful at a time, he drank it willingly.

The above incident illustrates the fact that each individual is a person in his own right. Many older persons have set ways which may seem unusual to the nurse, but the sooner such a quirk is recognized, the more successful will the nurse be in her total care of that patient.

Usually the oldster needs to be coaxed to drink enough fluids. An output of one liter or more indicates that his intake is sufficient for his needs. Obviously, the recording of intake and output is important.

In giving postoperative intravenous fluids, some surgeons prefer to give them slowly over a 24-hour period rather than more rapidly at 2 or 3 separate times. If this regimen is followed, it is wise to splint the patient's arm (unless a plastic cannula is used). The nurse should watch for any swelling or discomfort at the intravenous site.

Disorientation and Confusion. The older patient even in normal life may show evidences of disorientation and confusion as to time and space. Operation or injury may precipitate such a state in patients who heretofore have been mentally clear. The nurse must recognize the dangers of these mental changes and guard against injury or accident by the use of side rails and by careful observation. In particular, these patients must be watched to see that they do not remove dressings, infusion needles, suction tubes and catheters.

Postoperative Distention. Most often this is due to retention of swallowed air in the intestinal tract. This can be avoided by aspiration of the air from the stomach through a suction tube introduced through the nose and the esophagus into the gastric lumen. Suction may be provided in many ways, and in many cases is maintained until peristalsis is recovered, usually on the second or third day.

In older people, the sluggish peristalsis in the colon frequently results in incomplete evacuation and therefore retention of fecal material in the sigmoid colon and the rectum. The absorption of fluid produces a hard fecal mass which is irritating to the gut and often produces frequent small stools, a sort of pseudodiarrhea. Digital examination reveals a hard mass of fecal material in the rectum. When this mass is broken up by the finger and by enemas, the symptoms are relieved.

Incontinence. In the older person, there may be a loss, temporary or even permanent, of control over the bladder and the bowel,

resulting in incontinence. Often these symptoms are most apparent when the patient is below par, either following operation or after a debilitating illness or trauma. They often disappear as the patient recovers and returns toward his normal strength and vigor. Urinary incontinence is easily treated by the use of an indwelling catheter (Foley). Usually the catheter will be attached by tubing to a container for collecting urine, and often an irrigating apparatus is also used so that the bladder and catheter can be washed out with an antiseptic solution at intervals. Catheters are usually changed every 3 or 4 days, and particular attention must be paid to the technic of catheterization in order to avoid cystitis and other urinary complications. The problem is one of keeping the patient clean and avoiding complications which arise secondary to the moisture and the uncleanliness. In cases of fecal incontinence, thorough washing with soap and water followed by drying and a change of bed linen will go a long way toward the prevention of decubiti. Often absorbent disposable pads may be used to protect the bed and permit easy and frequent changes.

Pain. Enough drug to relieve pain but not enough to make it difficult for the patient to perform his exercises may be given. The older patient may show a marked sensitivity to the sedative drugs. Therefore, it is wise to give sedation in smaller than ordinary doses. This applies not only to the narcotics but also the barbiturates and similar drugs.

Exercise. Activity in as well as out of bed is essential to recovery. Bed exercises include turning from side to side, flexing and extending the legs and the arms, deep breathing and deliberate coughing. In getting out of bed, the patient should turn to his operated side and bend his knees up. As he swings his feet over the side of the bed, the nurse can assist him to a sitting position. A stool should be available for him to stand on for a few moments before he steps down. *Ambulation means that he walks, not sits in a chair.*

Even in the older patient early ambulation is the rule, but signs of fatigue should mean a return to bed. The period out of bed can be gradually increased as strength returns.

CONVALESCENCE, REHABILITATION AND RECREATION

Convalescence may be difficult because strength is regained slowly. Above all, the elder one needs a great deal of patience. He has a tendency to fret about his limitations. Some authorities advocate that one day be allowed for each decade of one's age for convalescence from acute illness. Patients often find this difficult to accept.

Every attempt should be made to maintain an interest in people or things. Diversional and recreational therapies are of invaluable help for the aged and deserve a generous part of the patient's time. All phases of the rehabilitative program must be within the realm of possibility. The older person must be encouraged to do things for himself in order to become self-sufficient. The nurse must refrain from becoming overly motherly in this respect.

Appearance. A great morale booster is to look well; to look well implies that one feels well. The older person may be neglectful of his appearance; hence, a bit of encouragement by the nurse may direct his attention to "how he looks" rather than "how he feels." An attractive hair-do brightens a woman's spirit; this may be done by simple brushing and combing, setting a wave or braiding long hair. A cleverly placed hair ribbon, flower or small ornament in the hair may bring compliments from those who come in contact with the elderly woman. Both men and women enjoy a new garment or a bit of color on their person. Even conservative men seem to like bright-colored pajamas. A small flower on the lapel of his bathrobe will brighten his spirits. A shave and a haircut do for a man what lipstick does for most women. Almost everyone finds the fragrance of certain dusting powders and colognes refreshing. This has special appeal if it is a scent that is in keeping with the individual's personality. Surely the nurse will be able to find some one thing that will help immeasurably to cheer her older patient.

Physical Activity. The dangers of prolonged bed rest, even prolonged sitting, are numerous and should be avoided even when the patient objects to a change. The rocking chair is more helpful than a straight or an overstuffed chair. The rocking chair is an inexpensive, easily obtainable therapeutic device that enables all but the most feeble to exercise with dignity at any time. Use of the calf and forearm muscles encourages venous return and increases cardiac output. Pulmonary ventilation is increased and hypostatic pulmonary congestion is discouraged. From the psychological point of view, rocking is socially acceptable; in such a chair, one can participate in home activities and be an integral part of the family.

Walking activities should be encouraged as soon as the patient is able and the physician approves. Instruction in the proper use of aids, such as a walker, crutches or a cane, must be given to the patient; and he should be taught why it is important to maintain proper body posture, and how to do it.

Learning. Mental as well as physical activity is the nucleus of successful rehabilitation. It must be emphasized that old people can learn; the learning process is not limited to the young. Hence, the oldster can learn to care for himself and can learn absorbing and interesting hobbies. It is for the nurse and all other members of the health team to teach and direct this potential learner. Instructions must be clear and complete. They must be repeated frequently enough to allow the patient to grasp them. He should be aware of the reasons for doing prescribed activities; many times the patient misinterprets such activities as measures to release the nurse from her many duties rather than accepting them as a means essential for his recovery. (See also Chap. 21, on rehabilitation nursing, p. 363.)

Recreation. In the words of Piersol and Bortz, "The society which fosters research to save human life cannot escape responsibility for the life thus extended. It is for science not only to add years to life, but more important, to add life to the years."*

Recreation is more than just having fun; it is fundamental to physical and mental well-being. No matter how old or disabled one becomes, the desire for the dignity that comes only through purposeful activity is never lost.

* Ann. Int. Med. 12:964, 1939.

Rusk* states that some surveys have shown that among older people who participate actively in Golden Age Clubs, day centers and similar programs, there are 50 per cent fewer visits to physicians' offices and clinics, 50 per cent fewer general hospital admissions and 800 per cent fewer psychiatric breakdowns than among persons of the same age not participating in active recreation programs.

As soon as the patient is capable of participating in any type of group activity or is willing to undertake some project on an individual basis, such should be planned. The nurse can enlist the help of others, such as occupational therapists, volunteer aides and members of the family, in the organizing of activities designed to occupy the patient's time pleasantly, maintain his enthusiasm and keep him in possession of his faculties and aware of his own personal worth. If a project is successful in this respect, one of the most important goals in the therapeutic progress will have been accomplished.

No plan for rehabilitation will be success-

* Rusk, H. A.: Recreation for the aged, The New York Times, p. 62, July 9, 1961.

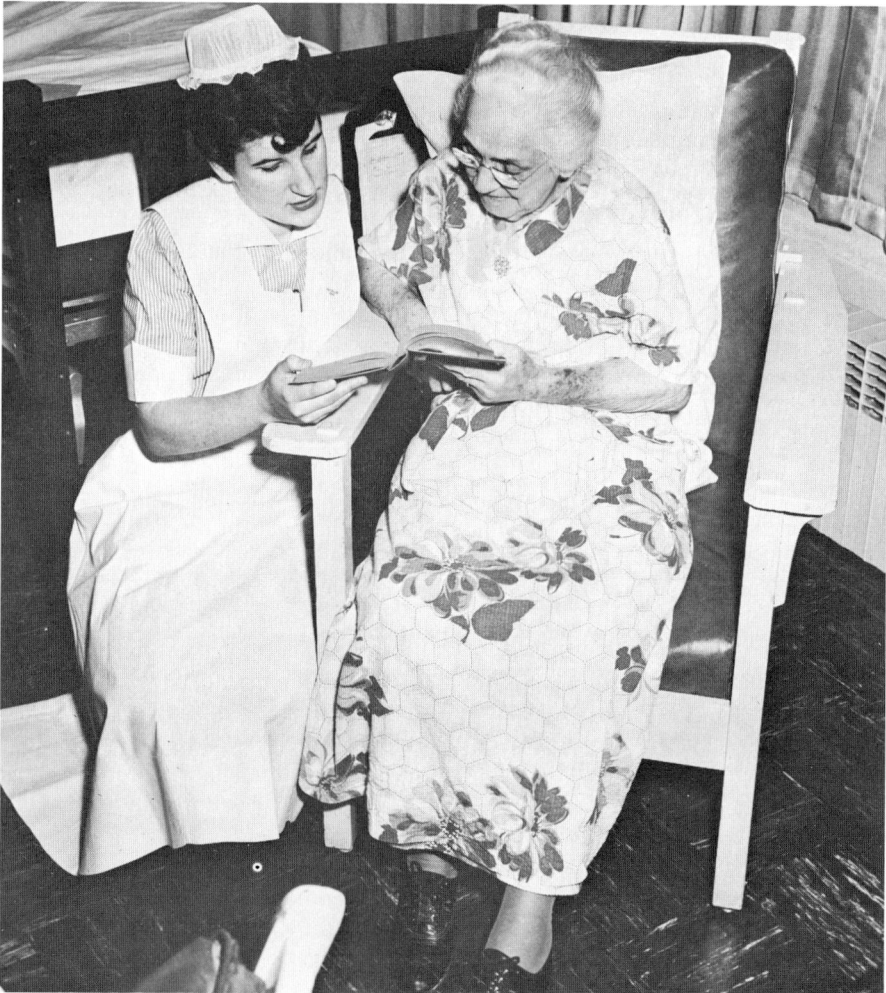

FIG. 103. Activity for the elderly person is essential for the morale and should be encouraged. (School of Nursing, Massachusetts Memorial Hospitals)

ful unless it is continued beyond the walls of the hospital. Continuity of care can be planned with the visiting nurse programs and other community agencies as well as the patient's own family. In many instances, the geriatric patient does not have a family to whom he can return. Real adjustments may have to be made. The smoother the transfer, the more graceful will be the resumption of normal living for the elderly.

LONG-TERM ILLNESS

The duration of an illness, depending on its course, its nature and the degree of disability, deserves serious consideration in the planning and the conduct of medical and nursing care. Such planning should be done by the nurse in collaboration with the physician and other co-workers, in order that she may be informed adequately and advised properly concerning her responsibility for the instruction and the rehabilitation of the patient and the re-education of his family.

In most cases, the adaptation of the patient to prolonged disability is accomplished without apparent difficulty. More important, however, is the quality of his ultimate readjustment to normal life following his recovery from organic disorders. The risk of chronic psychological invalidism never can be discounted, and its consequences are far from benign. At best, convalescence may be prolonged unduly, creating unnecessary hardships for the patient's family. At worst, the patient may be unwilling to assume the responsibilities he should accept and of which he is physically capable, obstinately resisting the loss of his passive and protected status. In either case, without capable instruction in the significance of the patient's attitudes and reactions, the family may be quite defenseless. The fostering of invalidism, which is frequently the unintended result of the family's attitude, seriously compounds the difficulties of rehabilitation and should be discouraged vigorously by those who are in a position to advise.

The treatment and the prevention of psychiatric disability in patients with chronic disease is essentially a problem of appropriate psychotherapy. The patient should be diverted continuously, by means of every available device, from his personal problems and discouraged from indulging in morbid self-absorption. Facilities should be made accessible for his intellectual stimulation, artistic satisfaction or productive accomplishment of any type that seems to be desirable and potentially effective. Occupational therapy, expertly conducted, should be incorporated into the program of treatment at the earliest opportunity and continued throughout convalescence. The requirements of individual patients are highly variable, but whatever the problems involved or therapeutic methods employed, the individuals responsible for their management must be acutely aware of the psychological complications that threaten, alert to any untoward developments of this character and, most important, sufficiently impressed by their own responsibilities in its prevention.

GRAVITY OF PROGNOSIS

What is in the mind of a patient suffering from a fatal disease? What are his hopes and fears? How nearly does he suspect intuitively the truth of the situation, and, if he suspects the truth, by what psychological mechanisms is he saved from despair? How specifically and in what detail should he be informed regarding his illness and its probable outcome? If he demands an accurate appraisal of his status and a true estimate as to the prognosis, should this be supplied? What is his family to be told? What are the responsibilities of the nurse as regards the transmission of diagnostic and prognostic information to the patient's family?

These and similar questions regularly confront physicians and nurses responsible for the care of the seriously ill. Some of them may be answered without equivocation, with a reasonable degree of certainty and without important reservations, while others, depending on the personal philosophy of the physician, the family and the status of a particular patient, may be answered in generalizations which, although basically valid, are open to a variety of interpretations.

First, as regards the nurse-patient and the nurse-family relationship, it may be stated unequivocally that whatever information is to be supplied concerning the diagnosis, whether or not it has been definitely established, never should be volunteered to the

SENIOR CITIZEN'S CHARTER

Rights of Senior Citizens:

Each of our Senior Citizens, regardless of race, color or creed, is entitled to:
1. The right to be useful.
2. The right to obtain employment, based on merit.
3. The right to freedom from want in old age.
4. The right to a fair share of the community's recreational, educational, and medical resources.
5. The right to obtain decent housing suited to needs of later years.
6. The right to the moral and financial support of one's family so far as is consistent with the best interest of the family.
7. The right to live independently, as one chooses.
8. The right to live and to die with dignity.
9. The right of access to all knowledge as available on how to improve the later years of life.

Obligations of the Aging:

The aging, by availing themselves of educational opportunities, should endeavor to assume the following obligations to the best of their ability:
1. The obligation of each citizen to prepare himself to become and resolve to remain active, alert, capable, self-supporting and useful so long as health and circumstances permit and to plan for ultimate retirement.
2. The obligation to learn and to apply sound principles of physical and mental health.
3. The obligation to seek and to develop potential avenues of service in the years after retirement.
4. The obligation to make available the benefits of his experience and knowledge.
5. The obligation to endeavor to make himself adaptable to the changes added years will bring.
6. The obligation to attempt to maintain such relationships with family, neighbors and friends as will make him a respected and valued counsellor throughout his later years.

From the 1961 White House Conference on Aging

patient or his family by the nurse, excepting as planned as a result of mutual discussions with the responsible physician. By the same token, whatever prognostications are offered by the nurse should be precisely as specific as his, and no more. Finally, any remarks of hers which bear on the possible implications of the diagnosis, prognosis or treatment should be made advisedly, in the light of the physician's known views and intentions. This admonition deserves considerable emphasis, for nothing is more destructive of confidence and morale than an impression of inconsistency, and nothing is more threatening to therapeutic success than confusion and distrust in the mind of the sick patient. Obviously, all of the statements and the actions of the nurse should be calculated to convey a sense of optimism; no matter how grave the situation or depressing the outlook, the nurse can lend a great deal of encouragement without exceeding either the bounds of reality or her professional responsibilities.

Normally, protective psychological mechanisms operate in patients with lethal disease and apparently to excellent effect, for very few such patients become acutely anxious or profoundly depressed, even when it is seemingly obvious that a fatal outcome is imminent. The precise nature of these mechanisms presumably differs, depending on the individual and the situation. A conversion of the patient's will to live to a complete acceptance of the idea of death, even a desire for death, may be one aspect of this process of psychological adaptation in cases with prolonged and painful illnesses, although in most instances there is no sign of a death wish. On the contrary, the evidence would suggest that the desire to live persists with great tenacity, ideas of death apparently being altogether excluded from awareness.

The question regarding the degree to which the physician and the nurse are justified in supporting this false but benign optimism, on the other hand, of disabusing the patient of his misconceptions, in practice proves to be very much less difficult than one would anticipate. Patients become aware of an unfavorable prognosis far earlier than expected—in fact, almost as soon as its fatal character is established—probably because the reassurance received thereafter lacks its former conviction. However, provided that he is satisfied with the professional conduct of his case, as soon as he recognizes the truth of the situation, he promptly abandons his insistent questions regarding the precise prospects, and his anxieties become focused on problems that are completely irrelevant or only indirectly related to his personal affliction. Rarely does such an individual request a categorical answer concerning prognosis if he expects an unfavorable reply. Interest in the disease itself continues overt and lively, to be sure, but its flavor is perhaps a little more academic in quality. The manifestations of the disease may be increasingly absorbing to the patient, but there is no apparent inclination on his part to discuss their real implications.

It is not often, therefore, that the physician or the nurse must decide how much of the tragic truth to tell; they seldom are asked. An occasional patient does persist in his direct questioning, apparently with logical reason, perhaps relating to his business plans or obligations to his family. Under these circumstances some physicians may feel justified in acceding, offering a complete evaluation of the case in detail and stating their conclusions in definite terms. It may be mentioned that the occasional result of this decision is a complete and unexpected shattering of the patient's morale.

Members of the patient's family and those of his associates who require explicit information, of course, must be made acquainted with the complete situation, and at least one member of the immediate family should be advised from the outset regarding all possible developments. If this is done, candid discussions concerning prognoses with the victims of hopeless disease are in no way justified. Optimism, valid or false, is to be strengthened, not destroyed, if the humane objective of medical care is to be served completely.

BIBLIOGRAPHY AND SUGGESTED READING

Books:

Buckley, B. R.: Nursing Care of the Aged, Madison, Wis., Publications Division, Univ. Wisconsin, 1962.

Field, M.: Patients are People, New York, Columbia Univ. Press, 1953.

Newton, K.: Geriatric Nursing, ed. 3, St. Louis, Mosby, 1960.

Rudd, T. C.: The Nursing of the Elderly Sick, Philadelphia, Lippincott, 1954.

Stieglitz, E. J.: Geriatric Medicine, ed. 3, Philadelphia, Lippincott, 1954.

————: The Second Forty Years, Philadelphia, Lippincott, 1946.

Worcester, A.: The Care of the Aged, the Dying and the Dead, ed. 2, Springfield, Ill., Thomas, 1940.

Articles:

Aring, C. D.: Senility, A.M.A. Arch. Int. Med. 100:519-528, 1957.

Austin, C. L.: The basic six needs of the aging, Nursing Outlook 59:138, 1959.

Batchelder, E. L.: Nutritional status and dietary habits of older people, J. Am. Dietet. A. 57:471-475, 1957.

Bayne, J. R. D.: Philosophy of geriatric care, Canad. Nurse 58:612-613, July, 1962.

Beal, J. M.: Basic principles in the surgical management of the aged, Geriatrics 14:269-273, 1959.

Blumenthal, G.: Emotional aspects of feeding the aged, J. Am. Dietet. A. 56:829-831, 1956.

Bueker, K.: Adolescents need attention, Am. J. Nursing 60:372-373, Mar. 1960.

Cameron, C., and Campbell, A. F.: Accident prevention for older people, Nursing Outlook 4:332-334, 1956.

Charles, D. C.: Outstanding characteristics of older patients, Am. J. Nursing 61:80-83, Nov. 1961.

Donahue, W.: The nurse and the geriatric patient, Nurs. Survey 1:5, April, 1962.

Green, J. J.: General physiology of aging, Geriatrics 14:318-331, May, 1959.

Gallagher, J. R., Heald, F. P., and Masland, R. P.: Recent contributions to adolescent medicine, New Eng. J. Med. 259:24-31, 74-81, 123-130, 1958.

Hall, B. H.: Mental health of senior citizens, Nurs. Outlook 56:206, 1956.

Knapp, M. E., and Owen, R. R.: Rehabilitation of the geriatric patient, Geriatrics 14:306-311, May, 1959.

Konzen, R. S.: Guide for geriatric care, Am. J. Nursing 57:1166-1167, 1957.

Lonergan, R. C.: As we grow older, Am. J. Nursing 56:736-737, 1956.

Newell, R. R.: What should we tell the patient? J. Chronic Dis. 7:52-57, 1958.

Roberts, D. W.: Care of the long-term patient, J. Chron. Dis. 1:53-62, 1955.

Schwartz, D.: Medication errors made by aged patient, Am. J. Nursing 62:51-53, Aug., 1962.

Schwartz, D., Wang, M., Zeitz, L., and Goss, M.: Problems of ambulation and traveling among elderly chronically ill clinic patients, Nursing Research 12:165-171, Summer, 1963.

Sheldon, J.: There are several aspects of aging that need investigation, Am. J. Nursing **57**:70, 1957.

Sholtis, L. A.: Nursing the elderly surgical patient, Am. J. Nursing **51**:726-728, 1951.

Soller, G. R.: The aging patient, Am. J. Nursing **62**:114-117, Nov., 1962.

Swartz, F. C.: Medicine's biggest battle-taming time, J.A.M.A. **164**:1477-1481, 1957.

Symposium: Problems of the mind in later life, Geriatrics **11**:137-179, April, 1956.

Warren, M.: Mental confusion in elderly persons, Geriatrics **14**:207-218, April, 1959.

Patient Teaching Aids

Pamphlets

Food Guide for Older Folks, Home and Garden Bulletin No. 17, Washington, D.C., U.S. Department of Agriculture, 1961.

Ross, M.: Is There a Grandparent in the House?, Washington, D.C., U.S. Department of Health, Education, and Welfare, no date.

Safety Hints for Elderly Persons, Chicago, National Safety Council, 1960.

The Older Person in the Home, Washington, D.C., U.S. Public Health Service Pub. No. 542.

National Agencies

National Council on Aging
345 East 46 Street
New York 17, New York

National Social Welfare Assembly
1790 Broadway
New York 19, New York

21

Principles and Practices of Rehabilitation Nursing

PHILOSOPHY OF REHABILITATION

It is never how high one rises that determines one's merit, but rather how far one has come, considering his difficulties.

Rutledge, Archibald: Valor in Nature, Think, June, 1956.

Rehabilitation is the process by which a disabled or ill patient is enabled to achieve his maximum possible physical and mental efficiency. How close he comes to achieving this goal will determine the degree to which he becomes a socially and economically independent member of society. Rehabilitation has been called the third phase of medicine, the first being preventive, the second diagnosis and treatment, the third convalescence and rehabilitation. Morrissey defines modern rehabilitation as a process of wholesome adjustment to a handicap by educating the patient to integrate all of his resources and to concentrate more on existing abilities than on the permanent disabilities with which he must live.

In the interval between World Wars I and II, rehabilitation efforts developed significant meaning. The first comprehensive program in rehabilitation was started in 1947 at the Bellevue Hospital in New York City by Dr. Howard Rusk. Since then programs have been developed in most medical centers. Many hospitals have elaborate departments; however, a successful program can be carried out even in a small hospital and with a minimum of personnel and equipment. A positive point of view plus dedication, pa-

tience and willingness to move through the many stages from inactivity to activity must be a part of the patient and of all those who work with him in achieving this goal.

Rehabilitation concerns not only the individual; it also concerns the nation. Early in 1962 the Department of Health, Education and Welfare launched a new approach in public welfare that stresses "services instead of support, rehabilitation instead of relief." The promotion of rehabilitation services and the family-centered approach will receive particular emphasis. States will be reimbursed for three-quarters of the costs, thereby providing an incentive to the individual states to provide more rehabilitation services for persons receiving welfare. The economic advantage of such an emphasis is readily apparent; instead of an individual receiving welfare aid, he will be rehabilitated into employment. Instead of being a parasite on society, he will be a contributor. The effect on the individual is to change him from a hopeless dependent to an active independent citizen.

In the hospital setting, the patient and his problems are evaluated and a program is set up to enable him to achieve self-sufficiency within the level of his capabilities and desires. His abilities are stressed rather than his disabilities. Since each patient has a different level of capability, the program is individualized. Through such a program the patient is motivated and helped to attain social interdependence and greater economic security.

THE REHABILITATION TEAM

Rehabilitation requires a team of persons working together and contributing specialized services that may be required to assist the patient. The team members meet in group sessions at frequent intervals to evaluate the patient's progress and make the necessary program changes. His *physician* has the responsibility of making the diagnosis so that therapy can be directed toward realistic goals; he directs the patient's therapeutic program. The *physiatrist* is a physician who is a specialist in physical medicine and rehabilitation. He tests the patient's physical functioning and supervises his rehabilitation program. The *psychologist* assesses the patient's motivation, values and attitudes toward his disability. He also may talk with the family to help them to cope with the problems that have arisen as a result of the patient's disability. Other counselors and therapists assist in this program. Vocational rehabilitation is the preparation of the disabled for useful employment. Through vocational rehabilitation the patient works toward economic independence. The *vocational counselor* tests him to determine his interests and aptitudes so that vocational training can be instituted. The *physical therapist* supports and supervises the patient during the prescribed exercise program. Using activities to develop skills that can be transferred to home and work situations, the *occupational therapist* devises practical projects for the patient to pursue that will develop his coordination and maintain his interest. The *social worker,* through contacts with the family, the community and the employment situation, gives advice to facilitate the adjustment of the patient to his social environment.

The Nurse in Rehabilitation

The nurse has a unique function on the rehabilitation team, giving rise to the art of rehabilitation nursing. Since the nurse (whether hospital, public health, industrial or school) spends so much more time with the patient than the other members of the team, she is able to note problems and needs, to offer support and to render care in a manner that no other member of the team is usually in a position to do. The nurse must support the therapy that is initiated by other members of the team. Her attitudes and understandings can either facilitate or hinder the rehabilitation program. Instead of doing things for the patient, her function is to *teach him to help himself.* As a member of the rehabilitation team, the nurse should:

1. Recognize the rehabilitation potential as dependent upon the individual and his environment.

2. Emotionally accept the individual with a disability.

3. Understand the functions and the skills of all members of the health team as a basis for effective cooperation.

4. Maintain good interpersonal relationship with other team members.

5. Assist in the promotion, the stimulation and the coordination of team-care programs.

6. Provide for the continuity of rehabilitative care, since she is in the best position to know what has been done, and why, and what the plans are for the future.

7. Know what resources are available within the hospital, as social service, vocational facilities, school program and volunteer services.

8. Know what community resources are available for continuity of care that will promote the maximum health and welfare of the patient and his family.*

To overcome the patient's disability, the nurse helps him learn to care for his daily needs, to walk or employ some other method of transportation, to use ordinary toilet facilities, to communicate with others, and to apply and care for his own artificial prosthetic devices. These functions appear simple, but it may take many hours or many weeks of training to accomplish the patient's therapeutic goal.

Rehabilitation is an integral part of nursing and *should begin with the initial contact with the patient.* Every major illness carries with it the threat of disability. If the patient is hospitalized with a burn and develops a contracture deformity, his recovery time will be delayed greatly. Disabilities are not static but tend to become worse, and some complications of inactivity can give the patient

* Adapted from material presented by the National League for Nursing, New York.

more pain and discomfort than the initial injury or disease.

The importance of rehabilitation often is underestimated. There are over 30 million disabled persons in the United States, and the aged population is steadily increasing. Every patient, regardless of his problem or diagnosis, has the right to rehabilitation services. Thus, rehabilitation is a large and increasing area of nursing responsibility. Though not all hospitals have departments of physical medicine and rehabilitation, *the principles of rehabilitation are basic to the care of all patients,* and the pages that follow point out how the nurse applies them.

PSYCHOLOGICAL IMPLICATIONS OF A DISABILITY

A physical disability often has a deep psychological significance to the patient. Physically a part of his body has deteriorated. He may have the shattering realization that he can do less than formerly. His shape and posture may have changed, as may have his state of mind. Even his position in society may be altered. He may classify himself as a member of a minority group. In short, he may feel that he is different.

Disability may spell hardship or even tragedy to the individual, depending on his occupation, cultural background and social status, and the support he receives from or provides for his family.

A person usually goes through a series of emotional reactions to a newly acquired disability. The first reaction may be that of denial. The patient may refuse to accept his new limitations and have a sometimes unjustified overconfidence in speedy recovery. His false hopes lead him to hear only what he wants to hear. He is likely to be self-centered and even childlike in his demands.

The patient may progress to a period of depression in which he appears to mourn for his lost function, or missing body part. This period of grief appears to be a necessary stage in making the required adaptations in living. He should not merely be encouraged blithefully to "cheer up." The nurse, simply with her attentive and ready-to-act presence, can transmit a feeling of caring to this patient.

In time the patient becomes more familiar with his condition and is able to tolerate it better. He revises his body image and modifies his former picture of himself. He is able to accept a degree of dependency and not resent being "waited upon." He begins to realize that hopelessness is futile and knows that he must adapt to the permanent aspects of the disability while relentlessly pursuing victory over temporary weaknesses. It is from this point in rehabilitation that the patient begins to look ahead and develop realistic goals for his future.

Some patients do not accept their disability; they waste emotional energy in rebelling futilely against unalterable damage. Others ignore it and will not put forth any effort to adapt for everyday life the abilities that survive the disease or the treatment. Still others may over-react and build a false reputation for being "cheerful and courageous." Although "ignoring" may seem healthy, often it includes a total rejection of the disability, which keeps the patient from doing the small things that will be helpful to him. These patients may require assistance from either a psychologist or a psychiatrist. The nurse has the responsibility of watching patient reactions to disability and of reporting them to the physician. She has the privilege of listening to the patient, encouraging him and sharing in his satisfactions and triumphs as he progresses in his program. It is through the support and the inspiration of the members of the rehabilitation team that the patient becomes all that he is capable of being.

PRINCIPLES AND PRACTICES OF REHABILITATION NURSING

The most common complications that threaten a patient with a prolonged illness or disability are contractures, decubitus ulcers and bladder and bowel problems.

When muscles are not used, they become shortened; such shortening produces a limitation on the range of motion (contracture). These deformities may be prevented if the causal conditions are understood properly and preventive measures are instituted early.

When tissues do not receive adequate nourishment and exercise, they tend to deteriorate and to atrophy. By initiating deliberate and proper measures, tissue damage

---

DEFINITIONS

Adduction—movement of a limb toward the body's center.

Abduction—movement away from midline of the body; turning outward.

Extension—when referring to an extremity means straightening out the joint.

Hyperextension—extension beyond the ordinary range.

Flexion—bending the various joints, such as the knee or the elbow, or the thigh on the trunk.

Dorsiflexion—bending backward.

Rotation—turning or movement of a part around its axis.

Internal: turning inward toward the center.

External: turning outward away from the center.

Pronation—turning downward.

Supination—turning upward.

---

and decubitus ulcers can be combated and prevented.

Bladder and bowel difficulties may result from disease, injury or shock. In many patients, refunctioning can be accomplished through individualized teaching and persistent attention to the establishment of regular function.

The major responsibilities of the nurse in rehabilitation are (1) to prevent deformities and complications; (2) to initiate, to teach and to support the patient (and his family when necessary) during the daily activities of living which include self-care; and (3) to refer the patient for proper follow-up care and supervision. Each of these categories will now be discussed in detail.

Prevention of Deformities and Complications

Deformities and complications of illness or injury often can be prevented by proper body position in bed, and by exercises.

Unless contraindicated, the patient should be turned frequently. The reasons for changing body positions are these: (1) to prevent contractures; (2) to stimulate circulation and to help to prevent thrombophlebitis, decubiti and edema of the extremities; (3) to promote lung expansion; (4) to promote drainage of respiratory secretions; (5) to relieve pressure on a body area.

The most common positions that the patient assumes in bed are the dorsal or supine, the side-lying or lateral, and the prone positions. The essential principles of body alignment necessary for maintaining these positions follow.

Dorsal or supine position

1. The head is in line with the spine, both laterally and anteroposteriorly.

2. The trunk is positioned so that flexion of the hips is minimized.

3. The arms are flexed at the elbow with the hands resting against the lateral abdomen.

4. The legs are extended with a small firm support under the popliteal area.

5. The heèls are suspended in a space between the mattress and the footboard.

6. The toes are pointed straight up.

7. Small towel rolls are placed under the greater trochanters in the hip joint areas.

Side-lying or lateral position

1. The head is in line with the spine.

2. The body is in alignment and is not twisted.

3. The uppermost hip joint is slightly forward and supported in a position of slight abduction.

4. A pillow supports the arm, which is flexed at both the elbow and the shoulder joints.

Prone position

1. The head is turned laterally and is in alignment with the rest of the body.

2. The arms are abducted and externally rotated at the shoulder joint; the elbows are flexed.

3. A small flat support is placed under the pelvis, extending from the level of the umbilicus to the upper third of the thigh.

4. The lower extremities remain in a neutral position.

5. The toes are suspended over the edge of the mattress.

Therapeutic Exercises

These exercises are prescribed by the physician and performed with the assistance and guidance of a physical therapist. If such a therapist is not available, the nurse may assist the patient. The objectives and goals of an exercise program are determined by the patient's condition. Exercise, when correctly done, assists in (1) maintaining and building muscle strength; (2) maintaining joint function; (3) preventing deformity; (4) stimulating circulation; and (5) building endurance. There are five types of exercise.

Static or Muscle Setting: An exercise performed by the patient.

PURPOSE: To maintain strength when a joint is immobilized.

ACTION: Contract or tighten the muscle as much as possible; hold for several seconds, then "let go" and relax. Breathe deeply.

Passive: An exercise carried out by the therapist or the nurse without assistance from the patient.

PURPOSE: To retain as much joint range of motion as possible; to maintain circulation.

ACTION: Stabilize the proximal joint and support the distal part. Move the joint smoothly, slowly, and gently through its full range of motion. Avoid producing pain.

Active Assistive: An exercise carried out by the patient with the assistance of the therapist or the nurse.

PURPOSE: To encourage normal muscle function.

ACTION: Support the distal part and encourage the patient to take the joint actively through its range of motion. Give as little assistance as is necessary to accomplish the action. Short periods of activity should be followed by adequate rest periods.

Active: An exercise accomplished by the patient without assistance.

PURPOSE: To encourage normal muscle function and preserve muscle strength.

ACTION: Active exercise when possible should be done against gravity. The joint is moved through full range of motion without assistance. (Make sure that the patient does not substitute another joint movement for the one intended.)

Resistive: An active exercise carried out by the patient working against resistance produced by either manual or mechanical means.

PURPOSE: To provide resistance in order to increase muscle power.

ACTION: The patient moves the joint through its range of motion while the therapist resists slightly at first and then progressively with increasing resistance. Sandbags and weights can be used and are applied at the distal point of the involved joint. The movements should be done smoothly.

Range-of-motion Exercises

Each joint of the body has a normal range of motion. In many musculoskeletal conditions the joints may lose their normal range, stiffen, and produce a permanent disability. If the range of motion is limited, the functions of the joint and the muscle that moves the joint are impaired. In order to prevent painful deformities, range-of-motion activities when permitted are carried out passively, with active assistance, or actively. Range-of-motion exercises are designed for either maintaining or increasing the maximum motion of a joint.

The patient must be in a comfortable position, lying supine with his arms to the side and his knees extended. Good body posture is to be maintained in each position assumed during the exercise. The bed should be high enough to permit the nurse to reach effectively the part to be exercised.

Unless otherwise ordered, a joint should be moved through its full range of motion about 5 times at least once every day. A joint should not be moved beyond its free range of motion. Therefore, the motion should be stopped at the point of pain. When muscle spasm is present, the joint should be moved slowly and to the point of resistance. Then a gentle steady pressure is exerted until the muscle relaxes.

In performing range-of-motion exercises, the bones above and below the joint to be moved are considered. For example, in taking the elbow through its range of motion, the humerus must be stabilized while the

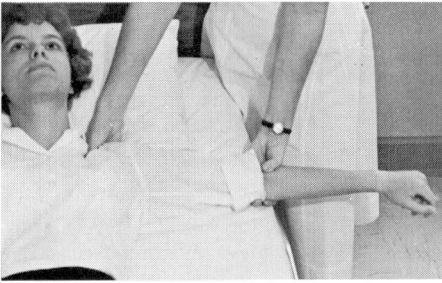

Abduction-adduction of the shoulder

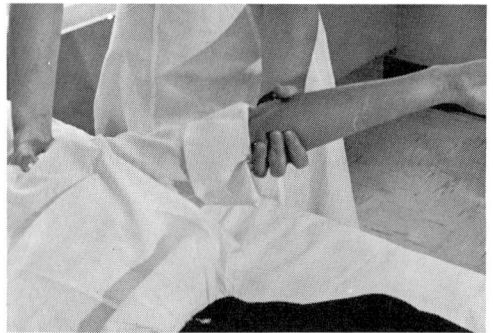

Hyperextension of the shoulder.

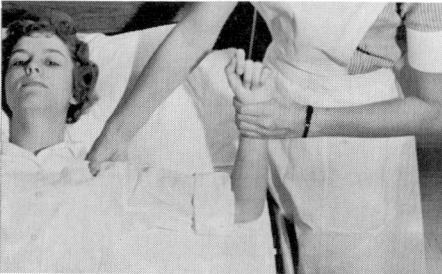

Internal-external rotation of the
shoulder (neutral position).

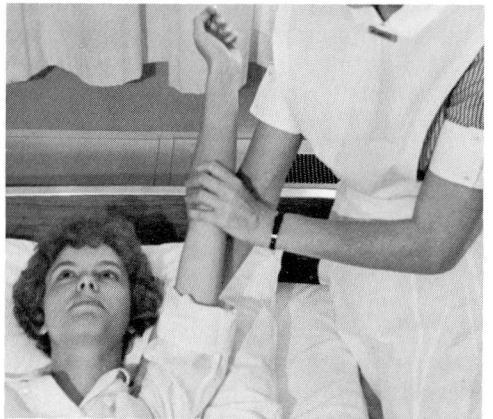

Flexion of the shoulder

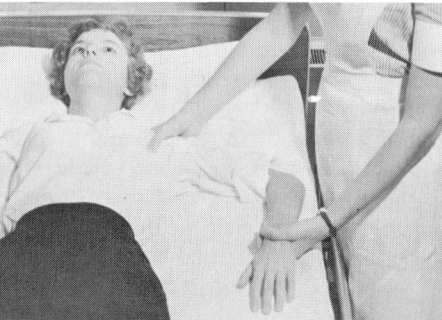

Internal rotation of the shoulder.

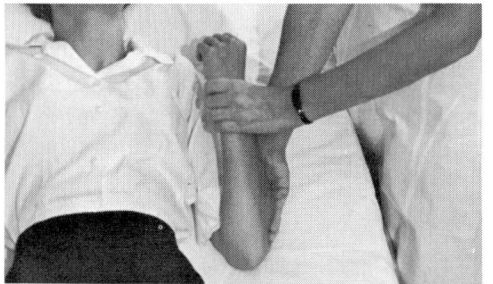

Flexion of the elbow.

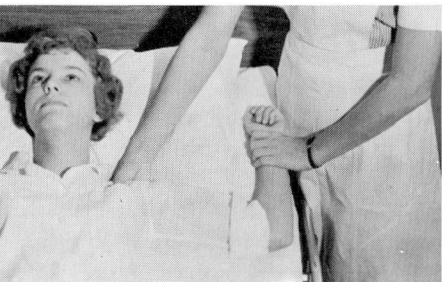

External rotation of the shoulder
(note: hand touches bed).

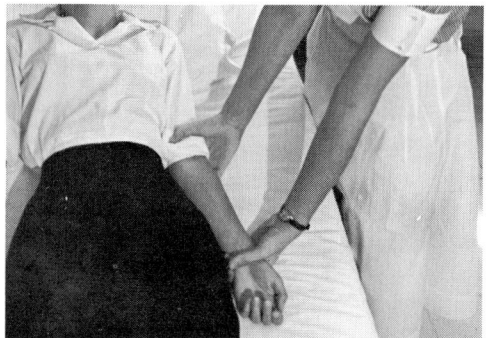

Extension of the elbow.

FIGURE 104

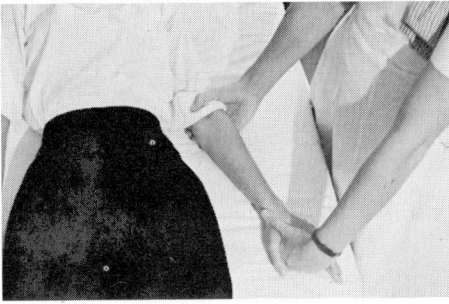
Pronation of the forearm.

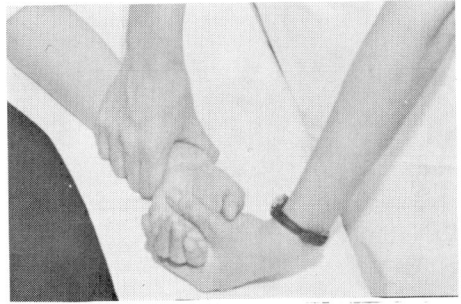
Ulnar-radial deviation.

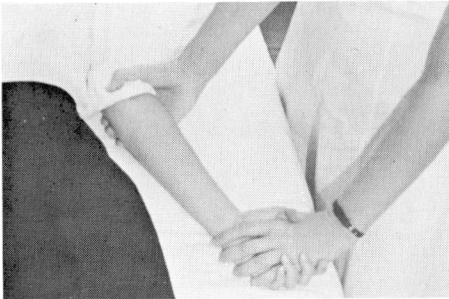
Supination of the forearm.

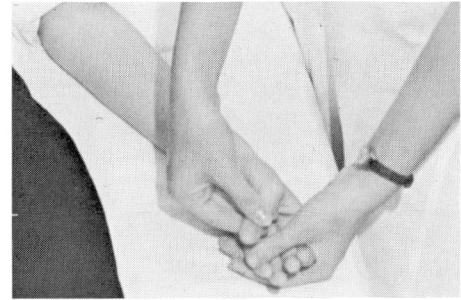
Thumb opposition.

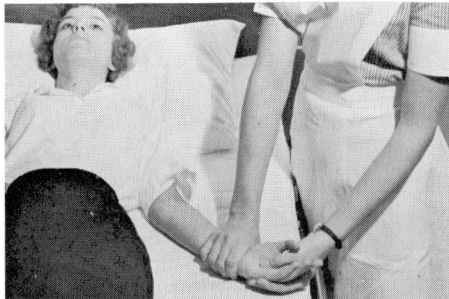
Extension of the wrist.

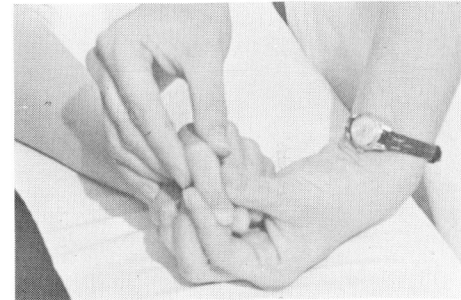
Flexion-extension of the fingers.

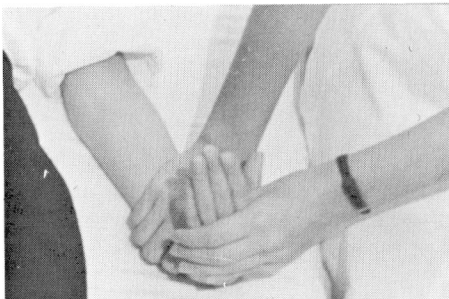
Flexion of the wrist.

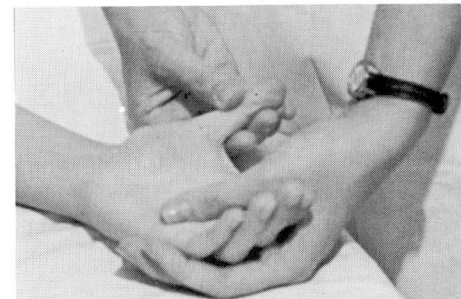
Abduction-adduction of the thumb.

FIGURE 104 (*Continued*)

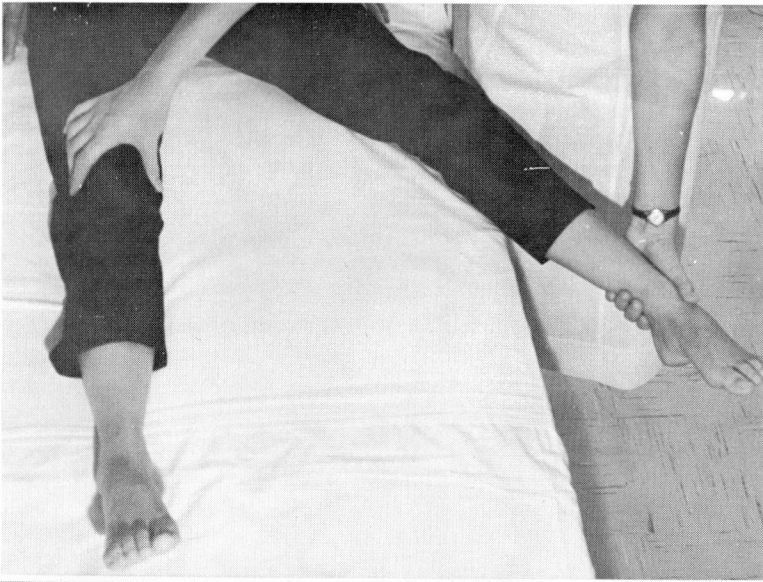

Abduction-adduction
of the hip.

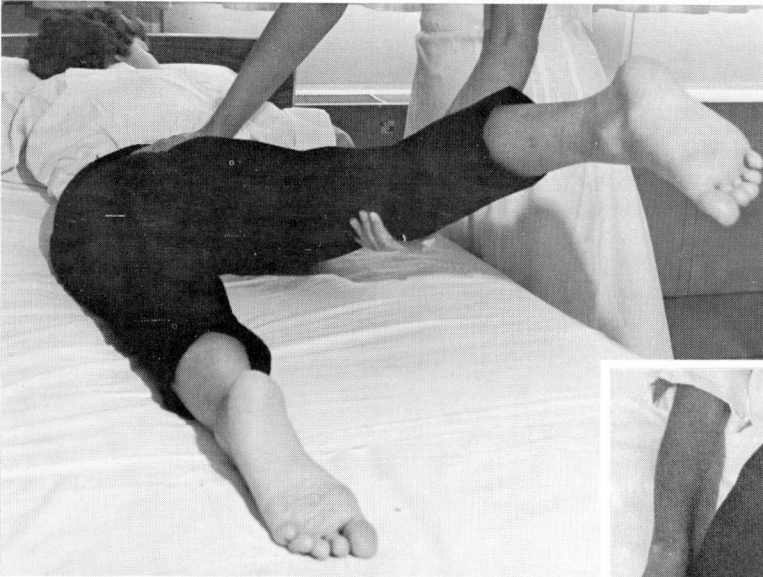

Hyperextension of
the hip.

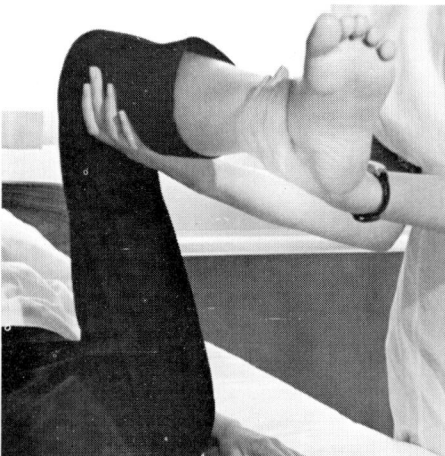

Flexion of the hip.

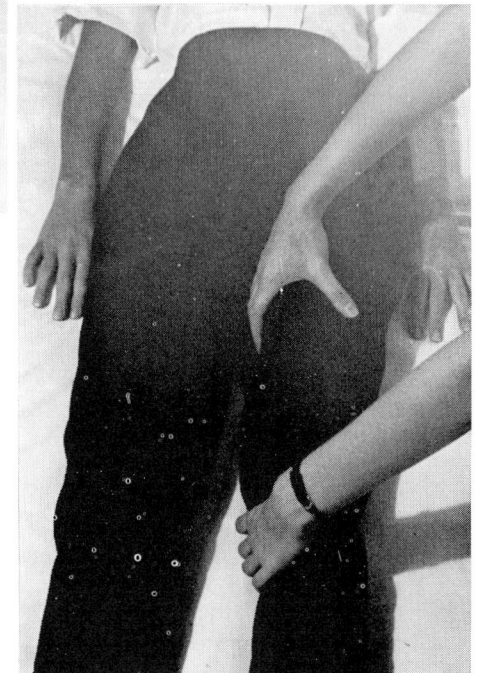

Internal-external rotation of the hip.

FIGURE 105

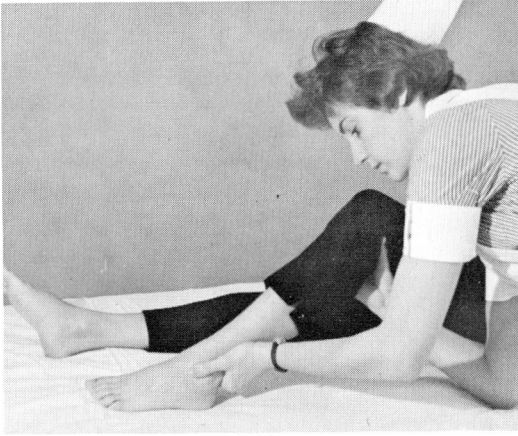

Flexion of the knee.

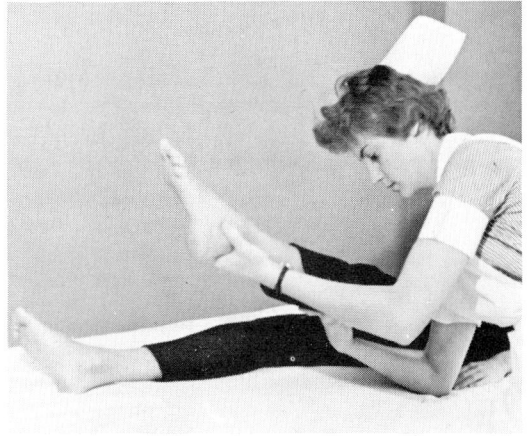

Extension of the knee.

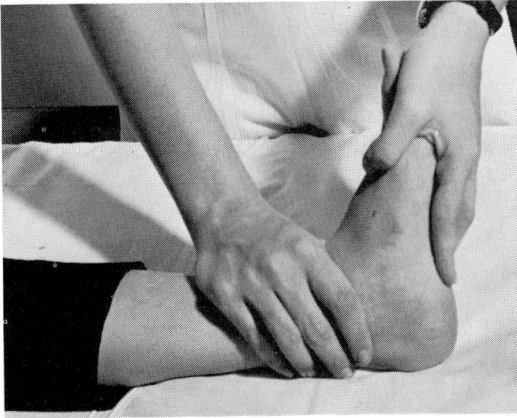

Dorsiflexion of the foot.

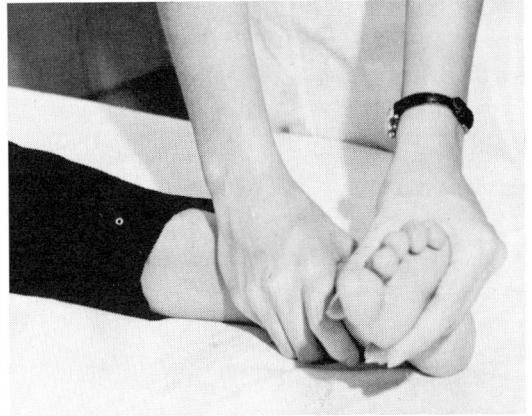

Inversion-eversion of the foot.

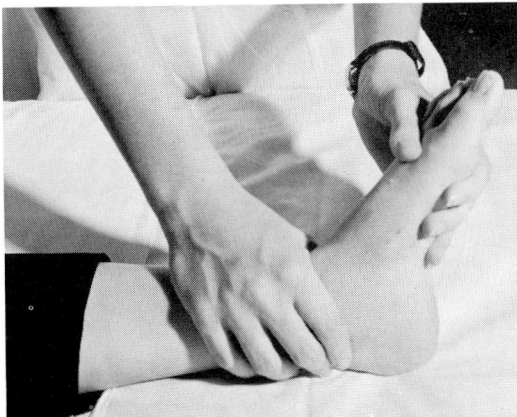

Plantar flexion of the foot.

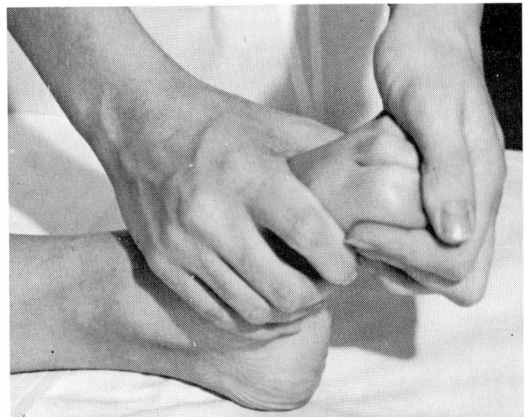

Flexion-extension of the toes.

FIGURE 105 (*continued*)

TABLE 14. Passive Range-of-Motion Exercises Adapted for Nursing

Joint	Normal Movement of Joint	Part to be Stabilized	Part to be Moved
Shoulder:	Flexion Extension Abduction Adduction Internal rotation External rotation Hyperextension (done in prone position)	Shoulder girdle	Arm
Elbow:	Flexion Extension Supination Pronation	Arm	Forearm
Wrist:	Flexion Extension Ulnar deviation Radial deviation	Forearm	Hand
Thumb:	Flexion Extension Abduction Adduction Opposition	Metacarpals and wrist	Metacarpo- phalangeal joint of thumb
Distal phalanx of thumb:	Flexion Extension	Proximal phalanx of thumb	Distal phalanx of thumb
Joints of fingers: metacarpophalangeal joints	Flexion Extension Abduction Adduction	Metacarpals of hand	Fingers
Interphalangeal joints	Flexion Extension	Proximal or middle phalanx	Middle and distal phalanx
Toes: Interphalangeal joints	Flexion Extension	Proximal or middle joint phalanx	Middle and distal phalanx
Toes: Metacarpophalangeal joints	Flexion Extension Adduction Abduction	Metatarsal	Proximal phalanx
Ankle:	Dorsiflexion Plantar flexion Eversion Inversion	Leg	Foot
Knee:	Flexion Extension	Thigh	Leg
Hip:	Flexion Extension Adduction Abduction Internal rotation External rotation Hyperextension (done in prone position)	Pelvis	Thigh
Neck:	Flexion Extension Rotation	Support head	Head

radius and the ulna are moved through their range of motion in the elbow joint.

Table 14 shows the normal movement of joints. To assist the nurse to learn logically the technic of range of motion, the name of the joint, the anatomic movements of the joint, the part to be stabilized, and the part to be moved are identified.

Fear and Pain. The ability of a patient to follow a pattern of exercises may be thwarted by *fear* and *pain*. These produce increased tensions and may result in muscle spasm and tightness of joint ligaments. If fear and pain are not relieved, they may lead to stiffness of joints, limitation in range of motion, muscle contractures and poorly coordinated muscle activity. For example: *pain* in the chest, as observed in chest and breast surgery, cardiac pain or burns of the thorax, frequently causes many patients to hold the arm close to the body, resting on the chest or abdominal wall with the elbow flexed. If permitted to continue for prolonged periods of time, this may result in tightness of the ligaments around the shoulder and elbow joints; and spasm of the large pectoral muscles and biceps may lead to adaptive shortening, tightening and contractures of these muscles. The weight of the arm on the chest and/or the abdomen restricts the expansive motion of the chest wall and muscles of respiration, which leads to inadequate ventilation.

Fear (as observed in patients who have had cardiac, chest or breast surgery, infections in the lungs and burns of the chest wall), often accounts for these individuals assuming protective positions that are restrictive in nature and prevent proper physiologic alignment.

Preventing External Rotation of the Hip

Patients who are in bed for periods of time may develop external rotation deformity of the hip. The hip is a ball-and-socket joint and has a tendency to rotate outward when the patient lies on his back. A trochanter

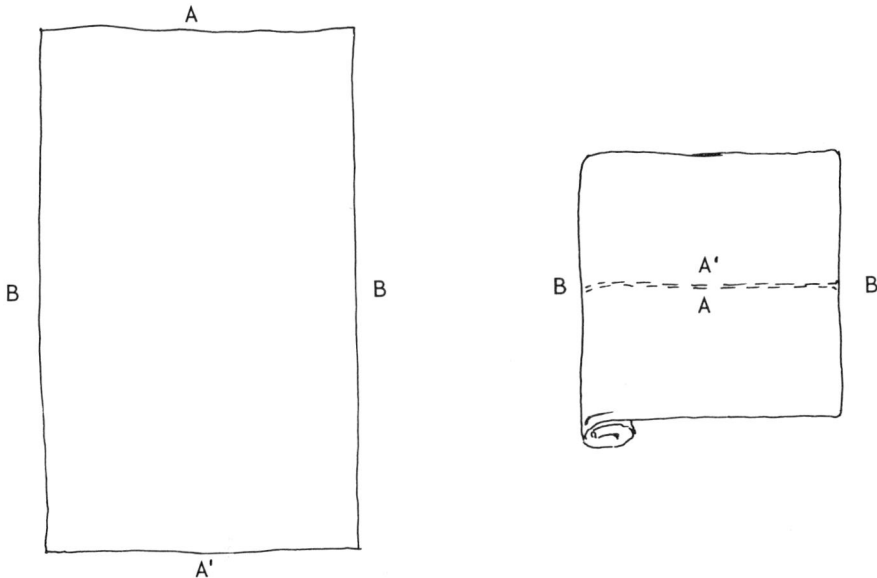

Fig. 106. To make a trochanter roll: Take both ends of the towel (A) and bring them to the center. The towel is now folded in half with the edges at the center. Turn the towel over so that the ends (A) are facing downward. Turn the patient on his side with his upper leg flexed. Place one side (B) of the towel in the midline of the buttock. The towel should extend from the crest of the ilium to the midthigh. Then place the patient in a dorsal position with his leg extended. Grasp the remaining side (B) of the towel and roll it in an underneath fashion until the entire roll is well under the patient's buttock. The roll should be taut and smooth. For the larger patient, a draw sheet or a bath blanket may be used.

roll extending from the crest of the ilium to the midthigh will prevent this deformity. With correct placement, the trochanter roll serves as a mechanical wedge under the projection of the greater trochanter.

Preventing Foot Drop (Plantar Flexion)

This is a deformity in which the foot is plantar flexed. If the condition continues without correction, the patient will walk on his toes without touching the ground with the heel of his foot. The deformity is caused by contracture of both the gastrocnemius and the soleus muscles. Prolonged bed rest, lack of exercise, incorrect positioning in bed, and the weight of the bedding forcing the toes into plantar flexion are factors that contribute to this crippling deformity. To prevent it, a footboard is used to keep the feet at right angles to the legs when the patient is in a supine position. The patient is encouraged to flex and then to extend (curl and stretch) his feet and toes frequently. The ankles should be moved clockwise and counterclockwise in a rotary motion several times each hour.

Preventing and Treating Decubiti

The prevention of decubitus ulcers (bedsores) is one of the most important consider-ations in the nursing care of patients. Such a sore is due to pressure that produces ischemia and consequently impaired nutrition to the tissues. This deprivation causes the cutaneous tissues to be broken or destroyed, and there is a progressive destruction of underlying soft tissue. The ulcer may be extremely painful and very slow to heal. Bacterial invasion and secondary infection are difficult to avoid. The lesion, if large enough, permits a continuous loss of serum which may deplete the circulating blood and the entire body of essential protein constituents.

Any patient who is stuporous, emaciated, incontinent, paralyzed, or whose treatment involves the immobilization of any portion of the body is in constant danger of developing a decubitus ulcer.

Essentials of Prevention. The best treatment of decubiti is prevention. The principles that underlie the nursing management are (1) to relieve or to remove pressure; (2) to stimulate the circulation; and (3) to keep the skin dry.

The patient needs frequent changes of position and the avoidance of positions that result in excessive local pressure. If possible, he should be taught and encouraged to turn himself. Bony prominences may be protected by inserting small pieces of foam

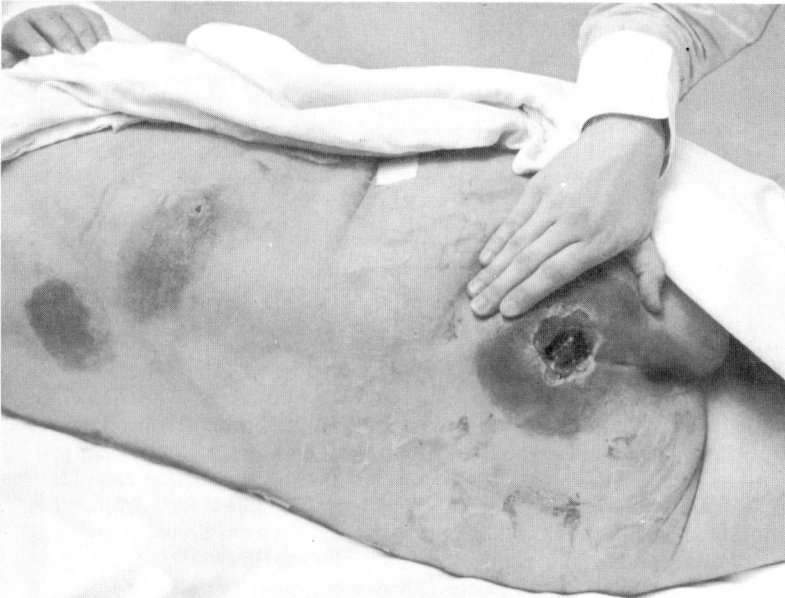

Fig. 107. Decubitus ulcer or bedsore over sacrum.

rubber beneath the sacrum, the trochanters, the heels, the elbows, the scapulae and the back of the head when there is pressure on these sites. The use of a footboard will remove the pressure of the bedding from the feet and the extremities. The alternating pressure pad mattress is especially valuable in conditions in which the patient cannot turn. The alternating inflation and deflation of the pad produces a constriction followed by a dilatation of the superficial blood vessels of the skin. By such action, pressure on any one part is reduced and an adequate blood supply is encouraged.

Since the stimulation of circulation relieves tissue ischemia, the forerunner of decubitus ulcers, the patient is encouraged to keep active. (Activity also stimulates the metabolic processes and helps to improve morale.) Frequent skin massage is useful as a means of stimulating the blood flow in the skin. A gentle circular motion is used around bony prominences and other vulnerable areas. If an abrasion is discovered, massage should be directed in ever-widening circles away from the lesion. Again, turning aids the circulation. The use of a rocking bed and a tilt table also aids in stimulating circulation.

Maceration of the skin by continuous moisture must be prevented by meticulous hygienic measures. The skin should be washed with a mild soap and water and blotted dry with a soft towel. The skin then is lubricated with an emollient lotion to keep it soft and pliable. It is desirable that the patient assist in caring for his skin. He should be taught to inspect it at frequent intervals for evidence of pressure. Foreign bodies should be kept out of the bed because they serve to irritate the skin. Foundation sheets should be tightly stretched to prevent wrinkles.

Treatment. If a decubitus ulcer develops, the essentials of care are to remove the pressure and to keep the area clean and dry. The metabolic processes are stimulated by keeping the patient as active as possible. Blood flow may be improved by gentle massage to the adjacent area. The patient is placed on a high protein diet. Plasma, blood, sugar and other nutrients have been employed to encourage healing of the wound. Many clinicians and investigators feel that proteolytic enzymes have a significant place in the management of these wounds. However, two factors are always necssary for the successful healing of a decubitus ulcer: (1) avoidance of further pressure, and (2) keeping the wound well débrided and clean.

For deep decubiti that refuse to heal by conservative means, some surgeons advocate excision of the ulcer and often of the underlying bony prominence, with plastic closure by skin and fat flaps.

Supporting the Patient in Daily Self-care

When a patient has a physical disability, the nurse helps him to make all types of adaptations in order to perform the self-care activities of daily living. This nursing practice requires common sense and a little ingenuity, for many patients do not perform these commonplace activities easily. Often a simple maneuver requires much concentration and the exertion of considerable effort.

Morrissey offers *three fundamental principles* which are relevant to all instruction *in self-care methods:** The first is that the nurse teaches and guides, but the patient is obliged to do the work alone. Secondly, motivation is an important factor; it is not possible to instruct and guide an unwilling patient. And third, there are individual differences in all people. Hence, self-care technics should be flexible and easily adjusted to the patient's needs.

By using an "Activities of Daily Living (A.D.L.) Sheet," (Fig. 108) to evaluate the ability of a patient to perform certain activities, it is possible to determine his limitations. Another advantage of such a guide is to show the patient how he is progressing from one time to the next; this may be a valuable morale booster. When a patient's progress can be demonstrated, there is a tendency for such evidence to be a source of motivation.

Before initiating an A.D.L. program, the nurse must understand the patient's medical condition, his functional capacity and therapeutic goal. She also must be familiar with every detail of his care. It is wise to know the patient's family background in order to

* Morrissey, A. B.: Rehabilitation Nursing, p. 144, New York, G. P. Putnam's Sons, 1950.

ACTIVITIES OF DAILY LIVING (A.D.L.) SHEET

Evaluation of the Patient's Functioning

	TOTAL ASSIST-ANCE	PARTIAL ASSIST-ANCE	INDE-PENDENT

Prescribed Activities:

Range of Motion

Positioning

Use of Tilt Table

   Degree

   How long

Exercises

   Breathing

   Balancing

   Crutch Training

   Parallel Bars

   Steps

Other Information:

Appliances or Prosthesis

Ambulation

Time Permitted Up

Bladder/Bowel Program

Bathing/Grooming Schedule

Speech Problems

Activities Being Learned

Name:

Diagnosis:

Doctor:

Functional Capabilities:

	TOTAL ASSIST-ANCE	PARTIAL ASSIST-ANCE	INDE-PENDENT
1. Flexes neck			
2. Raises hand to head			
3. Raises hand behind head			
4. Reaches out at shoulder level to side (laterally)			
5. Pronates/supinates forearm			
6. Grasps objects			
7. Begins grasp ability			
8. Closes fist			
9. Opens fist			
10. Flexes and extends knee joint			
11. Touches toes while seated			
12. Crosses foot over opposite knee while sitting (with or without help of hands)			
13. Transfers from sitting to standing (with or without holding to support)			
14. Walks			

FIG. 108. On the actual chart there is sufficient space left under each item for notes.

know how much support the family can give. An understanding of the educational background of the patient and the family members also will be helpful to the nurse.

The role of the nurse in A.D.L. is to teach, support and supervise the patient while he does these activities. An Activities of Daily Living program is started as soon as the rehabilitation process starts. The longer a muscle is in disuse, the weaker and more atrophied it becomes. The patient must learn that he will lose what he does not use.

Since there are many ways to teach a task, the following is offered as a guide:

Teaching the Activities of Daily Living

1. Ascertain what methods can be used to accomplish the task. (Example: There are several ways of putting on a given garment.)

2. Determine what the patient can do by watching him perform.

3. Ascertain the motions necessary for the accomplishment of the activity.

4. Encourage the patient to exercise the muscles necessary to perform the motions involved in the activity.

5. Select activities that encourage gross functional movements of the upper and lower extremities (e.g., bathing, holding larger objects).

6. Gradually include activities that use finer motions, e.g., buttoning clothes, eating with a spoon.

7. Increase the period of activity as rapidly as the patient can tolerate.

8. Perform and practice the activity in a real-life situation.

9. Encourage the patient to do every activity up to his maximum capabilities within the framework of his disability.

10. Support the patient by giving justifiable praise for effort put forth and for acts accomplished.

The A.D.L. Sheet is an information sheet for those who are taking care of the patient. The data on it serve to inform each member of the rehabilitation team what activities the patient can do. It also serves as an index of progress. For example, after it has been determined that the patient can bathe himself, this information is noted on the A.D.L. Sheet. The nurse who is responsible for the patient reviews this sheet at morning care time. She knows then what the patient is capable of doing and what activities he is learning. Thus the patient does not regress, because all members of the rehabilitation team are working toward the same goal.

The A.D.L. Sheet in Figure 108 assesses the motions of the patient. These activities are key goals. If the patient can sit up and raise his hands to his head, he probably can begin to bathe himself. By asking the patient to do certain motions the nurse can determine what activities the patient will be able to do.

If the patient has difficulty in performing the activity, an adaptation will have to be made. Perhaps a new method can be learned. If the patient cannot quite reach his head, perhaps he will be able to touch his head by leaning forward. Or, if the method cannot be changed, adaptive equipment (self-help devices) may be used—such as adding a long handle to a comb, "building up" the handle of a spoon, or a similar modification.

Assisting the Patient with Ambulation

Transfer Activities. As soon as the patient is able to bathe, feed and dress himself in bed, he is ready to learn to do these activities from a wheelchair. By this time, it is desirable that the patient be able to raise and move his body in different directions by means of a "push-up" exercise. However, the method of transferring from the bed to the wheelchair will depend on the individual's problems. If the muscles that the patient uses to lift himself off the bed are not strong enough to overcome the resistance of body weight, a polished light-weight board may be used to bridge the gap between the bed and the chair, and the patient slides across on it. This board (or bench) also may be used to transfer the patient from the chair to the toilet or the bathtub.

Before the patient is taught to transfer, he is evaluated to determine his ability to transfer from one area to another. The nurse demonstrates the technic of transfer and the patient then is ready to practice and perform this activity (Fig. 109).

Preparation for Ambulation. Regaining the ability to walk is a prime morale builder. To be prepared for ambulation—whether

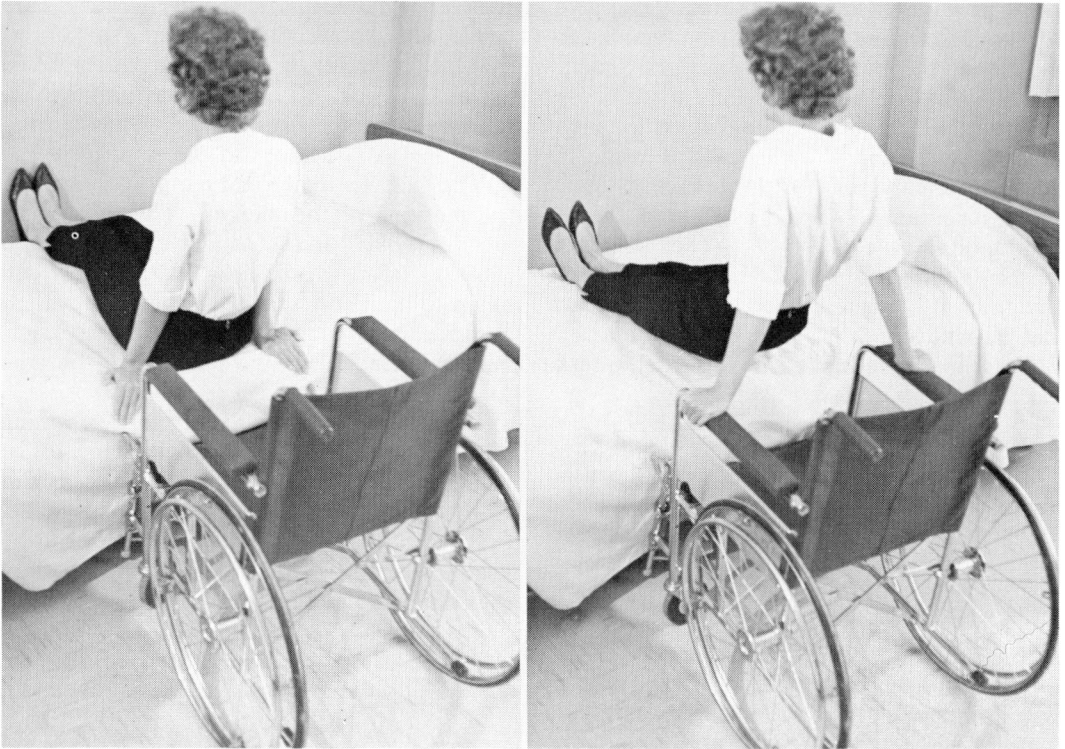

Fig. 109. A patient moves from her bed to a wheelchair. (*Left*) The wheelchair is placed facing the bed with the wheels locked and the pedals in the "down" position. (*Right*) The patient transfers her hands from the bed to the arms of the wheelchair, then lifts and pushes herself back into the chair.

with braces, cane or crutches—the patient must be strengthened and conditioned. *Exercise is the foundation of preparation.* By performing mat and parallel-bar exercises, the patient develops balance and coordination and strengthens his muscles. The following are preconditioning exercises that the nurse can teach and supervise.

To strengthen the muscles needed for ambulation, the *quadriceps setting* is used. The patient contracts the quadriceps muscle while attempting to push the popliteal area against the mattress and raising the heel. He maintains the muscle contracture until the count of five and relaxes for the count of five. He should repeat this exercise 10 to 15 times hourly. In the *gluteal setting,* he contracts or "pinches" the buttocks together until the count of five, relaxes for the count of five, and repeats.

To strengthen the muscles of the upper extremities, which are used for handling the cane, the crutches, and the walker employed in early ambulation, *sit-ups* are helpful. While in a sitting position, the patient raises his body from the chair by pushing his hands against the chair seat (or mattress). He also should be encouraged to do *push-ups* while in a prone position. Teach him to *raise arms* above his head and lower them in a slow, rhythmical manner while holding traction weights, gradually increasing the poundage of the weights. He can *strengthen his hands* by crumpling newspaper and squeezing a rubber ball. *Pull-ups* on a trapeze, lifting the body, is another effective conditioner.

Crutch-walking. In the treatment of most fractures of the lower extremity, of various forms of arthritis and after operations on the leg—especially after amputation—crutches provide a convenient method for getting from one place to another. Not an inherited skill, crutch-walking must be taught, and this learning process must begin early. It includes psychological preparation that can be developed long before the physical need is present. The individual needs of each patient must be considered and the methods of approach directed to them. The patient's age, his interests and his future intentions, as well as his prognosis, are essential factors.

Adjustable crutches are practical because the disease may make changes in the muscles and the joints, or because the patient may improve and progress to a different crutch base and gait.

To measure a standing patient for crutches, measure 1½ to 2 inches from the axillary fold to a position on the floor 4 inches in front of the patient and 6 inches to

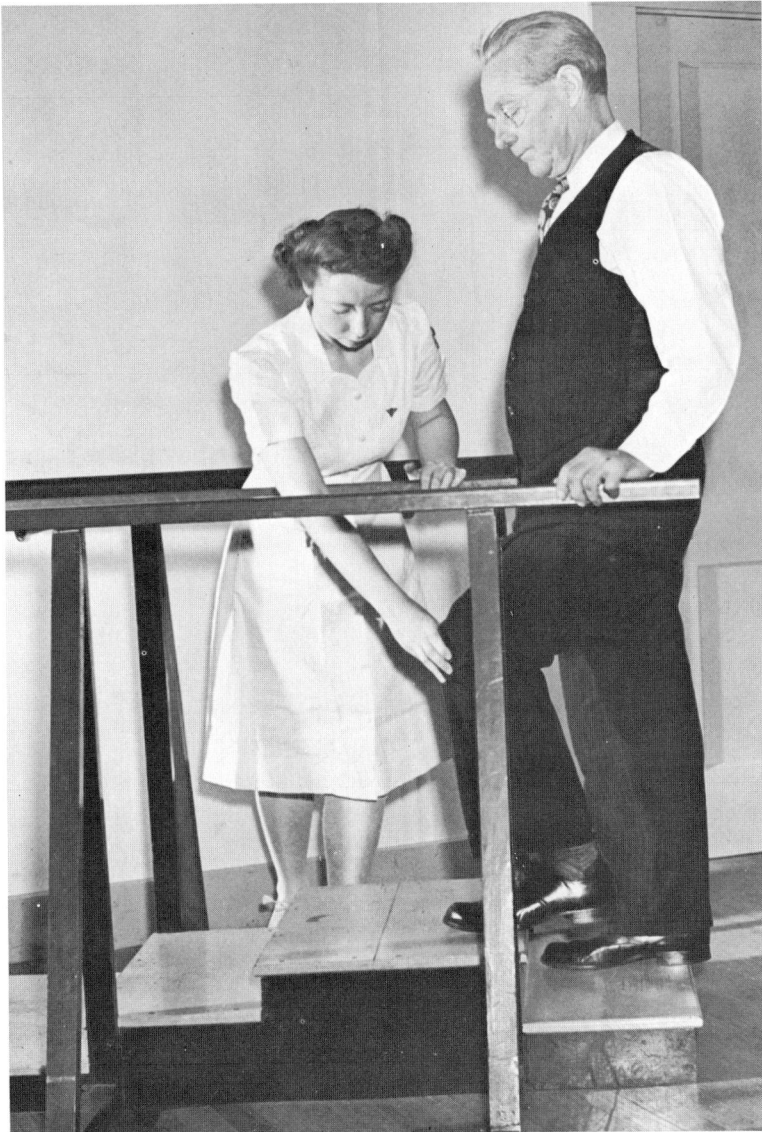

FIG. 110. Platform stairs with steadying guide rails help to restore confidence at the same time that the patient benefits from the exercise. (Liberty Mutual Insurance Co., Boston, Mass.)

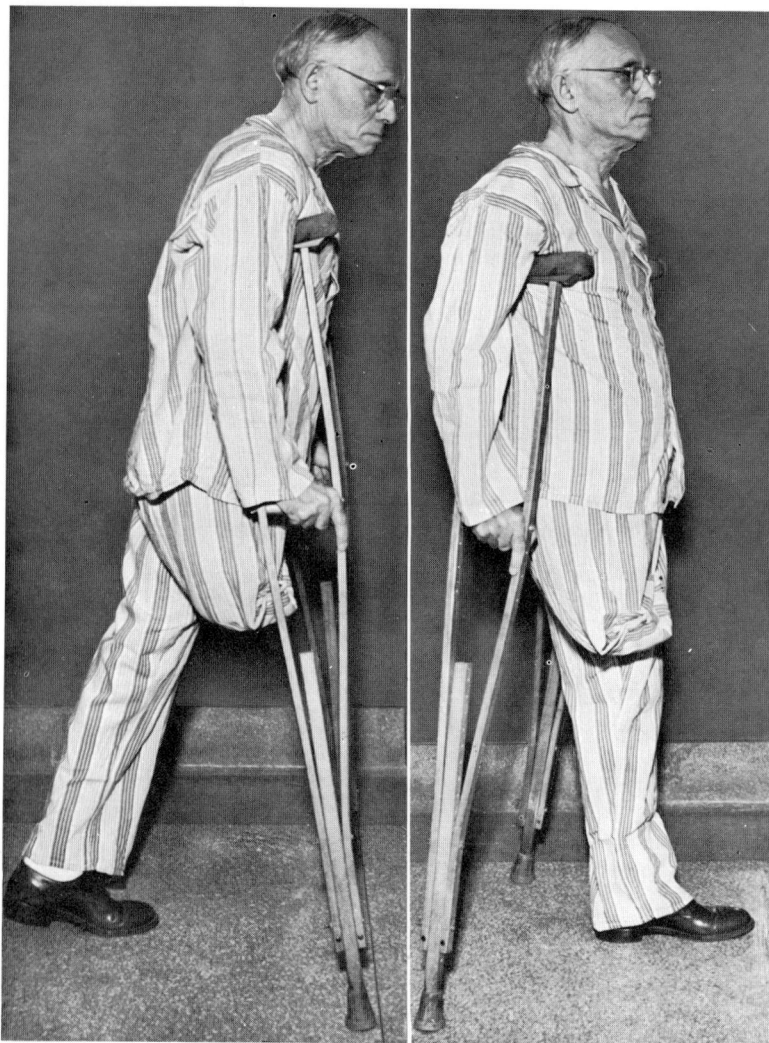

Fig. 111. Crutch-walking. (*Left*) Note that the patient's weight is borne not in the axilla but on the palm of the hand, with the arm extended. The weight of the patient's body should be inclined forward to be supported by the crutches.

the side of his toes. (This is merely an approximate measure. It is desirable to have a 2-finger width insertion between the axillary fold and the armpiece.)

If the patient has to be measured while lying down, measure from the anterior fold of the axilla to the sole of the foot, and then add 2 inches.

The handpiece should allow a 30° elbow flexion. The wrist should be extended, and the hand dorsiflexed.

The patient should wear shoes that fit well and have firm soles.

The crutches should be fitted with large rubber suction tips before measuring.

Good posture is essential to crutch walk-ing. Before trying to use crutches, the patient should learn to stand by a chair on the unaffected leg in order to achieve balance. The nurse explains and demonstrates to the patient how he should manipulate his crutches before he attempts to do so.

The *tripod position* is the basic crutch stance. The crutches rest approximately 8 to 10 inches in front and to the side of the patient's toes. This gives the strongest and most balanced support. Since, to provide stability, a greater height requires a broader base, a taller patient needs a wider base and a shorter patient a narrower base.

The patient must be taught to support his weight on the handpiece. If the weight is

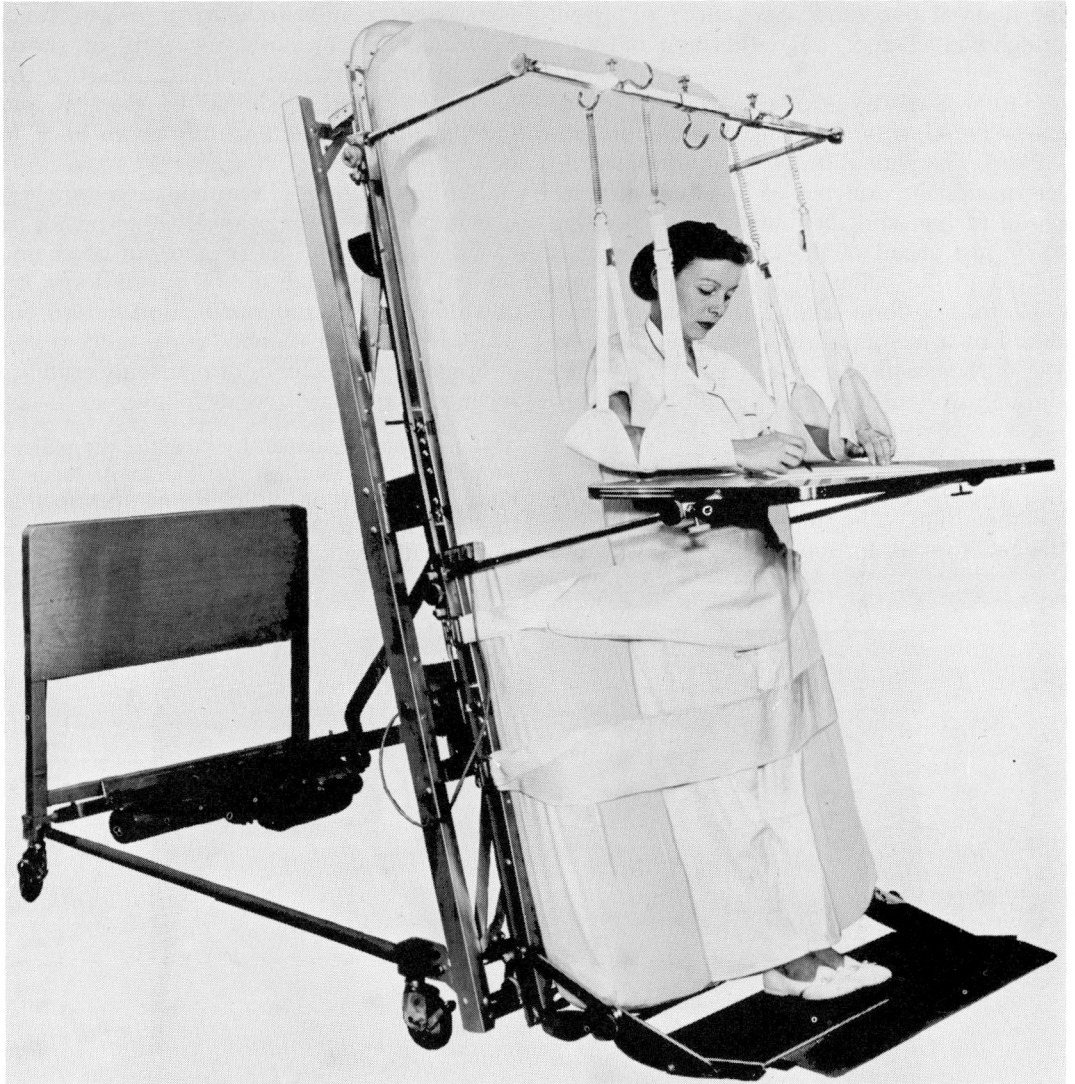

Fig. 112. A tilt bed, also called a tilt table.

borne on the axilla, the pressure of the crutch can damage the brachial plexus nerves and produce "crutch paralysis." A foam rubber pad on the underarm piece will relieve pressure on the upper arm and the thoracic cage.

Ability to shift body weight is the next step. The crutch gait selected depends on the nature of the patient's disability. The nurse must know how much (if any) weight can be placed on the affected side. She should know whether the crutches are being used for balance and support. The crutch

gait should be prescribed by the physician.

All gaits begin in the tripod position. The more common gaits are:

THE 4-POINT GAIT. This gait can be used when supported weight-bearing is permitted for both legs. It is safe and gives maximum balance because there are always 3 points of contact with the floor; hence it is slow because it requires constant shifting of weight. The sequence is to advance (1) right crutch, (2) left foot, (3) left crutch, (4) right foot.

THE 2-POINT GAIT. This gait is faster, since there are only 2 points of contact with the floor at one time. Sequence: (1) right crutch and left foot, (2) left crutch and right foot.

THE SWINGING-TO AND SWINGING-THROUGH GAITS. These gaits are more advanced. The patient bears weight on his good leg, places the crutches at an equal distance ahead of him and then swings to a position to or just ahead of the crutches. Weight is shifted to the palms of the hands and then back to the good leg. The elevation produced by a medium-heeled shoe on the good leg may permit the affected leg to swing through without touching the floor and without unnecessary flexion. It is desirable that the patient learn as many gaits as possible so that he may change his pattern when one gait tires him. The nurse should not permit patients to walk for too long, especially those who have been bedridden for a long time. Such signs as cyanosis, sweating or shortness of breath should be indications that the lesson on crutches should be stopped and the patient permitted to rest or go back to bed.

Before a patient is sent home on crutches, it is important to ascertain whether or not he can dress himself, get in and out of chairs, on and off the toilet, in and out of doors, up and down stairs and ramps, and in and out of a car, a taxi or a public conveyance.

Some of the technics of managing crutches have been standardized, as follows:

If the door is opened by pushing, the patient should get as close as possible to it, balance himself securely on crutches and feet so that the hand nearest the doorknob can be released, and turn the handle. The door is then pushed

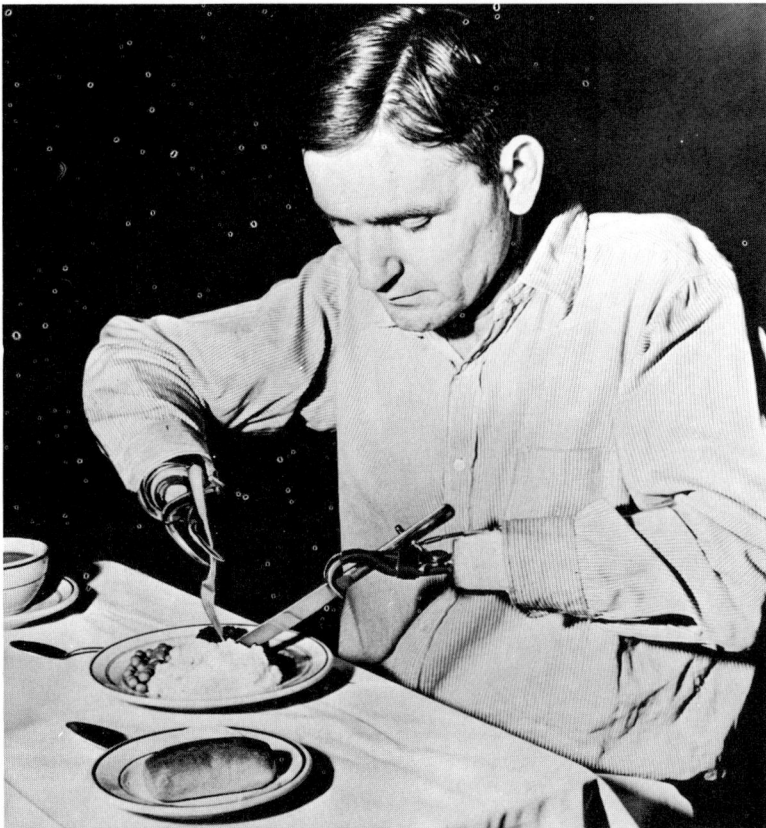

FIG. 113. This man, who is a bilateral arm amputee, is feeding himself by using mechanical prostheses. (Liberty Mutual Insurance Co., Boston, Mass.)

ajar and a crutch is quickly advanced to hold the gain. This operation is repeated until the patient, moving in progressive stages clears the door. Difficulties: getting close enough to the door; clearing the doorsill while advancing.

If the door must be opened by pulling, the above procedure is modified in that the patient stands to one side and pulls with the free hand.

Sitting down in and standing up from chair: These procedures are difficult. Soft, low chairs add to the difficulties. The technique should first be practiced with a fairly high chair equipped with arms and placed against the wall.

For standing up, one or both feet should be placed under the chair, not away from it. Grasping a hand piece of the crutch in each hand (or both hand pieces in one hand), the patient pushes down.

For sitting down, most techniques follow the practice of either falling or letting the body down into the chair, starting from a standing position with the patient's back to the chair. For the latter purpose, the crutches are grasped at the hand pieces for control; for the former method, the body is bent forward at the hips. Falling can be controlled to a certain extent, if muscular capacity allows, by gradually bending trunk forward, then knees, then placing hands on knees, and finally completing the forward bending of trunk until the body falls easily into the chair. Crutches may be previously placed against the chair, or be held passively during the change of position.*

The Use of the Tilt Table. Weight bearing on the long bones is essential to normal physiologic functioning. In order to prevent complications of inactivity, the upright position with weight bearing on the long bones is desirable at the earliest possible time. This position stimulates circulation to the lower extremities and prevents decalcification of the bones, thus aiding in the maintenance of normal acid-base balance and the prevention of renal calculi.

Some disabilities prevent patients from assuming an upright position by the usual methods. A tilt table or bed is a device that will permit this essential activity.

To assist the patient who has been in the recumbent position for a length of time, the nurse should consider the problems that may ensue when a standing position is assumed.

The position should be assumed progressively and gradually. Evaluation of the patient's tolerance may be made by observation of blood pressure, pulse and general appearance. To prevent some of the more common complications, such as orthostatic hypotension and edema of the lower extremities, elastic compression bandages on the lower extremities may be indicated.

Helping With Prosthetic and Orthotic Appliances

A *prosthesis* is an artificial replacement for a missing portion of the body. An *orthotic* device is an orthopedic appliance commonly termed a *brace*. A prosthetist or an orthotist fit these appliances only by prescription of the physician.†

Preprosthetic Care. The nurse performs a distinctive function in the preprosthetic phase of the patient's care. She sees the patient at the beginning of the disability and can help him to develop an attitude of realistic hopefulness. Her major function is to prevent deformities so that the time between the healing of the tissues and the fitting of the prosthesis is kept to a minimum. In the amputation of an extremity, she is responsible for bandaging the stump correctly, so that proper shrinkage and shaping of the stump occurs and the patient can be fitted more effectively with a prosthesis (see p. 1016).

Braces. The patient should be fitted for a brace according to the prescription of the physician. A brace is a support that protects weakened muscles, prevents and corrects anatomic deformities and controls involuntary muscle movements. The essential parts of leg braces are frames, hinges, joints, straps, belts and lining. In the upright frames, the hinges and the joints usually are made of steel. Often a brace may appear to be

---

* Gordon, E. E.: Multiple Sclerosis, Application of Rehabilitation Techniques (p. 29), National Multiple Sclerosis Society, New York, 1951.

† Specific prostheses are described later in this book, when the clinical conditions calling for them are discussed, e.g., limb prostheses for the amputee and a breast prosthesis for the patient who has had a radical mastectomy. Information concerning prosthetic and orthopedic appliances may be obtained also from The American Board for Certification in Orthotics and Prosthetics, Inc., 919 18th Street, N.W., Washington 6, D. C.

heavy; yet its weight is necessary in order to be safe, durable and effective.

In caring for a patient wearing a brace, the major responsibility of the nurse is to make certain that the patient wears the brace and that it is not applied too tightly. The following are the main points in the care of braces.

1. All locks should be opened once a week and cleaned with fine wire or a hairpin; place a drop of machine oil in each joint.

2. Repair leather when necessary. Little can be done about perspiration stains; however, washing the leather in lukewarm water, with saddle soap, will help to preserve the leather.

3. When not in use, it is well to lay the brace on a table or the floor in good alignment; hanging may cause it to distort its position.

4. Twisting of the brace may occur with use; check alignment frequently. The joints should coincide with the body joints.

5. Before putting a brace on, check carefully for worn areas, missing or loose screws and the condition of straps and buckles.

6. Pressure areas may occur if metal rubs the skin. After removing a brace, check the skin immediately for reddened areas.

7. Have the brace checked periodically.

Note: The patient himself should care for his brace when he is able.

Helping to Overcome Elimination Problems

Urinary and bowel incontinence in a patient is another problem that challenges the nurse's ingenuity. Bladder and bowel control are important functions of the body; social acceptance of the individual may be affected if he suffers from incontinence. Patients with various medical and surgical conditions have to be trained in regaining control of these functions.

Bladder Training. Tidal drainage, discussed on page 915, will condition or pretrain the bladder for activity that is not controlled by the central nervous system but is automatic. After tidal drainage is discontinued (or the indwelling catheter removed), the patient is ready for a bladder-training regimen. With the approval and the cooperation of the physician and with the willingness of the patient (who knows his habit patterns better than anyone else) a schedule is set up with definite times indicated for the patient to try to empty his bladder using either the bedpan or the toilet. The interval between voiding in the early phase of the training period is fairly short ($1\frac{1}{2}$ to 2 hours), but as the patient's bladder capacity increases, the interval is lengthened. A suggested procedure is to give a measured amount of fluid every 2 hours. After drinking, the patient waits for 30 minutes and then attempts to void. He gradually increases the period between voiding times. (It is best to give larger amounts of fluid at breakfast and to withhold fluids at bedtime.) The patient is encouraged to hold his urine until the specified voiding time. Usually, there is a relationship between drinking, eating, exercising, and voiding, and the alert patient soon can determine his own intake schedule. Regularity is the key to success. Bladder training for the paraplegic or quadraplegic patient is discussed further on pp. 971-975.

To assist in the act of voiding, the patient should either stand or sit with the thighs flexed and the feet and the back supported. Increasing intra-abdominal pressure by massage over the bladder or by leaning forward while sitting will help to initiate evacuation of the bladder.* The patient must approve of the program and have a sincere desire to establish control. It may take weeks to accomplish; patience and persistence on the part of both nurse and patient plus expressions of approval for even slight gains are necessary. The use of a diaper at any time is discouraged, since its psychological effect is one of regression rather than progression.

Bowel Training. The first essential to bowel training that requires reflex assistance is the *establishment of regularity*. Any attempts at evacuation should be done within 15 minutes of the same time daily. An active aid toward bowel evacuation is the stimulation of peristalsis. Therefore, the patient should establish his bowel evacuation time after a regularly scheduled meal. One of the best times is after breakfast. However, if the patient has a previously-established habit pattern, it should be followed.

* *See also:* Fuerst, E. V., and Wolff, L.: Fundamentals of Nursing, ed. 2, p. 380, Methods for Assisting the Process (voiding), Philadelphia, Lippincott, 1959.

Physical activity is another helpful aid to peristaltic activity and bowel movement. Unless contraindicated by other existing conditions, the diet should include adequate roughage and a fluid intake between 2,000 to 4,000 ml. daily. Prune juice or fig juice taken at the same time daily may be beneficial when constipation is a problem.

The reflex habit should be established by regularity early in the course of the patient's illness. It may be aided by mechanical means. About 30 minutes before the scheduled bowel time, a glycerine suppository is inserted into the rectum. After the scheduled interval, the patient is encouraged to attempt to have a bowel movement. If at all possible he should assume the normal position for defecation. Instruct him to bear down and to contract his abdominal muscles. The patient may be taught to apply pressure to the abdominal wall to assist with his defecation.

After this routine is well established, mechanical stimulation with the suppository probably will not be necessary, and in a few weeks the patient will be having regular daily bowel movements.

Patient Referral

The objective of a referral system is to maintain continuity of patient care as the patient is transferred from the hospital to his home or a convalescent home. Frequently the public health nurse is the case finder whose astute observations made the rehabilitation services possible to the patient. By visiting the patient in the hospital, the public health nurse is able to see what adjustments will have to be made in the home. She can help the family to select, to improvise, or to borrow the needed equipment from another agency. She determines what can be done to ease the family situation and can suggest ways in which adaptations in living arrangements can be made. After the patient returns to his home, the visiting or public health nurse makes sure that the patient does not "lose ground" and that he is able to maintain the independence that he gained in the hospital. The Activities of Daily Living Sheet is sent home with the patient so that the visiting nurse knows exactly what activities the patient can perform.

If the hospital has a home-care program, the home-care nurse acts as a liaison between the patient and the hospital to determine the need for continued nursing care.

The Office of Vocational Rehabilitation provides services whereby the disabled person is assisted in obtaining the help he needs to engage in remunerative work. These services are provided by state agencies and include diagnostic, medical, surgical, psychiatric and hospital services, and assistance in securing prosthetic appliances. There is a counseling, training, placement and follow-up service available to help the patient to select and attain a vocational objective.

The following is a selected list of agencies and organizations, both official and voluntary, that work with or for patients needing rehabilitation services.

Voluntary Agenices (Private Agencies)

American Legion
National Rehabilitation Program
1806 K Street, N.W.
Washington 6, D.C.

American Medical Association
Committee on Rehabilitation
535 N. Dearborn Street
Chicago 10, Illinois

American Occupational Therapy
    Association, Inc.
250 West 57th Street
New York 19, N.Y.

American Orthotics and Prosthetics
    Association
919 18th Street
Washington 6, D.C.

American Physical Therapy Association
1790 Broadway
New York 19, N.Y.

American Psychological Association
1333 16th Street, N.W.
Washington 6, D.C.

American Rehabilitation Committee, Inc.
28 East 21st Street
New York 10, N.Y.

Association for the Aid of Crippled Children
345 East 46th Street
New York 17, N.Y.

Disabled American Veterans, Inc.
5555 Ridge Avenue
Cincinnati 13, Ohio

Goodwill Industries of America, Inc.
1229 20th Street, N.W.
Washington 6, D.C.

International Society for the Rehabilitation
of the Disabled
701 First Avenue
New York 17, N.Y.

National Association for Mental Health, Inc.
10 Columbus Circle
New York 19, N.Y.

National Association of Social Workers, Inc.
1 Park Avenue
New York 16, N.Y.

National Foundation, Inc.
301 East 42nd Street
New York 17, N.Y.

National Rehabilitation Association
1025 Vermont Avenue, N.W.
Washington 5, D.C.

National Research Council of the
National Academy of Science
2101 Constitution Avenue
Washington 25, D.C.

National Society for Crippled Children and
Adults, Inc.
2023-55 West Ogden Avenue
Chicago 12, Illinois

Veterans of Foreign Wars of the
United States
National Rehabilitation Service
Room 610, Wire Building
1000 Vermont Avenue, N.W.
Washington 5, D.C.

World Rehabilitation Fund
400 East 34th Street
New York 16, N.Y.

Institute of Physical Medicine and
Rehabilitation
New York University—Bellevue Medical
Center
400 East 34th Street
New York 16, N.Y.

Federal Agencies

Department of Health, Education and
Welfare
Office of Vocational Rehabilitation
330 Independence Avenue, S.E.
Washington 3, D.C.

President's Committee on Employment of
the Physically Handicapped
U. S. Labor Building
Washington 25, D.C.

Veterans' Administration
Washington 25, D.C.

CLINICAL SITUATION

Mr. John Simpson is a 54-year-old patient hospitalized with a cerebral vascular accident. His right side is paralyzed. Before his illness he was employed as a janitor in an elementary school. On the second day of hospitalization, the physician indicates that Mr. Simpson can start in his program of activities of daily living. The nurse can teach all of the following activities:
Bathing
Changing position in bed
Sitting up in bed
Eating
Putting on clothing
Combing hair
Brushing hair
How should the nurse teach these activities? In what order should the activities be taught? Which activities have similar motions? How many different ways can these activities be performed?

**BIBLIOGRAPHY AND
SUGGESTED READING**

Books

Allgire, M., and Denny, R. R.: Nurses Can Give and Teach Rehabilitation, New York, Springer, 1960.

Anderson, M. N. (ed.): Clinical Prosthetics for Physicians and Therapists, Springfield, Ill., Thomas, 1959.

Buchwald, E.: Physical Rehabilitation for Daily Living, New York, McGraw-Hill, 1952.

Daniels, L., Williams, M., and Worthingham, C.: Muscle Testing, ed. 2, Philadelphia, Saunders, 1956.

Dunton, W. R., and Licht, S.: Occupational Therapy, Springfield, Ill., Thomas, 1957.

Fash, B.: Kinesiology in Nursing, New York, McGraw-Hill, 1952.

Garrett, J. F.: Psychological Aspects of Physical Disability, Rehabilitation Series No. 210, Washington, D.C., U.S. Dept. Health, Education and Welfare, 1952.

Morrissey, A. B.: Rehabilitation Nursing, New York, Putnam, 1951.

Knocke, F., and Knocke, L.: Orthopedic Nursing, Philadelphia, Davis, 1954.

Larson, C. B., and Gould, M.: Calderwood's Orthopedic Nursing, ed. 5, St. Louis, Mosby, 1961.

Lawton, E. B.: Activities of Daily Living for Physical Rehabilitation, New York, McGraw-Hill, 1963.

Rusk, H.: Rehabilitation Medicine, St. Louis, Mosby, 1958.

Terry, F. J., Benz, G. S., *et al.*: Principles and Techniques of Rehabilitation Nursing, ed. 2, St. Louis, Mosby, 1961.

Williams, M., and Worthingham, C.: Therapeutic Exercise, Philadelphia, Saunders, 1960.

Winters, M. C.: Protective Body Mechanics in Daily Life and in Nursing, Philadelphia, Saunders, 1952.

Articles

Deaver, G. G., Jerome, M. M., and Taylor, W. E.: Rehabilitation, Am. J. Nursing 59: 1278-1281, Sept., 1959.

Drake, M.: Rehabilitation, an added dimension in nursing care, Am. J. Nursing 60:1105-1106, Aug., 1960.

Gordon, E. B., *et al.*: A study of rehabilitation potential in nursing home patients over 65 years, J. Chronic Dis. 15:311-326, March, 1962.

Horner, A. L., and Jennings, M.: Before patients go home, Am. J. Nursing 61:62-63, June, 1961.

Knocke, L.: Crutch walking, Am. J. Nursing, 61:70-73, Oct., 1961.

Lineberger, M. I.: Children who need prostheses, Nurs. Outlook 7:28-30, Jan., 1959.

Madden, B. W., and Affeldt, T. E.: To prevent helplessness and deformities, Am. J. Nursing 62:59-61, Dec., 1962.

Miller, C. H., and Hamil, E. M.: Rehabilitating patients with chronic disease, Nurs. Outlook 6:324-325, June, 1958.

Nursing in Rehabilitation Services, Nursing Outlook 10: Sept., 1962.

Patton, C. J., and Barckley, V.: Almost all's right with their world, Nurs. Outlook 7:31-33, Jan., 1959.

Rusk, H.: Nursing in rehabilitation, Tomorrow's Nurse, Oct.-Nov., 1960.

Saunders, E., and Swinyard, C. A.: The public health nurses' role in rehabilitation, Nurs. Outlook 9:426-427, July, 1961.

Saxon, J.: Techniques for bowel and bladder training, Am. J. Nursing 62:69-71, Sept., 1962.

Smith, L. A.: An orthotist, prosthetist—what are they? Nurs. Outlook 7:34-35, Jan., 1959.

Verhonick, P.: A preliminary report of a study of decubitus ulcer care, Am. J. Nursing 61: 68-69, Aug., 1961.

PART TWO

Nursing Care of Patients With Specific Medical and Surgical Problems

22

Nursing in Conditions of the Nose and the Throat

The sole function of the respiratory system is to serve as a route of gaseous exchange between the atmosphere surrounding the body and the tissues within, so that the cells may have access to the oxygen that they require and a means of dissipating their waste carbon dioxide.

It is apparent that any abnormality involving the respiratory system that interferes with its primary function is a potential threat to every organ, tissue and cell in the body, since it can easily result in a general state of oxygen deficiency complicated by carbon dioxide poisoning. A certain amount of interference of this sort, impairing aeration, is one of the most common and important of the complications of respiratory diseases.

Conditions that interfere with this mechanism result in an incomplete oxygenation of the blood, or *hypoxemia.* Arterial blood no longer has its bright red color; it is a dark purplish red. The patient's skin takes on a bluish pallor (cyanosis), which is best noted in the nail beds, the lips and the tongue.

Hypoxemia may occur from circulatory difficulties, such as cardiac failure, congenital cardiac or vascular defects, pulmonary embolism and so forth. Certain drugs interfere with the oxygenation of the blood (sulfanilamide, acetanilid) and produce cyanosis.

Surveying a complete listing of respiratory diseases, the nurse is impressed by the unusually high proportion that are infectious. Indeed, infections of the upper respiratory tract, considered as a group, represent the most common of all illnesses. The explanation for this prevalence undoubtedly is related to the fact that the external surface of

the respiratory organs, including the alveolar walls, presents a very extensive area of exposure to the bacteria-laden atmosphere. Moreover, respiratory infections are spread far more readily than are other types of infections, owing to the rate at which virulent organisms are dispersed in the expired air of infected patients, with the obvious likelihood that these contaminants soon will enter numerous other respiratory tracts in the vicinity.

Consideration is given in this chapter to both major and minor problems that cause interference with the normal function of the upper respiratory tract. In this unit, the major objectives of study for the nurse are to understand the complications that may result from simple upper respiratory infections and to recognize her role in teaching individuals how to control the spread of upper respiratory infections.

ANATOMY OF THE UPPER RESPIRATORY TRACT

Nose. The nose has two passages, called *nares,* separated in the middle by the septum. These passages open externally through the anterior nostrils and posteriorly into the nasopharynx. Between these two openings the air passages expand into broad chambers, on the lateral sides of which are three turbinate bones and into which open the paranasal sinuses, cavities within the hollow bones that surround the nasal passages.

Paranasal Sinuses. These include the frontal sinuses, located in the lower forehead between and above the eyes; the ethmoidal group of sinuses, both anterior and posterior,

376

extending along the roof of the nostrils; the sphenoid sinuses, opening at the rear; and, located on either side of the nose, the maxillary sinuses, or antra. The same type of ciliated epithelium that lines the nasal passages also lines these paranasal sinuses.

Turbinate Bones. The turbinate bones, the name of which was suggested by their shell-like appearance, are adapted by shape and position to increase the mucous membrane surface of the nasal passages and to obstruct slightly the current of air flowing through them. The sense organs of smell are located in the olfactory membrane, which covers the roof of the nose and the superior turbinate bones.

The current of air entering the anterior nostrils is deflected upward to the roof of the nose, describing a circuitous route before it reaches the nasopharynx. Therefore, it comes into contact with a large surface of moist, warm, mucous membrane that catches practically all dust and germs in the inhaled air. This air is moistened and warmed to body temperature and brought into contact with sensitive nerves, some of which detect odors and others of which provoke sneezing to expel irritating dust.

Pharynx. The pharynx is the throat. It is limited below by the larynx and the upper end of the esophagus. Its upper extension is the nasopharynx, into which open the posterior nostrils and the eustachian tubes from the middle ears. The nose and the nasopharynx are lined with the same type of ciliated epithelium as the trachea and the bronchial tree; but the pharynx, which serves as both a respiratory and an alimentary passage, is lined with squamous (flat-celled) epithelium.

Tonsils. The tonsils are two almond-shaped bodies, one on each side at the back of the throat.

Adenoids. The adenoid, or pharyngeal tonsil, is located in the roof of the nasopharynx. The tonsils and the adenoids constitute only two of a ring of similar masses of lymphoid tissue which completely encircles the throat. These organs are important links in the chain of lymph nodes guarding the body from invasion by organisms entering the nose and the throat.

Larynx. The larynx is a cartilaginous epithelial-lined structure forming the upper extremity of the trachea. The vocal cords, controlled by muscular attachments, are mounted in its lumen. Over it, preventing the entry of ingested food or liquid, is attached a valve flap called the *epiglottis*. The whole function of the larynx is to permit vocalization. It is the "voice box."

THE PATIENT WITH PROBLEMS OF THE NOSE

Epistaxis (Nosebleed)

Epistaxis may result from injury or disease. It is due to the rupture of tiny, distended vessels in the mucous membrane of the anterior septum and is not uncommon in normal young persons. The usual cause of small nosebleeds is "picking" of the nose. Other local causes are deviated septum, perforated septum, cancer and trauma. Epistaxis may also occur as a symptom of acute rheumatic fever, acute sinusitis, arterial hypertension and hemorrhagic diseases.

Treatment. In providing emergency care, the nurse will recall that cessation of bleeding is aided by the maintenance of an elevated position of the trunk and by promoting vasoconstriction in the nasal mucous membrane. The patient might snuff iced water or pinch the soft outer portion of the nose against the midline septum for 5 or 10 minutes continuously. Other measures are the application of an ice collar to the neck or the instillation of a local vasoconstricting drug, such as Neo-Synephrine, into the nostril. Should these measures fail, the physician may find it necessary to apply Adrenalin or a cauterizing agent, such as silver nitrate solution or stick, to the bleeding point.

Often, however, the origin of the bleeding cannot be found. In these patients, after spraying the nose with cocaine and Adrenalin solutions, a rubber finger cot or the finger of a rubber glove may be inserted into the nostril, the open end being held with 3 or 4 hemostats while gauze packing is inserted. Pressure may be increased by moistening the gauze. The packing should be removed after 24 hours.

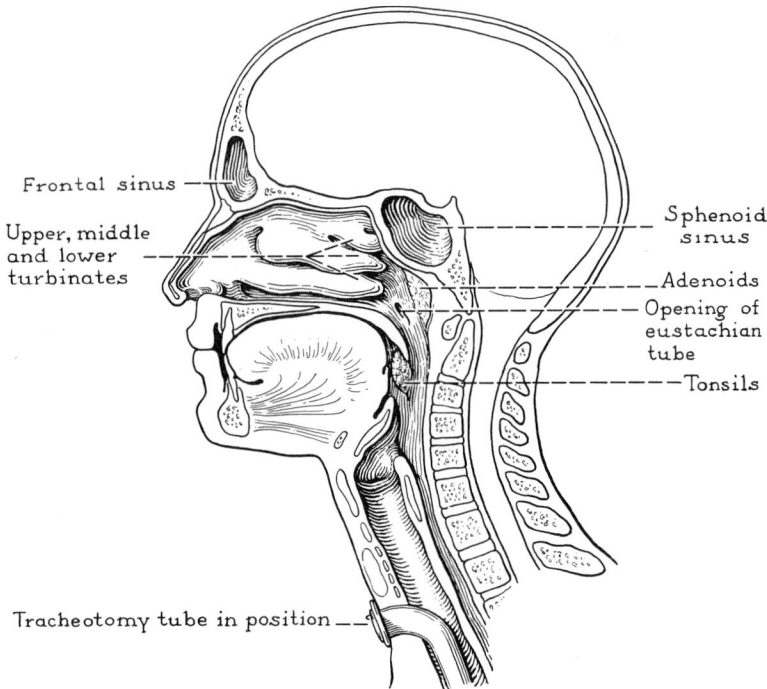

Frontal sinus

Upper, middle
and lower
turbinates

Sphenoid
sinus

Adenoids

Opening of
eustachian
tube

Tonsils

Tracheotomy tube in position

FIG. 114. Diagrammatic cross section drawing to show the parts of the upper respiratory tract and their relation to each other. In the lower part of the neck there is a tracheotomy tube in position.

Rhinitis

Rhinitis is an inflammatory lesion involving the mucous membrane of the nose. It is sometimes a manifestation of allergy, in which instance it is referred to as "vasomotor rhinitis," but usually is due to an infection. The most common variety of infection causing it is "coryza" (the common cold); it also is encountered with regularity in the early stages of measles and other specific viral infections.

In acute rhinitis, the nasal mucous membrane becomes congested, swollen and edematous. This quickly subsides, and the membrane returns to normal. After repeated attacks, however, particularly in cases which originate as a result of chronic sinusitis, this swelling becomes obstinate, and the patient has a "chronic catarrh." These persons say that they are "subject to colds." The fact is that, excluding the recurring attacks of allergic vasomotor rhinitis, their attacks are acute exacerbations of the same "cold." If continued, chronic rhinitis leads to the deposition of abnormally large amounts of connective tissue in the nasal mucous membrane, which greatly thickens it, and causes

the formation of spurs, polyps and hypertrophies on the nasal septum. Wasting or atrophy of the mucous membrane, the cartilage and the bones lining the nasal passages eventually may occur, with the result that these passages become large empty caverns, adhering to the walls of which is an abundant exudate emanating a disagreeable odor. This condition is called *ozena*.

The patient should be cautioned against blowing his nose too frequently or too hard. It should be done with the mouth open slightly while blowing through both nostrils to equalize the pressure.

Nasal Obstruction

Obstruction to the passage of air through the nostrils results frequently from a deflection of the nasal septum, hypertrophy of the turbinate bones or from the pressure of polyps—grapelike swellings that arise from the mucous membrane of the sinuses, especially the ethmoids. This obstruction also may lead to a condition of chronic infection of the nose and result in frequent attacks of nasopharyngitis. Very frequently the infection extends to the sinuses of the nose (mucous-lined cavities filled with air that drain normally into the nose). When sinusitis develops and the drainage from these cavities is obstructed by deformity or swelling within the nose, pain is experienced in the region of the affected sinus.

Treatment. The treatment of this condition requires the removal of the nasal obstruction, followed by measures to overcome whatever chronic infection exists. In many patients the underlying nasal allergy is the lesion requiring treatment. At times it is necessary to drain the nasal sinuses by radical operation. The operations performed depend on the type of nasal obstruction found. Usually they are performed with local anesthesia. This is obtained by introducing into the nostrils pledgets of cotton soaked in 10 per cent cocaine solution with Adrenalin. The nurse who assists the surgeon in operations on the nose and the throat must be extremely careful to identify the solutions of cocaine and procaine, for the toxic nature of cocaine when injected

hypodermically would make the mistake a most serious one.

If a deflection of the septum is the cause of the obstruction, the surgeon makes an incision in the mucous membrane and, after raising it from the bone, removes the deflected bone and cartilage with bone forceps. The mucosa then is allowed to fall back in place and is held there by tight packing. Generally the packing used is soaked in liquid petrolatum to facilitate its removal in from 24 to 36 hours. This operation is called commonly a *submucous resection.*

Nasal polyps are removed by clipping them at their base with a wire snare. Hypertrophied turbinates may be treated by astringent applications to shrink them up close to the side of the nose.

After these procedures, the head of the bed is elevated to promote drainage and to help to alleviate the patient's discomfort due to edema. Frequent oral hygiene should be given because the patient will be breathing through his mouth.

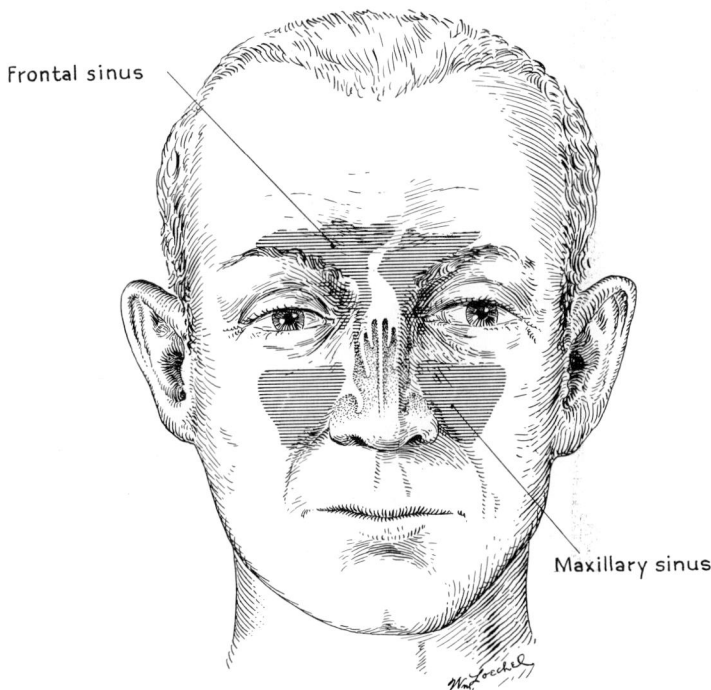

FIG. 115. Diagrammatic drawing to show position of nasal sinuses and their relation to facial structures.

Fractures of the Nose

Fractures of the nose usually result from direct violence. As a rule, they do not produce any serious consequences, but the deformity that may follow often gives rise to obstruction of the nasal air passages and to facial disfigurement.

Immediately after the injury there is usually considerable bleeding from the nose, both from the nostrils and into the pharynx. There is marked swelling of the soft tissues adjacent to the nose and, frequently, a definite deformity.

Treatment and Nursing Care. As a rule, the bleeding can be controlled by the application of cold compresses. A roentgenogram is helpful in determining the displacement of the fractured bones and in ruling out an extension of the fracture into the skull. With local cocainization of the nose or with intravenous anesthesia, it is possible usually to bring displaced fragments into alignment and then hold them by intranasal packing or external splints (Fig. 116). The important points in the reduction of the fracture are to reform the nasal passages and to realign the bones so as to prevent disfiguring deformity. After reduction, the swelling that occurs may be decreased by the application of ice compresses with the patient in the sitting position.

Plastic Surgery of the Nose

The nose is such a prominent organ of the face that its deformity may cause the patient considerable embarrassment. The deformity may result from congenital causes, from disease or from injury.

Deformities resulting from congenital causes often may be corrected by simple operations in which the nose is straightened or lengthened by either removing offending bone or supplying new tissue (usually costal cartilage). The incisions are so placed as to be inconspicuous. In deformities resulting from injury or disease, various types of plastic surgery may be employed. Skin, tube or sliding grafts may be used to cover the defects left by scars, malignancy or injuries. In some instances, especially in older people with malignancy, artificial appliances may be modeled and held in place with the rims of glasses. (See Reconstructive Surgery, p. 772.)

Nursing Care. After operation the patient usually is placed flat on his back with the head slightly elevated. Ice compresses are used frequently after operation to reduce bleeding, swelling and pain. Hemorrhage is the chief postoperative complication, and it must be remembered that the spitting up or the vomiting of blood that has run back into the pharynx is as much a symptom of nasal hemorrhage as is the flow at the nares. Fre-

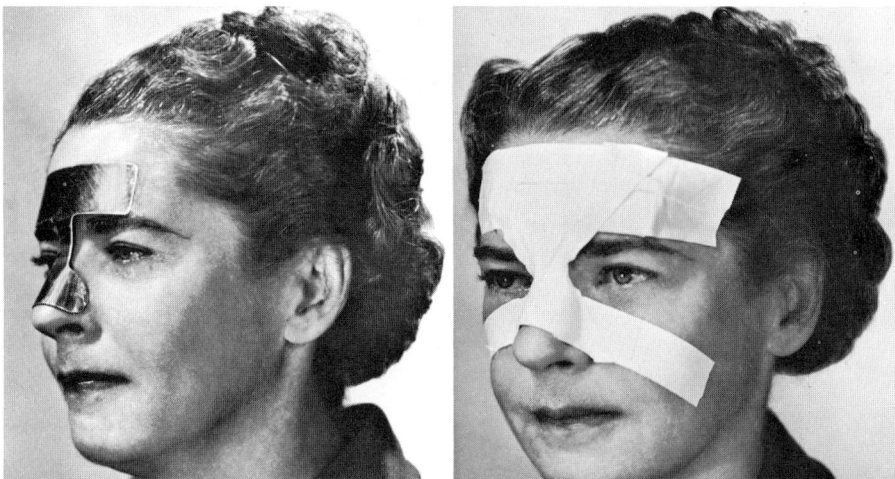

FIG. 116. Nasal splint occasionally used following fractures and plastic operations on the nose. It is an aluminum splint padded with foam rubber which can be held in place with adhesive. (V. Mueller & Co., Chicago, Ill.)

quent swallowing, followed by belching, often is indicative of bleeding that results in an accumulation of blood in the stomach.

In patients with whom local anesthesia has been used, the blood sometimes trickles down the throat, but the patient is not sufficiently aware of it to show a swallow reflex. If the bleeding is excessive or continuous, or if any of the constitutional signs of hemorrhage appear, the surgeon should be called, and the nurse should have ready for his use fresh packing, a light, a head mirror, a nasal speculum and packing forceps.

These patients may have a liquid diet on the day of operation and whatever they prefer after that. Sedatives often are necessary on the day and the night of operation, but after that there is little need of them. The patient is tempted often to blow his nose because of a full feeling, but if it is explained to him that this is because of the packing in his nose, he will be more patient. Packing is removed usually after 24 hours.

THE PATIENT WITH SINUSITIS

The sinuses are involved in a high proportion of upper respiratory tract infections. If their openings into the nasal passages are clear, the infections within them recover promptly; but if their drainage is obstructed by a deflected septum or by hypertrophied turbinates, spurs or polyps, the sinusitis may persist as a smoldering secondary infection or it may flare up into an acute suppurative process.

Acute Sinusitis

Acute sinusitis may be localized to one sinus or may involve several. If all are involved, the condition is called *pansinusitis.* The most prominent symptom of acute sinusitis is pain, the location of which is diagnostically important, and therefore should be noted by the nurse. In *frontal sinusitis,* the patient complains of frontal headache; in *ethmoidal sinusitis,* the pain is usually in or about the eyes; in *maxillary sinusitis,* pain is lateral to the nose and sometimes is accompanied by aching of the upper teeth of the corresponding side; in *sphenoidal sinusitis,* occipital headache may result. Nasal congestion and discharge are usually,

but not necessarily, present. The patient feels generally miserable, quite apart from pain. Fever, however, if present at all, is usually mild. This may be the case even in the presence of an acute suppurative infection, or "empyema" of a sinus. The most dangerous variety of sinusitis is empyema of a frontal sinus, because it may rupture posteriorly, producing a brain abscess.

The treatment of acute sinusitis is bed rest and the establishment of free drainage of the sinuses involved. This usually can be accomplished by nasal instillations or sprays of Neo-Synephrine (¼ per cent) or a similar vasoconstrictor drug. Depending on the type of infecting organism and the extent of the infection, the patient may be instructed to apply local therapy of this sort at intervals of from 1 to 4 hours until drainage is established. The use of penicillin usually speeds recovery and definitely diminishes the chance of complications which follow the extension of a bacterial sinusitis. One of the antihistaminic agents (e.g., Pyribenzamine or thenylpyramine fumarate) in oral doses (25 to 50 mg.) may be beneficial, at least symptomatically, in very early cases.

Chronic Sinusitis

Chronic sinusitis usually manifests itself by persistent nasal obstruction, due to discharge and edema of the nasal mucous membrane. The patient experiences cough, due to the constant dripping of the discharge backward into the nasopharynx, and headaches, which are apt to be most pronounced on awakening in the morning.

The treatment of chronic sinusitis usually is the use of vasoconstricting drugs locally, in the form of sprays or nose drops, in an effort to establish proper drainage. Structural deformities that obstruct the ostia of the sinus may require *surgical attention:* polyps may require excision or cauterization, a deflected septum may have to be removed or a narrowed ostium widened.

For drainage of the maxillary sinus, the incision is made along the upper gum line above the canine teeth (Caldwell-Luc operation). To drain the frontal sinus an incision is made through the inner third of the eyebrow.

Some victims of severe chronic sinusitis obtain relief only by moving to a dry climate.

THE PATIENT WITH PROBLEMS OF THE PHARYNX AND THE TONSILS

Pharyngitis

Acute Pharyngitis

Acute pharyngitis, caused by several viruses and bacteria, is a febrile inflammation of the throat. The pharyngeal membrane becomes fiery red; the lymphoid follicles of the throat and the tonsils become swollen and flecked with exudate, and there may be tender enlargement of the cervical lymph nodes. Uncomplicated virus infections usually recover promptly, within 3 to 6 days after the onset. But pharyngitis caused by certain of the more virulent bacteria, such as beta hemolytic streptococcus, hemolytic Staphylococcus aureus, influenza, or the diphtheria bacillus, is a more severe illness during the acute stage and far more important in the incidence of dangerous complications. These complications include sinusitis, otitis media, mastoiditis, cervical adenitis, rheumatic fever, nephritis and, in the case of infection by the diphtheria bacillus, paralysis. A throat culture is the chief means of determining the causative organism. When this is obtained, proper therapy can be prescribed.

Nursing Care. The patient should be kept in bed during the febrile stage of his illness. When he is ambulatory he needs periods of rest. Medical asepsis must be observed to prevent the spread of infection. Examine the skin once or twice daily for possible rash, because acute pharyngitis may precede some other communicable disease.

Aside from throat cultures, it may be necessary to secure nasal swabbings and blood cultures for further laboratory investigation to determine the nature of the causative organism.

Hot saline gargles or irrigations are employed, depending on the severity of the lesion and the degree of pain. Recognizing that the benefits of this treatment depend on the degree of heat that is applied, the nurse should ensure that the temperature of the solution is sufficiently high to be effective, i.e., approaching the limits of tolerance,

which vary with each individual patient but never exceed 120° F. A throat irrigation, properly performed, is the most effective means available for reducing spasm in the pharyngeal muscles and relieving soreness of the throat. However, unless the principle of the procedure and its technic are understood clearly by the patient, the results may be less than completely satisfactory. Patients for whom the throat irrigation is a new experience should have it explained in advance by the nurse.

Symptomatic relief in patients with severe sore throat also may be afforded by the application of an ice collar and by means of analgesic drugs, e.g., aspirin or acetophenetidin in doses of 0.3 to 0.6 Gm. given at 3-to-6-hour intervals and, if required, codeine sulfate, 15 to 30 mg. (0.25 to 0.5 Gr.), 3 or 4 times daily. Antitussive medication, in the form of codeine, Hycodan or Toryn (see p. 120), may be required to control a persistent and painful cough which often accompanies acute pharyngitis. One of the barbiturates, e.g., Nembutal (0.1 to 0.2 Gm.), may be prescribed as a soporific at bedtime.

If a bacterial etiology is suspected or demonstrated, treatment may include the administration of antimicrobial agents.

A liquid or soft solid diet is provided during the acute stage of the disease, depending on the patient's appetite and the degree of discomfort caused by swallowing.

The patient should be encouraged to drink to the limit of tolerance, the minimum intake during the febrile stage exceeding, if possible, 2,500 ml. each day. Success is often aided if the rationale of therapy is explained adequately to the patient. His personal tastes also need to be considered and indulged when possible.

Mouth care may add greatly to the patient's comfort and aid in preventing the development of fissures of the lips and pyoderma about the mouth in cases of bacterial infection.

Convalescent Care. Resumption of full activity should not be permitted until a period of time has elapsed which is at least equal to that of complete bed rest. Unusually conservative management is indicated in

FIG. 117. Views of oral pharynx. (A) Showing enlargement of the tonsils. (B) Showing peritonsillar abscess on the right-hand side.

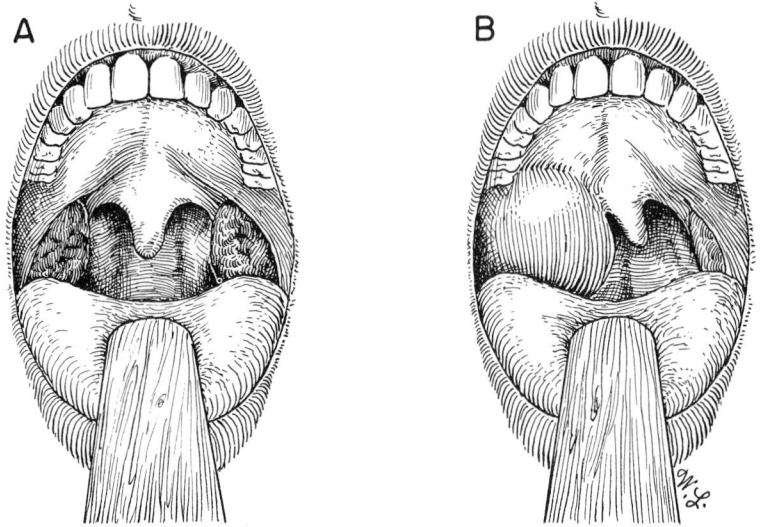

cases of hemolytic streptococcus infection in view of the possible development of complications such as nephritis and rheumatic fever, which may have their onset 2 or 3 weeks after the pharyngitis has subsided. Local extension of an apparently quiescent pharyngitis may develop in the form of sinusitis, otitis media, mastoiditis or cervical adenitis. Daily recording of morning and evening temperatures should be continued until convalescence is complete, and the patient or his family should be familiarized with symptoms that deserve investigation from the standpoint of a possible complication.

Chronic Pharyngitis

This disease is common in adults who work amid dusty surroundings, use the voice to excess and suffer from chronic cough. Its incidence also is high among habitual users of alcohol and tobacco.

Nasal congestion may be relieved by nasal instillations or sprays containing ephedrine sulfate, Neo-Synephrine or Tuamine sulfate in saline, and, in the early stages, one of the antihistaminic drugs such as Pyribenzamine, pyranisamine maleate or thenylpyramine fumarate in doses of from 25 to 30 mg. every 4 to 6 hours by mouth. The attendant malaise is controlled effectively by aspirin or acetophenetidin. Contact with others should be avoided, at least until the

fever has subsided completely, in order to prevent spreading the infection.

Three types of chronic pharyngitis are recognized: (1) hypertrophic, characterized by general thickening and congestion of the pharyngeal mucous membrane; (2) atrophic, probably a late stage of the above (this membrane is thin, whitish, glistening and, at

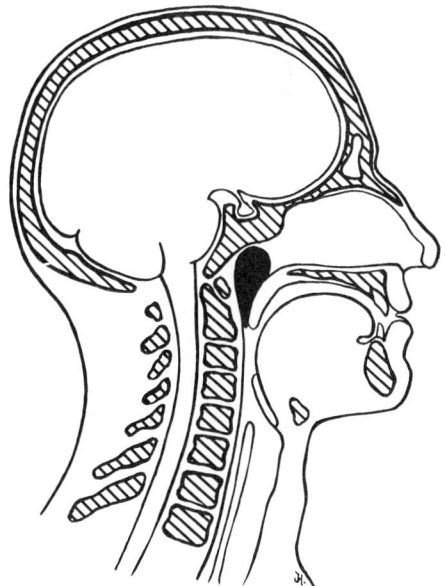

FIG. 118. Vertical section through the skull, showing a mass of adenoids in the nasopharynx.

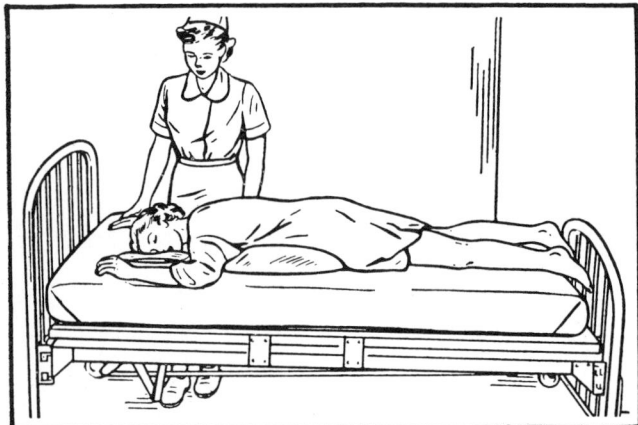

Fig. 119. Position following tonsillectomy which is comfortable and allows drainage of excretions from throat. (Winters, M. C.: Protective Body Mechanics in Daily Life and in Nursing, Philadelphia, Saunders)

times, wrinkled); and (3) chronic granular ("clergyman's sore throat"), with numerous swollen lymph follicles on the pharyngeal wall.

Patients with chronic pharyngitis complain of a constant sense of irritation or fullness in the throat, of mucus collecting in the throat and expelled by coughing and of difficulty in swallowing. While chronic pharyngitis is annoying, it seldom disturbs the general health.

Treatment. The treatment of chronic pharyngitis consists of the avoidance of alcohol and tobacco, resting the voice and the correction of any upper respiratory, pulmonary or cardiac condition that might be responsible for a chronic cough.

Diseases of the Tonsils and the Adenoids

Tonsils

The tonsils are two groups of lymphatic tissue situated one on each side of the oropharynx. They are frequently the seat of acute infectious processes and of chronic infection, constantly giving off toxins in small amounts. Therefore, they are considered one of the most common sites of focal infection, producing chronic systemic diseases such as chronic arthritis, nephritis and so forth. Furthermore, they often grow to such a size as to interfere with normal respiration, a condition that is spoken of as hypertrophy of the tonsils. (See Fig. 117.)

Frequent acute infections, chronic infections, hypertrophy—all are regarded as indications for the removal of the tonsils.

Tonsillectomy may be performed under local anesthesia with the patient in a sitting position or under general anesthesia with the patient in the dorsal position. The tongue is depressed and the tonsil is grasped with tenaculum forceps. The tonsil is freed by blunt and sharp dissection sufficient to allow the snare to encircle the remaining attachment, which is crushed and the tonsil is removed. Hemorrhage usually is controlled by pressure with small gauze sponges. Occasionally it is necessary to clamp and ligate the bleeding vessel. Often the blood is swallowed, or, if the patient is unconscious, it will run down into the stomach and not be recognized until the patient vomits copiously.

Adenoids

Acute adenoiditis. A common accompaniment of acute tonsillitis, enlargement of the adenoid is responsible for the nasal obstruction and, to a certain extent, the vertical headache commonly experienced in this infection.

Chronic adenoiditis. This is of particular importance because the adenoid, when hypertrophied, is in a position to obstruct the posterior nares and the eustachian tubes (Fig. 118). Adenoid hypertrophy may cause (1) mouth breathing, tendency to facial deformities, and crooked teeth, (2) earaches, running ears, and mastoid infection, (3) frequent head colds, bronchitis, (4) fetid breath, voice impairment, snoring and noisy respiration.

Extension of the infection to the middle ears, via the eustachian tubes, may result in acute otitis media, the potential complications of which include spontaneous rupture of the ear drums and further extension into the mastoid cells, causing acute mastoiditis; or the infection may reside in the middle ear as a chronic, low-grade smoldering process which eventually may lead to permanent deafness.

Because enlarged adenoids are the cause of a long list of symptoms, adenoidectomy is recommended as soon as the condition is discovered, even if this is in infancy. The treatment, of course, is operative removal, which is done usually in conjunction with a tonsillectomy.

Nursing Care for Tonsillectomy and Adenoidectomy

The chief danger after these operations is from hemorrhage; therefore, most surgeons require an evaluation of hemostasis before operation. Atropine always should be given before operation under general anesthesia to decrease the amount of mucous secretion. After operation, the patient should be placed in the dorsal or the sitting position, according to the wishes of the surgeon. For patients who have had general anesthesia, the most comfortable position is prone, with the head turned to the side to allow for drainage from the throat (Fig. 119). An ice collar should be applied and a basin and gauze provided for the expectoration of blood and mucus. Children are treated best by placing them in the prone position with the head turned to the side, so that secretion may drain from the mouth and the pharynx.

Bleeding may be bright red if the patient spits it out at once. Often, however, it is swallowed and becomes brown in color immediately, due to the action of the acid gastric juice. If the patient vomits large amounts of altered blood or spits bright blood at frequent intervals, or if the pulse rate increases gradually, the attending surgeon should be notified. The nurse should have in readiness for him a light, a head mirror, gauze, curved hemostats and a waste basin. Occasionally it may be necessary to suture or ligate the bleeding vessel. In such cases the patient must be taken to the operating room and given anesthesia.

If there is no bleeding, water and cracked ice may be given the patient as soon as desired. Acetylsalicylic acid, suspended in water as a gargle or given in chewing gum, sometimes is used to relieve discomfort. The diet should be liquid or semiliquid for several days, excluding orange or lemon juice and other acids. Ice cream, ice sherbet, gelatin desserts, custards, and Junkets are very acceptable foods, especially for children.

Home Instruction. The patient may be discharged from the hospital the day after the operation, but he should convalesce at home for several days. This means getting plenty of rest and resuming activity gradually. Any bleeding should be reported to the physician; secondary hemorrhage may occur about a week after operation.

Sulfonamides and Antibiotics. In all of these acute infections of the pharynx, sulfonamides and antibiotics are used. They are given prophylactically, as well as therapeutically, before and after surgical procedures on the pharynx and the larynx. (See p. 192.)

Peritonsillar Abscess (Quinsy)

Peritonsillar abscess, or quinsy, is an abscess that develops above the tonsil in the tissues of the anterior pillar and soft palate. As a rule, it is secondary to a tonsillar infection. The usual symptoms of an infection are present, together with such local symptoms as difficulty in swallowing (dysphagia), thickening of the voice, drooling and local pain. An examination shows marked swelling of the soft palate, often to the extent of half-occluding the orifice from the mouth into the pharynx.

Treatment. A considerable measure of relief may be obtained by throat irrigations or the frequent use of mouthwashes or gargles, using saline or alkaline solutions at a temperature of from 105° to 110° F. This treatment hastens the pointing of the process.

The abscess should be evacuated as soon as possible. The mucous membrane over the swelling first is painted with 10 per cent cocaine solution; then, after a small incision has been made, the points of a blunt hemostat are forced into the abscess pocket and opened as they are withdrawn. This operation is performed best with the patient in the sitting position, as it is easier then for him to expectorate the pus and the blood that accumulate in the pharynx. Almost immediate relief is experienced. After-treatment is warm gargles at intervals of 1 or 2 hours for from 24 to 36 hours.

Some laryngologists advocate bilateral tonsillectomy for acute peritonsillar abscess; they claim that this is necessary to prevent recurrences and eliminate unsuspected asymptomatic pockets of infection.

Antibiotics, usually penicillin, are extremely effective in the control of the infection in peritonsillar abscess. Given early in the course of the disease, the abscess may be aborted, and incision can be avoided. If antibiotics are not given until later, the abscess must be drained, but improvement in the inflammatory reaction is rapid.

THE PATIENT WITH PROBLEMS OF THE LARYNX

Laryngitis

Acute laryngitis is manifested by hoarseness or complete loss of the voice (aphonia) and by severe cough. The treatment is bed rest, steam inhalations and abstinence from talking and smoking. If the laryngitis is part of a more extensive respiratory infection due to a bacterial organism, or if it is severe, appropriate antibacterial chemotherapy should be instituted.

Chronic laryngitis, marked by persistent hoarseness, may follow repeated attacks of acute laryngitis. It is sometimes a complication of chronic sinusitis and chronic bronchitis. The condition also may be induced by the frequent inhalation of irritating gases, the excessive use of tobacco or alcohol or by the habitual overuse of the voice, as in the case of public speakers. Laryngoscopic examination is always indicated in a patient with chronic laryngitis in order to eliminate the possibility of tuberculosis or tumor of the larynx. The treatment of the condition is rest of the voice, elimination of any primary respiratory tract infection that may be present and restriction of smoking.

Laryngeal Obstruction

Edema of the Larynx

Edema of the larynx (or glottis) is a serious, often fatal, condition. The larynx is a stiff box which will not stretch, and the space within it between the vocal cords, through which the air must pass, is narrow. Swelling of the laryngeal mucous membrane, therefore, may close this orifice tightly, suffocating the patient. Edema of the glottis occurs rarely in patients with acute laryngitis, occasionally in cases of urticaria and more frequently in severe inflammations of the throat —for example, diphtheria, erysipelas and scarlet fever. It is an occasional cause of death in severe anaphylaxis (angioneurotic edema).

Laryngeal Spasm

Spasm of the muscles of the throat, the symptoms of which resemble those of edema of the glottis, occurs acutely in malnourished infants and young children suffering from rickets. The condition usually is explainable on the basis of a reduction in the blood calcium, or a combination of this factor and alkalosis, due, for example, to vomiting. These disturbances in the blood chemistry are prone to lead to muscle spasm or tetany (p. 826). Usually associated with the laryngeal spasm are spasmodic contractions of other muscle groups (spasmophilia). During the spasm the child struggles for breath; the face becomes blue, then, suddenly, the spasm is relieved and the child takes a deep breath with a crowing sound. For therapy, the administration of acidifying salts such as ammonium chloride and intravenous calcium lactate or calcium gluconate is indicated. The diet must be improved, supplemented with calcium and some adequate source of vitamin D.

Laryngeal Tuberculosis

The larynx is not infrequently attacked by tuberculosis. Patients so affected become hoarse, have a most persistent cough and suffer acute pain when they attempt to swallow (dysphagia). Treatment entails complete rest of the vocal cords for a prolonged period of time and a course of antibiotic therapy with streptomycin, para-aminosalicylic acid or isoniazid. Direct destruction of the lesion by electrocautery may be undertaken if chemotherapy is unavailing.

Cancer of the Larynx

Cancer of the larynx occurs in both men and women. It may occur as early as the

18th year, but usually it is seen in men of middle age or older. The early symptoms are hoarseness or discomfort in the region of the larynx; later, there may be pain, obstructed respiration, difficulty in swallowing, bleeding or swelling of the neck by tumor growth. Certain factors seem to be related to the development of cancer of the larynx: heavy smoking, vocal straining, chronic laryngitis, and family predisposition.

Treatment. In the early stages it can be cured in more than 80 per cent of patients by proper surgical removal. The operation of choice is (1) laryngofissure for the early case and (2) laryngectomy for the more advanced case.

LARYNGOFISSURE (THYROTOMY). This operation is the splitting of the thyroid cartilage of the larynx in the mid-line of the neck and the removal of the portion of the vocal cord that is involved in the tumor growth. After bleeding has been controlled, the neck is closed and is allowed to heal. Sometimes a tracheotomy tube is left in the trachea when the wound is closed, in which event it is removed usually after a few days. The patient is instructed not to use his voice until so ordered by his physician.

LARYNGECTOMY. In this operation the entire larynx is removed. The trachea opens permanently on the lower portion of the front of the neck. The opening of the larynx into the pharynx is closed by sutures.

Nursing Care. Inasmuch as surgery of the larynx is done most commonly for a tumor that may be malignant, the nurse often has a patient who is worried for many reasons: Will the surgeon be able to remove all the tumor? Is it cancer? Will I die? Will I choke? Will I ever speak again? Therefore, the psychological preparation of the patient is as important as the physical. If he is going to have a complete laryngectomy, he should know that he will lose his natural voice completely but that, with training, there are ways in which he can carry on a fairly normal conversation. Mouth hygiene prior to surgery is imperative. Usually antibiotics are ordered to reduce further the possibility of infection. In men, preoperative shaving includes the beard and the hair on the neck and the chest down to the nipple line.

Surgery can be done under local or general anesthesia. After operation the patient with a laryngofissure may have a tracheotomy tube. (See p. 389.) The physician may insert a naso-esophageal catheter (No. 16 French urethral catheter), and feedings are given under the same precautions that prevail in gastrostomy feedings. (See p. 608.) Oral feedings often are started on the first day after operation if acceptable to the patient. The tracheotomy tube is removed at the surgeon's discretion. This may be in 2 or 3 days.

In caring for a person with a total laryngectomy, it must be realized that the laryngectomy tube (which is shorter but has a larger diameter than the usual tracheotomy tube) is the only airway the patient has. The care of this tube is the same as for a tracheotomy tube. (See p. 389.) The patient should be observed for excessive coughing or hemoptysis. He should be told to avoid using his voice for the first few postoperative days. Communication can be done with a "magic slate." It is well to remember that he needs his right hand for writing; therefore the left arm is preferred for intravenous feedings.

A naso-esophageal catheter is passed by the physician after operation and liquid feedings are given. Thereafter the nurse is permitted to remove and pass this tube because there is no possibility of its getting into the trachea, the trachea now being sutured permanently to the skin as a tracheotomy. After a few days the patient can be taught to pass his own feeding tube. Good mouth hygiene must be followed rigidly. After about 7 days, when the incision has healed, the surgeon may allow the patient to begin oral feedings. Then he begins to develop his ability to belch. About an hour after he has eaten, the nurse can remind him to belch. Later this action, which at first is genuine, is transformed into simple explosions of air from the esophagus. At this point the speech pathologist progresses with him in an attempt to make his speech intelligible and as close to normal as is possible.

Antibiotics often are a part of treatment, as there is a possibility of incisional contamination. Vitamins may be given as supplemental feedings, and infusions often are necessary to keep up fluid, electrolyte and nutritional balance. The laryngectomy tube can be removed when the stoma is well healed; usually this is from 3 to 6 weeks postoperatively.

Rehabilitation. The partially laryngectomized patient has little difficulty, for in a matter of a few days his voice will improve. However, the completely laryngectomized patient often is depressed and needs encouragement. The rehabilitative management of this patient requires a team that includes the surgeon, the nurse, the patient's family, persons who have had laryngectomies, and the speech pathologist.

The patient should be referred to a speech pathologist before surgery. The physician describes the nature of the surgery and tells the patient that he will lose his ability to vocalize speech. He should be reassured that much can be done for him through a rehabilitation program. The speech pathologist reassures the patient that with speech therapy his sound source can be replaced with either laryngeal or esophageal speech or one of the artificial larynx methods. It is ideal for the patient to begin to learn laryngeal or esophageal speech preoperatively. In this way the patient can hear his "new" voice and ask questions concerning speech training.

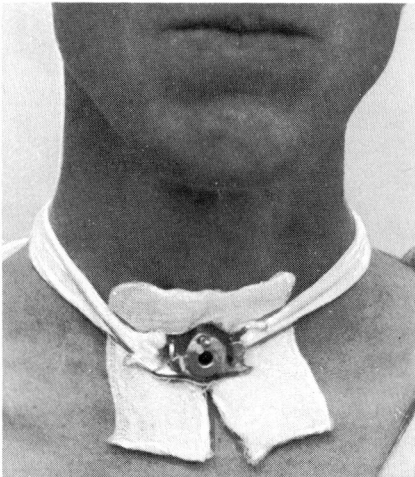

Fig. 120. Tracheotomy tube in use. After a few days the split dressing is changed to an unsplit one, and the tube is pushed through the dressing before it is inserted.

There are two methods of learning to speak after a laryngectomy: (1) The use of esophageal speech. By this method the individual swallows air and, by proper muscle control, can produce sounds on the return "belch" of air. Laryngectomized patients make the best teachers for other laryngectomized patients. Results are fairly satisfactory, in that the patient is able to talk with no unnatural equipment. However, the voice produced is hoarse and low pitched. (2) The use of an artificial larynx. A variety of artificial larynxes is available. One type is a vibrator powered by batteries. It is placed against the larynx. Another, also battery powered, utilizes a plastic tube that is inserted into the side and well to the back of the mouth. This device provides a continuous sound source in the mouth that the patient is able to modify by depressing or closing his mouth, changing the shape of his lips or moving his tongue.

Approximately 60 per cent of the patients are able to vocalize effectively using the laryngeal or the esophageal speech method.* Several patient-teaching booklets listed at the end of the chapter are helpful tools for patient use.

Aspirated Foreign Bodies

Foreign bodies frequently are aspirated into the pharynx, the larynx or the trachea, especially by children. They cause symptoms in two ways: by obstructing the air passages they cause difficulty in breathing that may lead to asphyxia; later they may be drawn farther down, entering the bronchi or one of their branches and causing symptoms of irritation, such as a croupy cough, bloody or mucous expectoration and paroxysms of dyspnea. The physical signs and roentgenograms confirm the diagnosis.

In emergencies, when the signs of asphyxia are evident, immediate treatment is necessary. Frequently, if the foreign body has

* During the past few years, at various places throughout the country, laryngectomees have been organizing into groups for the combined purposes of sociability and complete rehabilitation under such names as Lost Cord, New Speech, New Voice, Esophageal Speech, Nu Voice and Cured Cancer Clubs.

FIG. 121. Semidiagrammatic view showing tracheotomy tubes in place. Note the method of holding the tube in place by tape ties, which are inserted through openings in the outer tube and passed through slits in the tape so as to make a flat connection. Tracheotomy tube and inner tube are shown in place. An obturator, which is introduced into the outer tube when the tracheotomy tube is inserted, completes the tracheotomy set.

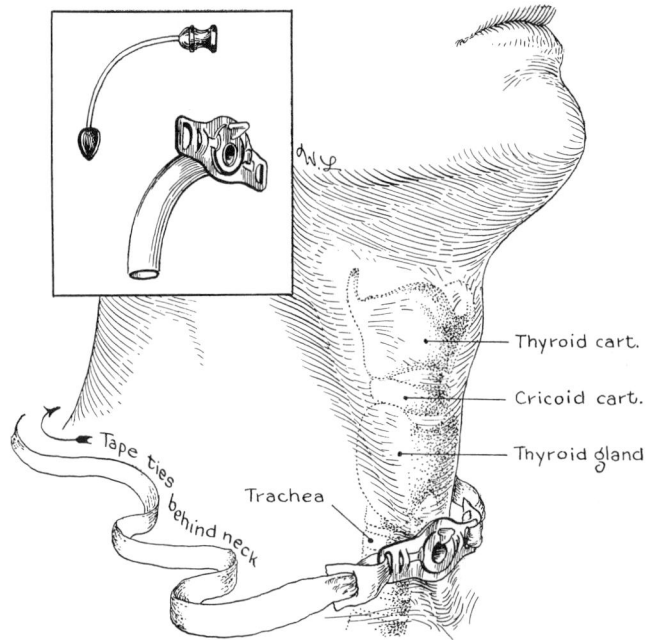

lodged in the pharynx, it may be dislodged by the finger. If the obstruction is in the larynx or the trachea, an immediate tracheotomy is necessary.

Tracheotomy and Tracheostomy

A *tracheotomy* is an operation in which an opening is made into the trachea through which the patient may breathe. It is performed because of obstruction of the air passage in the larynx from any cause—tumors, foreign bodies, diphtheritic membranes, paralysis of the vocal cords and edema of the glottis; also for obstruction occurring during or after operations on the neck. If the opening is a permanent one, the term *tracheostomy* is used.

The patient is placed on the table with the head hyper-extended, a median incision is made through the skin of the neck, the muscles are separated and retracted and the trachea is opened in a vertical direction. A sterile tracheotomy tube is inserted and held in place by tapes fastened round the patient's neck. Usually a square of sterile gauze is placed between the tube and the skin before the tape is tied (Fig. 120). The tubes of proper size should occupy half the cross-sectional area of the trachea (Fig. 121). They

are usually made of sterling silver (plastic is available). Each tube consists of three pieces: an outer cannula, to which the retaining tapes are fastened; an obturator, an olive-tipped, curved silver rod that is used to guide the cannula into the opening in the trachea; and an inner cannula that is inserted into the outer cannula after the withdrawal of the obturator.

Nursing Care

When emergencies arise in which a tracheotomy must be done, the life of the patient is at stake, and strict observance of aseptic technic and the psychological preparation of the patient are of secondary importance. However, there are instances in which there is time to explain the purpose of such surgery to the patient, with the result that he will adjust better to his situation after operation. He should realize that he will lose his voice temporarily, and that he will breathe by means of a tube in his trachea.

Immediate Postoperative Care. This patient should have a nurse in attendance for at least the first 24 hours after operation. If this is impossible, he should be placed near the nurse's station or in the intensive care unit, where he can be watched closely. Surgery was done to relieve obstruction; it is the responsibility of the nurse to keep the newly made opening patent. Another objective in nursing care is to alleviate the apprehension of the patient. It is a new experience for him, and often he has a real fear of asphyxiation.

Slightly blood-tinged mucus usually is the first kind of secretion to come through the tracheotomy tube. As time passes, the amount of blood that comes through should diminish and disappear. If it does not, this may indicate hemorrhage, and it should be reported. All secretions should be wiped away carefully and quickly before they are aspirated by the patient. An electric or a wall-suction apparatus should be on hand for aspiration. The receptacle for collecting secretions may have about 50 ml. of tap water in it to prevent tenacious mucus from adhering to the container, which would make it difficult to clean later. The rubber catheter connected to suction may be Size 8 or 10 for children and from 12 to 16 for adults. It should be cut diagonally at the tip and have 2 or 3 holes along the side. Suction should be gentle to avoid injuring delicate mucous membrane. Suction should be applied intermittently for periods of no longer than 5 seconds. Prolonged aspiration may produce a drop in the arterial oxygen concentration. Inefficient suctioning also will irritate the mucosa of the trachea. The nurse usually is permitted to introduce the catheter up to 5 inches, but deeper aspiration may be done by the physician. If complete removal of mucus is not done at frequent intervals, the dried secretions may cause obstruction. A towel spread bib-fashion across the chest and below the tube may help to keep the patient neat when secretions are profuse.

The inner cannula is removed gently by the nurse about every hour for the first day and less frequently after that. It is important to keep this tube clean to prevent encrustations and clogging. If the secretion is thick, instill about 5 drops of sterile water into the trachea through the tracheotomy tube before aspirating. (Care of the tube is explained later.) Before the inner cannula is replaced, the patient should be aspirated. *Generally, the outer cannula is not removed by the nurse.* However, if the patient has a tracheostomy, this may become her responsibility after about 10 days. Meanwhile, the surgeon changes the outer cannula as often as he feels that it is necessary.

A sterile dressing, 3 x 3 inches, is split to fit under the tapes and the shield of the tube so that the incision is covered (Fig. 120). This becomes soiled easily and should be replaced as often as is necessary. Care must be taken to prevent dislodging or moving the tube when this is done.

For a time after operation many surgeons cover the opening of the tube with a few layers of gauze moistened in warm saline solution. This tends to moisten the inspired air and to filter out dust, which function is performed in normal life by the nose and the pharynx. However, it will be more to the patient's comfort if the air in the room is kept moistened with steam or cold vapor than if moist gauze is used as mentioned, as this tends to prevent the evacuation of secretions.

The patient may have fluids during the day of operation and diet as tolerated after that if there are no other contraindications. Scrupulous mouth care is given before and after meals and whenever necessary. He may be placed in the semi-Fowler or sitting position. Morphine sulfate usually is not given as these patients are not in acute pain. Moreover, the drug is contraindicated because it depresses the cough reflex.

Paper and pencil should be kept near the patient so that he has a means of communication. He needs reassurance, especially during the first night, for he has a real fear that he will asphyxiate while he is asleep. A tap bell or electric cord signal should be within his reach.

Postoperative Complications. The nurse must realize that her responsibility to these patients lies not only in keeping a patent airway but also in recognizing untoward symptoms. Pulse and blood pressure should be checked at least every half hour during the first day to detect any signs of hemorrhage. This will not always be evident by oozing from the tracheotomy tube; bleeding may occur inwardly.

Increasing apprehension and restlessness

may indicate anoxemia. Perhaps the airway is becoming blocked and suctioning may relieve the symptoms. If not, call the physician. The character of respirations can be suggestive of difficulty. Any changes from the usual type of breathing may indicate a problem. If they are increasingly more rapid and seem to have concomitant wheezing or crowing, there may be an obstruction. *This also may be apparent if he has an indrawn appearance above the clavicles, in the suprasternal notch and in the epigastrium with each inspiration.* Color change from pallor to cyanosis is a symptom of respiratory embarrassment. If aspiration does not help, call the physician immediately.

Subcutaneous emphysema is a condition in which air escapes into the tissues. A puffiness is noted near the stoma as air escapes from the trachea. This may extend to the upper chest, the neck and the face. A crackling sensation may be detected on gentle pressure. With absorption of air by the tissues, this disappears in a few days. Wound infection can occur easily; therefore, good technic must be practiced in changing dressings and keeping the incision clean. If food or water leaks through the wound or the patient coughs or chokes immediately after eating or drinking, an esophageal fistula may have developed. This symptom should be reported to the surgeon at once. Occasionally, due to violent paroxysms of coughing or to poorly tied tapes, the tracheotomy tube may be expelled. The opening in the trachea will fall together and, unless immediate treatment is given, the patient may die from asphyxia. The nurse must remember in such an emergency that the Trousseau dilator or a hemostat will spread the tracheal wound and allow the patient to breathe until the duplicate tube can be inserted by another person.

Care of Tubes. Cold running water will remove much of the secretions from a tube. However, for more adherent mucus the following methods of cleaning are suggested:

Place the tube in a bowl with 2 per cent sterile soda bicarbonate solution. This will help to liquefy the secretions. Sterile saline also may be used. Pipe cleaners are effective; they are soft and will not injure the tube, yet the inner wire gives a degree of firmness. A 2-inch bandage on a piece of folded wire also can be used. Small test tube brushes are effective.

METAL TUBES. After a thorough cleaning, silver polish can be used to remove any tarnish. The cannula then is boiled or autoclaved and, finally, reinserted. Careful handling of tracheotomy tubes is important, because they are made of a soft metal and are damaged easily. A dented tube may fit poorly and cause trauma to the patient when an attempt is made to remove it. A part of one tube is not interchangeable with a similar part of another set of tubes. Therefore, each set of three parts must be kept intact.

PLASTIC NYLON TUBES. The care of these tubes is simplified, since they will not dent or tarnish. Furthermore, parts are interchangeable. Other decided advantages are that they are light in weight, will not frost in cold climates and can be boiled or autoclaved.

In preparing tapes for a tracheotomy tube, ¾-inch twill tape makes a strong set of ties. Each tie should be 16 inches long. About 1 inch from the end, a horizontal slit should be made. This end of the tie can be inserted through the side opening on the outer cannula, and the opposite end of the tie then can be threaded through the slit end and drawn tightly. This is more effective than to tie a knot to anchor the tape to the cannula, because a sizable knot can cause a pressure area on the neck of the patient. (Fig. 121.) Another method of securing a tape is to staple the short end to the long end.

Equipment at Bedside. The nurse who is caring for a tracheotomized patient should keep near at hand:

CLOSED STERILE TRAY CONTAINING:

Duplicate tracheotomy tubes with obturator

Trousseau dilator

Forceps

Scissors

2 retractors

Hemostat

Gauze sponges

Pair of sterile rubber gloves

OPEN TRAY CONTAINING:

A bowl of sterile saline solution (to flush catheter attached to suction)

A second rubber catheter

A container of clean split 3 x 3 gauze squares

The tube cleaning equipment may be kept here or at a near-by sink.

Teaching the Patient. The patient is taught to care for his own tracheotomy tube as soon as feasible. The nurse can instruct him concerning the parts of the instrument and how they function. With the use of a mirror, she can show him how to remove and how to insert the inner cannula. The care of this delicate instrument must be explained and demonstrated in detail, and the patient should repeat the demonstration to the nurse. If the patient is unable to care for himself, some member of the family will have to be taught before he is discharged.

Sometimes the insertion of a tracheotomy tube is a temporary procedure to tide the patient over an acute respiratory obstruction. In such cases the patient must return gradually to normal breathing. This is accomplished by producing a partial obstruction of the airway in the tracheotomy tube by the insertion of partial corks. When they are first inserted the patient must be watched constantly for signs of respiratory obstruction. If the patient tolerates a small cork, the opening may be decreased further by the use of larger ones until eventually the entire opening can be plugged. When the patient tolerates complete obstruction of the tracheotomy tube, it may be removed and the opening permitted to heal. This process is known as *decannulation*. During this process the nurse must inspect the corks carefully to see that they are not broken. As a rule, they are fixed to the tracheotomy tube with braided silk threads. The most suitable corks are those made of pure rubber ground down to fit the tube. In learning to talk, the patient may be permitted to use a cork to close the opening temporarily so that voice sounds will be produced more clearly. Often merely the placing of a finger over the tracheotomy opening will aid him when he talks. However, this must be cleared with the physician, for talking may be contraindicated if the larynx is to be at rest following disease or edema.

If the tracheotomy is permanent, the patient should be instructed regarding the danger of aspirating water. Therefore, he must not swim and he must exercise caution in taking a shower. So far as appearance is concerned, women can wear filigree made specially by a jeweler, or scarves, ties and so forth in such a way that the tracheotomy tube is not seen. Usually in a man the shirt will cover up the tracheotomy opening.

SPECIFIC INFECTIONS OF THE UPPER RESPIRATORY TRACT

Streptococcal Sore Throat

Ranking high among the most uncomfortable, debilitating and dangerous of the upper respiratory tract infections are those produced by the Group A streptococcus. This type of infection is characterized by the abrupt onset of sore throat, chilly sensations or frank chills, temperature elevations above 101°F., headache and general malaise. Children may experience acute abdominal pain, nausea and repeated vomiting during the acute phase of this infection. The pharynx is diffusely reddened; the tonsils and the tonsillar nodes beneath the angles of the mandible enlarge; the uvula becomes edematous. A patchy or confluent exudate covers the tonsils and the pharynx. The face is flushed, and individuals who are not immune to the exotoxin of the Group A streptococcus (i.e., who are "Dick positive") are likely to develop the typical rash of scarlet fever. The blood leukocyte count generally exceeds 12,000.

Nursing Care and Chemotherapy. The nursing care of patients with acute pharyngitis, including the type due to the hemolytic streptococcus, is discussed in detail on pages 382 to 383. Early chemotherapy in patients with hemolytic streptococcal infection is of the utmost importance from the standpoint of preventing its most serious complications— acute rheumatic fever and acute glomerulonephritis. Penicillin is the drug of choice, and the intramuscular route is the optimum method of administration. Antibiotics which

OUTLINE OF NURSING MANAGEMENT OF A PATIENT WITH AN UPPER RESPIRATORY OBSTRUCTION

Causes of obstruction:

Injury or disease at or above the level of the glottis
Diseases of the pharynx, the mouth, the neck or the trachea
Inability of the patient to clear his air passages of secretions

Symptoms:

Inspiratory dyspnea with stridor
Suprasternal retraction
Indrawing of epigastrium, supraclavicular and intercostal spaces
Cough
Increasing pulse and respiratory rates
Restlessness, apprehension and struggling
Hypotension
Progressive subcutaneous emphysema
Cyanosis (a late sign)

Nursing Objectives and Principles of Care

1. To open the airway until a permanent airway is established
   A. Assist with cricothyrotomy (incision through the cricoid and thyroid cartilages) if there is a complete airway obstruction
   B. Prepare for laryngoscopy to determine status of larynx
   C. Assist with bronchoscopy if larynx is clear
   D. Prepare patient for tracheostomy if indicated

2. To maintain a patent airway
   A. Keep the tube clear of secretions and crust formation by
      a. Suctioning efficiently to initiate vigorous coughing
      b. Cleaning the inner tube when indicated
      c. Humidification of the room with cold vapor, steam or a room humidifier
      d. Encouraging fluid intake to keep the patient well hydrated
      e. Keeping sedation at a minimum to avoid cough depression
   B. Observe constantly to ensure that the tube is in the trachea

3. To allay the apprehension of the patient and his family
   A. Explain the function of the tube
   B. Stay with the patient until he is able to communicate
   C. Teach the patient to suction his tube as soon as he is able to do so

4. To prevent and treat complications such as
   A. Respiratory arrest and cardiovascular collapse
      a. Start artificial respiration
      b. Place patient in Trendelenburg position
      c. Administer vasopressor drugs as ordered
   B. Atelectasis
      a. Prepare the patient for roentgenogram
      b. Secure equipment for aspiration of pleural space

may serve as adequate substitutes for penicillin, in the event of penicillin sensitivity, include erythromycin, tetracycline, chlortetracycline and oxytetracycline.

Vincent's Infection

This infection, commonly called "trench mouth," "Vincent's stomatitis" or "Vincent's angina," is generally considered to be due to a combination of two organisms, one a spirochete and the other a fusiform bacillus. It usually occurs in association with oral sepsis, as a secondary complication of dental caries and alveolar abscesses. Vincent's infection begins and spreads from the margins of the gums, especially those of the incisors of the lower jaw. The gums first become swollen and ooze blood; later their inflamed borders become necrotic and present against the teeth an ulcerated margin, which may spread even to the alveolar processes, causing necrosis of the bone and enlargement of the neighboring lymph nodes. Isolated ulcers, covered with a false membrane which may suggest diphtheria, often appear on the buccal surfaces, the tongue, the tonsils and the palate (see Plate 5).

Treatment. The food should be nutritious and of soft consistency. Hourly mouth washes or irrigations are indicated. These should consist of fluids rich in free oxygen, such as sodium perborate in 2 per cent solution. In mild cases, after the sloughs have separated, a paste of sodium perborate powder is applied repeatedly to the ulcers. Penicillin, given parenterally, is often effective in this condition.

Common Cold

The common cold, or acute coryza, commonest of all respiratory illness, is presumably a viral infection which affects predominantly the upper respiratory tract. Rarely serious in itself, it is nevertheless an important predisposing factor in relation to bacterial infections of the respiratory tract and sufficiently prevalent to warrant serious consideration as a problem in economics and public health. Following an incubation period of from 12 to 48 hours, a prodromal malaise and chilliness develop, during which time the nasal mucous membrane is con-

gested and dry. The patient begins to sneeze, and a thin, clear, irritating nasal discharge is exuded. The swollen mucous membrane now almost fills the normally narrow air passages and obstructs nasal respiration. The pressure causes headache and closes the orifices of the tear ducts. The supersensitive mucous membrane stimulates frequent sneezing to keep the nose open. During the ensuing 3 or 4 days, the serous discharge becomes purulent, after which the swelling and the exudation gradually subside and the "cold" abates. The infection frequently extends into the throat and the lower respiratory tract, so that what is initially a nasopharyngitis finally may develop into a pharyngitis, laryngitis, tracheitis or bronchitis.

Treatment. The patient with acute coryza should remain quiet, preferably in bed, until the acute stage has subsided. The importance of confinement, moreover, is not limited to the laity but extends equally to every nurse with an active respiratory infection. Indeed, this advice is peculiarly appropriate in the case of the nurse, for not only her own health but also the safety of her patients is at stake.

Symptomatic relief may be obtained with ¼ per cent Neo-Synephrine nasal sprays, hot saline throat gargles or irrigations and aspirin, which the physician may order. Measures for the prevention of the spread of this highly communicable infection include the use of disposable tissues to absorb nasal secretions and oral droplets that are expelled on coughing, sneezing or blowing the nose and a paper bag for the collection and incineration of these tissues.

Adenovirus Infections

The term "adenovirus" (glandular virus) refers to a group of viruses of which 23 distinct types have been identified. Of these, 3 have been implicated as being the cause of 2 specific respiratory infections in man. One has been labeled "nonbacterial pharyngitis," or "pharyngoconjunctival fever," and the other, "ARD" ("acute respiratory disease").

Pharyngoconjunctival fever, caused by Type 3 adenovirus, is characterized by high fever, which lasts from 1 to 10 days, sore throat, painful enlargement of lymph nodes in the neck and follicular conjunctivitis. The tonsils are enlarged and the throat is red. A patchy, grayish-white exudate may be present in the tonsillar crypts. ARD, which is attributable to adenovirus Types 4 and 7, is a somewhat milder infection. The fever is less marked, the throat less sore. Cervical nodes are less enlarged and are not tender. Conjunctivitis is lacking.

Laboratory data are similar in both infections. The leukocyte count is normal, and throat cultures fail to demonstrate any pathogenic strain of bacteria as the predominating organism. Both infections are self-limited, fail to respond to any type of specific therapy now available and are devoid of complications.

Herpes Simplex Infection

The herpes simplex virus most commonly produces the familiar *herpes labialis* (cold sore, fever blister or canker), but in children who are reacting to this virus for the first time, the infection may take the form of an acute herpetic gingivostomatitis. Small vesicles, single or clustered, may erupt on the lips, the tongue, the cheeks and the pharynx (Plate 5). These soon rupture, forming sore, shallow ulcers which are covered with a gray membrane. Herpes infections appear often in association with other febrile infections, such as pneumococcus pneumonia, meningococcic meningitis and malaria. The herpes virus does not yield in the slightest to any of the chemotherapeutic agents that have become available to date. However, some relief is experienced with supportive medications containing *Lactobacillus acidophilus* (e.g., Lactinex).

CLINICAL SITUATION: THE PATIENT WITH A TRACHEOSTOMY

Mr. C. R. was admitted from the Emergency Room after an automobile accident in which he sustained multiple injuries. As he was in a profound state of unconsciousness, a tracheostomy was performed as a means of reducing resistance to air flow and decreasing his respiratory effort.

1. The nurse should aspirate Mr. R's tracheostomy tube when
   A. Symptoms of hypoxemia develop.
   B. The respirations become noisy.
   C. The blood pressure begins to rise.
   D. The respirations become irregular.

2. The cough reflex has been called "the watch dog of the lungs." To assist in preserving the cough reflex, the nurse should
   A. Employ oxygen.
   B. Give the codeine as ordered.
   C. Employ tracheal aspiration.
   D. Give steam inhalations.

3. To prevent encrustations from occluding the tracheostomy tube, an important nursing action is to
   A. Direct humidified air toward the tracheostomy tube.
   B. Change the outer cannula when necessary.
   C. Institute measures to dehydrate the patient.
   D. Give the prescribed antibiotic as ordered.

4. The physician stated that "Mr. R. will have to be watched for symptoms of respiratory acidosis." The nurse would know that the patient was developing respiratory acidosis by the appearance of which of the following symptoms?
   A. Decreasing respirations and lethargy.
   B. Increasing anxiety and restlessness.
   C. Singultus and euphoria.
   D. Cachexia and stupor.

BIBLIOGRAPHY AND SUGGESTED READING

Bauer, W. D., Edwards, D. L., and McGavran, M. H.: A critical analysis of laryngectomy in the treatment of epidermoid carcinoma of the larynx, Cancer **15**:263-270, March-April, 1962.

Coleman, L. L.: Children need preparation for tonsillectomy, Nurs. World **130**:8-9, May, 1956.

Conley, J. J.: Tracheotomy, Am. J. Nurs. **52**:1078-1081, 1952.

Gardner, W. H.: They will talk again. Nurs. Outlook **1**:314-315, 1954.

Gardner, W. H., and Harris, H. E.: Aids and devices for laryngectomees, A.M.A. Arch. Otolaryng. **73**:145-152, 1961.

Goldman, H. B.: The clinical application of bioflavonoids in otolaryngology, Eye, Ear, Nose, Throat Monthly **35**:246-249, 1956.

Gilmore, S. I.: Rehabilitation after laryngectomy, Am. J. Nurs. **61:**79-81, June, 1961.

Heaver, L., White, W., and Goldstein, N.: Clinical experience in restoring oral communication to 274 laryngectomized patients by esophageal voice, J. Am. Geriat. Soc. **3:** Sept., 1955.

Holinger, P. H., Johnson, K. C., and Mansueto, M. D.: Cancer of the larynx and nursing care, Am. J. Nurs. **57:**738-743, 1957.

How a pre-tonsillectomy party prepares children for surgery, Hosp. Topics **34:**55-57, May, 1956.

Jackson, C. L., and Norris, C. M.: Cancer of the Larynx, CA **12:**2-7, Jan.-Feb., 1962.

Lubart, J.: Importance of adenoidectomy, Arch. Pediat. **77:**491–495, 1960.

Monteiro, L.: The patient had difficulty communicating, Am. J. Nurs. **62:**78-81, Jan., 1962.

Osmum, P.: Are your sure you have a cold? Am. J. Nurs. **52:**168-169, 1952.

————: Nosebleeds, Am. J. Nurs. **56:**1411-1413, 1956.

Reed, G. F.: The long-term follow-up care of laryngectomized patients, J.A.M.A. **175:**980-985, 1961.

Smith, A. V.: Improved tracheotomy techniques, Am. J. Nurs. **57:**1442, 1957.

Williams, H. N.: Speech rehabilitation of the laryngectomized patient, CA **4:**126-130, July-August, 1961.

Witten, C. L.: Nosebleed, G.P. **26:**98-100, Dec., 1962.

Patient-Teaching Aids and Information Sources

A Handbook of Nursing Care for Head and Neck Patients. A 9-page pocket-sized illustrated booklet for tracheostomy and laryngectomy patients, New York, Memorial Center for Cancer and Allied Diseases, The Nursing Division, 1954.

Cancer of the Mouth and Respiratory Tract. A pocket-sized 20-page pamphlet. Pamphlet No. 5, Washington, D.C., U. S. Government Printing Office, 1952.

Doehler, Mrs. Paul A.: Esophageal Speech, A Manual for Teachers (with a section for patients). (22 pages.) May be obtained from: The American Cancer Society (Mass. Div.), Inc., 138 Newberry St., Boston 16, Mass., 1956.

Hilyemeyer, R.: Meeting the nursing needs of the patient with total laryngectomy, Monograph 4: Technical Innovations in Health Care: Nursing Implications, New York, Am. Nurses, Assoc., 1962.

Hygiene for the Post-Laryngectomized Patient. A picture brochure, which is an excellent teaching aid. Connecticut State Dept. of Health, Hartford, Connecticut, 1960.

It's a Cold, Cold World, (Pamphlet T (b) 4876) New York, Metropolitan Life Insurance Co., 1953.

Rehabilitating Laryngectomees (pamphlet), New York, American Cancer Society, Inc., 1962.

Speech Rehabilitation following Laryngectomy. An 8-page brochure from the Clinical Service of the National Hospital for Speech Disorders, 61 Irving Place, New York 3, N. Y.

Waldrop, W. F., and Gould, M. A.: Your New Voice, (a 32-page booklet containing 13 lessons on how to use your new voice). Chicago, American Cancer Society, 1960.

Other Sources of Information for Patients After Laryngectomy:

American Speech and Hearing Association, Suite 532
1001 Connecticut Avenue, N.W.
Washington 6, D.C.

International Association of Laryngectomees
521 W. 57th Street
New York 19, New York

23

Patients With Medical and Surgical Conditions of the Chest

ANATOMY AND PHYSIOLOGY OF THE LUNGS

The cells of the body derive their necessary energy from the oxidation of food products furnished by the blood stream. For this process, as for any type of combustion, oxygen is required. As a result of oxidation in the body tissues, carbon dioxide is produced and must be removed from the cell as soon as formed. Deprived of oxygen and stifled by accumulated carbon dioxide, no body cell can survive.

Cells are supplied with oxygen and dispose of waste carbon dioxide through the medium of the circulating blood. No cell is far removed from a capillary, the thin walls of which present no barrier to the passage of water or dissolved gases. Interposed between the capillary and the cell membrane is a thin layer of tissue fluid, or lymph, from which the cells continuously extract oxygen. As a result, the oxygen tension outside the capillary is always lower than it is within, where it reflects the concentration of that gas passing inside the red blood cells. Thus,

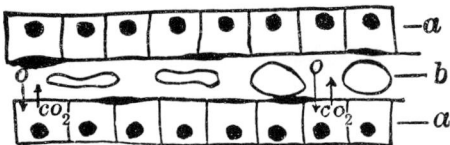

Fig. 122. Internal respiration. (a) Tissue cells. (b) Capillary through which blood is flowing. (The lymph spaces are omitted for the sake of clearness.) The interchange of oxygen and carbon dioxide is shown by arrows.

oxygen diffuses in solution from the capillary blood through the capillary wall, into the surrounding lymph, through the membrane of the tissue cell and into the contents of that cell. Diffusion of oxygen from blood to cells proceeds in this manner without interruption in all tissues of the body. The movement of carbon dioxide from cell to blood is accomplished by a similar process of diffusion, the dissolved gas moving continuously via the same route as the oxygen, but in the opposite direction (Fig. 122). As a result of these exchanges the arterial blood loses approximately one third of its oxygen, while its carbon dioxide content is increased by about one fifth. It has now become venous blood.

These relationships are demonstrated in Table 15, which shows the normal values for oxygen and carbon dioxide concentration in both arterial and venous blood.

The site at which venous blood again becomes arterial blood, i.e., where its oxygen deficit is restored and its excess carbon dioxide is removed, is in the capillaries of the lung. Here, following rapid diffusion of these gases through an extensive liquid-gas

TABLE 15. Comparison of the Gaseous Content of Both Arterial and Venous Blood.

	ARTERIAL	VENOUS
Oxygen content, vols. per cent (ml. O_2/100 ml. blood)	18 to 21	12 to 14
Oxygen saturation, per cent (O_2 content/O_2 capacity X 100)	94 to 96	60 to 80
Carbon dioxide content, vols. per cent (ml. CO_2/100 ml. blood)	50 to 55	62 to 65

397

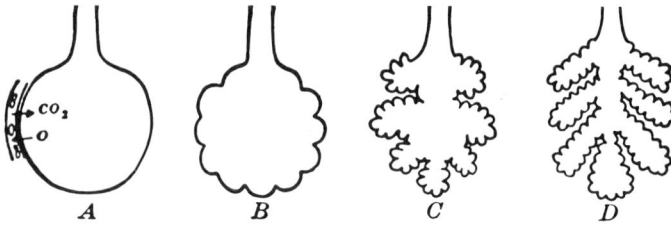

FIG. 123. The simple lungs of amphibians. (A) The simplest lung, showing a capillary in the wall and the interchange of oxygen and carbon dioxide. (B, C and D) More complex lungs, showing how an increase in respiratory surface is gained without any increase in the bulk of the lung as a whole.

interphase, the blood is approaching equilibrium with the air that we breathe.

The simplest type of lung (Fig. 123) is a narrow-mouthed sac lined with a thin membrane which contains an extensive network of capillaries. Gases diffuse easily and rapidly through this membrane. A simple structure of this type, although found in certain amphibians, is inadequate for man, who, because of his relatively large blood volume, requires a vast capillary system and a much more extensive respiratory surface.

The human lung is a composite organ, a collection of myriads of tiny lungs, each of which is separate and complete in itself. Figure 124 represents one of these functioning units. Each has a tiny bronchus, called a *bronchiole* (a), opening into a group of air sacs or *alveoli* (b).

The alveoli furnish the respiratory surface. They are small air sacs scarcely visible to the eye. Their elastic walls are lined by thin alveolar epithelial membrane, a single layer of flat epithelial cells through which gases easily diffuse. Included within these walls is a network of pulmonary capillaries. So numerous are these alveoli that if their walls, the respiratory surface, were united to form one big sheet, it would cover an area of over 90 square yards.

The bronchioles through which air enters and leaves the alveoli are lined with an epithelial membrane composed of ciliated columnar cells, i.e., tall cells whose free ends are covered with short "hairs," called *cilia* (Fig. 125). These cilia maintain a constant whipping motion, always in the same direction, sweeping out any foreign substance or excess of mucus. The bronchioles join to form larger and larger bronchi, so that all the bronchi and bronchioles in one lung represent branches of one primary bronchus (Fig. 126). The two primary bronchi then unite to form the trachea.

The lungs are elastic structures enclosed in an airtight chamber with distensible walls—the thorax. The movements of respiration involve the walls of the thorax and its floor, the diaphragm; their effect is alternately to increase and decrease the capacity of the chest. The lungs expand and contract passively, being so elastic that they can follow easily the changing volume of the thoracic cavity. The only open passage admitting air into the thorax is the trachea. When

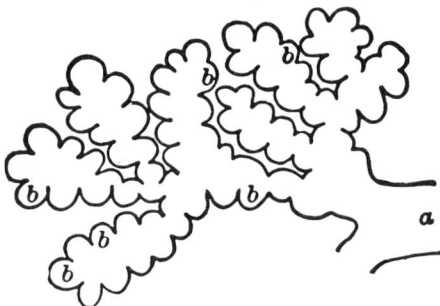

FIG. 124. One of the tiny lungs of which the lungs are composed. (a) Terminal bronchiole. (b) Air cells (alveoli).

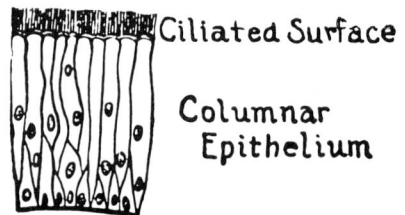

FIG. 125. Ciliated epithelium (cross section).

Fig. 126. The bronchial tree. The two lungs are represented as opened, showing the branches of the bronchi. The mottling of the left lung suggests the tiny lungs (Fig. 124) which reach the surface (much exaggerated). The terminal bronchioles and the smaller branches of the bronchi are not shown. The fine bronchi unite, forming larger and larger tubes until there is only one for each lung, the primary bronchus. The two primary bronchi unite to form the trachea.

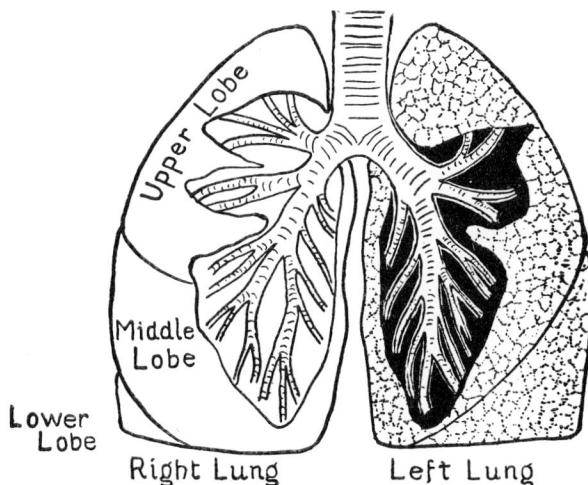

the capacity of the chest is increased, air must enter, due to the lowered pressure within. It passes through the trachea and the bronchi and inflates the lungs. When the chest collapses to its previous volume, the elastic lungs collapse with it, forcing the air out. In this fashion the entire lung is "ventilated," that is, each alveolus during inspiration receives a supply of fresh air which is expelled during the next expiration (Fig. 127).

The outer surfaces of the lung are enclosed by a smooth, slippery membrane called the *pleura*—which also extends to cover the interior wall of the thorax and the superior surface of the diaphragm. The pleura is always moistened by lymph, which allows the opposing pleural surfaces, i.e., the "parietal pleura" lining the thorax and the "visceral pleura" covering the lungs, to rub together freely and painlessly during respiration.

The mediastinum is the wall which divides the thoracic cavity into two halves. It is composed of two layers of pleura between which lie all of the thoracic structures except the lungs.

PATHOLOGIC PHYSIOLOGY OF RESPIRATION

Deficient Aeration. Interference with aeration, resulting in a reduction in blood oxygen and an abnormal increase in its carbon dioxide content, can be caused by abnormal respiratory movement, obstruction of

the respiratory tract or a reduction in the area of "respiratory surface," the area of alveolar epithelium where the blood-gas exchange occurs. Laboratory studies in such cases would reveal an abnormally low oxygen content of both arterial and venous blood in proportion to its oxygen capacity, whereas its carbon dioxide content would be elevated abnormally.

Symptoms and signs that immediately strike the nurse's attention and represent to her the picture of oxygen lack include the appearance of cyanosis, an increasing pulse rate, drowsiness or restlessness and, often, confusion. Carbon dioxide retention, if only moderate in degree, may or may not be accompanied by clinical manifestations, depending on the length of time this situation has existed and on the degree to which base (e.g., sodium) is available to neutralize

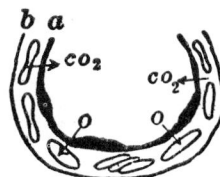

Fig. 127. External respiration. (a) The wall of an alveolus, consisting of one layer of cells through which gases, but not liquids, can pass. (b) A capillary. The arrows show the interchange of gases.

the excess carbonic acid. If sufficient sodium has been retained to keep the blood acidity within the physiologic range, i.e., at a pH level between 7.35 and 7.40, no symptoms referable to the excess carbon dioxide are to be expected. Such a patient is said to have "compensated acidosis."

In uncompensated respiratory acidosis the blood acidity is increased, i.e., the pH falls below 7.35. The most prominent sign associated with this metabolic disturbance in its early phases is hyperpnea, characterized by rapid, deep breathing. Long-standing carbon dioxide retention eventually reduces or eliminates altogether the sensitivity of the respiratory center to an elevation of carbon dioxide concentration in the blood, or to a lowering of the blood pH. Under these circumstances, oxygen deficiency becomes the principal respiratory stimulus. Such patients may display no hyperpnea; on the contrary, if their hypoxia is relieved by oxygen inhalation therapy their respiratory rate may decline to dangerously low levels, as described on page 190. An excess of carbon dioxide in the blood of any patient, regardless of his earlier status, is capable of producing coma and death.

Hyperventilation. An increase in the respiratory rate is a common finding in patients suffering from a wide variety of disorders, in most of which the respiratory center is hyperstimulated as a result of acidosis, hypoxia or by nervous reflexes from the lungs or elsewhere. In the vast majority of patients, an increased respiration serves a definite physiologic need by restoring an oxygen deficit or reducing an excess acidity by increasing carbon dioxide excretion; in such instances the term "hyperventilation," which suggests excessive respiration, is hardly applicable. True hyperventilation is encountered in patients with hysteria. Whatever its psychiatric implications in these cases, it is certainly without physiologic benefit to the patient, its principal effect, as described on pages 57 to 58, being to "wash out" carbon dioxide, with the result that the blood becomes too alkaline. This immediately induces a train of symptoms, including sensations of numbness, tingling of the arms and the legs, dizziness, faintness and abnor-

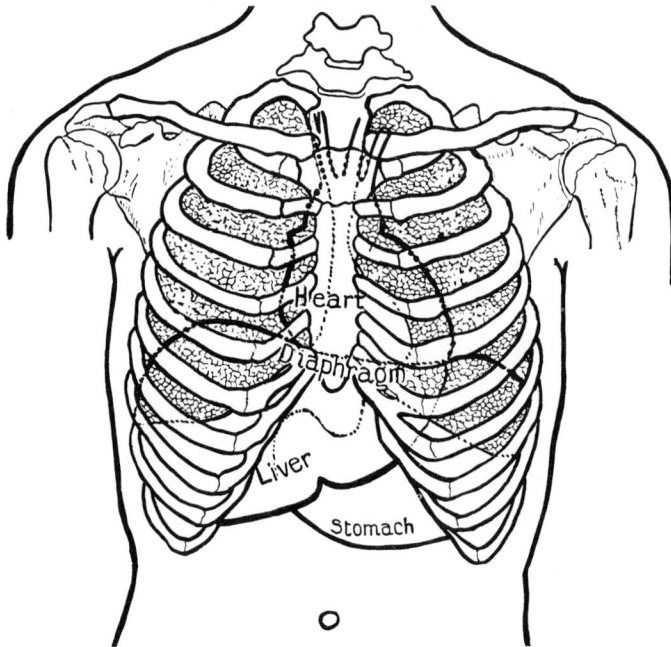

Fig. 128. Diagram of the thoracic and the upper abdominal organs.

mal contractility of the muscles, evidenced by spasmodic twitchings of the facial muscles and the extremities. These effects are entirely reversible, lasting only for the duration of the alkalosis, namely, until the hyperventilation has ceased.

Therapeutic measures which effectively restore the normal blood acidity, despite continuance of overbreathing, are inhalations of carbon dioxide-oxygen mixtures containing 10 per cent carbon dioxide, or having the patient inhale and exhale in a paper bag, causing him to rebreathe some of the carbon dioxide in his own expired air. However, such treatment is obviously without effect on the underlying disorder, which requires skilled psychiatric management.

DIAGNOSTIC STUDIES IN THORACIC CONDITIONS

Pulmonary Function Tests. These tests are done with a spirometer and are designed to determine how well the lung "ventilates," that is, its ability to take in oxygen and release carbon dioxide. In addition, tests are being perfected to determine how well oxygen and carbon dioxide are exchanged between the alveoli and the pulmonary capillary blood; this is called "diffusion." Several terms in common usage are of interest to the nurse:

Vital capacity is the maximum volume of air that can be expelled from the lungs by forceful effort following a maximum inspiration.

Residual volume is the volume of gas remaining in the lungs at the end of a maximum expiration.

Total lung capacity is the sum of the vital capacity and the residual volume.

Tidal volume is the amount of air inspired during each respiratory cycle when the patient is breathing naturally.

Minute volume is the amount of air inspired normally in one minute.

Maximum breathing capacity is the largest amount of air that can be breathed per minute by making the greatest possible voluntary effort.

These tests usually are done only on chest patients having borderline respiratory reserve. As a rule, no special preparation is

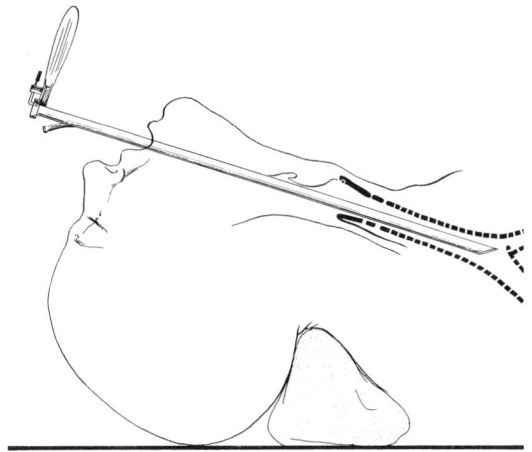

FIG. 129. Semidiagrammatic view shows the introduction of the bronchoscope.

required for these tests; the nurse can tell her patient that he is to have a breathing test. He follows the instructions of the physician as to whether to breathe normally, inhale deeply, etc.

Roentgenograms. *Roentgenograms and sectional roentgenograms* (laminogram, planogram or strategram) are a real aid to the physician and the surgeon in recognizing lung function, the relationship of the vital structures and suggestions of pathology (see page 101). Patience and cooperation on the part of the patient are desirable, and the nurse should endeavor to obtain them.

Bronchogram. A bronchogram is an x-ray examination of the bronchial tree after a radiopaque dye is instilled. Before the procedure, a sedative and atropine are given, and usually a meal is withheld to prevent aspiration from regurgitation. Cocaine or pontocaine in the form of a spray through the nose and the mouth will help to prevent gagging and coughing when the tube is passed nasally. After such a roentgenogram, food and fluids are withheld until the effects of the local anesthetic have worn off. The patient is placed on a regimen of postural drainage to allow the oily dye to be removed. Often because of the hazards of oil in the respiratory passages, he is sent home for two months before surgery is done.

Bronchoscopy and Esophagoscopy. When

a foreign body enters the smaller air passages in the lungs, it may obstruct the bronchi with a resulting obstruction of air in the portion of the lung supplied by them. This produces a partial collapse of the lung with pulmonary symptoms of cough, expectoration and so forth. Secondary infection often occurs with resultant formation of chronic pulmonary suppuration or abscess.

In many cases it will be possible to remove the foreign body and to relieve the patient's symptoms by means of *bronchoscopy*. By this method of treatment, a lighted rigid tube is inserted through the pharynx and the trachea into the bronchus containing the foreign body. After aspiration of the secretions, the foreign body may be removed with forceps. Many brilliant cures have been effected by this method of therapy, which demands the highest degree of skill and adequate equipment (Fig. 129).

Bronchoscopy also is used in the diagnosis and the treatment of many intrathoracic diseases. By means of this lighted tube, tumors of the air passages can be viewed and biopsied, secretions can be aspirated for study and medication is applied at times. In the study of some diseases of the lungs, such as bronchiectasis, radiopaque liquids are injected to outline the air passages on the x-ray film (*bronchogram*).

Esophagoscopy is the viewing of the interior of the esophagus through a lighted tube. It is used to remove foreign bodies, to inspect lesions of the esophagus, such as ulcers, diverticuli and tumors, and often to make a positive diagnosis by removing small bits of tissue for microscopic examination (biopsy).

NURSING CARE. Before bronchoscopy or esophagoscopy the patient must take nothing by mouth for at least 6 hours. Morphine sulfate or a similar drug usually is given adults. All removable dentures must be removed. He should be told what to expect so as to gain his cooperation. Many times, such a patient fears that he is to undergo real surgery. When he sees physicians and nurses garbed in operating masks and gowns, he may reasonably be upset.*

When the patient returns from the operat-

---

* The procedure may be done under local anesthesia using cocaine, Butyn Sulfate or Xylocaine or under a general anesthetic. During a bronchoscopic examination the nurse may assist the patient by "vocal anesthesia," informing him of the progress of the procedure and praising him for his helpful participation.

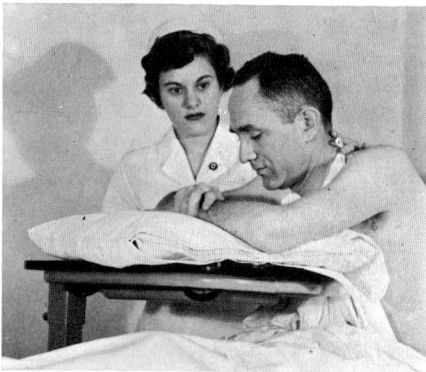

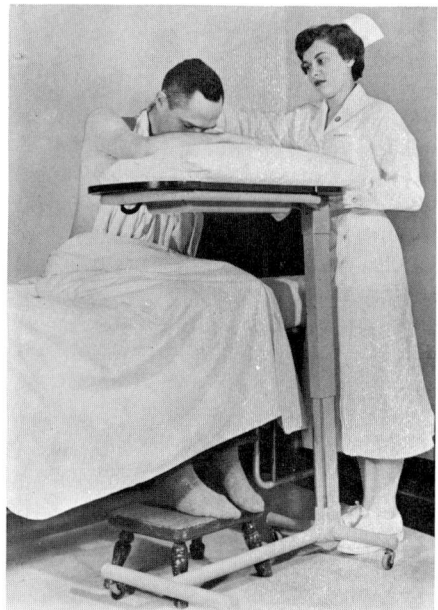

FIG. 130. Positions for thoracentesis. (*Top*) Patient in sitting position in bed with pillow over the bed table for support. (*Bottom*) Patient with feet over the side of the bed, using the bed table for support.

ing room the local anesthetic used in the throat may interfere with swallowing and cause him to choke. After bronchoscopy, cracked ice may be given during the first 2 hours. After the return of the cough or gag reflex, liquids may be given and, if the hypodermic does not cause nausea, the patient is permitted to return to the preoperative diet in about 6 hours. Difficulty in breathing, particularly in children, is looked for and reported promptly.

Until the local anesthesia has disappeared after esophagoscopy, care should be exercised in giving liquids. Determine whether the patient can cough before offering any fluids. Then, they may be given, if they are tolerated, and the patient is permitted to return to the preoperative diet in about 6 hours. Some discomfort on swallowing may occur, but marked discomfort should be reported promptly.

Thoracentesis. The aspiration of chest fluid may be a therapeutic or a diagnostic procedure. During the thoracentesis the nurse must maintain the proper position of her patient in order to minimize trauma. If the patient is able he should be placed in a sitting position, leaning on an overbed table to widen the intercostal spaces (Fig. 130). If the patient is unable to sit, place him on his unaffected side and help him to maintain his arm over his head. Inform the patient of every pressure movement, such as the application of cold antiseptic solution and the injection of procaine. Observe his respirations and general reaction to the procedure. Charting should include a description of the character and the amount of fluid removed and the patient's condition. Watch for coughing, blood-tinged sputum, and any change in his color, pulse or respiration.

Sputum Studies. For a sputum culture, the patient should be instructed to cough deeply so that a true specimen may be obtained for the sterile Petri dish. Often a qualitative study is done to determine whether the secretions are saliva, mucus or pus. Usually they separate into layers that are seen readily when a conical glass container is used. For quantitative studies, the patient is given a waxed pasteboard container into which to expectorate. This is weighed at the

end of 24 hours, and the amount and the character is described and charted. In disposing of such a specimen, sawdust is added to the container in order to absorb and minimize the spread of organisms, and then it is wrapped in paper and taken to the incinerator. To prevent odors, all sputum containers should be covered and concealed. Malodorous discarded mouth wipes should be removed, and there must be good ventilation in the room. Metal sputum containers should be cleaned thoroughly and sterilized frequently.

PROBLEMS OF PATIENTS WITH PULMONARY DISORDERS

Certain problems are encountered frequently in the care of patients with chest conditions. These relate to the occurrence of cough and expectoration, the necessity for mouth care, symptoms of dyspnea, chest pain and hemoptysis, and the presence of air or fluid in the pleural cavity.

Cough, Expectoration and Mouth Care

The stimulus producing a cough may arise from an infectious process or from an air irritant, such as smoke, smog, dust or a gas. "The cough is the watchdog of the lungs" and is the patient's chief protection against the accumulation of secretions in the bronchi and bronchioles. On the other hand, the presence of cough may indicate serious pulmonary disease. For example, it is one of the prominent symptoms of bronchogenic carcinoma. If the cough is harsh and loud, the patient probably has a disease of the trachea or large bronchi, while the presence of a painful, short, dry cough may indicate a lesion of the parenchyma or pleura.

A patient who coughs long enough will almost invariably expectorate sputum. The production of sputum is the reaction of the the lung to any constantly recurring irritant. The nurse should determine whether the sputum is associated with a nasal discharge. If there is a profuse amount of purulent sputum, the patient may have an overwhelming infectious process; whereas a gradual increase of sputum over a period of time may reveal the presence of chronic bronchitis or bronchiectasis. Pink-tinged

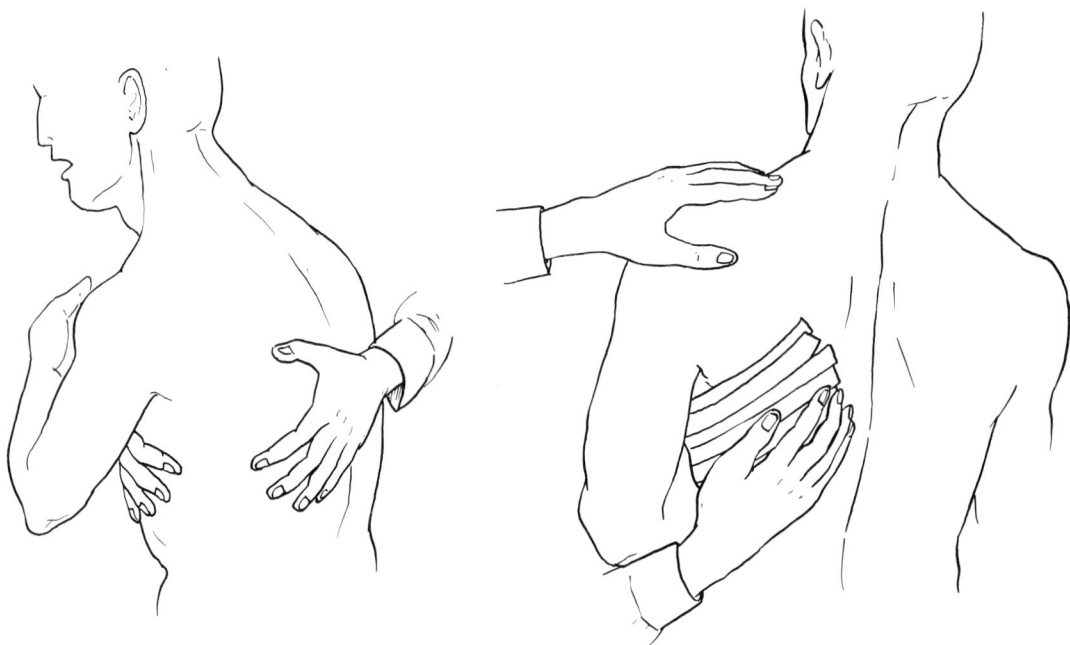

FIG. 131. (*Left* and *right*) Technics for support of incision while patient with thoracic surgery coughs. (See text.) (From Barrett, R. J., and Tuttle, W. M.: Preoperative and postoperative care of the thoracotomy patient, Surg. Clin. N. Am. **39:**1609)

mucoid sputum is suggestive of a lung tumor, and profuse frothy pink material may indicate pulmonary edema. The nurse's charting should be specific with respect to the amount, the odor, the character, and, if known, the source of the sputum.

Promotion of an Effective Cough Routine. Effective coughing is necessary for the mobilization and the removal of bronchial secretions and exudates. The promotion of vigorous coughing is essential for the patient undergoing thoracic surgery. Preoperatively he should be assured that coughing will not "break his incision open" and informed that he will be assisted to cough every hour.

If possible, the patient should be in a sitting position while coughing, and the nurse should stand behind him. The patient should be taught to cough into two tissues. Either of the following technics may be used:

1. The nurse's hands should support the chest incision anteriorly and posteriorly. The patient is instructed to take several deep breaths, inhale, and then to cough forcibly (Fig. 131, *left*).

2. With one hand, exert downward pressure on the shoulder of the affected side while firmly supporting beneath the wound with the other hand. The patient is instructed to take several deep breaths, inhale, and then cough forcibly (Fig. 131, *right*).

Mouth Care. The patient's appetite may be lessened because of the odor and the taste in his mouth that result from the frequent raising of sputum. Adequate mouth hygiene, proper environment and wise selections of food will stimulate his appetite. After careful cleansing and rinsing of the mouth, sputum cups and emesis basins should be removed before his meal arrives. Some foods, such as citrus juices, make the mouth feel fresher and the patient is then more receptive to the rest of the meal.

Dyspnea

Dyspnea, as discussed on page 58, is a symptom common to many pulmonary conditions, including tracheal or bronchial obstruction by inflammatory processes, tumors of the mediastinum or aspirated foreign bodies. Parenchymal lesions of the lung, as well as pulmonary atelectasis, reduce the vital capacity and therefore predispose to dyspnea. Respiration becomes shallower and more rapid if the lungs become congested or inflamed. In general, the acute diseases of the lungs produce a more severe grade of dyspnea than do the chronic diseases.

Therapeutic control of dyspnea depends on the success with which its cause can be eliminated. Alleviation of the symptom is achieved by placing the patient at rest and, in severe cases, by the administration of oxygen inhalation therapy.

Chest Pain

Chest pain associated with pulmonary conditions may be sharp, stabbing and intermittent, or dull, aching and persistent. It usually is felt on the side where the pathology is located, but it may be referred elsewhere, for example, to the neck, the back or the abdomen. Chest pain is experienced by most patients with pneumonia and pleurisy, and it is a common symptom of bronchogenic carcinoma.

Patients with pain of the pleuritic type are more comfortable when they can be persuaded to lie on the affected side, a posture that tends to "splint" the chest wall, restrict the expansions and the contractions of the lung and reduce the friction betwen the injured or diseased pleurae on that side. Pain associated with cough may be lessened by manual splinting of the rib cage, as illustrated in Figure 131.

Analgesic and antitussive medication in the form of codeine sulfate and Hycodan will alleviate the harrassing cough and reduce the pain of pleurisy. If the pain is severe, meperidine hydrochloride may be given intramuscularly in doses of 50 to 100 mg. at intervals of from 4 to 6 hours. On the other hand, because of its suppressive action on the respiratory center, morphine is used rarely or only with extreme caution in patients with chest disorders. For relief of extreme pain the physician may resort to regional anesthetic block, which is achieved by injecting procaine along the intercostal nerves supplying the painful area.

Hemoptysis

When a patient expectorates blood, the question at once arises as to its source. Has it come from the lungs, the nasopharynx or the stomach? Careful observation by the nurse, who may be the only witness to the episode, may be of great value in determining this point. The following points should be borne in mind as she makes and records her observations.

If the hemorrhage is in the stomach, the blood is vomited rather than coughed up—although with vomiting there is considerable coughing and vice versa. Blood from the lung is usually bright and frothy, whereas blood that has been in contact with gastric juice is sometimes so dark that it is referred to as "coffee-ground" material. Patients whose bloody sputum originates from the nose or the nasopharynx usually precede their expectoration with considerable sniffing, and blood may appear in the nares, The term *hemoptysis* is reserved for the coughing of blood arising from a pulmonary hemorrhage.

Hemoptysis occurs in many lung diseases, notably tuberculosis, bronchiectasis, lung abscess, pulmonary infarcts, tumors and pneumonia. It is a symptom of mitral stenosis due to rupture of a blood vessel somewhere in the congested pulmonary circuit. A careful history and physical examination are necessary to establish a diagnosis of the underlying disease. Careful roentgenologic examination is indicated. This may include fluoroscopy, stereoscopic plates and Lipiodol bronchograms. If the nature of the process is not evident, bronchoscopy should be performed without delay in order to rule out an early tumor growth, bronchiectasis, an abscess or a foreign body.

Nursing Care. A patient who has experienced a hemoptysis, whatever its cause, should be placed immediately at complete bed rest and his respiratory movements reduced to a minimum by every available means, including oxygen inhalation therapy and morphine sedation. Sandbags may be applied to the anterior chest to restrain its motion. If the hemorrhage is not controlled by these measures, an artificial pnemothorax may be induced in an effort to prevent as much mechanical expansion and contraction of bleeding lung tissue as possible. Transfusion may be required if peripheral vascular collapse ensues or if shock results from the loss of blood. Equipment for performing an emergency laryngoscopy and bronchoscopy should be in readiness for the removal of blood clots from the respiratory passages if the patient shows the initial signs of asphyxia.

The nurse must realize that hemoptysis is one of the most frightening of all the symptoms that patients experience. Fright promotes hyperventilation, which is the opposite desired, namely, a minimum of thoracic movement. Therefore, it is of the utmost

importance that she avert panic and maintain emotional equilibrium in her patient by presenting the appearance of untroubled calm herself, functioning swiftly, efficiently and with utmost assurance, betraying no hint of alarm, but radiating confidence and optimism.

Atelectasis

Pulmonary atelectasis, or collapse, may result from pressure on the lung tissue, confining its normal expansion on inspiration. Such pressure may be caused by a fluid ac-

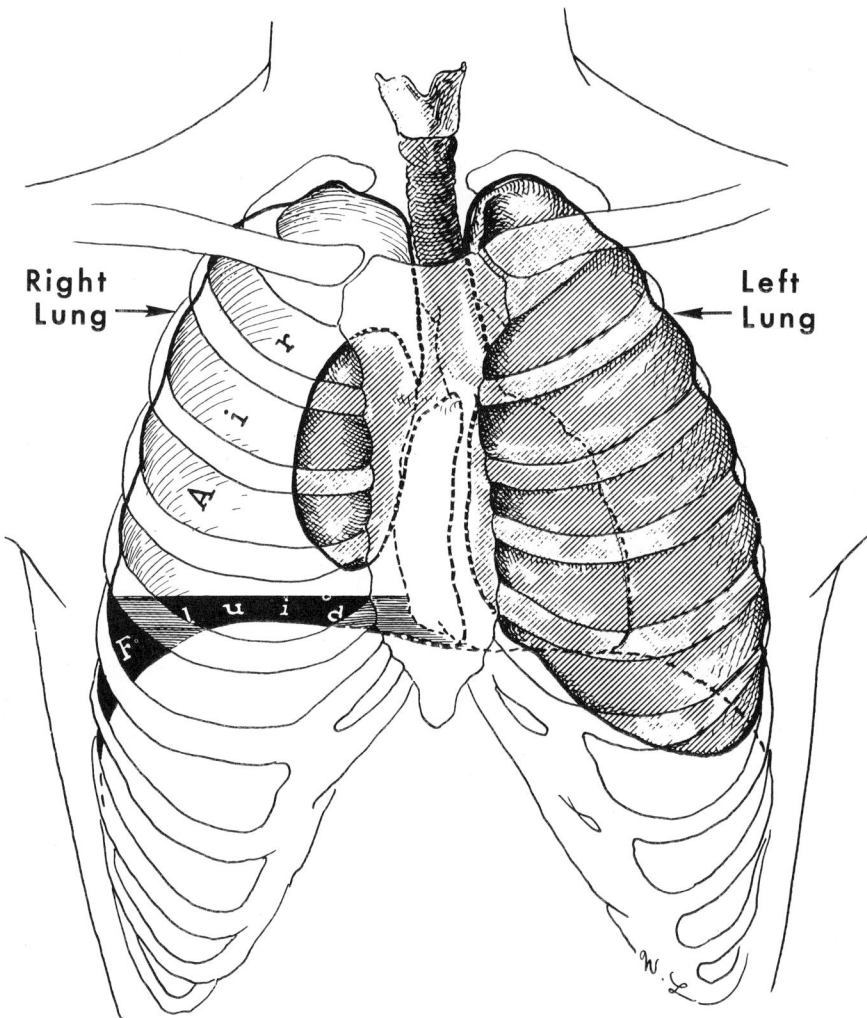

Fig. 132. Diagrammatic view of the chest cavity showing hydropneumothorax on the right side with atelectasis (collapse) of the right lung.

cumulation within the thorax (pleural effusion), by air in the pleural space (pneumothorax), by an extremely large heart or a pericardium distended with fluid (pericardial effusion). It may be due to a tumor growth within the thorax or to an elevated diaphragm displaced upward as the result of abdominal pressure. In such circumstances there is a crowding of the intrathoracic contents, and, since the spongy lung tissue is most compressible, it collapses without resistance. Where it is compressed it becomes airless, or atelectatic, and the efficiency of pulmonary function is reduced accordingly. Atelectasis of this type is encountered most often in cases of pleural effusion due to cardiac failure, or in pleural infection.

Another form of atelectasis is caused, not by external pressure, but by obstruction of a bronchus, the effect of which is to impede the passage of air to and from the alveoli communicating with it. The alveolar air thus trapped soon becomes absorbed into the blood stream, and, all external communication having been blocked, its replacement from the outside air is impossible. The net result is that the portion of lung so isolated becomes airless: it shrinks in size causing the remainder of the lung to overexpand (compensatory emphysema). Bronchial obstruction, in this way causing atelectasis, may follow inhalation of a foreign body. It may be due to a plug of thick exudate which is not, or cannot be, expelled by coughing. Thus, it occurs in severe bronchial asthma, due both to bronchiolar spasm and to plugging of the bronchi by a thick tenacious secretion. This is the usual mechanism producing the "massive collapse" occasionally observed postoperatively and in debilitated bedridden individuals. In these people there is likely to be long-continued respiratory depression, together with inadequate depth of respiratory excursion, and perhaps unusually profuse or poorly expectorated bronchial secretions. Tumors of the bronchi often make their presence known first by an atelectasis resulting from their obstructive growth.

Symptoms. If collapse occurs suddenly, and if sufficient lung tissue is involved, the following may be anticipated: marked dyspnea, cyanosis, prostration and pleural pain which usually is referred to the lower chest. Fever commonly occurs. Tachycardia and dyspnea are unusually prominent. The patient characteristically sits bolt upright in bed, his expression anxious, his color cyanotic and his respirations labored. The chest wall on the affected side moves little, if at all, whereas on the opposite side the excursion appears excessive. Examination reveals signs of displacement of all intrathoracic organs toward the side of the collapsed lung, which lacks resonance on percussion and radiance by roentgenograms. Lungs which have collapsed due to the obstruction of a bronchus should be re-expanded as rapidly as possible to avoid the common complications of pneumonia or lung abscess.

Treatment, Nursing Care and Prevention. If atelectasis has resulted from a pleural effusion or pressure pnemothorax, the fluid or air may be removed by needle aspiration. If bronchial obstruction is the cause, the nature of the obstruction must be ascertained and it should be relieved, if at all possible. To accomplish this, the respiratory center is stimulated to the maximum by means of carbon dioxide inhalations which may be administered at the bedside by the nurse, and also caffeine—particularly if morphine, a respiratory depressant, is to be used for the control of the pleural pain. The patient should be turned frequently and inverted intermittently in an effort to stimulate coughing. If these measures do not relieve the obstruction, prompt recourse should be had to bronchoscopy, which affords a most effective means of bronchial drainage and also of accurate diagnosis, both as regards location and nature of the obstructive lesion —exceedingly important in view of the possible presence of an aspirated foreign body. Antibiotic therapy should be given prophylactically in all cases of atelectasis, the objective being to forestall the development of a bacterial infection in the collapsed portion of the lung.

The incidence of postoperative pulmonary atelectasis has been reduced significantly as a result of the more conservative and judicious use of preoperative and postoperative sedation and by early ambulation of postoperative patients. Another important factor in its prevention is the stimulation of ventilation during and following operation by means of carbon dioxide inhalations, the purpose of which is to cause hyperventilation and, therefore, more adequate drainage of bronchial secretions. All stuporous, debilitated and heavily sedated patients should be turned frequently in bed, a procedure that affords increased respiratory excursion on the uppermost side.

Collections of Air and Fluid in the Pleural Cavity

Hydrothorax. Serous (nonpurulent) effusions may occur in such medical conditions as cardiac or renal failure, lung and pleural tumors and so forth. The presence of the fluid may so embarrass respiration as to require aspiration (thoracentesis). (See Fig. 130.)

Pneumothorax and Hemothorax. Air in the pleural cavity may occur spontaneously from rupture of a lung alveolus; it may be induced deliberately to collapse cavities and set the lung at rest, as in the treatment of tuberculosis; or it may arise from trauma, the air entering the pleural cavity through the resulting wound or from the injured lung. Bleeding usually accompanies such trauma, so that a hemopneumothorax results. Aspiration of the blood and air permits re-expansion of the lung and a return to a more physiologic state. In neglected cases or in those in which an infection has taken place, operation with removal of the clot and drainage is necessary.

Chylothorax. Injury to the thoracic duct or to other lymphatic radicals in the chest may permit the escape of lymph into the pleural cavity. The lymph from the thoracic duct, rich in fat absorbed from the intestines, is called *chyle,* and the condition is called *chylothorax.* Injuries to the lymphatic radicals may arise from trauma or from operations in the posterior thorax, such as esophagectomies or sympathectomies. Small leaks may heal spontaneously, but thoracentesis may be required to relieve respiratory embarrassment. If the leak continues, operative intervention is required to suture or ligate the injured vessel. Continued loss of chylous fluid ends fatally.

NURSING CARE OF THE PATIENT WITH CHEST SURGERY

In addition to a skillful operation, the success of chest surgery depends on good preparation before operation and intelligent observation and nursing care after operation.

Preoperatively, the emphasis is on (1) assisting the patient who is undergoing diagnostic studies, (2) reducing the number of organisms in the upper respiratory tract, (3) preparing the patient mentally and physically for the surgical program ahead and (4) acquainting the patient with some of the postoperative problems, such as coughing.

Postoperatively, the nurse is concerned with (1) maintaining a patent airway, (2) providing for maximum expansion of the remaining lung tissue, (3) recognizing early symptoms of untoward complications and (4) providing supportive and rehabilitative measures.

Preoperative Management

Psychological Aspects. Usually there are several days to the preoperative phase, which provides time for the nurse to talk with her patient. By listening to him, she may be able to discover how he really feels about his illness and the proposed treatment. He may reveal significant reactions: the fear of hemorrhage because of bloody sputum, the discomfort of a chronic cough and chest pain, the social stigma attached to a foul-smelling sputum, the fear of death because of dyspnea—all contribute to his psychological status. The nurse can help him to overcome many of his fears by correcting any false impressions, by offering reassurance in the capability of the surgical team and by reporting special problems to the appropriate services available.

General Preparation. This is a general evaluation of the patient to determine and to correct any associated problems, such as metabolic disturbances, dehydration, cardiac impairments, etc. If he is malnourished and has a history of weight loss, naturally he will be placed on a high-caloric, high-protein diet reinforced with vitamins. He is encouraged to be up and about to maintain good muscle tone. Blood tests, including sedimentation rate, are done. The patient is told that he will be required to cough postoperatively and that it may hurt to do so. He is also taught how to cough; the nurse emphasizes the importance of bringing up secretions. She also can tell him that he may be receiving oxygen therapy, and that this is routine to facilitate breathing. Also, blood transfusions may be given. He should know that such treatment does not necessarily mean that his condition is precarious.

Reduction of Organisms in Upper Respiratory Tract. MOUTH HYGIENE. Inasmuch as the mouth is a portal of entry for organisms into the respiratory tract, good oral care is a necessity. If the patient needs dental care, this should be reported to the physician. Brushing of the teeth must be done on rising in the morning, after each meal and before retiring.

POSTURAL DRAINAGE may be indicated in bronchiectasis and other chest conditions to bring up excess secretions. (See pp. 428-430.)

ANTIBIOTICS AND CHEMOTHERAPY. In addition to the above methods for reducing the number of organisms present, systemic antibiotic therapy and chemotherapy are used.

Immediate Preoperative Preparation. The night before surgery, the patient is given a mild sedative, after he has had the operative area shaved (see Fig. 39), and an enema, if ordered. The usual preparation immediately before surgery is done. In patients with suppurative diseases, atropine is withheld until postural drainage is done. Usually, chest surgical patients receive a larger amount of atropine than do abdominal surgical patients, so that secretions are minimized.

The anesthetic is administered by the endotracheal technic, and one anesthetic or a combination of anesthetic agents is used.

Operative Procedures

Pneumonectomy. The removal of an entire lung is done chiefly for cancer, but may be performed for extensive unilateral tuberculosis, multiple lung abscesses or bronchiectasis. A posterolateral or anterolateral thoracotomy incision is made with resection of one or two ribs. The pulmonary artery and the pulmonary vein are ligated and severed. The main bronchus is divided and sutured and the phrenic nerve on the involved side is crushed to allow the diaphragm to rise on the affected side so that the cavity that is left may be reduced.

Lobectomy. A lobe of lung is removed when the pathology is limited to this one area. This operation may be done for cysts, abscesses, benign tumors, tuberculosis or bronchiectasis. A thoracotomy incision is used, its exact location depending on the lobe to be resected. When the pleura is entered, the involved lung collapses and the main vessels and the bronchus are ligated and divided. After the lobe is removed, the remaining lobes of the lung are re-expanded. This patient usually has two chest catheters for drainage. The upper tube is for the removal of air; the lower one is for drainage of fluid.

Segmental Resection. Some lesions are confined to a segment of lung. Bronchopulmonary segments are subdivisions of the lung that function as individual units. They are held together by delicate connective tissue; disease processes may be limited to a single segment. Such an area can be removed, thereby allowing healthy functioning pulmonary tissue to remain. This is especially important in patients who have limited cardiorespiratory reserve; they need their undiseased segments.

A lingular segment of the upper lobe of left lung may have to be removed in which case the operation is called a *lingulectomy*.

Wedge Resection. This resection of a small, well-circumscribed lesion may be done without regard for the location of the intersegmental planes. The pleural cavity usually is drained because of the possibility of an air leak.

Postoperative Management

Reception of the Patient. During transfer of the patient to the recovery room or the patient's unit, it is extremely important to note that a patent airway is maintained. The patient usually is supine with his head turned to the side to allow for secretions to drain. Blood pressure, pulse and respirations are taken every 15 minutes for 2 or 3 hours, then at 30-minute intervals for the next several hours. Usually, these vital signs are taken hourly during the first night. Oxygen therapy is administered by tent or oropharyngeal catheter. It is used only as long as necessary. Beyond this time, it retards early ambulation and discourages coughing.

Position of the Patient. After the stabilization of the vital signs and the patient's return to consciousness, the head of his bed is elevated 30° to 45°. It is preferable not to use the Trendelenburg position, because the elevation of the diaphragm may interfere with ventilation. Adequate blood replacement usually takes care of shock. However, some surgeons feel that the Trendelenburg position should be used not only to combat shock but to facilitate postural drainage; therefore, the best advice is to check with

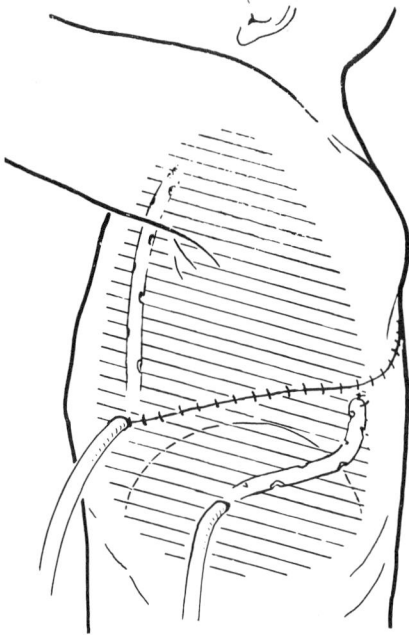

FIG. 133. Postoperative drainage of the chest. The upper drainage tube is used for the escape of air from leaks in the resected lung. The tip is anchored in the parietal pleura near the apex and brought out through the anterior end of the incision. The lower tube is usually for serosanguineous drainage. (Johnson, Julian, and Kirby, C. K.: Surgery of the Chest, p. 99, Chicago, Yr. Bk. Pub.)

the surgeon responsible for the particular patient.

The patient with a pneumonectomy should be turned hourly from the back to the operated side and not turned directly onto his unoperated side. Turning to the unoperated side is contraindicated because of the possibility of the spread of infection and additional strain on the already overtaxed remaining lung.

The patient with a lobectomy usually can be turned from the back to either side; however, some surgeons prefer that the patient not lie on the operated side so that optimum lung expansion can take place on that side.

For individuals who have had a segmental or a wedge resection, lying on the operated side is contraindicated, since it is desirable to have the remaining lung tissue on this side expand as much as possible.

Pain and the Use of Narcotics. Narcotics are used judiciously for these patients. Certainly their use must be individualized, for the threshold of pain varies from person to person. Many surgeons forbid the use of morphine in postoperative chest patients. On occasion, some of the intercostal nerves are injected or cut during the operation, thus reducing the problem of pain. The important point for the nurse to remember is that she wants her patient to be as comfortable as possible but does not want his cough reflex to be dulled.

Fluids and Nutrition. The patient usually receives a blood transfusion during the operation or immediately after it, and this is followed by infusion. The rate of flow should not be greater than 50 to 60 gtt./min. (unless ordered by the physician) because of the danger of pulmonary edema. The early symptoms of such a complication are cyanosis, dyspnea, rales and bubbling sounds in the chest, as well as frothy sputum. Such a condition must be reported to the physician immediately. Clear fluids may be given when the patient has responded to treatment and when no nausea is present. The next day and thereafter he may have solid foods as desired.

Adequate Air Exchange. Immediately after operation, many of these patients receive oxygen as a supportive measure. This

FIG. 134. (A) Water seal drainage alone has been found to be adequate in most patients. (B) Water seal suction may be used when a persistent air leak is present and cannot be controlled by drainage alone. (C) This demonstrates a useful arrangement for chest suction. The first trap bottle permits visualization of the fluid drainage. The second, in combination with the first bottle, can operate as a simple water seal. When the third bottle is added, the amount of suction can be measured by the depth of the tube under water. (Parts A & B are from: Blades, B.: Surgical Diseases of the Chest, p. 63, St. Louis, Mosby, 1961; (C) is from Roe, B. B.: The use and abuse of chest drainage, West. J. Surg., **61:**708, December, 1953)

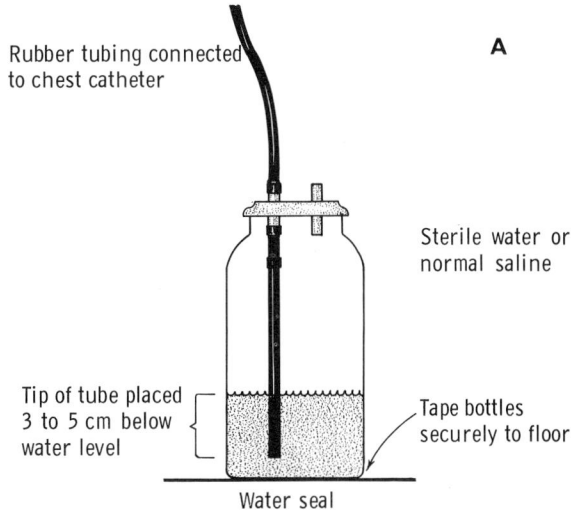

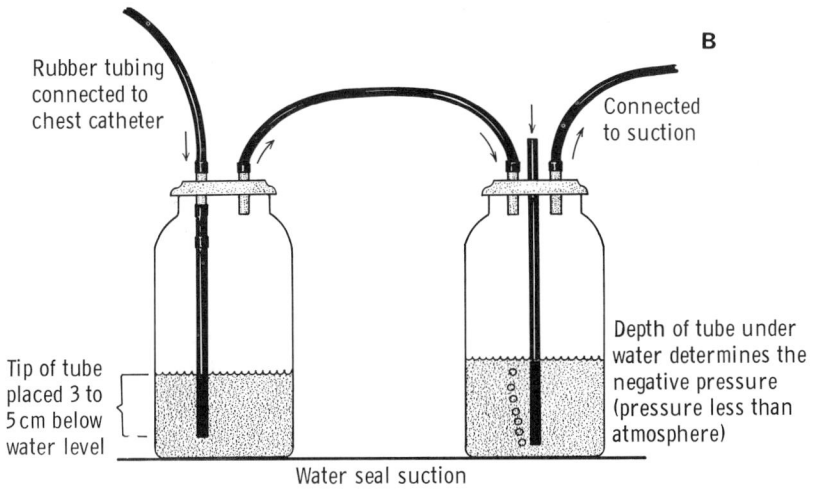

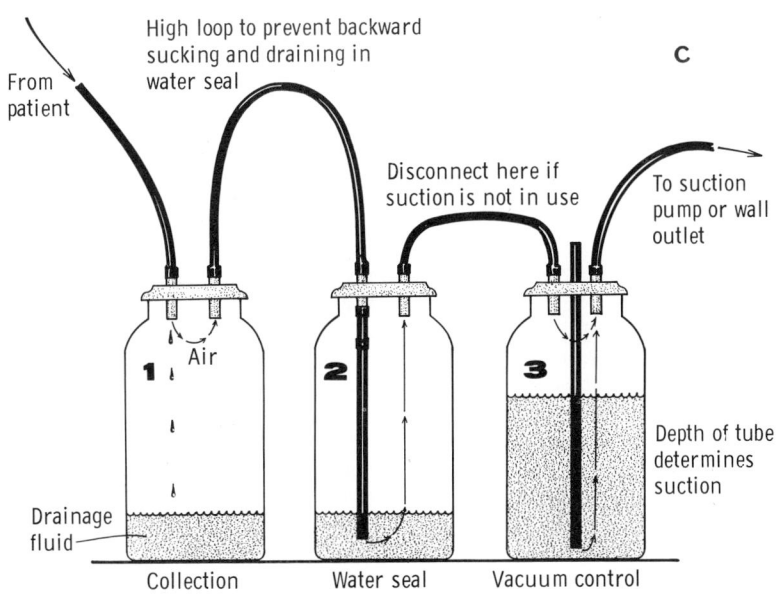

A

Rubber tubing connected to chest catheter

Sterile water or normal saline

Tip of tube placed 3 to 5 cm below water level

Tape bottles securely to floor

Water seal

B

Rubber tubing connected to chest catheter

Connected to suction

Tip of tube placed 3 to 5 cm below water level

Depth of tube under water determines the negative pressure (pressure less than atmosphere)

Water seal suction

C

High loop to prevent backward sucking and draining in water seal

From patient

Disconnect here if suction is not in use

To suction pump or wall outlet

Air

1

2

3

Depth of tube determines suction

Drainage fluid

Collection   Water seal   Vacuum control

GUIDE FOR THE USE OF WATER-SEALED CHEST DRAINAGE

PURPOSE:

An intrapleural drainage tube is used after any intrathoracic operative procedure. One or more chest catheters (usually No. 28 Fr. rubber tubes) are held in the pleural space in the posterior axillary line by suture to the chest wall. The purpose is:
1. To remove air and fluid from the thoracic cavity; and,
2. To facilitate re-expansion of the lung after surgery or trauma.

NURSING ACTIVITIES

Attach the drainage tube from the pleural cavity to tubing that leads to a long glass tube that ends under sterile water.

The glass tube should be approximately 1 inch below the water line. Mark the original fluid level on the bottle.

Fasten the tubing to the draw sheet so flow by gravity will occur. The tubing should not loop or interfere with movements of the patient.

Encourage good body alignment. When the patient is in the lateral position, place a sandbag on each side of the tubing to protect it from the weight of the patient's body.

Put the arm and the shoulder on the affected side through range-of-motion exercises several times daily.

"Milk" the tube at prescribed intervals.

Make sure that there is oscillation of fluid level in the tube:
  a. The oscillation of fluid level in the tube will stop when the lung has re-expanded.
  b. There may be cessation of oscillation before re-expansion due to blood clots and fibrin sealing off the tube.

Tape the part of the tube entering the drainage bottle to a tongue blade.

Encourage the patient to cough and deep-breathe.

Observe and report symptoms of respiratory embarrassment, pressure in the chest and symptoms of hemorrhage immediately.

Stabilize the drainage bottle within wooden blocks on the floor or in a special holder.

Caution visitors and personnel against handling equipment and/or displacing the bottle.

Clamp the patient's chest tube (close to the chest) immediately if the apparatus is damaged. Have this clamp available at the bedside at all times.

If the patient has to be transported to another area, place the drainage bottle below the chest level if he is lying on a stretcher and in his lap if he is in a wheelchair.

When assisting in removal of the tube:
  a. Give the analgesic as ordered as this is a moderately painful procedure.

RATIONALE UNDERLYING NURSING AND TREATMENT MEASURES:

Water-sealed drainage provides for the escape of air and fluid into a drainage bottle. The water acts as a seal and keeps air from being drawn back into the chest.

If the tube is submerged too deeply below the water level, a higher intrapleural pressure is required to expel air.

Kinking or looping or pressure on the drainage tubing can produce retrograde pressure, thus forcing drainage back into pleural cavity.

The patient's position should be changed frequently and the body kept in good alignment to prevent postural deformities and contractures.

Exercise helps to avoid ankylosis of the shoulder and assists in minimizing postoperative pain and discomfort.

"Milking" the tubes prevents them from becoming plugged with clots and fibrin.

Oscillation of the water level in the glass tube shows that there is effective communication between the pleural cavity and the drainage bottle.

Constant attention to maintain the patency of the tube will facilitate prompt expansion of the lung and minimize later complications.

This prevents kinking of the tube and resultant obstruction of drainage.

Coughing and deep breathing assist in raising the intrapleural pressure and in clearing the bronchi, expanding the lung and preventing atelectasis.

If any part of the apparatus is damaged, the closed system of drainage will be destroyed and the patient will be endangered by the attainment of atmospheric pressure in the pleural space and the resultant collapse of the lung.

The negative intrapleural pressure is not great enough to pull the fluid into the pleural cavity if the bottle is kept below the chest level.

During removal of the tube, the chief precaution is to avoid the entrance of air into the pleural cavity.

GUIDE FOR THE USE OF WATER-SEALED CHEST DRAINAGE *(Cont'd)*

NURSING ACTIVITIES *(Continued)*	RATIONAL UNDERLYING NURSING AND TREATMENT MEASURES: *(Continued)*
b. Ask the patient to exhale. The tube is withdrawn and a 2 x 2 gauze sponge is applied quickly and made air tight with snug-fitting adhesive.	
Wash hands thoroughly before and after handling the equipment.	Introduction of organisms during treatments can produce contamination of the pleural cavity.

is essential because of the diminished respiratory reserve due to decreased lung volume, blood loss and reduced blood pressure. The quality of respirations must be noted by the nurse. Dyspnea, cyanosis and acute chest pain suggest a tension pneumothorax and they should be reported immediately. The treatment would be an aspiration of the chest or thoracentesis, for which the nurse should be prepared.

The use of the blow bottle can be dangerous to a patient who has had extensive surgery because of the fear of blowing out a ligated section of the bronchial tree. Therefore, a blow bottle should be used only when it has been ordered specifically by the physician.

Suction and Drainage. Catheters are positioned strategically in the chest for postoperative connection to drainage bottles for two chief reasons: (1) to allow for the escape of air that otherwise might produce a pneumothorax, a shift of the mediastinum to the unoperated side or an emphysema and (2) to allow for the withdrawal of serosanguineous fluid (Figs. 133 and 134).

The important aspect of nursing attention is this: Be certain that the system is airtight and the tubes open. "Milking" the tubes will prevent plugging with clots or fibrin. Only enough suction tubing should be used to bridge the bottles and to extend to the wall and the patient, allowing leeway for the patient to turn. Excess tubing can be tripped over and often is caught behind the bed. A safety pin or a clip is effective in securing drainage tubing to the draw sheet; make sure that there are no kinks in the tubing. A trough can be made with the draw sheet so that the tubing is nestled and the safety pin does not constrict the tubing. Abdominal pads or small pillows around the tube to make a trough also will help.

The color, the consistency and the amount of drainage should be charted at least every 24 hours. In closed suction it is important to clamp the suction tubing before removing the drainage bottle to measure the contents.

Usually the catheters are removed in 2 or 3 days, providing that the remaining lung tissue is well expanded, that air leaks are eliminated and that the total fluid drainage is less than 75 ml. daily. Pneumonectomy patients usually do not have chest suction and drainage; however, if used, it is similar to that described above.

The Removal of Retained Secretions. This is undoubtedly the most important aspect of postoperative nursing care in the chest patient. It is imperative that he cough strongly enough to bring up secretions. He usually is taught to do this preoperatively and knows that he will have pain. The danger in retaining secretions is that of atelectasis and pneumonia. When mucus is thick and tenacious, inhalations of steam or bronchodilator aerosols may help. If the nurse is unsuccessful in getting her patient to bring up secretions or if he refuses to cough, an endotracheal aspiration must be done. Usually the surgeon does this; however, in many hospitals, this is becoming a nurse's responsibility.

Endotracheal Aspiration. A No. 16 rubber catheter, wall or electric suction, a square of gauze, tissue wipes and an emesis basin are all that is required for this procedure. The patient is instructed to sit upright. When he protrudes his tongue, it is grasped with a dry piece of gauze and pulled forward gently. Next, the tube is advanced through the nose until it reaches the glottis. Then the patient is instructed to inhale or cough, and the catheter is passed quickly into the trachea (Fig. 135). Inability of the patient to produce vocal sounds distinctly is the best evi-

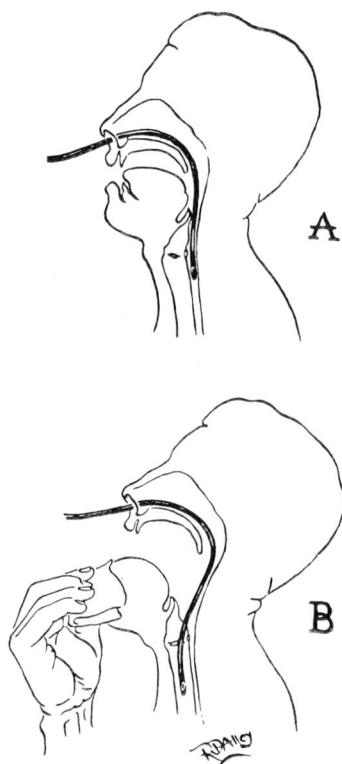

FIG. 135. Endotracheal aspiration. (A) Shows the tendency of the catheter normally to pass into the esophagus. (B) With the tongue and the epiglottis drawn forward, the plane of the glottic opening is more horizontally inclined, permitting ready passage of the catheter into the trachea. (Lindskog, G. E., and Liebow, A. A.: Thoracic Surgery and Related Pathology, p. 618, New York, Appleton)

the chest with the application of pads or a sandbag for further support. In some instances a type of skeletal traction may be employed to keep the chest wall from collapsing.

In general, the signs and the symptoms which should be reported to the surgeon immediately are cyanosis, dyspnea, pallor, acute chest pain, increase in pulse and respiratory rates, temperature elevation over 99° F., systolic blood pressure reading below 90 mm. and evidence of hemorrhage on the dressings.

Early Ambulation and Convalescence. If shock has been prevented adequately and the patient does not have heart disease or a limited cardiovascular reserve, he may get out of bed the evening of or the day after surgery. Drainage tubes and bottles may hinder this somewhat.

Breathing and postural exercises recommended by the surgeon and the physical therapist are begun a day or two after surgery to produce better lung ventilation, to restore motion and muscle tonus in the shoulder girdle and trunk and to maintain normal posture.

Roentgenograms are taken frequently to determine the patient's progress. If air or fluid accumulates in the chest, it will be necessary to aspirate by means of a thoracentesis.

For patients who have had surgery for lung cancer, the nurse will refer to the chapter on cancer nursing, p. 309.

Rehabilitative plans are made by the surgeon, the nurse, the patient, his family, the physical therapist and the medical social worker. The nurse will find the following points helpful in her suggestions to the patient:

1. Practice deep breathing exercises for the first few weeks at home.

2. Practice good body alignment by standing up straight with shoulders held back (preferably in front of a full-length mirror).

dence that the catheter is in the trachea. Then the catheter is connected to gentle suction. The catheter should be moved slowly up and down the trachea. The chief value of endotracheal aspiration is that it stimulates the cough reflex and produces violent coughing.

Complications. The nurse should be alert for *atelectasis* (page 406), *emphysema* (page 432), and *tension pneumothorax* (page 442). In patients from whom three or more ribs have been removed, there is a possibility of paradoxical chest motion.

Paradoxical chest motion (Fig. 136) can occur when the integrity of any portion of the thoracic bellows is lost, such as multiple rib fractures or removal of several ribs as in a thoracoplasty. The nurse should observe chest movements of her thoracic surgical patients. When she detects paradoxical motion, she should report it immediately, for if uncorrected, it may result in serious respiratory and circulatory impairment. Treatment usually consists of firm adhesive strapping of

FIG. 136. (A and B) Normally, on inspiration all portions of the thoracic cage move outward, and the diaphragms move downward. Motion is in the opposite direction on expiration. (C and D) When a portion of the chest wall becomes flexible as a result of losing its bony support, motion of the flexible area is controlled by the changing intrapleural pressures and is in a direction opposite to that of the normal positions of the chest wall. (Johnson, Julian, and Kirby, C. K.: Surgery of the Chest, p. 21, Chicago, Yr. Bk. Pub.)

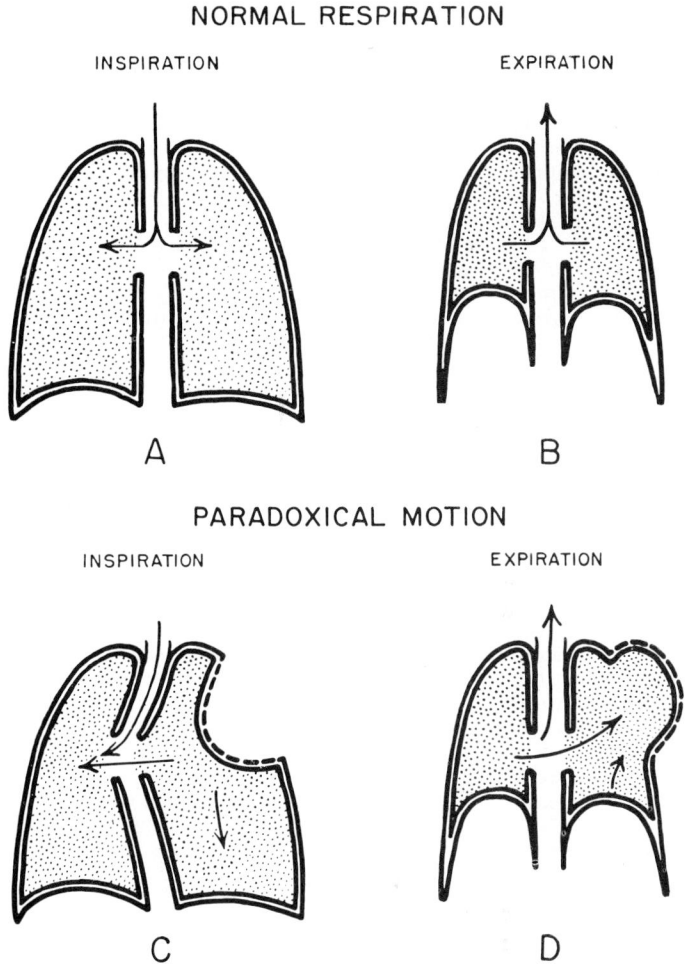

NORMAL RESPIRATION

INSPIRATION

EXPIRATION

A

B

PARADOXICAL MOTION

INSPIRATION

EXPIRATION

C

D

3. Practice exercises that he did while in the hospital.

4. Practice good oral hygiene by brushing teeth well and visiting his dentist frequently.

5. Remain away from crowds during upper respiratory epidemics.

6. Seek medical attention at the onset of an upper respiratory infection.

7. Avoid areas where the air is filled with dust, smoke, and irritating chemicals.

8. Avoid anything that may cause spasms of coughing.

9. Maintain good nutrition.

10. Obtain adequate rest.*

* Adapted from Bickford, E., and Budd, E.: Pulmonary resection. 2. Nursing care, Am. J. Nurs. **52**:40-43, 1952.

Rehabilitation of the Chest Patient

Rehabilitation should begin when the patient seeks help; consequently, rehabilitation measures are an integral part of his therapeutic program. Basic rehabilitation measures that are applicable to most patients with pulmonary conditions include (1) the promotion of an effective cough routine (see page 403); (2) activities to improve the efficiency of pulmonary function; and (3) skeletal exercises for the retraining of injured muscles and the prevention of deformities. The rehabilitation program is designed and adjusted to meet the needs of each individual patient. The nurse or the therapist observes the patient closely during his exercise program in order to evaluate his ability to toler-

SUMMARY OF THE MEDICAL AND NURSING MANAGEMENT
OF THE CHEST-SURGERY PATIENT

PREOPERATIVE OBJECTIVES: To ensure optimum patient condition for surgery.

I. *To improve ventilatory function:*
   A. Institute breathing exercises to improve respiratory efficiency.
   B. Improve condition of patients who have impaired pulmonary function.
      1. Administer Intermittent Positive Pressure Breathing treatments (page 435) and bronchodilating drugs.
      2. Control infections with antibiotics.

II. *To minimize pulmonary secretions:*
   A. Eliminate smoking to reduce pulmonary irritation.
   B. Maintain schedule of oral hygiene to reduce bacterial flora in mouth.
   C. Treat existing infections if present.
      1. Antibiotic therapy.
      2. Postural drainage to facilitate removal of secretions.
   D. Provide adequate hydration to reduce viscosity of secretions.

III. *To prepare the patient for the surgical experience by reassurance and explanation:*
   A. Orient the patient to the postoperative period.
      1. Function of the chest tube.
      2. Cough routine.
      3. Type of incision.
      4. Breathing and exercise program.
      5. Control of pain.
      6. Oxygen tent.
      7. Blood transfusion.
   B. Encourage expression of psychological and safety needs.

POSTOPERATIVE OBJECTIVES: To restore normal function as early as possible.

I. *To ensure proper expansion of the lung:*
   A. Promote coughing to clear airway.
   B. Water-sealed chest drainage to remove air and fluid from chest.
   C. Frequent changing of position to mobilize secretions.
   D. Breathing exercises to aid lung re-expansion.
   E. Careful pain control to facilitate coughing and deep breathing.
   F. Removal of tracheobronchial secretions if patient is unable to clear airway.
      1. Nasotracheal suction (mechanical stimulation of cough).
      2. Bronchoscopy.
      3. Tracheostomy.

II. *To restore normal range of motion and function of shoulder and trunk:*
   A. Skeletal exercises to promote abduction and mobilization of shoulder.
   B. Breathing exercises to immobilize the thorax.
   C. Ambulate as soon as pulmonary and circulatory systems are compensated.
   D. Encourage progressive activities according to development of fatigue.

III. *To anticipate and forestall possible complications:*
   A. Hypotension (during immediate postoperative period).
      1. Evaluate blood pressure and pulse carefully.
      2. Measure urinary volume.
      3. Have blood replacement available.
   B. Cardiac arrhythmias.
      1. Apical and radial pulse measurements.
      2. Have digitalis or quinidine available.
   C. Hemorrhage.
      1. Evaluate vital signs.
      2. Evaluate chest drainage.
      3. Have blood replacement available.
   D. Atelectasis.
      1. Prepare for bronchoscopic aspiration.
      2. Have oxygen available.
   E. Acute pulmonary edema.
      1. Careful regulation of intravenous fluids.
      2. Have parenteral digitalis, diuretics, and rotating tourniquet setup available.
   F. Respiratory insufficiency.
      1. Place patient in respirator for assisted ventilation.
      2. Prepare for tracheostomy.

ate the prescribed activity and evaluate his progress.

Promotion of Respiratory Efficiency

Patients with pulmonary problems should be maintained in correct recumbent, sitting and standing postures. Only one pillow should be permitted. The shoulders should be level, the hips and the shoulders aligned to prevent scoliosis.

Breathing Exercises. The rate, the depth and the rhythm of respirations are affected by the patient's emotional state. Many of these patients are anxious and apprehensive. Their tension causes further respiratory impairment, as tension and muscular stress increase metabolic demand. Assisting the patient to relax is part of the therapeutic program. Instruct him to contract and relax his muscles consciously without moving the part. (This is a form of isometric exercise: muscle relaxation and contraction affected without joint movement.) For example: "Contract the muscle of your left hand, let go, relax."

The purpose of breathing exercises is to obtain full movement of the diaphragm and to assist in lung re-expansion.

EXAMPLE: Place the patient in a recumbent position. Place one of his hands on his abdomen and the other on his upper chest. Instruct him to inhale through his nose, raising his abdomen against his hand. Exhale while pursing the lips and contracting the abdominal muscles, moving the abdomen inward. The chest should not move.

The contraction of the abdomen and the expiratory muscles against increased pressure obtained from pursed-mouth breathing assists in emptying the lungs and aids in the elevation of the diaphragm. As the patient is increasingly able to tolerate this exercise, 8 to 10 pounds of sandbags can be placed on his abdomen to increase the intra-abdomi-

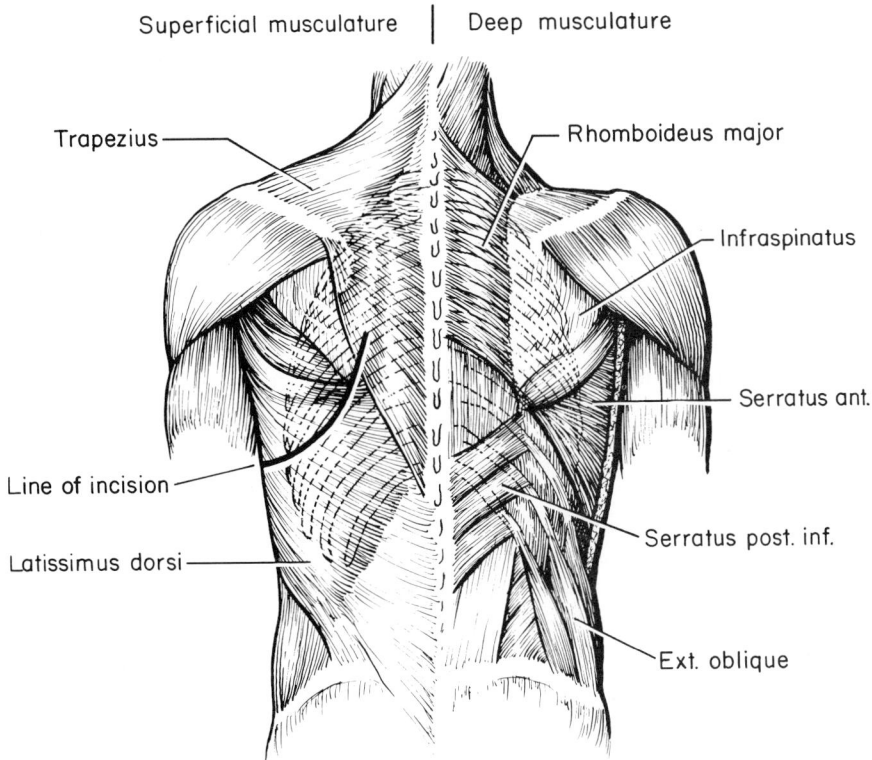

FIG. 137. Muscles affected by thoracotomy. Rehabilitation should be planned in relation to the action of the muscle involved.

Muscle Affected by Thoracotomy	Function	Activities to Restore Function
Trapezius	Promotes arm extension, abduction and reach extension.	Extend the arm up and back, out to the side and back, down at the side and back.
Rhomboideus major	Adducts and slightly elevates scapula.	Place hands in small of back. Push elbows as far back as possible.
Latissimus dorsi	Depresses the shoulder.	Sit erect in an armchair; place the hands on the arms of the chair directly opposite either side of the body. Press down on hands, consciously pulling the abdomen in and stretching up from the waist. Inhale while raising the body until the elbows are extended completely. Hold this position a moment, and begin exhaling while lowering the body slowly to the original position.
Serratus anterior	Rotates scapula and fixes it against the rib cage.	Reach over head and "push" in an upward and outward motion.

nal pressure. This aids exhalation. The exercise is repeated 10 to 15 times and is performed at least 3 times daily.

Patients with emphysema have air trapped in the alveoli. Therefore they are encouraged to inhale quickly and exhale slowly. Raising the arms during inspiration and returning them to the sides while tightening the abdominal muscles during exhalation will also improve expiration.

Skeletal Exercises. Figure 137 shows the muscles that are affected by the most common thoracic surgical procedures. In order to perform chest surgery, the muscle groups that make up the shoulder girdle and maintain trunk posture are transected. If the muscles on one side of the body are affected, the contralateral muscles (those on the other side) become stronger and can produce deformity.

The patient's joint range should be measured preoperatively to help to determine the postoperative goal. The patient needs to be reassured that the exercises will help to prevent deformity of the trunk and the upper extremities. Other objectives of skeletal exercises before and after thoracic surgical procedures are to assist in maintaining a normal range of motion of the involved joints, to gain maximum pulmonary function and to improve the patient's posture.

The patient's shoulder should be taken through a full range of motion on the operative side in order to prevent frozen shoulder. The nurse should do this several times daily. It is desirable for the patient to participate in this activity at least 6 times daily as soon as his condition permits.

The exercises shown above may be done by the patient as soon as the surgeon permits. They should be stopped as soon as pain and fatigue begin. Other activities may be added as the patient's condition improves and he is ready for them.

When the patient is able to perform these exercises without shortness of breath, he can progress from lying to sitting, then to standing and walking posture. Bending forward while walking helps forced expirations. Each procedure is introduced in sequence. The patient should be shown the exercise, encouraged to practice it with supervision, and then instructed to rest. A patient with a productive cough should evacuate his sputum before beginning the exercises. Breathing exercises will not only strengthen the diaphragm, the lower rib cage and the abdominal muscles, but also they will help the patient to increase his activities gradually without shortness of breath. The emphasis on any breathing exercises should be placed on improving expiration.

THE PATIENT WITH A PULMONARY INFECTION

Acute Tracheobronchitis

An acute inflammation of the mucous membranes of the trachea and the bronchial tree, acute tracheobronchitis often follows infections of the upper respiratory tract. A patient with a viral infection has a lessened resistance and can readily develop a secondary bacterial infection. The adequate treatment of upper respiratory infections is one of the major factors in the prevention of acute bronchitis. Inhalation of physical and chemical irritants, gases, or other air contaminants is also an important cause of acute bronchial irritations.

The patient's symptoms result from the mucopurulent sputum that is secreted by the hyperemic edematous mucosa of the bronchi. The patient has a dry, irritating cough and expectorates a scanty amount of mucoid sputum at first. He complains of sternal soreness from coughing, has fever, headache and general malaise. As the infection progresses, the sputum is more profuse and purulent, and the cough becomes looser. Acute tracheobronchitis can be a serious disease in very young children. The child is acutely ill and may have noisy strident respirations with intercostal retraction. Strict nursing vigilance and prompt action are required if these symptoms of respiratory obstruction appear.

Medical and Nursing Management. The treatment is largely symptomatic. Therefore, the nurse's observations are important in determining the therapeutic plan. The patient is placed on bed rest. Moist heat to the chest will relieve the soreness and pain, and hot drinks may prove soothing. Cool vapor therapy or steam inhalations are beneficial in relieving the laryngeal and tracheal irritation. Increasing the vapor pressure (moisture content) in the air will reduce irritation.

Cough depressants should not be given, or given only with caution, when the cough becomes productive. An expectorant, such as potassium iodide, may be given and the fluid intake increased to "thin" the viscous and tenacious secretions. Usually recovery will ensue within 7 to 10 days. Antibacterial chemotherapy may be ordered if the patient does not improve promptly.

A primary nursing function is to caution the patient against overexertion and chilling, which can induce a relapse or extension of the infection. Aged individuals are prone to develop bronchopneumonia as a complication. They are not always able to cough effectively and therefore tend to retain the mucopurulent exudate. These patients should be turned and should assume the sitting position at frequent intervals. Adequate opportunity for convalescence should be provided after the acute infection subsides, in order to avoid its recurrence.

Chronic Bronchitis

Chronic bronchitis is a progressive and potentially serious disease. The patient's major problem is the protracted and abundant production of inflammatory exudate that fills and obstructs his bronchioles and is responsible for his persistent, productive cough and shortness of breath. Alveoli adjacent to the affected bronchioles may

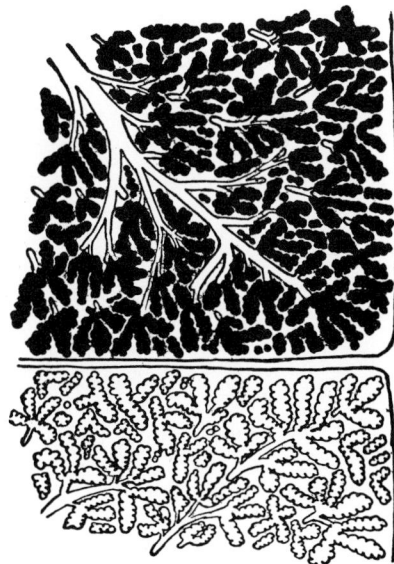

FIG. 138. The adjacent margins of two lobes of the lung. The lower lobe is normal; the upper is the seat of a lobar pneumonia. Note that the air cells are filled by the exudate, but the bronchi are free.

become damaged and fibrosed. In time, irreversible lung changes may occur, with resultant emphysema or bronchiectasis.

This disorder may follow an acute respiratory infection, such as pneumonia or influenza. It is encountered in individuals whose occupation exposes them to irritating gases and smoke. Heavy tobacco smokers exhibit a high incidence of chronic bronchitis. The disease is most prevalent among middle-aged and elderly men—individuals who are especially vulnerable to recurrent attacks of acute bronchitis.

Because of the disabling nature of chronic bronchitis, the nurse should direct every effort toward its prevention. All patients with acute upper respiratory infections should receive proper treatment and adequate convalescence. Symptomatic individuals should stop smoking; air irritants of other types should be avoided whenever possible.

The main objective in the treatment of chronic bronchitis is the control of acute infections that threaten the lungs. Patients who are especially vulnerable should receive appropriate antimicrobial chemotherapy in the early stage of every febrile respiratory infection. To facilitate the removal of bronchial exudates, and to supply aerosolized medication most effectively, intermittent positive pressure breathing (page 435) may be instituted. In some cases that are complicated by an underlying bronchiectasis, postural drainage is beneficial. Basically, the medical treatment and the nursing management of patients who have chronic bronchitis or pulmonary emphysema (page 432) are very similar.

Pneumonia

The term *pneumonia* refers to a partial solidification of the lung, due to the filling of the alveoli with an inflammatory exudate in response to an infection or, less commonly, to a chemical irritant. Pneumonia is classified according to its causative agent, if known: for example, as a *bacterial, viral,* or *lipid pneumonia.* If a substantial portion of

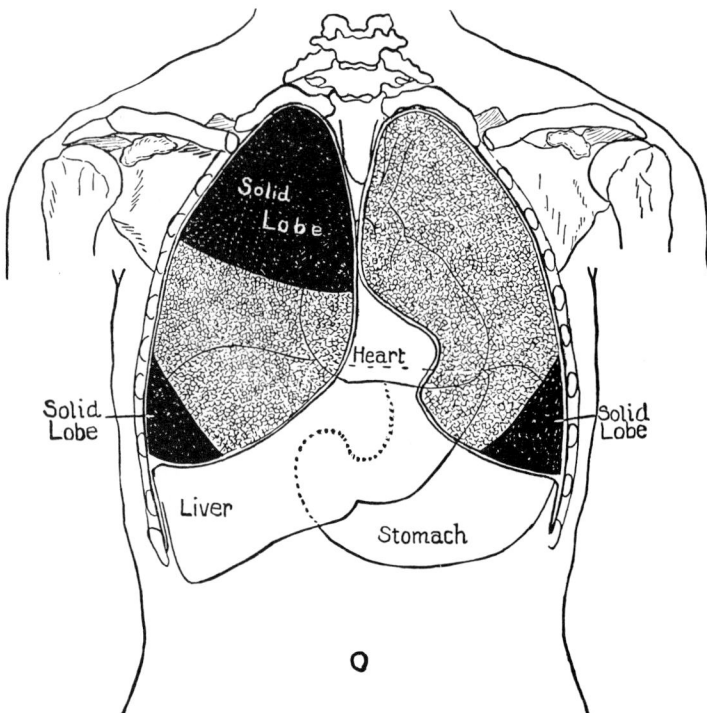

FIG. 139. Lungs with pneumonia involving the right upper and lower and the left lower lobes. (Only the tips of the lower lobes can be seen in a front view such as this.)

one or more lobes is involved, the disease is referred to as *lobar pneumonia*. *Bronchopneumonia* implies that the pneumonic process is distributed in patchy fashion, having originated in one or more localized areas within the bronchi and extended to the adjacent lung parenchyma.

Prevention. The nurse should be acquainted with various factors and circumstances that commonly predispose to the development of pneumonia, so that she may be alert to the possibility of its occurrence and assist most effectively in its prevention. Aged individuals, patients with chronic bronchitis or emphysema, patients with cardiac failure and pulmonary congestion, and patients who are debilitated are prime candidates for pneumonia. Individuals who are intoxicated chronically are peculiarly susceptible to this infection and, if acquired, the course of pneumonia in the alcoholic patient is likely to be unusually severe.

Any patient who is permitted to lie passively for prolonged periods in bed, relatively immobile and breathing shallowly, is highly vulnerable to the risk of bronchopneumonia. The likelihood of its development is increased markedly if the patient is unable to cough effectively because of debility, prostration or shock, or as a result of sedation with a cough-suppressing drug. Any condition that promotes the retention of secretions in the bronchi predisposes to pneumonia. Aspiration of foreign material into the lungs during a period of unconsciousness, e.g., during anesthesia, is very likely to be followed by bronchopneumonia.

Bronchopneumonia, as a postoperative complication, is a potential threat in every case. There is a danger that the patient's cough reflex may be overly suppressed by drug sedation, or that coughing may be inhibited by the production of pain at the operative site. In the latter instance, the patient should be encouraged to cough as vigorously as possible while the nurse "splints" his incision in the manner illustrated in Figure 131. Any patient scheduled to receive a sedative drug, particularly one of the opium alkaloids, should be observed closely from the standpoint of respiratory rate and depth before the drug is given; and

its administration should be withheld if respiratory depression is apparent, for respiratory depression predisposes to the pooling of bronchial secretions and, therefore, to the development of pneumonia. Postoperative pneumonia should be anticipated in the elderly patient and its development forestalled by frequent changes of his position. The observation of slow and shallow breathing may warrant the repeated administration, to such a patient, of carbon dioxide at hourly intervals or oftener. An important prophylactic measure, which is widely applicable, is the frequent suctioning of secretions from the mouths of patients who are unconscious or otherwise helpless, thereby reducing the likelihood that this material may be aspirated, accumulate in the lungs and induce bronchopneumonia.

Bacterial Pneumonia

Etiology. Bacterial pneumonia is most prevalent during the winter and spring months, when upper respiratory infections are most common.

The infecting agents most often responsible for this disease are the *pneumococci,* capsulated diplococci, of which there are at least 35 distinct immunologic types. Some of these predominate in certain localities at certain seasons, some are almost certain constant inhabitants of the normal upper respiratory tract. Organisms much less frequently involved include *Staphylococcus aureus, Klebsiella pneumoniae (Bacillus mucosus-capsulatus,* Friedländer's bacillus), *Streptococcus hemolyticus,* and *Hemophilus influenzae.*

Symptoms and Signs. The onset of acute pneumococcal pneumonia is precipitous. Previously well, the patient is suddenly prostrated by a sharp pain in the chest which prevents him from taking a deep breath. He is seized with a severe chill. The temperature rises rapidly and within a few hours reaches a level of 104° to 106° F. The pulse is rapid and bounding. The cheeks are flushed, the eyes bright and the lips cyanotic. The respiration is rapid; the nostrils dilate with each inspiration, and each expiration is punctuated with a grunt. The dyspnea may become extreme, and, although not truly orthopneic, the patient prefers to be propped up in bed because of his cough, which is short, painful and incessant.

The mental symptoms may be so pronounced as to overshadow all others, dominating the clinical picture completely. The patient may exhibit a restless, excited delirium. In such patients, who can least afford a delay in treatment, the diagnosis of pneumonia may be overlooked for a time, unless the nurse is unusually observant and alert to spot whatever clue might be at hand, such as a fleck of bloody sputum on the bedclothes or a transient chill.

Initially, the sputum may be clear; occasionally it is frankly bloody. But eventually, in the typical case, it becomes rusty in color and so tenacious that it can be expectorated only with such difficulty that the nurse may be obliged to wipe it from the mouth. (The nurse is reminded to adhere to the principles of medical asepsis in caring for these patients.) Bacteriologic examination of this material reveals the infective agent.

The blood leukocyte count usually becomes elevated during the first or second day, ranging during the acute stages from 20,000 to 30,000 per cubic millimeter, a finding which is a great help in diagnosis. The blood culture frequently is positive in the early stages before therapy is begun.

Treatment and Nursing Management. If the patient with bacterial pneumonia is treated promptly and appropriately, the infection, in most cases, is controlled quickly. Antimicrobial chemotherapy is instituted without delay, usually in the form of penicillin administered by intramuscular injection. Depending on the identity of the infecting organism isolated from the sputum, throat or blood cultures, and its drug sensitivity, as determined *in vitro* in the microbiology laboratory, another antibiotic or a sulfonamide drug may be substituted for penicillin.

The patient is placed on bed rest until the infection shows signs of clearing. Although specific isolation precautions generally are unnecessary, visitors should be restricted to members of the immediate family. The arrangement of the bed should provide maximum comfort and optimum respiratory efficiency, the orthopneic or semi-orthopneic position being preferred if dyspnea is severe. The least possible disturbance should attend the treatments and examinations that are carried out during the early, acute stage of the illness. The patient must be protected from drafts and, as a further precaution against chilling, dry linen should be substituted at once for garments or bedding dampened by perspiration.

OXYGEN. Oxygen inhalation therapy is indicated if the patient is cyanotic, dyspneic, or complains of pain on breathing, or if breathing appears to require undue effort. Under these conditions an oxygen tent or mask offers more than physiologic support: it brings both relief from pain and rest.

ANALGESIC AND ANTITUSSIVE MEDICATION. Codeine sulfate or Hycodan will alleviate the harrassing cough and reduce the pain of pleurisy. If pain is severe, Demerol may be given subcutaneously in 50- to 100-mg. doses at intervals of 4 to 6 hours; morphine, on the other hand, because of its suppressive action on the respiratory center, generally is considered as being contraindicated in patients with acute pneumonia.

The antipyretic drugs are useful in controlling general malaise and muscular pains; on the other hand, if the temperature is markedly elevated, the diaphoretic (sweat stimulating) action of these agents may only add to his discomfort. It must not be forgotten that numerous physical devices are available which may be as efficacious as the analgesic drugs and at the same time lack their undesirable side-effects; for example, the febrile patient with pneumonia may obtain quite as effective relief from tepid sponges as with any of the drugs previously enumerated.

The combination of oxygen deficiency, high fever and toxicity associated with pneumonia may precipitate an acute anxiety state, delirium or disorientation. Should the patient develop these symptoms, sedation, possibly in the form of intramuscular paraldehyde (6 to 10 ml.) may be ordered. Tepid sponges will exert a quieting effect and tend to reduce the fever. Restraints should be avoided; an excited patient will resist these vigorously, with the result that he may become thoroughly exhausted and severely febrile. Quiet conversation with the patient, arranging for a member of his family to stay with him or allowing him to sit in a chair often will help him through this phase.

ANTIDISTENTION THERAPY. Abdominal distention is a frequent complication of pneumonia in severely toxic cases. It is not merely a source of great discomfort, but it impairs the efficiency of respiration by elevating the diaphragm and limiting its excursion. Measures indicated for its relief include the repeated administration of small saline enemas (2 pints), the insertion of a rectal tube, the application of moist heat to the abdominal wall and the subcutaneous injection of Prostigmin methylsulfate or Prostigmin bromide (0.5 to 1.0 mg. given at 4-hour intervals).

SOPORIFICS. Chloral hydrate is perhaps the least objectionable of all hypnotic agents in treating patients with acute pneumonia; mental aberrations due to cerebral hypoxia are less apt to occur in patients treated with this soporific than with other drugs in common use. The barbiturates are efficacious and likewise without ill effect in the majority of patients.

NUTRITION. The food selection for patients with pneumonia is limited to liquids and soft solid foods of high caloric value until the appetite is restored and a more liberal regimen is possible.

HYDRATION. Adequate hydration is important during the febrile period, when evaporation of moisture from the skin is increased. Adequate hydration is also of value in the stimulation of respiratory tract secretion. Milk, because of its nutritious qualities, is especially recommended; its caloric value may be increased by the addition of lactose, which cannot ferment in the gastrointestinal tract and, therefore, does not contribute to abdominal distention.

Patients with pneumonia complicated by congestive heart failure must not receive an unlimited quantity of fluids, and the sodium intake must be curtailed rigidly. Hydration of these patients demands the most careful supervision, for there is grave danger that fluid will accumulate to dangerous excess in the tissues, particularly in the lungs, producing pulmonary edema and, quite possibly, death.

ELIMINATION. The use of cathartics is rarely warranted in pneumonia, fecal retention being avoided quite readily in most patients by means of low saline enemas.

MOUTH CARE. Cleansing of the mouth, with particular attention to the tongue and the lips, should be performed conscientiously as long as the patient is febrile and dehydrated and the sputum is purulent. The importance of oral hygiene is even greater if there are herpetic sores about the mouth, which cause a great deal of discomfort in a high proportion of pneumonia patients.

COMMUNICABLE DISEASE PRECAUTIONS. Measures to prevent the spread of the patient's infection should be carried out by the nurse with all due sense of responsibility. The infective organisms can become disseminated by means of air-borne droplets or through contact with articles contaminated by the patient's respiratory secretions. The hands should be washed thoroughly after each manual contact with the patient or his immediate environs. Mouth wipes, paper bags and disposable sputum cups should be used exclusively and should be wrapped securely and burned without delay. The patient should be instructed to turn away from those at his bedside while coughing. The risk of contagion, regardless of the type of pneumonia or the stage of treatment, cannot be neglected as long as fever persists.

In so far as it is possible, visitors should be excluded during this phase, and any who are admitted should receive instructions regarding protective measures to be adopted.

Clinical Examinations and Records. The temperature, the pulse and the respiration should be examined at 4-hour intervals, and the blood pressure should be measured at least once daily during the acute stage; these data should be charted promptly and the record kept easily accessible at all times. Included on the chart should be data relative to the daily fluid intake and the number of stools each day.

Diagnostic Tests. In addition to routine blood, urine and stool examinations, blood cultures are taken and sputum specimens collected for bacteriologic study. It is essential that the sputum obtained for laboratory examination consist of material that is coughed from the depth of the bronchial tree and diluted as little as possible by saliva. If coughing is inhibited by pleural pain, the maneuver may be assisted by turning the patient on the affected side. An x-ray examination of the chest is indicated in every patient as soon as it can be performed. Personnel assigned to take portable bedside roentgenograms should be acquainted with the risk of infection and properly versed in the protective methods to be followed. An electrocardiogram also may be requested if the character or the rate of the pulse is abnormal or if there is any evidence of heart disease from the past history or the physical examination.

Complications. A spread of the pneumonic process or its failure to resolve may occur if the lungs are invaded by a species of bacteria against which the patient has not acquired an adequate immunity. Another explanation for these complications is the development, by the bacteria, of an acquired resistance to the particular agent that is employed in therapy, the effectiveness of which for that organism is, therefore, lost. Fortunately, however, bacterial resistance does not extend to all drugs and antibiotics that are available, and cure usually can be obtained by means of a suitable substitution of another agent.

Empyema, an accumulation of infected fluid in the pleural space, is now a relatively uncommon development with the advent of modern therapy. Its treatment and prevention are accomplished by chemotherapy alone, unless the empyema fluid is unusually viscid, in which case thoracotomy and mechanical drainage may also be required.

Septicemia following invasion of the blood stream may result in meningitis, endocarditis, purulent arthritis or other localized infections. A pneumococcal infection may invade one of the paranasal sinuses, causing acute sinusitis, or it may enter the middle ear, resulting in acute otitis media. All infectious complications of pneumonia, as mentioned above, are entirely preventable and responsive to treatment with the same type of specific therapy that is effective in clearing the antecedent pneumonic process.

Atelectasis, "collapse" of the lung, is perhaps the most important of the non-infectious complications of pneumonia. It is caused by the obstruction of a bronchus with accumulated secretions which fail to be expelled before all of the alveolar air in the distal portion of the lung has been absorbed completely by the blood stream. This complication is prevented by avoiding unnecessary sedation of the patient, so that the cough reflex never is greatly impaired, and by wisdom in the restriction of his activity so that he is never too immobile or immobilized for too long a period while acutely ill.

The appearance of *shock* in a patient with pneumonia is an ominous development. This complication is encountered chiefly in patients who have received no specific treatment; have been treated too little or too late; have received chemotherapy to which the infecting organism is resistant; or whose pneumonia is complicated by another debilitating illness. To combat peripheral collapse and maintain the arterial blood pressure, a vasoconstrictor agent such as Metaraminol bitartrate is given intravenously in the form of a constant infusion, and at a rate that is readjusted constantly in accordance with the pressure response. Corticosteroid drugs, such as hydrocortisone or dexamethasone, may be administered parenterally to combat shock and toxicity in patients with pneumonia who are extremely ill and in apparent danger of succumbing to the infection.

Primary Atypical Pneumonia (Viral pneumonia; acute interstitial pneumonitis)

Primary atypical pneumonia is an acute respiratory disease characterized by the appearance of an inflammatory pulmonary infiltration. It is generally believed to be viral in origin although no specific agent has been demonstrated. The inflammatory process spreads throughout the entire respiratory tract including the bronchioles. Generally it has the characteristics of a bronchopneumonia.

Usually the patient has had an upper respiratory infection, and the onset of his pneumonic symptoms is gradual. The predominant symptom is a harrassing and non-productive cough. After a few days, mucoid or mucopurulent sputum is expectorated.

Fig. 140. Diagram of the chest of a patient with pleurisy with effusion (on the right side). Note that the lung above the fluid is compressed, the heart and the trachea are pushed to the left, and the liver is lower than normal.

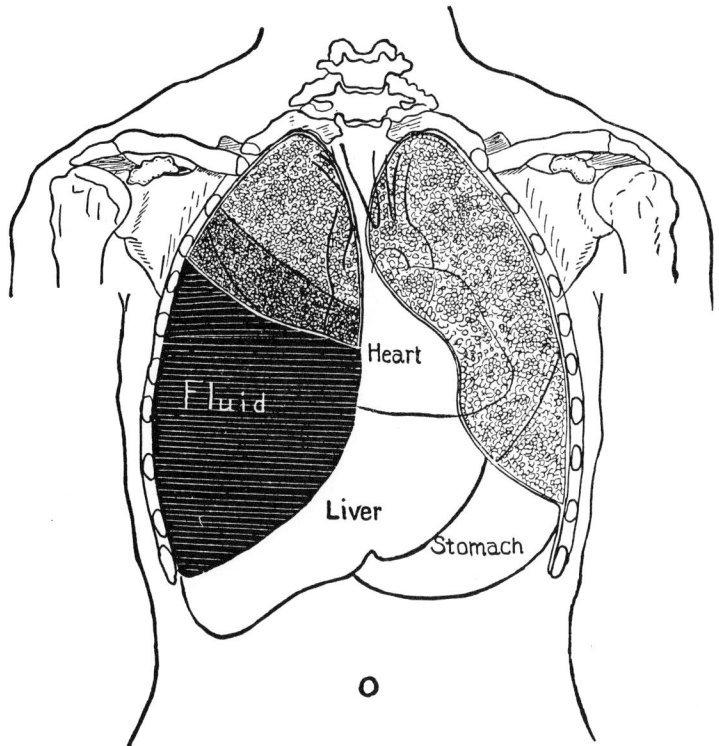

The patient complains of headache that is aggravated by the cough. Malaise, chilliness, and fatigue are present. There is moderate remittent fever that clears over a period of days, rather than hours. The temperature falls by lysis. The acute stage of the illness runs its course over a 1- to 3-week period. The patient's convalescence usually is prolonged.

The diagnosis of primary atypical pneumonia is frequently uncertain. Therefore, the nurse's observations are especially important. Although no specific laboratory test exists for viral pneumonia, in over one-half of the patients cold hemagglutinins will appear in the patient's serum sometime during the course of the illness, probably reflecting an immune response.

The objective of nursing care is to promote the patient's rest and comfort. He should be placed in a single room and protected from activities that produce fatigue. At this time there is no specific treatment for viral diseases of the respiratory tract, but it must be kept in mind that the patient can have a mixed infection. The tetracycline drugs sometimes are given to patients who have a prolonged febrile course. The nursing care and treatment (with the exception of antibacterial therapy) is the same as that given to the patient who has a bacterial pneumonia.

Pleurisy

If a small area of pleural surface becomes infected, each breath at once becomes painful; hence, the patient, in order to diminish the rubbing movement of these two surfaces, holds that side as quiet as he can and takes the shallowest breaths possible. Since the inflamed area is covered by a thin sheet of fibrin, this disease is called *fibrinous* (or dry) *pleurisy*.

Symptoms. Fibrinous pleurisy usually begins with a chill and fever, a sharp cutting pain on each deep breath, often called a *stitch in the side,* and a short, painful, nonproductive cough. These symptoms may continue for a few hours or days. Many cases are tuberculous in origin, pleurisy often being the patient's first evidence of this disease. Pleurisy also occurs in association with lobar pneumonia and pulmonary infarcts. Careful x-ray and sputum examinations are indicated in order to discover the underlying condition.

Treatment and Nursing Care. The patient should be kept at bed rest until the fever subsides and as comfortable as possible with such agents and devices as those discussed in relation to the bacterial pneumonias, depending on the specific indications in each particular case. Inasmuch as this patient has real pain on inspiration, the nurse can offer suggestions to make him more comfortable. Instruct him to lie on the affected side in order to splint the chest wall; this will lessen the stretch of the pleura. The nurse or the patient can use the hand to splint the rib cage when the patient must cough. Often he is apprehensive and needs empathy and the comfort measures that the nurse can provide. Patients with an apparently spontaneous fibrinous pleurisy should be treated with a view to preventing the further development of any tuberculosis present.

Pleural Effusions

Pleurisy with effusion sometimes begins as a fibrinous pleurisy, but in the majority of patients the onset is so insidious that the patient scarcely realizes its presence. Gradually he becomes pale, short of breath, easily fatigued, loses weight and strength and, sometimes, but not always, has a slight dry cough. Many a person with such symptoms continues at work until he is so tired that he must stop, whereupon the doctor often finds one of the pleural cavities almost full of fluid (Fig. 140).

This type of pleurisy is usually tuberculous, but a few cases are due to infections by other organisms which cause empyema.

Symptoms. On inspection, the affected side looks distended, does not move on respiration and is flat on percussion. The heart is visibly moved to the more normal side, which is seen to make unusually wide respiratory excursions, since one lung must do the work of both. The presence of the fluid is demonstrated clearly on roentgenograms. Some of it should be removed at once by thoracentesis for examination. Of the fluid that is aspirated, some should be cultured on the usual bacteriologic media, some injected into a guinea pig to demonstrate the presence or absence of tubercle bacilli and some studied (cytologically) in a search for possible tumor cells indicating carcinoma of the pleura. The fluid may be clear, straw-colored and sterile on culture. Such findings suggest tuberculosis as the cause of the pleurisy. Fluid containing blood may be found in patients with tuberculous pleurisy, patients with malignant tumors involving the pleura and patients who have a pulmonary infarction. Sufficient fluid should be removed often enough through a large needle to keep the patient comfortable. The patient should be guarded against further progress of any tuberculous lesion present.

Nursing Care. Care of patients with pleural effusion entails the enforcement of bed rest with restriction of physical activity as long as fever persists and the provision of a nutritious diet reinforced with dietary supplements, as indicated. It is the nurse's responsibility to prepare the patient, mentally and physically, for thoracentesis and to assist the physician in its performance.

Empyema Thoracis (Pyothorax)

Acute Empyema Thoracis is a collection of pus in the pleural cavity. It occurs as a result of pneumonia or injury to the chest wall, and is most frequent in children. The usual history is of an acute pneumonia, in which a septic temperature persists or develops after the crisis has occurred. The patient is extremely ill, often with sufficient dyspnea to require a sitting posture (orthopnea) in order to obtain relief. Roentgenograms, which are of considerable aid to the surgeon, must be taken in the upright position.

Treatment. The causative organisms are identified, and the appropriate antibiotic is administered. A regimen of intermittent aspiration and instillation of antibiotics is tried. The use of fibrinolytic enzymes such as trypsin, streptokinase and streptodornase seems to be effective in dissolving fibrin clots and decreasing the viscosity of pus. However, if the patient still has a temperature elevation after a week or 10 days, and the cavity is not well on the way to obliteration, surgical drainage is done.

Operations. The operations are of two types. In the first type, an effort is made to drain the pleural cavity without permitting the entrance of air into it. This is spoken of often as *closed drainage.* In the second type, drainage of the empyema cavity is accomplished by the removal of a section of rib, which permits an opening into the pleural collection. This is spoken of as *open drainage or thoracotomy,* and is used in cases with thick pus.*

When the pus is thick, indicating an empyema of long duration, the pus cavity usually is fairly well walled off, and the danger of collapse of the lung is not so great.

After an operation for empyema, the chief consideration in the recovery of the patient is the collapse of the empyema cavity by expansion of the lung. To this end the patients are instructed to breathe deeply every hour; they are urged to blow into a spirometer or a blow bottle, using the increased intrapulmonary pressure thus developed to expand the lung.

These patients should be allowed out of bed as soon as possible, usually after from 7 to 10 days. They may sit in a wheel chair and outdoors in the sun if this is possible. A high caloric diet is given, especially high in carbohydrates, protein and vitamins. The chief nursing challenge is to encourage this patient to meet his nutritional needs. Attractive trays with small servings offered frequently and any other ways of tempting him to eat should be employed.

As soon as the drainage has decreased sufficiently, the tube may be removed from the chest and the wound is covered by simple gauze dressings. The convalescence should be passed as much as possible in the open air and sunlight.

Lung Abscess

This term refers to a localized necrotic lesion characterized by cavity formation. In the initial stages this cavity in the lung may or may not communicate with a bronchus; eventually, however, it becomes surrounded or "encapsulated" by a wall of fibrous tissue,

* If the inflammation has been of long standing, an exudate can form over the lung and interfere with its normal expansion. This will have to be removed surgically (decortication).

except at one or two points where the necrotic process extends until it reaches the lumen of some bronchus or the pleural space and establishes, thereby, a communication with the respiratory tract, the pleural cavity or both. In the first instance, its purulent contents are evacuated continuously in the form of sputum, whereas if a pleural exit is accessible, empyema results; if both types of communication are furnished, the case becomes one of "bronchopleural fistula."

Etiology. A lung abscess may occur as the sequela of an infected pulmonary infarct or of bacterial pneumonia. There are many situations, however, in which bacterial infection plays no etiologic role, the origin instead being a lung tumor or an aspirated foreign body impacted in a bronchus.

Prevention. All individuals who are responsible for the care and training of children should be taught to recognize the importance of lung abscess as a dangerous disease, but one that is preventable inasmuch as its most important cause in childhood is the careless handling of small objects, such as coins, whistles, thimbles, buttons, etc., which should be kept out of the mouths of children as much as possible. If aspiration of a foreign body occurs, it is imperative that medical advice be sought at once so that bronchoscopic examinations may be conducted at the earliest possible moment.

Course. Many patients experience fever at first, and, for a time, this is their only symptom, but as soon as a bronchial communication is established, allowing the abscess to drain, the symptoms are progressively more severe and the infection is increasingly productive of sputum that is both purulent and foul. Fever mounts, emaciation becomes pronounced, and, unless therapy is effective, death soon may intervene.

Symptoms. After the early, relatively asymptomatic stages have passed, the diagnosis of lung abscess is fairly self-evident from the course it runs. In addition to the physical findings in the chest, clubbing of the fingers (hypertrophic pulmonary osteoarthropathy) may supply a helpful clue. Confirmation may be obtained from the x-ray examination or by direct bronchoscopic visualization, a procedure that is almost always indicated because the possibility of a foreign body in the lung cannot be excluded otherwise.

Preoperative Treatment and Nursing Care

A lung abscess will heal if the cavity can be emptied of its contents completely and at frequent intervals. This objective may be accomplished by means of postural drainage, by aspiration through a bronchoscope or by open drainage through a chest wall incision, i.e., "open thoracotomy." The first method suffices in the majority of patients.

Patients with chronic lung abscesses whose

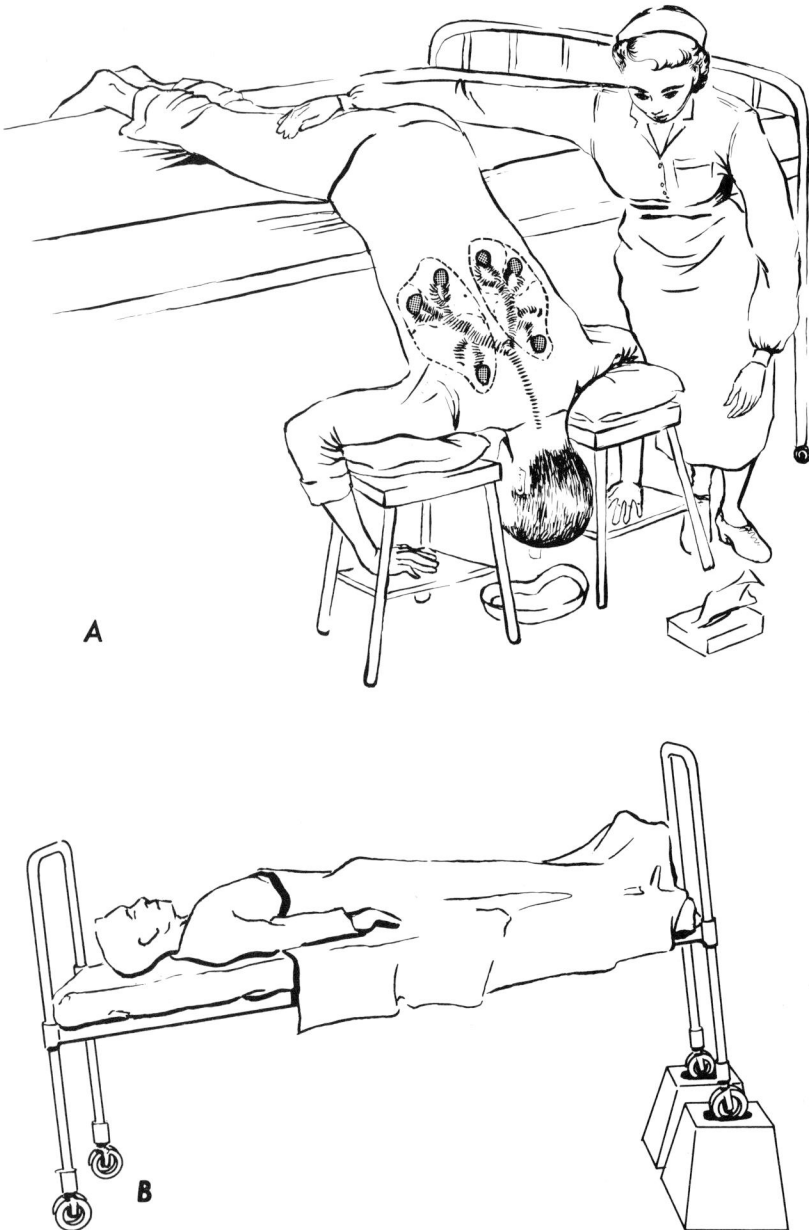

FIG. 141. (A) This position for postural drainage is good for the lowest lobes, fairly good for the middle lobe but inadequate for the upper lobes. (B) This head-low position is good for drainage from the lower halves of each lung.

lungs have become honeycombed with multiple fibrotic hardwalled cavities after a prolonged putrid infection can be restored to health only by the complete removal of the process by lobectomy or pneumonectomy. Before the operation the patient must be prepared adequately with antibacterial chemotherapy, blood transfusions and dietary measures in order to reduce the operative risk to a minimum.

Drug Therapy. A combination of drugs usually is employed in the treatment of lung abscess in recognition of the fact that a variety of organisms may be involved, some of which may be relatively unresponsive to any single agent. An acceptable combination, for example, is sulfadiazine by mouth and penicillin by parenteral injection or in combination with streptomycin. A more important consideration, however, is the ade-

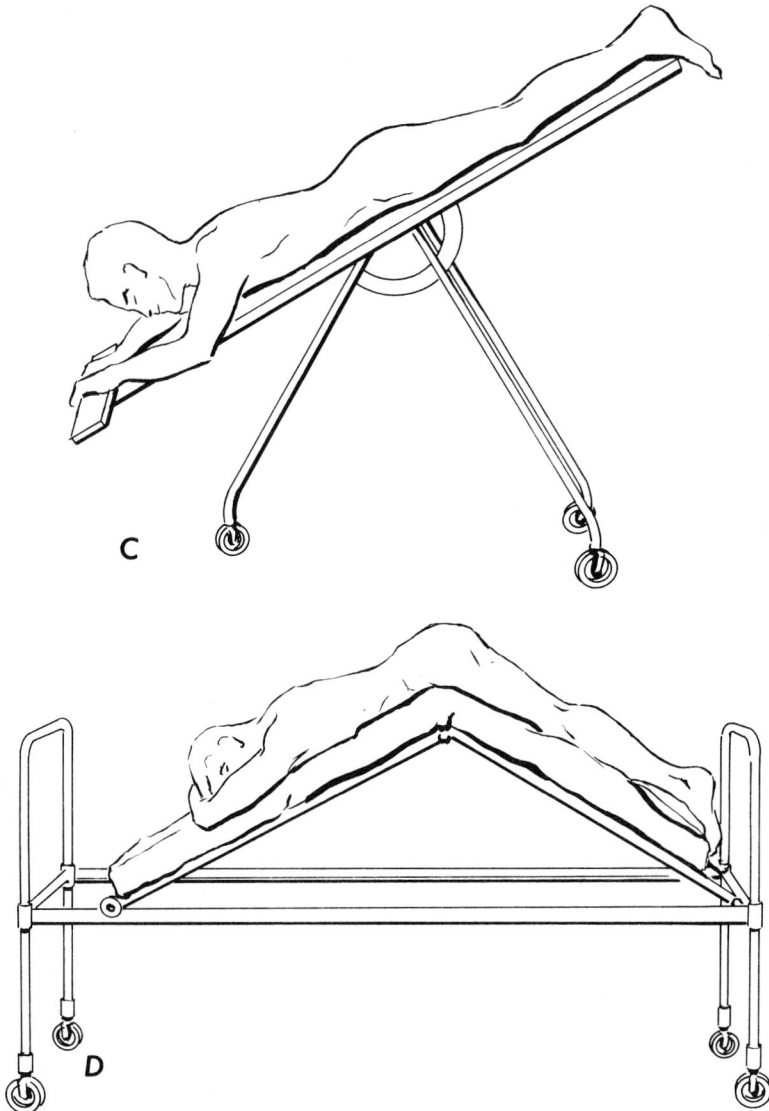

FIG. 141 (*Continued*). (C) A tilt table can be used for draining the lower halves of each lung and is particularly useful in draining posterior lesions. (D) When the patient's bed can be adjusted to provide this position, it is a comfortable one; however, it is effective in draining the lower lung only and inadequate for the upper lobes.

quacy with which drainage is accomplished, whatever the means employed.

Terpin hydrate or hydriodic acid syrup (only if tuberculosis has been excluded) may be used. Codeine should be given only if definitely indicated, and only on a temporary basis to relieve an exhausting cough.

Postural Drainage. This is accomplished by placing the patient in a position so that the head and the thorax are dependent in relation to the rest of the trunk. The patient may simply flex his body over the side of the bed, head and shoulders hanging as close to the floor as possible, while his legs, held by the nurse, remain supported on the bed. A chair or a foot-stool of the proper height beside the bed provides a stable support. Resting his weight on his hands or elbows, the patient can maneuver himself into an optimal position, namely, the position which has been found by the patient to yield a most prompt and copious expectoration. Evacuation of the abscess is aided by coughing, which, therefore, should be encouraged. The frequency and the duration of postural drainage are decided on the basis of the volume of sputum ejected on each occasion, averaging from 5 to 10 minutes every 2 to 4 hours, and taking into account the patient's need for rest and his resistance to fatigue. Because of the exhausting character of the procedure, no period of drainage should exceed 10 minutes. During each performance the patient's color and pulse should be examined repeatedly by the nurse for signs of suffocation or peripheral circulatory collapse requiring immediate resumption of the horizontal position.

Satisfactory drainage can be accomplished in some patients with less arduous effort. For example, the patient may lie prone, with head and shoulders dependent, on a bed which has been elevated at one end to an angle of 20 degrees from the horizontal. Or, the patient may lie prone, with head at the foot of a bed which has been angulated to the maximum knee-rest position.

If the sputum is foul-smelling, this procedure may well be carried out in a room away from other patients. Deodorizers should be used. Paper wipes and a bag for their disposition must be available. After postural drainage, it is refreshing for the patient to brush his teeth and use a mouthwash; he then should rest in bed for a half hour.

The effectiveness of postural drainage is estimated on the basis of the clinical signs: the course of the fever, pulse and respiration; the changes in appetite; the alterations in the body weight and in the patient's sense of well-being. Its efficiency is best determined by estimating the proportion of exudate remaining in the abscess cavity at the conclusion of the drainage, as seen by roentgenograms, or as actually obtained by direct suction through a bronchoscope. If suction through a bronchoscope proves to be a rewarding procedure, it too should be scheduled routinely at intervals of from 1 to 3 days.

Surgery

Surgical intervention is indicated only when both postural and bronchoscopic drainage have proved to be inadequate as judged by the repeated failure to empty the cavity completely.

Postoperative Nursing Care

After surgery there is usually a somewhat prolonged period of drainage before the wound closes entirely. In many cases, it may be necessary for some person in the family to change the simple dressings frequently enough to prevent excoriation of the skin and an offensive odor. Therefore, it is advisable frequently to give instructions in the method of dressing the wound and to demonstrate it. If possible, these patients are placed under the supervision of a public health nurse or some community agency that will help the family to meet any problems that may arise as a result of the care and the needs of these patients.

Bronchiectasis

Bronchiectasis is the permanent dilatation of one or several bronchi (Fig. 142). Some cases are congenital, more result from chronic bronchitis, and many cases originate in attacks of severe influenza or whooping cough, especially if the attacks occur in adult life. In the majority of patients several bronchi, usually of the lower lobes, are affected. The dilatation may be cylindrical—that is, tubular—or there may develop one or more saclike cavities containing several ounces of pus.

The condition results from weakening of the bronchial walls by chronic infection. The walls become permanently distended by severe coughing. The infection extends to the peribronchial tissues, so that in the case of saccular bronchiectasis each dilated tube virtually amounts to a lung abscess, the exudate of which drains freely through the bronchus.

Symptoms. Characteristic symptoms of bronchiectasis include chronic cough and the production of foul sputum in copious amounts. A high percentage of patients with this disease experience hemoptysis. Clubbing of the fingers is very common. The patient is likely to be subject to repeated episodes of pulmonary infection.

Most cases of bronchiectasis pass unrecognized, being mistaken for simple chronic bronchitis. A definite clue is offered by the prolonged history of productive cough, with a sputum consistently negative for tubercle bacilli. The diagnosis is established on the basis of the roentgenogram of the chest taken after the instillation of Lipiodol (a radi-opaque iodide in an oil base) through the trachea into the bronchi. Direct bronchoscopy occasionally is valuable in determining the location and the extent of the disease.

Treatment. There is no satisfactory method available for collapsing a bronchiectatic cavity; therefore, the cavity fails to heal on conservative therapy. The only definitive therapy is surgical removal; it may be necessary to remove a segment of a lobe (segmental resection), a lobe (lobectomy) or an entire lung (pneumonectomy).

Segmental resection is the removal of an anatomic subdivision of a pulmonary lobe. The chief advantage is that only diseased tissue is removed, with greater conservation of healthy lung tissue. Bronchography aids in the delineation of the segment.

Postoperatively, 2 tubes from the chest of the patient are connected to water-seal controlled suction. Air from air leaks following segmental resection is removed by this method, and the remaining lung is maintained in a more expanded state. Suction is discontinued in 2 or 3 days. (Preoperative and postoperative nursing care for segmental resection is the same as for any chest surgical patient, as discussed earlier in this chapter.)

The immediate prognosis with surgical

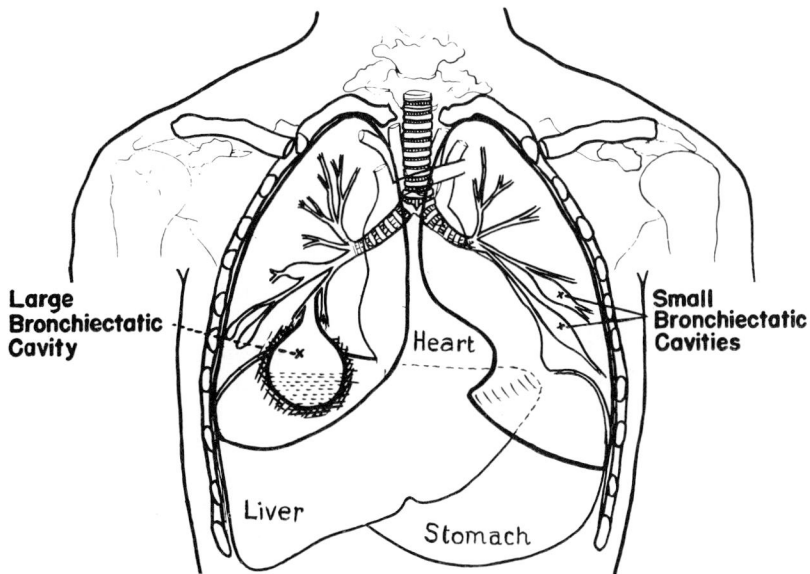

FIG. 142. Lungs affected by bronciectasis.

treatment is good, even in the case of bilateral operations, and with recovery, the patient is cured completely of a most disagreeable and often incapacitating chronic disease. The operation is preceded by a period of preparation, which is exceedingly important. The object of this is to eradicate as far as possible the pulmonary infection and to improve the general condition of the patient, who may be extremely debilitated as a result of the disease. The infection is treated by frequent drainage of the cavity. This is accomplished by means of postural therapy or, if the abscess is suitably situated, by direct suction through a bronchoscope. A course of chemotherapy, combining the administration of sulfadiazine or chlortetracycline by mouth and penicillin by injections, should be started before the operation and continued in the postoperative period. The patient's general condition is improved by a liberal nutritious diet. If anemia is present, transfusions of whole blood are indicated.

Prevention depends on the avoidance of pertussis, accomplished by prophylactic immunization in childhood; on adequate management of chronic bronchitis; and on the successful treatment of pneumonia.

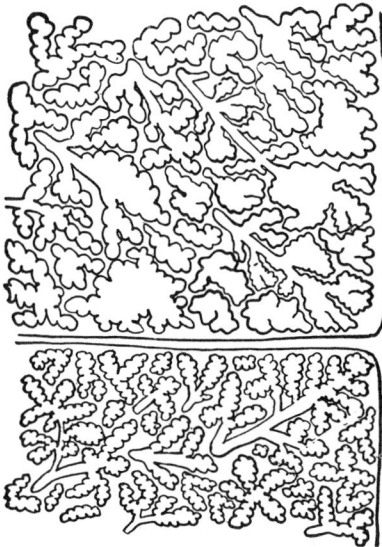

FIG. 143. Emphysema of the lung. Above is a portion of an emphysematous lobe; below, for comparison, is represented a portion of a normal lobe.

THE PATIENT WITH PULMONARY EMPHYSEMA

Emphysema, or "blowing up of the lungs," is a common respiratory problem in our aging population. In this condition there is dilatation of all of the finer air passages and dilatation and coalescence (fusing together) of the alveoli (Fig. 143). The alveolus is the site in the lung where venous blood and environmental air complete the process of gas exchange. In order for gas exchange to be effective, the alveoli must be adequately ventilated with air. Interference with alveolar ventilation may occur if there is bronchial obstruction or in conditions in which there is uneven expansion of the lungs with poor air distribution. Common conditions causing impaired alveolar ventilation are bronchial asthma, chronic bronchitis and pulmonary emphysema.

Emphysema results in *marked increase in airway resistance,* which is especially noted during and at the end of expiration. In order to get air into and out of the lungs, negative pressure is required during inspiration and an adequate level of positive pressure must be attained and maintained during expiration. The rest position is one of inflation. Instead of being an involuntary act, expiration becomes a muscular act. The patient becomes increasingly short of breath, the chest becomes rigid, and the ribs are fixed at their joints. This accounts for the "barrel chest" of many of these patients.

There is a continuous reduction of the vital capacity. Full deflation becomes increasingly difficult, and finally impossible. The alveoli, long distended, begin to break down, a process accelerated by recurrent infections. As the walls of the alveoli are destroyed, the internal surface of the lungs, i.e., the area available for the exchange of oxygen and carbon dioxide between the atmosphere and the blood, continually decreases. There is interference with carbon-dioxide diffusion and the increased carbon-dioxide concentration stimulates respiratory activity in lungs that are already overworked and handicapped. This causes a mild to severe pulmonary acidosis. There is also impairment of oxygen diffusion with inadequate oxygen saturation of the venous blood.

As the alveolar walls continue to rupture, the pulmonary capillary bed is reduced. The pulmonary blood flow is speeded and the right ventricle is forced to maintain a higher blood pressure in the pulmonary artery. Right-sided heart failure is one of the complications of emphysema.

Symptoms. Due to the inefficient mechanics of respiration and the impaired gaseous interchange between the alveolar air and the blood through the fibrotic alveolar walls, the arterial blood is poorly oxygenated. Dyspnea and varying degrees of redness and cyanosis follow. The patient complains of increasing shortness of breath on exertion and constant fatigue. The emphysematous lung is not contracted on expiration, and the bronchioles are not effectively emptied of their secretions. The patient readily develops inflammatory reactions and infections due to the pooling of these secretions. Hence, violent productive cough is a usual and persistent symptom. In fact it is not unusual for the patient to develop rib fractures from cough. The sputum is usually thick and mucoid in character. One complication of this disease, if not controlled, is right ventricular strain due to the increased resistance to blood flow through the pulmonary vessels. The presence of leg edema (dependent edema) or pain in the region of the liver suggests the development of cardiac failure.

Nursing Observations. The nurse's observations and charting should reveal an understanding of the patient and his disease. What are the pulse and the respiratory rates? Are the respirations even? Does the patient contract his abdominal muscles during inspiration? Are the accessory muscles of respiration

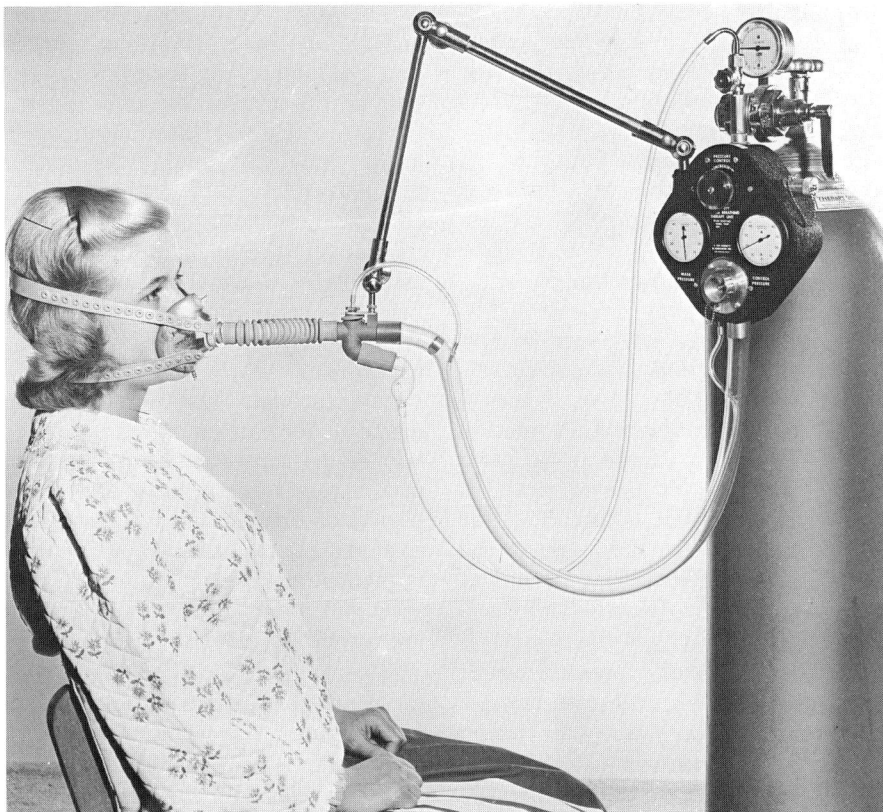

FIG. 144. Medication administered by intermittent positive pressure (Bennett). The drug may be administered continuously or intermittently. (Winthrop Laboratories and Bennett Respiration Products, Inc.)

used? Does exertion increase the dyspnea? Is cyanosis evident? Are the patient's neck veins engorged? Is he coughing? What is the color and consistency of the sputum? What is the status of the patient's sensorium? Is there increasing stupor and apprehension? At what times during the day does he complain most of fatigue and shortness of breath?

Treatment and Nursing Care

Preventive measures designed to forestall the development and progression of this disease must be recognized by the nurse.

Obstructive adenoids and chronically infected tonsils should be removed in early youth, and all attacks of bronchitis and bronchial asthma should be treated adequately. Adolescents should be discouraged from smoking. Smokers should be advised to stop smoking immediately.

Patients with emphysema should be informed unequivocally that, for them, smoking is contraindicated. They should restrict themselves to a life of moderate activity, ideally in a climate with minimal shifts in temperature and humidity.

The aim of the treatment of emphysema is to decrease airway resistance so that it is easier for the patient to breathe. This is accomplished by:

1. Relieving bronchospasm and promoting bronchial drainage; and,

2. Preventing and treating promptly episodes of bronchial infection (these are overlapping in their effects).

Relief of Bronchospasm and Promotion of Bronchial Drainage. Patients respond differently to a therapeutic program, and it may take a period of trial to ascertain the most effective treatment for the patient. Oral preparations containing ephedrine or similar bronchodilating drugs are beneficial to certain patients. Aminophylline (500 mg.) is effective orally or in rectal suppositories. If the patient is too dyspneic and ill to tolerate oral medication, aminophylline (250 to 500 mg.) is given slowly intravenously. Epinephrine 1:1000 (0.5 to 1 ml.) subcutaneously may afford relief. To clear the air passages of bronchial secretions, expectorants may be ordered. The iodides assist in lessening the

viscosity of the sputum. If the sputum is thick and purulent, enzymes such as trypsin or Streptokinase serve to liquefy the secretion by digestion.

Aerosol solutions of bronchodilator drugs given by intermittent positive pressure on inspiration produce maximal bronchodilatation in many patients. Solutions of isoproterenol (Isuprel) and phenylephrine hydrochloride (Neo-Synephrine) are effective. Intermittent positive pressure breathing helps by reducing airway resistance, relieving bronchospasm, mobilizing bronchial secretions, and increasing alveolar ventilation with little effort by the patient. Oxygen is forced into the lungs and accumulated carbon dioxide is flushed out of the residual air spaces. The improvement of the oxygen saturation of the arterial blood and a reduction of its carbon dioxide content assists in relieving the patient's hypoxia and gives considerable relief from constant respiratory fatigue.

The nurse must understand the proper use and maintenance of various types of inhalation equipment. It is impossible to teach a patient the use of an intermittent positive pressure breathing machine unless the nurse knows how to assemble the machine properly and quickly. Several types of these machines are available, and she should familiarize herself with them. She can practice the assembly of the machine and actually use it herself several times (without medication). If an emphysematous patient is taught these procedures poorly, the treatment program suffers through loss of the patient's confidence in the nurses and the physician. The cost of the aerosolized bronchodilators when used from 3 to 4 times daily over a long period of time is high. It is wasteful of the patient's efforts and money if the procedure is ineffective.

Management. Patients with emphysema are prone to develop bronchial infections. The prevention and the prompt treatment of these are two of the most important aspects of emphysema therapy. The cough associated with acute bronchitis introduces a vicious cycle, with further trauma and damage to the lungs, further progression of symptoms and further increase in susceptibility to bronchial infection. The patient

INTERMITTENT POSITIVE PRESSURE BREATHING (IPPB.) UNIT

The intermittent positive pressure breathing (inspiration) unit is a piece of equipment that supplies air or oxygen under increased pressure during inspiration.

NURSING ACTIVITIES:	RATIONALE UNDERLYING THE NURSING MANAGEMENT AND TREATMENT:
Explain the procedure to the patient.	Proper explanation of the procedure will help to insure the patient's cooperation.
Take the blood pressure and the pulse before and after inhalation using bronchodilator drugs on patients for the first time.	Bronchodilators accelerate cardiac action. They produce precordial distress, palpitation, dizziness, and nausea.
The patient should be sitting or in a semi-Fowler's position.	The diaphragmatic excursion is greater in this position.
Turn on the oxygen cylinder.	This is a pressure-operated machine whose source of pressure may be supplied from a cylinder of oxygen, a cylinder of compressed air, a pipe line, or a motor-driven air compressor.
Place the prescribed medicine in the nebulizer.	The volume of medication is gauged to give a treatment lasting 15 to 20 minutes. Notify the doctor if the medication is nebulized too quickly.
Select the pressure prescribed. Cover the mouthpiece with a paper towel to ascertain when the predetermined pressure is reached.	Each unit should be tested to see whether the pre-determined setting is accomplished before treating the patient.
Turn on the nebulizer control to produce a fine spray.	Adequate fog and particle size is essential to sufficient medication distribution.
Adjust the mask or the mouthpiece on the patient. If the patient objects to the nose clip, instruct him to hold his nose. After several treatments, the patient can train himself to do without the nose clip.	The mask or mouthpiece must constitute a closed circuit, if the unit is to cycle. (If the patient exhales through the nose while using the mouthpiece, the unit will not reach the desired pressure.)
The patient should place his hands on his diaphragm while breathing, concentrating on causing motion with the diaphragm rather than with the chest muscles.	This type of breathing encourages good diaphragmatic motion and reduces residual air volume.
Instruct the patient to make only a slight inspiratory effort, i.e., breathe as passively as possible.	A slight inspiratory effort will activate the positive pressure phase, and the lungs will be inflated with a rapid rate of flow until the predetermined pressure is reached.
The patient should exhale using a gently forced expiration.	After the lungs are inflated, the flow of gas ceases and allows the patient to exhale without any assistance from the machine.
Encourage the patient to continue this type of breathing until all the medication is given.	The medication should be completely nebulized to ensure treatment effectiveness.

should be instructed to report to the physician immediately if his sputum becomes discolored, for purulent expectoration is evidence of infection. He should be taught that any worsening of his symptoms—for example, increased tightness of the chest or increase in dyspnea—also is suggestive of infection and should be reported.

In many instances, breathing exercises succeed in improving pulmonary ventilation. These are designed to alter the patient's breathing pattern from the thoracic type, characteristic of emphysema, to the lower costal and diaphragmatic type, favoring efficiency and conserving effort (see p. 417).

The patient may be ambulant and active within the limits of his ability, unless otherwise ordered. Ambulation prevents weakness and loss of muscle tone and aids morale.

A patient with emphysema has definite periods of the day when his exercise tolerance is decreased. This is especially true on arising in the morning, because bronchial secretions and edema collect in the lungs during the night while he is lying supine. He often will be unable to shave or to wash. Activities requiring the arms to be supported above the level of the thorax may produce distress. These activities may be tolerated better after he has been up and moving around for an hour or more. Therefore, he has the right to participate in planning his nursing care with the nurse and determining the best time for bathing and shaving. A hot beverage on arising will assist him to expectorate and will shorten the period of disability noted on arising.

Another period of increased disability occurs immediately after meals, particularly the evening meal. Fatigue from the day's activities coupled with abdominal distention combine to limit his exercise tolerance. The patient's chief complaint at this time is fatigue. This is another way of saying, "I am dyspneic": dyspnea is the underlying cause of his fatigue.

The patient should be instructed to avoid excessive heat and cold. Heat increases the body temperature, hence raises the oxygen requirements of the body; cold tends to promote bronchospasm. High altitudes aggravate the hypoxia; dusty areas stimulate bronchospasm.

One of the major teaching factors is to help the patient to accept realistic long-range goals. If he is severely disabled, the objective of treatment is to preserve his present pulmonary function and relieve his symptoms as much as possible. If his disease is mild, the objective is to increase his exercise tolerance and prevent further loss of pulmonary function. The patient has to be told what to expect. He and those caring for him need patience to achieve these goals.

A patient with moderately advanced emphysema may have chronic respiratory acidosis. Therefore, he should be placed in oxygen only by direct order of the physician, and the amount and the method of oxygenation should be prescribed specifically. Since his respiratory center has become unresponsive to carbon dioxide, as opposed to the normal individual, the only remaining stimulus to which this center responds is arterial hypoxia, or low oxygen tension. If arterial hypoxia is abruptly terminated by the administration of high concentrations of inhaled oxygen, the respiratory center may cease to function. Symptoms of respiratory acidosis appear, including forgetfulness, increasing stupor, apprehension, a feeling of claustrophobia (if the patient is in an oxygen tent) and coma. However, oxygen often can be administered safely in this situation by *gradually* increasing the oxygen concentration. This will *slowly* correct arterial hypoxia, allowing the respiratory center to regain at least some of its original sensitivity to the stimulating effects of normal physiologic levels of carbon dioxide.

THE PATIENT WITH A PULMONARY EMBOLUS

Pulmonary infarction follows the closure of a pulmonary artery by a blood clot; the clot may arise in the pulmonary artery itself, due to an adjacent pneumonia, or it may be swept as an embolus into the pulmonary circulation from a large peripheral vein—particularly a leg or a pelvic vein. The plugging of a large pulmonary vessel may cause sudden death. Closure of a medium-sized branch of a pulmonary artery in previously normal persons will not necessarily cause any ill effects whatever, but in patients with chronic passive congestion an infarcted area develops, which quickly becomes infiltrated by blood escaping from the neighboring capillaries.

Symptoms. Characteristic of pulmonary embolism are the sudden onset of chest pain, cough which is productive of bright red sputum, rapid and shallow respirations, tachycardia and fever. If much of the lung is involved, the patient may become markedly cyanotic, and death may occur promptly, the terminal picture resembling that of coronary thrombosis. On the other hand, the symptoms may consist merely of fever and slight tachypnea in mild cases, and a chest roentgenogram may be required to differentiate the case from one of bronchopneumonia.

Treatment. No direct therapeutic approach is possible other than embolectomy, which is rarely indicated and rarely possible. Anticoagulant therapy should be instituted at once, employing intravenous heparin, for its immediate effect, and Dicumarol, by mouth, for continuous anticoagulant activity,

after 2 to 3 days. In all cases oxygen administration and the use of morphine are used.

Prevention and Nurse's Responsibility. Since any patient with thrombosis of the leg or pelvic veins is a candidate for a pulmonary embolism, the procedure of tying off a thrombosed vein above the thrombus is often carried out. This may involve ligation of the femoral or iliac veins, or even the inferior vena cava. The most important aspect of prevention, however, lies in forestalling the formation of thrombi in these peripheral veins, hence the importance of mobilizing patients from their beds as soon as safety permits.

The wearing of elastic stockings has decided value in preventing thromboembolic disease, for its effect is to curtail venous pooling, thereby reducing the likelihood of ischemic damage to venous endothelium, hence venous thrombosis, in the lower extremities, the site of clotting in 90 per cent of cases. Many hospitals now require all

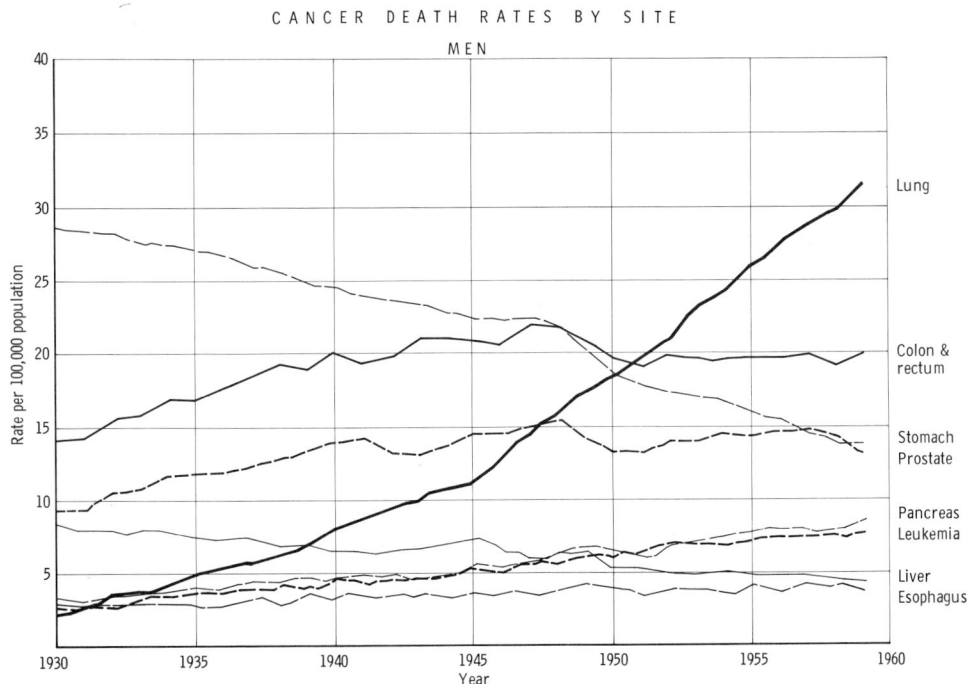

FIG. 145. Cancer death rates by site. The lung cancer death rate for males rose from 3.6 per 100,000 population in 1930 to approximately 32.5 in 1960, while death rates for other sites remained fairly level or actually decreased. It is estimated that about 41,000 Americans, 35,500 men and 5,500 women, will die of lung cancer in 1963. (Adapted from: 1963 Cancer Facts and Figures, p. 10, New York, American Cancer Society)

bed patients to wear elastic stockings at all times, unless specifically contraindicated. Among the few contraindications are the presence of active thrombophlebitis in one or both lower extremities and the existence of inflammatory or ulcerative skin lesions on a leg or a foot. As long as the patient is confined in bed, active leg exercises should be undertaken under the supervision of the nurse. If active exercise is not practicable, and if the physician so prescribes, the nurse may provide passive exercise in the form of alternate flexion and extension of the knees and raising and lowering of the bed frame beneath the legs in order to avoid prolonged venous stasis.

Heparin and Dicumarol are of prophylactic value in many conditions which are un-

usually susceptible to the development of thromboembolic disorders. Often these patients have a history of peripheral vascular disease, recent myocardial infarction, and pelvic infection. Other patients who must be watched for pulmonary infarction and embolism are those who have undergone prolonged operative procedures and those with malignant neoplastic diseases.

PATIENTS WITH TUMORS OF THE CHEST

A chest tumor may be *primary,* that is, it may arise within the lung or the mediastinum; or it may represent a metastasis from a primary tumor site elsewhere. Metastatic tumors of the lungs are not rare, since the blood stream brings to them free cancer

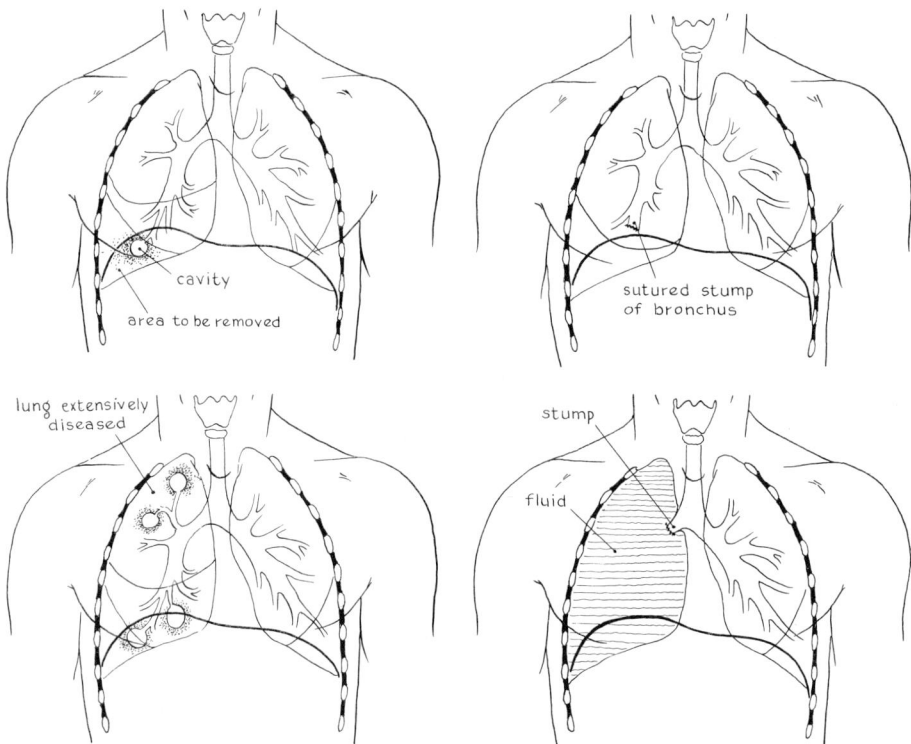

Fig. 146. Diagrammatic drawings show lobectomy and pneumonectomy for lesions of the lung. The lesions shown are abscesses or tuberculous cavities, but the same operations may be done for bronchiectatic cavities or for lung tumors. (*Top, left*) Lesion in the lower lobe of the right lung and (*top, right*) appearance after lobectomy. (*Bottom, left*) Multiple areas of disease in the right lung. These may be tuberculous cavities, an abscess cavity, a bronchiectatic cavity, or a lung tumor. (*Bottom, right*) Appearance after removal of the entire lung—pneumonectomy.

cells from primary cancers elsewhere in the body. Such tumors grow in and between the alveoli and the bronchi, which they push apart in their growth, often for a long time causing few or no symptoms. If, however, a nodule grows just beneath the pleura, the affected pleural cavity fills with fluid (often bloody), which, if removed, quickly collects again.

Primary tumors of the lung may be benign or malignant. In the majority of patients, at least, they arise from the bronchial epithelium. If they are benign they are known as *bronchial adenomas,* if malignant, *bronchiogenic carcinomas.* The effects they produce on the patient are exceedingly variable, depending entirely on their location and the nature of their growth. Benign adenomas are apt to bleed, giving rise to repeated hemoptyses. Also, by obstructing a bronchus, they may cause emphysema or atelectasis of the lobe with which the bronchus communicates. The malignant carcinoma, in addition to causing bleeding and bronchial obstruction, spreads to involve other portions of the lung tissue, and frequently other organs as well, notably the lymph nodes of the mediastinum and the neck, the liver, the adrenal glands and the bones. By direct extension it may invade a pulmonary vein, a portion of the vena cava or the heart itself, giving rise to symptoms attributable to the resultant circulatory disturbance.

Cancer of the Lung

Cancer of the lung is proving to be an increasingly common tumor in the male population, and statistically it now is a leading cause of death in white males (Fig. 145). There is suggestive evidence which links this cancer to excessive cigarette smoking, and there are many statistics which would seem to confirm this impression. Lung tumors appear to come from the lining membrane of the larger air passages and occur much more often in men of 40 years of age and beyond. Early symptoms are a cough and a wheeze. Then the tumor produces most commonly a chronic cough, often associated with pain or discomfort in the chest, some dyspnea on exertion and sputum that often contains streaks of blood. The diagnosis is made by a combination of diagnostic methods. Usually the roentgenogram shows a definite tumor mass, and by bronchoscopy one may remove sections of the tumor or examine the secretions for tumor cells.

Treatment. In the treatment of carcinoma of the lung, it may be necessary to remove a lobe or all of one lung in order to remove the disease process. These operations are spoken of as *lobectomy* when only one lobe is removed or *pneumonectomy* when an entire lung is removed. (See Fig. 146.) Such operations are performed under endotracheal anesthesia; as a rule, a wide incision is made between the ribs to expose the pedicle of the lung. After the diseased tissue is removed, the chest wall is closed tightly and often a drainage tube is inserted into the pleural cavity. This tube may or may not be used for airtight suction or water-seal drainage but, in any event, it must be kept airtight unless otherwise ordered. The surgeon may make an intrathoracic injection of penicillin and/or streptomycin in the post-pneumonectomy patient for a few days.

Tumors of the Mediastinum

Benign mediastinal tumors, comparatively rare, include the following types: adenoma of the thyroid, fibroma, lipoma, chondroma, myoma and cysts. The majority of primary mediastinal malignant tumors are sarcomas which arise in the thymus or mediastinal lymph nodes. The carcinomas found in this region usually are secondary to those of the breast or the gastrointestinal tract, but rare primary ones arise in the esophagus, the trachea, a bronchus, the thymus or an accessory thyroid gland.

Cysts of the mediastinum usually are small when benign. Dermoid cysts occasionally develop, and these may ulcerate into the air passages.

Symptoms. Nearly all the symptoms of mediastinal tumors are due to the pressure of the mass against important intrathoracic organs. Among these pressure symptoms are bulging of the chest wall; orthopnea, an early sign due to pressure against the trachea, a main bronchus, the recurrent laryngeal nerve or the lung; cardiac palpitation, anginal attacks and various other circulatory disturb-

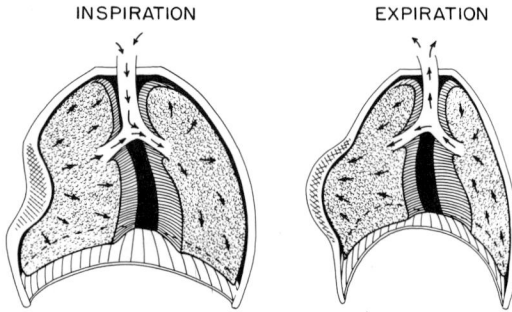

INSPIRATION   EXPIRATION

Fig. 147. Paradoxical motion of chest wall occurs with multiple rib fractures. (*Left*) On inspiration, the softened portion of the chest wall moves inward, uncoordinated with the rest of the chest wall. When the unaffected lung inspires, the portion of the lung underlying the defect expires, resulting in cross-breathing or in-breathing. The mediastinum also shifts toward the unaffected side. (*Right*) On expiration, the reverse occurs, as indicated by arrows. (Strieder, J. W.: GP **13**:75-85)

ances; cyanosis; swelling of the face, the neck and the upper extremities, and the marked distention of the veins of the neck and the chest wall, evidence of the closure of large veins of the mediastinum by thrombi; and dysphagia, due to pressure against the esophagus. The fingers may become clubbed.

Diagnosis. Roentgenograms are of great value in the diagnosis of mediastinal tumors and cysts, yet even with the aid of the fluoroscope and roentgenokymogram it may be difficult to distinguish between a mediastinal abscess, tumor and aortic aneurysm. The biopsy of an enlarged lymph node removed from above the clavicle or in the axilla may reveal the diagnosis. Blood studies are of value in excluding leukemia, and sputum examinations aid in ruling out tuberculosis, while the presence of teeth and hair in the sputum indicates that the tumor is a dermoid cyst.

Treatment. With the exception of intrathoracic goiters and cysts, few mediastinal tumors can be removed by operation. Fibroid tumors occasionally are removed by x-ray irradiation. This irradiation also often retards the growth of carcinomas, yields

quite favorable results in cases of lymphosarcoma and usually gives prompt but temporary relief in cases of Hodgkin's disease, Hodgkin's sarcoma or lymphatic leukemia.

THE PATIENT WITH AN ASPIRATED FOREIGN BODY IN THE LUNG

Foreign bodies not infrequently are aspirated into the lung, especially by children. The object lodges more commonly in the right main bronchus, as it is more vertical than the left (see Fig. 126). The complete closure of a bronchus by a foreign body may result in sudden death. However, the usual result is that the lobes communicating with the occluded bronchus collapse as the air contained in them becomes absorbed in the blood stream.

A small solid object such as a pin, a tack or a tooth in a bronchus causes trouble, not from the obstruction of a bronchus, but from infection. For a short time following the aspiration there may be symptoms of choking, gagging and coughing. But these symptoms, often mild, abate and for a time become forgotten. For weeks the only suggestion of trouble may be a persistent cough. Such substances as peanuts, grains of corn, etc., on the other hand, produce a severe bronchitis with high irregular fever and all the symptoms and signs of a severe pneumonitis. Whether the foreign body is composed of organic or inorganic material, signs of obstructive emphysema, atelectasis or lung abscess eventually appear.

Treatment. The prognosis is serious unless the foreign body is removed early, for rarely is it coughed up spontaneously. Therefore, bronchoscopy is indicated when this diagnosis is suspected. When removed early, aspirated foreign bodies rarely give rise to complications.

Prevention is of the utmost importance and consists in teaching children not to put small toys, coins, buttons, pencil caps and such articles in their mouths. Open safety pins should never be put on a pillow near a baby, nor should a child be permitted to play with a button box. Parents require considerable education in such details of child training, and no small part of their responsibility

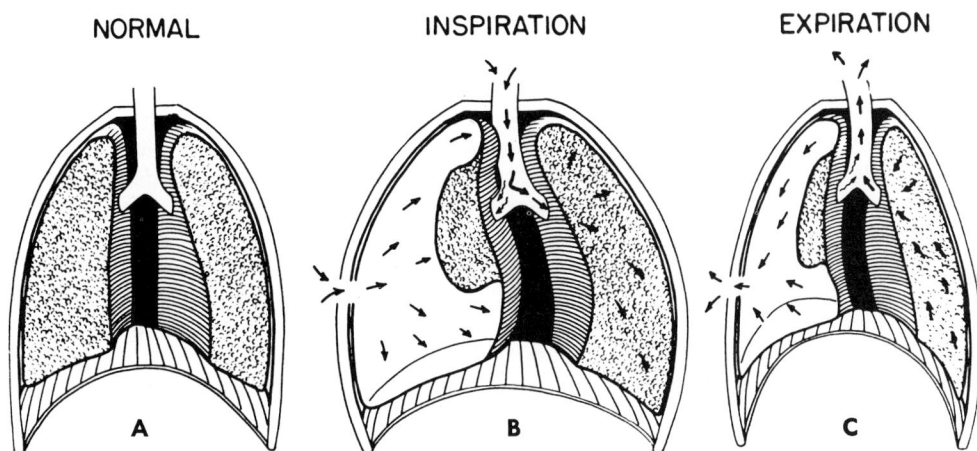

NORMAL   INSPIRATION   EXPIRATION

A   B   C

FIG. 148. Open pneumothorax and mediastinal flutter. (A) Normal lung. (B) The mediastinum shifts toward the unaffected side on inspiration and, as noted by arrows, air rushes into pleural cavity. Air may enter the unaffected lung through the trachea, but the collapsed lung can take little or no air. (C) On expiration, the reverse is true. The mediastinum swings back toward midline and air escapes through the thoracic wound. Air also can leave the normal lung on expiration, but the collapsed lung contributes very little to either phase of respiration. (Streider, J. W.: GP **13**:75-85)

in this regard is the example that they set for their offspring.

THE PATIENT WITH CHEST INJURIES

Injuries to the chest may cause minor or serious disturbance of cardiorespiratory function, depending on which part of the complex mechanism is involved. Thus, a fall against the side of a bath tub may fracture one or two ribs with painful but rather slight disturbance of respiratory function, whereas an automobile accident in which the driver of the car is thrown against the steering wheel may cause a crush of the chest with cardiac and lung injuries that may be rapidly fatal. In the treatment of injuries to the chest, efforts are made to correct the disturbances of cardiorespiratory function caused by the trauma.

Closed or Crush Injuries. Simple fracture of one or two ribs is a painful injury; and because of pain with respiration, there is some degree of limitation of respiratory excursion. Pain can be relieved occasionally by chest strapping, but more commonly a local anesthetic is injected at the fracture site, or is used to block the intercostal nerves that transmit painful sensations from that area.

When the chest is crushed between two objects, multiple fractures of each of several ribs may occur, so that one portion of the chest wall no longer has a bony connection with the rest of the rib cage. This is called "stove-in" or "flail" chest. During attempted respiration, the detached part of the chest wall shows a paradoxical movement, being pulled in on inspiration and blown out on expiration (Fig. 147). This impairs the normal mechanics of respiration enough to jeopardize ventilation seriously. Various methods of stabilizing the chest wall may be used to overcome the paradoxical movement of the injured area during respiration. These may include traction with weights and pulleys applied through wires, or towel clips applied to the broken portions of the ribs (Fig. 148).

In addition, these more severe injuries usually are accompanied by the collection of blood in the chest cavity (hemothorax) from torn intercostal vessels or from lacerations of the lungs, or the escape of air from the injured lung into the pleural cavity (pneumothorax). Often, both blood and air are found in the chest cavity (hemopneumothorax). The lung on that side of the chest is compressed, thus interfering with its normal function. Needle aspiration of the blood and/or air allows the lung to re-expand and again perform its function in respiration.

Tension Pneumothorax. In some patients, air may be drawn into the pleural space from the injured lung, or through a small hole in the chest wall. In either case, the air that enters the chest cavity with each inspiration is trapped there: it cannot be expelled through the air passage or small hole in the chest wall. A tension thus is built up in the chest, which produces a collapse of the lung and even may push the heart and the great vessels toward the normal side of the chest, thus not only interfering with respiration but also with the circulatory function. Relief of this "tension pneumothorax" must be looked on as an emergency measure. A tube must be inserted into the chest to which suction is applied, to withdraw the air in the pleural space and thus relieve the tension (Fig. 149).

Sucking Wounds. Open pneumothorax implies an opening in the chest wall large

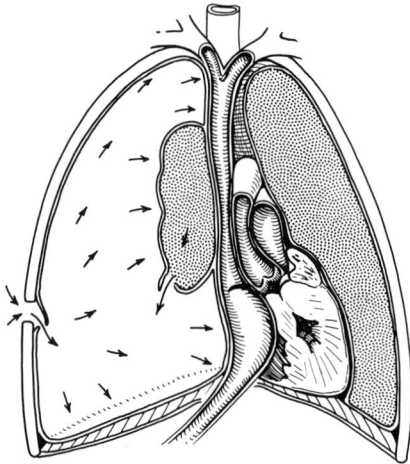

Fig. 149. Two mechanisms of tension pneumothorax. Closed tension pneumothorax occurs with rupture of the lung; air may escape into the pleural cavity during inspiration. Open tension pneumothorax occurs with a valvular type of opening through the chest wall to outside air. Note compression of contralateral lung and interference with venous return to the heart through venae cavae. (Streider, J. W.: GP 13:75-85)

enough for air to pass freely in and out of the thoracic cavity with each attempted respiration. The rush of air through the hole in the chest wall produces a sucking sound, and such injuries are termed "sucking wounds" of the chest. In such patients not only is the lung collapsed, but the structures of the mediastinum (heart and great vessels) are pushed toward the uninjured side with each inspiration and in the opposite direction with expiration. This is termed "mediastinal flutter," and it produces serious embarrassment of circulatory function. To stop the flow of air through the opening in the chest wall is lifesaving. In such an emergency, anything may be used that is large enough to fill the hole, (towel, handkerchief). In the hospital, the opening is plugged by sealing it with gauze impregnated with petroleum jelly.

Wet-Lung Syndrome. Almost every major injury to the thorax is associated with the "wet-lung" syndrome. This syndrome is due to several factors, all of which interfere with the normal passage of air into the lung. They include an increase in tracheobronchial secretions, blood in the tracheobronchial tree, an inability to cough up these secretions because of pain, and ineffectual cough due to the mechanical effects of the injury. In addition, atelectasis of a lung or part of a lung often occurs as a result of the obstructed airway, all of which adds to the difficulty of blood oxygenation. Cyanosis and dyspnea with rattling, labored respiration are associated symptoms. If the airway cannot be cleared by catheter suction or bronchoscopy, a tracheostomy often is performed. This permits the frequent aspiration of retained secretions that is a most important part of the nursing care of these patients. (See Tracheotomy Care, p. 389.)

Cardiac Tamponade. Blows on the anterior chest, stab wounds and crush injuries may cause bleeding into the pericardial sac, with resultant compression of the heart. When the heart is unable to function normally, the patient exhibits cyanosis and dyspnea, the pulse becomes weak, the blood pressure falls, and there may be loss of consciousness from lack of cerebral circulation. Decompression of the pericardium by needle aspiration or by operation permits heart action to be resumed. If the bleeding is due to a wound of the heart, the wound must be closed by suture.

Subcutaneous Emphysema. When the lung or the air passages are injured, air may enter the tissue planes and pass for some distance under the skin. The tissues give a crackling sensation when palpated, and the subcutaneous air produces an alarming appearance with face, neck, body, and scrotum misshapen by subcutaneous air. Fortunately, subcutaneous emphysema is of itself not a serious complication. The subcutaneous air is spontaneously absorbed, if the underlying air leak is treated or stops spontaneously.

General Considerations and Nursing Care

Most patients with severe chest injuries are in a state of shock for a time. This is treated by intravenous fluids, blood, etc. (See Treatment of Shock, p. 296.)

Pain must be treated cautiously to avoid a depression of the cough reflex. Perhaps meperidine hydrochloride (Demerol) rather than morphine is better in this regard. Older people are especially prone to respiratory depression from morphine or other depressants. Nerve block may be used effectively.

Many injuries involving the chest also may have associated abdominal and other injuries that will require treatment and close observation by both the doctor and the nurse.

Principles of nursing care are essentially those discussed on pages 408 to 418.

CLINICAL SITUATIONS

A. 1. Mr. John Lyles, a 36-year-old laborer, was admitted to the hospital from the Emergency Service with a diagnosis of lobar pneumonia. Which group of symptoms would you expect this patient to present?

a. High fever, chest pain, short incessant cough.

b. Dyspnea, paradoxical chest motion, carphologia.

c. Rusty sputum, deep full respirations, afebrile.

d. Expiratory grunt, delirium, bradycardia.

2. The nursing staff was admonished to watch for symptoms of complications. These would include:

a. Moist warm skin and increasing dyspnea.

b. Fall in temperature and rapid, thready pulse.

c. Drowsiness and a dicrotic pulse.

d. Elevation of temperature, and slow, bounding pulse.

3. The doctor orders oxygen to be given Mr. Lyles if necessary. Signs of oxygen want would include all of the following *except*

a. Restlessness and apprehension.

b. A change in the pulse rate.

c. Constriction of the pupils.

d. Dyspnea and cyanosis.

B. 1. Mr. Howard Wright, 62 years old, has been in the hospital for a week undergoing diagnostic studies. He has a tentative diagnosis of cancer of the lung (right). Mr. Wright had a bronchoscopic examination. After this procedure, the primary responsibility of the nurse is to

a. Withhold fluids until a cough reflex is demonstrated.

b. Elevate the head to facilitate breathing.

c. Take the blood pressure every 15 minutes until stable.

d. Watch for subclavicular retraction.

2. On the 8th day after admission, a right lobectomy was performed. Immediately after the patient was returned to his room, water-sealed chest drainage was employed. In caring for closed drainage, the *most* important single factor involved in the nursing care of this patient is to

a. Label the drainage bottle.

b. Allow no outside air in the circuit.

c. Measure all drainage.

d. Measure the degree of tube oscillation.

3. The purpose of closed chest drainage (water-sealed) is to

a. Allow air and fluid to escape.

b. Prevent a spontaneous pneumothorax.

c. Reduce the possibility of paradoxical respiratory motion.

d. Prevent chest fluid from causing retrograde pressure on the wound.

PLAN OF NURSING CARE

Name: Mr. John Shanahan   **Diagnosis:** Emphysema   **Age:** 58

Occupation: Coal miner—retired   **Marital Status:** Married   **Religion:** Protestant

Principles Underlying Treatment: Decrease airway resistance

Therapeutic Plan: Achromycin   250 mg. q. 4 h.
Chymotrypsin   10,000 Units buccally q.i.d.
(Isuprel 1:200 4 gtt.)
(Neo-Synephrine 1% 14 gtt.)
    by IPPB (inspiration) @ 20 lbs. pressure, t.i.d.
Soft diet
No smoking

Nursing Problem: Patient becomes frustrated when he is dyspneic

Objective of Care: To increase patient's exercise tolerance
To teach patient how to do A.D.L. without expending too much effort
To help patient develop realistic goals for his future

APPRAISAL OF PATIENT NEEDS:

1. Patient quite dyspneic in early morning and early evening (will not eat breakfast).

2. Patient becomes quite anxious during IPPB treatments.

3. He becomes depressed during visiting hours (he is 150 miles from his home) and does not have visitors frequently.

4. Greater exercise tolerance is noted in patient around noon.

5. He would like to "go back to the mines for part-time work."

Nursing Activities to Meet Needs:

(Student is encouraged to list these activities before checking the answers on page 458.)

1.

2.

3.

4.

5.

BIBLIOGRAPHY AND SUGGESTED READING

Books

Banyai, A. L. L. (ed.): Nontuberculous Diseases of the Chest, Springfield, Ill., Thomas, 1954.
Blades, B.: Surgical Disease of Chest, St. Louis, Mosby, 1961.
Comroe, J. H. *et al.*: The Lung—Clinical Physiology and Pulmonary Function Tests, Chicago, Yearbook, 1955.
Hinshaw, J. C., and Garland, L. H.: Diseases of the Chest, Philadelphia, Saunders, 1956.
Johnson, J., and Kirby, C. K.: Surgery of the Chest, ed. 2, Chicago, Yearbook, 1958.
Lindskog, G. E., and Liebow, A. A.: Thoracic Surgery and Related Pathology, New York, Appleton, 1953.
Naclerio, E. A. (ed.): Bronchopulmonary Disease, New York, Hoeber, 1957.

Articles

Creighton, H., and Coulter, Jr., W. W.: The whys of a pulmonary function test, Am. J. Nurs. **60:**1771-1774, 1960.
Creighton, H., and Peabody, Sr., J. W.: Inflammatory diseases of the pleura, Am. J. Nurs. **59:**346-348, 1959.
Davies, D. F., and Davies, A. H.: Lung cancer: cigarette smoking as a cause, Am. J. Nurs. **61:**65-69, April, 1961.
Hadley, F., and Bordicks, K.: When a patient has a respiratory difficulty, Am. J. Nurs. **62:** 64-67, Oct., 1962.
Hebert, W. M.: Crushing injuries of the chest, Am. J. Nurs. **59:**678-681, 1959.
Hobby, A. W.: Cough, its pathology and management, Am. J. Nurs. **89:**285-293, Feb., 1955.
MacVicar, J.: Exercises before and after surgery, Am. J. Nurs. **62:**61-63, Jan., 1962.

McClure, E. J., and Leighton, L. A.: Pulmonary emphysema, Am J. Nurs. **57:**594-598, 1957.

Robinson, F. N.: Nursing care of the patient with pulmonary emphysema, Am. J. Nurs. **63:**92-96, Sept., 1963.

Schlesinger, E. M.: Nursing the patient with a crushed chest, Am. J. Nurs. **59:**682-684, May, 1959.

Stephan, P. J.: Nebulization under intermittent positive pressure, Am. J. Nurs. **57:**1158-1160, 1957.

Williams, M. H.: Pulmonary emphysema, Am. J. Nurs. **63:**88-91, Sept., 1963.

Journals

The American Review of Respiratory Diseases: Official Journal of the American Thoracic Society, published by the National Tuberculosis Assoication, New York, N.Y.

Diseases of the Chest: The official periodical of the American College of Chest Physicians.

Bulletin

Medical Bulletin on Tobacco: Pub. quarterly by Am. Pub. Health Assoc., Am. Heart Assoc., Am. Cancer Soc., and Nat. Tuber. Assoc., Room 712, 1790 Broadway, New York 19, N. Y.

Patient-Teaching Aids

Cancer of the Mouth and the Respiratory Tract, Washington, D.C., U.S. Pub. Health Serv., Pub. No. 427, 1959.

Haas, A.: Essentials of Living with Pulmonary Emphysema, a 45-page illustrated booklet, Patient Pub. No. 4, The Institute of Physical Medicine and Rehabilitation, New York University Medical Center, N. Y.

How to Breathe Better. An Instruction Manual published by the Oklahoma Allergy Clinic, Pasteur Medical Bldg., N.W. 10th St., Oklahoma City, Oklahoma.

McGrady, P.: Cigarettes and Health, Washington, D.C., U.S. Pub. Affairs Pamphlet No. 220A, 1960.

National Tuberculosis Association has published useful pamphlets on these topics: Chronic Bronchitis, The Facts, 1962; Chronic Cough, The Facts, 1962; Emphysema, The Facts, 1962; Influenza, The Facts, 1962; Pleurisy, The Facts, 1962; Pneumonia, The Facts, 1962; Shortness of Breath, The Facts, 1962.

Saltman, J.: Emphysema, Washington, D.C., U.S. Pub. Affairs Pamphlet No. 326, 1962.

The Air We Live In; The Health Effects of Air Pollution, Washington, D.C., U.S. Pub. Health Service Pub. No. 640.

The Lungs in Health and Disease. A pamphlet. Chicago, Ill., American Medical Association.

To Smoke or Not To Smoke. New York, American Cancer Society.

24

Patients With
Pulmonary Tuberculosis

CLINICAL MANIFESTATIONS

Tuberculosis is a term that refers to all tissue changes for which the tubercle bacillus can be held responsible and denotes all disease entities that are based on those pathologic changes. Since this bacillus can establish itself in almost every type of human tissue, and since there is no organ system which it cannot colonize, the clinical manifestations of tuberculosis are extremely numerous and varied. Commonest, by far, of all variants of this infection is pulmonary tuberculosis, in which there is involvement of some portion of the lung parenchyma, together with the bronchi and the bronchioles within it, the mediastinal nodes which drain it and the pleura which covers it. In other patients the principal site of involvement is in the upper respiratory tract, as in cases of tuberculous tonsillitis and laryngitis. The most prominent lesion may be a tuberculous laryngitis. Lymph nodes which guard the lymphatic drainage may become infected, producing the picture of tuberculous adenitis. Organisms which are swallowed and later absorbed from the small bowel may localize in the mesenteric or retroperitoneal lymphatic system, giving rise to tuberculous mesenteric adenitis or peritonitis and later tuberculous ileitis or splenitis or renal tuberculosis. The infection may spread from retroperitoneal to mediastinal nodes, producing tuberculous mediastinitis, pleuritis or pericarditis. From lymph nodes in the neck, the mediastinum or the retroperitoneum the infection may extend to the spine, causing tuberculous osteomyelitis with resultant vertebral collapse and deforming kyphosis, or may enter the spinal canal and infect the meninges, producing tuberculous meningitis.

Transported via the blood stream, which it has many opportunities to enter, the tubercle bacillus finds access to and may localize within the brain, forming a "tuberculoma"; cause tuberculous uveitis; or when in a joint, produce tuberculous arthritis. Or it may implant and grow simultaneously in hundreds of sites throughout the body, which is the situation in "miliary tuberculosis."

Mycobacterium tuberculosis, the tubercle bacillus, can be recognized partly from its size and shape, but particularly from the color-fast quality which it exhibits when stained by a certain method, i.e., its "acid-fast" quality. The variant called *Bacillus humanus* is responsible for 99 per cent of all fatal cases of pulmonary tuberculosis, as well as for about 40 per cent of the cases of tuberculosis of other organs. It is spread for the most part by the sputum of patients with pulmonary tuberculosis and infects other persons through the mucous membranes of the nose, the throat, the tonsils and the bronchial tree. *Bacillus bovinus* reaches man—particularly babies—in the raw milk of infected cows. Swallowed, it invades the body through the mucous membrane of the lower third of the small intestine. This bacillus causes about 50 per cent of all cases of tuberculosis of the lymph nodes, the bones, the joints, the serous sacs and the meninges of the central nervous system, and it also may infect the lung. In contrast with the majority of infectious diseases, the germ of tuberculosis, once it has gained a foothold in the body, is likely to remain there quiescent for years after the forces of immunity have controlled the original infection. If, during this quiescent period, the resistance of the host is weakened, the germ at once begins to multiply, causing any one of many tuberculous diseases. If the patient's body proves able to recover from this illness, then the tubercle bacilli again become dormant.

Pathology. Tuberculosis is one of the so-called *granulomatous* diseases; that is, when the organism invades normal tissues, these form in response to it a new tissue, masses of which are called *infectious granulomas.* The tubercle (little tumor), the characteristic lesion of tuberculosis, is a tiny spherical infectious granuloma just large enough to be seen with the naked eye. Another more diffuse and equally characteristic tissue reaction also occurs in response to the tubercle bacillus.

Tubercle bacilli, swept along by the lymph and blood streams, lodge in susceptible tissues in small clumps. The neighboring tissue cells quickly accumulate around each of these, forming a protective wall that checks their further spread and may kill them. If immunity is successful, after a long time the germs die, and the tubercle becomes transformed into a tiny mass of fibrous tissue. At the same time, the tissue of the tubercle may become necrotic and transformed into a cheesy mass, a process known as *caseation.* If this occurs, the germs are liberated from the imprisonment and lymph sweeps them into the surrounding tissues, which respond by enclosing these freed germs in new tubercles. In this way, the original miliary (like millet seeds) tubercle grows into larger and larger irregular masses, some as large as a fist.

The fate of the patient depends on which of these two processes prevails. If the tissue barriers survive, then the imprisoned tubercle bacilli cease to multiply and may die. Lime salts from the blood are deposited in the dead caseous material, and scar tissue forms around the infected area, which remains throughout life as a healed calcified mass. However, if the germs survive and are freed from the tubercle, they multiply and are swept along by the lymph stream into the neighboring tissues and by the blood stream into other organs, where they lodge and repeat the same process.

MILIARY TUBERCULOSIS

Miliary tuberculosis is the result of blood stream invasion by the tubercle bacillus. It is the most serious form of tuberculosis. The origin of the bacilli which flood the blood stream is either some chronic focus that has ulcerated into a blood vessel or multitudes of miliary tubercles lining the inner surface of the thoracic duct. The germs, poured from these foci into the blood stream, are carried throughout the body and locate throughout all tissues, everywhere inducing tubercle formation. Definite evidence of this tubercle formation almost always is found on x-ray examination of the lungs. Another location of diagnostic importance is the choroid of the eye, where these tubercles become visible on ophthalmic inspection.

The clinical course of miliary tuberculosis is varied, depending on which organs are involved earliest and most severely. The usual picture is one of prolonged, high, irregular fever without chills and gradually progressive inanition, weight loss and prostration. At first there may be no localizing signs except for splenomegaly, anemia and leukopenia, or at least the absence of leukocytosis, which distinguishes it from most other bacteremias. Within a few weeks, however, a roentgenogram of the chest reveals small densities scattered diffusely throughout both lung fields; these are the miliary tubercles, which gradually increase in size. Very few physical signs may be elicited on physical examination of the chest, but at this stage the patient suffers from a severe harassing cough, dyspnea and cyanosis. Treatment is precisely as described for pulmonary tuberculosis.

CHRONIC PULMONARY TUBERCULOSIS

Tissues respond to the invading tubercle bacillus in different ways, depending on the degree of immunity possessed by the patient and the degree of inflammatory reaction provoked by the organism and its products. Let us assume that a few tubercle bacilli, recently inhaled, have lodged and gained a foothold in the wall of one of the bronchi. It is usually one of the smaller bronchi near the periphery of the lung that is infected. The usual reaction is the prompt formation of clusters of tubercles around these bacterial clumps. Some of the organisms escape into the lymph ducts that drain this area of lung

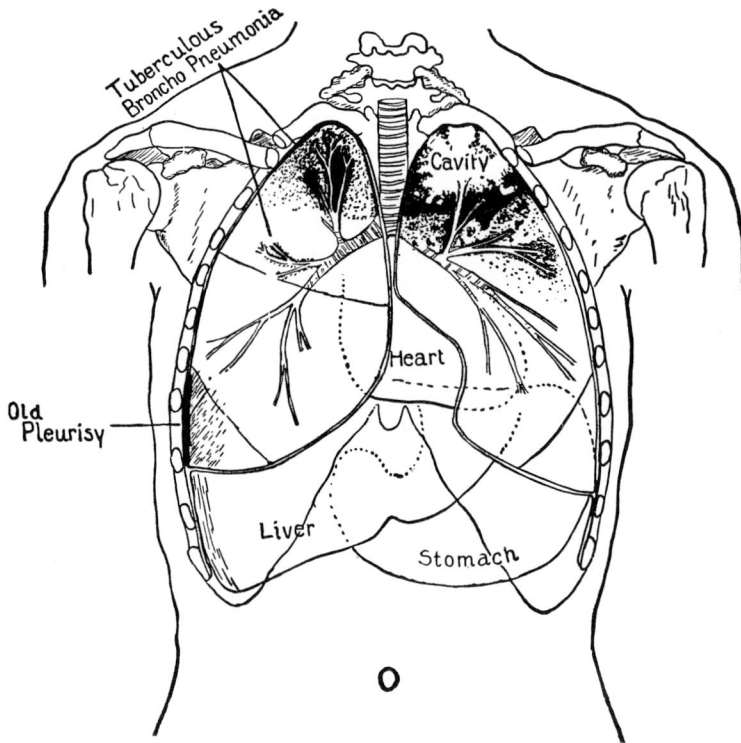

FIG. 150. A diagram of a chest showing tuberculous lesions. The oldest lesion is the patch of thickened pleura in the right lower axilla; the most recent is the slight bronchopneumonia in both upper lobes. At the apex of the left upper lobe is a cavity. Scattered miliary tubercles are represented in both lungs.

and are trapped in the hilar lymph node with which the duct communicates. The imprisoned bacteria gradually die, the tubercles in the lung tissue and in the infected lymph node become necrotic, and calcium becomes deposited in the caseous tissue. The end-result is a healed primary tuberculosis, manifested by a calcified nodule (the Ghon tubercle) at the site of the original infection and a calcified node at the corresponding hilus, a combination known as the *Ghon complex*. Subsequent invasions by the tubercle bacillus will be met more promptly, and, in most cases, unless the infecting dose is large, the organisms will never have a chance to multiply or spread. In America, a large, although decreasing, percentage (less than 20 per cent) of all persons contract such a lesion. The infection rarely gives rise to a single symptom or sign other than x-ray evidence of the Ghon complex.

Individuals who have experienced a primary tuberculous infection are sensitized or allergic to the chemical constituents of the organism. Henceforth, contact with the bacillus, whether it is alive or killed, produces an acute local tissue inflammation. This is the basis of the tuberculin test, in which a suspension of ground-up killed tubercle bacilli obtained from a culture is injected into the skin. If the patient is allergic —that is, has at one time had a tuberculous infection—a local skin inflammation results (p. 450); whereas if there is no allergy, no reaction whatever is obtained.

A similar inflammatory reaction develops in the lung of a person who has been sensitized previously to the tubercle bacillus, if this lung is invaded later by more organisms than his immune processes can handle at the time. In contrast with the relatively bland, silent, primary type of pulmonary tuberculosis, the course of the reinfection type is complicated by necrosis with resulting ulceration of the infected lung tissue. Clusters of tubercles, as in the primary type of tuberculosis, form at once around the nests of organisms, but now, due to the tissue sensitivity, these become surrounded by zones of inflammatory reaction. The alveoli in the area become filled with exudate; in other words, a tuberculous bronchopneumonia develops.

The tuberculous tissue in this area gradually becomes caseous and ulcerates into a bronchus, causing a cavity (Fig. 150). At the same time, as the ulcerations heal, considerable scar tissue forms locally, especially around the cavities. The pleura over the infected lobe, more often an upper lobe, becomes inflamed, then thickened and retracted by scar tissue.

This cycle of inflammatory bronchopneumonia proceeds to ulceration with cavitation, followed by scarring. Unless the process can be arrested, it spreads slowly downward toward the hilum and later extends into adjacent lobes. The activity of the process may be very prolonged and characterized by long remissions, when the case may appear to be arrested, only to be followed by periods of renewed activity.

Depending on whether the predominant pathologic feature of the infection is ulceration or fibrosis, a case is designated as *chronic ulcerative pulmonary tuberculosis* or *chronic fibroid tuberculosis*. Fibroid tuberculosis is that form of the infection in which the healing process is sufficient to prevent gross caseation of the tuberculous areas yet cannot halt the infection. The result is a gradual transformation of a lobe, or of the entire lung, into a mass of fibrous tissue. The pleurae become thick and adherent, and the bronchi dilated, their walls pulled apart by the contracting scar tissue in the lung, while the chest on the affected side becomes shrunken, the spine curved laterally.

Symptoms and Course

Chronic pulmonary tuberculosis is insidious in its onset and course—so insidious that its diagnosis may be missed for a long time.

The early symptoms seldom suggest the lungs as the seat of the disease. Often the patient notices first that he is losing weight; that, although he feels very well on rising in the morning, he fatigues a little more easily than previously, especially in the afternoon. He becomes a trifle pale, his appetite gradually fails, and he may suffer from "indigestion." He gradually acquires a cough, or at any rate he "clears his throat" every morning. His temperature, although normal in the morning, is definitely elevated each afternoon (Fig. 151).

With the progress of the disease, the anorexia, the "indigestion," may be marked. Abdominal pain or even vomiting may occur after meals. The cough, for weeks passed off as bronchitis or a cigarette cough, gradually becomes more troublesome, and the sputum increases. There is no longer doubt as to the afternoon fever; the patient has night sweats. Loss of weight and strength is rapid.

Hemoptysis (hemorrhage from the lungs) is frequent in pulmonary tuberculosis. It may be the first symptom noticed by the patient. These hemorrhages, due to ulceration of an artery, may be profuse, even fatal. They occur unexpectedly and quite independent of exertion or activity. In fact, they may occur during sleep.

The course of chronic, ulcerative pulmonary tuberculosis is marked by ups and downs. Now the healing process gains the ascendancy and the patient feels better; now the ulcerative process progresses and he feels worse. So it goes for months and years, until either the disease stops or an acute exacerbation of the trouble, such as tuberculous bronchopneumonia, enters the scene. Many are the cases of chronic tuberculosis in which

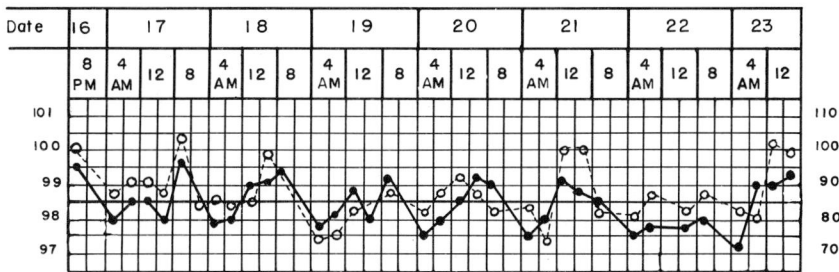

FIG. 151. Chart showing the afternoon fever of tuberculosis.

the cavity formation is arrested and the patient is able to continue at his occupation for many years. In the past such patients were largely responsible for the spread of this disease.

Diagnosis

All patients with a history of unexplained weight loss, fatigability, fever, chronic cough or chest pain deserve careful study to rule out pulmonary tuberculosis. The added history of contact with tuberculous individuals, previous pleurisy or hemoptysis is extremely suggestive. The physical signs, if present at all, may be those of pneumonitis, perhaps with contraction, of one or both upper lobes.

The most important single examination is roentgenography of the chest, by which means even minimal tuberculous lesions can be identified and their activity gauged to a certain extent. The sputum, especially the morning sputum, and the fasting gastric contents should be examined repeatedly, both microscopically, after concentrating them and applying the acidfast stain to the concentrate, and by special methods of culture which favor the growth of the tubercle bacillus in an artificial medium. The intraperitoneal inoculation of guinea pigs with concentrated sputum and gastric washings also is recommended as an additional check in the bacteriologic "screening" investigation.

Tuberculin Testing. The *Mantoux test* involves the inoculation of tubercle bacillus extract ("tuberculin") into the skin of the forearm on its inner aspect. The material is injected as superficially as possible beneath the skin surface, with needle bevel up (Fig. 152). Either of two substances may be used: "Purified Protein Derivative" (PPD.) or "Old Tuberculin" (OT.). After a lapse of from 48 to 72 hours the site of injection is examined for the presence or absence of an inflammatory response, which is evaluated on the basis of the extent of induration. An area of induration measuring 5 mm. or more in diameter is interpreted as a positive reaction. This reaction, in a patient with active tuberculosis, may be very intense; therefore, if a patient is suspected of having an active infection it is customary to initiate the test with an injection of very dilute ("first strength") PPD., repeating the procedure with successively higher doses of the material if negative reactions are obtained.

The *Heaf test* employs an automatic skin-puncturing device, as follows: A concentrated solution of tuberculin is placed on an area of skin that has been cleansed with acetone and driven into the skin mechanically by means of an apparatus incorporating a battery of needles arranged in a circle. The detection of 4 or more points of palpable induration at puncture sites signifies a positive reaction.

In the *"patch test"* the tuberculin is not introduced beneath the skin but is held in contact with its surface by means of an adhesive tape, which usually is placed on the back, between the scapulae. The patch test is considered less reliable than the intradermal tests, yielding the highest percentage of false-positive and false-negative results of all the tuberculin tests available.

A positive tuberculin test indicates that a patient has had contact with the tubercle bacillus, but yields little information regarding the activity of the infection. In general, the more intense the reaction, the greater the likelihood of an active infection. A negative test is even more valuable diagnostically, for it practically rules out the presence of active tuberculosis excepting in patients with miliary tuberculosis, who may lose their capacity to react to tuberculin, and in patients who are receiving one of the corticosteroid drugs, whose tests may become negative in the face of an active infection.

Management of Pulmonary Tuberculosis

Basic Concepts and Objectives

The recent advent of effective chemotherapy has resulted in a complete reversal of earlier concepts regarding the treatment, the nursing care and the rehabilitation of patients with tuberculosis. Before drugs became available, the therapeutic keynote was rest—physical, mental and emotional rest for the patient, and immobility for his diseased lung. The average hospital stay was well over 400 days. (Now it is approximately 180 to 200 days.) The psychological complications that are inherent in "rest," not to mention the physical deterioration that it induces, created a tremendous problem of rehabilitation, which was complicated further by the economic and vocational problems that were the inevitable product of very prolonged hospitalization.

The situation now is very different. Hospitalization of patients with active pulmonary tuberculosis still is highly desirable, although no longer an absolute prerequisite of adequate care. However, rest has been eliminated from the program, not because it has become unnecessary, but because it is regarded as being positively undesirable, tending to protect the tubercle bacillus rather than the patient. By the same token, all surgical procedures and other maneuvers designed to immobilize and collapse the tuberculous lung have been abandoned, including artificial pneumothorax, phrenicotomy, phrenic nerve crush operations and thoracoplasties of all types. Tuberculosis surgery now is more important than before, but it is of a different design and done with different intent: it is employed to re-expand lungs that are compressed and collapsed by contracted pleura or to remove lesions that have succeeded in harboring viable tubercle bacilli in the face of vigorous chemotherapy.

The rationale of the new surgical approach and the changed concepts regarding rest versus activity in tuberculous patients are readily understood if the following facts are appreciated. First, whereas there are several drugs to which the tubercle bacillus is susceptible, there is none to which it cannot develop resistance if conditions permit—specifically, conditions that allow it to metabolize for a time in the presence of the drug in low concentrations. Second, there is a tendency for blood vessels in tuberculous tissue to become thrombosed and obliterated, with the result that the involved tissue becomes ischemic and necrotic—an excellent nutrient medium for the tubercle bacillus and, moreover, one that isolates it from the blood stream and the lethal charge it is carrying. Third, although the organisms are ingested by tissue macrophages, they are not digested and destroyed; on the contrary, the tubercle bacilli find themselves in the safest possible place, i.e., enclosed within a membrane that is impenetrable to streptomycin. Fourth, the pathologic changes associated with tuberculosis are such as to cause stricture and finally complete stenosis of the smaller bronchi and the bronchioles; as a result, the necrotic lung tissue cannot evacuate itself, i.e., spontaneous drainage of these lesions becomes impossible.

The virtue of activity, as opposed to rest, then, is to promote drainage of the necrotic lesion, to mobilize the infective organisms, to flush them from their shelters into the open, so to speak, where the drug concentration is high—not allow them to remain sequestered in areas of low drug concentration, where they may survive long enough to acquire drug resistance. The justification for radical resection of a lesion that fails to heal promptly in response to chemotherapy is clear; namely, failure to heal, under these circumstances, may be construed as being evidence that the organisms contained in it have succeeded in becoming resistant, carrying the implication that the tissue that sheltered them when they were more vulnerable would afford no less protection in the future, should a different drug be tried, and that intensification of chemotherapy would have no effect other than to improve bacterial resistance.

Hospitalization and Communicable Disease Precautions

Tuberculosis patients should be hospitalized for proof of diagnosis, evaluation of the extent of pathology and to determine the responsiveness of the tubercle bacillus to chemotherapy. Further objectives of hospitalization are to protect the patient from serious drug toxicity or allergy, to isolate him while he is contagious and to perform surgery as soon as the indications are clear.

If patients are physically able, they should have bathroom privileges and walk to meals, assuming that there are dining-room facilities for ambulant patients. At other times their activities should be reduced to a minimum as long as tuberculous activity is manifest.

Patients with "open" tuberculosis, i.e., active and communicable because of the production of infective sputum, must be segregated, preferably in a sanatorium, and cared for by individuals trained in the practice of isolation technics. Instructions must be provided regarding the precautions that are necessary for the protection of others, including the necessity for covering the mouth and the nose while coughing or sneezing, for disposing carefully and quickly of tissues contaminated by sputum or other secretions, for making use of a paper bag pinned to the bed and for depositing the sputum in a closed sputum cup. Salivary secretion should not be spread over pens, pencils, bobbypins or stamps. Those individuals who are obliged to expose themselves to the risk of infection through contact with actively infected patients or materials that are contaminated by infective secretions never should relax their precautions for their own protection. They should use well-designed masks worn properly when in the vicinity of these patients and take pains to avoid unnecessary contact with the patient or objects in their immediate vicinity; when such contact is necessary, they should use a protective gown during the period of contact, and carefully wash their hands after the removal of the gown and the conclusion of the contact.

Visitors must be educated thoroughly in the practice of these precautions.

Nursing Care of Patients
With Pulmonary Tuberculosis

The activity of a tuberculous infection is gauged by changes in the body temperature, the pulse rate and the body weight. Therefore, all of these must be measured at appropriate intervals and charted.

The malaise attending high fever may be relieved effectively by the application of cool sponge baths. The discomfort of night sweats is reduced by the wearing of flannel night clothes, which should be replaced at once when damp.

Cough may be alleviated by steam inhalations. The inhalation may be prepared, for example, by boiling at the bedside a solution containing creosote, turpentine and benzoin tincture in equal parts, one teaspoonful of this mixture being added to one pint of water. Sedation should not be employed with the view of abolishing cough altogether, for a certain amount of coughing is necessary for the removal of exudate from the infected lung. Moreover, the use of narcotic agents,

even codeine, in chronic tuberculosis, as in any chronic disease, is hazardous because of the danger of addiction.

Hemoptysis. If hemorrhage occurs, the patient, if up and about, should be put to bed at once and immobilized as completely as possible. He should lie on the infected side, and the thoracic movement should be confined with sandbags or whatever device is immediately available. Morphine sulfate, 12 to 16 mg. ($\frac{1}{6}$ to $\frac{1}{4}$ gr.), may be given at 4-hour intervals if necessary to control pain, dyspnea and anxiety, and oxygen inhalations should be started on the appearance of cyanosis or dyspnea of increasing severity. If hypotension or "shock" appears, blood transfusions should be administered. Penicillin therapy should be started as prophylactic against the secondary development of bacterial pneumonia.

The color of the blood produced during the hemorrhage should be noted by the nurse and described carefully to the physician in the event that she is reporting the occurrence by telephone. If it is bright red, the bleeding is probably venous in origin and very likely will cease spontaneously. Under these conditions, sedation is not only unnecessary but also undesirable, for it impairs the evacuation of the blood from the bronchi. Blockage of the bronchi leads to the development of atelectasis, with the danger of fatal pneumonia in the collapsed lung.

Antituberculosis Chemotherapy

Isoniazid (INH), para-aminosalicylic acid (PAS) and streptomycin are the antimicrobials used most often in the treatment of tuberculosis at the present time. The following principles govern their use:

1. Two of these agents, or all three, usually are given in combination, in an effort to prevent the development of drug resistance.

2. Whatever drug combination is selected, isoniazid usually is included. (INH and PAS are generally considered to represent the combination of choice.)

3. Antituberculous chemotherapy, barring complications, is administered without interruption for a minimum of at least 12 months, or even for 24 months, in order to prevent relapse or the emergence of drug resistance.

Table 16 gives the details concerning the

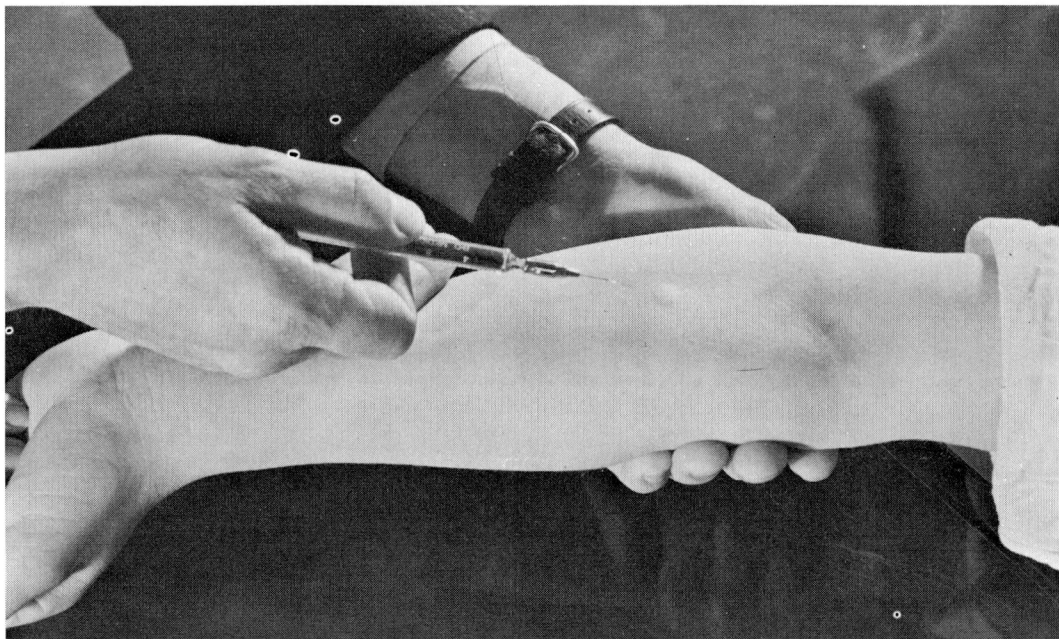

FIG. 152. The Mantoux Test. Using a tuberculin syringe and a subcutaneous needle with the bevel up, tubercle bacillus extract has been injected into the skin of the forearm. (National Tuberculosis Association, New York, N. Y.)

administration of the antituberculous drugs as well as the nursing implications associated with each of these agents.

Surgery in Pulmonary Tuberculosis

Segmental resection (removal of a portion of a lobe), lobectomy (a complete lobe) and pneumonectomy (entire lung) are carried out for the purpose of eliminating lesions that show little promise of yielding to chemotherapy, based on the persistence of positive sputum cultures after 3 months or more of combined drug treatment, or when it becomes evident that certain factors exist which would favor the reactivation of a quiescent lesion, such as cavitation, extensive caseation, bronchiectasis or bronchial stenosis (see p. 449). Other indications for surgery would be the discovery of renewed tuberculous activity after concluding a course of chemotherapy, or the necessity of removing a pleura that had become contracted following pleural effusions, or an earlier pneumothorax by a procedure known as "decortication" (described later), in order to permit the lung to re-expand and resume normal function.

Thoracoplasty with Pulmonary Resection. When lobectomy or pneumonectomy is performed for tuberculosis, some surgeons prefer to do a thoracoplasty in 3 to 6 weeks. In unusually good operative risks, these procedures can be done at the same time. The purpose of doing a rib resection is to prevent overdistention of the remaining lung tissue. The possibility of bronchopleural fistula and tuberculous empyema is lessened. Usually 4 ribs are removed following lobectomy and 6 or 7 following pneumonectomy.

Drainage Operations. Drainage procedures are used for palliation in patients who are quite ill. The *Monaldi* method is performed by inserting a catheter into the abscess or cavity through a cannula. After insertion, the catheter is attached to water-seal drainage. A *cavernostomy* is done by resecting a rib and incising the chest wall into the lung. Open wound drainage means that the dressings must be changed at least daily. *Empyema drainage* also can be done. This has been described on page 427.

Decortication of the Lung. Decortication is the surgical removal of fibrinous deposit

TABLE 16. Chemotherapeutic Agents Used in the Treatment of Tuberculosis

Drug	Customary Dosage	Therapeutic Considerations	Nursing Implications
ISONIAZID (INH)	300 mg., or 4 to 5 mg. per kilo. of body weight—daily by mouth	INH may be used alone in treatment of mild infections, e.g., asymptomatic primary tuberculosis. When INH is prescribed in high dosage, pyridoxine usually is given as an adjunct to prevent peripheral neuritis.	Observe patient for symptoms of numbness, tingling and weakness in the extremities, which are indicative of a complicating polyneuritis.
PARA-AMINO-SALICYLIC ACID (PAS)	12 Grams daily in divided doses—by mouth	Enhances effectiveness of INH and streptomycin.	Drug should be given with meals. Epigastric distress and diarrhea are common. Fever and skin rash may develop. For dyspepsia, offer milk (not antacids, which inactivate PAS). Stress importance of continuing PAS in face of minor complications.
STREPTOMYCIN	1 Gram 2 or 3 times weekly—intramuscularly	Highly effective during febrile, exudative stage of pulmonary tuberculosis, but effective for only limited period of time.	Be alert for, and report promptly, symptoms indicating ototoxicity: i.e., tinnitus, deafness, vertigo, or an unsteady gait. Watch for allergic skin reaction.

on the pleura that prevents re-expansion of the lung and has resulted from prolonged pneumothorax and tuberculous empyema. It is done in selected cases when there is little likelihood of reactivation of the disease and where healthy lung tissue can be re-expanded. The care preoperatively and postoperatively is the same as that described in Chapter 23, "Patients with Medical and Surgical Conditions of the Chest," pages 408 to 417.

Preoperative Nursing Care

An understanding of the mental problems of this patient is essential. When one realizes that he usually has a history of illness of a year or more, that he may have been in a sanatorium for a long while, and that he probably has had his hopes raised innumer-

able times only to be blasted when therapy failed, one is more tolerant of his reactions. He must be made to realize that a thoracoplasty is not an immediate cure, and that convalescence is slow. The socio-economic factors cannot be neglected. In addition, the patient usually is on isolation precautions. Some physicians prefer to have their patients raise as much sputum as possible about 30 minutes before operation. This may be done by postural drainage or by coughing voluntarily. The shaving of the chest and the remaining preparation is the same as that for other chest surgical patients.

Postoperative Nursing Care

Postoperative care is directed toward preventing many possible complications—for example, shock, hemorrhage, respiratory and circulatory collapse, paradoxical motion, the spread of infection, wound infection and deformity. The patient is kept in the Trendelenburg position until he is conscious and his vital signs are satisfactory. He should be turned from his back to the operated side every second hour and encouraged to cough in an effort to bring up secretions. Often the tight adhesive strapping is not sufficient to allay the patient's fears when he coughs, and it is necessary for the nurse to splint the wound with the palm of her hand or her forearm. During this postoperative period, the nurse must be on the alert for signs that suggest a retention of secretions such as "wet" inspirations and expirations after coughing, increasing dyspnea and a temperature elevation. If this occurs, the physician should be notified and an endotracheal aspiration tray made available. Every effort must be exerted to prevent atelectasis, not only because of the resultant obstruction of a portion of the lung but also because of the likelihood of spread of infection.

Paradoxical motion is one of the complications that can occur in the postoperative thoracoplasty patient (see Fig. 136). By applying external pressure, this phenomenon can be controlled. Sandbags that weigh about 5 lb. can be applied beneath the clavicle. Unfortunately, they are cumbersome and difficult to keep in place. Some surgeons prefer to apply thick gauze pads beneath the clavicle and in the axilla. They are held in place by 2-inch adhesive strips applied over the back and the shoulders so that skin tension will be distributed widely. Blistering from adhesive must be guarded against.

Physical Therapy. Passive and then active movements of the arm on the affected side should be started on the day of operation and continued after that on instructions from the physician and the physical therapist. Proper body posture with adequate support of the back, the shoulders and the arm must be maintained. A Balkan frame with a trapezelike bar provides an excellent means for the patient to move in bed with a desirable amount of exercise. Often the patient favors the operated side by lifting the arm with the opposite hand, by rotating the trunk instead of the head and by drooping his shoulder

protectively. Without a doubt this leads to scoliosis and a crippling posture, and it must be prevented. In all efforts at rehabilitation, the patient must express a desire and a willingness to help himself. After the second or the third stage of thoracoplasty, a small, firm pillow may be placed in the axilla on the operated side. This will increase collapse of the thoracic wall and prevent scoliosis. Some physicians prefer to have the patient use a chest sling, which is a piece of canvas from about 12 to 15 inches wide and 3 feet long. A hammock is formed to encase the patient as he lies on his operated side. By counteracting weights (pulley system) he is lifted from the bed, thus utilizing body weight to produce further collapse. He remains in this position for only a few minutes at first, after which the time gradually is increased to 30 minutes 3 times a day.

The successful care of this patient includes special emphasis on good mouth hygiene, plenty of fresh air, adequate nutrition, proper exercise and an optimistic frame of mind. Diversional occupational therapy that is prescribed carefully is essential because of the long period of essentially inactive convalescence. Frequently, this rehabilitative and "resting" stage can be spent at home.

Convalescent Care of the Tuberculous Patient

One of the most important aspects of nursing care in pulmonary tuberculosis is guiding the patient through his convalescence. A program of convalescence and rehabilitation is designed for each individual patient, tailored to meet his specific and unique requirements, and subject to constant readjustment as progress permits or circumstances require. Among the many controlling factors in this program are the course of his body temperature, pulse rate and respiratory rate; the amount and character of his sputum; his appetite and weight; his general health; and his sense of wellbeing.

One of the most important, and perhaps most difficult, of the nurse's responsibilities in relation to the convalescent care of the patient with pulmonary tuberculosis is to assist in combating the psychological in-

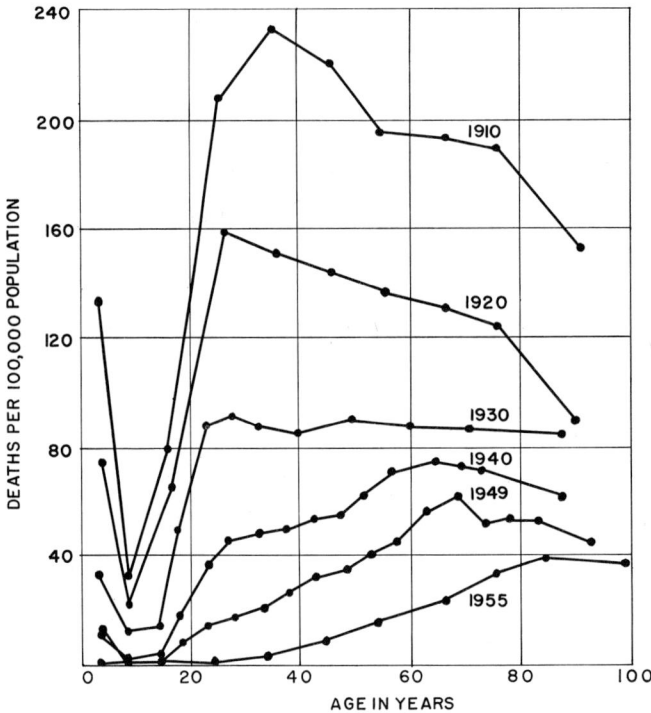

FIG. 153. Tuberculosis mortality rates in the U. S., showing the relative and absolute figures at various ages, comparing the similar age in the contemporary population. (Anderson, G. W.: Am. Rev. Tuberc. **67**:123)

validism that is so apt to result from any prolonged illness. His interest in outside pursuits and activities should be stimulated and his self-reliance encouraged.

Education of the Patient. The patient should be instructed in reading a thermometer and in the correct method of measuring the body weight. He must understand the importance of a complete physical examination, including roentgenograms of the chest, every 6 months for a minimum of 2 years after his discharge. The patient and his family should be instructed carefully in regard to possible complications, including hemorrhage, pleurisy and other untoward symptoms that are indicative of a possible recurrence of tuberculous activity. Literature concerning tuberculosis should be made available to the patient in order to improve his insight and knowledge of the disease.

Public Health and Prevention

Children exposed to individuals with active tuberculosis should be examined annually. Individuals who are positive reactors should have annual tuberculin tests and roentgenograms of the chest. During adolescence when they are most vulnerable, when old infections are particularly apt to become reactivated and new ones acquired, vigilance must be redoubled. Examinations should be arranged on the development of any suggestive symptom, such as unexplained weight loss, anorexia, pain in the chest or cough.

Due to the tuberculin testing of cattle and the pasteurization of milk, infection by drinking contaminated milk has become rare in this country.

It is to be anticipated that chemotherapy more effective than that now available will be developed, and the importance of tuberculosis as a public health hazard then may dwindle into insignificance. However, that day is not as yet at hand, and until it is, the general public must be kept fully aware of their duties and responsibilities for the prevention of tuberculosis. Whereas the death rate from tuberculosis has declined at a gratifying rate (Fig. 153), the number of new cases developing per annum has not changed very much in recent years. There are an estimated 250,000 known as well as unknown active cases of tuberculosis in the United States today. Moreover, the new cases are just as far advanced as they were before the advent of chemotherapy. Although children, particularly in adolescence, are susceptible to the disease, age is no barrier to its development; frequently, tuberculosis of the lungs and other organs is acquired in late life. Therefore, the necessity for careful examination, preferably on a routine basis, is obvious.

An important advance in tuberculosis prophylaxis is the opportunity which is becoming increasingly available for roentgenographic examination of the chest without cost; this is accomplished on a mass scale by means of photofluorograms, entailing the photographing of the fluoroscopic image while the chest is irradiated. With facilities of this type available, failure to be examined cannot be excused on the grounds of economy, nor, in fact, on any other basis.

Tuberculosis associations and health departments are working diligently to eradicate tuberculosis. It has been their experience that certain groups should receive top priority in case detection programs, among them persons who are or have been closely associated with patients with tuberculosis. A recent public health study revealed that almost 40 times more tuberculosis is found among contacts than is found among the general population.

Another susceptible group is comprised of known suspects who have symptoms suggesting tuberculous activity. Inactive cases should be followed closely, for they may become active again. Patients newly admitted to hospitals should be screened routinely for tuberculosis. Foodhandlers, a notoriously transient group, show a high tuberculosis rate. Tuberculosis testing in schools and child health clinics and community surveys for tuberculosis also are valuable in case finding.

The vaccine BCG. (bacille Calmette-Guérin) is given sometimes to nonreactors to tuberculin. It appears to be safe but does not offer measurable or absolute protection against tuberculosis. Its use is restricted to persons who are tuberculin negative, as it does not benefit persons who have already been infected and thus are positive tuberculin reactors.

The National Tuberculosis Association is a voluntary nonprofit public health agency dedicated to the prevention and the elimination of tuberculosis and other respiratory diseases and the improvement of health. The Association's official publications are the *Bulletin,* which disseminates information about tuberculosis and respiratory diseases to lay and professional groups, and *The American Review of Respiratory Diseases,* a journal for professional readers.

CLINICAL SITUATION

Indicate the best answer:

1. Tuberculosis may run a rapid course or be a slowly progressive disorder. Early in the course of the infection the patient is likely to
   A. Have no physical complaints.
   B. Complain of drenching night sweats.
   C. Have an episode of hemoptysis.
   D. Run an intermittent fever.

2. Tuberculous lesions develop most commonly in the
   A. Upper lobes.
   B. Lung parenchyma.
   C. Glands around the hilus.
   D. Lower lobes.

3. The Mantoux intracutaneous test is "read" by which of the following criteria?
   A. Area of erythema.
   B. Amount of pain at the site.
   C. Number of blebs at the site.
   D. Area of induration.

4. The most accurate tuberculin test is considered to be the
   A. Multiple puncture test.
   B. Intracutaneous test.
   C. Patch test.
   D. Scratch test.

5. Several combinations of antimicrobials are being used in the treatment of tuberculosis. Of the following, which is the most effective member of an antimicrobial combination?
   A. Para-aminosalicylic acid.
   B. Streptomycin.
   C. Isoniazid
   D. Viomycin.

BIBLIOGRAPHY AND SUGGESTED READING

Books and Pamphlets

Allen, J. C.: A Psychodynamic Approach of the Nurse in Combating Denial of the Disease— Tuberculosis; Monograph 12, Nursing Approaches to the Denial of Illness, New York, American Nurses' Association, 1962.

The Treatment of Tuberculosis and the Management of Tuberculosis Infection, Richmond, Va., Virginia Tuberculosis Association, 1962.

Publications of the
National Tuberculosis Association

The Chemotherapy of Tuberculosis, 1960; Diagnostic Standards and Classification of Tuberculosis, 1961; Goals and Standards for Eliminating Tuberculosis, 1960; How to Find Tuberculosis, 1962; Introduction to Respiratory Diseases, 1961; Safer Ways in Nursing, A Guide to Precautions in the Care of Patients (with tuberculosis and other respiratory diseases), 1962; South, Jean: Tuberculosis Handbook for Public Health Nurses, 1959; The Tuberculin Test, 1962.

Articles

American Thoracic Society: Tuberculosis control programs for nurses, nursing students and hospital personnel, Nurs. Outlook **9**:36-37, Jan., 1961.

Bullough, B.: Where should isolation stop? Am. J. Nurs. **62**:86-89, Oct., 1962.

Creighton, H., and Gabriella, Sister: Group teaching in Cajun country, Nurs. Outlook **9**:736-738, Dec., 1961.

Dickson, W., Jr.: Toward the elimination of tuberculosis, Nurs. Outlook **9**:630-632, Oct., 1961.

Feldman, F.: How to use the tuberculin test, Am. J. Nurs. **59**:856-859, June, 1959.

Frenay, M. C.: Drugs in tuberculosis control, Am. J. Nurs. **61**:82-85, April, 1961.

Gibson, F. J., and Taylor, R. M.: Selective case-finding in tuberculosis, Nurs. Outlook **7**:641-643, Nov., 1959.

Kressler, A.: Teaching patients with tuberculosis, Am. J. Nurs. **59**:1116-1118, Aug., 1959.

Merrick, M.: Building morale in a tuberculosis hospital, Am. J. Nurs. **61**:95, Nov., 1961.

Novak, M. L.: Social and emotional problems of patients with tuberculosis, Nurs. Outlook **6**:210-211, April, 1958.

Pamplona, P. A., and South, J.: The Arden House conference on tuberculosis, Nurs. Outlook **9**:30-35, Jan., 1961.

Richie, J.: A tuberculosis patient who refuses care, Nurs. Outlook **8**:621-623, Nov., 1960.

Spahn, C. H.: Tuberculosis or coccidiodomycosis? Nurs. Outlook **8**:25-27, Jan., 1960.

Weiss, M.: Chemotherapy and tuberculosis, Am. J. Nurs. **59**:1711-1714, Dec., 1959.

Wilson, A. B.: The big push to eliminate tuberculosis, Am. J. Nurs. **61**:110-112, Oct., 1961.

Patient-Teaching Aids and
Sources of Information

The Development of Present Knowledge about Tuberculosis. A pamphlet pub. by U. S. Dept. of Health, Education, and Welfare, No. 33-A of the Health Information Series, 1961.

Tuberculosis. Health Information Series, No. 30. A pamphlet by the U. S. Dept. of Health, Education and Welfare, 1963.

Additional information available from:
The National Tuberculosis Association
1790 Broadway
New York 19, New York

Tuberculosis Nursing Advisory Service
National League for Nursing
2 Park Avenue
New York 16, New York

U. S. Department of Health,
Education and Welfare
Public Health Service
Washington, D. C.

World Health Organization
Palais des Nations
Geneva, Switzerland

Answers to PLAN OF NURSING CARE (p. 444)

Nursing Activities to Meet Needs

1. Offer hot beverage at 7 A.M.
   Order breakfast tray at 9 A.M.
   Have him give his own bath at 11 A.M.
   (Observe and note which phase of the bath causes him to become fatigued.)

2. Stay with patient during IPPB treatment and offer encouragement.

3. Gray ladies in to see patient several times daily.

4. Call physical therapist to supervise his walking-breathing exercises.
   Remind him of his breathing exercises.

5. Vocational rehabilitation consultant to be called in order to evaluate his needs. Check with physician to see when he can do evaluation tests for future employment.

Unit IX. Nursing Care in Hematologic and Cardiovascular Disorders

ORIENTATION

The circulatory system, which includes the heart, the vascular channels and the blood, supplies the equipment and the mechanisms required for "internal respiration," the process by which a state of equilibrium is maintained among all cells within the body and the atmosphere surrounding it, for the nutrition of those cells and the disposal of their metabolic wastes and for the defense of the body as a whole against invading micro-organisms. The formed elements of the blood, and the disorders which affect these predominantly, are discussed in Chapter 25, the vascular channels through which the blood is pumped are considered in Chapter 26, and the pump itself, the heart, in Chapter 27.

Of the disease conditions affecting the circulatory system, the first to be presented are the hematologic disorders, each one of which is potentially of vital importance to every cell of the body. Included in this group are some disorders that predominantly affect the red cells, which may be too few or too many. White cells likewise may be either excessive in number or dangerously depleted, and several abnormalities are encountered that are responsible for spontaneous hemorrhages.

From a clinical standpoint, the reader will note a close resemblance among the various blood dyscrasias, irrespective of differences in their etiology or fundamental character. The symptoms of anemia, for example, for which there are many possible causes, are much the same in all cases. Similarly, as regards thrombocytopenic purpura (excessive bleeding due to a deficiency of blood platelets), the same type of purpura results whether platelet depression is due to a poison, an abnormal antibody, a malignant tumor in the bone marrow or an atomic bomb.

Cardiovascular diseases are discussed in two principal categories: those in which there is an interference with the efficiency of the heart as a pump, resulting in heart failure, or a disturbance of its own blood supply, causing anginal pain; and the so-called "occlusive peripheral vascular diseases" with disturbances of blood flow in some localized area, for example, an extremity. Regarding circulatory disorders in general, particularly those in which the heart or the blood vessels are damaged structurally, there appears to be one outstanding difference between these and most other types of disease: the reparative processes seldom lead to complete restoration of function, as in other tissues; consequently, permanent invalidism of some degree is a common complication of most vascular diseases and is one of the most important considerations in their treatment.

Cardiovascular disease, directly or indirectly, accounts for more deaths in our population than all other causes combined and is responsible for more than three times as many deaths as the second leading cause, cancer. Its lethal significance at all ages, the extent to which its importance increases in successively older age groups and the formidable threat to survival it poses during the latter decades are amply documented in Table 17.

TABLE 17. Relative Frequency of Cardiovascular Deaths in Different Age Groups of the Population, Expressed as Per Cent of All Deaths in Each Group

Age Group (Years)	Cardiovascular Deaths (%)
5	7
5–24	8
25–44	28
45–64	52
65–74	62
75 and over	71

25

Patients With Hematologic Disorders

THE CELLULAR COMPONENTS OF NORMAL BLOOD

Erythrocytes

The red cells, or *erythrocytes,* comprise the vast majority of all blood cells and are chiefly responsible for the color of this liquid tissue. Approximately 5 million erythrocytes are contained in 1 cu. mm. of blood, i.e., a drop about the size of the head of a very small pin. The normal red cell is a biconcave disk, its configuration resembling that of a soft ball compressed firmly between two fingers. The principal function of this cell is to transport oxygen and carbon dioxide. This is accomplished through the agency of an iron-containing pigment, *hemoglobin,* which accounts for 95 per cent of the mass of the cells, and the total concentration of which is normally about 15 Gm. per 100 ml. of whole blood. Hemoglobin has a great tendency to combine with oxygen, this affinity being such that when the two are in brief contact they unite to form *oxyhemoglobin,* the pigment accounting for the bright red color of arterial blood. However, this combination is a weak one, for oxyhemoglobin readily releases its oxygen when exposed to concentrations of oxygen lower than its own. The affinity of hemoglobin for oxygen, and the reversible nature of their combination, together explain the mechanism of oxygen transport in the body and the role of the red cell in this mechanism.

The red blood corpuscles are produced in red bone marrow, the tissue which also provides the blood with most of its leukocytes and all of its platelets. In infants the marrow of all the bones is red, but as the child grows older, about the time of puberty, fatty tissue (fat marrow) replaces the red marrow of the long bones. Hence, the red corpuscles of normal adults are formed only in the short and flat bones, such as the ribs, the sternum, the skull, the vertebrae and the bones of the hands and the feet. In certain types of anemia accompanied by an increased rate of blood production, great increases occur in the amount and the activity of the red bone marrow, which may replace, temporarily or permanently, the fatty marrow.

Red blood corpuscles in normal blood have no nuclei. From the primitive stem cells in red bone marrow arise *erythroblasts,* nucleated cells that in the process of maturing accumulate hemoglobin. The nucleus becomes small and dark (*normoblast*), then disappears, and the cell is known as a *reticulocyte.* The final step in maturation consists in the loss of all darkly staining substances and shrinkage to normal size.

For the proper evolution and maturation of red cells, the bone marrow requires iron, vitamin B_{12}, pyridoxine and doubtless a host of other nutrients, both organic and inorganic. Iron is needed for hemoglobin formation. If the amount of iron absorbed from the gastrointestinal tract is insufficient to meet the increased requirements imposed by growth, or to compensate for the loss as incurred as a result of bleeding, red cell maturation becomes faulty at the normoblast stage. Many of these cells, unable to incorporate hemoglobin in their cytoplasm, fail to develop further and never leave the marrow but disintegrate in situ, those which do mature fully and succeed in entering the circulating blood being abnormally small and containing less than the normal complement of hemoglobin. Vitamin B_{12} is absorbed from the gastrointestinal tract following the ingestion of certain foods, especially skeletal muscle, milk and eggs, by individuals possessing normal gastric juice. This vitamin is necessary for the evolution of red cells from their precursor cells in the marrow. Deficiency in this substance produces a disease called "pernicious anemia," characterized by abnormally large and misshapen red cells.

Leukocytes

The leukocytes, or white blood cells, normally are present in a concentration of between 5,000 and 10,000 cells in each cu. mm. of whole blood; in other words, there is one white cell for every 500 to 1,000 red cells. The leukocytes, unlike adult erythrocytes, contain no hemoglobin, but they do possess a nucleus; moreover, they are capable of active movement. Major categories of leukocytes include the granulocytic series, lymphocytes, monocytes and plasma cells. The numerical distribution of these cells and the morphologic features that distinguish each variety have been described in Chapter 6.

Blood Platelets

Blood platelets, or *thrombocytes,* the smallest and most fragile of the formed blood elements, are small particles devoid of nuclei that arise as a result of a fragmentation process, or "budding," from giant cells in the bone marrow called *megakaryocytes.* There are approximately 250,000 to 500,000 platelets per 1 cu. mm. of blood.

Platelet morphology, platelet tests and the role of platelets in hemostasis have been discussed fully in Chapter 6.

THE ANEMIC PATIENT

The term *anemia* signifies an abnormally low number of red blood cells or a decreased concentration of hemoglobin in the circulating blood. Anemias are classified on the basis of the mechanism responsible for their development. Possible mechanisms include loss of red cells as a result of bleeding; loss of red cells through excessive hemolysis, in

the case of the hemolytic anemias; and inadequate erythropoiesis (red cell production), the basis of the so-called "aregenerative" anemias.

Aregenerative Anemias

An aregenerative anemia, as this designation implies, is one that is attributable basically to failure by the bone marrow to release new red cells at a rate sufficient to maintain the red cell count and hemoglobin concentration at normal levels, assuming red cell loss to be within normal limits (i.e., approximately 1 per cent per day through senescence) or only moderately increased (as a result of hemorrhage or hemolysis). Under the stimulus of anemia, normal bone marrow, amply furnished with the necessary nutrients, is capable of at least a 6-fold increase in red cell production above that of the normal, nonanemic individual. In other words, red cell regeneration should keep pace with red cell loss, even if the latter were as much as 6 per cent per day, and no anemia should develop. Barring a greater rate of loss, or one of the deficiency states to be discussed presently, any anemia that might develop may be termed *aregenerative.* (This type of anemia also is designated as *hypoplastic* and *refractory* anemia; *hypoplastic* signifying subnormal or inadequate formation, and *refractory* referring to the fact that the anemia fails to respond to the administration of nutrients that are therapeutically effective in deficiency anemias.)

The aregenerative anemias are characterized by a reduction in the concentration of circulating reticulocytes, a manifestation of reduced bone marrow activity. Leukocyte and platelet counts, which also reflect marrow activity, likewise tend to be low. Such anemias occur as a result of nutritional deficiency, toxic bone marrow inhibition and physical injury of, and mechanical interference with, the bone marrow. Frequently the cause is unknown.

Aregenerative anemias of intrinsic origin arise as a result of chronic infections, such as active rheumatic fever, osteomyelitis or tuberculosis. The hemoglobin production in these cases often falls below red cell production, so that the anemia may be of the hypochromic type. The white count is often persistently elevated; the platelets may be elevated or reduced. Medications are of no avail in controlling this type of anemia until the infection has become quiescent. Nor, conversely, will anemias primarily due to lack of iron or some other specific nutrient respond adequately to these preparations if active infection is present.

The anemia of nephritis with nitrogen retention is another common example of toxic anemia of intrinsic origin. The anemia is usually of the normocytic normochromic variety but may be macrocytic. The platelets and the white cells are normal. Again, no response to marrow stimulants can be expected until renal function has been restored to normal.

Anemia may result from physical injury to the bone marrow, such as occasionally occurs in chronic exposure to x-ray or radioactive materials. Sometimes it is caused by mechanical interference with blood formation (myelophthisic anemia): for example, by leukocyte-forming bone marrow tissue such as is encountered in the leukemias, plasmoma and myeloma; by bone marrow invasion by metastatic carcinoma; by Hodgkin's disease of the bone marrow; or by infiltration with cells containing abnormal lipoid accumulations (xanthomatoses). Bone marrow function may be disturbed or destroyed by overgrowth of the surrounding bone cortex (osteosclerotic anemia), which results in fibrosis of the blood-forming organs. Bone marrow fibrosis is the end stage of many bone marrow disturbances, and occasionally it occurs without known cause.

Occasionally the process of blood formation may be taken over by the spleen, which becomes a site of so-called "myeloid metaplasia." This organ and, to a lesser extent, the liver of this patient may become greatly enlarged as a result of extensive proliferation of marrowlike tissue.

Deficiency Anemias

Iron Deficiency

In individuals who are iron deficient, the blood hemoglobin and the red blood cell count are reduced. The hemoglobin is reduced more than is the number of red cells, and for this reason the latter tend to be small and relatively devoid of pigment, i.e., "hypochromic." Hypochromia is the hallmark of iron deficiency. The cause of this deficiency is failure of the patient to ingest, or absorb, sufficient dietary iron to compensate for the iron requirements associated with body growth or for the loss of iron that attends bleeding, whether the bleeding is physiologic (e.g., menstrual) or pathologic.

Of all the deficiency states to which human beings are subject, iron deficiency is by far the commonest, and the hypochromic anemia of iron deficiency is more than twice as prevalent as all other types of anemia combined. This is true, despite the fact that the total loss of iron from all sources (in the sweat and the bile, and in cells desquamated from the lining of the gastrointestinal tract) in the normal individual who is not bleeding is exceedingly small in amount: between 0.5 and 1.5 mg. per day; and it is true even though the average diet furnishes from 10 to 15 mg. of iron each day. The reason becomes clear in the light of the following facts.

Less than 10 per cent of all iron that is ingested, including food iron plus any iron supplements that might be taken, is absorbed. This means that the diet alone, however well-rounded and ample, is unlikely to supply the body with more than 1.0 to 1.5 mg. of the mineral each day, which is little more than enough to satisfy the requirements of a normal male who is experiencing no blood loss (and is not subject to menstrual bleeding), has incurred no iron deficit from hemorrhages in the past and who is not in a period of rapid growth. Iron loss due to bleeding is calculated on the basis of 1 mg. iron per ml. of red cells, or 1 ml. per approximately 2.5 ml. of whole blood. Thus, the menstrual bleeding of a normal woman, which amounts to between 35 and 70 ml. every 28 days, on the average, adds 0.5 to 1.0 mg. to her average daily iron loss, and the total amount lost equals or exceeds the amount she is absorbing from her diet. Small wonder that the majority of growing adolescent girls are iron deficient! During childbearing the mother contributes approximately 400 mg. of iron to the fetus and 150 mg. to the placenta, and loses an additional 175 mg. through postpartum hemorrhage; in other words, she loses an average of about 2.7 mg. of iron per day throughout pregnancy. The additional iron requirement imposed by growth averages about 0.5 mg. per day from infancy to age 20.

It follows from these data that the normal male should subsist satisfactorily, from the standpoint of his iron needs, on a normal diet alone, without benefit of iron supplements. The development of iron-deficiency anemia in a male is prima-facie evidence of either: (1) faulty diet during childhood or adolescence; (2) a gastrointestinal disorder leading to malabsorption; or (3) most likely of all, he has lost blood recently or has bled sometime in the past. As for the female, the development of iron-deficiency anemia during adolescence is almost inevitable and, as a result of pregnancy, entirely inevitable in the absence of iron therapy.

Symptoms of iron-deficiency anemia, if mild, may be limited to pallor, fatigue and dyspnea on exertion. If severe, e.g., with hemoglobin values of less than 8 grams per 100 ml. of blood, the patient may complain of marked weakness and fatigability, breathlessness and cardiac palpitation. The tongue may become sore, and the nails brittle and spoon-shaped. Sometimes extreme difficulty in swallowing (Plummer-Vinson syndrome) is experienced, due to pharyngeal edema and ulceration. The diagnosis is based on the morphology of the red cells, which are hypochromic, microcytic and reduced in number; and on the finding of a low serum iron (hypoferremia), which may be as little as 10 micrograms per 100 ml. of blood or less, as compared with a normal value of between 50 and 150 micrograms. Just as important as confirming the diagnosis of iron deficiency is establishing its cause, which means, unless the cause is self-evident, a search for a source of blood loss, especially gastrointestinal bleeding.

Treatment. In the absence of active bleeding, infection or some other inflammatory process, or uremia, iron deficiency can be corrected and the blood picture restored to normal by the administration of an iron salt in adequate amount. Among the preparations used most commonly are ferrous sulfate, given in a daily dose of 0.9 to 1.2 Gm. (15 to 20 gr.); ferrous gluconate, 1.5 to 2.0 Gm. (24 to 30 gr.) daily; and ferric ammonium citrate, 6 Gm. (90 gr.) each day. Iron preparations suitable for parenteral injection include a dextran complex (Imferon) and a polysaccharide of iron (Feojectin) that are available for intramuscular and intravenous administration, respectively. These are useful in treating patients who are susceptible to gastrointestinal bleeding, or whose gastrointestinal absorption is impaired, as well as those, comprising about 20 per cent of iron-deficient patients, who seem unable to tolerate iron salts when ingested in effective doses.

Nursing Responsibilities in Iron Therapy. With respect to the oral feeding of iron salts, it is important to recognize that all of these, without exception, are gastric irritants. Therefore, they should be given in divided doses with, or shortly after, meals rather than on an empty stomach. The nurse should educate the patient who is receiving large doses of iron to anticipate a certain amount of dyspepsia from time to time and impress him with the fact that such symptoms carry no serious implications but rather serve as a guide in the regulation of dosage and schedule of treatment.

Since ferrous sulfate (which is extremely black) is formed in the intestines, iron salts alter the color of the stools, contributing a tarry color which suggests the presence of digested blood. The patient should be informed with regard to the color changes to be expected and reassured as to their benign character.

Ferrous sulfate is apt to deposit on the teeth and the gums. Hence, the nurse should urge the patient to cleanse the teeth frequently and with regularity, and those receiving liquid preparations of iron should be advised to use a straw for that purpose.

Pernicious Anemia (Vitamin B₁₂ Deficiency)

Pernicious anemia is a disease of adults that has a definite familial incidence and is characterized by macrocytic anemia, gastrointestinal disturbances, neurologic abnormalities typical of combined system disease, gastric achylia, a course marked by progressively severe relapses and ultimate death, without specific therapy, and the capacity to respond to the parenteral administration of vitamin B_{12}. The basic cause of this deficiency state is a defect in the gastric secretory function, the gastric juice being devoid of a material (intrinsic factor) that is necessary for the absorption of B_{12} (extrinsic factor) from the intestine.

Symptoms. Physical weakness during its entire course is one of the most conspicuous features of this disease. Usually it is the first symptom and finally it dominates the picture. This weakness is due to the anemia, which also causes the pallor, the dyspnea and the cardiac palpitation usually present. Gastrointestinal symptoms (sore mouth with smooth red "beefy" tongue, loss of appetite, indigestion, abdominal pain and recurring diarrhea or constipation) are conspicuous. Neurologic symptoms develop in a high proportion of untreated cases. These include tingling, numbness or burning pain involving the hands and the feet and a loss of position sense.

The red cells vary greatly, not only in size, but also in shape (poikilocytosis). Some are oval, some sausage-shaped, while others are distorted beyond description. In the stages of remission, whether spontaneous or as a result of treatment, the reticulocytes, nucleated red cells, platelets and leukocytes, all low in relapse, become elevated. Megaloblasts, the precursors of the normoblasts, rarely appear in the circulating blood.

In years past this disease was characterized by spontaneous remissions, for which no adequate cause could be assigned, and during which practically all the symptoms disappeared. Such remissions would be followed by relapses, the third or the fourth of which usually ended fatally.

Specific Treatment. Treatment of pernicious anemia consists in the administration, by parenteral injection, of vitamin B_{12} (cyanocobalamine).

Patients in full relapse customarily receive B_{12} in doses totaling between 100 and 1,000 micrograms each week during the first month, the vitamin being injected into the deltoid at daily (or weekly) intervals in the form of a solution containing 100 or 1,000 micrograms per ml.

Maintenance therapy, in the form of regular injections of vitamin B_{12}, must be continued throughout the remainder of the patient's life. One hundred micrograms, supplied at monthly intervals, satisfies completely the requirements of most patients for this vitamin, full hematologic remission being maintained and neurologic complications failing to appear, or existing lesions to progress, on this regimen. A small proportion of patients require more frequent injections in order to remain in optimum status; for such patients, from 100 to 200 micrograms may be injected at 2-week intervals.

Patients with pernicious anemia, in contrast with those with diabetes who receive insulin (see p. 828), are rarely encouraged or permitted to administer their own injections. Responsibility for the administration of therapy should always be retained by a physician or a clinic in order to be absolutely certain that it will never be discontinued. The intervals between injections are very long—not 24 hours, but from 2 to 4 weeks—and the lag period before the onset of relapse, if treatment is interrupted, is not 2 to 4 days, but may be from 1 to 2 years, or longer; and relapse, when it occurs, as it will, develops most insidiously, often with neurologic complications that are incapacitating and may not be reversed by resumption of therapy at this stage. The diabetic patient has a daily chore to perform, if he requires insulin; if he neglects his chore he soon feels unwell and is reminded. If his need continues to be disregarded he will become very ill and very uncomfortable, as he knows, or soon will learn. The patient with pernicious anemia feels absolutely well, and is absolutely well, while receiving therapy. He continues to feel well, even after months of neglect. With progression of relapse and advancing combined system disease there is interference with cerebration and distortion of mood, the net result of which is to lessen, rather than promote, the likelihood of medical consultation and resumption of therapy. An absolute and lifelong therapeutic requirement, such as B_{12} is for the pernicious anemia patient, calls for strong therapeutic safeguards which are lacking in a program of self-medication that is left to the discretion of a patient who becomes indiscrete without medication!

Nursing Care. A patient with pernicious

anemia who is sufficiently ill to require hospitalization, whose red count, for example, is less than 1.5 million, should be placed at bed rest until a satisfactory response to therapy has begun. A certain amount of activity outside the bed, including bathroom privileges and brief periods of sitting in a chair each day, usually is permissible and is to be recommended unless there is severe neurologic involvement of an incapacitating sort. Patients with this disease are unusually sensitive to cold, requiring extra blankets and obtaining comfort from flannel bedclothes. Footboards or cradles likewise may be an aid to comfort by protecting the extremities from the pressure of weighty linen.

The use of mechanical devices to prevent the patient from falling out of bed are to be recommended if there is evidence of mental deterioration due to combined system disease. Sensory disturbances, such as numbness of the hands and the feet, necessitate caution in applying hot-water bottles. Close observation of such patients by the nurse, as in any case of advanced cerebral disease, is an obvious necessity.

The mouth, especially the teeth and the gums, requires careful attention in elderly patients and those with severe glossitis. Special mouth care is supplied at regular intervals to maintain cleanliness of the oral cavity.

Involvement of the bladder and the rectal sphincters may complicate the problems of nursing care in cases of advanced combined system disease. If there is neurogenic paralysis of the bladder, tidal drainage may be instituted in an effort to stimulate spontaneous evacuation of that organ.

The temperature, the pulse and the respirations are examined and charted at least twice each day, and, until the red count decidedly improves or exceeds 2.0 million per cu. mm., a blood pressure examination is indicated each day.

A well-balanced diet is offered in which muscle meat, fish, milk and eggs are provided amply.

SYMPTOMATIC AND SUPPORTIVE THERAPY. Transfusions of whole blood or red cells may be required in order to increase the red cell count to safe levels during the interval between the start of the treatment and the onset of remission. The patient should be observed continuously during transfusion, since pyrogenic reactions may be extraordinarily violent and have proved to be fatal in severely anemic individuals. The nurse should report immediately any change in pulse rate or arterial pressure, as well as any evidence of chilling, fever or unusual symptoms of any type during or following transfusion. If a reaction occurs during the procedure, the infusion should be halted immediately by the nurse without waiting for instructions. She should then report the event to the physician and proceed to assemble equipment for whatever specimens he might desire to obtain.

A patient having a chill should be made as comfortable as possible with extra blankets, warm drinking fluids and whatever analgesic drugs may be prescribed.

Dyspepsia, if present, may be treated by means of hydrochloric acid given after meals, well diluted in a glass of water and sipped through a drinking tube, a treatment to be omitted as soon as a therapeutic response has been obtained, when this symptom can be expected to disappear spontaneously.

DIAGNOSTIC TESTS. Complete hematologic studies, including a sternal aspiration biopsy, are performed soon after admission and may be repeated at frequent intervals during hospitalization. A vitamin B$_{12}$ absorption test (p. 109) may be required X-ray examinations of the stomach (upper G.I. series) and of the colon (barium enema) are indicated in order to rule out neoplastic disease in the gastrointestinal tract, the incidence of which is increased in pernicious anemia.

It will be the responsibility of the nurse to prepare the patient for these examinations, both through explanation and actual preparation of equipment and surroundings, and to secure specimens as required.

Convalescent Care. As soon as a therapeutic remission is well under way, i.e., approximately 3 weeks after treatment is started, and the red cell count is well over 2 million, an increasing amount of activity is permitted, its limits depending chiefly on the patient's cardiovascular status and the degree of neurologic disability. Various degrees of flaccid and spastic paralysis may be present, for which appropriate physiotherapy is indicated, including massage, passive exercises and a complete program of progressive muscle re-education.

Mental Health. Excluding the patients in whom there is cerebral involvement, there are no problems entailing psychotherapy that are peculiar to pernicious anemia. The incidence of mental deterioration or senility is unusually high, owing to the complication of combined system disease and to the age distribution characteristic of these patients.

Education and Prevention. The one educational problem of prime importance in connection with this disease is that of teaching patients the need for continued medical observation and treatment, apparent cure notwithstanding. The risks of therapeutic neglect should be stressed with conviction but without occasioning unnecessary alarm. Assurance can be offered that the prognosis is excellent when therapy is adequate, although the complete reversal of severe neurologic disabilities already present cannot be guaranteed. The patient treated early and without interruption should not only live out his normal life expectancy but also should enjoy as good health as he might have in the complete absence of pernicious anemia.

Folic Acid Deficiency

Other forms of anemia that are similar, but etiologically unrelated, to pernicious anemia are the macrocytic anemias of sprue and other malabsorption syndromes (page 152); "pernicious anemia of infancy"; and "pernicious anemia of pregnancy." Gastric carcinoma, postoperative defects of the gastrointestinal tract, fish tapeworm infestation and severe chronic liver disease may also produce a pernicious anemia-like picture, including a macrocytic anemia. Some of these patients are, in fact, deficient in B_{12}, owing to failure of the latter to be absorbed in adequate quantities, as in pernicious anemia. However, the majority lack folic acid (pteroyl glutamic acid) and respond promptly to the oral administration of this vitamin in daily quantities of from 5 to 15 mg.

HEMOLYTIC DISORDERS

Excessive red cell destruction, the mark of a hemolytic disorder, gives rise to anemia, an increased concentration of free bilirubin in the plasma, the presence, in rare instances, of free hemoglobin in the plasma and the urine and an increased number of reticulocytes in the circulating blood.

The blood pictures characteristic of hemolytic anemias show normal or slightly enlarged red cells, numerous reticulocytes and nucleated red cells, increased platelets and polymorphonuclear leukocytosis, all indicative of intense bone marrow activity; there is also elevation of the plasma pigments, owing to the increased rate at which hemoglobin is liberated from the red cells and converted into bilirubin.

Infections, chiefly those associated with bacteremia (particularly with the *Streptococcus haemolyticus, Staphylococcus aureus,* the meningococcus and gas bacilli), malaria and *Bartonella* infections frequently cause increased blood destruction. There are numerous poisons that injure red cells, making them abnormally fragile and thus causing acute hemolytic anemia; some of these are aniline, nitrobenzene, trinitrotoluene and phenylhydrazine. Certain chemicals, including some drugs in common use, are nonhemolytic for the majority of persons but cause rapid blood destruction when ingested by individuals with an hereditary deficiency of the red cell enzyme "G-6-PD" (glucose-6-phosphate dehydrogenase); those susceptible to this hemolytic disorder include about 10 per cent of the Negro population. Among the drugs capable of inducing hemolysis under these conditions are certain antimalarial agents, such as primiquine; sulfonilamide; aspirin and phenacetin; and one food item, the Fava bean, responsible for the acute hemolytic disease known as "favism." In one hemolytic disorder, i.e., hemolytic disease of the newborn, the injurious agent is a blood group specific red cell antibody that is produced by the mother who has been immunized by the red cells of her offspring in utero, the antibody gaining entrance to the fetal circulation during gestation.

Red cell lysis, in the majority of patients with hemolytic disease (and in normal individuals), does not occur in the freely circulating blood but within the phagocytic cells of the reticuloendothelial system, notably those of the spleen and the liver. Liberation of hemoglobin into the plasma does not result from this type of hemolysis. However, destruction of red cells in the circulating blood is reflected by the appearance of hemoglobin in the plasma (hemoglobinemia) and, if the concentration of the pigment in the plasma becomes sufficiently high, it appears in the urine as well (hemoglobinuria). A description follows of two important examples of hemolytic disease without intravascular hemolysis, which are characterized, therefore, by jaundice but not by hemoglobinemia or hemoglobinuria.

Acquired Hemolytic Jaundice

This disease, otherwise known as "autoimmune hemolytic disease," is believed to represent one of the disorders of immunity, the patient's reticuloendothelial system having been stimulated to produce antibodies which tend to react with his own erythrocytes. The latter become coated with globulins and as a result tend to clump together. Aggregate masses of these cells become trapped in the sinusoids of the spleen, where they are easy prey for the phagocytic cells that are so abundant in that organ and are cannibalized en masse.

Clinically, acquired hemolytic jaundice is characterized by periods of exacerbations and remissions occurring over months or years. Its course often is marked by "crises" when massive blood destruction occurs, with death sometimes resulting from a precipitous and profound anemia.

Treatment. Treatment consists in the administration of steroids and, in most patients, splenectomy. The use of steroid hormones, including details of their administration, is described in Chapter 38. Complete remissions are to be expected in cases of acquired hemolytic jaundice in response to prednisone (Meticorten, Deltasone, Deltra, Paracort) or prednisolone (Meticortelone, Delta-Cortef, Hydeltra, Paracortol) in oral doses totaling 20 to 100 mg. per day, or dexamethasone (Decadron, Deronil) in doses of 3 to 15 mg. per day. Upon discontinuance of steroid therapy, however, the hemolytic state returns, and this continues to be the situation in almost all cases until the spleen is removed. Accordingly, splenectomy is indicated as soon as the hemolytic rate has been

reduced to normal by steroids. In the absence of the spleen, the site at which a large proportion of the destructive antibody is produced and hemolysis takes place, a prolonged remission is likely. Subsequent recurrences are not uncommon, but the severity of these attacks is relatively mild and their control, by steroids, relatively easy.

The diagnosis of acquired hemolytic jaundice is established by the demonstration that the red cells agglutinate spontaneously in a high-protein medium and that their membrane is layered with globulin, as evidenced by a positive Coombs' test (see p. 90).

Hereditary Spherocytosis

Included among the more common varieties of chronic hemolytic anemia is a type known as hereditary spherocytosis, or congenital hemolytic jaundice, which is due to an inherent defect in the red cell structure, namely, a shortage of membrane in proportion to cell contents. As a result, these cells cannot adopt the normal configuration, i.e., that of a biconcave disk, but must be spheroidal in shape. Abnormally thick and relatively inflexible, these "spherocytes" tend to become trapped in the splenic sinusoids where they are destroyed by phagocytes.

The condition is characterized clinically by anemia, reticulocytosis, jaundice, splenic enlargement and a family history of a hemolytic anemia. The diagnosis of hereditary spherocytosis depends on the detection of spherocytes in the blood smear and on the demonstration of an abnormal fragility test (see p. 92) which reflects their spheroidicity. Blood destruction is reduced to normal and the patient cured symptomatically by removal of the spleen.

Hemoglobinurias

The urine of patients with hemoglobinuria is red or dark brown, due to the presence, not of red blood cells, but of hemoglobin or its oxidation products, methemoglobin or hemosiderin. The cause of hemoglobinuria, as stated above, is intravascular hemolysis, i.e., the destruction of erythrocytes in the circulating blood stream, with the escape of hemoglobin into the plasma and thence into the urine. Hemoglobinuria almost always accompanies toxic hemolysis, as seen in patients, with or without G-6-PD deficiency, who have ingested one of the agents listed above. A rare individual may induce the symptom by walking or marching ("march hemoglobinuria"), but not by other types of activity.

Paroxysmal Cold Hemoglobinuria, with Cold Hemolysins. This condition is marked by the occurrence of hemoglobinuria after exposure to cold and is based on the presence in the plasma of a hemolytic red cell antibody that produces its effect when blood is chilled and then warmed again. Plasma containing such a hemolysin will lyse normal cells as well as the patient's cells under these circumstances. This disorder occurs as a rare complication of late syphilis, and its recognition is based on the patient's description of attacks in which the urine suddenly changes color, becoming dark red for a brief period, then clears again. The attacks themselves may begin within a few minutes or several hours after the chilling and are ushered in by malaise, pains in the head, the abdomen or the legs, chills and fever. The condition clears up with cure of the syphilitic infection.

Paroxysmal Cold Hemoglobinuria, with Cold Agglutinins. Abnormal hemolysis in these patients is attributable to a cold agglutinin in the plasma, which occasionally appears in the course of virus pneumonia. Because of this antibody, red cells are spontaneously agglutinated when the blood is cooled. Agglutination renders the red cells especially vulnerable to mechanical destruction in the circulation. In both conditions there are signs of hemolysis, including the appearance of free hemoglobin in the urine, when the patient has been exposed to cold.

Paroxysmal Nocturnal Hemoglobinuria. This is a rare disease in which the red cells are defective, having the abnormal property of hemolyzing when the blood becomes slightly more acid than usual, as happens in sleep. Its treatment consists of transfusions, large volumes of washed red cells being supplied in rapid succession. Temporary reduction of the hemolytic rate may follow this maneuver.

HEMOGLOBINOPATHIES

Both excessive hemolysis and subnormal rates of hemoglobin production are respon-

sible for anemia in patients with hemoglobinopathy, i.e., patients in whom there is an hereditary defect in the structure of the hemoglobin molecule. Two important diseases that are based on such a defect are sickle cell anemia and thalassemia.

Sickle Cell Anemia

Sickle cell disease (hemoglobin S disease) is a hereditary disease appearing almost exclusively in Negroes. Its name refers to the crescentic shape which the red cells acquire when exposed to low oxygen tensions (see p. 89), a characteristic that renders this disease unique. When sickle cell disease occurs in the heterozygous state (i.e., based on a single defective gene, inherited from one parent), the condition is completely devoid of symptoms, causes no ill-health or disability throughout life and is designated as "sickling trait." Sickle cell anemia (homozygous S disease), on the other hand, based on a defective gene from both parents, is a definite disease entity, characterized by excessive hemolysis, anemia and jaundice. Such patients are subject to frequent attacks of abdominal, muscular and joint pain, which are presumed to be due to jamming of the circulation by sickled red cells. There is no effective treatment for this disorder, other than red cell transfusions to control hemolytic crises. Transfusions also are indicated as a prophylactic measure before the delivery of pregnant females with S disease.

Thalassemia

Thalassemia major, or Cooley's anemia, is a relatively uncommon hereditary disease affecting persons of Mediterranean origin. Its features include a severe chronic hemolytic anemia, marked enlargement of the liver and the spleen and jaundice. The red cells are small and hypochromic, as in severe iron deficiency; however, in contrast with the latter, serum iron values are normal or high in thalassemia. Diagnostic signs in this disease include the finding of an increased concentration of fetal hemoglobin and the demonstration of an abnormal type of hemoglobin (A_2) on electrophoretic analysis (see pp. 88 and 89). No treatment is available, other than symptomatic replacement of red cells by transfusion.

Thalassemia minor, or "Cooley's trait," is

devoid of symptoms or signs except for the laboratory findings of defective red cells, the latter being abnormally small and the concentration of intracellular hemoglobin markedly reduced. This deficiency of hemoglobin sometimes is compensated for by a proportionate increase in the red cell count, the level of which may constantly exceed 6 or 7 million per cu. mm. When the condition exists merely as a trait, it is presumed to have been transmitted from one parent only, whereas Cooley's anemia presumably reflects the inheritance of this defect from both parents.

Other Hemoglobinopathies

The red cells of thalassemia patients, containing hemoglobins A_2 and F (fetal hemoglobin) and hemoglobin S disease, represent but two of a group that totals at least 8 hereditary disorders of molecular structure involving hemoglobin. In addition to hemoglobins A_2, F, S and normal hemoglobin (A), 6 other forms of human hemoglobins have been identified, each of which has been assigned as the cause of a hemolytic disorder. These likewise are designated by letter; they include hemoglobins C, D, E, H, I and J. Their differentiation is described on page 89. From the clinical standpoint, each is characterized by hemolytic anemia, red cell hypochromia and the presence of target cells (see p. 87). Commonest of the group (barring S disease) is hemoglobin C disease, which in the heterozygous form affects 2 to 3 per cent of American Negroes. One in 6,000 Negroes has homozygous C disease, which is comparable in severity and similar in its manifestations to mildly or moderately severe S disease.

THE PATIENT WITH TOXIC BONE MARROW DEPRESSION

Anemia due to toxic inhibition of the bone marrow may result from exposure to any of a variety of chemical substances, including some that are employed as therapeutic agents. The character of the peripheral blood reflects inactive marrow, as evidenced by a reduction in the output of all formed elements arising from that source, including erythrocytes, leukocytes and platelets. The red cells are decreased in number but are of normal size and contain a normal amount of hemoglobin. The number of circulating reticulocytes is less than normal, distinguishing this type of anemia from those due to excessive hemolysis. Certain specific marrow poisons are responsible for characteristic changes in red cell morphology, which may aid in establishing specific diagnoses. For example, one of the features of lead poisoning is the appearance of stippled red cells in the peripheral blood and the development of a tendency on the part of the red cell to disintegrate when subjected to mechanical trauma, i.e., demonstrating an increased "mechanical fragility."

A depression in the white cell count and the platelet count may be expected to occur in association with toxic anemias of this type, and the degree to which these elements are affected corresponds in general to the grade of anemia. If platelet deficiency is severe, the patient will experience epistaxes and other hemorrhagic complications. Purpuric lesions are almost certain to appear; when they do, the nurse will observe that they are most prominent in areas of friction and pressure. Laboratory studies will demonstrate a prolongation of bleeding time, impaired clot retraction and increased capillary fragility. Of the white cells, those in the granulocyte series are principally, or exclusively, affected, the lymphocytes being affected last and least. If granulopenia is severe, the danger of sepsis becomes grave, and death is almost inevitable unless averted by vigorous and well-selected chemotherapy, as discussed on page 470.

Marrow poisons capable of inhibiting the production of red cells, white cells and platelets alike in any individual include benzol, nitrogen mustard, urethane, myleran, arsenic, antifolic compounds and gold salts. Despite their toxicity, the last have been used in cases of rheumatoid arthritis, on the basis of the empiric observation that their intravenous use is occasionally followed by a period of improvement in these cases. The remaining compounds are useful to a varying extent because of, rather than despite, their toxic properties, i.e., their specific ability to kill young cells, which is a desirable objective in one disease caused by a rapid and unregulated overgrowth of cells, namely, leukemia.

Certain drugs and chemicals exhibit a toxic effect on the marrow that is limited to one or two of its production activities. Lead, for example, is very prone to produce anemia and may cause a depression in the output of granulocytes but is not expected to cause thrombocytopenia. Moreover, there are drugs which cause hypoplastic syndromes of greater or lesser severity and with varying degrees of frequency, but cause it only in susceptible individuals. Those who are susceptible are described as having a "drug idiosyncrasy" with respect to the particular agent responsible for their marrow failure. Among the drugs having a tendency to produce such an idiosyncrasy, with refractory anemia one of its prominent manifestations, are chloramphenicol (Chloromycetin), an important antibiotic drug, and Mesantoin, an anticonvulsant used widely in the treatment of epilepsy.

Treatment. Whole-blood or red cell transfusions usually are required at frequent intervals, and perhaps indefinitely, in order to maintain the concentration of hemoglobin and the red count at an efficient level in patients with marked depression of marrow activity. If the hypoplastic syndrome also includes marked thrombocytopenia it may be decided to furnish platelets by using blood donors who have those elements in great excess because of polycythemia vera, but such therapy is of limited value and restricted application, as will be discussed later. If granulopenia is present and sufficiently marked to impair the patient's defenses against infection, antibacterial chemotherapy is strongly indicated as a prophylactic measure. The administration of one of the corticosteroid drugs, e.g., prednisone or dexamethasone, is warranted in cases showing evidence of severe marrow damage, on the basis that an antigen-antibody reaction might be involved and is responsible for an idiosyncrasy reaction on the part of the marrow, in which event the disease process might well subside in response to these agents. If a drug idiosyncrasy has been identified, in fact, as the cause of hypoplastic anemia in a given case, it is imperative that every step be taken that will ensure the patient against repetition of the noxious exposure.

Leukopenia and Agranulocytosis

The outstanding feature of marrow failure, in some cases, is a reduction in the total leukocyte count, rather than anemia, attributable to failure of the circulating granulocytes to be replaced as rapidly as they are lost from the blood. The life span of the granulocyte is approximately one fifteenth that of the red cell; thus, any impairment of marrow production which affects all marrow products equally will be reflected by granulopenia, even agranulocytosis (complete absence of granulocytes), long before anemia becomes apparent.

Leukopenia has many possible causes, including viral infections, overwhelming bacterial sepsis and neoplastic diseases of the bone marrow, particularly leukopenic or "aleukemic" leukemia. However, the most common etiology is drug toxicity, for numerous chemical agents, including some used in medical treatment, are capable of suppressing bone marrow activity and decreasing the production of white cells. Among these are included benzene, amidopyrine, sulfapyridine, Mesantoin, gold (given by injection), nitrogen mustard, urethane, radiophosphorus (P^{32}) and many others. No clinical manifestations are to be expected as a result of leukopenia per se unless the reduction in the granulocytes is extremely marked; in this event the patient becomes susceptible to bacterial infections. Infection of the throat, or "agranulocytic angina," is the most dangerous of these complications; the throat becomes increasingly sore and eventually gangrenous, accompanying which are all of the manifestations of a systemic infection. Without treatment, death may be anticipated within 1 to 3 days, but with appropriate antibacterial chemotherapy the process usually can be controlled.

Prevention. Because of their known susceptibility to throat and other infections, patients with marked granulopenia or "agranulocytosis" routinely are given a prophylactic course of antibiotic (e.g., penicillin) therapy, whether or not an infectious complication has arisen, pending the reappearance of polymorphonuclear leukocytes in the blood.

Treatment and Nursing Care. Patients

with agranulocytosis receive vigorous anti-bacterial chemotherapy, utilizing whatever antibiotic agent or agents that might be indicated on the basis of the bacteriologic findings. A drug, or combination of drugs, having the widest possible range of antibacterial effect is desired in such cases, i.e., chlortetracycline, oxytetracycline or penicillin in combination with streptomycin. A trial of steroid therapy, employing prednisone or dexamethasone by mouth, is justified in the hope of eliminating any abnormal antigen-antibody reaction that might be responsible for the marrow disturbance.

Hot saline irrigations of the throat are employed to keep it clear of necrotic detritus and exudate. Comfort is provided by supplying an ice collar and whatever analgesic, antipyretic and sedative drugs may be indicated. Blood transfusions usually are given as a supportive measure, but they do not correct the basic deficiency, that of circulating granulocytes. The essence of treatment, apart from eradicating the infection, is to eliminate, if possible, the factor responsible for the bone marrow depression. Spontaneous restoration of its function, except in the case of neoplastic diseases, often occurs in time, i.e., within 2 or 3 weeks, if death from infection can be averted.

THE PATIENT WITH POLYCYTHEMIA

Polycythemia vera is characterized by a persistent and marked elevation of red cell count, hemoglobin and hematocrit, associated with increased granulocytes and platelet production, chronic cyanosis and splenomegaly. The cause of this disease is unknown; many regard it as an example of malignant overgrowth of the marrow.

Persons who are middle-aged and older are affected predominantly. Their complaints include headaches, indigestion, pain in the legs and sometimes mental confusion. These people are apt to have peptic ulcers which often bleed and arterial and venous thromboses (cerebral, coronary, mesenteric, etc.). The spleen usually is enlarged and often is the site of infarction. The total blood volume, as well as the concentration of red blood cells and hemoglobin, is increased. The cause of death most often is

severe hemorrhage in the gastrointestinal tract or coronary thrombosis.

The treatment of polycythemia vera consists of repeated large venesections, x-ray irradiation of the long bones or the intravenous injection of radioactive phosphorus (a form of internal radiation). Nitrogen mustard (HN_2) and Myleran (busulfan) also are capable of producing prolonged clinical remissions in this disease.

Secondary polycythemia, or erythremia, is characterized by an abnormal elevation of the red cell count and occurs in several unrelated conditions, all resulting in poor oxygenation of the blood, hence hyperstimulation of the bone marrow. It occurs physiologically at high altitudes where the oxygen tension in the atmosphere is low, in association with congenital heart disease and in pulmonary emphysema, which conditions are marked by chronic cyanosis.

Treatment to reduce the red cell count generally is unwarranted in secondary polycythemia since the latter develops as a compensatory mechanism designed to improve the delivery of oxygen to the body tissues. However, some patients receive symptomatic benefit from venesections and are treated accordingly.

PATIENTS WITH LEUKEMIA AND LYMPHOMA

Leukemia (white blood) is a term that originally was applied to a few cases in which the blood appeared milky at necropsy. Since such a condition can arise only when the leukocyte count almost or quite equals that of the red cells, it means that the leukocyte count must be about 1,000,000 per cu. mm. and the anemia profound. Only one disease can produce it, the one we still call *leukemia*. (However, in the great majority of cases of this disease the blood is red, since the leukocyte count seldom rises above 500,000 per cu. mm.)

Several varieties of leukemia are recognized; they all are characterized by the presence of immature leukocytes of one type or another in the peripheral blood and by extensive hyperplasia (overgrowth) of the tissue producing that particular cell. The most common are the myelogenous, lymphatic and monocytic leukemias, these terms specifying, in each case, the type of cell involved.

Acute Leukemia

The clinical course of leukemia may be fulminating, progressing rapidly to a fatal termination within a few weeks. This form of the disease is labeled as "acute," versus "chronic," leukemia, when the duration is measured in years. The acute leukemias are encountered most often in children and young adults. Regardless of the cell type, i.e., whether lymphatic, myelogenous, monocytic or "stem cell" (the most primitive, undifferentiated type), all present many characteristics in common. The onset is typically very sudden, manifested by an acute tonsillitis, furunculosis or the appearance of an abscess in the mouth or the skin. The total course may be limited to a few days or weeks and is marked by a high fever. Hemorrhagic features appear early and may include bleeding from the gums, the nose, the stomach and the rectum, as well as hemorrhages into the skin and into the fundus of the eyes. Swelling and gangrenous ulceration of the gums, the cheeks, the jaw and the tonsils likewise are common.

Acute leukemia is an important disease to keep in mind, since it may be mistaken for diphtheria, scurvy, purpura, typhoid fever, rheumatic fever or some specific type of anemia. The diagnosis is established readily by the finding of blood leukocytes predominantly or exclusively primitive in type, a lowering of the red cell count and a marked reduction of platelets.

Treatment and nursing care in this condition, together with that in other forms of leukemia and the lymphomas, are described on page 474.

Monocytic Leukemia

This is a type of acute leukemia in which the white cell count usually varies from 15,000 to 50,000 per cu. mm. but may exceed 100,000; from 70 to 90 per cent of these cells are young monocytes. Enlargement of the liver, the spleen and the lymph nodes seldom is marked. This condition usually occurs in association with infections in the mouth. It generally starts with pallor, lassitude, fever and a rapidly developing anemia and is followed in a few months by ulceration of the gums and a necrotic stomatitis, during which the patient fails rapidly.

Chronic Myelogenous and Lymphatic Leukemias

Chronic Myelogenous Leukemia. This is a condition characterized by white cell counts ranging from 100,000 to 1,000,000 per cu. mm.; a high percentage of these leukocytes are immature cells. The condition is associated with a great enlargement of the spleen and the liver but little swelling of the lymph nodes. Chronic myelogenous leukemia may appear at any period of life, most often between the ages of 25 and 40. The onset of this disease is usually gradual and insidious. Many patients accidentally discover a tumor (the spleen) in the abdomen, or complain of dragging sensations due to the weight of this organ. The long bones (the tibias, the ribs and the sternum, in particular), due to their invasion by the abnormal marrow, often become spontaneously painful and tender on pressure. Death usually occurs within 3 to 5 years after the initial onset of the disease, due to general exhaustion, severe anemia, hemorrhage or secondary infection.

Chronic Lymphatic Leukemia. Occurring most frequently between the ages of 45 and 60, this leukemia is characterized by a greatly increased leukocyte count, over 90 per cent of the cells being mature lymphocytes. The onset is typically insidious, with symptoms which closely resemble those of the myelogenous type. For months the only significant physical sign may be the gradual appearance of a generalized lymph node enlargement. Subsequent developments include the appearance of anemia, fever, cachexia and hemorrhagic features, all of which are apt to be more pronounced than in myelogenous type leukemia.

Leukemic infiltrations appear in the retinae of the eyes and in the skin, which may become pruritic and bronzed. Ascitic and pleural effusions are not uncommon, the latter occasionally chylous because of the pressure of enlarged nodes on the thoracic duct.

Myeloma

Myeloma, "multiple myeloma," "myelomatosis" (or "plasma cell leukemia") is another tumor of reticuloendothelial tissue which tends to localize in the bone marrow, invading and destroying the surrounding bones and shedding the characteristic plasma cell, or "plasmacyte," into the blood stream. As in other types of leukemia, the clinical picture may include enlargement of the lymph nodes, the spleen and the liver, as well as anemia and hemorrhagic phenomena. Study of the peripheral blood reveals the presence of plasmacytes (small mononuclear cells with round nuclei and dark-blue-staining cytoplasm) and a reduction of both red cells and platelets. Further indications of the diagnosis are obtained from the findings of an increased concentration of globulin in the plasma and the presence of an unusual protein in the urine (Bence-Jones proteinuria). (See also p. 71.)

Lymphomas

The lymphomas are included among the neoplastic diseases of the blood-forming organs. They are characterized by the wild and unregulated growth of cells arising from reticuloendothelial tissues, and all are capable of spreading to and infiltrating other tissues and organs. The most characteristic feature of lymphoma, clinically, is lymph node enlargement, but in its advanced stage, any of these tumors may become disseminated throughout the body. Even the blood may be invaded, in which event the case becomes one of leukemia by definition, since the malignant reticuloendothelial cell is basically of the same category as are the primitive blood leukocytes.

The mildest form, termed "Hodgkin's paragranuloma," carries a relatively good prognosis as regards life expectancy and therapeutic response. Hodgkin's granuloma is less benign but hardly can be classed as a highly malignant disease, since therapeutic remissions have been known to last for periods extending from 5 to 15 years, whereas Hodgkin's sarcoma and reticulum cell sarcoma are highly invasive and rapid in their growth.

Hodgkin's granuloma is the most common variety of lymphoma. It usually begins as a painless enlargement of the lymph nodes on one side of the neck, which becomes increasingly conspicuous. However, for months generalized pruritus may be the first and only symptom and later is often a most distressing one. The individual nodes remain firm and discrete (that is, they do not soften and do

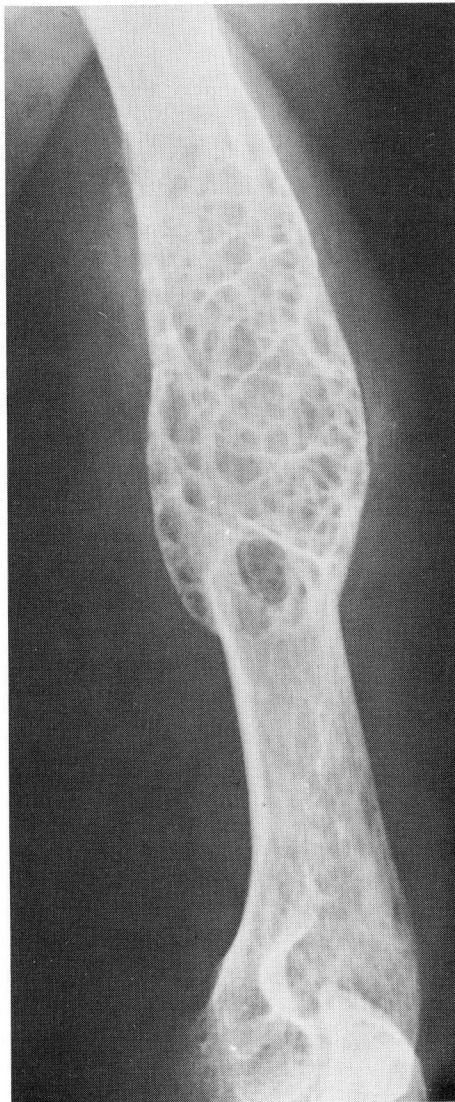

Fig. 154. Bone destruction, decalcification and tumor formation in humerus, from myelomatosis. (J. F. Ross, M.D., Los Angeles)

not fuse) and they are seldom tender and painful. Soon the lymph nodes of other regions, usually the other side of the neck, also enlarge in the same manner. The mediastinal and retroperitoneal lymph nodes may also enlarge, causing severe pressure symptoms: pressure against the trachea causing dyspnea; the esophagus, dysphagia; the nerves, laryngeal paralysis, and brachial, lumbar or sacral neuralgias; the veins, edema of one or both extremities and effusions into the pleura or peritoneum; and the bile duct, obstructive jaundice. Later the spleen may become palpable, and the liver may enlarge. In some patients the first nodes to enlarge are those of one axilla or of one groin. Occasionally, the disease starts in mediastinal or peritoneal nodes and may remain limited to them. In still other cases the enlargement of the spleen is the only conspicuous lesion.

Sooner or later a progressive anemia develops. A leukocytosis often is observed with an abnormally high polymorphonuclear and an elevated eosinophil count. About half the patients have a slight fever, but with a temperature seldom above 101° F. However, the patients with mediastinal and abdominal involvement present a remarkable intermittent fever. The temperature, for periods of from 3 to 14 days, goes as high as 104° F., returning to normal within a few weeks. Untreated, this disease is progressive in its course; the patient loses weight, becomes cachectic, the anemia becomes marked, anasarca appears, the blood pressure falls, and in from 1 to 3 years death is likely to ensue. However, suitable treatment may prolong life appreciably.

Nursing Care and Treatment

The principal objectives of therapy in patients with leukemia and lymphoma are: (1) to halt or to retard the overgrowth of the malignant cells as completely and for as long a time as possible in order to forestall or eliminate damage to normal tissues and organs; (2) to compensate for whatever damage may be caused by the abnormal growth and to protect the patient from the consequences of this damage; and (3) to provide symptomatic relief from whatever pain and discomfort may be associated with the disease. The direct attack on the malignant tissue may employ irradiation, chemotherapeutic or surgical measures, or any combination of these, depending on the character of the illness. The surgical approach is useful in a very small proportion of cases —those in which the process appears to be confined to a single region of the body, from which its complete removal seems a reasonable possibility. The methodology, the clinical effects and the complications of radiation therapy and chemotherapy, as applied in cases of leukemia and lymphoma, as well as the nursing problems associated with these treatments, are discussed in detail in Chapter 19.

Supportive and protective measures are very important in the treatment of patients with leukemia and lymphoma, including the correction of anemia and the control of infection, to which these patients are peculiarly subject. The instructions issued to the patient by the nurse regarding the prevention of infection can be extremely helpful in accomplishing this objective. The only effective antianemic therapy in these patients in the transfusion of whole blood or red cell concentrates. Infections are treated by chemotherapy and other auxiliary measures according to their type and location. The hemorrhagic complications of bone marrow disease, mainly due to platelet deficiency, are unresponsive to present-day treatments other than blood transfusion for the restoration of blood loss.

Symptomatic Treatment. The malignant disorders under discussion are capable of producing any and all types of symptoms demanding therapeutic measures for their relief. Pain may originate in soft tissues anywhere in the body, due to the encroachment of glandular swellings that are associated with most leukemias and lymphomas. If superficial and well localized, these pains may respond to simple measures, such as the application of cold compresses, but chief reliance usually must be placed on the analgesic drugs, such as codeine sulfate or phosphate in doses of 15 to 60 mg. (0.25 to 0.5 gr.); morphine sulphate, 10 to 30 mg. (0.17 to 0.5 gr.); or one of the more effective morphine substitutes, such as meperidine hydrochloride (50 to 200 mg.) or methadon hydrochloride (amidone hydrochloride), the latter being given orally in doses ranging from 2 to 10 mg. at from 3- to 4-hour intervals, as required.

Respiratory difficulties that are caused by tumors in the neck and the mediastinum may be ameliorated by placing the patient in a semi-orthopneic position, oxygen inhalations being required in patients with marked obstruction of the trachea or the bronchi. Control of a distressing or intractable cough may necessitate the use of sedatives, such as codeine, Hycodan or other opiates, depending on the indications. Areas of the skin that have been exposed to x-ray irradiation are likely to be sensitive and should be protected from unnecessary pressure or friction. If a patient complains of pruritus or exhibits excoriations, his nails should be trimmed and an antipruritic lotion, e.g., Quotane Hydrochloride, applied.

Hydration and nutrition must be furnished by parenteral routes to a considerable proportion of patients, and the value of these measures as symptomatic therapy is incalculable, especially in patients who are extremely ill. Patients suffering from abdominal lymph node enlargement are especially prone to lose their appetites completely, posing an almost insurmountable problem from the standpoint of oral feeding. Hygienic measures are mandatory in the care of these, as in all, sick patients; the details of these measures depend on the character of the individual case and on the ingenuity of the nurse.

Mycosis Fungoides

Mycosis fungoides is regarded as a variant of the lymphoma group of diseases, most closely allied with Hodgkin's granuloma. Although the lymph nodes, the liver and the spleen are involved as well, the skin is the site of its most prominent manifestation throughout the entire illness.

The course of this disease, like that of the other lymphomas, is characterized by remissions and exacerbations. It begins as a generalized severe itching which may last for years; this is followed by a stage of eruptions of erythematous urticarial eczematous or psoriasislike lesions. These eruptions come and go, possibly for years, before any of the typical tumors appear, and they also continue to some degree throughout the entire course of the disease. The swellings characteristic of this disease arise from some of the above-mentioned lesions, which become indurated and more and more fungoidal until they are mushroom-like growths, vivid scarlet or purplish in color, varying in size from that of a cherry to that of an egg, or even an orange. The body may be covered with such lesions. At first these appear and disappear alternately, but later they become more permanent, more or less confluent. Some of them break down, forming crateriform ulcers. For years the patient's general health seems unaffected, although the skin manifestations appear tempestuous; later the patient becomes weaker, cachectic and dies.

Treatment. X-ray irradiation, nitrogen mustard (HN_2) and radiophosphorus (P^{32}) have demonstrated about an equal degree of effectiveness. Remissions lasting for periods of a few months have been induced by each of these therapeutic agents.

THE PATIENT WITH A BLEEDING DISORDER

Protection of the body against excessive and lethal blood loss is afforded by several mechanisms. Thus, hemorrhage from a large lacerated vessel is retarded as a result of an abrupt lowering of the arterial blood pressure, i.e., "shock," which reduces the rate of blood flow throughout the body and, therefore, reduces the rate of its escape. Further protection also may be furnished by compression of the leaking vessel by the swelling mass of blood (hematoma) surrounding the vessel. Complete and permanent sealing of the latter, however, is accomplished through the clotting of the blood, an adherent gel-like mass, produced as described on page 91, effectively controlling most types of hemorrhage. Another phenomenon of protective value, occurring before clotting, is the aggregation of platelets at the point of vascular rupture. Masses of these tiny, sticky blood elements apparently form a temporary plug at this site, mechanically impeding the escape of blood, meanwhile liberating the material responsible for starting the formation of a clot precisely where a clot is needed most urgently. Finally, a factor of great importance in the prevention of bleeding is the normal resistance of blood vessels to mechanical rupture, i.e., by the pressure of blood exerted from within the vessel or traumatic pressures exerted from the outside.

Based on a disturbance of one or another of these factors—the clotting properties of the blood, the availability of platelets and the stamina of the blood vessels—a variety of disorders are encountered which are characterized, in common, by an abnormal tendency to bleed. These will be discussed in three major categories: those classed as vascular purpura, marked by the spontaneous rupture of small vessels which presumably are defective or injured; those attributable to a deficiency of platelets; and those which are related to the existence of a clotting defect.

Vascular Purpuras

Purpura is the term applied to small hemorrhages in the skin and the mucous membranes; they occur spontaneously as an isolated phenomenon or as an accompaniment of obvious disease. The smallest hemorrhages, pinhead in size, are called "petechiae," whereas larger hemorrhagic lesions are described as "ecchymoses." Both types occur as the result of vascular rupture, permitting the leakage of blood into the subcutaneous tissue of the mucous membranes. In one type, called "symptomatic" or "secondary" purpura, this bleeding is quite unrelated to any intrinsic defect of the blood vessels; certain types of blood stream infections, for example, meningococcemia and subacute bacterial endocarditis, exhibit this phenomenon due to direct damage to the vascular walls by the infectious agent. Another group of patients exhibiting this type of purpura are those with severe arterial hypertension and "easy bruisings," perhaps due to an abnormal degree of pressure in the fragile capillary circuits when the blood flow within these vessels is increased, as may occur as a result of a blow, exposure to heat or following the release of a tourniquet on an extremity. Other examples of vascular purpura, the mechanism of which is even more obscure, are found in cachectic individuals and in patients with uremia.

Anaphylactoid Purpura. This represents yet another type of vascular purpura, the clinical features of which are somewhat more complex and comprise a distinct entity. Among its numerous manifestations are various skin lesions, purpuric and otherwise, and episodes of arthritis, abdominal pain, hematuria, gastrointestinal hemorrhages and fever. These attacks recur for years, and each attack lasts for several weeks. The leakage of blood vessels at localized points throughout the system apparently is responsible for the principal complications of anaphylactoid purpura, the basic cause of which, however, is obscure. Generally it has been regarded as an allergic disorder. Steroid therapy often is effective.

Familial Hemorrhagic Telangiectasia. This is a hereditary disorder manifested by an abnormal tendency to bleed and become bruised. Localized aggregations of dilated capillaries may be observed in the skin and in the mucous membranes of the nose or the mouth. They also may be present in the gastric mucosa, explaining certain cases of gastrointestinal bleeding. Whether the characteristic lesions are present or absent, there may be a generalized decrease in capillary "resistance," as evidenced by the abnormal ease with which the vessels are ruptured by minor traumas. However, the precise nature of the defect is obscure, and the condition does not respond to any proved method of treatment.

Toxic Purpura. This condition has been observed after exposure to certain drugs and poisons, including aniline, certain arsenicals, Sedormid (a soporific) and snake venom. Some of these toxic cases present the features of thrombocytopenic purpura, but others are explained more readily on the basis of blood vessel damage.

Platelet-Deficiency Disorders

Thrombocytopenic Purpura. A reduction in the number of circulating platelets (thrombopenia) below a critical level (approximately 20,000 per mm.) inevitably is followed by the appearance of spontaneous hemorrhages in the skin, the mucous membranes and the internal organs and is responsible for prolonged bleeding from small lacerations on the body surface. Death may occur as a result of hemorrhage in the brain. Thrombopenia, as a complication of certain diseases, already has been discussed, e.g., in relation to toxic depression and neoplastic invasion of the bone marrow. Cases of this type are labeled "secondary thrombocytopenia."

Treatment of secondary thrombocytopenia often is not rewarded by improvement unless the basic defect can be corrected. A transient increase in circulating platelets may follow a transfusion of blood from a donor with polycythemia vera, if the blood is given immediately after collection, using injection equipment that is completely devoid of unprotected glass, steel or rubber surfaces. Donor platelets may survive for 5 or 6 days at first, but their life expectancy is shorter after each succeeding transfusion, so that replacement therapy becomes ineffective and must be abandoned. Splenectomy is similarly without benefit in the majority of these cases whose fundamental problem is failure of the marrow to produce platelets whether the spleen is present or absent.

Idiopathic Thrombocytopenic Purpura. This disease, like acquired hemolytic jaundice, represents a disorder of immunity, for the present evidence indicates that the mechanism responsible for the platelet deficiency in these patients is based on the presence of a platelet antibody. The condition is characterized clinically by its early onset, which usually precedes puberty; its sex distribution, occurring most commonly in females; and the manner in which it progresses, its course being marked by remissions and exacerbations over periods of many years. It responds to steroid therapy and to splenectomy precisely as does acquired hemolytic jaundice. Steroids enable a patient with either disease to be subjected to splenectomy with equal impunity and equally favorable prognosis.

The role of these formed elements in the mechanism of clot formation has been well established, but whether or not the clotting defect associated with thrombocytopenia can explain all of its hemorrhagic manifestations is debatable. Most of these suggest that some abnormality of the blood vessels themselves causes a structural weakness of their walls.

This "weakness" is presumed to reflect not a structural defect in the vessels themselves but the absence of a mobile defense barrier which the platelets provide. The barrier consists of plugs and films which normally are constructed with great rapidity by platelets and form by a process of agglutination at sites where the vessel wall is lacerated or damaged by distention.

The hemorrhagic disorders now to be discussed are attributable solely to defective clotting, the basis of which, in each instance, is the lack of some blood constituent that is involved specifically in the process of coagulation.

Clotting Defects

Hemophilia and Hemophilic States

Hemophilia is a rare disorder, limited exclusively to males who are popularly known as "bleeders." Whenever and wherever these individuals are struck, a large bruise is apt to appear, and any small cut or scratch of the skin may result in a hemorrhage that may last for several hours or days. They may bleed to death as a result of epistaxis following a blow on the nose, or from hemorrhage of the gums following a tooth extraction. Purpuric hemorrhages of the type observed in thrombocytopenic purpura are unusual, but internal hemorrhages are common, one of the characteristic bleeding sites, for example, being the weight-bearing joints, the result of which is an ankylosing type of arthritis, one of the most constant features of this disease. Hematuria, gastrointestinal bleeding and hematoma formation between muscle groups likewise are characteristic of hemophilia. The abnormality usually manifests itself in early childhood and lasts throughout life.

Blood clotting is retarded greatly in this disease, the coagulation time being prolonged far beyond the maximum limits of normal (10 to 12 minutes), often to as long as an hour or longer. The bleeding time, measured by the duration of blood oozing from a small prick in the skin, however, is within the normal range (3 to 6 minutes), and the number of circulating platelets is likewise normal. The clotting defect is attributable to the absence of one of the plasma proteins required for normal clotting, namely one of the thromboplastin precursors, AHG (antihemophilic globulin) or PTC (plasma thromboplastin component). Its absence is an inherited abnormality which invariably is transmitted from mother to son: the inherited trait, in other words, is sex-linked. For example, if Mr. A. is a bleeder, none of his children, either his sons or daughters, will be bleeders, and their descendants will also be spared; his sister's sons, on the other hand, may be affected. The disease is transmitted only through the women of the family, and yet none of these women is a bleeder.

Treatment. The best emergency measure for the control of hemorrhage from an oozing skin wound is the direct application to the cut of some tissue juice extract or even a fresh piece of meat. However, definitive treatment consists of replacing the missing factor by transfusions of fresh whole blood or plasma or of intravenous injections of purified "antihemophilic globulin" extracted from normal human plasma. As a result of these procedures, the clotting time is reduced to near normal for several hours, and the hemorrhagic tendency consequently is abolished for a time. The same treatment is indicated as a prophylactic measure in these patients preparatory to any operative procedure that may be contemplated, including dental extractions. This form of replacement almost always is effective; however, hemophiliacs have been encountered who are apparently "sensitized" (i.e., produce antibodies) against the clotting factor which they lack and, therefore, are completely unresponsive to treatment, just as Rh-negative individuals, lacking the Rh factor themselves, can be sensitized by repeated transfusions of Rh-positive blood and, as a result, eliminate Rh-positive donor cells almost as rapidly as they are injected.

It rarely happens that an individual, usually an adult female, develops a condition that is precisely similar to hemophilia in all respects except for its etiology and pathogenesis. The cause of this hemophilialike disorder is related to the production of an auto-immune antibody which has a specific neutralizing effect on thromboplastin. This development occurs spontaneously, for reasons unknown, sometimes in close relation to parturition during the postpartum period. Treatment is highly inefficient because of the destructive effect of the antibody on therapeutic agents containing antihemophilic globulin, and the prognosis is quite unpredictable. Deaths have occurred in these patients, despite massive doses of this substance and vigorous treatment with steroids.

Hypoprothrombinemia

Prothrombin, as previously discussed, likewise is essential for the clotting process. This substance is produced in the liver from one of the fat-soluble vitamins, vitamin K. Our main supply of K is synthesized by the bacteria which reside in the intestine. Normal prothrombin activity in the blood depends on adequate absorption of this vitamin from the gastrointestinal tract and on adequate liver function for its conversion. Therefore, prothrombin deficiency may arise as a result of diarrhea, from a lack of bile in the gastrointestinal tract (necessary for normal fat absorption) due to biliary tract obstruction, from a gastrointestinal disorder of any other type which interferes with the digestion or absorption of food products or as a result of liver disease. The principal manifestation of prothrombin deficiency, as observed in patients with hemophilia, is prolonged hemorrhage from blood vessels that are damaged by trauma or disease, which explains the characteristic occurrence of ecchymoses, hematuria, gastrointestinal bleeding and postoperative hemorrhages.

Hemorrhagic Disease of the Newborn. Sometimes spontaneous bleeding is observed in infancy during the first 10 days of life, with the development of ecchymoses into the skin or, following an operative delivery, hematomas at the sites where forceps were applied. In severe cases, there also may be hemorrhage from the umbilical stump, into the gastrointestinal tract, into the brain and elsewhere. The cause of the disorder is vitamin K deficiency, the basis for which is a similar deficiency in the mother.

Dicumarol Toxicity. Dicumarol is a drug which is often employed medicinally for the express purpose of inducing a partial depression of prothrombin activity, its action blocking the conversion of vitamin K to prothrombin by the liver. Properly applied, Dicumarol therapy need never give rise to a hemorrhagic disorder but should merely inhibit, as intended, the formation of clots within blood vessels. In excessive dosage, however, it produces the complete picture of prothrombin deficiency, with consequences that often prove to be extremely dangerous.

Treatment. Hypoprothrombinemia, if due to vitamin K deficiency, responds to treatment with any of several preparations that are available for oral or parenteral administration. However, when corrective measures are urgently required, particularly in patients with liver disease or Dicumarol toxicity, the effective treatment requires the direct replacement of prothrombin by means of transfusion, purified preparations of prothrombin being unavailable as yet.

Deficiency of Prothrombin Conversion Accelerators

Hemorrhagic disorders have occurred as a result of deficiency states involving both factors responsible for accelerating the conversion of prothrombin to thrombin, i.e., the stable factor, or "serum prothrombin conversion accelerator" (SPCA) and the labile factor. The net result of such a deficiency is precisely equivalent to that caused by a lack of prothrombin itself. Treatment consists in the injection of plasma (or whole blood). Unless it can be established that the stable, rather than the labile, factor is involved, it is wise to employ fresh blood in these transfusions, since the labile compound rapidly becomes inert during storage.

Hypofibrinogenemia

Fibrinogen, the precursor of fibrin (the substance of the clot), may be deficient due to an inherited trait (congenital fibrinopenia), eclampsia or prolonged surgical procedures attended by massive hemorrhages that deplete the available supply of this factor in the circulating blood. The result, as in other clotting defects, is a hemorrhagic diathesis with uncontrollable bleeding from all sites where there is blood vessel damage, traumatic or otherwise. Effective treatment is possible by means of whole blood or plasma transfusions, or, preferably, by injections of purified fibrinogen fractionated from human plasma.

Fibrinolysis. A phenomenon in which clots form and then spontaneously dissolve, fibrinolysis is responsible for a serious hemorrhagic disorder, one clinically identical with that of fibrinogen deficiency, which, in effect, this is. Its occurrence, fortunately rare, is observed in the course of prolonged surgical operations in patients who have severe blood loss and have experienced oligemic shock or following trauma. Solution of the clot is due to the action of a proteolytic enzyme, "plasmin," a normal blood constituent, the enzymatic properties of which normally are held in check and never released except under certain circumstances, when efficient removal of thrombi or hematoma obviously requires the liquidation of fibrin. However, in this hemorrhagic disorder plasmin activity, instead of being confined to a restricted area, extends throughout the body. The only treatment of possible avail is the intravenous injection of large quantities of concentrated fibrinogen, since whole blood or plasma cannot possibly be administered in sufficient quantities or with sufficient speed to compensate for its rapid destruction by the abnormal enzymatic activity.

SPLENECTOMY

The spleen, the largest lymphoid organ in the body, is situated in the upper left portion of the abdomen under the diaphragm. It becomes of interest surgically when it is injured or diseased. Not infrequently splenic rupture is produced with severe injury to the left loin and the upper left abdomen. In such patients, rapid hemorrhage from the highly vascular organ makes splenectomy necessary. In hemolytic jaundice and in some other diseases of the blood (purpura, splenic anemia, leukemia and so forth), removal of the spleen often is of value as a therapeutic measure.

Splenectomy is not a difficult operation when the spleen is small but, when the organ is hypertrophied and surrounded by many adhesions, its removal is more difficult. Hemorrhage and abdominal distention are the most frequent postoperative complications. The nursing care of such patients is

COMMON PROBLEMS OF PATIENTS WITH BLOOD DISORDERS

The Problem	Nursing Management
Fatigue and weakness	Plan nursing care to conserve the patient's strength. Give frequent rest periods. Encourage ambulation activities as tolerated. Avoid disturbing activities and noise. Encourage optimum nutrition.
Hemorrhagic tendencies	Keep the patient at rest during the bleeding episodes. Apply gentle pressure to the bleeding sites. Apply cold compresses to the bleeding sites when indicated. Do not disturb clots. Use small gauge needles when administering medications by injection. Support the patient during transfusion therapy. Observe for symptoms of internal bleeding. Have a tracheostomy set available for the patient who is bleeding from the mouth or the throat.
Ulcerative lesions of the tongue, the gums, and/or the mucous membranes	Avoid irritating foods and beverages. Give frequent oral hygiene with mild, cool mouthwash solutions. Use applicators or soft-bristled toothbrush. Keep the lips lubricated. Give mouth care both before and after meals.
Dyspnea	Elevate the head of the bed. Use pillows to support the patient in the orthopneic position. Administer oxygen when indicated. Prevent unnecessary exertion. Avoid gas-forming foods.
Bone and joint pains	Relieve pressure of bedding by using a cradle. Administer either hot or cold compresses as ordered. Provide for joint immobilization when ordered.
Fever	Administer cool sponges. Give antipyretic drugs as ordered. Encourage fluid intake unless contraindicated. Maintain a cool environmental temperature.
Pruritus and/or skin eruptions	Keep the patient's fingernails short. Use soap sparingly. Apply emollient lotions in skin care.
Anxiety of the patient and his family	Explain the nature, the discomforts and the limitations of activity associated with the diagnostic procedures and treatments. Offer the patient the service of listening. Have an empathetic attitude. Promote the patient's relaxation and comfort. Remember the patient's individual preferences. Encourage the family to participate in the patient's care (as desired). Create a comfortable atmosphere for the family to visit with the patient.

the same as for those who have undergone laparotomy. It should be remembered that surgery for disease of the spleen is fraught with much danger because of the serious associated diseases of the liver and the blood. Rupture of the spleen is associated frequently with other severe injuries that increase the gravity of the case. After splenectomy, the majority of patients have a constant temperature that at times is as high as 101° for ten days or so. Occasionally deficient wound healing and dehiscence of the wound follow the operation.

Enlarged spleen (splenomegaly) often causes such discomfort or disability as to justify its removal. In these patients a snugly fitted abdominal binder helps to prevent postoperative overdistention of the stomach and the intestines. Prostigmine or Pitressin administered hypodermically is of value in this connection.

CLINICAL SITUATIONS

A. The Patient With Pernicious Anemia

Mrs. C. P., a 46-year-old bank clerk, is admitted to the hospital complaining of general malaise, digestive disturbances and a slight muscle tremor. Her diagnosis is pernicious anemia.

1. Pernicious anemia is caused by
    A. A virus that destroys the erythrocyte factor in bone marrow.
    B. The presence of an enzyme in the gastric mucosa.
    C. A deficiency of iron and protein in the diet.
    D. Failure to absorb the intrinsic factor.

2. In addition to hematologic studies, the diagnostic test most likely to be ordered for Mrs. P. is
    A. Guaiac test.
    B. Sternal puncture.
    C. Liver biopsy.
    D. Gastric analysis.

3. The patient with pernicious anemia who does not follow treatment adequately is most apt to develop
    A. Aplastic anemia.

B. Degenerative changes in the spinal cord.
    C. Stomach carcinoma.
    D. Hypoplasia of the bone marrow.

4. While teaching Mrs. P. about her condition, the most important factor for the nurse to stress is
    A. The importance of frequent blood evaluations.
    B. The need for vitamin B_{12} during her entire lifetime.
    C. To avoid persons with infectious diseases.
    D. To ensure adequate iron and protein intake.

B. The Patient With Leukemia

Mr. H. B., age 38, is admitted to the medical unit with a diagnosis of acute leukemia.

1. Assuming that each of the following factors is present in Mr. B's history, which one is most frequently associated with this disease?
    A. Chronic osteomyelitis.
    B. Acute glomerulonephritis.
    C. Acute throat infections.
    D. Chronic peptic ulcer.

2. One of the objectives of the medical management of Mr. B. is to correct the complications of the leukemic process. This is accomplished by
    A. Treatment of glandular swelling.
    B. Use of analgesic drugs.
    C. Administration of antibiotics.
    D. Treatment of anemia.

3. Mr. B. has frequent small hemorrhages from his gums, nose and rectum. This hemorrhagic complication is due to
    A. Bone marrow hypoplasia.
    B. Platelet deficiency.
    C. Radiation therapy.
    D. Previous chemotherapy.

4. If serious bone marrow depression occurs as a result of the therapy, Mr. B. will be prepared for
    A. X-ray therapy.
    B. Folic acid.
    C. Blood transfusions.
    D. Vitamin B_{12} injections.

BIBLIOGRAPHY AND SUGGESTED READING

Articles

Condit, P. T., and Eliel, L. P.: Effects of large infrequent doses of Amethopterin on acute leukemia in children, J.A.M.A. **172:**451-453, 1960.

Dalldorf, G.: Lymphomas of African children, J.A.M.A. **181:**1026-1028, 1962.

Ellison, R. R., *et al.:* Comparative study of 6-chloropurine and 6-mercaptopurine in acute leukemia in adults, Ann. Intern. Med. **51:**322-338, 1959.

Fouts, P. J., *et al.:* Absorption of radioactive B_{12} in patients with pernicious anemia after long-term oral and parenteral therapy, Ann. Intern. Med. **52:**29-43, 1960.

Fritz, R. D., *et al.:* The association of fatal intracranial hemorrhage and 'blastic crisis' in patients with acute leukemia, New Eng. J. Med. **261:**59-64, 1959.

McIntyre, P. H.: Total body irradiation, Am. J. Nurs. **61:**62-64, Sept., 1961.

Murray, R., *et al.:* Leukemia in children exposed to ionizing radiation, New Eng. J. Med. **261:** 585-589, 1959.

O'Kell, R. T.: Understanding the hemophilias— A, B, and C, Am. J. Nurs. **62:**101-102, June, 1962.

Registry on Blood Dyscrasias (Council on Drugs), J.A.M.A. **179:**888-890, 1962.

Scharfman, W. B., *et al.:* Idiopathic thrombocytopenic purpura, J.A.M.A. **172:**1875-1884, 1960.

Wintrobe, M. M.: Blood dyscrasias, Am. J. Nurs. **60:**496-500, April, 1960.

Patient-Teaching Aids and Sources of Information

Anemia. Pub. No. 167, Public Health Service, Washington, D. C., U. S. Dept. Health, Education and Welfare, 1962.

Blood and the Rh Factor. Pub. No. 790, Public Health Service, Washington, D. C., U. S. Dept. Health, Education and Welfare, 1960.

The Story of Blood. Pamphlet from The American Red Cross, Washington, D. C., 1963.

26

Patients With Vascular Disorders

VASCULAR ANATOMY AND PHYSIOLOGY

Blood vessels are of three types: arteries, capillaries and veins.

Blood Vessels

Arteries. The arteries carry the blood from the left heart to all parts of the body (Fig. 155). Their walls, necessarily thick and strong, since the column of blood within them is under high pressure, are made up of three layers. The inner layer, the intima, is a thin membrane covered by a single layer of flat endothelial cells and provides a surface suitable for contact with the flowing blood. The middle layer, the media, on which the strength and caliber of the vessel depend, is a thick strong coat made up of muscle fibers mingled with strands and sheets of strong elastic tissue. The outside coat, the adventitia, is a thick layer of connective tissue which binds the artery to the structures through which it courses.

Capillaries. As the artery, by dividing, becomes smaller and smaller, first the adventitia disappears, and the media becomes progressively thinner. Finally, after repeated divisions, the tiny artery, called an *arteriole,* breaks up into a group of tiny tubes with walls of but a single layer of cells. Such a vessel is a capillary, a tube about $\frac{1}{32}$ inch long and just wide enough for red corpuscles to pass through in single or double file (Fig. 156).

The nourishment and oxygen carried by the blood cannot pass through the walls of the arteries and the veins, but it can pass through those of capillaries, which consist of one layer of intimal cells. During the brief second that the blood slowly traverses the capillary, there is a quick exchange of gases and dissolved substances between the blood in this vessel and tissue lymph. In this way the tissue cells receive a fresh supply of food and oxygen and rid themselves of their special products, as well as all waste matter resulting from their cellular metabolism (Fig. 157).

There are myriads of capillaries in the tissues. Could all the capillaries in the body be joined end to end to form one single tube, it would stretch for thousands of miles. Several are in the near vicinity of each tissue cell; in fact, each actively functioning cell is literally surrounded by capillaries. Not all of the same group are open at the same time; the number of such vessels open and functioning in a given area is closely related to the needs of that area. It appears to depend on the concentration of certain cellular products in the vicinity and also on the activity of the autonomic nerve fibers, which have an important influence on their caliber.

Veins. At the distal ends of the capillaries begin the smallest veins (venules). These, by uniting, become larger and larger and their walls thicker. Even the largest veins are thin. The 3 layers are present, but the smooth muscle layer is inconspicuous compared with that in the walls of arteries of the same size; there is no need for such a heavy muscle layer because the blood within them is under much lower pressure. The larger veins are equipped with valves to prevent pooling and backflow of blood into areas which they drain.

The Systemic Circulation

If we trace a blood cell in its journey starting at the aortic valve (Fig. 158, point n), we find that when it leaves the heart it enters the aorta, passes into one of the many branches of this, thence through smaller and smaller arteries until it enters a capillary—in a muscle, for example. After passing through this capillary, b, it enters a small vein, o, whence it moves on through larger and larger veins until finally it enters the vena cava, c, which carries it to the right atrium, d, of the heart, and thence into the right ventricle.

Pulmonary Circulation. It then enters the pulmonary circulation. The right ventricle pumps it through the pulmonary artery, p, into the lungs, f, where it passes through one of the capillaries in the wall of an alveolus and then enters a pulmonary vein, q, thence into the left atrium, g, and from this into the left ventricle, h, where is located the aortic valve whence it started.

Portal Circulation. Other corpuscles take a somewhat more complex route. From the aorta they enter the mesenteric arteries, m, and through their branches finally reach the capillaries of the intestinal wall, i. Passing through them they enter mesenteric veins, and then on into the portal vein, j, which carries them to the liver. Here they must pass through a second capillary, k, and then on into the hepatic vein, l, to the vena cava and to the right side of the heart. The journey of this second corpuscle has included a trip through the portal system.

The Lymphatic System

The lymphatic system is another set of tubes which ramify throughout most of the body. The vessels of this system start as lymph capillaries draining tissue spaces. These unite to form the lymph vessels, which in turn pass through lymph nodes and finally empty into the large thoracic duct which joins the jugular vein on the left side of the neck. The lymphatic system of the abdominal cavity maintains a steady flow of digested fatty food (chyle) from the intestinal mucosa to the thoracic duct. In other parts of the body its function is more regional; the

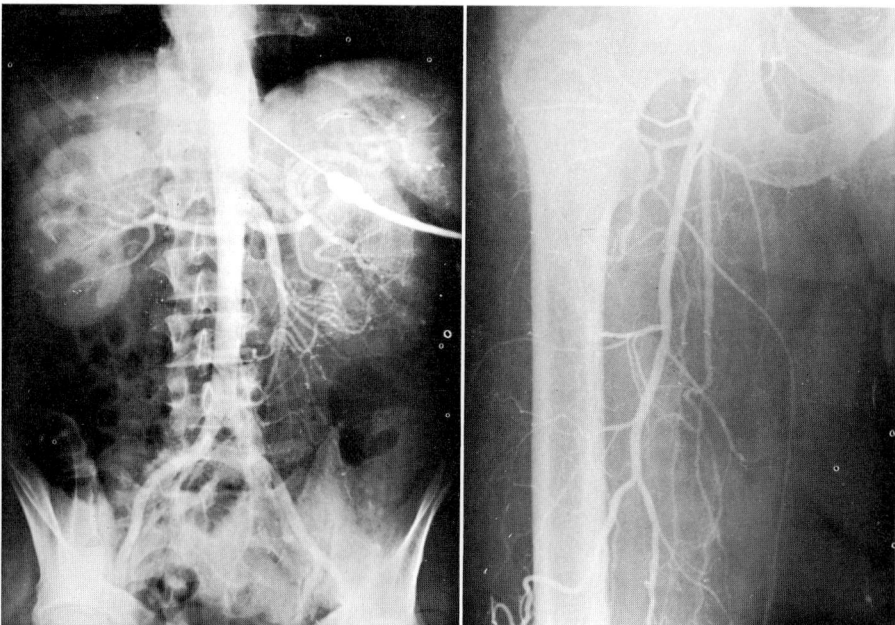

Fig. 155. Arteriography. *(Left)* Demonstrating the x-ray appearance of the abdomen immediately following the injection of contrast medium into the abdominal aorta, which is visible together with its major branches and the kidneys. *(Right)* X-ray view of the thigh, after this aortic injection, showing the femoral artery and its branches. (Richard Chute, M.D., Boston)

lymphatic vessels of the head, for example, empty into clusters of lymph nodes located in the neck, and those of the extremities, into nodes in the axillae and the groin.

PATIENTS WITH DISORDERS OF THE ARTERIES AND THE VEINS

Thrombophlebitis and Thrombo-embolism

A *thrombus* is a blood clot formed within the lumen of a blood vessel, which it partly or completely closes (Fig. 159). If it occurs on the wall of one of the cavities of the heart it is called a mural thrombus. The vessel thus occluded is said to be thrombosed, and the condition is called *thrombosis*. It is believed that the blood will not clot spontaneously within a vessel unless its intimal surface has sustained some damage. It may be injured by trauma, degenerated by arteriosclerotic changes or inflamed. Inflammation may result from direct infection. On the spot of injured intima, platelets first collect. These, disintegrating, liberate substances which cause fibrin formation, the latter entangling the blood cells, with a thrombus as the result.

An *embolus* is usually a thrombus or a fragment of a thrombus which breaks away from the point where it formed, is swept on in the blood stream through the arteries, comes to one too small for it to pass through and plugs it tightly (Fig. 160). This process is called *embolism*. The majority of emboli are fragments of thrombi formed on the walls of the cavities of the heart and on the edges of the heart valve. Others are fragments of thrombi in veins, especially from thrombi laden with germs, as in cases of in-fectious phlebitis. An embolus from a vein or from the right heart may travel to the lungs and occlude a branch of the pulmonary artery; one from a pulmonary vein, the left heart; from a large artery will plug a small systemic artery. Where the embolus stops, it again becomes a thrombus. Apart from thrombi, emboli may consist of bubbles of air (air embolism), plugs of fat (fat embolism) or, in short, any foreign body in the blood stream.

The effects of embolism will depend on what vessel is closed and on what tissues become deprived of their blood supply.

There are two types of arteries: those that communicate (anastomose) with some of the finer branches of nearby arteries (Fig. 161), and those which do not, the latter termed end-arteries. If an end-artery becomes plugged, all circulation along that channel stops, and the tissue which that artery feeds becomes necrotic. But if the vessel closed is not an end-artery, then, when it is closed, the arteries which anastomose with it will send blood through the communicating branches into the artery beyond the obstruction, and so keep alive the tissues which the closed artery formerly fed (Fig. 162). The small anastomosing arteries at once begin to grow larger and larger until they are able to carry all the blood necessary. Then we say a sufficient collateral arterial circulation has been established.

Phlebitis. Inflammation of the walls of veins occurs following direct injuries (such as a perforating wound or a bruise) to a vein, as an extension of an infection of the tissues surrounding the vessel, as a result of continuous pressure against the vein by a

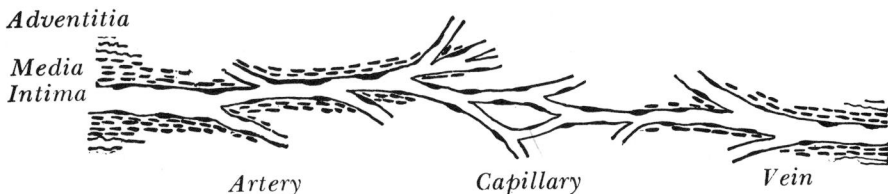

FIG. 156. Diagram of an artery, a capillary and a vein. Note how the walls of the artery "thin out" until the wall of the capillary is only the intima, a single layer of cells. (Of course the transitions from artery to capillary, etc., are actually very much more gradual.) (×300)

tumor or aneurysm and, as we shall see, as a common complication of varicose veins. The condition is apt to arise in circumstances which promote stasis in the leg veins. Thus, it is not an uncommon complication of late pregnancy and should be anticipated in all patients who must be in bed for a prolonged period. For each bedfast patient, whether postoperative, postpartum or ill with any condition which significantly reduces muscular movement, provision must be made for adequate venous drainage from the lower extremities, whether by active or passive leg exercises or by postural changes. A thrombus is likely to form at the infected point; also, thrombosis not due to infection often is the reason for the development of secondary phlebitis where previously there had been none.

Thrombophlebitis. This term is applied to the condition in which a clot forms in a vein, either secondary to phlebitis or due to partial obstruction of the vein. The danger in this situation is that the clot, or a portion of it, may become detached and be swept into the pulmonary circulation, producing embolism.

The most common sites of thrombophlebitis, as has been discussed, are the leg and the pelvic veins. There may be few or no symptoms referable to the local condition, the first intimation of its presence being unexplained fever or pulmonary embolism. Thrombophlebitis involving the leg veins, however, ordinarily causes some pain and tenderness in the thigh or the lower leg and a certain degree of swelling of the limb. Treat-

ment, in the case of femoral thrombophlebitis, consists in bed rest, with the affected limb elevated. If there has been evidence of pulmonary embolism, both femoral veins or the vena cava may be ligated to prevent further escape of clots which might give rise to a fatal pulmonary embolism.

Anticoagulant Therapy

Anticoagulant therapy is used almost routinely in these patients, the administration of both heparin and Dicumarol being started at

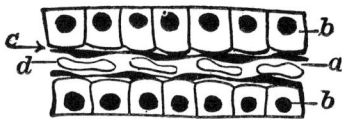

FIG. 157. A capillary and the cells which it furnishes with food and oxygen and whose excreta it removes. (a) Lumen of capillary. (b) Tissue cells. (c) Lymph space between cells and capillary wall. (d) Red blood cells represented as squeezing through the narrow capillary. (×600)

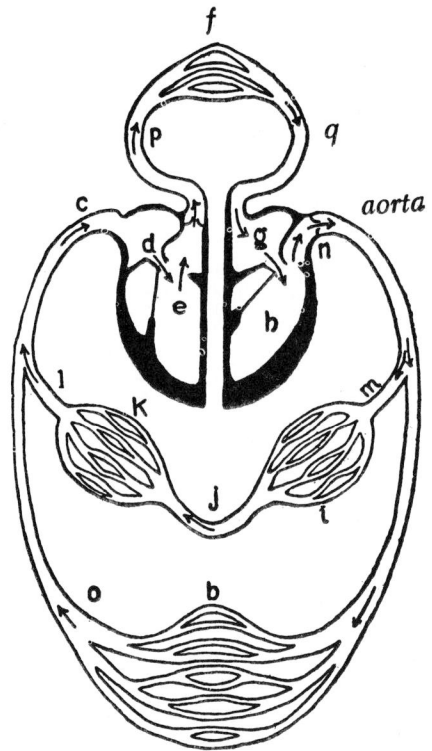

FIG. 158. Diagram of the circulation of the blood. (b) The capillaries of the systemic circulation (e.g., muscles, brain). (c) Vena cava. (d) Right auricle. (e) Right ventricle. (f) Capillaries of the lung. (g) Left auricle. (h) Left ventricle. (i) Capillaries of the stomach and the intestine. (j) The portal vein. (k) Capillaries of the liver. (l) Hepatic vein. (m) Mesenteric artery. (n) Aortic valves. (o) A vein anywhere in the body except the lungs or abdominal viscera. (p) Pulmonary artery. (q) Pulmonary vein.

the earliest possible moment after the thrombotic process is discovered. Heparin or Dicumarol may be given with the object of delaying clotting of the blood, both as a preventive measure in postoperative patients and to forestall the extension of a thrombus once it has formed.

Measures for the prevention or reduction of blood clotting within the vascular system are indicated in cases of thrombophlebitis, pulmonary embolism, coronary thrombosis and, in fact, for any active thrombotic or embolic process. The usual treatment consists of the administration, singly or in combination, of heparin or Dicumarol, which reduces the normal activity of the clotting mechanism. Heparin interferes with the clotting reaction at many points, but primarily it acts as an antagonist to thrombin; Dicumarol blocks the formation of prothrombin from vitamin K, a conversion normally taking place in the liver.

As a therapeutic agent, each of these drugs has its advantages and disadvantages. Heparin is prompt and predictable in its effects but requires an injection technic for its administration. Dicumarol, on the other hand, although far more economical of expense and effort and suitable for oral administration, frequently is disadvantageous because of the prolonged lag period (2 to 3 days) between its ingestion and the appearance of its effect and because of the unpredictable duration of its anticoagulant action, the latter sometimes persisting for as long as 3 weeks. An alternative agent that resembles Dicumarol in its effect on prothrombin formation but achieves this effect more rapidly and is more susceptible to close regulation is phenindione or Hedulin.

Patients to be "heparinized" first are tested for clotting efficiency by a determination of the clotting time. Heparin then is injected, preferably by the intramuscular route, in a dosage of from 50 to 100 mg. Four hours later the clotting time is determined again; if it is prolonged, the test is repeated after 2 hours. If no residual heparin effect is demonstrable at that time, the initial dose is considered suitable for continued repetition at intervals of 6 hours thereafter. If, on the other hand, no clotting delay is discovered 4 hours after the intial injection, a larger quantity of the drug is given promptly; the effectiveness of this, from the standpoint of duration, again is tested as described above. This measure of "heparin tolerance" is repeated until the proper dosage is established, e.g., one that maintains a prolonged clotting time for a 5- to 6-hour period and permits, therefore, a convenient scheduling of injections.

Dicumarol is given orally in an initial dose of from 200 to 300 mg., the patient previously having been tested for prothrombin activity by a measurement of the prothrombin clotting time. A second dose, somewhat smaller, is given on the following day. Subsequent doses are adjusted on the basis of daily prothrombin determinations, the average dosage requirement being from 50 to 100 mg. per day.

The principal complication of anti-coagulant therapy with either drug is the occurrence of spontaneous bleeding anywhere in the body. The earliest evidence of a hemorrhagic diathesis is obtained on routine examination of the urine, evidence of bleeding from the kidneys (microscopic hematuria) being one of the first signs of danger. The effects of heparin can be abolished very promptly by the intravenous injection of protamine sulfate, the dosage of which should be approximately double that of the

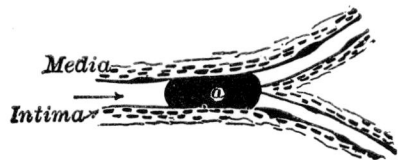

Fig. 160. An embolus plugging a small artery. The embolus (a) is forced along by the blood stream until it reaches a bifurcation of the vessel—here it stops.

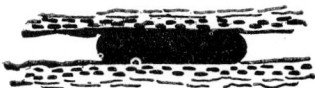

Fig. 159. A small artery plugged by a thrombus.

heparin given on the previous dose. The elimination of Dicumarol or Hedulin activity is relatively more difficult and will continue to be so until purified injectable human prothrombin is available generally. The most effective measure is the transfusion of fresh whole blood or plasma. Vitamin K_1 (Mephyton) is also capable of restoring the prothrombin activity to normal.

Surgery

In many patients with advancing age, the peripheral arteries become plugged with arteriosclerotic material (see p. 491), or they may be blocked by emboli arising from the heart in various forms of cardiac disease. In either case the blood flow to the periphery, usually the feet, is obstructed, and either sudden or gradual reduction of circulation occurs, with changes such as cyanosis or blanching and gangrene and pain of the toes and the feet. It is possible by study of the circulation with special x-ray technics (aortography and arteriography) to determine what type of disease is present in the arteries. In many patients, it may be possible to remove the obstructing area or to bypass it so that blood again can flow from above to the lower portion of the artery, mostly in the leg. When the artery is obstructed by an embolus in cardiac disease, the embolus usually lodges where the artery divides, and in such patients a direct and almost immediate attack is made on the obstruction. The artery is opened and the obstructing embolus is removed, after which the artery is resutured.

In patients whose obstruction is due to arteriosclerosis, arteriography will show the

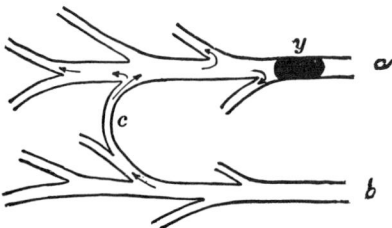

Fig. 161. Anastomosing arteries (a and b) are connected by an anastomotic branch (c). If a is plugged by the thrombus (y), the circulation in a will be maintained by b.

site of the obstruction. Occasionally it is possible to remove the obstructed area in the vessel and resuture the vessel (endarterectomy). More often, however, the obstruction is bypassed by introducing a graft consisting of a vein or a synthetic material into the circulation above the obstruction and carrying it downward to anastomose it, end-to-side, below the obstruction (Fig. 163). In this way blood flow again is brought into the lower leg, and many cases of impending gangrene can be averted.

Of course, there are dangers associated with this type of surgery. In many patients it is unsuccessful because the vessels of the lower leg are so filled with atheromatous material that they are not able to carry the blood flow to the foot and the toes. In such patients, despite the successful bypass, an amputation may become necessary. In spite of the difficulties of this type of surgery, excellent results are obtained in a certain group of patients who are spared amputation, at least for the time being.

Nursing Care. It is not unusual for a nurse to have a patient who during his convalescence complains of pain in the calf of the leg that is aggravated when the foot is dorsiflexed (Homan's sign). She must be aware of the fact that this may be a symptom of phlebothrombosis, and that, to avoid dislodging a thrombus, she should not massage the part. She should keep the patient in bed and notify the physician.

When a ligation is to be done or a clot is to be removed, the nurse must know what area or areas are to be prepared. A common method employed by some surgeons to indicate the site is to make an X on the skin with an applicator stick dipped in methylene blue. For a femoral ligation, the inguinal and, possibly, the pubic areas should be shaved on the side that is affected.

Postoperative care is according to the orders given by the surgeon. The operative dressing must be examined for signs of hemorrhage. In addition, the nurse must realize that the patient may have a serious circulatory difficulty. It is important to check the pulse and the blood pressure and also to pay attention to any mention of pain or numbness in an extremity or pain in the chest. In any circulatory problem the patient as a whole must be considered.

Prevention

The use of anticoagulant drugs for the prevention of thrombo-embolic diseases or to limit their extension if already present, has been discussed. The importance of early ambulation and systematic exercises for the patient at bed rest, as a means of avoiding venous stasis in the lower extremities, has been emphasized.

Deep-breathing exercises are beneficial, as they produce in the thorax increased negative pressure, which assists in emptying the large veins.

One further approach to prophylaxis is the use of elastic stockings extending to the knee, which are prescribed for patients on a regimen of restricted activity, particularly those who are confined to bed (Fig. 164). These stockings, by exerting a sustained, evenly distributed pressure over the entire surface of the calves, reduce the caliber of the veins of the lower extremities, with the result that venous blood flow is speeded, and any tendency toward stagnation or pooling of blood in that area is reduced or abolished. It is important for the nurse to note that any type of stocking, including the elastic type, can be converted into a tourniquet if applied incorrectly, i.e., rolled tightly at the top, and consequently produce stasis instead of reducing it. Obviously, this must be avoided, and the nurse must satisfy herself that her patients so understand.

These stockings should be removed for a brief interval at least twice daily. While they are off, the nurse should inspect the skin for signs of irritation and examine the calves for possible tenderness. If any skin changes or signs of tenderness are observed, these should be reported at once.

The Postphlebitic Leg

As a result of the block of the deep veins in phlebitis, the superficial veins often dilate to take over the return of venous blood from the leg. The clot in the deep vein is canalized and partly absorbed in time, so that the deep veins again may partly function. However, the valves of the vein usually are destroyed by the phlebitis; thus, blood may pass downward toward the foot when the patient is in the erect position. This results in a chronic venous stasis with associated

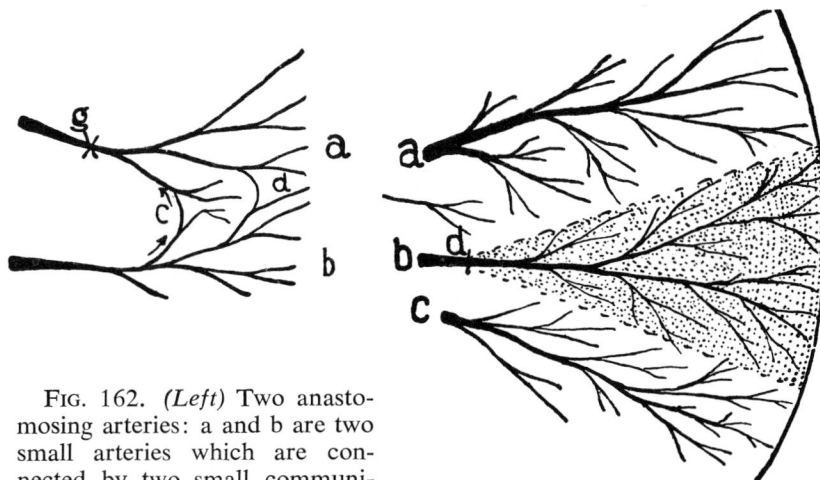

FIG. 162. *(Left)* Two anastomosing arteries: a and b are two small arteries which are connected by two small communicating branches or anastomoses (c and d). If a should become plugged at g, the circulation through a would not stop, but the blood would flow from b through c and d into the branches of a. *(Right)* End-arteries and an infarct: a, b and c are three small arteries which have no communicating branches. If b becomes plugged at d, then all the tissue supplied with nourishment by b must die. This dead area is an infarct (the dotted triangle).

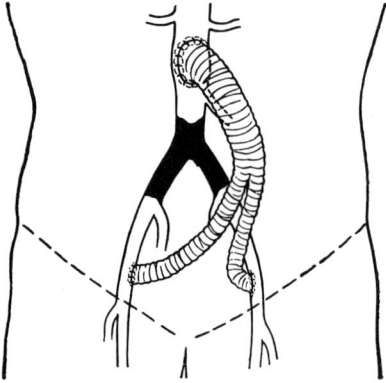

FIG. 163. A diagram of aortobilateral iliac bypass prosthesis. (Jordan G. L.: Atherosclerotic lesions of the aorta and peripheral arteries, Med. Sci. **12**:209)

changes: discoloration, swelling and ulceration (Fig. 165). The treatment of this type of venous stasis is much more difficult than that resulting from varicosities of only the superficial veins. In some patients there may be no superficial venous enlargement visible or palpable.

Various measures have been suggested in the attempt to remove the venous stasis. These include ligation of the superficial femoral veins and ligation of the saphenous (long and short), if these are varicosed. Most often a more conservative method of therapy is applied, consisting largely of methods to prevent venous stasis by providing external pressure and gravity drainage of venous blood. In order to impress the patient with the necessity for thwarting venous stasis and swelling of the legs, certain rules

have been suggested for the patient with phlebitis. These are:

1. Prevent swelling by constant wearing of elastic stockings. These should be put on the first thing upon arising and worn until going to bed at night. The only time the stockings should be removed is when bathing.

2. Mere standing produces increased venous stasis; therefore, some slight exercise should be attempted, such as walking, moving the toes in the shoes, etc. In the year following the attack of phlebitis, the legs should be elevated to a horizontal position on a chair at least 5 minutes out of every 2 hours.

3. At least 2 or 3 times a day the legs should be elevated above the head by lying down. With the leg elevated on the back of a sofa or even against the wall while the patient is lying on his back, the venous blood is drained by gravity from the part. Whenever possible, the leg should be elevated on another chair when sitting down.

4. At night, the foot of the bed should be elevated 6 or 8 inches to permit venous drainage by gravity to take place.

5. Patients with irritation of the skin of the leg should apply bland, oily lotions to prevent scaling and dryness.

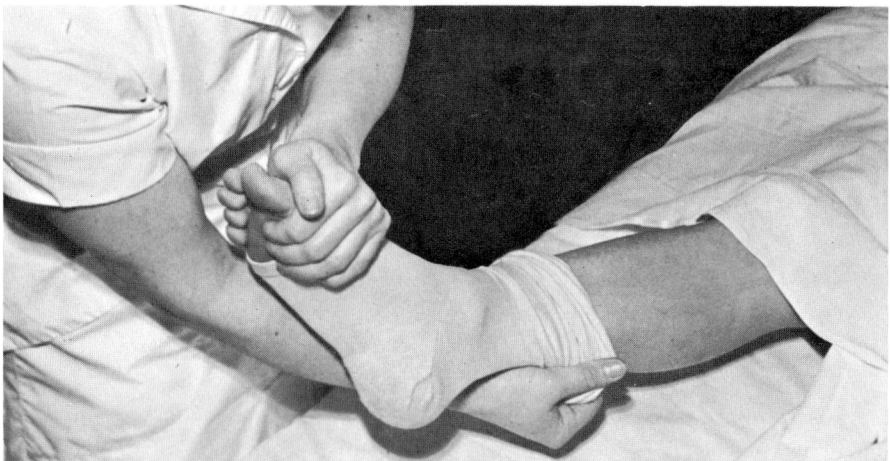

FIG. 164. Application of elastic stocking.

6. Finally, the patient should be careful to avoid all trauma, bruising, scratching or other forms of injury to the skin of the leg and the foot.

If these suggestions are carried out repeatedly, it is possible to avoid many of the complications that otherwise appear in the postphlebitic leg.

Arteriosclerosis Obliterans

Arteriosclerosis, or hardening of the arteries, is the disease that indirectly kills the majority of all men beyond middle life. Its symptoms do not arise from the diseased arteries themselves, but are those of the heart, the kidneys, the brain, etc., whose functions, because of it, are disturbed.

The most common direct results of arteriosclerosis are the narrowing, the closure by thrombosis and the rupture of the smaller arteries (Figs. 166 and 167). Its indirect results are malnutrition, with subsequent fibrosis of the organs which the sclerotic arteries supply with blood. All actively functioning tissue cells require an abundant supply of food and oxygen and are sensitive to any reduction in the supply of these. If such reductions are severe and permanent, these cells undergo ischemic necrosis and are replaced by fibrous tissue, which requires much less food. Hence, malnourished organs become sclerotic and, in time, since scar tissue contracts, more or less contracted. Thus arise the degenerative areas in the brain, in the heart's weak myocardium and in the small contracted kidneys.

When the long arteries of the extremities are affected by arteriosclerosis, the blood supply may be insufficient to maintain the tissues in a viable state, and gangrene (complete death of the tissue) occurs (Fig. 168). This change usually affects the toes and the feet. Usually gangrene is of the dry type, a mummification. Frequently, however, the gangrenous area becomes infected secondarily and produces marked systemic, as well as local, symptoms.

Arteriosclerosis affects the entire arterial tree in varying degrees, with some organs developing more fibrosis than others. Since the myocardium and the kidneys furnish the most significant symptoms of this malady, the majority of patients are grouped under the term cardiovascular-renal diseases.

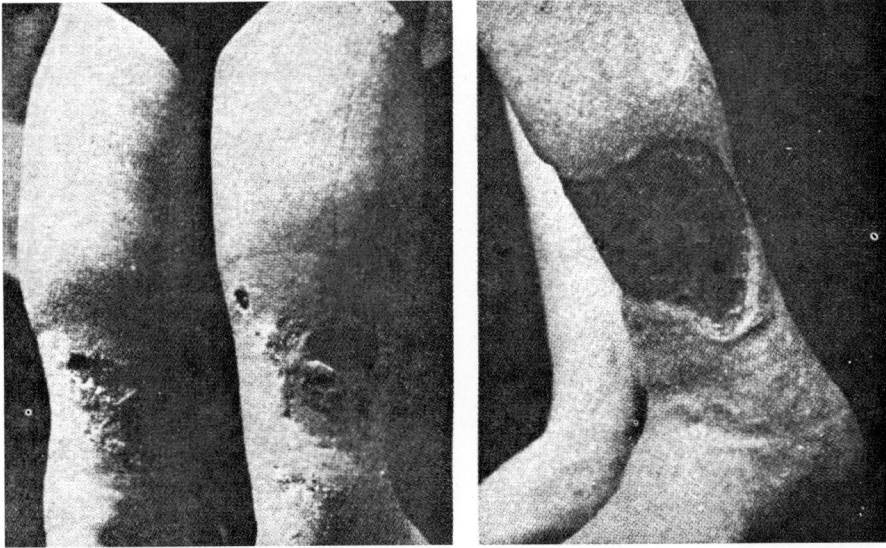

FIG. 165. *(Left)* Relatively early stage of the ulceration in a thrombophlebitic process. *(Right)* Late stage of ulceration following thrombophlebitic edema. Note the punched-out edges of the ulcer with marked induration and fibrosis around its edge.

Etiology. A moderate degree of arteriosclerosis is considered by some authorities as an inevitable evidence of the aging of the vessels, almost as normal for elderly persons as is white hair. However, this is not a fair statement of the case. Many an elderly person has soft vessels, and a few young men have marked arteriosclerosis. It commonly is associated with diabetes mellitus, chronic nephritis and arterial hypertension.

Some investigators believe that the condition is due to a disease of lipid metabolism or to over-ingestion of cholesterol-containing foodstuffs. The tendency to arteriosclerosis is a definitely inheritable condition. The statement has been made that almost 70 per cent of all patients who develop this condition early in life give a history of the disease among several generations of their family. At present the factors most stressed are a hereditary tendency, metabolic disturbances and factors related to arterial hypertension.

Symptoms. The symptoms of arteriosclerosis are mentioned in the descriptions of the various diseases of the organs which it injures.

Prognosis. The prognosis for the patient depends on the location of the weakest spot in his arterial tree.

Management. The management of arteriosclerosis must be individualized, since no two patients are affected alike. Although a damaged artery cannot be repaired, nevertheless, by early treatment, the destructive processes often can be reduced, and the

organ dysfunctions already created may be relieved in part. The patient should not retire from the business world lest he lose all initiative. He should, however, avoid strenuous or fatiguing efforts, should rest each day at noon, should retire early, take long vacations and treat all minor illnesses as serious.

When the toes and the feet are involved, preventive measures, such as keeping the feet clean and wearing loose shoes, should be taken. There is rarely any treatment of any value for the arteriosclerotic patient with gangrene, except removal of the gangrenous parts. In such cases, in order to obtain a wound that will heal, it is necessary that a high amputation be performed, usually through the thigh. (See Amputation, p. 1014.)

Arteriosclerotic patients, as a rule, have a variety of symptoms attributable to several organ systems, as one might expect in the case of a generalized vascular disease. Of the organ systems that suffer most as a result of generalized arteriosclerosis and whose dysfunction gives rise to the most disagreeable and dangerous symptoms, five feature most prominently: the brain, the heart, the gastrointestinal tract, the kidneys and the muscles of the extremities. The proportionate involvement of each organ system varies widely from patient to patient, and the therapeutic problems to which each gives rise are discussed in detail in the sections of the book devoted to the patient with diseases of that particular system.

Surgery. Because the ischemia produced by the arteriosclerosis of the larger vessels is associated often with a spasm of the smaller, less-involved peripheral vessels, attempts have been made to increase the peripheral circulation by dividing the sympathetic nerve

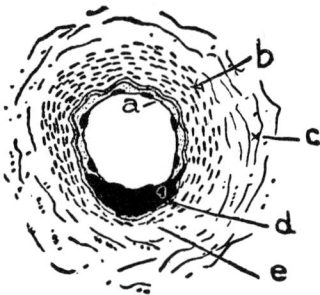

FIG. 166. Cross section of artery through an arteriosclerotic patch. (a) Intima. (b) Media. (c) Adventitia. (d) Arteriosclerotic patch. (e) Atrophied media.

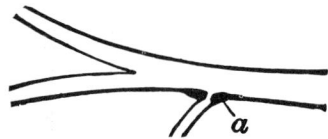

FIG. 167. Arteriosclerosis. A small patch of arteriosclerosis (a) partially is occluding the mouth of a small branch artery.

supply to these vessels. This procedure, *sympathectomy,* releases the contraction of the arterials and permits an increased peripheral blood supply.

Other types of surgery helpful to many patients with arteriosclerosis (or thromboembolism) are discussed on page 488.

Hypertensive Vascular Disease

Hypertensive vascular disease is an all-inclusive term referring to the damage sustained by the heart, the blood vessels and the tissues dependent on those vessels, as a result of hypertension. Whereas the basic causes of the disorder are obscure for the most part, the mechanism directly responsible for an increase in arterial pressure is well known. This involves the sustained constriction of arterioles throughout the entire body, brought about by a continuous contraction of the smooth muscle fibers in the vessel walls. Epinephrine, the hormone produced by the adrenal medulla, is capable of causing such constriction, and excessive continuous secretion of that hormone in patients with pheochromocytoma (p. 844) is one important, though rare, cause of chronic arterial hypertension. Renin, a chemical agent released from kidneys when the renal blood supply is reduced, accounts for arterial hypertension in patients with kidney lesions of various types. The condition is also associated with certain endocrine disorders, including hyperthyroidism, basophilic adenoma of the pituitary and tumors of the adrenal cortex.

With respect to 95 per cent of hypertensive patients, however, the cause of their disease is not understood. One assumes that their pressure-regulating mechanisms, for reasons unknown, operate at a setting that is altered and abnormally high. As a result, all regulatory apparatus concerned with the caliber of arterioles cooperates in maintaining an increased vascular tone and, consequently, an increased arterial pressure. The vessel walls inevitably thicken. If the tension is excessive and blood flow reduced sufficiently, the tissues that are served by those vessels, and the vessels themselves, will be damaged. The damage that is most serious from the standpoint of the patient's health and survival is that which occurs in the heart, the brain and the kidneys, where vascular spasm and vascular leakage interfere most vitally.

Patients with essential hypertension exhibit a variable increase in both diastolic and systolic pressures. After periods of rest and in response to sedation, these pressures tend to subside toward normal levels but do not decline as much as would normally be observed. Conversely, stimuli that normally produce a rise in blood pressure, such as emotional stress, exertion or exposure to cold, cause a much greater rise in these patients.

Their symptomatic complaints are very

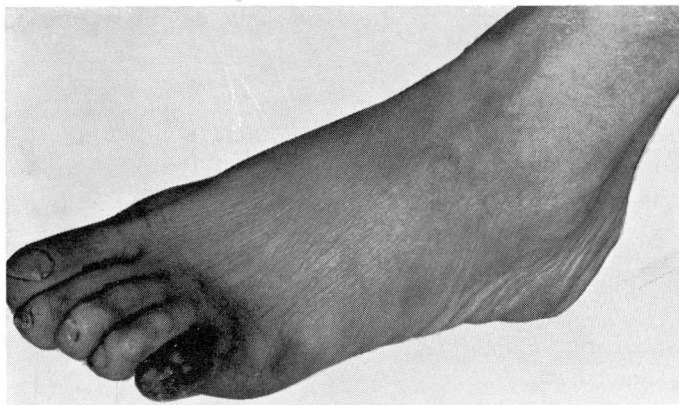

FIG. 168. Diabetic gangrene.

likely to include headache, emotional irritability, dizziness, palpitation, visual disturbances and nose bleeds. The ultimate course is determined in each patient by the distribution of organ damage, i.e., what organs are affected and how seriously. When it is the heart, the patient will experience angina, congestive heart failure and myocardial infarcts; when there is cerebral damage, mental changes will occur, possibly lapses of consciousness and, eventually, exitus as a result of cerebral thrombosis or hemorrhage; or, if significant renal damage has occurred, the patient will experience hematuria, and signs of kidney failure will develop terminating in uremia.

With respect to duration of symptoms and the rate of progress, essential hypertension is an extremely variable disease. The severest cases, which usually terminate fatally within a period of 2 to 3 years, or less, are said to have "malignant hypertension." In sharp contrast with this picture is the most common type of case in which symptoms dependent on hypertension are mild or altogether lacking for many years and are apt to terminate after 10 to 20 years, or longer, as a result of some other disease altogether.

Treatment

Mild hypertensive vascular disease requires very little medical attention, which usually is limited to general advice pertaining to overweight, overexertion and overexcitement. If hypertension is severe and if organ damage is not considered to be excessive or irreversible, surgical ablation of large portions of the sympathetic nervous system may be undertaken, for example, by means of bilateral dorsolumbar sympathectomy. A more conservative measure, perhaps, is the prescription of a low sodium diet. This helps to prevent edema due to sodium retention. When followed rigorously, this is effective, but the dietary restrictions that such a regimen must impose are tolerated by very few individuals and are quite impractical on a long-term basis.

Antihypertensive Drugs. Happily, great advances have been made during recent years in the chemotherapeutic approach to arterial hypertension, and a considerable variety of agents now are available which can be ad-

ministered singly, or in combination, with substantial benefit to the majority of patients with this disease. These drugs are selected, and their dosage adjusted, on an individual basis in each case, with the object of achieving a gradual restoration of normotensive pressure levels, while subjecting the patient to the least possible risk and producing a minimum of side-effects.

First to be administered, in most cases, is one of the Rauwolfia Serpentina drugs, for example, Raudixin, in an intital dose of 50 mg.; Rauwiloid, 2 mg.; reserpine (Serpasil, Serpiloid, Reserpoid, Sandril), rescinnamine (Rescamine, Moderil) or deserpidine (Harmonyl), 0.1 mg., 1 to 4 times daily. These doses may be doubled gradually, but within a period of from 1 to 3 months the minimal effective dose should be sought in order to avoid mental depression, insomnia or nightmares.

Enhancement of the Rauwolfia Serpentina effect, if desired, may be obtained by adding an extract of veratrum, for example, Veriloid (2 mg.) or Vergitryl (1 unit), protoveratrine derivatives of veratrum, such as Provell or Veralba (0.25 mg.) or pure protoveratrine A (Protalba, 0.1 mg.), given 3 or 4 times a day. The dosage in each instance may be increased somewhat, if necessary, but not without risking the production of nausea and undesirable degrees of hypotension.

Another drug that may be selected as a supplement to Rauwolfia Serpentina is hydralazine hydrochloride (Apresoline), given in a starting dose of 10 mg. 4 times a day. This dose may be increased tenfold with reasonable safety; however, larger amounts have produced a toxic syndrome with clinical and laboratory features similar to those of disseminated lupus erythematosus. A fourth type of antihypertensive agent, and one of the most promising to date, is an oral diuretic, chlorothiazide (Diuril), which is given in a dose of 125 mg., and eventually 500 mg., 3 times a day. In order to avoid marked potassium depletion on this regimen, the patient should receive potassium regularly as a dietary supplement. A fifth class of hypotensive drugs is comprised of the ganglionic blocking agents, exemplified by pentolinium tartrate (Ansolysen), which is given in a dose of 20 mg., 2 to 4 times a day. Al-

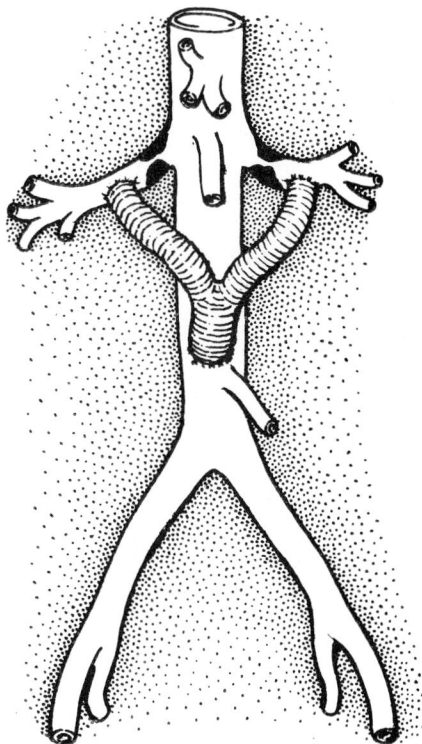

FIG. 169. A diagrammatic illustration showing a synthetic graft (shaded area) from the aorta to the renal arteries beyond the obstruction (blackened area). By such revascularization of the kidney, significant improvement has been noted in selected patients with severe hypertension.

though extremely potent, from the standpoint of reducing arterial hypertension, their usefulness is limited sharply by the narrowness of the margin between their effective and their toxic doses.

Patients receiving ganglionic blocking agents should have their blood pressure taken while they are standing, as these drugs produce orthostatic hypotension.

General precautions that are applicable generally to patients on antihypertensive chemotherapy include the following:

Gastric secretion tends to increase, and peptic ulcers may become reactivated or develop anew in response to this type of chemotherapy; accordingly, antacids often are prescribed in conjunction with these drugs.

Weight gain is likely to occur, particularly in response to Rauwolfia Serpentina or reserpine; in view of this possibility, a low-fat diet may be prescribed for recipients of these particular drugs.

Hot weather, a febrile illness or dehydration from any cause tend to enhance the potency of antihypertensive drugs; accordingly their dosage should be reduced automatically under these circumstances.

The soporific effect of antihypertensive drug therapy should be countered not by administering a "psychic energizer" (see p. 136) but by lowering the dosage of the offending drug.

The patient with hypertension should have his intake and output measured and recorded during the time he is hospitalized. Serial blood pressure evaluations are made on each arm in order to determine if primary hypertension is present. The patient is observed for headache, dizziness, visual disturbances, chest pain and tingling or numbness of the arms. He is usually more comfortable when the head of his bed is elevated.

Intelligent patients often become expert in managing their own chemotherapy and, depending on the level of intelligence, may be encouraged to do so. Some physicians teach their hypertensive patients to take their own blood pressures, as a basis for regulating drug dosage; others find this to be unnecessary and regard it as undesirable.

Revascularizing of the Kidney. One of the advances in the surgical treatment of hypertension has been the discovery that vascular abnormalities of the renal arteries, usually arteriosclerotic in type, can be corrected by operation. With the injection of a radiopaque dye into the aorta (aortography) it is possible to demonstrate a narrowing of the renal artery and reduction of renal blood flow in about 20 per cent of the patients with severe hypertension. Revascularization of the kidney via synthetic grafts from the aorta to the renal artery beyond the obstruction has restored the blood pressure to normal in about half the patients who were operated on by Dr. DeBakey and his group at Baylor College of Medicine. In another 8 to 10 per cent the hypertension was reduced.

Nursing care relating to hypertensive vascular disease is discussed in detail in those sections devoted to the treatment of coronary heart disease and congestive heart failure.

Thromboangiitis Obliterans
(Buerger's Disease)

Buerger's disease is a recurring inflammation in the arteries and the veins of the extremities, usually of the lower extremities, and results in thrombus formation and occlusion of the vessels. The cause of the condition is not known, but it is believed by many to be of bacterial origin because of the acute stages of the disease.

It occurs primarily in men between the ages of 25 and 45, and there is considerable evidence that smoking is a factor, if not in the etiology at least in the progress of the disease. As a rule, the patient appears for treatment when the disease has affected so many of the vessels of the extremity as to reduce the peripheral arterial circulation. He complains of cramps in the legs after exercise, which are relieved by inactivity (intermittent claudication); often there is considerable burning pain. As the disease progresses, definite cyanosis of the part appears when it is dependent, and ulceration with gangrene occurs, especially about the nails and the toes.

Treatment. The treatment must be started early. The main objects are to improve the blood flow to the extremities, to reduce their blood requirement and to protect them from trauma and infection, to which they are dangerously susceptible.

Scrupulous attention to cleanliness is essential: daily washing of the feet with bland soap and warm water is desirable. After washing, the feet are dried with the aid of rubbing alcohol, patted with a soft nontraumatizing towel and powdered. Clean socks or stockings should be worn each day or changed as often as necessary. The patient should massage the extremities with a bland lubricating oil each day. Circumstances predisposing to trauma and infection must be strictly avoided. Shoes and stockings should be fitted accurately, and the feet protected adequately from cold and, similarly, from the incautious exposure to heat provided by mechanical warming devices or hot water. Caustic antiseptics, such as iodine or phenol and its derivatives, never should be applied to the feet if the peripheral circulation is inadequate, for tissue necrosis develops easily under these conditions. The patient must restrain himself from performing feats of minor surgery on corns and calluses. Caution must be exercised in the cutting of the toenails, which should be trimmed squarely. Circular garters and rolled stockings are to be avoided. Medical attention is indicated on the initial appearance of color changes in the feet, the development of a blister, an abrasion or infection, or changes in sensation, such as tingling, burning, numbness or pain.

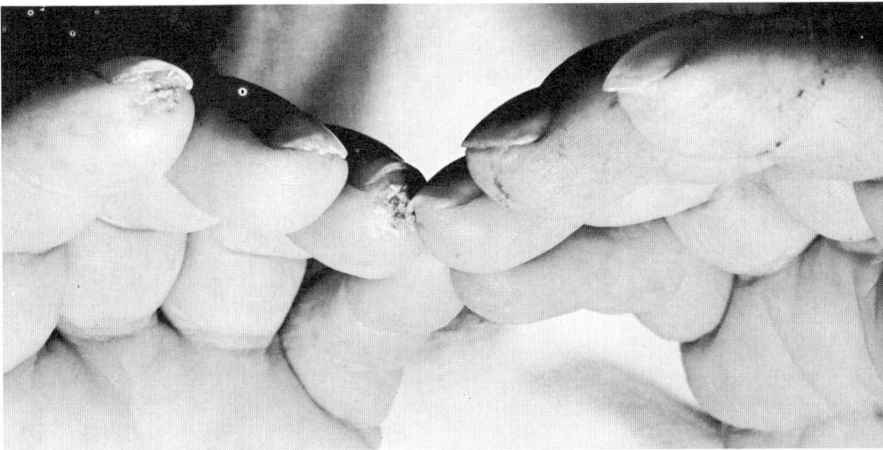

FIG. 170. Raynaud's disease. Note necrosis of tissue of fingertips.

The use of tobacco is forbidden for patients with Buerger's disease.

For patients with peripheral vascular disease with intermittent claudication, exercises are prescribed which are designed to promote the development of collateral circulation in the affected limbs. These exercises involve alternate raising and lowering the legs in timed cycles, the rate and the duration of the exercises being regulated specifically for each individual patient on the basis of changes in the color of the skin and subjective sensations of discomfort.

It is important to remember that in no case of acute local circulatory insufficiency, whether due to an embolus or to intrinsic arterial disease, should heat be applied to the affected extremity. Heat merely increases tissue metabolism and raises the requirement for oxygenated blood, which demand cannot be fulfilled. Some clinics even pack the extremity in ice, reporting resultant relief of pain and occasional halting of a gangrenous process.

It has been found worth while, in many types of peripheral obliterative arterial disease involving the legs, to perform a temporary sympathetic block by injecting the lumbar sympathetic ganglia and cords with procaine. The proportion of patients who respond to this abolishment of the vasoconstricting influence of the sympathetic nervous

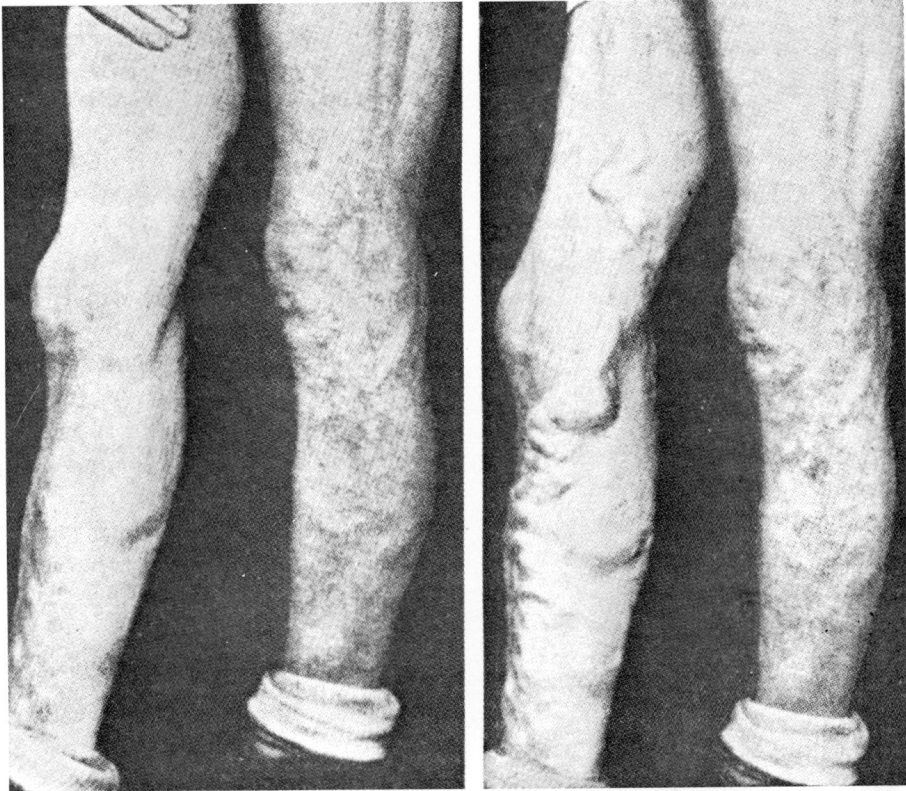

Fig. 171. A patient with varicose veins. *(Left)* The patient was placed on a bed with the leg elevated so as to drain the blood from the superficial veins. Manual pressure then was applied over the uppermost portion of the vein and the patient was asked to stand. Note that, with hand compressing the upper portion of the vein no veins are seen in the lower leg. *(Right)* Hand pressure has been removed from the upper portion of the thigh, and the veins have filled up rapidly. This indicates incompetence of the valves, which permits the backward flow of blood in veins. This is a positive Trendelenburg test.

system has been striking. Cold, cyanotic, painful legs with circulation impaired as a result of arteriosclerosis, as well as by inflammatory arterial disease, occasionally have returned to a much more normal state immediately after this test procedure. If definitely favorable, a lumbar sympathectomy may be performed for a more permanent effect. In the late stages of the disease, after gangrene has appeared because of deficient circulation, amputation may be necessary. Occasionally, conservative measures may be practiced after desensitization of the part involved by injecting alcohol into the sensory nerves. However, the disease is a progressive one, and often the amputation of a single toe must be followed by amputation of another, until eventually it is necessary to amputate a foot or a leg (p. 1014).

Raynaud's Disease

Raynaud's disease is found most often in young people between the ages of 18 and 30; it affects the female more often than the

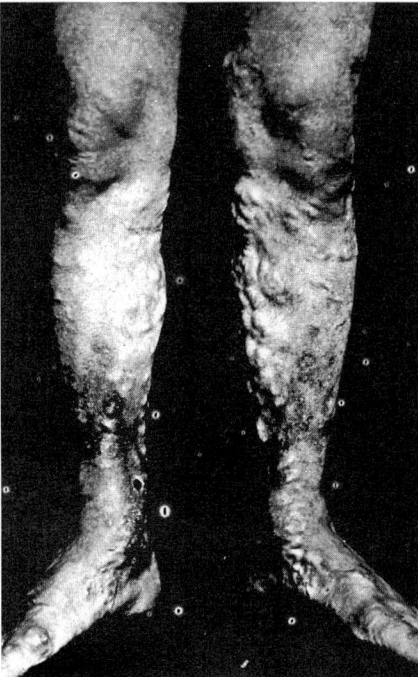

FIG. 172. Varicose ulcers at usual
locations.

male. It is characterized by a blanched, almost deathlike, appearance of symmetrical parts of the extremities—that is, both hands (Fig. 170) or both feet or all four members —or by local asphyxia, which produces a marked purplish color in the extremities involved. These phenomena are brought about by some disturbance in the vasomotor mechanism to the part, which produces spasms of the arteries, and they seem to be initiated by exposure to cold. When they occur frequently, they cause nutritional changes in the part and gangrene appears in areas— most often the fingertips — and sometimes large parts of the member are involved. The disease occurs in an attack from which the patient may recover, but the recurrence of the attack is not infrequent.

Treatment. In mild cases without gangrene, conservative therapy, such as protection from cold, and at times fever therapy by intravenous typhoid vaccine, may be found to be helpful. In marked cases, however, an interruption of the sympathetic nerves by removal of the sympathetic ganglia or division of their branches is the only method of affording much improvement. These ganglia are located either in the upper part of the thorax and lower neck for the upper extremity or along the vertebral column behind the peritoneum for the lower extremity. The operation for removal of these ganglia is spoken of as a *sympathetic ganglionectomy*.

Varicose Veins

The blood flow in the veins is maintained in a direction toward the heart by a series of cup-shaped valves. A deficiency of these valves may be produced by disease, as in phlebitis, or by long-standing distention, due to back pressure on the veins, as in pregnancy, or to long periods of being in the erect position. When the valves become deficient, the veins dilate gradually. This phenomenon occurs almost always in the lower extremities, and the veins most affected are those that lie in the subcutaneous fatty tissues, especially the long saphenous vein. (Fig. 171.)

The dilatation of this vein produces a venous stasis with secondary edema, replacement fibrosis in the subcutaneous fatty tissue, pigmentation of the skin and, because of these changes, a lowered resistance to infection and to trauma. The symptoms produced most often are disfigurement due to the large size of the vein, easy fatigue of the part, a heavy feeling, cramps in the legs at night and, often, pain during the menstrual period. The veins may occur at any age, but they appear most commonly in women after pregnancy. If varicose veins are untreated, the changes in the lower leg mentioned above may appear. Repeated attacks of inflammation are not uncommon and ulceration may develop.

Treatment. In the treatment of varicose veins, it is essential to remove the hydrostatic pressure of the column of blood in the veins. This can be done by a ligation of the saphenous vein in the upper part of the thigh.

Then the dilated saphenous vein with its incompetent valves is removed by a procedure called "stripping." A metal or plastic stripper is inserted into the lower end of the vein in the groin and is threaded down the leg toward the knee and the ankle. If the vein is not too tortuous (twisted) it may be possible to thread the stripper through the entire vein down to the ankle. In other patients the stripper may be caught in vein pockets in the thigh or the leg. An incision is made at the lowermost point of the stripper, and the end of the stripper is pulled out of the vein. By tying the vein to the stripper and pulling downward, the vein is pulled out of its location in the subcutaneous tissues. Pressure along the course of the vein is all that is necessary to control bleeding. After several incisions are made, excision of tortuous veins may be necessary in addition. The legs are dressed with gauze and elastic adhesive bandages. The veins which then remain may be closed by the injection of sclerosing substances, such as sodium morrhuate. These produce a local chemical thrombosis that closes the veins and in most cases relieves the symptoms.

Varicose Ulcers

The prolonged venous stasis and edema seen in patients with varicose veins result in a gradual replacement of subcutaneous fatty tissue by fibrous tissue. The skin becomes discolored and, on pressure, is firm and brawny. These tissues have a poor resistance to infection, so that minor trauma and abrasions result in ulcerations that tend not only to remain but to enlarge and progress (Fig. 172). The ulcers are surrounded by an area of hard edema and frequently are characterized by a burning pain. In advanced cases, the ulcers may progress to involve the entire circumference of the leg. They are seen most often in patients who have had a previous phlebitis.

When varicose veins have progressed to ulceration, supportive therapy of some type is of value, in addition to the treatment of the veins themselves. This support may be given by elastic bandages or stockings, but can probably be accomplished best by the use of a gelatin paste (Unna's) boot.* This is applied over the ulcer, involving usually the foot and extending upward as far as the knee. With this treatment most ulcers will heal.

The thin epithelium that eventually heals the ulcer is traumatized easily, and recurrence of ulceration is not infrequent. In many patients, a better and more permanent healing may be obtained by excision of the fibrous subcutaneous tissue and the application of skin grafts.

It is recognized that the underlying cause for the ulcer is venous stasis due to varicose veins. Therefore, after the ulcer has been "cleaned up" by appropriate treatment, a definite attack usually is made on the varicose veins, and by ligation and/or stripping, they are removed. Rapid healing of the

---

* *Unna's Paste for Gelatin Boots:* Unna's gelatin mixture is a frequently used supporting dressing, especially on the lower leg. It is prepared in a double boiler as follows: gelatin 200 Gm., zinc oxide pulv. 100 Gm., glycerin 400 ml., hot water 375 ml. Dissolve the gelatin in the hot water. Mix the glycerin and the zinc oxide powder until smooth, then add to the dissolved gelatin. Cook in the double boiler for one half hour. This makes enough paste for 4 or 5 boots. The skin is painted and a layer of gauze bandage applied, followed by more paste and more bandage until the desired thickness is obtained, usually 2 or 3 layers. The boot is changed every 1 to 2 weeks. After application, the patient should remain nearby for at least an hour in order that circulation can be checked. If the toes are warm, normal in color and show no signs of edema, he may be discharged.

ulcer usually takes place as soon as the venous stasis is removed.

Nursing Care. This patient usually is ambulatory after surgery; however, the nurse is expected to check circulation in his operated leg occasionally. If edema or other circulatory disturbances are noted, the patient is put to bed, and his leg is elevated.

The nurse can emphasize several points in her contact with these patients. Circular garters must be avoided. When sitting, the patient should not cross his legs, as this may impair circulation. The patient should avoid standing for long periods of time. If the extremities swell, the condition can be alleviated by proper elevation and support of the legs. He can be taught how to apply and to care for elastic bandages. Also, he should take precautions to avoid trauma, as leg ulcers and infections do not heal easily.

NURSING CARE OF THE PATIENT WITH A PERIPHERAL VASCULAR PROBLEM

Psychosocial Problems

Much of the progress made by patients with peripheral vascular conditions depends on nursing care. The problems of these individuals may appear minor compared with those of other patients, and, as a result, often they are neglected; yet they may have long histories of circulatory difficulties and are depressed and greatly in need of help.

Treatment may be a long slow process; this in itself can become discouraging. Usually this patient is past 50 and perhaps has other physical problems. Peripheral vascular diseases are chronic or soon become chronic. All avenues that may be sources of worry to this person should be explored and relieved inasmuch as emotional disturbances aggravate vascular disturbances.

Physical Problems

Effect of Temperature. Changes in atmospheric temperature have greater effect on a patient with a vascular disease than on the healthy person. Warmth is desirable in order to provide or maintain optimum circulation to the extremities. This should be achieved by warm clothing rather than by the use of hot water bottles, electric pads or hot baths. The effect of these physical measures may be

damaging before the individual is aware of it, because of impaired nerve function. Exposure to chilling must be avoided, for this can cause vasoconstriction and result in further restriction of the circulation to a diseased extremity. Therefore, in cold weather adequate clothing should be worn.

Cleanliness and Prevention of Infection. By practicing sound hygienic habits and keeping the body clean, many problems can be avoided. However, as one ages, skin and vascular changes indicate that changes in care are needed. Vigorous rubbing of the skin after a bath must be replaced by gentle rubbing or patting. Since dryness occurs more freqently, superfatted soaps with a mild detergent action should be used instead of harsh soaps (see p. 745). After a warm bath, softening lotions or creams should be applied gently to the skin.

Care of the Feet. The nurse and the physician are responsible for instructing the patient in this connection. It must be realized that the chief objective is to protect him from foot trauma. Each night the feet should be washed with neutral soap and warm water. They must be dried thoroughly, but not roughly. Lanolin or petrolatum can be used to prevent drying and cracking of the skin. Lamb's wool placed between the toes helps to prevent irritation. Woolen socks can be worn in winter and white cotton socks in warm weather. A clean pair should be available every day. Bed socks may be worn, but hot-water bottles or electric heating pads should not be used. The patient must be instructed not to use strong antiseptics, such as tincture of iodine, Lysol and so forth. Corns and calluses require expert care. The trimming of toenails is done best after a footbath; they should be trimmed straight across. The patient also should be instructed not to cross his knees when sitting. Any signs of blister, ingrowing toenail, infection and so forth must be reported to the physician.

Methods of Improving Circulation

If postural exercises are prescribed, the patient should elevate the extremities for a minute and then place them in a dependent position until the rubor or cyanosis becomes maximum, then lie with them in the horizontal position for a minute. These time intervals may be changed according to the disease, the condition of the patient and his ability to continue them. Again, it is important to emphasize that if the leg is to be elevated, the object (such as a bed cradle or an inverted chair) on which the part is resting must be padded to prevent injury to the limb.

Buerger-Allen Exercises. With the patient lying flat in bed, the legs are elevated above the level of the heart for 2 minutes. Then sitting on the edge of the bed with the legs dependent, he exercises the feet for 3 minutes. He then lies flat for 5 minutes. This may vary from patient to patient.

Contrast Baths. Cold water is placed in one tub and warm water in another. The temperature of the water in each tub should be prescribed by the doctor, and the tubs should be large enough to immerse both extremities at once to the middle of the leg. The feet and the legs are immersed in the water in each container alternately for 1 minute during a period of about 15 minutes. This procedure may be repeated 2 or 3 times a day. After the prescribed time of treatment, the feet are dried carefully and lubricated with a bland cream, such as lanolin.

The Sanders Oscillating Bed. A method of administering passive postural exercises to allow for the intermittent filling and emptying of capillaries, venules and arterioles is the use of the Sanders oscillating bed. The bed is set on a rocker operated by a motor so that it tilts on its long axis at regular intervals. The intervals may be adjusted according to the needs of the patient and the wishes of the physician. The patient can be taught to operate the switch; he may stop the bed for his meals or treatments. This method of administering passive postural exercises may be carried out day and night. It is claimed by some to have produced relief of the pain resulting from being in one position too long and of the pain associated with ulcers and gangrene. It may be used in the treatment of arteriosclerosis, thromboangiitis obliterans and, in minor degree, of arterial embolism.

Dressings

If it is desirable to treat an extremity with moist dressings and there are no open wounds, this can be done with surgically clean gauze and solution. However, if there is an ulcer or an open infection, strict asepsis must be followed. In this case, use sterile gloves rather than attempt to change or apply dressings with forceps. The extremity must be supported adequately when bandage dressings are removed or applied. Often the surgeon will débride necrotic tissue and irrigate the wound. Petrolatum gauze or plain dressings moistened with saline at room temperature may be applied. If only some parts of an extremity are to receive moistened dressings, the best way to prevent areas from becoming wet is to apply petrolatum. A plastic wrapping can secure the dressings in place, but it should not be held in place with a constricting bandage.

Nutritional and Drug Therapy. A diet high in protein is desirable to prevent tissue breakdown. Vitamins, particularly B and C, also are needed. Obesity should be avoided, inasmuch as excess weight increases congestion and affects proper functioning of the heart which, in turn, affects circulation. A balanced and varied diet that maintains a desirable weight for the patient, provides less fat, more protein and a good selection of fruits and vegetables is recommended. The patient with diabetes mellitus would require special dietary care. Strict asepsis would have to be observed in the administration of hypodermic medication.

Drug therapy consists mainly of vasodilators to dilate blood vessels and anticoagulants to lessen the tendency of the blood to coagulate. Vasodilators are given to combat vasospasm, relieve obstruction in an artery due to a thrombus, or to aid circulation when vessels are narrowed by disease, for example, arteriosclerosis. Anticoagulants are used in the treatment of thrombosis and prophylactically in patients that are suspected of developing thrombosis or thrombophlebitis.

Smoking

As a rule, tobacco in any form is denied these patients. Vessel spasm definitely is related to smoking. A major nursing problem is to help the physician to convince many avid smokers of the need to stop this habit. Otherwise, there is little hope for improvement of the vascular condition.

THE PATIENT WITH PERIPHERAL VASCULAR PROBLEMS

Objectives and Principles of Medical and Nursing Management

SYMPTOMS

Intermittent claudication
Differences in skin temperature, size and color of the extremity
Tingling and numbness of toes
Trophic changes

THE PROBLEM:

1. Peripheral arterial insufficiency of the extremities represents only one part of the disease that affects other parts of the body.

2. A patient's arteriosclerosis is usually advanced before his symptoms become apparent.

3. The end-result of uncontrolled circulatory impairment is gangrene.

MANAGEMENT:

I. To remove all vasoconstricting factors:
  A. Encourage the patient to abstain completely from tobacco.
  B. Instruct the patient to avoid wearing circular garters and constricting girdles or belts.
  C. Avoid experiences which are emotionally upsetting to the patient.
  D. Keep the patient as comfortable as possible with the prescribed analgesic drugs.

II. To increase peripheral blood flow to the extremities:
  A. The patient should sleep with the head of the bed elevated.
  B. Encourage the patient to take warm baths.
  C. Teach the patient that heat to the feet by means other than warm clothing is contraindicated.
  D. Give vasodilating drugs as ordered.
  E. Increase collateral circulation:
    1. Engage in passive and active exercises as indicated.
    2. Progressively increase walking time.

III. To decrease the metabolic demands of the body:
  A. Prevent injury and infection.
  B. Teach the patient hygienic care of his feet.
  C. Keep the patient on bed rest if ulceration or gangrene is present.
  D. The patient must avoid exposure to cold.
  E. He must reduce physical activity to allowed limits.

IV. To prepare for surgical procedures that will increase circulation:
  A. Sympathectomy.
  B. Bypass graft procedures.
  C. Thrombo-endarterectomy.

THE PATIENT WITH A LYMPHATIC CONDITION

Tuberculosis of Lymph Nodes

The local spread of tuberculosis almost entirely is through the lymph channels. Hence the nodes which filter the lymph flowing from the portals of entry for tubercle bacilli are the first tissues actually to become infected, and the condition which arises in them is called *tuberculous adenitis.* Lymph nodes thus diseased often swell to the size of Lima beans or larger, and, since these nodes nearly always are arranged in groups, large swellings may develop. These nodes may heal and return to their normal size, but always with a caseated area at their center which eventually becomes impregnated with lime salts. (Such calcified nodes bear witness throughout life that once they were tuberculous.) Occasionally, this tuberculous inflammation extends to tissues surrounding the infected nodes, matting them together into one caseous necrotic mass—a tuberculous abscess.

Tuberculosis can involve simultaneously practically all the lymph nodes of the body, but this condition is rare. Usually it is a regional condition, only those nodes that receive the germs through some portal of entry or that drain some tuberculous focus being infected. The groups of nodes most frequently involved in primary infections are the cervical, the mediastinal and the mesenteric glands.

Tuberculous Cervical Lymphadenitis. Formerly called *scrofula,* this is the most common form of tuberculosis of children between the ages of 3 and 7. The portal of entry of the germs usually is the tonsils. Early in the disease the individual nodes in the group may be distinguishable by palpation, but later they become matted together and often become necrotic. Such abscesses, breaking through the skin, explain the running sores in the neck which remain open for months and leave, as they heal, the ugly scars so conspicuous throughout life.

Tuberculous Mediastinal Lymphadenitis. The tracheobronchial (mediastinal) lymph nodes, draining the tracheal and bronchial mucous membranes, when tuberculous cause few or no local symptoms unless an abscess forms or unless they become sufficiently large to exert pressure. When they exert pressure on the trachea, they cause paroxysms of coughing; when on the blood vessels or nerves in the mediastinum, they cause distention of the veins of the chest wall and other symptoms.

Tuberculous Mesenteric Lymphadenitis. Tuberculosis of the lymph nodes of the mesentery and of those behind the peritoneal cavity draining the intestines is a common disease of young children infected by milk from tuberculous cows. In some patients these nodes suppurate; in others, they form large masses in the abdomen (mesenteric tabes). In all, if extensive, they produce a gradual loss of weight and strength, a distention of the abdomen and diarrhea, with passage of thin, offensive, fatty stools.

Necrosis of tuberculous mesenteric lymph nodes produces tuberculous peritonitis.

Treatment and Nursing Care

The treatment of tuberculous lymphadenitis, in whatever region it develops, employs the same general measures and embodies precisely the same principles as those prescribed in connection with pulmonary tuberculosis. Tuberculous abscesses involving the cervical nodes are incised or aspirated. Chemotherapy employing streptomycin with para-aminosalicylic acid as an adjunct has proved to be effective in many types of lymph node tuberculosis.

Lymphangitis and Lymphadenitis

Lymphangitis is an acute inflammation of the lymphatic channels. It arises most commonly from a focus of infection in an extremity. Usually it is caused by the Streptococcus. The characteristic red streaks that extend up the arm or the leg from an infected wound outline the course of the lymphatics as they drain toward nodes in the elbow or the axilla in the arm or the knee or the groin in the leg. The presence of a lymphangitis indicates that the infection has not become localized, but is extending at least to the lymph nodes, and, in some patients, it may progress and involve the blood stream (septicemia). The absorption of toxins produces high fever, often chills, in addition to the local symptoms of pain, tenderness and swelling along the lymphatics involved. The lymph nodes in the course of the lymphatic channels also become enlarged, red and tender (acute lymphadenitis), and often become necrotic and form an abscess (suppurative lymphadenitis). The nodes involved most often are those in the groin, the axilla or the cervical region. Also lymphadenitis occurs frequently without any signs of a preceding lymphangitis, due to bacteria that have lodged in the lymph nodes from lymph drained from a focus of infection. The same signs (redness and swelling) and symptoms (pain, tenderness and fever) as already mentioned for acute lymphadenitis are present. Here, again, abscess formation may take place.

Lymphangitis and acute lymphadenitis now are not of serious import, because these infections are caused nearly always by organisms (Streptococcus and Staphylococcus) that are brought under control rapidly by the sulfa drugs and the antibiotics. The part affected is treated usually by rest, elevation and the application of hot moist dressings, but the rapid response to penicillin and/or sulfadiazine usually makes this treatment unnecessary after a very short time. If necrosis has resulted in abscess formation, incision and drainage become necessary.

Acute Cervical Adenitis. This acute infection of the lymphatic glands of the neck is usually secondary to an infection in the mouth, the pharynx or the scalp.

This condition occurs very frequently in children, and the prophylactic treatment should be directed toward preventing infection in these areas or removing it should it occur. School nurses and public health nurses especially should inspect the teeth and the tonsils of children under their care and should recommend appropriate prophylactic treatment. Pediculosis of the scalp (lice) is a very common cause of infection of the posterior group of glands. These parasites should be looked for in every patient with "glands of the neck," and parasiticides should be applied in all positive or suspicious cases.

The patients develop a swelling of one side of the neck that is markedly tender and edematous. The systemic signs, which in the case of children usually are marked, are those of

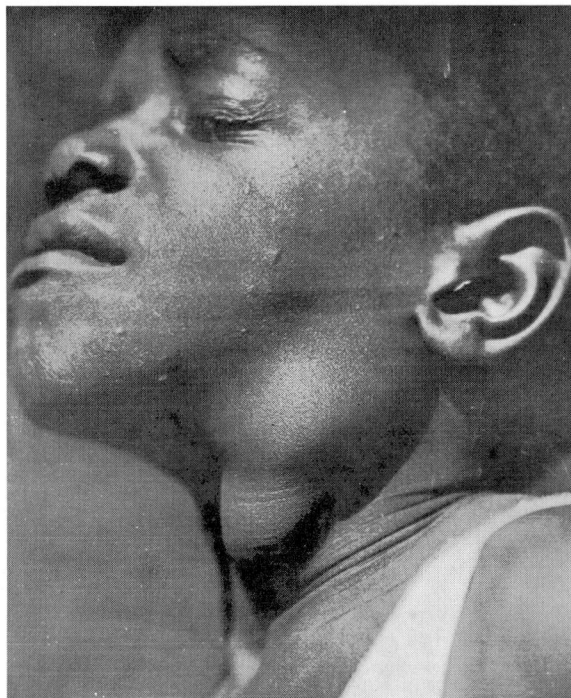

Fig. 173. Tuberculous cervical adenitis.

an acute infection. The process often goes on to abscess formation and spontaneous rupture if the swelling is not incised.

TREATMENT. The treatment in the early stages comprises attention to the focus of infection, the use of penicillin intramuscularly and the application of warm moist dressings or poultices. If an abscess forms, incision and drainage are required. Frequently the hot moist applications are continued for several days after operation.

Lymphedema—Elephantiasis

An obstruction to the lymph flow in the extremities produces a chronic swelling of the part, especially if it is in a dependent position. The obstruction may be in both the lymph nodes and the lymphatic vessels, and at times it is seen in the arm after a radical mastectomy for carcinoma, and in the leg in association with varicose veins or a chronic phlebitis (Fig. 174). In the latter case the lymph block usually is due to a chronic lymphangitis. Lymph block due to a parasite (filaria) is seen frequently in the tropics. When chronic swelling is present, there are frequent bouts of acute infection characterized by high fever and chills. These lead to a chronic fibrosis and a thickening of the subcutaneous tissues and hypertrophy of the skin. To this condition of chronic swelling of the extremity, which recedes only slightly with elevation, is given the name *elephantiasis*.

The swelling of lymphedema may be prevented by the application of elastic bandages or stockings. Often elephantiasis produces such marked disability that surgical relief is sought. The thickened fibrosed subcutaneous fat and much of the excess skin are cut away, along with the fascia overlying the muscles. Skin grafts are cut from the tissue removed and applied to the exposed muscles. By removing the subcutaneous tissue in which the fluid collects, the part is brought back to normal size and to normal function.

In the postoperative care of these patients, pressure dressings are applied to hold the skin grafts in place until they attach themselves to the underlying muscles.

Nursing Care. A block to the lymphatic flow in an extremity means that the part involved may be traumatized easily. Before operation, the arm or the leg is supported on a pillow and bandaged. Some surgeons order diuretics to help in reducing edema. Sulfa drugs and penicillin may be given prophylactically. The part is washed carefully with soap and water before surgery. In the postoperative care of these patients, transfusions usually are necessary to prevent the shock that may arise from the long operative procedure and rather profuse blood loss. The extremity is elevated for at least 2 weeks and then is lowered gradually. If it is a leg, weight is borne only with support. Precautions to avoid injury must be observed carefully.

CLINICAL SITUATION

Five days after a hysterectomy, Mrs. J. developed thrombophlebitis of the right leg.

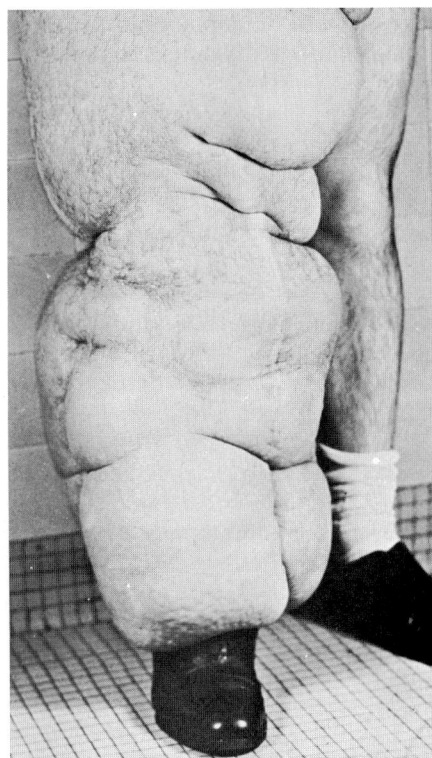

FIG. 174. An example of marked elephantiasis of the right leg. The scar denotes site of a previous attempt at operative reduction of the elephantiasis.

1. Which action on the part of the nurse reveals the greatest understanding?

A. Place heat over the affected leg immediately.

B. Keep the patient at rest and call the doctor.

C. Elevate the leg and apply a pressure bandage.

D. Elevate the leg and prepare an anticoagulant.

2. Of the following signs, which is characteristic of thrombophlebitis?

A. The veins fill from above to below, rather than from below to above.

B. The foot is blanched when it is lowered and there is delayed filling when the leg is raised.

C. There is pain in the calf of the leg when the foot is dorsiflexed.

D. There is pain in the calf muscles when exercised that is relieved with rest.

3. Which of the following symptoms should the nurse be particularly alert for in a patient with thrombophlebitis?

A. Respiratory difficulty, hemoptysis and sudden chest pain.

B. Swelling of the dorsum of the foot and back pain.

C. Redness, swelling, and pain of the affected leg.

D. Intermittent claudication relieved with rest.

4. Mrs. J. has been employed as a clerk typist. Which suggestion about her work habits should a nurse offer to help to prevent the recurrence of this condition?

A. Put her feet on a foot stool while working at her desk.

B. Exercise her legs at regular intervals by crossing and uncrossing them.

C. Drink only decaffeinated coffee at coffee break and lunch.

D. Walk around the office at periodic intervals.

BIBLIOGRAPHY AND SUGGESTED READING

Articles

Agrifoglio, G., and Edwards, E. A.: Surgical treatment of varicose veins, J.A.M.A. **178:** 906-911, 1961.

Anlyan, W. G. *et al.:* Fibrinolytic agents in surgical practice, J.A.M.A. **175:**290-292, 1961.

Breault, M.: Phlebitis, Canad. Nurse **57:**640-643, 1961.

Buetow, I. A.: Nursing care in lymphedema, Am. J. Nurs. **56:**1550-1552, 1956.

Harpuder, K.: Rehabilitation of patients with arterial disease of limbs, Geriatrics **10:**451-455, 1955.

Kritchevsky, D.: Cholesterol and atherosclerosis, Am. J. Clin. Nutr. **10:**269-276, 1962.

Latham, H. C.: Thrombophlebitis, Am. J. Nurs. **63:**122-126, Sept., 1963.

Marple, C. D., and McIntyre, M. J.: Anticoagulant therapy—medical aspects and nursing care, Am. J. Nurs. **56:**875-879, July, 1956.

Myers, T. T.: Results and technic of stripping operations for varicose veins, J.A.M.A. **163:** 12, 1957.

Pratt, G. H.: Lymphedema, Am. J. Nurs. **56:** 1548-1549, 1956.

Quint, J. C.: Nursing the patient with endarterectomy, Am. J. Nurs. **58:** 996-998, 1958.

Schweisheimer, E.: Raynaud's syndrome, Canad. Nurse **51:**774-775, 1955.

Sensenig, D. M., and Morson, B. J.: Buerger's disease, Am. J. Nurs. **57:**337-340, 1957.

Patient-Teaching Aids and Information

Varicose Veins. An 11-page informative pamphlet, New York, American Heart Association, 1961.

Varicose Veins. Publication No. 154, Washington, D. C., U. S. Dept. Health, Education and Welfare, 1959.

27

Patients With Conditions of the Heart

THE NURSE AND HER CARDIAC PATIENT

Cardiovascular disease, heart disease in particular, is the number one health problem of our society, ranking first as a cause of death in the United States. Concerning this group of diseases fear and misunderstanding are rife, much of which can be alleviated, or clarified, by well-informed nurses.

Safe and effective nursing care in cardiac conditions requires a thorough appreciation of the pathologic and physiologic processes that are involved. And, if the nurse is to contribute materially toward the recovery of her cardiac patients, she must understand clearly the rationale of the treatment that is prescribed for them.

The major concern of the patient with heart disease is his symptoms. Whereas these vary to a considerable extent from patient to patient, most of them, if cardiovascular in origin, are likely to be included in this brief list: fatigue, chest pain, dyspnea, orthopnea, cough, palpitation, edema and cyanosis. Symptomatic relief is largely a nursing problem; it is the initial objective of nursing. But objectives change as the patient's problems and needs change. With the passage of time therapeutic priorities must be revised in accordance with these needs. Facets of nursing care to be considered, apart from observation, identification, interpretation and relief of symptoms, include the teaching of methods for the prevention of symptomatic recurrences, and the instruction of patients regarding health measures that are designed to retard the progression of heart disease. One important nursing goal is to equip the patient with knowledge and inspiration to participate effectively in his own plan of care.

To provide the nurse with a sound factual basis for her concepts regarding various cardiac conditions she is likely to encounter, and to acquaint her with some of the many specific nursing problems that will confront her in connection with heart-disease patients, this chapter has been designed.

ANATOMIC FEATURES OF THE HEART AND NORMAL CARDIAC FUNCTION

The heart is a hollow muscular pump which forces the blood on by contractions, called *beats* or, better, *systoles*. The only visible evidence of these is a slight outward thrust of the apex of the left ventricle, called the *apex beat*, usually seen at a point just below the medial to the left nipple in the 4th or 5th costal interspace (Fig. 175). Each systole is followed by a period of rest, called its *diastole*, during which the heart wall is relaxed. So that the blood may always be pumped in the right direction, the heart is provided with valves. Thus, when the right ventricle contracts, it forces the blood through the pulmonic orifice into the pulmonary artery, since the tricuspid valve prevents its regurgitation into the right atrium, whence it came. The heart contraction over, the blood in the pulmonary artery cannot flow back into the right ventricle, now in diastole, since the pulmonic valve closes to prevent this. In a similar manner, on the left side of the heart, the mitral valve prevents any backflow from the left ventricle into the atrium, and the aortic valve its return into the left ventricle. These valves are membranes of wonderful strength, yet almost as thin as heavy paper. The edges of the mitral and tricuspid valves are anchored by fine but very strong threads called *chordae tendineae*.

The ability and the tendency to contract are inherent in all parts of the heart wall (myocardium). Cut the ventricle entirely free from the rest of the heart and under proper conditions it will contract regularly, about 28 times per minute. The walls of the atria also can beat independently and do so at a faster rate than the walls of the ventricles.

The Pacemaker and Conduction System

The heart has a pacemaker, the sino-atrial node, located in the right atrial wall near the opening of the superior vena cava, where, normally, all its beats start. It is through this node that certain nervous centers in the brain control the rate of the heartbeat. Through sympathetic nerve fibers they hasten it, and through fibers in the vagus nerve they slow it. It is the balance of these two nerve systems controlling the sino-atrial node that determines the rate of the heartbeat.

Normally every muscular contraction of the heart, therefore every heartbeat and pulse wave, occurs specifically in response to a single electrical impulse that has been generated by, and originated in, this node, serving as the *pacemaker*. Each of these impulses travels simultaneously through the atrial walls, exciting their immediate contraction, and through a special bundle of nerve fibers ("bundle of His") to the atrioventricular (A.V.) node. Here transmission is delayed for about one-tenth of a second and its pathway divides, two separate nerve

bundles and their communicating fibers conducting the impulse from the A.V. node to the right and the left ventricles, respectively, distributing it throughout their walls and stimulating them to contract.

Thus, entailed in each heartbeat is an orderly, precisely timed sequence of events, as follows: an electrical discharge emanates from the sino-atrial (S.A.) node, in immediate response to which the two atria contract and empty their contents into the corresponding ventricles, which at that instant are in open communication and a state of relaxation. After an interval of .07 to .10 seconds, the two ventricles contract simultaneously: the right ejects its contents (systemic venous blood from the superior and inferior vena cavae, via the right atrium) into the pulmonary arterial circuit; and the left ejects oxygenated blood from the pulmonary circuit (delivered from the pulmonary veins by the left atrium) into the aorta and the systemic circulation.

TESTS OF CARDIAC FUNCTION AND DIAGNOSTIC AIDS IN CARDIAC DISEASE

In order to determine accurately the nature and the exact location of cardiovascular defects, many studies are done. To begin with, a complete history of the patient is taken from his birth to the present. The physical examination includes fluoroscopy and x-ray study of the chest to determine heart size and chamber enlargement. Tests for the evaluation of cardiac function include measurements of the systemic venous pressure, pulmonary circulation time and vital capacity; electrocardiography; roentgenographic examination of the chest; and cardiac catheterization (see Chap. 6, p. 95).

CARDIAC ARRHYTHMIAS

The rate and the rhythm of the heartbeat depend on the speed and the regularity with which electrical impulses are generated by the pacemaker—normally the S.A. node—and on the functional integrity of the conduction system that distributes these impulses through the myocardium. The activity of this node, as previously pointed out, is subject to the influence of the autonomic nervous system. Moreover, it responds to

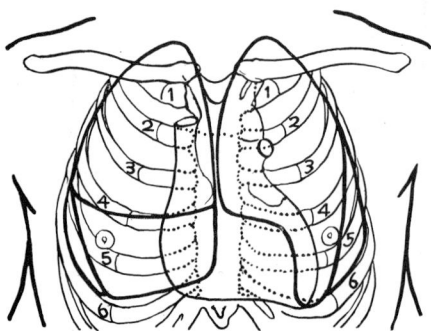

FIG. 175. Outline of the heart relative to the ribs and the lung margins.

chemical changes in the blood and is highly susceptible to the action of several drugs. Its normal activity may be altered, and its conduction pathways interrupted, as a result of local disease. And its function as a pacemaker can be usurped by the A.V. node or by some other "hyperirritable" focus elsewhere in the conduction system. Moreover, heart muscle has the ability to contract on its own, without benefit of nervous control; this property becomes important in patients with complete heart-block, whose ventricles beat at a slow, unvarying pace, approximately 28 beats per minute, or the so-called "idio-ventricular rate." Factors such as these, affecting the production or the distribution of pacemaking impulses, may speed or slow the heart rate, producing tachycardia or bradycardia, respectively, or disrupt its rhythm, i.e., cause an arrhythmia. (The term *arrhythmia,* as it commonly is applied, refers to abnormalities of heart rate, as well as to irregularities of rhythm.)

The existence of an arrhythmia may or may not be responsible for symptoms; it may or may not represent a manifestation of serious underlying heart disease; and it may or may not jeopardize, per se, the health and the safety of the patient. How various arrhythmias differ with respect to clinical features, complications and clinical significance will become evident from a perusal of the following sections, in which certain of the more common and important types are described.

Ectopic Beats

The most common cardiac irregularity is that caused by ectopic beats (called also *premature beats* or *extrasystoles*). While the heart is contracting regularly, and all of its beats are originating in the sino-atrial node, some overirritable portion of the wall of the atrium or the ventricle suddenly starts an abnormal contraction called an *extrasystole.* Each extrasystole follows very soon, but not immediately, after one of the regular beats. It cannot follow immediately. No stimulus can arouse the ventricle then, for each contraction uses up all the available energy of the myocardium. This brief period is called the *refractory phase* of the beat. The extrasystole and the beat which it follows occur so close together that the patient usually feels them as one, but with the stethoscope, both can be heard. Because of the refractory phase following the extrasystole, the heart cannot respond to the next regular stimulus from the node, and, therefore, it rests quietly until the regular stimulus, next in order to the unanswered one, produces its beat. The patient is conscious that his heart missed a beat, but usually he complains, not of the unusually long pause, but of the beat following it. This, since the ventricle has become overdistended with blood during the interval, is a very strong one. He says that the heart "jumped," "turned over," "jarred the whole body."

Premature beats often occur in cases of heart disease, but the patient usually is unconscious of such premature beats. The extrasystoles that patients complain of are those of hearts organically normal and usually mean merely that the patient is nervous, smokes too much, eats too fast, etc.

Paroxysmal Atrial Tachycardia

In the condition called *paroxysmal tachycardia,* the heart suddenly doubles or trebles the number of its systoles per minute, continues at this rate for a while and then, just as suddenly, resumes its normal speed. Such attacks of regular, rapid heart action, during which the heart is not under the control of the sino-atrial node, may last for minutes, hours or even days in otherwise healthy persons. Similar attacks of tachycardia occur in patients with valvular heart disease, and these are often of more serious consequence. How much patients suffer from such attacks depends on the personality of the individual. All patients feel exhausted and have shortness of breath while the attacks last, often a sense of fluttering under the sternum and possibly a peculiar feeling of apprehension; but the majority suffer no serious distress. A few, however, have pronounced cardiac palpitation and even severe anginal pains. As far as can be determined, these painful attacks are in no way different from those of patients who disregard them.

The cause of paroxysmal tachycardia is not known, but the chances are that some spot in the wall of the atrium, less often in that of the ventricle, is hyperirritable from birth and occasionally usurps for a while the function of the sino-atrial node as the heart's pacemaker. This condition really has little or no serious importance.

Treatment. Sometimes the patient can abort an attack of paroxysmal tachycardia by attempting to swallow a large piece of dry bread crust, or by pressing his finger against his eyeballs or over the carotid sinus (located just below the angle of the jaw). These maneuvers may not succeed, in which case ipecac sirup should be taken in amounts of 1 or 2 drams (4 or 8 ml.), or Pronestyl Hydrochloride (procaine amide), in doses of 0.25 or 0.50 Gm.

Atrial Fibrillation

Atrial fibrillation, indicated by a pulse that is irregular in force and rhythm, develops in the following conditions: in about one half of all patients with severe cardiac disease, in hyperthyroidism, in acute fevers, sometimes in digitalis intoxication and in patients with arteriosclerotic and hypertensive heart disease. The condition may be continuous or it may occur for limited periods of time only (paroxysmal fibrillation).

The presence of atrial fibrillation means that the sino-atrial node has entirely lost control of the heart rhythm and that several parts of the atrial wall are being stimulated to contract simultaneously and with great rapidity, with the result that the atrium merely quivers, that is, fibrillates. An atrium beating in this manner sends a confused medley of stimuli to the ventricle, which responds as strongly and to as many impulses as possible.

In atrial fibrillation, all grades of irregularity in force and rhythm are seen. Some are so severe that the condition is called *delirium cordis;* others are so mild that the condition can be detected only on electrocardiograms. Physical activity always increases the irregularity of a fibrillating heart. This is an important point in diagnosis, since it excludes the somewhat similar irregularity due to the presence of numerous extrasystoles, for these are usually abolished by exercise.

The ventricle, which may receive as many as 500 stimuli per minute, races at excessive speed—so rapidly that it does not have time to fill adequately between successive beats. This inadequacy leads to a reduction in cardiac output. The heart rate at the apex may range from 180 to 220 beats per minute, but because of gross variations in stroke volume, there usually is a pulse deficit.

Treatment. The object of treatment is to protect the ventricles and improve their efficiency by reducing the rate of their contractions. This is accomplished by digitalis, a drug that stimulates the vagus nerve and retards the rate of atrioventricular conduction, thus blocking most of the stimuli originating in the quivering atria. An attempt may be made to restore the cardiac rhythm to normal by the administration of Pronestyl Hydrochloride (procaine amide) or quinidine, which reduce the electrical excitability of the myocardium, prolong the refractory period that follows each stimulus, and slow electrical conduction, thereby limiting the spread of these stimuli. It is important to bear in mind that the fibrillating atrium is a favored site for the formation and lodgement of a thrombus; and should it harbor such a thrombus, restoration of its rhythm to normal may cause the clot to be dislodged and then propelled into the pulmonary or systemic circulation with consequences, such as pulmonary or cerebral infarction, that potentially are fatal.

Atrial Flutter

This disturbance of heart action is characterized by a tachycardia of the atrium, this

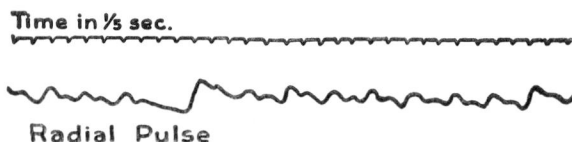

FIG. 176. Atrial flutter.

chamber beating perhaps from 300 to 400 times a minute, while the ventricle, protected by a greater or lesser degree of heart-block, responds regularly to each second or third atrial contraction. The result is a regular pulse rate, seldom over 150 per minute and usually nearer 100, which changes suddenly, often doubling or halving its rate (Fig. 176). Fainting spells are common. This condition may resemble fibrillation, which possibly is due to a similar mechanism, since they often alternate. It is seen commonly in elderly persons, in whom it may persist for months or years with few or no symptoms other than palpitation.

Treatment. The best treatment of flutter is digitalis in sufficiently large doses to cause a higher degree of heart-block. Fibrillation then may ensue, and restoration of normal rhythm may be induced with quinidine.

Heart-Block

Heart-block results from disturbances of the atrioventricular bundle which keep some (partial block) or all (complete block) of the stimuli from the atria from reaching the ventricles. In cases of partial block, if each second stimulus is blocked, the pulse is regular but slow; if each third or each fourth stimulus fails to pass, a bigeminal or trigeminal pulse is observed. However, as a rule, the result of partial heart-block is an irregular pulse. The diagnosis is made best from electrocardiograph records, which show that some atrial beats meet with no response from the ventricles.

Complete heart-block implies complete independence of the atrial and ventricular contractions, the bundle of His having become impassable for stimuli. The block may be temporary or permanent; if permanent, the ventricles may initiate and control their own contractions for many years, beating at a regular pace but slowly, about 28 beats per minute, which is characteristic of the idioventricular rhythm. However, such stability is the exception rather than the rule for the majority of patients with lesions involving the bundle exhibit a variety of ventricular arrhythmias and tend to shift from one to another. Associated with each shift may be a temporary cessation of cardiac output, followed at once by a precipitous fall

of the arterial pressure to 0. With halting of the cerebral blood flow, his brain rapidly becoming hypoxic, the patient loses consciousness and may exhibit a convulsive seizure. Barring prompt resumption of effective ventricular contractions, death is inevitable. Such an episode is termed a "Stokes-Adams attack" and its recurrence is the hallmark of "Stokes-Adams disease" (or syndrome). (See below.)

Transient complete heart-block may be induced with large doses of digitalis and its analogues, quinidine and certain poisons. In patients with "carotid sinus sensitivity" it may be produced by overstimulation of the vagus. Moreover, it may develop in the course of acute rheumatic fever or diphtheria. Complete block, which may be permanent, can result from damage to the bundle of His by an impinging, invasive or ulcerative lesion in the septum, such as a gumma or a tumor. However, it most often follows an occlusion of the posterior coronary artery, which provides this bundle with its principle blood supply.

Treatment. The treatment of heart-block is to remove the cause, if possible—drug toxicity, diphtheria, etc. If the block is complete and permanent, and the idioventricular rhythm is firmly established, no symptoms are produced and no treatment is indicated. However, when the block is attended by episodic arrhythmias and Stokes-Adams attacks, treatment decidedly is indicated and is available. Therapy may involve the administration of drugs, the application of an external pacemaker, the installing of an electrical pacemaker within the lumen of the right ventricle or the implantation of a cardiac pacer directly on the wall of the left ventricle. The medical, surgical and nursing implications of Stokes-Adams disease (syndrome) will now be considered in detail.

Stokes-Adams Disease

As a result of arteriosclerotic coronary artery disease or after myocardial infarction, tissue necrosis may occur, and scars form, in a location that coincides with the pathways of the electrical impulses from the S.A. node, interrupting their conduction and producing an atrioventricular block. The conduction defect produces unpredictable disturbances of ventricular rhythm that are manifested by either a slow idioventricular rhythm, ventricular standstill, ventricular tachycardia, or ventricular fibrillation. The block may be transient or permanent, partial or complete. The resultant reduction in cardiac output produces cerebral ischemia and presents as dizziness, syncope, convulsions, or death. This is Stokes-Adams disease, and the attacks are referred to as Stokes-Adams attacks. Once the conduction defect has taken place these patients must be treated vigorously by drugs to increase the ventricular rate. Such drugs as Isuprel, which is sympathomimetic, and atropine, which is parasympatholytic, are very helpful in increasing the rate for adequate cardiac output. However, even with vigorous medical management life expectancy is probably less than 2 years.

Because the life-endangering defect is the disturbance in ventricular rhythm, some other source of stimuli must be used to sustain an adequate ventricular rate. This has become possible through direct electrical stimulation of the myocardium, utilizing an external source of electricity and transmitting the impulses through skin electrodes, intracardiac electrodes, or electrodes implanted directly on the ventricular muscle. Stokes-Adams disease is the major indication for external pacing of the heart. Another is

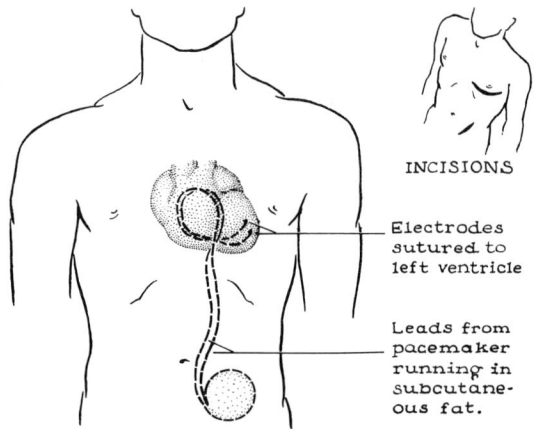

FIG. 178. Permanent pacemaker placed subcutaneously through incisions shown in insert.

a somewhat similar conduction defect that sometimes occurs as a complication of open-heart surgery of the interventricular septum; depending on whether the conduction tissue is destroyed, or merely damaged, the heart will require permanent or temporary external pacing.

External Cardiac Pacing

Patients with Stokes-Adams attacks are admitted to the hospital immediately and placed on a medical program. Electrodes are attached to the chest wall overlying the heart and connected to a monitoring system. The monitoring system contains an oscilloscope, an external pacemaker, and a defibrillator. The oscilloscope allows constant observation of the electrocardiograph pattern, the pacemaker starts automatically when the impulses from the heart cease, and the defibrillator is used to stop ventricular fibrillation. If the response to the medical program is unsatisfactory the external pacemaker will run almost constantly. Since a high voltage is necessary to pace the heart through the chest wall, it is very painful and distressing, and a low voltage system must be substituted of which the patient is not conscious.

The Intraventricular Pacemaker

The patient is taken to fluoroscopy with the monitoring system, and a cardiac electrode is passed into the right ventricle of the

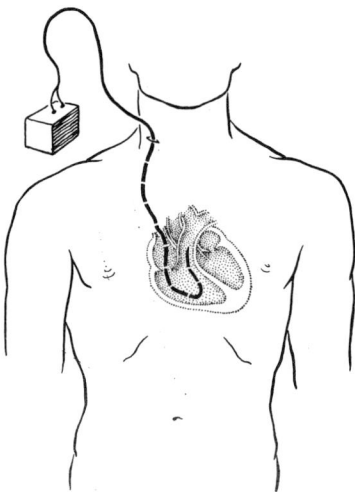

FIG. 177. Temporary pacemaker inserted into the heart through the jugular vein.

heart via the anterior jugular vein in the right side of the neck or via the median antecubital vein at the volar surface of the right elbow (Fig. 177). This electrode is similar to a cardiac catheter but has 2 electrodes within and 2 connections remaining on the outside. The 2 connections are attached to a low voltage (10 to 12 v.), external transistorized battery. This battery produces a current of about 2 milliamperes and is capable of pacing the heart without sensation to the patient. Since the impulse is transmitted to the heart through the column of blood, an attempt is made to place the tip near the pulmonary artery, where the column is narrowest.

Although this electrode may be used for extended periods of time, even up to several years, the disadvantages are that the patient must be kept on anticoagulants, sepsis may occur where the electrode enters the skin, and it is cumbersome for the patient to manage. However, it allows adequate time for studying the patient, for the heart to recover from its insult, and for obtaining an implantable pacemaker from the factory.

Ideally, the implantable pacemaker should emit its impulses in response to the S.A. node and thus be under control of the autonomic nervous system. Such a unit will soon be available and will require implanting 2 electrodes on the atrium and 2 on the ventricle. However, we are at present using a pacemaker that has a preset rate of choice and that requires implanting only the 2 electrodes on the ventricle. The electrodes are made of platinum and are designed to resist corrosion as well as breakage due to torsion. The battery is composed of transistors and has a life of 5 years.

Surgical Implantation of the Myocardial Pacer

Preoperative Preparation of the Patient. The discussion thus far has dealt with the stabilization of the patient in preparation for surgical implantation of a pacemaker. Substantially, this represents the preoperative preparation of the patient. After the introduction of the intracardiac electrode, the heart rate can be varied by turning a control on the low voltage pacemaker. In this way studies can reveal the heart rate that will produce maximum cardiac output and this is the rate then chosen for the ordered pacemaker.

Though the heart is under control of the intracardiac electrode, it is still wise to suppress vagal tone. Therefore, atropine, gr. 1/50 (1.2 mg.), should be used along with an adequate dose of morphine or Demerol Hydrochloride as preoperative medication.

Operative Procedure. Figure 178 provides a schematic representation of the scope of the procedure. An oblique left abdominal incision below the belt line provides a pocket in the subcutaneous tissues for the pacemaker. A tunnel made with a sterile sigmoidoscope allows the electrodes to be passed from the abdominal incision subcutaneously to the thoracic incision. Finally, an incision in the left 5th interspace allows adequate exposure of the heart and a point of entrance for the electrodes to be implanted on the left ventricle.

With the patient supine, the left 5th interspace is entered from the sternum to the posterior axillary line. The intercostal space is opened with a Burford retractor for adequate exposure. With the lung packed off posteriorly, the phrenic nerve is identified on the pericardium, which is opened anterior to the nerve. The pericardium is held open with stay sutures and the coronary vessels identified on the left ventricle. At this point, the abdominal pocket is made and the pacemaker inserted. The electrodes are passed through the sigmoidoscope (that was used to make a tunnel from the abdominal to the thoracic incision) and then into the pericardium in readiness for implantation. A bare area on the left ventricle, devoid of coronary vessels, is chosen for the site of implantation. The electrode plates are placed side by side about 1 to 2 cm. apart. The tip of the electrode projects from the plate and is inserted into a hole in the epicardium made by a sharp-pointed knife. There are 4 perforations on the electrode plates that are used to suture them into position. After the second electrode is secured, the pacemaker functions immediately, so the external unit must be disconnected simultaneously. The sutured electrodes then are secured additionally by a patch of Ivalon sponge, which fills the space between the electrodes and the pericardium. The pericardium then is closed loosely to allow for drainage, and a small

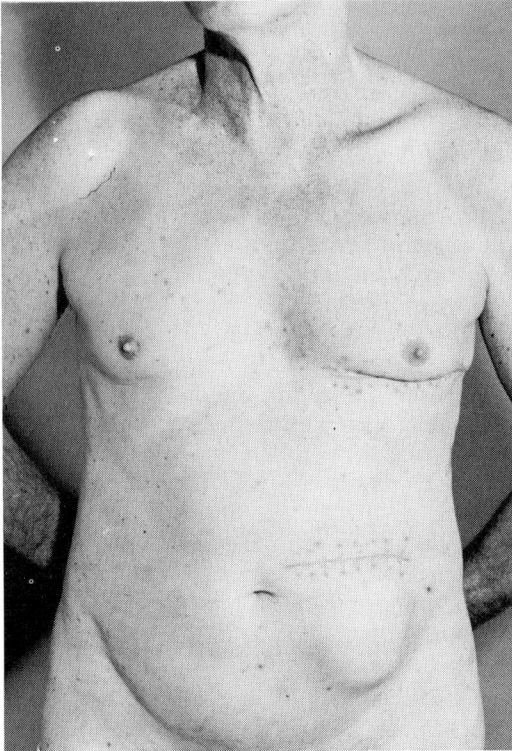

FIG. 179. Photograph of patient with implanted pacemaker. (Chardack, W. M., et al.: Treatment of complete heart block with an implantable and self-contained pacemaker, Fig. 8, Bull. Soc. int. chir. **4**:420)

amount of redundancy is provided for the electrodes to avoid tension. Finally, the thoracic and abdominal incisions are closed without drainage to avoid any possible contamination.

Postoperative Care. In the majority of patients the heart will respond only to the impulses of the pacemaker and therefore at the built-in rate. This rate does not vary with exercise or excitement and will remain the same except that body heat will increase it several beats during the first few days. However, sometimes the heart still produces beats of its own and this results in extrasystoles. If the latter are excessive it may be necessary to suppress the intrinsic beats with appropriate drugs, such as procaine amide and quinidine. Eventually, the implanted pacemaker takes over completely, and the medications may be stopped.

These patients are permitted liquids by mouth the night of surgery; are permitted out of bed on the first day postoperatively; and the average postoperative hospitalization is from 8 to 10 days. Daily electrocardiograms are taken to evaluate the health of the myocardium, and interval chest roentgenograms are filmed to assure that full expansion of the left lung has taken place and to check for possible pleural effusion.

Specialized Nursing Care

The cardiac arrest that ocurs in Stokes-Adams attacks can be reversed quickly by pounding on the sternum or by external cardiac massage (see page 515). Here, perhaps more than in any other field, nursing care makes the difference between life and death. Therefore, nurses must learn to administer external cardiac massage to sustain the patient until the external pacemaker can be applied.

After installation of the intracardiac electrode the patient's pulse must be watched very carefully until the optimum voltage and rate is determined. Because the impulse is transmitted through a column of blood rather than directly to the myocardium, the heart does not respond to every impulse until the voltage and the rate controls are optimally fixed.

Before the open operation these patients need tremendous reassurance. They realize that their hearts are diseased and therefore are frightened by the thought of a heart operation. However, this fear is managed best by acquainting them with the fact that the risk of surgery is less than the risk of their disease.

After installation of the pacemaker they are relatively out of danger, but close attention again must be given to vital signs. As mentioned before, we must look for extrasystoles resulting from intrinsic beats and control them early, for they may result in ventricular fibrillation.

Complications

The major complication following pacemaker implantation is, of course, a faulty unit that ceases to function. Under these circumstances the patient is treated as in a Stokes-Adams attack with external massage, external pacemaker, and a medical program until

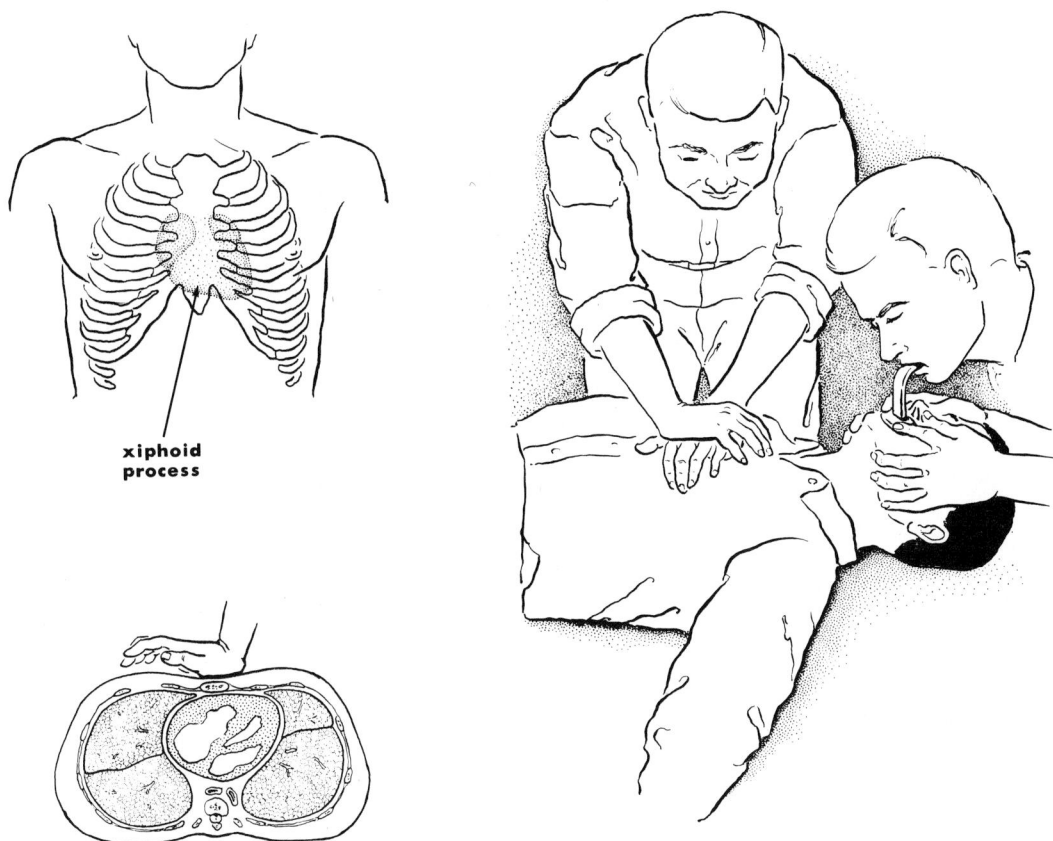

xiphoid
process

FIG. 180. Closed-chest cardiac massage.

the defect is corrected or a new pacemaker can be implanted.

Cardiac Arrest and Resuscitation

Cardiac arrest is defined as the sudden, unexpected cessation of the heartbeat. All heart action may stop, or asynchronized muscular twitchings (ventricular fibrillation) may occur. The incidence of cardiac arrest in the operating room varies, but is thought to approximate 1 in 1,200 operations. The factors that play a major role in the etiology of arrest are the following: anoxia caused by airway obstruction; inadequate ventilation; anesthetic depression; hypotension; retention of CO_2 (hypercapnia); coronary occlusion and myocardial infarction; and neurogenic reflexes. Outside of the operating room, cardiac arrest may result from drowning, electric shock, carbon monoxide and other types of poisoning, drug reactions, and suffocation.

There is a 4-minute interval between the cessation of circulation and the appearance of irreversible brain damage. During this period, the diagnosis of arrest must be made and the circulation must be restored. *The most reliable sign of arrest is the absence of a carotid pulsation.* Valuable time should not be wasted taking the blood pressure, or listening for the heartbeat. Restoration of circulation can be accomplished by either closed-chest massage, or open-chest massage. Whichever method is used, the lungs must be ventilated by mouth-to-mouth breathing, or by insufflation of oxygen through a pharyngeal or an endotracheal tube.

Closed-Chest Massage

Closed-chest cardiac massage can be applied under almost any conditions, if necessary, in or out of the hospital. Instructions for its performance are the following:

1. Place the patient supine on a firm surface.

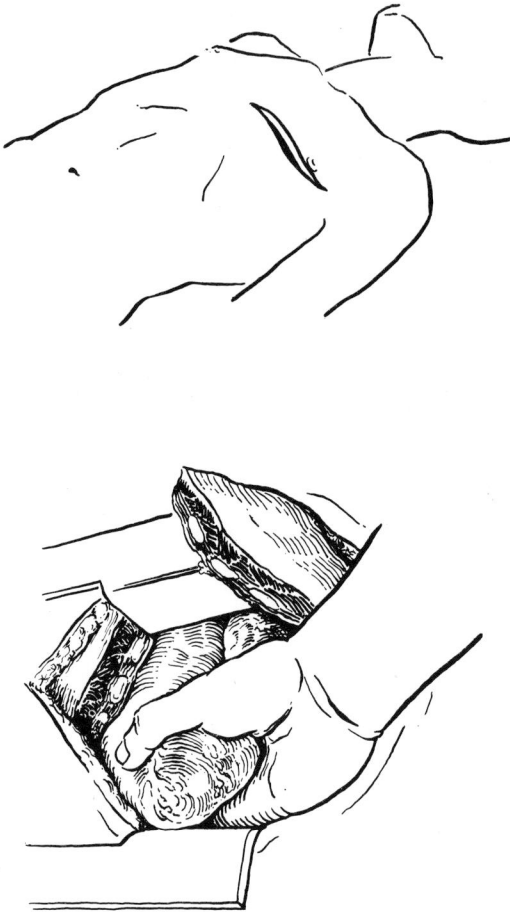

Fig. 181. Open-chest cardiac massage after incision in 4th intercostal space as shown.

2. Kneel or stand at right angles to the patient's trunk.

3. Have an assistant start rescue breathing (Fig. 180, right). If no second person is available, stop cardiac massage every 30 seconds for 10 seconds, so that you may ventilate the patient's lungs with 3 or 4 deep breaths.

4. Locate the xiphoid process (Fig. 180, top left), and over it place the heel of one hand (Fig. 180, bottom left). Place the heel of the other hand directly over the heel of the lower hand (Fig. 180, right).

5. Apply firm pressure directly downward, displacing the sternum backward toward the vertebral column. (Make sure that the fingers are not constricting any portion of the chest,

and that only the heel of the hand is used.) Exert sufficient pressure to enable another observer to palpate a pulse in the carotid artery. Relax and reapply pressure.

6. Exert downward pressure at a rate of about 50 to 60 times a minute and in rhythmic fashion. Sternal compressions and pulmonary ventilations should be coordinated, the ratio between these rates being approximately 4 to 1.

7. Continue ventilation and massage until the heart beat is restored and peripheral pulsations are detected, or until other therapy can be instituted.

NOTE: During this procedure an electrocardiogram to record the electrical activity of the heart should be obtained. If ventricular fibrillation is detected, defibrillation may be accomplished by means of an electric current (440 volts for 0.25 seconds) delivered through 2 electrodes placed on the chest wall.

Open-Chest Massage

The left chest is entered through the 4th interspace anteriorly (Fig. 181). The ribs are separated, and the heart is grasped in the palm of the hand. Cardiac pumping, avoiding finger pressure, is carried out rapidly (80 to 100 times per minute). If the heart is fibrillating, defibrillation is performed by placing the electrodes directly on the heart.

Use of Drugs

The administration of drugs serves as a useful adjunct to both external and open cardiac resuscitation. An advantage of the open method is the fact that the heart can be visualized and the effect of the drug observed. Epinephrine (0.1 to 0.2 ml. of 1:1,000 solution) is injected into the ventricle, when the heart is "flabby" and has exhibited no response to massage after 5 minutes. If the heart is responding somewhat, 0.2 mg. of isoproterenol hydrochloride is injected into the ventricle. If there is no response, 20 ml. of molar lactate can be given into the ventricle, or 10 ml. of a 10 per cent solution of calcium gluconate can be given intravenously.

Intravenous Fluid Therapy

Concurrent with pulmonary oxygen exchange and cardiac massage, the intravenous administration of fluid and blood is important.

Postresuscitation Measures

After cardiac resuscitation, close observation of the vital signs is important because of the high incidence of recurrent arrest. A wire electrode connected to a pacemaker may be inserted into the heart muscle to provide an electrical stimulus to cause cardiac contraction in the event that a rearrest occurs. Adequate pulmonary ventilation must be maintained. Oxygen therapy is administered. Tracheal aspiartion may be helpful. When bronchial secretions cannot be cleared by coughing or aspiration, a tracheotomy is performed.

The patient's temperature is taken hourly; a rapid rise usually indicates cerebral damage. The usual cooling measures are employed if necessary, e.g., alcohol sponges. Whole blood is preferred to replace blood volume. Complications that may occur are acute cerebral edema, pneumothorax and wound infection.

Nursing of Patients with Cardiac Arrhythmias

Not infrequently the nurse is the first to recognize the existence of an arrhythmia, based on her examination of a patient's pulse. Examination of a pulse never should become "routine." The nurse invariably should seek to correlate its rate, rhythm and character with other facets of her patient's condition. In so doing, she cannot fail to improve her acuity as a clinical observer and, thus, she will add continuously and materially to her accumulating stores of knowledge.

Nurses should be diarists, recording everything of significance that they observe. Of all members of the health team they are the ones who spend the most time with the patient and, as a result, are in the best position to acquire significant data. For example, their recorded description of a patient's appearance and behavior during an episode of arrhythmia very often proves invaluable and, in many instances, this information otherwise is unobtainable.

The pulse should be counted carefully for at least 1 full minute. Variations in force and frequency, as well as general character-istics and overall rate, should be noted. If an abnormality is detected, it should be reported without delay. The carotid pulse should be counted in addition to the radial pulse, and, if an arrhythmia is suspected, the apical pulse rate should be measured by auscultation as well. It must be borne in mind that abnormal beats may not be detectable at the wrist, since a very weak pulse wave often fails to reach the periphery and, in this event, the apical and radial rates will not correspond. Both must be counted simultaneously but independently by 2 observers for no less than 1 minute, in order to determine the degree to which they differ quantitatively, i.e., the pulse deficit. The greater the deficit, the less efficient the ventricular contractions are assumed to be, and the less favorable the clinical evaluation of cardiac function.

The electrocardiogram is of great value in establishing the type of rhythmic disturbance that is present. This recording is most informative during the course of an arrhythmic episode. Arrhythmias are prone to be transient and elusive. Should the nurse discover evidence of such a disorder in a patient previously free of cardiac arrhythmia, or in whom a diagnosis of arrhythmia has not been established with certainty, she is quite entitled—indeed, she is obligated—to request an electrocardiogram, assuming that agency regulations permit. The nurse explains to the patient the basic principles of the electrocardiogram and its application in his particular case.

If the patient's arrhythmia is of a transient variety, as is likely to be the case, he should remain in bed most of the time until the episode is terminated. Obviously, it is unnecessary to alert the patient to all facts and facets of his cardiac disturbance, to which he otherwise might remain oblivious. However, most patients with an arrhythmia complain of palpitation, shortness of breath, dizziness and precordial pain, and they are prone to be anxious. Anxiety tends to beget more symptoms, which promote increased anxiety with further aggravation of symptoms, etc., etc., until fear and anxiety far outweigh the actual gravity of the organic disorder. From the standpoint of this patient's cardiac status, as well as his comfort, it is important that this vicious cycle be broken. Broken it can be, and readily, by a display on the part of the nurse of an attitude that at once expresses confidence and composure, that evinces understanding and implies capability; an attitude that is founded securely on clinical experience, sound education and detailed knowledge of the problem, and an attitude to which this knowledge lends the necessary conviction.

PATIENTS WITH CORONARY ARTERY DISEASE

Coronary Arteriosclerosis

Commonest of all the disorders of the heart is coronary arteriosclerosis or, more specifically, atherosclerosis. This disease produces degeneration and fibrosis of the myocardium and eventual cardiac failure. Or it may cause more acute episodes of myocardial hypoxia that are manifested by attacks of angina pectoris and that lead eventually to acute myocardial infarction. Atherosclerosis, the prevailing type of arteriosclerosis, begins with fatty degeneration of the vascular intima, a process that subsequently extends to involve also the media. Waxy cholesterol plaques become deposited on the inner lining of the arteries, interfering with the absorption of nutrients by the endothelial cells that compose the lining, and obstructing the blood flow by their protrusion into the lumen of the vessel. The vascular endothelium in involved areas becomes necrotic, then scarred, further compromising the lumen and impeding the flow of blood. At sites such as these, where the lumen is narrow and the walls rough, there is a great tendency for clots to form, which explains the fact that intravascular coagulation, followed by thromboembolic disease, is among the most important complications of atherosclerosis (and among the most important of all the diseases to which man is heir!).

A second form of arteriosclerosis, a product of chronic arterial hypertension, is characterized by thickening and calcification of the arterial media, converting the vessel into a relatively inflexible tube with a very narrow lumen. Patients with hypertension exhibit such changes with regularity and with consequences that may be benign or serious, depending on the location and the extent of the sclerotic changes and their distribution throughout the body, i.e., what organs are involved predominantly.

Coronary arteriosclerosis, irrespective of type, produces symptoms and complications through narrowing of the arterial lumena, and obstruction of blood flow therein. This impediment to blood flow persists and progresses, to the extreme detriment of all tissue cells that depend for their survival on the native components of blood and on various other constituents that it transports. In greatest jeopardy are the cells that require more than the average amount of oxygen, dextrose, amino acids, or other nutrients—such as, for example, the brain, the kidneys and the heart muscle. Myocardial cells, deprived of their customary and normal supply of nutrients and oxygen, undergo degeneration and eventually are replaced by fibrocytes, the harbingers of scarring. Altered in structure, its functional efficiency forever impaired, the heart eventually must fail.

The cardinal symptom of relative myocardial hypoxia is pain of cardiac origin. This is also the outstanding feature of the angina pectoris syndrome, as well as an early, prominent manifestation of myocardial infarction.

Angina Pectoris

Angina pectoris is a syndrome that is featured by paroxysms of pain in the anterior chest, produced as a result of insufficient coronary blood flow and myocardial hypoxia. This may be a purely relative matter: i.e., in the face of constant coronary flow in an individual previously without symptoms, acute myocardial hypoxia, with the classic symptoms of angina pectoris and with characteristic changes on electrocardiogram, may occur at any time as a result of any number of factors, especially the following: physical exertion, especially exertion of an unaccustomed type; strong emotion; exposure to cold; or a meal that is unusual in timing or content. The majority of patients with angina pectoris are males over 45, who ostensibly had been in excellent health and considered themselves to be perfectly fit.

The pain varies greatly in severity, from a sense of mere upper substernal pressure to pain that is agonizing. If severe and typical, it starts over the precordium and the upper sternum, radiates to the left shoulder and sometimes down the inner surface of the arm to the elbow, the wrist, and even to the 5th and ulnar aspect of the 4th fingers. Occasionally it seems to start in the throat, hence the name *angina*. In some cases it is reflected to the right shoulder; in others, to the upper abdomen, in which case it may simulate gallstones. When it is at all severe, the patient at once immobilizes himself. He cannot do otherwise; he cannot speak, his face is ashen, and he is covered with clammy sweat. With rest, the attack passes off completely, leaving him comfortable. Along with the physical pain, the patient also suffers a mental agony, a sense of impending death. This apprehension is so characteristic that when it occurs alone, as it sometimes does, it is sufficient for diagnosis.

Treatment. The basic program of care for the patient with angina pectoris embodies 3 aspects: (1) the amelioration of symptoms during attacks; (2) the abortion of attacks, or curtailment of their duration; and, (3) prevention of recurrences. Each patient must be evaluated and treated on an individual basis.

During an anginal attack the presence of a capable, knowledgable and understanding nurse is definitely beneficial from the therapeutic standpoint, tending, as it does, to allay apprehension, therefore helping to reduce a tachycardia or an elevation of arterial pressure that, if present, might tend to promote or prolong myocardial hypoxia.

The pain of an acute anginal attack usually is controlled with 1 or 2 tablets of nitroglycerin (glyceryl trinitrate), containing from 1/200 to 1/50 grain and placed under the tongue or in the buccal pouch. Its action is rapid and, in most patients, very effective. The patient should be reassured as to the nonhabituating qualities of the drug and cautioned to carry it with him at all times. For some patients the inhalation of amyl nitrite is equally effective. This agent, a liquid, is stored and distributed in tiny sealed glass tubes, which may be broken in a handkerchief and inhaled, as needed. Peritrate (pentaerythritol tetranitrate) may be prescribed as a prophylactic device, hoping to prevent attacks.

If a patient senses that an attack is imminent he should cease all unnecessary movement, the objective being to reduce to a minimum the oxygen requirements of his ischemic myocardium, hoping that its needs can be met by the limited supply presently available and the impending attack thereby averted.

There are patients whose attacks occur predominantly in the morning. This peculiar predilection obviously calls for a change in the schedule of daily activities. As a first step, the patient should plan to rise earlier each morning so that he may complete his shaving, washing and dressing in a more leisurely fashion and, hopefully, may maintain this unhurried pace throughout the entire day — performing his scheduled tasks and meeting whatever commitments he has without haste or a sense of pressure. Sound advice for any patient with angina pectoris would be to initiate all movements with deliberation; avoid exposure to cold; avoid tobacco; eat regularly but lightly; and, if overweight, correct obesity.

If the patient is in the hospital, the nurse can observe with care and record all facets of his activity, with particular regard for the activities that have been found to precede and may precipitate attacks of anginal pain. When do attacks tend to occur? Shortly following a meal? After engaging in certain activities? After physical activity in general? After visits from members of the family, or others? The answers to these questions, ascertained from observation, can provide valuable clues to the conduct of an effective convalescent program and a basis for designing a logical program of prevention.

As a group, patients with angina pectoris are inclined to be tense and fearful, especially if they have lived with their diagnosis for a short time only and as yet do not comprehend or are unwilling to accept its implications. There are favorable aspects to every situation—including our patient's—however bleak it may appear. Of these, he needs to be made aware and reminded constantly. Moreover, he should be encouraged to participate actively, and as soon as possible, in a systematic program of convalescence and prevention—a program that is calculated to bolster and sustain his morale, restore self-confidence and foster independence. Its major objective and its principal effort, to which the nurse is a most important contributor, is his education. Education of the cardiac patient, conducted on a fairly sophisticated level, is designed to acquaint him with the basic nature of his illness and to furnish him with the facts he needs if he is to reorganize his living habits in a way that is effective, i.e., that will reduce the frequency and the severity of the anginal attacks, delay the progress of the underlying disease and help to protect him from other complications.

Myocardial Infarction

This term refers to the process by which myocardial tissue is destroyed in regions of the heart that are deprived of their blood supply after closure of the coronary artery or one of its branches either by a thrombus or through obstruction of the vessel lumen by atherosclerosis.

The majority of patients with myocardial infarction are men over 50 with arteriosclerosis of the coronary vessels and often with arterial hypertension. In a typical case the pain starts suddenly, usually over the lower sternal region and the upper abdomen, and is continuous; but it may increase steadily in severity until it becomes almost unendurable. It is a heavy viselike pain which may radiate to the shoulders and down the arms, usually the left. Unlike the pain of true angina, it begins spontaneously (not following effort, emotional upset, etc.), does not immobilize the patient, persists for hours or days and is relieved neither by rest nor by nitrites. The pulse may become very rapid, irregular and feeble, even imperceptible, and the heart may dilate. Gallop rhythm (accentuated third heart sound making the three heart sounds similar to those of a galloping horse) often develops. Because of the abdominal pain and vomiting, the condition of these patients often is diagnosed as an acute indigestion. It is important to note that about 10 per cent of the patients with acute myocardial infarction, diagnosed on the basis of subsequent electrocardiograms, deny having experienced any pain or discomfort whatever. These are the so-called "silent coronaries."

From the first, the patient with a severe occlusion is in shock; his color is ashen, he breaks out in a clammy sweat and in a few minutes is confined to bed. Vomiting is common. In a few hours his temperature rises, his blood pressure falls to an unusually low point, the leukocyte count rises to 15,000 or 20,000. Changes are seen with great regularity in the electrocardiogram; changes testifying not only to the presence, but also to the location, of the infarct.

Prognosis. The possibility of recovery will depend on the size of the infarct. Some patients die instantly, others in a few minutes or hours. Other patients live a few days, often from 4 to 10, and then die either from softening and rupture of the infarcted area of the heartwall or from myocardial failure. Others suffer from embolus during the following week. (The inner surface of the infarcted area of the heart wall will be covered by a blood clot, fragments of which may break loose.) About 50 per cent will recover from the acute attack. A small infarct may heal with scar formation, leaving the patient fairly well, but a second occlusion often occurs later, or the patient develops heart failure.

Treatment and Nursing Care

Medical management and nursing care of the patient with myocardial infarction are designed to: (1) alleviate shock; (2) relieve pain; (3) rest the myocardium; (4) prevent complications; (5) achieve physiologic and functional rehabilitation; and (6) halt the progression of arteriosclerosis, the lesion that is basically responsible for the myocardial infarct.

Shock. The patient is admitted to the nursing unit as an emergency, probably via stretcher and in a state of shock. The same principles of nursing care that are applicable in other shock states are likewise appropriate in the care of this patient. The sitting position may further depress the arterial pressure; therefore, he should not be obliged or permitted to adopt it. Unnecessary movements on his part should be discouraged; he should be lifted from the stretcher to the bed.

The patient's pulse and respiratory rates should be measured at frequent intervals, as a guide to the progress of his vascular collapse. Shock must be treated with vigor; the longer it persists, the greater the peril to the patient.

If the patient is severely hypotensive, an intravenous infusion of dextrose solution may be started. This will serve as a vehicle for the injection of a vasopressor drug, such as Levophed or Aramine and a route of administration that will permit the most precise regulation of dosage. The nurse, under the direct supervision of the physician, can readjust the flow rate as often as necessary in accordance with fluctuations in the blood pressure until such time as the pressure has become stabilized at a normotensive level.

Pain and Hypoxia. Narcotics are given to alleviate pain and apprehension. If pain is only moderately intense, it should respond to intramuscular Demerol; if severe, its control may require intravenous morphine. The wise nurse will take the precaution of measuring the patient's blood pressure and counting the pulse and the respiratory rates before administering these narcotics, for they may depress further the arterial pressure of a patient who already is hypotensive. If pain persists despite analgesic medication, or if the patient appears to become increasingly restless, complains of headache or exhibits pronounced tachycardia, it may be assumed that he is suffering from hypoxia and is a candidate for oxygen inhalation therapy.

Rest. The key element in the treatment and the nursing care of patients with myocardial infarction is rest—physical rest and emotional rest—which should be as nearly complete as can be arranged and should be continued until the circulatory status has been restored to normal and the area of infarction has healed, i.e., no less than 3 to 6 weeks.

The patient should be spared every unnecessary physical exertion. This may create difficulties in the case of a patient who insists on taking care of himself. During the acute stage the patient should be disturbed as little as possible during the hours of sleep, so that maximum rest will be afforded each day. Visits from casual acquaintances and business associates should be deferred, and close friends and relatives, who *are* admitted, should be instructed to avoid lengthy and controversial discussions.

Contrary to prevailing concepts, the recumbent position is not necessarily the posture of choice from the standpoint of cardiac rest. On the contrary, the work of the heart appears to be at a minimum when the patient—especially the elderly patient—is sitting in a chair. This observation is the basis for the "armchair" treatment of heart failure ("Armchair treatment" does not mean ambulation; it means *rest in an armchair!*)

Ambulation usually is not permitted until 3 or 4 weeks have elapsed after an episode of infarction. The precise time when a particular patient may ambulate is dictated by many considerations and is determined on the basis of the total clinical picture. Moreover, physical exertion is not the sole factor that increases the work of the heart. Others, quite as important from the standpoint of the myocardial burden, include obesity, which should be brought under control, speedily and permanently; arterial hypertension, which, if severe and persistent, should be accorded topmost priority in treatment; anemia, which should be corrected without delay, by whatever means are appropriate; and tobacco smoking, which stimulates peripheral and coronary vasoconstriction and tachycardia and, therefore, should be avoided.

Diet. The diet may be liquid, soft or regular, depending on the patient's circulatory status and comfort. In general, high residue and fermentative foods should be avoided and small feedings supplied at frequent intervals during this acute stage. Cardiac failure is an indication for the restriction of both sodium and fluid intake.

Prevention of Complications. The patient's prognosis may be jeopardized by the advent, during the initial 2 weeks, of any one of several complications, including thromboembolism, congestive failure, an arrhythmia, and myocardial rupture. To be on the alert for any such development is an important nursing responsibility.

THROMBOEMBOLISM. Clots tend to form on the interior wall of an infarcted ventricle. From these so-called "mural thrombi" embolic material is likely to separate and find its way into the pulmonary or systemic circulation. Other and more common sources of emboli in patients with myocardial infarction are the leg veins, where blood flow, owing to muscular inactivity and reduced cardiac output, is likely to be sluggish. Phlebothrombosis in the legs may be prevented by the application of elastic stockings, and by the performance of leg exercises, including frequent and repeated flexion of the feet and the toes. Another prophylactic measure of value is the administration of an anticoagulant drug, such as Dicumarol, which inhibits clot formation by reducing the production of factors responsible for the evolution of thrombin. The responsible nurse will see to it that the anticoagulant medication is withheld on each occasion until the daily prothrombin clotting time has been reported by the laboratory, and will inform the physician at once if the results of the test are not within the desired range.

CONGESTIVE FAILURE. This complication ensues if myocardial damage is so extensive that cardiac efficiency is impaired, i.e., to the point that ventricular emptying is incomplete and cardiac output is inadequate. The nurse must be on the outlook for the premonitory symptoms of dyspnea and edema —symptoms that may presage the rapid onset of serious pulmonary edema. In an effort to avoid excessive fluid retention, the physician is likely to restrict routinely the sodium intake of all of his patients with a myocardial infarction. (The treatment of congestive heart failure is discussed on page 541.)

CARDIAC ARRHYTHMIAS. This kind of complication is especially common following posterior myocardial infarcts, inasmuch as the posterior coronary artery furnishes the principal blood supply to the conduction system of the heart. To ensure that an arrhythmia will not fail to be detected, and detected at the earliest possible moment, the pulse should be counted at frequent intervals, preferably by auscultation at the apex and for no less than 1 full minute. The occurrence of extrasystoles and dropped beats, ordinarily considered of minor import, should be viewed with concern in a patient with a fresh myocardial infarct, for it may signal the onset of a more serious arrhythmia. Any change in the rate, the rhythm, the volume or the character of the patient's pulse

should be reported in detail and without delay.

MYOCARDIAL RUPTURE. Another complication, likewise a hazard during the first 2 weeks after an infarct, is myocardial rupture, which is almost always fatal. This is most apt to occur in patients with severe hypertension. Of course, the risk is increased by factors or circumstances that tend to elevate the systolic arterial pressure—some of which can be avoided or at least moderated. Among these factors are vigorous coughing and straining at stool which, from the standpoint of arterial pressure, are as stressful as weight lifting or even more so.

Certain general rules for living are usually prescribed by the physician at this stage, the character of which must vary widely from patient to patient, owing to marked differences in practicalities and individual personalities. The nature of these instructions will be decided by the physician, ideally after joint discussion with the nurse whose familiarity with the patient as a person lends great significance to her views of his long-term management. Questions that will pertain may concern such matters as requirements for rest, criteria for controlling activities, recommendations as to diet and the use of tobacco. In relation to smoking, it may be pointed out that most sudden deaths that occur in individuals with a past history of a myocardial infarction are due to cardiac arrhythmia, notably ventricular fibrillation, and that most of the individuals so afflicted are habitually heavy smokers. Logically, any individual who has sustained a myocardial infarct is well advised to eliminate the use of tobacco.

The patient's progress is followed with the aid of repeated electrocardiograms and determinations of the erythrocyte-sedimentation rate. His cardiac function is estimated on the basis of his symptoms and physical signs. Gradually his self-confidence should be built up, and a mode of living should be established, with respect to work, recreation and hobbies, that will enable him to live a useful, happy and active life within the limits of his health.

Control of Arteriosclerosis. Obviously, since myocardial infarcts are the result of coronary artery obstruction and since the cause of the latter is usually atherosclerosis, every possible effort should be made to arrest the progress of this vascular lesion. To be sure, atherosclerosis is a multifactorial disease with its occurrence and course dependent on a hereditary predisposition and influenced greatly by the existence of uncontrolled diabetes, obesity or arterial hypertension. Persistent elevation of the blood cholesterol with excessive proportions of saturated, relative to unsaturated, fats in the diet also may be implicated in its pathogenesis. Some of these factors are amenable to control. For example, either diabetes or arterial hypertension, if present, should be managed under constant medical supervision.

The obese patient should lose weight until an optimum nutritional status is attained, a goal that is unlikely to be achieved and, ideally, should not be attempted without the advice and the guidance of a physician. The role of saturated versus unsaturated fatty acids in the diet and of the blood cholesterol level are as yet uncertain but, conceivably, may be of great significance in the genesis of atherosclerosis. Therefore, although medical opinions may vary in this regard, it is very important for the patient who has had a myocardial infarct to accept without reservations and abide meticulously by any dietary restrictions that his physician may choose to impose.

Rehabilitation. The nurse can assist the patient toward his goal of independence even when he is on strict bed rest. This assistance is given by asking the patient's preference in small matters and by directing his thinking toward the time when he will be active again. His questions must be answered truthfully and his confidence built in those who are responsible for his care. These are positive approaches in preventing the patient from becoming a cardiac cripple.

It has been shown that with narrowing of the coronary arteries there is an associated growth of collateral vessels. It takes time for the patient to develop an adequate collateral (secondary) circulation after a myocardial infarction. As the collateral vessels develop, the oxygen supply to the myocardium is increased, and the patient is gradually permitted to return to normal activities. It is desirable to train the patient for each added activity. If the patient has to climb stairs, he should start with a few steps at a time and each day gradually increase the number until he can tolerate a full flight of steps.

The same principle applies to any activity that the patient must attempt in his job. The work situation is analyzed, and the patient is trained and conditioned for each new activity, such as walking the distance to the bus, lifting objects and so forth. The patient is cautioned to stop before he becomes fatigued. The amount of work that he is usually able to assume depends on his occupation as well as the severity of the attack. Most patients can return to a full work status if they can learn to live within their cardiac reserve. Achieving this means stopping activities before becoming fatigued. The nurse has a role in restoring the patient's confidence and helping him to adopt this new philosophy.

PATIENTS WITH ENDOCARDIAL DISEASE

The endocardium is the endothelial layer of tissue that lines the heart's cavities and covers the flaps of its valves. Of the diseases that affect it, the majority represent various types and stages of inflammation, i.e., *endocarditis,* or its aftermath. They include: (1) rheumatic endocarditis, one of the many complications of acute rheumatic fever; (2) bacterial endocarditis, produced by direct bacterial invasion of the endocardium, particularly that portion covering the valve leaflets; and, (3) chronic valvular heart disease, based on structural deformities of the heart valves, either of congenital origin or acquired as a result of either rheumatic or bacterial endocarditis in the past. Whenever an area of endocardium becomes inflamed, for whatever reason, there forms at that site a fibrin clot, called a *vegetation.* In time this clot becomes converted into a mass of scar tissue. The scarred endocardium becomes thickened, stiffened, contracted and deformed. A fringe of vegetations ranging along the free margins of the valve flaps, marking the site of earlier erosions, repre-

MANAGEMENT OF THE PATIENT WITH ACUTE MYOCARDIAL INFARCTION

NURSING MEASURES

RATIONALE AND IMPLICATIONS

1. Provide complete rest.

Strict, continuous bed rest is required initially. Later, if cardiac damage is slight and nonprogressive, patient may rest in armchair.

The objective is to reduce to a minimum the frequency and the vigor of cardiac contractions, thereby lowering the oxygen requirements of the damaged and ischemic myocardium thus:
(1) relieving anginal pain;
(2) preventing further ischemic damage;
(3) preventing cardiac failure; and,
(4) avoiding myocardial rupture.

2. Relieve suffering.

Supply analgesic medication, within prescribed limits, as frequently and amply as necessary to control pain.

Pain associated with myocardial infarct is likely to be agonizing and difficult to relieve. Oxygen inhalation may enhance the effectiveness of narcotic drugs.

Display attentiveness and an attitude of reassurance.

Pain often is attended by fear of impending death, emotional agitation and physical restlessness, which tend to elevate the arterial blood pressure and increase cardiac work.

3. Make clinical observations to evaluate progress and to detect complications:

A. Measure and record the arterial blood pressure at frequent intervals.

Arterial hypotension usually reflects myocardial weakness and cardiogenic shock, requiring vasopressor therapy.

B. Measure and evaluate frequently the rate, the rhythm and the quality of the pulse. Determine the ventricular rate by auscultation at cardiac apex, by radial palpation, or both simultaneously (2 observers) for the presence and the degree of pulse deficit.

Tachycardia may signify an incipient cardiogenic shock.
A pulse irregularity may presage a dangerous arrhythmia—such as cardiac standstill or ventricular fibrillation.
A pulse deficit indicates atrial fibrillation and the need for digitalization.

C. Observe the rate and the character of respirations.

Tachypnea may reflect pulmonary congestion, signifying congestive heart failure; oligopnea may indicate that the patient has been oversedated with a respiratory-depressing opiate drug.

D. Measure and record daily urine output.

The urine volume provides a rough guide as to the state of the water balance, a measure of renal function and a clue to the development of congestive failure.

E. Observe color of skin, lips and nailbeds for evidence of cyanosis.

Appearance of cyanosis may be a clue to the development of pulmonary congestion and edema, manifestations of congestive heart failure. Oxygen therapy is certain to be prescribed. Application of tourniquets and a phlebotomy may speedily become necessary. Rapid digitalization and the injection of a mercurial diuretic may be indicated.

MANAGEMENT OF THE PATIENT WITH ACUTE MYOCARDIAL INFARCTION
(Continued)

4. Be ready for the following resuscitative measures:

A. Administration of oxygen by tent, oropharyngeal. catheter or positive pressure technic.

Oxygen inhalation, especially in the presence of pulmonary congestion, tends to reduce respiratory exertion and cardiac output, therefore helping to relieve pain and to protect the myocardium. Oxygenation by positive pressure technic is indicated in desperate situations, such as are created by ventricular standstill or fibrillation.

B. Administration of vasopressor drug (e.g. Levophed, Aramine, etc.).

Vasopressor therapy is likely to be administered by constant intravenous injection, the dosage of drug being regulated on the basis of arterial pressure fluctuations as observed and recorded by the nurse.

C. Know the location and be ready to make available without delay the cardiac pacer (artificial pacemaker).

Resumption of coordinated ventricular contractions and survival of the patient with cardiac arrest or ventricular fibrillation will depend on prompt application of external electric stimuli by the pacemaker.

5. Take steps to prevent thromboembolic complications.

A. The position of the patient at complete bed rest must be changed frequently. Request him to flex his toes repeatedly and forcefully.

These measures are designed to expel venous blood from the lower extremities, where the flow is apt to be most sluggish and intravascular coagulation is most apt to occur.

B. See that elastic stockings, if prescribed, are worn continuously and correctly.

Properly applied, these stockings reduce the volume of the venous channels in the legs, thereby inceasing the venous flow rate and helping to prevent venous pooling. They should extend above the knee; should *not* be rolled at the top. If improperly applied, their effect will be to obstruct, rather than to facilitate, venous return from the calves.

C. Administer anticoagulant medication as prescribed.

Inhibition of clotting is intended to reduce risk of clot formation in the legs, on the damaged wall of the heart, or elsewhere. This is a common occurrence in patients with myocardial infarction and as a source of emboli is responsible for many fatalities.

The dosage of anticoagulant is regulated on the basis of a daily clotting test, the results of which should be obtained promptly and relayed to the physician, as indicated.

MANAGEMENT OF THE PATIENT WITH ACUTE MYOCARDIAL INFARCTION
(Continued)

NURSING MEASURES	RATIONALE AND IMPLICATIONS
6. Supply a modified diet and assist with meals.	A low (i.e. approx. 1,000) calorie soft diet usually is prescribed, to avoid stimulating the gastrointestinal tract unnecessarily and minimize abdominal distention—the effect of which is to impede respiratory movements and impair pulmonary ventilation.
7. Facilitate elimination, promoting regular, effortless defecation through the administration of mild laxatives and low enemata, as indicated. Substitute bedside commode for bedpan, if permissible, and if the patient's cardiac status warrants.	Straining at stool produces sharp elevations of arterial blood pressure, straining the left ventricle and increasing the risk of myocardial rupture.

---

sents the basic lesion of endocarditis and is the forerunner of chronic valvular heart disease.

Rheumatic Endocarditis

Rheumatic fever is a disease—a preventable disease—that usually has its onset in childhood following a hemolytic streptococcus infection. Whereas the most prominent symptom of rheumatic fever is polyarthritis, the most serious damage occurs in the heart, where every structural component is likely to be the site of an inflammatory reaction. The heart damage and the joint lesions as well,

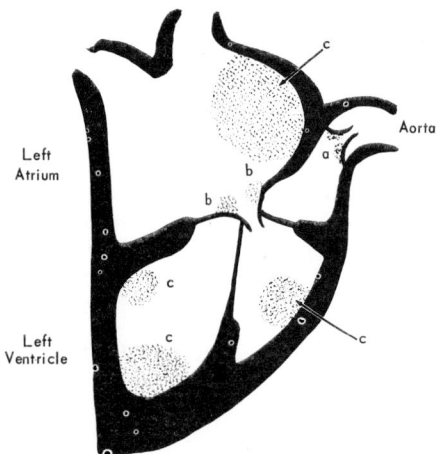

FIG. 182. The vegetations of acute endocarditis in their most common locations. (a) Vegetations on the aortic valve (ventricular surface of flaps). (b) On the mitral valve (atrial surface of flaps). (c) Mural thrombi.

are not infectious in origin, in the sense that these tissues are invaded and directly damaged by destructive organisms; rather, they represent a sensitivity phenomenon, occurring in response to prior contact with a bacterium: specifically, the *beta hemolytic streptococcus*. Blood leukocytes accumulate in the affected tissues to form nodules, which eventually are replaced by scars. The myocardium is certain to be involved in this inflammatory process, i.e., *rheumatic myocarditis* develops, which temporarily weakens the contractile power of the heart. The pericardium likewise is affected, i.e., *rheumatic pericarditis* also occurs during the acute illness. These myocardial and pericardial complications usually are without serious sequelae; on the other hand, the effects of *rheumatic endocarditis* are permanent and often crippling.

Rheumatic endocarditis anatomically manifests itself first by tiny translucent vegetations, which resemble beads about the size of the head of a pin, arranged in a row along the free margins of the valve flaps. These tiny beads look harmless enough and may disappear without injuring the valve flaps, but more often their results are serious. They are the starting point of a process that gradually thickens the flaps after years, rendering them just a little shorter, just a little thicker than normal, just a little shriveled along their edges — not much, but enough to prevent them from closing the orifice of the valve perfectly. Hence a leak develops; the valve is said to be "incompetent." In other patients the inflamed margins of the valve flaps become interadherent, with the result that the valve orifice is narrowed, or "stenotic."

A very small percentage of patients die as the immediate result of acute rheumatic fever; when death does occur at this stage, usually it is due to acute myocarditis. Most patients recover with gratifying speed and their recovery ostensibly is complete. However, although free of symptoms, the patient is left with certain permanent residuals in the form of valvular deformities. The extent of cardiac damage, or even its existence, may not have been apparent on clinical examinations during the acute phase of the disease. Eventually, however, the heart murmurs that are characteristic of valvular stenosis, incompetence, or both, become audible on auscultation and, in some patients, even detectable as "thrills" on palpation. The myocardium usually can compensate for these valvular defects very well for a time, despite its increased burden. As long as it can do so, the patient will remain in apparent good health. However, sooner or later it will fail to compensate — and decompensation, when it occurs, will be signaled by the manifestations of congestive heart failure, described on page 540.

Treatment. The patient with rheumatic endocarditis should be confined to bed as long as he is febrile and remain quiet thereafter until the erythrocyte sedimentation rate (a fair though nonspecific index of rheumatic activity) returns to normal. Salicylates customarily are prescribed in large doses, and invariably to good effect, so far as the elimination of fever and arthritis are concerned. However, neither these nor any other drugs appear to affect the development or the progress of rheumatic endocarditis.

The patient with rheumatic endocarditis, whose valve function is faulty but whose disease is quiescent, does not require therapy as long as his heart pumps effectively. Nevertheless, he faces the threat of recurrent attacks of acute rheumatic fever; of bacterial endocarditis; of embolism from vegetations or mural thrombi in the heart; and of eventual cardiac failure. The relation between valvular disease and congestive heart failure is discussed on page 529; the treatment of heart failure, on page 541.

Prevention. Unfortunately, rheumatic fever is prone to recur, unless recurrence is forestalled by prophylactic antimicrobial therapy, and each attack renders the patient more susceptible to a subsequent recurrence. Furthermore, each attack adds to the valvular damage already present, further impairing cardiac function and hastening the advent of eventual decompensation. Obviously, it is in the area of prevention that the medical team can make its most significant contribution to the welfare of the patient with rheumatic endocarditis.

The nurse should be familiar with the symptoms of streptococcal pharyngitis and aware of its role in relation to rheumatic fever, so that she may be convincingly emphatic in her instructions to individuals so afflicted—especially individuals with a past history of rheumatic fever. Early and effective treatment of streptococcal infections, including streptococcal pharyngitis, has been shown to prevent the onset, as well as the recurrence, of acute rheumatic fever as an aftermath. Rheumatic fever subjects must be especially wary of contact with persons with symptoms suggesting bacterial pharyngitis, or who are known to have contracted a streptococcal infection within a period of 3 months. Any patient with evidence of bacterial pharyngitis should be regarded as a candidate for antibiotic therapy, pending the results of a throat culture. Moreover, every patient with a history of rheumatic fever should receive monthly prophylactic injections of penicillin, in order to avoid another streptococcal infection. On the occasion of his monthly visit the nurse should reiterate the reasons for prophylaxis and emphasize the importance of continuing it indefinitely. The patient must recognize and should accept the fact that he is a "rheumatic fever patient," and as such can lead a normal life only if he is willing to submit to certain limitations and inconveniences. In relation to this facet of his education, the nurse is in a position to play a very important role.

Bacterial Endocarditis

Subacute bacterial endocarditis is a febrile disease resulting from infection of a heart valve that has been damaged by rheumatic fever, or one that is abnormal by virtue of a congenital defect. The incidence of this disease is highest among individuals between the ages of 20 and 40.

Subacute bacterial endocarditis is caused by streptococci of the *viridans* group, organisms of low virulence that normally inhabit the mouth and the gastrointestinal tract. Characteristically, 1 to 3 weeks before the onset of his illness the patient has had a bacterial pharyngitis or has been subjected to a dental extraction, or to oral, genitourinary or rectal surgery—procedures that almost invariably are attended by transient bacteremia. Such bacteremias are extremely common, and ordinarily are harmless, thanks to the protective activities of the reticuloendothelial system. However, on heart valves that are abnormally vascularized or otherwise altered by prior disease, blood-borne bacteria are prone to lodge—and there they thrive. As they multiply they cause the valve leaflets to become eroded; on these erosions, fibrin is deposited and vegetations form, in accordance with the sequence described above. The bacteria themselves become enmeshed in a network of fibrin that, in turn, forms a barricade against the phagocytic cells and immune antibodies in the circulating blood thereby protecting them from destruction and ensuring their continuing growth.

The onset of subacute bacterial endocarditis usually is insidious and seldom can be dated with precision. Typical symptoms include weakness, malaise and intermittent fever, with alternating chills and sweats. A unique feature of the disease is the appearance of small painful swellings, called "Osler's nodes," on the tips or lateral borders of the fingers and toes. Petechial hemorrhages are to be found on the skin and the conjunctivae. Clubbing of the fingers is common. If the disease runs a protracted course the patient loses a substantial amount of weight and becomes very anemic. His complexion acquires a "cafe-au-lait" hue as a result of the anemia. The pulse rate is accelerated. A mild leukocytosis is present, and a bacteremia usually can be demonstrated by means of a blood culture.

As the blood courses through his heart, vegetations may separate from the diseased valve and be carried to distant sites in the body. Embolic fragments from this source, or from a mural thrombus in the heart, may lodge in the kidneys, the brain or elsewhere, including myocardium, often with serious and occasionally lethal consequences.

Acute bacterial endocarditis differs from the subacute variety only with respect to the infecting organism, which is relatively virulent (e.g., the hemolytic streptococcus, *Staphylococcus aureus,* the pneumococcus or the gonococcus), and the clinical course, which progresses more rapidly and is relatively stormy. The most conspicuous symptoms are those of sepsis: high fever, chills, prostration and marked leukocytosis.

Treatment. The basic objective of therapy is to eradicate the invading organisms. This is accomplished by the administration of an antimicrobial drug, one selected on the basis of blood cultures and the sensitivity tests that are applied to the organism isolated from these cultures. Penicillin, given in massive doses (e.g., 2 million units or

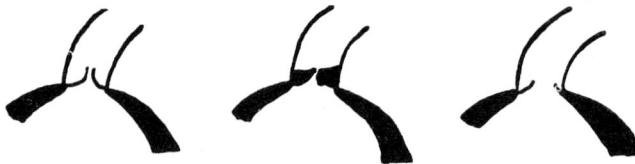

FIG. 183. The aortic valve. *(Left)* Normal valve. *(Center)* The flaps of the valve are so thickened by vegetation that the orifice of the aorta is partially occluded; this is aortic stenosis. *(Right)* The valve flaps are so torn that they cannot close the orifice; this is aortic insufficiency.

more intramuscularly or intravenously each day for 4 to 6 weeks) sufficiently early in the course of the infection, is curative in most patients. The selection and the administration of antimicrobial agents, including penicillin, are discussed on pages 192 to 195.

Whereas eradication of the infection usually can be achieved, thanks to modern antibacterial chemotherapy, the valvular damage it has produced is irreparable, and the ultimate prognosis of the patient who has been "cured" of bacterial endocarditis will depend to a large extent on the degree to which his cardiac efficiency has been impaired.

Chronic Valvular Heart Disease

If the heart muscle remains strong, the circulatory apparatus can adjust itself efficiently even though a valve is injured badly. The details of such adjustment, called *compensatory changes,* include modifications in the rate and the character of the heartbeat, changes in the blood pressure, hypertrophy of the myocardium, a redistribution of the blood in the body, etc., all changes that lessen the untoward results of the valve defect.

Aortic Stenosis

Narrowing of the orifice between the left ventricle and the aorta (Fig. 183) is a lesion found most frequently in elderly men. Often it is the result of arteriosclerosis or rheumatic fever. The flaps of the aortic valve fuse and partially close the opening between the heart and the aorta. The left ventricle overcomes this obstruction to circulation by contracting more slowly, but with greater energy than normal, forcibly squeezing the blood through the very small hole. The first heart sound, therefore, is a long-drawn rough and vibrating *r-r-r-r-rub-dub.* If one rests the hand over the aortic area, he feels a vibration which is the most intense of all cardiac thrills and which resembles the purring of a cat.

The pulse is slow in rate and small in volume; the pulse pressure is low. Because the blood is squeezed slowly into the aorta, the ascent of each pulse wave is gradual and its apex is rounded (Fig. 184 A).

To compensate for this condition, the left ventricle shows the strain by a thickening of the muscle wall. Other signs and symptoms are dizziness and fainting because of reduced blood volume to the brain, anginal-type pain in the chest because of lessened blood supply to the heart, and a low blood-pulse pressure because of diminished blood flow. Once these symptoms develop, surgery should be considered.

This condition, being primarily rheumatic in origin, is associated with mitral valve disease in over half of the patients. Hence, a mitral commissurotomy may be done at the same time.

Treatment. The fused aortic valves are spread apart with an instrument introduced through a stab wound in the left ventricle or by enlarging the valve from above, through the aorta, with a knife or a dilator.

If the stenosis becomes more marked or if the myocardium becomes weakened, a break in compensation eventually occurs. The left ventricle dilates, and signs of congestive heart failure appear.

Aortic Insufficiency (Regurgitation)

Aortic regurgitation is caused by inflammatory lesions that deform the flaps so that they fail to seal perfectly the aortic orifice during diastole. This valvular defect is occasionally the result of endocarditis of the

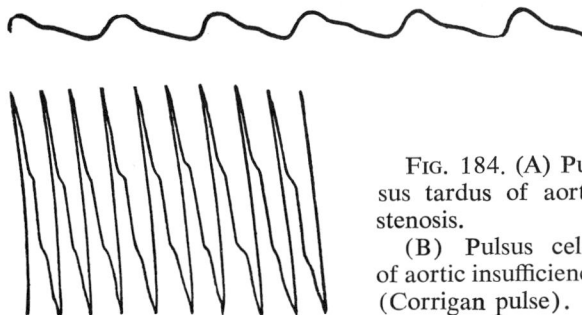

FIG. 184. (A) Pulsus tardus of aortic stenosis.
(B) Pulsus celer of aortic insufficiency (Corrigan pulse).

rheumatic type or the bacterial type, but is commonly due to syphilis.

Because of the leak in the aortic valve during diastole, some of the blood in the aorta, always under high pressure, hisses back into the left ventricle, which must handle both that which the left atrium normally delivers into it through the mitral orifice and that returning from the aorta. The left ventricle dilates to accommodate this increased volume, hypertrophies in order to be able to expel it, and does so with more than normal force, thus raising the systolic blood pressure. By another reflex the cardiovascular system tends to become accommodated: the peripheral arterioles become relaxed, so that the peripheral resistance is lessened and the diastolic pressure greatly lowered. The pulse pressure is considerably increased in these cases, and one of the characteristic signs of the disease is the Corrigan pulse, described on page 60 (Fig. 184 B). The nature of the pulse wave is quite unmistakable, and the capillary pulse is pronounced. The diagnosis often can be made when shaking hands because of the throb of the entire hand.

Compensation may remain excellent for a long time, but when the left ventricle dilates because of weakness, a relative mitral insufficiency arises and a train of events leading to cardiac failure is initiated.

If the damaged aortic valve could be completely replaced, the problem would be corrected. Hufnagel devised a plastic ball which allows blood to flow in only one direction. It is placed in the aorta distal to the subclavian artery, where it prevents backflow beyond the valve. This has been used in moderate and severe cases; it is palliative and prevents regurgitation of about 70 per cent of the cardiac output. Newer valves are being tested successfully and will soon be used on patients with milder forms of aortic insufficiency.

Mitral Stenosis

Mitral stenosis is by far the most common of the cardiac lesions that are produced by acute rheumatic fever and is considered the typical lesion. It has been estimated that nearly 1,000,000 persons in the United States have mitral stenosis. In this disorder, acute rheumatic endocarditis has glued the mitral valve flaps (commissures) together and, by shortening the chordae tendineae, has pulled the flap edges almost down to the tips of the papillary muscles, thus greatly narrowing the mitral orifice. Normally, one should be able to put three fingers through this orifice with ease, but in well-marked cases of stenosis one can hardly pass a lead pencil through it. The left ventricle is not affected, but the left atrium has great difficulty in emptying itself through the narrow orifice into the ventricle. Therefore it dilates and hypertrophies. Since no valve protects the pulmonary veins from a backward flow from this atrium, the pulmonary circulation becomes markedly congested. As a result of the abnormally high pulmonary arterial pressure that must be maintained by the right ventricle, it is subjected to an unfunctional strain and eventually fails.

Patients with mitral stenosis are prone to be cyanotic, short of breath, to cough and to suffer from "bronchitis." Hemoptysis is a common symptom. The pulse is small in

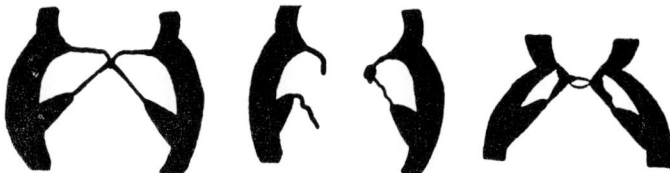

FIG. 185. The mitral valve. *(Left)* The normal valve. *(Center)* The valve flaps are shrunken and torn so that they cannot close the orifice; this is mitral insufficiency. *(Right)* The valve flaps are so thickened that the orifice is partially occluded; the small circle represents the maximum orifice in some extreme cases; this is mitral stenosis.

volume and often irregular because of fibrillation. The apex beat is in about normal position and not conspicuous on inspection; but on palpation, the shock of the first sound is felt as a characteristic sudden tap, like that of a hammer. At this point also, over an area of not more than an inch in diameter, is felt and heard a characteristic purring crescendo thrill, due to the atrial systole. This, steadily increasing in intensity, ends in the above-mentioned sudden tap. In many patients this thrill appears only after exercise. At the pulmonary area one feels a similar tap, but this is the shock of the second sound.

Commissurotomy for Mitral Stenosis. When left atrial enlargement develops in a patient with mitral stenosis, as shown by roentgenograms, and the patient experiences fatigue and dyspnea on exertion, early operation usually is indicated. In selected patients, it is possible for the surgeon to free the thickened and fused valve flaps by fracturing them with his index finger (finger-fracture method) or by cutting them with a special knife (Fig. 186).

In this surgery, it is necessary for the pleura and the pericardium to be opened after making an incision through the 3rd or the 4th interspace. Procaine is infiltrated around the base of the left atrial (auricular) appendage, and a purse-string suture is applied. When the tip of the appendage is excised, the surgeon is able to insert his finger; by tightening the purse-string suture there is little blood loss while the surgeon fractures or cuts the commissures. When the surgeon withdraws his finger, immediately the purse-string suture is closed tightly.

Mitral Insufficiency

The typical mitral lesion of rheumatic origin produces not only stenosis but also incompetence of that valve (see Fig. 185).

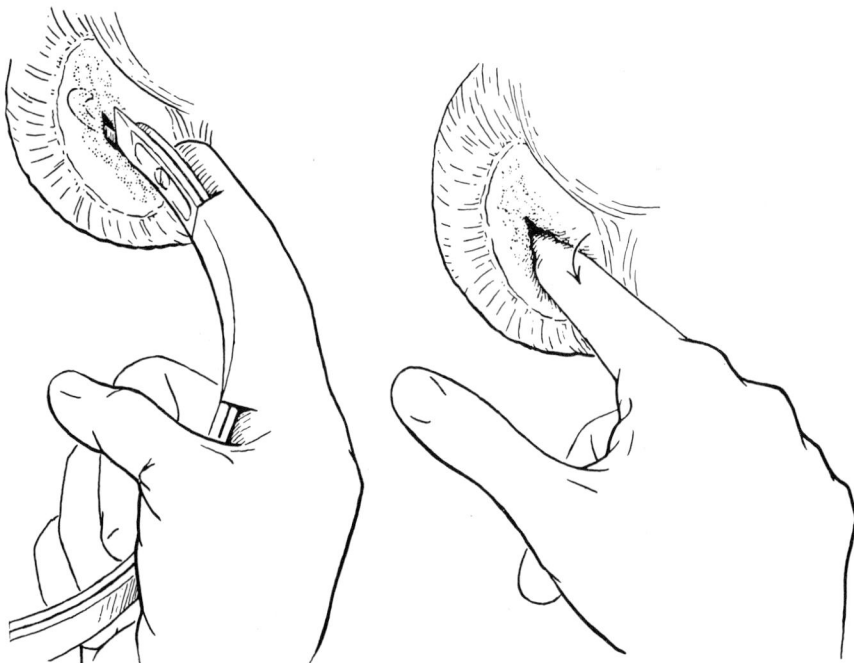

FIG. 186. Mitral commissurotomy. *(Left)* A drawing of the special knife used in cutting commissures. The surgeon wears two gloves on his operating hand; the outer glove is cut in two places to accommodate the knife. *(Right)* Illustrates the finger fracture method of breaking the fibrous bands at the ends of the mitral valve. (Johnson, J., and Kirby, C. K.: Surgery of the Chest, p. 329, Chicago, Yr. Bk. Pub.)

Shortening or tearing of one or both of the mitral valve flaps prevents the perfect closure of the mitral orifice, while the powerful left ventricle is forcing the blood into the aorta. Then at each beat the left ventricle will force some of the blood back into its atrium; this blood will add to the blood then beginning to flow into this chamber from the lungs. The left atrium must dilate and hypertrophy. This backward flow of blood from the ventricle also checks the current of blood flowing under low pressure from the lungs, which, therefore, become congested, and this, in turn, throws an extra strain on the right ventricle. Therefore, the result of even a slight mitral leak always involves both lungs and the right ventricle.

Patients with mitral insufficiency are always just a trifle cyanotic; after exertion they actually become blue. Even while compensation is good, palpitation of the heart, shortness of breath on exertion and cough due to chronic passive pulmonary congestion are common symptoms. The pulse may be regular and of good volume, but not infrequently it becomes irregular, either as a result of extrasystoles of fibrillation, which may persist indefinitely.

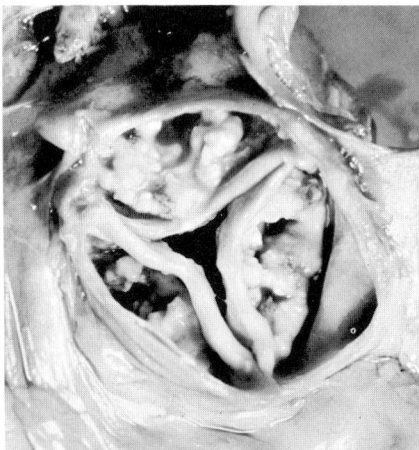

FIG. 187. Rheumatic endocarditis, tricuspid valve. The margins of the 3 valve flaps are thickened, beaded and interadherent, and the flaps themselves are covered with a profusion of calcified vegetation. (Charles S. Sommers, M.D., Boston)

Various surgical measures are used in attempts to improve the competence of this valve.

Tricuspid Lesions

Tricuspid insufficiency, the result of disease of the tricuspid valve flaps, occurs rarely, though more often in children than in adults. The usual cause is severe rheumatic endocarditis (Fig. 187).

Symptoms. The symptoms of tricuspid insufficiency are marked. At each beat the right ventricle forces blood in two directions: through the pulmonary valve, the normal direction, and back through the leaking tricuspid valve into the right atrium. The flow of venous blood from the systemic circulation is impeded, causing signs of general cyanosis and overfilling of all the veins of the body. A pulse wave similar to that sent by the left ventricle throughout the arterial tree may be transmitted into the larger veins. Therefore, the liver, now swollen to perhaps 2 or 3 times its normal size, pulsates. The walls of the stomach and the intestines, the kidneys and other abdominal organs, since they are turgid with venous blood, cannot function well and give rise to symptoms of chronic passive congestion. The skin of the legs and the dependent portions of the body becomes edematous. Fluid collects in the abdominal cavity (ascites) and in the pleural cavities (hydrothorax). If the heart can compensate again, circulation will improve at once, the congestion of the various organs will be relieved, and all symptoms due to it will disappear.

Lesions of the Pulmonary Valve

Pulmonary valve disease with both insufficiency and stenosis is due to congenital malformations. It is rarely seen except in children since, for the most part, it is incompatible with prolonged life.

PATIENTS WITH MYOCARDITIS

The heart is a muscle, hence its efficiency depends on the health of its individual muscle fibers. When this is good, the heart can function well in spite of severe valvular injuries; when it is poor, life is in jeopardy.

Acute myocarditis, or acute inflammation

of the cardiac muscle tissue, occasionally resembles other inflammations in that an inflammatory exudate is present, as in cases secondary to an acute endocarditis or pericarditis. But usually it appears itself as an acute degeneration of the heart muscle fibers, which are replaced later by fibrous tissue cells.

Etiology. Acute myocarditis may develop as a complication of many acute infections, including diphtheria and typhoid fever, and one caused by a virus of the Coxsackie group. By far the commonest cause, however, is *beta hemolytic streptococcus,* Lancefield, type A infection, following which myocarditis may occur as a late complication, 2 to 3 weeks after the acute febrile phase. This is the so-called "rheumatic myocarditis," a constant feature of acute rheumatic fever. Another type, a toxic form of myocarditis, eventually occurs in severe hyperthyroidism.

The symptoms of acute myocarditis usually are indefinite. Often the first evidence of its presence is suddenly developing cardiac dilatation with heart failure, which may rapidly lead to death. In other cases, its presence is suggested by breathlessness, a low blood pressure, disturbances of rate and rhythm and evidences of cardiac enlargement.

Management. The main requirement is complete rest in bed, for sudden death may follow the slightest exertion of the body. Every attempt is made to anticipate the patient's needs and wishes. He is fed, bathed, lifted and turned so that his strength may be conserved. The necessity for such assistance is explained to the patient, with emphasis on the fact that it is but a temporary need that will be eliminated as soon as the inflammatory process subsides. Digitalis and caffeine may be employed as circulatory stimulants.

Convalescence. The convalescence should be prolonged and carefully guarded, for heart failure often occurs after the patient seems to be practically well.

PATIENTS WITH PERICARDITIS

Pericarditis, as its name implies, refers to an inflammation of the pericardium, the membranous sac enveloping the heart. This inflammation may be due to infection by organisms brought to it by way of the blood stream in the course of a bacteremia or by extension of an infectious process involving an adjacent organ, such as a tuberculous lymph node, an infected pleura or a mediastinal abscess. It appears often in the course of acute rheumatic heart disease that is the result of infection. Noninfectious pericardial inflammation occurs in uremia and occasionally in coronary thrombosis over the area of myocardial infarction. Acute benign idiopathic pericarditis is an inflammatory lesion of uncertain etiology, possibly caused by a virus, possibly representing an allergic phenomenon, its only complicating feature being an occasional tendency to recur.

The patient may complain of chest pain and dyspnea. Pain, if present, varies from mild to severe. Usually it is felt in the central substernal region, radiating to the shoulder and the neck. It is likely to be aggravated by respiration, thus demonstrating its pleural origin. (Infectious pericarditis nearly always is accompanied by acute pleuritis.) In the course of her observations the nurse should attempt to discover whether or not the pain is influenced by respiratory movements, with or without the actual passage of air; by flexion, extension or rotation of the spine, including the neck, or by movements of the shoulders and the arms; by coughing; or by swallowing. Notation of these relationships may be very helpful in establishing a diagnosis. Typically in acute pericarditis the pain is increased by respiration (with passage of air), by coughing and, occasionally, by swallowing; it is uninfluenced by posture or other movements.

Dyspnea occurs as a result of compression of the bronchi or the parenchyma of the lung by the distended pericardium. The patient obviously is ill, in distress, restless and anxious; his complexion is pale or cyanotic or both. He prefers to adopt a forward-leaning or a sitting posture. Pericarditis per se often gives rise to no signs other than fever and the production of a friction rub that is audible on auscultation and is synchronous with the heartbeat.

Pericardial Effusion. This may accompany the general anasarca of nephrosis or advanced congestive heart failure. In this type of case, the fluid is noninfected and is of low specific gravity and protein content. However, in pericarditis due to infections other than tuberculosis, the fluid is likely to be purulent, and from it the organism can be cultured. Blood occasionally finds its way into the sac (hemopericardium) as a result of traumatic injury, tumor of the pericardium or dissecting aneurysm. When caring for a patient who has sustained an automobile accident, ascertain whether his chest impinged on the steering wheel, and report this information. It should be borne in mind that hemopericardium may follow any chest injury, even in the absence of external laceration or rib cage fracture.

Whatever the character of the fluid, if it accumulates in sufficient amount, the heart action is embarrassed. The blood pressure drops and fluctuates with respiration (pulsus paradoxicus), being lowest on inspiration, at which phase the pulse may be imperceptible. The venous pressure tends to rise, as is evident by the development of engorged neck veins and generalized edema. The heart sounds become feeble in intensity, there are signs of cardiac enlargement and compression of the left lung posteriorly. This is a life-threatening situation, demanding close and constant observation. These should include hourly measurements of the arterial pressure and pulse rate, for on the course of these vital signs hinges the decision regarding the need for pericardial paracentesis.

To improve the cardiac function, if it becomes impaired seriously, a pericardial tap is performed, all the available fluid being aspirated through a needle inserted usually near the apex. Tapping may have to be performed repeatedly and at frequent intervals, depending on the speed of fluid reaccumulation. The type of pericarditis most apt to require frequent tapping and eventual surgical removal of the pericardium is the tuberculous variety. Purulent exudates may require open drainage through a surgical chest wall incision.

Patients with bacterial infections of the pericardium are treated with the antimicrobial agent of choice for each particular patient, based on identification and sensitivity tests.

Chronic Constrictive Pericarditis. Usually of tuberculous origin, this disease is a chronic inflammatory thickening of the pericardium with an obliteration of the pericardial space. Often the adherent pericardium becomes calcified. The heart action is much embarrassed by this tough, unyielding enclosure, and edema, ascites and hepatic enlargement result. The fixation of the heart to the pericardium often produces a retraction of the chest wall with every heartbeat. Surgical removal of the constricting diseased pericardium (pericardectomy) is the only treatment of any benefit. This is done by cutting away the overlying costal cartilages and excising carefully the thickened covering of the heart.

PATIENTS WITH AORTIC DISEASE

Aortitis

Aortitis is arteritis of the aorta, its arch being particularly affected. There are two types of this disease—the arteriosclerotic and the luetic. Both cause pain, dilatation or aneurysm of this vessel and aortic-valve insufficiency.

Arteriosclerotic Aortitis

Aortitis of the arteriosclerotic type, which is but a part of general arteriosclerosis, usually appears after the age of 60. In this, the entire surface of the intima degenerates and becomes sclerosed.

Luetic Aortitis

Luetic aortitis, unlike the arteriosclerotic type, usually begins before the age of 50. It starts at the root of the aorta and spreads in the form of a few discrete patches scattered over an otherwise normal intima. Its symptoms often are unusually severe, yet in some patients they are entirely absent.

Symptoms. The most common symptoms of luetic aortitis are sensations of substernal oppression or weight, or viselike feelings of constriction of the chest, or attacks of pain, often agonizing. There are characteristic sudden attacks of dyspnea (often called *asthma*) which start abruptly, are agonizing, last from 5 to 15 minutes and are accompanied by rapid pulse rate, high blood pressure, deep cyanosis and profuse sweating.

Diagnosis. Luetic aortitis should be thought of in all cases of lues, even though no symptoms suggest its presence, and especially if vigorous antiluetic treatment has failed to reverse a positive serologic reaction. The condition often is discovered unexpectedly on roentgenograms. The presence of aortic insufficiency without an associated mitral lesion, paroxysmal dyspnea, anginal attacks and the development of an aortic aneurysm all suggest this diagnosis.

Prognosis. Of untreated patients, over two thirds die within 1 year after the characteristic symptoms appear. While luetic aortitis in large measure can be prevented by early and adequate antiluetic therapy, and can be arrested by specific treatment, the damage never can be repaired entirely.

Aortic Aneurysms

Nature and Classification of Aneurysms

Since arteries are elastic tubes filled with blood flowing under high pressure, should the wall of a vessel gradually become weak and yet not burst, it will become distended at the weakened point. Such local distention is described as an *aneurysm*. Very small aneurysms due to local infection are designated as *mycotic aneurysms*. An aneurysm which is somewhat larger, but still limited in extent, projecting from one side of the vessel only is called a *saccular aneurysm* (Fig. 188). If the whole artery becomes dilated, a *fusiform aneurysm* develops (Fig. 189). A wall of scar tissue at once begins to form around the developing aneurysmal sac, but never quite rapidly enough, hence there arises a slowly growing, pulsating tumor

filled with blood communicating with the lumen of the vessel.

Possible causes for local weakness of the arterial wall that may result in aneurysm include local trauma by knife or missile, a local infection either pyogenic or luetic, and arteriosclerosis. Some spots may have been congenitally weak. This is true in the case of most cerebral aneurysms.

About 90 per cent of aortic aneurysms are located within the thorax, and the majority of these are on the aortic arch. The cause in most patients is syphilis, though a certain percentage of aneurysms of the fusiform type are due to arteriosclerosis.

Subjective Symptoms. Some aortic aneurysms give symptoms so slight that for a time the condition is not suspected, but all eventually make their presence known by symptoms of congestive heart failure or the pressure that the pulsating tumor exerts against other intrathoracic organs. Pain is the most prominent pressure symptom. This may be constant and boring in character, due to the erosion of a vertebra or rib by the pressure of the pulsating sac, or intermittent and neuralgic, due to pressure against nerves. Other conspicuous symptoms are dyspnea, the result of the pressure of the sac against the

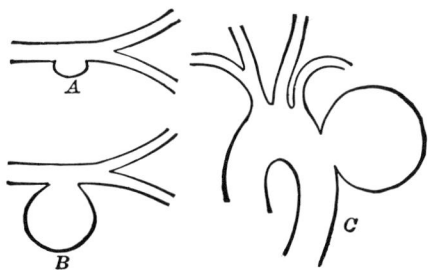

FIG. 188. Saccular aneurysms. (A) A small saccular aneurysm. (B) A later stage of A. (C) A saccular aneurysm of the arch of the aorta, a very common and often huge form which often may be several inches in diameter.

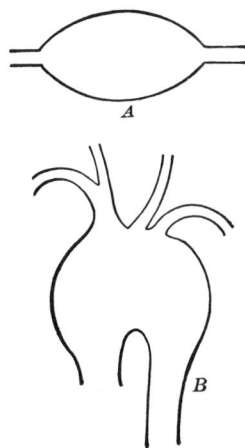

FIG. 189. Fusiform aneurysms. (A) A fusiform aneurysm of a small artery. (B) Fusiform aneurysm of the arch of the aorta, the commonest form. This also is called a diffuse aneurysm, or a dilatation of the arch.

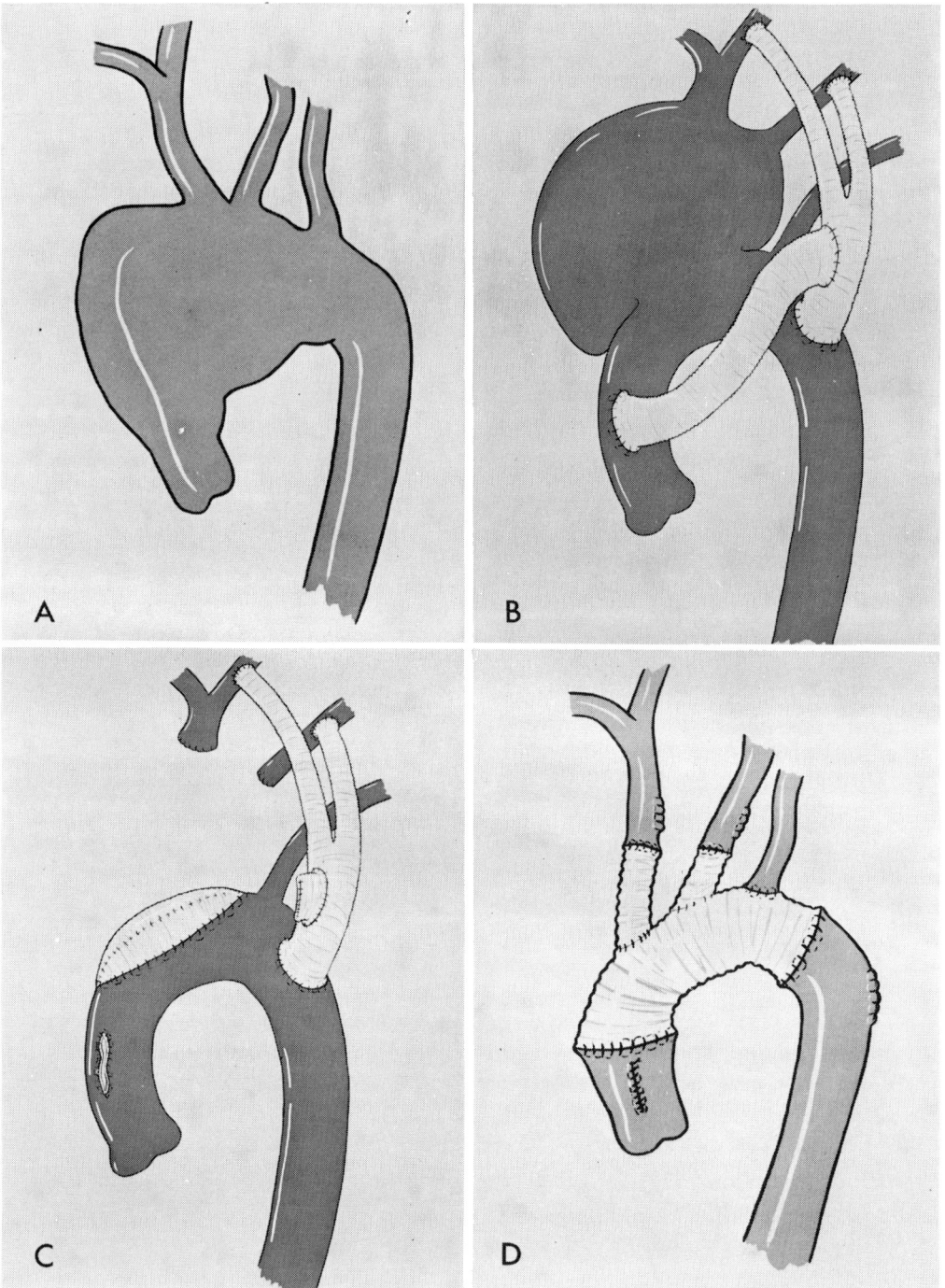

Fig. 190. (A) Drawing illustrating location and extent of aneurysm. (B) Drawing illustrating method of treatment utilizing temporary bypass graft to maintain normal aortic circulation during excision of aneurysm. (C) Drawing illustrating completed procedure with patch graft angioplasty to repair excised segment of aortic arch and conversion of temporary bypass graft to innominate and left common carotid arteries into the permanent graft. (D) Method of treatment utilizing still another form of temporary bypass grafts to maintain normal aortic circulation during excision and graft replacement of aneurysm. (DeBakey, M. E.: Changing concepts in vascular surgery, Figs. 12B, 12E, 13C and 13D, J. Cardiov. Surg. 1:3-44)

trachea, a main bronchus or the lung itself; cough, frequently paroxysmal and with brassy quality ("goose cough"); hoarseness, weakness of the voice or complete aphonia (evidences of pressure against the left recurrent laryngeal nerve); and dysphagia, due to impingement against the esophagus. In cases of luetic aneurysm, the patient is also likely to suffer from angina and paroxysmal dyspnea, a consequence of the luetic aortitis which caused the aneurysm.

Objective Symptoms. Dilated superficial veins on the chest, the neck or the arms, edematous areas on the chest wall and often cyanosis are evidence that large veins in the chest are being compressed. The pupils of the eyes may be unequal because of pressure against the cervical sympathetic chain.

Tracheal tug is due to adhesions between the sac and the trachea. The pulses at the two wrists will differ markedly if the aneurysm impedes the blood flow into the left subclavian artery. An abnormal pulsation usually can be seen on the chest wall over the aneurysm, and occasionally the sac itself protrudes as a tumor under the skin, which means that it has eroded through the ribs.

Diagnosis. The diagnosis of most aneurysms is made readily on fluoroscopic examination, which reveals a pulsating tumor. Nevertheless, mediastinal tumor, lung tumor and enlarged mediastinal lymph nodes occasionally are difficult to exclude. In such cases a positive serologic reaction is a great help.*

* A more accurate diagnosis is made by injecting radiopaque solution into the heart or the aorta. This angioaortogram permits a visualization of the vessels and of the aneurysm.

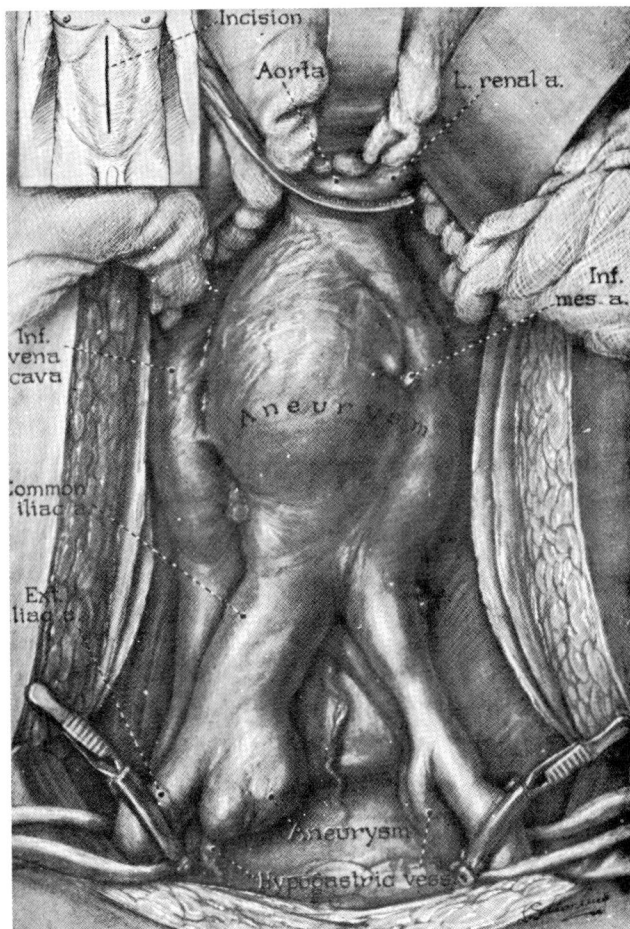

Fig. 191. Aneurysm of the abdominal aorta as seen at laparotomy. (Bahnson, Henry: Considerations in the excision of aortic aneurysms, Ann. Surg. **138**:381)

Treatment. The prognosis for the patient with an advanced aneurysm is poor, and death from the serious effects of compression or from rupture is inevitable without treatment. However, with modern surgery it is now possible to remove the aneurysm and restore vascular continuity. Aneurysms of the aortic arch are the most complicated and difficult to treat (Fig. 190).

Aneurysm of the Abdominal Aorta

This aneurysm (Fig. 191) presents a palpable mass with a definitely expansile pulsation, produces a constant, severe, boring pain and causes a number of other pressure symptoms as well. The pressure of the pulsatile mass may erode the vertebral bodies. Untreated, the eventual outcome is rupture

and sudden death. Medical treatment has nothing to offer these patients.

Surgery for aneurysm of the abdominal aorta is rapidly becoming the accepted method of treatment. When time permits, the aneurysm is outlined by injecting into the aorta a radiopaque dye (aortogram). The roentgenogram taken after the injection shows the size and the extent of the aneurysm. Surgical excision of the section of the aorta involved in the aneurysmal disease is carried out with replacement of the excised segment by a homograph or an artificial Dacron vessel (Fig. 192). This type of surgery is not always successful because most of the patients are in the older age group and the vascular tract is widely diseased in addition to the area of aneurysm. However, since

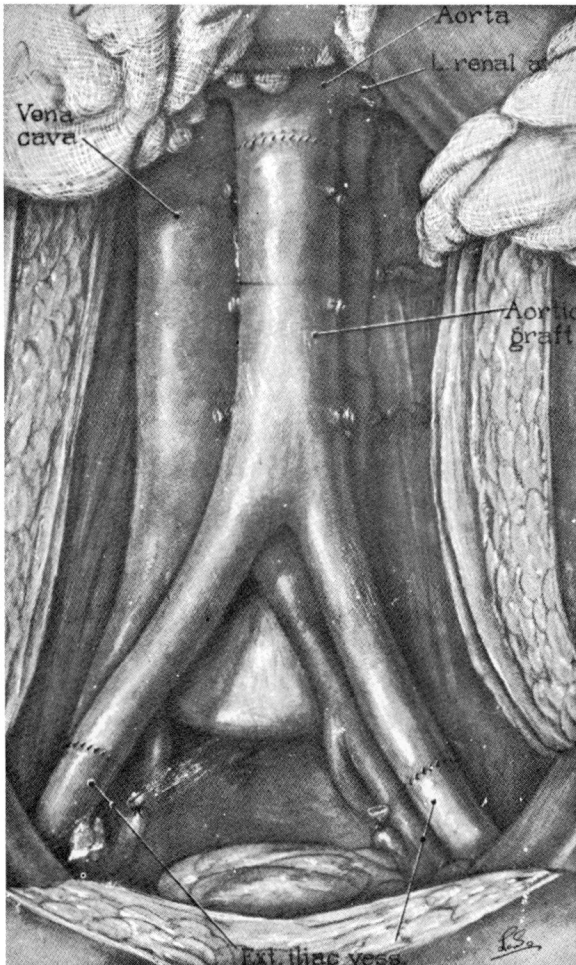

FIG. 192. The aortic homograft has been sutured to the aorta just below the renal arteries and to the two external iliac arteries. (Bahnson, Henry: Considerations in the excision of aortic aneurysms, Ann. of Surg. **138**:382)

no other treatment offers any benefit, the patient is compelled to take the risk. Surgeons even are attempting to remove recently ruptured aneurysms. It is understandable that the risk is much greater in such patients and the prognosis less favorable.

Dissecting Aneurysm of the Aorta

On rare occasions an aorta diseased by arteriosclerosis develops a tear in its intima. This permits blood to dissect its way into the substance of the aortic wall. This wall then may be split apart by the blood, which of course is under pressure, with the resultant formation of a large hematoma in the wall, the layers of which may be ripped apart for a considerable distance. Such dissection leads to compression and occlusion of the arteries branching from the aorta in the area involved by the process. The rip occurs most commonly in the region of the arch. The dissection of the aorta may progress backward in the direction of the heart, closing off the mouths of the coronary arteries and leading to hemopericardium. Or, it may extend in the opposite direction, causing occlusion of the arteries supplying the gastrointestinal tract, the kidneys, the spinal cord and even the legs. This is one of the most catastrophic accidents that can involve the cardiovascular system, and recovery from it is rare. It is diagnosed on the basis of signs and symptoms closely resembling those of coronary occlusion (p. 520), but with signs in addition due to multiple occlusions of the aortic branches. In this type of aneurysm, as well as in cases of the syphilitic variety, a definitive diagnosis is made by aortography.

Surgical Therapy. Although the prognosis is not good, the lives of many patients with dissecting aneurysms of the aorta may be saved by excising the aorta involved in the aneurysm and replacing the segment of vessel with a Dacron graft (Fig. 193).

Aortic Thrombosis (Leriche's Syndrome)

Gradual occlusion of the abdominal aorta and the iliac arteries was first described by Leriche and has been recognized in recent years by the injection of radiopaque dye into

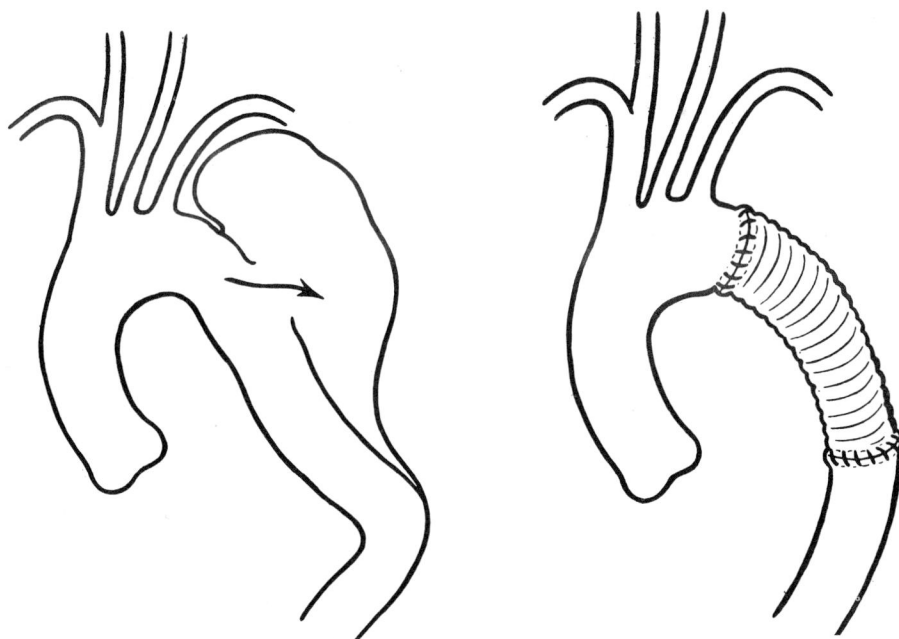

FIG. 193. *(Left)* Drawing illustrating location and extent of dissecting aneurysm. *(Right)* Drawing illustrating method of treatment by excision and graft replacement. (DeBakey, M. E.: Changing concepts in vascular surgery, Figs. 16C and 16F, J. Cardiov. Surg. **1**:3-44)

the aorta (aortography). This occlusion of the distal aorta is more common in men and results occasionally from an embolus but more often from gradually increasing arteriosclerotic changes in the lower portion of the aorta. The symptoms occur characteristically in early middle age; because of the poor circulation in the extremities, there is extreme fatiguability in the lower extremities and loss of sexual function. Atrophy of the lower extremities is a late symptom.

Treatment consists of excision of the diseased portion of the aorta, with replacement of this area by a graft.

THE PATIENT IN CONGESTIVE HEART FAILURE

The majority of patients with heart disease sooner or later display the combination of symptoms and signs that we recognize as the syndrome of congestive heart failure. The manner of its onset, its predominant features and its course vary considerably from one individual to another, depending on the nature of the cardiac disorder, the clinical status of the patient and the factors that have led to its occurrence. There are many possible predisposing factors: for example, the myocardium may have been subjected to severe and prolonged strain as a result of systemic or pulmonary arterial hypertension or due to the presence of valvular disease. On the other hand, the myocardium may have been weakened by the advent of an acute myocarditis, an arrhythmia, or a myocardial infarct.

The clinical manifestations of congestive heart failure stem primarily from 3 major alterations of circulatory dynamics, derangements that are common to most of these patients: (1) the cardiac output is diminished to the extent that vital organs no longer are profused adequately with arterial blood, their oxygen and nutritional requirements fail to be met and they suffer from deprivation; (2) the pulmonary vascular bed no longer is emptied efficiently by the left atrium and ventricle, with the result that the pulmonary vessels become engorged, pulmonary hypertension develops, and pulmonary edema may supervene; (3) blood returning to the heart from the periphery is not dispatched onward into the pulmonary vessels rapidly enough to avoid congestion in the systemic veins and venules; the venous pressure rises, the liver and other organs become congested and fluid escapes through the walls of engorged capillaries to form dependent edema and ascites.

When the blood supply to the kidneys is reduced, glomerular filtration is decreased, and tubular reabsorption increased, with the result that excessive amounts of sodium and water are retained in the body. This is the situation in congestive heart failure, renal blood flow becoming diminished in these patients as a consequence of a reduction in cardiac output. Moreover, the abnormal tendency to retain water is exaggerated through the action of aldosterone, an adrenal hormone that enhances tubular reabsorption of sodium and therefore promotes the formation of edema. Production of this hormone is increased in patients with congestive heart failure. Impairment of renal blood flow eventually leads to other and more serious abnormalities of kidney function, as evidenced by albuminuria and azotemia (nitrogen retention, or uremia).

Pulmonary engorgement impairs respiratory efficiency and is responsible for dyspnea in these patients. In the ambulatory patient, breathlessness is most severe at night after he has retired. It is at this time that his blood volume, already somewhat excessive, will have been further augmented by edema fluid reabsorbed from the legs, and will be at its maximum. His venous pressure is maximal and pulmonary congestion is most extreme. This sequence of events is responsible for attacks of so-called "paroxysmal nocturnal dyspnea." In addition to dyspnea, the patient in failure is likely to cough a good deal, and may even experience hemoptysis. However, the most dramatic and most dangerous complication of pulmonary congestion is pulmonary edema, discussed on page 545.

Failure of the systemic venous blood to be propelled with normal rapidity into and through the pulmonary circulation results in an increase in the systemic venous pressure and venous stasis. Peripheral edema forms, owing to the escape of fluid from engorged capillaries and venules. The liver and other splanchnic organs become congested, and ascitic fluid may accumulate, following venous hypertension and vascular engorgement.

Splanchnic congestion impairs the appetite and promotes gaseous abdominal distention. Consequently, nutrition suffers and tissue substance is lost, although weight loss may be obscured by the edema.

Impairment of cerebral blood flow and reduced oxygenation of the arterial blood together explain some of the neurologic complications of congestive heart failure, including symptoms of physical exhaustion and undue fatigue, difficulty in mental activity, impairment of memory, excessive drowsiness (or insomnia), and even hallucinations and delirium.

Heart failure does not necessarily involve both ventricles simultaneously, or equally. For a time one of these may perform far below its normal level of efficiency, while the other remains relatively unaffected. Whether the right or the left ventricle is affected earlier depends on the nature of the circumstances responsible for the failure. For example, with the advent of congestive heart failure in a patient with arterial hypertension, whose left ventricle has been subjected to undue strain for many years, the left ventricle loses its efficiency earlier and to a greater extent than does the right. As long as this disparity exists, more blood is delivered into the pulmonary circulation by the right ventricle than is removed by the left, with the result that the patient experiences symptoms of pulmonary congestion and is a candidate for the development of pulmonary edema. This is the situation in so-called "left ventricular failure."

When the strain is imposed predominantly on the right ventricle, as in patients with long-standing pulmonary disease and pulmonary hypertension, the output from the right ventricle is reduced before that of the left, and to a more marked degree. The manifestations of failure under these circumstances will be most prominent in the splanchnic area and the distal extremities, appearing in the form of dependent edema, hepatic engorgement and ascites, i.e., the picture of "right-sided failure." Failure of either ventricle is followed inevitably, and within a brief period of time, by equal impairment of the other.

Management of Congestive Failure

The basic objectives in the treatment of patients with congestive failure are (1) to reduce the cardiac load by lessening the tissue demand for blood and by eliminating factors that tend to stimulate cardiac activity unnecessarily; (2) to reinforce the action of the heart, improving its effectiveness as a pump and thereby delivering more blood to the tissues; and (3) to eliminate the excessive accumulation of body water.

Rest

If the cardiac load is to be decreased, it is essential that the patient have both physical and emotional rest. Rest lessens the tissue demand for oxygen, and for the supply and the removal of metabolites in general. The patient may be impressed by the importance of this therapeutic approach when he hears that each day of complete rest spares the heart approximately 25,000 contractions.

Body Alignment. In order to secure proper rest, the body should be in proper alignment. A semirecumbent position, with a pillow placed longitudinally under the back, is restful. Moreover, in this position the venous return to the heart and the lungs is reduced, pulmonary congestion is alleviated, and impingement of the liver on the diaphragm is minimized. A footboard should support the feet in order to avoid footdrop. The lower arms should be supported with pillows to eliminate the constant pull of their weight on the shoulder muscles, which is very tiring. The orthopneic patient may sit on the side of his bed with his feet propped up on a chair, his head and arms resting on an over-the-bed table, and his lumbosacral spine supported by a pillow. The patient with pulmonary congestion rests comfortably in an arm chair, a position that is especially advantageous because it tends, more than any other, to reduce the shift of fluid from the periphery to the lungs. The patient who spends the entire day in an armchair finds that lying in bed with his head elevated provides a welcome change at night.

Hygienic Care. Although, during the acute stage of congestive failure, a partial bath may suffice and may be the extent of bathing permissible, a full bath each day is to be preferred as a source of relaxation and as a circulatory stimulant.

The nurse must be ever conscious of the fact that prolonged immobility, combined with the presence of tissue edema, favors the development of decubiti. Nursing measures to forestall this complication include frequent massaging of the skin with emollient lotions, the placing of foam rubber wedges under bony prominences and areas of tenderness, and placing the patient on an alternating pressure pad mattress.

Promoting Sleep. Patients in congestive failure are unusually prone to be restless and anxious at night. A quiet, well-ventilated room predisposes to sound sleep. To some patients, the presence of a member of the family provides the necessary reassurance. Others are relieved of their anxiety and insomnia by illumination of the bedroom throughout the night. They should be observed repeatedly for possible respiratory arrhythmia, such as Cheyne-Stokes respirations, indicating a disturbance in the function of the respiratory center. If such an arrhythmia is discovered, it may be worthwhile to test the effect of oxygen inhalations, administered briefly each night just before retirement.

Soporific drugs have a definite place in the care of the patient with congestive heart failure and insomnia. Paraldehyde and chloral hydrate are among the safest of the soporific agents, and are as likely as any to be effective. It should be recalled that the patient with hepatic congestion is unable to detoxify drugs with normal rapidity, and should be medicated with unusual caution. As a result of cerebral hypoxia, with superimposed nitrogen retention, he may react unfavorably to soporific drugs, becoming confused and increasingly anxious in response to medication. Such a patient should not be restrained; restraints are likely to be resisted, and resistance inevitably will increase the cardiac load. If he insists on getting out of bed he should be installed comfortably in an armchair. As his cerebral and systemic circulation improve, the quality of his sleep will improve.

Rest is not possible without relaxation. Emotional stress produces vasoconstriction, elevates the arterial pressure and speeds the heart. Relaxation may be secured by avoiding situations that tend to promote anxiety and agitation. Patients who are particularly prone to be tense should be maintained in a less reactive, even drowsy, state, in order to eliminate any emotional stimuli that would exact unnecessary and undesirable demands on the heart.

Pain of cardiac origin is relieved effectively by one or more tablets of nitroglycerine placed under the tongue, or by inhalations of amyl nitrite. Theobromine sodium salicylate and aminophylline are of value in some cases.

Digitalis Therapy. In order to strengthen the heart, digitalis or another cardiac glucoside of comparable type may be prescribed. The effect of these drugs is to increase the force of systolic contractions and, if atrial fibrillation is present, to slow the ventricular rate (see page 510). The usual dosage schedule specifies the administration of 1 unit of digitalis every 6 hours until a physiologic level is attained. The full dosage of this preparation is usually 1 unit per 10 pounds (5 kg.) of body weight. If the cardiac failure seems severe, the initial doses may be as much as 8 units, 6 hours apart, until the full therapeutic effects of digitalis have been obtained, or such toxic effects of this drug, such as depression, nausea or disturbances of heart rhythm, e.g., bigeminal pulse, appear. Later, a daily maintenance dose of 1 unit is given. Digitoxin, of which 0.1 mg. is equivalent to 0.1 Gm. (1 unit) of digitalis, may be prescribed in lieu of the latter.

Diet

The optimum diet for most patients with congestive heart failure is low in bulk, caloric value, fat and sodium. The average patient in this group, being somewhat overweight and relatively inactive, can subsist quite satisfactorily on a low-energy diet. Since abdominal distention elevates the diaphragm and interferes with respiration, gas-forming foods should be avoided. Small, frequent feedings are perferable to large bulky meals for the same reason. However, the most important consideration with respect to the diet is its sodium content, for the amount of sodium in the body determines the degree of its hydration; restriction of sodium intake is the key to success in the prevention and treatment of over-hydration, or edema. The diet prescription should specify the precise weight of sodium that may be ingested each day, usually 500 to 600 mg. in contrast with 2 to 4 Gm., which is the average daily intake of a normal individual on an unrestricted diet. (Modification of the normal diet for sodium restriction is demonstrated in Table 5, page 150.)

The patient must be taught the purposes and the principles of sodium restriction, equipped with food tables listing items of low sodium and high sodium content and given specific instructions regarding the use of these tables. Merely to supply vague generalizations on the subject of meal planning will only serve to de-emphasize its importance. Obviously, before the nurse can consider herself in a position to impart this instruction to her patients, she herself must possess a reasonable knowledge of the subject.

Diuresis

If edema is not controlled adequately by sodium restriction and digitalization alone, one or more diuretic drugs may be prescribed. Widely used for this purpose is chlorothiazide (Diuril). Aldactone (spironolactone), a drug that specifically blocks the action of the hormone aldosterone (see page 840), is an effective oral diuretic agent that is given in average daily adult doses of 400 mg., especially when used in combination with Diuril or one of the organic mercurial diuretics. Inherent in its diuretic action is the tendency of Aldactone to cause potassium retention, because of which it must be used with caution, or withheld, in patients with elevated blood-potassium levels (hyperkalemia). The organic mercurial drugs promote the urinary excretion of sodium, and therefore water. Certain of these, for example, Neohydrin, are effective by mouth; others, like Mercuhydrin, must be given intramuscularly, subcutaneously or intravenously. As much as 3,000 to 5,000 ml. of urine may be excreted in response to a single mercurial injection. As a basis for evaluating the effectiveness of therapy, patients receiving diuretic drugs should be weighed daily at the same hour, and these measurements should be entered in the permanent hospital record.

A voluminous diuresis entails many voidings in rapid succession, which may prove quite taxing for the sick patient. In order to minimize fatigue and conserve his energy the patient who is debilitated or very ill should be assisted on and off the bedpan, and between voidings his sacrum should be supported with a pillow or a foam rubber wedge.

Before diuretic therapy is commenced, the possibility of a urinary tract obstruction must be excluded. The elderly male patient should be treated with special vigilance, inasmuch as the incidence of urethral obstruction due to prostatic hypertrophy is high among such individuals. Signs of bladder distention should be sought routinely by palpation of the abdomen in the midline, just above the symphysis pubis.

Large and repeated diureses can lead to potassium depletion. This poses new problems for the cardiac patient, for among the complications of hypokalemia are marked weakening of cardiac contractions and the precipitation of digitalis toxicity in individuals receiving digitalis, thereby increasing the likelihood of a dangerous arrhythmia (see page 510). To lessen the risk of hypokalemia and its attendant complications, patients receiving diuretic drugs should also be supplied with potassium salts as a supplement.

Regulation of Fluid Intake. The total amount of fluids should be limited, since an excess of water, unless the sodium intake is restricted carefully, is retained in the body, increasing the edema and adding to the burden of the heart. The daily total volume of all fluids ingested, which should be measured and charted, in general should be from 1,500 to 2,000 ml. in 24 hours. The patient may become interested in recording the amounts of fluids ingested. This may help him to restrict liquids and permit adequate spacing of fluid intake during the course of 24 hours. On a low sodium diet, the cardiac patient may be allowed water in excess of this amount, even 3 L. and more, since without sodium to hold it in the tissues it is rapidly excreted through the kidneys. In fact, water, in the absence of sodium chloride, often acts as an excellent diuretic. The fluid intake is regulated best to correspond to the urine output, fluids for each day being calculated on the basis of the total urinary excretion for the previous 24 hours. Charting of the fluid balance daily, together with daily weighing of the patient (at the same time), is an excellent and simple way of determining the progress of the cardiac and renal function (Fig. 194). In this way, the tendency to water retention, which indicates increased cardiac insufficiency or renal failure, is recognized early; and, similarly, diuresis, indicating improvement in the function of these systems is estimated quantitatively.

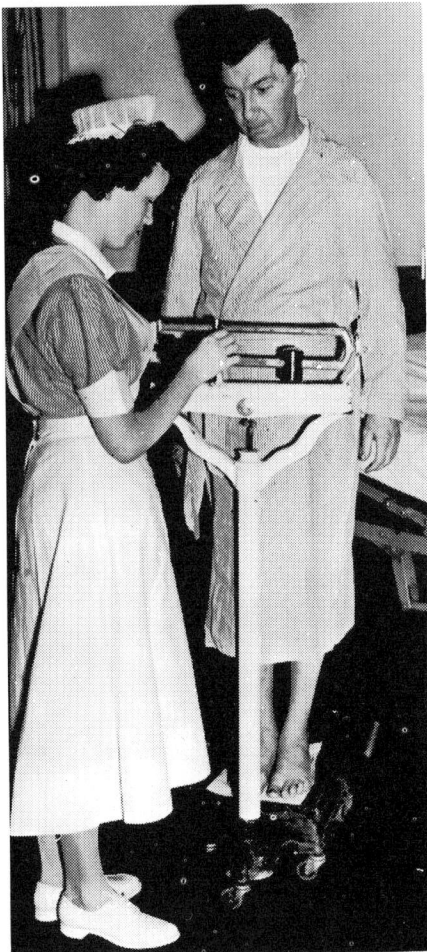

Fig. 194. The body weight of the patient with cardiac, renal or hepatic disease should be measured and recorded at the same time daily, for it serves as an accurate reflection of his fluid balance and provides important information with respect to his clinical progress.

Evacuation. The bowels are kept as nearly empty as possible of gas as well as solids by the use of such cathartics as compound licorice powder, cascara and mineral oil. The importance of this is twofold; it aids in the elimination of water from the intestine and facilitates the passage of stools. Straining at stool involves considerable muscular effort which, for these patients, may prove to be very dangerous.

It often happens that patients with lesser grades of cardiac decompensation are kept in bed too long and kept much too quiet. Also, that after a prolonged stay in bed, the severe cases are not re-educated carefully and deliberately enough to physical activity. The patient with fever, of course, should remain quietly in bed until his temperature remains normal, but for those without fever, there are definite advantages in allowing mild exercise. This exercise, however, should be planned carefully. At first it is ideal for the patient, lying flat on his back or propped up in bed, systematically to engage in free-arm and free-leg movements. Later, he is allowed to sit in a chair and then to walk for increasing distances. Mild exercise improves muscle tone and aids in venous return. The pulse response to sitting up and walking is observed carefully and recorded in the nurse's notes.

Mental Diversion. This aspect of treatment is especially important in patients who have experienced a complete reversal of mode of life, from normal strenuous activity to almost complete inactivity for an appreciable period of time. The patient's interests must be distracted from his own fears and symptoms, which are apt to be alarming enough, and projected into the surrounding environment. As his strength improves and more activity is permitted, he should be encouraged to become increasingly self-reliant and to perform whatever functions, such as eating, bathing and reading, as seem possible and desirable. These activities in themselves usually are diverting enough, at least for a time. Other and more pleasurable pursuits also should be made possible, such as access to a radio or television set, a library and equipment for some creative project; and new interests should be cultivated, the possibilities for which are endless.

Prevention. Careful child health examinations in school in the presence of the parent, with careful follow-up, will lead to early discovery of heart lesions. Care for these children may be provided in special classrooms. The family case method of study of rheumatic fever patients has been a new and useful technic in medical centers.

The economic loss to the community and to the individual as a result of heart disease is tremendous. It is felt that perhaps some of this loss may be prevented by the careful management of patients in the early stages of the disease. Many forms of heart disease do not prevent patients from anticipating years of usefulness to themselves and to society if they follow a mode of living within their cardiac reserve.

The child will have problems of adjustment to make as he returns to school. Exercise and the pressure of school work may be fatiguing, and careful planning by parents, teachers and all responsible persons is necessary. Some states have Vocational Rehabilitation counselors assigned to work primarily with cardiovascular patients. An adult guidance service attempts to estimate vocational possibilities.

THE PATIENT WITH ACUTE PULMONARY EDEMA

Pulmonary edema represents the ultimate stage of pulmonary congestion, in which fluid has leaked through the capillary walls and is permeating the airways, giving rise to dyspnea of dramatic severity. Pulmonary congestion, it will be recalled, comes about when the pulmonary vascular bed has received more blood from the right ventricle than the left can accommodate and remove. The slightest imbalance between inflow on the right and outflow on the left side of the heart may have drastic consequences: for example, if with each heartbeat the right ventricle pumps out just one more drop of blood than the left, within the space of only 3 hours the pulmonary blood volume will have expanded 500 ml.!

Most patients with pulmonary edema have chronic heart disease of a type that imposes a strain preponderantly on the left ventricle, such as arterial hypertension or aortic valvular disease. The development of this complication signifies that cardiac function has become grossly inadequate. Terminally the pulmonary capillaries, engorged with an excess of blood which the left ventricle has been incompetent to disgorge, no longer are able to retain their contents. Fluid, first serous and later bloody, escapes into the adjacent alveoli, through the communicating bronchioles and bronchi and thence, mixed with air and churned by respiratory agitation, out of the mouth and the nostrils, producing the ominous "death rattle."

But death from pulmonary edema is by no means inevitable. If appropriate measures are taken, and taken promptly, many attacks can be aborted, and many patients will survive this complication to benefit from measures directed against its return. Fortunately, pulmonary edema usually does not develop precipitously, but is preceded by the premonitory symptoms of pulmonary congestion. Moreover, even after it has become well established it usually does not progress to a fatal termination with lightning rapidity; its course may occupy a period of many minutes, even hours, during which treatment may prove to be effective.

The typical attack of pulmonary edema occurs at night after the patient has been recumbent for a few hours. Recumbency increases the venous return to the heart and favors the resorption of edema fluid from the legs. The circulating blood becomes diluted, and its volume expands. The venous pressure mounts and the right atrium fills with increasing rapidity. There is a corresponding increase in the right ventricular output, which eventually surpasses the output from the left ventricle. The pulmonary vessels become engorged with blood, and proceed to leak. Meanwhile the patient has been increasingly restless, oppressed with anxiety and unable to sleep. His complexion is grey; his hands are cold and moist; his nail beds become cyanotic. He has been coughing incessantly and producing increasing quantities of mucoid sputum. As his pulmonary edema progresses his anxiety becomes more acute. He is confused, then stuporous. He breathes noisily and moistly, nearly suffocated by the blood-tinged frothy fluid which now is pouring into his bronchi and trachea. He literally is drowning in his own secretions. The situation is precarious and demands immediate action.

Treatment

The prime objectives of therapy, simply stated, are the following: (1) to reduce the right atrial inflow of systemic venous blood; and (2) to increase the left ventricular outflow.

To retard the venous return to the heart, i.e., the right atrial inflow, the patient is placed in the near-upright orthopneic position, head and shoulders up, feet and legs down, thus favoring the pooling of blood in dependent portions of the body. As long as, and to the extent that, blood accumulates in the periphery, correspondingly less blood returns to the heart. An attempt is made to reduce the blood volume and increase the oncotic pressure of the blood (hence render it less susceptible to leakage) through dehydration and, to this end, diuretics are administered in the form of Mercuhydrin or Diuril injections, or both.

Phlebotomy. One of the most effective means available for lowering the venous pressure, hence reducing the venous return to the heart, is the rapid withdrawal of from 500 to 700 ml. of blood from a peripheral vein (i.e., a phlebotomy, or venesection). The resulting decrease in venous return is accompanied by a corresponding decline in the right ventricular output. Accordingly, the pulmonary artery pressure drops, the pulmonary vessels become less congested and the lung capillaries, no longer congested, reabsorb the fluid that has escaped. The

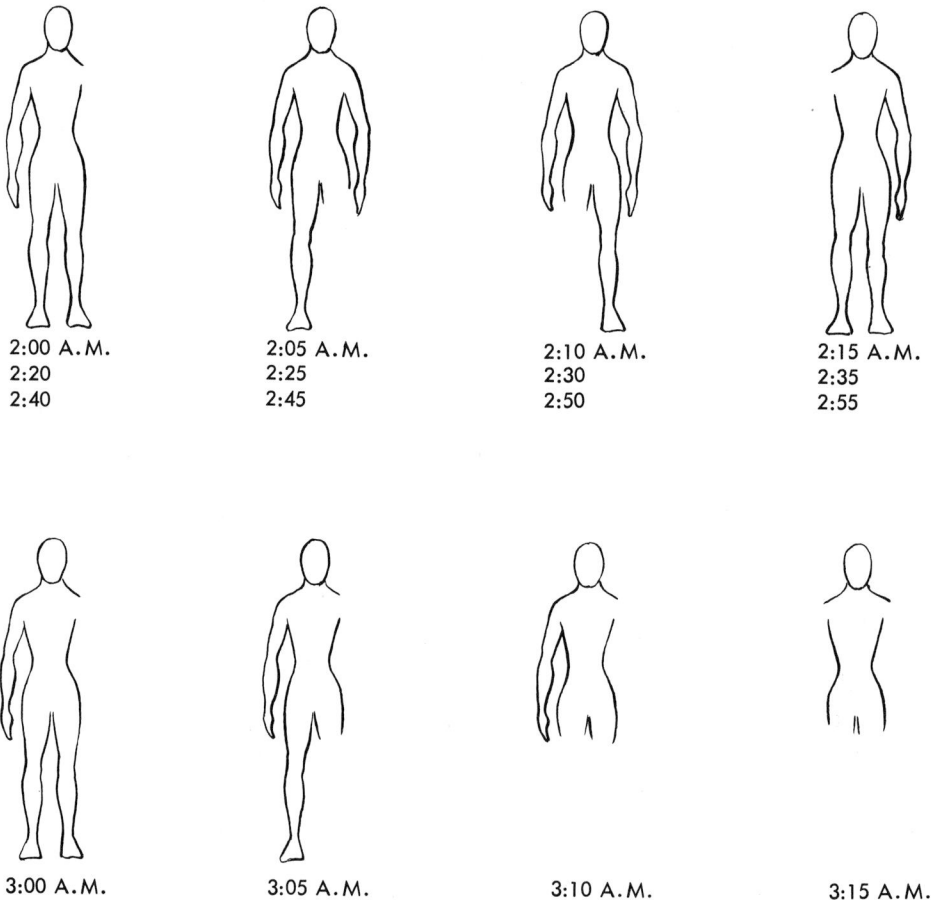

2:00 A.M.   2:05 A.M.   2:10 A.M.   2:15 A.M.
2:20   2:25   2:30   2:35
2:40   2:45   2:50   2:55

3:00 A.M.   3:05 A.M.   3:10 A.M.   3:15 A.M.

Fig. 195. Rotating tourniquet technic. Timing of compression and release of extremities and the sequence of rotation and sequence of removal of tourniquets during a course of tourniquet therapy which was prescribed for 1 hour starting at 2 A.M.

edema clears; the immediate danger has passed. The efficacy and technical simplicity of phlebotomy commend its use in the management of pulmonary edema of all types. All that is required is a standard blood donor set, a supply of which should always be readily available to the clinical staff, plus a reasonable familiarity with its use. The only important contraindication to this procedure is the presence of marked anemia.

Rotating Tourniquets. Another therapeutic measure that achieves essentially the same objectives as does phlebotomy consists in the production of venous stasis in the extremities by either applying tourniquets or inflating pneumatic cuffs around the upper arms and legs, the immediate effect of which is equivalent to removing about 1,000 ml. of circulating blood. Ideally, 4 sphygmomanometer cuffs are employed for this purpose since these permit the regulation of compression precisely as desired: i.e., to a point slightly above the level of diastolic pressure. In lieu of cuffs, 4 rubber tubes (2 feet long, with an outside diameter of ⁵⁄₁₆ to 1½ inches) may be used; these are tightened sufficiently to cause venous congestion without obliterating the arterial pulse. If this procedure is to be accomplished safely and with maximum benefit the tourniquet tension on every extremity and on every application must be correct. Moreover, the timing of their application and release must adhere rigidly to a schedule which insures that 3 of the 4 extremities are compressed and 1 is free at all times throughout the procedure; that no extremity is compressed continuously for periods of longer than 15 minutes; and that no less than 5 minutes shall intervene between consecutive periods of compression applied to the same extremity. The proper routine is depicted in Figure 195. The 15 minute limitation on continuous stasis, and the specification regarding periods of release, are intended to reduce the risks of phlebothrombosis and fatal pulmonary embolism, to which patients in congestive heart failure are uniquely predisposed and which are increased decidedly as a result of the injudicious application of tourniquets. Patients who are to receive this treatment should be reassured as to its nature and purpose; otherwise, they are certain to be disturbed by the attending discomforts and alarmed by the cyanotic discoloration of their congested extremities. The multiplicity of duties and activities involved in tourniquet therapy is sufficient to engage the full attention of one individual, and the importance of the procedure is such as to warrant its assignment as the sole responsibility for the time being of one member of the team.

Oxygen. Oxygen may be administered by tent or by mask—the mask permitting delivery of the gas under slight positive pressure and possibly more effectively. Because of their relatively low density and viscosity, helium-oxygen mixtures are breathed with less effort than 100 per cent oxygen or oxygen diluted with atmospheric air; hence, they may be employed to advantage in the treatment of pulmonary edema. If the respiratory passages are obstructed by foamy edema fluid, the oxygen may be bubbled through 95 per cent ethyl alcohol or 2-ethyl-hexanol, which exert an antifoaming action.

Drugs. In order to improve the contractile force and increase the output of the left ventricle the patient is digitalized, as described on page 542. In addition to strengthening the heart action, steps are taken to reduce to a minimum those factors that tend to stimulate cardiac output. Morphine is given subcutaneously, intramuscularly or intravenously in 15 to 30 mg. doses to relieve anxiety, pain and dyspnea. It must be realized that dyspnea per se involves a great deal of muscular effort, and from the standpoint of pulmonary ventilation is a most unrewarding activity. Thus, the more rapid and shallow the respirations become, the more oxygen is consumed by the respiratory muscles, whereas this type of breathing contributes very little more, if any, to the oxygenation of the blood than does the slower, quieter and deeper type of respiration. A reduction of the respiratory rate is one of the important objectives behind the administration of morphine. Excessive respiratory depression, on the other hand, is a complication to be guarded against and watched for carefully in patients receiving that drug.

Allaying of Anxiety. This is a most important consideration in treating patients with pulmonary edema, a cardinal feature of which is basic, primitive fear—fear that is self-intensifying and that tends in itself to intensify the severity of the condition. Apropos of the patient's apprehension and need for reassurance, the nurse must never forget that her patient, however oblivious to his surroundings he may appear, nevertheless may be capable of perceiving and responding to actions, words and appearances that to him represent either a favorable omen or are of ominous significance, to which many a recovered patient can testify. She must not be too quick to assume that he no longer is eligible for, or capable of benefiting from, her reassuring words and acts.

Prevention

As in the case with most medical and surgical complications, pulmonary edema is easier to prevent than to treat. Thus, if recognized in its early stages when the presenting symptoms and signs are solely those of pulmonary congestion, the situation may be corrected by relatively simple measures. These include: (1) vertical positioning of the patient to restore ventricular balance; (2) digitalization to improve myocardial efficiency, and, (3) the elimination of exertional and emotional stress to reduce the left ventricular load. The long-range approach to the prevention of pulmonary edema must be directed at its precursor, namely, pulmonary congestion, the prevention of which depends on the lightening of this load by a variety of means which have already been discussed—including the prevention of overhydration and elimination of edema, the curtailment of physical activity, the correction of obesity and the control of arterial hypertension, if present. Surgical valvuloplasty, presently to be discussed, may be performed to eliminate or to compensate for valvular defects that limit the flow of blood into or out of the left ventricle, thereby impairing the cardiac output and predisposing the patient to the development of pulmonary congestion and edema.

A final point, and one that is especially important in relation to the role of the nurse in this prophylaxis, concerns the problem of iatrogenic (physician-produced, or therapeutically induced) pulmonary edema precipated by the administration of parenteral fluids too rapidly or in too great a volume. Intravenous infusions tend to elevate the venous pressure and increase the venous return. Given injudiciously to patients with little or no cardiac reserve, such injections readily initiate pulmonary edema. Accordingly, when intravenous fluids are given to elderly patients, or to patients with known cardiac disability, they should be administered at a slow, measured rate, the recipient having been placed and supported in the orthopneic position and kept under close observation throughout the procedure.

CARDIOVASCULAR SURGERY
Historical Survey

Surgery of the heart has made rapid strides in the last decade; however, experimental work was reported at the beginning of the 20th century. In 1896 Rehn reported the first successful repair of a lacerated right ventricle. In 1923 Cutler, Levine and Beck performed the first selective surgery for mitral stenosis, and in 1938 Dr. Robert Gross did the first ligation of a patent ductus arteriosus. The excision of a coarctation of the aorta and reconstruction by primary anastomosis was performed successfully by Dr. Gross in Boston and Dr. Crafoord in Stockholm in 1945. Dr. Charles P. Bailey did a successful mitral commissurotomy in June, 1946. Dr. Alfred Blalock and Dr. Helen Taussig of Baltimore improved the circulation of "Blue babies" (the problem of tetralogy of Fallot) by shunting the blood into the pulmonary circulation after anastomosing the right subclavian artery to the right pulmonary artery. Dr. William Potts modified this technic by anastomosing the left pulmonary artery to the aorta.

Operations were being performed around the heart, but intracardiac surgery was impeded because there was no means for working within the heart in a dry field. Finally, in 1952 Floyd John Lewis, in Minneapolis, used hypothermia to close the first atrial septal defect by direct approach. It is known that if the heart stops for about 4 minutes and oxygenated blood is not pumped to the

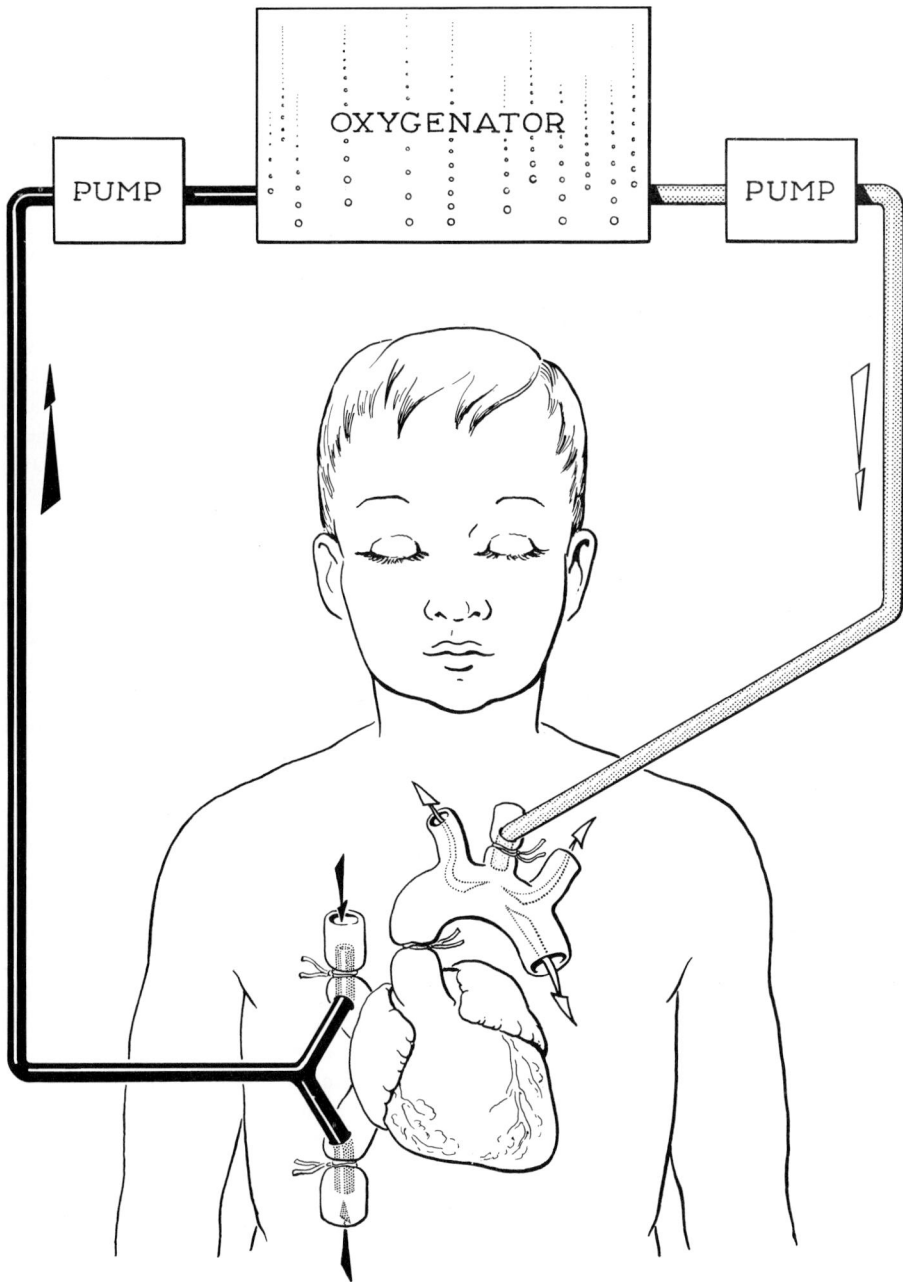

FIG. 196. Diagrammatic drawing to show the use of a pump oxygenator in operations upon the heart. Blood is collected from the inferior and the superior venae cavae and drawn through a pump into the oxygenator, which is a substitute for the lung. Then it is pumped into the lesser circulation, into the aorta. Thus the systemic circulation is maintained while the blood flow through the heart is shut off. This enables operations on the heart such as repair of intra-atrial and intra-ventricular defects.

brain at normal temperatures, the patient will suffer irreparable brain damage. If the patient's general temperature is lowered, the length of time which the brain can be deprived of oxygenated blood can be prolonged to about 8 minutes without such damage. However, the difficulty with hypothermia is that when the patient's temperature gets down to about 80°F., the likelihood of ventricular fibrillation is great. The correction of this is relatively easy in the warm heart, which has no abnormalities, but in abnormal cooled hearts, restoration may be very difficult. What was still needed was a pumping device to take over the functions of both heart and lungs for as long as was necessary to operate. After many years of work, John Gibbon of Philadelphia used a "heart-lung" machine in 1953 during an operation to repair an atrial septal defect; the pump oxygenator worked for 26 minutes during surgery.

The "heart-lung" machine is being refined, simplified and popularized. Meanwhile, C. Walton Lillehei, of Minnesota, developed the ingenious idea of using a donor, especially the father, for a child, to perform as a heart and lungs to do the work of the patient during the operation. However, this risks two lives instead of one.

Whereas early "heart-lung" machines oxygenated the blood by a process known as "filming" (letting it run thin over a flat surface), De Wall suggested bubbling oxygen through the blood and defoaming it to get rid of excess bubbles. The De Wall oxygenator is one of the most popular. Some surgeons still refuse to use "bubbled" blood because of the possibility of introducing an air embolus into the circulatory system.

Open-heart surgery can now be done successfully, employing the "heart-lung" machine. To prevent the heart from beating and moving during surgery, potassium citrate is injected into the atrium after the "heart-lung" machine takes over its function. Following surgery on the heart, blood flows through, washing out the chemical, and the heart resumes its beat spontaneously.

Heart surgeons can now correct an impressive number of defects, including patent ducts, coarctation of the aorta, aortic aneurysms, atrial and ventricular defects, and scarred, leaking and stenosed heart valves.

The most common of all heart defects continues to defy the surgeon's efforts: reduced or blocked blood flow through the coronary arteries. Claude Beck has attempted to restore blood supply by irritating the pericardial sac, by scraping it with an abrader or dusting irritant asbestos powder into the sac. Hufnagel revived an operation (first done by an Italian surgeon about 20 to 30 years ago) which consists of cutting and tying off both mammary arteries, thus shunting blood over into the coronaries. In 1956 Bailey attacked the problem of the diseased coronary arteries by reaming out the diseased portion.

Aids to Open-Heart Surgery

The scope of intracardiac surgery has been limited in the past by the inability to visualize lesions inside the chambers of the heart. The use of hypothermia, the pump oxygenator and a variety of available grafts has made this kind of surgery possible. The nurse can best appreciate these contributions by understanding how they are used.

Hypothermia. With the use of technics which lower body temperature, the amount of anesthetic agent can be reduced, the danger of surgical shock lessened and the time that such vital organs as the brain and the spinal cord can be deprived, without damage, of their blood supply can be lengthened; also, blood loss is reduced. The disadvantages of hypothermia are cardiac standstill or ventricular fibrillation, which are difficult to correct when the patient has been cooled. For this reason cardiac hypothermia is used less frequently since the advent of the pump oxygenator.

Pump Oxygenator ("Heart-Lung" Machine). The pump oxygenator takes over the functions of the heart and the lung during surgical intervention on the heart. By diverting venous blood (coming into the right atria via the superior and the inferior venae cavae) into the oxygenator, providing the means of oxygenation of the blood and pumping it back into the arterial system via the femoral or the subclavian artery, the heart-lung machine achieves the functions of these major organs of the body (Fig. 196).

An anterior thoracotomy incision is made by entering the 3rd or the 4th intercostal spaces, and the pericardium is incised. Tape tourniquets are passed about the superior and the inferior venae cavae, and plastic catheters are inserted, through which blood is drawn into the pump oxygenator. Into the right or the left femoral artery in the groin, a catheter is passed upward into the iliac artery for the return of oxygenated blood from the machine into the circulatory system.

Two types of pumps are in use and several kinds of oxygenators. The process of oxygenating the blood may be done by filming, bubbling or by a membrane interphase. Most methods will provide satisfactory oxygenation and carbon dioxide elimination.

After the heart is emptied of blood, usually potassium citrate is injected to arrest the beat. The heart may be open for periods up to 60 minutes; however, most defects can be repaired in less than 15 or 20 minutes.

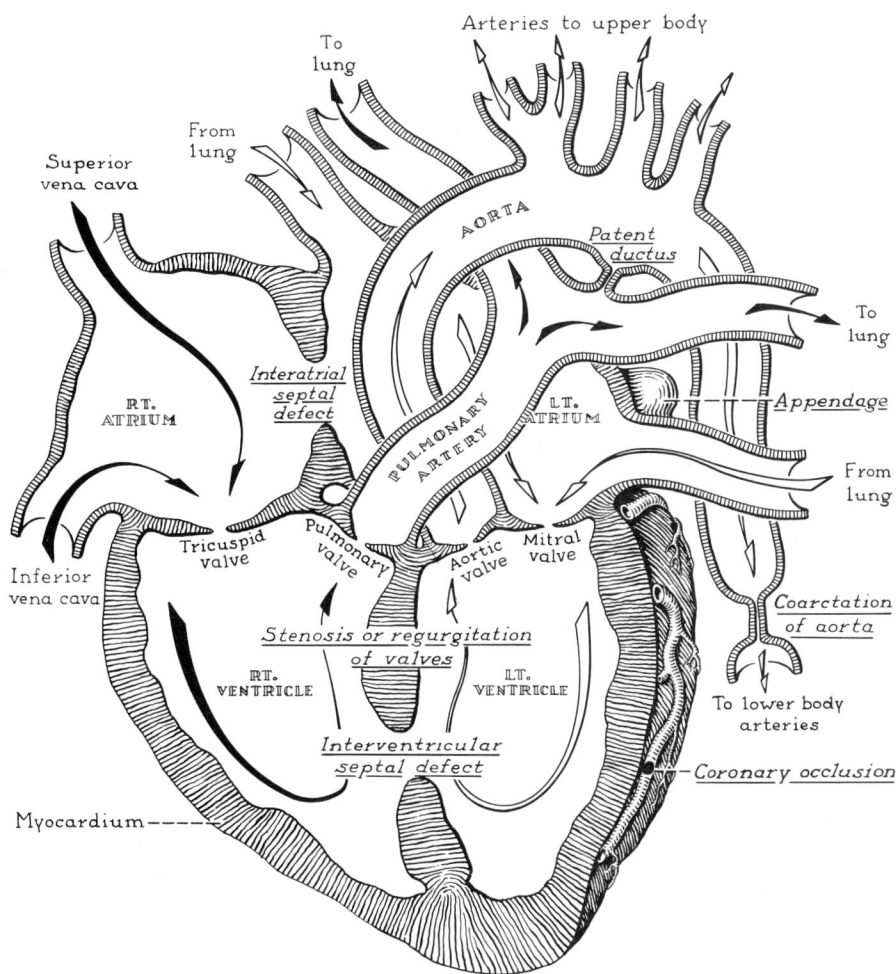

FIG. 197. Diagrammatic drawing showing heart and large vessels and the various defects which might be treated surgically. The defects which require surgical therapy are described in the text. The heart has as a prime objective the propulsion of an adequate volume of blood through two systems, the pulmonic and the systemic. The flow through these two systems must be balanced exactly, since any disequilibrium results in the accumulation of fluid on one side or the other.

Grafts. By grafts, one usually means blood-vessel grafts. At the turn of the century, a femoral artery was replaced by a femoral artery of another person. Viability of a graft was thought to be important, but this is no longer true. A blood vessel may be obtained for use as a graft under sterile or unsterile conditions. If unsterile, it may be sterilized by radiation, ethylene oxide or a chemical disinfectant.

A graft may be preserved by freezing it very rapidly to avoid damaging it and then drying it by drawing out all the moisture in a vacuum. A freeze-dried graft may be kept in a sealed container for several years. When it is needed, the graft is dropped into a saline solution, where it soon becomes flexible, pliable and similar to its original state.

Today grafts are available as tubes and patches made of polyvinyl (Ivalon) sponge, Vinyon, nylon, Orlon and Dacron.

Classification of Heart and Great Vessel Surgery

I. Intracardiac Surgery
   A. Congenital conditions
      Pulmonary stenosis
      Tetralogy of Fallot
      Tricuspid stenosis
      Septal defects—atrial and ventricular
   B. Surgical treatment of acquired heart conditions
      Trauma
      Inflammation
      Mitral stenosis
      Mitral insufficiency
      Aortic stenosis
      Aortic insufficiency
   C. Cardiac standstill and resuscitation
II. Surgery of the blood vessels
      Patent ductus arteriosus
      Coarctation of the aorta
      Aortic aneurysms
      Aortic thrombosis (Leriche's syndrome)
      Splenorenal and portacaval anastomosis

Surgery for Congenital Heart Disease

This term may describe some defect in the development of this organ or a prenatal lesion resulting from endocarditis acquired during intra-uterine life. Persons thus afflicted are not numerous, since the majority of babies born with heart lesions soon die, but a few survive even to adult life.

Anomalies due to defective development of the heart are numerous in variety. Some affect its position only. In some persons, the heart lies in the right instead of the left half of the chest (dextrocardia). Such abnormalities in position may affect the heart and the large blood vessels only, or all the viscera of the abdomen also may be inverted (situs inversus). Such persons may be quite healthy.

Defects in the development of the heart itself are much more serious. In general, each of these represents the persistence of some feature normal to this organ at some stage of its development. The most common of these defects is an open ductus arteriosus.

Open Ductus Arteriosus (Fig. 198). Normally in fetal life the ductus arteriosus is open between the pulmonary artery and the arch of the aorta, such being essential to life in utero. This should close soon after birth but, if closure does not occur, the patient usually will show signs of its abnormal existence in the form of retarded or seriously restricted growth, hypertrophic heart, a subsequent streptococcic endocarditis and, at times, aneurysmal dilatation, embolus and so forth. To prevent these occurrences, the duct may be closed by suture or ligature. The best time for such a ligation is between the ages of 4 and 12. In recent years the trend has been toward division of the ductus, which when done by a skillful surgeon is relatively easy and safe. The surgical approach for this must be through the chest and the pleural cavity; therefore, all preoperative, operative and postoperative nursing precautions for chest surgery must be observed.

Pulmonary Stenosis. This is a congenital narrowing of the pulmonary artery at its exit from the heart. It leads to an inadequate flow of blood through the lungs. The treatment is to enlarge the opening so that there is an adequate blood flow from the right heart to the lungs.

Tetralogy of Fallot. When pulmonary stenosis is accompanied by a defect of the interventricular septum, a shift of the aorta to the right side and a hypertrophy of the right ventricle, the condition is called *tetralogy of Fallot*. Children so affected are spoken of as *blue babies*.

Clinical signs of *tetralogy of Fallot* are cyanosis and "clubbing" of fingers, a heart of normal size, a murmur at the base, and no pulmonic second sound. Exercise tolerance of the individual shows marked variation. Operation is indicated when the primary difficulty is lack of circulation to the lungs, and cyanosis.

Two methods now are used in the treatment of tetralogy of Fallot. The Blalock and Taussig method of directing blood to the lungs is by an anastomosis between the pulmonary artery and one of the aortic branches, such as the left subclavian, the left common carotid or the innominate. The Potts method is a direct anastomosis between the aorta itself and the pulmonary artery. This will increase the flow of blood through the lungs and relieve the cyanosis. Results of surgery are very satisfactory. The color becomes pinker, the blood becomes thinner, the "clubbing" of fingers and toes begins to

disappear, and the patient becomes stronger and more active.

Septal Defects. The walls (septa) separating the atria and the ventricles of the heart also are subject to congenital defects that can be corrected often by surgery.

ATRIAL DEFECTS. The clinical picture presented by the patient with an atrial septal defect is variable. Inhibition of growth, dyspnea, limitation of activity and systolic murmur may be apparent in large septal defects. Cardiac catheterization is the most reliable technic for making a final diagnosis. A large defect usually will lead to progressive cardiac enlargement, increased pulmonary flow and eventual right heart failure.

The repair of atrial septal defects is to close the opening extending between the right (venous) and the left (arterial) sides of the heart. This may be done in various ways. At times, it may be done by suturing a part of the heart wall into the hole; in other instances, by entering the heart and directly closing the opening by suture or by the use of a patch of plastic material sutured into place to close the hole.

VENTRICULAR DEFECT. In the patient with this defect, the flow of blood is from left to right because of higher pressure in the

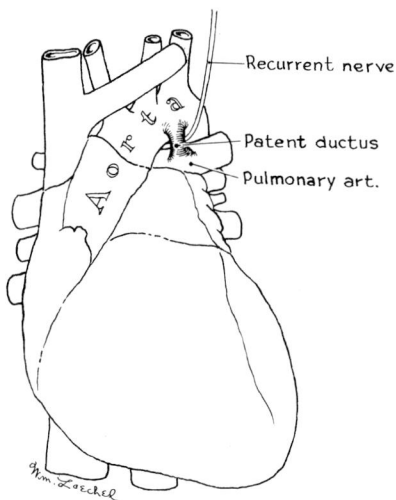

FIG. 198. Diagrammatic drawing of the heart and the great vessels, showing patent ductus arteriosus. This is a congenital communication between the aorta and the pulmonary artery. It closes as a rule. However, when it remains open, often it is necessary to close it surgically.

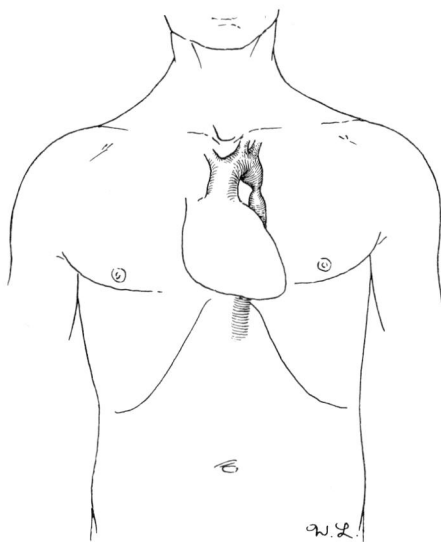

FIG. 199. Diagrammatic view to show the narrowing of the aorta in the usual position found in coarctation of the aorta.

left ventricle; hence, the patient is not cyanotic. The chief symptom appears to be a loud systolic murmur over the base of the heart. Cardiac catheterization is the most conclusive diagnostic procedure. The treatment obviously is to close the defect; however, this has been far from satisfactory by the closed method. With open-heart technic, the technical problems will no doubt be overcome.

Coarctation of the Aorta. About one fourth of all patients affected by this congenital narrowing of the aorta live relatively normal lives; however, most patients begin to show symptoms as they approach adolescence. Hypertension is noted in the upper extremities and lower pressure in the lower extermities, often so low that a pulse is not palpable in the vessels. The chief difficulty is that as such an individual grows older, extreme hypertension can occur in the upper part of the body, causing headache, cerebrovascular accidents, rupture of the aorta and death. The life expectancy at birth of a patient with coarctation of the aorta is estimated at 32 years or less.

This condition, which occurs twice as often in males as in females, can be corrected surgically in one of two ways. The coarctation can be removed, and the two ends of the vessel can be anastomosed. At times, this is impossible because of an inelastic aorta or because the defect may involve a long section of the aorta. In these patients, it is necessary to use a graft. The ideal time for surgery is from ages 8 to 16. Before the age of 8 the vessel is too small, and after 16, degenerative changes begin to take place in the arterial walls.

CARDIOVASCULAR SURGICAL NURSING

Cardiovascular surgical nursing is challenging, dramatic and demanding. Progress in recent years has been great. Whereas many patients will be remarkably improved by an operation, many other patients, for one reason or another, will not be eligible for surgery. It is important for the nurse to recognize that, as in any other kind of surgery, the patient is evaluated and treated on an individual basis. Many of these patients know much about heart disease and their own history; therefore, it is necessary for the nurse to be well informed in order to interpret, teach and care for her patient in keeping with his needs.

Observation of the patient is perhaps even more important in cardiovascular nursing than in other clinical areas. By knowing the patient preoperatively, she will know his habits, his preoccupations and interests, his activity limitations, his worries and the place he assumes in his family. She will recognize changes in mood and personality shifts. Circulatory and respiratory changes often occur rapidly; therefore, the nature and the effect of such signs and symptoms must be reported accurately and intelligently to the physician.

Auditory as well as visual signs may be significant. A change in the character of breathing may be heard, or a "different" sound may be detected as the nurse listens with a stethoscope against the patient's chest. In this kind of nursing, it is essential that she become familiar with heart-and-lung sounds; any opportunity which presents itself for her to "listen" with a stethoscope should be seized. The sense of feeling is another important avenue of perception. The rhythm and the nature of the pulse elicited in places other than the wrist have clinical value.

Socioeconomic aspects are major considerations which are reflected in the care and the treatment of the cardiac surgical patient. Usually, he has had a long medical history leading up to the decision that perhaps surgery can help. He may have consultations, travel some distance to a cardiac surgical clinic and have preliminary checkups prior to his admission to a hospital, where at least 2 weeks are spent undergoing various diagnostic tests. This is costly. Then the decision is reached regarding the treatment of choice. If it is surgical, aside from the usual charges, the patient may need at least a dozen pints of blood for the "heart-lung" machine, special medications which are varied and expensive, intensive nursing care for at least the first 5 postoperative days and many roentgenograms and laboratory studies. Upon discharge from the hospital, it is not uncommon for the patient to be asked to stay at a nearby hotel within walking distance of the cardiac clinic for about a week, during which time additional evaluation is done, and more concrete individual advice is given regarding future activity of the patient. Health insurance may cover a part of the financial burden; however, much must be assumed by the patient and his family.

The concern, the support and the value of the family must never be minimized in the early or long-range plans for the individual patient. The nurse is in a strong position to assist the patient-family relationship as she teaches, interprets, encourages and understands their many problems.

Preoperative Care

Only those aspects of nursing care which are unique to the cardiovascular surgical patient will be mentioned. (The principles outlined in Part I of this text would obtain throughout.)

Regardless of the publicity and the frequency with which heart surgery is being performed today, the individual about to face such an operation is worried and concerned. He needs to know that he is in competent hands. Meeting his emotional and spiritual needs is a vital part of his preparation; his postoperative progress depends on it.

In addition to diagnostic tests, the preoperative cardiovascular patient will have complete blood studies and chest roentgenograms. He will have his blood pressure taken and the apical-radial pulse rate noted every 4 hours; he is also weighed daily. This is done in order to establish a base line or guide as to the level at which these indices are normal for each particular patient. As for the dietary regimen, he may be on a restricted sodium diet, depending upon the degree of congestive failure. Depending on his needs, his diet is planned to achieve optimum nutritional levels. The need for diuretics and digitalis are evaluated at this time.

Preoperative Instruction of the Patient

1. **Mouth Care.** Good mouth hygiene must be emphasized in order to minimize the number of pathogenic organisms in the respiratory tract.

2. **General Hygiene.** Daily bathing is essential; many preoperative cardiac patients have edema; therefore, a clean healthy skin is necessary to prevent tissue breakdown. Nails should be trimmed; if nail polish is

used it should be colorless, since cyanosis and capillary fluctuation may not be detected with opaque polish. Likewise, makeup should not be applied the day of surgery, so that skin color changes may be noted more readily.

3. **Coughing and Deep Breathing.** These activities are extremely important for proper aeration of the lungs postoperatively. The patient should be encouraged to practice coughing effectively by (1) taking a deep breath, (2) tightening the stomach muscles and (3) exploding the cough.

This may be the ideal time to acquaint the patient with the use of the respirator (Bennett, Dotco or whatever type is used in the local hospital) in anticipation of the possible need for positive-pressure or intermittent-positive-pressure breathing (p. 435) postoperatively.

4. **A planned "talk"** about what to expect postoperatively, such as the reason for chest tubes, oxygen therapy, fluid and drug therapy, turning and so forth, is given informally and individually to each patient. This will help greatly in the postoperative period. At this time, any questions the patient might have are answered or referred to the physician, the social worker or the person who can supply the answer.

Immediate Preoperative Nursing Care

Over and above the routine immediate preparation, the wrists and the ankles may be shaved in anticipation of a "cut-down." This is performed early on the day of surgery; a plastic catheter is used to cannulate the vein, and a blunted 15-gauge or 18-gauge needle is used to connect the plastic tube to the intravenous set. A "cut-down" is done so that easy access to a vein may be always present.

A nasogastric tube may be inserted before surgery to prevent abdominal distention and nausea postoperatively. Before administering the preoperative medication, a record should be made of the patient's blood pressure, temperature, pulse and respiration. Any unusual change in these signs should be reported to the surgeon. A Foley catheter may be ordered for insertion into the urinary bladder; this may be done after the patient is anesthetized.

Postoperative Care

In general, all postoperative patients who have had heart and great vessel surgery are cared for in the same manner as chest surgical patients, with the possible exception of the coronary artery surgical patient. When it is realized that death resulting from heart surgery occurs more frequently in the first 48 hours postoperatively and not on the operating table, the nurse will be impressed by the necessity for expert and effective care.

Vital Signs. The apical-radial pulse, blood pressure and respiration are taken every 5 to 10 minutes until stable, usually for 6 to 8 hours. It is important to keep the blood pressure at desirable levels to prevent irreversible shock and damage to the heart, the brain, the kidneys and the liver. Postoperative care of patients with mitral or aortic commissurotomy tolerate lowered blood pressures such as 80 or 90 without ill effects. However, should the systolic pressure fall below 80, it may be necessary for the physician to administer neosynephrine or some other vasopressor drug.

If hypotension persists, a thrombus may be blocking a graft or anastomosis site. Other problems that may result from hypotension are cerebral ischemia, myocardial infarction and renal shutdown.

The blood pressure of patients who have had coronary artery surgery (revascularization surgery) must be watched more closely. Their blood pressure ought to be maintained not lower than 10 points below the preoperative level.

With an increase in blood pressure, the anastomosis or graft may disrupt. Pain or activity may cause an increase in pressure and should be controlled by medication. A safe range in blood pressure is from 20 mm. above to 20 mm. below the normal systolic reading.

Volume and rhythm of pulse should be noted as well as the rate. Pulse irregularity must be reported, since it may be indicative of fibrillation and subsequent cardiac arrest.

It is important in the immediate postoperative period to check the peripheral pulse because of the hazard of peripheral emboli, particularly in patients who have had mitral valve surgery.

However, there are patients whose peripheral pulses are not expected immediately postoperatively, and this information should be made known to the nurse by the surgeon. Peripheral pulses need not be counted but simply verified as to their presence. Check points are the temporal artery, the radial artery, the posterior tibial artery and the dorsalis pedis artery. If these pulses are not detected, check the next proximal pulse.

The physician should be notified of any temperature over 102° F., inasmuch as this causes extra work for the heart. Lower temperatures ranging from 94° to 97° F. ought to be reported also, since this may indicate shock or cardiac decompensation. In raising body temperature, an electric blanket may be used at the request of the surgeon; hot water bottles should *not* be used.

General Observation. Cyanosis must be watched for and corrected. The lighting in the unit should allow for optimum observation of nail beds, lips and skin. Blanching or mottling in the extremities may indicate embolic phenomenon, especially when accompanied by numbness, tingling, loss of motion and/or pain. Report the least suspicious sign to the physician at once.

Venous distention of the neck may be noted as the patient regains consciousness. This results from straining due to chest pain, discomfort and even the presence of the endotracheal tube; eventually, it will disappear.

Check surgical dressings, especially posteriorly, for signs of hemorrhage or constriction.

Maintaining Patency and Function of Equipment. This includes the intravenous infusion, nasogastric tube connected to its suction machine, Foley catheter attached to a drainage tube and bottle, and proper function of the water-sealed chest drainage. Two Kelly clamps should be available near the water-seal drainage equipment to be used in the event of accidental disconnection. (These are discussed in more detail on pp. 412, 557.)

Maintaining a Patent Airway

Retained Secretions. This is a common problem in thoracic and cardiac postoperative surgical patients. Signs include apprehension, perspiration, rapid pulse, dyspnea, cyanosis, a "wet" cough, if any, and wet noisy respirations. A steady rise in temperature and pulse is often a sign of retained secretions and, possibly, of atelectasis. If secretions are not removed, atelectasis and cardiac failure result; this is inexcusable.

Coughing must be done in such a way that secretions down deep are brought up and expelled. The nurse can assist the patient by splinting the chest with her hands or arms. It has been found helpful to support the upper abdomen when encouraging the patient to cough. If secretions cannot be brought out in this way, endotracheal suctioning must be done. At times it may be necessary to perform a bronchoscopy or a tracheotomy.

Aerosol therapy using a mucolytic agent such as Isuprel* also aids in the removal of secretions. Sadove states that "through its surface action wetting characteristics and its thinning action Isuprel aids in the control and elimination of secretions. With supersaturation the secretions are maintained liquid and the cilia can function more efficiently with greater ease of movement of the less viscid secretions; therefore, secretions may be brought to the area where they can stimulate the cough reflex and be eliminated. The cough reflex is more effective on these thinned and watery secretions and the pain and trauma of the paroxysmal bouts of coughing are reduced."

Positioning and Turning. Usually, the patient is kept flat in bed until the systolic blood pressure is over 100 mm. Hg. Before the head of the bed is raised, the blood pressure should be taken and repeated 5 minutes after the new position is assumed. If the blood pressure has dropped, lower the patient and wait for at least 30 minutes before elevating again.

Patients who have had mitral, aortic or congenital heart surgery, usually may be turned from side to side every 2 hours and placed in semisitting position; however, check with physician for individual specific orders. Postoperative coronary artery surgical patients are usually kept quiet on their backs for 48 hours. Turning these patients even 15° may cause a marked drop in blood

* Winthrop Laboratories, Inc.

Emergency Cart

To provide immediate care for the patient in the first minutes of respiratory or cardiac collapse or of severe hemorrhage, a freely movable table which contains the following items should be located within easy access to postoperative cardiovascular patients:

Portable oxygen tank with equipment for administering oxygen
Hand-operated resuscitator (bellows)
Intravenous and "cut-down" tray with plasma expander and other prepared solutions
Tracheostomy set containing an assortment of tracheostomy tubes
Tray containing emergency drugs, sterile syringes and needles
Defibrillator and pacemaker equipment
Emergency instrument tray for thoracotomy in event of cardiac arrest— sterile gloves
Bronchoscopy set and battery box
Laryngoscope

---

pressure. After 48 hours, they may turn from the back to the right side every 2 hours. Patients who have had mammary artery implants are never turned to the left side, because of interference with lung expansion and the possibility of herniation of the heart from its pericardial sac.

The bed never should be elevated at the knees without a written order from the surgeon. Such a position after surgery on the descending aorta or vessels of the legs may produce thrombosis by inhibiting the flow of blood through the lower extremities.

Oxygen Therapy. For ease of ventilation of the lungs, oxygen is given by face mask at 8 liters per minute until the patient has fully reacted. Then oxygen by oropharyngeal catheter is administered at approximately 6 liters per minute. Proper positioning of the tube is important as well as frequent cleaning of the tube.

Drainage Systems

Water-sealed Drainage. A catheter is introduced through a stab wound in the lower part of the chest. An extension of this catheter with its distal end placed under a fluid level will permit excess air and fluid to drain from the pleural space but will allow nothing to re-enter. Another reason for chest drainage is to maintain subatmospheric pressure in the pleural cavity. The drainage bottle must be secured at the side of the bed, and a clamp must be available at all times to close the tube near the chest wall in the event of accidental disconnection of tubing or suction bottle.

Watch for excessive drainage of blood. It is usual to expect 400 to 500 ml. of serosanguineous drainage in 24 hours, following mitral commissurotomy, and up to 1,200 ml. in 24 hours for mammary artery implant. If there is no drainage, fluid may be accumulating in the thorax, with ultimate cardiac embarrassment.

For valvular surgical patients, drainage tubes usually are removed in 24 hours. Patients with mammary implants retain their drainage tubes longer.

To prevent clots from forming in the tubes, they are milked or stripped as necessary. This may be done by hand or with an especially designed chest tube stripper (Mueller).

A suggested method of noting the amount of drainage in a given period of time is to place an inch-wide strip of adhesive tape vertically on the drainage bottle. A line is drawn on the tape at hourly intervals to indicate the level of drainage at that time.

Gastrointestinal Nasosuction (Wangensteen). A common occurrence with postoperative cardiac surgical patients is paralytic ileus. Often as a result of trauma to the vagus nerve during surgery, there is a temporary inability of the stomach to empty properly, and gastric dilatation results. For patients who have had surgery for coronary artery insufficiency, the stomach must be kept deflated to relieve pressure on the heart and help to prevent angulation of the implanted artery; this may occur when the heart is pushed upward by a distended stomach. For these reasons, gastrointestinal suction is used.

Pointers on General Postoperative Care

Pain. Patients have a considerable amount of chest pain postoperatively, due mostly to rib retraction during surgery. Demerol Hydrochloride (50-100 mgm. every 3 to 4 hours) is given during the first 24 to 48 hours after surgery. The patient must be evaluated carefully so that enough medication may be given to keep him fairly comfortable and yet not more than is necessary, which would depress him generally and his cough reflex specifically.

The nurse is challenged to keep the patient as comfortable as possible by changing his position, supporting dependent parts, splinting his chest as he coughs, etc., before resorting to narcotics. When such medications are used, less than the average dose is given; the patient is observed for undue depressant effect. Narcotic antagonist drugs are available (Lorfan and Nalline) should this occur.

Thereafter, it is advisable to decrease the amount and the frequency of sedation and attempt to determine the cause of restlessness if possible, such as oxygen want, fear, position discomfort and so forth.

Diet—Fluids. Fluids are given as soon as tolerated; they should not be too hot or too cold, for this may set up cardiac irregularities. Since fruit juices cause nausea, omit them in the beginning. A return to soft and normal diet is done as soon as the patient wishes. The one exception is the surgical patient who has had coronary-artery surgery. Food should be postponed until abdominal cramps and the passage of gas have passed.

The nurse should be aware that cardiac patients may exhibit unusual thirst and drink large quantities of fluids. In instances of fluid retention, it may be necessary to restrict fluid intake. Since fluid balance in the cardiac patient is of extreme importance, all fluid intake and output must be recorded. Also, it may be necessary to weigh the patient daily.

Postoperative Exercises. Deep breathing is encouraged to ventilate and expand the lungs. It is carried out deliberately, slowly and quietly through the nose. The patient must not become overtired. After the first 24 hours, patients are encouraged to move. A "pull" can be made from a double thickness of muslin (approx. 3 yds. long and 4" wide). By doubling this to form a loop which is placed around the foot end (center) of the bed, the ends can be drawn through the loop, thereby securing it. The ends serve as a "pull" for the patient; these can be tied together in a knot to facilitate grasping.*

Patients have a tendency toward left shoulder pain which will result in "a frozen left shoulder" unless combated vigorously throughout the postoperative period. These patients must be urged to move their left shoulder freely, starting soon after operation. This does not mean passive motion by moving their left arm with their right arm. It means active motion of left hand—combing hair, reaching for various objects, buttoning neck buttons and so forth.

When surgery has not involved the lower extremities, leg exercises (flexion and extension) should be performed every 2 hours postoperatively.

Medications. Antibiotics are given routinely postoperatively to help prevent infections. Such therapy is usually maintained for 10 to 12 days in order to minimize any tendency for reactivation of rheumatic fever. Vitamin supplements are added as soon as solid food is tolerated. Digitalis may or may not be ordered, as determined by the cardiologist. Quinidine is usually given to convert atrial fibrillation to normal sinus rhythm.

First Postoperative Day. A portable upright chest plate is taken to determine the rate of lung expansion and to detect fluid collection, pneumothorax or emphysema.

A hematocrit, a red blood count and a hemoglobin test are done to indicate the degree of blood loss during surgery. Also, a routine urinalysis is done.

Complications. Although the first 48 hours are most critical, it is several days before the patient has really passed the danger point. The usual complications are: (1) *respiratory:* hypoxia, respiratory failure, pneumothorax, atelectasis, (2) *circulatory:* hemorrhage, arterial insufficiency, (3) *renal shutdown.* In addition, there may be problems of fluid imbalance, muscle spasm, hiccup, pain, worry and apprehension. Each of these discomforts or complications have been described in Chapter 18. The nurse caring for a patient who has had heart surgery needs to be aware that these problems can occur; she is in a position to detect early symptoms and to ward off major difficulties by prompt attention and action.

Psychological Aspects. On the whole, patients who have had explanations preoperatively and an opportunity to talk out their fears, anxieties and concerns seem to make a better adjustment to the postoperative phase of their treatment.

States of depression in the postoperative cardiac patient have ranged from mild, transient depression to a full-blown depression with suicidal tendencies. Those patients with transient personality changes resulting from their reluctance to leave the shelter of a "cardiac life" require special understanding and support. For varying lengths of time, these people have been sick and have held the center of attention in the family circle. After surgery, a weaning process must start.†

Convalescence

From the 5th to the 8th days, the patient may be allowed to dangle his feet, then gradually be allowed out of bed until full mobilization is reached by the 12th to the 14th day. This is determined by the physician on an individual basis.

* We have made an exercising rod which helps the patient to strengthen his arms and chest muscles and, at the same time, permits him to raise himself to a sitting position in bed. The exerciser is made by drilling a hole through the center of an 8-inch piece of broom handle. Through the hole we thread and tie one end of a piece of clothesline, 50 inches long, then tie its other end to the foot of the bed in the center. The rod-piece is kept near the patient so that he can grasp it. He uses both hands or one and then the other, to pull himself up. Sister M. Xavier, R.N., Saint Luke's Hospital, New Bern, N. C. (Trading Post—American Journal of Nursing), **55:**1092, 1955.

† Bolton and Bailey studied 1,500 patients in an attempt to determine if there were some particularly characteristic preoperative elements which would be of significant help in predicting the likelihood of patients' developing postoperative psychoses. Results: There seems to be no relationship to sex, age, severity of heart disease, duration of failure, or complications of surgery which would lead to cerebral ischemia. However, postoperative psychoses occurred more frequently in cases of acquired heart disease which had a dynamically significant mitral insufficiency. Bolton, H. E., and Bailey, C. P.: Psychosomatic Aspects of Cardiovascular Surgery *in* Cantor, A. J., and Foxe, A. N.: Psychosomatic Aspects of Surgery, p. 40, New York, Grune, 1956.

Tests are done on the day prior to discharge for comparison with the preoperative studies and with future studies. Changes can be noted that are indicative of the success of the operative procedure. These tests are also useful in determining future medical treatment, the nature of activities and the type of diet.

Instructions for Convalescence
*After Operation**

Patients, regardless of the ease with which they tolerate surgery, should set aside a minimum of 8 weeks for convalescence. This period should be devoted to the recovery of strength depleted by the previous illness and the rigors of hospitalization.

During the first week exercise is limited to walking for short periods in the morning and the afternoon. This should be done on level ground in the home or outside for 15 or 20 minutes. Shorter periods are advised if fatigue develops. Stair-climbing is permitted, but since this requires a greater output of energy, it should be done slowly and only when necessary.

The remainder of the waking day is spent out of bed and in relaxing activities such as reading, painting, knitting, writing or speaking with visitors. A nap after the noon meal is beneficial. Showers or tub baths may be taken from the start. It is necessary to avoid drafts and to keep warm in order to prevent respiratory infections; 10 hours of sleep is the minimum requirement, and it is wise to retire before 11 o'clock.

After the first week, exercise is more liberal. Walking can be continued for longer periods. Regular rest will prevent unusual fatigue. Patients may enjoy a leisurely drive, although they should refrain from doing their own driving for several weeks.

Usually, an unrestricted diet is prescribed. Meals are to be ample, eaten with leisure and followed by a half hour of relaxation. In instances where partial improvement rather than complete cure has been accomplished, continued sodium restriction may be necessary for 3 months, sometimes indefinitely.

At the conclusion of the first 2 weeks of home care, the patient should be able to attend to all his duties without unusual fatigue or difficulty. Shortness of breath and ankle swelling should not be present. Persistence of these complaints requires medical care.

Pain in the area of the incision is common for a varying length of time. Occasionally, the discomfort is a bandlike tightness or numbness. Although an annoying complaint, it is not a serious one and is readily controlled with such simple drugs as aspirin. A gradual subsidence of this distress will be noted after the first several weeks, although damp weather and other climatic changes occasionally cause its return.

It is most important to guard against infection of any type. A common cold may develop into a serious illness if ignored. To prevent upper respiratory infections, avoid fatigue, exposure and direct contact with persons already infected. If, despite these precautions, respiratory infection should occur, bed rest, warmth and prompt medical care must be instituted immediately in a patient with rheumatic heart disease.

A suitable antibiotic must be taken before and after any dental extraction. It is necessary to consult one's physician for the drug of choice before such dental work is undertaken.

A decision to return to a full working status must await a complete evaluation of the patient's cardiac condition. This is generally scheduled at the end of the 8-week period following operation.

Women with household responsibilities have generally undertaken light duties, such as dusting and cooking, prior to the 8-week examination. However, approval for full household duty should await the result of this medical review.

In re-establishing a routine of life, sound habits must be formed. Health cannot be bought with a single stroke of the surgeon's knife. Exhausting routines may wipe out the benefits already won. Sensible adjustments have been made by people of all temperaments and walks of life. Cardiac surgery cannot erase all the consequences of years of illness. It remains for the patient to regulate his life sensibly in order to protect the gains this modern miracle of treatment has made possible.

* Bailey Thoracic Clinic: *Your New Way to Health,* a brochure for patient instruction.

ROLE OF THE NURSE IN PREVENTING HEART DISEASE

In the course of her contacts with patients and their families the nurse is likely to encounter many individuals with cardiovascular symptoms who have not sought, but obviously need, diagnostic, therapeutic or preventive services. As an informed case-finder she will be particularly alert for symptoms of edema and shortness of breath. Whenever she hears an individual blame his exertional dyspnea on a "cold," "too many cigarettes" or "old age," the nurse, who realizes that dyspnea never is normal, will attempt to convince him of the importance of securing immediate medical attention.

The nurse should instruct parents regarding the potential dangers that are associated with tonsillitis and pharyngitis. Were every patient with streptococcal pharyngitis to receive prompt and adequate treatment with penicillin, rheumatic fever would virtually cease to exist. The nurse has an important role in the instruction of patients who have had rheumatic fever, which should stress the purpose and the importance of continuing antibiotic prophylaxis for an indefinite period of time.

How may the nurse be an effective case-finder for congenital heart disease? It is important that she serve in this role, for by so doing she can make a major contribution to its early diagnosis. Early diagnosis is the key to the successful treatment of congenital heart disease, which is most likely to be accomplished by early surgery: i.e., surgery carried out before the patient develops pulmonary hypertension. With the school nurse and the public health nurse continually on the lookout for children who become cyanotic or unduly breathless on exertion, this diagnostic possibility is not likely to be overlooked. Moreover, familiar as she is with the normal patterns of body growth and development, the nurse will be quick to perceive the possibility of congenital heart disease in a child who appears not to be developing normally. Should she encounter an individual who is in the first trimester of pregnancy and has just been exposed to German measles, she should undertake to advise an immediate visit to the doctor for prophylactic injections of gamma globulin, for the evidence indicates that if this particular infection is contracted at this stage of pregnancy the offspring is more likely to be afflicted with congenital defects than otherwise would be the case.

Syphilitic aortitis and aortic aneurysm are preventable. The nurse who participates in the treatment of patients with early syphilis must educate these individuals concerning the potential long-range effects of this infection that are avoidable if the disease is eradicated completely by adequate therapy. She will stress to the patient the desirability of complete cooperation with his physicians throughout the follow-up period, and until such time as he may receive his final discharge from the clinic.

Of course, obese individuals should be encouraged to correct their nutritional status. Weight reduction assumes an over-riding importance for the individual who is overweight if, in addition, he has arterial hypertension or coronary artery disease—and he should be instructed accordingly. Convincing evidence has accumulated that points to an association between cigarette smoking and deaths from the complications of coronary heart disease. Any cigarette smoker with symptoms of angina pectoris or with a history of myocardial infarction should be informed of this relationship in no uncertain terms, and strongly urged to discontinue the use of tobacco forthwith. Whatever success the nurse may have in assisting the patient toward this objective represents an exceedingly important contribution to the prevention of heart disease.

Patients who repeatedly return to their physician or hospital in a recurrent state of cardiac decompensation need continuing re-evaluation and repeated preventive teaching. A detailed description of the previous day's meals should be requested on the occasion of each visit, in order to determine to what extent he has been adhering to his low-sodium diet. Although meticulous about his diet, does he relieve his dyspepsia with antacid powders which contain sodium? Is he keeping track of his weight to detect water retention and help to control edema? These and many other considerations bear repeated discussion. Repetition is essential to the process of learning; it likewise is an important principle in preventive teaching.

CLINICAL SITUATIONS

Coarctation of Aorta

Jake Kessler did not know he had a congenital anomaly of the aorta until a physical examination revealed an unusually high blood pressure (left arm), whereas the pulse in his lower extremities proved to be absent. The 17-year-old high school student submitted to a repair of his coarctation with the consent and the encouragement of his parents.

1. If untreated, coarctation of the aorta may cause
   A. Cerebrovascular accidents.
   B. A fusion of the commissures.
   C. Atresia of the aorta.
   D. Rupture of the aorta.

2. Correction of a coarctation of the aorta can be done by
   A. Anastomosing the pulmonary artery with one of the aortic branches.
   B. Cutting the fibrotic thickened area with a special knife.
   C. Introducing fine wire into the affected area.
   D. Excising the constricted area and repairing the defect with a graft.

3. Postoperative chest pain which persists for some time is an indication that
   A. Surgery has been effective.
   B. Surgery has not been effective.
   C. Postoperative complications are present.
   D. May be disregarded and will disappear.

The Patient With Myocardial Infarction

1. The principal objective underlying the treatment of a patient after a myocardial infarction is to
   A. Lower his cholesterol intake.
   B. Insure a blood supply to the ischemic muscle.
   C. Increase his chlorides and lower his potassium level.
   D. Decrease his cardiac reserve to rest the heart.

2. An acute myocardial infarction requires expert medical and nursing supervision. The outcome of this disease depends on all of the following *except*
   A. The prevention of shock due to loss of body fluids.
   B. The prevention of a continued hypertension.
   C. The capability of injured muscle to recover.
   D. The prevention of complications.

3. A blood test that is useful in determining when physical activity can be increased after a myocardial infarction is (a) (an)
   A. Erythrocyte sedimentation rate.
   B. Prothrombin clotting time.
   C. Blood urea nitrogen.
   D. Blood transaminase.

4. The nursing care of a patient with congestive heart failure should primarily be directed toward
   A. Insuring accurate intake and output.
   B. Supplying adequate nourishment.
   C. Securing optimum rest.
   D. Elevating the edematous extremities.

5. Edema is most effectively controlled in patients with heart failure by
   A. Proper positioning.
   B. Fluid restriction.
   C. Administration of heart depressants.
   D. Restriction of sodium intake.

6. Heart-block often follows an occlusion of the posterior coronary artery. In which area of the heart does this condition originate?
   A. Sinoatrial node.
   B. Bicuspid valve.
   C. Atrioventricular bundle.
   D. Mitral valve.

BIBLIOGRAPHY AND SUGGESTED READING

Books

Bailey, C. P.: Surgery of the Heart, Clinical Symposia, Vol. 10, No. 5, Summit, New Jersey, Ciba Pharmaceutical Prod. Inc., Sept.-Oct., 1958.

Bramwell, C.: A Clinical Introduction to Heart Disease, London, Oxford, 1959.

Committee on Pharmacy and Pharmaceuticals: American Hospital Formulary Service, Hamilton, Illinois, Hamilton Press, Inc., 1961.

Friedberg, C.: Diseases of the Heart, ed. 2, Philadelphia, Saunders, 1956.

Harrison, T. R. (ed.): Principles of Internal Medicine, ed. 3, New York, McGraw-Hill, 1958.

Johnson, J., and Kirby, C. K.: Surgery of the Chest, ed. 2, Chicago, Yr. Bk. Pub., 1958.

Largey, L. B.: Knowledge, understanding and skill necessary to meet the nursing needs of the adult patient who has undergone open-heart surgery, Monograph 3: Technical Innovations in Health Care: Nursing Implications, American Nurses' Association, 1962.

Levine, S.: Clinical Heart Disease, ed. 5, Philadelphia, Saunders, 1958.

Luisada, A. A.: Cardiology: An Encyclopedia of the Cardiovascular System, vol. 3, New York, Blakison-McGraw, 1959.

Mattingly, C. B. (ed.): Cardiovascular Disease Nursing, Washington, D.C., Catholic Univ. America, 1960.

McCombs, R. P.: Internal Medicine, ed. 2, Chicago, Yr. Bk. Pub., 1960.

Modell, W., *et. al.:* Handbook of Cardiology for Nursing, ed. 4, New York, Springer, 1961.

Natof, H. E., and Sadove, M. S.: Cardiovascular Collapse in the Operating Room, Philadelphia, Lippincott, 1958.

Peddie, G. H., and Brush, F. E.: Cardio-vascular Surgery, A Manual for Nurses, New York, Putnam, 1961.

Ritchie, M.: The nurse's responsibility in cardiac arrest, Monograph 3: Technical Innovations in Health Care: Nursing Implications, American Nurses' Association, 1962.

Rhodes, I. B.: Discussion—nursing care for open-heart surgery, Monograph 3: Technical Innovations in Health Care: Nursing Implications, American Nurses' Association, 1962.

White, P. D.: Heart Disease, New York, Macmillan, 1951.

Articles

American Heart Association: Cigarette smoking and cardiovascular diseases, Circulation **22:**160-166, 1960.

Aynes, E. A.: Tetralogy—a study of growing importance, Nurs. Outlook **8:**38-40, 1960.

Bear, A. F.: Aortic aneurysm, Am. J. Nurs. **60:**858-859, June, 1960.

Briggs, L., and Mortenson, J. D.: Nursing care of the patient with a prosthetic heart valve, Am. J. Nurs. **63:**66-70, Oct., 1963.

Closed chest cardiac resuscitation—professional and legal implications for nurses, Am. J. Nurs. **62:**94-95, May, 1962.

Corrie, R., Welsh, J. D., Saeger, Jr., A. L. and Sommer, L.: Comprehensive care for the rheumatic heart patient, Nurs. World **133:**8-11, Feb. 1959.

Crawley, M.: Care of the patient with myocardial infarction, Am. J. Nurs. **61:**68-70, Feb., 1961.

Creighton, H.: The nurse's role in cardiac catheterization, Nurs. World **133:**25-28, Feb., 1959.

Cross, C. J.: Back to work after myocardial infarction, Am. J. Nurs. **62:**58-61, Feb., 1962.

Dean, W.: Measuring venous blood pressure, Am. J. Nurs. **63:**70-72, Oct. 1963.

Elliott, F. C., and Winchell, P.: Heart catheterization and angiocardiography, Am. J. Nurs. **60:**1418-1422, Oct., 1960.

Gazes, P. C. and Boone, J. A.: External or closed-chest cardiac massage, report of two cases, J.A.M.A. **176:**621-622, May 20, 1961.

Hadley, B. J. and Wenhold, B. K.: The private duty nurse teaches cardiac care, Am. J. Nurs. **62:**50-53, Jan., 1962.

Hashim, S. A.: The relation of diet to atherosclerosis and infarction, Am. J. Nurs. **60:**348-352, March, 1960.

Hayter, J.: Acute myocardial infarction, Am. J. Nurs. **59:**1602-1604, Nov., 1959.

Heap, B.: Sodium restricted diets, Am. J. Nurs. **60:**206-209, Feb., 1960.

Keller, M., and Segner, E. F.: When heart and hands are overburdened, Am. J. Nurs. **62:**92-94, Jan., 1962.

Keller, N. W.: Acute pericarditis, Med. Times **86:**39-53, 1958.

Kelly, A. E. and Gensini, G. G.: Coronary arteriography, Am. J. Nurs. **62:**86-90, Feb., 1962.

Klassen, G. A.: Stokes-Adams syndrome, Canad. Nurse **58:**34-36, Jan., 1962.

Klose, L. M. and Whalen, R. E.: What patients undergoing cardiac catheterization feared, Am. J. Nurs. **62:**112-114, Oct., 1962.

Kouwenhoven, W. B., Jude, J., and Knickerbocker, G. G.: Closed-chest cardiac massage, J.A.M.A. **173:**1064-1067, 1960.

Kritchevsky, D.: Cholesterol and atherosclerosis, Am. J. Clin. Nutr. **10:**269-276, April, 1962.

Martin, D. M., Case, F. G., and Miller, A. C.: Nursing care of the patient with an abdominal aortic aneurysm, Am. J. Nurs. **59:**60-62, Jan. 1959.

More than two hands (editorial), Am. J. Nurs. **61:**43, July, 1961.

Nicholson, M.: Nursing care in Stokes-Adams syndrome, Canad. Nurse **58:**37-42, Jan., 1962.

Rusk, H. A., and Gertler, M. M.: Rehabilitation in congestive heart failure, Circulation **21:**444-447, 1960.

Safar, P., Brown, T. C., Holtey, W. J., and Wilder, R. J.: Ventilation and circulation with closed-chest cardiac massage in man, J.A.M.A. **176:**574-576, May 20, 1961.

von Marpurgo, D. M., and Gauder, P. J.: Co-ordinated action in cardiac arrest, Am. J. Nurs. **62:**91-93, May, 1962.

White, J.: Closed-chest cardiac massage, Am. J. Nurs. **61:**57-59, July, 1961.

White, P. D.: The nursing of patients with cardiovascular diseases, Tomorrow's Nurse **2:**6-10, Feb.-March, 1961.

Wood, E. C.: Understanding the patient with heart disease, Nurs. Outlook **7:**90-92, Feb., 1959.

Patient-Teaching Aids

A Club for Mended Hearts: Nurs. Outlook **5:**163, 1957.

American Heart Association, 44 E. 23 St., New York 10:

A booklet listing films, filmstrips, slides and transcriptions is available.

A booklet listing teaching aids for the patient is available.

Some particularly good booklets:

How the Doctor Examines Your Heart

If Your Child has a Congenital Heart Defect

Food for your Heart—A Manual for Patient and Physician

Heart Attack

High Blood Pressure

Strokes (A Guide for the Family)

The Facts About Employment and Heart Disease

The Heart of the Home. A pamphlet to Encourage the Homemaker to Apply Time- and Energy-Saving Principles.

Varicose Veins. An 11-page pamphlet.

Your Sodium-Restricted Diet. (Three booklets—one for strict, one for moderate, and one for mild restriction.)

Public Affairs Pamphlets, 419 New Jersey Ave., S.E., Washington 3:

Blakeslee, A. L.: How to Live with Heart Trouble, No. 184

————: Know your Heart, No. 137

Ogg, E.: Good News for Stroke Victims, No. 259

Taubenhaus, M.: Rheumatic Fever, No. 126A

Ross Laboratories: Columbus 16, Ohio.

Congenital Heart Abnormalities, No. 7. A 57-page illustrated outline, with a study guide giving a diagrammatic presentation of the heart anomalies.

U. S. Dept. of Health, Education, & Welfare, Public Health Service Publications:

The Circulatory System, No. 482. A 59-page illustrated guide for nursing education.

Little Strikes, No. 689

Strike Back at Stroke, No. 596. A 37-page illustrated and informative booklet describing what can be done for the stroke patient.

Other good pamphlets are:

Coronary Artery Disease, No. 145

Heart Disease, No. 45

Hypertension, No. 146

Rheumatic Heart Disease, No. 144

Unit X. Nursing Care of Patients
With Digestive Disorders

ORIENTATION

Scope of Gastroenterology

Unit Ten is concerned with the gastrointestinal canal and two abdominal organs, the liver and the pancreas, which communicate with it and are indispensable for its normal digestive functions. Abnormalities of this tract are numerous and exemplify every type of major pathology that has been described in connection with other organ systems. Congenital, inflammatory, infectious, traumatic and neoplastic lesions have been encountered in every portion and at every site along its 25-foot length. In common with many other organ systems, it is subject to circulatory disturbances, faulty nervous control and senescence.

Quite apart from the multiplicity of organic diseases to which the gastrointestinal tract is heir, there are many extrinsic factors—some related to disease, others not—which can interfere with its normal functions and produce symptoms duplicating those of intrinsic gastrointestinal disease. An anxiety state, for example, often finds its chief expression in the syndrome of functional indigestion or motor disturbance of the intestine. Moreover, certain organic diseases have been ascribed to emotional imbalances. Peptic ulcer and chronic ulcerative colitis, for example, have been explained on a psychogenic basis by many observers. Such diseases are commonly referred to as "psychosomatic" disorders, a terminology which underlines, so to speak, the importance of the mind-body relationship in their pathogenesis. Regarding the importance of this relationship, there can be no doubt, for, regardless of their fundamental etiology, their severity, course and outcome are influenced greatly by the mental health of the patient.

The nurse should be thoroughly cognizant of the relation between the level of her patient's mood and his appetite and bowel function, and between his sensory awareness and the manner in which he interprets sensations. She must also recognize the importance of her own attitude toward the patient and his complaints as an influential factor capable of modifying his symptoms in either direction. Her display of genuine tolerance and sympathetic interest toward the patient is often the key to his cooperation, and if that is obtained the major obstacle to therapeutic success has been removed.

Anatomy and Function of the Gastrointestinal Tract

The gastrointestinal canal is a tube, about 25 ft. in length, through which the food passes and is subjected to the action of various digestive fluids (Fig. 200). All solid food, to get within the body, must first be liquefied, for only liquids can be absorbed into the blood vessels and the lymphatics in the stomach and the intestine.

Constituents of food, even though in liquid form, in most cases must first be modified chemically before they can be absorbed.

Carbohydrates. Although our daily diet contains many different sugars and starches, practically the only carbohydrate which the tissue cells utilize as fuel is glucose (dextrose), of which there is little in our food. Therefore, all carbohydrates eaten, if they are to be used, first must be changed into glucose. The bulk of the carbohydrate in fruits and vegetables is in the form of starch, although the riper, the softer and the sweeter these foods are, the more of their starches are in sugar form—for the plants store their carbohydrates in the form of starches and, like the human body, transform them into sugar before they metabolize them. Before they are absorbed, all starches, which are relatively insoluble, must be changed into sugars. All the complex sugars first must be broken down to simple sugars, like glucose, levulose and galactose, and all of these must be converted or "inverted" into glucose.

Fats. Most of the fats in our food are liquid at body temperature but are insoluble in water. All fats are combinations of glycerin and various fatty acids. This combination is split up by digestion. The glycerin thus set free is easily absorbed as such, while the fatty acids promptly unite with alkalies to form true soaps, which likewise are absorbed easily. Most of our food fat, however, is not split thus, but instead is divided, by the action of the bile salts, into microscopic globules. In other words, it is emulsified, and emulsions, as well as solutions, are able to pass through the intestinal mucous membrane into its lymphatic vessels.

Proteins. These are complex materials that are not absorbed until they have been split into single fatty acids, glucose and amino acids, all of which are absorbed readily. Having passed through the mucous membrane of the intestinal wall, many are resynthesized into complex compounds. The glycerin and fatty acids may be reunited to form fats of a different character, and the amino acid products of protein digestion, circulating in the blood, are resynthesized into the particular proteins of which the body cells are composed.

Oral Digestion

All foods receive their preparation for digestion in the mouth, and starch digestion actually begins there. The solid foods are ground into pulp by the teeth, which makes gastric digestion easier; and in the mouth they are mixed with saliva containing ptyalin, an enzyme which initiates starch digestion. The food may be in the mouth for but a few seconds, but this salivary digestion continues until the acid of the gastric juice has destroyed the ptyalin. Foods should be well masticated. There is much truth in the

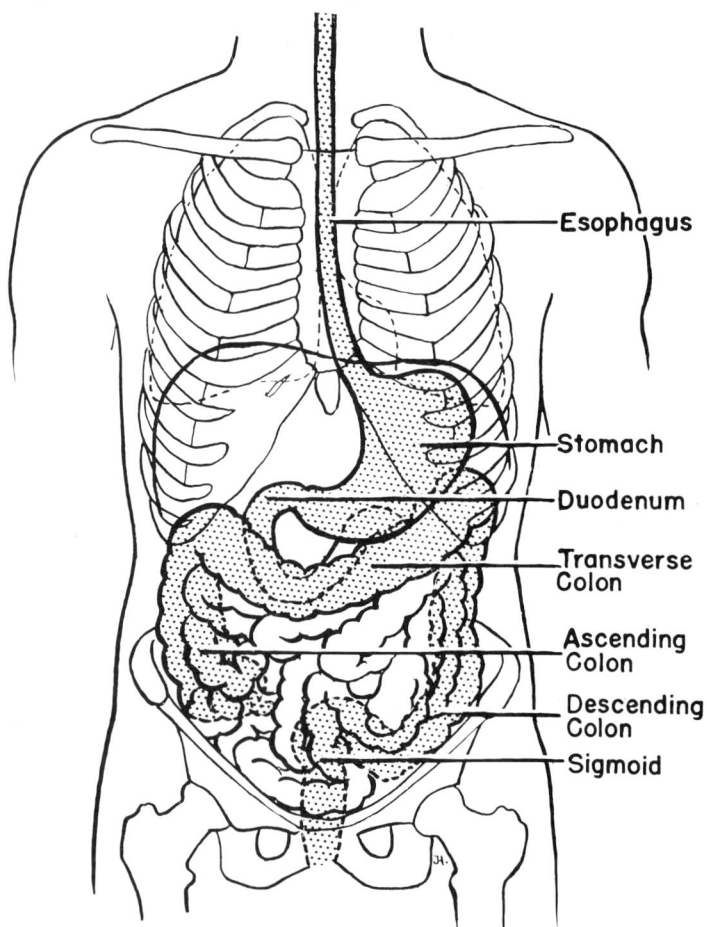

Fig. 200. Diagram showing the position of the digestive organs.

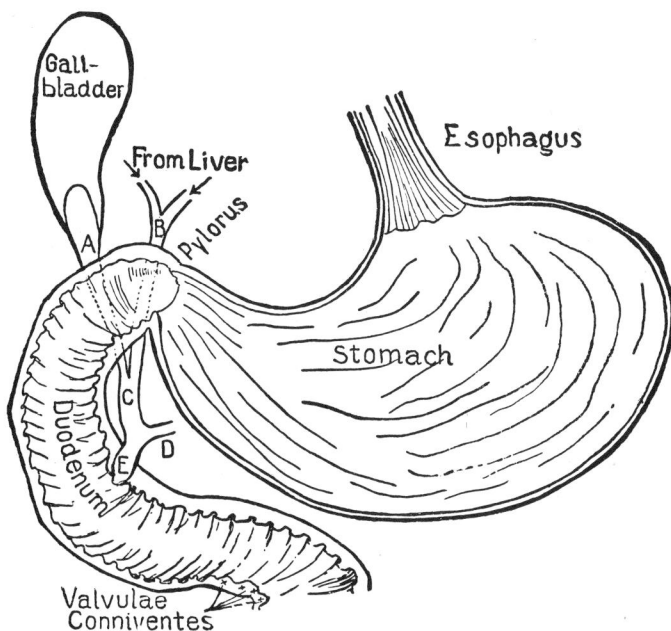

FIG. 201. The normal stomach, the duodenum and the bile ducts. (A) The beginning of the cystic duct. (B) The hepatic duct. (C) The common bile duct. (D) The pancreatic duct. (E) The ampulla of Vater.

old proverb that "food well chewed is half digested," for the smaller the particles of meat and vegetables that are swallowed, the more accessible is the food to the digestive juices. Moreover, thorough mastication is desirable because it stimulates the secretion of gastric juice.

Swallowing. A complex motor act involving highly coordinated contractions of the tongue and the pharynx, swallowing propels the food from the mouth into the esophagus.

The Esophagus

The esophagus is a muscular tube about 9 in. long, equipped with both circular and longitudinal muscle fibers. It conducts the ingested material into the stomach, wavelike contractions of its wall expressing its contents into the gastric reservoir.

The Stomach

The stomach is a distensible pouch situated between the esophagus and the duodenum (Fig. 201). During a meal it distends to become a large hollow receptacle capable of holding about 1,500 ml. The organ is situated in the upper abdomen, almost entirely on the left side of the body, for the most part tucked away beneath the ribs. The lesser curvature, or upper margin, of the stomach is from 3 to 6 in. long. The greater curvature is considerably longer, its length depending on the degree of gastric distention. At its widest point the stomach, when full, measures from 4 to 5 in. There are two orifices to the stomach: the cardiac orifice, its inlet, and the pylorus, its outlet. Both orifices are ringed with muscle tissue by which they can be closed.

Gastric Juice. The gastric mucosa secretes each day several hundred milliliters of a clear, colorless liquid, the function of which is to start the digestion of the food proteins. Gastric juice contains pepsin, an enzyme which splits and dissolves proteins; hydrochloric acid, necessary for this peptic digestion; and rennin, the effect of which is to clot milk and thereby prevent its absorption before it has been digested properly by the intestinal enzymes.

Gastric secretion normally is stimulated in one of two ways: first, through the nervous system; and, second, by chemical substances from the food which are absorbed into the gastrointestinal mucosa. The earlier stimulus of secretion is psychic; it is a response to the odor, the appearance and the taste of appetizing food. When we do not enjoy our food, or when we are under some mental stress, the secretion of gastric juice is inhibited and digestion gets a bad start.

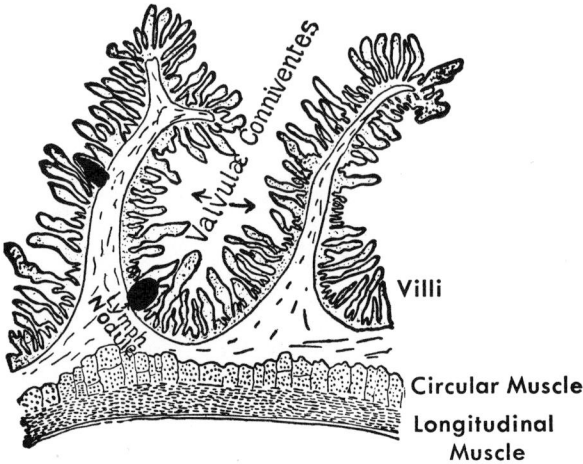

FIG. 202. A section through the wall of the small intestine (jejunum) made parallel with the length of the bowel, showing the folds of the mucosa and the villi on the folds (magnified).

Equally important is the secretion of gastric juice stimulated by a hormone, *gastrin*. This hormone is produced by the mucosa of the antrum, and is carried by the blood stream to the acid-pepsin producing cells of the body of the stomach. Gastrin is produced when the antrum is distended with food, and by certain products of protein digestion.

Practically no food is absorbed in the stomach; all is passed on into the duodenum, there to become exposed and acted on by the pancreatic juice and the bile.

The Duodenum

The duodenum is a muscular tube about 12 in. long and forms the upper end of the small intestine. The stomach communicates with the duodenum via the pylorus. Also, the common bile duct and the pancreatic duct enter the duodenum at a point from 8 to 10 cm. below the pylorus.

The first food swallowed enters an empty stomach. At once the pylorus closes tightly. If the proper stimulus is present, the walls of the stomach soon begin to pour out gastric juice, and a gentle churning movement (gastric peristalsis) begins, the effect of which is to mix the food thoroughly with the juice. As the mass of food is pressed toward the pylorus, the liquid portion (chyle) is allowed to enter the duodenum, but the food that is still solid is retained in the stomach until it is liquefied by the mechanical action of peristalsis and the chemical effects of the gastric

juice. This process normally requires from 1 to 6 hours. If, at the end of a few hours, any solid masses of food remain, they are forced on, through the pylorus, by powerful expulsive stomach contractions.

Pancreatic Juice. The pancreatic duct opens into the duodenum approximately 10 cm. distal to the pylorus. Through this duct is secreted a digestive juice containing three enzymes: trypsin, lipase and amylase. Trypsin is a powerful proteolytic enzyme which digests proteins more rapidly and completely than pepsin. In contrast with pepsin, trypsin acts, not in an acid, but in an alkaline medium. It is manufactured in the pancreas as trypsinogen, which has no digestive power — otherwise, the pancreas and its duct would themselves be digested. It acquires its potency in contact with the mucous membrane of the duodenum, owing to another enzyme, enterokinase. Amylase, or diastase, is practically the same as the ptyalin of saliva. Its function is to break down starches and complicated sugars in food to the simple sugars: glucose, levulose, etc. Lipase, or steapsin, is an enzyme that splits fat into its two components, glycerin and fatty acids. In childhood, the pancreatic juice also contains lactase, important in the digestion of milk sugar.

Bile. This liquid, which is secreted by the liver, also enters the duodenum at this point (Fig. 201E). Many of its constituents are waste products, no longer of use to the body, but bile also contains alkalies, which help to neutralize the acid from the stomach and form soluble soaps from the fatty acids that are liberated from food fats as a result of the action of lipase. The bile salts are important in the emulsification and absorption of fats and fat-soluble vitamins from the intestine. Bile is formed almost continuously, but most of it is formed during digestion. Some of it is stored in concentrated form in the gall-bladder, which serves as a reserve tank. It probably is this stored bile which enters the duodenum first when intestinal digestion begins.

The Intestine

The intestine is a muscular tube, approximately 20 feet long, extending from the pylorus to the anus. The first 12 inches beyond the pylorus comprise the duodenum, which has been discussed. The proximal two fifths of the small intestine beyond the duodenum is called the jejunum (Fig. 202), the lower three fifths, the ileum. The ileum opens into the colon or large bowel, and just below this juncture of ileum and colon, at a point which is protected by the ileocecal valve, the *vermiform appendix* is connected.

The colon (Fig. 200) is about 5 ft. long. It starts as a pouch, called the *cecum,* into the side of which the ileum and the appendix open. It then ascends upward toward the liver as the *ascending colon,* crosses the abdomen as the *transverse colon,* descends into the left flank as the *descending colon* and terminates in a short curve, called the *sigmoid flexure,* which leads into the rectum.

Along the whole length of the small intestine is secreted a fluid containing several enzymes, the function of which is to complete the chemical process of digestion. These include enterokinase, already mentioned as the activator of trypsinogen; secretin, the substance that stimulates the pancreas to secrete its digestive juice; erepsin, that completes the enzymatic breakdown of proteins which was initiated by pepsin and trypsin; and a carbohydrate-splitting enzyme for each simple sugar: maltase, to invert maltose into dextrose; invertase for the inversion of cane sugar into dextrose and levulose; and lactase to convert milk sugar into dextrose.

Thorough mixing of the chyle—the liquefied food masses—with the digestive fluid is accomplished by rhythmic peristaltic contractions of the muscular intestinal wall that split up the masses and churn them repeatedly for several minutes in small segments of the bowel. At intervals during this process, the chyle is propelled onward through the intestine by peristaltic waves running longitudinally along its entire length. One layer of muscle fibers of the intestinal wall is arranged as a ring round the bowel lumen; when this contracts, the lumen is constricted. Another layer of fibers runs parallel with the lumen; when this contracts, the intestinal loop is shortened. These two movements, passing in orderly succession down the bowel, and coordinated so that they push its contents along, are called peristaltic waves (Fig. 203).

As the digested material courses through the small intestine, the utilizable portion is absorbed through its lining and enters the lymph vessels and the blood vessels in the wall of the intestine. The mucous membrane lining the bowel wall is thrown into folds and has a surface much like velvet, being covered completely with fingerlike processes known as *villi* which vastly increase its absorbing surface. By the time the chyle reaches the ileocecal valve, practically all that is of value has been absorbed. That which is left is the indigestible part of the food, consisting largely of cellulose, some of the constituents of the bile and the intestinal fluids, many epithelial cells thrown off from the intestinal wall and, finally, vast numbers of the bacteria which grow in the intestine, eventually comprising at least one fifth of the solid feces.

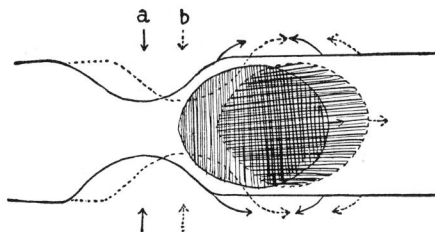

FIG. 203. Diagram of a peristaltic wave. In the bowel is a bolus of food. The solid line (a) represents the beginning of the wave; the dotted line (b) represents the wave a moment later.

28

Patients With Conditions of the Lips, the Mouth and the Esophagus

CONDITIONS OF THE LIPS

Trauma

Wounds of the face and the lips rarely become infected, because of the rich blood supply of that region. If an accidental wound is cleaned and sutured early, healing is rapid. This is the case also in the event of an intentional wound of the surgeon's making. Dressings are both unnecessary and conspicuous. The wounds are sutured best with silk or nylon and painted with Whitehead's varnish. Primary healing occurs without much scarring.

Congenital Deformities

Harelip. Harelip and cleft palate are deformities that result from embryonal maldevelopment. Harelip may appear in any form from a mere notch on the lip border to a deep fissure that may extend up to the nostril. The deformity may be unilateral or bilateral. If the malformation is marked, the child should be operated on as soon as possible after birth. Operation is borne well at that early age, but if treatment is delayed the baby becomes a poorer surgical risk because of loss of weight and strength due to his inability to nurse properly.

The operation is performed with the child on his back, the head being allowed to hang over the operating table and rest in the lap of the surgeon. In this way blood and mucus escape easily without being aspirated or swallowed. The easiest way to handle the baby is to roll him in a small blanket, binding the legs and the arms to his sides. The operation is a simple suturing together of the tissues of the lip to make it possible for the child to nurse.

After the operation, nursing should not be allowed for from 5 to 6 days, but mother's milk or formula should be fed by a medicine dropper. The tip of the medicine dropper should be protected by a small rubber tube and placed in the corner of the infant's mouth. In this way there will be less strain on the suture line by sucking. The physical needs of the baby should be met so as to keep crying to a minimum: crying produces tension on the incision.

Cleft Palate. This deformity is associated frequently with harelip. The cleft may involve only the soft palate. However, it may extend through the hard palate and even involve one or both nostrils. Such children cannot talk or eat properly and an operation is required. This is done best in their second year. Flaps of periosteum and mucous membrane are formed and sutured together to close the defect. The harelip frequently is corrected at the same time. The excess of the red border is excised and the tissues of the lips are joined by one of several methods of plastic operations. The suture line is sealed with Whitehead's varnish and tension is removed from the sutures by the application across the lip of an adhesive strapping that tends to hold the cheeks together, or by adhesive strips placed around the lips. Another procedure for closing cleft palate is that of making a prosthesis to replace missing or inadequate parts. Each patient must be evaluated as an individual to determine which is best for him—surgery or a prosthesis; many times, it is both.

Nursing Care

The success of the operation depends in large measure on the care that these children receive both before and after operation. In no circumstances is it advisable to operate on these patients in the presence of an infection of the nasopharynx or the tonsils.

Asepsis of the mouth cannot be attained, but a high degree of cleanliness is possible, and the extreme vascularity of these tissues usually ensures healing in spite of the bacterial flora that is present always. Both before and after operation the nose and the mouth should be sprayed or swabbed at frequent intervals with mild alkaline antiseptic solutions (liquor antisepticus alkalinus or Dobell's solution). Each feeding should be followed by a thorough cleansing of the mouth. The stitches on the inner and the outer parts of the lip may be swabbed carefully with a cotton applicator dipped in hydrogen peroxide to free the incision of milk or serum. If the wound is kept clean and free of infection, the cosmetic results are better.

Immediately after operation the danger is from asphyxia. To avoid this danger the child should be placed on his side with the head low, so that vomitus, blood and mucus may drain easily from the mouth. The tongue may fall back frequently and obstruct the pharynx. This may be prevented by affixing to the cheek, with an adhesive strip, the silk thread drawn through the tongue at the time of operation. As soon as the child has recovered consciousness, the thread may be removed.

Dyspnea may occur when the operation has brought about a considerable narrowing of the nostrils. The nurse should watch such children carefully and depress the lower lip with a strip of adhesive until the child becomes accustomed to the new condition. Arm restraints may be necessary to prevent him from touching his face and injuring the suture line. These may be made of padded splints and placed so that the elbow cannot be flexed. They should be removed every 4 hours to massage both arms. The child's position should be changed to avoid pulmonary complications.

If a child with both harelip and cleft palate has had only the harelip repaired, his mother must be instructed as to how to care for him until the second operation is performed. She should learn the most effective way of feeding her child and of protecting him from respiratory infections. The long-range postoperative care of a child who has had such repairs will include teaching him to enunciate properly. This calls for tact and patience from all concerned.

Epithelioma

Cancer of the lip, usually called *epithelioma,* occurs most frequently on the lower lip in men as a chronic ulcer. It grows rapidly, develops into a foul crater and soon produces secondary growths in the glands of the neck.

Treatment. The treatment of this disease, if begun early, is wide excision of the growth, frequently with removal at the same time of the glands of the neck. If treated late, the lesion is removed locally by electrodesiccation, combined with radiation of the glands of the neck.

Nursing Care

The nursing care of the patient in the early stages is to give mouthwashes and keep the lesion or wound as clean as possible. Feeding often is a problem. Liquid and soft foods should be served attractively in amounts sufficient to enable the patient to gain strength and weight.

The inoperable cases are pitiable, both before and after electrodesiccation. The growth is painful and foul-smelling. Such people cannot eat, saliva drools over the lips or the lesion, and after months of suffering, death comes usually from cachexia or secondary hemorrhage. The nurse should try to make the last days of such patients as comfortable as possible. They need kindness and understanding. They should have meticulous mouth care and the benefit of deodorants. The frequent use of sedatives is necessary.

CONDITIONS OF THE MOUTH

Oral Infections

Ludwig's Angina. This is an acute septic inflammation of the tissues of the floor and the submaxillary region of the mouth and of the submaxillary region of the neck. Its onset is sudden: the patient has difficulty in talking and swallowing, he has pain and salivation and, finally, dyspnea. The patient is profoundly toxic, but does not exhibit the high temperature and the leukocytosis that might be expected. Death may occur suddenly due to edema of the glottis that produces asphyxia or to intense toxemia.

TREATMENT. The treatment is early incision with drainage, then the application of hot wet dressings to the neck and the use of hot mouthwashes. If dyspnea develops, a tracheotomy must be performed. The nurse must watch these patients closely for respiratory difficulty, stertorous (noisy) breathing, cyanosis or rapid increase in swelling. These symptoms are the early signs of beginning respiratory obstruction. Early treatment with penicillin often is able to abort the infection and to ward off serious complications.

Alveolar Abscess. This usually is a sequela of dental infection. It begins with a moderate tenderness and swelling of the gums, which if untreated leads to a swelling of the whole side of the face with extreme tenderness and inability to open the mouth fully. Frequently the abscess points on the cheek side of the infected tooth, and pus may be expressed from that area by gentle pressure.

TREATMENT. The abscess must be opened by an incision on the outside of the gum that extends down to the jaw bone. A drainage tube usually is inserted for a few days. The postoperative care is the administration of hot antiseptic mouthwashes at 2-hour intervals, except when the patient is asleep. This treatment should be continued until the swelling subsides. External heat also hastens

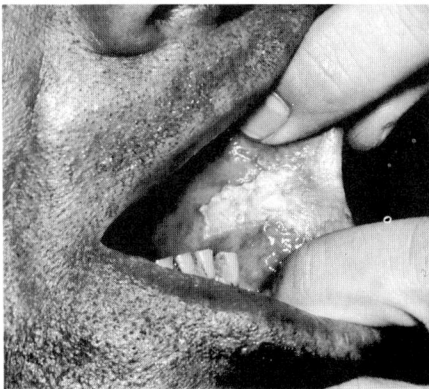

FIG. 204. Leukoplakia.

the subsidence of the infection and relieves pain and soreness to a large extent. The patient should be encouraged to expectorate and not to swallow the foul pus that collects in the mouth. A sputum cup or basin always should be within easy reach.

Abnormalities of the Salivary Glands

Acute Inflammation. Inflammation of the salivary glands is the essential lesion of mumps. Due usually to a staphylococcal infection affecting one or a few glands, most often one parotid, inflammation occurs as a serious complication of several acute infectious diseases, such as typhoid fever, typhus fever and pneumonia. It is most apt to occur in elderly acutely ill and debilitated individuals whose salivary glands, because of general dehydration, fail to secrete sufficiently and whose parched mouths offer poor defense against invasion of the parotid ducts by pathogenic organisms.

In all the above-mentioned conditions, except mumps, the onset of this complication is sudden, with an exacerbation of the fever and of the symptoms of the primary condition. The gland swells, becomes tense and tender, pain is felt in the ear, and there is interference with swallowing. The swelling rapidly increases, the overlying skin soon becomes red and shiny, and in a few days fluctuation often is present.

TREATMENT AND NURSING CARE. At the onset of the swelling, an icebag may be applied over the affected gland, and chemotherapy may be instituted with penicillin or one of the sulfonamides. A suppurating gland may require incision and drainage. Proper hydration of the patient, by the parenteral route if necessary, and adequate mouth care offer the best chance of preventing this complication.

Syphilis causes both acute and gummatous parotitis. In all cases of these two luetic conditions the gland swells gradually and there is salivation. However, there is seldom any pain, and there is little tendency to suppuration. All patients respond readily to antiluetic therapy.

Salivary Calculus (Sialolithiasis). In two thirds of all cases involving one submaxillary gland, this abnormality follows bacterial infections of the gland or stricture of its duct because of trauma or inflammation. These stones are composed mainly of calcium oxalate. If located within the gland, they are irregularly lobulated and vary in diameter from 3 to 30 mm. Stones in the duct are small and oval.

Calculi within the salivary gland cause no symptoms unless infection arises; but a calculus that obstructs the gland's duct causes sudden, local and often colicky pain, which is suddenly relieved by a gush of saliva. Where this condition exists, the gland is swollen and quite tender, the stone itself often is palpable and its shadow may be seen on roentgenograms. The calculus should be excised.

Tumors. Neoplasms of almost any type, but the great majority of them malignant, develop in salivary glands, and in 75 per cent of all patients in one parotid. They may remain small and quiescent for years, then suddenly begin to increase in size.

The best treatment of parotid tumor is the early and complete excision of the mass, followed by irradiation of the area involved. Local recurrences are common; the recurrent growth usually is more malignant than the original one.

Cancer

Leukoplakia buccalis (also called "smoker's patch") and the related *keratosis labialis* are seen in middle-aged adults, more than 80 per cent of them men. These conditions are characterized early by the appearance of one or two small, thin, often crinkled, pearly patches on the mucous membrane of the tongue, the mouth, or both, due to keratinization of the mucosa and sclerosis of its underlying tissue (Fig. 204). In time, most of the tongue and the mouth may become covered by a creamy white, thick, fissured or papillomatous mucous membrane which desquamates from time to time, leaving a beefy-red base. This condition results from chronic irritation by carious, infected or poorly repaired teeth, by tobacco and by highly spiced foods. Occasionally it is due to lues. Not infrequently, cancers start in the keratinized patches.

Carcinoma may arise in any part of the mouth. However, it appears most frequently on tongue, cheek and lip. Often the individual feels a roughened area with his tongue. In tobacco chewers, the mucous membrane of the cheek is the commonest site. A jagged tooth may be the source.

Carcinoma of the tongue occurs most frequently in men of or past middle age. The lesion is found usually on the lateral margin. It begins as a small ulcer that does not heal. The growth spreads rapidly to the lymph nodes of the neck. The earliest symptom is pain or soreness of the tongue on eating hot or highly seasoned foods. Later, pain develops on swallowing even liquids. Earache, face ache and toothache become almost constant. Speech becomes difficult and salivation occurs. Unable to eat or sleep because of the pain, the patient loses weight and strength rapidly. Death results usually from aspiration pneumonia due to inability to swallow normally, from toxemia caused by septic absorption from the foul, ulcerating growth or from hemorrhage from the growth.

Treatment and Nursing Care

The only cure is surgery following early recognition of the condition. The enlargement of lymph nodes indicates metastases. This may necessitate more extensive surgical dissection combined with radium and x-ray therapy. When the tongue is involved, it is necessary often to perform a *hemiglossectomy* or a *glossectomy*.

The care of the mouth is extremely important for the welfare of the patient. The type of nursing care given in these serious and often offensive conditions is an index frequently of the efficiency of the nurse. If the patient is conscious and able to help himself, the nurse can teach him how to keep his mouth clean. She must remind him and keep him supplied with a toothbrush or gauze-padded tongue depressor, as well as a mouthwash.

The general physical condition of a person often is reflected in his mouth. Therefore, good nutritional levels must be maintained. If the breath has a foul odor, the nurse must encourage and assist the patient with his oral hygiene before and after each feeding. Often a bad taste in the mouth spoils the taste of food and limits the intake of nourishment. If the patient is a mouth-breather, he needs more mouth attention than the average per-

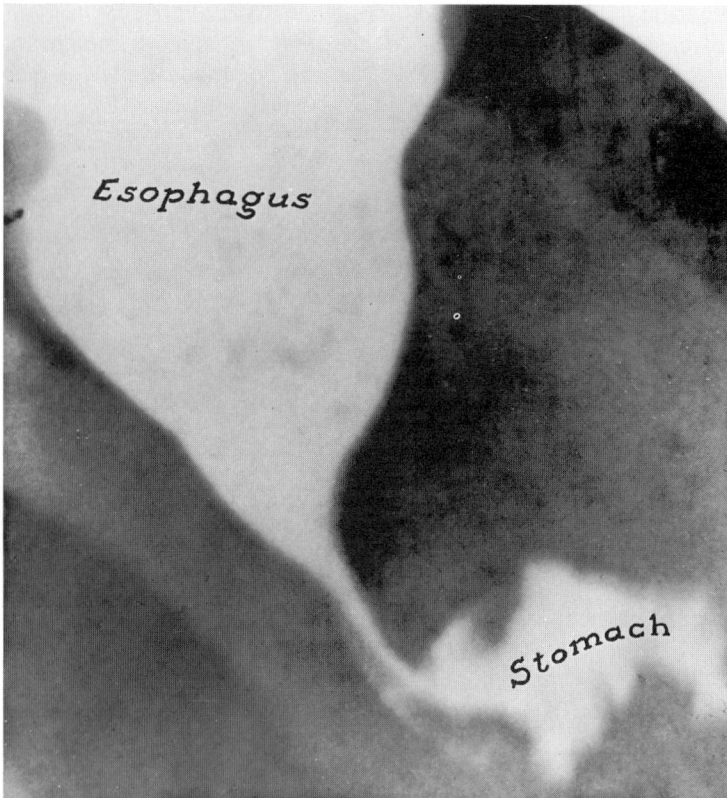

Fig. 205. The area of the lower esophagus and the upper stomach to show the marked narrowing in a case of achalasia. Note the marked dilatation of the esophagus above the narrowed area, the very markedly constricted lower esophagus and the small amount of barium which passed through this area into the stomach.

son. The use of swabs of mineral oil with lemon juice is refreshing. Lanolin applied to dry and cracking lips is soothing.

Dentures must be removed frequently and cleaned. Before they are replaced, the mouth also should be cleaned. Often care is given to the teeth, but the "furred" or coated tongue is neglected and bad breath continues. In the unconscious patient, the nurse is wholly responsible for maintaining good mouth hygiene. The use of a special mouth tray with all necessary applicator sticks, padded tongue depressors, mouthwashes, lubricants and so forth encourages frequent mouth attention.

Individuals with mouth lesions may have feeding problems. The use of a paper or plastic straw, a glass tube or a teaspoon may be effective. The Breck feeder, so frequently employed with children, may be of use. Food should be soft or liquid and nonirritating; i.e., not too hot or too cold and not highly seasoned. It should be served attractively to tempt the patient to take it. Small, frequent feedings are more desirable than large, less frequent ones. The desires as well as the nutritional needs of the patient should be taken into consideration. If he is not able to take anything by mouth, it may be necessary to feed him by means of a nasogastric tube. Before feedings are given, the position of the tube must be checked by injecting slowly, drop by drop, 1 or 2 ml. of saline. If the tube is in the esophagus, as it should be, the patient should have no reaction. If it is in the trachea, he will cough violently. The care of this tube is similar to that of a gastrostomy tube. (See p. 608.)

If the lesion is such that the patient salivates constantly, this may be relieved somewhat by inserting a gauze wick in the corner of the mouth. The saliva that drops from the end of the wick may be caught in a small basin. Another way of removing mouth secretions is by the use of a small rubber catheter attached to a suction apparatus. Mouth

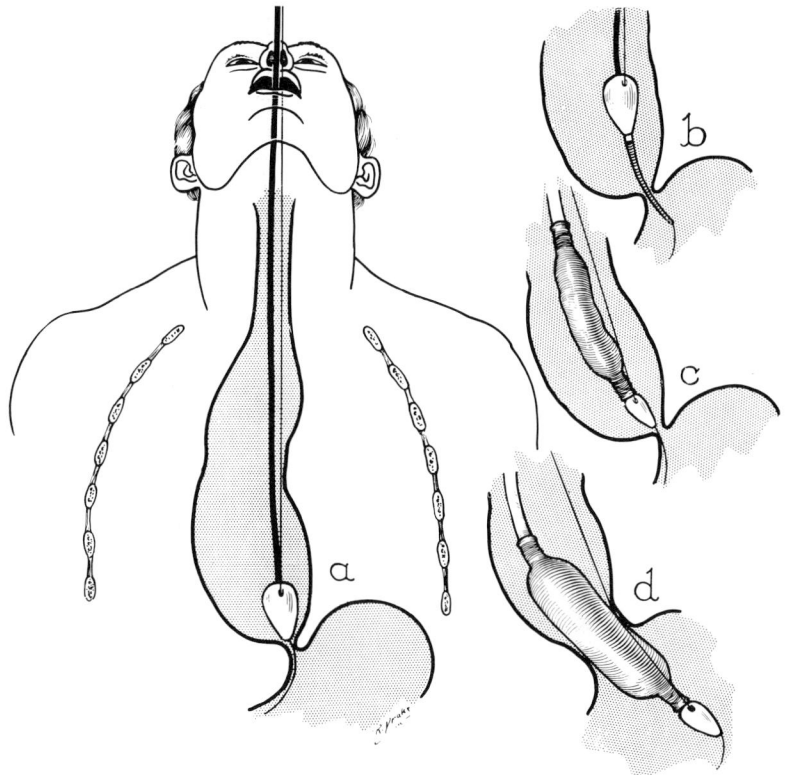

FIG. 206. Dilatation of the lower esophagus with rubber balloon technic in cases of cardiospasm (achalasia). The dilator is passed, guided by a previously swallowed thread, into the upper stomach. When the balloon is in proper position it is distended by pressure sufficient to dilate the narrowed area of the esophagus. (Olsen, Ellis and Creamer: Achalasia of the cardia, Am. J. Surg. **93**:299-307)

wipes, as well as a paper bag attached to the bed or the bedside stand to receive soiled tissues, always should be on hand. An effective way of holding dressings of the mouth or the lower jaw in place is by the use of a face mask. The strings can be tied at the top of the head.

To combat odors, the doctor may order such oxidizing agents for a mouthwash as potassium permanganate 1:10,000, hydrogen peroxide in half strength, sodium perborate and so forth. In addition, for patients with malodorous cancer lesions, a room deodorant may be used. Many effective kinds are available. Good room ventilation must be maintained. In extensive mouth sores, a power spray can clean wounds effectively and necrotic tissue can be removed more easily. If radium is used, the usual radium precautions are observed. When radium needles are implanted, each needle has a thread attached to it. The patient should know upon waking that these are present and that they are not to be removed. The power spray is effective in cleansing the mouth

when these are in place. Radium may be implanted in a moulage (molded dental compound), and this may be applied to some part of the mouth for a specific length of time. It is usually permissible to remove the mold for meals and at night. When it is reinserted, it is important for the nurse to note that it is in its proper position. (For care of radium, see p. 317.)

Speech often is interfered with or is difficult. Simply to supply the patient with a pad of paper and a pencil or "magic slate" may make a tremendous difference in his depressed condition. Often these patients are reluctant to associate with other patients; they prefer to be alone. If there are 2 or more patients with a similar condition, they can help each other. It is easier for them, and for others, if they have their meals apart from other patients. Kindness, attention to cleanliness and keeping the patient comfortable are the keynotes of the nursing care of these patients. The doctor's orders regarding special treatments, diet and medications must be followed. In advanced malignant cases, the nurse should be on guard for hemorrhage, respiratory obstruction and wound infection.

Follow-up and Home Care. Before the patient leaves the hospital, facilities for home care should be checked. When appliances such as a food blender, a suction machine and a vaporizer are necessary, the social worker may have to arrange for their purchase or loan. The patient, or a member of his family, must be instructed in meeting his needs. The importance of follow-up visits to the physician, clinic or outpatient department must be stressed.

CONDITIONS OF THE ESOPHAGUS

The esophagus is the mucus-lined tube that leads from the pharynx through the chest to the stomach.

Congenital Anomalies

The most common congenital malformation of the esophagus is *atresia* (absence or closure of the passage). The esophagus may end in a blind pouch and the remaining portion may be connected with the trachea and produce a tracheo-esophageal fistula. Many variations of malformation have been found. It is detected usually in the infant when he regurgitates on taking fluids, becomes cyanotic and chokes as the fluids escape from the nose and the mouth. The only treatment is surgical repair in the first few days of life. This usually includes a temporary gastrostomy. Besides the problem of caring for a very young infant after a thoracic operation, the nurse must recognize the importance of feeding and maintaining fluid balance. The major threats postoperatively are: (1) aspiration of feedings; (2) atelectasis; and (3) pneumonitis.

Trauma

The esophagus is not an uncommon site of injury. Stab or bullet wounds of neck and chest often produce such injury. Swallowed foreign bodies—dentures, fish bones, safety pins and so forth—may injure the esophagus as well as obstruct its lumen. Usually, foreign bodies can be removed with the aid of the esophagoscope. The injuries to the esophagus are the more serious part of the problem, because they may lead to deep cervical or mediastinal abscess, or to stricture formations. Drainage of such abscesses requires a thoracic exposure.

Chemical Burns. Stricture of the esophagus also occurs, usually in children, after chemical burns.

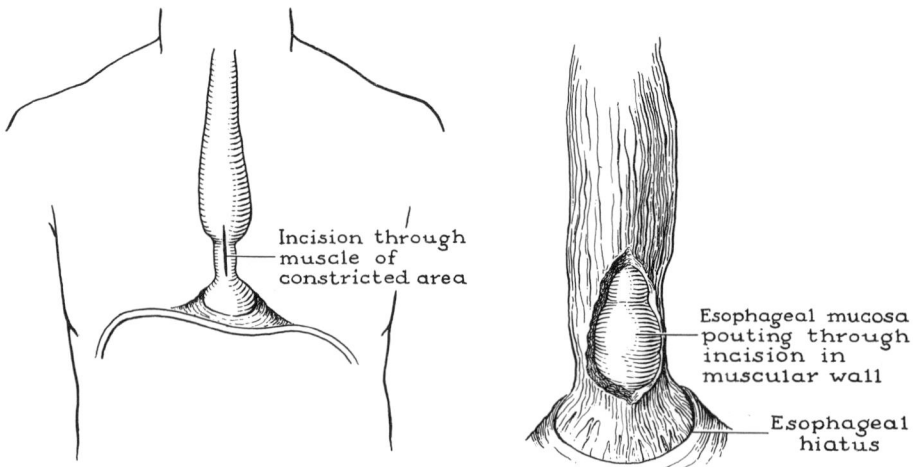

FIG. 207. Diagrammatic drawing to show the method of treatment of achalasia. The esophagus is approached from in front on the left side. An incision is made through the muscularis of the esophagus sufficiently to allow a pouting of the esophageal mucosa. Separation of the muscular fibers relieves the narrowing at the lower end of the esophagus and permits the patient again to swallow normally.

FIG. 208. Paraesophageal hiatus hernia. The arrow indicates the site of the opening in the diaphragm through which the cardiac end of the stomach has passed, to become displaced into the thorax.

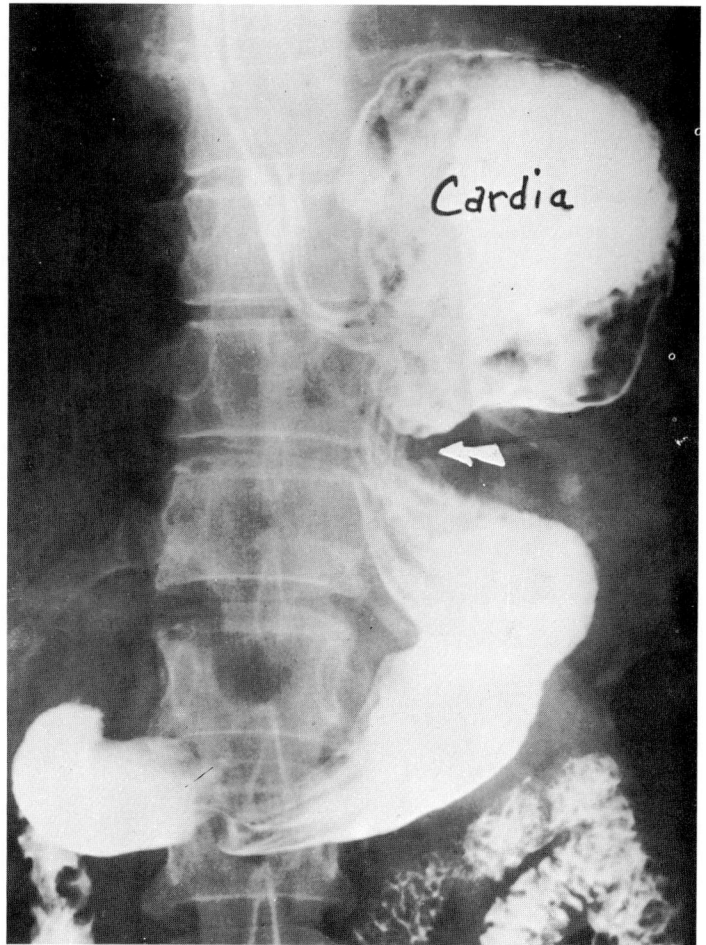

The acute chemical burn of the esophagus has associated severe burns of the lips, the mouth and the pharynx with pain on swallowing and, sometimes, difficulty in respiration due either to swelling in the throat or a collection of mucus in the pharynx. Many are profoundly toxic. If the patient is able to swallow, fluids should be given in small quantities at a time. Secretions should be aspirated from the pharynx if respiration is embarrassed. The necessity for high fluid intake may require administration by the intravenous route.

When the acute stage subsides, the patient may swallow normally for a time, but usually multiple stricture levels form in the esophagus. These may be dilated by the retrograde bouginage method of Tucker. A gastrostomy opening is made and a braided silk string is inserted into the esophagus.

One end is brought out through the gastrostomy opening and the other end through the nose. The two ends are tied together and form a complete loop. Dilatation is obtained by pulling larger and larger bougies upward through the esophagus by means of the string. It is important that this string be left in place at all times. The gastrostomy is kept open by means of a gastrostomy tube, through which feedings may be given if necessary. Dressings around this tube should be changed whenever soiled. The tube should be changed daily to prevent irritation about the wound. (See Gastrostomy, p. 608.)

Cardiospasm (Achalasia of the Cardia)

Cardiospasm or *achalasia* is a term used to denote benign stenosis of the lower end of the esophagus. This is usually associated with a lack of peristaltic activity in the esophagus itself and often with a failure of the cardiac sphincter of the stomach to open. Narrowing of the esophagus just below the stomach results in a gradually increasing dilatation of the esophagus in the upper chest, and the symptoms produced are those of difficulty in swallowing. The patient has a sensation of food sticking in the lower portion of the esophagus, and as the condition progresses, regurgitation of the food is com-

mon, sometimes spontaneously and other times brought on by the patient because of the discomfort that is produced by the prolonged distention of the esophagus with food stuffs that will not pass into the stomach. The cause of this condition is believed to be due to a degeneration of the nerves that go to the involuntary muscles of the esophagus. The condition is diagnosed by roentgenograms (Fig. 205) which show the marked

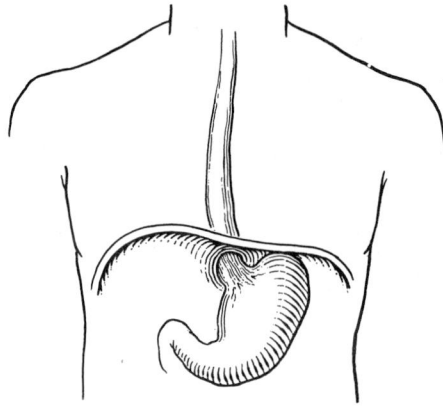

Normal position of
esophagus and stomach

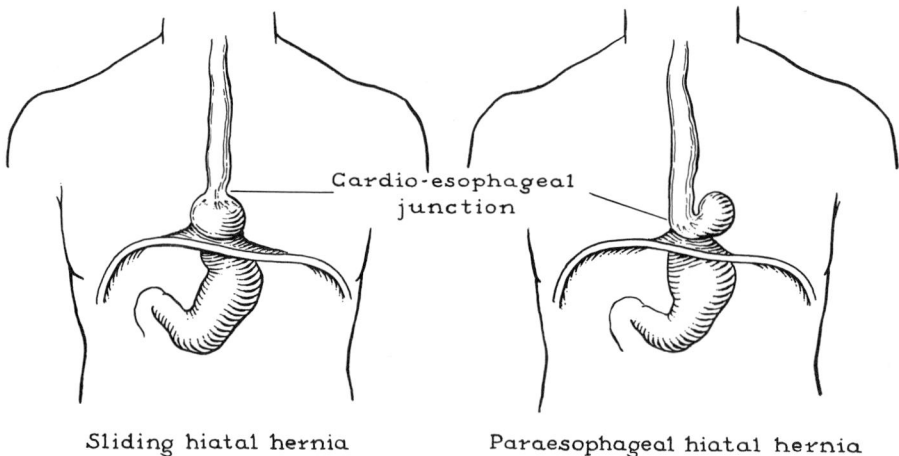

Cardio-esophageal
junction

Sliding hiatal hernia   Paraesophageal hiatal hernia

Fig. 209. Diagrammatic drawings to show the anatomy of hiatal hernia of the two types. The sliding type of hernia with the short esophagus passes directly through the esophageal hiatus. In the paraesophageal type, the cardio-esophageal junction is in approximately its normal position, but a mass of the cardiac end of the stomach passes through the hiatal hernia beside the esophagus.

dilatation of the esophagus and the narrowing of its lower end.

The treatment of achalasia is divided into two parts: nonsurgical and surgical. The nonsurgical therapy, stretching of the narrowed area of the esophagus, is accomplished by the distention of a bag placed in this area through the mouth (Fig. 206). This bag (Plummer) is passed along a previously swallowed thread which leads into the stomach. Hydrostatic dilatation usually gives good results in about 60 per cent of the patients, but the dilatation which is required may result in a rupture of the esophagus in a small number of cases. The surgical treatment (Fig. 207) consists in a division of the muscular fibers which enclose the narrowed area of the esophagus, allowing the mucosa to pouch out through the divided area in the muscle layers. This permits food to be swallowed without obstruction, and the operation is used with very good results. The operation is spoken of as *esophagomyotomy* and is reserved usually for the later and more resistant lesions, whereas dilatation is more often practiced in early lesions.

Nursing Care

The operation of esophagomyotomy is most often performed through the chest, and the nursing care is that used for any patient who has had a previous thoracotomy. In the immediate postoperative period, a tube drainage is often introduced into the chest and is placed in through an underwater drain or suction. The tube is usually removed after the 2nd or the 3rd day. The usual discomfort that is noted with patients with thoracotomy wounds must be kept in mind and appropriate sedatives given. Frequent turning of the patient is imperative so that both lungs may become well aerated in the immediate postoperative period. After 2 or 3 days the patient is started on fluids by mouth, and the diet is gradually increased so that by the 7th or the 8th day soft foods may be taken with ease.

Hiatus Hernia

The esophagus enters the abdomen through an opening in the diaphragm to empty, at its lower end, into the upper part of the stomach. The opening in the diaphragm normally encircles the esophagus tightly; therefore, the stomach lies within the abdomen completely. In a condition known as *hiatus* (or *hiatal*) *hernia,* the opening in the diaphragm through which the esophagus passes, becomes enlarged, and part of the upper stomach tends to come up into the

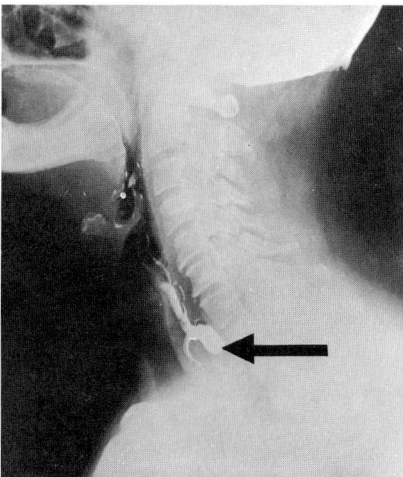

FIG. 210. Diverticulum of the esophagus. Roentgenogram showing the appearance of an esophageal diverticulum. Note the retention of barium in the diverticulum.

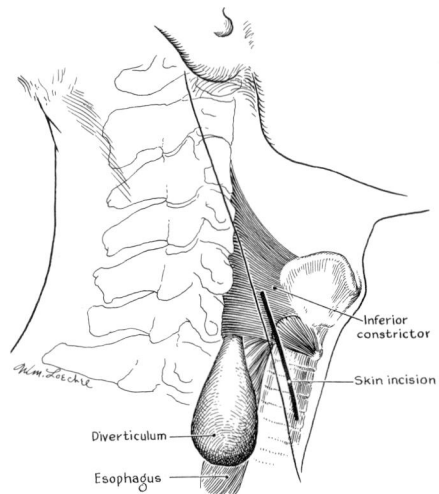

FIG. 211. Diagrammatic drawing shows how diverticulum projects through the muscles of the upper portion of the pharynx.

lower portion of the thorax. This complication may be present in many patients without giving any symptoms, but there is often a feeling of fullness in the lower chest and a splashing sound noted in the substernal area in patients in whom the hiatal hernia is large. In addition, the gastric juice produced by the stomach mucosa tends to be loculated in the portion of the stomach above the diaphragm, and for this reason ulcerations and bleeding occur in this group of patients. Finally, the erosive action of the gastric juice on the stomach and the lower esophagus may produce a condition known as esophagitis, with the production of pain and discomfort in the substernal area.

All of these symptoms produce an uncomfortable and often very ill patient if bleeding is a factor.

In those hernias that are found accidentally in the x-ray examination (Fig. 208) and do not produce symptoms, no treatment is

necessary. Many of these hernias are of the sliding type in which the stomach tends to extend into the chest when the patient is lying down, but it goes back into the abdomen when the patient is erect (Fig. 209). In those patients in whom the hernia is present constantly, and even in the sliding type of hernia in patients in whom symptoms appear, surgical correction of the abnormality is necessary. The operation is one in which the stomach is replaced into the abdomen and the enlarged esophageal opening is made smaller so that the stomach cannot extend above the diaphragm. This operation may be performed from the abdomen, in which case the stomach is pulled down, and the crura of the diaphragm are brought together behind the esophagus. In other instances the operation may be performed through the left chest, separating the ribs. The esophagus is identified, and the herniated portion of the stomach is pulled down into the abdomen,

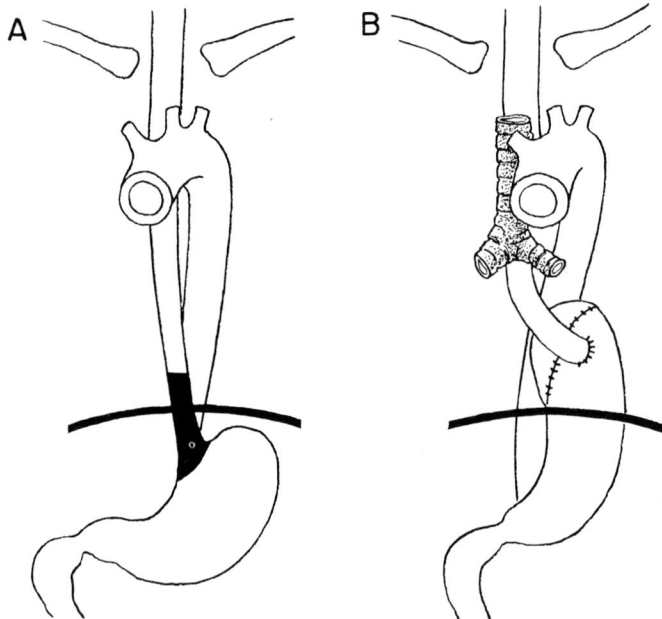

FIG. 212. (A) Black portion of esophagus indicates carcinoma. (B) Relations of the viscera after resection of a carcinoma of the lower fourth of the thoracic segment and the abdominal segment of the esophagus. The proximal esophagus is relatively long and a large segment of the stomach, including the lesser curvature, the cardia and the fundus, has been resected. The anastomosis lies in the lower portion of the mediastinum.

and again the esophageal opening in the diaphragm narrowed by sutures from above.

Nursing Care

The immediate postoperative care of these patients is that used for any thoracotomy or laparotomy. In patients with thoracotomy a chest tube is often introduced, which is placed in underwater drainage or suction. The drain is usually taken out in a day or two, after the lung has completely expanded. The patient is given fluids and food on the 2nd or 3rd day after operation, and gradually increasing amounts of food are given as tolerated by the patient. In some individuals edema at the site where the esophagus passes through the diaphragmatic hiatus may give some delay in food intake for a time, but usually this subsides without incidence in 2 or 3 days.

Esophageal Diverticulum

A *diverticulum* of the esophagus is an outpouching of the wall of this structure, usually in the cervical region and on the posterior aspect (Figs. 210, 211). The patients notice first a sensation of difficulty in swallowing, with fullness in the neck, and often they state that it feels as though their food stops before it gets into the stomach. The operable variety is due to a weakness in the wall, and the pouch appears on one side of the neck. It causes symptoms by becoming filled with food, which is regurgitated later.

These diverticula may be removed surgically. After operation, the nurse must feed the patient through a nasogastric tube that usually is inserted at the time of operation. The feedings may include any liquid, but a careful record of their kind, amount and character must be kept in order that the surgeon may know that the patient is receiving sufficient calories. After each feeding, the tube should be irrigated carefully with water. The wound also must be watched carefully for evidences of leakage from the esophagus and a developing fistula.

Nursing Care

When a patient has difficulty in swallowing, it is usual to limit his diet to those foods that pass more easily. Blenderized meals supplemented with vitamins are usually ordered. Sometimes these patients are the victims of unbalanced diets and unbalanced fluid levels. Often they express a fear of cancer. Preoperative preparation by the surgeon and the nurse is directed toward getting them into optimum physical and mental condition. Food and/or fluids high in vitamin and protein content are given. Diagnostic tests, such as esophagoscopy and roentgenograms, are carried out. The nurse should explain the procedure to the patient before he is taken for such an examination so as to allay his fears. After an esophagoscopy the patient may complain of a sore throat. This passes in a few hours with mild sedation. A day or two before the operation a silk string usually is swallowed by the patient. This enables the esophagoscopist to follow more readily into the esophagus with his scope and eliminates the danger of rupture of the diverticulum. The lighted scope makes the surgery much simpler. A Levin tube is threaded through the scope and into the stomach before the scope is removed. The anesthesia used may be local or inhalation. The patient often is out of bed on the day of operation. After operation for transthoracic esophagectomy, the patient may be given oxygen therapy to facilitate breathing and to prevent hypoxemia. The nursing care in this most serious condition follows the general principles employed in thoracic surgery.

Carcinoma of the Esophagus

Carcinoma of the esophagus is a disease that occurs in older people, and more often in men. It is characterized by a gradually increasing difficulty in swallowing. At first only solid food gives trouble but, as the growth progresses and the obstruction becomes more complete, even liquids cannot pass into the stomach. Regurgitation of food and saliva occur, and there is a progressive loss of weight and strength due to starvation. The diagnosis is confirmed by x-ray examination and by esophagoscopy. Bronchoscopy usually is performed also, especially in tumors of the middle and the upper third of the esophagus, to determine whether the trachea has been involved by the tumor and to help in determining whether the lesion can be removed.

Surgical removal of the growth is the only hope of cure. This can be accomplished by an approach through the thorax or through the abdomen and the thorax for lower esophageal lesions. The portion of the esophagus containing the growth is removed, and the continuity of the gastrointestinal tract is reformed by bringing the stomach into the chest and implanting the proximal end of the

esophagus into it (Fig. 212). The chest is closed after insertion in the pleural cavity of a drain that is led under water or is attached to a suction apparatus.

Lesions in the middle and the upper thirds of the esophagus, particularly, are often not suitable for surgical excision. However, in some clinics success has been reported in which a tunnel is created beneath the ster-

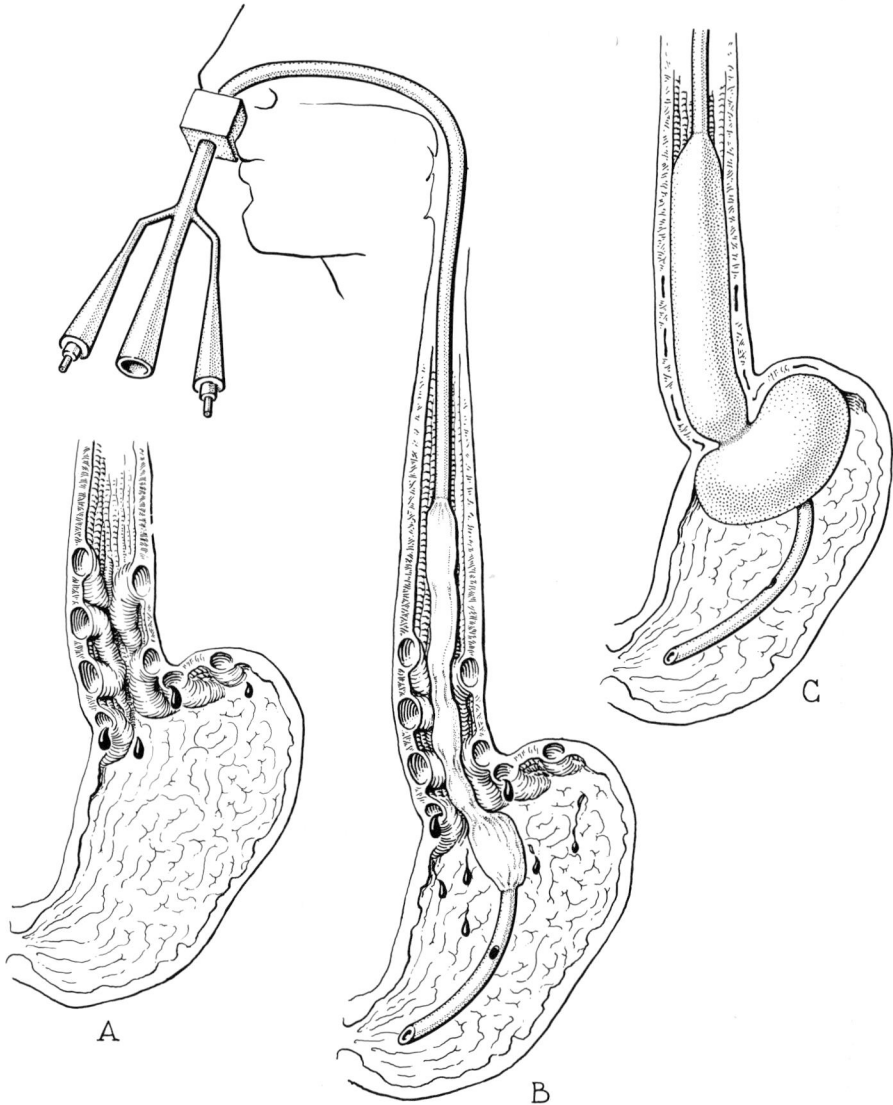

Fig. 213. Diagrammatic drawing to show esophageal varices and their treatment by a compressing balloon tube (Blakemore). (A) Dilated veins of the lower esophagus. (B) The tube is in place in the stomach and the lower esophagus but is not inflated. (C) Inflation of the tube and the compression of the veins which can be obtained by distention of the balloon. See Figure 213 D.

num and a resected segment of either jejunum or colon replaces the diseased esophagus. A palliative procedure in which a plastic tube is introduced through a cervical incision has been done with resultant symptomatic relief, improvement in nutrition and amelioration of psychological symptoms.

If the growth is found to be inoperable either before or at operation, a gastrostomy often is performed as a palliative procedure to permit the administration of food and fluids (see Gastrostomy Care, p. 608).

Nursing Care

Frequently it takes many days to prepare these patients for surgery. Numerous laboratory tests are required of blood protein, hemoglobin and so forth to determine the patient's physiologic status, and an effort is made to correct the deficiencies by the parenteral administration of blood, fluids, amino acids, electrolytes and vitamins. These measures, in addition to roentgenograms and esophagoscopic studies, may be somewhat troublesome to an older patient. A sympathetic and understanding nurse can do much to make the patient understand the necessity and the value of the various procedures.

In the postoperative phase, the fundamentals of care are similar to those used in gastric and thoracic surgery. The patient usually is placed in an oxygen tent. He must be turned frequently and encouraged to take deep breaths. Even so, by the second day there may be an accumulation of blood and serous fluid in the pleural cavity that necessitates a thoracentesis.

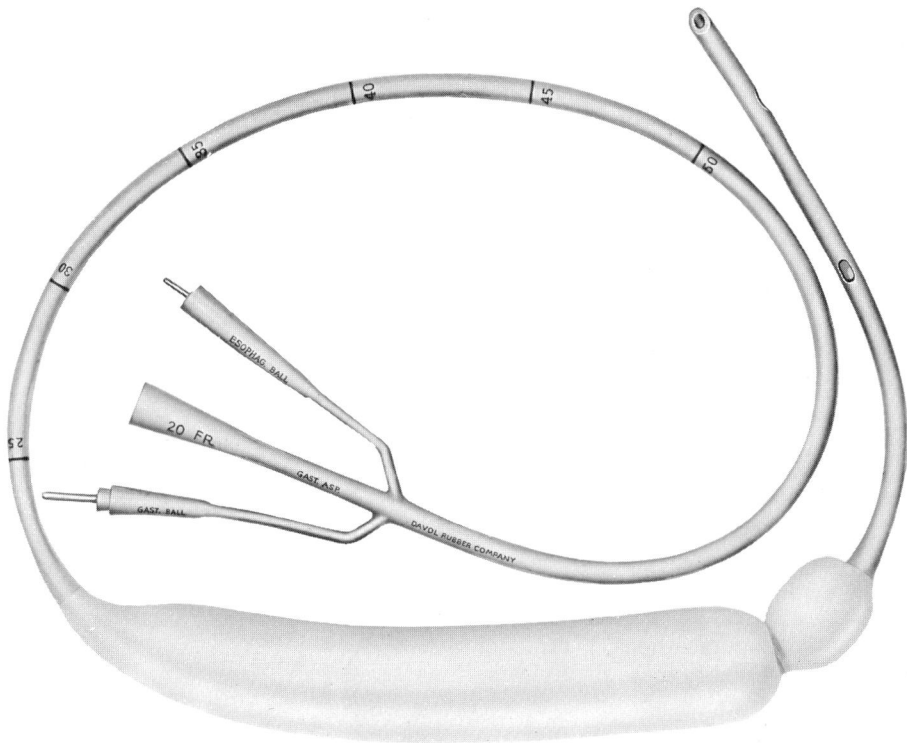

FIG. 213 D. Blakemore tube for the compression treatment of bleeding from esophageal varices. The tube consists of a central tube which is extended into the stomach, a balloon which is inflated in the upper end of the stomach and a longer balloon which is used to produce pressure in the lower portion of the esophagus. The tube which comes with the balloons has 3 parts, one of which goes to the gastric balloon, another to the esophageal balloon and the middle one extends through the balloon into the stomach for purposes of aspiration. The method by which the tube is used is shown on the facing page. (Davol Rubber Company)

In surgery of the esophagus, a nasal catheter usually is inserted in the esophagus as far as the esophagogastric anastomosis or through it. This must be attached to a continuous suction apparatus. It is removed within 3 to 5 days, and fluids may be given by mouth in increasing amounts. Soft foods are added gradually. Intravenous blood and fluids must be continued for several days after operation until the patient is able to take sufficient food and fluids by mouth. Penicillin usually is given prophylactically for several days preoperatively and after surgery.

Home Care. The needs of the patient will be determined by his medical condition, the method necessary for feeding, his degree of self-sufficiency, the family situation and the economic factors affecting his care. The plan for his discharge and home care should be started early in the postoperative period. This includes teaching the feeding procedure, care of the equipment and choice of foods and how to supplement them to meet his nutritional needs. The aid of a medical social worker, as well as a visiting nurse, may be necessary to follow the patient in his early adjustment out of the hospital.

Bleeding Esophageal Varices

Esophageal varices are dilated tortuous veins usually found in the submucosa of the lower esophagus; however, they may extend well up into the esophagus and into the stomach. Such a condition nearly always is caused by portal hypertension which, in turn, is due to obstruction of the portal venous circulation within the substance of a cirrhotic liver.

Esophageal varices should be suspected in the presence of hematemesis and melena, especially in the patient who has been addicted to alcohol. Usually these dilated veins cause no symptoms unless the mucosa over them becomes ulcerated. Then massive hemorrhage takes place, which if not controlled may result in death.

Treatment. The patient with bleeding varices is seriously ill. To control the hemorrhage, pressure is exerted on the cardiac portion of the stomach and against the bleeding varices by a balloon tamponade (Sengstaken-Blakemore tube, Fig. 213). Bleeding also is treated by sedation and complete rest of the esophagus (parenteral feedings). Straining and vomiting must be prevented. Gastric suction usually is employed to keep the stomach as empty as possible. The patient complains of severe thirst, which may be relieved by frequent oral hygiene and ice chips if permitted. The nurse must keep close surveillance on the patient's blood pressure. Vitamin K therapy and multiple blood transfusions often are indicated. A quiet environment and calm reassurance by doctor and nurse will help to relieve the patient's anxiety.

Surgical procedures that may be employed are (1) injection of sclerosing drugs via the esophagoscope; (2) direct surgical ligation of varices; and (3) portacaval and splenorenal venous shunt operations.

CLINICAL SITUATION

Mr. Z. has had a hiatus hernia treated by esophagoscopy.

1. Fluids should be withheld until
   A. The roentgenograms have been read.
   B. Salivation appears normal.
   C. Peristalsis is audible.
   D. The gag reflex has returned.

2. Inspection of his mouth is an important part of gastrointestinal evaluation. Leukoplakia is considered to be
   A. Symptomatic of Vitamin B deficiency.
   B. An early form of cancer of the tongue.
   C. A precancerous lesion.
   D. Diagnostic of leukemia.

3. Mr. Z. may have many vague complaints. One of the most common symptoms of hiatus hernia is
   A. Hematemesis.
   B. Epigastric distress.
   C. Progressive hoarseness.
   D. Polyphagia.

4. One of the principles underlying medical management of Mr. Z. is to
   A. Decrease intra-abdominal pressure.
   B. Increase the amount of food intake.
   C. Liberalize the fat intake.
   D. Assume a recumbent position after meals.

BIBLIOGRAPHY AND SUGGESTED READING

Books

Merendino, K. A.: Esophagus *in* Harkins, H. N., *et al.:* Surgery—Principles and Practice, ed. 2, pp. 637-659, Philadelphia, Lippincott, 1961.

Articles

Breed, J. E., and Carroll, W. W.: Radiocobalt treatment of lip cancer, Mod. Med. **25:**87-88, Aug. 15, 1957.

CA, Bulletin of Cancer Progress. A complete issue devoted to oral cancer, **9:**110-144, July-Aug., 1959.

Ciba Clinical Symposia. Diseases of the Esophagus, **8:** (complete issue), Jan.-Feb., 1956.

Cunningham, L. M.: The patient with ruptured esophageal varices, Am. J. Nurs. **62:**69-71, December, 1962.

DeVries, P. A., and Barrett, A. C.: Care of the infant with an esophageal anomaly, Am. J. Nurs. **61:**51-53, June, 1961.

Farr, H. W.: Cancer of the tongue, Am. J. Nurs. **57:**1314-1317, 1957.

Ginsberg, M. K.: A study of oral hygiene nursing care, Am. J. Nurs. **61:**67-69, Oct., 1961.

Heimlich, H. J., and Greenless, T. W.: Carcinoma of the esophagus, J.A.M.A. **161:**192-195, 1956.

Hislop, R.: Nursing care of patients with mouth or throat cancer, Am. J. Nurs. **57:**1317-1319, 1957.

MacCollum, D. W., *et al.:* Habilitation of the cleft palate patient, New Eng. J. Med. **254:** 299-307, 1956.

Mackler, S. A., and Mayer, R. M.: Palliation of esophageal obstruction due to carcinoma with a permanent intraluminal tube, J. Thorac. Cardiov. Surg. **28:**431-443, 1954.

Randall, P.: The management of cleft lip and cleft palate patients, Am. J. Med. Sci. **233:** 204-219, 1957.

Zuidema, G. D., and Klein, M. K.: A new esophagus, Am. J. Nurs. **61:**69-72, Sept., 1961.

Patient-Teaching Aids and Information

Pamphlet materials available from:
American Dental Association
222 E. Superior Street
Chicago 11, Ill.

A source of material for patient teaching:
Cancer Nursing. A Manual for Public Health Nurses, American Cancer Soc., 1950.
  1. Head and Neck. Oral Cancer, Control of odors, irrigations, dressings, nasal feedings, pp. 33-38.
  2. Liquid diets—suggestions for liquid feedings, menus, pp. 82-84.
  3. Smooth diet for mouth cases, p. 87.

Film: Oral Cancer—The Problem of Early Diagnosis.
  (16 mm. sound, color, 33 min.) Available on loan from state health departments and state divisions of American Cancer Society.

29

Patients With Gastric and Intestinal Problems

TERMINOLOGY AND TOPOGRAPHY

Before studying specific diseases and operations, the nurse should be familiar with the prefixes denoting abdominal organs and the suffixes used to denote the diseases of or operations on these organs.

Suffixes used to denote the names of diseases and operations are:

itis—inflammation of—as *appendicitis,* an inflammation of the appendix.

otomy—to make a cut into—as *gastrotomy,* to make an opening into the stomach.

ostomy—to make a mouth or opening into —as *cystostomy,* to insert a tube into the urinary bladder.

ectomy—to cut or remove—as *salpingectomy,* to remove the fallopian tube.

pexy—to sew up in position—as *nephropexy,* to sew the kidney up in position.

orrhaphy—to repair a defect—as *herniorrhaphy,* to repair a hernial defect.

plasty—to improve by changing the position of the tissue—as *pyloroplasty,* an operation to enlarge the pyloric opening of the stomach.

(See also the appendix.)

Abdominal Topography. For purposes of convenience in description, the abdomen has been divided into nine regions by imaginary lines, as illustrated in Figure 214.

The abdominal cavity normally contains a small amount of fluid that lubricates the peritoneal surfaces. This cavity is lined with a thin, glistening membrane called the *peritoneum.* This structure covers all the abdominal organs, forming folds between which the coils of intestine are located. Some organs (such as the liver, the pancreas, the kidney and the urinary bladder) are not covered completely by peritoneum; hence inflammations of these structures may not always involve the general abdominal cavity

Organs	Prefix	
Stomach	*Gastr*	*Gastritis*—inflammation of stomach
Pylorus	*Pylor*	*Pylorectomy*—removal of pyloric end of stomach
Liver	*Hepa*	*Hepatitis*—inflammation of liver
Gallbladder	*Cholecyst*	*Cholecystitis*—inflammation of gallbladder
Common bile duct	*Choledoch*	*Choledochitis*—inflammation of common bile duct
Small intestine	*Enter*	*Enteritis*—inflammation of intestine
Colon	*Col*	*Colitis*—inflammation of large colon
Appendix	*Appendic*	*Appendicitis*—inflammation of appendix
Urinary bladder	*Cyst*	*Cystitis*—inflammation of urinary bladder
Fallopian tube	*Salping*	*Salpingitis*—inflammation of fallopian tube
Ovary	*Oophor*	*Oophoritis*—inflammation of ovary
Pelvis of kidney	*Pyel*	*Pyelitis*—inflammation of pelvis of kidney
Kidney	*Nephr*	*Nephritis*—inflammation of kidney
Rupture	*Herni*	*Herniorrhaphy*—repair of hernia
Loin or abdomen	*Lapar*	*Laparotomy*—incision in the abdomen

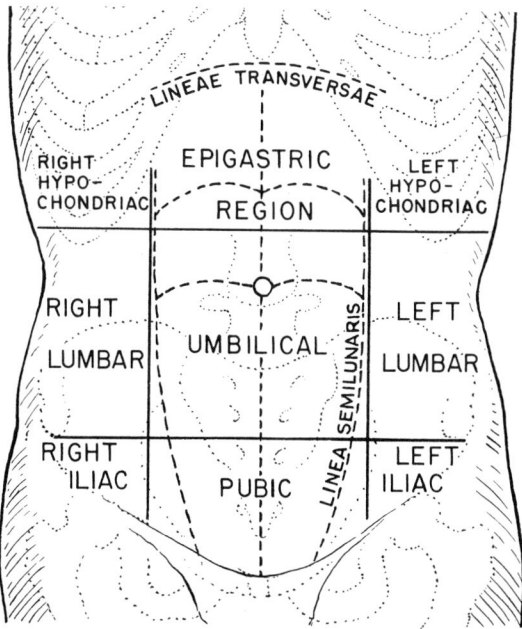

FIG. 214. Regions of the abdomen.

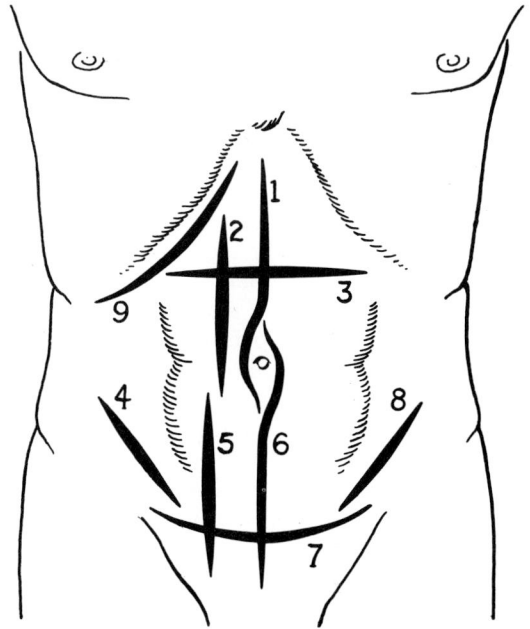

FIG. 215. Diagram to show the various abdominal incisions which are used. (1) Upper midline incision. (2) Upper right rectus incision. (3) Transverse incision in the upper abdomen. (4) Gridiron incision on the right. (5) Lower right rectus incision. (6) Lower midline incision. (7) Pfannenstiel incision. (8) Left gridiron incision. (9) Subcostal incision.

but may develop into retroperitoneal extensions or abscesses.

Abdominal Incisions

Laparotomy or *abdominal section* are terms used to describe any operation that involves opening the abdominal cavity. The gridiron or the McBurney incision (Fig. 215) is the simplest. It opens the abdomen through a small wound made by spreading the fibers of the muscles through which it passes. This incision is suitable especially for operations upon the appendix, and, as it has the advantage of being closed without tension, it makes a firm wound in which hernias rarely form.

More widely useful, however, are the vertical incisions made in the midline or to either side of it. These are made to pass between or through the rectus muscles. Many other types of incisions may be made. These vary, depending on the preference of the surgeon.

Precautions. In making abdominal incisions, the wound always is protected from skin contamination by the fastening of towels, gauze sponges or plastic material to its edge. Bleeding points are caught and ligated as they appear, and the tissues are divided layer by layer as they are encountered.

In all operations on the gastrointestinal tract, the surgeon makes an opening into a tube filled with many kinds of bacterial life. Because of the highly acid juices of the stomach, the upper intestine and the stomach are believed to contain less bacteria than the lower. Nevertheless, whenever the intestinal tract is opened, there is danger of the spread of infection from it into the peritoneal cavity unless strict precautions are taken. Moist sponges are placed round the portion through which the incision is to be made, and all tissues not directly implicated in the operation are covered as completely as possible. Rubber-covered clamps may be placed on the intestine in order to prevent the escape of its contents. When the incision in the intestine has been made, the contents of the opened loop are sponged out and the sponges are discarded.

When the openings in the intestines have been closed, all instruments, needles, sutures, scissors and so forth that have been used are removed from the operating table. Soiled sponges are discarded after the suture line has been mopped off with moist gauze, and fresh sterile towels or covers are placed about the operative field. The surgeon's gloves and those of his assistants should be changed before the operation is continued.

These precautions are taken in every gastrointestinal operation and are observed rigidly in operations on the large intestine, where infection is found most commonly. Closure is made in the reverse order, and each layer is united accurately until the wound has been closed. As a general rule, sutures are not placed in fat or muscles, but only in the firm aponeurotic layers, which are able to hold the wound closed until healing has taken place. Reinforcing, "stay" or tension sutures of heavy silk or wire often are employed to give added strength and to prevent the formation of dead space in the wound.

THE ROLE OF THE NURSE IN GASTROINTESTINAL DIAGNOSIS

One of the most interesting aspects of gastroenterology is the problem of clinical diagnosis in patients with digestive complaints. Part of the diagnostic difficulty arises from the fact that, despite the large array of etiologic possibilities, the number of symptoms referable to the digestive system that are distinctive and of diagnostic value is surprisingly limited; dysphagia, anorexia, nausea, vomiting, hematemesis, melena, constipation, diarrhea and abdominal pain comprise practically the entire list. Therefore, unusual importance attaches to the precise quality of each symptom presented, its mode of onset, its duration, the timing of its recurrences, its relation to meals and other events and the character of associated symptoms.

The observant, well-informed nurse can contribute materially to the diagnosis in many cases of digestive-tract disease and in most cases with functional disturbances of the gastrointestinal tract, for she is in an admirable position to observe and discuss with the patient those symptoms that are potentially so informative.

Given the proper tools, the correct diagnostic approach and the expert collaboration of the nurse, the physician usually can establish a diagnosis. Correct gastroenterologic diagnoses are rewarding indeed, for in no other category of disease is correct treatment more urgently required, and in none are opportunities for benefit or cure so numerous.

Because of the elusive nature of many gastrointestinal disorders the patient under investigation is likely to be subjected to a battery of complicated tests, including repeated roentgenographic studies after the ingestion and the rectal instillation of barium, the collection and the examination of numerous stool specimens, intubation of the stomach or the small bowel and aspiration of their contents, and usually one or more endoscopic procedures as well. Preparation of the patient for each gastrointestinal roentgenologic study involves fasting, catharsis, retention enemas and colonic irrigations. His muscles sore from lying on many hard narrow examining tables, with "gas pains" from hunger, tired and probably anxious, the patient may have a few new complaints to impart after his rigorous work-up, and small wonder!

Each examination should be explained carefully to the patient in advance. During the procedure he expects and deserves the full attention of the attending doctor and nurse, whose conversation should be calculated to alleviate his anxiety and elicit his full cooperation.

Stool examinations and gastric analysis have been described (pages 95 and 96, respectively), and the responsibilities of the nurse in relation to these tests have been discussed. Preparations for roentgenologic examinations involving the barium meals and barium enemas are specified on page 105. Barium, incidently, predisposes to constipation and eventually fecal impaction, prevention of which is a very important consideration in the care of any patient who is undergoing these studies.

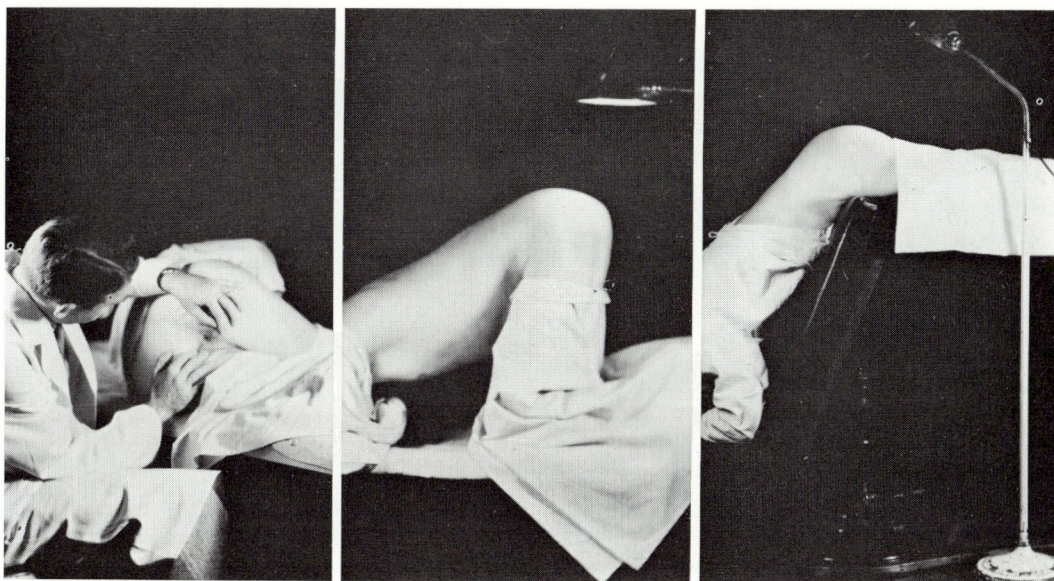

FIG. 216. (*Left*) Lateral, or Sims's position for examination of the anal region and the lower rectum. (*Center*) Knee-chest position for examination of the anal canal and the lower rectum. (*Right*) Position on the proctoscopic table for examination of the anal canal and the lower rectum.

The Rectal Examination

Visual inspection and digital examination of the anus and the rectum are indispensable for detection and identification of lesions involving these structures. Moreover, rectal examination is extremely useful in the diagnosis, or for the exclusion, of many intra-abdominal and pelvic conditions, including appendicitis, diverticulitis, salpingitis, tumors of the ovary, the uterus and the colon, and prostatic lesions of various types.

As the first step, the buttocks are spread apart with gauze pads or tissue wipes, and the anus and the perianal area are surveyed for fistulas, hemorrhoids, abscesses, fissures and other abnormalities. Next, with his examining index finger covered with a glove or a finger cot, the physician procedes to palpate the anal orifice and the rectum. The nurse should ensure that the requisite items are at hand, including a nonsterile glove or finger cot, lubricant, tissue wipes and a light source. During the procedure she should station herself at the patient's side to lend support and reassurance and to help him to assume the positions necessary for this examination.

Rectal examinations frequently are carried out in the lateral (Sims's) position (Fig. 216). The patient, draped with a sheet, lies on his left side (if the physician is right-handed), lower leg extended and upper leg flexed on the abdomen.

Anoscopy, Proctoscopy and Sigmoidoscopy. By means of tubular instruments that incorporate small electric lights, the lumen of the lower bowel may be viewed directly. The anoscope is employed to examine the anal canal; proctoscopes and sigmoidoscopes, to inspect the rectum and the sigmoid, respectively, for evidence of ulceration, tumors, polyps or other pathology. It goes without saying, that such an examination requires that the lower bowel be empty of feces; to this end, a cleansing soapsuds enema should be given at least 2 hours before endoscopy. Nevertheless, fecal material may remain to obstruct the examiner's view; to wipe it away, long swabs with generous cotton tips must be available.

The patient to be 'scoped assumes the knee-chest position (Fig. 216), resting on his knees, feet extending over the edge of the bed or the examining table. Knees

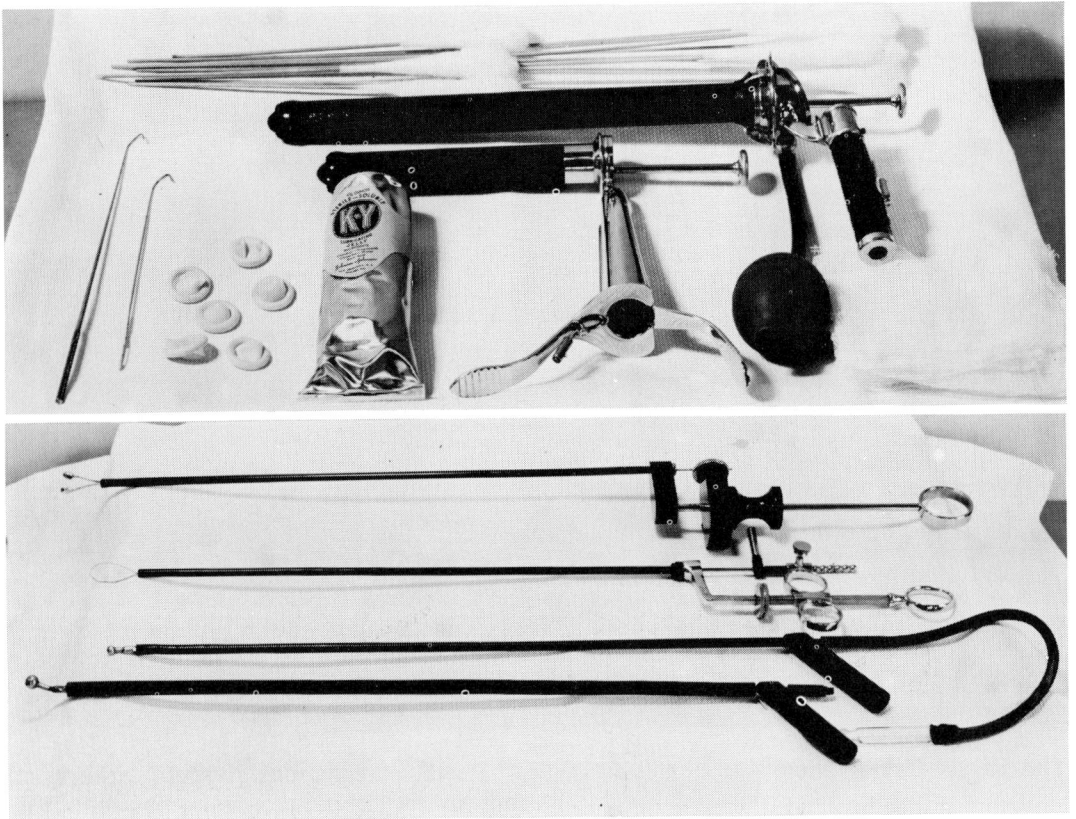

FIG. 217. (*Top*) Tray for anal and rectal examinations. The tray contains hooked probes, finger cots, lubricant, lighted anoscope and proctoscope, waste cotton and cotton swabs 16 in. and 8 in. long. (*Bottom*) Accessory instruments frequently used: biopsy forceps, electrosnare and suction electrodes with straight and curved tips.

spread apart to give steady support, the patient leans over, and rests the side of his face on the bed or the table, with his forearms on either side of the head and his hands placed on top of the other above the head. His back is now inclined at about a 45-degree angle and he is in proper position for the introduction of an anoscope, procto- scope or sigmoidoscope. Maximum convenience and comfort are afforded by a table that has been especially designed for rectal endoscopy: the so-called "proctoscopic table," which tilts the patient into the optimum position.

Many offices and hospitals are equipped with special rooms that are designed and

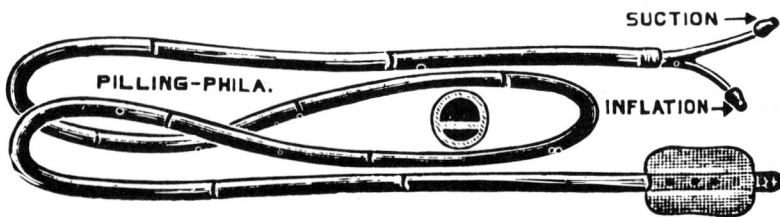

FIG. 218. Miller-Abbott tube.

PLATE 1

SUGAR

CLINITEST

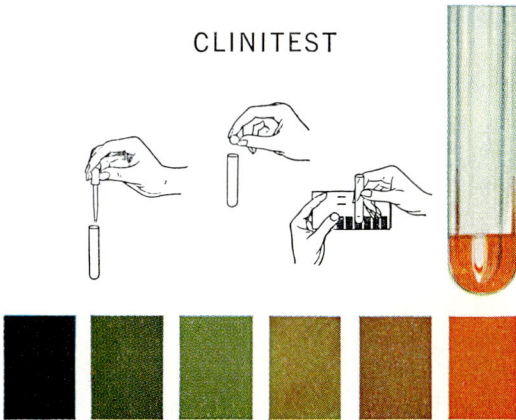

BILIRUBIN

ICTOTEST

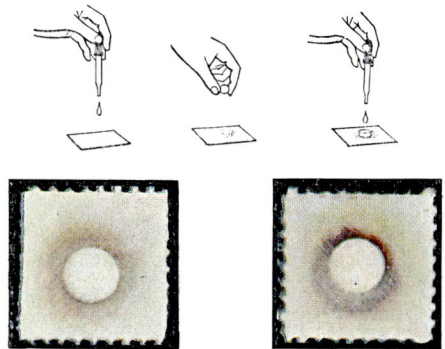

BLOOD

OCCULTEST

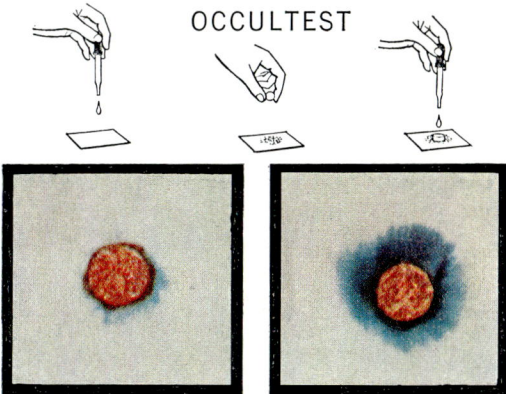

KETONE BODIES

ACETEST

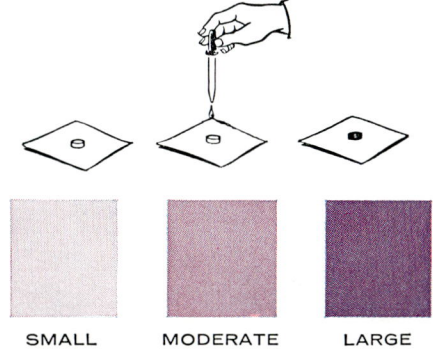

PROTEIN and GLUCOSE

URISTIX

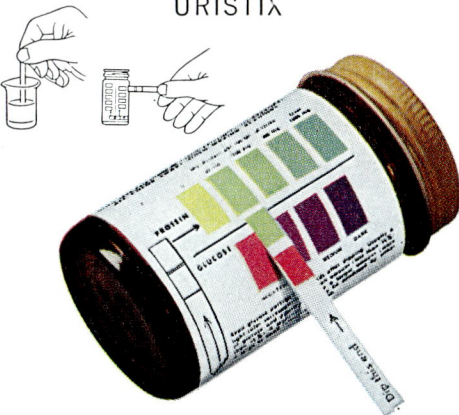

PHENYLKETONE

PHENISTIX

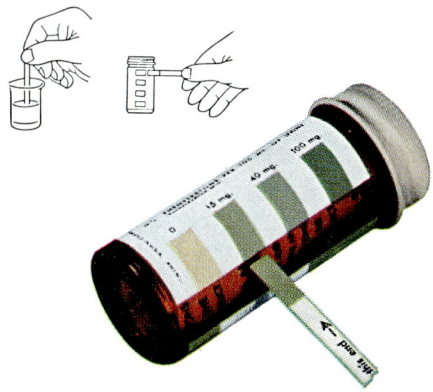

Tests for abnormal urine constituents.

PLATE 2

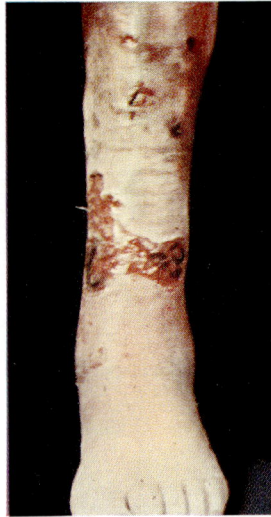

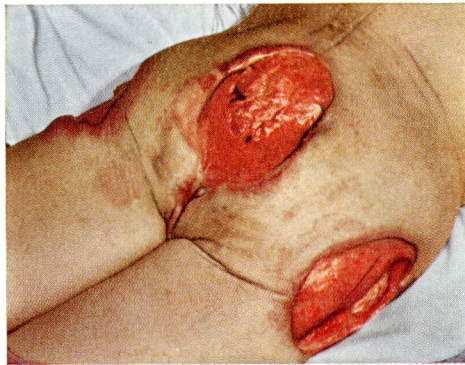

Ischemic necrosis of the skin. (*Top*) A "stasis ulcer," occurring as a complication of venous pooling and tissue edema in a leg with varicose veins. (*Bottom*) Multiple, extremely extensive decubitus ulcers that have developed in vulnerable pressure areas as a result of prolonged ischemia and as a direct consequence of failure to sustain peripheral blood flow in a debilitated, paralyzed patient. (Herbert Mescon, M.D., Boston)

PLATE 3

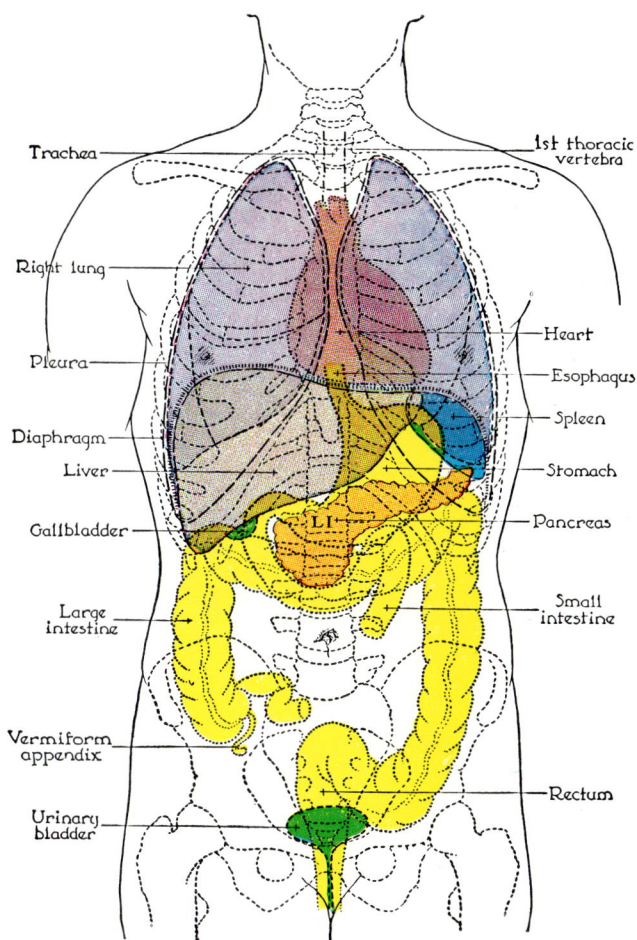

Location of the principal organs. This diagrammatic representation shows the position of the organs in relation to the surface of the body, as well as the skeletal framework. The kidneys (not shown) are behind the stomach, one on each side of the spine. (Eliason: First Aid in Emergencies, Philadelphia, Lippincott)

Plate 4

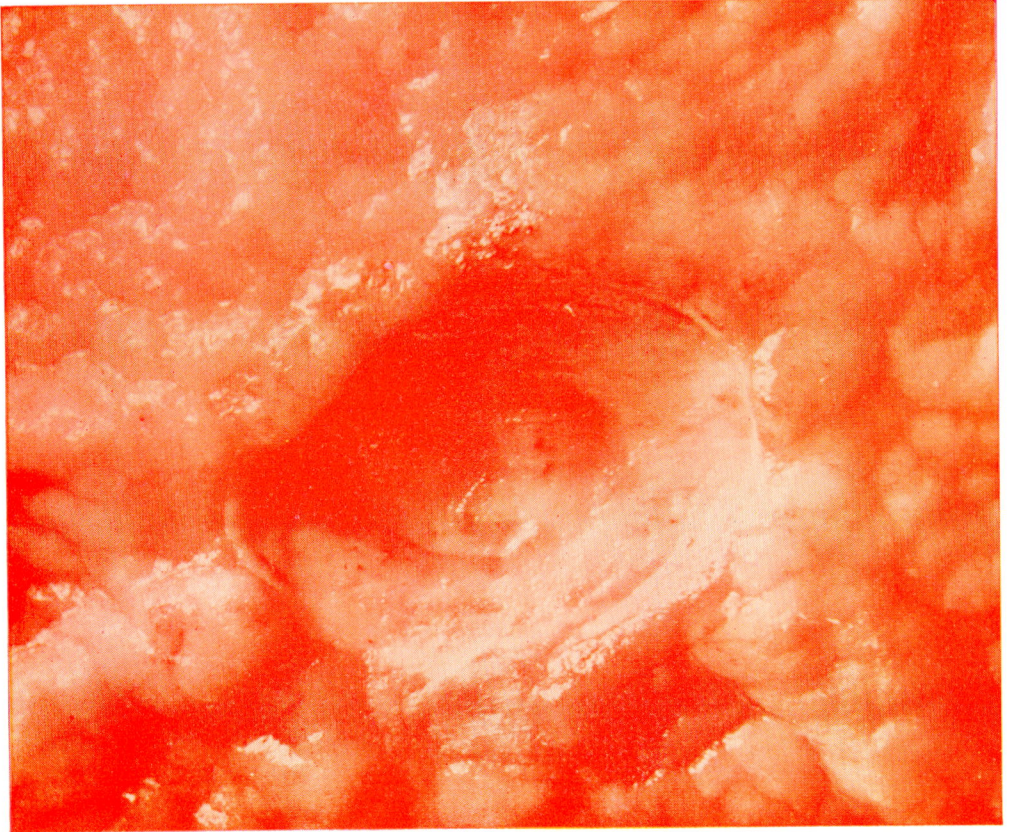

A well-defined gastric ulcer. (From L. Kraeer Ferguson, M.D.)

PLATE 5

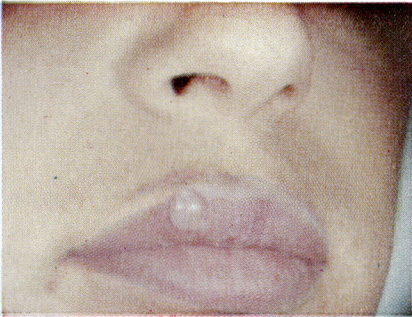

Herpetic vesicle of the lip.

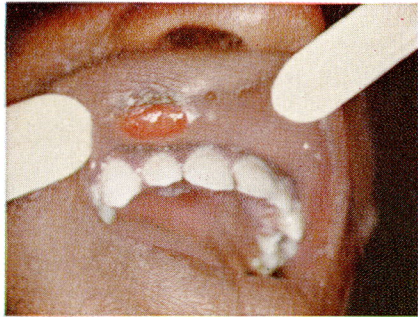

Chancre of the upper lip.

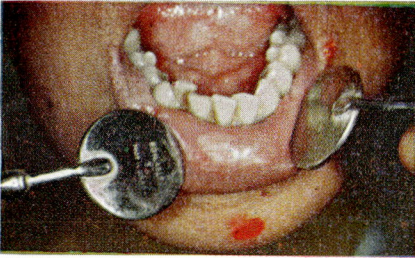

Oral and dermal manifestations of
acute syphilis.

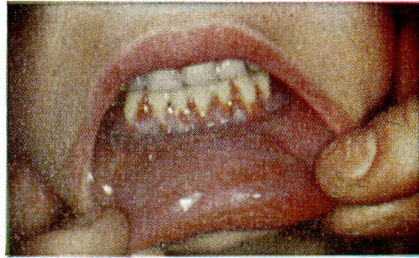

Tuberculous lesions of mucosa
and gums.

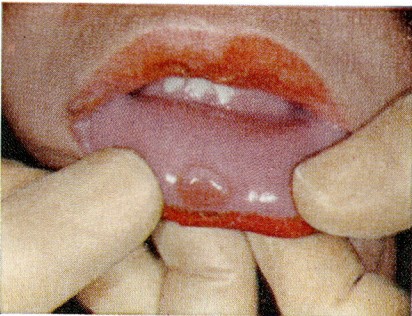

A syphilitic patch on the oral mucosa.

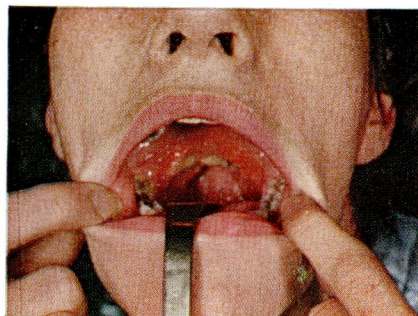

Vincent's angina.

(Burket, L. W.: Oral Medicine, ed. 3, Philadelphia, Lippincott)

PLATE 6

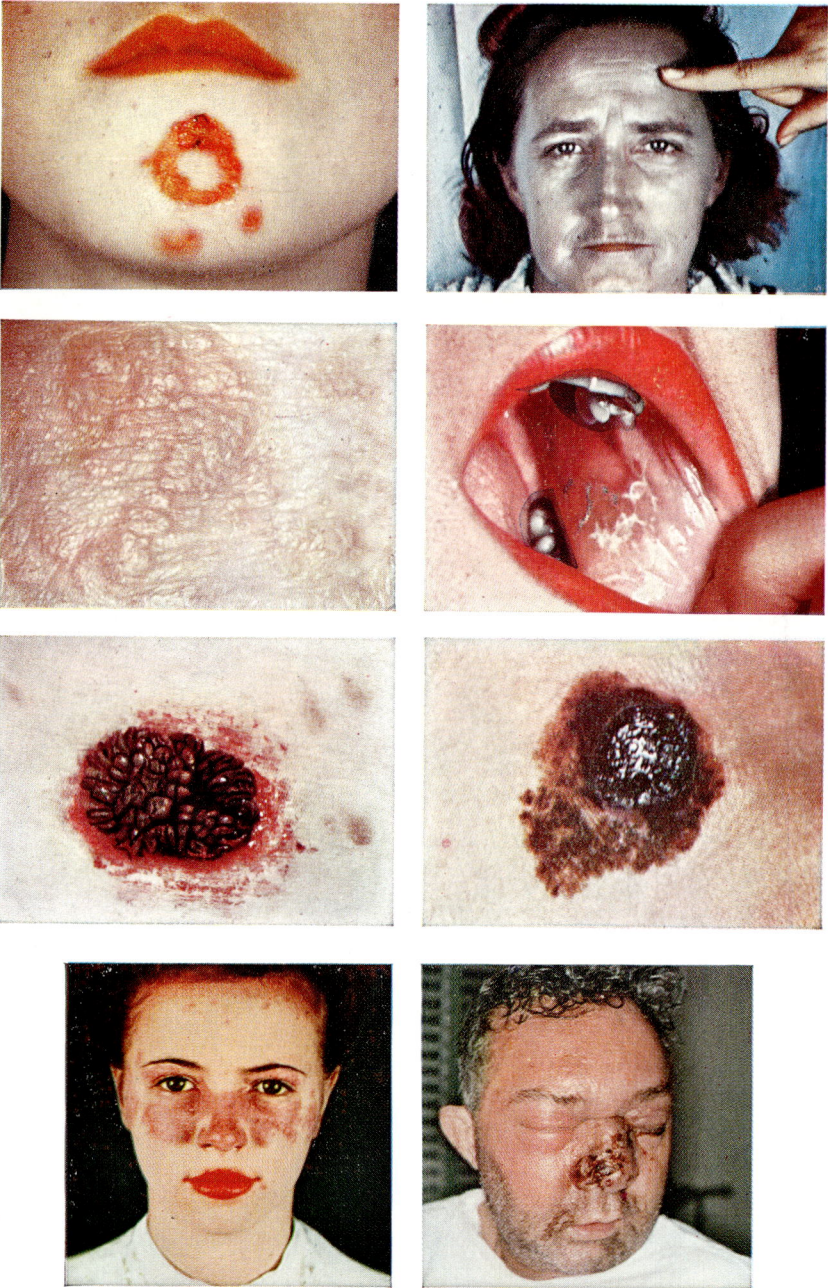

Left (top to bottom). Impetigo contagiosa; lichen planus of skin; benign warty mole; lupus erythematosus. Right (top to bottom). Argyria; lichen planus of buccal mucosa; malignant melanotic sarcoma; erysipelas. (Herbert Mescon, M.D., Boston)

PLATE 7

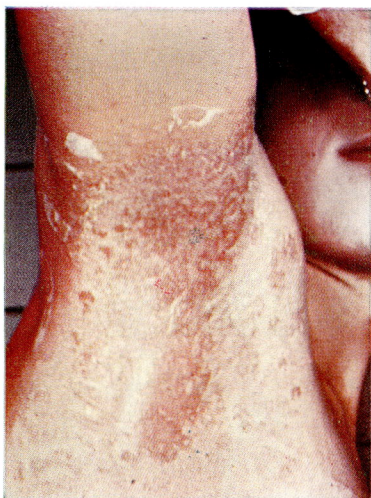

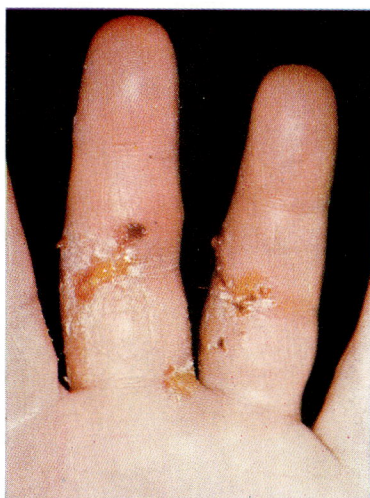

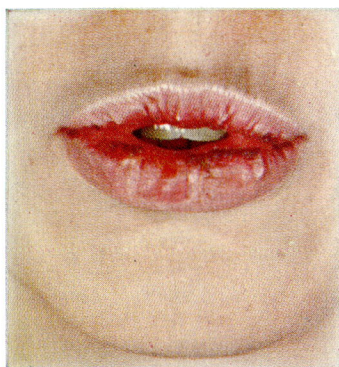

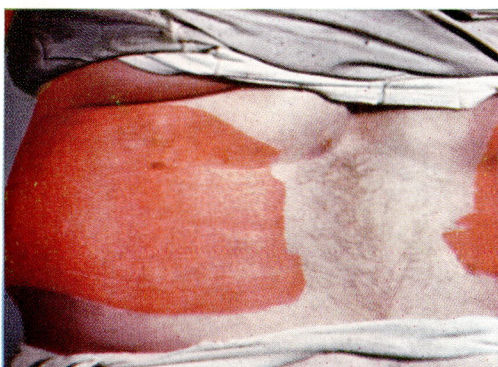

Contact dermatitis exhibited by four sensitized individuals, and occurring as a manifestation of skin allergy in response to a specific antigen, i.e., a cream deodorant *(upper left)*; a soap *(upper right)*; lipstick *(lower left)*; and adhesive plaster *(lower right)*. (Herbert Mescon, M.D., Boston)

PLATE 8

STAGES IN PROGRESSIVE HEALING OF SECOND- AND THIRD-DEGREE BURNS

(From "Management of the Cocoanut Grove Burns at the Massachusetts General Hospital.")

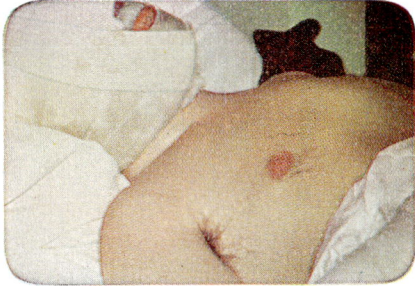

A

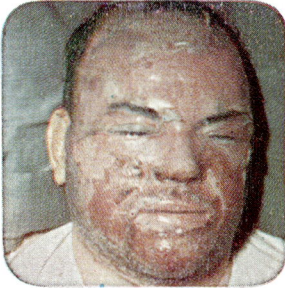

B

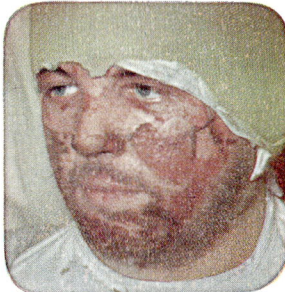

C

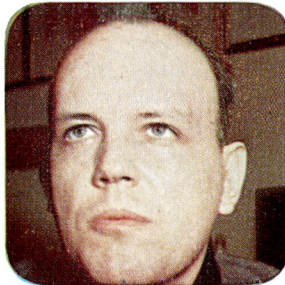

D

(A) 3rd day. Massive subcutaneous edema. Fluid, expressed from burns by pressure dressing, gravitated downward.

(B) 7th day. Edema despite pressure dressing. Some destroyed skin and dry serum still present and uninfected.

(C) 9th day; edema diminished; skin still weeping; crusts have re-formed. Some skin débris.

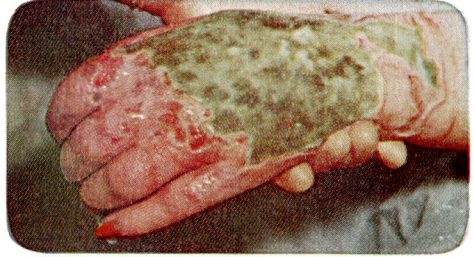

E

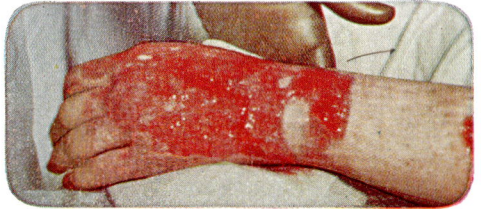

F

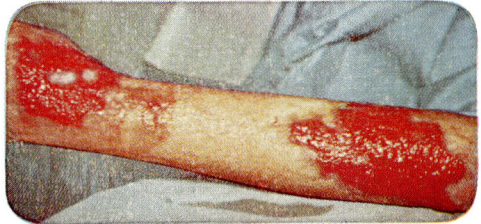

G

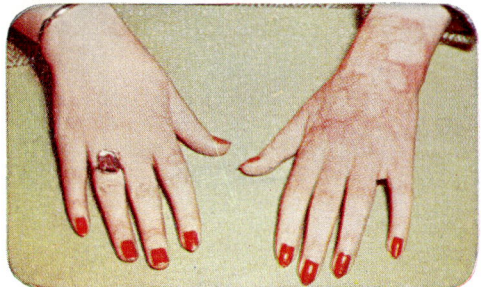

H

(D) 55th day. Absence of scarring; return to normal contours. Scalp healed without grafting.

(E) 19th day. Slough still in place. Skin immediately adjacent normal; no evidence of infection.

(F) 30th day. Most of the slough has separated. Granulations are edematous; infection is minimal.

(G) 51st day, the day of grafting. Note healthy appearance of granulations and islands of viable skin in center of raw surface on back of hand.

(H) Final view of hands at 3½ months.

PLATE 9

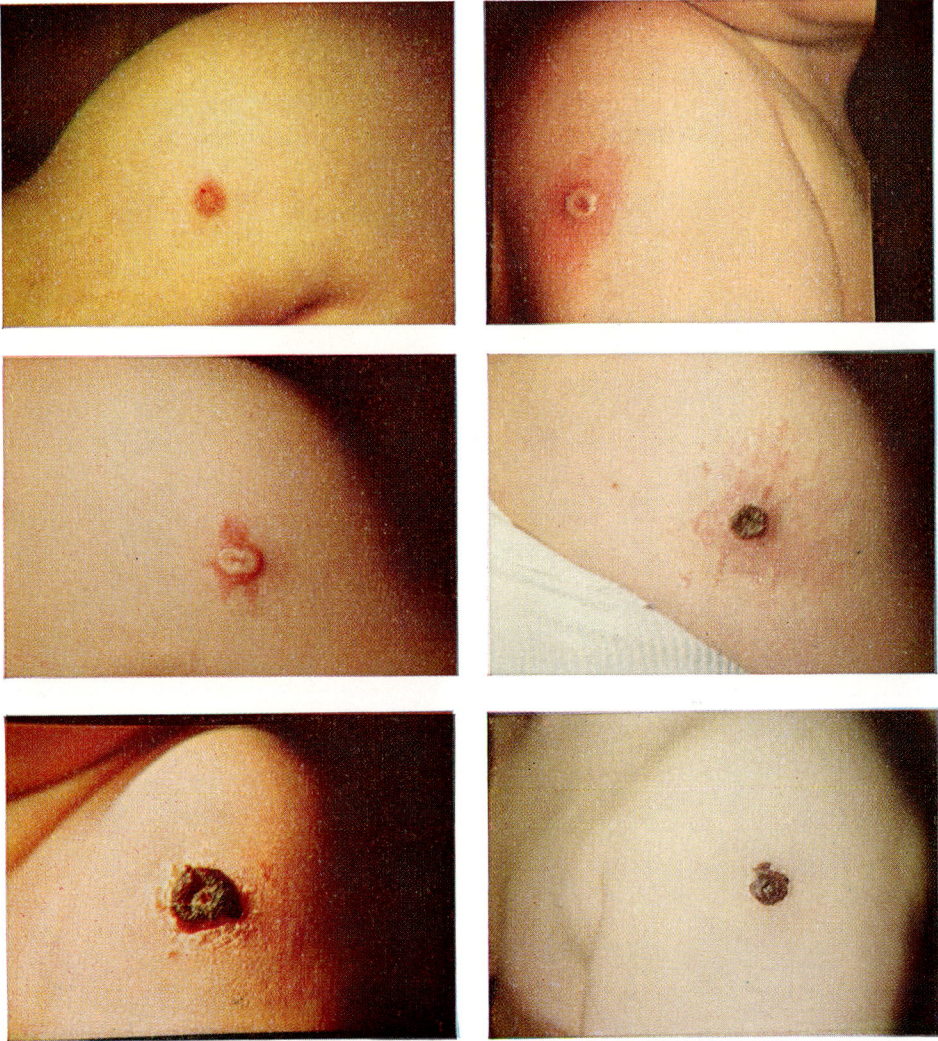

Evolution of vaccinia. (*Top, left*) Day 3. (*Top, right*) Day 6. (*Center, left*) Day 9. (*Center, right*) Day 15. (*Bottom, left*) Day 20. (*Bottom, right*) Day 30.

PLATE 10

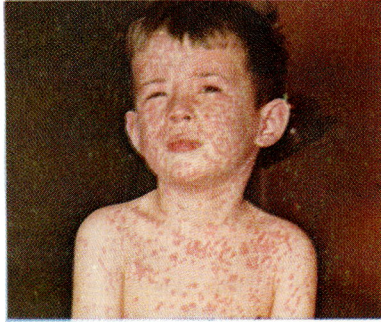

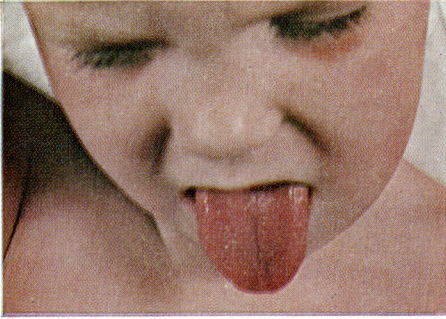

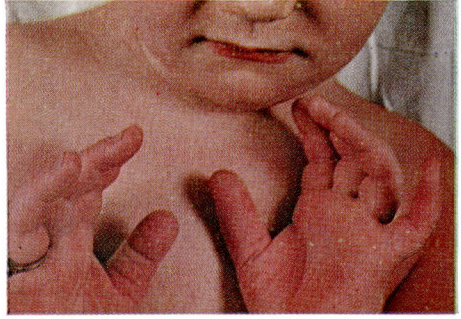

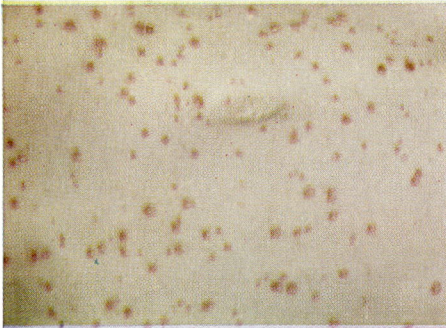

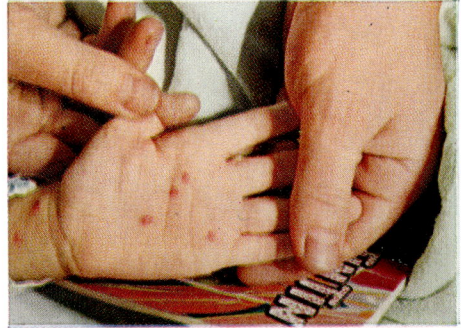

(Top) Measles rash. (Center, left and right) Strawberry tongue and exanthema of scarlet fever. (Bottom, left and right) Rash of chickenpox.

PLATE 11

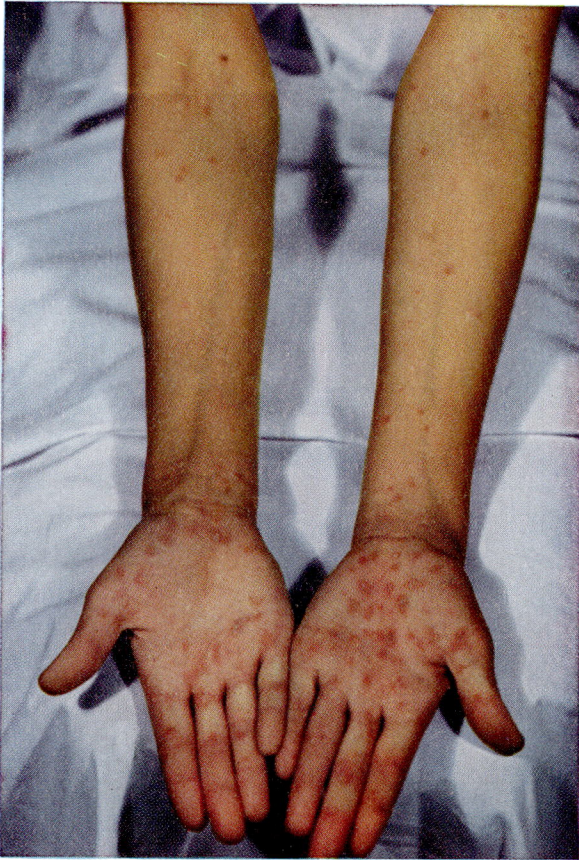

Secondary stage of early syphilis—maculopapular rash. (Kampmeier, R. H.: Essentials of Syphilology, Philadelphia, Lippincott)

outfitted primarily for proctoscopy. These include facilities for applying suction through long tubes that are introduced through the scope to remove any secretion, exudate, blood or excreta that might be obstructing the area of observation. After each use these tubes must be cleansed thoroughly by aspirating water through them, and the collecting bottles should be emptied and cleaned likewise.

As part of the endoscopic examination, one or more small pieces of tissue may be removed for histologic study, a procedure referred to as a "biopsy." This is done with small biting forceps introduced through the proctoscope. If present, rectal and sigmoidal polyps may be removed through the proctoscope by means of a wire snare with which to grasp the pedicle, or stalk, and an electrocoagulating current to sever it and to prevent bleeding. It is extremely important that all tissue that is excised by the endoscopist be placed immediately in moist gauze or in an appropriate receptacle, labeled correctly and legibly, then delivered without delay to the pathology laboratory.

GASTRIC AND INTESTINAL INTUBATION

Tubes inserted into the stomach and the intestine are used to aspirate the contents of these organs in the active and prophylactic treatment of many intra-abdominal lesions. The nasogastric catheter or so-called short tube is introduced through the nose or the mouth into the stomach. By aspiration, the gas and the fluids that collect in the stomach may be removed. It is especially valuable in the postoperative care of many patients

after abdominal operations and especially in the treatment of vomiting postoperatively. The long tubes or double lumen tubes are rubber tubes which are introduced through the stomach into the intestinal tract. They are used to aspirate the intestinal content and so to prevent gas and fluid distention of the coils of intestine. The long tubes are the Miller-Abbott, the Harris and the Cantor tubes. These are used in the active treatment of intestinal obstruction, especially that of the small intestine. They also are used prophylactically, being inserted the night before operation to prevent obstruction after abdominal operation. By their use the intestine is threaded on the tube and so shortened and held together compactly, making it relatively easier to pack off the intestine at the time of operation on the colon. Usually, the tubes are allowed to remain in place after operation until peristalsis is resumed, as shown by the passage of gas by rectum. Intubation usually is practiced in the treatment of all forms of intestinal obstruction, but it is especially effective in paralytic ileus and in postoperative obstruction. These patients can be given liquid nourishment by mouth with the tube still functioning.

Types and Use of Gastrointestinal Tubes

Miller-Abbott Tube. This is a double lumen, No. 16 Fr. 10-ft. tube: one lumen of the tube is used to inflate the balloon at the end of the tube; the other, entirely independent, is used for aspiration (Fig. 218). Before inserting the tube, the balloon should be tested, its capacity measured and then deflated completely. The tube should be lubricated sparingly and chilled well before the

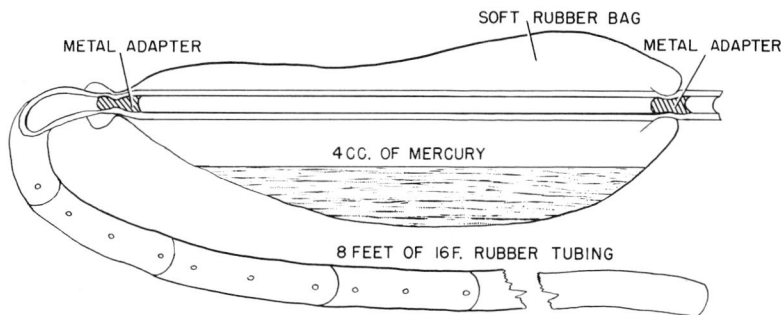

FIG. 219. Harris tube.

doctor inserts the tip through the patient's nose. Markings on the tube indicate the distance it has been passed.

Harris Tube. This is a single-lumen mercury-weighted tube of about 6 ft., and a lumen of 14 on the French scale. This tube has a metal tip that is introduced first into the nostril after having been lubricated. The mercury-weighted bag follows. The weight of the mercury carries the bag by gravity. As this is a single lumen tube that is used wholly for suction and irrigating, there is no difficulty in irrigating it. Usually a Y-tube is attached to the end of the tube, so that the suction apparatus is attached to one side, and an outlet with a clamp is available on the other side for irrigating purposes (Fig. 219).

Cantor Tube. The Cantor tube is 10 ft. long and No. 18 Fr. Its distinguishing feature is that it is larger and has the mercury-filled bag at the extreme end of the rubber tubing (Fig. 220).

To Introduce Nasogastric Tube and Attachment of Suction Apparatus:

1. The nasogastric tube is prepared for use by sterilizing and placing it in a basin containing cracked ice for at least 5 minutes.

After lubricating the end of the tube with water-soluble jelly, the nurse assists the patient to hyperextend his head while the surgeon introduces the tube through the nostril. The nurse should provide the adhesive fixation for use when the tube has been inserted the required distance.

2. The nasogastric catheter is attached to the tube leading to the trap bottle, usually by a Y tube. The other end of the Y tube is attached to a small piece of rubber tubing closed by a clamp. Through this tube irrigations of the nasogastric catheter may be accomplished (Fig. 222).

3. The tube line from the nose to the trap bottle is fixed in position on the bed so that there will be no pulling upon it. This may be accomplished by a safety pin through the bed sheet or by adhesive-tape loops that may be tied or pinned to the bed.

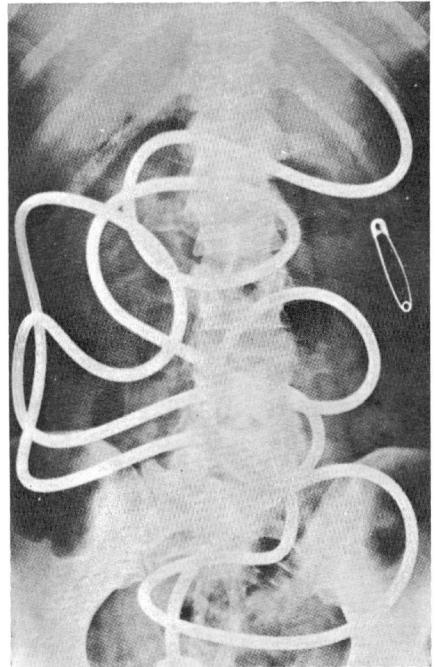

Fig. 221. Miller-Abbott tube in use. Note the balloon at the end of the tube, which has been distended with mercury. The tube has threaded its way down the intestinal tract, and, by suction on the end of the tube, the intestine has been decompressed.

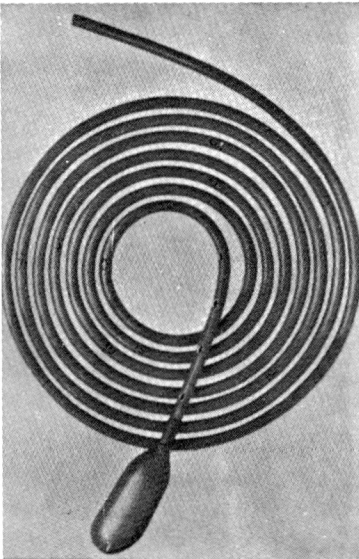

Fig. 220. Cantor tube. (Davol Rubber Co., Providence, R. I.)

To Irrigate Nasogastric Catheter:

Keep the nasogastric catheter open by the injection of a measured small amount of water or saline through the Y tube connection, using a Luer-tip or Asepto syringe. When fluid is injected, the tubing on the other side of the Y connection leading to the trap bottle should be clamped. Suction should not be made with a syringe unless ordered.

To Maintain Adequate Intake:

While gastric-suction drainage is in use, an adequate parenteral intake should be maintained. The amount and the type of fluids are prescribed by the surgeon.

To Keep Accurate Records of:

1. Drainage, amount and type, every 12 hours.
2. Amount of fluid instilled by irrigation of the nasogastric catheter and the amount of water taken by mouth.
3. Amount and character of vomitus, if any.
4. Duration of any period in which the suction apparatus did not appear to function.
5. Effects produced by the treatment.

Nursing Care of Intubated Patients

Before the patient is intubated, it is wise for the nurse or the doctor to explain the treatment and its purpose. A cooperative patient adds much to the success of the procedure. He may be allowed to sit up, and a towel can be spread bib-fashion over his chest. Tissue wipes should be available. The patient ought to be screened from other patients, and the doctor should have adequate light. Often the physician will swab the nostril and spray the oropharynx with

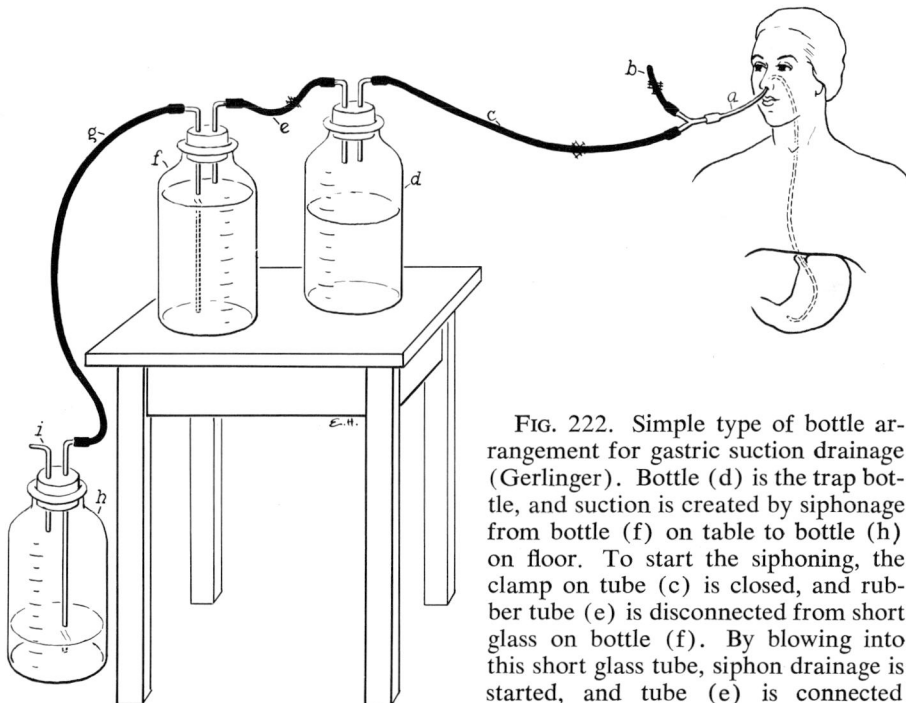

FIG. 222. Simple type of bottle arrangement for gastric suction drainage (Gerlinger). Bottle (d) is the trap bottle, and suction is created by siphonage from bottle (f) on table to bottle (h) on floor. To start the siphoning, the clamp on tube (c) is closed, and rubber tube (e) is disconnected from short glass on bottle (f). By blowing into this short glass tube, siphon drainage is started, and tube (e) is connected again. When bottle (f) becomes empty, it is replaced simply by bottle (h), which now is full, and, after blowing into tube (i) to begin siphonage, tube (e) is attached, and suction drainage is continued. If the exchange between bottles (f) and (h) is made before the water level in bottle (f) gets below the level in the long glass tube, the siphonage already established will be maintained and will not have to be restarted. During exchange of bottles (f) and (h), the clamp on tube (e) is closed. When emptying trap bottle (d), clamps on tubes (c) and (e) are closed.

pontocaine to dull the nasal passage and the gag reflex and make the procedure more tolerable. Encouraging the patient to breathe through his mouth often helps, as does swallowing of water if permitted.

When the tube is passed to the desired distance, the nurse should fasten the catheter to the nose with adhesive tape. A minimum amount of adhesive for the maximum effect should be used. The tube then is connected to the suction apparatus. Enough leeway should be allowed to permit the patient to turn without risk of dislodging the tube. Rigid mouth and nostril hygiene must be followed in caring for these patients, as these tubes may be in place for several days. Applicator sticks dipped in water can be used to clean the nose. This can be followed by mineral oil. Frequent mouth attention is comforting. If the nasal and pharyngeal mucosa is excessively dry, steam inhalations may be beneficial. Throat lozenges, an ice collar, chewing gum (if permitted) and frequent movement also assist in relieving discomfort.

When it is desirable to remove the tube, it is necessary to deflate the balloon and withdraw it gently and slowly for about 6 to 8 inches at intervals of 10 minutes until the tip reaches the esophagus, when the remainder is withdrawn rapidly out of the nostril. Should the tube not come out easily, force should not be used—the physician should be notified. As it is withdrawn, the tube should be concealed in a towel, for it is not a pleasant spectacle and may cause the patient to vomit. After its removal the patient will be grateful for good mouth care.

Gastrointestinal tubes must be cleaned thoroughly with plain water, then by soapy water. The balloon should be removed and discarded. A syringe can be used to force the solution through the tube. Organic solvents, such as alcohol or benzine, should not be used—they weaken rubber. The entire tube should be immersed in a disinfecting solution for 10 minutes. After a thorough rinsing, the tube should be hung to dry in such a way that there are no angulations in it. As rubber tubing may retain an unpleasant odor, the tube can be soaked in lavender water for a few minutes if necessary. Before the tube is used again, a new balloon or bag

should be attached. Some are attached by rubber cement and others are tied with black silk. Instructions for replacement of bags come with the tube.

PROBLEMS RELATED TO THE STOMACH AND THE DUODENUM

Functional Disturbances

Indigestion. As a result of disturbed nervous control of the stomach or of disease elsewhere in the body, many individuals suffer intensely from "indigestion," although their stomachs are without a trace of disease. Abdominal pain is the most common complaint of these individuals. This pain is usually in the upper abdomen and it usually is associated with eating, occurring during or immediately after a meal. Its character may be described as crampy, it may be a feeling of fullness, distention or burning. The types of food that cause the most discomfort are apt to be fatty foods, probably because they remain in the stomach longest and because these patients commonly have an abnormal aversion to fatty foods. Coarse vegetables and highly seasoned foods likewise cause considerable distress. Alkalies, such as sodium bicarbonate, afford only partial relief or perhaps none at all. The basis for the abdominal distress is obviously the patient's own normal gastric peristaltic movements. These anxious and hypersensitive individuals gradually have become acutely conscious of sensations which normally are not noticed, and they are interpreted as pain.

Psychic Vomiting. This is a common symptom in persons with an anxiety neurosis and may be exhibited by any normal individual in a tense situation. Such vomiting may be only occasional or it may be frequent— after every meal. Usually the amount vomited is very small, so small that the nutrition is not in the least disturbed, which is an important diagnostic point; but some severely neurotic individuals develop persistent vomiting to such a degree that they eventually starve to death. The usual neurotic vomiting is not preceded by nausea; the patient simply regurgitates his food and expectorates. Children sometimes learn the trick and are proud of it.

Aerophagia (Air Swallowing). This is not

an unusual symptom of nervous persons. It may appear in attacks lasting for hours. Some individuals eructate large amounts of air with a loud and impressive noise. One may wonder at the source of the air, but by watching we observe that unconsciously they are continually swallowing it, and then, as if by design, attract attention by noisy eructation. The physician can successfully thwart the patient in the performance of this feat by insisting that a cork or some other object be held between the teeth; this renders air swallowing more difficult.

In most psycho-neurotic individuals the gastric symptoms form only a part of the neurotic picture, but, in some patients, severe stomach symptoms overshadow all others and require careful study to rule out organic gastrointestinal disease. The fact that the patient is manifestly neurotic or hysterical, however, does not prove that his gastric symptoms are functional, for a nervous individual has the same chance of contracting gallbladder disease or carcinoma of the stomach as have more stable individuals. All possible diagnostic methods should be employed before a definite diagnosis of functional indigestion has been decided upon. Nervous dyspepsia is diagnosed incorrectly in many cases, not only of organic gastrointestinal disease, but also of unsuspected tuberculosis, cardiac decompensation, uremia, pernicious anemia and atypical migraine. Too much care cannot be taken.

Pylorospasm. In this disturbance, the muscle closing the orifice between the stomach and the duodenum, instead of relaxing, contracts vigorously and painfully at the time that the stomach wall is contracting. The result is upper abdominal pain, occasionally very severe. This usually is due to the presence of a small peptic ulcer near the pylorus.

Hyperacidity. The so-called *heartburn acid eructation,* etc., are due to reverse peristalsis. Because of spasm of the pylorus, reverse peristalsis churns the gastric juice to the cardiac end of the stomach, whence it is forced up the esophagus and into the pharynx where it can be tasted.

Gastritis

Acute Gastritis. This is a complaint so common that its symptoms need not be described in detail. Often it is due to some dietary indiscretion. The individual eats too much or too rapidly or eats food which is noxious because it is too highly seasoned or infected. Acute gastritis also may be the first sign of an acute systemic infection. However, the best examples of acute gastritis are those due to alcohol, to overindulgence in salicylates and to uremia.

The gastric mucous membrane of a stomach that is the seat of acute gastritis is red and swollen and secretes a paucity of gastric juice containing very little acid but much mucus. The patient has uncomfortable feelings in his abdomen, with headache, lassitude, nausea, often vomiting and hiccuping. The vomiting relieves him considerably, for it removes the irritating substances. The tongue is coated, and the flow of saliva is increased. If the irritating food is not vomited but reaches the bowel, colic and diarrhea may be the result. As a rule, the patient is well in about 1 day, although he may not have much appetite for the next 2 or 3 days.

Treatment consists in the parenteral administration of glucose and saline as long as the vomiting persists. When the patient is able to take nourishment by mouth, a bland diet, perhaps supplemented by alkalies, is offered.

Chronic Gastritis. In early cases of chronic gastritis, the mucous membrane of the stomach is thickened and its rugae are prominent. As time passes, both its lining and its walls become thinned and its secretion lessens in quantity and in quality, eventually consisting almost entirely of mucus and water.

One of the important causes of chronic gastritis is chronic uremia. Among the local causes of gastritis are benign and malignant ulcers of the stomach and cirrhosis of the liver complicated by portal hypertension, the latter causing the chronic congestion of the stomach wall.

The diagnosis is established on upper gastrointestinal x-ray series and by gastric analysis.

Symptoms of chronic gastritis vary greatly. The appetite may be poor (anorexia) or too good (bulimia); there is usually some distress ("heartburn") after eating, and often there are eructations of gas. The taste in the mouth is bad; there is usually considerable nausea and perhaps some vomiting, especially early in the morning.

Treatment consists of having the patient eat only easily digested, properly prepared food and chew it well; and, since the muscles of the stomach are weakened, he should eat only small amounts at a time and, therefore, eat more frequently.

The diet may consist entirely of milk for a few days, subsequently replaced by a soft diet such as is described on page 598. Whatever special treatment might be indicated depends on the basic cause of the gastritis in each individual patient.

Peptic Ulcer

A peptic ulcer is an excavation formed in the mucosal wall of the stomach, in the pylorus or in the duodenum, and is due to the erosion of a circumscribed area of its mucous membrane (Fig. 223). This erosion may extend as deeply as the muscle layers or through the muscle to the peritoneum. Peptic ulcers are more apt to be in the duodenum than in the stomach, but, whether on the gastric or on the duodenal side, most of them occur near the pylorus, a few being situated in the pylorus itself. As a rule, they occur singly, but there may be a number of them present at once.

The etiology of peptic ulcer is poorly understood. The disease occurs with the greatest frequency between the ages of 20 and 40, but it has been observed in childhood, even in infancy. It seems to develop in persons who are emotionally tense, but whether this is the cause or the effect of the condition is uncertain. Important predisposing factors associated with recurrence of activity in peptic ulcer include emotional stress, excessive smoking and the season of the year, for this disease tends to appear and recur most commonly in the spring and the fall.

Symptoms

Pain. As a rule, the patient with peptic ulcer complains of pain, or a gnawing sensation, sharply localized in the midepigastrium. The pain recurs from 1 to 3 hours after meals and becomes progressively more severe toward the end of the day. This pain typically is relieved quite promptly by food or alkalies, either of which neutralizes the free acid in contact with the ulcer. If the patient takes neither food nor alkali, the pain gradually wears off as the secretion of acid stops and it empties into the intestine. The

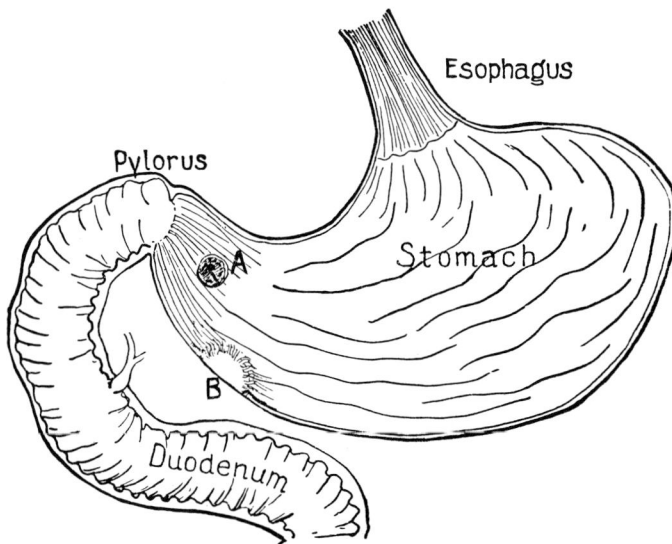

Fig. 223. Ulcers of the stomach. (A) A small punched-out ulcer near the pylorus. (B) A large ulcer cut across.

character of the pain may be described as a dull, burning sensation, a feeling of emptiness or gnawing pain so severe that the patient is in agony. Some relief is obtained by local pressure on the epigastrium. Sharply localized tenderness can be elicited by gentle pressure in the epigastrium at or near the midline.

Vomiting. This is the second classic symptom of peptic ulcer. It is due to pyloric obstruction, as a result of muscular spasm of the pylorus or of mechanical obstruction. The latter may be due to scarring or to acute swelling of the inflamed mucous membrane adjacent to the acute ulcer. The vomiting may or may not be preceded by nausea; usually it follows a bout of severe pain, which is relieved by ejection of the acid gastric contents.

Hemorrhage. Manifested by hematemesis, melena, or both, hemorrhage is the common complication of peptic ulcer. Occasionally this appears without any antecedent history of dyspepsia. A large amount of blood, even 2 or 3 qts., may be vomited. The patient may become almost exsanguinated, and rapid blood replacement may be required to save his life. When the hemorrhage is of large proportions, most of the blood is vomited; when small, much or all of the blood may be passed in the stools, which, due to the digested hemoglobin, appear tarry black. Chemical tests (benzidine, guaiac or orthotolidine) are necessary to detect occult blood which does not alter the gross appearance of the stools, since this type of melena is decidedly more common than gross hemorrhages from the bowel.

Perforation. Perforation of a peptic ulcer may occur unexpectedly, without much evidence of preceding indigestion. Perforation into the free peritoneal cavity is one of the abdominal catastrophes, and the symptoms and signs are those of an acute surgical abdomen. The typical history is that of sudden severe upper abdominal pain, persisting and increasing in intensity, accompanied by vomiting and collapse. The abdomen is extremely tender and board-like in rigidity, and signs of shock develop. Immediate surgical intervention is indicated, for the perforation must be closed as quickly as possible.

Study of Patients with Peptic Ulcer

The nurse plays a large role in the study of patients with peptic ulcer. Since an ulcer usually bleeds, at least in small amounts, the appearance of blood in the stools is an important diagnostic finding. The stools should be collected as requested by the physician. Frequently, it is important to avoid food containing meats for a period of time before stool collection for occult blood.

A great deal of information of value both to the internist and to the surgeon concerns the secretion of gastric acid. In ulcer of the duodenum especially, this secretion is more than normal, and its acid content is very high. For this reason, an analysis of the gastric juice obtained by aspiration of the juice through a tube is an important diagnostic procedure. Often, stimulation of the acid is carried out by using injections of histamine.

There are many technics for gastric analysis. The type that is preferred by the physician in charge is the one that the nurse should follow. Careful collection and marking of the aspirates at intervals are necessary.

Ulcer Management and Nursing Care

The nurse must familiarize herself with every detail of the treatment prescribed for her patient and with the rationale of this treatment. Orders must be carried out punctiliously and in a manner calculated to make them acceptable to the patient. This is usually accomplished by a show of confidence and understanding, by making every effort to accommodate his likes and dislikes within the limits prescribed and by dint of rational detailed explanations when indicated. His day-to-day response to treatment should be observed with care and recorded for the information of the physician.

Acute peptic ulcer is treated most effectively by putting the patient at strict bed rest, sedating him comfortably and neutralizing the gastric juice at frequent and regular intervals with milk drinks and alkaline powders. Ideally, bed rest should continue until the patient is continuously free of pain and is eating normally. Sleep should be re-enforced by sedative drugs to the extent that is necessary to overcome wakefulness. Frequent changes of position, the use of pillows and bed cradles for comfort, quiet surroundings, protection from oversolicitous visitors and prompt responses to his requests will do much to ensure complete rest for the patient. The diet and the medication schedule require the closest cooperation on the part of patient and nurse, for it is extremely important that they be followed rigorously. Ulcer pain, as has been stated, can be agonizing, and the responsibility for its relief necessarily devolves on the nurse, who must see that the patient receives his feedings on time.

The main objective of treatment at this stage is to protect the ulcer from exposure to acid gastric juice. This is accomplished effectively by administering from 2 to 4 Gm. of calcium carbonate hourly. This agent does not produce alkalosis, and its constipating effect is relieved by an occasional dose of magnesium carbonate. In addition to the antacid compounds, one of the many anticholinergic drugs usually is given to suppress gastric secretion or to delay gastric emptying and, thereby, increase the effectiveness of the antacid compound. Among the antisecretory drugs are atropine or belladonna, Banthine and Prantal Methylsulfate. Banthine, in a dose of 0.2 mg. per Kg., is similar in effectiveness and toxicity to Prantal, given I.M. in doses of 0.1 mg. per Kg. of body weight. Both are preferable to atropine and belladonna from the standpoint of toxic side-effects, but the latter are similar in quality, regardless of which particular agent is used. Symptoms of toxicity for which the nurse should be alert include dryness of the mouth and the throat, excessive thirst, difficulty in swallowing, flushed dry skin, rapid pulse and respiration, dilated pupils and emotional excitement.

Milk and cream given regularly at 1-hour or 2-hour intervals may comprise the entire diet for the first few days. During this period the nurse will be responsible for giving the patient his feedings. If he proves to be reliable, the ingredients of his diet may be left at his bedside. The nurse should avoid leaving an excess of milk, which may have an opportunity to sour. The responsibility for seeing to it that the patient takes these feedings still rests with the nurse. A patient on such a regimen may become uncooperative be-cause of dissatisfaction with his diet, and, if so, it may be modified to include milk, with or without cream, ice cream or the bland liquids. The patient and his family should be educated in the reasons for, as well as details of, his ulcer regimen to assure their maximum cooperation. The present trend in ulcer therapy is toward greater latitude in the choice of the dietary constituents, the emphasis being placed on regular feedings rather than on antacid and antispasmodic agents.

Therapy during the night is scheduled in such a manner that sleep will not be curtailed, but at the same time periods of fasting will not exceed 2 or 3 hours, for many of these patients secrete gastric juice continuously day and night.

Sedative drugs are an important part of the therapeutic program for patients with acute peptic ulcer. These may be prescribed on a regular schedule. The patient may become quite drowsy, in which event he will require close supervision when ambulatory, as well as protective rails on his bed, in order to avoid injury. Heavily sedated patients should be turned frequently and should be required to wear elastic stockings constantly as a prophylactic measure for the prevention of thrombophlebitis.

In a few days, after the pain has been controlled, a regular schedule of frequent bland feedings is inaugurated, supplemented by powders or other neutralizing substances as needed. Ideally, the stomach at no time is overloaded; at no time is free acid present in excess or peristalsis vigorous. Dilute orange juice will supply vitamin C (ascorbic acid), which is otherwise lacking in the diet. As progress is made from the simple milk diet, trays must be served attractively and with attention to specific preferences so that the patient will eat with enthusiasm all that is given him. The food should be of bland character, containing all the essential constituents in proper balance, and it should not provoke the secretion of gastric juice or be monotonous. This diet usually should be continued for several weeks after discharge, even after all symptoms have disappeared.

The emotional make-up of the patient with ulcer reflects immaturity, insecurity and frustration. Such individuals are inclined to be irritable and demanding and to take offense easily. The nurse must recognize that her patient has fashioned some very concrete problems as a conscious basis for his anxiety. These he is eager to discuss with the nurse during her unhurried contacts with him, and such discussions afford him satisfaction and relief. Indeed, her very presence, as she responds to his many calls, brings relief. If the nurse is aware of her therapeutic role in relation to her patient she will not be annoyed by his repeated signals.

It is a well-known fact that many patients with acute ulcer symptoms, due to proved ulcer, derive complete temporary relief from nothing more than severance of all connections with environmental anxiety-producing factors—unfavorable diet and hygienic conditions notwithstanding. Such a solution is rarely practicable, however, for environments, particularly internal emotional environments, are not easily shed. Freedom from ulcer recurrences is favored by adherence to a sound hygienic routine of living, which implies regularity of habits in general, moderation in all pursuits, adequate rest daily, ample relaxation, good diet discipline and, at least in this instance, abstinence from smoking. Beneficial alterations of stress situations frequently are possible through wise counseling by the physician (in some cases aided by a psychiatrist) of the patient and the patient's family. The basis of such counsel may be established by the observation of a nurse who has been able to elicit pertinent information in this connection. An increased food budget may be required to provide an adequate bland diet for the patient. (Extra food expense can be eliminated, or held to a minimum, by providing standard family items which have been processed with a sieve or a "blender," or by using commercial baby foods, flavored to taste and served warm.) Ulcers are prone to recur, despite medical and surgical measures, if the patient must return to the same environment to face the same problems that earlier had played a contributory role in their production.

Treatment of pyloric obstruction, developing in the course of acute peptic ulcer, may require repeated gastric aspirations in addition to the milk and alkalies. If the signs of obstruction persist over a period of a few days despite adequate medical care, surgical intervention becomes necessary.

Hemorrhage, which can be massive and fatal, requires the speedy application of measures designed to halt the bleeding and then to replace the lost blood. Small, frequent, bland feedings are provided to prevent hunger contractions. Demerol hydrochloride may be indicated if the patient is extremely restless or in pain. Whole-blood and/or plasma transfusions are employed to keep the circulating blood volume at a safe level. One does not wait for a drop of blood pressure before embarking on transfusion therapy if there are signs of tachycardia, sweating and coldness of the extremities.

The nurse plays an important role in observing and reporting these symptoms immediately, then carrying out the procedures indicated in cases of oligemic shock, as outlined on page 297.

Surgical Treatment of Peptic Ulcer

Although most patients with peptic ulcer respond to medical treatment, complications may develop that demand surgical therapy. These complications are perforation, hemorrhage, obstruction to the pylorus, or inability to control the ulcer pain by medical means—a complication most often described as "intractability." The purpose of operation is to relieve complications. Since the ulcers are believed to result from the acid pepsin of the stomach, the operations are designed to lower the production of acid by the stomach to a point at which further ulcerations will not occur. This is done either by removing a large part of the acid-forming cells of the stomach, usually the distal two thirds or three quarters, or by removing the acid-stimulating mechanism of the stomach, i.e., dividing the vagus nerves and removing the antral portion of the stomach. The excessive gastric acid is produced in duodenal ulcer largely by stimulation that arrives over the vagus nerves. The antral portion of the stomach also stimulates acid production by way of the hormone *gastrin* produced in its mucosal layer and absorbed into the blood stream and carried to the acid-producing cells of the stomach. By removing these two stimulating factors, acid secretion is reduced to a minimum.

Preoperative Nursing Care. Often the cause of the ulcer will not be removed by surgical intervention alone. Constant fear or worry may be disturbing the individual. Only when this factor is eliminated can the best results be looked for. The surgeon and the nurse must realize that the "psyche" has much influence over the "soma," and all efforts to allay the apprehension and the fears of the patient should be employed. Perhaps an immediate preoperative worry is fear of the anesthesia or of malignancy. As these patients have a long illness, they are discouraged frequently and often are helped by spiritual therapy. Economic and social factors may have influenced the patient to such an extent that long hours of work, no recreation, tension, fatigue, etc., have contributed in good measure to his illness. The nurse might seek these factors tactfully in an effort to aid the physician as he directs treatment so that a recurrence of the patient's ulcer might be eliminated.

The patient has laboratory analyses, roentgenologic series and a general physical check-up before surgery is attempted. The function of the nurse is to prepare her patient for each of these diagnostic measures by explaining their nature and significance to him. Specific physical preparation will be prescribed by the physician.

Before operation is begun on the upper intestinal tract, special care should be paid to the hygiene of the mouth. The teeth of these patients usually are bad, and the nurse should urge frequent mouthwashes and a thorough brushing of the teeth at least 3 times daily.

The nutritional and fluid needs of the patient are of major importance. In those patients with pyloric obstruction, there usually is prolonged vomiting with resultant weight and fluid loss. Every effort must be made to restore an adequate nutritional level and to maintain an optimal fluid and electrolyte balance. Again, the nurse plays a key role in helping her patient to achieve a satisfactory preoperative status so that postoperative hazards are kept at a minimum.

Gastric suction through a nasogastric tube is used often to empty the stomach, especially in patients with pyloric obstruction, and a Levin tube often is inserted before the patient goes to the operating room; this is left in place for operative and postoperative use. It is important that the colon be empty when the patient comes to surgery. Usually this is insured by an enema the day before operation. If gastrointestinal roentgenograms have been made shortly before the day of operation, it is most important that the patient have enemas to remove completely the barium that may remain in the colon. The nurse should report it when the enema returns still show the whitish color of barium in the fecal material. The patient usually is limited to full fluids during the 24-hour period preceding surgery. The abdomen should be prepared from the nipple line to the symphysis (see Fig. 39C, p. 210), although the incision usually is made in the upper right quadrant or the midline.

Operative Treatment. In patients whose bleeding is the outstanding symptom, there usually is a period of transfusion in preparation for the operative procedure. This is especially important in older patients in whom recurrence of hemorrhage often ends fatally. In these patients, the ulcer-bearing area is removed and the vessels leading to the area are ligated. As a rule, this entails a subtotal gastrectomy with removal of the ulcerated area in the duodenum. An end-to-side type of anastomosis is performed between the end of the stomach and the jejunum.

An almost immediate operation must be performed on those patients who reach the hospital with ulcers that are perforated and draining gastric or intestinal contents into the abdominal cavity. The abdomen is opened and the perforation through the ulcer is sutured and overlaid with omentum. In a few patients it may be necessary also to perform an anastomosis between the stomach and the jejunum. Ulcers complicated by a gradually increasing closure of the pyloric opening of the stomach occur usually in older people. In these individuals, a conservative type of operation—posterior gastrojejunostomy—may be used (Fig. 224, *Top left*).

It is difficult to distinguish benign ulcers of the stomach from cancer of the stomach.

Therefore, many surgeons are of the opinion that most large gastric ulcers should be treated by operation.

Usually the operation consists of an excision of the entire pyloric portion of the stomach, as much as three fourths of the stomach proper often being removed with the ulcer. The end of the duodenum is closed. The opening in the stomach then is sutured partially and the remaining opening is sutured to the side of the jejunum (Fig. 224, *Top, right* and *Bottom, left*).

In the case of intractable ulcer not amenable to any type of medicinal or other conservative treatment, the foregoing operation is advised. In this type of operation it is hoped, in both gastric and duodenal ulcers, not only to remove the ulcer-bearing areas in both the duodenum and the stomach but to reduce the acid pepsin secretion of the stomach to a level that will prevent the appearance later of ulcers on the margin of the stoma or even in the jejunum.

VAGOTOMY is performed in many of these cases. In this operation, both vagus nerves are sectioned along the lower esophagus either above or below the diaphragm. This abolishes the nervous factor in acid pepsin secretion, which is especially important in the causation of duodenal ulcers. Vagotomy usually is performed with a gastroenterostomy or a gastric resection.

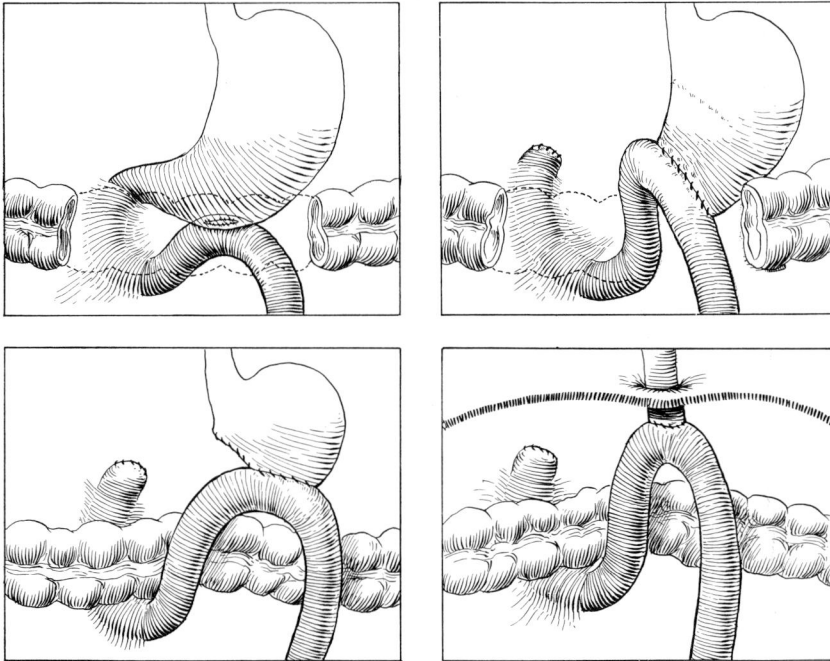

FIG. 224. Diagrammatic drawings to show types of gastric operations. (*Top, left*) Posterior gastrojejunostomy. The jejunum is sutured to the stomach behind the colon, which has been cut away to show the anastomosis. (*Top, right*) Subtotal gastric resection with posterior gastrojejunostomy. The resected portion includes the first part of the duodenum, the pylorus and from two thirds to three quarters of the stomach. The stump of the duodenum is closed by suture, and the side of the jejunum is anastomosed to the end of the stomach (Polya) posterior to the colon. (*Bottom, left*) Subtotal gastric resection with anterior gastrojejunostomy (Hofmeister type). The resection is as in B. The anastomosis is made anterior to the colon, the side of the jejunum is anastomosed to part of the cut end of the stomach, and the rest is closed by sutures. (*Bottom, right*) Total gastrectomy. The entire stomach is removed and the esophagus is anastomosed to a loop of jejunum under the diaphragm.

Gastric Cooling and Freezing

For some time in the treatment of bleeding gastric and duodenal lesions, cold has been used. Once it was used as ice-water lavage of the stomach. More recently Dr. O. H. Wangensteen has used actual cooling and freezing not only in the treatment of bleeding from the stomach, the duodenum, or esophageal varices but also in treating the ulcer itself. Cooling and freezing has been accomplished by the introduction into the stomach of a balloon into which is passed a cooling solution. This solution may be circulated for several days. Particular care must be taken that the special machine available for this sort of treatment is not tampered with, because of danger from overcooling or rupture of the stomach by overdistention of the balloon. This method of treatment is by no means generally accepted, but at this writing it offers a method of rapidly controlling gastric, duodenal and esophageal hemorrhage. Frequently it gives only temporary control of the bleeding, and operation may be necessary.

Discharge and Home Care

Patients who have been operated on for peptic ulcer often need instruction as to their diet for months and even years after operation, because, even though the ulcer has been removed, secondary ulcers sometimes occur. The best way to prevent these is to reduce the amount of the acidity of the gastric juice and to avoid coarse foods. Therefore, patients are instructed to avoid foods that tend to stimulate acid secretion in the stomach. Such foods are as follows:

All acids, e.g., vinegar, pickles, sour foods.

Raw fruits, e.g., apples, grapes, lemons, oranges.

Meat-stock soups, e.g., bouillon, consommé.

Condiments and spices, e.g., excess of chili and black pepper, mustard, horseradish, cloves, nutmeg.

Concentrated sweets, e.g., honey, molasses, candy.

Coarse foods, e.g., nuts, corn, cabbage.

For the first 6 months, the patient may require 6 small meals a day because of his reduced gastric capacity. He must avoid overeating.

Merely to hand a patient awaiting discharge from hospital a diet list is not sufficient preparation. He should be brought to realize that emotional factors have a definite effect on food digestion. The need for peace of mind is so important; both he and his family should know this. If some of his problems remain unsolved, perhaps the medical social worker can help. The patient must realize that he is a responsible partner in his own treatment.

The patient should resume normal activities and responsibilities gradually. Time should be allowed daily for rest periods; these should follow each meal to promote good digestion. Good habits of sleeping and relaxing should be formed. Finally, moderation in all activities must be practiced. Follow-up visits to the physician are an important part of convalescent care.

Congenital Hypertrophic Pyloric Stenosis

This condition, which is characterized by hypertrophy of the circular muscle fibers of the pyloric sphincter at the outlet of the stomach, requires surgical treatment more frequently than does any other condition during the first few months of life. Its cause is not understood definitely, but spasm of the pyloric muscle, in addition to edema of the mucous membrane from mechanical irritation of curds, would seem to be the main factors in its development. Heredity also appears to play a part in the etiology. The first-born male child is the one affected most frequently.

Diagnosis. Vomiting, which appears in the 2nd or the 3rd week of life, is the most constant symptom. As vomiting continues, the infant loses weight, dehydration appears and the stools become scanty. Peristaltic waves may be seen going from left to right across the upper abdomen during feeding. Palpation usually will reveal a small tumor mass in the right upper quadrant of the abdomen. The administration of a thin barium meal will show gastric retention and confirm the diagnosis.

Treatment and Nursing Care

Dehydration, acidosis, electrolyte imbalance and anemia must be corrected by adequate parenteral fluids, saline, glucose and

PRINCIPLES OF MEDICAL AND NURSING MANAGEMENT OF THE PATIENT WITH A PEPTIC ULCER

Major Problems
  A. Pain and dyspepsia
  B. Anxiety and emotional distress
  C. Promotion of physical and emotional rest
  D. Prevention of complications

Objectives
  1. To assure mental and physical rest:
     A. Bed rest to remove patient from stressful environment
     B. Written nursing-care plan to provide for optimum coordinated care
     C. Sedatives and soporific medications to promote relaxation and sleep
     D. Medications and dietary feedings given on time

  2. To rest the motor and secretory activities of the stomach through a therapeutic diet:
     A. Bland protein and fat foods to neutralize acidity
     B. Small feedings to rest the gastrointestinal tract
     C. Frequent feedings to absorb excess acid
     D. Nonstimulating foods to avoid irritation of the gastric mucosa
     E. Progression to nutritionally adequate diet as rapidly as possible

  3. To relieve pain and discomfort and promote healing:
     A. Antacid drugs given to neutralize gastric secretions and afford symptomatic relief
     B. Anticholinergic drugs given to decrease gastric motility and reduce volume of gastric secretions
     C. Adequate hydration to relieve side-effects of anticholinergic drugs
     D. Therapeutic diet as ordered

  4. To assist the patient to accept and follow his therapeutic program:
     A. Demonstrate interest in patient and eliminate factors producing anxiety.
     B. Teach importance of taking prescribed medication and diet on time.
     C. Assist patient to develop insight into causes of his tension and frustration.
     D. Implement and reinforce instructions issued by the doctor.
     E. Teach the importance of moderation in all activities.
     F. Encourage the elimination of smoking.
     G. Stress the value of psychiatric interviews if prescribed.

  5. To recognize the complications of peptic ulcer:
     A. Perforation
        1. Assist with transfusion to treat shock.
        2. Prepare to institute nasogastric suction to remove gastrointestinal secretions.
        3. Give drugs to control pain.
        4. Prepare patient for immediate surgery.

     B. Hemorrhage
        1. Prepare for prompt and rapid transfusion for blood replacement.
        2. Administer sedation to allay anxiety and keep patient at rest.
        3. Assist with gastric intubation for aspiration of stomach contents.
        4. Evaluate clinical response to blood replacement.
        5. Observe continuously to maintain blood pressure at physiologic level.
        6. Observe urinary volume.
        7. Observe stools for melena.
        8. Prepare for surgical intervention if indicated.

blood. Transverse division of the hypertrophied circular pyloric muscle fibers to increase the diameter of the constricted area is the treatment of choice. This procedure is known as *pyloromyotomy* or the *Fredet-Ramstedt operation* (see Fig. 225). Prior to operation the stomach contents should be aspirated with a small rubber catheter passed through the nose. The catheter is left in place during the operation to keep the stomach deflated at all times. Body heat of the infant must be conserved by keeping him well wrapped up while going to surgery. Preoperative medication consists usually of appropriate doses of atropine. Open-drop ether is the anesthesia of choice.

The postoperative care is important in the recovery of these severely ill infants. Feedings are begun as soon as the baby has recovered from anesthesia. Water is given first in 1-ounce quantities every 2 hours. This is followed by whey and increasing amounts of breast milk or formula, as indicated in the individual case. After from 10 to 14 days a normal feeding regimen should be attained. The nurse must observe her very young patient carefully for any signs or symptoms which might be suggestive of complications as otitis media, wound infection, evisceration and pneumonia. Fluid and electrolyte balance must be maintained and anemia corrected as indicated.

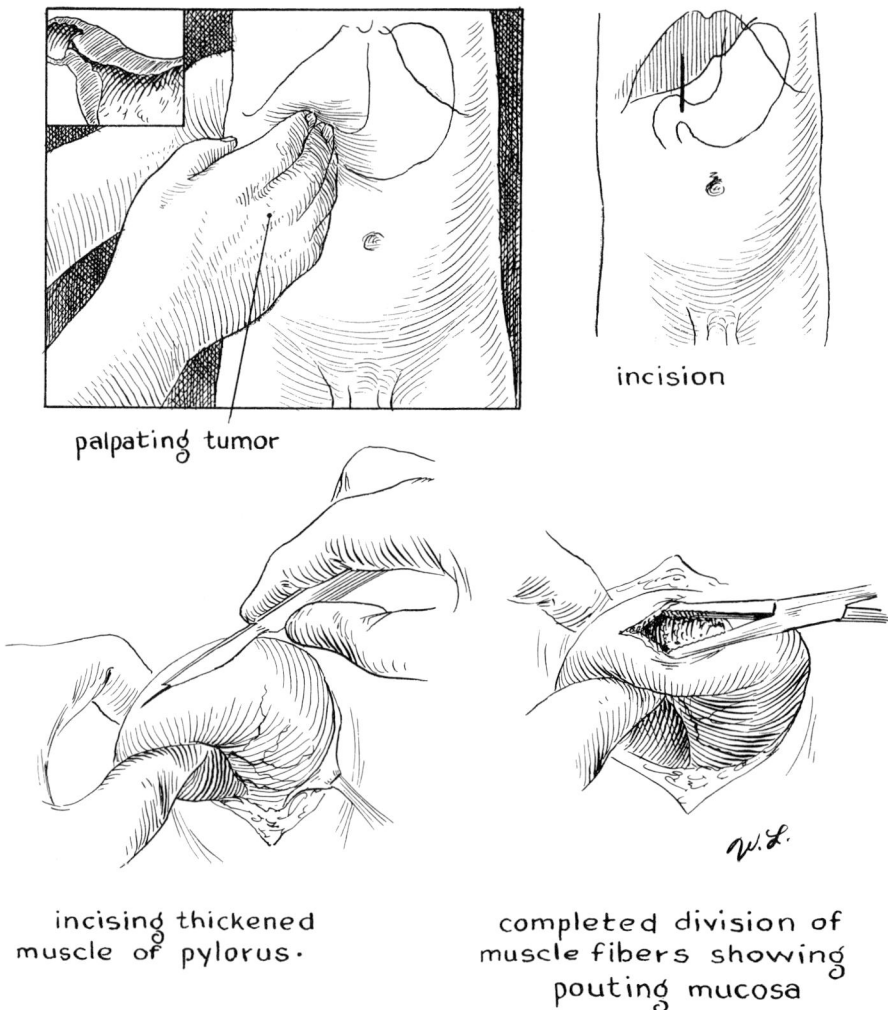

palpating tumor

incision

incising thickened muscle of pylorus.

completed division of muscle fibers showing pouting mucosa

FIG. 225. Ramstedt operation for congenital hypertrophic pyloric stenosis.

During hospitalization of the patient, the surgeon and the nurse should attempt to alleviate undue concern by the parents. A mother faces an emotional struggle that may be as difficult to treat as the organic disease of the child. These are situations in which the nurse can give assurance and encouragement. The results of surgery are very gratifying. Most large series of cases report a mortality of less than 1 per cent.

Gastric Cancer

Cancer of the stomach, a disease that still accounts for more than 20,000 annual deaths in the United States, is typically a disease of middle age. It occurs chiefly in persons over 40, but is seen occasionally in younger people. The most common type of neoplasm of the stomach is carcinoma (Fig. 226); sarcomata and lymphomata are relatively rare.

Symptoms and Diagnosis

The early symptoms of this disease are often indefinite, since most of these tumors start on the lesser curvature, where they cause little disturbance to the gastric functions. Other malignancies follow chronic ulcers. Later, after they have spread to the cardiac orifice, or especially to the pylorus,

the suffering may be distressing; but this is due not to the cancer as such, but to disturbance in gastric motility. Weight loss, weakness, anemia and sometimes icterus appear late in the disease. Pain in gastric cancer, as in cancer in almost all other parts of the body, is a late symptom. Whereas pain is, to the average layman, a sensitive indicator of disturbed physiology or disease, it is ironic that pain rarely warns the individual who has cancer while there is still an opportunity of curing it.

The most important early symptoms are a progressive loss of appetite; the appearance of, or change in, gastrointestinal symptoms that have been increasingly apparent for a matter of weeks or months only; and the appearance of blood in the stools. If the tumor causes obstruction at the cardiac orifice, vomiting or a feeling of fullness will immediately follow the meal. If it is near the pylorus it will eventually obstruct this channel, and vomiting will become a prominent symptom. A certain number of patients apparently have experienced no symptoms attributable to gastric disease, but, having died for some other reason, are found at necropsy to have cancer of the stomach.

The dyspepsia mentioned is by far the

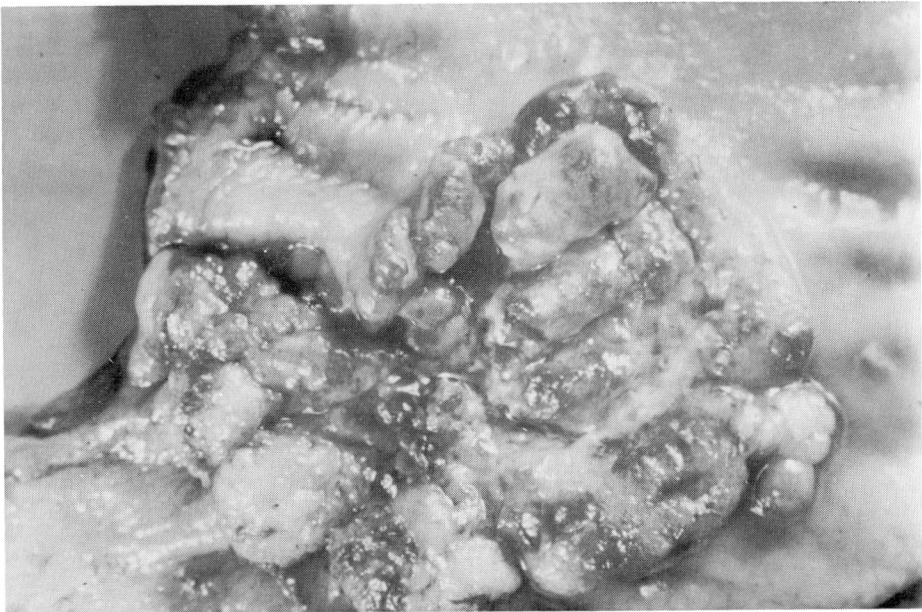

FIG. 226. Gastric carcinoma.

most important of all early symptoms. If two persons were to describe their dyspepsia in much the same words, but one were to say his trouble began when he was a young man and had been present more or less ever since, while the other were to declare that he had had a normal digestion until he was 40 years old or more, it would be reasonable to postulate, tentatively, that the former has no cancer, while the latter may have one. If, in addition to this unprecedented development of dyspepsia, he has lost weight and strength and has become rather pale, we may be more confident of the suspected diagnosis.

Another important symptom occasionally present is the vomiting of coffee-ground vomitus. The blood which leaks slowly from the cancer (large hemorrhages are rare in patients with cancer) is altered chemically and forms small clots or precipitates; therefore, the vomitus acquires that appearance. The patient may not vomit, but one may con-stantly find traces of blood in the stools if these are examined chemically by the guaiac or benzidine test. This is a very early valuable sign of a cancer anywhere along the gastrointestinal canal, but it is by no means confined to patients with malignancy, bleeding being a common complication of benign peptic ulcer as well.

If we examine the gastric juice, we find quite early that there is no free hydrochloric acid present. Often we do find some lactic acid formed from the gastric contents within 1 hour after the meal. Cytologic examination of the sediment from a centrifuged specimen of gastric juice examined by the Papanicolaou technic may show the presence of carcinoma cells; if so, the diagnosis is established. Sometimes the cancer is palpable especially if it is located near the pylorus. Operation usually is justified. We may find also in the abdomen other tumors, metastases of this gastric malignancy. The metastases

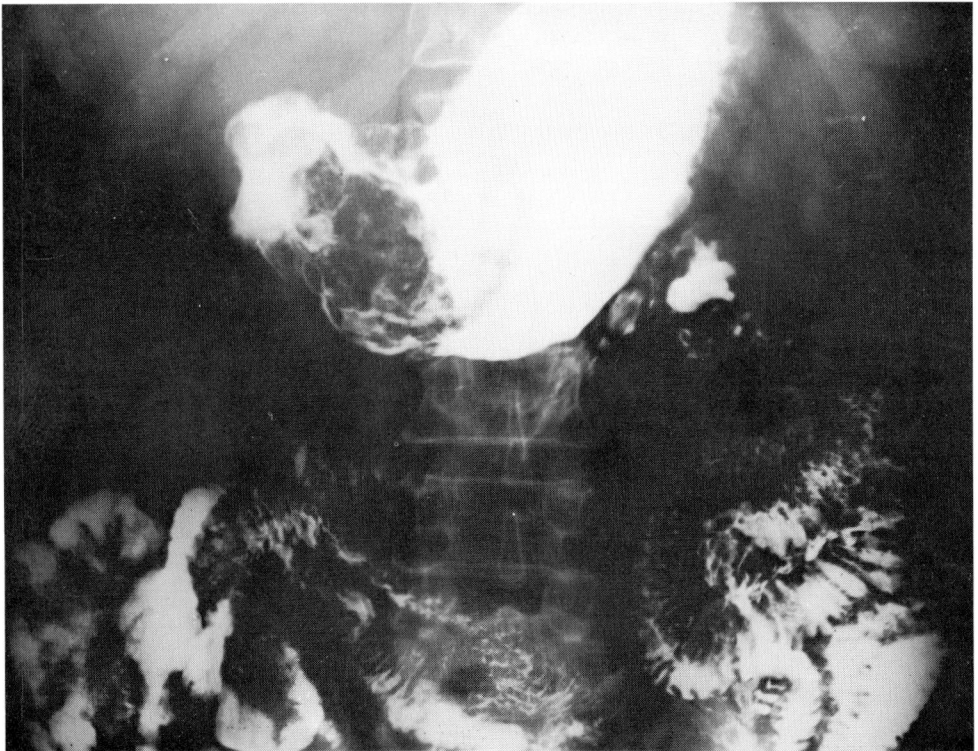

Fig. 227. Roèntgenogram of carcinoma of the stomach. Note how the normal outline of the stomach is deformed by displacement of barium meal at the site of large gastric carcinoma.

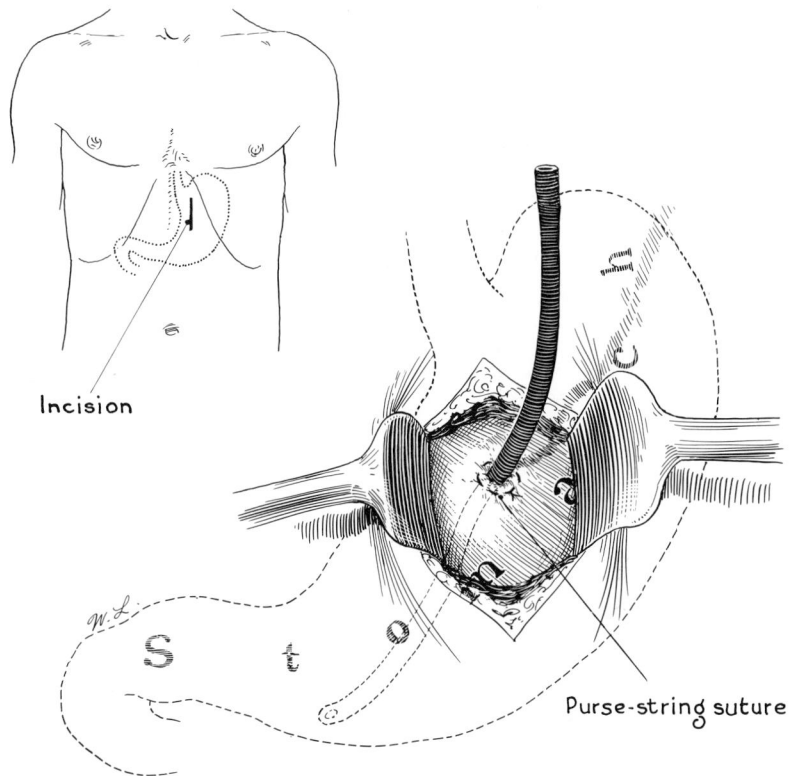

are most apt to be located on the surface of the liver, in the skin at the umbilicus, in the left supraclavicular node, etc. In the early diagnosis of gastric cancer, roentgenologic, fluoroscopic and gastroscopic examinations are most valuable, as they often demonstrate the trouble before other signs appear. Dyspepsia of more than 4 weeks duration in any person over 40 calls for complete roentgenographic examination of the gastrointestinal tract, for no other single method offers a comparable means of diagnosing gastric cancer at a curable stage.

Treatment

At this writing there is no successful treatment of gastric carcinoma except removal of the tumor. This type of tumor does not respond to x-ray therapy or to any chemotherapeutic agents. Since surgery is the only method of therapy and since it is impossible to determine before operation the extent of the tumor and whether it can be cured, all patients with carcinoma of the stomach, with few exceptions, must be operated on. If the

tumor can be removed while it is still localized to the stomach, many patients can be cured. If the tumor has spread beyond the area that can be excised surgically, cure cannot be effected. However, in many of these patients, effective palliation may be obtained by resection of the tumor. Although a radical operation is necessary to remove gastric cancer and the area to which it may have spread, as a rule some part of the stomach can be preserved. However, in some patients the entire tumor can be removed only by total gastrectomy. (See Fig. 224, *Bottom, right.*) If a radical subtotal gastrectomy has been performed, the stump of the stomach is anastomosed to the jejunum, as in the gastrectomy for ulcer. When total gastrectomy is performed, gastrointestinal continuity is restored by an anastomosis between the ends of the esophagus and the jejunum, or sometimes a part of the colon may be interposed between the esophagus and the small intestine to act as a substitute stomach.

These patients should receive preparation similar to that for operation on peptic ulcers.

Blood transfusions often are needed before, during and after operation. Gastric suction drainage usually is employed to empty the stomach both preoperatively and postoperatively.

Some of the complications that may follow gastrectomy are shock, hemorrhage, vomiting, peritonitis, obstruction, hiccup, parotitis, pulmonary embolus and phlebitis. For a full description, see pages 295 to 308.

Gastrostomy

This operation, in which a permanent opening is made into the stomach, is performed for the purpose of administering food and fluids when an impermeable stricture of the esophagus exists. The esophageal stricture may be due to scar-tissue contracture. In children, it occurs often as a result of lye burns, and in older people it is due most frequently to a carcinomatous growth.

Preoperative Preparation. The purpose of the operative procedure should be explained to the patient so that he will have a better understanding of his postoperative course. Fluids are administered by vein; the nature of the fluids is determined by the fluid, the electrolyte and the nutritional needs of the patient.

Operation. The anterior gastric wall is grasped through the left rectus incision, and a tube is inserted into the stomach. This tube, usually a No. 20 or a No. 22 rubber catheter, is held in place by sutures placed round it. The end of the tube is brought through the wound to the anterior abdominal wall and clamped.

Postoperative Nursing Care

The psychological care of this patient is as important as his physical and nutritional care. The observing nurse will note his reactions and handle the situation accordingly.

The patient may be given fluids (10 per cent glucose solution is best) through the tube at once if he is much dehydrated. At first only an ounce or two at a time is given, but the amount is increased gradually until, by the end of the 2nd day, from 6 to 8 ounces may be given at one time provided this quantity is tolerated.

Tube Feedings. There have been several recent innovations in the preparation of tube feedings. Powdered feedings that are easily liquefied are commercially available. Since the advent of the food blender, a normal diet can be liquefied and fed through a tube. Blenderized tube feedings allow the patient to follow his usual diet pattern and thus are psychologically more acceptable. Good bowel function is promoted, since the fiber and residue content are similar to that of a normal diet.

Warm milk, cream, eggs, sugar, olive oil, broths and so forth may be given through the tube. The nurse may prepare a tray containing a funnel to which a rubber tubing and a glass adapter are attached. This would be attached to the gastrostomy tube at the time of feeding. Water at room temperature should be available and used to precede and follow the feeding. The feeding should be warmed by placing it in a basin of water. Feedings never should be given directly from the refrigerator. When fluid first is poured into the tubing, the receptacle should be tilted so that air will escape from the tubing and not enter the stomach and produce distention. The feeding should be allowed to flow into the stomach by gravity. The flow can be regulated by raising or lowering the receptacle. Force never should be used. If there seems to be an obstruction, stop the feeding and report the condition to the surgeon.

The diet mixture may be divided into 4 feedings for the day and 3 for the night. They must be given very slowly. If the patient becomes nauseated, the fats must be decreased in amount and then increased gradually until the caloric requirement again is met. Water should be given as ordered through the tube.

Feedings should be recorded carefully as to amount of fluid and contents, in order that the surgeon may know whether the patient is obtaining enough to satisfy his caloric, nutritional and fluid requirements. After each feeding, the tube should be irrigated with warm water and clamped. Neglect of this procedure may cause the catheter to become clogged. The nurse in charge of a patient with a gastrostomy always should have a duplicate tube sterilized and ready for use. After 5 or 6 days, the tube may be removed if loose, and a fresh one, lubricated with petrolatum, inserted. Thereafter the tube is held in place by a thin strip of adhesive which first is twisted about the tube and then firmly attached to the abdomen. A small dressing is applied over the tube and the whole is held in place by a firm abdominal binder. Thereafter the tube should be changed every 2 or 3 days, and adults should be taught how to do this for themselves. Once the opening into the stomach has been established, there is no possibility or necessity for a sterile technic in changing and introducing a gastrostomy tube. The tube should be clean but not necessarily sterile. The patient should learn also how to feed himself and should know what foods may be taken.

The skin about a gastrostomy opening requires special care. Sooner or later it may become irritated due to the action of gastric juices which leak out around the tube. If uncared for, the skin becomes macerated, red, raw and painful. Daily dressing of the wound will avert this in large measure. However, it is well to apply some bland ointment, such as zinc oxide or petrolatum, to the area about the tube.

After several weeks, the tube may be removed and inserted only for feedings. Between times, the gastrostomy opening may be protected by a small gauze pad that is held in place by adhesive.

Postoperative Complications and Nursing Problems After Gastric Resection

Shock has been mentioned as a complication, especially in very ill patients. The restoration of normal temperature and the administration of fluids are the prophylactic measures necessary in every case. For symptoms and treatment of shock, see Chapter 18, Postoperative Complications, pages 296 to 298.

Vomiting may occur once or twice after operations on the stomach. The vomitus usually is composed of a dark, bloody fluid. Usually, nausea and vomiting disappear after 8 or 10 hours. If vomiting continues after the first 24 hours, it is due probably to blood retained in the stomach. A change of position or a glass of warm water or sodium bicarbonate solution may aid in draining the stomach or inducing vomiting.

The nasogastric tube often is inserted to provide continuous gastric drainage by suction.

Hemorrhage is occasionally a complication after gastric operations. The patient exhibits the usual signs (Chap. 18) and usually continues to vomit bright blood in considerable amounts. Emergency treatment is the administration of morphine and the placing of an icecap on the abdomen. Adrenalin hydrochloride solution may be given in water or saline by mouth for its effect in producing vasoconstriction. The nurse should be prepared for the intravenous injection of saline or blood.

Pulmonary Complications frequently follow upper abdominal incisions because of the tendency to shallow respiration. Therefore, the nurse should urge the patient to breathe deeply several times each hour when awake in order to obtain full aeration of the lungs. A change in position, turning the patient from side to side, also is an aid in preventing these complications.

The *dumping syndrome* is a label loosely applied to postoperative symptoms that come on after eating. It is probable that it results from a rapid emptying of gastric contents into the small intestine, which has been anastomosed to the gastric stump. Symptoms are varied and may consist of palpitation, sweating, a feeling of faintness and weakness which may last only a few minutes or for as long as 30 minutes, even forcing the patient to lie down for a time.

There may be several causes for these symptoms, including a small gastric remnant remaining after the operation, the large opening from the gastric stump into the jejunum and the ingestion of food high in carbohydrates and electrolytes which have to be diluted in the jejunum before absorption can take place. The ingestion of fluid at mealtime is another factor in the rapid emptying of the stomach into the jejunum. The symptoms which occur are probably brought about by rapid distention of the jejunal loop anastomosed to the stomach and a withdrawal of water from the circulating blood volume into the jejunum to dilute the high concentration of electrolytes and sugars. Most patients with "dumping syndrome" recognize that meals high in sugars and salt produce these symptoms;

consequently, they avoid these foods. They also have found that a dry meal (without liquids) reduces the appearance of "dumping" symptoms. Surgeons are attempting to reduce "dumping" by formation of smaller stomas and larger gastric stumps. On rare occasions, reoperation may be necessary to correct this syndrome.

Vitamin B$_{12}$ Deficiency. Total gastrectomy brings to an abrupt, complete and final halt the production of "intrinsic factor," the gastric secretion that is required for the absorption of Vitamin B$_{12}$ from the gastrointestinal tract. (See page 151.) Therefore, unless this vitamin is supplied by parenteral injection and continues to be supplied by that route throughout his life, the patient inevitably will suffer from vitamin B$_{12}$ deficiency, his status in time becoming identical to that of a patient with pernicious anemia in relapse. All of the manifestations of pernicious anemia, including macrocytic anemia and combined system disease, may be expected to develop within a period of 5 years or less, to progress in severity thereafter and, in the absence of therapy, to prove fatal. This complication is avoided by the regular monthly intramuscular injection of from 100 to 200 micrograms of B$_{12}$, a regimen that should be started without delay after gastrectomy.

Nursing Care After Gastric Surgery

In the operating room the administration of fluids is begun by transfusion and infusion, as much as from 2,500 to 3,000 ml. being given daily for the first 2 or 3 days. This is one of the best methods of warding off postoperative shock, a condition especially prone to develop in patients who have undergone operation for bleeding, perforated ulcer or cancer.

When recovery from anesthesia is complete, the patient is placed in the Fowler position, as this favors drainage of the stomach. Change of position from one side to the other at frequent intervals tends to prevent postoperative pulmonary and vascular complications. Nothing is given these patients by mouth for at least 24 hours. This precaution is taken to allow the suture line to seal off thoroughly and thus minimize the

danger of leakage and peritonitis. Antibiotic and vitamin therapy are instituted parenterally. To relieve dryness of the mouth during this period, mouth-washes should be given at frequent intervals. To allow the patient to moisten his lips with ice that is enclosed in a piece of gauze often is refreshing. The nurse also can use an applicator stick dipped in mineral oil and lemon juice to swab dry lips. Very often a nasogastric tube attached to a suction apparatus is used to remove mucus, liquids, blood, gas and materials that accumulate in the stomach during the first 24 to 48 hours after operation. Repeated irrigation of the tube with syringe and physiologic saline or Ringer's solution may be needed to keep the tube open. The amount of solution used should be charted. With the nasogastric tube it is important for the nurse to give care to the nostrils. An applicator stick moistened with water and followed by an applicator stick dipped in mineral oil can be used to clean the nostril.

When the surgeon orders fluids, they should be given warm and sparingly at first. Beginning with 1 or 2 drams every half hour, the amount is increased gradually until 3 or 4 ounces is being taken. Warm tea with sugar and lemon is very acceptable. Cold fluids usually cause distress. If the patient does not vomit, more fluid may be given by mouth. On the 3rd or 4th day, milk and other bland liquids may be added to the diet, and on the 5th day a routine diet should be instituted. Should the patient vomit, eruct or hiccup at any time, the intake should be stopped and instructions requested.

After radical resections of the stomach in the treatment of carcinoma, the remaining gastric stump may be extremely small; after total gastrectomy, there is no gastric reservoir at all. The nutrition of these patients is the important postoperative therapy. Since they cannot eat large meals, frequent smaller ones are necessary. They should be high in caloric value, with foods that do not require much churning for digestion. This means a diet rather high in eggs, milk, butter and cream. If vegetables are taken, they should be pureed or soft. Fruits should be stewed or finely chewed.

PRINCIPLES OF NURSING MANAGEMENT OF A PATIENT WITH A GASTRIC RESECTION

Major Problems
1. Postoperative pain and discomfort
2. Maintenance of adequate nutrition
3. Prevention of complications

Objectives
1. To relieve the patient of pain and discomfort:
   A. Frequent turning for comfort and the prevention of pulmonary and vascular complications
   B. Meticulous oral hygiene to counteract mouth dryness
   C. Analgesics or narcotics for pain control
   D. Parenteral antibiotics for prevention of infection
   E. Oral fluids withheld until ordered (sealing of suture line)
   F. Gastric suction to remove liquids, blood and gas in stomach
2. To promote adequate nutrition:
   A. Intravenous fluids to prevent shock and maintain optimum fluid and electrolyte balance
   B. Oral fluids when audible bowel sounds are present
   C. Fluids to be increased according to patient's tolerance
   D. Bland diet with vitamin supplements as indicated by patient's condition
   E. Supplementary iron-vitamin therapy to insure adequate intake
   F. Avoidance of foods that may initiate development of "dumping syndrome"
3. To develop an awareness of complications that may follow gastric surgery:
   A. Shock
      1. Evaluate drainage from dressing and drainage bottle.
      2. Evaluate blood pressure, pulse and respiratory rates.
      3. Give blood and fluid replacement at time ordered.
   B. Hemorrhage
      1. Watch drainage for presence of blood.
      2. Evaluate blood pressure, pulse and respiratory rates.
      3. Start blood replacement if indicated.
   C. Pulmonary complications
      1. Encourage deep breathing and coughing to counteract voluntary diaphragm splinting.
      2. Promote frequent turning and moving to mobilize bronchial secretions.
      3. Ambulate when ordered to increase respiratory exchange.
   D. Thrombosis and embolism
      1. Encourage participation in self-care activities to increase circulation.
      2. Encourage early ambulation to minimize stasis of venous blood.
      3. Use elastic stockings as indicated to prevent venous stasis.
      4. Check dressing and binders for tightness that impairs circulation.
   E. Wound evisceration
      1. Use abdominal binders if ordered for support.
      2. Prevent distention and wound infection.
      3. Support incision when coughing.
      4. Promote good nutrition.
      5. Inspect dressing frequently.
   F. "Dumping syndrome"
      1. Teach patient to avoid eating large meals.
      2. Avoid hot, cold, salty, or highly concentrated carbohydrate foods.
      3. Take fluids between meals.
      4. Avoid liquids with meals.
      5. Eliminate sweets from the diet.
      6. Eat regularly, slowly and in a relaxed environment.
      7. Lie down after meals.
4. To promote the rehabilitation of the patient:
   A. Help him to modify his environmental stresses.
   B. Encourage him to remain under medical supervision.
   C. Advise adequate caloric intake after discharge from the hospital.
   D. Weigh regularly.

PROBLEMS INVOLVING THE SMALL AND THE LARGE BOWEL

Chronic Constipation

Constipation is a term which describes an abnormal infrequency of defecation, also abnormal dryness of the stools. Most normal persons have one bowel movement a day. Some, however, go 2, 3 or 4 days without a movement; their stools are normally moist, and they suffer no discomfort. On the other hand, some constipated persons, at times, have a diarrhea of liquid stools, due to the irritation caused by the presence in the colon of hard, dry fecal masses. Such stools contain a good deal of mucus, secreted by glands in the colon in response to these irritating masses. The rectum, in severe constipation, may become impacted, that is, filled with masses of hard feces which must be removed by the fingers or first softened by instillations of oil before they can be washed out by an enema.

There are few organic causes of chronic constipation. The most important of these are morphine addiction, lead poisoning and cancer of the large bowel, a condition in which constipation usually alternates with diarrhea. Painful hemorrhoids and anal fissures, by inducing rectal spasm, also may lead to temporary constipation. Other factors that predispose to its development include limitation of muscular exercise, unfamiliar diet, weakness, debility and fatigue.

By far the most common type of constipation is on a functional, rather than organic, basis. Many patients develop a habit constipation because of the careless or neurotic habit of delaying each bowel movement as long as possible. The rectal mucous membrane and musculature become insensitive to the presence of fecal masses, and consequently the stimulus required to produce the necessary peristaltic rush for defecation becomes increasingly greater. The initial effect of this fecal retention, or hoarding, is to produce irritability of the colon, which, at this stage, goes frequently into spasm, especially after meals, giving rise to colicky mid-abdominal or low-abdominal pains. Eventually, after several years, perhaps, the colon loses muscular tone; it is

essentially unresponsive to normal stimuli. The patient may be said to have *atonic constipation,* whereas in the earlier stage the condition is sometimes referred to as *spastic constipation,* although they should not be regarded as separate entities.

Teaching the Patient. In simple or functional constipation, the role of the nurse is that of assisting with the re-education of the patient. The physiology of defecation should be explained carefully, with particular emphasis on the importance of heeding promptly the urge to defecate. Instruct the patient to have a regular time for defecation, preferably after a meal. Thinking about the act of defecation, i.e., "auto-suggestion," may be an aid in initiating the reflex. A small footstool to promote flexion of the thighs will insure an optimum posture during defecation.

Patients who worry about having a *daily* bowel movement need reassurance. Carefully explain that some healthy persons have a bowel movement 3 times daily while others do so only 2 or 3 times a week. Knowing that some of the food eaten may normally remain in the intestinal tract 48 hours after ingestion will help the patient to understand and accept the fact that a daily bowel evacuation is not always necessary. The use of laxatives should be discontinued. If the feces remain too long in the rectum and become dehydrated, and hardened, the patient may be instructed to take 2 or 3 ounces of warm oil in the form of a rectal instillation at bed time. A small enema of physiologic saline the next morning should help to alleviate this condition.

The patient must know what constitutes a normal diet. When teaching the patient, emphasize the similarities between his prescribed diet and the normal diet. In general, a high-residue, high-fiber diet is prescribed for atonic constipation; a bland or low residue diet is indicated for the patient with an irritable colon. Approximately the same amount of foods should be eaten at each meal, and the patient should ingest 2 liters of fluid daily (or more if he perspires freely).

It takes time to break bad habits and form new ones. It takes time to teach the patient.

Remember that repetition is one of the laws of learning. The wise use of every patient contact to help the patient to adjust to his new regimen of treatment will do much to help to develop a nurse who is worthy of the patient's confidence.

Acute Constipation

Acute constipation, in contrast with the chronic variety, always indicates an acute and, frequently, a serious disorder. The symptom may prompt one to order a laxative, but it must be remembered that acute constipation may be an early symptom of acute appendicitis, and that a purge given in this condition may well produce perforation of the inflamed appendix. A similar situation exists in typhoid fever. In general, one should not prescribe a cathartic for fever, nausea or pain merely because the bowels fail to move; and, before such medication is offered, it must be quite clear that no inflammatory disease of the intestinal tract is present.

Enemas are relatively safe as regards the possible perforation of an inflammatory lesion of the bowel, provided that they are administered with extreme caution. Dextrose or saline solutions, or water alone, may be instilled, but nothing more irritating than these, and the nurse should be prepared to halt the irrigation at once if pain is induced or increased in the slightest degree.

Complications and Nursing Implications of Constipation

The maintenance of elimination is basic to the care of every patient. The mechanical difficulties and the physical discomforts associated with defecation and micturition that harass the bed patient are widely known to the medical profession and the laity alike. It is doubtful, however, whether this aspect of medical and nursing care is generally recognized as a problem of considerable magnitude, the implications of which, in some instances, are far from trivial. The effort entailed in defecation is considerable. With the use of a bedpan the muscular strain is inevitably greater, and when constipation is imposed in addition, the performance of this function can be extremely fatiguing, if not altogether exhausting. This is a serious consideration in the management of patients with congestive heart failure, which may be dangerously aggravated in patients with recent myocardial infarction and susceptibility to cardiac rupture, and in those with arterial hypertension.

Straining at stool has a striking effect on the arterial blood pressure. During the period of active straining, the flow of venous blood in the chest is temporarily impeded due to an increase in intrathoracic pressure which tends to collapse the large veins in the chest. The atria and the ventricles receive less blood, and consequently less is delivered by the systolic contractions of the left ventricle; the cardiac output is decreased, and there is a transient drop in arterial pressure. Almost immediately after this period of hypotension, a rise in arterial pressure occurs; the pressure is elevated momentarily to a point far exceeding the original level (the so-called "rebound" phenomenon). In patients with arterial hypertension, this compensatory reaction may be exaggerated greatly, and the peaks of pressure attained may be dangerously high—sufficient, indeed, to rupture a major artery in the brain or elsewhere. It is not possible to make other than a rough estimate of the frequency with which the act of defecation is the terminal event and brings on death due to vascular accidents which are the result of straining at stool. The danger is not sufficiently appreciated, however, particularly in patients with vascular diseases of the type described. Inasmuch as straining is promoted by constipation, the latter cannot be dismissed as altogether inconsequential; on the contrary, it must be concluded that the regularity and the consistency of the stools, as well as the mechanical aspects of defecation, are matters of prime concern.

To facilitate elimination, the patient should assume the normal position for defecation. In most instances there is less strain to the patient if he can be assisted to a bedside commode. A bedpan placed on a chair will suffice if a commode is not available. Or the patient may be seated on the bedpan at the side of the bed with his feet supported on a chair. If he cannot sit up, a small support should be placed under the lumbosacral curve to minimize strain and increase his comfort while using the bedpan.

Other nursing measures to promote gastrointestinal elimination include ensuring an adequate fluid and food intake, adhering to the patient's established defecation time, and the administration of enemas, suppositories, and medications prescribed by the physician.

The Primary Malabsorption States

The above term is applied to three closely related conditions: namely, tropical sprue, idiopathic steatorrhea (nontropical sprue) and celiac disease. Tropical and nontropical sprue are diseases of adults; in clinical manifestations and pathologic changes, the two conditions are very similar. However, their geographic incidence and their causes differ and they respond to different treatments. Celiac disease is limited to childhood but resembles idiopathic steatorrhea in all other respects, and probably represents the juvenile phase of that disease.

The pathologic defect is similar in all three conditions. The principal lesion involves the intestinal mucosa, especially the intestinal villae, which become severely blunted or are lost altogether. As a result, the absorptive surface within the small bowel is substantially reduced in area and food absorption is correspondingly impaired.

Patients with the malabsorption syndrome, if neglected, become weak and emaciated due to starvation. Failing to absorb the fat-soluble vitamins A, D and K (Chap. 9) they must anticipate the development of the corresponding avitaminoses. Manifestations of abnormal bleeding are likely to appear as a result of K deficiency and hypoprothrombinemia (p. 478). Anemia develops, which is of the macrocytic type characteristic of folic-acid deficiency (p. 466). Impaired absorption of calcium may be responsible for gradual demineralization of the skeleton and, in the case of children with celiac disease, for the stunting of growth. Moreover, calcium deficiency may lead to extreme neuromuscular hyperirritability, including attacks of hypocalcemic tetany (p. 826).

The basic factor in the pathogenesis of idiopathic steatorrhea and celiac disease is a specific and profound intolerance to a protein substance (gluten) contained in wheat, rye and barley. A constituent of gluten, *gliadin,* for reasons that are not clear, exerts toxic effects on the intestinal mucosa, damaging or destroying its villi and crippling its function. The familial incidence of these disorders, which is increased, suggests that a hereditary factor, i.e., an inborn error of metabolism, may be involved, and that enzymatic activities governing the digestion of gliadin may be affected. In any case, the elimination of gluten from the patient's diet is followed by striking clinical improvement. His diarrhea ceases and his nutritional status is restored to normal. This gratifying remission may be expected to last as long as the patient remains on a gluten-free diet, and no longer. Unfortunately, the total exclusion of gluten is difficult to accomplish, since this substance is incorporated into many foods as a binder and filler. It is contained in almost every bakery product, "wheat-free" or otherwise, and is an ingredient of other foodstuffs as well, including some brands of ice cream.

The factors primarily responsible for the onset and the progression of tropical sprue have not as yet been clarified. Its clinical course appears to be unaffected by the presence or the absence of gliadin in the diet; hence gliadin intolerance seemingly plays no role in its pathogenesis. Of greatest benefit in this condition is the administration of folic acid, which usually is prescribed in 5 mg. doses by mouth, 3 times each day until a remission is established, and once daily thereafter for a period of from 4 to 6 months. The beneficial effects of folic acid in patients with tropical sprue appear with such regularity and on occasion are so striking as to suggest that this particular malabsorption syndrome may be attributable to, as well as productive of, folic-acid deficiency.

Diarrhea

Diarrhea is one of the cardinal symptoms of small-bowel disease. It is a condition in which there is unusual frequency of bowel movements, as well as changes in the amount, the character and the consistency of the stools. In acute cases the stools are grayish-brown, foul smelling and filled with undigested particles of food and mucus. The patient complains of abdominal cramps, distention, intestinal rumbling (borborygmus), anorexia and thirst. Painful spasms of the anus may attend each defecation.

Diarrhea and its associated symptoms occur in a variety of disorders. The efficient nurse will facilitate the diagnosis in each case by recording her discerning observations, including the patient's symptoms, behavior and remarks. Accurate description of abnormal stools is of great importance in diagnosis. For example, watery stools are characteristic of small-bowel disease, whereas loose, semisolid stools are associated more often with disorders of the colon. Voluminous, greasy stools suggest intestinal malabsorption, and the presence of mucus and pus in the stools denotes inflammatory enteritis or colitis.

Acute. Most acute diarrheas are due to the stimulating effect of some irritant on intestinal peristalsis. The irritant stimulating the diarrhea may arise from a localized infection or ulceration in the intestinal wall, due, for example, to a carcinoma, a diverticulitis or a tuberculous lesion. The irritant may be chemical. Castor oil, after it has been acted upon by the digestive juice, is an example of a mild intestinal irritant, as are most of the vegetable cathartics. Certain unripe fruits, which cause crampy diarrhea, likewise belong in this category.

The inflammatory response to these mild irritants is slight; little or no mucous membrane lining is destroyed on exposure to them unless their concentration in the intestinal fluid is excessive. Their chief effect is to produce hyperemia (vascular dilatation, with local increase in blood flow, in other words, blushing) of the intestinal mucosa and increase in mucous secretion. There also occurs a motor response of hyperperistalsis, which persists until the irritant is excreted. This explains the symptoms of crampy diarrhea. Some chemicals, such as mercuric chloride, are extremely caustic. They cause intense circulatory congestion of the intestinal walls and necrosis of its lining membrane, which separates away in shreds. The unfortunate individual who ingests such a caustic experiences severe crampy diarrhea with persistent passage of liquid bloody stools. The eventual outcome, usually, is death.

Infectious. By far the most common intestinal irritants are the products of certain bacteria, whether their growth occurred in the intestine or in the food before it was eaten. In the case of the enteric pathogens, the organisms causing bacillary dysentery, bacterial growth with release of the irritating toxins takes place in the intestine. On the other hand, practically all cases of food poisoning, or ptomaine poisoning, are due to the ingestion of food heavily contaminated and already containing the toxin. *Staphylococcus aureus,* for example, if given an opportunity to grow in food, produces an exotoxin that is extremely irritating to the intestinal tract.

Whether the gastrointestinal tract is exposed to toxins introduced in food or produced by bacteria growing within the intestine, an infectious enterocolitis is produced. The inflammatory response may vary from mild hyperemia and hypermotility of the gastrointestinal tract to severe inflammation of the intestine, depending on the virulence of the infecting organism and the amount of toxin liberated. Clinically, except for the presence of diarrhea, there is little similarity between a case of food poisoning due to the ingestion of food containing bacterial toxins and a case of bacillary dysentery. The diarrhea in food poisoning is explosive in onset, develops within a very few hours following the toxic meal and, except in severe cases, will subside within 1 or 2 days—as soon as the toxin is excreted and the inflammatory response subsides. There is little or no fever, and usually the only associated symptoms are those directly attributable to the diarrhea, namely, dehydration and weakness. Dysentery, due to the growth of gastrointestinal pathogens within the gastrointestinal tract, on the other hand, develops with a more gradual onset, persists for several days or weeks, and there are striking constitutional symptoms in addition to the diarrhea. These clinical differences are quite understandable when it is realized that in the infectious diarrheas a bacterial invasion of the intestinal mucosa is involved. Then, not only must the bacterial toxins be excreted or destroyed, but also the bacteria themselves must be eradicated, and this takes considerably longer.

Diagnosis

The diagnosis of an acute diarrhea is based on the course of the disease: the type of onset and progression, the presence or absence of fever and a study of the stools, which are examined for bacteria as well as for blood and pus. In cases of possible infection, the suspected food is tested by bacteriologic cultures. It is very important to remember that diarrhea often is present in various systemic infections. It may be the initial misleading complaint in certain of the exanthemata before the appearance of the rash, and it may complicate or mask such conditions as mastoiditis, pneumonia and pyelitis, especially in children.

Treatment

Patients with acute diarrhea are placed at bed rest until the episode has terminated. They may be treated with a sedative drug, such as a barbiturate, or with a more powerful opiate, for example, paregoric or opium tincture. Fluid and electrolyte replacement, orally or parenterally, is an extremely important measure, symptomatically as well as supportively. During the acute stages very little is prescribed by mouth other than water, bouillon (for its salt content) and milk, the last furnishing water, electrolytes and also calories. Potassium replacement, accomplished by the parenteral injections of an appropriate electrolyte solution (pp. 168,

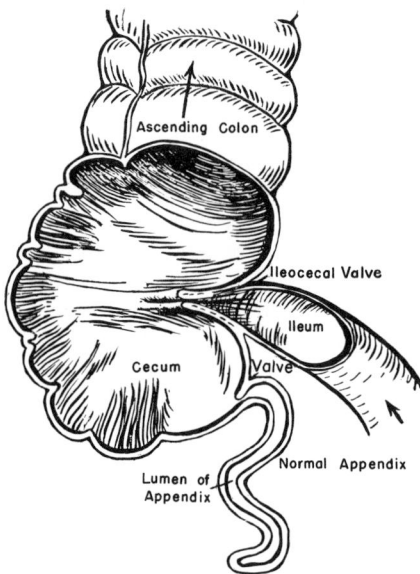

FIG. 229. The normal cecum, showing the ileocecal valve and the vermiform appendix.

169), is necessary in very severe diarrheal disorders, particularly in infants and young children. Sulfonamide chemotherapy, with sulfadiazine or Gantrisin, may be indicated in infectious cases.

Prevention

All cases of acute diarrhea should be treated as potentially infective until they are proved otherwise. If the diarrhea is of infectious origin, those caring for the patient should determine whether there is any diarrhea among his family and neighbors. Ask him about his recent sources of food and water. Every nurse is a case finder. By reporting a larger than usual number of cases of diarrhea, she assists the local health officer to discover whether an epidemic is starting in the community.

Proper precautions to avoid the spread of the disease through contamination of the hands, the clothing, the bed linen, etc., with feces or vomitus are specified in the next section.

Diarrhea always should be regarded as a potential risk under conditions of crowding; outbreaks occur with particular frequency in institutions such as prisons, boarding schools and army camps, in trailer camps and even in hospitals, unless sanitary precautions are observed rigidly and constantly. Precautions include ensuring that proper storage and refrigeration facilities are available and are used for the handling of all fresh fruits and meats. Meat products should be cooked thoroughly, and all cooked meats should be refrigerated immediately unless they are consumed promptly. Milk and milk products should be refrigerated constantly and protected against exposure. The food items which are particularly prone to infection and provide the best environment for bacterial growth include custards and cream fillings, such as are prepared in éclairs, cream pies, layer cakes, cream puffs, etc. Such materials should be cooked thoroughly and then be brought to refrigerator temperature immediately unless they are to be eaten within a very few hours after cooking.

Isolation Technic and Precautions

The following precautions should be observed meticulously, not only in this, but also in other communicable enteric infec-

Fig. 230. Acute appendicitis, gangrene of the appendix, perforation and spreading peritonitis. In this case, the appendix was not removed, and the inflammation spreads to the surrounding loops of bowel. An abscess will form in the shaded area, or the inflammation may spread through the entire peritoneal cavity.

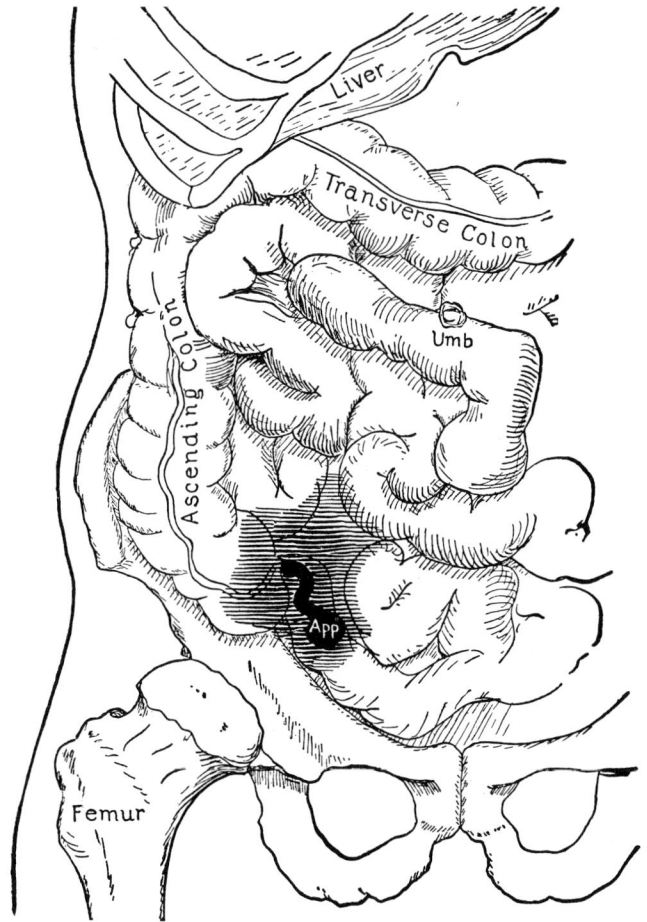

tions, including enteritis due to *Salmonella* infection and dysentery of all types.

Screening. The patient's room should be completely screened against the entry of flies and other insects; if the patient is treated in an open ward, the area adjacent to his bed should be framed and screened.

Linens. All nurses, doctors, and other hospital personnel in contact with the patient should wear gowns and scrub their hands with soap and running water after each contact. All bed linen and clothing should be collected in an individual precaution bag and sterilized by autoclaving, by boiling or by soaking for 1 hour in a 5 per cent formalin or 2 per cent cresol solution.

Dishes. All dishes, trays and eating utensils should be sterilized after use by boiling for 15 minutes. Uneaten food is collected in a paper bag and burned in the incinerator.

Dejecta. Depending on the nature of the

equipment for sterilizing bedpans and their contents, the following procedures may be adopted.

All feces should be sterilized in the bedpan by completely covering them with 5 per cent cresol or 10 per cent formalin solution for from 30 to 60 minutes. Formed feces should be broken up with a stick to facilitate adequate exposure to the antiseptic. Urine and bath water similarly should be exposed to these antiseptic solutions. Dejecta never should be discarded into toilets without previous sterilization, for flies may have access to the material itself or to the water in the bowl, which has become contaminated and is infective. (These measures are unnecessary if city sewage automatic bedpan washing equipment of the type delivering water sprayed at high temperature is available.)

Miscellaneous Items. Each patient should be equipped with his own individual ther-

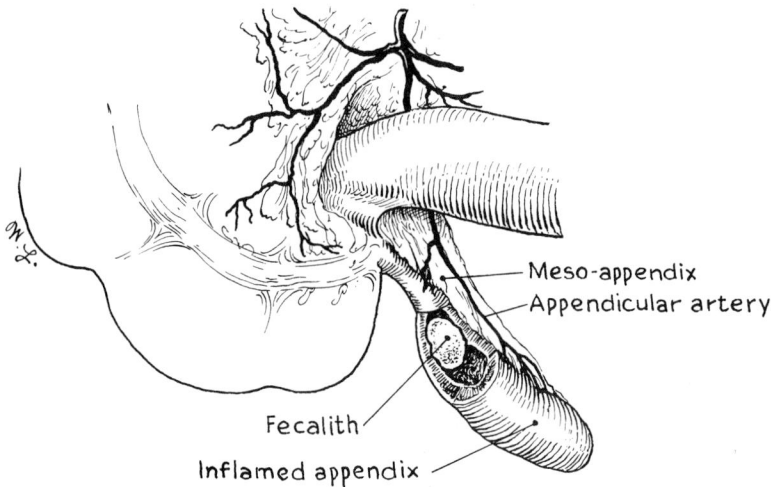

Meso-appendix
Appendicular artery
Fecalith
Inflamed appendix

mometer, bedpan, basin, urinal and toilet articles. Wastes, wipes, etc., are collected in paper bags and disposed of by burning in an incinerator.

Visitors. Nonprofessional visits should be kept to a minimum, and all persons admitted should be obliged to wear gowns and observe precautions as instructed, i.e., refrain from touching the patient, his bed, bedside table or any object which the patient has handled or is within his reach.

Home Nursing

Precautions to be observed in caring for patients with infectious enteritis in the home include the following.

Linens should be boiled for 30 minutes or soaked for 1 hour in a 2 per cent Lysol solution.

Liquid waste and excreta should be collected in a special container, allowed to stand for 1 hour with equal parts of 5 per cent chlorinated lime solution and then emptied. Bedpans and urinals may be soaked for 1 hour in a 2 per cent Lysol or a 5 per cent chlorinated lime solution.

Public Health Teaching

Proper housekeeping, especially in kitchen maintenance, is obviously very important in the prevention of epidemic diarrhea. All materials used in the preparation and the serving of food must be cleansed rigorously and kept in immaculate condition. All food handlers should receive detailed instructions

in hygienic principles and practices and, on the development of any illness that is potentially infectious, should be relieved of their duties immediately.

Regional Enteritis

Regional enteritis, or terminal ileitis, is an inflammatory disease of the small bowel, the cause of which is obscure. The lesion is one of chronic granulomatous inflammation involving initially the terminal ileum, but later extending throughout the small intestine, and leading to obstruction or perforation of the bowel. It is a relatively uncommon disease. Of those individuals afflicted with it, most are in the younger age group.

Characteristically, there occur symptoms of diarrhea and recurrent, cramping, right-sided abdominal pains, the location and character of which frequently lead to a mistaken diagnosis of acute appendicitis. On physical examination, a tender mass may be felt in the right lower abdomen. Important in diagnosis are typical roentgenologic findings on gastrointestinal series indicating localized areas of spasm in the small bowel.

Treatment. Treatment, which is successful in only about half the cases, consists of surgical resection of the involved intestine. Even if the inflammation seems to be confined to the portion of bowel removed, this procedure by no means ensures that there will be no recurrence and spread of the process.

Steroid drugs, by virtue of their nonspecific anti-inflammatory action, are useful in controlling acute exacerbations of this disease and in avoiding their recurrence.

Appendicitis

The appendix is a small tube about 4 in. long and as large around as the little finger. Its structure is similar to that of the ileum. One end of it is closed and the other opens into the cecum just below the ileocecal valve (Fig. 229). No definite function can be assigned to it in man. It fills with food and empties as regularly as does the cecum, of which it is a part. It empties inefficiently, however, and its lumen is very small, so that it is prone to become obstructed and is particularly vulnerable to infection, or appendicitis.

Symptoms. Acute appendicitis starts typically with a progressively severe generalized or upper abdominal pain, which, within a few hours, becomes localized in the right lower quadrant of the abdomen. This pain usually is accompanied by a low-grade fever and often by vomiting. At McBurney's point, located halfway between the umbilicus and the anterior spine, one expects to find local tenderness on pressure and some rigidity of the lower portion of the right rectus muscle. A moderate leukocytosis is often present.

Just how much tenderness there will be, how much muscle spasm, whether or not there is constipation or diarrhea, etc., depend not so much on the severity of the appendical infection as on the location of the appendix. If the appendix curls around behind the cecum (retrocecal appendix), pain and tenderness may be felt in the lumbar region; if its tip is in the pelvis, these signs may be elicited only on rectal examination. Pain on defecation suggests that its tip is against the rectum; pain on micturition, that it is near the bladder or impinges on the ureter. Eventually, the inflamed appendix fills with pus and then is apt to perforate. Once ruptured, the pain is relieved temporarily, and for a short time the patient feels much better. However, the symptoms soon recur and increase in severity as a local abscess forms or general peritonitis develops (Fig. 230).

The symptoms of acute appendicitis in a child are not nearly as definite as they are in adults. The attack begins with pain, usually slight, which soon disappears. A few hours later the symptoms become more definite, but even then the child may not seem to be seriously ill. Fever is often slight. Whereas there may be exquisite tenderness of the abdomen, rigidity is less marked than it is in older patients. Vomiting, however, begins earlier and is more persistent than in adults, and sudden perforation often occurs unexpectedly in apparently mild cases.

Complications. If the appendix can be removed before inflammation has progressed to the point of perforation, there is no further trouble. The abdomen can be closed at once, and the patient can be out of the hospital in a week or less. However, if perforation has occurred, the patient may develop generalized peritonitis (p. 622), or an appendiceal abscess may result, in which case the surrounding loops of bowel become adherent and wall off the spreading peritonitis. A certain number of patients having appendicitis, on whom operation was performed too late or not at all, develop the dangerous complication of pylephlebitis, that is, a spread of the infection into the portal venous system, thence to the liver, where abscesses develop. This complication is to be suspected in a patient with chills, fever and jaundice following an attack of abdominal pain suggestive of appendicitis.

Nonoperative Treatment. Operation is always indicated if acute appendicitis is suspected, unless there is good evidence that perforation has occurred recently and a generalized peritonitis has developed. In this case the patient is treated conservatively with parenteral electrolyte and amino acid solutions, gastric suction, drainage and antibiotics, in the expectation that the infection will localize and be susceptible to surgical drainage. As long as the question of operation is undecided, morphine is withheld, even in the face of moderate suffering, because it may mask the patient's symptoms. After the decision has been made, he may be sedated comfortably.

Operative Treatment

Preparation for Operation. This depends entirely on the length of time spent in the hospital before operation. If an emergency operation is necessary, shaving of the abdomen, voiding by the patient and the administration of the prescribed hypodermic injection are required. Usually an enema is not given but, if one is ordered, it is given low and slowly. Chemotherapy and/or antibiotics are administered before and after surgery.

Appendectomy. If the patient has been suffering from acute abdominal pain, he accepts the operation as a means of relief. This acceptance of surgery makes his anesthetic and postanesthetic course a relatively easy one. The operation may be performed under nitrous oxide, ether, spinal or local anesthesia. The usual incisions are the McBurney, the muscle-splitting or the gridiron and the lower right rectus incision (Fig. 215). After the peritoneum has been opened, the appendix is brought into the wound and its mesentery is ligated with a catgut ligature. The appendix is freed and a purse-string suture is inserted round its base. After cutting through the organ at its base between clamps or ligatures, using the electrocautery or a knife followed by pure phenol and alcohol, the stump is inverted and the purse-string is tied. The appendix, the knife, the hemostats and the forceps used when the appendix was severed no longer are sterile, and they should be discarded. Sponges used to protect the wound and intestine also should be removed from the table. If the appendix has perforated and caused an abscess or a peritonitis, drainage tubes must be inserted.

Postoperative Nursing Care

Appendectomy Without Drainage. As soon as the patient recovers from the anesthesia he should be placed in the Fowler position. Morphine, from 0.016 Gm. to 0.011 Gm. (gr. ¼-⅙), may be given at intervals of 3 or 4 hours. Fluid should be given by vein for the first 12 hours but, if there is no nausea at the end of from 6 to 8 hours, water or hot tea may be given by mouth in increasing amounts. Fluids and food may be given as desired the day after operation. An enema is given on the morning of the 3rd day. The stitches are removed from the incision between the 5th and the 7th days.

After removal of the appendix a complication that at times is annoying is the inability to void. The patient may be allowed to stand with support or to sit on the edge of the bed with the feet on a chair. In this manner, the necessity for catheterization may be averted.

Appendectomy With Drainage. The treatment of patients after an appendectomy requiring drainage is complicated by local or general peritonitis. They should be placed in strict Fowler position as soon as they recover from the anesthetic and treatment for peritonitis should be instituted as described fully on page 622. These patients should be watched carefully for many days for signs of intestinal obstruction and secondary hemorrhage. Secondary abscesses may form in the pelvis, under the diaphragm or in the liver. These cause an elevation of temperature and pulse rate with an increase in the leukocyte count. A fecal fistula, with the discharge of feces through the drainage tract, develops at times. The complication arises most often after the drainage of an appendiceal abscess. The attention of the surgeon should be drawn to feces on the dressings.

Diverticulosis and Diverticulitis

A *diverticulum* is a sacular dilatation, a blind passage, so to speak, leading from the lumen of the gut. An abnormal example is Meckel's diverticulum, an outpocketing of the ileum. Diverticula, in fact, may occur anywhere along the course of the gastrointestinal tract, from the esophagus to the rectum. These defects may be congenital. They may be the result of local degeneration and weakening of the muscular wall, or they may be due to mechanical factors, such as a constant pulling on the intestinal wall from without or pressure from within its lumen. An individual who possesses diverticula is said to have *diverticulosis*.

Diverticula of the large bowel occur in from 3 to 10 per cent of adults. When present, they are usually multiple and tend rather to involve the distal portions of the colon. In contrast with Meckel's diverticulum, the colonic diverticula are rarely congenital defects, but are acquired, usually during adulthood. The cause of the diverticula is thought to be herniation of the lining mucous membrane through defects in the muscular layer of the colon, this herniation arising as a result of chronic overdistention of the bowel. Whatever their cause, large bowel diverticula are more apt to cause trouble than those situated in the small intestine. Whereas the contents of the latter are fluid in consistency, the material passing through the colon becomes increasingly firm and viscid, and diverticula located in the region where the fecal matter is most dehydrated, namely, in the sigmoid and the descending colon, are most apt to become obstructed. Obstruction of a diverticulum, as in the case of the appendix, leads to infection and inflammation. This is referred to as *diverticulitis.*

Diverticulitis usually occurs in patients over 40 years of age. It is by no means rare. It has been estimated that approximately a third of the patients with diverticulosis at one time or another experience diverticulitis. The condition may occur in acute attacks or it may persist as a long-continued, smoldering infection. Inflammation of a diverticulum, if its obstruction continues, tends to spread to the surrounding bowel wall, giving rise to irritability and spasticity of the colon. If the infection is unusually severe, perforation of the colon can occur, with resultant peritonitis; or, if the inflammation is less acute and more slowly progressive, the result may be extensive scarring and abscess formation involving the bowel wall and eventually producing some degree of lower intestinal obstruction. Complications of this severity fortunately are rarely seen.

The most common symptom of a moderately severe acute diverticulitis is crampy pain in the left lower quadrant of the abdomen, with associated flatulence, slight nausea and a low-grade fever. Milder grades of the condition may give rise only to bouts of soreness, mild cramps in the lower abdomen and irregularity of bowel habit. Hemorrhage occurs in from 10 to 20 per cent of the cases. The bleeding is not persistent but may be massive. The diagnosis is made on the basis of fluoroscopic and x-ray findings with a barium enema. Direct visualization by means of sigmoidoscopy occasionally is helpful.

Treatment and Nursing Care. The treatment and the nursing care of acute diverticulitis consist of the elimination of roughage from the diet, hot applications to the lower abdomen and repeated warm-saline enemas. Systemic and, more especially, the surface-acting antimicrobials are of great value. Those most commonly used are the so-called bowel antiseptics, such as sulfathalidine and neomycin. These drugs reduce the bacterial flora of the bowel, diminish the bulk of the stool and soften the fecal mass so that it traverses more easily the area of inflammatory obstruction.

Surgery is reserved for cases complicated by colonic perforation, obstruction, abscesses or fistulae. A very important aspect of the treatment is prevention of recurrences. To this end, patients who have experienced diverticulitis should, henceforth, restrict themselves to a low-residue diet, eliminating particularly the coarser cereals and vegetables. It is especially important that they establish a regular bowel habit. To promote regular and complete evacuation, an adequate fluid intake should be maintained, and mild laxation should be employed whenever necessary.

Meckel's Diverticulum

Meckel's diverticulum is a congenital abnormality, consisting of a blind tube, comparable with the appendix, which usually opens into the distal ileum near the ileocecal valve. It represents a remnant of a fetal structure, the omphalomesenteric duct, which in fetal life connects the embryonic yolk sac with the digestive tract. A portion of this duct persists as a diverticulum in approximately 2 per cent of the population. It is more common in men than in women. It usually opens into the ileum at a point from 1 to 3 ft. proximal to the ileocecal valve. Most diverticula are less than 4 in. long, although on rare occasions they may even exceed 3 ft. in length.

The importance of Meckel's diverticulum lies in the fact that its mucosal lining not infrequently is composed in part of aberrant, or misplaced, tissue—tissue characteristic of another portion of the gastrointestinal tract. It may, for example, contain gastric or jejunal mucosa, or even pancreatic tissue. Such aberrant tissues tend to ulcerate. Thus, the diverticulum may give rise to gastrointestinal hemorrhage—its most common manifestation in childhood; it may become inflamed and lead to intestinal obstruction; or it may perforate, causing peritonitis (see below).

The most common symptoms of a diseased Meckel's diverticulum are abdominal pain, typically umbilical in location, or the passage of stools containing blood. This blood is not apt to be tarry black, as in the case of a slowly bleeding gastric or upper intestinal lesion, nor yet bright red, as would be expected from a colonic hemorrhage; but, rather a dark crimson color. The treatment is surgical excision of the diverticulum.

Peritonitis

Peritonitis is inflammation of the peritoneal cavity. Usually it is due to bacterial infection, the organisms coming from disease of the gastrointestinal tract, the internal genital organs of the female and, less often, from outside by injury or by extension of inflammation from an extraperitoneal organ such as the kidney.

Symptoms depend, of course, on the location and the extent of the inflammation, and these in turn are determined by the disease causing the peritonitis. At first a diffuse, colicky type of pain is felt. This tends to become constant, localized and more intense near the site of the process. The area of the abdomen affected becomes extremely tender and the muscles become rigid. Usually, nausea and vomiting occur and peristalsis is diminished. The temperature and the pulse rate increase, and almost always there is an elevation of the leukocyte count. These early signs and symptoms of peritonitis also are the symptoms of the disease causing the condition.

Treatment and Nursing Care

Treatment is directed toward removing the cause: if this is an acutely inflamed appendix, an appendectomy is performed; if it is a ruptured duodenal ulcer, the opening in the duodenum is closed; and so on.

If the cause of the peritonitis is removed at an early stage, the inflammation subsides and the patient recovers. Frequently, however, the inflammation is not localized and the whole abdominal cavity becomes involved. The patient is acutely ill. He has severe pain and must be treated gently. Treatment and nursing care are concerned with combating the infection, establishing and eliminating the cause of the peritonitis, and making the patient as comfortable as possible.

Nothing is given by mouth; therefore, good mouth hygiene must be carried out by the nurse. Fluids of saline and glucose are administered by vein in an attempt to establish an adequate fluid level and to ensure an adequate urinary output both before and after operation. This is important, for many toxins are thrown off in this way. The effectiveness of this regimen can be attained only by the accurate recording of fluid intake and output by the nurse. This includes the measuring and the recording of vomitus. The antibiotics, especially penicillin and streptomycin or chlortetracycline or oxytetracycline, may be given parenterally. Usually penicillin and streptomycin are administered intramuscularly, whereas chlortetracycline or oxytetracycline may be given in intravenous solutions.

It is essential that the nurse observe and record symptoms accurately. Her description of the nature, the location and the shifts of pain in the abdomen is very important. She may do much in establishing confidence and hope in the patient, who realizes very often the seriousness of his condition.

When he has recovered from the anesthetic after operation, the patient is placed in the Fowler position to facilitate drainage. Nothing is given by mouth and he continues to receive fluids by vein. To prevent vomiting and distention, a gastrointestinal tube is passed through the nose into the stomach and/or the duodenum. This tube is connected to wall or Wangensteen suction and must be checked by the nurse to see that it works properly. Obviously, it will be necessary to give care to the nose and the mouth to keep the patient comfortable. Cotton applicators dipped in water or mineral oil are effective in cleaning the nose. The use of a toothbrush and a mouthwash by the patient is refreshing. Mineral oil with lemon juice is pleasant as a lubricant for dry lips.

Drains are inserted frequently during the

operation, and it is essential that the nurse observe and record the character of the drainage. Care must be taken in moving and in turning the patient to prevent dislodging or removing the drains accidentally. When the temperature and the pulse rate fall, the abdomen becomes soft, peristaltic sounds return and the patient begins to pass gas and have bowel movements, the peritonitis is subsiding. Food and fluids can be given by mouth in increasing amounts and parenteral fluids are reduced.

Two or the most common complications that must be watched for are wound evisceration and abscess formation. Any suggestion from the patient that an area of the abdomen is tender or painful or "feels as if something just gave way" should be reported to the surgeon.

Intestinal Tuberculosis

Primary tuberculous infections of the bowel wall are rare; the majority of cases develop as a complication of pulmonary tuberculosis. The disease spreads in the lymph channels of the intestinal wall, forming a ring of tubercles, which, coalescing, form an encircling ulcer in its mucous membrane. Tuberculous intestinal ulcers give few informative symptoms: merely chronic indigestion, with more or less flatulence, and diarrhea, but little pain. X-ray examination of the small and the large bowel is of great aid in the diagnosis of this disease. The treatment is that of tuberculosis in general.

Tuberculous Peritonitis

This infection presumably reaches the peritoneal cavity from caseous mesenteric lymph nodes. There are three forms of the disease: acute tuberculous peritonitis, peritonitis with effusion and adhesive peritonitis. Usually, however, one speaks merely of a "wet" and a "dry" form.

Symptoms. Acute tuberculous peritonitis rarely develops as abruptly as the acute pyogenic types described above. The pain usually is less severe, local tenderness and muscle spasm are more vague, the patient is less ill, and he tends to improve progressively. Indeed, in most patients, the local symptoms and signs are few or absent altogether; often the only physical sign elicited

is immobility of the abdominal wall during respiration, a sign that is quite suggestive of this disease. On palpation, the abdomen feels doughy rather than rigid. An irregular fever is characteristic, and either diarrhea or constipation may be present.

The "wet" form of the disease, in addition to the symptoms just described, is characterized by a striking distention of the abdomen, caused by a large amount of free fluid in the peritoneal cavity, and also by tympanites (gaseous distention of the intestines).

In the adhesive form of tuberculous peritonitis, the peritoneal cavity largely becomes obliterated by adhesions. There may be present large masses consisting of caseous tuberculous exudate walled in between the viscera, all of the bowel bound together into one mass, the omentum thickened and rolled up into a mass, visceral organs encased in a thick shell of tuberculous tissue or collections of clear fluid exudate encapsulated in various parts of the abdominal cavity. While these lesions are developing, patients may have varying degrees of malaise, loss of weight and strength, fever and anemia.

Treatment. Tuberculous peritonitis of all types improves following a regimen of chemotherapy and rest such as has been described for tuberculous infections in general.

Chronic Ulcerative Colitis

Chronic ulcerative colitis is a disease in which a patchy necrosis and desquamation of the colonic epithelium develop. This process involves the entire large colon in most cases. The cause is unknown, but it is considered by some possibly to represent an example of psychosomatic disease. There may be several precipitating factors, the net effect of which is a self-pepetuating destructive infection of the mucosal lining of the large intestine. The usual signs and symptoms are the frequent passage of bloody stools containing pus, abdominal cramps, fever, anemia and weight loss. It is a serious disease, and the mortality rate is high. Even mild cases are apt to recur for years. In the diagnosis of chronic ulcerative colitis, dysentery, due to the common intestinal organisms, and especially *Endamoeba histolytica*

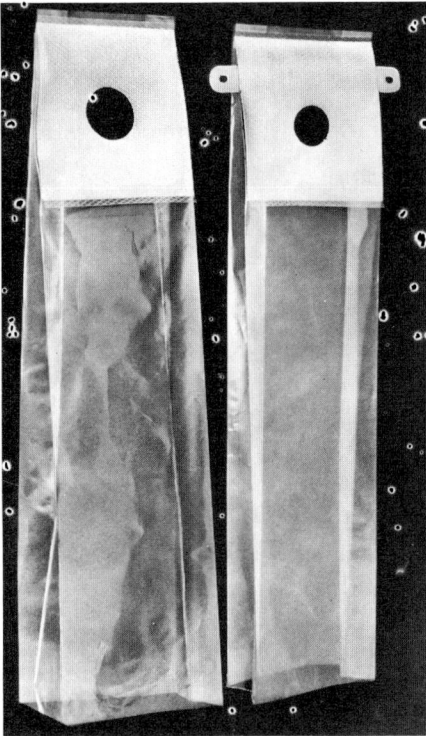

FIG. 232. Plastic disposable ileostomy bags (Bongort) with adhesive facing. The opening can be cut to meet the needs of the individual patient. The bag on the right has tabs through which twill tapes can be fastened and tied around the body for additional security. (United Surgical Supplies Co.)

other diseases of the colon with similar symptoms.

Treatment and Nursing Care

The patient with acute ulcerative colitis is placed at bed rest and given sedative drugs, i.e., barbiturates, in sufficient dosage to ensure constant drowsiness for several days, and paregoric, or intramuscular injections of magnesium sulfate. The purpose of this sedation is to reduce to a minimum the colonic peristalsis, i.e., to rest the infected bowel. It is continued until the stools approach normal frequency and consistency. Meanwhile, the patient is watched carefully for signs of colonic perforation, a calamitous complication of this disease. The patient is nourished and maintained in a state of good hydration with a soft or liquid diet. Parenteral fluids with vitamin supplements added, as well as blood transfusions, are adminis-

infection, must be ruled out by careful stool examination. Sigmoidoscopy and barium enema x-ray examination are of diagnostic value in distinguishing this condition from

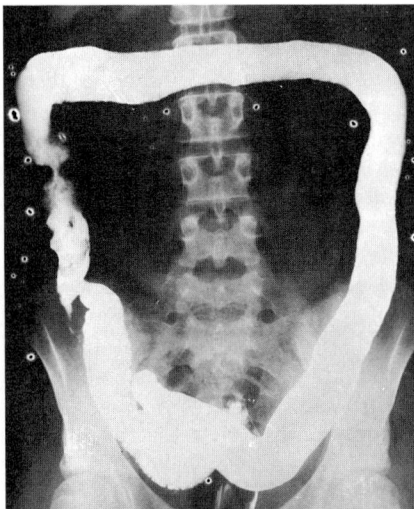

FIG. 233. Roentgenogram of colon in ulcerative colitis. The bowel has become a semirigid tube as a result of the long-standing inflammatory process.

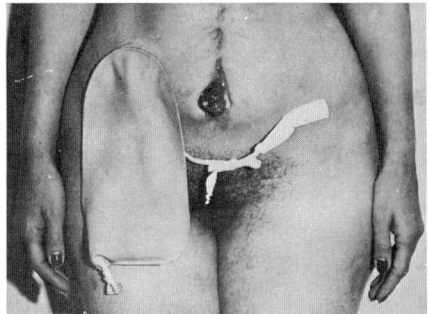

FIG. 234. Patient with ileostomy wearing a Rutzen bag. This patient has had a subtotal colectomy. Because of ulcerative colitis, the colon has been removed from the cecum to the sigmoid. The sigmoid is seen implanted in the midline wound. The secretions of the ileum are caught in the rubber bag, which is cemented to the skin. The rubber band closes a spigotlike extension at the lower end of the bag. Removal of the band permits drainage of the secretions into the toilet. See also Fig. 243.

FIG. 235. Diagrammatic drawing that shows an *inguinal* hernia. Note that the sac of the hernia is a continuation of the peritoneum of the abdomen and that the hernial contents are intestine, omentum or other abdominal contents that pass through the hernial opening into the hernial sac.

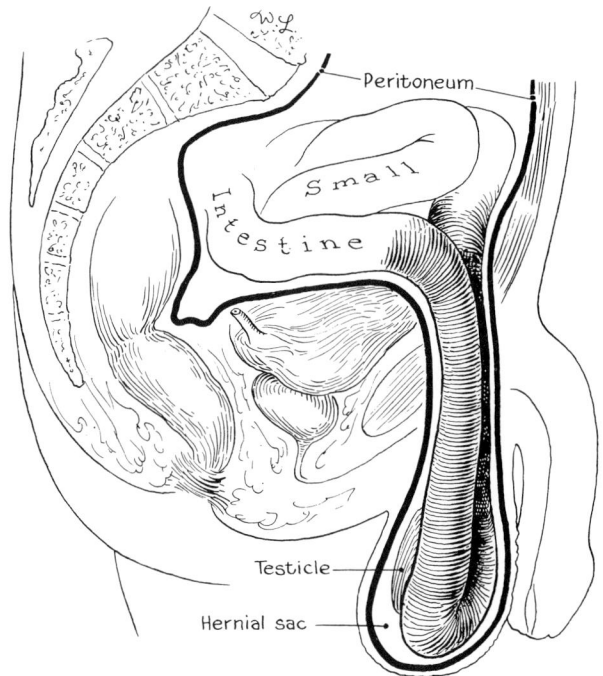

tered as indicated. Anodyne suppositories will relieve painful rectal spasms produced by frequent diarrheal stools.

Temporary remissions have followed the administration of steroids; therefore, this form of therapy deserves trial if standard measures prove to be unsuccessful.

Operative Treatment. A prolonged period of preparation with intensive fluid, blood and protein replacement is necessary before operation is attempted. Chemotherapy and antibiotics are useful adjuncts.

The operations performed are directed toward diverting the flow of the intestinal contents from the diseased portion of the colon. If the disease involves only the distal colon, a *colostomy* (p. 635) in the transverse colon may be performed. If the whole colon is involved, an *ileostomy* (opening of the terminal ileum on the abdominal wall) must be performed. Usually it is necessary to remove the diseased colon (colectomy).

PREOPERATIVE CARE. For a patient with ulcerative colitis the preoperative care should include an understanding of the problems faced by the patient. These may be social and emotional, as well as physical; they may have resulted from or contributed to the diseased condition. His personality

may be affected by innumerable factors. Let him know that his complaints are understood. Fear and anxiety accompanies diarrhea. Any patient who is suffering from the discomforts of frequent bowel movements and rectal soreness will be anxious, discouraged, and depressed. The patient with this condition is often a hypersensitive individual. Encourage him to talk and ventilate his feelings. This in an outlet for emotional tension. Listen to the matters that may be disturbing him. Direct the attention to the individual patient, not to his bowel condition. The nurse's evident interest in the patient will aid in gaining his confidence, which is an important part of his preoperative treatment.

Usually, the patient is on a low residue diet offered frequently in small feedings. He may receive iron for secondary anemia and antibiotics to reduce bacterial growth in the intestinal tract. All other preoperative measures are similar to general abdominal surgery.

POSTOPERATIVE CARE. If it is known before operation that a patient is to have an ileostomy, it is well to begin psychological preparation at that time. The acceptance of an ileostomy is often difficult, and the patient deserves all the support which can be given to him. It is necessary to develop in him a point of view that an ileostomy is a challenge; if accepted with courage he can master it and proceed to live normally and happily. This is difficult to bring about in many individuals, and the task of developing a proper attitude in the patient becomes a challenge for the nurse. Other patients who have had ileostomies are an excellent source of help to this patient.

The opening of the small intestine on the abdomen discharges continuously the liquid contents of the small intestine. Because these discharges contain digestive enzymes, they are highly irritating to the skin of the abdomen. As soon as operation is completed, a temporary plastic bag with an adhesive facing is placed over the ileostomy and firmly pressed onto surrounding skin. The contents

draining from the ileostomy are thus kept from coming in contact with skin and are collected and measured as the bag becomes full. After the ileostomy has had a chance to heal, a permanent rubber bag is obtained and held in place on the skin with rubber cement.

Because these patients lose much fluid and food in the early postoperative period, an accurate record of fluid intake, urinary output and rectal discharges is necessary to help the surgeon to gauge the fluid needs of the patient. Fluids, blood and amino acid are given in large amounts until the patient becomes accustomed to the new digestive arrangement.

Such patients probably are the most difficult of all to nurse. Their prolonged illness makes them irritable, weak and, at times, psychopathic. The nurse must recognize that

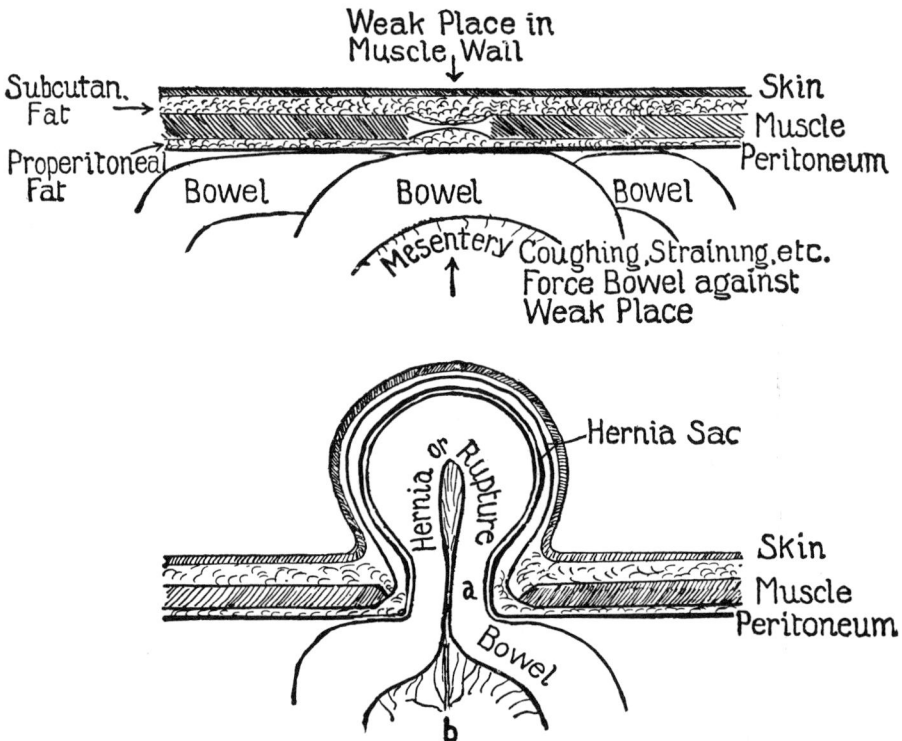

FIG. 236. *Ventral* or *incisional* hernia. The weak place in the muscle wall pictured above might be any one of the "rings" of the abdominal wall, naturally weak since through it some blood vessel, etc., passes through the abdominal wall. (a) The neck of the sac, the point where the bowel is pinched by the ring of muscle. (b) The artery supplying the loop of bowel with blood; it, of course, is occluded if the pressure of the ring is great.

this behavior often is a result of complex socioeconomic pressures. She must be consistent in expressing sincere friendliness and exhibiting a nonjudgmental attitude. Operation often results in an almost immediate change in their mental outlook and, as soon as they learn to care for their ileostomies, they become normal, affable and attractive people. A patient, sympathetic and tolerant nurse is most important in the recovery of these patients.

Mesenteric Thrombosis

If one of the larger arteries supplying the intestine becomes plugged, that segment of the bowel supplied by this artery soon will become gangrenous; in other words, intestinal infarction occurs. Mesenteric thrombosis is most common in individuals past middle age who are suffering from generalized arteriosclerosis. Sclerosis of the mesenteric arteries, as in the case of the coronary or the cerebral arteries, predisposes to thrombosis of these vessels. Another cause of their sudden occlusion is embolism, for example, from a mural thrombus in the heart or from an endocarditis.

The symptoms of mesenteric thrombosis are sudden severe diffuse abdominal pain, distention, shock, which is often profound, and passage of blood in the stools.

Treatment. Treatment of the condition is a surgical emergency. Unless the infarcted portion of the bowel is removed promptly, intestinal perforation surely will occur through the gangrenous wall, with fatal peritonitis as the end-result.

Abdominal Hernia

A *hernia* (spoken of by the laity as "rupture") is a protrusion of a viscus through the wall of the cavity in which it is naturally contained. This definition may apply to any part of the body; for instance, the protrusion of the brain after a subtemporal decompression is called *cerebral hernia*. However, in general, the term is applied to the protrusion of an abdominal viscus through an opening in the abdominal wall. The weakness may be congenital, i.e., failure to close of one or more of the openings in the abdominal wall normally found in the fetus; or it may be acquired, due to prolonged

strain on the abdominal muscles or after illness or operation.

The hernial sac is formed by an outpouching of the peritoneum and may contain large or small intestine, omentum and, occasionally, the bladder. When the hernia first is formed, the sac is filled only when the patient is on his feet, the contents returning to the abdominal cavity as soon as he lies down.

Types. There are four types of abdominal hernia. The most common type is the *inguinal* (Fig. 235). This hernia is due to a weakness of the abdominal wall at the point through which the spermatic cord emerges in the male and the round ligament in the female. Through this opening the hernia extends down the inguinal canal and often into the scrotum or the labia. It is common in the male, and it may appear at any age.

Femoral hernia appears below Poupart's ligament (i.e., below the groin) as a round bulge. It is more frequent in women.

Umbilical hernia results from failure of the umbilical orifice to close. It is most common in fat women and in children as a protrusion at or slightly below the umbilicus.

Ventral or *incisional* hernias (Fig. 236) occur due to a weakness of the abdominal wall. They are due most frequently to previous operations in which drainage was necessary, complete closure of the tissues being impossible. Weakened by infection, only a slight bulge results at first, but this increases gradually in size until a definite hernial sac is produced.

There are many other forms of hernia, some of which occur inside the abdominal cavity. Such a hernia is spoken of as *internal* hernia.

Complications. As times goes on, adhesions form between the sac and its contents, so that the hernia becomes *irreducible*. Any hernia, whether previously reducible or not, may at any time become incarcerated or strangulated. An *incarcerated* hernia is one in which the intestinal flow is obstructed completely. In a *strangulated* hernia the contents not only are irreducible, but the blood and the intestinal flow through the intestine in the hernia are stopped completely. This condition obtains when the loop of intestine in the sac becomes twisted; swelling occurs and a constriction is produced at the neck of the sac. The result then is an acute intestinal obstruction, plus the added danger of gangrene of the bowel. The symptoms are pain at the site of strangulation, followed by colicky abdominal pain, vomiting, and swelling of the hernial sac.

Treatment

Surgical. In most cases the hernia should be repaired by operation; otherwise, it is in continual danger of strangulation. When this occurs, operation becomes imperative, and it is attended invariably by considerable risk.

The operation comprises removal of the hernial sac after dissecting it free from surrounding structures, replacing its contents in the abdominal cavity and ligating it at the neck. The muscle and the fascial layers then are sewed together firmly over the hernial orifice to prevent a recurrence. In the repair of large hernias, tantalum gauze mesh has been implanted. Tantalum is an inert element which when woven into a gauze or a screen is malleable and strong and produces minimum tissue reaction. When a strangulation has occurred, the operation is complicated by the intestinal obstruction and injury to the bowel.

Mechanical. In infants, a hernia may at times be helped by the application of a truss, an appliance having a pad that is held snugly in the hernial orifice and should keep a reducible hernia reduced. A truss also may be used in the treatment of a hernia in adults when, because of age, or disease, it seems inadvisable to subject the patient to the risk of an operation. A truss does not cure a hernia; it simply prevents the abdominal contents from entering the hernial sac.

Preoperative Nursing Care

In emergency conditions of strangulated or incarcerated hernia, the nurse will prepare her patient as in any other acute surgical problem. However, most patients are individuals who are in good physical condition and are having a herniorrhaphy as elective surgery. The patient may be prompted by the knowledge that an unrepaired hernia may become a serious emergency, or he may have difficulty securing employment because of this condition.

The suprapubic region and the anterior surface of the upper thigh should be shaved carefully. It is important for the patient not

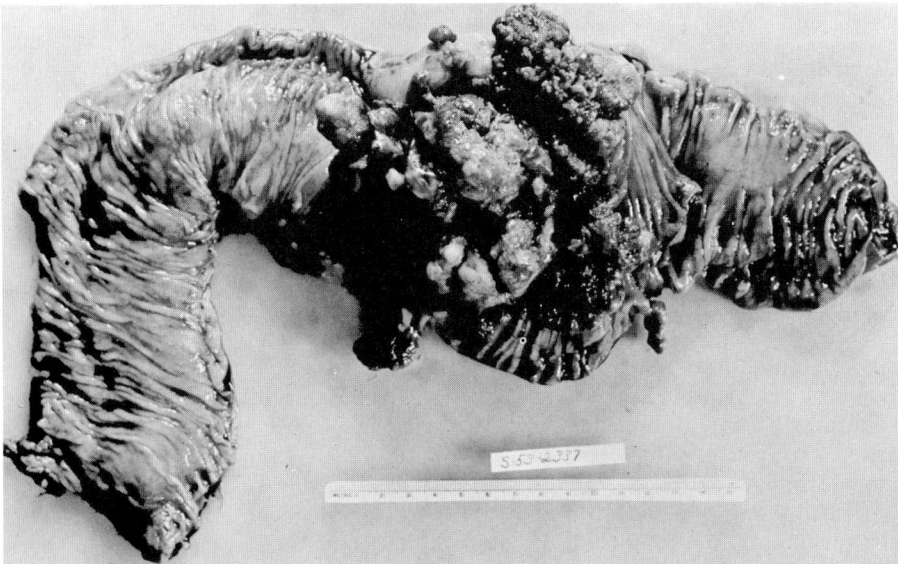

Fig. 237. Carcinoma of the colon. The transverse colon was resected and opened by a longitudinal cut, which exposed the mucosal lining and demonstrated a large fungating tumor mass. (Russell P. Sherwin, M.D.)

to have a cold or a cough. Such a strain may break the sutures and defeat the purpose of surgery. When he goes to the operating room, his bladder must be empty to prevent accidental injury during the surgical repair.

Nursing Care After Herniorrhaphy

Prolonged bed rest is not necessary after such operations, and in many cases patients are allowed out of bed a day or two after operation. In the event of edema and swelling of the scrotum, bed rest may be prolonged somewhat, and a suspensory bandage or a jock strap may be necessary to give support and to provide pressure.

The chief complication to be watched for in connection with the repair of a hernia is the retention of urine. The patient may have problems in voiding after spinal anesthesia and surgical handling of the bladder. When these patients may not stand or sit up and, if conservative measures fail to give relief, catheterization must be performed.

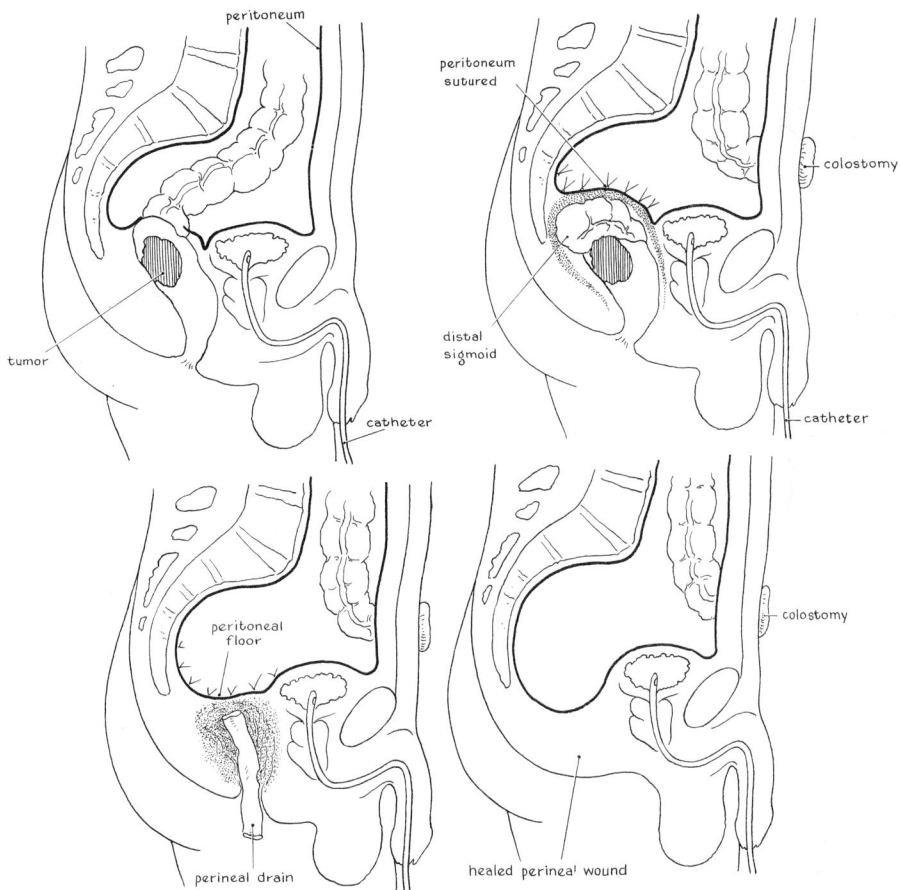

FIG. 238. Diagrammatic representation of abdominoperineal resection for carcinoma of rectum. (*Top, left*) Tumor in rectum. (*Top, right*) At operation, the sigmoid first is divided and a colostomy is established. The distal bowel has been dissected free to a point below the pelvic peritoneum. The pelvic peritoneum is sutured over the closed end of the distal sigmoid and rectum. The perineal resection includes removal of the rectum and free portion of the sigmoid from below. (*Bottom, left*) The perineum is closed loosely about drains placed beneath the peritoneum in the hollow of the sacrum. (*Bottom, right*) The final result after healing.

Infection, or at least an imperfect healing, is all too frequent in these wounds. The elevation of temperature several days after operation or soreness in the operative region should lead to the discovery of the trouble. If early remedial measures are taken, the patient's convalescence is not delayed.

The patient should be instructed specifically as to his activity after leaving the hospital. As a rule, athletics and extremes of exertion are not permitted for at least 6 or 8 weeks after the operation.

Tumors of the Intestine

Tumors of the small intestine, as in the case of duodenal tumors, are rare. Lipomata (fatty tumors), fibromata (connective tissue tumors), angiomata (blood vessel tumors), and carcinoid (carcinomalike) tumors are all benign in character. Some of these may take the form of polyps projecting into the intestinal lumen. Their chief importance lies in the fact that they may give rise to intussusception (p. 632). Sarcoma and lymphosarcoma—malignant tumors of connective tissue and lymphoid tissue, respectively—may arise in the small bowel, producing intestinal hemorrhage or obstruction.

Tumors of the colon, on the other hand, are relatively common. Benign polyps are much more common in the large than in the small intestine. They may be very numerous. When multiple, the condition is referred to as polyposis—often, apparently, a congenital abnormality. These polyps not infrequently become cancerous.

Cancer of the colon (Fig. 237) and the rectum always arises from the epithelium lining the intestine. The effects produced depend largely on its location. As in the case of cancer elsewhere in the gastrointestinal tract, the chief symptoms are the passage of blood in the stools, anemia, obstruction and perforation. A suddenly developing obstruction may be the first symptom of cancer involving the colon anywhere between the cecum and the sigmoid, for in this region, where the bowel contents are liquid, a slowly developing obstruction will not become evident until the lumen is practically closed. Cancer of the sigmoid and the rectum causes earlier symptoms of partial obstruction, with constipation alternating with diarrhea, lower abdominal crampy pains and distention. Any patient with a history of inexplicable change in bowel habit and the passage of blood in the stools should be studied carefully to rule out cancer of the large bowel. The possibility that a rectal carcinoma exists, detectable but still asymptomatic, and still operable, is one important reason for the inclusion of a rectal examination as part of every routine physical examination. Helpful additional symptoms, often present, are those of progressive weakness, anorexia, weight loss, anemia and lower abdominal pain. The most important diagnostic procedures are the abdominal and rectal examinations, sigmoidoscopy, repeated examination of the stools for the presence of blood, determination of the blood-hemoglobin concentration for the question of anemia and, usually the most conclusive of all, the barium roentgenologic examination.

Preparation for Operation. This includes the shaving of the abdomen and the perineum, and rectal irrigation that is continued until the fluid returns clear. Usually a high caloric, low residue diet is given for several days before operation if time and the patient's condition permit. If an emergency does not exist, these patients are prepared for several days by being given intestinal antiseptics of the sulfa group (sulfasuxidine or sulfathalidine) and the antibiotics Achromycin and neomycin. These are given by mouth to reduce the bacterial content of the colon and to soften and decrease the bulk of the contents of the colon. The nurse should pay attention to any mention of pain and its location. She also should record fluid losses, such as would occur by vomiting and diarrhea. This will aid the surgeon in regulating the fluid intake and maintaining proper balance. Preoperative intestinal intubation with a Miller-Abbott or Cantor tube facilitates the performance of intestinal surgery and minimizes postoperative distention. In the event that there is any possibility of a permanent colostomy, the patient should be informed of it by the surgeon, and he should be assured that it can be handled effectively and need not interfere with his usual social and business life. He should be assured also that he need not develop into a dependent person. This mental preparation of the patient is an extremely important part of his preoperative care.

The patient is sent to the operating room with an indwelling (Foley) catheter in place.

Operative Treatment. This will depend on the position and the extent of the cancer. When the tumor can be removed, the involved colon is excised for some distance on each side of the growth to remove the tumor and the area of its lymphatic spread. If distant (liver) metastasis has occurred, the tumor may be excised for palliation but without hope of cure. The intestine may be reunited by an *enterocolostomy* or by an end-to-end anastomosis of the colon. When the growth is situated low in the sigmoid or the rectum, the colon is cut above the growth and brought out through the abdominal wall,

forming thus an abdominal anus, called a *colostomy*. The growth then is removed from below by a perineal incision. (*Abdominoperineal resection,* Fig. 238.)

In the event that the tumor has spread and involves surrounding vital structures, it is considered to be inoperable. When the growth in the rectum or the sigmoid is inoperable, and especially when symptoms of partial or complete obstruction are present, a colostomy may be performed. A loop of the colon, near the junction of the descending colon and the sigmoid, is brought out of the abdomen through a lower left rectus incision and maintained in place by a glass rod or rubber tube inserted underneath the loop. If the obstruction is complete, the loop may be drained by the insertion of a rubber tube

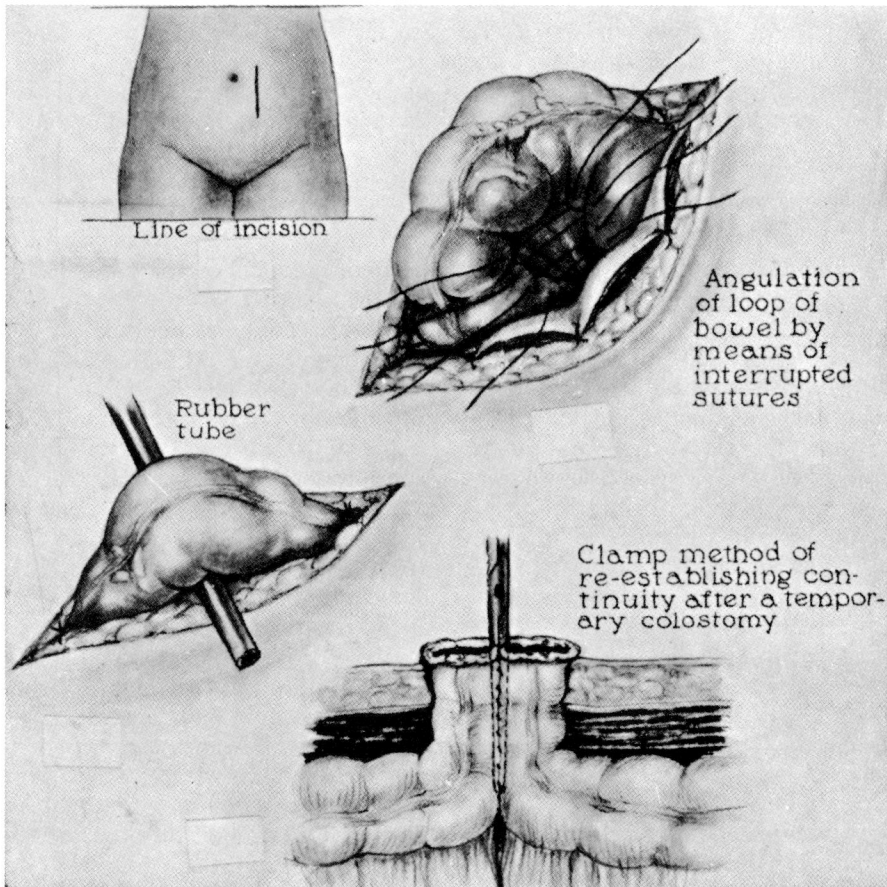

FIG. 239. (*Left*) Steps in simple loop colostomy. (*Right*) Steps in a Mikulicz temporary colostomy. After the latter procedure the colostomy is closed.

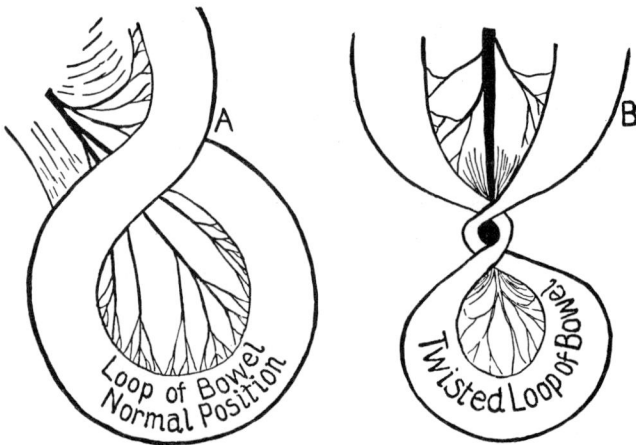

FIG. 240. Intestinal obstruction caused by a twist of a loop. (A) The normal position of a loop. (B) The result of a twist. This will occlude the bowel and also, by pressure, will close the blood vessels in the mesentery, causing the death of the bowel beyond the twist.

or by the use of a right-angled glass tube called a Paul's tube, which is held in the intestine by a purse-string suture. When the obstruction is incomplete, the colostomy loop is allowed to remain unopened for several days to permit the peritoneal cavity to become thoroughly sealed off. During this time the patient is given a clear diet. The intestine is opened by electrocautery, as hemorrhage is slight after its use.

Intestinal Obstruction

Intestinal obstruction results if, for any reason, the intestinal contents are prevented from flowing normally along the bowel. Obstruction may be partial, or it may be complete. Its seriousness depends on the region of bowel that is affected, the degree to which the lumen is occluded and, especially, on the degree to which the blood circulation in the bowel wall is disturbed. Small bowel obstruction is always serious, for, in consequence of persistent vomiting, it leads to profound disturbances in the electrolyte balance of the body: first, to alkalosis, from the loss of the gastric hydrochloric acid; then, to profound dehydration and acidosis, due to the loss of water and sodium from the small intestine. If the obstruction is only partial and develops slowly, the symptoms are relatively mild. Large bowel obstruction, even if complete, is also comparatively undramatic, provided that the blood supply to the colon is not disturbed.

Causes

Intestinal obstruction occasionally results from a foreign body lodged in the bowel. This may be false teeth, jewelry, a large fruit stone, a gallstone, a mass of parasitic worms, etc. In other cases, a stricture of the bowel is the result of the contracting scar of an ulcer in its wall, due, for example, to tuberculosis. The intestine may become pinched in a peritoneal pocket (hernia) or there may be peritoneal adhesions. A loop of intestine may become twisted about itself (volvulus) (Fig. 240) or may tie itself into a true knot.

Hernia (pp. 627-630) is one of the most common and important causes of intestinal obstruction.

Intussusception is another cause of intestinal obstruction. In this condition, the bowel, above a certain point, pushes itself into the bowel below that point, much as a telescope is shortened by pushing one section into the next (Fig. 241). This likewise occurs through peristalsis. The point at which intussusception most commonly develops is at or near the ileocecal valve. The telescoping, or invagination, also may start at the point of attachment of a tumor in the colon—particularly a pedunculated tumor— as a result of its becoming engaged by a peristaltic wave and propelled along the colon, dragging into the lumen that portion of the wall to which its pedicle is attached. When intussusception starts at the ileocecal valve, the terminal portion of the small bowel may invaginate its way down the whole length of the large bowel and protrude at the anus. Any child who has been seized with pain in the abdomen and then passes

FIG. 241. Intussusception. The bowel is represented as working its way down within itself. Of course, the mesentery containing the blood vessels to the bowel wall also is dragged down. Should these vessels become closed by the pressure produced at the point of invagination, death of the inner portion of the loop would result.

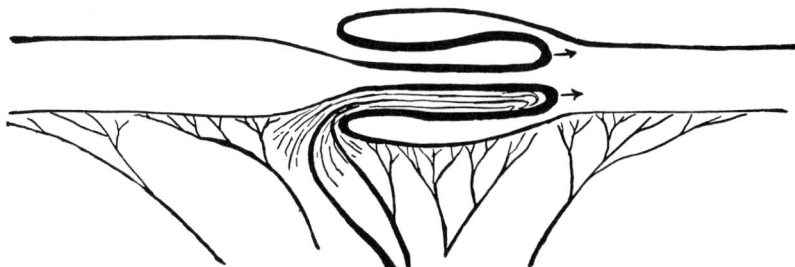

blood and mucus in the stools should be examined with the possibility of intussusception in mind.

Postoperative Adhesions. After abdominal operation, there are many areas produced which are not completely healed within the abdomen, and to these areas loops of intestine may become adherent. The attachment of these loops of small intestine via inflammatory adhesions usually is only temporary and of no particular moment. However, occasionally these inflammatory adhesions may produce a kinking of an intestinal loop, which causes obstruction of the intestinal flow. This intestinal obstruction usually appears on the 3rd or 4th day after operation, when peristalsis normally is resumed and when food and fluids are being given to the patient for the first time. The symptoms are typical of any intestinal obstruction— crampy abdominal pain, distention, vomiting, etc.

In most cases of postoperative inflammatory obstruction, the difficulty may be relieved by intestinal intubation. By decompressing the bowel above the site of the obstruction, the inflammation is permitted to subside, and the obstruction is relieved. When the obstruction cannot be relieved by this conservative means, a reoperation may be necessary to free the adherent intestine and to permit the intestinal flow to be resumed.

Paralytic Ileus. Occasionally after abdominal operations, after operations on the kidney and, frequently, in cases of peritonitis, peristaltic movement becomes paralyzed due to traumatic or toxic affection of the nerves that have to do with the intestinal movement. This results in a distention of the intestine with gas, produced by decomposition of the intestinal contents or by the swallowing of air. The lack of peristalsis results in an accumulation of this gas in the intestine, causing distention. Few or no peristaltic sounds can be heard, and the patient may be extremely uncomfortable, if not in marked pain. This condition is spoken of as *paralytic ileus* to distinguish it from *organic ileus,* which is caused by an organic obstruction of the intestine. Relief of the distention associated with paralytic ileus often is obtained by intestinal intubation (see below).

Symptoms of Intestinal Obstruction

The initial symptom of small bowel obstruction is usually pain, wavelike in character. Constipation ensues. The patient may pass blood and mucus, but no fecal matter and no flatus. Vomiting occurs. This is often characteristic. If the obstruction is complete, the peristaltic waves become extremely vigorous and assume a reverse direction, the intestinal contents being propelled toward the mouth instead of toward the rectum. If the obstruction is in the ileum or distal to it, fecal vomiting takes place. First, the patient vomits the stomach contents, then the bile-stained contents of the duodenum and the jejunum and, finally, with each paroxysm of pain the darker, fecal-like contents of the ileum are ejected. Soon, due to the loss of water, sodium and chlorides in the vomitus, the unmistakable signs of dehydration become evident. The patient complains of intense thirst, drowsiness, generalized malaise and aching. The tongue and the mucous membranes become parched; the face acquires a pinched appearance. The abdomen becomes distended, and the lower the obstruction in the gastrointestinal tract, the more marked is the distention. If the situation is allowed to continue uncorrected, shock appears, due to dehydration and loss of plasma volume. The patient is prostrated; the pulse becomes increasingly weak and rapid; the temperature and the blood pressure are lowered; the skin is pale, cold and clammy. At this point, death may supervene rapidly.

Lower intestinal obstruction differs clinically from the small bowel type in that the symptoms develop and progress relatively slowly. This difference is due to the fact that the colon is able to absorb its fluid contents; and, it can distend to a considerable degree beyond its normal full capacity. In patients with an obstruction in the sigmoid or the rectum, constipation may be the only symptom for days. Eventually the abdomen becomes markedly distended; loops of large bowel become visibly outlined through the abdomen wall, and the patient suffers from crampy lower abdominal pain. Finally, fecal vomiting develops, and the terminal features are essentially those of ileum obstruction. In patients with fecal impaction there is no shock.

Treatment and Nursing Care. Most cases of intestinal obstruction are surgical problems. From the medical standpoint, it is essential that the conditions be recognized. They must not be confused with other, more benign, causes of constipation, vomiting, abdominal pain and distention. A purgative never is given to a patient suspected of having obstruction, for this will seriously aggravate the situation.

The most important criteria by which obstruction is distinguished, as such, include the existence, location and character of pain, the presence of distention and the occurrence of flatus or defecation. The eliciting of this type of evidence is within the scope of the nurse's responsibility.

In addition, she must measure, record and chart 4-hour temperatures, pulse rates and blood pressure readings as well as fluid intake and output. Any stool that might be passed, or a portion thereof, is to be saved for direct inspection by the physician as well as to be tested for the presence of occult blood. Arrangements for that test as well as for urinalysis, hemoglobin measurements and blood cell counts should be made promptly on request by the physician or automatically on her own initiative if circumstances warrant it in this type of emergency.

If the disorder is an incarcerated external hernia, an attempt may be made to reduce it, not by applying pressure to the extruded mass, but simply by having the patient lie flat on his back with knees flexed and with an icepack placed continuously over the mass. This position, and cold, may cause the edema and swelling of the incarcerated bowel to subside, allowing the loop to escape back through the ring or opening into which it has worked itself. If reduction does not occur, prompt surgical intervention is necessary.

Preoperative Care. Before attempting surgery on an ill patient with intestinal obstruction, steps are taken to correct the dehydration and to decompress the dilated bowel. Adequate amounts of physiologic saline solution with dextrose are given intravenously to replace the sodium, chloride and water lost in the vomitus and to supply nourishment. Decompression is accomplished by intubating the small intestine with a Miller-Abbott tube, for example, and constantly aspirating the fluid and gaseous contents, employing constant suction siphonage.

Preoperative preparation is the giving of a small enema and the shaving of the entire abdomen. These measures often are supplemented by decompression of the intestine by the use of suction attached to a Miller-Abbott, a Cantor or a Harris tube. The tubes frequently become clogged and must be irrigated by the nurse at frequent intervals. Extreme care must be exercised in irrigating the Miller-Abbott tube, in that the irrigating solution must be introduced into the portion marked "Suction." The other lumen leads to the distensible rubber bag and serious accidents have occurred (rupture of the intestine) when, by mistake, the nurses have introduced into the bag fluid meant for irrigation.

Surgery. The surgical treatment of intestinal obstruction depends largely on the cause of the obstruction. In the most common causes of obstruction, such as strangulated hernia, obstruction by adhesive bands, and so forth, the operation consists of repair of the hernia or division of the band to which the intestine is attached. In some hernias, it may be necessary to remove the portion of bowel which has become strangulated and perform an anastomosis. Operation for intestinal obstruction may be simple or complicated, depending on the duration of the obstruction and the condition of the intestine as found at operation. In occasional patients, intestinal intubation may not be sufficient to decompress the bowel. In these cases, it is not uncommon to introduce a catheter into the distended intestine. This catheter is brought out through the abdominal wall, usually through a separate incision, to decompress the intestine and is spoken of as a *tube enterostomy.*

When the large intestine becomes obstructed, usually by cancer, it is frequently necessary to relieve the colonic obstruction before it is possible to resect the cancer itself. This is done by inserting a large tube into the cecum (cecostomy) or by making an opening in the colon above the site of the obstruction by bringing a loop of colon up to the skin surface. When this is opened, the obstruction is relieved and the tumor can be treated at a later time. This operation a called a *loop colostomy.*

Postoperative Care. After operation, fluids must be given these patients in large amounts. An accurately kept intake and output record is essential, since it is information that the surgeon must have if the nutritional needs of the patient are to be met. If an enterostomy has been performed, a bottle should be attached to the side of the bed and a tube connected with the enterostomy tube, inserted in it. If peristalsis is active and the tube has been placed properly in the bowel, a considerable amount (from 500 to 1,000 ml. of fecal fluid should drain away in the first 12 to 15 hours after operation. Frequently the fenestra of the enterostomy tube becomes clogged by fecal masses and, obviously, the drainage will cease until the tube is cleared. The nurse should observe the amount of drainage accumulating in the collection bottle and, if there is no increase in the quantity of fluid for several hours, she should regard it as an indication that the tube has clogged. Many surgeons make sure that the fenestra remains open by having the nurse inject a half ounce of warm saline solution into the enterostomy or colostomy tube at intervals of from 2 to 3 hours. The skin about the enterostomy is protected by strips of petrolatum gauze, aluminum paint or zinc ointment. Again it is emphasized that an accurate record must be kept on these patients.

Care and Teaching of the Patient With a Colostomy

From the point of view of safety, the permanent colostomy, as we know it today, is a lifesaving procedure that is compatible with active participation in social and business life, and as such its drawbacks pale into insignificance. A philosophical acceptance of this and readjustment of one's daily habits are not achieved in one day, but getting used to this, as to any other handicap, can be accomplished by being put on the right track and facing each day with courage, optimism, and determination.

Responsibility of the Nurse

A *colostomy* (a temporary or permanent opening of the colon through the abdominal wall) is, as we have seen, used often in the treatment of ulcerative colitis, tumors of the colon, and some intestinal obstructions. The nurse cannot teach effectively if all facets of the problem facing a patient with a colostomy are not known; if, on the other hand, she has a broad understanding of colostomy care but does not know her patient, again she will fail. To give adequate support, care and instruction to this patient, the nurse must know not only basic information, but also she must know her patient. What does he think, feel, express, suppress, desire, fear and so forth? In her daily contacts with the patient who has a colostomy, valuable rapport can be establised to facilitate his adjustment. The nurse must understand and practice the psychology and the principles of learning as they apply to each particular individual.

In presenting this section, the major prob-

* Dubois, E. C.: Hints on the management of a colostomy, Am. J. Nursing **55**:72, 1955.

lems usually experienced by this patient will be discussed:

Psychological Preparation
Regulation of Function
　　Selection of Appropriate Diet
Choice of Suitable Equipment or Appliance
Hygienic Measures

Psychological Preparation

Thousands of people who have colostomies are engaged actively in business today. With the improvement of surgical and nursing procedures, and the assistance of patients who have "lived" with their colostomies, it is now possible to give intelligent assistance to the person about to have a colostomy or an ileostomy.

The support and the teaching of a patient must be individualized. Therefore, the same approach may not be appropriate for all patients. Before operation, some may find that a simple line drawing illustrating the nature and the function of the lower intestinal tract is helpful. By this means the deviations necessary for his particular situation can be explained. For others, having another patient who has had a colostomy talk to them presents a comfortable opportunity for the expressions of fears and doubts. In still other situations, some surgeons believe that a minimal amount of explanation should be given the patient preoperatively; simply telling a patient that he will have major surgery in order to correct his problem is sufficient. In other words, the extent of psychological preparation must be approached on a personal basis.

The patient needs to know what a colostomy is and how it functions; he should know that it need not hamper his way of living and that with patience, as well as some trial-and-error methods, he will be able to manage, control and master it.

As in the care of any other surgical patient, the nurse must know the plan of care to be followed, and she must know her patient. During the interval of preoperative

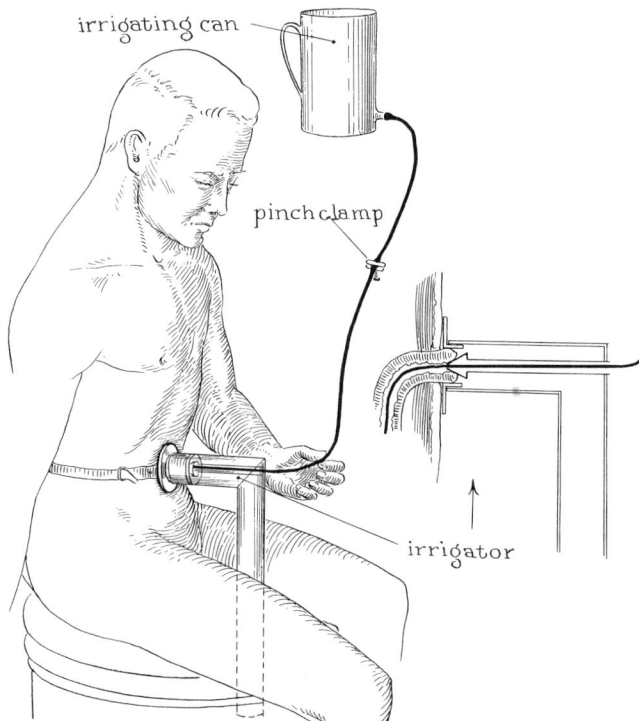

Fig. 242. Diagrammatic drawing showing patient with apparatus useful in the home irrigation of colostomy.

care she should encourage the patient to talk out his concerns and fears; in this way the nurse will be able to direct and help him.

Postoperatively, many surgeons are getting the patient out of bed on the first postoperative day, and he is encouraged to care for his colostomy from the very first irrigation. The return to normal diet is more rapid, and every effort is made to encourage him to live as he did before his operation. Psychologically, this appears to de-emphasize the abnormality of the situation.

It is well to remember that this is a strange and new experience for the patient. Most likely he has never seen an incision under surgical dressings and, less likely, a colostomy. The shock of this first sight may be minimized if he has seen drawings and perhaps a picture or two of the anatomy involved.

Regulation of Function of a Colostomy

The colostomy is opened on the 2nd or the 3rd postoperative day by the surgeon, and often there is an evacuation of loose stools. In anticipation of this the nurse will have protected the bedding with a rubber sheet covered with a towel, and she will have an emesis basin positioned at the side of the patient.

Necessary equipment:

    Irrigating set (2 quart can or bag, tubing, adapter)
    Catheter, clamp, colostomy irrigator
    Solution at 105° F.
    Petrolatum to lubricate catheter
    Toilet tissue to clean around colostomy before and after irrigation
    Newspaper or paper bag to receive soiled dressings
    A place to set or hang the irrigating container
    Dressings or cover for colostomy following irrigation

In the first irrigations of the colon the amount of solution varies from 250 ml. to 1,000 ml. These irrigations are done to cleanse the intestinal tract of gas, mucus and feces. From this time on an attempt is made to establish regularity of evacuation, and it becomes a nursing responsibility. Such a procedure is similar to the conventional enema. A No. 16 or a No. 18 catheter may be used with the enema can. The pa-

tient may sit up in bed, or, if permissible, he may sit in a chair before the toilet in the bathroom. A rubber sheet can be used as a trough leading into the toilet bowl. The patient is encouraged to watch the procedure as performed by the nurse. She should do it slowly and answer his questions. The catheter, lubricated with petrolatum to reduce friction, is inserted from 2 to 3 inches at first, and the solution is allowed to run in. The catheter then can be inserted gently up to from 6 to 8 inches. At first, only about 500 ml. of solution is given, and this may be increased gradually every day up to 1,500 ml. The temperature of the solution is about 105° F., and the irrigating can is placed about 18″ to 24″ above the level of the colostomy opening. The purpose of the irrigation is to empty the distal bowel of fecal material. As distention of the colon is an effective stimulus for bowel evacuation, the irrigating solution should be introduced in such amount and with such pressure as to distend the bowel and give the patient a feeling of fullness. If the patient complains of cramps, the level of the can may be lowered to lessen the force of the flow. The patient should be taught that the rate of flow of solution varies with the pressure and the caliber of tube. Pressure depends on height; therefore, when increased pressure is desired, the container of solution may be raised and vice versa. Solutions may be soapy solution, plain water or saline. The irrigation may be given daily, every other day or every 3 days according to the experience of the patient. Some patients prefer to take a warm bath after an irrigation. This promotes a feeling of cleanliness and relaxation. During the irrigation, when done at home, it may be pleasant and diverting to have a radio nearby. While waiting for the return flow, it may be an opportune time to read. (The entire procedure usually takes between 45 minutes and 1 hour.) Nothing but flatus and a slight amount of mucus should escape from the colostomy between irrigations. Attention should be paid to the time of day the procedure is carried out. It should fit into the post-hospital routine of the individual. For a businessman, perhaps the most convenient time would be in the evening; for a housewife, it may be the middle of the morning. The establishment of definite habits will be appreciated by the patient. As soon as he is able to do his own irrigation, the patient should be encouraged to do so. However, the nurse should assist the patient when he begins self-care, to prevent discouragement and frustration. The teaching sessions should proceed at the patient's pace, and it is desirable to have a family member present to learn this procedure. Written instructions will be helpful in the teaching-learning process.

"Wet" colostomies are those through which both urine and feces are excreted because of transplantation of ureters into the colon. These colostomies are never irrigated, because of the danger that contaminated material will be forced into the ureters and produce infection.

In a double-barrel colostomy, there are two openings, the proximal and distal segments of colon. The proximal portion is the functioning colon, whereas the distal end is irrigated only to keep it clean and free of mucus. If there is an obstruction in this section, it may be necessary to siphon the fluid. In case the cancer has not been removed, it is well to irrigate the lower loop, from anus to colostomy, every 2 or 3 days, to remove the irritating mucus that collects. If the growth has been removed by the perineal route, the wound should be watched carefully for signs of hemorrhage. The close proximity of the wound to the sacrum necessitates a frequent change of dressings in order to keep the area clean and dry.

The perineal wound usually contains a drain or packing that is removed gradually so that on about the 7th day all drains are out. There usually are sloughing bits of tissue that must come away for the following week or 10 days. This process is hastened by mechanical irrigation of the wound. An irrigating can with 1:5,000 potassium permanganate solution and a soft rubber catheter at the tip facilitates this procedure, which should be carried out at least once daily until the wound is clean. The nurse often gives these irrigations. During the procedure it is important to protect the bed with an extra rubber sheet and absorbent pads, and it may be well to time the irrigation so that it can be performed before the patient receives morning care.

Selection of Appropriate Diet

After a liquid diet, the physician usually orders a low-residue diet. It is necessary to begin with a strict diet, but later it can be more liberal as indicated below.

Colostomy Diet No. 1. Used in the hospital while first gaining control and at any time later when loose movements occur.

Breakfast: Large portion of cream of wheat with boiled milk, and sugar if desired; 2 hard-boiled eggs; dry toast; 1 glass of boiled milk
Lunch: Creamed soups (creamed lettuce soup 3 or 4 times a week); creamed fish or meat; baked or mashed potato; boiled rice or custard
Dinner: Meat or fish, creamed whenever possible; escalloped vegetable—no spinach or carrots; soft pudding, custard or junket

Colostomy Diet No. 2. Used after gaining control in the hospital (2 weeks) and continued for 2 months at home.

Cereals—cream of wheat, farina, strained oatmeal, puffed wheat or rice
Eggs—any way except fried
Breads—white, plain or toasted; soda crackers
Soups of all kinds except tomato or corn, not highly seasoned
Potato and Substitutes — baked, mashed, creamed or boiled potato; macaroni; spaghetti; noodles; boiled rice
Meats and Substitutes—roast beef or lamb; broiled steak or lamb chop; oven-baked bacon
    Stewed, creamed, boiled or baked chicken
    Cheese, cottage and cream (white)
    Fish, broiled, baked or creamed
Desserts—Jello, junket, custard, tapioca and cornstarch pudding, plain ice cream, plain cake, sponge and angel cake, plain cookies

Colostomy Diet No. 3. Added to No. 2 after 2 months if control is still effective.

Raw lettuce and celery
Fruits—bananas, canned pears, peaches, apricots, applesauce, baked apple (no skin)
Vegetables—asparagus, beets, green beans, carrots, squash, peas, spinach
Orange juice
AVOID: spices, highly seasoned foods, fried foods, raw fruits and vegetables, gas-forming foods such as onions, turnips, cabbage family, beans, nuts, melons, carbonated drinks, iced-drinks. Also avoid overeating and eating at odd times.

The patient will be able to tell that certain foods interfere with control and these should be eliminated. It becomes an individual matter.

Choice and Care of Suitable Equipment

Early in the postoperative care of the colostomy or ileostomy patient, the use of a plastic stoma bag is effective in preventing skin irritation and reducing offensive odors. Such protection is relatively inexpensive, since the bags are disposable.

Various types of irrigating sets are available. They are made of plastic material and rubber that permit the patient to insert a catheter through a transparent plastic cover directly into the colostomy. When fluid returns, it is directed downward through a tube into a pail or into the commode. This makes it possible for the patient to care for himself at the toilet in the bathroom. The surgeon may recommend equipment to use, or the patient may have an opportunity to examine several kinds and select the type most likely to meet his needs. Commercially made equipment is convenient but not essential. Improvised sets can be made from disposable infusion equipment; the patient can take this home for use there.

Colostomy bags (Fig. 243) may be worn immediately after irrigation; then a change to a simple dressing may be effective. Patients are instructed in the care and the cleaning of equipment to prolong its life and keep it free of odors. Cleaning by soap or a detergent and water and exposing it to fresh air usually is sufficient; however, it may still be necessary to deodorize the appliance; liquid deodorizers are available to use in washing and soaking equipment. The other aspect of the problem is the control of odors arising from the body excreta as they collect in the appliance. Readily soluble deodorizing tablets may be inserted in plastic or rubber bags, or putting a few drops of chlorophyll solution into the bag will help in the control of odors. Powdered charcoal also may be sprinkled into the bag to absorb odors.

As a rule, colostomy bags are not necessary. As soon as the patient has learned a routine for his irrigation, bags may be dispensed with, and a simple dressing of disposable tissue often covered with Saran wrap is held in place by an elastic belt or girdle. Except for the escape of gas and a slight amount of mucus, nothing comes from the colostomy opening between irrigations; therefore, the inconvenience of a colostomy bag is unnecessary.

Hygienic Measures

In general, the patient needs to be reminded that good health practices will aid materially his feeling of well-being and his

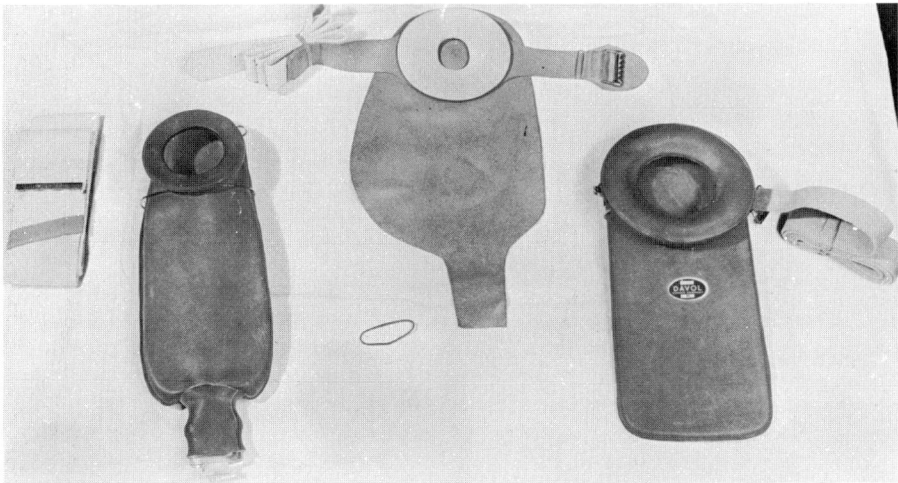

Fig. 243. Various types of bags that collect intestinal secretions. The bags on the left and on the right are the common types of colostomy bags. The bag in the center is the Rutzen type, which is cemented to the skin. This is used when the secretions are more liquid, as in the case of an ileostomy or an ascending colostomy.

positive adjustment to his colostomy. His diet should be adequate and well-balanced; laxatives are never used. Lastly, it is valuable to observe a habit for doing certain activities at a certain time each day, e.g., mealtime, irrigation time, bedtime and so forth.

Skin Care. Soap and water should be used to clean the skin. Dry thoroughly. Consult the physician before trying skin medications.

RECTAL AND ANAL CONDITIONS

Ischiorectal abscess is located in the fatty tissue beside the anus. Usually it is caused by infection from the rectum. Treatment consists of incision and drainage. Packing is inserted, and this demands daily changing. The first dressing of these wounds may be extremely painful; therefore, it is well to protect the edges of wounds with petrolatum gauze and to loosen the packing before removing it, by soaking it with peroxide of hydrogen. These wounds are allowed to heal by granulation. Bowel movements should be formed rather than liquid or soft. Cathartics or mineral oil are not usually used.

Fistula in ano is a tiny tubular tract that has its skin opening beside the anus and goes from there by a tortuous route into the anal canal. Pus is leaking constantly from the cutaneous opening, making it necessary for the patient to wear a protective pad.

Three or 4 hours before operation, the perineum should be shaved and the lower bowel evacuated thoroughly, several warm soapsuds enemas being used. The patient

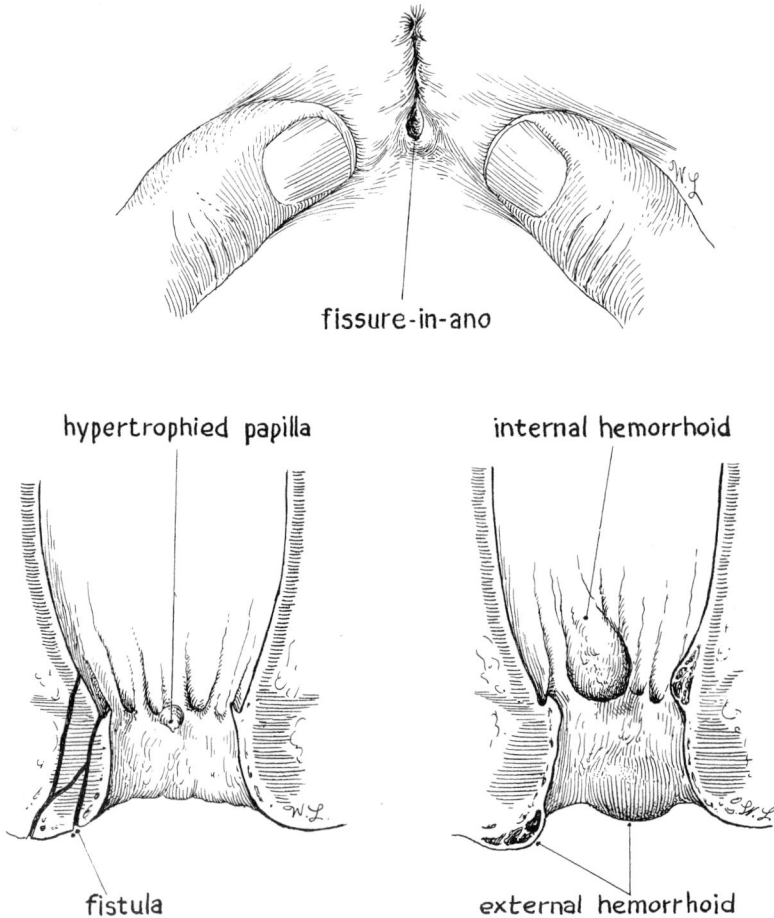

FIG. 244. Various types of anal lesions.

should be allowed to evacuate the enemas on a commode. The last enema should return clear and should be evacuated entirely.

For operation, the patient usually is placed in the lithotomy position, and the sinus tract is identified by inserting a probe into it or by injecting the tract with methylene blue solution. The fistula then may be dissected out or laid open by an incision from its rectal opening to its outlet. The wound is packed with gauze.

Postoperative treatment and complications are the same as those following hemorrhoidectomy (p. 693).

Fissure in ano is a longitudinal ulcer in the anal canal. It is associated frequently with constipation, and its most pronounced symptom is excruciating pain when the bowels move. The same preoperative preparation as for fistula in ano is indicated. Several types of operations may be performed: in some cases the anal sphincter is dilated and the fissure is excised; in others, a part of the external sphincter is divided. This gives a paralysis of the external sphincter with consequent relief of spasm and permits the ulcer to heal. When there is a large overhanging sentinel hemorrhoid, excision of the ulcer and of the hemorrhoid is performed.

Hemorrhoids or *piles* is the name given to masses of skin or mucosa over dilated veins in the anal canal. They occur in two locations. Those occurring above the internal sphincter are called *internal hemor-*

rhoids and those appearing outside the external sphincter *external hemorrhoids.* They cause itching, bleeding at stool and pain. Internal hemorrhoids prolapse frequently through the sphincter and cause considerable discomfort. If the blood within them clots and becomes infected, they grow painful and are said to be *thrombosed.*

The preoperative treatment is that described for fistula in ano.

The operation usually is digital dilatation of the rectal sphincter and removal of the hemorrhoids by the use of a clamp and cautery or by ligation and excision. After completion of the operative procedures, a small rubber tube, often covered with petrolatum gauze, may be inserted through the sphincter to permit the escape of flatus, and also of blood if there should be any hemorrhage. Instead of the rubber tube, some surgeons place pieces of Gelfoam or Oxycel gauze over the anal wounds. Dressings in such cases are held in place by a T-binder.

A **pilonidal cyst** is found in the intergluteal cleft on the posterior surface of the lower sacrum. It is thought by some to be formed by an infolding of epithelial tissue beneath the skin, which may communicate with the skin surface through one or several small sinus openings. Hair frequently is seen protruding from these openings, and this gives the cyst its name—*pilonidal*—a nest of hair. The cysts rarely give symptoms until adolescence or early adult life, when infection produces an irritating drainage or

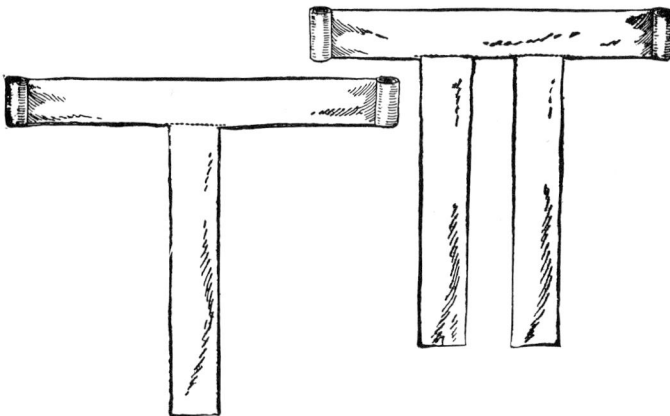

Fig. 245. (*Left*) T-bandage or T-binder. (*Right*) Four-tailed bandage.

an abscess. Trauma appears to play a part in producing the inflammatory reaction in these cysts.

In the early stages of the inflammation, the infection may be controlled by antibiotic therapy. Once an abscess has formed, as in cases of a hair-containing sinus, surgery is indicated. When an abscess is present, incision and drainage are performed. Usually, however, because the abscesses tend to recur or form secondary sinuses that cause irritating drainage, radical excision of the cyst is necessary. In patients with hair-containing sinuses without marked inflammatory reaction, operation is necessary for the same reason. The entire cyst and the secondary sinus tracts are excised. In many cases the resulting defect may be sutured, but in some the defect may be so large that it cannot be closed entirely, and it is allowed to heal by granulation.

The nursing care of these patients presents no problem. In those with abscess, hot moist applications are used frequently. After excision of the cyst, the care is that of any superficial wound. For the first few days, this patient often is more comfortable lying on his abdomen or side with a pillow between his legs. Most patients may be allowed out of bed a few days after operation, and their postoperative care is carried out in the doctor's office.

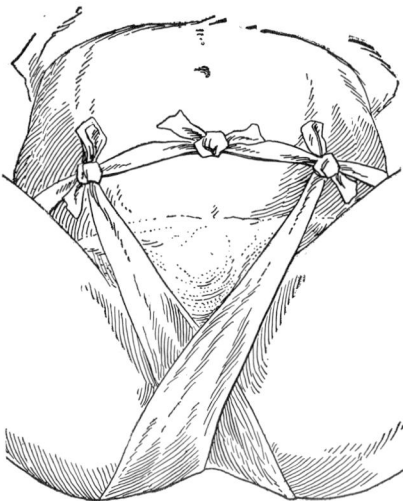

Fig. 246. Modified T-bandage of perineum applied.

Nursing Care in Rectal and Anal Surgery

Unusual finesse is required of the nurse in caring for patients with rectal problems. Such people often are sensitive and embarrassed and need someone on whom they can rely. The effect of emotional upset is seen when such a patient is to have a rectal examination by the doctor. He is not relaxed and cooperative. When the nurse and the physician secure the confidence of the patient, he is helped easily.

Position. The patient may be placed in the dorsal recumbent position with the knees flexed. An effective drape can be made by using a sheet or a bath blanket. A corner of the sheet is used to cover one leg and the opposite corner the other leg. Of the remaining 2 corners, one covers the torso, and the other falls over the perineum and can be lifted easily at the time of the examination. Such draping prevents undue exposure, which is appreciated by the patient (Figs. 280 and 281).

Another comfortable position that is used frequently is Sims's lateral. The upper leg should be flexed sharply and the lower leg flexed less sharply for best positioning. Also, it is most desirable to have the buttocks well over to the side of the bed. The anus may be exposed by folding back a small section of the sheet. The knee-chest position allows the best exposure, but it is not the most comfortable one. The patient rests on his knees and chest with thighs vertical. The arms usually are above the head and give partial support. The patient's head should be turned so that the side of the face rests on the bed. Draping may be done with 2 sheets, 1 for the upper and 1 for the lower part of the body, or with a large sheet with an opening in the center. For any digital rectal examination, the physician needs a rubber glove or a finger cot and lubricant.

Special Care. The perineum is shaved carefully before surgery. This may vary with the nature of the operation. Usually a lower bowel irrigation is ordered, which should be given at least 2 hours prior to surgery. The skin area should be cleaned as thoroughly as possible.

After operation, the nurse should see to it that the perineum is irrigated with warm water after each bowel movement and after each voiding in the case of female patients. Liberal use of analgesics for the first 24 hours may be necessary. Voiding can be a problem; therefore, all methods to encourage voluntary micturition should be tried before resorting to catheterization.

Caution. After hemorrhoidectomy, hemorrhage may occur from the veins that were cut. If a rubber tube has been inserted through the sphincter after operation, evidence of bleeding should be apparent on the dressings. If, however, the patient feels faint, restless and anxious, and the pulse rate increases, the nurse should recognize internal or concealed hemorrhage and give appropriate treatment until the surgeon can be obtained.

After rectal operations, patients usually are allowed out of bed to void, even on the day of operation and may be up and about without difficulty the next day. A foam-rubber ring will increase greatly the patient's sitting comfort.

Pain is relieved greatly in these patients by the application of moist heat. This may be applied in the form of hot compresses or hot sitz baths 3 or 4 times daily and especially after each bowel movement. An ice cap to the head or over the heart will help to prevent the faint feeling experienced by many patients during sitz baths. Mineral oil may be ordered. Some surgeons prefer that a warm oil retention enema be given when the patient feels a desire to defecate; a soapsuds enema given through a catheter may be prescribed if there has been no bowel movement by the 3rd day after operation. The food preferred by the patient is given usually.

Discharge. When it is time for the patient to be discharged from the hospital, he should know how to take sitz baths and how to test the temperature of the water. Sitz baths may be given in a bathtub, which necessitates the application of very warm water 3 or 4 times a day. If this tends to make some post-operative patients weak, sitz baths may be given by employing a bath basin or some large container with enough water to cover the perineum. The patient should be informed about his diet and made aware of the significance of proper eating habits. Also, he ought to know what laxatives he can take safely and why exercise is important. The surgeon usually outlines a schedule in detail to cover the daily routine. This can be reviewed for the patient by the nurse.

CLINICAL SITUATIONS

(Questions 1 to 3 relate to the care of Mr. R. B., a patient on the medical unit, admitted with a diagnosis of peptic ulcer.)

1. Mr. B. was taken to the X-ray Department for roentgenograms of the upper and lower gastrointestinal tract. After a barium series, the nurse should be alert for what complication?
   A. Borborygmus
   B. Impaction
   C. Peritonitis
   D. Melena

2. Mr. B. has been placed on a diet consisting of 3 ounces of milk and cream every hour. The main objective of this diet is to
   A. Aid in tissue repair.
   B. Increase the patient's strength.
   C. Neutralize the gastric acidity.
   D. Control the nausea.

3. The physician left order for Pro-Banthine 30 mg., b.i.d. to be given to Mr. B. The physiologic action of this drug is to
   A. Decrease gastric motility and secretion.
   B. Prevent secondary infection.
   C. Neutralize free hydrochloric acid.
   D. Promote the digestive process.

4. A patient suddenly complains of nausea and pain around the umbilicus radiating to the right lower quadrant. Which of the following actions by the nurse may be indicated?
   A. Heat to localize the infection.
   B. Cold to inhibit the inflammatory process.
   C. Neither heat nor cold, as both may be dangerous.
   D. Alternate heat and cold to stimulate circulation.

5. Which is the most desirable position for a patient with peritonitis?
   A. Supine with knees flexed.
   B. Left lateral.
   C. Trendelenburg.
   D. Fowler's position.

6. The first symptom indicative of a perforation of a duodenal ulcer is
   A. Sudden severe pain in epigastrium.
   B. Projectile vomiting of "coffee-ground" material.
   C. Rectal hemorrhage.
   D. Rigid "boardlike" abdomen.

(Questions 7 to 9 relate to Mrs. S. J., 68, who has been hospitalized with a diagnosis of cancer of the lower bowel.)

7. In cancer of the colon the nurse would expect the patient to complain of
   A. Pain relieved by eating.
   B. Abdominal pain after a fatty meal.
   C. A change in bowel habits.
   D. Vague digestive symptoms.

8. The primary reason for giving neomycin sulfate or sulfasuxidine before colon resection is to
   A. Fight any secondary infection that may be present.
   B. Serve as a urinary antiseptic.
   C. Decrease peristalsis in the large intestines.
   D. Destroy intestinal bacteria.

9. A colostomy was performed on Mrs. J. The most important aspect of nursing after a colostomy is
   A. Psychological reassurance and teaching self-care.
   B. Regulation of diet to form liquid stools.
   C. Keeping the patient well-sedated and relaxed.
   D. Irrigating the perineal wound.

BIBLIOGRAPHY AND SUGGESTED READING

Books

Cecil, R. L., and Loeb, R. F.: Textbook of Medicine, ed. 10, Philadelphia, Saunders, 1959.
Harkins, H. N., *et al.:* Surgery—Principles and Practice, ed. 2, Philadelphia, Lippincott, 1961.

Articles

Stomach and Small Intestines

Bachrach, W. H.: Physiology and pathologic physiology of the stomach, Ciba Sympos. **11**, Jan.-Feb., 1959.
Crohn, B. B.: Current status of therapy in regional ileitis, J.A.M.A. **166:**1479-1480, 1958.
Crow, B.: Bleeding duodenal ulcer, Canad. Nurse **57:**635-639, July, 1961.
Cummins, A. J.: Use and abuse of anticholinergic drugs in the management of gastrointestinal disease, Ann. Intern. Med. **46:**352-358, 1957.
Farris, J. M., and Smith, G. N.: Vagotomy and pyloroplasty, Ann. Surg. **152:**416-429, Sept., 1960.
Gardner, F. H.: Tropical sprue, New Eng. J. Med. **258:**791-796 and 835-842, 1958.
Harridge, W. H.: Treatment for perforated peptic ulcer, Surg. Clin. N. Amer. **41:**37-42, 1961.
Jay, A. N.: Is it indigestion? Am. J. Nurs. **58:**1552-1553, 1958.
Klug, T. J., Ellensohn, J. A., and Zollinger, R. M.: Gastric resection, Am. J. Nurs. **61:**73-76, Dec., 1961.
Landau, E., *et al.:* Partial gastrectomy for duodenal ulcer; comparison of late results in relation to the indication for surgery, New Eng. J. Med. **264:**428-430, 1961.
Magruder, L., and Rauch, M. K.: Nursing care in gastric resection, Am. J. Nurs. **61:**76-77, Dec., 1961.
Mehnert, J. H., *et al.:* A clinical evaluation of postoperative nasal gastric suction, Surg. Gynec. Obstet. **109:**607-612, Nov., 1959.
Woldman, E. E.: Peptic ulcer, Am. J. Nurs. **59:**222-223, 1959.

Appendix

Bonilla, K. B., *et al.:* Experiences with management of the ruptured appendix, Am. J. Surg. **102:**439-443, Sept., 1961.
Palumbo, L. T.: Appendicitis—is it on the wane? Am. J. Surg. **98:**702-703, Nov., 1959.

Colon

Blacketer, L.: Anna, a 12 year old with colitis, Am. J. Nurs. **62:**106-107, Feb., 1962.
Buckwalter, J. A.: Abdomino-perineal resection morbidity, Arch. Surg. **74:**770-779, 1957.
Dericks, V. C.: Rehabilitation of patients with ileostomy, Am. J. Nurs. **61:**48-51, May, 1961.
Hallburg, J. C.: The patient with surgery of the colon, Am. J. Nurs. **61:**64-66, 1961.
Inexpensive colostomy irrigation equipment, Am. J. Nurs. **58:**844, 1958.
Ingles, T., and Campbell, E.: The patient with a colostomy, Am. J. Nurs. **58:**1544-1546, 1958.
Levin, B. G.: For more effective shigellosis control, Am. J. Nurs. **61:**104-108, Nov., 1961.
Machella, T. E.: Problems in ulcerative colitis, Am. J. Med. **13:**760, 1952.

Medical and Surgical Treatment of Ulcerative Colitis, Ciba Sympos. **7,** July-Aug., 1955.

Samp, R. J.: The results of a questionnaire survey of colostomy patients, Surg. Gynec. Obstet. **105:**491-497, 1957.

Sarvajic, J.: Current concepts in the management of ulcerative colitis, Nurs. World **133:** 25-29, June, 1959 and **133:**23-27, July, 1959.

Steigmann, F.: Are laxatives necessary? Am. J. Nurs. **62:**90-93, Oct., 1962.

Wolfman, E. F., Jr., and Flotte, C. T.: Carcinoma of the colon and rectum, Am. J. Nurs. **61:**60-63, March, 1961.

Hernia and Hemorrhoids

Hansen, D. E.: Abdominal hernia, Am. J. Nurs. **61:**102-104, March, 1961.

Holmes, G. W., and Dobrushin, D. J.: Diaphragmatic hernia, Am. J. Nurs. **56:**183-186, 1956.

Rowland, P.: Nursing care in hemorrhoidectomy, Canad. Nurse **55:**123-128, 1959.

Patient-Teaching Aids and Information

Conditions of the Abdomen

Andresen, A. F. R.: Here's What Indigestion Means. An 8-page pamphlet, American Medical Association.

Film: Gastrointestinal Cancer, The Problem of Early Diagnosis (16 mm., sound, color, 33 min.) Available from State Health or State Cancer Society.

Tonkin, R. D.: The Story of Peptic Ulcer, Philadelphia, Saunders, 1957.

What You Should Know About Healing Your Ulcer. A 21-page booklet by members of the staff of New York Hospital-Cornell Medical Center. Available from Wyeth Laboratories, Inc., Radnor, Pa.

Colostomy

Booklet of Instructions for Persons with a Colostomy, The New York Hospital, New York, N. Y.

A Colostomy? A 12-page brochure prepared by the 1955 Nursing Class, Dept. of Nursing, University of Kansas Medical Center (Kansas City, Kans.). This is described by Theresa Hanlon in Am. J. Nursing **54:**1517-1518, 1954.

Care of Your Colostomy. A 19-page source book of information, American Cancer Society.

Chart and pamphlets on colostomy care: United Surgical Supplies Co.

Inexpensive colostomy irrigation equipment, Am. J. Nursing **58:**844, 1958.

Manual for Ileostomy Patients, ed. 3, 1955. A 53-page pamphlet, QT, Inc., Boston.

The C and I Newsletter, published monthly by the Colostomy and Ileostomy Rehabilitation Guild, Inc.

30

Patients With Disorders of the Liver and the Biliary Tract

NORMAL STRUCTURE AND FUNCTION

The liver is a large organ, weighing about 1,500 Gm., or 3 lbs. Most of it is located behind the ribs in the upper right-hand portion of the abdominal cavity (Fig. 247). It is made up of a myriad of small units called *lobules,* each just large enough to be visible with the naked eye and all similar in size, shape and function.

Each lobule has somewhat the shape of a thimble. It is composed of liver cells and vessels (Figs. 248 and 249). Through its center runs a tiny tributary to the hepatic vein, which carries the blood to the heart. Along the periphery of each lobule course 3 or 4 tiny branches of the portal vein, which conducts the blood from the digestive organs to the liver. These portal and hepatic veins are connected by a multitude of small capillaries, and around these the liver cells are arranged. The liver thus is composed of multitudes of cells, and on one side or several sides of each of these a capillary is situated. Through these capillaries flows practically all the blood from the stomach, the intestines, the pancreas and the spleen, so that every bit of nourishment that is absorbed from the gastrointestinal tract into the blood has to come into close contact with these liver cells.

There is another type of cell in the liver, likewise situated close beside the capillaries, namely, Kupffer's cells. These are phagocytic cells and belong to the reticuloendothelial tissue, distributed also in other organs throughout the body, especially in the spleen, the bone marrow and the lymph nodes. The function of these Kupffer cells appears to be in part the engulfing of particulate matter in the blood, including defective or old red blood cells ready to be retired from circulation. The hemoglobin from the red cells is split chemically; its iron-containing fraction is conserved for the formation of more hemoglobin, and the rest is converted into bile pigment.

Within the liver cells start tiny bile ducts, or canaliculi, which unite between the rows of liver cells to form larger ducts comparable in size with blood capillaries. These in turn unite and course along between the liver lobules, forming still larger ducts which eventually lead into the large hepatic duct, a tube about 2 inches in length and ¼ inch in diameter. Beneath the liver is the gallbladder, a pouch that can hold from 30 to 50 ml. of bile. Connected to the gallbladder is a duct, called the *cystic duct,* which is about ½ inch in length and ⅛ inch in diameter. The hepatic duct and the cystic duct unite to form the common bile duct, a tube about 3 inches long and about ¼ inch in diameter, which terminates in the duodenum. The hepatic duct; its continuation, the common bile duct; its offshoot, the cystic duct; and the gallbladder all together comprise what is referred to as the biliary tract (Fig. 253).

The functions of the liver are numerous and varied. This organ receives via the portal vein all the blood returning from the gastrointestinal tract—blood which carries all the products of carbohydrate and protein digestion. The digested carbohydrate arrives in the liver in the form of glucose. Here it is converted into glycogen, or animal starch, and is stored (glycogenesis) as such. From this storage depot of glycogen a constant supply of carbohydrate is released into the blood stream (glycogenolysis)—again in the form of glucose—the rate of its release varying according to the changing body requirements. Most of it eventually will serve as body fuel, being metabolized in the tissues to provide heat and energy; some is transformed again into glycogen and stored in the muscle tissues; the rest is converted into fat and stored by special cells (fat cells) located chiefly in the subcutaneous tissues and within the abdominal cavity. The liver also is capable of manufacturing glucose from non-carbohydrate sources, such as proteins, fats and lactates (glucogenesis), so that the body is not solely dependent on food as a source of this substance.

The liver likewise plays an important role in protein metabolism. Here the amino acids derived from foods lose their amine groups and are incorporated into new proteins. Among these are many of the plasma proteins, including fibrinogen, prothrombin, the prothrombin accelerators and albumin. Just as in the case of carbohydrate, a certain amount of protein is stored in utilizable form in the liver, to be available as required. Moreover, it is in the liver that certain poi-

sonous nitrogenous by-products of protein digestion and metabolism are converted into nontoxic substances. For example, ammonia bodies are returned to the blood from the liver as urea, which is not poisonous; the urea is cleared from the blood stream by the kidneys, which excrete it into the urine.

The liver plays a key role in the metabolism of fatty acids as well as ketone bodies. It prepares for the body, stores for it and supplies it with numerous other essential substances via the blood stream. One such material is necessary for the normal development of the immature red blood cell in the bone marrow. This substance is vitamin B_{12} (cyanocobalamine), and its deficiency leads to the development of pernicious anemia (p. 463). The liver is concerned in the manufacture and the storage of other vitamins, including vitamins A and D, as well as many components of the B complex. Certain metals, such as iron and copper, are stored in the liver. It is also one site of formation of the specific immune antibodies which protect the body from infectious agents and their toxins.

The liver secretes glucose, urea, maturation factor, vitamins, etc., into the blood

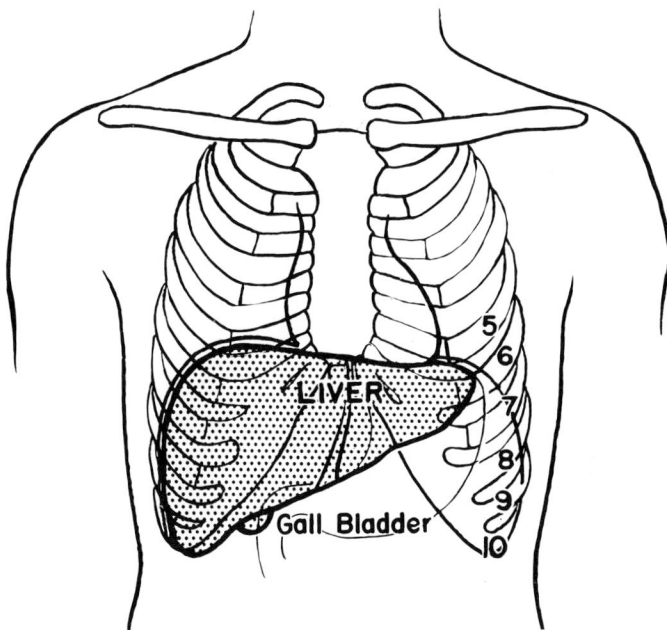

FIG. 247. Outline of the liver, anterior view.

stream. They are collected from the liver cells into the adjacent blood capillaries, which, in the center of each liver lobule, connect with a branch of the hepatic vein. This drains into the inferior vena cava, which conducts the blood directly to the heart. Hence they arrive in the general cir-culation and are available to all the body tissues. This mode of secretion by an organ —namely, into the blood—is termed *internal secretion.*

In addition to being an organ of internal secretion, the liver is also an excretory organ, its excretory product being the bile. Bile formation by the liver is taking place constantly. Its excretion into the gastrointestinal tract is not continuous, however, but intermittent. Between meals most of the bile produced by the liver is diverted into the gallbladder, where a large proportion of its water is absorbed, the final solution being from 5 to 10 times more concentrated than that originally secreted by the liver. Following a period of fasting, as soon as fatty food passes through the pylorus from the stomach, the gallbladder empties this reserve of concentrated bile through the cystic duct, via the common bile duct, into the duodenum (Fig. 253).

The function of bile as a digestive fluid already has been described. Its role in intestinal digestion is to aid in the enzymatic transformation of fats into soluble soaps by causing them to emulsify, that is, break up into a suspension of very small globules

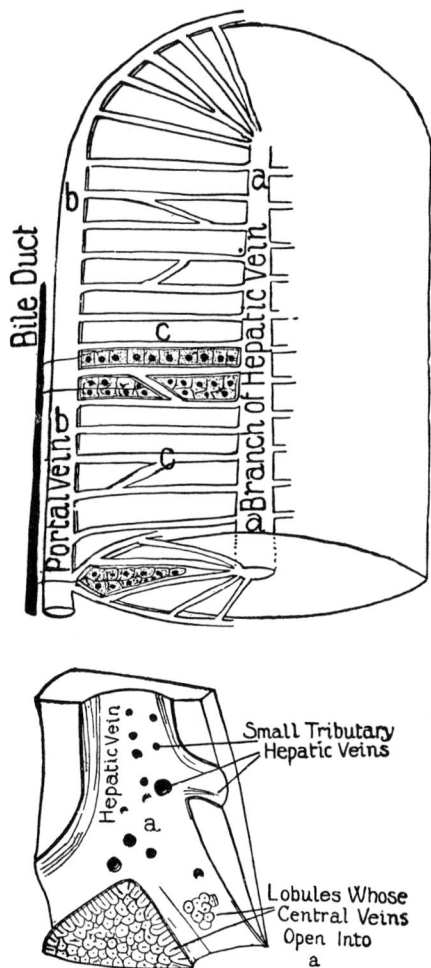

FIG. 248. (*Top*) A small fragment of liver, very slightly magnified. The cut was made along a small hepatic vein. In the lower portion the lobules are represented. (*Bottom*) One liver lobule, in vertical section. The blood flows from *b,* a branch of the portal vein, through the capillaries, *c,* to *a,* a branch of the hepatic vein. While in the capillaries it comes in contact with the liver cells. From these cells start the bile capillaries which flow to the bile duct.

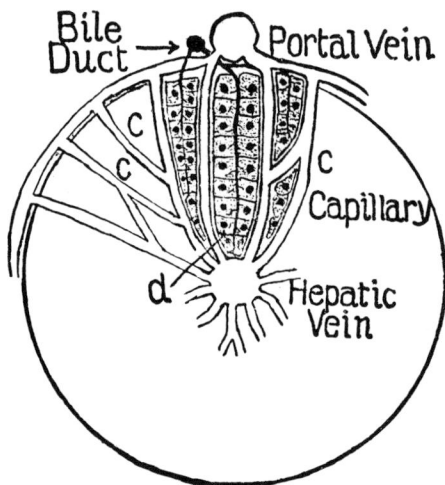

FIG. 249. One liver lobule in cross section. The blood flows from the branch of the portal vein through the capillaries (c) to the branch of the hepatic vein. While in the capillaries it comes in contact with the liver cells (d). In these cells arise the tiny bile capillaries which empty into the bile duct.

which are more readily attacked by the fat-splitting enzymes in the intestinal fluid.

Bile also serves as a vehicle for the removal of various substances which the liver cells clear from the blood, including bilirubin and urobilinogen.

Bilirubin is a pigment derived from hemoglobin. A by-product of hemolysis, this pigment constantly is being formed and introduced into the blood stream by histiocytic cells engaged in the phagocytosis of outworn or defective erythrocytes. Attached to albumin, bilirubin circulates in the plasma until it comes in contact with a liver cell which promptly absorbs it, separates it from its albumin attachment, conjugates it with glycuronic acid and secretes it, along with other bile constituents, into the adjacent bile canaliculus. Thence, via a succession of communicating channels within the liver and the hepatic ducts outside the liver, the bilirubin glucuronide escapes through the common bile duct into the duodenum. Subsequently, while in transit through the intestines, this pigment becomes converted into urobilinogen and most of it makes a direct exit from the body as fecal urobilinogen. However, some urobilinogen is absorbed through the intestinal mucosa into the blood; of this, a portion is excreted by the kidneys as urine urobilinogen, while the remainder is secreted by the liver cells into the bile and returns once again to the gastrointestinal tract.

THE JAUNDICED PATIENT

When for any reason the bilirubin concentration in the blood becomes abnormally increased, all the body tissues, including the sclerae and the skin, become tinged with a yellow or a greenish-yellow color. This condition is called *jaundice*. There are three types of jaundice: (1) hemolytic jaundice, which is attributable to an abnormally high concentration of bilirubin in the blood, the amount exceeding the capacity of normal liver cells to excrete it; (2) hepatocellular jaundice, due to the inability of diseased liver cells to clear normal amounts of bilirubin from the blood; and (3) obstructive jaundice, caused by an impeded or interrupted flow of bile through the external ducts draining the liver (extrahepatic obstruction) or through their radicles within the liver parenchyma (intrahepatic obstruction).

Hemolytic jaundice is the result of an abnormally great destruction of the red blood cells, the effect of which is to flood the plasma with bilirubin so rapidly that the liver, although functioning perfectly normally, cannot excrete this pigment as rapidly as it is formed. This is the type of jaundice that is encountered in patients with hereditary spherocytosis (p. 467), autoimmune hemolytic anemia (p. 466), erythroblastosis fetalis, hemolytic transfusion reactions (p. 182) and other hemolytic disorders. The bilirubin in the blood of these patients is of the unconjugated or "free" type. Fecal and urine urobilinogen are increased; on the other hand, their urine is free of bilirubin. Patients with this type of jaundice, unless their hyperbilirubinemia is extreme, do not experience symptoms or complications as a result of the jaundice *per se*. However, very prolonged jaundice, even if mild, predisposes to the formation of "pigment stones" in the gallbladder, and extremely severe jaundice—e.g., in patients with levels of free bilirubin above 20 to 25 mg. per cent—is attended by a definite risk of serious brain-stem damage, as exemplified by the kernicterus of severe, untreated hemolytic disease of the newborn (p. 466).

Hepatocellular jaundice is always the result of a diffuse, widespread (although not necessarily serious) liver impairment, and it reflects the failure of the liver cells to clear bilirubin from the blood in normal fashion. This type of jaundice in very mild form is a common finding in normal infants at birth and for a day or two postpartum, or until the liver of the newly born has acquired the ability to conjugate bilirubin and excrete it at the requisite pace.

Hepatocellular jaundice of lifelong duration occurs as one manifestation of liver dysfunction in the so-called "Dubin Johnson syndrome," which is based on an inborn error of metabolism affecting liver cells; other features of the syndrome include abdominal pain, weakness, nausea and vomiting, and various alterations in blood chemistry. Another disorder marked by lifelong jaundice of a similar type is Gilbert's disease, which is due, not to liver cell dysfunction, but to the congenital absence of a substance (transferin) required to transport plasma bilirubin within the liver cells where it can be conjugated. These patients, despite blood bilirubin levels of as high as 5 mg. per cent, are otherwise normal and generally remain in good health.

Not only hepatocellular jaundice but other and often considerably more profound derangements of liver function are encountered in patients with epidemic hepatitis (p. 653), homologous serum jaundice (p. 654), hepatic cirrhosis (p. 655) and hepatic toxicity. For example, such dysfunction has followed the administration of certain drugs, including cinchophen and others. Extremely serious—indeed, often lethal—liver damage regularly is associated with arsenic, phosphorus and carbon tetrachloride poisoning.

Patients with hepatocellular jaundice are clinically ill, depending on the extent to which their liver function is disturbed; this may be very little, or it may be profound. As for laboratory manifestations, both free and conjugated bilirubin are likely to be increased in the blood, for an element of intrahepatic obstruction usually is present as well as faulty clearance of bilirubin by the sick liver cells. Urine urobilinogen is apt to be increased, and fecal urobilinogen, decreased. The urine is prone to be dark and foamy owing to the presence of bilirubin, and the stools are light or clay-colored, owing to its absence.

Obstructive jaundice of the extrahepatic type may be caused by plugging of the bile duct by a gallstone (Fig. 253), by an inflammatory process, by a tumor, or by an enlarged gland pressing on it. Or the obstruction may involve the small bile ducts within the liver substance (i.e., intrahepatic obstruction), caused, for example, by pressure on these channels from inflammatory swelling of the liver substance or by an inflammatory exudate within the ducts themselves. Intrahepatic obstruction due to stasis and inspissation of bile within the canaliculi is an occasional occurrence following the ingestion of certain drugs, which accordingly are referred to as "cholestatic" agents. These include phenothiazine (e.g., Sparine, Trilafon, etc.); phenothiazine derivatives (e.g., Thorazine); sulfonamide drugs; tolbutamide (Orinase) and other antidia-

betic drugs; arsphenamine; thiouracil; and p-aminobenzoic acid (PAB). Whether the obstruction is intrahepatic or extrahepatic, and whatever its cause may be, if bile cannot flow normally into the intestine, but is dammed back in the liver substance, it is reabsorbed into the blood and there carried over the entire body, staining the skin and the sclerae; it is excreted in the urine, which becomes a deep orange color and foamy in appearance. Because of the decreased amount of bile in the intestinal tract, the stools become white or clay-colored. The skin may itch intensely, requiring repeated starch baths and oil inunctions. Dyspepsia, and especially an intolerance to fatty foods, may develop temporarily, due to impairment of fat digestion in the absence of intestinal bile.

SPECIAL PROBLEMS OF PATIENTS WITH DISORDERS OF THE LIVER

The complications of liver disease are numerous and varied. In many instances their ultimate effects are incapacitating or lethal; their advent is ominous, and their treatment is notoriously difficult. Among the most important of these complications are severe gastrointestinal hemorrhages and excessive water retention with ascites and edema, the result of circulatory changes within the diseased liver leading to portal hypertension; impairment of the central and peripheral nervous systems and abnormal bleeding tendencies, attributable to the inability of malfunctioning liver cells to metabolize certain vitamins; and hepatic coma, reflecting the incomplete metabolism of protein fragments by the diseased liver.

Portal Hypertension

One set of problems, largely limited to patients with hepatic cirrhosis, arises as a result of obstruction to the flow of portal venous blood through the liver, the effect of which is to elevate the blood pressure throughout the entire portal venous system. Portal hypertension accounts for the formation of esophageal, gastric and hemorrhoidal varicosities, which are prone to rupture and often are the source of massive hemorrhages from the upper gastrointestinal tract and the rectum, as described on page 656. Portal

LIVER BIOPSY AND THE ROLE OF THE NURSE

There are many types of jaundice, and for each there are many possible causes. To distinguish one form from another and to discover its cause is often impossible solely on the basis of the clinical examination plus a battery of liver function, hematologic and other routine laboratory tests. A procedure that often is very helpful in such cases, and one that facilitates greatly the diagnosis of most hepatic disorders, is the liver biopsy, i.e., the sampling of liver tissue by needle aspiration for purposes of histologic study. The responsibilities of the nurse in relation to liver biopsy and the rationale of her participation in this procedure are summarized below:

NURSING ACTIVITIES

RATIONALE

Ascertain in advance that hemostasis tests have been requisitioned, completed and reported, and that compatible donor blood is available.

Many patients with liver disease have clotting defects and are abnormally prone to bleed.

Measure and record the patient's pulse, respirations and arterial pressure immediately prior to biopsy.

Prebiopsy values provide a basis on which to compare his vital signs and evaluate his status following the procedure.

Describe to the patient in advance:
1. Steps contemplated
2. Sensations expected
3. After-effects anticipated
4. Restrictions of activity to be imposed afterward

Explanations serve to allay his fears, to ensure his cooperation and to reinforce his instruction.

Give support to the patient during the procedure.

The proximity of an understanding nurse enhances comfort and promotes a sense of security.

Expose the right side of the patient's abdomen.

The skin at the site of penetration will be disinfected and infiltrated with local anesthetic.

Instruct the patient to inhale and exhale deeply several times, finally to exhale and to hold his breath at the end of expiration.

Holding the breath immobilizes the chest wall and the diaphragm; penetration of the diaphragm thereby is avoided, and the risk of lacerating the liver is minimized.

The physician promptly introduces the biopsy needle via the transthoracic (intercostal) or transabdominal (subcostal) route, penetrates the liver, aspirates and withdraws. The entire procedure is completed within 5 to 10 seconds.

Breathing may now resume.

Immediately following the biopsy, assist the patient to turn on his right side, place a pillow under his costal margin and caution him to remain in this position, recumbent and immobile, for several hours.

In this position the liver capsule at the site of penetration is compressed against the chest wall, and the escape of blood or bile through the perforation is impeded.

LIVER BIOPSY AND THE ROLE OF THE NURSE (Continued)

NURSING ACTIVITIES	RATIONALE
Measure and record the patient's pulse and respiratory rates and his arterial pressure at 10- to 20-minute intervals for the prescribed period of time, or until his status proves to be stable, and his condition has been pronounced to be satisfactory. Be alert to detect and to report promptly any increase in pulse rate or any decrease in arterial pressure, any complaint of pain or manifestations of apprehension.	These signs may indicate the presence and the progress of hepatic bleeding or bile peritonitis, the most frequent complications of liver biopsy.

hypertension accounts also for the large accumulations of fluid (ascites) in the abdominal cavity that are characteristic of patients with cirrhosis. As ascites forms, the volume of extracellular fluid throughout the body shrinks; in response to this shrinkage, the adrenal glands are stimulated to secrete increased quantities of the hormone aldosterone, which in turn causes the kidneys to retain sodium and water to excess and is responsible for the generalized edema of cirrhosis. The management of gastrointestinal hemorrhage, ascites and edema in patients with liver disease and portal hypertension will be discussed later in this chapter.

Avitaminoses

A second group of complications that are common to patients with severe chronic liver disease of all types is caused by failure of damaged liver cells to make certain vitamins available in an active form to the body. Among the specific deficiency states that occur on this basis are vitamin A deficiency (p. 151); beriberi (p. 152), polyneuritis (p. 152) and Wernicke-Korsakoff psychosis, all attributable to a deficiency of thiamine; skin and mucous membrane lesions characteristic of riboflavin deficiency (p. 152); "rum fits," which probably are due to pyridoxine deficiency; hypoprothrombinemia (p. 478), characterized by spontaneous bleeding and ecchymoses, due to vitamin K deficiency; the hemorrhagic lesions of scurvy (p. 153), i.e., vitamin C deficiency; and the macrocytic anemia of folic acid deficiency (pp. 152, 466). The threat of these avita-

minoses provides the rationale for supplementing the diet of every patient with chronic liver disease with ample quantities of vitamins A, B complex, C and K.

Hepatic Coma

Hepatic coma, one of the dreaded complications of liver disease and a manifestation of profound liver failure, in essence is ammonia intoxication. Its principal manifestations are those of brain dysfunction and damage. It is caused by failure of the liver cells to detoxify (by converting to urea) the ammonia that constantly is entering the blood stream as a result of its absorption from the gastrointestinal tract, its production by metabolizing kidney tissue, and its liberation from contracting muscle cells.

Clinical Features. The earliest symptoms of hepatic coma, i.e., the manifestations of impending coma, include minor mental aberrations and motor disturbances. The patient appears to be slightly confused; he becomes untidy; there is a faraway look in his eye; he tends to drowse during the day and to wander at night; and he may exhibit a coarse, or "flapping" tremor, especially of the hands. In a more advanced stage there are gross disturbances of consciousness, and the patient is completely disoriented with respect to time and place. With further progression of the disorder he lapses into frank coma and is likely to succumb.

Aggravating and Precipitating Factors. As indicated above, the major—and probably the key—factor in the pathogenesis of liver coma is the accumulation of ammonia in the blood. The largest source of blood ammonia is the enzymatic and bacterial digestion of proteins (including dietary and blood proteins) in the gastrointestinal tract. Ammonia from this source is *increased* as a result of gastrointestinal bleeding; a high protein diet; the ingestion of ammonium salts (e.g., ammonium chloride, prescribed as a diuretic); bacterial growth in the small bowel; and uremia. On the other hand, gastrointestinal ammonia is *decreased* by elimination of protein from the diet and by the administration of bowel sterilizing antibiotics, such as neomycin sulfate, kanamycin sulfate and chlortetracycline.

Ammonia is supplied also by the kidneys as they carry out the deamination of various amino acids. Ammonia from the kidney is *increased* following the administration of diuretics, such as chlorothiazide, and steroid drugs; following the restriction of dietary sodium; and in patients with potassium depletion. Ammonia from muscle tissue is *increased* during exercise.

As might be anticipated in part from the foregoing comments, liver coma may be induced in susceptible patients as a consequence of any of the following: gastrointestinal bleeding; any infection, especially an enteric infection; a surgical procedure; any acute disturbance in water and electrolyte balance, especially hyponatremia (sodium depletion), hypokalemia (potassium depletion) and water intoxication; the administration of diuretic agents, such as acetazolamide (Diamox) or chlorothiazide (Diuril); the ingestion (or injection) of ammonium salts; and protein feedings.

Nursing Management. The patient with impending hepatic coma should be observed several times each day from the standpoint of his neurologic status. A daily record should be kept of his handwriting and his performance in arithmetic. His fluid intake and output and, if feasible, his body weight should be charted each day. His vital signs should be measured and recorded every 4 hours. Evidences suggesting pulmonary or other infection should be sought frequently and carefully, and reported promptly, if observed.

If it becomes apparent that liver coma is indeed impending, the patient's protein intake will be reduced sharply, or eliminated altogether for the time being, and an antibiotic drug will be prescribed for sterilization of the bowel (e.g., chlortetracycline, neomycin sulfate or kanamycin sulfate, 6 to 8 Gm. orally on the 1st day and 4 Gm. daily thereafter). Sedative and analgesic drugs, if prescribed at all, will be administered to this patient in very conservative doses and under very close observation.

VIRAL HEPATITIS

Epidemic Hepatitis

Sometimes referred to as catarrhal jaundice, this is an infectious disease of the liver cells caused by an ultramicroscopic virus. The mode of its transmission is probably through the ingestion of foods or liquids infected by the virus, although a respiratory mode of transmission has not been excluded. As is the case in homologous serum jaundice (p. 654), the infection can be acquired as a result of an inoculation, e.g., a blood transfusion. The incubation period is estimated to be between 3 and 4 weeks.

The course of the illness is prolonged, lasting from 4 to 8 weeks, and is characterized chiefly by jaundice, which at its peak may be intense. Symptoms of a mild upper respiratory infection, with low-grade fever, may be present for a few days at the onset, even before the jaundice becomes apparent. Indigestion is present to a varying degree, marked by vague epigastric distress, anorexia, nausea, heartburn and flatulence. These symptoms tend to clear as soon as the jaundice reaches its peak—perhaps 10 days after its original appearance. The liver and the spleen are often moderately enlarged for a few days after the onset; otherwise, apart from the jaundice, there are few physical signs to be elicited.

Treatment and Nursing Care. Bed rest during the acute stage and the provision of a diet that is both acceptable and nutritious are part of the treatment and nursing care. During the period of anorexia the patient should receive frequent small feedings, supplemented, as needed, by intravenous infusions of glucose. As soon as his appetite is restored, he should be placed on a diet which provides approximately 3,000 calories and about 150 Gm. each of protein and fat. He should be well hydrated, receiving much of his fluid in the form of sweetened fruit juices.

Prognosis. Recovery from epidemic hepatitis is the rule; a rare case progresses to an acute liver necrosis (acute yellow atrophy), terminating in cirrhosis of the liver or even death.

Prevention. Epidemic hepatitis can be prevented by the administration of gamma globulin given intramuscularly in a dose of 0.01 ml. per pound of body weight during the period of incubation if this treatment is instituted within a period of a few days following exposure.

Homologous Serum Jaundice

This disease, the importance of which was recognized during World War II, occasionally follows the therapeutic or prophylactic injection of materials containing human serum, such as convalescent serum, certain vaccines and whole blood or plasma. Clinically, the disease closely resembles epidemic hepatitis. However, the incubation period is relatively much longer: between 2 and 6 months. The mortality is appreciable, ranging from 0.1 to 10 per cent, depending on the infective dose and the condition of the patient.

Symptoms and signs include, in addition to jaundice, dyspepsia, abdominal pain, generalized aching, malaise and weakness. The liver usually is enlarged, and splenomegaly is common. In contrast with epidemic hepatitis, respiratory symptoms are minimal or absent, and the occurrence of fever is rare.

Treatment and Nursing Care. It is important that bed rest be continued until the progress of the hepatitis has definitely subsided, and, subsequently, the patient should be restricted in his activities until the hepatic enlargement and the elevation of serum bilirubin have disappeared. Adequate nutrition should be maintained and supplemental nutrients provided by the administration of ample quantities of vitamin B complex, carbohydrates and proteins. Other therapeutic measures employed to control the dyspeptic symptoms and general malaise include the use of salicylates, alkalies, belladonna and mild barbiturate soporifics.

Convalescence may be prolonged, complete symptomatic recovery sometimes requiring as long as from 3 to 4 months. During this stage, gradual restoration of physical activity is permitted and encouraged following complete clearing of the jaundice.

Preventive. Individuals receiving infected blood or blood derivatives are protected from homologous serum jaundice by the concomitant injection of gamma globulin. However, infective blood donors cannot be identified with certainty, and supplies of gamma globulin are far from sufficient to permit its routine use in conjunction with every transfusion. The use of disposable syringes, needles and lancets reduces the risk of spreading this infection from one patient to another in the process of collecting blood samples or administering parenteral therapy.

TOXIC HEPATITIS

There are several chemicals which are liver poisons, producing, when taken by mouth or injected parenterally, acute liver cell necrosis or toxic hepatitis. The chemicals most commonly implicated in this disease are arsenic, chloroform, carbon tetrachloride, phosphorus and gold compounds.

The milder cases of toxic hepatitis closely resemble those of epidemic hepatitis, being quite comparable in symptoms, signs and course. However, a considerable proportion of cases unfortunately progress to the stage of acute liver necrosis or acute yellow atrophy. Within a few days the jaundice becomes extremely intense. The fever mounts; the patient becomes deeply toxic and prostrated. Vomiting may be persistent, the vomitus containing blood. Hemorrhages appear under the skin. Delirium, coma and convulsions develop, and within a few days the patient usually dies.

There is little to be done in the line of treatment, except to provide comfort, supply repeated blood transfusions and intravenous glucose and saline solutions. A few patients recover, only to develop cirrhosis.

LIVER ABSCESSES

The liver is a sieve through which flows all the blood returning from the gastrointestinal tract. Whenever an abscess develops anywhere along this tract, there is danger that an infected embolus will be transported

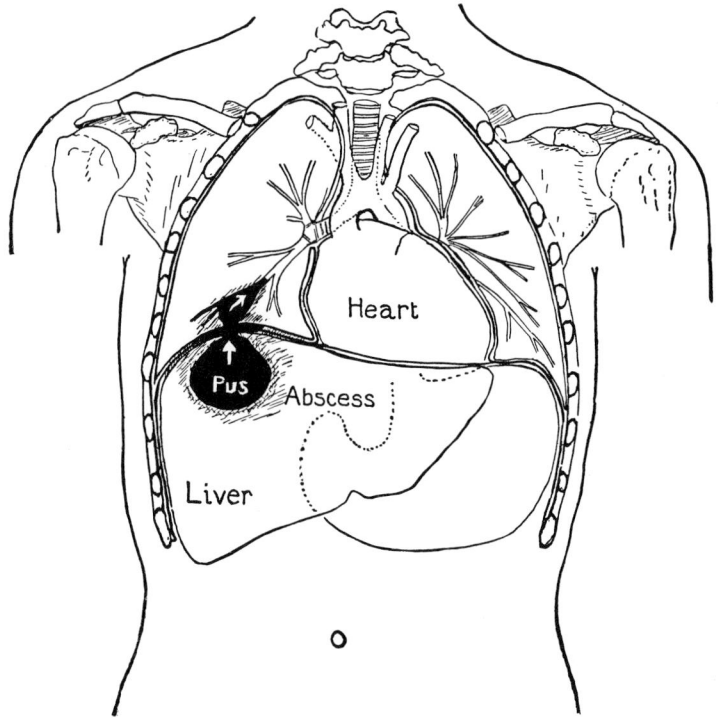

FIG. 250. Diagram of an abscess of the liver perforating through the lung into a bronchus. The preceding inflammation will have obliterated the peritoneal and the pleural cavities in the path of the abscess.

via the portal venous system to the liver, and that secondary abscess formation will take place in that organ. Moreover, in patients with bacteremia, organisms may be carried via the hepatic artery to the liver and lodge there. Most bacteria promptly are engulfed and destroyed, but occasionally some gain a foothold and multiply. The bacterial toxins destroy the neighboring liver cells, and the necrotic tissue produced serves as a protective wall for the organisms. Meanwhile, leukocytes migrate into the infected area. The result is an abscess cavity full of a liquid containing living and dead leukocytes, liquefied liver cells and bacteria (Fig. 250). Pyogenic abscesses of this type are usually multiple and small. The liver may be fairly honeycombed by them. The result is an extremely serious disease, manifested by high fever, chills alternating with sweats, jaundice, painful enlargement of the liver, anemia, toxemia and eventual death. Specific chemotherapy will be given in such cases, depending on the identity of the infective agent, as described in Chapter 13.

Liver abscesses may be due to several kinds of bacteria and to a fungus (actinomy-cosis). The commonest agent, however, is a protozoan, *Entamoeba histolytica,* one of the most important causes of dysentery.

HEPATIC CIRRHOSIS

Portal Cirrhosis

Portal cirrhosis is a disease characterized by episodes of necrosis involving the liver cells, sometimes occurring repeatedly throughout the course of the disease. The destroyed liver cells are replaced by scar tissue, the amount of which in time may exceed that of the functioning liver tissue. The disease usually has a particularly insidious onset and a very protracted course, occasionally proceeding over a period of 30 or more years.

The basic mechanism responsible for the development of cirrhosis is yet to be described. It occurs with greatest frequency among alcoholics. However, many explain the role of alcohol in the production of cirrhosis on the basis of nutritional deficiency with reduced protein intake rather than on alcohol toxicity, and certainly some cases are observed among the abstemious.

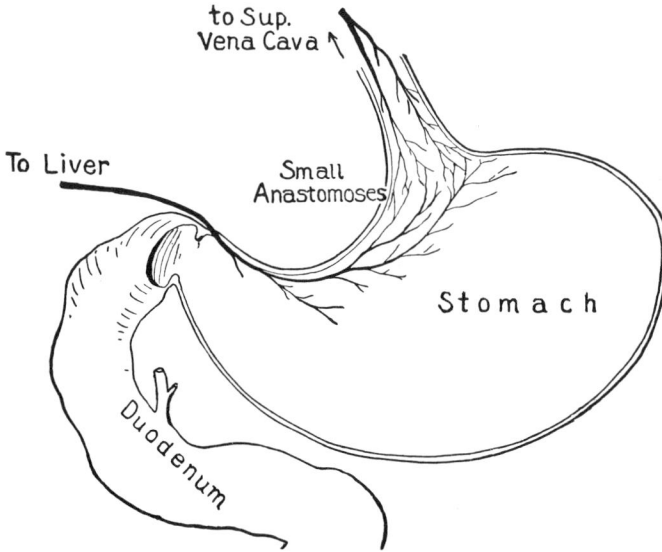

FIG. 251. Diagram of the stomach, showing the venous circulation at the lesser curvature. It will be seen that the blood in the veins of the esophagus flows upward and empties into the superior vena cava without flowing through the liver, and that the blood in the veins of the lesser curvature of the stomach flows toward the pylorus and then through the liver. These two sets of veins are united by fine anastomoses.

The liver early in the disease is apt to be large, its cells loaded with fat; later, as the replacing scar tissue contracts, it becomes small. Also, its surface often becomes rough, because the scar tissue within it is disposed in coarse bundles, which by contracting pull in the capsule at certain points and cause the islands of residual normal tissue and of new regenerating liver tissue to project in little lumps. Hence arose the term *hobnail liver.*

Symptoms. The early symptoms of cirrhosis, associated with a temporarily acute hepatitis, include anorexia, nausea, vomiting, jaundice and fever. These symptoms may clear up in the course of days or weeks, not to reappear for many years; or they may recur frequently, and eventually with the addition of others characteristic of the later stages of the disease.

The late symptoms are due partly to chronic failure of liver function and partly to obstruction of the portal circulation. Practically all the blood from the digestive organs is collected in the portal veins and carried to the liver. Since these cirrhotic livers do not allow it free passage, it is dammed back into the spleen and the gastrointestinal tract, with the result that these organs become the seat of chronic passive congestion; that is, they are stagnant with blood and so cannot function properly. Such patients are apt to have chronic dyspepsia and changes in bowel habit, with constipation or diarrhea. There is a gradual weight loss. The spleen becomes congested (Banti's syndrome). Fluid may accumulate in the peritoneal cavity (ascites), in which event a dehydration regimen is instituted. This involves the reduction of sodium intake to approximately 200 mg. daily; restriction of fluids, if the serum sodium is low; administration of an oral diuretic drug, such as Hydrodiuril, and possibly injections of a mercurial diuretic, such as Mercuhydrin. Spironolactone (Aldactone), an aldosterone-blocking agent, also may be supplied to reinforce the action of these diuretics. Occasionally, it is necessary to resort to abdominal paracentesis (see p. 658).

At certain points in the abdomen the portal circulation anastomoses with the general circulation, and through these channels some portal blood can flow to the heart without first passing through the liver (Fig. 251). One of the points of collateral circulation is at the cardiac orifice of the stomach. The blood from the esophagus flows directly to the heart; that from the stomach flows to the liver. Veins always anastomose, so that blood here can choose between these two routes. When there is obstruction to the portal circulation, as in cirrhosis, portal hypertension develops, and, because of its increased pressure, a portion of the blood in the gastric veins escapes through the

FIG. 252. Diagram of the stomach, showing the venous circulation of the lesser circulation of the lesser curvature in a severe case of cirrhosis of the liver. The current of blood now will flow toward the esophagus, and the fine anastomoses will be distended into varices. These have thin walls and rupture, causing profuse hemorrhages into the stomach.

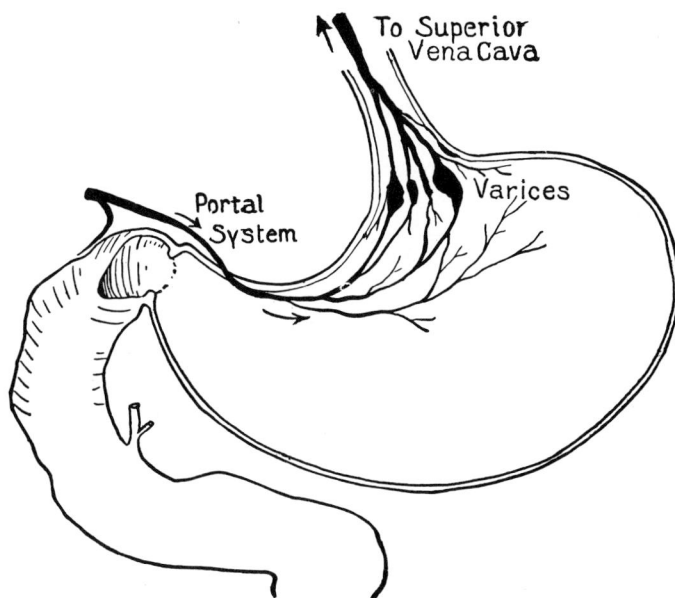

esophageal veins. Unfortunately, however, these veins become distended, forming esophageal varices, the thin walls of which often rupture (Fig. 252). Thus, about 25 per cent of patients with cirrhosis experience small hematemeses, while some have profuse hemorrhages from the stomach.

Within the lower rectum there is a point at which the portal and the general circulations meet. In cirrhosis of the liver, venous varices form here, also. These are known as hemorrhoids. These, too, may rupture and cause severe hemorrhages. Of course, hemorrhoids are common, but in the majority of cases they are due to simple constipation. They involve the external hemorrhoidal veins (external hemorrhoids), which usually thrombose before they bleed. However, in cirrhosis it is the internal hemorrhoidal veins which dilate. Blood is less apt to clot in them, so that when they rupture they bleed severely.

Other late symptoms of cirrhosis are attributable to chronic failure of liver function. The concentration of plasma albumin is lowered, predisposing to the formation of edema. Because of inadequate formation, utilization and storage of certain vitamins, notably vitamins A, C and K, signs of their deficiency frequently are encountered—particularly hemorrhagic phenomena associated with vitamin K deficiency. Chronic gastritis

and poor gastrointestinal function, together with the factors of poor diet and impaired liver function, account for a deficiency type of anemia likewise often associated with this disease.

Therefore, the chief signs of portal cirrhosis are fever, jaundice, gastrointestinal disturbances and enlargement of the liver in the early stages. Later in the disease this organ becomes smaller and nodular, the spleen enlarges, ascites appears, jaundice recurs, distended veins develop at the anastomotic points described above, and spider telangiectases (dilated superficial arterioles resembling little bluish-red spiders) appear in the skin of the face and the trunk. As the case progresses, edema, anemia, purpura and signs of polyvitaminosis are likely to appear. The patient may die in liver failure, experiencing increasing weakness, wasting and depression and finally delirium, coma and convulsions.

Treatment and Nursing Care. The cirrhotic patient who has no ascites or edema and exhibits no signs of impending coma should receive a normal, adequate diet supplemented by vitamins of the B complex and others, as indicated (including vitamins A, C and K). Patients with prolonged or severe anorexia, or those who are vomiting or eating poorly for any reason, can be fed by tube with milk and enough added starch hydrolysate (e.g., Dextri-Maltose, Dexin, etc.) to satisfy their caloric requirements. Patients with diarrhea and fatty stools (steatorrhea) should receive pancreatin as a dietary supplement, and if this is supplied, they probably will tolerate and absorb a normal diet.

The cirrhotic patient with ascites and edema should restrict his sodium intake to 200 to 500 mg. daily but maintain a normal protein, caloric and vitamin intake. Table salt, salty foods, salted butter and margarine and all the ordinary canned and frozen foods should be avoided. Liberal use should be made of powdered low-sodium milk and milk products. If water accumulation is not controlled on this regimen the salt restriction must be more stringent, i.e., the daily sodium allowance should be reduced to 200 mg. and diuretics administered, as indicated previously.

The cirrhotic patient with signs of impending or advancing coma should receive temporarily a low-protein or protein-free diet, but a high caloric intake should be maintained, and supplementary vitamins and minerals should be supplied (e.g., liquid potassium, if the serum potassium is normal or low, and if renal function is normal). As soon as the situation permits, the protein intake should be restored to normal or above.

The ill cirrhotic patient requires the careful attention of the nurse. His weight and his fluid intake and output volumes must be measured and recorded daily. His position in bed should be adjusted for maximum respiratory efficiency, which is especially important if ascites is marked. Skin care must be observed meticulously because of the presence of subcutaneous edema and the relative immobility of the patient.

Accumulations of ascitic fluid often lessen or disappear in response to the dehydration program outlined above. To conserve the patient's body proteins, abdominal paracentesis is avoided for as long as possible. However, if the abdomen of the patient is tightly distended with fluid, and if the ascites shows no evidence of becoming reduced as a result of a low sodium intake, diuretics and spironolactone, the mechanical removal of the fluid is justified, provided that each aspiration is limited to 3 to 5 liters.

Preparatory to that procedure the patient is placed in the upright position on the edge of the bed, fully supported, with his feet resting on a stool and one arm fitted with a sphygmomanometer cuff. The trocar is introduced with sterile precautions through a stab wound in the midline below the umbilicus, and the fluid is drained through an effluent tube into a container.

The nurse will have prepared the patient for the treatment by supplying the necessary information, instructions and reassurance. *She will be sure to have the patient void as completely as possible just prior to paracentesis.* Sterile equipment and appropriate receptacles will have been made ready. During the procedure itself the nurse will help the patient to maintain the proper posture and will observe him closely for evidence of vascular collapse, such as the appearance of pallor, increase in pulse rate or a decline in blood pressure, the latter having been recorded at frequent intervals from the beginning of the procedure.

The procedure having been concluded and the patient restored to his original recumbent position, the nurse will take the responsibility for proper disposal of the equipment and the ascitic fluid. The amount collected should be measured and recorded, and samples of the fluid, properly labeled, should be sent to appropriate laboratories for examination of the cellular sediment, its specific gravity, protein concentration and bacterial content.

Hematemesis, with a profuse hemorrhage from an eroded esophageal varix, is not an uncommon complication of cirrhosis in its later stages. This is due to the marked portal hypertension which results from the long-standing cirrhosis. The treatment of hemorrhage from the esophageal veins by compression with a balloon is described on p. 584. However, balloon compression of the bleeding varices is only a temporary expedient, and usually some more definitive treatment must be given to prevent recurring hemorrhage in these cases. In some patients the veins are attacked directly through a thoracotomy incision. The esophagus is incised, and the dilated veins are oversewn with catgut sutures. This procedure gives a more definite compression of the veins and may stop the hemorrhage at the time, but it has no corrective effect on the portal hypertension.

SURGICAL BY-PASS PROCEDURES. In the present-day treatment of portal hypertension, certain by-pass procedures have been used to divert the blood from the portal system into the vena cava. The most common procedure is to create an anastomosis between the portal vein and the inferior vena cava, which is spoken of as a *portacaval anastomosis*. As a result of shunting portal blood into the vena cava, the pressure in the portal system is decreased, and consequently the danger from hemorrhage from esophageal and gastric varices is reduced. When the portal vein because of thrombosis or for other reasons cannot be used, a shunt may be made between the splenic vein and the left renal vein (*splenorenal shunt*). Some surgeons prefer this shunt to the portacaval shunt, even though the portal vein could be used.

Both of these operations are rather extensive procedures and are not always successful because of secondary clotting in the veins used for the shunt. Nevertheless, this method is the only one by which a lowering of pressure in the portal system may be brought about, and since hemorrhages from the esophageal varices are often fatal, many of these relatively poor-risk patients must be subjected to these attempts to save their lives. The postoperative care of these patients is the care of patients with any abdominal operation, but care is complicated by the treatment of the cirrhotic liver, which is the main problem in the recovery of these patients.

AT THE TIME OF DISCHARGE the patient will receive detailed instructions, in part from the nurse, principally relating to his dietary habits. Of utmost importance is the exclusion of alcohol completely and permanently from his diet, a fact of which he doubtless is well aware. However, if he is to succeed in abstaining completely and permanently, he will need all the help he can possibly muster from the most skilled psychiatrist, the most admired and trusted religious adviser and the most effective group in this therapeutic field, Alcoholics Anonymous. Sodium restriction will have to continue for a considerable period of time, if not permanently; if this diet is to be followed correctly, he will require written instructions. The nurse will see that these are provided.

Biliary Cirrhosis

A less common cause of cirrhosis is ascending infection of the biliary tract (cholangitis), with spread of the infection from the gallbladder by way of the hepatic duct to the small bile ducts in the liver substance. That portion of the liver chiefly involved, therefore, consists of the portal and the periportal spaces, where the bile canaliculi of each lobule communicate to form the liver bile ducts. These areas become the site of inflammation, and the bile ducts become occluded with inspissated bile and pus. An attempt is made by the liver to form new bile channels; hence, there is an overgrowth of tissue made up largely of disconnected, newly formed bile ducts and surrounded by scar tissue.

Symptoms and signs of this disease include intermittent jaundice and fever and the finding of an enlarged, hard, irregular liver, which eventually becomes atrophic. The treatment is the same as that described for portal cirrhosis, i.e., the treatment of any form of chronic liver insufficiency and, when indicated, surgical treatment designed to eradicate the biliary tract infection.

Other types of cirrhosis include those of healed subacute yellow atrophy, syphilis of the liver and hemochromatosis, in which there occurs a pigment deposition with associated scarring not only of the liver but also of the pancreas and other organs.

HEPATIC TUMORS

Few cancers originate in the liver, and those which are primary in that organ usually start in the bile ducts. However, metastases are found in the liver in about one half of all late cancer cases. The primary growth may be almost anywhere, and since the blood stream and the lymphatics from the body cavities nearly all reach the liver, malignant tumors anywhere in the trunk are likely to reach this organ eventually. Moreover, the liver apparently is an ideal place for these malignant cells to take root and to grow. Often the first evidence of a cancer in an abdominal organ is the appearance of one of its liver metastases, and, unless exploratory operation or necropsy is performed, the primary growth never may be discovered.

Diagnosis of malignant disease of the liver is made, regardless of the location of the

THE PATIENT WITH PORTAL CIRRHOSIS

PROBLEMS	NURSING IMPLICATIONS
Anorexia	Encourage patient to eat meals and supplementary feedings
	Offer frequent small feedings
	Give attention to esthetic factors and attractive trays at mealtime
	Eliminate alcohol
Nausea and vomiting	Oral hygiene before meals
	Ice collar for nausea
	Tube feedings, as required
Weight loss and fatigue	Continuous encouragement of intake of high-protein, high-calorie diet
	Give supplementary vitamins (A, B complex, C and K)
	Parenteral fluids as ordered
	Conserve patient's energy
Abdominal pain	Bed rest to protect liver
	Antispasmodics and mild sedatives
	Encourage patient to eat slowly and chew thoroughly
	Observe, record and report presence and character of pain
Hematemesis	Be alert for symptoms of anxiety, epigastric fullness, weakness and restlessness
	Observe for presence of bleeding and shock
	Record vital signs at frequent intervals
	Keep patient quiet and limit activity
	Observe during blood transfusions
	Assist physician in passage of tube for esophageal balloon tamponade
	Measure and record nature, time and amount of vomitus
	Give meticulous oral hygiene
	Maintain patient in fasting state if indicated
	Administer vitamin K as ordered
	Stay in constant attendance during episodes of bleeding
	Offer cold liquids by mouth when bleeding stops (if ordered)
Melena	Observe each stool for color, consistency and amount
Constipation	Ensure adequate fluid and food intake
	Encourage abdominal exercises
Diarrhea	Increase fluid intake
	Give medications as ordered
Jaundice	Note and record varying degrees of jaundice of the skin and the sclerae.
	Relieve pruritus with good skin care, bathing without soap and massage with emollient lotions
	Keep patient's fingernails short to prevent skin excoriation from scratching
	Give empathetic attention to patient's complaints and problems
Edema of extremities	Restrict sodium
	Administer diuretics as ordered
	Give careful attention and care to skin
	Turn and change position frequently
	Elevate extremities at intervals
	Weigh patient daily
	Record intake and output
	Passive range-of-motion exercises
	Small foam rubber supports under heels, malleoli, etc.
	Careful control of rate of flow of intravenous infusions

THE PATIENT WITH PORTAL CIRRHOSIS (Continued)

PROBLEMS	NURSING IMPLICATIONS
Ascites	Assist patient during paracentesis:
	1. Have him void before procedure
	2. Position correctly and use pillow support
	3. Record both the amount and the character of fluid aspirated
	4. Check dressing for fluid seepage and evidence of wound infection
	5. Protect puncture site with dry dressings
	Give diuretics, potassium and protein supplements as ordered
	Restrict sodium
	Record intake and output
	Give careful attention to skin
	Elevate head of bed to facilitate breathing
	Give pillow support under costal margin when in side-lying positions
	Observe for symptoms of impending coma
Hydrothorax and dyspnea	Elevate head of bed
	Conserve patient's strength
	Change position at intervals
	Assist patient during thoracentesis:
	1. Support and maintain position during procedure
	2. Record both the amount and the character of fluid aspirated
	3. Observe for evidence of coughing, increasing dyspnea and/or pulse rate
Fever	Record temperature regularly
	Encourage fluid intake
	Give cool sponges for elevated temperature
	Supply icecap to head as ordered
	Give antibiotics as ordered
	Avoid exposure to infections
	Keep patient at rest
	Note urinary volume and concentration
Hemorrhagic manifestations: ecchymosis, epistaxis, petechiae, and bleeding gums	Avoid trauma
	Maintain safe environment
	Avoid forceful blowing of nose
	Prevent trauma to gums from tooth brushing
	Encourage intake of foods with high content of vitamin C
	Apply cold compresses where indicated
	Record location of bleeding sites
	Avoid constrictive clothing
	Use small gauge needles for injections
Increasing stupor: mental changes, lethargy, hallucinations, and hepatic coma	Restrict dietary protein
	Give small frequent feeding of carbohydrates
	Protect from infection
	Keep environment warm and draft-free
	Pad the side-rails of the bed
	Limit visitors
	Supply careful nursing surveillance to ensure patient's safety
	Avoid narcotics and barbiturates
	Arouse at intervals
	Give sensitive nursing care during terminal phase

Fig. 253. Diagrammatic drawing showing the biliary ducts and the gallbladder. The diagram indicates, in black, common areas in which stones are found. It is evident that stones lying in the gallbladder and the cystic duct do not cause an obstruction of the flow of bile from the liver into the duodenum. Stones that lodge in the common duct or the ampulla of Vater obstruct the common bile duct and thus are associated with an absorption of bile pigment that produces jaundice.

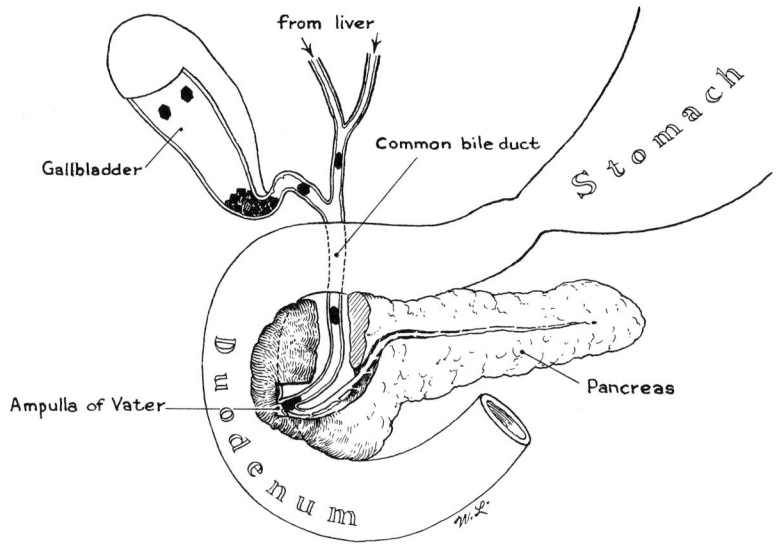

primary tumor, when there is a recent loss of weight, loss of strength and anemia (the last being the commonest early symptoms of any cancer which interferes with nutrition), together with rapid enlargement of the liver, which on palpation presents an irregular surface. Jaundice is present only if the larger bile ducts are occluded by the pressure of malignant nodules in the hilum of the liver. Ascites occurs only if such nodules obstruct the portal veins, or if tumor tissue is seeded in the peritoneal cavity. The only treatment is palliative.

THE PATIENT WITH GALLBLADDER DISEASE AND BILIARY OBSTRUCTION

Gallbladder Disease

Patients suffering from gallbladder disease who need the most frequent attention are those who have gallstones (cholelithiasis). These calculi form very commonly in the gallbladder because of infection or the precipitation of bile constituents (bile salts and cholesterol). They appear to form most frequently in women who have borne children and usually in the obese individual. The presence of the stones generally indicates some dysfunction of the gallbladder, and the disease is spoken of as chronic gallbladder disease.

Symptoms. Two types of symptoms arise,

those due to disease of the gallbladder itself, with indigestion, chronic pain in the upper right abdomen and distention after eating, and those due to obstruction of the bile passages (especially the cystic duct) by a gallstone. This occurrence causes excruciating upper right abdominal pain that radiates to the back or the right shoulder and usually is associated with vomiting and nausea. These symptoms generally are so severe as to require morphine hypodermically. Such attacks are given the name of *biliary colic*.

Diagnosis. In the diagnosis of these chronic forms of gallbladder disease, considerable information may be obtained by the *cholecystogram* (p. 103). A dye is given, either by mouth or intravenously, which is excreted in the bile by the liver. Normally, the gallbladder shadow, as outlined, may be seen on the roentgenogram, and the shadow gradually decreases in size and becomes more dense as the dye is concentrated by fluid absorption. Finally, the normal gallbladder is able to empty part of its contents if a fatty meal is taken. A fatty meal is used to stimulate the gallbladder to contract in order to obtain better visualization. The diseased gallbladder is indicated by a very faint shadow, which does not become concentrated and does not empty when a fatty meal is eaten (Graham-Cole test).

A *duodenal drainage* with examination of

the bile for crystals and pus cells is another diagnostic procedure.

At times the gallbladder may be the seat of an acute infection that causes acute pain, tenderness and rigidity of the upper right abdomen, associated with nausea and vomiting and the usual signs of an acute inflammation. This condition is spoken of as *acute cholecystitis*. If the gallbladder is found to be filled with pus, there is said to be an *empyema* of the gallbladder.

Treatment. Surgical treatment is demanded for the relief of long-continued symptoms, for the removal of the cause of biliary colic and in patients who have acute cholecystitis.

Preparation for a simple gallbladder operation is the same as for any upper abdominal laparotomy. Patients may be placed on the operating table with the upper abdomen raised somewhat by an air pillow or sandbag to make exposure easier.

CHOLECYSTOSTOMY. This is an operation performed for the relief of certain cases of acute cholecystitis and of chronic gallbladder disease. The gallbladder is opened, the stones and the bile or the pus are removed, and a tube is sutured in the opening for drainage. As soon as the patient is returned to bed, the nurse should connect this tube to a drainage bottle placed at the side of the bed. Failure to perform this duty may result in the leakage of bile round the tube and its escape into the peritoneal cavity.

CHOLECYSTECTOMY. This is the operation by which the gallbladder is removed after ligation of the cystic duct and artery. The operation is performed in most cases of acute and chronic cholecystitis.

CHOLEDOCHOTOMY. In this operation an incision is made into the common duct for removal of stones. After the stones have been evacuated, a tube usually is inserted into the duct for drainage. The gallbladder also contains stones as a rule. A cholecystectomy is performed.

When the common duct is obstructed because of the pressure of an inoperable carcinoma of the head of the pancreas, an operation is performed that will lead the bile into the intestinal tract by a different route.

Biliary Obstruction

Not infrequently a gallstone may pass from the gallbladder through the cystic duct and lodge in the common bile duct; or the head of the pancreas, through which the common duct passes, may be the seat of a carcinoma. Either condition may obstruct the flow of bile into the duodenum and result in the following characteristic symptoms.

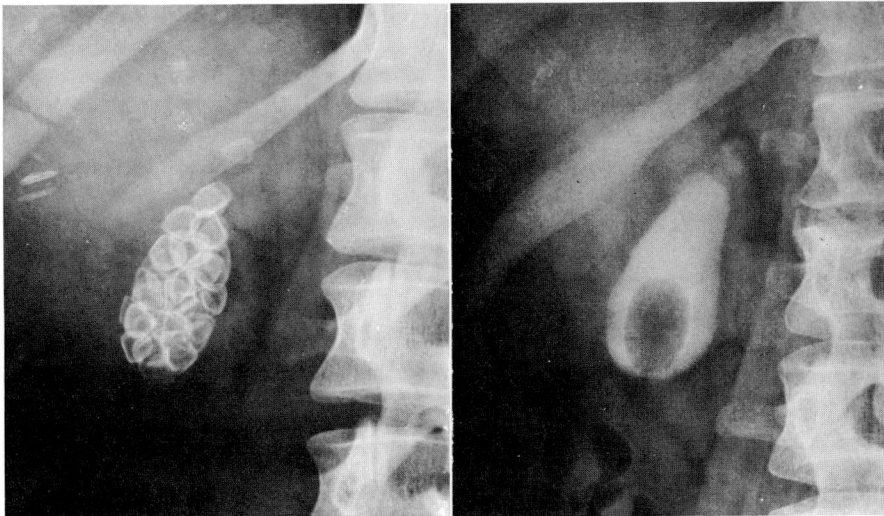

FIG. 254. (*Left*) Gallstones that show in a roentgenogram, due to calcification in their content. (*Right*) Single nonopaque gallstone shown as a negative shadow by displacing dye in cholecystogram.

The bile, no longer carried to the duodenum, is absorbed by the blood and gives the skin and the tissues a yellow color known as *jaundice*. The excretion of the bile pigments in some measure from the blood by the kidneys gives the urine a very dark color. The feces, no longer colored with bile pigments, are grayish, like putty, and usually are spoken of as clay-colored. There frequently is marked itching of the skin, and nausea occurs after eating fatty foods, because there is a marked disturbance of the digestion and absorption of fats when bile does not flow into the duodenum. Various laboratory tests of the blood (icteric index, van den Bergh, serum bilirubin, etc.) indicate the degree of pigment retention and therefore the depth of jaundice.

Operations on patients with obstructive jaundice are most serious, because there is always marked damage to the liver, and there is the added danger of hemorrhage. Therefore, these patients should receive special preparation. The diet should be low in fats and high in protein and carbohydrate. Frequently it is wise to administer protein solution intravenously for a day or two before operation.

It is well known that the hemorrhagic tendency in jaundice is due to a deficient formation of the prothrombin. This is an important factor in the clotting of blood, which becomes deficient in jaundice because of inadequate absorption of the fat-soluble vitamin K. Often the blood prothrombin may be raised adequately by administration of vitamin K, or a new supply may be added to the patient's blood by transfusion. Carbohydrates are given in large amounts by mouth and intravenously to build up the glycogen stores in the liver. The nurse should note the color of the urine and the stools and send specimens of these excreta to be examined for bile pigments. The operations performed depend on the cause of the biliary obstruction.

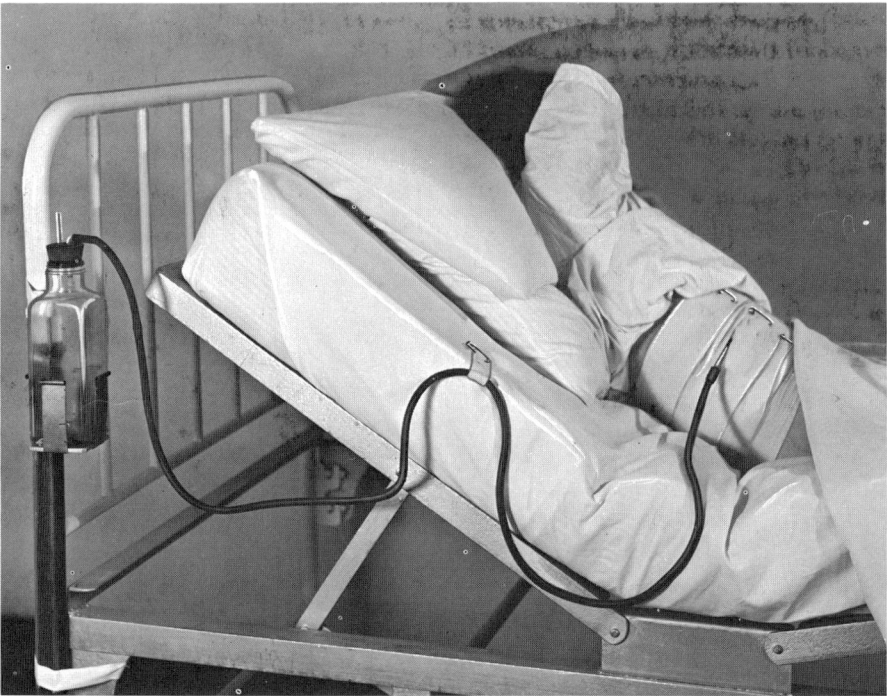

FIG. 255. Cholecystostomy. Note the drainage bottle attached to bedpost and also the drainage tube anchored to the bed by adhesive. The height of the bottle is adjusted as ordered by the surgeon. The height of the drainage bottle is determined by the rapidity of decompression desired.

FIG. 256. Diagrammatic drawing showing the situation after an operation in which the gallbladder has been removed and a T-tube introduced into the common duct. A hemostat holds the ligated end of the cystic duct. The tube has been sutured in place in the common duct and led out through the wound.

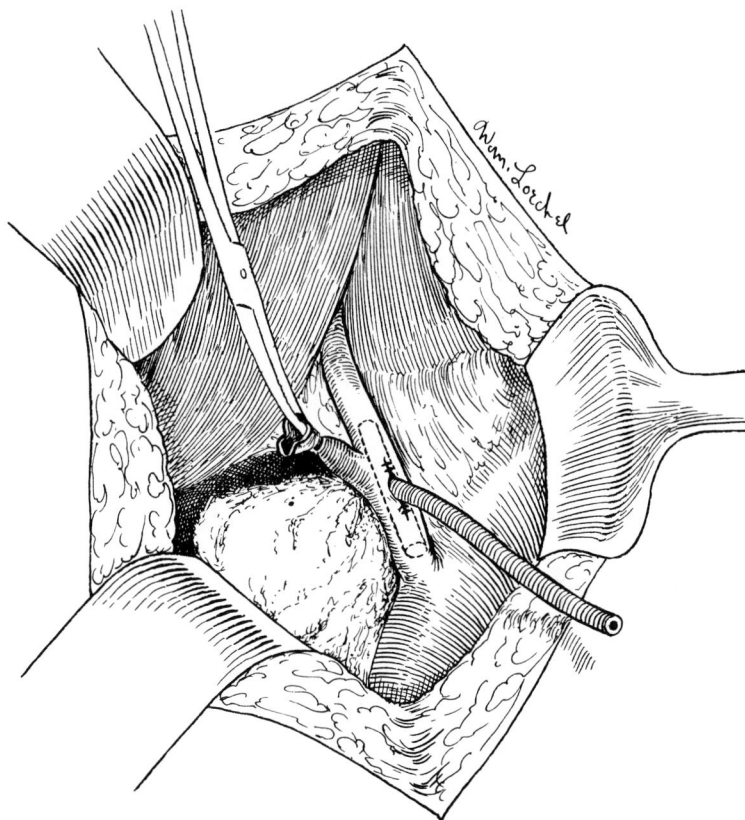

Nursing Care after Operations on the Biliary Tract. As soon as recovery from anesthesia has occurred, the patient is placed in the Fowler position. The usual treatment for any laparotomy is indicated, i.e., fluids by vein and gastric-suction drainage if vomiting occurs; water and other fluids may be given in 24 hours and an enema and a soft diet after 72 hours.

As mentioned before, in patients with cholecystostomy or choledochostomy the drainage tubes must be connected immediately to a drainage bottle or bottles. In addition, tubing should be fastened to the dressings or to the bottom sheet with enough leeway for the patient to move without dislodging it (see Fig. 255). In order to prevent total loss of bile, the drainage tube or collecting bottle may be elevated above the level of the abdomen, so that bile will drain through the apparatus only if pressure develops in the duct system. The bile collected should be measured and recorded every 24 hours, its color and character being charted.

After 5 or 6 days of drainage, the tubes may be clamped for an hour before and after each meal, the purpose being to deliver bile to the duodenum to aid in digestion. The nurse must exercise special care in turning or lifting these patients not to dislodge the tubes. Within 7 to 10 days the drainage tubes are removed from the gallbladder or common bile duct. Bile may continue to drain from the drainage tract in considerable quantities for a time and necessitate frequent change of the outer dressings and protection of the skin from irritation.

In all patients with biliary drainage, the stools should be observed daily and their color recorded. At frequent intervals specimens of both urine and feces should be sent to the laboratory for examination for bile pigments. In this way the surgeon is able to tell that the bile pigment is disappearing from the blood and is draining again into the duodenum. A careful record of fluid intake and output should be kept and totaled for each 24 hours.

The diet of these patients should be low in fats and therefore high in carbohydrates and proteins. The patients themselves usually will refuse to eat fatty foods because of the nausea that follows. Vitamin K administration is continued after the operation.

These patients are especially prone to pulmonary complications, as are all patients with upper abdominal incisions. They should be taught to take 10 deep breaths every hour to aerate the lungs fully. Activating these individuals by getting them out of bed as early as permissible will reduce the likelihood of thrombophlebitis and pulmonary atelectasis, complications to which the more obese patient is unusually susceptible.

CLINICAL SITUATIONS

(Questions 1 to 5 relate to Mr. J. J., a 55-year-old male, who is being treated on the Medical Unit for cirrhosis of the liver.)

1. Following a liver biopsy on Mr. J., the nurse knows that there may be serious complications. Which symptom indicates difficulty?
    A. Inability to void.
    B. Rapid, thready pulse.
    C. Labored respirations.
    D. Progressive jaundice.

2. Immediately preceding paracentesis, the nurse should prepare the patient by
    A. Having him fast.
    B. Asking him to void.
    C. Keeping him well-sedated.
    D. Having him lie in a supine position.

3. Mr. J. becomes extremely restless. Which of the following is the safest drug to administer to this patient?
    A. Thorazine.
    B. Sodium phenobarbital.
    C. Paraldehyde.
    D. Morphine.

4. The most important nursing measure in caring for the patient with cirrhosis of the liver is to
    A. Promote absolute bed rest.
    B. Use measures to relieve pruritis.
    C. Ensure optimum nutrition.
    D. Avoid fatty foods.

5. Mr. J. had vomited 350 ml. of bright red blood, which his physician stated was the result of a ruptured esophageal varicosity.

Which of the following may occur after an esophageal hemorrhage?
    A. Lower abdominal pain.
    B. Rectal bleeding.
    C. Proteinuria.
    D. Cheyne-Stokes respirations.

(Questions 6 to 8 relate to Mrs. M. J., an obese, 40-year-old housewife, who has been admitted to the Surgical Unit with severe jaundice.)

6. Mrs. J.'s roentgenograms reveal that she has gallbladder pathology. The jaundice is most likely to be due to a stone lodged in the
    A. Gallbladder.
    B. Duodenum.
    C. Cystic duct.
    D. Common bile duct.

7. A cholecystogram using radiopaque tablets was ordered for Mrs. J. The purpose of this test is to
    A. Test the function of the liver.
    B. Determine the patency of the duodenum.
    C. Visualize the gallbladder.
    D. Test for biliary flow.

8. Following a cholecystectomy, the nurse should make frequent observations of the patient, knowing that the most likely complication is apt to be
    A. Pneumonia.
    B. Oliguria.
    C. Ascites.
    D. Tenesmus.

9. Which of the following statements is true concerning epidemic hepatitis and homologous serum jaundice?
    A. Serum hepatitis has a longer incubation period.
    B. The diseases are easily distinguishable after onset.
    C. The virus of epidemic hepatitis is found only in the feces.
    D. Each type produces immunity against both kinds of viral hepatitis.

10. Homologous serum hepatitis may be prevented by the
    A. Use of pooled plasma.
    B. Irradiation of blood.
    C. Proper sterilization of needles and syringes.

D. Prophylactic administration of gamma globulin.

BIBLIOGRAPHY AND SUGGESTED READING

Gallbladder

Kellen, N. J.: Cholecystitis and cholecystectomy, Canad. Nurse **51:**548-552, 1955.

Palumbo, L. T., and Fisk, J. E.: Present-day treatment of diseases of the biliary tract and nursing care of the patient with surgery of the biliary tract, Am. J. Nurs. **60:**50-55, Jan., 1960.

Liver

Davidson, C. S.: Diet in the treatment of liver disease, Am. J. Med. **25:**690-697, 1958.

Editorial: Therapy of ascites in patients with cirrhosis of the liver, A.M.A. Arch. Intern. Med. **92:**603-605, 1953.

Gellis, S. S., and Hsia, D. Y.: Viral hepatitis, New Eng. J. Med. **249:**400-408, 1953.

Gordon, E. S.: The treatment of cirrhosis of the liver, A.M.A. Arch. Intern. Med. **97:**340-350, 1956.

Hanger, F. M.: Current status of therapy of infectious hepatitis, J.A.M.A. **165:**1696-1699, 1957.

Leibowitz, S.: Hospital precautions against spread of acute viral hepatitis, J.A.M.A. **167:** 1474-1476, 1958.

Point, W. W.: Jaundice, Am. J. Nurs. **58:**556-557, 1958.

Ward, R., *et al.:* Infectious hepatitis, New Eng. J. Med. **258:**407-416, 1958.

Watson, C.: Current status of treatment of cirrhosis of the liver, J.A.M.A. **166:**764-771, 1958.

31

Patients With Disorders of the Pancreas

The pancreas is a very important gland that has to do with the digestion of food elements and the metabolism of sugar in the body. It lies across the upper abdomen behind the peritoneum and the stomach. Its external secretion, containing enzymes that are needed for the digestion of carbohydrates (amylase), proteins (trypsin) and fats (lipase), is delivered into the duodenum at the ampulla of Vater near the entrance of the common bile duct (Fig. 257). The stimulus for its production is the presence of food in the duodenum, in response to which a hormone (secretin) is liberated into the blood stream and carried to the pancreas, causing the latter to secrete. Pancreatic secretion is stimulated also by nerve impulses transmitted via the vagus nerves.

In addition to this external secretion, the pancreas produces an internal secretion, or endocrine substance, *insulin*. This hormone is manufactured by small collections of cells scattered throughout the pancreas called the "islands of Langerhans," and is absorbed directly into the blood stream. Insulin is required for the utilization of carbohydrate (sugar) by the body. (See p. 672.)

Both the internal and the external secretions of the pancreas are indispensable for normal body function. Any interruption of the production or interference in the delivery of the external secretion produces severe digestive and nutritional disturbances. Any shortage of insulin causes serious disturbance of carbohydrate metabolism.

THE PATIENT WITH ACUTE PANCREATITIS

Acute pancreatitis is brought about by the digestion of this organ by the very enzymes it produces, principally trypsin. Exactly how this autodigestion gets started is not known with certainty. However, in view of the frequent association of pancreatitis with gallbladder disease, it is believed that gallstones entering the common bile duct and lodging at the ampulla of Vater may obstruct the flow of pancreatic juice, or cause a reflux of bile from the common duct into the pancreatic duct, activating the powerful pancreatic enzymes within the gland. (Normally, these remain in an inactive form until the pancreatic juice reaches the lumen of the duodenum.) Another etiologic factor in this disease appears to be the excessive ingestion of alcohol; at any rate, a definite relationship can be established between alcoholic intake and the onset of symptoms in many cases of acute pancreatitis.

Two forms of acute pancreatitis are encountered: acute edematous (or interstitial) pancreatitis, and acute necrotic (or hemorrhagic) pancreatitis.

Acute Interstitial Pancreatitis. This condition is characterized by an edematous swelling of the gland and the escape of its enzymes into the surrounding tissues and the peritoneal cavity. Pancreatic lipase produces fat necrosis in the omentum, and the peritoneal fluid increases due to the irritating effect of these digestive enzymes. Symptoms of the disease are due to this irritation; they include: abdominal and back pain, nausea, vomiting and tenderness across the upper abdomen. The definitive diagnostic test for acute pancreatitis is the estimation of blood amylase, which early in the disease increases in amount.

Since the pathologic process responsible for this disease is autodigestion of the pan-

Fig. 257. Diagram of some of the abdominal organs. The stomach and the liver, which normally cover these organs, are not represented. (a) Hepatic duct. (b) Cystic duct. (c) Common duct; the arrow is in the ampulla of Vater. (d) Pancreatic duct, which is represented as exposed.

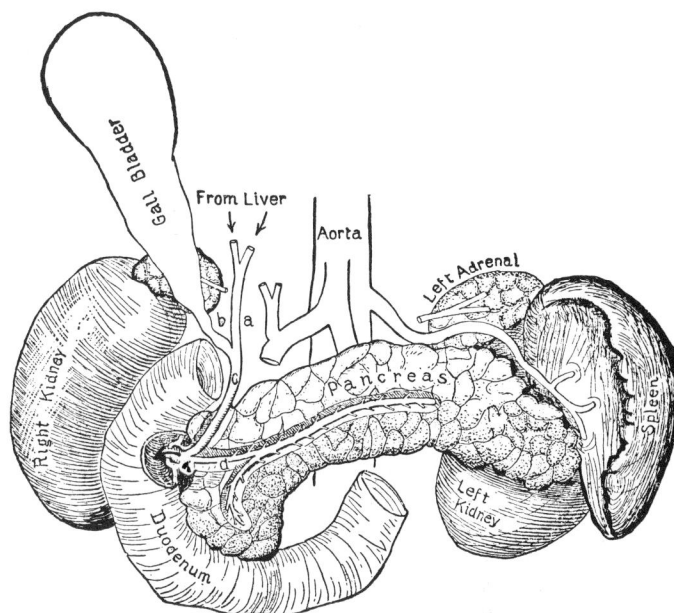

creas, an attempt is made to decrease the production of these enzymes. Oral feedings are interrupted to control the formation of secretin. Atropine or Banthine is administered to block the nerve impulses that stimulate pancreatic secretion. The patient is maintained on parenteral fluids. Morphine or Demerol is given to relieve pain. Most attacks of acute interstitial pancreatitis are self-limited and may be expected to subside in 3 or 4 days.

Acute Hemorrhagic Pancreatitis. Acute hemorrhagic (or necrotic) pancreatitis perhaps represents merely a more advanced form of acute interstitial pancreatitis. Enzymatic digestion of the gland is more widespread and complete. The tissue becomes necrotic, and the damage extends to its vascular radicles with the result that blood escapes into the substance of the pancreas and beyond into the retroperitoneal tissues. Symptoms are severe, consisting of pain in the upper abdomen and back, nausea, vomiting and the development of shock with hypotension, tachycardia, cold, clammy skin, and cyanosis. The diagnosis is established on the basis of an elevated blood amylase level plus the clinical picture.

Treatment consists of the measures recommended for acute interstitial pancreatitis plus those indicated for shock (p. 296).

They include intravenous fluids, blood transfusion, antibiotics, and drugs for the relief of pain. Careful nursing observation is extremely important.

If the patient survives the initial shock, pancreatic necrosis often leads to the formation of secondary abscesses in the region of the gland, which are manifested clinically by mounting fever and leukocytosis. Such abscesses must be drained surgically during the later stages of the disease. Drainage is likely to be profuse and long-standing, so that these patients are certain to require close observation and constant care for a considerable period of time.

THE PATIENT WITH CHRONIC PANCREATITIS

After repeated attacks of acute interstitial pancreatitis, or, in some instances, after the prolonged use of alcohol in large amounts, patients may develop a chronic fibrosis of the pancreatic gland itself, with obstruction of its ducts and destruction of its secreting cells. This type of pancreatitis is prone to appear in adult men and is characterized by recurring attacks of severe upper abdominal and back pain, accompanied by vomiting. Attacks often are so painful that morphine, even in large doses, does not provide relief. As the disease progresses, these patients may become addicted to opiates. Because of the destruction of the gland by fibrosis, the pancreatic secretions may be deficient in amount; or obstruction of the ducts by fibrosis may prevent the pancreatic juice from entering the duodenum and playing its role in digestion. As a result, the digestion of foodstuffs, especially proteins and fats, is disrupted. The stools become frequent, frothy (or soap-like) and foul-smelling, owing to the presence of partially hydrolyzed fat, a condition referred to as "steatorrhea." As the disease progresses, calcifications of the gland may occur, and calcium stones may form within the ducts.

The treatment of chronic pancreatitis depends on its probable cause in each particular patient. When it develops in association with gallbladder disease, efforts are made to relieve the difficulty by operating on the biliary tract, exploring the common duct and removing the stones; usually, the gallbladder is removed at the same time. In addition, an attempt is made to improve the drainage of the common bile duct and the pancreatic duct by dividing the sphincter of Oddi, a muscle that is located at the ampulla of Vater (this operation is known as a "sphincterotomy"). The nursing care after such an operation is the same as that indicated for all patients undergoing biliary tract surgery. A T-tube usually is placed in the common bile duct, which involves the necessity for a drainage bottle to collect the bile postoperatively.

In the absence of evidence indicating biliary tract disease, the most common cause of chronic pancreatitis is chronic alcoholism. In such patients, the pancreas becomes markedly fibrotic, to the extent that the pancreatic ducts may be obstructed. In some patients the obstruction may be relieved by sphincterotomy, but in others, the obstruction is located within the confines of the gland itself and therefore is not amenable to this procedure. Other possible approaches include opening the pancreatic duct and placing the entire gland inside a loop of jejunum; or the tail of the pancreas may be removed and the remaining stump sutured into the end of a loop of jejunum. These somewhat complicated operations are performed with the object of draining the pancreatic juice via a route that by-passes the obstruction in the ductal system.

Despite these operative procedures the patient is likely to continue having pain and digestive difficulties from his pancreatitis unless he abstains completely from the use of alcohol. This point should be emphasized by the nurse in the course of her instruction of the patient and his family.

THE PATIENT WITH PANCREATIC CYSTS

As a result of the local necrosis that occurs at the time of acute pancreatitis, collections of fluid may form in the vicinity of the pancreas. These become walled off by fibrous tissue and are called pancreatic cysts. They are the commonest type of pancreatic cyst, most other types developing as a result of congenital anomalies.

Pancreatic cysts may attain considerable size. Because of their location behind the posterior peritoneum, when they enlarge they impinge on and displace the stomach or the colon, which are adjacent. Eventually, through pressure or secondary infection, they are likely to produce symptoms, in which event they must be drained. Drainage may be established into the gastrointestinal tract or through the skin surface. In the latter instance, the drainage is likely to be profuse and damaging to tissue, due to its enzyme content. Hence, steps must be taken to protect the skin in areas adjacent to the drainage site to prevent excoriation. Ointments will protect the skin provided that they are applied before excoriation takes place. Another method of protecting the skin involves the constant aspiration of juice from the drainage tract by means of a suction apparatus, so that enyzme contact is avoided. This method demands a great deal of nursing attention to be sure that the suction tube does not become dislodged from the drainage tract and that the entire apparatus functions properly without interruption.

THE PATIENT WITH PANCREATIC TUMORS

Carcinoma of the Pancreas

Cancer may arise in any portion of the pancreas: in the head, the body or the tail,

Fig. 258. Drawings which show types of operations for carcinoma of the pancreas. (A) Indicates the end-result for resection of the carcinoma of the head of the pancreas or the ampulla of Vater. The common duct is sutured to the end of the jejunum, and the remaining portion of the pancreas and the end of the stomach are sutured to the side of the jejunum. (B) Shows lines that indicate the amount of tissue removed. (C) An alternate method of treatment when an inoperable tumor of the head of the pancreas has been found. In such cases the bile may be permitted to flow again into the intestine by anastomosing the jejunum to the gallbladder. In addition, an accessory operation between the loops of jejunum has been performed.

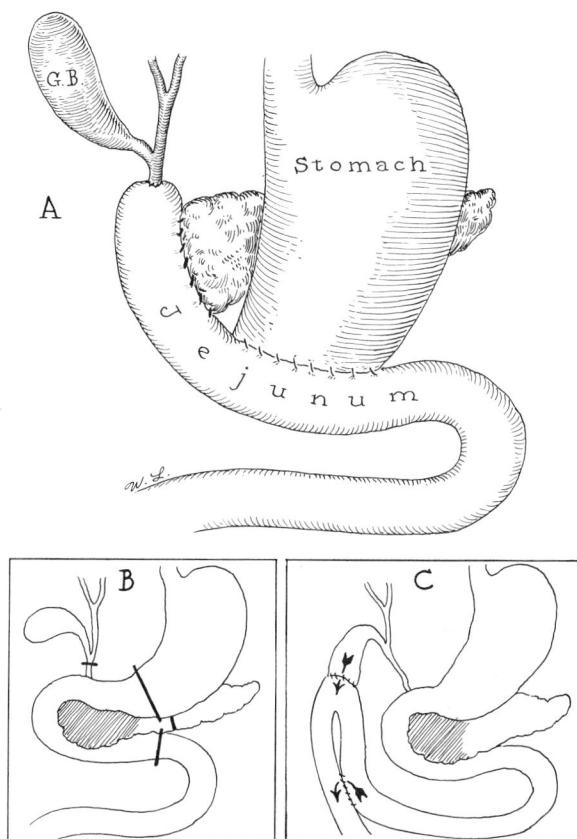

producing symptoms and signs that vary depending on the location of the lesion and whether or not functioning, insulin-secreting pancreatic islet cells are involved. Tumors that originate in the head of the pancreas—decidedly the most common location—give rise to a distinctive clinical picture and will be discussed separately. Functioning islet cell tumors, whether benign (adenomata) or malignant (carcinomata) are responsible for the syndrome of hyperinsulinism, and are described on page 672. With these exceptions, carcinoma of the pancreas is notoriously lacking in clear-cut, characteristic symptomatology, and because of its rather nondescript features, patients with this form of cancer often are denied the advantages of an early diagnosis.

Diagnosis. Common to all types of pancreatic carcinoma are symptoms of rapid, profound, progressive and inexplicable weight loss; vague, ill-defined, upper or midabdominal discomfort which is totally unrelated to any gastrointestinal function and is difficult to describe; and a boring pain in the midback that is unrelated to posture or activity. Most likely to prove helpful in diagnosis is the gastrointestinal roentgenographic examination, which may demonstrate deformities in adjacent viscera caused by the impinging pancreatic mass. A very important clue, when present, is the development of signs that indicate insulin deficiency—glycosuria, hyperglycemia, and abnormal glucose tolerance.

Treatment. Therapy usually is limited to palliative measures. Definitive surgical treatment, i.e., total excision of the lesion, often is not applicable because of the extensive character of the growth when it is finally diagnosed, for by this time, widespread metastases—especially to the liver, the lungs, and the bones—are likely to have developed.

Tumors of the Head of the Pancreas

Tumors in this region are detected by the

fact that they obstruct the common bile duct where it passes through the head of the pancreas to join the pancreatic duct and empty at the ampulla of Vater into the duodenum. Obstruction to the flow of bile produces jaundice, clay-colored stools and dark urine. This disease usually occurs in older, thin men. It must be differentiated from the jaundice due to a biliary obstruction caused by a gallstone in the common duct, which usually is intermittent and appears typically in obese individuals, most often women, who have had previous symptoms of gallbladder disease. The tumors producing the obstruction may arise from the pancreas, from the common bile duct or from the ampulla of Vater.

Operation is indicated in these patients, first to be sure that the jaundice is not due to an impacted gallstone, which can be removed with relative ease. If a tumor is found, it may be removed if it has not invaded many of the important structures adjacent to it (portal vein, superior mesenteric artery). The operation entails removal of the head of the pancreas, the duodenum and adjacent stomach and the distal part of the common bile duct. The stomach, the cut end of the pancreas and the common bile duct then are anastomosed to the jejunum. This operation, first suggested by Whipple, may be done in either 1 or 2 stages. It has resulted in the cure of many patients with cancer of the ampulla and the bile ducts, but unhappily it is only palliative in most cases of carcinoma of the head of the pancreas. When excision of the tumor cannot be performed, the jaundice may be relieved by diverting the bile flow into the jejunum. This is done by anastomosing the jejunum to the gallbladder (cholecystojejunostomy).

Nursing Care. When these patients come to the hospital, they are in such a poor nutritional and physical state that a fairly long period of preparation is necessary before operation can be attempted. Various liver and pancreatic function studies are carried out, vitamin K is given to restore the blood prothrombin activity, and diets high in protein often are given with pancreatic enzymes. Blood transfusions frequently are used as well.

Because of the extensive surgery performed, much depends on the nursing care after operation. This differs little from that after any upper abdominal operation, except that these patients are poor surgical risks, and therefore they need intensive nursing attention during the immediate postoperative period.

Pancreatic Islet Tumors

In the pancreas are located the islands of Langerhans, small nests of cells that secrete directly into the blood stream and, therefore, are part of the glands of internal secretion (endocrines). The secretion, insulin, has to do with the metabolism of sugar, and a deficient secretion produces diabetes. Tumors of these cells produce a hypersecretion of insulin, so that the body sugar is used up too rapidly. The fall of the blood sugar level (hypoglycemia) produces symptoms of weakness, mental confusion and even convulsions. These may be relieved almost immediately by taking sugar by mouth or by intravenous glucose.

Once the diagnosis of a tumor of the islet cells has been made, surgical treatment with removal of the tumor usually is recommended. The tumors may be benign adenomas, or they may be malignant. Complete removal results usually in a most dramatic cure. In some patients the symptoms may not be produced by an actual tumor of the islet cells but by a simple hypertrophy of this tissue. In such cases a partial *pancreatectomy*—removal of the tail and part of the body of the pancreas—is performed.

Nursing Care. In preparing these patients for operation the nurse must be on the watch for symptoms of hypoglycemia and be ready to give sugar, usually orange juice with sugar, should they appear. After operation, the nursing care is the same as that following any upper abdominal operation.

Ulcerogenic (Zollinger-Ellison) Tumors

Some tumors of the islands of Langerhans are associated with a hypersecretion of gastric acid that produces ulcers in the stomach, the duodenum and even the jejunum. The hypersecretion is so great that even after partial gastric resection there still may be enough acid to produce further ulceration.

When a marked tendency to develop gastric and duodenal ulcers is noted, an ulcerogenic tumor of the islands of Langerhans is suspected. These tumors, which may be benign or malignant, are treated when possible by excision. Frequently, however, because of extension beyond the pancreas, removal is not possible. In many cases, a total gastrectomy may be necessary to reduce the secretion of gastric acid sufficiently to prevent further ulceration.

BIBLIOGRAPHY AND SUGGESTED READING

Anderson, D. H.: Cystic fibrosis of the pancreas, J. Chronic Dis. 7:58, 1958.

Birnbaum, D., and Kleeberg, J.: Carcinoma of the pancreas, Ann. Intern. Med. 48:1171-1184, 1958.

Ciba Clinical Symposia: Diseases of the Pancreas, vol. 9, no. 2, Mar.-Apr., 1957.

Howard, M. A.: Surgical aspects of jaundice, Am. J. Surg. 92:532-537, 1956.

Raskin, H. F.: Carcinoma of the pancreas, bilary tract, and liver, CA 11:137-148, July-Aug., 1961; and 11:166-179, Sept.-Oct., 1961.

Shallenberger, P. L., and Kapp, D. F.: Acute pancreatitis, Ann. Intern. Med. 48:1185-1193, 1958.

Unit XI. Nursing in Conditions Involving the Kidneys, the Urinary Tract and the Reproductive System

ORIENTATION

The kidneys and their drainage channels, the urinary tract, together comprise the renal system. This organ assembly is mainly responsible for extracting the soluble metabolites from the blood and removing them from the body. Another and related aspect of its excretory function is the regulation of the water content and the electrolyte composition of the body fluids; the inorganic ions are excreted in the urine or retained in the body, depending on their individual concentrations in the plasma. Constant precision of operation on the part of the renal system is an absolute requirement for good health; in fact, if its functions are interrupted for more than a few days, death is inevitable. Details regarding the mechanisms of normal kidney function are poorly understood, and, insofar as diseases of the kidney are concerned, medical knowledge is quite as imperfect. The anatomic structure of this organ and its physiologic activities are discussed in the introductory paragraphs of Chapter 32; the remainder of the chapter is concerned with problems associated with disorders of the renal system.

In common with other organs of the body, the kidneys are affected seriously by any factor which impedes the flow of blood through its substance. The slightest change in the renal circulation, however transient, is reflected at once by alterations in the volume and the composition of the urine. The nurse is well aware that an episode of oligemic shock lasting only 2 or 3 hours is sufficient to depress kidney function, and if shock is allowed to continue uncorrected or incompletely corrected a little longer, the patient may never survive the damage to his kidneys.

Most of the diseases in which the kidneys are seriously and chronically involved are circulatory diseases, based on pathologic changes in the renal blood vessels causing a reduction of blood supply. Kidney failure, as might be expected, is common in patients with arteriosclerotic and hypertensive vascular disease, the renal situation in these cases being but one aspect of a generalized process. Glomerulonephritis (Bright's disease), in which renal insufficiency is most profound, also can be regarded as a vascular disease, one in which the pathologic process, in the early stages at least, is confined principally to the renal capillaries. In general, the type of tissue damage that is characteristically produced by vascular disease is extremely disruptive of organ function, and recovery, if it occurs at all, is seldom complete. Classic examples of its deleterious effects are to be found in patients with vascular disease of the kidney, who are notable for their susceptibility to renal failure, the duration of their ailment and the gravity of their prognosis.

The clinical features of kidney disease depend chiefly on the presence or the absence of renal insufficiency, renal infection and arterial hypertension, one of its most important complications. Renal failure is reflected in the syndrome of uremia, a complicated situation clinically, with therapeutic problems as challenging for the nurse as any encountered in clinical practice. These problems are related to the failure of toxic metabolites to be excreted, the excess accumulation of certain materials in the blood, and the spillage of others that are essential to the body economy.

Infections of the kidney, causing diffuse inflammatory reactions or the formation of abscesses, are invariably serious because of their local destructiveness, their tendency to become widespread, and the occurrence of damaging complications. Stones and deforming scars which originate in an infection may interfere with urinary drainage. Moreover, permanent alterations of the renal blood vessels in pyelonephritis, a type of kidney infection, may be responsible for impairment of kidney function and also for chronic, incapacitating arterial hypertension. Fortunately, most urinary infections are responsive to modern anti-bacterial chemotherapy if treatment is selected appropriately and applied correctly. Obviously, a prerequisite for proper treatment is the collection of urine specimens correctly, i.e., without bacterial contamination, in order to permit the accurate identification of the infecting organism. The collection and the testing of urine samples, as well as special tests for evaluating renal function, are discussed in detail in Chapter 6 (pp. 65 to 77).

32

Patients With Renal and Genitourinary Problems

NORMAL STRUCTURE AND FUNCTION

The kidneys are paired organs, each weighing approximately 125 Gm., located in a position lateral to the bodies of the lower thoracic vertebrae a few centimeters to the right and the left of the midline. Anteriorly, they are separated from the abdominal cavity and its contents by layers of peritoneum; posteriorly, they are shielded by the lower thoracic wall. Each, essentially a duplicate of the other, is composed of minute structural units; functionally, they may be regarded as little kidneys. To understand one of these renal units is to understand the whole kidney.

Each renal unit is constructed of living cells arranged in the form of a tube, or *tubule*. Figure 259 represents the upper end of one of these tubules. Its wall is constructed with renal epithelial cells, on the outer side of which is a fine network of capillaries (b), through which blood is constantly flowing.

At its upper end this tubule swells into a hollow ball called Bowman's capsule (c). At the pole of this ball, which is opposite the point where the tubule enters, the wall is pushed in, much as a child can push one half of a rubber ball into the other half, by a knot of capillaries, the glomerulus (d). These glomeruli can be seen by the naked eye only as red dots about the size of a pinprick. The wall of this hollow ball is lined with flat epithelial cells quite unlike those lining the tubule. The tube, when it leaves the capsule (Fig. 260), is quite tortuous and is called the *proximal convoluted tubule* (c). It then makes a long straight loop, the loop

of Henle (Fig. 261, d), which again becomes convoluted (e), after which it opens into a long straight tube, the *collecting tubule* (f), which grows larger and larger in its course.

The capillaries of the glomerulus, all of which branched from one vessel (Fig. 259, e)—a branch of the renal artery—unite again into one vessel (f), which leaves the capsule, passes down the tubule and again is divided into the network of capillaries (b), mentioned above as surrounding the tubule.

Through the walls of the capillaries of each glomerulus pour out into its capsule, by a process quite similar to simple filtration, most of the constituents of the urine, and this fluid passes down the tubule.

Some of the substances which the glomeruli filter out are of use to the body, and these the convoluted tubules absorb back into the blood stream. Much of the water is reabsorbed through the tubular walls. A portion of the tubule contributes to the formation of urine by secreting materials derived from the blood into the fluid passing through its lumen. The urine, as finally formed, flows down to the open end of the tubule into the pelvis of the kidney.

The capillaries surrounding the tubules reunite to form the renal vein, the blood of which now is practically free of waste. A large amount of blood flows through the kidneys, nearly 10 times as much as through any other organ of the same weight. In this way the kidney is continuously purifying the entire volume of blood.

Cortex. This is the most important part of the kidney, because all the important structures of the kidney are here. It is a

676

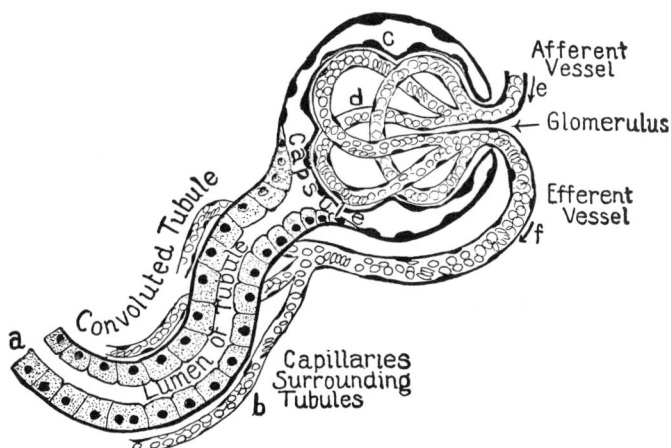

Fig. 259. Upper end of a convoluted tubule, together with a glomerulus. (a) Convoluted tubule. (b) The capillaries surrounding a tubule. (c) Bowman's capsule. (d) The capillaries which make up the glomerulus. (e) The afferent artery which divides into the capillaries (d). (f) The efferent artery which divides into the capillaries (b)—these capillaries (b) unite to form the renal veins.

zone from about 4 to 6 mm. in thickness. In it the glomeruli are arranged on little vertical arteries, like bunches of grapes, and between these rows of glomeruli are the con-

voluted tubes. The loops of Henle and the collecting tubules together comprise pyramidal-shaped structures called *pyramids,* the apices of which project into the drainage portion of the kidney.

Pelvis. The pelvis is a sac with several fingerlike outpocketings extending into the substances of the kidney; these are called *calyces,* and into them the collecting tubules open. Distally, the pelvis becomes constricted to form the ureter, and this empties into the urinary bladder. The urine, there-

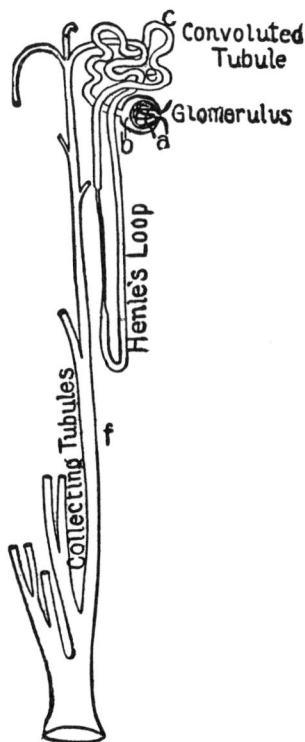

Fig. 260. The "unit" of the kidney. (a) Glomerulus. (b) Capsule. (c) Convoluted tubule. (f) Collecting tubule.

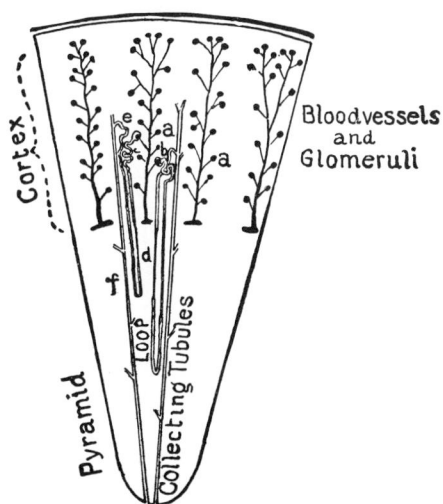

Fig. 261. Scheme of one pyramid. (a) Glomeruli arranged like a bunch of grapes on the artery. (b and e) Proximal convoluted tubules. (d) Loop of Henle. (f) Collecting tubule.

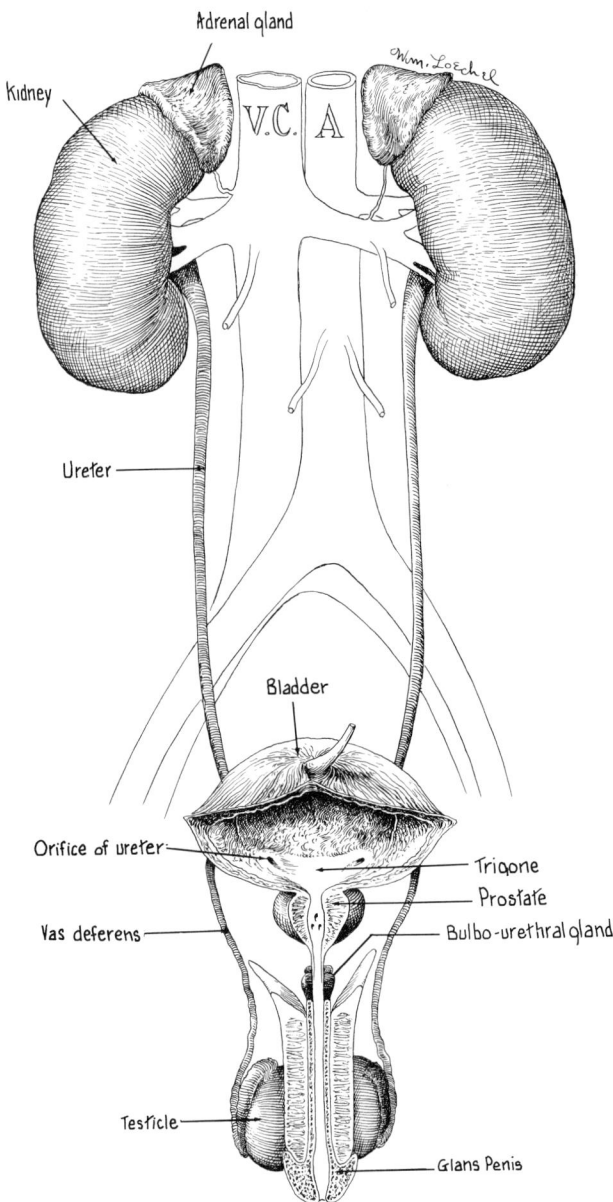

FIG. 262. Diagrammatic view of the genitourinary tract and the male reproductive system. Note the position of the adrenal gland in relation to the kidney. The pelvis of the kidney lies somewhat obscured by the renal vessels. (V.C.) Vena Cava. (A) Aorta.

fore, flows down the tubes into the pelvis of the kidney, and then down the ureter to the bladder.

EXAMINATION OF THE PATIENT

Visualization (Roentgenograms)

Roentgenograms are used to study the urinary tract in many ways. The direct examination ("flat plate") is used to determine the size and the position of the kidneys and

to visualize stones in the kidney, the ureter and the bladder (Fig. 268). Various organic compounds of iodine, when given intravenously, are excreted rapidly by the kidney in the urine. The presence of these compounds makes the urine-producing parts of the urinary tract opaque to the x-rays, so that they can be delineated on the x-ray film (*intravenous pyelogram, urogram* or occasionally mentioned as K.U.B., kidney-ureter-bladder). (See Fig. 267.) This is not only a method of outlining the urinary passages but also a test of kidney function. The position of the ureters is often marked by taking an x-ray film with ureteral catheters in place. Less frequently, the kidney pelvis and the ureters are studied by the injection of radiopaque solutions through ureteral catheters (*retrograde pyelogram*) or into the bladder through urethral catheters (*cystogram*).

Hypaque or Renografin are the most commonly used radiopaque substances. When the physician injects such a contrast medium, the patient may have a feeling of warmth, a salty taste in his mouth and flushing of the face. This soon passes as the patient is encouraged to take deep breaths. Should the patient exhibit further signs of sensitivity or untoward reaction, the physician should be notified.

By direct palpation it is frequently possible to determine the size and the movabil-ity of the kidneys. By rectal examination in the male, the prostate gland may be palpated digitally as a part of the study of the urinary difficulty that occurs when it hypertrophies in older men.

Cystoscopy

A direct method of study is by direct vision and catheterization of the ureters. This is performed through a cystoscope, which is inserted through the urethra into the bladder. By distending the bladder with sterile water, illumination from a small electric bulb permits visualization of the bladder wall and of the ureteral orifices. Small catheters may be threaded through these orifices into the ureters up to the kidney pelves to collect urine from each kidney separately for analysis and bacteriologic study. They also outline the course of the ureters in x-ray studies.

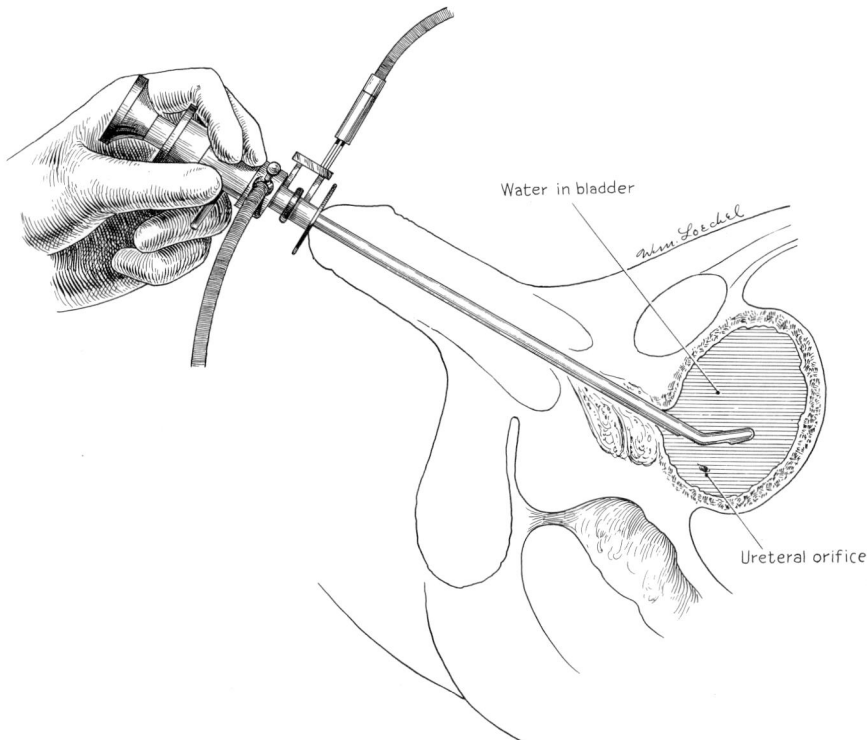

Water in bladder

Ureteral orifice

FIG. 263. Diagrammatic view of cystoscope introduced into the bladder in the male. The upper cord contains electricity for the light at the distal end of the cystoscope. The lower tubing leads from a reservoir of sterile water that is used to inflate the bladder. Of course, the entire procedure of cystoscopy is a sterile one.

Often it is the nurse who is called on to explain the meaning of a cystoscopic examination to her patient. This is a real part of preparation, because if he has no idea of the type of procedure that is to take place, his fears undoubtedly will make him tense. The preparation usually includes his drinking 1 or 2 glasses of water before going to the examining department. Often a sedative plus the instillation of a local anesthetic into the bladder may be sufficient; however, depending on the patient, it may be necessary to use spinal or general anesthesia. Since this is a sterile procedure, complete aseptic technic must be carried out.

The cystoscope is a delicate, expensive instrument that has many lenses and a small light bulb. It must be handled carefully; most cystoscopes cannot be sterilized by heat, but recently heat-resistant scopes have been made. In selecting a chemical for disinfection, the nurse must be sure that it will not react with the cement that holds the lenses in place. An aqueous germicide, such as Zephiran Chloride 1:1,000, is effective if the scope is clean and dry before immersion. Ureteral catheters that are made of plastic material can be sterilized by autoclaving. If they are made of French woven fabric, they must be disinfected with a germicide. Thorough rinsing after chemical disinfection must be carried out to prevent chemical burns of the bladder mucosa or the ureteral walls. Sterile-packaged disposable ureteral catheters now are available.

When a cystoscopy is performed, sterile water or saline may be used as an irrigating fluid to distend the bladder. Following such an examination, most patients prefer to remain in bed for the rest of the day. If there is any pain, a sedative may help. The application of a hot-water bottle to the lower abdomen is soothing. Fluids should be taken liberally.

Aortography

An outline of the kidney circulation is made possible by the injection of radiopaque material into the aorta near the renal arteries. This injection is made through a long needle that is introduced through the back while the patient is on the x-ray table; roentgenograms are made immediately. The kidney circulation thus visualized is often of great diagnostic value in searching for tumors, cysts and other renal disease.

PROBLEMS ENCOUNTERED

Retention

Retention is failure to expel the urine from the bladder. The patient is said to have residual urine when urine remains in the bladder after voiding. The problem of retention may arise in any postoperative, acutely ill, elderly or bedridden patient. The patient may develop infection as a result of retention and may even have impairment of renal function. The nurse must be on guard for symptoms of retention, or they may be overlooked. The patient may not be able to void or may have urinary frequency, dribbling or straining when voiding. Also, he may have the sensation that he has not emptied his bladder. A patient with a long-standing prostatic obstruction may accommodate to this discomfort, and if it has had a gradual onset, he will not seek help until he is forced to do so by the problem of acute retention.

How can the nurse determine if a patient has retention? By observation of the patient. The nurse should assume a position in which she can view the suprapubic area at eye level. A mass in the suprapubic area that is either visible or palpable may be a sign of retention.

The nurse should measure the volume of output in a given single voiding. Frequent voiding in small amounts may be indicative of urinary retention. Nursing measures, such as proper positioning to encourage micturition, offering fluids, placing the patient's hands in warm water, etc., should be used to assist the patient to void.

Catheterization is indicated following certain genitourinary operations, in bladder obstruction, in the performance of certain diagnostic tests, and when the patient is unable to void. However, catheterization can lead to urinary tract infection. To safeguard the patient, the following points of care are essential in urethral catheter management: (1) strict surgical asepsis should be employed; (2) the catheter should be smaller than the external urinary meatus to help to minimize trauma; (3) the catheter should be lubricated well with an appropriate lubricant; and (4) the catheter should be passed gently and skillfully.

A bladder that has been overdistended has a weakened resistance and is easily invaded by bacteria.

Frequency and Dysuria

The nurse often encounters the problems of frequency and dysuria (painful or difficult urination) in caring for patients with genitourinary conditions. Among the most common causes of frequency and dysuria are infections of the genitourinary tract. The patient complains of frequent urination accompanied by a burning sensation. To help the physician to find the cause and to eradicate the infection, the nurse must be specific in determining the time when the patient's discomfort occurs. When does the burning occur? Before voiding? During voiding? After voiding? Urethritis frequently causes burning during the act of voiding, whereas trigonitis may produce burning both before and after urination. Interstitial cystitis may cause urinary frequency and pain in the genital area. Dysuria associated with fever and chill usually is indicative of prostatitis or an infection in the upper urinary tract. Colicky pains suggest a stone or other obstruction of the urinary tract. Recording all available information associated with the patient's symptoms will help to assure a more accurate diagnosis.

Hematuria

Hematuria (blood in the urine) is a symptom of a large number of disorders that may be from systemic conditions or from localized diseases of the genitourinary tract. Acute fevers, chronic infections, blood dyscrasias and renal calculi are just a few of the causes of this condition. Hematuria associated with dysuria and frequency is encountered in acute urinary infections, whereas painless hematuria may be the first sign of a malignancy.

The presence of hematuria should be reported immediately to the physician, as it is a symptom of conditions that must be diagnosed and treated promptly. Sometimes the hematuria is microscopic, and the urine will appear to be essentially normal. When bleeding is occurring in the kidney, the urine mixes with blood as it passes down the ureter and when voided appears to be smoky. Hemorrhage occurring along the urinary tract will produce gross hematuria.

Urinary Incontinence

Urinary incontinence presents many social and psychological problems. It may result from an inflammatory condition (cystitis) and be of a temporary nature, or it may result from a more serious neurologic condition (paraplegia) and be permanent. Usually, the patient's problems with incontinence will lessen when he is making progress in other activities of daily living, such as walking. Most patients with urinary incontinence can be conditioned to gain urinary control through systematic habit-training or by the establishment of an automatic bladder. Such a program will require more nursing time than changing the patient's wet bed but the rewards of seeing a patient lose his fear of embarrassment will far outnumber the problems associated with his rehabilitation. The rehabilitation of a patient with urinary incontinence is discussed on pages 370 and 915.

NURSING RESPONSIBILITIES

Observations

The nurse's role in the treatment of renal disease entails a number of difficult problems and responsibilities. To accomplish it properly, she must equip herself with a great many facts pertaining to clinical observation, pharmacology, therapeutics, medical technology, dietetics, fluid balance and electrolyte metabolism, and she must, of course, be exceedingly well-versed in the practice of medical and surgical nursing. She must become familiar with the significance of a great many tests and with the methodology of these tests—at least to the extent of knowing what type of specimen is required in each instance, and how it should be collected, contained, preserved and stored. She must understand the significance and realize the importance of an accurate intake and output chart and daily record of the body weight as criteria for evaluating her patient's progress in response to therapy. She should understand the rationale behind each of several special diets. Drug therapy might involve the use of any one of several antibacterial agents, spasmolytic drugs, hypotensive drugs, analgesic drugs, sedative drugs, opiates, digitalis, alkaloids and diuretics. Unusual psychological disturbances of organic, as well as emotional, origin will confront her very often, and her powers of clinical observation will be challenged by a great variety of symptoms and signs that reflect pathology in every organ system in the body.

Fluid and Electrolytic Balance

A major nursing problem in caring for patients with renal disorders is the maintenance of the fluid and the electrolyte balance. The nurse must be astute in observing these patients and absolutely accurate in the recording of data. Every patient will have a fluid intake-output chart on which the nurse will record all fluids ingested, regardless of their route, and the urine excreted. A 4-hour temperature chart and daily weight chart also will be kept to assist the doctor in calculating the amount of fluid that the patient may receive. Other factors to be noted on the patient's record are complaints of thirst, signs of dehydration, e.g., excessive thirst, parched lips and tongue, dry and loose skin. Edema also should be reported if and when observed. Any directions regarding the intake of fluids or loss thereof must be understood thoroughly by the nurse and painstakingly explained in detail to other members of the team caring for the patient. In supervising intravenous therapy, the nurse will be responsible for adjusting the flow rate in accordance with the physician's orders. In order to keep a check on the electrolyte balance, the doctor will order repeated blood examinations. The nurse must prepare the patient for this testing by explaining that these studies are necessary to help the doctor to plan the treatment of the condition and to be certain that the needed elements in the blood are maintained at a satisfactory level.

Maintaining Adequate Drainage

It is necessary for the patient with a disease of the urinary system to have proper drainage of waste products. A regulated diet and medications will aid in establishing the desired chemical and electrolyte balance, whereas proper balance between intake and output aids in providing the necessary dilution and elimination of waste products.

Drainage of the urinary system is accomplished usually by the use of catheters, whether inserted directly into the kidney pelvis, the ureter or the bladder. The specific purpose for which a catheter is used, as well as the length of time it will be in place, establishes the criteria for selecting the proper catheter. The nurse should know where and why a catheter is used in each patient. Catheters come in an array of sizes and lengths and may have one or more openings placed in various positions near the tip. A catheter may be made of hard or soft rubber, woven fabric, metal, glass or plastic. The tip may be opened or closed; its shape may be mushroom (Pezzer), winged (Malecot) or simply round and blunted.

A catheter may drain directly into dressings or, more commonly, be attached to an adapter and drainage tubing which leads to a receptacle. Principles of physics having to do with gravity, fluid flow and pressure need to be reviewed in order to maintain adequate and safe outflow of drainage for the patient.

Improper drainage will occur when (1) kinks or twists exist in the tubing, (2) loops collect pools of drainage, and (3) any part of the system has been cleaned improperly, and deposits have accumulated.*

Disposable plastic drainage sets are available which obviate the need for cleaning and reusing equipment. Drainage bottles should be cleaned daily. If tops are used, and an air vent is provided on drainage bottles, odors can be controlled.

A catheter or drainage tubing may become clogged by a blood clot or a mucous plug. To check the patency of the system, the catheter may be disconnected from the connecting tube and observed for free-flowing drainage. If none appears, offer the patient 2 glasses of fluid to drink and recheck the catheter as described in 30 minutes. If

---

* After use, clean catheters by soaking in cold water and a detergent. Force 5 per cent acetic acid through the lumens to dissolve urate crystals; use hydrogen peroxide to dissolve dried blood. Rinse thoroughly before sterilizing.

drainage does not appear, irrigate the catheter (if there is an order); otherwise, notify the physician.

When an indwelling catheter is desired, the Foley catheter is preferred. This catheter has an inflatable rubber bag near its tip. After it is inserted into the bladder, the bag is inflated with water or air. The inflated bag is too large to pass through the vesical orifice, and the catheter will remain in the bladder without other fixation until the rubber bag is deflated. The nurse will note that one outlet of the catheter leads to the bag. Before these catheters are sterilized for use, she must check the bags to see that they do not leak. The bag is inflated to the desired amount (usually 5 ml.) by the physician after he inserts the catheter. A clamp, a rubber band or a "self-seal" is used to keep the fluid from running out of the bag. Most catheters used today are disposable and come in sterile packages. (See Fig. 264.)

The Foley catheter may be 2-way or 3-way. The 2-way catheter allows for drainage from one channel. The other outlet is for the purpose of inflating the bag. The 3-way catheter allows saline to flow into the bladder by one route and to return to the drainage bottle by the other channel. The larger of these two pathways is for drainage. The third opening is to permit water or air to inflate the bag near the tip of the catheter. The 3-way Foley catheter can allow for constant bladder irrigation. The flow of saline is regulated so that the number of drops per minute can be seen in the glass Murphy drip. Usually, from 30 to 60 drops are sufficient per minute.

PROBLEMS AFFECTING THE KIDNEYS

Acute Renal Failure

Renal failure results from damage to the kidneys. It may develop slowly or suddenly. Acute renal failure, which is manifested by sudden oliguria or anuria, may be caused by acute glomerulonephritis; by shock, which produces tubular ischemia and impaired renal circulation; by chemical poisoning (carbon-tetrachloride) or drug poisoning (salicylates). Following severe transfusion reactions, the hemoglobin filtering through the kidney glomeruli becomes concentrated

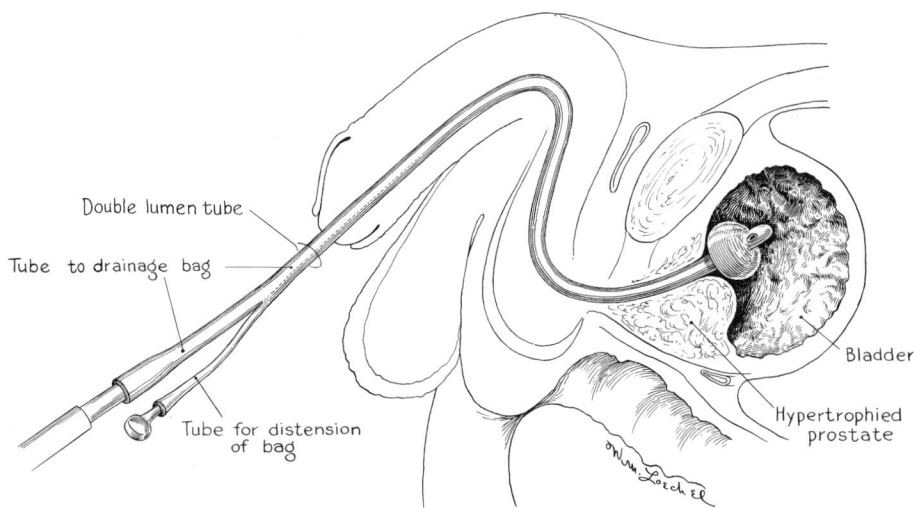

Fig. 264. Diagrammatic drawing to show Foley catheter in place. This is a two-way catheter. One part leads to the drainage bottle; the other part, shown plugged with a peg, is used to inflate the rubber balloon at the end of the catheter. After a known amount of air or water is injected into the balloon, the tube is plugged with a peg or folded upon itself and held with a rubber band to prevent the escape of the medium from distending the bag. Only when the catheter is withdrawn is this tube opened.

in the kidney tubules to such a degree that precipitation occurs and may impair or halt the excretion of urine. Renal failure also follows burns, crushing injuries and infections, such as septic abortions. The kidneys become swollen and edematous, and the epithelial cells in the tubules may undergo necrosis.

The patient appears to be critically ill. He is lethargic with persistent nausea, vomiting, and diarrhea; his skin and mucous membranes are dry from dehydration; his breath may have the odor of urine. Drowsiness, headache, muscle twitching and convulsions are the central nervous system manifestations that are present in varying degrees. The urinary output is scanty and has a low specific gravity. All tests show depressed renal function; there is an elevation of the blood urea nitrogen, nonprotein nitrogen and serum potassium levels.

The kidney has a remarkable ability to recover from insult. Therefore, the objectives of treatment are to remove the cause and then to maintain the patient in as normal a state as possible, so that the repair of renal tissue and the restoration of renal function can take place.

During the oliguric state the fluid intake is adjusted to provide *only* for the body needs. The nurse keeps a careful record of intake and output and the patient's daily weight. To maintain the fluid balance, the patient is given approximately 400 ml. of fluid daily, plus the amount lost from urine, vomitus, perspiration, etc. Since the patient is not excreting the end products of catabolism, there is an excessive accumulation of these products in the blood. Therefore, the diet given is low in protein and high in pure carbohydrates to aid in preventing ketosis and to minimize protein breakdown. Testosterone (25 to 50 mg. daily) also may be given to minimize protein catabolism.

If the serum potassium reaches a dangerous level (6 mEq. per liter), cation-exchange resins are given orally or by retention enema to decrease the serum potassium.

Since sepsis is a serious complication, all measures to provide environmental asepsis are instituted. No one with a cold or an infection should be permitted in the patient's room. He should be turned frequently to help prevent pulmonary and skin complications. The nurse must watch for circulatory complications (pulmonary edema) that may develop from the excessive accumulation of body fluids. The elevation of serum potassium can produce cardiac arrhythmias and cardiac standstill. There may be a tendency to erythrocyte destruction, impaired red blood cell formation and platelet deficiencies. The patient should be watched for evidences of bleeding.

The oliguric phase of acute renal failure may last from 12 to 14 days and is followed by the diuretic phase. The patient begins to increase his urinary output until he is voiding 2,000 to 2,500 ml. daily. Blood chemistry evaluations are made to determine the amount of sodium, potassium and water needed for replacement. After the diuretic phase, the patient is placed on a high-protein and high-caloric diet. He is encouraged to resume his activities gradually, since he will have muscular weakness from excessive catabolism.

Dialysis. If the patient with renal failure does not respond to conservative methods of treatment, some method of dialysis may be performed to remove the waste products and to maintain the patient until renal recovery takes place. Methods of dialysis include hemodialysis and peritoneal dialysis. The main indication for dialysis is a high and rising level of serum potassium.

There are several types of equipment used. Each uses the principle of a cellophane membrane that is placed between the patient's blood and a wash solution. The cellophane membrane has pores that are similar to those of the glomerular capillaries. Blood is removed from the patient's radial or brachial artery and pumped through the cellophane tube immersed in the rinsing fluid or bath of electrolyte solution. The nonprotein nitrogen retention products pass through the semipermeable membrane of the cellophane tube into the bath fluid. Thus the end products of protein catabolism, water and exogenous poisons are removed from the blood. The blood continuously recirculates from the patient through the dialyzing tube for a period of 4 to 7 hours. The temperature-controlled bath is changed intermittently to avoid the accumulation of toxins.

After this treatment the patient is watched for evidences of bleeding, as most patients are heparinized before dialysis to prevent the blood from clotting during the procedure. The cutdown site is observed for signs of phlebitis. The patient's vital signs as well as the volume and the appearance of his urine are recorded and reported.

Peritoneal Dialysis. Hemodialysis requires a trained team and an effective dialyzing machine. When these are not available, or when the patient's condition does not permit transportation to a dialyzing center, peritoneal dialysis can be used. In this technic an appropriate sterile dialyzing fluid is introduced into the peritoneal cavity at intervals. The surface area of the peritoneum acts as the semipermeable membrane. Several liters are infused rapidly by needle paracentesis and a plastic catheter. The fluid generally remains in the peritoneal cavity for 1 hour and then is drained by siphonage. As soon as the peritoneal cavity is emptied, fresh solution is reinfused. A dialysis may require from 20 to 25 such exchanges, and the procedure usually takes from 12 to 36 hours.

The nurse should have the patient empty his bladder before the treatment is started. During peritoneal dialysis his vital signs are taken and recorded regularly. The nurse observes and records the appearance of the drainage fluids, the patient's general condition, and the volume of the intake and the output.

Chronic Renal Failure

Every nurse should be acquainted with the characteristic signs of renal failure, including the early signs. Although sometimes its onset is sudden, in the majority of patients it begins with one or more of a group of symptoms—lethargy, headache, drowsiness, vomiting, restlessness, mental wandering, foul breath, etc.—which may persist for weeks. If active treatment is begun then, the renal failure may disappear. Otherwise, these symptoms become more marked, and others appear: the patient gradually or suddenly becomes increasingly more and more drowsy; the respiration becomes Cheyne-

Stokes in character; a deep coma develops, often with convulsions, which may be mere muscle twitchings or severe spasms quite similar to those of epilepsy. A white powdery substance, composed chiefly of urates, appears on the skin, the "uremic frost." Unless treatment is successful, death soon follows.

Treatment and Nursing Care. The treatment and nursing care of renal failure should be prompt and vigorous; therefore, the nurse must report immediately any signs that she might observe. By the administration of sodium chloride intravenously (approximately 8 Gm. daily by mouth or the equivalent in parenterally administered fluid), an attempt is made to maintain the alkaline reserve which is rapidly being depleted by the accumulated acids not being excreted normally; by means of forcing fluids and intravenous hypertonic glucose solution an attempt is made to stimulate diuresis. Fluid and salt intake may be restricted to reduce the accumulation of fluid in the tissues. A careful record of intake and output must be maintained, and any change in the urinary output must be reported immediately. These patients should have very special protection from infections. No one should be allowed contact with a patient who has the slightest indication of an upper respiratory infection. This first sign of a cold, or even a suspicion on the part of the patient that he might be acquiring a cold, should be reported to the physician at once. All usual nursing measures should be carried out meticulously, especially those designed to protect him from chilling.

Early evidences of cerebral irritation should be reported at once. These may vary from slight twitching or headache to delirium. The patient must be protected from self-injury during involuntary movements, and it is advisable to pad metal crib beds or use canvas sides for the bed, which should be in place whenever the patient is not under direct observation. The onset of convulsions should be recorded, as well as their duration, course, extent and general effect on the patient. The doctor should be notified at once, and suitable therapy should be initiated. Magnesium sulfate injected intramuscularly or intravenously has beneficial effects both as a sedative for the central nervous system and as a diuretic. Lumbar puncture, draining the spinal fluid if it is under pressure, will afford temporary relief. Such treatment may restore the patient to consciousness, and, if so, the immediate danger is past.

Acute Glomerulonephritis

Glomerulonephritis, or Bright's disease, refers to a disease in which the kidneys are seriously damaged and partially destroyed by an inflammatory process that originates as an immune response on the part of the kidneys. The stimulus of that reaction in most cases is a beta hemolytic streptococcus infection of the throat, which ordinarily precedes the onset of the nephritis by an interval of 2 to 3 weeks. It is assumed that the kidney receives its first exposure to the bacterial antigens in the form of toxins which are excreted into the urine. In glomerulonephritis all of the renal tissues are badly injured, and they react to their injuries by progressive inflammatory, degenerative and healing processes. All the several renal tissues—glomeruli, tubules, blood vessels and stroma—are affected in every form of glomerulonephritis, but in each the tissues are involved in varying degrees.

All nephritic changes leave their scars. The process, once started, tends to progress, and the dangers of exacerbations are great. The striking clinical picture of late glomerulonephritis is less often the endstage of one continuous process of long duration than it is the result of a series of repeated injuries extending over a period of years.

In acute glomerulonephritis the kidneys are large, swollen, fatty and congested. An exudate of blood plasma, red corpuscles and leukocytes escapes from the capillaries and infiltrates the kidney substance. The renal cells are so injured that they cannot do their work properly; many of them die.

Acute glomerulonephritis is predominantly a disease of youth. The cases which seem to have developed later are usually acute exacerbations of a quiescent glomerulonephritis already present. Acute glomerulonephritis in children usually develops in association with an acute upper respiratory infection, tonsillitis, scarlet fever or, indeed, any of the hemolytic streptococcal infections.

It may appear also as a complication of infection caused by other organisms, particularly the hemolytic *Staphylococcus aureus*. The time relation is usually quite constant, that is, the infection precedes the first of the nephritic signs by approximately 2 weeks.

Symptoms. The symptoms of acute glomerulonephritis are extremely variable. Sometimes the disease begins suddenly, and even violently, with fever, occasionally accompanied by a chill, headache, dizziness, nausea and vomiting, pains in the back, rapidly progressive swelling of the face and the feet—and such weakness that the patient cannot walk. The symptoms are seldom as definite as this, and acute glomerulonephritis is a good illustration of a dangerous disease which sometimes progresses to serious damage before the person suspects that he is sick. The child may feel merely tired, complain of headache and show only slight edema of the eyelids, while his urine shows every sign of a severe acute glomerulonephritis.

On the other hand, the acute exacerbations and unsuspected chronic glomerulonephritis may be mistaken for primary acute attacks. Although often uremic convulsions or sudden death may be the first indication of the chronic glomerulonephritis, yet the condition, which has been developing for years, may be manifested first by an acute attack that the patient believes to be his first. In the majority of cases, however, patients with acute exacerbations have from the first noticed that both ankles swell a little, that the face is pale, and that the eyelids are a little puffy. Otherwise, they may feel so well that they convince themselves that these signs are unimportant. Some of these patients have visual disturbances for a while, yet without evident lesions in the eyes; most develop a retinal hemorrhage or an albuminuric retinitis. In severe cases symptoms of psychosis, stupor, vomiting, convulsions and coma may develop. The arterial blood pressure usually is elevated.

The urine will be scanty and bloody; there may even be none (anuria) for a day or two. Usually, however, the patient early in the disease passes from 50 to 200 ml. daily of a highly colored cloudy urine with a specific gravity between 1.020 and 1.025 (that is, low, considering the total amount) and with a thick sediment of red blood cells, leukocytes and all kinds of casts. This urine contains large amounts of albumin.

As the patient improves, the amount of urine increases, whereas the albumin and the sediment diminish. Occasionally, perhaps oftener than we realize, the patient recovers entirely. Some patients become severely uremic and progress to a fatal termination within weeks or months, despite every form of therapy that can be offered; others, after a period of apparent recovery, insidiously develop chronic glomerulonephritis.

Treatment and Nursing Care. The treatment and nursing care of acute glomerulonephritis, or an acute flare-up of a more chronic condition, should begin with rest. This includes not only physical rest in bed but also the elimination of all worry and all causes of discomfort and restlessness. Evidences of cerebral edema indicate prompt spinal fluid drainage and dehydrating measures: parenteral magnesium sulfate acts as an excellent diuretic, as well as a sedative for the central nervous system, in patients with convulsions.

Pulmonary edema may occur as a result of fluid retention and cardiac failure, the basis for the latter in many patients being the rapid development of arterial hypertension, which subjects the left ventricle to a very real and unaccustomed strain. Its treatment varies in no essential respect from the routines applied in other types of cases, except for the use of mercurial diuretics, which are considered to be contraindicated in acute glomerulonephritis. The patient should be sedated, placed in an orthopneic position and digitalized, oxygen inhalations being supplied, if necessary. The patient should be in a warm, well-ventilated room, protected from drafts. The sodium and the water intake should be reduced to a minimum, and the stools should be kept loose with saline cathartics.

DIET. In order to rest the kidney during the acute phase, the diet is low in protein. The intake of sodium is also limited, depending on the degree of edema present. The intake of fluids likewise should be restricted, a maximum volume of 1,200 ml. per day being permissible, depending on the degree

of water retention, until signs of progressive recovery are evident. The chief source of nutrition in this early period may be foods composed largely of carbohydrates and fats. Thirst may be relieved by ice water, sipped in small amounts or furnished as a mouth rinse. With improvement in the patient's renal status, many of these restrictions may be relaxed, and his personal preferences and reactions may be heeded more closely in the planning of his diet.

DETAILED CARE. An accurate daily record of the patient's weight, fluid intake and urinary output is of value in estimating the renal function and as a basis for rational therapy. The total amount and the frequency of voided specimens are recorded faithfully by the nurse daily, and samples are saved for laboratory examination, which includes the determination of specific gravity, albumin and constituents of the sediment.

The condition of the skin and the surface membranes is important. Bath water should be sufficiently warm to bring a glow to the skin. Fresh air is desirable, but chilling definitely is to be avoided. Frequent massaging of the skin and changing of the patient's position in bed are recommended strongly. If there has been marked weight loss, debility or edema, skin care is of greater importance because of the susceptibility of such patients to acquire decubitus ulcers. Oral hygiene never must be neglected.

Regular elimination is ensured by means of mineral oil and, if necessary, tap-water enemas.

A detailed therapeutic regimen is to be anticipated in these patients. The nurse must assist in securing the complete cooperation of the patient and ensure that treatments are carried out properly. She may be involved in special diagnostic procedures, including the P.S.P. urine excretion test, urine concentration, blood chemistry examinations, intravenous or retrograde pyelograms, cardiovascular function tests and others. She must also watch the patient for signs of complications such as cardiac failure, pulmonary edema or cerebral edema. These patients will have their vital signs recorded every 4 hours and any significant change reported immediately.

Convalescence. When the patient loses

his edema, and the urine is free from albumin, casts and red blood cells, he is allowed to sit up, then to get out of bed (wrapped warmly), and thenceforth to become increasingly active. However, he should avoid overexertion and exposure to cold for years. Should he contract a respiratory infection, he should go to bed and treat it seriously. A woman who has had glomerulonephritis requires special observation and attention during pregnancy.

Prevention. Prevention of glomerulonephritis may be a matter primarily of avoidance of upper respiratory infections, as well as other acute and chronic infections, and of giving adequate treatment, should they occur. It includes the control of the spread of these diseases by early reporting, isolation, use of prophylactic immunizations and antibiotic treatment, wherever indicated.

Social Aspects. The social significance devolves from the prolonged convalescence and continued ill health, which constitute economic problems. These patients have difficulty in securing insurance policies, for life expectancy in the nephritic group as a whole is materially shortened.

Chronic Glomerulonephritis

Chronic glomerulonephritis is assumed to have its onset in the same manner as does the acute form of the disease and to represent a milder type of antigen-antibody reaction, but one so mild that it can be overlooked easily. After repeated occurrences of these reactions the kidneys are reduced to as little as one fifth of their normal size, consisting largely of fibrous tissue. Their cortex shrinks to a layer of from 1 to 2 mm. in thickness, and in some areas it is gone entirely. The surface of the kidney is rough, for the renal tissue disappears in irregular patches, and bands of scar tissue by contracting distort the remaining cortex. The glomeruli suffer greatly. Many of them, and their convoluted tubes as well, have disappeared. The branches of the renal artery are thickened.

Symptoms. The symptoms of chronic glomerulonephritis are variable. Some patients with severe grades of this disease have no symptoms at all for a long time. They may discover their condition as the result of an application for life insurance, when the blood pressure is found to be elevated. Or it may be suggested during a routine eye examination, when vascular changes or hemorrhages are found. The first intimation others have is a sudden, severe nosebleed, a stroke, paralysis or uremic convulsion. Most patients merely notice that their feet are slightly swollen at night, but never markedly, unless an acute exacerbation of the nephritis is in progress. The majority of all patients have also such general symptoms as loss of weight and strength, increasing irritability and nocturia. Headaches, dizziness and digestive disturbances are common.

If these patients are examined carefully, it is likely that the heart will be found to be considerably enlarged, the arteries sclerotic and tortuous, the blood pressure high, and the radial artery resistant because of the arteriosclerosis. Epistaxis, hemorrhages from the lungs and the kidneys and into the retina and the cerebrum are common.

Later in the disease these patients do not "feel well"; they lose weight and strength; they have severe headaches, shortness of breath and dyspnea at night, suggesting bronchial asthma. Still later, Cheyne-Stokes respiration and the symptoms of chronic congestion of the gastrointestinal canal may appear. The heart dilates, fibrillates, pulsus alternans and anginal pains appear, all of which indicate that the damaged heart cannot maintain an adequate output against such high arterial pressure. Various grades of edema develop, depending on the degree to which plasma albumin is decreased and on the severity of heart failure.

The examination of the eye grounds is most important. These patients complain of black spots before their eyes, flashes of light, dimness of vision and transitory blindness. On examination, thickening of the retinal arteries is seen, also retinal hemorrhages and exudates, and edema of the disks. The skin is dry, with a tendency to eczema and pruritus. Cachexia, with secondary anemia, is common. Later, cardiac edema, often confused with renal edema, and the symptoms of renal failure may appear.

Among the common symptoms of chronic glomerulonephritis are polyuria, frequent micturition, particularly at night, and a fixation of a specific gravity of the urine, that is, the urine does not show the normal variability of concentration due to what is eaten, drunk or done, but regardless of the patient's activities, it is all of practically the same composition. It never contains more than a trace of albumin, except during the occasional acute exacerbations, and this may be absent for weeks or be present only in the afternoon. Also, the urine contains so few casts that they may be difficult to find. Occasionally, red blood cells appear in the urine. Early in many cases the renal function tests indicate abnormal function: the inulin-Diodrast clearance demonstrates the defect earliest. Eventually, there is evidence of marked renal decompensation by even the grossest tests.

In the so-called *nephrotic stage* of chronic glomerulonephritis the picture is striking. The skin has a pale, pasty color; often the whole body is swollen with edema, and almost always the face, the lower extremities and the dependent parts are so affected. The eyes are almost closed by the puffed lids, edema of the retina may interfere with vision, and the limbs appear to be twice their normal size. Often the finger can be pushed fully a quarter of an inch into the skin of the

legs. This is referred to as *pitting edema.* Let an extremity hang down over the side of the bed, and more water accumulates, making it still larger. The fluid collects in the portion of the body that is in the lowest position. This is called *dependent edema.* These patients are truly "waterlogged." Fluid collects also in the abdominal cavity (ascites), which greatly distends the abdomen. It appears in one or both pleural cavities (hydrothorax, fluid in the chest); the patient is short of breath and must sit upright (orthopnea). Fluid may collect in the pericardial sac (pericarditis with effusion), and the patient is in consequence short of breath, cyanotic and has a weak pulse, especially during inspiration (paradoxical pulse). Repeated chest taps may be necessary to relieve the dyspnea.

Prognosis. The prognosis at this stage of the disease is poor. A few patients will improve, and they may enjoy fair health for many years. However, the great majority fail progressively and die in 1 or 2 years, often in a uremic condition.

Of importance in judging the progress of the disease is the weight, the red blood cell counts (there is danger of progressive anemia) and the blood pressure. One should

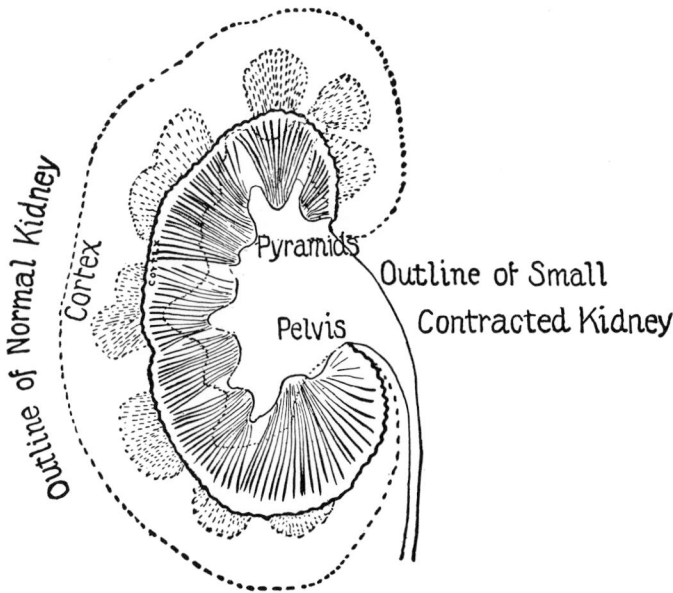

Fig. 265. Nephrosclerosis.

watch also the blood urea nitrogen and phenolsulfonphthalein curves.

Treatment and Nursing Care. The treatment of the ambulatory patient with chronic nephritis is entirely nonspecific and symptomatic, depending on the situation that presents itself at any given time. Thus, if hypertension is present, treatment is directed toward sparing the cardiovascular system; if chronic uremia is developing, toward readjustment of the diet and the fluid intake in an effort to maintain as normal a metabolic situation as possible. If there is apparent chronic renal tract infection, a possible factor in producing glomerulonephritis, steps should be taken to detect it and to treat it. This condition is apt to last from 10 to 15 years, and the patient naturally would insist on remaining active. Reasonable compromises must be made in the management of each patient; not only should the factors which are apt to precipitate acute exacerbations of his illness be borne in mind but also the total welfare of the individual.

Colds are to be avoided, and any infection of the nose, the throat or the mouth should be treated carefully. Climate is most important. A warm, agreeable one may prolong life considerably. Moderate exercise in the open air is important. Hydrotherapy in the form of warm baths gives great comfort. The heart condition must be watched, and cardiac efficiency improved. Constipation should be avoided. The rule for this patient's life is "temperance in all things."

Treatment of patients with marked edema presents many difficulties. The patient is elevated in bed and made as comfortable as possible. He should be encouraged to drink as much fluid as he can eliminate, the weight being carefully followed for evidence of increasing fluid retention. Sodium restriction, however, is extremely important. The nurse should watch for all symptoms which suggest renal failure. Assistance should be secured in moving or lifting the patient so that he is protected from an accidental fall, and so that he may be relieved of any exertion in turning. There should be no tugging or undue pressure on edematous areas.

If there is evidence of cardiac failure, digitalis is given to aid the heart. If anemia is present, the patient should receive iron, although little response will be forthcoming so long as renal failure continues.

If the nonprotein nitrogen blood level is normal, the diet should contain protein in excess of 80 Gm. daily because of the theo-

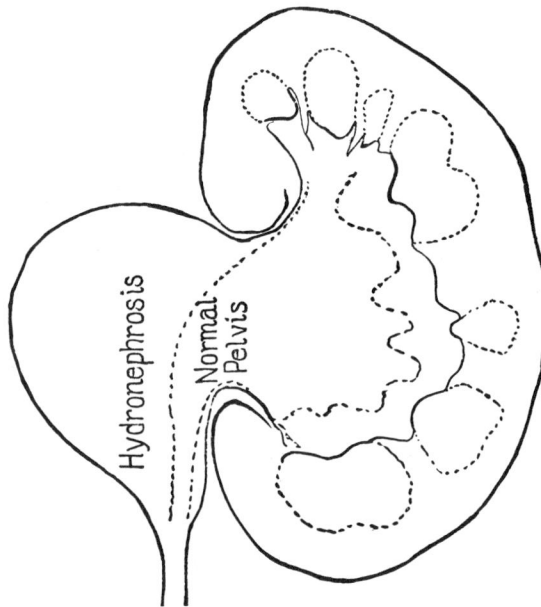

FIG. 266. Hydronephrosis.

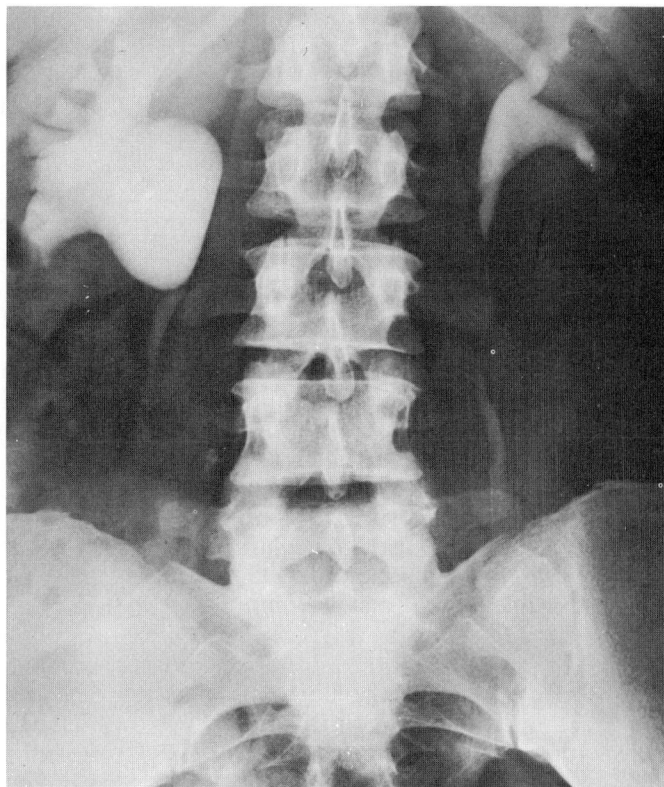

retic value of a normal high-protein intake as a means of combating hypoproteinemia. Because of the proteinuria, the diet is high in protein to make up for this protein loss. The amount of protein intake depends on the degree of proteinuria present.

Nephrosclerosis

Nephrosclerosis is hardening or sclerosis of the kidney and usually is seen as a result of renal hypertension.

Malignant nephrosclerosis, as opposed to benign nephrosclerosis, though different in degree, merely represents the situation presented in the section headed Chronic Glomerulonephritis. Patients with the malignant type progress rapidly to a fatal termination through the stages of albuminuria, increasing hypertension, failing renal function, and eyeground changes and die usually within a few months. The factor responsible for this termination may be uremia, congestive heart failure due to hypertensive heart disease, or a cerebral accident. It occurs most com-

monly from the 3rd to the 5th decade. So far as one can state at the present time, it is a generalized vascular disease that starts in the kidney and finally involves the entire vascular tree. It is always difficult to decide to what extent the vascular damage is responsible for, and to what extent it is a result of, the hypertension.

Cases of benign nephrosclerosis (Fig. 265) are most apt to be found in older age groups. These individuals rarely complain of renal symptoms, although for years the urine has a low and fixed specific gravity and contains a small amount of albumin and an occasional hyaline or granular cast. Only late in the disease does renal insufficiency appear. This type of renal disease is the result of a peculiar type of renal arteriosclerosis, which in a patchy manner produces wedge-shaped areas where glomeruli and tubules have largely disappeared, alternating with other areas where the renal units are practically intact—indeed, are able to function more actively than normal. The diffuse glomerular changes and the evidences of inflammation seen in glomerulonephritis are absent.

Hydronephrosis

Obstruction to the normal flow of urine will produce a damming up of urine with a resultant back pressure on the kidney. If the obstruction is in the urethra or the bladder, the back pressure affects both kidneys, but if the obstruction is in the ureter, due to stone or kink, only one kidney is damaged.

The pelvis of the kidney (including the calyces) is the wide sac into which the urine from the pyramids is poured, and by narrowing to a small tube it becomes the ureter. The pelvis has thin walls whose inner surface is lined with the same type of mucous membrane as the ureter and the bladder.

The pelvis of the kidney and its calyces will be distended by the partly dammed-back urine when the ureter is somewhat obstructed.

If in such a case no inflammation is present and the fluid is clear, the condition is called *hydronephrosis* (Figs 266, 267).

To cause dilatation of the pelvis of the kidney, the obstruction of urine must be gradual, partial or intermittent, but not sudden and total, for such would cause immediate anuria and therefore no distention at all of the pelvis.

Partial or intermittent obstruction may be due to a renal stone which has formed in the renal pelvis but has dropped into the ureter and blocked it. Again, the obstruction may be due to a tumor of some other abdominal or pelvic organ pressing on the ureter, or to bands of scar tissue resulting from an abscess or inflammation near the ureter, which pinch it. The disorder may be due to an odd angle at which the ureter leaves the renal pelvis, or to an unusual position of the kidney, favoring a ureteral twist or kink. In elderly males the most common cause is urethral obstruction at the bladder outlet by an enlarged prostate.

Whatever the cause, if the fluid accumulates intermittently in the renal pelvis, it distends this and its calyces. If the obstructions are frequent, and the pressure which develops is high, in time atrophy of the kidney results, which causes the kidney to spread out into a thin cystlike shell. If, however, the pressure of the fluid is never very high, the kidney may not suffer much, although its dilated pelvis may almost fill the whole abdomen. In cases of hydronephrosis, the patient may scracely know of his trouble, or he may have pains which are severe only when the fluid in the pelvis is under pressure.

Treatment. The treatment is to discover the cause of the obstruction and, if possible, to remove it. Sometimes the urine must be drained by catheter or by operation. If the cause is a tumor or bands of adhesions, removal is indicated. If the cause is benign prostatic hypertrophy, the prostate may have to be extirpated, partially or wholly, depending on the patient's condition and the degree of obstruction. When one kidney only is involved, and its function is nil, nephrectomy may be performed.

Nephroptosis

Nephroptosis, or movable kidney, is a condition found chiefly in thin, long-waisted women from 30 to 50 years of age. The pad of fat which normally surrounds the kidney is absent. The posture is usually poor, and the abdominal muscles are relaxed, the result of which produces a weakness and a dragging pain in the loin. At times the kidney may sag so that it almost reaches the pelvis when the patient stands (floating kidney). This abnormal movability may produce torsion or kinks in the ureter; acute pain, nausea and vomiting, and at times chills and fever may be produced by this obstruction to the ureter. These attacks are known as *Dietl's crises*. The attack often may be relieved by having the patient lie down with a pillow placed under the hips or by manipulating the kidney.

Treatment. The treatment of the condition is directed toward building up the general health. Belts often are applied to give abdominal support. One attack of Dietl's crisis warrants a complete urologic study (cystoscopy, pyelography, urography). If obstruction or infection is present from a ptotic kidney, operative intervention may be necessary. The kidney is fixed in position by sutures in an operation called *nephropexy*.

Urinary Tract Infections and Pyelonephritis

There is some basis for every case of urinary tract infection. The majority are ascending infections, and the infection is favored by some mechanical defect, such as a congenital anomaly or a ureteral stone in the urinary tract, which produces stasis of urine. Permanent correction of this situation in many patients must entail more than mere temporary sterilization of the urine; it will necessitate careful search for and, if possible, removal of the mechanical defect.

Pyelitis signifies infection of the kidney pelvis. Pyelonephritis is a bacterial infection of one or both kidneys that affects both the interstitial renal tissue and the renal pelvis.

The walls of the renal pelvis are lined internally with a mucous membrane that continues down the ureter to the bladder. When inflamed, this mucous membrane swells, its surface cells are discarded, its blood vessels become congested and may bleed, and pus pours out into the pelvis. When the disease is chronic, practically all this mucous membrane is destroyed, and then the pelvis is like any other abscess. Later, the ureter may become obstructed, and then the pus sac may become distended to large size (*pyonephrosis*). Such an abscess may rupture, or the pus within it may thicken into a solid mass.

In kidney infections the urine at first is cloudy because of the abundance of epithelial cells, mucus, pus and blood, and also, when its reaction is alkaline, because of the phosphate precipitate. When the cause is tuberculosis, however, the pyuria is acid. Some patients with pyelitis may on one day void a perfectly clear urine, since the ureter from the diseased pelvis is blocked. Therefore, no kidney trouble is suspected. Then on the next day the urine may contain pus which has escaped from the diseased side. Should one kidney be entirely destroyed by disease, the other kidney, if normal, is quite able to do the work of both.

The causes of infection are many. They include infection by *E. coli* especially, also *M. tuberculosis* and other pyogenic bacteria. One must remember that bacteria (and some of them quite virulent ones) frequently get into the body and are circulated by the blood stream to the kidneys; these they sometimes, but not always, infect. However, the kidney's resistance to these organisms may be lowered by any condition that imposes an obstruction to its urinary drainage: a stone in its pelvis; a renal cancer; a twist in, or a tumor pressing on, the ureter; any congenital abnormality of the ureter or the bladder; or an enlarged prostate obstructing the urethra. In another very important group of cases an inflammation starts in the bladder and travels up the ureter to the pelvis. Pyelitis is most common in young girls and in pregnant women. Its greatest importance lies in the possible complication of this disease by pyelonephritis, wherein the infection spreads to the kidney, with occasionally serious results.

Symptoms. The symptoms of pyelitis and pyelonephritis vary greatly. In many patients they are spectacular, with high fever, a high leukocyte count and severe chills. In others there will be pain in the back due to the distention of the pelvis, but this is rare. In still other cases, however, there are no conspicuous symptoms.

Diagnosis. The diagnosis is made from repeated systematic examinations of the urine, combined with cystoscopy, to be certain that both ureters are functioning. In all cases the urine should be examined for tubercle bacilli, and a roentgenogram should be taken to see if there is ureteral obstruction, or if the renal pelvis contains a stone.

Treatment. The treatment will depend on the cause.

Any obstruction of the urinary system must be corrected, as these conditions will perpetuate the infection. If no obstruction is present, a high fluid intake is encouraged to prevent urinary stasis.

A urine culture is obtained to find the pathogens. The sensitivity test helps in the selection of an appropriate antibiotic. Throughout the course of treatment it is necessary to obtain repeated urine cultures and sensitivity tests as a given antibiotic may lose its effectiveness.

Specific antibiotic therapy (Furadantin, penicillin, streptomycin, Chloromycetin) is continued until the infection is eliminated completely. The sulfonamides, with an unusually wide range of activity, ease of administration and ready availability, are employed extensively with this type of patient, the usual dosage being approximately equivalent to 1 Gm. per liter of urine output per day.

Carbuncle of the Kidney

Carbuncle of the kidney is an infection of hematogenous origin which is caused usually by the staphylococcus. It usually follows a cutaneous boil or carbuncle and is characterized by fever, malaise, and dull pain in the region of the kidney. This type of infection, if recognized, usually subsides with chemotherapy and penicillin.

Perinephric Abscess

Perinephric abscess is an abscess in the fatty tissue about the kidney which may arise secondary to an infection of the kidney or as a hematogenous infection originating in foci elsewhere in the body. The symptoms often are acute in onset, with chills, fever, high leukocytosis and other signs of suppuration. Locally, there is tenderness posteriorly in the loin.

Treatment. The treatment consists of incision and drainage of the abscess by a lumbar incision. The use of suitable antibiotics is a standard procedure.

In the postoperative care the nurse should place the patient in the dorsal position. Because the drainage often is profuse, frequent changes of the outer dressings may be necessary.

Tuberculosis of the Kidney and the Genitourinary Tract

Clinically, tuberculosis of the kidney is uncommon, although microscopic lesions in the kidney are encountered not infrequently. However, such lesions cause few or no symptoms. The majority of cases with renal tuberculosis are due to extension of the infection to the kidney via the blood stream. At first the symptoms are mild; there is usually a slight afternoon fever and a loss of weight and appetite. The process of tuberculosis generally starts in one of the renal pyramids; ulceration into the kidney pelvis follows; the germs are carried down with the urine into the bladder; the bladder is likely to become infected, with destruction of the ureterovesicle valve on the other side following, thereby presenting an opportunity for ascending infection of the previously healthy kidney.

Tuberculosis of the lower genitourinary tract is almost always secondary to renal tuberculosis, the infection having been propagated downward. Tuberculosis of the female genital tract is not necessarily a complication of urinary tract tuberculosis, but in the male, tuberculous epididymitis and prostatitis are almost invariably preceded by bladder involvement.

Tuberculosis of the urinary bladder is practically never a primary infection but an extension to the bladder of tuberculosis of a kidney or of the genital tract. This disease gives rise to several small ulcers, the majority of them near the trigone. The symptoms of bladder tuberculosis are those of cystitis in general but with an unusual degree of bladder irritability and frequent hematuria.

Symptoms. The clinical picture of renal tuberculosis is that of pyelitis: a urine containing pus, blood and also tubercle bacilli, that may be discovered only through guinea pig inoculation of the suspected urine. Suggestive early symptoms of this disease are a urine, increased in amount, that contains considerable pus and yet is acid in reaction (in nearly all other pyurias the urine is alkaline), and early and frequent renal hemorrhage into the urine. The symptoms of pain, dysuria and urinary frequency, when they occur, are due to bladder infection. Symptoms of bladder irritability (viz., frequency of urination, nocturia) are a later manifestation of the disease.

Treatment. The current trend is toward medical treatment rather than surgery. The treatment of a patient having renal tuberculosis consists of the combined administration of streptomycin, 1 Gm. biweekly, para-aminosalicylic acid, 12 Gm. daily, or 0.15 to 0.30 Gm. of isoniazid daily, together with the measures previously described as applicable to tuberculosis in general. For extensive unilateral renal tuberculosis, nephrectomy is the treatment of choice.

Renal Calculi

Stones are formed in the urinary tract due to the deposits of the crystalline substances (uric acid, calcium phosphate and oxalate) excreted in the urine. They may be found anywhere from the kidney to the bladder and vary in size from mere granular deposits, called sand or gravel, to stones as large as an orange found in the bladder.

When the stones block the flow of urine, hydronephrosis develops, and the constant

FIG. 268. Flat plate of the abdomen, showing a large calculus in the left kidney.

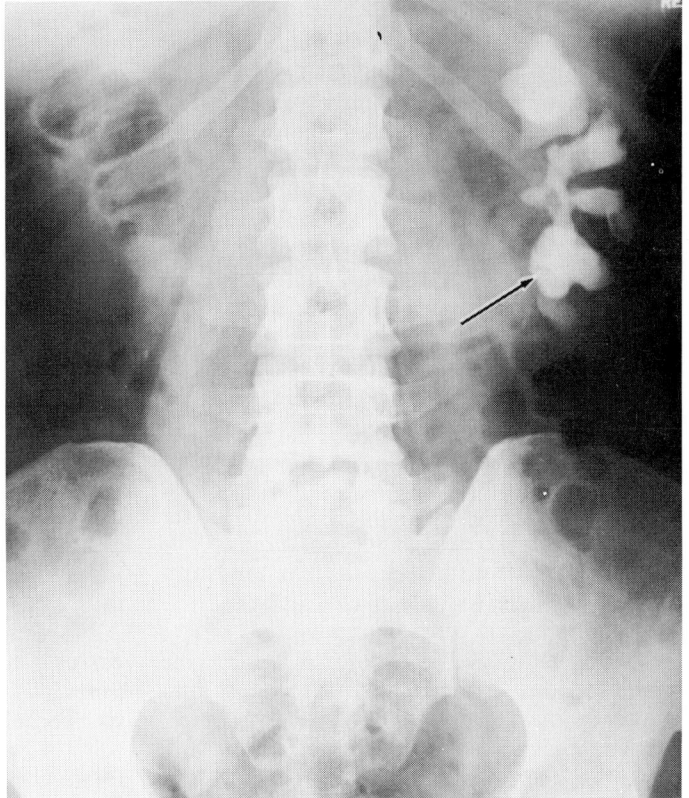

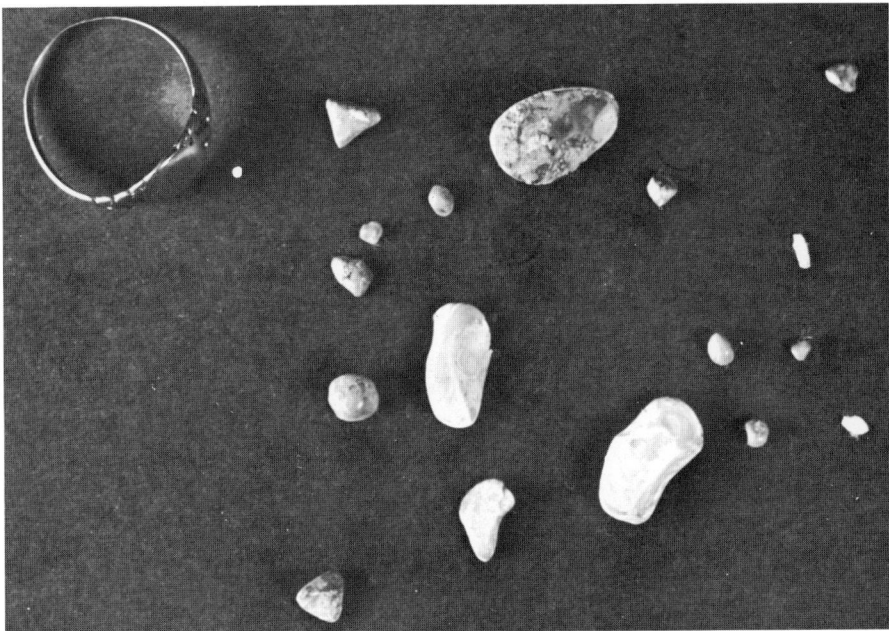

FIG. 269. A varied assortment of renal calculi, recovered from a uretal diverticulum. A finger ring is shown as a standard for comparison of size. (Richard Chute, M.D., Boston)

irritation of the stone may be followed by a secondary infection, causing pyelonephritis, cystitis and so forth.

Stones in the kidney may produce few symptoms; usually, however, there is a dull ache in the loin, and the patient passes increased amounts of urine containing blood and pus cells. If the pain suddenly becomes acute, the loin is exquisitely tender, and nausea and vomiting appear, the patient has an attack of *renal colic* (Figs. 268, 269).

When stones lodge in the ureter, acute shocking colicky pain is experienced, referred down the thigh and to the genitalia. There is usually a frequent desire to void, but very little urine is passed, and it usually contains blood because of the abrasive action of the stone as urine is passed. This group of symptoms is called *ureteral colic.* The diagnosis is confirmed by intravenous urogram and/or retrograde pyelography.

Urinary calculi must be removed to relieve recurring attacks of pain and to prevent the more serious secondary disease that their presence may lead to (hydronephrosis, secondary infection). If the stone is in the kidney, the operation performed may be a *ne-phrotomy* (simple incision into the kidney with removal of the stone), or nephrectomy, if the kidney is functionless due to infection or hydronephrosis. Stones in the kidney pelvis are removed by a *pyelotomy,* in the ureter by *ureterotomy,* and in the bladder by *cystotomy.* Sometimes an instrument is inserted through the urethra into the bladder, and the stone is crushed in the jaws of this instrument. Such an operation is called a *litholapaxy.* (See Fig. 270.)

Treatment and Nursing Care. Active treatment must be instituted for renal and ureteral colic. The objective of treatment is to relieve the pain until its cause can be removed. Morphine or meperidine hydrochloride will allay the pain. Hot baths also are useful. Unless the patient is vomiting, fluids are forced, as this treatment tends to increase the hydrostatic pressure behind the stone and thus to assist it in its downward passage.

No time should be lost by the nurse in carrying out these treatments, because at times the pain suffered by these patients is so excruciating that shock and syncope result. A patient will be grateful for any relief. Cystoscopic examination and passage of a

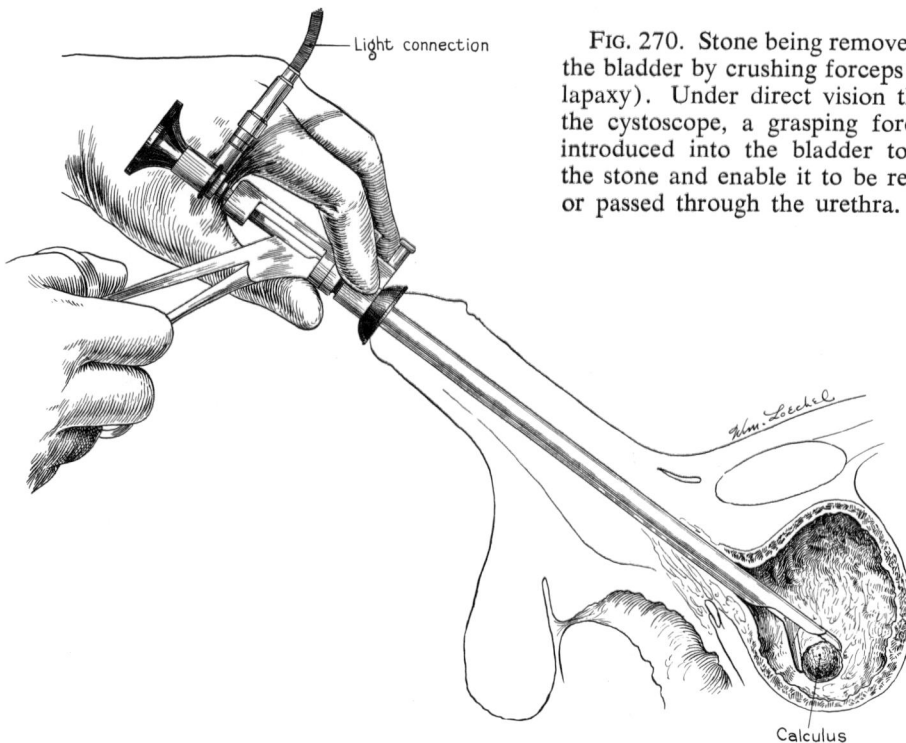

— Light connection

FIG. 270. Stone being removed from the bladder by crushing forceps (litholapaxy). Under direct vision through the cystoscope, a grasping forceps is introduced into the bladder to crush the stone and enable it to be removed or passed through the urethra.

Calculus

small ureteral catheter past the obstructive stone, whether in ureter or renal pelvis, will immediately relieve back pressure upon the kidney and alleviate the intense agony. Whether this is done or not, the nursing care of patients with calculi require constant watchfulness for the spontaneous passage of a stone. All urine should be strained through gauze, as uric acid stones may crumble. When stones are recovered, the physician will have them analyzed and then will prescribe a suitable diet to help to prevent further stone formation. Most stones consist of calcium oxalate or phosphate, and in such cases an acid ash diet may be given. Clots should be crushed and the sides of the urinal inspected for clinging stones. The lodgment of a stone in the ureter may at times cause complete suppression of urine, a condition termed *calculous anuria*. Unless this condition is relieved, renal failure develops, and death rapidly follows. If no urine is excreted within 36 hours, immediate operation is indicated. If the location of the stone is known, it may be searched for and removed; otherwise, the diseased kidney is incised and drained, and the stone is removed at a later operation when the patient is in better condition.

Discharge Instructions. Inasmuch as urinary calculi may recur, it is necessary for the patient to understand this possibility and to follow a regimen of prophylaxis. This consists of maintaining a high fluid intake, avoiding infections, since toxins are eliminated via the kidney, and adhering to certain dietary restrictions. Food high in calcium should be avoided.

For patients who are inclined to develop phosphatic calculi, a limited amount of phosphorous should be ingested. To offset excess phosphorus, aluminum hydroxide gel often is ordered, since it combines with the excess phosphorus, causing it to be excreted through the intestinal tract rather than the urinary system.

Renal Tumors and Cysts

Malignant tumors of the kidney may arise from embryonal rests of adrenal tissue in the kidney, hypernephroma, or from malignant degeneration of renal tissue. The usual symptom which first calls attention to the tumor is painless hematuria. Such a sign should be investigated immediately, for it may be the only early clue. Roentgen study usually confirms the diagnosis, and nephrectomy is performed if the tumor is operable. Often roentgen therapy is used in addition and as a palliative measure in inoperable tumors.

Cysts of the kidney may be multiple (polycystic) or single. Polycystic disease usually is congenital and involves both kidneys; therefore, it is only treated by surgery if infection occurs within the cysts. Solitary cysts often attain large size and are removed; the defect in the kidney is repaired.

Congenital Anomalies

Congenital anomalies of the kidney are not uncommon. Occasionally, there is fusion of the two, forming what is called a horseshoe kidney. One kidney may be small and deformed and often is nonfunctioning. Abnormal vessels to the kidney may kink the ureter. Not infrequently there may be a double ureter or congenital stricture of the ureter. The treatment of these anomalies is necessary only if they cause symptoms, but it goes without saying that before renal surgery is attempted, it is important to know that the other kidney is present and functioning.

Kidney Trauma

Various types of crushing injuries of the loin may injure the kidney, producing tears in its structure. The appearance of blood in the urine following an injury to the loin is highly suggestive of an injury to the kidney; therefore, a urinalysis always must be made.

In minor injuries to the kidney, healing may take place with conservative measures, such as the application of cold and firm adhesive support to the loin. When the kidney is injured sufficiently to cause hemorrhage of considerable amount, operation may be necessary. The damaged kidney usually has to be removed, although on occasions it is possible to repair it.

THE PATIENT HAVING KIDNEY SURGERY

Nursing Care—Preoperative and Postoperative

All operations on the kidney should be attempted only after a period of study and preparation. Fluids should be given in large amounts to promote increased excretion of waste products before the time of operation.

The preparation is described on pages 210 to 211. Usually, the incision is made in the loin, and the shaving should extend past the spine posteriorly and beyond the midline anteriorly, above the rib margin and well below the iliac crest. Apprehension should be allayed by gaining the confidence of the patient. Often the loss of a kidney may give the impression to him that he will be an invalid the rest of his life. This is not true in most instances, because normal function may be maintained by a single kidney.

The patient is placed on the operating table with a sand or an air pillow under the loin of the unaffected side. The upper extremity corresponding to the side to be operated upon is extended to increase the size of the loin space. The lower extremity is flexed. The kidney is first exposed by an oblique incision, then delivered into the wound, and the appropriate operation is performed.

The general nursing care after operation is much the same as that after a laparotomy. It is important for the patient to move to prevent chest and peripheral vascular complications. Adequate fluids should be given by vein, and by mouth when nausea ceases. An accurate intake and output chart should be kept. A normal diet may be given to these patients as soon as peristaltic activity is present. This is best indicated by passage of gas. Following such operations as nephrotomy, pyelotomy and ureterotomy, urine may drain from the wound for a time. This should not be mistaken by the nurse for hemorrhage. Often following these operations, drainage tubes have been placed directly in the kidney, the pelvis or the ureter; these will naturally divert the urine and keep the wound drier. The nurse should watch these tubes carefully after operation to see that there is no blockage, as from blood clot. Often following a nephrostomy, a surgeon will request periodic irrigation of the drainage tube. This is usually about 10 ml. of saline, inasmuch as the area to be irrigated is a small one. The nurse must be cautious in turning the patient on the operated side when a drainage tube is in place. A small pillow placed on either side of the tube will make a trough

so that the tubing will not bend on itself. The character of the drainage and the number of milliliters eliminated should be tabulated every 12 to 24 hours. Frequent changing of these dressings is necessary to prevent maceration of the skin and the offensive urinous odor which is embarrassing to the patient and all concerned. The Montgomery strap dressing is conveniently used in this connection.

Occasionally, clamps are left in the incision following nephrectomy, because it may be impossible to ligate the renal vessels. On examination of the operative site the nurse may see the handles of these instruments extending from the dressings over the wound. In no circumstances should the clamps be dislodged. Obviously, such a patient is not permitted to lie on the operative side. Pillows placed strategically add to the comfort of this patient.

Following a nephropexy, the patient usually is placed in such a position that his chest is lower than his hips to facilitate the adherence of the kidney to its new position.

Drug therapy to combat infection may include penicillin and streptomycin. The nurse is expected to be able to recognize the toxic manifestations of these agents and to report such an occurrence to the physician.

When a patient who has had a kidney operation is ready for discharge, it is important that he know what his posthospital care should be. If he still has drainage tubes in place which must be irrigated, as is true of a nephrostomy, he or some member of his family should be taught the care of this dressing and treatment. For postoperative nephrectomy, it is imperative that he refrain from lifting heavy objects for the first year.

Complications

Hemorrhage. Following nephrotomy and nephrectomy, the patient should be watched carefully for signs of hemorrhage. When inspecting the dressings, the nurse should remember that the ooze usually collects at the back and not on the anterior dressings. The constitutional signs of hemorrhage—an increasing pulse rate, restlessness and sweating —have been mentioned in Chapter 18. Because of the large vessels ligated, hemorrhages due to slipping of a ligature may be rapidly fatal. Therefore, the nurse should not hesitate to call the surgeon should the slightest suspicion of this complication arise.

Abdominal Distention. This complication occurs not infrequently after operations on the kidney and the ureter and is thought to be due to a reflex paralysis of intestinal peristalsis. In a weakened patient, the symptom may become very distressing, even causing embarrassment of the heart and respiration.

For relief of the abdominal distention, decompression by the use of a nasogastric tube gives rapid relief. The tube may be removed as soon as normal peristalsis and passage of gas are apparent.

Pain. Pain similar to renal colic is often a distressing symptom after operations on the kidney and the ureter. It is due commonly to the passage of clotted blood down the ureter. This symptom is usually of short duration but demands adequate doses of narcotics for its relief.

PROBLEMS AFFECTING THE BLADDER

The bladder is a muscular sac lined with mucous membrane, lying behind the symphysis pubis and covered above by peritoneum. It receives the urine from the ureters, and when it is sufficiently distended (the normal bladder capacity is about 500 ml.), sensations of discomfort are experienced. When the sphincters of the bladder are relaxed (voluntarily) urine is discharged via the urethra. This channel is short in the female, not more than 4 cm. (1½ in.) long, so that infection of the bladder by this route is not uncommon. In the male the urethra is much longer, passing through the prostate gland and the penis (Fig. 272).

Congenital Malformations

These occur occasionally in this region, resulting in the absence of the anterior wall of the bladder. This condition, known as *exstrophy* of the bladder, often is associated with other congenital defects, hernia and deformities of the urethra and the penis in the male (epispadias). Two methods have been used in the treatment of exstrophy. In one a plastic operation attempts to form a bladder, and in the other the ureters are severed at a point above their entrance into the bladder and are implanted into the rectum or the sigmoid.

Bladder Injuries

Injury to the bladder may occur with a fracture of the symphysis pubis, and occasionally in drunken individuals from kicks or blows in the lower abdomen when the bladder is full. The immediate result is extravasation of urine into the retropubic space or the peritoneum with pain, shock and an inability to void. What urine is obtained either by voiding or by catheter contains blood. If a rupture of the bladder is suspected, a cystogram will confirm the diagnosis. Early operative repair of the injured bladder is indicated. The patient will have an indwelling catheter for approximately 10 days following surgery.

Cystitis

This is an inflammation of the urinary bladder that may be introduced from external sources or from the kidneys via the urine. A very frequent cause of infection from external cause is unsterile catheterization. In hospital practice, cystitis occurs more frequently in women, probably due to the short urethra and to the fact that catheterization is performed with an improper technic. The latter factor may be avoided by careful attention to the details of sterility and asepsis.

The cardinal symptoms of cystitis are 3 in number: (1) pain in the region of the bladder, which may be constant or only during urination; (2) frequency of urination; and (3) changes (pus and often blood) in the composition of the urine.

Treatment. Pain and burning on urination may be alleviated somewhat by making the urine alkaline by the administration of sodium bicarbonate or sodium citrate gr. 20 (1.3 Gm.) 3 or 4 times daily. Urinary antiseptics often are employed. These are usually sulfonamides (Gantrisin, specifically), streptomycin, tetracycline derivatives or chloramphenicol, depending on the organism.

These measures, combined with a bland diet and a large amount of fluids, usually suffice to relieve the patient.

A urinary analgesic such as Pyridium will help to allay discomfort. Warm baths also are useful.

When the cystitis is caused by a stone in the bladder or by some obstruction to the urethra, as a hypertrophied prostate or a stricture, an operation frequently is necessary to drain the bladder (cystostomy). This operation is discussed later.

The Female Patient With Urinary Infection

The female urethra is quite vulnerable to bacterial invasion, for in women, unless the personal hygiene of the patient is observed stringently, organisms migrating from the intestinal contents may gain ready entrance to the bladder and infect the urinary tract. If the infection remains confined to the bladder, it is termed "cystitis"; if the kidneys also are infected, the designations of "pyelitis" or "pyelonephritis" are applied, depending on whether the kidney pelves alone or both pelvis and parenchyma of these organs are involved.

Clinical evidences of urinary tract infection include symptoms of urinary frequency, urgency and dysuria. Back pain also is to be expected if there is involvement of the ureters and the kidneys. Fever is a common and occasionally the sole clinical manifestation of the disease. Indeed, this is so often the case that the preliminary investigation of obscure fever invariably should include a search for pus in the urine, irrespective of the presence or the absence of symptoms indicative of urinary tract involvement.

Prevention and Nursing Care. This complication is almost entirely a problem of personal hygiene and nursing care. Although urinary infection in essence is quite simple, its requirements are very strict, namely, the complete removal of fecal material from the perineum following each defecation and during intervening periods the constant maintenance of thorough cleanliness of the perineum with respect to fecal contamination. It must be recognized that the technics of perineal care customarily employed by healthy ambulatory girls and women may become totally inadequate during illness and bed confinement. Efficient lavage under these conditions is relatively difficult, even for patients who are not greatly incapacitated. Emphatic instructions must be issued by the nurse regarding the importance of thorough ablution and the necessity for careful cleansing of the perianal region with soap and water after each defecation. More-over, if there ever is reason to doubt the capacity of a patient to complete her own hygiene, the performance of this function must be undertaken personally by the nurse as one of the most important responsibilities associated with the care of the bed patient.

Urinary infections of the type described are ordinarily of brief duration, provided that there is no underlying renal disorder and no urinary obstruction, and assuming that the immune mechanisms are intact, and that repeated reinfection does not occur. Recovery is not invariably prompt and spontaneous, however, and the response of the infection to therapy may be very stubborn, particularly if there is an associated pyelonephritis.

Treatment. Therapy consists in the ample provision of fluids, i.e., 3 or more quarts daily, unless this degree of hydration is contraindicated on other grounds, to assure a voluminous urine output. Specific chemotherapy with sulfonamides, streptomycin or another antibiotic agent, administered singly or in combination, is indicated.

Bladder Tumors

Tumors of the bladder occur commonly in older individuals. They arise as a cauliflowerlike growth in the bladder mucous membrane. Bleeding occurs when the tumor is traumatized by the contraction of the bladder in urination. A tumor is suspected when there is hematuria, frequency and dysuria, and the diagnosis is confirmed by direct examination of the bladder wall through the cystoscope.

Most tumors are small and are treated by electrocoagulation of the growth through a cystoscope. After irrigation of the bladder, it is distended with water or saline, and the coagulating needle is placed in the growth. Excellent results are reported by this method of treatment.

Neurogenic Bladder

The management of the neurogenic bladder is discussed on page 915.

THE PATIENT WITH URINARY DIVERSION

Common Methods of Urinary Diversion

The most common methods of urinary diversion are: (1) bringing the detached ureter through the abdominal wall and attaching it to an opening in the skin; this ureteral terminal ("bud") extends 1 ml. above the skin level and is surrounded by periureteral tissue in order to maintain maximum blood supply (Fig. 271 B); and (2) introducing the ureter into the sigmoid, which allows urine to flow through the colon and out of the rectum (ureterosigmoidostomy). (See Fig. 271 D.) The advantages of the cutaneous ureterostomy over the sigmoid implant are several: the procedure is relatively simple from the surgeon's point of view, the danger of fecal contamination is eliminated, postoperative hydronephrosis is avoided, and there is an absence of an electrolyte imbalance from reabsorption of urine from the bowel. Still another advantage is the accessibility of the kidneys for irrigation and study. The disadvantages of cutaneous ureterostomy are the necessity of wearing leg urinals, the possibility of stenosis of the implanted ureter if catheters are not used continuously, the necessity of taking care of catheters if used, and the cumbersome apparatus and the ever-present possibility of leakage.

The ureters also may be transplanted to a section of terminal ileum, one end of which is brought to the abdominal wall as an ileostomy opening (Fig. 271 E). The loop of ileum is a simple conduit of urine from the ureters to the surface, and it is more convenient than a cutaneous ureterostomy, because an ileostomy bag may be used to collect the urinary excretion (p. 639).

Nursing Care

The Patient With Cutaneous Ureterostomy. The deviations from routine care have to do with intelligent and satisfactory management of the mechanical and the physical problems involved and with strengthening the psychological adjustment of the patient, helping him to accept this permanent condition in as healthy a spirit as possible.

The cutaneous opening may be single, if only one ureter is involved, or double, if both are implanted. Various types of apparatus are available which in principle are similar to those used in the care and the management of an ileostomy. Skin care is essential, and the maintenance of a functioning aperture is vital. Since in many instances there is a danger of stenosis, indwelling catheters may be used. The patient must learn the sterile procedure involved in sterilizing and inserting a ureteral catheter. The important point is to position it properly: if the openings at the tip are inserted too far in the kidney pelvis, the catheter will be beyond the source of urine; it will not drain. Likewise, if it is not inserted far enough, the openings of the catheter may be occluded by the wall of the ureter, and the catheter will not drain.

Commercial apparatus is available in which a cap can be cemented to the skin surrounding the cutaneous "bud," and then the domelike covering is connected by rubber tubing to a rubber urinal worn on the leg. Specific instructions on the application and the care of apparatus accompany the apparatus.*

The Patient With Ureterosigmoidostomy. Psychological preparation of the patient with bladder malignancy is important. The usual preoperative regimen is followed, and in addition the patient may be on a liquid diet for about 5 days preoperatively, so that the colon may be kept clean. Sulfathalidine or oral neomycin sulfate may be given to lessen the number of intestinal organisms. The patient should be told that hereafter he will be voiding by rectum.

Postoperatively, a drainage tube may be in place in the rectum. Irrigations of this tube may be ordered at frequent intervals. Force never should be used because of the danger of introducing an infection into the newly implanted ureters.

Reassurance and encouragement should be a part of the care of the patient, for this is a new experience. When the rectal drain is removed, the patient will begin to learn to control his rectal sphincter. At first, urination will be frequent, and bedding may have to be changed. With patience, greater control will be gained, and he will be able to ask for the bedpan "just in time." An understanding nurse can help this patient greatly.

---

* Singer Ureterostomy Appliance, C. R. Bard, Summit, N. J., Whitmore Ureterostomy Set, United Surgical Supply Co., Port Chester, N. Y.

The student is referred to a nursing care study of a patient who had both a colostomy and a ureterostomy: Priest, P. I., and McCann, V. H.: Home care for Mrs. Murphy, Amer. J. Nurs. 57:1578-1580, 1957.

Kidney

Bladder

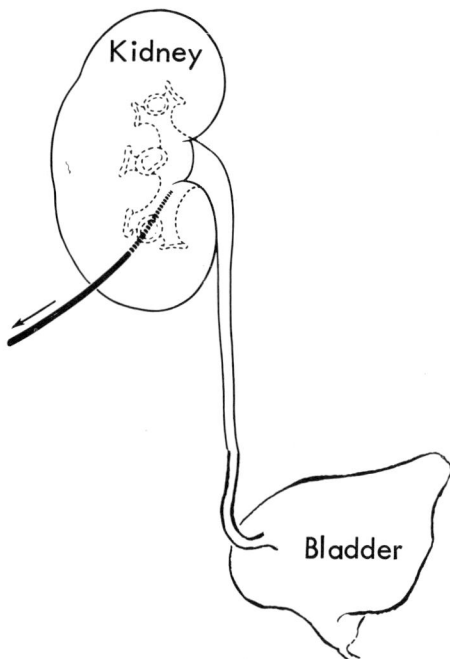

Nephrostomy. Indication for this is urinary obstruction in the lower urinary tract (prostate and prostatic obstructions, etc.) and in some cases of renal calculi in which the calculus is removed instead of performing a nephrectomy. Problems of the patient: chronic urinary infection; chronic pyelonephritis; renal deterioration; accidental dislodgement of the tube.

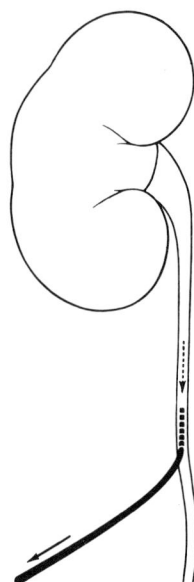

Ureterostomy. This is performed for stricture of the ureter and inflammatory obstruction. Problems of the patient: obstruction of ureter; ureteral stricture; periureteral abscess; leakage around appliance.

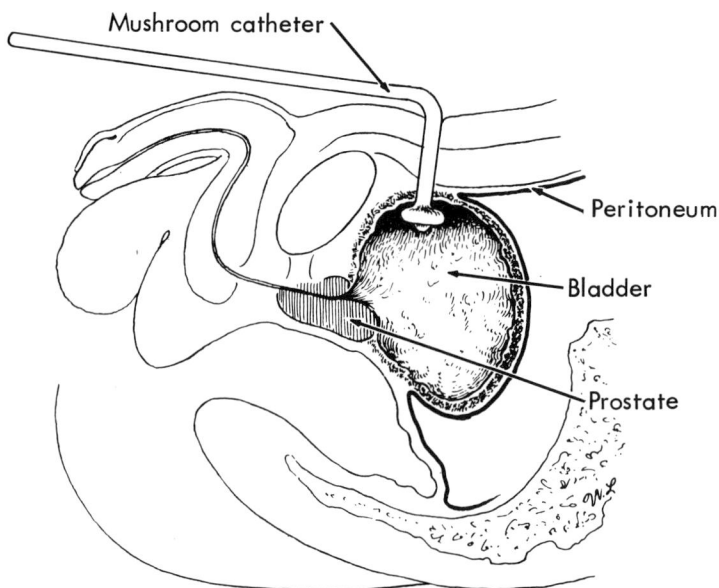

Mushroom catheter

Peritoneum

Bladder

Prostate

Cystostomy. Performed for obstruction of outlet of the bladder by prostatis or prostatic carcinoma; following the removal of stones from the bladder; and in some cases of chronic cystitis. Problems of the patient: chronic infection of the bladder; stone formation.

Fig. 271. Methods of urinary diversion. Problem-solving activity: the major problem of the patient who has a urinary diversion operation is chronic infection and its sequelae. What are the underlying reasons for each of these problems? What measures may be

Ureterosigmoidostomy. This is performed for congenital malformations of the bladder (exstrophy of the bladder) and in some patients with carcinoma of the bladder and pelvic organs not involving the rectum. Problems of the patient: chronic and recurring infection of the urinary tract; reabsorption of urinary electrolytes; malignancy at the site of ureter implantation.

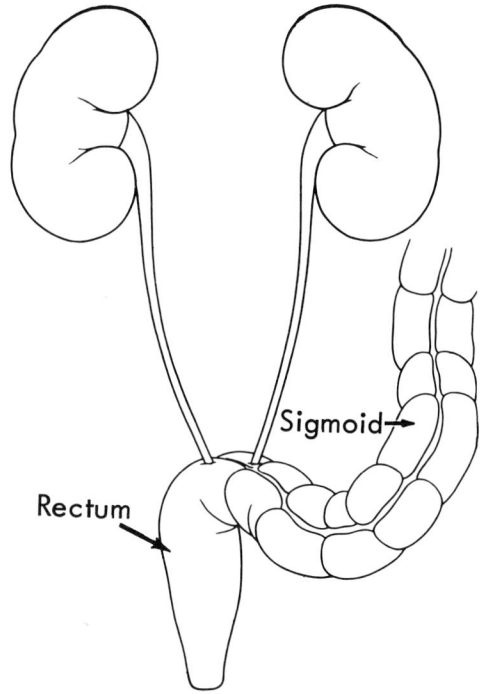

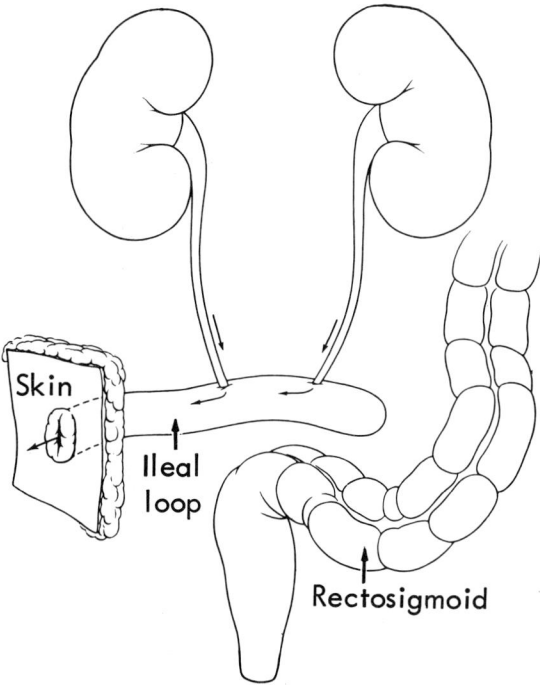

Ileal conduit. Performed when the bladder is removed for cancer of organs involving the bladder. In many instances the rectum also is removed, so that ureterosigmoidostomy could not be used. Problems of the patient: permanent ileostomy appliance must be worn; stricture development at the implant site.

FIG. 271 (*cont.*)
taken by the physician to treat the patient? What are the functions of the nurse in caring for these patients? (Bloom, J., and Merrill, J. P.: Review of methods of urinary diversion, G. P. **23:**91-97)

The Patient With an Ileal Conduit. Urinary resection in cases of cancer of the pelvis, or in other conditions in which the ureters become blocked, or in cases in which a total cystectomy must be performed often requires some form of urinary diversion. This can be accomplished in some cases by introduction of the ureter into the rectum or the sigmoid; or the urine is diverted by implanting the ureter into a loop of ileum, which is led out through the abdominal wall as an ileostomy (Fig. 271 E). This loop of ileum is known as an *ileal conduit*. It is a short piece of ileum that has been removed from the intestinal flow. The bowel continuity is obtained by anastomosis of the remaining ileum. Urine is collected in an ileostomy bag cemented to the abdominal wall. When the patient returns from the operating room, the ileostomy bag already has been applied. This is connected to a drainage tube and bottle. The nurse should measure and record the urinary volume hourly. The ileostomy appliance usually remains in place as long as it watertight, and then it is changed. Eventually, a permanent rubber or plastic bag is used. The skin around the stoma may become irritated due to the secretion from the ileum or to urinary leakage. Therefore, it is important that the nurse inspect the application of the bag to be sure this irritation does not occur. Occasionally, tincture of benzoin is used on the skin before applying the bag (p. 639).

The remaining care of the patient is essentially the same as for any intestinal resection. As soon as bowel function resumes (as indicated by the passage of gas), the patient may have food and fluids by mouth, but until that time fluids and electrolytes are given intravenously.

The Patient With a Cystostomy. An operation whereby the bladder may be drained through an abdominal wound (suprapubic cystostomy) is indicated in the treatment of diseases causing obstruction of the urethra (prostatic hypertrophy, occasionally stricture) and for the removal of calculi and tumors from the bladder (Fig. 271 C).

In preparation for the operation the abdomen and the upper thighs should be shaved. This is the one abdominal operation in which it is not necessary to have the patient void immediately before operation. The patients often are aged and weakened by disease; hence, the operation frequently is performed under local or spinal anesthesia. The bladder is filled with fluid to carry the peritoneum upward, and the patient is placed in the Trendelenburg position. An opening is made into the bladder below the peritoneum, and the appropriate operation is performed within the bladder. Then a drainage tube is inserted and the bladder wall is closed round it.

The postoperative nursing care has much to do with the success of the operation. Especially in cases of prostatic hypertrophy, the patients are usually aged and rather poor operative risks. Pulse and blood pressure must be checked every half hour for the first 2 hours and then less frequently if stable. Shock is not an uncommon postoperative complication. Fluids must be given by vein and by mouth until at least 2,500 to 3,000 ml. are taken daily. The diet should be soft at first and increased accordingly. Since old patients are prone to pulmonary complications, the nurse should turn the patient frequently from side to side and urge him to take deep breaths every hour. After 24 hours the head and the shoulders should be elevated. Skin care is an important adjunct to good nursing care in these patients. Frequent washing of the skin with soap and water and the application of petrolatum or zinc oxide ointment will prevent excoriation.

The chief attention of the nurse, of course, should be directed toward keeping the patient and the bed dry. When a tube has been inserted into the bladder, it may be attached to a bottle at the side of the bed. With constant suction, the urine which collects in the bladder is removed and caught in a drainage bottle. This helps to prevent odors and keeps the patient dry, but it must be inspected frequently by the nurse. In many cases, when this appliance is not available, a very satisfactory dressing may be made from a large square of rubber tissue with a small opening cut in the center. Liquid adhesive is applied to the abdomen about the cystostomy opening, and the rubber tissue is sealed to the skin. One sterile dressing and two sterile pads of absorbent cotton are placed over the opening, and the rubber is folded over them. The whole dressing is secured by several Montgomery straps. These dressings should be changed every half hour for the first 48 hours, then hourly, and after that p.r.n., depending on the fluid intake. It is very important to prevent the dressings from becoming saturated.

CONVALESCENCE. A cystostomy may be temporary or permanent, depending on the original purpose of the operation. The patient often is sensitive about the "bottle and tube" which he carries with him. If he is with other similar patients, the inconvenience and the awkwardness do not seem so great. However, if he is by himself or on a floor where he is the only one with such a device, diversional activity should be sought that will meet his particular interests.

Odors will not be a problem if the drainage tubing and the bottle are changed daily. They must be cleaned thoroughly with soap and water.

For the patient who is going home with a cystostomy, the use of a rubber or a plastic urinal is effective. This is an oval-shaped bladder. To one end of the bag a rubber or a plastic tubing is attached that can be connected to the drainage tube in the patient. The other end has a screw cap. The bag can be strapped to the inner aspect of the thigh or the calf in male patients or to the thigh in female patients. When it fills, it is quite easy to empty into the toilet by unscrewing the cap. The patient should be instructed regarding adequate cleaning of the bag with soap and water to prevent odors. At night he may use the drainage bottle at the side of the bed as the collecting unit; during this time the bag can be exposed to fresh air.

PROBLEMS AFFECTING THE URETHRA

Caruncle

A caruncle is a small, red, extremely vascular polypoid growth situated just within, and protruding from, the external urethral meatus of women, probably the result of long-continued infection or irritation of the mucosa at this point. On rare occasions it causes no subjective symptoms. As a rule it is acutely sensitive, causing a local burning

pain exaggerated by exertion and frequency of urination, which is exquisitely painful. The caruncle should be removed by fulguration, clamp and cautery or excision.

Urethritis

Urethritis, or inflammation of the urethra, in the majority of patients is due to gonorrhea (see p. 1080). Nongonorrheal urethritis may represent the extension of a chronic pyogenic prostatitis or follow direct injury to the urethra by instrumentation. (Never is it produced by strains, injuries or soiled toilet seats.) Nongonorrheal urethritis generally heals promptly, leaving no sequelae.

The symptoms of acute gonorrheal urethritis are frequency, burning urination, and, a discharge, which in the male is abundant and creamy but in the female, relatively scanty. In the discharge of acute cases the gonococcus easily is demonstrated; but in the very scanty discharge of more chronic infections this organism may be difficult to find, although it is always present.

The gonorrheal infection always involves the tissues around the urethra, often causing stricture, and around the glands about the external genitalia, causing abscesses. It may spread to the bladder, causing cystitis; to the cervix of the uterus; to the fallopian tubes, causing the great majority of cases of pelvic abscess; and occasionally to the peritoneal cavity, giving rise to peritonitis. The gonococcus carried by the blood stream causes one type of infectious arthritis, one form of acute bacterial endocarditis and certain skin diseases.

Urethral Strictures

A urethral stricture is a narrowing of the lumen of the urethra. Strictures result from inflammation or trauma of the urethra. They produce symptoms of obstruction and retention of urine. One of the most common causes of inflammation is that produced by the gonococcus organism. It is important for the nurse to know if the disease is in its infectious stage, and if it is, to take the necessary precautions.

Treatment. The treatment may be palliative (gradual dilatation of the narrowed area with metal sounds) or operative (incision of the stricture—urethrotomy). If the stricture has become so small as to prevent the passage of a catheter, several small filiform bougies are used in search of the opening. When one bougie passes beyond the stricture into the bladder, it is fixed in place, and urine will drain from the bladder beside it. The stricture then can be dilated to larger size by the passage of a larger sound following behind the filiform as a guide. Sometimes a suprapubic cystostomy must be performed. The postoperative treatment of these cases is similar to that described for cystostomy, page 704.

PROBLEMS RELATED TO THE MALE REPRODUCTIVE SYSTEM

In the male, several organs serve both as parts of the urinary tract and of the reproductive system (Fig. 272). Disease of these organs may produce functional abnormalities of either or both systems. For this reason diseases of the entire reproductive system in the male usually are treated by the urologist.

Anatomy and Physiology

The structures included in the male reproductive system (Fig. 272) are the testes, the vas deferens and the seminal vesicles, the penis, and certain accessory glands, such as the prostate gland and Cowper's gland. The testes are formed in embryonal life within the abdominal cavity near the kidney. During the last month of fetal life, they descend posterior to the peritoneum, to pierce the abdominal wall in the groin and to progress along the inguinal canal into the scrotum. In this descent, they are accompanied by blood vessels, lymphatics, nerves and ducts, which, along with supporting and investing tissue, make up the spermatic cord. This cord extends from the internal inguinal ring through the abdominal wall and the inguinal canal to the scrotum. As the testes descend into the scrotum, a tubular process of peritoneum accompanies them. This normally is obliterated, the only remaining portion being that which covers the testes, the *tunica vaginalis*. (When this peritoneal process does not obliterate but remains open

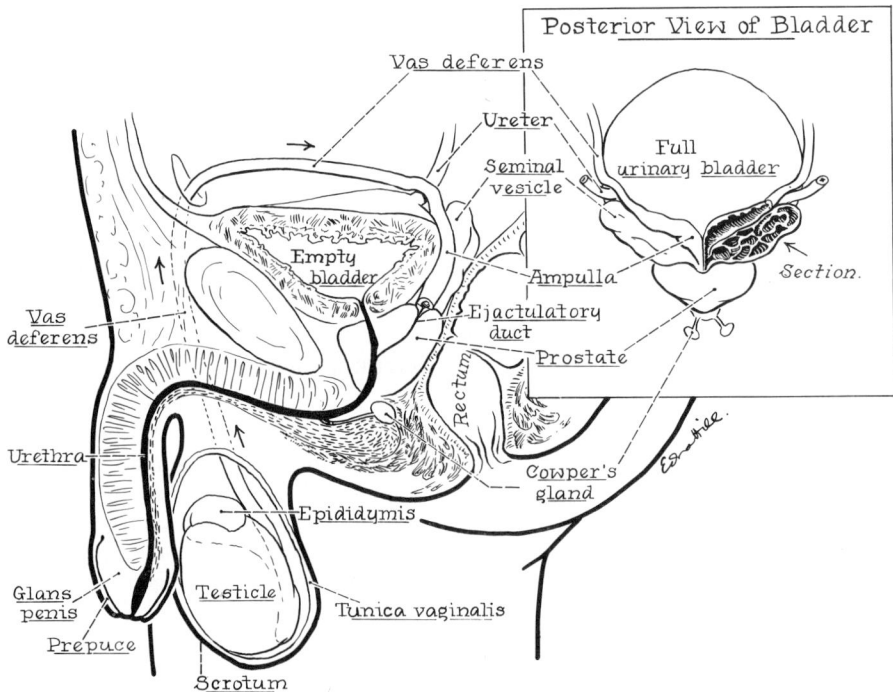

FIG. 272. Semidiagrammatic drawing showing anatomy of male reproductive system.

into the abdominal cavity, a potential sac remains into which abdominal contents may enter to form an indirect inguinal hernia.)

The testes proper consist of numerous seminiferous tubules in which are formed the male reproductive elements, the spermatozoa. These are transmitted by a system of collecting tubules into the epididymis, which is a hoodlike structure lying on the testes and containing tortuous ducts that lead into the vas deferens. This firm tubular structure passes upward through the inguinal canal to enter the abdominal cavity behind the peritoneum and then extends downward toward the base of the bladder. An outpouching from this structure is the seminal vesicle, which acts as a reservoir for the secretion of the testes. The tract is continued as the ejaculatory duct, which then passes through the prostate gland to enter the urethra. The secretion of the testes is carried by this pathway to the end of the penis in the reproductive act.

The testes have a dual function. The pri-

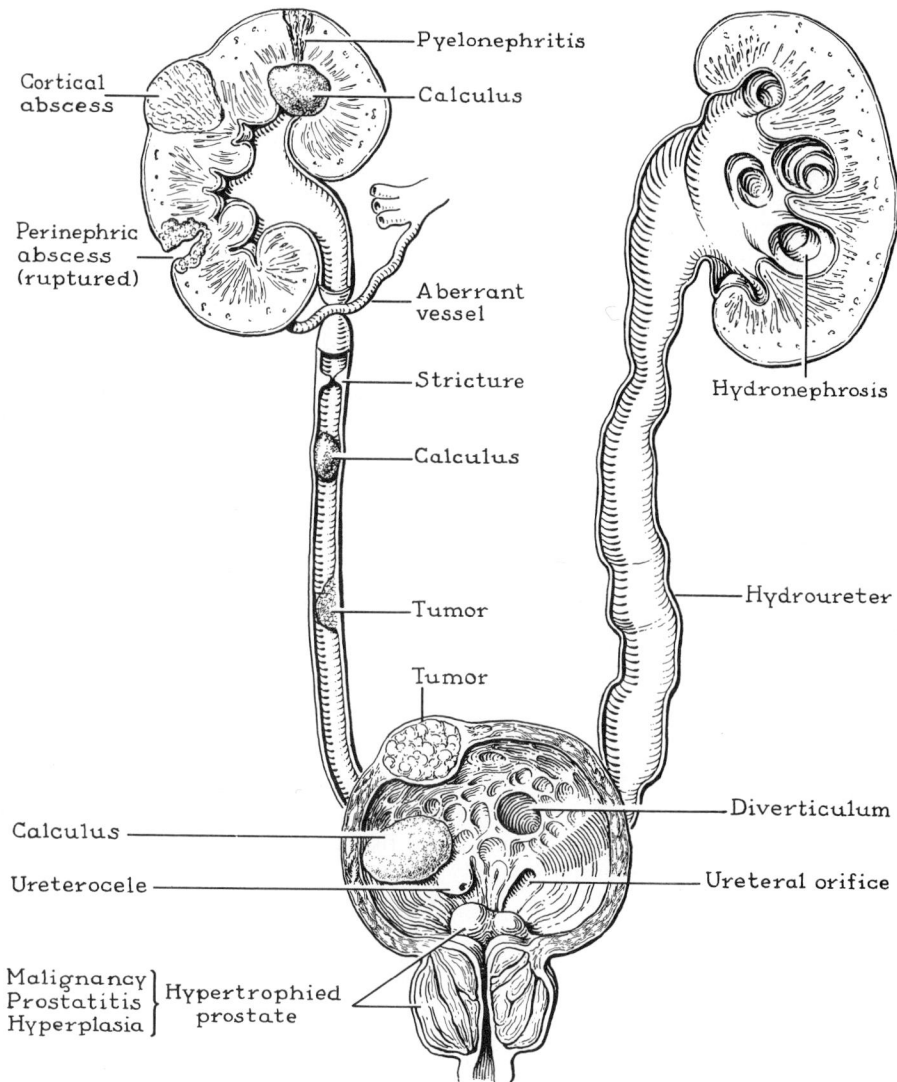

Fig. 273. Commonly encountered male urogenital problems.

mary function is reproduction, the formation of spermatozoa from the germinal cells of the seminiferous tubules. However, the testes are also important glands of internal secretion. This secretion is produced by the so-called interstitial cells and is called the male sex hormone. It has to do with the preservation of the male sex qualities.

The prostate gland lies just below the neck of the bladder. It surrounds the urethra posteriorly and laterally and is traversed by the ejaculatory duct, the continuation of the vas deferens. This gland produces a secretion which is chemically and physiologically suitable to the needs of the spermatozoa in their passage from the genital glands.

The penis has a dual function of being the organ of copulation and of urination. Anatomically, it consists of a glans penis, a body and a root. The glans penis is the soft rounded portion at the end which retains its soft structure even when erect. The urethra opens at the extremity of the glans. The glans normally is covered or protected by an elongation of the skin of the penis—the foreskin—which may be reflected to expose the glans. The body of the penis is composed of erectile tissues that contain numerous blood vessels which may become distended during sexual excitement. Through it passes the urethra, which extends from the bladder through the prostate to the end of the penis.

Congenital Malformations. Many disturbances of normal growth may occur. The most common is a failure of the testes to descend into the scrotum. This condition is called *cryptorchism*. The testes may remain within the abdomen, may pass through the abdominal wall but be arrested in the inguinal canal, or may pass through the external abdominal ring but not descend into the scrotum. In almost all cases of undescended testicle, there is a potential if not a concomitant indirect inguinal hernia. In addition, the testicle not in the normal position may atrophy, and there is some evidence that such an organ may undergo malignant degeneration. In many boys the testicle may descend spontaneously shortly after puberty, and in other instances the descent may be brought about by hormonal therapy. In patients in whom the testicle does not descend normally, an operation often is performed to place it in the scrotum.

Failure of the urethra to form normally in the penis is known as *hypospadias* when the urethral opening is on the lower wall of the penis; when it is a groove on its upper surface, the condition is called *epispadias*. These anatomic abnormalities may be repaired by various types of plastic operations. Unfortunately, all too often two or more attempts at repair are necessary, but frequently with good results.

Psychosocial Aspects of Care

The patient with a genitourinary problem deserves understanding and a dignified approach by the nurse in all her contacts with him. In many instances he is sensitive and embarrassed, and sometimes he even possesses a sense of guilt. His dignity, sensitivity and confidence can be maintained on a wholesome plane by the proper response and conduct of the nurse.

In caring for the male patient the successful nurse needs to know male psychology. She should be aware of the position her patient occupies in his family and community. Early in her contact with the elderly urologic patient, she should note all evidences of the aging process, such as hearing, chewing, habits and posture, especially in bed. By careful observation the nurse is able to determine his attitude toward life and toward his incapacity. Then from her evaluation she is able to know and to help him as an individual. At the same time she is equipped better to interpret the needs of the patient to the physician.

Conditions Affecting the Penis

Gonorrhea occurs as a result of an infection with the gonococcus, which penetrates the tissues of the urethra as a result of sexual exposure. The time elapsing from the moment of infection until the development of disease may be from 2 to 7 days, and sometimes longer. The infection produces a marked purulent, usually painful urethral discharge. At first the anterior portion of the urethra is invaded, but not infrequently the infection extends posteriorly to involve the prostate and to extend along the vas deferens to produce infection in the seminal vesicles and in the epididymis. The disease is diagnosed by the examination of a stained smear of the pus from the urethra. The gonococcus appears as a bean-shaped organism in pairs lying within the pus cells and staining in a characteristic manner (see p. 1066).

Early treatment of the infection is most likely to prevent development of the complications of gonorrhea. It must not be forgotten that the transmission of the infection from the urethra to the eyes may produce a very marked ophthalmia (see p. 864). Penicillin prophylaxis and therapy have given excellent results.

Penile ulceration may be of several types, but because of the danger of chancre (syphilis), all lesions are considered to be syphilitic until proved otherwise. Diagnosis is made by a combination of history of the disease, a microscopic examination of a darkfield specimen removed from the lesions, and a blood serology examination. The treatment of penile ulceration varies greatly, depending on the cause of the ulceration. It is not started until the diagnosis is made.

Chancre is a firm ulceration which is the primary lesion of syphilis. It occurs as a result of sexual exposure. Local treatment usually is unnecessary other than a mild antiseptic and a protective dressing, the main portion of the treatment being confined to systemic measures that usually result in a rapid healing of the local lesion. Penicillin produces a rapid cure.

Chancroid is an ulceration produced by a mixed infection, usually associated with marked lymphadenopathy in the groin. Treatment often necessitates circumcision and cauterization of the ulceration.

Balanitis is an ulceration produced by a spirochete and a fusiform bacillus commonly found in the oral cavities. These organisms are largely anaerobic; therefore, the infection always occurs under the foreskin. Circumcision, cauterizing or oxidizing antiseptics frequently are used in the therapy.

Herpes of the glans penis begins as a small blister which produces secondary ulceration. This is not a venereal disease, and the ulcerations heal rapidly under protective dressing or with a mild antiseptic treatment.

Phimosis is a condition in which the foreskin is narrowed so that it cannot be re-tracted over the glans. It may be corrected by circumcision. The operation consists in the removal of the foreskin so that the glans penis is not covered. Many infants and adults are circumcised for hygienic or therapeutic reasons.

Carcinoma of the penis occurs in the skin of the penis and rarely, if ever, occurs in circumcised individuals. It represents about 3 per cent of all skin cancer. Local treatment or complete amputation of the penis may be necessary.

Conditions Affecting the Testes and Adjacent Structures

Undescended testis is a common congenital defect. The normal testis originates from embryonic tissue near the kidney, and as the fetus develops the testis moves downward into its normal position in the scrotum. If the testis does not descend, hormone therapy and/or surgery (*orchidopexy*) are employed to secure proper positioning.

In orchidopexy an incision is made over the inguinal canal, and the testis is brought down and placed into the scrotum. To maintain proper position of the testis, traction may be applied to the thigh by means of a suture drawn from the lower end of the scrotum.

Epididymitis is due to an infection by pyogenic organisms or tubercle bacilli. It usually is secondary to prostatitis or infections in the seminal vesicles and the urethra. It may be a complication of gonorrhea. The infection passes upward through the urethra and the ejaculatory duct, and thence along the vas deferens to the epididymis.

The patient complains of pain and soreness in the inguinal canal along the course of the vas deferens and then develops pain and swelling in the scrotum and the groin. The epididymis becomes swollen and extremely painful; the temperature is elevated.

The patient should be placed on bed rest with the scrotum elevated to prevent tension on the spermatic cord. A scrotal support will accomplish this. Heat applications produce hyperemia and help to allay the infection. Antibiotics may be indicated.

Orchitis is an inflammation of the testes that may occur as a result of some systemic infection. In addition, torsion of the spermatic cord or severe trauma may be factors in the production of orchitis. The symptoms are characteristic. The testicle becomes swollen, tense and painful, and the condition often is accompanied by a high temperature, nausea and other systemic symptoms. The marked swelling inside the dense capsule of the testes may be sufficient to shut off the blood supply to the organ, so that gangrene of the testes is not infrequent. The sudden cessation of pain is a symptom of this complication.

Rest, elevation and the application of hot and cold compresses are the usual local measures. The general systemic infection causing the local lesion should be cared for. If suppuration occurs, incision and drainage often are necessary.

Tumors of the testicle usually occur in the adult during the years of greatest sexual activity. They are almost always malignant and most frequently arise as the result of congenital abnormalities in the testis itself. The tumors tend to metastasize early to distant areas. The symptoms appear very gradually with a gradual swelling of the testicle, followed by backache, pain in the abdomen, loss of weight, and general weakness. The metastatic growth may be more marked than the local testicular one. The enlargement of the testicle without pain is a significant diagnostic finding.

Removal of the testicle, followed by irradiation and retroperitoneal lymph node dissection is the accepted method of therapy.

Hydrocele is a collection of fluid in the tunica vaginalis. It may be acute or chronic. The acute type occurs in association with acute infectious diseases of the epididymis or as a result of local trauma or of a systemic infectious disease, such as mumps. This type of hydrocele usually disappears spontaneously with improvement in the causative disease, and no local treatment is necessary. Chronic hydrocele is that which occurs as a result of a low-grade infection of the testes or the epididymis. It may occur also without any evident infection of these structures. The tunica vaginalis becomes widely distended with fluid; this lesion is differentiated from a hernia by the fact that it transmits light when transilluminated.

Treatment of the chronic type of hydrocele is sought because of the inconvenience of the large scrotal mass. Palliative therapy may consist of simple aspiration of the fluid;

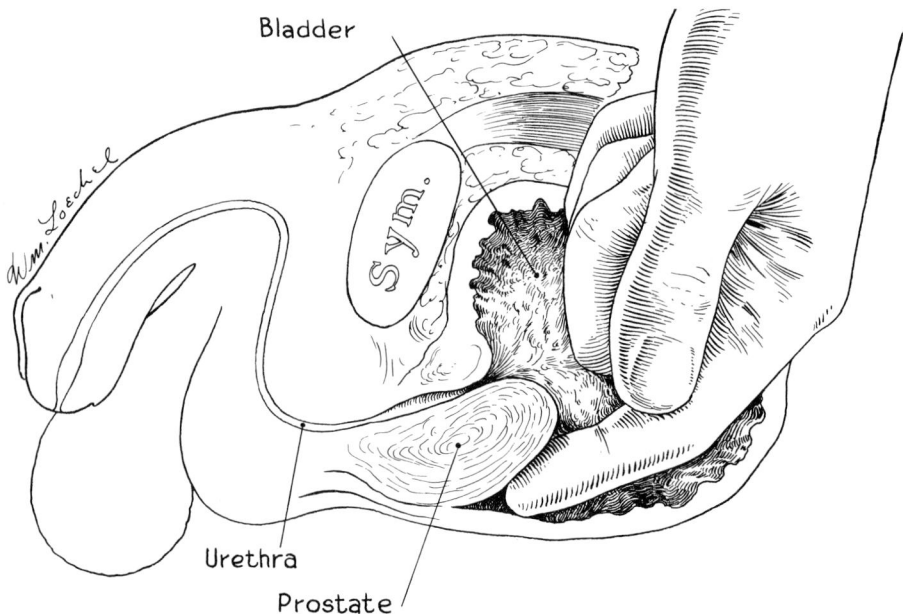

FIG. 274. Diagrammatic drawing to show how the prostate is shelled out of its bed with the finger in suprapubic prostatectomy.

this usually results in a reaccumulation of the fluid, so that frequent aspirations are necessary.

In the surgical treatment of hydrocele, an incision is made through the wall of the scrotum down to the distended tunica vaginalis. The sac is opened and excised or everted around the testicle. In the postoperative care of these patients, a suspensory bandage usually is worn for a period of time. Such a support is made commercially and is obtainable in the pharmacy. However, gauze, muslin or adhesive suspensories can be improvised.

Varicocele is a dilatation, elongation and tortuosity of the veins of the spermatic cord. This occurs most frequently in the veins on the left side in young adults. Very few if any subjective symptoms may be produced by the enlargement of the spermatic vein, and as a rule no treatment is required. When pain, tenderness and discomfort in the inguinal region are symptoms, therapy may be instituted. This usually consists in excision of the enlarged veins. In the postoperative care of these patients, a suspensory bandage is worn for a time.

Conditions of the Prostate

Benign Prostatic Hypertrophy. In many patients past 50 years of age the prostate gland enlarges, extending upward into the bladder and producing obstruction to the outflow of urine by encroaching on the vesical orifice. This condition is known as enlargement of the prostate, or prostatic hypertrophy. Since this produces an obstruction to the flow of urine, a gradual dilatation of the ureters (hydro-ureter) and kidneys (hydronephrosis) results. The hypertrophied lobe extends upward into the bladder and forms a pouch which retains urine. This pouch is not emptied when voiding takes place, and the remaining urine (called residual urine) decomposes and may produce calculi or a cystitis. Considerable difficulty and frequency in urination develop gradually, and finally the patient is unable to void at all.

Carcinoma of the Prostate. Cancer of the prostate occurs in patients in the older age group. The symptoms may or may not be marked. If the neoplasm is large enough to encroach on the bladder neck or to cause obstruction of urine, then the patient has the same signs as those noted in benign prostatic hypertrophy. However, many prostatic carcinomas are extremely malignant with few local symptoms and yet are widely disseminated. Metastases occur in bone, brain and lungs. On rectal examination, the prostate usually is found to be "stony hard" and fixed. Symptoms due to metastases are backache, loss of weight, loss of appetite and anemia. These can be alleviated and improved by castration and estrogen administration or by both.

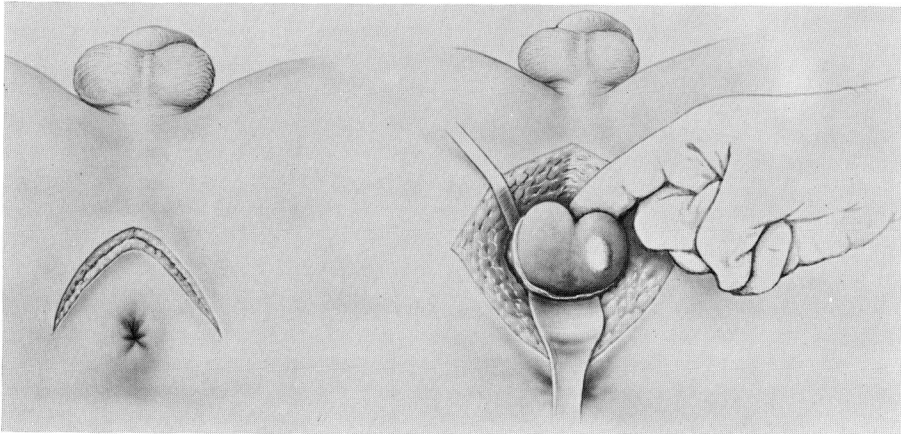

Fig. 275. Diagrammatic drawing to show the incision and how the prostate gland is removed in perineal prostatectomy. (John K. Lattimer, M.D., and Merck Sharp & Dohme, Division of Merck & Co., Inc.)

Treatment for Benign Hypertrophy and Cancer of the Prostate. If a patient is admitted as an emergency because he is unable to void, the physician immediately tries to catheterize him. The ordinary rubber catheter frequently will be too soft and pliable to pass through the urethra into the bladder. A thin wire, called a *stylet,* then can be introduced into the catheter which will prevent the catheter from collapsing when resistance is met. The surgeon often employs a catheter coated with wax whose end is upturned to form a slight angle (called a coudé-woven catheter).

In obstinate cases metal catheters must be employed. These have a curve more marked than the ordinary, called the *prostatic curve.* Sometimes, a suprapubic cystostomy is necessary to give adequate drainage (Fig. 271 C). Treatment depends on the extent of disease. If the cancer has not invaded the capsule, then total radical prostatectomy by perineal or retropubic method

is the procedure of choice. If metastases are present, or the process has invaded beyond the capsule, and the patient is having symptoms of urinary obstruction, then transurethral resection to allow an adequate channel for the passage of urine is indicated.

Preoperative Nursing Care. Estimation of kidney function, the administration of fluids in large quantities, and constant drainage of the bladder by an inlying catheter are important parts of this regimen. During this time the nurse is able to help her elderly patient to adjust to his environment. By conversation and observation she will note his idiosyncrasies, physical incapacities and mental attitude. The nurse should attempt to make his adjustment to surgery and its implications as smooth as possible. Any complications, such as cardiac and pulmonary, must be investigated before the patient has surgery. If the urinary obstruction has been nearly complete for a considerable period, a marked distention of the bladder occurs. If

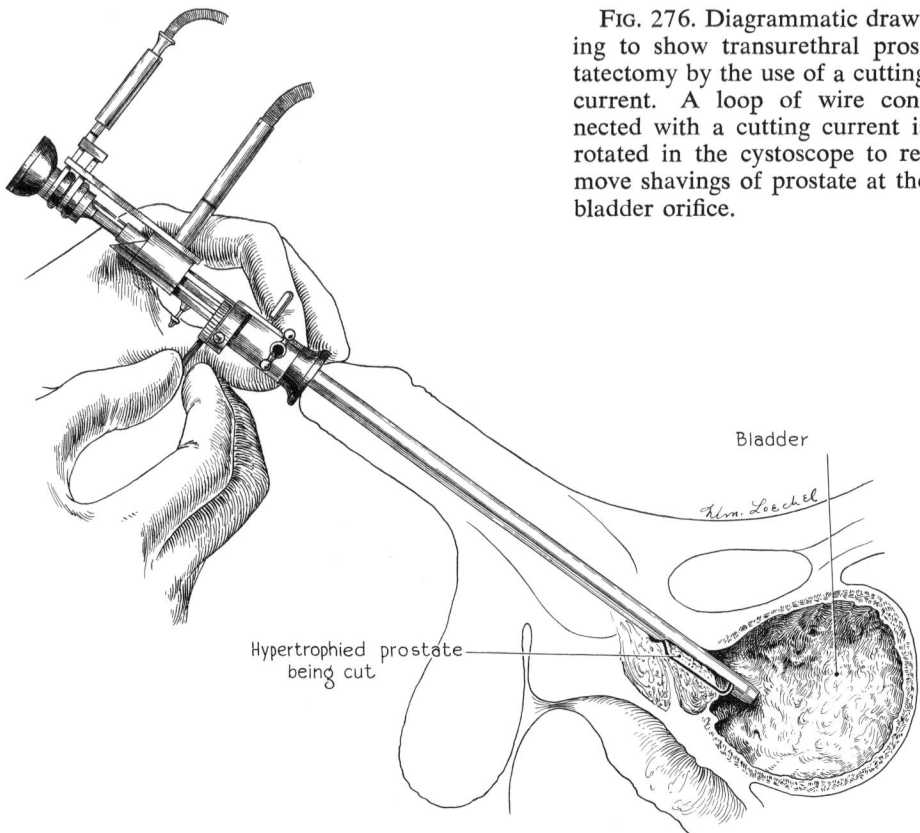

Fig. 276. Diagrammatic drawing to show transurethral prostatectomy by the use of a cutting current. A loop of wire connected with a cutting current is rotated in the cystoscope to remove shavings of prostate at the bladder orifice.

Bladder

Hypertrophied prostate being cut

urine is relieved too suddenly, the patient may go into shock because of hemorrhage, or a renal shutdown may occur, producing uremia. For these reasons it may be desirable to remove urine gradually over a period of several days. The simplest method is to connect a urethral catheter or drainage tube with a Y-tube suspended on a bedside rack. Urine flows over the suspended Y-tube into the collecting bottle. At intervals the tubing is lowered until *bladder decompression* is accomplished.

In addition to one of the temporary measures (suprapubic cystostomy or indwelling catheter) to make the patient comfortable prior to major surgery, he is encouraged to take fluids and to eat a high-caloric diet. Eggnogs can be given between meals. Attention must be given to his own personal preferences and habits if he is to accept surgery favorably.

Prostatectomy. When the tests of the kidney show that the function has returned more nearly to the normal level, the patient is considered to be ready for operation. Four different approaches are possible in removing the hypertrophied fibroadenomatous portion of the prostate gland. The gland may be removed through an abdominal wound, a *suprapubic prostatectomy.* An opening is made into the bladder, and the gland is removed from above (Fig. 274). Such an approach can be used for a gland of any size, and few complications occur, although blood loss may be greater than with other methods. Another disadvantage is that an abdominal incision is required with the concomitant hazards of any major surgical procedure.

In *perineal prostatectomy,* the gland is removed through an incision in the perineum (Fig. 275). This approach is practicable when other approaches are blocked. It is good when open biopsy is needed. Postoperatively, the wound is contaminated easily because of the position of the incision. Incontinence, impotence or rectal injury are more likely as sequelae.

Instruments have been devised with an ocular and operating system which can be introduced through the urethra to the prostate. Under direct vision small pieces of obstructing gland tissue can be removed with an electric wire. This is called *transurethral*

resection of the prostate (Fig. 276). The real advantage of this method is that there is no incision. It may be used for glands up to moderate size, and it is ideal for most poor-risk patients with small glands. This approach usually means a shorter hospital stay; however, strictures are more frequent, and repeat operations are more likely.

Another technic is to make a low abdominal incision and approach the prostate gland between the pubic arch and the bladder (without entering the bladder). This is called *retropubic prostatectomy.* This is suitable for large glands high in the pelvis. Blood loss is controlled more easily; however, inflammation of the pubic bone (osteitis pubis) is more likely.

Postoperative Nursing Care. As soon as the patient returns from the operating room, the nurse should check his pulse and his blood pressure, because the *immediate dangers following prostatectomy are shock and hemorrhage.* Bleeding may occur from the bed of the prostate, so that before completion of the operation many surgeons pack the cavity or produce pressure on the walls by distending a small rubber bag attached to a tube which leads out through the urethra. In the suprapubic approach the packing or the bag is removed later through the abdominal wound. In spite of these precautions, the nurse must watch the patient carefully for signs of hemorrhage.

The drainage tube is connected to a piece of sterile plastic or rubber tubing placed in a drainage bottle near the patient's bed. At least every hour the nurse should inspect the urethral catheter for signs of obstruction. Any indications of kinking or compression of the drainage tubing must be avoided. A loop in the tubing may cause fluid to collect, thereby obstructing the flow. If the patient complains of pain, the nurse should check the drainage tubing and correct any obstruction before administering an analgesic.

An intake of fluids up to 3,000 ml. daily is encouraged. Obviously, an intake and output record is necessary. How rapidly a patient returns to a normal diet depends on the individual patient. Most patients are allowed bathroom privileges on their 2nd postoperative day.

Following perineal prostatectomy, the sur-

TABLE 18. Comparison of Surgical Approaches for Prostatectomy

The operation of choice depends on (1) the size of the gland, (2) the location of the gland, (3) the age of patient, (4) the condition of patient, and (5) the presence of associated diseases

	Advantages	Disadvantages	Nursing Implications
Transurethral	Safer for surgical risk patient Shorter period of hospitalization and convalescence Useful for smaller gland Lower mortality rate	Requires highly skilled operator Not indicated for greatly enlarged prostate Recurrent obstruction may develop. Delayed bleeding may occur.	Watch for evidence of hemorrhage (drainage in bottle). Observe for symptoms of urethral stricture (dysuria, straining, small urinary stream).
Suprapubic	Technically simple. Offers wider area of exploration Permits exploration for cancerous lymph nodes Allows more complete removal of obstructing gland Permits treatment of associated lesions in bladder	Requires surgical approach through the bladder Control of hemorrhage difficult Urinary leakage around suprapubic tube Convalescence more prolonged and uncomfortable	Watch for indications of shock. Observe for hemorrhage. Give meticulous aseptic attention to area around suprapubic tube.
Perineal	Offers direct anatomic approach Permits gravity drainage Particularly efficacious for radical cancer therapy Allows hemostasis under direct vision Low mortality rate Less incidence of shock	Higher postoperative incidence of impotency and urinary incontinency Problem of damage to rectum Restricted operative field	Use drainage pads and bath towels to absorb excess urinary drainage. Secure foam rubber ring for patient comfort.
Retropubic	Most versatile procedure Permits easier control of hemorrhage Shorter period of convalesence	Cannot treat associated pathology in bladder Increased incidence of osteitis pubis	Watch for evidences of hemorrhage.

geon will change the dressing on the 1st day postoperatively; after that it may become the nurse's responsibility. Careful aseptic technic must be practiced, for the possibilities of infection are great. Dressings can be held in place by a double-tailed T-binder (Figs. 245, 246). The tails can cross over the incision to give double thickness, and then each tail is drawn up on either side of the scrotum to the waistline and fastened. Rectal temperatures should not be taken, and a rectal tube should be used only on specific order by the physician. Any signs of oozing, infection, tenderness or pain should be reported.

Rehabilitation. As the days pass and drainage tubes are removed, the patient often shows signs of discouragement and depression because he is not able to gain control of his bladder immediately. There may be urinary frequency after the catheter is removed.

The following exercise is helpful for regaining urinary control. Tense the perineal muscles by pressing the buttocks together; hold this position; relax. This exercise, done 10 to 20 times each hour, can be performed while the patient is sitting or standing. It is important for him to know that regaining urinary control is a gradual process, and that even though he may be discharged from the hospital with "dribbling," it gradually should diminish. His wife or some other responsible member of the family should be told of his condition. It is well for the family to realize that he should be encouraged to do as much for himself as possible. He needs mental stimulus to prevent boredom, despondency and physical lassitude. On the other hand, he must refrain from strenuous exercise, and he should avoid alcohol for at least a month. If any bleeding is detected, he should be advised to call his physician immediately.

When a cystostomy has been performed, the nursing care discussed on page 704 should be given carefully.

CLINICAL SITUATION

The Patient With a Prostatectomy

Mr. J. A. is a 72-year-old patient who for the past 6 months has been experiencing increasing urinary retention. He is hospitalized with a diagnosis of prostatic hypertrophy.

1. Since prostatic carcinoma is curable when it is detected early, the nurse should teach male patients over 40 to have periodic
   A. Rectal examinations.
   B. Cystoscopic examinations.
   C. Treatments with hormones.
   D. Renal function studies.

2. The physician performed a cystoscopic examination on Mr. A. Immediately following a cystoscopy all of the following may be considered to be normal *except*
   A. Low back pain.
   B. Burning upon voiding.
   C. Gross hematuria.
   D. Pink-tinged urine.

3. The diagnosis was confirmed, and Mr. A was taken to the operating room for a transurethral prostatectomy. The most frequently encountered complication following this operation is
   A. Urinary retention.
   B. Hemorrhage.
   C. Dysuria.
   D. Low backache.

4. Mr. A. has an indwelling catheter attached to straight drainage. To prevent a secondary bladder infection from developing, the nurse should
   A. Keep the drainage bottle emptied.
   B. Have the area around the meatus and the catheter cleansed frequently.
   C. Use measures to acidify the urine.
   D. Clamp the catheter at hourly intervals.

BIBLIOGRAPHY AND SUGGESTED READING

Ansell, J. S.: Nephrectomy and nephrostomy, Am. J. Nurs. **58:**1394-1396, Oct., 1958.

Barnes, R. W., and Purdey, A. H.: Prostatic tumors, Am. J. Nurs. **56:**982-987, June, 1956.

Chute, R.: Preoperative and postoperative care of aged patients undergoing urological surgery. J.A.M.A. **148:**184-187, 1952.

Corcoran, A. C.: Renal failure, Am. J. Nurs. **56:**768-770, June, 1956.

Cox, C. E., and Hinman, Jr., F.: Incidence of bacteremia with indwelling catheter in normal bladders, J.A.M.A. **178:**919-921, 1961.

Creevy, C. D.: Ileac diversion of the urine, Am. J. Nurs. **59:**530-533, Apr., 1959.

Hand, J. R.: Infections of the urinary tract, Am. J. Nurs. **57:**1008-1010, Aug., 1957.

Heckel, N. J.: Kidney stones—their etiology and treatment, Am. J. Nurs. **55:**194-197, Feb., 1955.

Jackson, A. F.: Cancer of the bladder, Am. J. Nurs. **58:**249-250, Feb., 1958.

Kaplan, S. A., and Callison, C.: Nephrosis in children, Am. J. Nurs. **56:**300-303, Mar., 1956.

Kleeman, C. R., Hewitt, W., and Guze, L. B.: Pyelonephritis, J.A.M.A. **173:**257-259, 1960.

Littlepage, S.: Genitourinary injuries—nursing care, Am. J. Nurs. **55:**973-974, 1955.

Lubash, G. D.: Dialysis with the artificial kidney, Nurs. World **132:**10-13, Oct., 1958.

MacLean, M. M., *et al.*: Hemodialysis and the artificial kidney, Am. J. Nurs. **58:**1672-1675, Dec., 1958.

Meyerson, C.: A congenital anomaly of the urinary bladder, Am. J. Nurs. **62:**86-88, Jan., 1962.

Mossholder, I. B.: When the patient has a radical retropubic prostatectomy, Am. J. Nurs. **62:**101-104, July, 1962.

Obermeyer, W. B.: Crotch care, Am. J. Nurs. **57:**618-620, 1957.

Parker, D.: Treatment of urinary tract infection, J.A.M.A. **154:**972-974, 1954.

Reams, G. B., and Powell, E. J.: Postoperative catheterization—yes or no? Am. J. Nurs. **60:**371, Mar., 1960.

Spence, H. M.: Genitourinary injuries, Am. J. Nurs. **55:**970-973, 1955.

Taufic, M. R.: Nursing the patient after nephrectomy, Am. J. Nurs. **58:**1397-1398, 1958.

Thompson, G.: After renal surgery, Am. J. Nurs. **61:**106-107, Sept., 1961.

Tollefson, D. M.: Nursing care of the patient with an ileac diversion of the urine, Am. J. Nurs. **59:**534-536, Apr., 1959.

Twiss, M. R., and Maxwell, M. H.: Peritoneal dialysis, Am. J. Nurs. **59:**1560-1563, 1959.

Patient-Teaching Aids and Information

Anatomy for the Patient. A 20-page pamphlet with many schematic drawings illustrating anatomy, pathology and therapy. Schering Corporation, Bloomfield, N. J.

Cancer of the Genitourinary System, No. 6 in Cancer Series, Supt. of Documents, U. S. Govt. Printing Office, Washington, D. C.

Home Care for the Patient after Urological Surgery (Cutaneous ureterostomy), Nursing Division, Memorial Center, 444 E. 68th St., New York 21, N. Y.

Pads of instruction tear sheets available from Pharmaceutical Division, Homemakers' Products Corporation:

1. Home Care of the Bedridden Incontinent.
2. Instructions for Care of the Ambulatory Incontinent.

Pamphlets on sex education available from:

1. American Medical Association.
2. National Education Assocation.

33

Female Patients With Conditions of the Reproductive System

THE FEMALE ORGANS OF REPRODUCTION

The nursing of the gynecologic patient requires a certain knowledge of the anatomy of the female organs. The external genitalia (vulva) are enclosed by the *labia majora,* two thick folds of tissue. They extend above from the hairy eminence over the pubic bones and the mons pubis and are united below by a fold of tissue called the *posterior commissure.* The *labia minora* are two smaller lips of tissue covered with delicate skin within the labia majora. They unite above to form a partial covering for the *clitoris,* a highly sensitive organ made up of erectile tissue. Between the labia minora, below and posterior to the clitoris, is the external urinary meatus, the external opening of the short (1½ in.) female urethra. Below this orifice is a larger opening, the vaginal orifice, made smaller in the virgin by the *hymen,* a thin fold of tissue stretched across the lower part of the entrance to the vagina (Figs. 277, 278). It disappears commonly after childbirth.

On each side of the vaginal orifice is located a *Bartholin's gland,* a small bean-sized gland that empties its mucous secretion by a small duct, the orifice of which is to be found within the labia minora, external to the hymen.

The tissue between the external genitals and the anus is called the *perineum.*

The *vagina* is the canal lined with mucous membrane, about 3 or 4 inches long, that extends downward and forward from the uterus to the vulva. Anterior to it are the bladder and the urethra, and below it lies the rectum. The anterior and the posterior walls normally lie in contact with one another. The upper part of the vagina, called the *fornix,* surrounds the *cervix* or the neck of the uterus (Fig. 279).

The *uterus* is a pear-shaped muscular organ that in the virgin is about 3 inches long and about 2 inches wide at its upper part. Its walls are about ½ inch thick. It is divided into a narrow neck or cervix that projects into the vagina and a larger upper part, the *fundus* or body, that is covered posteriorly and partly anteriorly by peritoneum. It lies posterior to the bladder and is held in position in the pelvic cavity by several ligaments. The *round ligaments* extend anteriorly and laterally to the internal inguinal ring and down the inguinal canal, where they blend with the tissues of the labia majora. The *broad ligaments* are folds of peritoneum extending from the lateral pelvic walls and enveloping the fallopian tubes. The uterosacral ligaments extend posteriorly to the sacrum, and the uterovesical ligaments pass anteriorly. The cavity of the uterus is triangular in the fundus. It narrows to a small canal in the cervix that has a constriction at each end, the external and the internal os. The upper lateral parts of the uterus are called the *cornua.* From them extend outward the oviducts or fallopian tubes, the lumen of which is continuous internally with the uterine cavity.

The *ovaries* lie behind the broad ligaments, behind and below the tubes (Figs. 278, 279). They are oval-shaped bodies, about 1 inch to 2 inches long, and they contain thousands of tiny egg cells or ova. The ovaries and the fallopian tubes are called the *adnexae.*

The ovary, which normally contains from 30,000 to 40,000 ova, remains quiescent in early life, but at the time of puberty, usually between the 12th and the 14th years, a new function appears. The ova begin to ripen or mature, enlarging as a sort of cyst known as a *graafian follicle*. The cyst enlarges till it reaches the surface of the ovary, where rupture occurs, and the ovum is discharged into the peritoneal cavity. This function of periodic discharge of matured ova is called *ovulation*. The ovum usually finds its way into the fallopian tube, where it is carried to the uterus. If it meets a spermatozoon, the male reproduction cell, a union occurs, and *conception* takes place. Following the discharge of the ovum, the cells of the graafian follicle undergo a rapid change. Gradually they become yellow in color (the corpus luteum) and produce a secretion that has the function

of preparing the uterus for the reception of the fertilized ovum.

If conception does not occur, the ovum dies, and the mucous membrane lining the uterus (the endometrium), which has become thickened and congested, becomes hemorrhagic. The upper layer of lining cells and the blood that appears in the uterine cavity are discharged through the cervix and the vagina. This flow of blood, mixed with mucus and cells, which occurs as a rule every 28 days during the sexual life of females, is called *menstruation*. The period of flow lasts usually from 4 to 5 days, during which time from about 50 to 60 ml. of blood is lost. After the cessation of the menstrual flow the endometrium returns to an inactive state until stimulated again by ovulation. It is

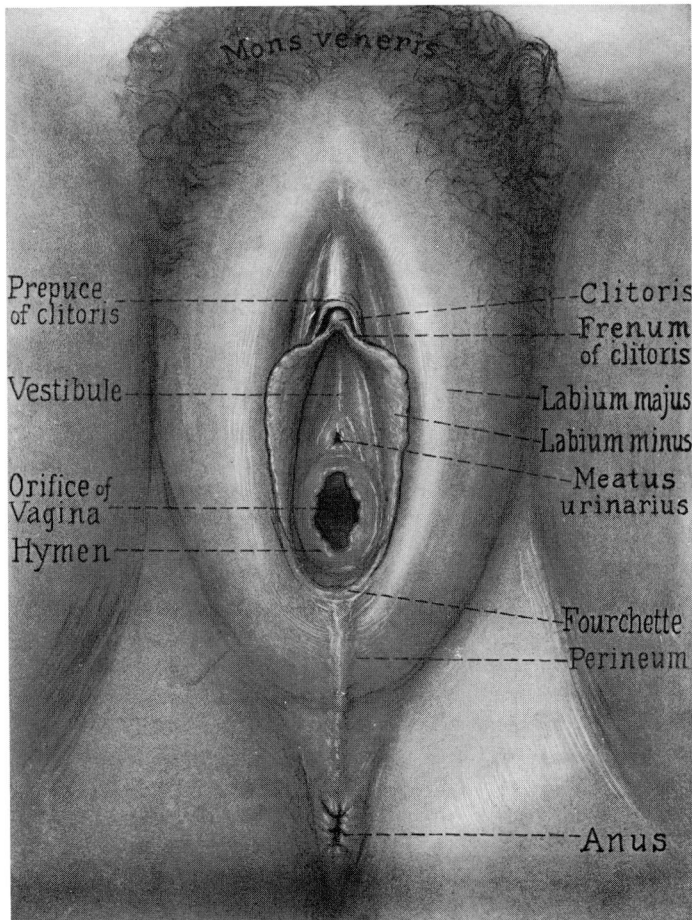

Fig. 277. External genitalia in the female.

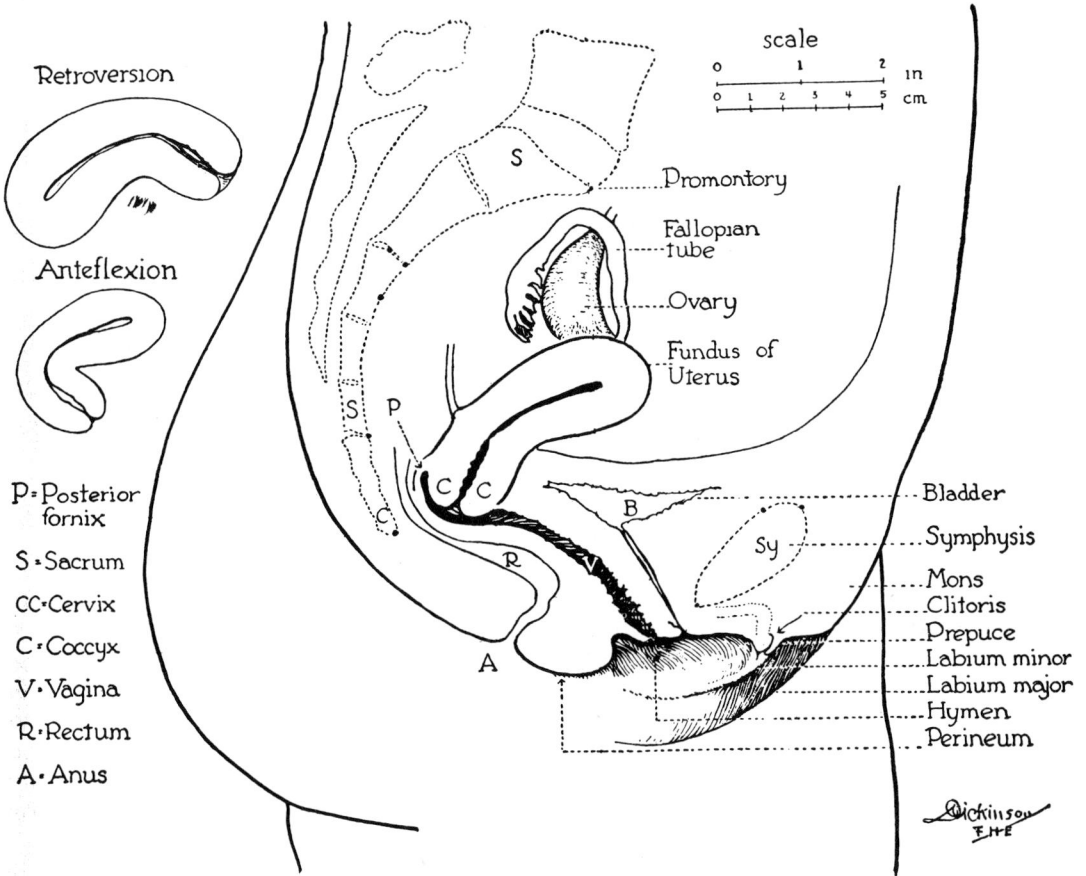

Fig. 278. Female pelvis and contents, standing, median section. (Robert L. Dickinson, M.D., New York City)

believed that ovulation usually occurs mid-way between menstrual periods. During the menstrual periods there is often a physical as well as a mental depression.

Between the ages of 45 and 50 years, there is in most women a cessation of the menstrual flow. This period, called the *menopause* (change of life, climacteric), is associated with atrophy of the breasts and genital organs and sometimes with psychic and vascular disturbances. It is at this time that uterine and breast cancers most often appear. If ovarian secretion is terminated suddenly by removal of the ovaries or by irradiation, an artificial menopause may be induced. This may produce even more marked symptoms than the normal menopause. Substitution endocrine therapy often is helpful to tide the

patient over this distressing period of physiologic readjustment.

GYNECOLOGIC EXAMINATION OF THE PATIENT

The patient who is to have a gynecologic examination often has many fears and worries. She needs reassurance, understanding and tactful regard for her emotional as well as her physical problems. Preparation includes voiding and evacuation of the bowels. Sufficient clothing should be removed to allow adequate exposure of the genitalia. All bands about the waist must be loosened and the girdle should be removed to permit examination of the abdomen. In preparation for the examination and in placing the patient on the examining table, the nurse should take spe-

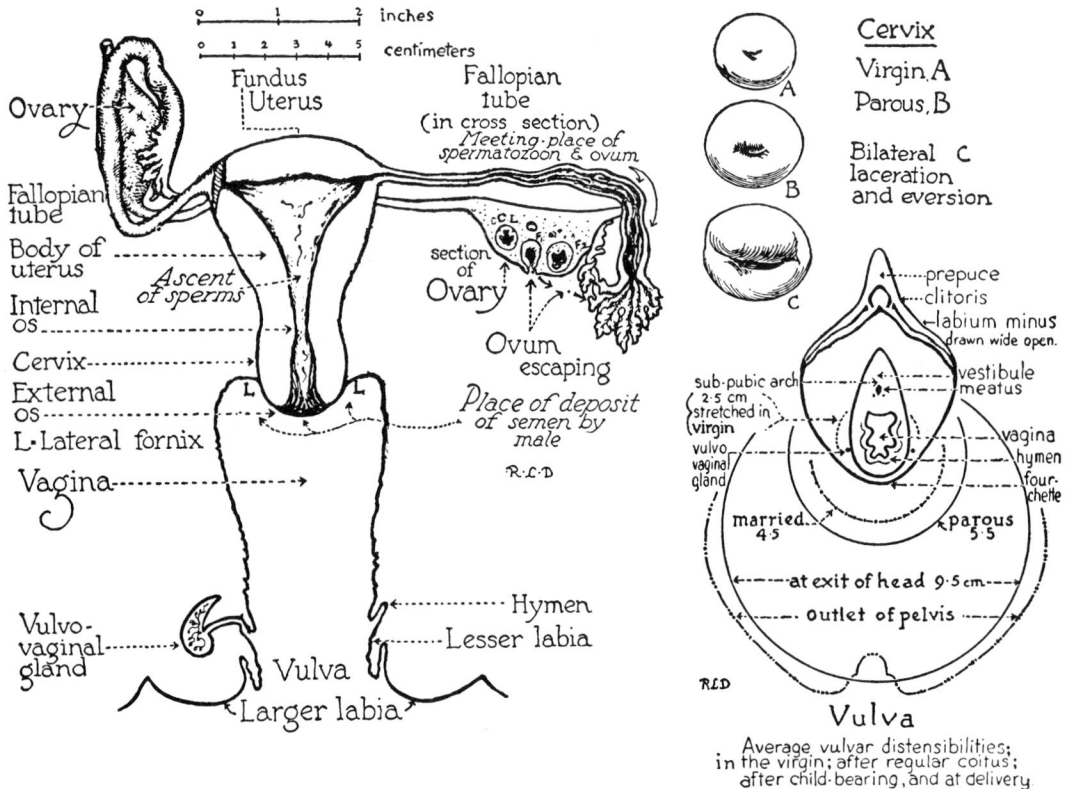

FIG. 279. Diagram of internal genitals. (*Left*) the ovary and the tube in true position; (*right*) spread out and cut in two to show inside structure. (Robert L. Dickinson, M.D., New York City)

cial precautions to avoid exposing the patient. The nurse should be in attendance during the examination.

Positioning the Patient

The examination of the patient for a gynecologic condition is made best with the patient on the examining table. Three positions are employed commonly for these examinations. The most common is the dorsal position, with the knees and the hips flexed and the heels resting in foot rests. A sheet is draped diagonally over the patient (Figs. 280, 281), the lower corner being caught in the hands and gathered up so as to expose the vulva. A small towel then may be used to cover the exposed parts until the physician is ready to make the examination (Fig. 282).

In Sims's position the patient lies on one side, usually the left, with her left arm behind her back. The right (uppermost) thigh and the knee are flexed as fully as possible,

and the left leg is partly flexed. A sheet then is draped over the lower extremities and the hips in such a way as to expose the genitalia (Fig. 283).

In the knee-chest position the patient kneels on the table so that the feet extend over the end. The knees should be separated and the thighs at right angles to the table. The head is turned to one side, and the arms grasp the sides of the table; the chest and the side of the face rest on a soft pillow (Fig. 284).

If for any reason an examining table is not available, or the patient cannot be moved conveniently, these positions may be assumed in bed. Many physicians prefer to make the examination in the dorsal position with the patient across the bed, the hips extending slightly over the edge and the feet on the examiner's knees or on two chairs placed beside the bed. The cross-bed position must be used if instruments are to be used in making the examination. A sheet drape is used to cover the patient in the same way as for the table examinations.

The Examination

This includes first an inspection of the external genitalia, then an examination of the vagina and the cervix, the speculum being used to expose the parts. Finally, a bimanual examination is made by inserting one or two fingers of the left hand in the vaginal canal and palpating the abdomen with the right hand. In this way the uterus and the adnexa may be more or less accurately examined.

Cytologic Test for Cancer (Papanicolaou). This test is done for the purpose of diagnosing genital cancer. It comprises the aspirating or the swabbing of vaginal secretions from the posterior fornix and making a smear on a glass slide. The secretion usually is "fixed" immediately by immersing the slide in equal parts of 95 per cent alcohol and ether. The patient should be instructed not to take a douche before this examination, as such a treatment will wash away cellular deposits.

The pathologist examines and interprets the cytologic smear. The classification for cytologic findings as suggested by Papanicolaou is as follows:

Class 1. Absence of atypical or abnormal cells.

Class 2. Atypical cytology but no evidence of malignancy.

Class 3. Cytology suggestive of, but not conclusive for, malignancy.

Class 4. Cytology strongly suggestive of malignancy.

Class 5. Cytology conclusive for malignancy.*

The finding of an abnormal smear (with the exception of Class 5) does not necessarily mean that the patient has cancer but points out that additional procedures, such as punch biopsies or a dilatation and curettage, are indicated. The patient will be grateful for this explanation.

Dilatation and Curettage

A dilatation and curettage (D and C) is the widening of the cervical canal with a dila-

* Papanicolaou, G. N.: Atlas of Exfoliative Cytology, Cambridge (Mass.), Harvard, 1954.

tor and the scraping of the uterine endometrium with a curette. It is done to secure endometrial or endocervical tissue for cytologic examination, to control abnormal uterine bleeding and as a therapeutic measure for incomplete abortion.

For this procedure the patient usually is sent to the operating room, preoperative preparation being determined by the nature of the anesthetic agent. With the patient in the lithotomy position, the cervix is dilated with an instrument and scrapings of the endometrium are obtained by means of a curette. Tissue for biopsy also may be obtained by cutting with an electric needle or by using a punch biopsy forceps. After operation the patient usually prefers to rest the remainder of the day. Her diet is what she desires.

The nurse should watch for evidences of excessive vaginal bleeding. The patient may experience difficulty in voiding after the operative procedure, which may result in urinary retention. The urine is measured following the first few voidings after surgery. Discomfort in the form of pelvic and low back pain is usually relieved by mild analgesics.

Hysterosalpingogram

A hysterosalpingogram is an x-ray study of the uterus and the fallopian tubes after the injection of a contrast media. This diagnostic procedure is done to study sterility problems, to evaluate tubal patency and to determine the presence of pathology in the uterine cavity.

The patient is placed in the lithotomy position, and the cervix is exposed with a bivalved speculum. A cannula is inserted into the cervix, and radiopaque dye is injected into the uterine cavity and the tubes. X-ray films are taken to show the path and the distribution of the contrast materials.

Pelvic Pneumoperitoneum (Nitrous Oxide Gynecogram)

This is a diagnostic procedure for the visualization of the female reproductive organs. Nitrous oxide gas is injected approximately 2 inches below the umbilicus into the pelvic cavity. This gas surrounds the organs of the pelvic cavity and thus outlines them on x-ray negatives. By changing the patient's position on the table the gas is displaced to all areas

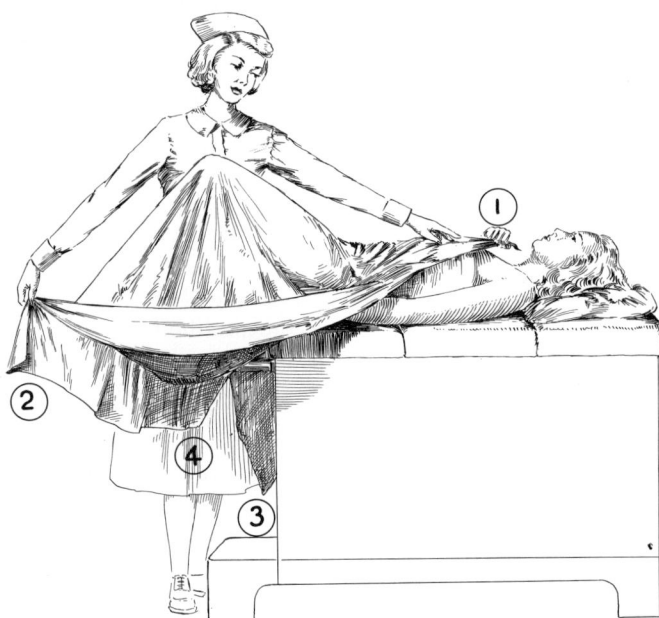

FIGURE 280

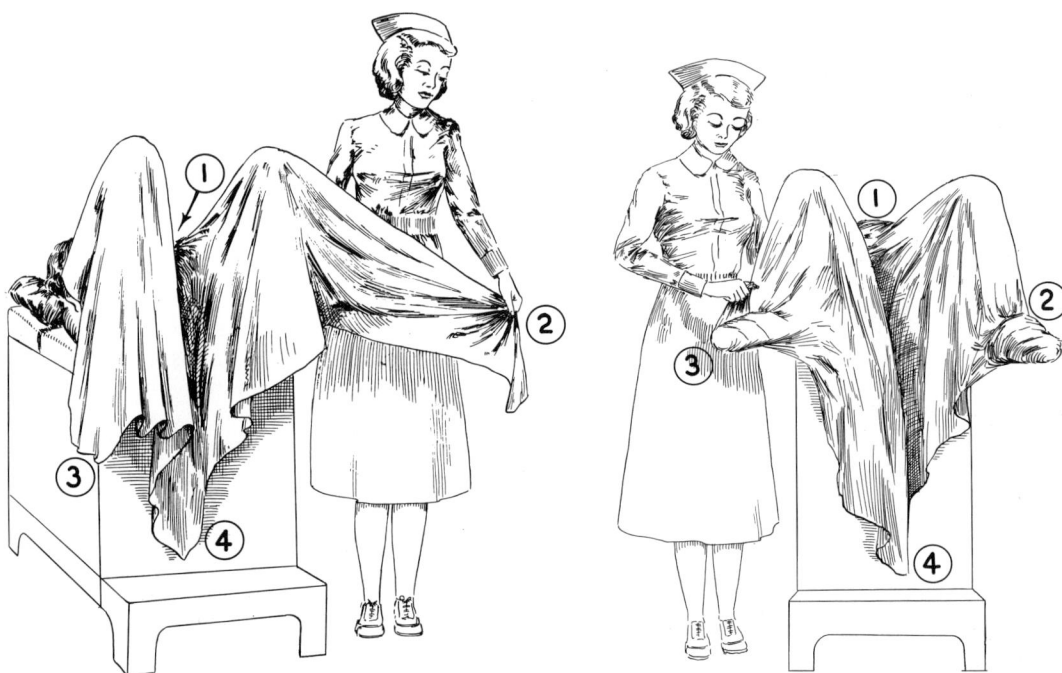

FIGURE 281

FIGS. 280, 281. Showing successive steps in draping for gynecologic examination. Note that the sheet is secured by wrapping the feet with corners 2 and 3.

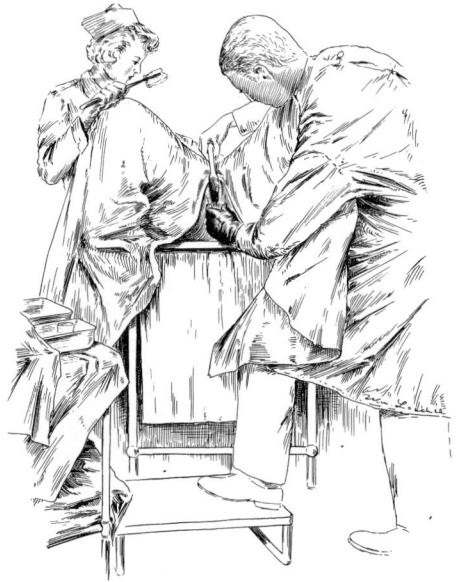

Fig. 282. Gynecologic examination. Dorsal position on examining table.

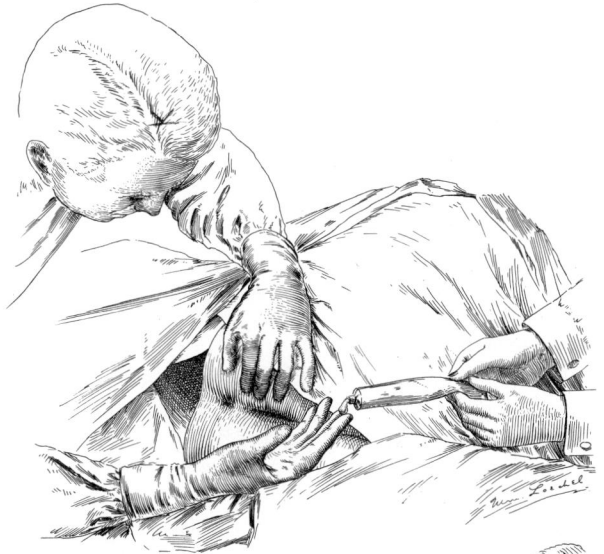

Fig. 283. Gynecologic examination in bed. Sim's position.

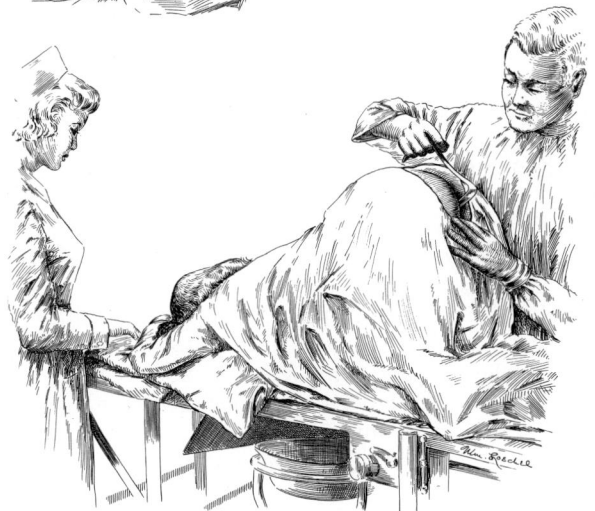

Fig. 284. Gynecologic examination. Knee-chest position.

of the pelvic cavity. Originally intended as a diagnostic aid for the detection of Stein-Leventhal syndrome (polycystic ovaries), this test now is used to find other pelvic disorders.

The patient is informed that she will experience a feeling of fullness during the gas injection, which will be followed by a sensation of pressure under the diaphragm. She also may have spasmodic pains in the right shoulder due to nerve irritation of the diaphragm from the gas displacement.

After the gynecogram the patient is placed in a Trendelenburg position for approximately 2 hours. This will help to relieve the shoulder spasm. A mild analgesic usually is all that is necessary to relieve any other discomfort.

DISTURBANCES OF MENSTRUATION

There is a definite interrelation between the hormonal secretions of the ovary, the thyroid and the pituitary glands. A disturbance of this relationship by an increased or decreased function of one or more of these glands may have an influence on the menstrual function. This is probably the most common cause of menstrual disturbances.

Dysmenorrhea

Dysmenorrhea, or painful menstruation, is a common condition found most often in unmarried women. The pain probably is due to uterine spasm. This may be caused by a narrowing of the cervical canal but is more probably a result of endocrine gland dysfunction. The symptoms, acute cramplike pains in the lower abdomen, often associated with headache and vomiting, are most severe during the first day of the period. Pregnancy and childbirth often cure the condition.

Treatment. The treatment of dysmenorrhea may be medical, surgical and/or psychological. The medical treatment of dysmenorrhea is moderate exercise and the use of analgesics, sedatives, or mild antispasmodics. The patient should be encouraged to eat a nutritious diet as this helps to promote the proper function of hormones. Fatigue should be avoided, and emotional upsets should be investigated and corrected, as these factors tend to lower the pain threshold.

Patients who have severe dysmenorrhea may be helped by hormone therapy.

In the surgical treatment an effort is made to correct the conditions causing the narrowing of the cervical canal. Displacements of the uterus (pp. 736-737) are corrected, and the cervical canal is dilated or stretched. Some physicians prescribe pelvic exercises, and others have treated the condition by cutting nerve fibers (presacral neurectomy).

Amenorrhea

Amenorrhea, or the absence of menstrual flow, occurs normally during pregnancy and lactation. However, extreme anxiety, acute or chronic disease, anemia or disease of the ductless glands (especially the thyroid and the pituitary) and certain ovarian tumors (particularly arrhenoblastomas) may cause amenorrhea.

Treatment. The treatment is directed toward the correction of the cause. Often there is a pituitary or thyroid dysfunction in the background that may be helped by appropriate measures.

Menorrhagia

Menorrhagia is excessive bleeding at the time of the regular menstrual flow. Its cause in early life may be due to endocrine disturbances, but menorrhagia with increase in duration of the menstrual periods in later life usually is due to inflammatory disturbances or tumors of the uterus.

Metrorrhagia

Metrorrhagia is the appearance of blood from the uterus between the regular menstrual periods or after the menopause. It is always the symptom of some disease, often cancer or benign tumors of the uterus; therefore, it merits early diagnosis and treatment.

THE MENOPAUSAL STATE

This period of a woman's life, usually occurring between the ages of 42 and 52, marks the end of her active reproductive life. Menstruation then ceases, and as a result of the complete cessation of activity on the part of the ovaries, the reproductive organs and the mammary glands atrophy. No more ova develop and no ovarian hormones are produced. A similar situation prevails earlier if the ovaries are removed or destroyed by irradiation, giving rise to the artificial menopause. From the medical point of view this period is of concern because of certain more general manifestations—some temporary, some permanent—that may appear.

Usually, the menopause starts gradually and is recognized by the change in menstruation. The monthly flow becomes smaller in amount, then irregular and finally ceases. Often, the time between periods gets longer—there may be a lapse of several months between them. Any prolonged menstrual flow or bleeding between periods should be reported to the physician promptly.

Before and during these changes in the monthly periods certain symptoms may appear, e.g., hot or warm flushes, dizziness, weakness, nervousness, insomnia. Many women have very mild symptoms; some have none at all; with a few the discomfort is very severe.

The symptoms are caused by the disappearance of the female sex hormone that the ovaries produce. The same symptoms occur when the ovaries are removed surgically because of disease (surgical menopause). After a period of months, or even a year or two, the body adjusts itself, and the symptoms disappear. While this adjustment is taking place, hot flushes, etc., can appear.

Modern medical treatment is very successful in relieving the symptoms of the menopause. The physician gives his patient medication containing the ovarian hormone (or chemicals which act like it). In other words, he puts back into her body what nature is no longer producing. The treatment is continued until her body adjusts itself, and hot flushes and other symptoms disappear. Treatment is necessary for a period of several months to a year or even two years. Medical care at this time also helps to correct the cause of nervousness and low spirits that often go along with menopause. Mental depression is not at all unusual at this time. Sometimes, it becomes so deep that even an everyday problem seems too much to cope with.

The menopause is not a complete change of life. The normal sex urges remain, and women retain their usual reaction to sex long after the menopause. There is nothing abnormal about the change of life and nothing unusual about the continuation of happy marital relations afterward.

Many women enjoy better health after the menopause than they have had for years. This is especially true with persons who have always suffered pain during their menstrual periods.

Patient Education and Treatment

The physician and the nurse should take the time to explain to the patient that the cessation of the menses is a normal physiologic function that is not necessarily accompanied by extreme nervous symptoms and various illnesses. Measures should be taken to promote her general health. Since many patients are in the menopausal age group, the following factors should be stressed in patient teaching:

The climacteric period is normal and self-limiting.

Overfatigue and environmental problems exaggerate the symptoms.

Interest and participation in outside activities help to absorb anxiety and to lessen tension.

A nutritious diet and avoidance of overweight will improve the physical condition.

The menopause does not mean a termination of the sex life.

An annual physical examination is essential to the maintenance of continuing good health.

The majority of patients will respond to a program of education, reassurance, modification of their living habits, and an improved regimen of health. In some patients mild sedatives and tranquilizers are necessary to control nervousness and to counteract depression. If hot flushes and sweats make the patient miserable, replacement therapy in the form of estrin is given. Short courses of estrogen therapy (diethylstilbestrol 0.5 mg. daily) will relieve the patient's symptoms and assist her during this period of physiologic adjustment. This drug also will produce re-epithelialization of the reproductive tract and relieve the itching and the burning of atrophic vaginitis.

THE PATIENT WITH A GYNECOLOGIC PROBLEM

The nurse is in a key position to teach and to advise girls and women regarding the principles of good health and personal hygiene. The reproductive system, like any other part of the anatomy, will function well if the body has adequate nutrition, exercise, rest and elimination. Teaching extends into the area of social diseases as well as prenatal and postnatal care. Complications can be prevented if proper medical care and supervision are available. The nurse is in a unique position to acquaint the lay person with the normal physiologic processes of menstruation and menopause. Many difficulties encountered by the young girl or the middle-aged woman usually can be corrected quite easily; if allowed to go untreated, they may cause irreparable damage. Danger signals which every woman should report to her physician are spotting, irregular or excessive bleeding or any bleeding after menopause. Persistent painful menstruation, leukorrhea and urinary disturbances also ought to be investigated. Many of these early signs can be corrected simply and permanently. An annual pelvic examination is especially important for the woman who is past 30 years of age. The broad public health implications are a necessary part of gynecologic nursing.

The gynecologic patient often calls for more understanding than other patients, because in addition to physical conditions there are many emotional factors governing the situation. She may resent any reference to her genitourinary system, feeling that she is suspected of questionable social or sexual habits. A real fear of venereal disease or of cancer may exist. All or any of these thoughts may manifest themselves in her conversation with the nurse, who by an understanding attitude can do much to dispel such anxieties.

Mixed emotional upsets can result from other fears. The suggestion of surgery as a means of treatment may raise a fear of disturbance of the reproductive process. Perhaps an explanation of the anatomy and the proposed treatment will clarify the situation. Any intention of sterilization must be explained carefully to the patient and her husband by the physician. Perhaps religious belief is more important to a patient than physical treatment. The decision rests with the patient, and, when it is made, it must be respected and supported.

Psychic factors may present themselves at the menopausal period. The loss of the reproductive capacity may cause disappointment if the woman has had no children. For a woman with a grown family, it may mean that she feels there is no further need for her. Present methods of mass production have left the individual with much less to do than formerly, and leisure time may hang heavily on her hands. But the nurse will continue to practice the principles of good nursing care and bend her energies to helping her patient to orient herself to any change that may be necessary for her to make at this period.

Special Nursing Considerations

Because many gynecologic diseases may be caused by highly infective organisms, especially the gonococcus, it is absolutely imperative that all instruments and equipment (catheters, douche nozzles, bedpans, rectal tubes and so forth) used in the treatment be sterilized both before and after their use. The nurse may protect herself by the use of rubber gloves, which should be cleansed and resterilized after treating each patient. If gloves are not available, or the procedure does not require their use, it is wise to scrub the hands thoroughly, especially after having had anything to do with an infected patient. When possible, dressings, perineal pads and so forth should be handled with forceps, and the forceps should be sterilized after use.

The spread of an infection from one patient to another or to the nurse is evidence of extreme laxity and carelessness in the nursing personnel, and its possibility should be constantly in mind in gynecologic work.

A second admonition to the gynecologic nurse is this: never talk about your patient or her disease. Gynecologic conditions often are of such a personal and a private nature that no patient would wish her nurse to tell other nurses, friends, or even her own family, the details of her operation or treatment. All such questions must be referred to the surgeon in charge of the patient. He alone is responsible. It is up to him to decide what information to give concerning his patient and which person should get it.

Preparation of Patient for Gynecologic Operations

This differs little from the details described for the preparation of a patient for a laparotomy. The lower half of the abdomen and the pubic and the perineal regions should be carefully shaved and cleansed with soap and water. The bowels and the bladder should be empty before the patient is sent to the operating room. This is most important.

Douches are common therapeutic measures in the treatment of patients with gynecologic diseases. They are used both before and after operation and are of two types: vulvar and vaginal.

Vulvar irrigations are indicated chiefly after operations on the perineum. They should be given after each urination or bowel movement in an effort to keep the incision free from infection. The patient should be brought to the side of the bed and placed on the bedpan in the dorsal position, with the knees apart and the labia separated. The bed should be protected by placing a rubber or plastic sheet under the pan. Warmed sterile water then is poured gently over the vulva from a sterile pitcher. The area is dried with sterile gauze or cotton, and a sterile dressing or pad is applied and held in place with a T-binder.

Vaginal douches are used therapeutically to cleanse or disinfect the vagina and adjacent parts both before and after operation. They may be used also to soothe inflamed tissues and to stimulate relaxed tissues. Occasionally, hot or cold douches are indicated in the treatment of oozing from the parts.

The patient is prepared for a vaginal douche in the same manner as for a vulvar douche.

Commonly used solutions include sterile water, normal saline, and boric acid solution.

Douches should be given at a temperature of 110° F. or as ordered. To give the douche, the patient is placed in the dorsal position on the bedpan and covered to prevent chilling. The tube leading from the douche bag is clamped, and the end of the tube with the douche nozzle is inserted into the reservoir, which then is hung on the standard. The reservoir should be not more than 2 feet above the level of the patient's hips. The nurse then puts on the sterile gloves, and, separating the labia with the thumb and the forefinger of the left hand, cleans the vaginal orifice and inserts the douche nozzle gently into the vagina for a distance of 2 inches, the tip being directed toward the hollow of the sacrum. The clamp then is removed from the tube, and the solution is allowed to flow. Pressure should be avoided to prevent douche fluid refluxing through the uterus and the tubes. The solution can be allowed to flow intermittently until at least 1 liter of solution has been used. The treatment should not be done hastily if therapeutic benefits are to be achieved. It should take from 20 to 30 minutes. At this time the nozzle may be removed, and the patient should be asked to strain as if trying to move the bowels. This act tends to expel the fluid remaining in the vagina. The bedpan then is removed, and the parts are dried with cotton. The patient should be instructed to remain flat on her back for at least an hour after a hot douche. After the douche has been completed, the apparatus should be cleansed and sterilized again, including the bedpan.

Vaginal antiseptic jellies have been available for local application since the advent of chemotherapy, sulfa and penicillin jellies. By means of an applicator, the patient is able to administer such medication. Creams or jellies can be used before and after operation, and in many instances they are substituted for the therapeutic and cleansing douche. It may be necessary for the patient to wear a perineal pad during the course of the application.

CONDITIONS OF EXTERNAL GENITALIA AND VAGINA

Vulvitis and Abscess of Bartholin's Glands

Vulvitis, an inflammation of the vulva, may occur as a result of uncleanliness or irritating discharges, but most often it is the result of a gonorrheal infection. The infecting organism, the gonococcus,

is infectious only in the moist state and grows only on moist surfaces. Under dry conditions it soon dies. Gonorrhea is therefore an almost purely contagious disease and is rarely transferred indirectly except in the case of young children. With this last exception, gonorrhea of the genitals is transmitted almost exclusively by sexual contact. (Graves)

The symptoms of the disease may be very slight, but in the typical case the patient complains of a constant burning pain that is worse during urination and defecation. The genitalia become red and edematous, and

Table 19. The Patient With a Vaginal Infection

Condition	Cause	Signs and Symptoms	Objectives of Treatment
Trichomonas vaginalis	Trichomonas vaginalis	Inflammation of vaginal epithelium, producing burning and itching Greenish-yellow or yellowish-white vaginal discharge	To remove exudate, relieve inflammation, restore acidity and reestablish normal bacterial flora: vinegar or pHisoHex douches; insert Floraquin tablets To destroy infective protozoa: insert chlortetracycline capsules q. 2 n. x 7
Monilial infection	Candida albicans (fungus)	Inflammation of vaginal epithelium producing itching, reddish irritation White cheeselike discharge clinging to epithelium	To eradicate the fungus: Local applications of gentian violet; Myco-statin vaginal supposi-tories To relieve other causative factors: Stop antibiotic therapy; determine if diabetes or other systemic disease is present
Infection of Bartholin's gland	Escherichia coli Trichomonas vaginalis Staphlyococcus Streptococcus Gonococcus	Erythema around Bartholin's gland Swelling and edema Development of Bartholin's abscess	To drain the abscess: Antibiotic therapy; surgical drainage; excision of gland in patients with chronic bartholinitis
Cervicitis— acute and chronic	Gonorrhea Streptococcus Many pathogenic bacteria	Profuse purulent vaginal discharge Backache Urinary frequency and urgency	To determine the cause: Cytologic examination of cervical smear To eradicate the gonococcus, if present: Penicillin, 600,000 units daily, or chloromycetin therapy if indicated To eradicate other causes: cervical cauterization
Postmenopausal vaginitis (atrophic vaginitis)	Lack of estrin effects	Loss of redness, tissue folds, and epithelial covering of the vagina Itching and burning	To provide estrogen therapy for vaginal epithelializa-tion: Topical estrogen therapy; improve nutrition

there is a profuse purulent exudate in which the gonococci may be found by examination of a smear.

The infection usually involves Bartholin's gland, the glands in the floor of the urethra and those in the cervix of the uterus. Not infrequently, the infection of Bartholin's gland leads to the formation of an abscess (vulvovaginal) that is characterized by more acute throbbing pain and swelling between the labia.

In the treatment of such a condition, the antibiotics (especially penicillin) are most effective. Not infrequently, the inflammatory reaction may subside, but there usually is a recurrence later if the gland is not excised. The duct of the gland often may be occluded after subsidence of the inflammation. As the gland continues to secrete, a Bartholin's cyst is formed. These cysts usually are removed surgically.

Once the acute stage of the infection has passed, the disease tends to become chronic. The organisms lurk in the infected glands, and the patient becomes a constant source of infection for others, often innocent persons. She is likely to have recrudescences of the disease with extension of the infection to the uterus, the fallopian tubes and even the peritoneal cavity. (For additional treatment see Acute Salpingitis, p. 738).

Vaginitis

Vaginitis is an inflammation of the lining of the vaginal wall. *Trichomonas vaginalis* and *Candida albicans* are two very common parasitic invaders. They produce intense itching and characteristic discharges.

Trichomonas vaginalis can be controlled by using Floraquin, which restores the glycogen, the *Lactobacillus acidophilus* and the acidity which are characteristics of normal vaginal tissue. A more recent treatment is the insertion of gelatin capsules of chlortetracycline every other night for a period of 2 weeks. *Candida albicans* is treated successfully by swabbing with gentian violet. Certain medicated jellies are also effective and more convenient to apply.

Gonorrheal Vulvovaginitis

This occurs often in infants and in little girls by indirect infection through towels, diapers, thermometers and the hands of attendants. It is not uncommon for an epidemic of this disease to occur in babies' and children's wards in hospitals or institutions; for this reason, every female child admitted to such an institution should be examined and a smear taken from the vulva for microscopic examination.

The treatment of acute gonorrheal vulvitis and vulvovaginitis is carried out best with the patient in bed. Soft diet, especially plenty of fluids, and urinary antiseptics comprise the early treatment. Female sex hormone has been used with success. This may be given hypodermically or by vaginal suppositories. Penicillin is used with excellent results.

The nurse must employ every possible precaution against spreading the infection to other patients by instruments, dressings, bedpans and towels, and, in addition, especially in children, care must be taken against infecting the eyes. (See p. 864.)

Leukorrhea

Leukorrhea is the name given to a whitish or yellowish vaginal discharge. It may be the result of one or more vaginal or uterine diseases, acute or chronic infections, lacerations of the cervix and neoplasms.

The nursing care comprises cleansing antiseptic douches. Correction of the cause of the discharge is necessary for cure.

Condylomata

Condylomata are warty papillary excrescences that appear on the external genitalia. They are the result of irritation and infection. There are two usual types. Those of the pointed type are associated with gonorrhea; the flat condylomata usually are considered to be syphilitic in origin. The condylomata of themselves cause few symptoms, but nearly always there is an associated leukorrheal discharge that causes maceration and irritation.

Kraurosis and Leukoplakia

Kraurosis is a disease of the vulva in which the skin over these structures becomes thin and white and easily fissured. As the disease advances, the structure of the vulva may be shrunken and leathery in appearance. The chief symptom is marked itching. Often it leads to the development of cancer of the vulva.

Ovarian extract, antihistaminics and vitamin A have been used with some success in the treatment of these patients, but often in advanced cases vulvectomy is performed.

Leukoplakia is a somewhat similar condition characterized by grayish-white patchy thickening of the vulvar skin with itching and burning. It is treated as is kraurosis.

Cystocele

Cystocele is a downward displacement of the bladder toward the vaginal orifice (Fig. 285). It is caused occasionally by tissue weakness, but most often it is a result of injuries received during childbirth. The condition appears as a bulging downward of the anterior vaginal wall that causes a sense of pelvic pressure, easy fatigue and often such urinary symptoms as incontinence, frequency and urgency of urination.

The treatment of the condition is surgical, the operation for the repair of the anterior vaginal wall being termed *anterior colporrhaphy*. Perineal exercises sometimes are prescribed and help to strengthen the weakened muscles. These are more effective in the early stages of a cystocele.

Rectocele and Lacerations of Perineum

Injuries to the muscles and the tissues of the pelvic floor frequently occur at the time of childbirth. Due to tears in muscles below the vagina, the rectum may pouch upward, pushing the posterior wall of the vagina in front of it. This condition is termed a *rectocele* (Fig. 286). The lacerations may extend at times so as to sever completely the fibers of the anal sphincter (complete tear). The symptoms of this condition are similar to those given for cystocele, substituting for the urinary symptoms those of constipation and incontinence of gas and liquid feces in patients with complete tears.

The operation for the repair of these patients is called a *perineorrhaphy* or a *posterior colporrhaphy*. Anterior and posterior colporrhaphies often are classed together under the term *plastic operations*.

Nursing Care after Perineal Operations.

The patient always is urged to void within a few hours after operation, and every 4 to 8 hours thereafter. The bladder should not be allowed to accumulate more than 5 ounces of urine for the first few days, especially after operations for cystocele and complete tear. If the patient does not void within the above period, or if she feels uncomfortable or has pain in the region of the bladder before 6 hours, catheterization should be performed. Some physicians prefer to have an indwelling catheter in the patient for 2 to 4 days. There are various other methods of bladder care.

After each urination or bowel movement, the perineum should be irrigated with warm sterile saline (see vulvar douche, p. 727) and the area dried with sterile cotton.

There are several methods used in caring

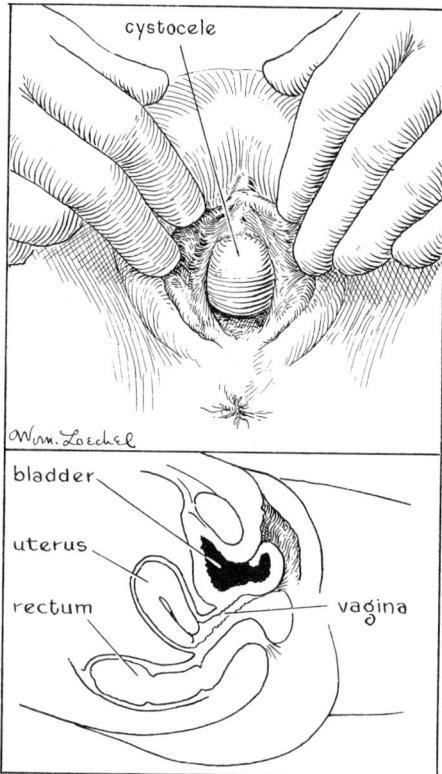

Fig. 285. Cystocele. Relaxation of the anterior vaginal wall permits downward bulge of bladder on straining.

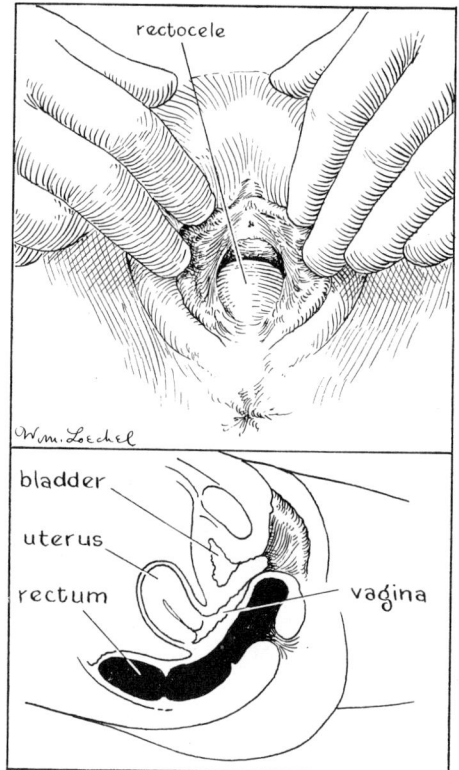

Fig. 286. Rectocele. Relaxation of the posterior vaginal wall permits bulging of the rectum with the vagina on straining.

for the stitches: one in which the stitches are left alone until healing occurs, i.e., for 5 to 10 days, and daily vaginal douches of sterile saline given thereafter during the period of convalescence; the other, the wet method, in which small douches of sterile saline are given twice daily, beginning on the day after operation and continuing throughout convalescence. Commercially available sprays containing a combination of antiseptic and anesthetic solutions are soothing and effective. Of course, the method to be used depends on the preference of the surgeon.

The routine postoperative care is much like that after an abdominal operation. The patient is placed in bed with the head and the knees elevated slightly. Liquid diet (many surgeons omit milk) is given on the first day and then a full diet as soon as desired.

Patients after operations for a complete perineal laceration (through the rectal sphincter) require special care and attention. The bladder should be emptied by catheterization if the patient is having discomfort. The patient should be kept flat in bed with the head raised on a pillow. Most surgeons prefer that the patient have no bowel movements for 5 to 7 days. A rectal tube should not be introduced during this period, and enemas never are used. Liquid diet without milk is given, and, in order to reduce peristalsis and "lock the bowels," opium pills or tincture of opium (15 minims) may be administered. On the 6th or the 7th day the bowels are opened by giving 1 ounce of mineral oil, followed at the first inclination for a bowel movement by a small oil enema (3 or 4 ounces) that should be retained for a few minutes.

Throughout the convalescence of all patients who have had plastic surgery, liquid petrolatum or other stool-softening agent is given each night after a soft diet is begun.

CONDITIONS OF THE UTERUS

Lacerations of the Cervix

Lacerations of the cervix often occur as a result of childbirth. When healing takes place, a considerable portion of the mucous membrane, which normally lies in the cervical canal, is everted. It practically always becomes infected and causes an annoying leukorrhea. Most surgeons believe that cervical lacerations predispose to cancer of the cervix, and for this reason these lacerations should be repaired, particularly in the 5th decade, the time when cancer is most likely to occur.

Endocervicitis

Endocervicitis is an inflammation of the mucosa and the glands of the cervix. In the majority of cases the inflammation is caused by the ordinary pyogenic organisms, but gonorrheal infection of the glands occurs not infrequently. The chief symptom is a thick purulent leukorrheal discharge, at times associated with sacral backache, low abdominal pain and disturbances in menstruation.

Palliative treatment consists of douches and the application of antiseptics to the cervix, but often a cure is effected only after destroying the cervical glands with a cautery or excising the diseased tissue. Bacitracin in combination with penicillin is proving to be effective in the treatment of chronic cervicitis and cervical erosion.

Cancer of the Cervix

Cancer of the cervix is the second most common cancer of women. It may occur at any age, but it is most common between the ages of 30 to 50. This disease is almost always curable in its preinvasive state. Early cancer of the cervix is usually asymptomatic. Therefore, to discover the disease early, every woman over 35 years of age should have a thorough gynecologic examination yearly.

Cancer of the cervix is found most often in patients who have had children. Chronic infections and erosions of the cervix seem to play a significant part in its development. It may become a large cauliflowerlike growth or a deep, ulcerating crater before giving many symptoms of its presence.

The following classification has been widely accepted. In studying this chart one has the sobering realization that the prognosis of the patient with Stage 4 cancer of the cervix is poor, and that the patient's problems are many.

The two chief symptoms of early carcinoma are leukorrhea and irregular vaginal

---

INTERNATIONAL CLASSIFICATION OF CARCINOMA
OF THE UTERINE CERVIX

Stage 0. Carcinoma in situ. The carcinoma is limited to the epithelial layer with no evidence of invasion.

Stage 1. The carcinoma is confined strictly to the cervix.

Stage 2. Parametrial cancer. The carcinoma infiltrates the parametrium on one or both sides, but does not invade the pelvic wall.

Stage 2. Vaginal cancer. The carcinoma infiltrates the vagina, but does not involve the lower third.

Stage 2. Corpus cancer. The endocervical carcinoma has spread to the corpus.

Stage 3. Parametrial cancer. The carcinomatous infiltration of the parametrium invades the pelvic wall on either one or both sides. On rectal examination, no cancer-free space is found between the tumor and the pelvic wall.

Stage 3. Vaginal cancer. The carcinoma involves the lower third of the vagina.

Stage 3. Isolated pelvic metastases. Isolated carcinomatous metastases are palpable on the pelvic wall (irrespective of the extent of the primary cervical growth).

Stage 4. Bladder extension. The carcinoma involves the bladder; determined by cystoscopic examination or by the presence of a vesicovaginal fistula.

Stage 4. Rectal extension. The carcinoma involves the rectum.

Stage 4. Distant spread. The carcinoma spreads outside the true pelvis (below the vaginal inlet, above the pelvic brim and now includes distant metastases to other organs).

---

bleeding or spotting. For a long time the leukorrhea may be the only abnormal symptom. The discharge increases gradually in amount, becomes watery and, finally, dark and foul-smelling because of necrosis and infection of the tumor mass. The bleeding occurs at irregular intervals, between the periods or after the menopause (metrorrhagia). It may be very slight, just enough to spot the undergarments, and it is noted usually after some form of trauma (intercourse, douching or defecation). As the disease continues, the bleeding may become constant and increase in amount.

As the cancer advances, the tissues outside the cervix are invaded, including the lymph glands anterior to the sacrum. The nerves in this region become involved, so that there is excruciating pain in the back and the legs that is relieved only by large doses of narcotics. The final picture is one of extreme emaciation and anemia, often with irregular fever due to secondary infection and abscesses in the ulcerating mass.

In situ cancer of the cervix is confined to the mucosal layer of the cervix. If the patient is of the childbearing age, the surgeon may perform an extensive conization, a procedure in which the substance of the cervix surrounding the entire length of the cervical canal is dissected free of its epithelial coverings and removed, like the core of an apple, together with the involved mucosa. Following this procedure, however, the patient will have to have periodic cytologic smears and close follow-up supervision. In the majority of patients a simple hysterectomy is preferred for cancer in situ.

Patients with more extensive cancer usually are treated with radiation therapy. Radium or radioactive cobalt is introduced into the endocervical canal for a period of time as prescribed by the radiotherapist. This treatment may be supplemented by external radiation therapy with supervoltage machines directed over the pelvis in an effort to eliminate the spread of cancer via the lymphatic system. A protective shield is placed over the intracavitary area receiving radium. The therapy is individualized ac-

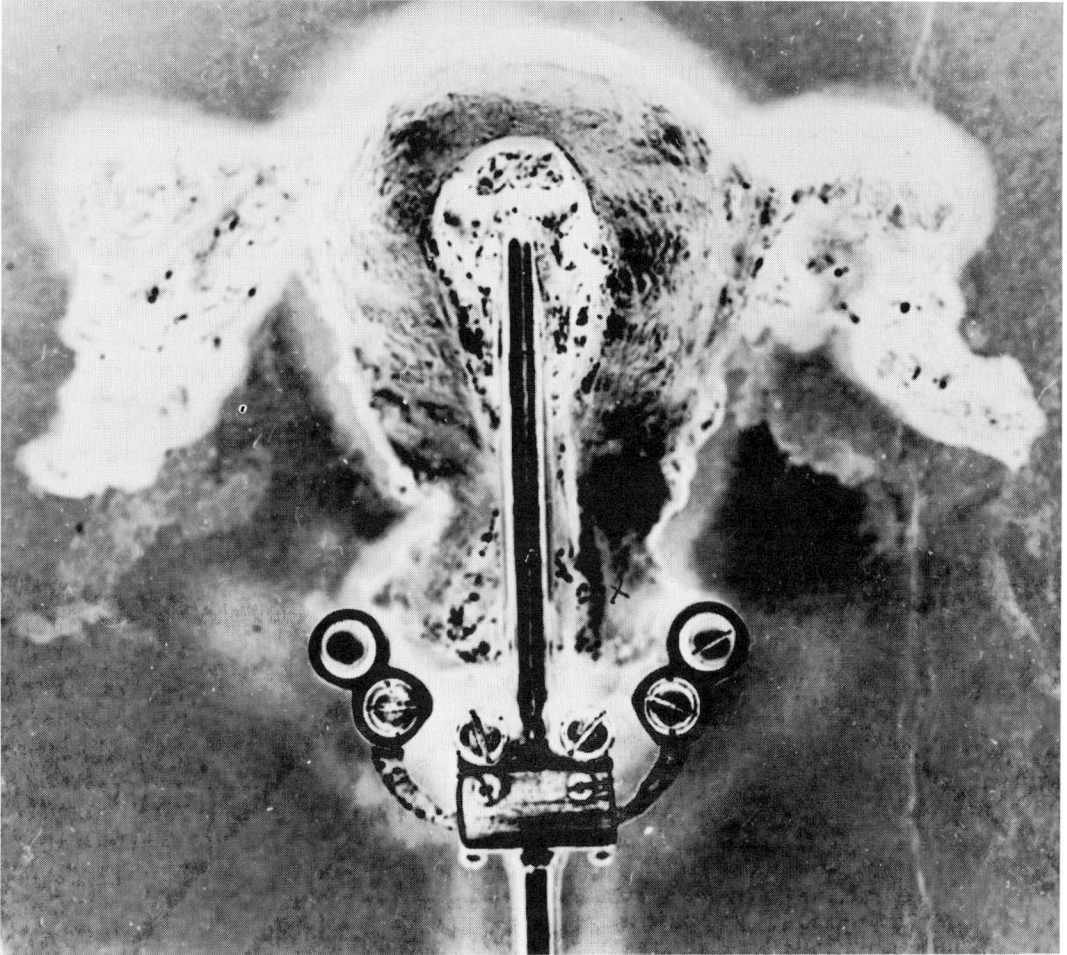

FIG. 287. Sagittal section through the uterus showing an Ernst applicator in treatment position. Gauze packing usually is placed on the anterior and the posterior sides of the applicator to hold it firmly in position. This may produce a sensation of pressure in the bladder and the rectum. (Radium Chemical Co., Inc., New York, N. Y.)

cording to the patient's stage of disease and her response and tolerance for radiation.

Radical surgery is advocated by some authorities especially when a patient is unable to withstand the effects of radiation or has a radiation-resistant cancer. The type of surgery may vary from a radical hysterectomy with bilateral dissection of nodes to a total exenteration of the pelvic organs. The latter operation is performed occasionally when distant metastasis has not occurred, and the disease is confined to the pelvis. The pelvic lymph nodes, the uterus, the vagina, the bladder, and the rectum are removed; the urinary stream is diverted into an isolated ileal loop or to the skin surface of the abdomen. The patient and her husband are advised before the operation about the permanent colostomy stoma and the diversion of the urinary stream.

Radiation Therapy. Several applicators are manufactured for radiation treatment of carcinoma of the cervix and the uterus. The Ernst applicator is one of those most commonly used for cervical carcinoma. It consists of a central portion (tandem) that is inserted into the uterus. The tandem contains from 1 to 3 radium tubes. Surrounding the cervix in the vaginal vault are radium-loaded capsules called *ovoids*. The ovoids and the intrauterine tandem are fixed together in one applicator. Different sections of the tandem and the ovoids are loaded with tubes of radium in the Radiotherapy Department and transported to the operating room in a long-handled lead cart.

An indwelling catheter is inserted to keep the bladder empty. Under anesthesia the cervix is dilated in the same manner as in a dilatation and curettage. The applicator is inserted, the tandem being placed in the uterus and the ovoids in the vaginal vault (Fig. 287). Then vaginal packing is inserted to maintain the position of the applicator. The objective of treatment at this time is to keep the tandem and the ovoids at certain anatomic points so that the radiation will remain at a fixed dosage and not be changed during the hours of treatment.

Nursing the Patient Receiving Radium Treatment. *While the radium is in place, all nursing measures are geared to keeping the radium applicator in the uterine canal and to prevent a change in the position of the applicator during the course of treatment.* Usually, the patient is on a low-residue diet to prevent the bowels from moving and possibly dislodging the radium. The nurse should inspect the catheter frequently to make sure that it is draining properly. *The chief hazard of improper drainage is that the bladder may become distended and be in the path of radiation.*

The patient is observed for evidence of temperature elevation, nausea or vomiting. These symptoms should be reported to the physician, as often they are indicative of radium sickness. Although antiemetic drugs may be given to the patient at this time, the radiotherapist usually modifies the dosage schedule, as these symptoms may indicate that the patient is reaching her point of tissue tolerance. These patients often have poor appetites and need to be encouraged to eat and to drink.

The nurse must remember to protect herself from excessive radiation. While appearing unhurried, she should care for the patient's needs in as efficient manner as possible. Hence, visits to the patient should not be aimless, and these nurse-patient contacts should provide opportunity for the patient to talk, relieving her anxiety and fear.

At the end of the prescribed period (the nurse should know the duration of the application), she should notify the surgeon in charge that it is time for the removal of the radium. Sterile gloves, long forceps and a waste basin should be provided for his use.

A linen bag is kept in the patient's unit, and any soiled linen is stored there until the radium has been removed and accounted for.

Radium is the most expensive metal in common use today. The tiny amount used in the application often is valued at thousands of dollars, so that extreme care is necessary in handling the tubes after their removal from a patient. The number of tubes applied should be noted on the operating sheet, and the nurse should be sure that the same number is removed. After removal from the filters, the tubes should be placed in small lead or brass bottles supplied for the purpose and taken immediately to the hospital repository. Burns may be obtained by an overdosage; that is, by not removing the radium at the end of the prescribed time or by too frequent handling of radium tubes. For this reason they should be removed promptly from the patient at the end of the prescribed period and handled not directly but with long forceps, preferably behind a lead shield. After the patient has had the radium removed, usually she is given a cleansing enema, and then she may be out of bed. (See p. 317, Radiation Therapy.)

Unfortunately, before x-rays can reach the tissue which requires treatment, they must pass through healthy tissue. The skin is especially vulnerable, and caution must be practiced to avoid burns. The skin is kept dry; the use of soap on irradiated areas is avoided. When areas of erythema occur, a bland ointment such as aloe vera ointment or white petrolatum may relieve the irritation. No ointment should be used unless ordered by the physician. With the use of supervoltage x-ray units, large tumorcidal doses can be given with less skin reaction.

Following large doses of x-rays, the patient may show anorexia, nausea and vomiting. Diarrhea and tenesmus are symptoms of radiation injury to the intestine. These symptoms should be reported to the physi-

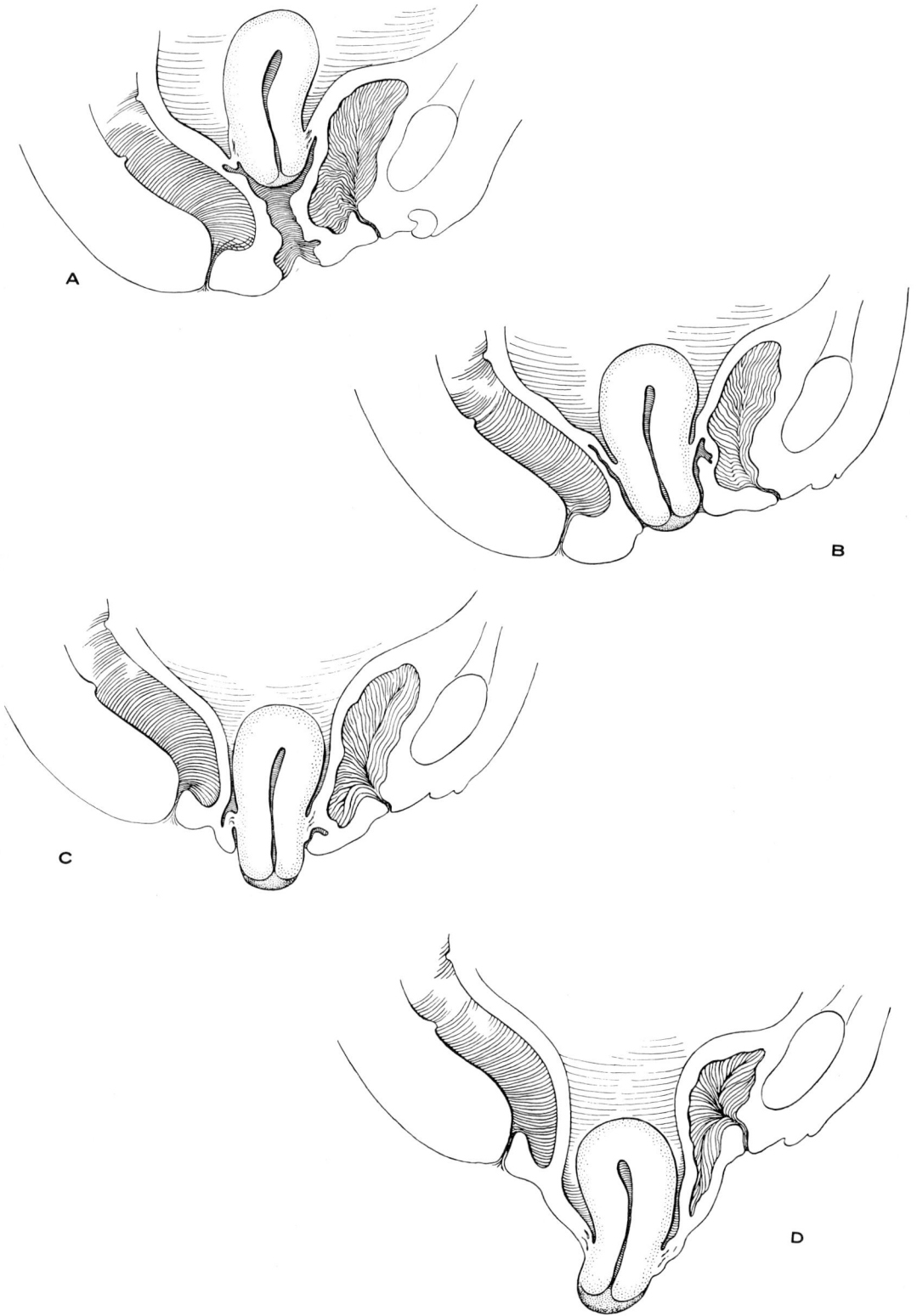

FIG. 288. (A) First-degree prolapse of the uterus and the vagina. (B) Second-degree prolapse. (C) Third-degree prolapse. (D) Procidentia. (Gray, L. A.: Prolapse of the uterus and vagina, Postgrad. Med. **30**:208-209)

cian, who will decide whether treatment should continue.

During treatment the nurse should encourage her patient to drink citrus-fruit juices. Small, frequent servings may be more appetizing than large servings. Pyridoxine orally is helpful in minimizing discomfort.

Nursing the Patient with Advanced Cancer of the Cervix. Unfortunately, not every patient will be seen by a physician and treated early. Only palliative treatment is suitable when the disease is advanced. The patient's major problems will arise from pain, vaginal bleeding and a foul-smelling discharge, intestinal obstruction, and urinary or fecal fistulae.

Mild analgesics, such as salicylates, will provide symptomatic relief at first, and later in the course of the disease, opiates will be necessary. Radiation therapy may help to control the pain. If not, a chordotomy may be effective.

Bleeding may be controlled by external or internal radiation, the insertion of local packing into the uterus, or by a bilateral hypogastric artery ligation. The malodorous discharge that is so distressing to the patient may be relieved by cleansing douches. Anti-

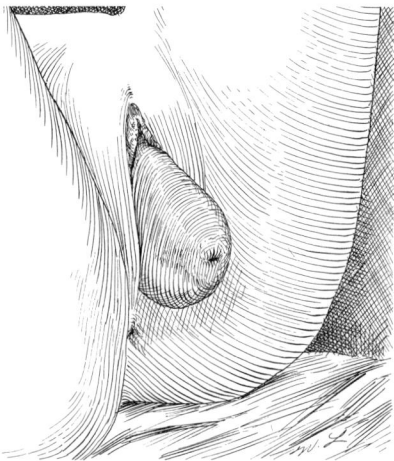

FIG. 289. Procidentia uteri. This is really a vaginal hernia caused by relaxation of the uterine ligaments. The vagina turns inside out and protrudes through the vulva. The opening in the center of the prolapsed vagina is the cervix.

biotic therapy will allay secondary infection. The soiled perineal pads should be changed frequently, wrapped in paper, and removed from the room immediately.

When an intestinal obstruction occurs, a colostomy may be necessary. Surgery or radiation therapy may cause the formation of urinary or fecal fistulae. If operative repair is not feasible, a diversion of the urinary or the fecal stream may be done. (See page 700.)

The nurse must be able to cope with the despair and the despondency manifested by these patients. It is important that the nurse help the patient to feel that her case is not "hopeless," and that she is not being neglected. Keeping the environment cheerful, promoting the intake of a nutritious diet, and encouraging the family to give extra little attentions will help to brighten the patient's day and to raise her morale.

Displacements of the Uterus

The uterus lies normally with the cervix at right angles to the long axis of the vagina and with the body inclined slightly forward. However, it is freely movable, owing to the requirements of pregnancy. The strain of this physiologic function, the formation of adhesions or a weakening of its natural supports may produce changes in the normal position that usually cause no trouble to the patient but may give rise to many troublesome symptoms.

Backward Displacements. The backward displacements (retroversion and retroflexion) may give rise to such symptoms as backache, a sense of pelvic pressure, easy fatigue, and leukorrheal discharge. More retrograde displacements are asymptomatic rather than symptomatic.

The treatment of backward displacements is surgical only if the condition is incapacitating. The uterus is brought forward into its normal position by way of an abdominal incision and maintained by shortening its ligaments. Some patients with retroversion may be treated by the use of pessaries. These are S-shaped instruments of hard rubber or crystal-clear Plexiglas that keep the uterus forward by exerting pressure on ligaments attached to the posterior wall of the cervix. They are of great value as a test of the patient's symptoms and often effect a cure. Pessaries must be removed and cleaned by the surgeon at frequent intervals.

Prolapse and Procidentia. Due to the weakening of the supports of the uterus, most often brought about by childbirth, the uterus may work its way down the vaginal canal (prolapse; Fig. 288 A, B, C) and even appear outside the vaginal orifice (procidentia; Figs. 288 D, 289). In its descent the uterus pulls with it the vaginal walls and even the bladder and the rectum. The symptoms caused are similar to those mentioned for backward displacements, plus urinary symptoms (incontinence and retention) from displacement of the bladder.

The best treatment is operative; the uterus is sutured back into place. In patients after the menopause the uterus may be removed (hysterectomy). Many patients may be treated by pessaries when, because of age or disease, operation is not feasible.

Patients with prolapse or procidentia should be kept flat in bed for 2 or 3 days with a vaginal pack or a pessary in place. This treatment serves to take the tension off the strained ligaments and allows the surgeon to proceed with greater ease.

Anterior Displacements. Anterior displacements of the uterus may give no symptoms, but often they are associated with dysmenorrhea or sterility, or both.

Treatment may be operative. Or a stem pessary may be used, a rubber or glass rod being introduced into the uterus for about 6 weeks to hold it in position.

Myomata or Fibroid Tumors

Myomatous or fibroid tumors of the uterus are benign tumors arising from the muscle tissue of the uterus. They are very common, occurring in at least 40 per cent of all women (Graves). They develop slowly between the ages of 25 and 40, and often they attain large size after this period. They produce symptoms due to pressure on surrounding organs—pain, backache, constipation and urinary symptoms—and they often cause menorrhagia, metrorrhagia and even sterility.

Vaginal Hysterectomy. Removal of the uterus in most patients is carried out through an abdominal incision. This is especially true when the operation is performed for either benign or malignant tumor, or in cases in which the uterus has to be removed because of disease in the ovary or the fallopian tubes. In most of these patients the entire uterus is removed surgically although the uterus occasionally is amputated above the cervix. In older individuals and especially in individuals in whom prolapse has occurred, the uterus may be removed through the vagina. The abdomen is not entered in the vaginal hysterectomy, but the entire procedure is carried out through the vagina. In these patients either the uterus alone may be removed, or the uterus including the fallopian tubes and the ovaries may be taken away. Postoperative care of such patients is similar to that of those patients who have had plastic surgical procedures performed.

Treatment and Nursing Care. The treatment of uterine fibroids depends to a large extent on their size and location. As a rule, large tumors producing pressure symptoms should be removed. Usually, the uterus is removed (hysterectomy), the ovaries being preserved, if possible. If the tumor is small, it may be removed (myomectomy), the wound in the uterus being closed. This is the procedure of choice in young women. If the tumor is producing excessive bleeding, the uterus and the tumor are removed (hysteromyomectomy). In some patients radium or roentgen treatment is successful in reducing the size of the tumor and in checking the menorrhagia.

The postoperative care of a patient after removal of the uterus is similar to that of a patient having a laporotomy.

During a hysterectomy the bladder is manipulated and dislodged from its usual position. An indwelling catheter drains the bladder during the operative procedure. After the catheter is removed, the urinary output of the patient is measured to determine that no residual urine is present.

The nurse must be alert for any symptoms suggestive of thrombosis or embolism, as these complications may occur following pelvic surgery. Early ambulation and the use of elastic compression bandages, plus constant vigilance, can reduce this hazard.

In patients in whom there is anemia due to the loss of blood caused by the tumor, convalescence may be hastened by a high-protein diet supplemented by iron salts. If the tumor has been so large as to produce marked relaxation of the abdominal walls, often it is wise to advise the patient to wear an abdominal support or a girdle for a time after the operation. For these patients the surgeon usually will order the application of an abdominal binder after surgery, to be worn until the support is obtained.

Cancer of the Fundus

Cancer of the fundus of the uterus is seen only about one eighth as often as cancer of the cervix. About 50 per cent of all patients with postmenopausal bleeding have cancer of the fundus. Its progress is slow, metastasis occurs later, and the symptom of irregular vaginal bleeding often appears early enough in the disease to allow cure by the removal of the uterus. In late cases, radium and roentgen rays are the usual therapeutic measures.

CONDITIONS OF OVARIES AND BROAD LIGAMENTS

Ovarian Cysts and Tumors

The ovary is a frequent site for the development of cysts. These may be simply pathologic enlargements of normal ovarian constituents, cysts of the graafian follicle or corpus luteum, or they may arise from abnormal growth of ovarian epithelium, when they are to be considered to be as benign tumors with a possibility of becoming malignant.

Dermoid cysts are tumors that are believed to arise from parts of the ovum that disappear normally as ripening (maturation) takes place. As their origin is unsettled, all that can be said is that they are tumors made up of undifferentiated embryonal cells. They are slow-growing and at operation are found to contain a thick yellow sebaceous material arising from a skin lining. Hair, teeth, bone, brain, eyes and many other tissues often are found in a rudimentary state within these cysts.

Endometriosis and Endometrial Cysts

With each menstrual period the epithelial cells that line the uterus are discharged through the cervix into the vagina. Occasionally, these cells may find their way through the fallopian tubes into the peritoneal cavity, where they may be implanted on adjacent structures, usually the ovary, but occasionally on the sigmoid and the pelvic peritoneum. The implanted cells react to hormone stimulation in the same manner as do the normal cells lining the uterus, i.e., by hemorrhagic desquamation. In the ovary this process leads to cyst formation. The cysts gradually enlarge with degenerated bloody material, chocolate in color, which gives these cysts their name "chocolate cysts." They often require removal.

When the cysts are small and uncomplicated, few symptoms are produced. When the cysts become large or are fixed in the pelvis, symptoms develop due to pressure on the surrounding structures: constipation due to pressure on the rectum and the sigmoid; edema of the legs due to pressure on the veins; backache and pain in the legs due to pressure on the nerves. Large tumors produce a marked distention of the abdomen, often larger than that due to pregnancy. Gradual emaciation occurs, and the patient takes on a characteristic drawn, haggard look, commonly referred to as the "ovarian facies."

If the tumor is pedunculated, it may become twisted and give rise to acute sudden pain, often shocking in its severity.

Treatment and Nursing Care

The treatment of ovarian cysts is surgical removal. However, if malignant degeneration has taken place, with invasion of the abdomen and emaciation (general carcinomatosis), operation is of little benefit. The patient may be given roentgen therapy and testosterone. The abdomen may be tapped to relieve distention from ascites.

The postoperative nursing care after cystectomy needs no special mention, except for one particular. The marked decrease in intra-abdominal pressure incidental to the removal of a large cyst often leads to considerable abdominal distention. This complication may be prevented to some extent by the application of a pad and an abdominal binder.

CONDITIONS OF FALLOPIAN TUBES

Acute Salpingitis

Acute salpingitis (acute inflammation of the fallopian tubes) may be due to infection by streptococci or staphylococci but most commonly by the gonococcus. This organism reaches the tubes via the uterus, and the pus formed may escape from the abdominal opening and involve the ovary and the peritoneum of the pelvis. The extension of the inflammation gives it the name *pelvic inflammatory disease*. As the acute process subsides, widespread adhesions may form between the intestines, the ovaries, the tubes, and sometimes even within the tubes themselves. These tubal adhesions are frequent causes of sterility and ectopic pregnancy.

The symptoms of acute salpingitis arise somewhat suddenly, and often a considerable time after the primary infection. There is an acute attack of abdominal pain, associated with tenderness across the lower abdomen, moderate fever and, usually, vomiting. With symptoms more pronounced on the right side, the diagnosis of the disease must be differentiated from appendicitis.

Treatment and Nursing Care

It has been found by experience that the inflammation tends to subside under conservative treatment. Penicillin, the sulfa drugs and erythromycin have been used with great success in producing an early subsidence of the acute inflammation. Therefore, these patients are placed in the Fowler position and given hot vaginal douches twice daily and hot applications to the abdomen. Within 1 to 4 weeks the acute symptoms subside, and the patient enters into the stage of chronic pelvic inflammatory disease. The residual adhesions may produce a variety of symptoms—pelvic pain, disturbances of menstruation, constipation, sterility, neuroses and so forth. However, many patients recover completely after one or two attacks if reinfection is prevented. Patients with large bilateral masses may be cured completely and even have children.

In young women, operation is deferred as long as possible. Surgical intervention is considered only when symptoms persist after douching, rest, continence and diathermy have been tried.

The surgical treatment of these patients is to free adhesions and remove as much of the pelvic organs as seems to be beyond repair. Very frequently a removal of the uterus with both tubes and ovaries—bilateral salpingo-oophorectomy and hysterectomy—is necessary to effect a cure.

The nursing care of these patients presents no special difficulty. The douches in the acute stage should be given at 120° F., and usually 4 liters of the prescribed solution will be used. The nurse should bear constantly in mind the necessity for observing strict precautions against infection when caring for these patients (see p. 726).

After operation the chief complications are distention (see Chap. 18), constipation and urinary retention.

Ectopic Pregnancy

Ectopic pregnancy is a pregnancy in which the fertilized ovum does not reach the cavity of the uterus but becomes caught and embedded in the fallopian tube or, occasionally, in the ovary or the abdomen. As the fertilized ovum increases in size, the tube becomes more and more distended until finally, from 4 to 6 weeks after conception has occurred, rupture takes place, and the ovum is discharged into the abdominal cavity. The symptoms may start with attacks of colicky pain on the affected side due to distention of the fallopian tube. When tubal rupture occurs, the patient experiences agonizing pain, faintness, shock and air hunger. It is recognized at once that the patient is desperately ill; all the signs of hemorrhage—rapid, thready pulse, subnormal temperature, restlessness, pallor, sweating—are in evidence. By vaginal examination the surgeon is able to feel a large mass of clotted blood that has collected in the pelvis behind the uterus.

The treatment of ectopic pregnancy always is surgical—removal of the tube (salpingectomy), and the ovary if necessary, on the affected side. However, many patients are in such a shocked condition that immediate operation cannot be performed. Measures then should be instituted to combat the shock and hemorrhage (see Chap. 18) by elevation of the foot of the bed, transfusions and so forth. When the operation is performed early, practically all such patients recover with remarkable rapidity, but without operation the mortality is 60 to 70 per cent.

After operation the treatment is the same as that for any laparotomy, plus transfusions to combat the acute anemia.

Considerations in Infertility

Infertility is the inability to conceive. It may be remedied. However, should the condition persist, it is referred to as *sterility*. It becomes a gynecologic condition, because it may be caused by many gynecologic diseases, among which may be mentioned displacements and tumors of the uterus, genital infantilism and inflammations.

The treatment of these conditions varies with the causative disease. In arriving at the correct diagnosis, the *Rubin test* often is used. This procedure is to determine the patency of the fallopian tubes, which so frequently become closed after inflammation, especially of the gonorrheal type. A gas (oxygen or carbon dioxide) introduced into the uterus through a cannula should escape under normal conditions through the tubes into the abdominal cavity. If no gas escapes, the tubes are believed to be closed and point to the probable cause of sterility. Lipiodol, a radiopaque substance, often is used to determine the site of tubal obstruction. This oily material is introduced through the uterus to fill the tubes. Then an x-ray picture is taken to show the outline of the tubal lumen (salpingogram).

As the secretions of the endocrine glands, especially the thyroid and the pituitary, are so closely related to ovarian function, the investigations often include a basal metabolic test and an examination of the urine for the female sex hormone. It is known that sterility often is due to a hypofunction of the thyroid, the pituitary and the ovary.

It should be stated that extensive investigations of the female should not be attempted until the husband has been examined. In about 35 per cent of sterile marriages the male is at fault.

The treatment of sterility is a difficult matter, because it may be caused by a combination of several factors. Efforts are made to build up the general health of the patient, supplying the lacking glandular hormones as indicated. Operative treatments include removal of obstructions and plastic operations to restore tubal patency.

PELVIC EXENTERATION

Radical Pelvic Surgery

Pelvic exenteration or evisceration may be performed when other forms of therapy prove to be ineffective in checking the spread of cancer. These patients are selected carefully on the basis of their likelihood to survive the surgery as well as to adjust to and accept the imposed limitations.

Anterior pelvic exenteration is the removal of the bladder and lower part of the ureters. In addition, in women the vagina, the adnexa, the pelvic lymph nodes and the pelvic peritoneum are removed. The ureters are implanted in the colon or the small intestines.

Posterior pelvic exenteration is the removal of the colon and the rectum. In addition, in women the uterus, the vagina and the adnexa are removed. The pelvic lymph nodes may or may not be excised.

Total pelvic exenteration is the removal of the rectum, the distal sigmoid colon, the urinary bladder, the distal portion of the ureters and the internal iliac artery and vein. In addition, in the female all pelvic reproductive organs, lymph nodes, and the entire pelvic floor, including the pelvic peritoneum, levator muscles, and perineum are removed. Both urinary and fecal diversion are necessary in this procedure; hence, the patient will have a colostomy, and a substitute bladder will be made from a segment of ileum.

Nursing Care

This is a patient who in all probability has faced surgery before and is aware of most of the physical preparation required before going to the operating room. However, the most important preparation is psychological. The needs of this patient are courage, the ability to realize what is about to happen to her, and the fortitude to be able to accept it. Her consent to have the operation may be given without question, since it may be clearly evident that this is a lifesaving procedure.

However, the full impact of adjustment may come several days postoperatively. Expressions of the patient may offer clues to her feelings that will give direction to subsequent care. Usually, the patient's reaction takes one of three courses. (1) She may adjust very well without any abnormal complications. (2) She may become depressed, listless, and wish to die. (This reaction may be altered with antidepressant medications.

Meanwhile, the nurse continues to emphasize the *positive* features of the patient's future.) (3) There may be an insidious reaction in which the patient exalts her disfigurement, assuming an almost martyrlike pose. By being preoccupied with herself and centering her attention on her disability, she may show pettiness, be selfish in her demands, and withdraw interest from her family. The nurse's hope here is to try to turn the patient's thoughts from herself to others and to direct the patient to see her body in its proper perspective, focusing more attention on the intact parts.

This patient requires intensive care postoperatively. Because satisfactory body function is dependent on adequate fluid balance, particular attention needs to be given to an accurate intake and output record. Proper functioning of the gastrointestinal tract may take several days. The nurse is referred to colostomy and ileostomy care on pages 635 to 640. Likewise, in the care of a patient with radical surgery, the likelihood of complications is greater; therefore, the nurse will need to be aware of the signs and the symptoms of postoperative complications as well as the ways and means of avoiding such problems.

Teaching and rehabilitation are a continuous part of the care of the patient with a pelvic exenteration. This should be gradual, moving from the simple to the more complex. The family should be included as the convalescence of the patient continues. Cognizance of the patient's own reaction and day-by-day progress is observed carefully; encouragement and understanding go a long way in helping her to achieve as many goals as possible.

CLINICAL SITUATION

Mrs. Jones, a 40-year-old housewife, has had a history of moderate leukorrhea and vaginal spotting between menstrual periods. She is concerned that she may have cancer.

1. The most frequently encountered symptom of early carcinoma of the cervix is
   A. Pain.
   B. Vaginal discharge.
   C. Dyspareunia.
   D. Intermenstrual bleeding.

2. The usual diagnostic test for carcinoma of the cervix is done. The most frequently used diagnostic procedure is the
   A. Rubin test.
   B. Cytological smear.
   C. Hysterosalpingogram.
   D. Frei test.

3. After further studies the pathologist reported that Mrs. Jones has invasive carcinoma of the cervix. The surgeon and the radiotherapist elected to treat her with intercavitary and external radiation. The aim of radiation therapy is to
   A. Alleviate the patient's symptoms as a palliative measure.
   B. Irradiate the adjacent pelvic organs.
   C. Protect the regional lymph nodes from ionizing radiation.
   D. Destroy the cancer at both the primary and the metastatic sites.

4. The nurse should report symptoms of radiation sickness, as some modification may have to be made in Mrs. Jones's treatment. Symptoms of radiation sickness include
   A. Skin irritation.
   B. Loss of weight.
   C. Nausea and vomiting.
   D. Altered libido.

PROBLEM-SOLVING ACTIVITY

Review the International Classification of Cancer of the Uterine Cervix (p. 732).

1. What are the major problems of the patient that the nurse will encounter while caring for a patient with Stage 3 and Stage 4 cancer of the cervix?

2. What treatment and nursing measures will be necessary to relieve the patient's symptoms and help to promote her comfort?

BIBLIOGRAPHY AND SUGGESTED READING

Books

Meigs, J.: Surgical Treatment of Cancer of the Cervix, New York, Grune, 1954.
Parker, E.: The Seven Ages of Woman, Baltimore, Johns Hopkins Press, 1960.
Parsons, L., and Sommers, S. C.: Gynecology, Philadelphia, Saunders, 1962.

Articles

Anderson, N. J.: Nursing care after vulvectomy, Am. J. Nurs. **60:**668, 1960.

Bourgeault, O. A.: The feminine hygiene question, Am. J. Nurs. **56:**1021, 1956.

Brunschwig, A., and Daniel, W.: Total and anterior pelvic exenteration, Surg. Gynec. Obstet. **99:**324-330, 1954.

Butcher, Jr., H. R., and Spjut, H. J.: An evaluation of pelvic exenteration for advanced carcinoma of the lower colon, Cancer **12:** 681-687, 1959.

Christopherson, W. M., *et al.:* Control of cervical cancer, J.A.M.A. **182:**179-182, 1962.

Douglas, R. G., and Sweeney, W. J.: Exenteration operations in the treatment of advanced pelvic cancer, Am. J. Obstet. Gynec. **73:** 1169-1182, 1957.

Ennis, E. H.: An effective drug for trichomoniasis, Obstet. Gynec. (NY) **19:**592-594, 1962.

Fay, A. B.: Dysmenorrhea, Am. J. Nurs. **63:**77-79, Feb., 1963.

Glynn, R.: Vaginal pH and the effect of douching, Obstet. Gynec. (NY) **20:**369-372, 1962.

Hofmeister, F. J., and Reik, R. P.: Vulvectomy, Am. J. Nurs. **60:**666-667, May, 1960.

Kozinn, D. J., and Taschdjian, C. L.: Candidiasis, Am. J. Nurs. **61:**52-54, Jan., 1961.

Lammert, A. C.: The menopause, Am. J. Nurs. **62:**56-57, Feb., 1962.

Manfredonia, G.: Radiation therapy for cancer of the cervix, Am. J. Nurs. **59:**513-515, 1959.

Menaker, J. S., and Powers, K. D.: Management of primary dysmenorrhea, Obstet. Gynec. (NY) **20:**66-71, 1962.

Menaker, J. S.: When menstruation is painful, Am. J. Nurs. **62:**94-96, Sept., 1962.

Miller, O.: Nursing care after pelvic exenteration, Am. J. Nurs. **62:**106-107, May, 1962.

Parsons, L., and Taymor, M. L.: Longevity following pelvic exenteration for cancer of the cervix, Am. J. Obstet. Gynec. **70:**774-785, 1955.

Riva, H. L., *et al.:* Ectopic pregnancy, Obstet. Gynec. (NY) **20:**189-198, 1962.

Schmitz, H. E., *et al.:* The technique of synchronous abdominoperineal pelvic exenteration, Surg. Gynec. Obstet. **108:**351-356, 1959.

Sherman, A. I., and Woolf, R. B.: An endocrine basis for endometrial carcinoma, Am. J. Obstet. Gynec. **77:**233-242, 1959.

Unpublished paper: Murphy, Christopher, Jr., J., Wyman, A. C., and DeVries, J. E.: Nitrous oxide gynecography, Alexandria Hospital, Alexandria, Virginia.

Patient-Teaching Aids and Information

Cervical Cytology for Nurses. A 17-page handbook on clinical procedures, Public Health Service Pub. No. 798, Washington, D. C., U. S. Dept. of Health, Educ. and Welfare, 1960.

Cytology and cancer of the cervix. A 9-page pamphlet available from American Cancer Society, 1958.

Educational materials, charts, booklets and films on menstrual hygiene available from Personal Products Corp., Milltown, N. J.; Tampax, Inc., 161 E. 42nd St., New York 17, N. Y.; Kimberly-Clark Corp., Education Department, Neenah, Wis.

Film: Uterine Cancer: The Problem of Early Diagnosis (16 mm. color, sound, 21 min.). Available from State Health Dept. or State Division of Cancer Society.

If You Only Knew. A pamphlet describing the problem of uterine cancer, American Cancer Society.

Menopause, Pub. Health Service Pub. No. 179, Washington, D. C., U. S. Govt. Printing Office.

Pelvic anatomy for the patient. A 20-page illustrated brochure, Schering Corporation, Bloomfield, N. J.

Vaginal Cytology Aids Early Diagnosis of Unsuspected Cancer. A folded pamphlet describing a vaginal smear, American Cancer Society.

Voluntary Agency

American Cancer Society, Inc.
521 West 57th St.,
New York 19, N. Y.

34

Patients With Dermatologic Problems

NORMAL SKIN

The skin, far from being a simple structure, is, in fact, an unusually complex assembly of distinctive tissues as highly specific and varied in their functions as any tissue in the body. Its outer surface consists of cells, stratified in layers like paving brick— an extraordinarily resistant protective covering through which chemicals or bacteria of any sort penetrate with difficulty. It is further protected by the oily and slightly acid secretions of the sebaceous glands, the effect of which is to limit sharply the opportunity for growth and colonization of bacteria.

Underlying this tough outer layer is the so-called *subcutaneous tissue,* which is comprised not of one homogeneous tissue but of several tissues. These include glandular, vascular, nervous, fat and muscular tissues, all supported and maintained in proper relation to one another by means of fibrous and elastic connective tissue. Therefore, one must regard the skin not as a single organ but as a group of organs, each responsive to its own particular stimuli and each vulnerable to the same noxious influences which threaten it elsewhere in the body.

Many skin lesions originate as a result of some injurious contact in the external environment, such as an infective organism, a toxic chemical or physical trauma. Others, while owing their origin to some external factor, actually represent damage caused by response to that agent rather than by the activity of the agent itself. This agent for most individuals might be completely harmless, but for the patient who reacts in this manner, on contact, it is far from harmless. A damaging reaction of this sort may take the form of a local inflammatory lesion, an ulcer or an abscess and accounts for a substantial proportion of all such lesions.

The nurse, whose professional work involves intimate and frequent association with dermatologic patients, is soon impressed by the importance of emotional stress as a factor influencing the state of the skin, the appearance of skin lesions and the progress of those lesions. The emotions apparently exert their influence through the autonomic nervous system which controls the caliber of the skin vessels. Recognizing that dilatation of an arteriole must lower the resistance to blood flow through that vessel, it follows that the blood pressure in the distal capillaries must increase, indeed, as much as tenfold. It is not difficult to imagine that such great pressures can produce a plasma leakage and/or hemorrhage through the capillary wall, causing lesions that damage or destroy the overlying skin.

Pruritus—the itch—is clearly instrumental in prolonging and aggravating skin lesions and, perhaps, in producing them as well, by compelling the patient to scratch. The pathologic physiology of itching and scratching is understood poorly, but the importance of the emotions in that symptom complex is abundantly clear.

There is very little constancy or uniformity in dermatologic practice as regards the details of therapeutic procedures. Therefore, instead of describing particular treatments at length and in great detail, only basic principles of therapy are stressed: principles which can be accepted, on the whole, as valid and which are obviously important in the planning and the execution of treatment and nursing care of dermatologic patients.

PROBLEMS OF THE DERMATOLOGIC PATIENT

Psychological Aspects

The nurse should accustom herself as quickly as possible to the less attractive aspects of dermatologic disease and overcome as completely as possible her personal (and natural) sense of repugnance when in close proximity to her patients. Conscious effort in that direction will make such contact progressively easier. She must never betray a reluctance to touch her patient, which would only add to his anxiety, frustration and humiliation, but must cultivate an attitude that promotes a sense of security and tends to restore optimism.

Patients with skin disease frequently are embarrassed and self-conscious as a result of unattractive or disfiguring lesions or because of the necessary display of conspicuous dressings. Also, there may be a depressive reaction to the constant sense of being scrutinized by observers who might be repelled by, or fearful of, the disease and frustration because of its protracted course. These psychological aspects of dermatologic practice require expert management on the part of the attending nurses, who must exhibit an understanding and unending patience and offer tireless encouragement to their patients.

Persistent pruritus, with resultant sleeplessness, may be a potent contributing factor in an anxiety state, which, in turn, inevitably reinforces the discomfort and fatigue.

Pruritus

Pruritus, or itching, is a symptom of many skin diseases, such as eczema, urticaria, etc., but it occurs also in the absence of any evident skin lesion. Thus, it is an important first indication of such serious diseases as diabetes mellitus, leukemia, mycosis fungoides, carcinoma or tuberculosis. Many cases are accompanied by gastrointestinal symptoms. Other forms appear in pregnancy, arteriosclerosis and renal, hepatic and thyroid diseases. The dry skin, particularly that of elderly persons, often itches intensely. Pruritus may be due to certain medicines taken internally, the external application of certain drugs, cold water, strong soaps and dyes and the use of woolen undergarments. Among the secondary results of pruritus which are due to scratching are excoriations, erythema, wheals, furunculosis and increased pigmentation.

Treatment. The cause of the pruritus, if known, should be removed. In some instances, patients are relieved by changing from a meat to a vegetable diet; in others, by substituting silk or cotton for woolen or nylon underwear. Soothing baths may contain sodium bicarbonate, starch, bran or menthol, the water at first tepid and then cooled, and the skin dried without rubbing. Phenol (about 2%) and menthol lotions (0.25 to 0.5%) are cooling drugs that can be applied externally.

Pruritus of *the anal and the genital regions* may be an accompaniment of local irritants, such as scabies and lice; local lesions, such as hemorrhoids; nicotinic-acid deficiency (pellagra, see Chap. 9); infection with certain fungi and yeasts and pinworm infestation. It occurs also in conditions such as diabetes mellitus, the anemias, hyperthyroidism and pregnancy.

The treatment is removal of the local cause, use of the soothing applications mentioned above, sitz baths and local heat or x-ray therapy. Pruritus may be controlled by bed rest and sedation, the frequent application of cold wet dressings, the use of starch or oatmeal baths and lotions or ointments containing menthol or phenol. Corticosteroids in ointment form have proved to be effective in some patients with itching. Excessive warmth should be avoided, bed covers being reduced to the minimum number consistent with comfort and safety, and the room kept cool. The patient should be urged to avoid scratching; if he cannot desist, or excoriates himself while asleep, he may need to wear mitts and receive heavy sedation.

Dermatalgia

This condition is often associated with neurogenic hyperesthesias. It is characterized by the presence of spontaneous burning, stinging, pricking or darting pains of the skin for which no demonstrable cause can be found. Sometimes it is general, although more acute over the hairy regions, but usually it is localized. It is not rarely a complaint of otherwise normal middle-aged women, in whom it may be constant or intermittent (but generally more severe during the night).

NURSING RESPONSIBILITIES IN DERMATOLOGY

Clinical Observations

Many systemic conditions may be accompanied by dermatologic manifestations. In fact, any patient hospitalized with a medical or surgical condition may suddenly develop itching and a rash. The nurse must be able to describe the dermatosis (abnormal condition of the skin) clearly and in detail. The following questions are pertinent: What is the color of the lesion? Is there redness, heat, pain or swelling? Is the eruption macular, papular, scaling or oozing? How large an area is involved? When did the patient first notice the eruption? How does he describe his sensations? Are there itching, burning, tingling or crawling sensations, or is there a loss of sensation? Was the appearance of the eruption related to the intake of food? What drugs is the patient receiving that might possibly have caused this reaction?

Primary lesions which do not produce a break in the skin include the following:

Macule—a spot on the skin that is not raised or depressed

Papule—a solid elevation of the skin

Vesicle—an elevation in the skin that is filled with serum

Pustule—an elevation in the skin that contains pus

Wheal—an area of transitory edema in the skin

Secondary lesions which break the skin include scales, crusts, excoriations, fissures and ulcers.

Care of the Skin

It is to be remembered that even skin that is perfectly normal is vulnerable to damage by the blandest of soaps unless the soap is completely removed by rinsing before the skin is dry. If soap remains in an area of skin that tends to be moist, the damage is greater and occurs more promptly. Residual soap is an important predisposing factor and, perhaps, the principal cause of such common lesions as "diaper rash" in infants and "athlete's foot." It may be pointed out, in this connection, that any substance on prolonged contact with moist skin can excite an inflammatory reaction which will result in lysis and desquamation of the skin in the area of contact. There is one, and only one, outstanding exception to this rule, namely, water.

Principles of Dermatologic Therapy

There is very little constancy or standardization in dermatologic therapy, and there is much variation among clinics in the nursing technics prescribed. In the following paragraphs it is proposed to offer no precise description of any particular type of treatment but, rather, to include certain general principles which are regarded as being important in the nursing care of patients with skin diseases.

In hospitals where patients are bathed as a matter of routine on admission, specific exceptions must be made of those presenting skin lesions. Some skin disorders are markedly aggravated by soap and water, and, for this reason, the procedure is postponed until ordered by the physician. Alternate modes of cleansing may be indicated, and the technic will depend on the character of the disease.

Skin that is denuded in the slightest, whether the area of desquamation is large or small, is excessively prone to damage by chemical means and, also, as a result of trauma. The friction of a towel, if applied with vigor, is sufficient to excite a brisk inflammatory response which will cause any existing lesion to flare up and increase in extent. Thus, the essence of skin care and protection in bathing a patient with abnormal skin is to ensure the complete removal of the soap when rinsing, then dry the area gently with a soft cloth and light touch.

The use of pledgets saturated in olive oil aids in loosening crusts, removing exudates or freeing an adherent dry dressing. The last mentioned also may be saturated with sterile physiologic salt solution or dilute (3%) hydrogen peroxide, which softens it and permits it to be pulled away gently.

Skin lesions which might conceivably be infectious should be regarded strictly as such, and proper precautions should be observed until the diagnosis is established. Rubber or disposable polyethylene gloves are worn by the nurse and the physician. (Oil causes rubber to deteriorate rapidly; therefore, if this is used on the patient, the gloves must be cleansed promptly.) Dressings removed from infected skin should be enclosed securely in paper wraps and burned as soon as possible.

Wet Dressings

Wet dressings are employed for many types of lesions. Due to water evaporation, wet dressings have a cooling effect and relieve inflammation, burning and itching. They are especially helpful for oozing, crusting types of skin conditions. Characteristic types of solutions, occasionally indicated, include physiologic saline, aluminum acetate (usually 0.5%), boric acid, magnesium sulfate (approximately 3%) and potassium permanganate (perhaps 1:4,000). These should be prepared in sterile water. For certain patients it is desirable to keep the dressing warm; for others, cool. Some dressings must be covered to prevent evaporation, whereas most are allowed to remain open. The *open dressing* requires frequent changing, for evaporation will, of course, be rapid.

The closed dressing is changed less frequently, and there is always a danger that it will cause not only softening but actual maceration of the underlying skin. Moisture is maintained satisfactorily by the use of fluffs in abundance, gauze roll or abdominal gauze. Cotton should not be applied directly adjacent to the skin. However, it retains moisture quite efficiently and, because of this property, is a useful component of a wet dressing if employed in thin sheaths between layers of gauze. Areas of normal skin that may be exposed to moisture for any extended period first should be coated with petroleum jelly, a silicone oil or zinc oxide paste.

Preparation of Wet Dressings. A dressing may be rinsed in the appropriate solution before application (this is the preferable procedure if warmth is desired), or the solution may be added—for example, with an Asepto syringe—after it is in place. Care must be taken lest the dressings become excessively soaked, and the solution runs over into non-infected areas. Sterile towels hold them in place. They may be protected further by plastic film secured with bandage, if necessary. So arranged, the temperature of the dressing is maintained for several hours. The use of external heating appliances is not only unnecessary but undesirable, for the danger of burning the skin is very real.

Remoistening of the dressing may be accomplished by removing the protective cloaks and pouring solution over the gauze, or the gauze may be removed completely, immersed again in the solution and then reapplied. If the remoistening is done without removal of the gauze, sterile water is alternated with the solution, particularly if the solution is that of a metallic salt, for evaporation causes it to become continuously more concentrated. If an exudate is present, the dressing should, of course, be changed completely at frequent intervals. A stocking may be converted into a convenient wet dressing for the leg, and a glove similarly prepared for the hand. Face lesions should be dressed with gauze fashioned into a mask and applied in several thicknesses. If wet dressings are required to cover extensive areas of skin, flannel pajamas soaked in the solution serve as a useful form of dressing. The full bath may be used as a total wet dressing if it is desirable to treat the whole skin surface, care being observed to avoid chilling.

Therapeutic Baths

Baths are useful as a means of applying medications to large areas of the skin, removing crusts and scales and relieving itching that accompanies acute dermatoses.

Dermatologic Medications and Dressings

Medications in the form of powders, lotions, creams and ointments are used to treat skin lesions. In general, lotions and emulsions are used for the more acute dermatoses

TYPES OF BATHS*	USES
1. Potassium permanganate baths (1 tsp. crystals to tub of warm water)	1. Oxidizing, disinfecting and deodorizing. Useful particularly in exudative, vesicular and bullous dermatoses.
2. Tar baths	2. Antipruritic, mildly keratolytic. Coal tar and oil of cade emulsions are most frequently used. They are valuable in the chronic dermatoses.
3. Colloid baths	3. Soothing bland baths are used to calm and relieve irritated, inflamed or pruritic skin conditions. They are usually prepared from cornstarch, oatmeal or colloidal oatmeal. Colloidal oatmeal requires no boiling to extract the colloid.
4. Emollient baths	4. These baths include emollient oils to soften and lubricate dry, scaly or lichenified skin.

* Franks, A. G.: Dermatologic uses of baths, Am. Pract. 9(No. 12): 1998-2000, 1958.

when large areas of skin are involved. Lotions exert a cooling action through water evaporation. They also have a protective effect and are applied easily with a soft paintbrush. Powders are dusted on the skin with a shaker or with cotton sponges. Although their medicinal action is brief, powders absorb moisture and reduce friction between the skin and the bedding. Pastes are mixtures of powders and ointments and are used in inflammatory conditions. Ointments retard water loss and are preferred in the more chronic or localized skin conditions. Pastes and ointments are applied with a wooden tongue depressor (Fig. 290). The patient should be taught to apply them gently but thoroughly.

Many of these topical applications are greasy and require a covering with dressings to prevent soilage of clothing. If it is to be satisfactory, a dressing must be comfortable as well as protective. Plastic film is advantageous because it is thin and adapts itself readily to anatomic structures of all shapes and sizes. (See Fig. 291, *top* and *bottom*.) Stretchable cotton dressings (Surgitube, Tubegauze) likewise are excellent covering materials.

Disposable polyethylene gloves make acceptable coverings for patients who require finger and hand dressings. When large body areas require covering, disposable diapers are useful. The plastic side is placed next to the skin and the diaper is held in place by being pinned to the underclothing.*

The patient with a dermatologic problem has to take an active part in his treatment. He must be able to apply and remove his medications and dressings. Therefore, he must be indoctrinated fully regarding treatment technics and the observations he is expected to report to his physician. In short, he participates in his own therapy as an assistant to the physician and the nurse.

PIGMENTARY DISORDERS

Skin Color. The color of the skin of the general body surface is best judged by that of the face, where, as a rule, all pigment abnormalities are most accentuated. Excluding pathologic pigments, such as methemoglobin or silver, its color depends on the amount of skin pigment present, the opacity of the epidermis, the quantity of blood circulating in the superficial vessels per unit of skin area (this determines the so-called *complexion*) and on the hemoglobin content of the blood.

The different shades of color of the various human races, as well as of healthy individuals of the same race, and the great majority of abnormal pigmentations due to

* Witten, V. H., and Sulzberger, M. B.: Newer dermatologic methods for using corticosteroids more efficaciously, Med. Clin. N. Am. 45:857-868, 1961.

disease all depend on quantitative changes in one pigment, i.e., melanin. The regions normally most pigmented are those exposed to the sun and the wind, such as the face and the hands, certain hairy regions, such as the axillae, the genitalia and the perineum, the linea alba and the areolae of the nipples.

A physiologic increase in pigmentation follows exposure to the sun (tan), which also increases the number and depth of color of any exposed pigmented areas (for example, freckles) already present. Pathologic increase in pigmentation may be general or local. If general, it is always deepest over those regions normally darkest. If the pigmentation is deep brown or black, the terms *melasma* or *melanoderma* are used.

Chloasma

Local areas of pathologic pigmentation on a skin otherwise normal, particularly of women, is called *chloasma*. These are fairly

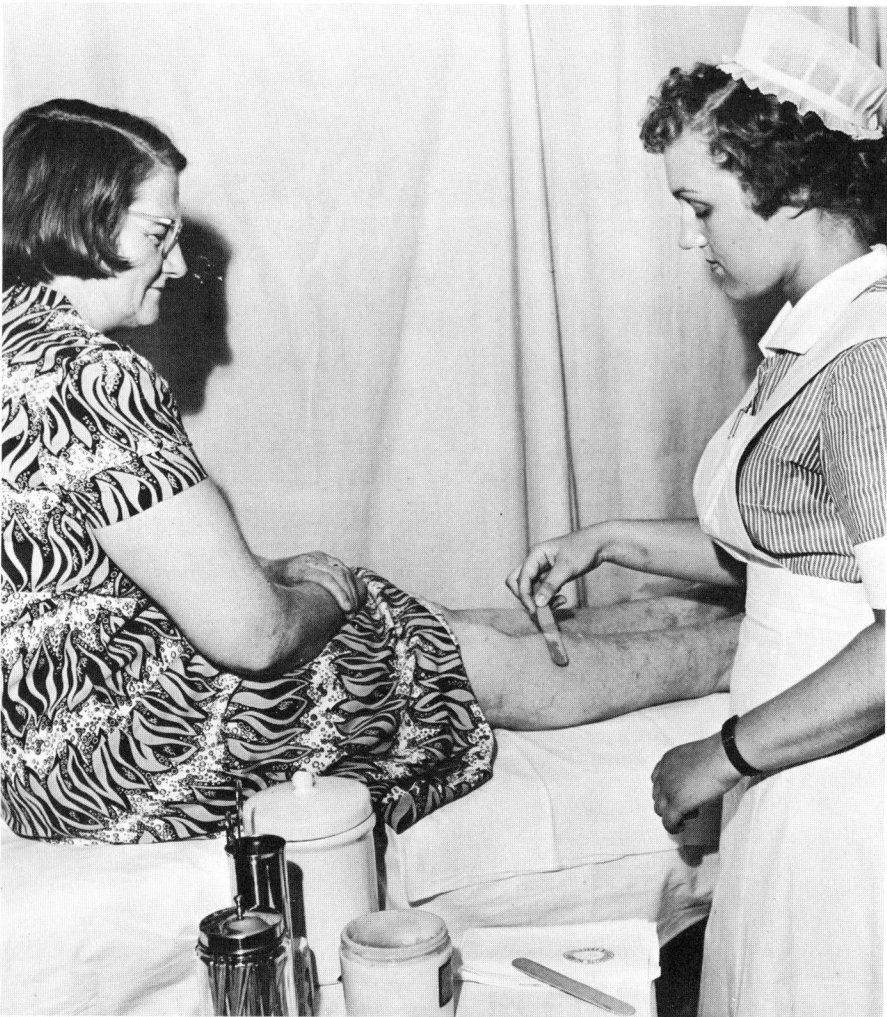

FIG. 290. The nurse is showing the patient how to apply an even coating of skin ointment to an area of dermatitis on her legs. She also will be taught how to cleanse her hands in advance, how to prepare and protect the equipment she uses and how to apply the dressing that will cover the lesion.

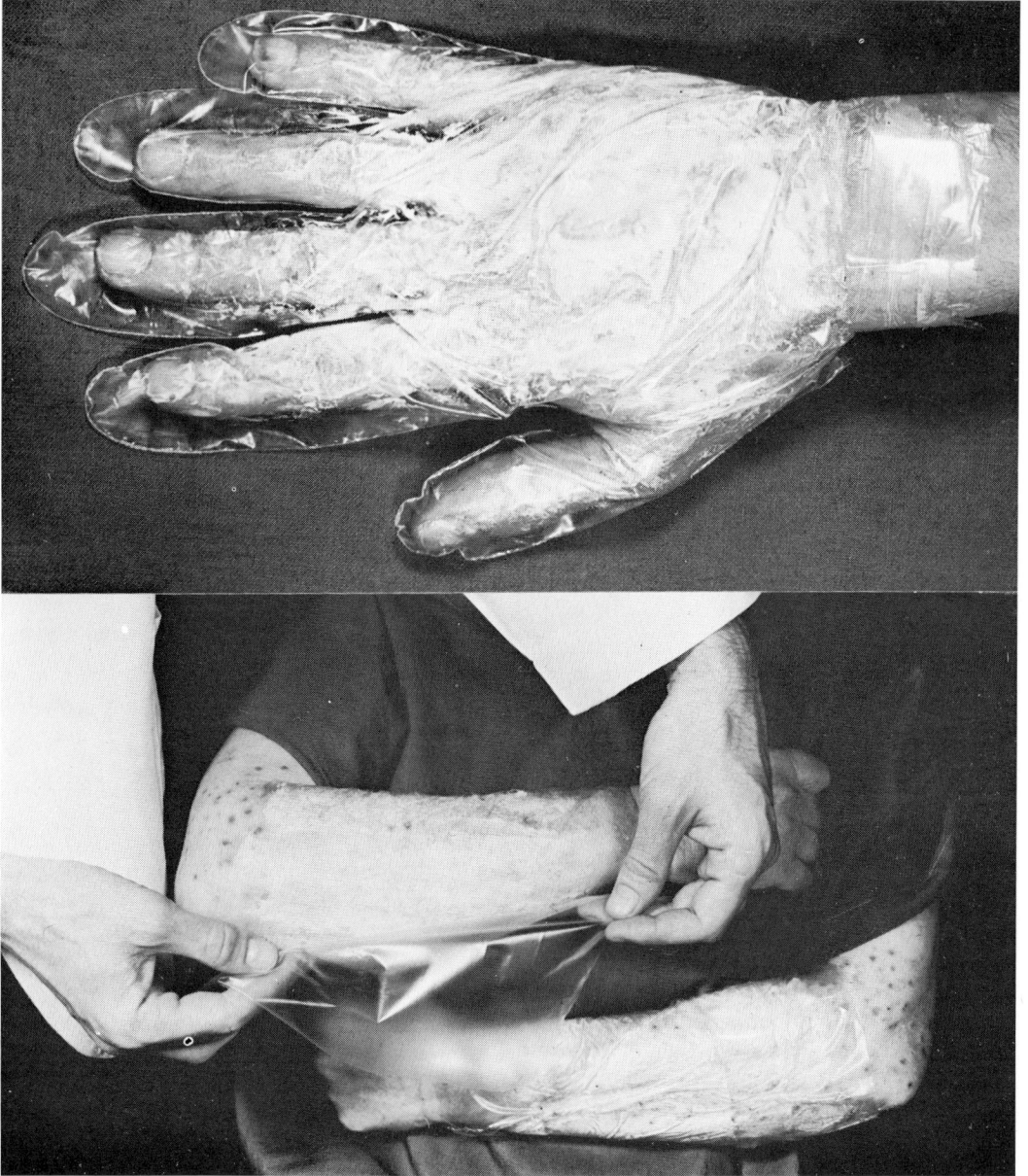

FIG. 291. *(Top)* The use of a thin plastic occlusive dressing over the hand assures better contact of medication with the skin lesion and is convenient and less cumbersome for the patient. *(Bottom)* After the affected areas have been cleansed and a layer of prescribed ointment or cream applied, the arm is covered with the occlusion dressing, fastened with adhesive or cellophane tape and wrapped with a lightweight cotton dressing to hold the plastic dressing in place. (Eli Lilly, Indianapolis, Indiana)

well-defined patches of various sizes, shapes and shades of yellowish-brown, brown or black discolorations. They are most numerous on the forehead but appear also on the breasts, the abdomen and elsewhere. Chloasma usually develops between the ages of 25 and 50 years. Sometimes it is apparently related to changes in the endocrine balance.

During pregnancy, there is usually an increased pigmentation of the linea alba and areolae of the nipples, yet some pregnant women develop a true chloasma gravidarum, which may be the first sign of their condition. This may appear either as a uniform pigmentation of the entire body, or as dark patches, irregular in size and shape, which become more and more conspicuous until after delivery.

The treatment of hyperpigmented areas depends on the cause. The patient must be studied carefully for signs of metabolic disease. Often the skillful use of bleaching preparations (containing salicylic acid or bichloride of mercury), peeling off the epidermis, improves the patient's appearance; but speedy recurrence of hyperpigmentation in the same area is not unusual.

Local Pigmentation. This results from intense cutaneous hyperemia, such as the chloasma toxicum, due to mustard plasters and blisters, and the chloasma caloricum, due to sunburn, heat and overexposures to roentgen rays. Chloasma traumaticum is due to irritation and friction of the skin. It may be caused by a truss or be due to scratching, as in cases of pediculosis corporis. Or any chronic itchy skin disease such as eczema and dermatitis herpetiformis may be the cause.

Melanoderma. Extreme pigmentation of the skin, normal in the Negro, may develop in connection with various organic and systemic diseases such as tuberculosis of the lungs and the peritoneum, but it reaches its most extreme grade in Addison's disease and vagabonds' disease (morbus erronum), the latter due to lice and dirt. In Von Recklinghausen's disease, the pigment may be marked enough to suggest Addison's disease. And, finally, an intense melanoderma appears occasionally in pernicious anemia and chronic heart disease.

Albinism

Albinism is due to a congenital lack of the normal skin pigment. The entire body surface may be affected or only certain regions. In the case of a complete albino, the entire skin is milky white or has a faint pinkish tinge, the hair is white or yellowish white, the irises of the eyes are pale blue, and the pupils are pink (owing to the lack of pigment in the choroid coat). This is a definitely inheritable congenital defect. Partial albinos have one, a few or many milky-white areas of various sizes and shapes scattered over the body surface. There is no treatment for this condition.

Vitiligo

Vitiligo (acquired patchy leukoderma) is a condition characterized by the presence on the skin, otherwise normal in texture, of circumscribed, irregular-shaped patches of milky-white areas surrounded by a zone of increased pigmentation. This zone makes them most conspicuous, especially during the summer, when sunburn darkens it. Any hair on these patches may retain or lose its pigment. The patches tend to increase in size, and, in time, they may cover almost the entire body surface. In some cases, however, they disappear.

There is no effective treatment known.

SECRETORY DISORDERS

Sweat and sebum inhibit the growth of bacteria, and serve to defend the skin against bacterial invasion.

Disturbances of sweat secretion produce increased or decreased moistness of the skin, best judged by the condition over the chest or the axillae, since that of the hands and the feet is controlled by other factors. (Thus cold, wet hands often indicate emotional hyperexcitability.) In general, a moist skin is also a warm skin, and a dry skin is chilly. However, diaphoresis and vasomotor dilatation are not always associated: hence, the cold sweats; the warm dry skin of the person who has drunk very little water or has lost much by profuse diarrhea, vomiting or polyuria; and the very hot and dry skin peculiar to some febrile states.

Anhidrosis and Hyperhidrosis

Anhidrosis (Absence of Sweating). This is normal to some persons whose skin is always dry, particularly in winter. Anhidrosis is a feature of certain chronic skin diseases such as icthyosis, eczema, pityriasis rubra pilaris, anesthetic leprosy, scleroderma or keloidal growths. A temporary anhidrosis accompanies profound emotional depression. It is a symptom of the action of certain drugs. A persistent suppression of sweat secretion is a symptom of myxedema, diabetes mellitus, diabetes insipidus and chronic nephritis. Localized suppression of sweat secretion is the rule over areas of subcutaneous edema and has been observed over skin areas where the nerves have been injured.

TREATMENT. The primary disease should be treated, but, with the exception of cases of myxedema and diabetes, the only relief of anhidrosis is from oily applications to the skin.

Hyperhidrosis. Normally, temporary hyperhidrosis (excessive sweating) is associated with subcutaneous hyperemia. It may be due to exercise, exposure to heat and exposure to certain light rays; but a cold sweat often accompanies fright, shock or very severe pain such as that of angina pectoris. Temporary hyperhidrosis is a response to the action of certain drugs, such as pilocarpine, ammonium acetate and various coal-tar products (the so-called *antipyretics*).

Persisting hyperhidrosis, increased still more by hot weather and physical exertion, is natural to some persons. It affects the general body surface, but always is marked in those regions where sweating normally is most active.

In certain diseases of the central nervous system, excessive sweating occurs over limited areas, as over half the face or on one side of the body. Profuse general sweating, most marked over the head, the face and the neck, is one of the sequelae of epidemic encephalitis.

TREATMENT. For excessive sweating, applications of an antiseptic solution (benzalkonium chloride) will lessen the odor and the discomfort. Sedatives are helpful to some patients.

Bromidrosis

Skin secretion with heavy penetrating odor, usually, but not always, associated with hyperhidrosis, is a characteristic peculiar to some persons. The treatment is essentially the same as for hyperhidrosis.

Miliaria

Miliaria (prickly heat) is an acute, mildly inflammatory eruption of discrete but closely crowded tiny red papules and vesicles which are smaller than a pinhead and are associated with more or less prickling, burning or itching.

Miliaria appears suddenly over the whole body or over limited portions. It occurs during periods of high temperature and high humidity in individuals who perspire freely.

Treatment. The underlying principle of treatment of miliaria is to reduce the factors which favor perspiration. To accomplish this the patient should bathe in cool water using a mild soap, and the skin should be patted dry. He should wear loose fitting cotton underclothing and avoid heat-producing foods and beverages and vigorous exercises. The application of a bland talcum powder may help to enhance the evaporation of perspiration. Staying in a cool environment with a low humidity offers considerable relief.

Miliaria Crystallina (Sudamina)

Miliaria crystallina is a disorder of sweat glands caused by the retention of sweat. There is a noninflammatory eruption on the face and the chest of small superficial vesicles with clear contents (sudamina), their appearance suggesting dewdrops on the skin. These vesicles vary in size from that of a pinpoint to that of a pinhead. Usually, they are thickly set but they always remain discrete. Sudamina are particularly common in acute rheumatic fever and debilitating illnesses.

Pompholyx

Pompholyx is an inflammatory affection of the skin of the palms and the soles and between the fingers and the toes. It is characterized by the appearance of crops of tiny vesicles, deep in the skin, associated with profuse sweating, burning and itching. As a rule, the distribution of the lesions is bilateral and roughly symmetrical. Attacks generally last a couple of weeks, but, because of the tendency to relapse, pompholyx may persist for long periods. It appears in association with acute anxiety states, for example, in students before an examination.

This is a self-limiting condition, usually disappearing with the easing of emotional stress. Aluminum acetate powder, locally applied, may be helpful.

SEBORRHEIC DERMATOSES

Seborrhea

The result of functional hyperactivity of the sebaceous glands, *seborrhea,* is a condition normal to some persons. It presents itself as a sallow, greasy condition of the skin, especially of the forehead, the nose and the scalp, the last mentioned often being covered with thin, dirty scales of dried secretions. It is seen most often in brunettes in association with coarse skin and prominent plugged follicles and in women with hypertrichosis. The importance of this condition, apart from its appearance, is that it predisposes the skin to several scaling diseases, among them seborrheic eczema, acne vulgaris and seborrheic warts. Seborrhea may be improved much with weak sulfur or salicylic acid. If this fails, ultraviolet irradiation should be tried.

The tiny white cystic nodules appearing on the face, especially under the eyes, in many cases of seborrhea are called *milia.* These are removed by puncturing and pressing out the enclosed material.

Acne Vulgaris

Acne vulgaris is a common chronic inflammatory disorder of the skin, characterized by the presence of blackheads, papules, pustules, cysts and nodules (Fig. 292). It appears most often on the face, the back, the chest and the upper arms.

Although acne is a local skin disease, its course is determined by the internal secretions, the general health and the diet. It usually appears between the ages of 12 and 30, but is worse at puberty and during adolescence, perhaps because at that age certain of the glands of the body are hyperactive, and these apparently influence the secretions of the sebaceous glands. This relation is also manifest during menstruation. Acne is worse also during periods of constipation and, perhaps, when the diet contains an excess of carbohydrates.

Treatment. The objectives of treatment are (1) to prevent follicular obstruction; (2) to clear secondary infections and reduce inflammation, and (3) to eliminate factors which may predispose to acne.

Comedones. The earliest and commonest lesions of acne are comedones, or blackheads, which are the result of increased secretion and concentration of sebum (the natural oil of the skin). Blackheads act as

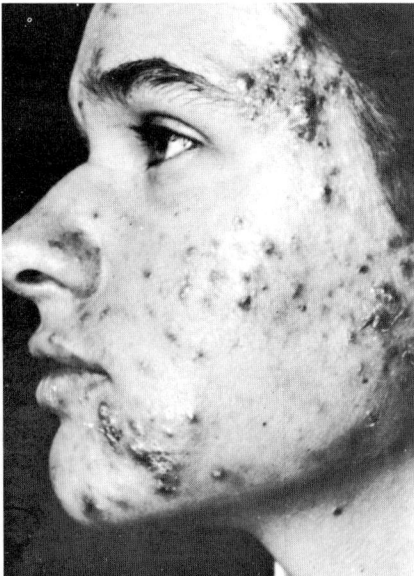

FIG. 292. Acne vulgaris. (Ralph E. McDonnell, M.D., New Haven)

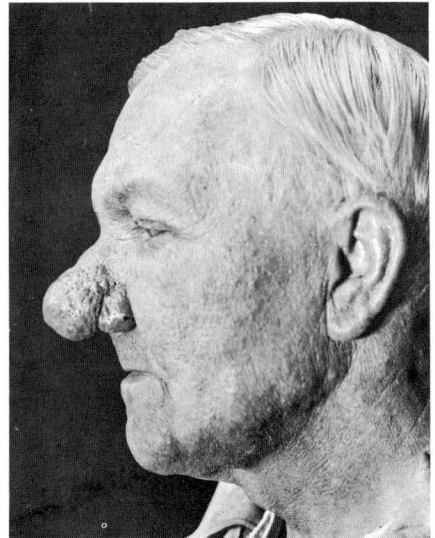

FIG. 293. Rhinophyma. (Ralph E. McDonnell, M.D., New Haven)

foreign bodies in the skin, setting up an inflammation which produces papules (papular acne), and these infections transform into pustules which, healing, may leave scars.

Blackheads are treated effectively by a thorough cleansing of the skin, morning and night, with green soap tincture; then, having expressed the comedones, 3 per cent salicylic acid in alcohol is applied. Ultraviolet light is useful in acne of the superficial acute inflammatory type without conspicuous comedones. In mild cases of this type, it is advisable to attempt the cure by hygienic measures, ultraviolet light and the application of sulfathiazole or sulfadiazine ointment or other antiseptic applications. Life in the fresh air and sunshine is beneficial.

Patients with acne may develop secondary infections which can produce pustular or cystic forms of acne. To control secondary infection and subsequent scarring, antibiotics may be given.

Foods that are known to be acnegenic (chocolate, seafood, sharp cheeses and nuts) should be avoided. Some drugs, especially those containing iodides and bromides, cause follicular irritation and, therefore, may aggravate acne. If the patient is under undue nervous tension, sebum production increases and the acne becomes worse. The problems of the teen-aged patient should be taken seriously by those caring for him. He needs understanding, reassurance and support. He must be cautioned not to squeeze blackheads, as this activity can produce scarring. Blackheads should be removed with a comedo extractor by the physician and not by the patient or anyone else.

Acne Rosacea

Rosacea is a chronic disturbance of the flush areas of the face (malar surfaces of cheeks, nose and chin) which leads to permanent hyperemia and the development of acneiform lesions, telangiectasis and hypertrophy of the skin; that of the nose results in rhinophyma (Fig. 293).

It begins as a continuous hyperemia of these areas. In time this tends to become a deeper red or a purplish red in color, the superficial capillaries becoming chronically dilated (telangiectatic). Inflammatory papules or acnelike pustules appear in the congested area. The skin of the nose is congested, coarsened and, finally, thickened by large nodular masses covered with pitted scars. It is seen most often in chronic alcoholics and may be a sign of vitamin deficiency.

Treatment. In the early stages of rosacea, the process may be halted by careful avoidance of factors causing facial hyperemia, such as overindulgence in alcohol, overexposure to sun or uncleanliness about the face. In the second stage, with venules permanently dilated and papules or pustules present, the dilated vessels should be treated by electrolysis, and the papules should be touched with a small high-frequency spark.

The best treatment for rhinophyma is the removal of the nodules on the nose by surgical diathermy or curettement under local anesthesia.

TRAUMATIC DERMATOSES

Skin Injuries

Erythema hyperaemicum is due to exposure to heat and, if repeated often enough, results in pigmentation.

Erythema traumaticum, due to bandages or a tightly fitting truss or garter, is definitely local, as is also that which represents the first stage of a bedsore (erythema paratrimma).

Erythema venenatum is the local erythema produced by the external application of various mineral and vegetable substances, such as mustard, arnica, strong soap, dyestuffs and certain plants. All are due to arteriolar vasodilatation in the affected areas. If sufficiently prolonged, all lead to brownish pigmentation locally.

Erythema intertrigo, or chafing, is hyperemia of opposing skin surfaces, such as at the axillae, folds of the neck, between the thighs or beneath the breasts. This is seen chiefly in children, fat persons and those not clean, but also in those who bathe too often, using irritating soaps. This may lead to an abrasion of the skin, but it disappears promptly after the part is cleansed and talcum powder is applied. If neglected, however, it may become a true dermatitis or an eczema.

Cold Injury

Frostbite, or freezing of the soft tissues of an exposed part, renders the skin pallid and insensitive. Later, in first-degree cases, it becomes red, swollen, edematous and tender. If more severe, it is studded with vesicles and bullae which last for several days; while, in the severest cases, the affected part becomes gangrenous and sloughs. The frostbitten part should be warmed slowly, not rubbed. Intravenous heparin may be used to prevent intravascular clotting in the affected area.

Chilblain. Chilblain of the hands and the feet, which may or may not have followed a previous frostbite, is a localized bluish-red erythema, often accompanied by burning, itching or tenderness. It tends to recur frequently each winter, following even slight exposures to cold. The skin during the attack feels cold and often is clammy from excessive sweating.

TREATMENT. The treatment of chilblain is to improve the circulation of the part by regular exercise and to raise the general health through ensuring adequate nutrition. In winter, woolen socks or gloves should be worn, and the whole body should be protected adequately against the cold.

Radiation Dermatitis

Moderate exposure of the skin to x-rays (such as used in roentgen-ray therapy) produces dryness with the loss of the hair; somewhat longer exposure results in a peculiar erythemalike sunburn. Earlier, the exposed area may have been edematous for a few days or weeks. Following overexposure, the red edematous skin soon becomes studded by vesicles or, when the redness begins to fade, by a slight brawny exfoliation. Later, it may be covered by telangiectatic blood vessels. The skin of the hands of those who are constantly exposed to x-rays becomes first erythematous and then pigmented, wrinkled and atrophic; the nails are brittle and thin. Keratoses appear. These may later develop into carcinomata.

Definite burns due to unfiltered x-rays usually appear in from 5 to 7 days, and those due to filtered x-rays or radium in

from 2 to 6 weeks following the exposure. In such cases the initial erythema continues longer and is accompanied by the sensation of warmth, burning or itching. Later, a dry, sluggish but often very tender ulcer develops. As a rule, it is shallow, has a slightly inflamed border and is covered with a tough, rather adherent, grayish, leathery crust. This ulcer shows little or no tendency to heal. Judicious encouragement to patients taking x-ray treatments is sometimes indicated, for a few are fearful in anticipation. The eyes should be closed while treatment is being received about the face.

During the entire course of treatments, the skin should be protected from strong irritants, including excessive exposure to sunlight. No ointments or lotions should be used on a field of irradiation without permission from the radiotherapist. Certain generalized systemic reactions may follow intensive irradiation therapy. These include generalized malaise, muscular aches and pains, anoxia, nausea and vomiting. These effects are noted and studied. If severe and definitely related to this treatment, the x-ray dosage may have to be reduced.

Factitious Dermatitis

Factitious dermatitis is any self-inflicted injury to the skin produced by hysterical persons or malingerers, who usually use chemical irritants and caustics. The lesion may be erythematous, vesicular, hemorrhagic or ulcerative, according to the method used. Superficial gangrenous lesions suggest this condition.

Such lesions, seldom numerous, develop on parts easily reached by the patient's hands. Their distribution does not correspond to that of ordinary cutaneous diseases. Often they are present on one side of the body only. Usually they are more or less linear, are sharply defined and have an artificial look. As a rule, they appear in crops, new ones appearing suddenly and the older ones persisting too long (since they are purposely kept irritated). If covered with a fixed dressing, however, they vanish promptly, and any new lesion will appear elsewhere.

INFECTIONS AND INFESTATIONS OF THE SKIN

Bacterial Infections

Furuncles. The staphylococcus is a common inhabitant of the skin surface and the circulating air. Frequently it causes surface infections by invading a hair follicle or the duct of a gland. The infection may be a very slight one, characterized by a small, red, raised, painful "pimple" that may subside very rapidly with the drainage of a tiny drop of pus. Frequently, however, the infection may progress and involve the skin and the subcutaneous fatty tissue in a tense, raised, reddened mound termed a *furuncle* and known familiarly as a boil. The hardened area of induration is the body's effort to localize the infection. The bacteria produce a necrosis of the invaded tissues, and, in a few days, the characteristic pointing appears and the boil is said by the laity to "come to a head."

TREATMENT AND NURSING CARE. If treated conservatively, the body may control the infection by eventual evacuation of the central necrotic core and the pus contained in this necrotic center. Hot moist applications will hasten this process. These may be applied in the form of hot compresses or poultices. In the conservative treatment of staphylococcic infections it is important not to rupture or destroy the protective wall of induration that has localized the infection. Therefore, the boil or pimple should never be squeezed, and it is well, when possible, to apply a splint to immobilize the part and thus protect the wall from being destroyed by movement. This procedure relieves the pain, as movement of the part produces tension on the infected area.

Local applications of neomycin or bacitracin ointment may help to limit the spread of the infection. If spreading still occurs or if the area of involvement poses a risk of complications (see below), systemic antibiotic therapy is indicated, employing Methicillin, Oxacillin or another of the agents that are effective against the staphylococcus, the selection of drug being governed in each case by the results of sensitivity studies.

Sometimes a furuncle is so intensely painful that it is wise not to wait for localization and spontaneous evacuation of the necrotic material. In such cases a crucial incision may be made through the area of infection to permit relief of tension and more direct evacuation of the pus and slough.

Special precautions must be taken with boils on the face, for this skin area drains directly into the cranial venous sinuses. Sinus thrombosis, with fatal pyemia, has been known to develop after manipulation of a boil in this location. Bed rest is advised for patients having boils on nose, lip, groin, perineum or about the anal region, and a course of chemotherapy is indicated to control the spread of the infection.

Carbuncles are staphylococcic infections similar to a boil, except that the infection spreads widely in the subcutaneous fatty tissues, producing numerous sites of pointing and, therefore, a much more extensive area of acute inflammation. Carbuncles appear most commonly in areas in which the skin is thick and the subcutaneous tissues are more fibrous; therefore, they are seen most frequently on the back of the neck and less frequently on the back and other parts of the body. They are more apt to occur in older and debilitated people, and they are especially frequent in diabetics. So frequent is this latter association that every patient past middle age with a carbuncle should be suspected of diabetes until it is disproved. In carbuncles, the extensive inflammation frequently is not associated with a complete walling-off of the the infection, so that absorption with production of high fever, leukocytosis and even the extension of the infection to the blood stream may occur.

TREATMENT AND NURSING CARE. In many cases a carbuncle may subside very rapidly by the administration of the antibiotic to which the infecting organism is sensitive. The antibiotic must be continued until the infective process is controlled. If the process already has gone on to form pus, incision and drainage may be necessary.

In caring for patients with carbuncles, the nurse must consider not only the surgical lesion but also the general care of an extremely toxic patient. Furthermore, since many of these patients are diabetic, the question of diet, the administration of insulin and intravenous glucose and the complications of diabetes, such as keto-acidosis, must be borne in mind.

Carbuncle of the upper lip is an unusually serious disease because of the danger of thrombosis and embolism of the veins of the face and the nose. Some of these vessels drain into the cavernous sinus, a large venous channel in the skull, and an extension of the process in that direction is attended with grave consequences. Some surgeons recommend early incision in the treatment of such patients but, since the advent of penicillin, incision rarely is necessary and by the use of this drug in large doses at regular intervals the danger of spreading infections usually is controlled. The nurse never should attempt to squeeze the lesion because of the danger of breaking the protective wall and thus producing an extension of the process. Rapid death may result from an intracranial extension causing septicemia or meningitis. Therefore, this apparently minor condition must be regarded as a very serious disease with a potentially high mortality.

Impetigo contagiosa is the name given the superficial staphylococcal or streptococcal cutaneous infections of the face and the hands which produce golden circular crusts loosely adherent to the skin (Plate 7). The lesions begin as discrete thin-walled vesicles and bullae, which rapidly become pustular and then dry, forming the above-mentioned crusts. These, easily removed, leave smooth, red, moist surfaces, on which other crusts soon form.

Impetigo contagiosa is seen at all ages, but particularly among undernourished children living under poor hygienic conditions. It is contagious and is transferred to other parts of the patient's body, as well as to other persons, by fingers or towels soiled with the exudate of the lesions. It is acquired by children in schools and by adults in barber shops, beauty shops, Turkish baths or swimming pools. Often it appears secondary to pediculosis capitis, scabies, cold sores, insect bites, poison ivy or eczema.

TREATMENT AND NURSING CARE. Strict cleanliness is imperative to prevent the spread of the disease and, also, to protect children. To hasten the curative process, the crusts first may be sponged with hydrogen peroxide, softened with olive oil and then removed by forceps. Topical ointments (bacitracin, neomycin, or polymyxin) are then applied. Care must be taken lest the disease be spread from one skin area to another or from one patient to another. Each patient should be instructed to keep his own towels and boil them before laundering. Children with this condition are excluded from school. Printed directions for hygienic care are distributed to these patients in skin clinics.

Infections of the Hand. MINOR INJURIES. There are many cuts, pricks and abrasions of the skin which may occur anywhere on the body but most often on hands and fingers. Although these wounds are potentially infected, they rarely become seats of infection if ordinary precautions are taken. Mechanical cleansing with soap and tap water and protection with a Band-aid or other form of dressing are usually all that is required to permit healing without infection. Antiseptics may be used if desired, but their role in preventing infection is much less important than is ordinary washing with soap and water.

Infections of the fingers and the hand are of extreme importance to the nurse, not only because she must know how to take care of these lesions but also because there are frequent accidents in nursing that may lead to a development of these infections in the nurse herself. Therefore, it is important that she know the cause and, especially, the prophylactic treatment of these infections, because they may lead to serious disability, if not to fatal consequences.

Since almost all of these hand and finger inflammations are due to infection, it is important to identify the organism and to determine its sensitivity to the antibiotics. In the treatment of these infections, the appropriate anitbiotic properly administered will permit rapid subsidence of the inflammatory process; it may abort the infection in some cases, and in other well-established infections it will hasten its resolution.

PARONYCHIA (runaround) is a common pyogenic infection involving the folds of tis-

FIG. 294. Paronychia or runaround. The infection lies between the soft tissues and the side of the nail. Drainage by inserting the tip of a scalpel along the edge of the nail is customary surgery.

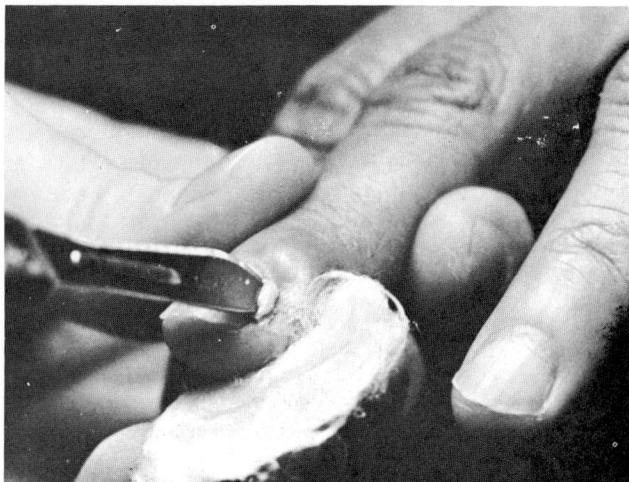

sue under the fingernail. It results most often from an infection of a hangnail and is seen frequently after manicuring. The infection extends between the soft tissues and the nail on the dorsum of the fingertip and forms a tense, painful, throbbing area of inflammation at the side of the nail. If the infection is allowed to go untreated, it may progress underneath the eponychium (cuticle) and then invade the space underneath the base of the nail. This gives this infection its common name.

Cleanliness of the hands and careful care of the nails are the best prophylaxis against paronychia. If the infection does occur, it is treated by hot soaks and by lifting up the soft tissues from the edge of the nail with the tip of a scalpel (Fig. 294). Once the pus is evacuated, the inflammation usually will subside with the use of hot moist applications.

INFECTIONS OF THE PULP OF THE FINGERTIP usually are the result of a puncture wound, the stick of a pin or a needle, when bacteria are carried into the layers of the skin or into the fatty tissues underlying it. When the infection lies between the layers of the skin, the abscess which is formed is spoken of as an *epidermal abscess*. This lesion is diagnosed easily, because it forms a small, tender, blisterlike mound at the site of the pinprick. Puncture and removal of the overlying skin may be performed without anesthesia, exposing the true skin below.

In workmen and in others in whom the surface skin is thick, the infection may not progress to the surface so readily and, instead, it may perforate through the true skin and invade the subcutaneous fatty tissues. This process is known as a *collar-button abscess*, one abscess cavity lying between layers of the skin connected by a narrow tract and a second abscess lying below the skin. In the treatment of such abscesses it is important naturally to drain both the superficial and the deep collection by incision.

FELON (DISTAL CLOSED SPACE INFECTION). The most common and serious type of infection of the fingertip is that due to the streptococcus in the pulp of the finger. There usually is a history of needleprick or pinprick or some other form of puncture, followed several days later by throbbing pain, which may be of such intensity as to prevent sleep. The swelling and the edema produced by the infection may be sufficient to impair or shut off completely the arterial supply to the soft tissue, so that rapid necrosis and even invasion of the bone may occur. The resulting disability often is great because of the extreme importance of the fingertips in the use of the hand and the fingers.

Treatment. Early incision and drainage will prevent the progress of the necrosis; therefore, wide incision often is practiced for what may appear to be a relatively small area of infection. It is surprising to note that radical incision is conservative therapy when dealing with infections of the pulp of the finger.

After incision, the wound is held open by rubber dam or gauze drainage and immobilized by an appropriate splint. Warm moist dressings are used until the area of slough has separated entirely, after which time healing may be permitted to take place.

Prophylaxis. In the prophylaxis of fingertip infections, the nurse who has pricked her finger with a needle or a pin should report it to the head nurse at once. Frequently, a slight enlargement of the incision or cauterization of the needle puncture with phenol may abort a serious infection. If throbbing pain becomes a prominent symptom, no time should be wasted in consulting a surgeon. The appropriate antibiotic must be administered.

INFECTIONS OF TENDON SHEATHS—TENOSYNOVITIS (WHITLOW). Infections of the tendon sheaths on the palmar surface of the hand occur most frequently from puncture wounds. Most often they are caused by the streptococcus. They are serious, because they may lead to a rapid destruction of the tendon itself and, therefore, to a marked finger and hand disability. An infection may involve the sheaths of the tendons in the fingers and the thumb; it may invade the fascial spaces of the hand, or it may advance along the tendon sheaths of the thumb and the fifth finger and invade the bursal space through which the tendons pass at the wrist. It produces a tense swelling of the involved finger with extreme pain when motion is attempted.

Treatment. Early incision and drainage are necessary to prevent necrosis of the tendon. Petrolatum gauze usually is laid in the wound to provide drainage.

The specific antibiotic is administered. In the early phases of the infection it may prevent necrosis and the necessity for incision. After incision, it is used to prevent extension of the infection and to hasten healing.

POSTOPERATIVE NURSING CARE. In the postoperative care of these patients, the nurse usually finds the part bandaged and on a splint, and for a time hot moist applications are applied through the dressings directly or through tubes fastened in them.

The nurse must be extremely careful to carry out a sterile technic in moistening the dressings because of the danger of producing a mixed infection which usually is associated with the extension of the inflammatory process. Elevation of the part must be enforced to reduce the inflammatory edema and to give comfort to the patient. This usually is accomplished by means of pillows, which should be protected with a plastic cover. (See p. 26, Hot Wet Dressing.)

After the acute inflammatory process has been controlled, the infected hand often may be treated in a warm saline bath 2 or 3 times daily. The basin and the solution should be sterilized and the solution placed in the basin at a temperature as warm as the patient can stand comfortably. This temperature is maintained as well as possible by adding more solution at intervals. The bath usually is continued for at least 30 minutes. Its purpose is to apply heat to aid in the discharge of the necrotic materials from the wound. After removal from the bath the hand is placed in a sterile towel, and dry heat may be continued by the use of an electric light in a bed cradle. The nurse must be careful to avoid scalding or burning.

Skin Tuberculosis. LUPUS VULGARIS IS the most common type of cutaneous tuberculosis. It appears as reddish-brown patches in which minute translucent nodules of apple-jelly color can be seen embedded deeply in the infiltrated cutis. These patches leave deforming scars on healing. The disease, which usually begins during childhood, develops in most cases on exposed portions of the body—particularly on the face, where the skin probably has become inoculated by dirty fingernails contaminated with the organisms of bovine tuberculosis.

Types. The atrophic type of lupus vulgaris forms a smooth, flat, slightly depressed or slightly elevated patch composed of white scar tissue enclosing "apple-jelly nodules." The hypertrophic type, most common on moist areas near the body orifices, is a warty vegetative growth, often crusted or producing an exudate. The ulcerative type produces ragged, deep, indolent and occasionally very tender ulcers covered by vegetations which are crusted and produce a purulent exudate. This last type occasionally appears in association with scrofuloderma, hence in cases of tuberculous lymph glands, bones or other structures. Patches of all these types present acute exacerbations, during which they become markedly edematous and hypertrophied, and are accompanied by lymphangitis or lymphadenitis.

Lupus vulgaris in time may greatly deform the nose, the lobe of the ear and the upper lip. The patches on the trunk and the extremities may become serpiginous or gyrate, while those on the hands and the feet may cause marked destruction, warty thickenings or elephantiasic enlargement. The patches on the mucous membranes appear as circumscribed, grayish, macerated or granulating areas, while those on the tongue are irregular, deep, painful fissures, sometimes associated with great enlargement of this organ.

SCROFULODERMA is the term applied to all tuberculous skin lesions which are direct extensions of deeper tuberculous processes. It develops over scrofulous cervical lymph nodes and surrounding the orifices of sinuses from tuberculous bones and joints. These lesions are oval-shaped or linear-shaped ulcerations with undermined edges; the ulcerations are covered with reddish granulations which often are crusted, are more or less edematous and produce considerable exudate. Healing, they leave hypertrophic scars and cicatricial bands.

TREATMENT. Antituberculous chemotherapy, described in detail in Chapter 24 (page 452), is applicable and used to good effect in patients with tuberculosis of the skin. General supportive care is important, with special heed to the nutritional and hygienic needs of the patient.

Fungus Infections

Fungi (low forms of plants) cause many common and important skin lesions; those that are circular in shape are known as *ringworm*. These infections are highly communicable. The diagnosis is made by identifying the fungus under the microscope.

Epidermophytosis (Athlete's Foot). The most common infection presumed to be due to a fungus is that involving the feet (particularly the skin between the small toes) and, less frequently, the hands. Clinically, this malady is characterized by sogginess and scaling of the skin in the affected area, accompanied by intense itching. The infecting fungus is to be found practically wherever human bare feet tread. Infection is more likely to occur if the feet are not dried thoroughly after bathing. The condition can become exceedingly severe, spreading to involve almost the entire sole of the foot. Lymphangitis and extension to the inguinal lymph nodes may occur. Actually, there is little proof that the fungus is anything but a benign saprophytic inhabitant of these moist and often bacterially infected areas.

TREATMENT AND NURSING CARE. The infected area must be kept clean and dry. Never apply the towel used on the feet to other parts of the body; use a paper towel, if necessary, for infected feet. Fresh socks should be worn daily. Drying applications— for instance, potassium permanganate soaks followed by talcum powder—should be used at least twice daily. Preparations containing undecylenic acid or its salts are useful in this condition. Use paper slippers or bath clogs and burn them at frequent intervals to avoid reinfection.

Ringworm. TINEA CAPITIS. Ringworm of the scalp is a contagious disease of the scalp caused by parasitic fungi. It appears as circular patches of erythema, crusts or tiny pustules. The hairs on the patch, invaded by the fungus, break off at or near the surface of the cuticle, leaving the area more or less bald. If the infection invades the deeper layers of the skin, it produces boggy patches and abscesses. This condition is called *kerion*.

Treatment. Griseofulvin is an oral antifungal agent that acts systemically to inhibit the growth of the fungi. It is specific for common fungus infections of the hair, the skin and the nails. The hair should be kept short and shampooed at frequent intervals. Local antifungal preparations may be rubbed in the scalp. A clean stocking cap should be used at night.

Nursing Care. A comb which may be boiled frequently should be used. Cut hair should be removed carefully with forceps, collected and destroyed because of the condition's infectiousness.

TINEA CIRCINATA. Typical ringworm of

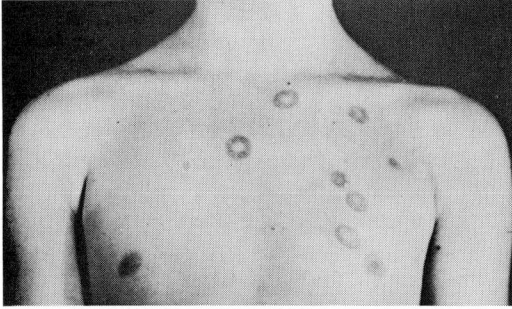

FIG. 295. Tinea circinata. This boy contracted the lesions by carrying a kitten under his shirt. (Paterson, D., and Mc-Creary, J. F.: Pediatrics, p. 439, Philadelphia, Lippincott)

the nonhairy surfaces presents from 1 to 10 small slightly elevated, somewhat scaly hyperemic patches, with advancing borders which are sharply outlined against the surrounding skin and the gradually clearing centers. When these reach from one to several inches in diameter, they may remain practically stationary for a long time, then spontaneously fade. The coalescence of several rings may form a large convoluted patch.

TINEA SYCOSIS (BARBER'S ITCH). This may present itself as areas of skin covered either by deep nodular and suppurative or by superficial scaly lesions, over which the hairs become loose and brittle and fall out, leaving partially bald patches. The confluent patches of the deep type produce diffuse boggy infiltrations with abscesses.

Treatment and Nursing Care. This is essentially the same as that for tinea capitis. Griseofulvin is helpful in this condition.

Parasitic Infestations

Pediculosis. Three varieties of lice (pediculi) infest man, and their very itchy bites are the cause of many skin troubles.

THE HEAD LOUSE, *Pediculus capitis,* lives on the scalp, its eggs (nits) attached to the hair. Its bite causes an intense itching, and the scratching, thus induced, leads to infection which produces impetigo, furunculosis and enlarged cervical lymph nodes. Dermatitis of the ears and neck in children is suggestive of this condition.

Treatment and Nursing Care. The application of benzyl benzoate emulsion to the scalp and the hair is effective. The next day the hair is shampooed. The treatment may have to be repeated if the infestation is severe.

THE BODY LOUSE, *Pediculus corporis,* lives chiefly in the seams of undergarments, to which it clings as it pierces the skin with its proboscis. Its bites cause characteristic minute hemorrhagic points and, on sensitive skins, evanescent wheals. Among the secondary lesions produced are hyperemia, parallel linear scratches, a slight degree of eczema and, in persistent cases, a general pigmentation which sometimes is as dark as that in Addison's disease. The skin most affected is that with which the clothing comes into closest contact, as around the neck, across the shoulders and the upper back,

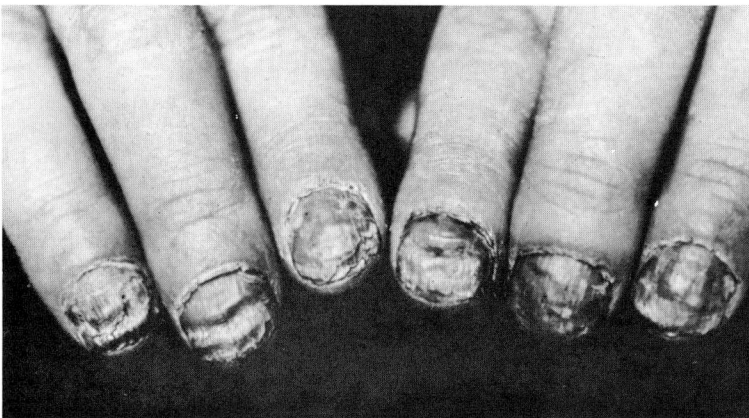

FIG. 296. Fungus infection of the fingernails. (Ralph E. McDonnell, M.D., New Haven)

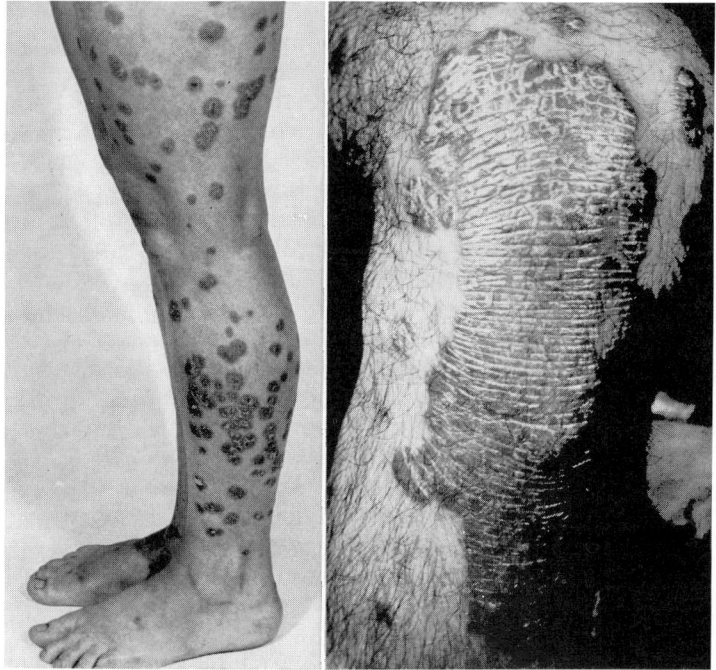

FIG. 297. Psoriasis of the leg and the knee. (Sauer, G. C.: Manual of Skin Diseases, p. 84, Philadelphia, Lippincott)

around the waist, over the sacrum and down the outside of the thighs. This louse is destroyed by boiling the undergarments. If boiling is impracticable (e.g., of various synthetic fibers), spraying the garment with 10 per cent DDT powder destroys the lice.

PUBIC LICE, *Pediculus pubis,* limit themselves to regions where the hair is short and stiff, such as the pubic region, the axillae, the beard and even the eyebrows and the eyelashes. The result of their bites and the scratching they induce includes excoriations, papules, pustules and other inflammatory lesions, sometimes severe enough to cause eczema.

The infected region should be shaved, washed thoroughly and treated with benzyl benzoate.

Scabies (The Itch) is a contagious skin disease due to the itch mite (*Sarcoptes scabiei*).

The characteristic lesion of scabies is the insect's burrow, a slightly elevated, tortuous or straight threadlike row of dark gray or blackish dots from ⅛ to ½ inch long. These burrows are found most often in the interdigital spaces, on the flexor surface of the wrists and about the breasts. The itching of

scabies, slight during the day, is usually intense at night after the patient retires, since the increased warmth of the skin rouses the parasites to greater activity. Secondary skin lesions, quite common, include itchy papules, vesicles and pustules, characteristically pres-

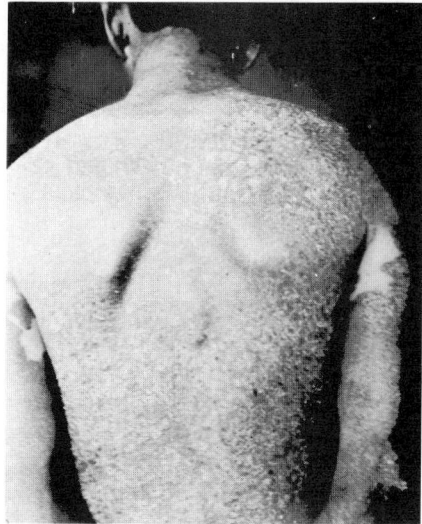

FIG. 298. Exfoliative dermatitis. (Ralph E. McDonnell, M.D., New Haven)

ent on the palms of the hands, on the wrists, about the elbows, in the axillae, on the lower abdomen and on the legs. In long-neglected cases a true eczema or impetigo may develop, especially on the hands and the forearms and in the axillary folds.

TREATMENT. Benzyl benzoate is applied topically and allowed to remain on the skin 24 hours. Following this application the patient bathes and changes his clothing and bedding.

Bedbugs. The bites of the bedbug (*Cimex lectularius*) produce purpuric spots often in irregular clusters of 3, 4 or more. Such groups sometimes are covered with a blood crust, but more often with inflammatory papules or wheal-like lesions. The legs, particularly the ankles, are the regions most often bitten. Menthol or phenol ointments have a soothing effect. Elimination of the insect may be accomplished by impregnating the bed with powder containing DDT and pyrethrins and spraying the walls and the floor with a similar solution. This problem seldom is encountered since metal beds have replaced the older wooden frames.

DERMATOSES OF UNKNOWN OR NONSPECIFIC ETIOLOGY

Erythema Multiforme

Erythema multiforme is an acute inflammatory skin eruption of bright red or purple-red macules, papules or bullae, symmetrically distributed, which appears rather suddenly and involves especially the upper part of the face, the neck, the forearms, the legs and the dorsal surfaces of the hands and the feet. This eruption fades after a few weeks, leaving no sequelae.

Two types, a maculopapular and a vesicobullous, are recognized. The dominant lesions of the former are well defined, bright red, but often, also, bluish and yellowish, have rounded edematous macules, or flat-topped papules, which have a tendency to spread peripherally and to fuse, forming complex patterns. The vesicobullous type, most common on the extremities, occurs as discrete or grouped vesicles or bullae, each surrounded by a hyperemic ring. Corticosteroid therapy is useful in the more severe forms. It is fortunately a benign and self-limited disease.

Erythema Nodosum

Erythema nodosum, a disease closely related to erythema multiforme, starts with mild constitutional symptoms such as fever, malaise and pains in the muscles and the joints. Then a crop of from 2 to 6 painful nodules appears on the extensor surfaces of both legs—rarely, elsewhere. These develop rapidly, reaching from 1 to 5 cm. in diameter. The skin covering them is bright red, smooth and shiny. From the appearance of these angry-looking nodules, one would expect them to suppurate, but they seldom do. After they reach full growth, they involute spontaneously, but, because of the appearance of fresh lesions, the course of the affection may extend over several weeks.

Erythema nodosum is a disease of youth, often associated with acute and chronic infections, perhaps most often with acute rheumatic fever. Many cases appear to fall into the group of so-called *anaphylactoid purpura,* which is essentially a vascular disease causing exudative as well as hemorrhagic phenomena throughout the body. No specific treatment is available.

Psoriasis

Psoriasis is an eruption of circular patches of all sizes, sharply defined against the normal skin and covered with abundant dry, silvery scales (Fig. 297). Scrape off these scales and one exposes the dark red base of the lesion covered with a thin white membrane which, if scratched, bleeds. These patches are not moist and never itch. They enlarge slowly, until, after many months, by coalescing they form extensive irregularly shaped patches.

Psoriasis appears most often on the extensor surfaces of the arms and the legs (especially about the knees and the elbows), on the scalp and the ears and over the sacrum. The face, the back of the hands, the palms and the soles are seldom affected; the tongue and the mucous membranes, never. Psoriasis per se causes no subjective symptoms, nor does it affect the general health. There is a hereditary predisposition to this disease. The condition, however, not infrequently is accompanied by rheumatoid arthritis. It has a marked tendency to improve and then recur, even throughout life; yet many cases stop spontaneously.

Treatment. The treatment of psoriasis is unsatisfactory. The physical health of the patient, and particularly his emotional life, should receive proper attention. Tar ointments combined with carefully graded doses of ultraviolet light sometimes clear the skin temporarily. It is most important that the patient be told how to care for his chronic disease, how to scrape the scales without introducing secondary infection and to obtain as much exposure to sunlight as possible.

Exfoliative Dermatitis

Generalized exfoliative dermatitis is characterized by a universal, obstinate, very itchy scaling of the skin, often accompanied by the loss of hair and nails (Fig. 298). It may develop as a primary condition. It may arise secondary to other chronic skin diseases, such as eczema and psoriasis, particularly if these are treated with irritating ointments over a long period of time.

This condition starts acutely as either a patchy or generalized erythematous eruption accompanied by fever, malaise and, occasionally, gastrointestinal symptoms (possibly due to similar lesions involving the gastrointestinal epithelium). The skin color changes from pink to dark red, then after a week the characteristic exfoliation begins, usually in the form of thin flakes which leave the underlying skin smooth and red, new scales forming as the older ones exfoliate. Relapses are the rule. Death, perhaps the result of secondary infection, occasionally occurs.

Treatment and Nursing Care. The treatment of this condition is most unsatisfactory; it includes bed rest and soothing applications to the skin. Corticosteroids lessen the severity of exacerbations and give the patient considerable relief. The patient is likely to become extremely irritable. In response, however, his nurse should be calm, good-natured, reassuring and sympathetic. She must carefully avoid exhibiting any trace of revulsion excited by his appearance, for he will be quick to detect unfavorable reactions on her part.

Pemphigus

Pemphigus (blister) is the term applied to a group of skin diseases, the lesions of which are bullae (round or oval watery blebs, i.e., blisters) of various sizes, some over an inch in diameter, which arise from a normal or only slightly reddened skin. Pemphigus is thought by some to be due to bacterial or virus infections; by others, to nerve dysfunctions. Still others are agreed that the cause is unknown.

Pemphigus (the common type) is a disease of adults, especially of those who are debilitated; its chief feature is crops of bullae, varying in size from that of a pea to that of a small egg, scattered over the body. Each bleb lasts from a few days to 2 weeks and then becomes a crust which falls off, leaving no scar and only slight pigmentation. This disease may continue for years, with long periods of freedom from lesions; but more often it presents a succession of acute exacerbations separated by intervals of a few weeks or longer, during which only a few scattered blebs are present. The mouth and the throat sometimes are involved and, in rare cases, the conjunctivae. The epidermis over the bullae in some cases is fragile and readily broken; hence, with spread of the eruption the entire body surface eventually becomes red, raw, edematous and foul smelling.

Treatment. The treatment of pemphigus is, first of all, to build up the general health with a high protein and high caloric diet and to keep the skin protected against secondary infections. There is a significant loss, through the skin, of tissue fluids and, therefore, of sodium chloride. This salt loss is responsible for many of the constitutional symptoms associated with the disease and must be combated with administration of adequate saline, parenterally or otherwise. The steroid hormones are effective in the disease, and their use here is fully justified.

Chemotherapy for the control of secondary infection is indicated. Plasma and whole-blood transfusion may be used to maintain the blood volume, as well as the hemoglobin and plasma protein concentrations.

Wet dressings or mild antiseptic lotions are protective and soothing. Patients with large areas of blistering have a characteristic odor that is lessened when secondary infection is controlled. Meticulous oral hygiene is important, for lesions in the mouth are common in pemphigus and add greatly to the patient's misery. The patient is usually depressed. The nurse should strive to give him the small but important "extras" that serve to lift the morale.

Pityriasis Rosea

Pityriasis (branlike; scaly) rosea, a skin disease of children and young adults, is a mild inflammatory disease of unknown cause characterized by an eruption of slightly raised and rather scaly round or ring-shaped lesions which early are pink but later salmon red in color. These lesions vary in size from that of a small pea to that of a 25-cent piece and are symmetrically distributed on the sides of the trunk, the back, the upper arms and the thighs, with special predilection for the axillae and the groin. They seldom appear on the face.

This eruption begins as a single lesion, the "herald patch," followed, after a week, by a general eruption which spreads rapidly. After from 3 to 10 weeks, this eruption disappears spontaneously. There are no constitutional symptoms. Some believe foods to be responsible; others consider it due to a skin parasite.

Treatment. This disease is self-limited and usually of only a few weeks' duration. For comfort during this period, a mild antipruritic, such as calamine lotion, may be indicated.

Lichen Planus

Lichen planus is an inflammatory disease of the skin and the mucous membranes, of unknown cause, characterized by a very itchy eruption of flat papules. It is most marked on the flexor surfaces of the extremities. Much of the body surface may be covered, but the face, the palms and the soles always remain free. The papules are flat, glistening, have a characteristic bluish-lavender color, are polygonal in shape and vary from a pinhead to a small pea in size. Their sides usually are perpendicular, and their centers are slightly depressed, scaly or covered by a network of glistening white striae. They are arranged in irregular annular and linear patches, separated by the natural lines of the skin, which they exaggerate and to which they give the appearance of a mosaic cut by crisscross lines. The central depression of some of the large papules is large enough to produce ringlike forms; other papules resemble warts. This eruption sometimes appears on the buccal mucosa several weeks before the skin becomes involved (see Plate 7).

Treatment. The treatment of lichen planus is nonspecific. Steroids relieve the itching by suppressing the inflammation but will not affect the lesions themselves. Antipruritic lotions and soothing ointments contribute greatly to the patient's comfort. Although it is a protracted disease, with or without treatment, eventually it clears completely.

Neurodermatitis

Neurodermatitis (lichen simplex chronicus) is the term applied to certain cutaneous diseases, the most conspicuous feature of which is thickening and congestion of the skin locally (but sometimes generally), the surface of which becomes a mosaic of flat, shiny, more or less angular, slightly elevated areas separated by exaggerated furrows. This process is called lichenification. In some cases, however, the eruption is decidedly papular, resembling lichen planus; in others, the patches of thickened skin are excoriated and slightly scaly or moist; on rare occasions they are nodular. The regions usually involved are the face, the back and the sides of the neck and the angle of the elbow and the knee, but the entire body may be covered.

Treatment. The first consideration in these cases of neurodermatitis is the control of the pruritus, accomplished as described on page 744.

Dermatitis Herpetiformis

Dermatitis herpetiformis is a chronic itchy eruption, the lesions of which are erythematous, papular, vesicular, pustular and, on rare occasions, hemorrhagic, possibly all present on the same skin. They appear always in clusters (a point necessary for diagnosis) and leave pigmented spots and, sometimes, scars after healing. The regions most often affected are the posterior axillary folds, the buttocks, the abdomen and the forearms. A marked (as much as 40%) eosinophilia of the blood is present, which is important in diagnosis. The general health may be undisturbed. This disease is attributed to focal infections, to intestinal disorders and to emotional disturbances. In other words, the etiology is unknown. Uncertain, likewise, is the prognosis for any given patient, as relapse is prone to occur despite all known therapy.

Treatment. The treatment of dermatitis herpetiformis is symptomatic, consisting of measures to improve the general health, especially from the hygienic and nutritional points of view. The administration of sulfapyridine has reportedly met with success. Phenolized calamine lotion and alkaline baths are soothing. Excoriated areas require protection against secondary infection, for which purpose sulfonamide and polymyxin-B (Neosporin) ointments are useful.

SYSTEMIC DISEASES WITH DERMATOLOGIC MANIFESTATIONS

Disseminated Lupus Erythematosus

Disseminated lupus erythematosus (D.L.E.) is a chronic inflammatory disease which affects nearly every organ system in the body, including the skin. Skin lesions are among the earliest, commonest, most obvious and most characteristic manifestations, and, therefore, are most likely to bring the patient to the attention of the physician. The etiology of this condition is not understood; its clinical and pathologic features, its course, its response to corticosteroid therapy and some of the laboratory findings associated with it suggest that it may be a disease based on auto-immunity.

Lupus erythematosus attacks persons predominantly of the younger age group and chiefly those of the female sex. Outstanding clinical characteristics include long-continued, low-grade fever; arthritis, akin to rheumatoid arthritis (page 1022); a skin rash with butterfly distribution involving the face (Plate 7); telangiectasis of the vessels in the nail beds; anemia, leukopenia; thrombocytopenia, similar to that in idiopathic thrombocytopenic purpura (page 477); and evidences of nephritis, notably proteinuria, pyuria and signs of renal insufficiency. A sterile endocarditis often develops, and cardiac failure is not infrequent. The disease is characterized by remissions and exacerbations. One factor which may produce the latter is exposure to sunlight. A fatal termination, due to renal failure, is to be anticipated eventually, but a specific prognosis is impossible, so variable is its course. It is possible to control the disease indefinitely and fairly satisfactorily by the administration of steroid hormones. Salicylates and the antimalarial drug chloroquine likewise are useful for symptomatic relief and retardation of the progression of lupus, but eradication of the process has yet to be achieved.

Of some diagnostic value is the observation of phagocytosis of leukocytes by other leukocytes in preparations which contain these cells in high concentration. This phenomenon is the basis of the so-called "L.E. test." Lupus erythematosus occurs without signs of systemic involvement, manifested only by a butterfly rash on the face, which is probably related in its pathogenesis to the disseminated form.

Dermatomyositis

This is a disease of unknown origin, characterized by a nonsuppurative inflammation of certain muscles, which become infiltrated with serum and collections of small round cells, while the muscle fibers present all varieties and degrees of degeneration. It is seen in young adults apparently in the best of health.

The onset of this malady is gradual, with vague prodromal symptoms which may persist for weeks. Then severe pain develops. This is definitely localized in certain muscles and spreads to others, group by group, until all may become involved. Usually there is a low-grade fever, with sweats, the appearance of subcutaneous edema and a dermatitis (erythematous, urticarial or eczematous) which may be general or confined to the skin overlying the muscles involved. This dermatitis eventually disappears, leaving the skin pigmented. On palpation the affected muscles have a characteristic hardness. The spleen may be enlarged. This disease and disseminated lupus erythematosus have much in common clinically and pathologically and, while the etiology of neither is understood, both may represent disorders of immunity.

Prognosis. Acute dermatomyositis runs its course in from 1 to 8 weeks. Subacute cases continue for months, periods of improvement alternating with relapses. Contractures may follow this condition. Over one half of all cases have proved to be fatal, either because of suffocation, produced by the involvement of the muscles of mastication and respiration, or because of bronchopneumonia.

Treatment. Rest in bed is essential. The pains may be relieved by the salicylates. Electrical stimulation of the muscles, followed by massage and gymnastic exercises, has some value in the prevention of atrophy and contractures and in preserving muscle function. The corticosteroid drugs, as in lupus, have proved beneficial in some cases.

Periarteritis Nodosa

This condition, possibly another example of auto-immunity, attacks persons of all ages and both sexes. In this disease the arteries, particularly the arterioles, are attacked by localized inflammatorylike processes, resulting in aneurysmal dilatation of these vessels and circulatory embarrassment to the parts which they supply. The clinical manifestations commonly encountered are quite similar to those enumerated in the foregoing description of lupus erythematosus disseminatus. The patient is prone to exhibit signs of prolonged fever, hypertension, nephritis, peripheral neuritis, palpable nodules along the arterial trunks and eosinophilia. Infrequently, aneurysms appear. These are the result of focal weakening of the arterial wall. They are most likely to develop in the abdomen. Periarteritis is apt to run a course of several years' duration, death finally occurring as a result of either renal decompensation or hypertension.

It has been noted that many patients had experienced allergic phenomena in response to sulfonamide therapy at some time prior to the development of the disease, which lends further emphasis to the importance of avoiding the use of such agents, unless based on specific indications.

Treatment. The treatment of patients with lupus erythematosus and periarteritis nodosa involves nothing specific. Dramatic, though temporary, remissions have been obtained by treatment with steroid hormones (p. 841).

Scleroderma (Progressive Systemic Sclerosis)

Scleroderma, as its alternate name implies, is not merely a skin disease, or "hardness of the skin" alone, but a disease in which there is progressive "hardening" throughout the

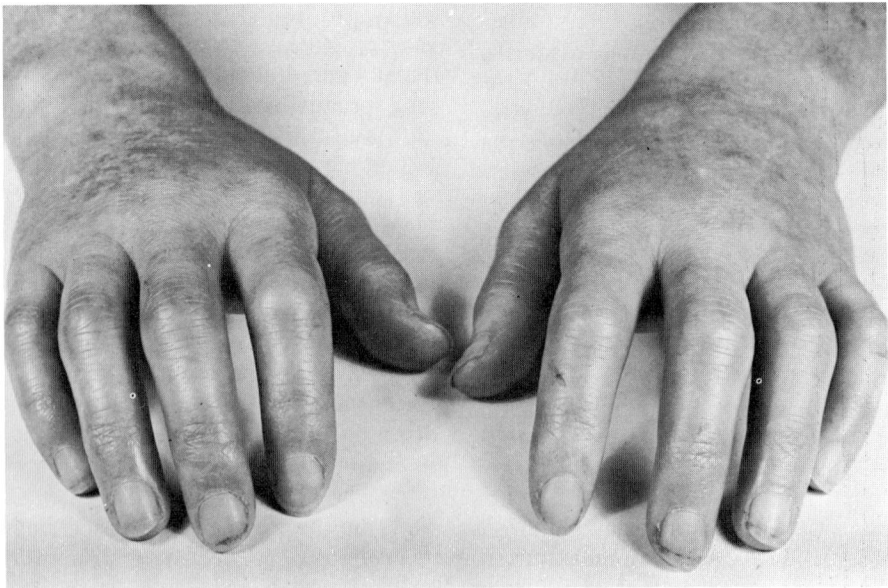

Fig. 299. Scleroderma. (Henry M. Lemon, M.D., Boston)

body. Specifically, this is a disease in which the connective tissues throughout the body slowly, but surely, become scarred and rigid. The basis for the common term, by which it is best known, is the fact that the superficial lesions are easily visible and remain the most prominent manifestation in the majority of patients.

The disease starts insidiously on the face and the hands, where the skin acquires a tense, waxy, wrinkle-free bound-down appearance, as illustrated in Figure 299. The skin and the subcutaneous tissues become increasingly hard and rigid and cannot be pinched up from the subjacent structures (hidebound). Wrinkles and lines are obliterated. The skin is dry (since sweat secretion over the involved region is suppressed), sometimes harsh and scaly and sometimes smooth. It is hairless and more or less bronzed.

The face becomes masklike, immobile and expressionless, and the mouth is rigid. The buccal mucous membrane likewise may be affected. Sometimes the teeth loosen and fall out. For years these changes may remain localized in the hands and the feet, but the condition spreads slowly: the limbs become stiff, immobile and shrunken; the fingers, semiflexed, immobile and useless; the hands, clawlike. The tense skin of the chest seriously restrains respiration. Similar changes affect the skin of the lower leg. This also presents wartlike hypertrophies.

The changes within the body are not visible directly but are vastly more important than those which are visible. The heart muscle becomes fibrotic, causing dyspnea; the esophagus is hardened, interfering with swallowing; the lungs are scarred, impeding respiration; there are digestive disturbances, due to hardening of the intestine; and a variety of other disturbances, including Raynaud's phenomenon and arthritis.

Scleroderma and disseminated lupus erythematosis are very much alike, clinically and pathologically, both involving the same structures in approximately the same way. Both are regarded as disorders of immunity, the result of an antigen-antibody reaction within the mesenchymal (connective tissue and bone) tissues.

No known treatment is effective in this condition, reliance, therefore, having to be placed on general supportive treatment.

Sarcoidosis

Sarcoid is the term given to groups of firm, elastic, subcutaneous, nodular infiltrations of the skin, some tiny, others even 2 or 3 cm. in diameter. On microscopic examination these are found to be comprised of multiple granulomas, which, except for the complete absence of necrosis, resemble the lesions of tuberculosis. They occur most often on the face and the external surfaces of the arms and the shoulders, but the larger types are on the trunk. The epidermis overlying these nodules is changed little. Only the largest of them break down or produce an exudate. Eventually they heal, leaving little or no scarring.

Although sarcoidosis is generally thought of as a skin disease, the skin, in fact, is but one of many organs involved in this strange process; indeed, the skin manifestations may appear only late, if at all. The complete clinical picture, not found as a rule, would include, in addition to the cutaneous lesions, the features of chronic, low-grade fever with little or no constitutional reactions; lymph gland enlargement, which may be generalized in distribution; iritis and uveitis, which may progress to blindness; splenomegaly; moderate anemia; the x-ray findings (usually chance) of spotty nodular areas of density throughout both lung fields, associated with which are few or no physical signs, excepting in the most severe cases, when venous return to the heart is obstructed by the fibrotic process, producing cor pulmonale; and cystic bone changes, most often involving the small bones of the hands.

The etiology of sarcoidosis has not been established as yet. No bacterial agent or virus has been proved to be responsible.

The Kveim Test. Of considerable diagnostic aid in connection with these patients is a skin test which involves the intracutaneous inoculation of homogenized sarcoidal tissue from a patient with this disease. Four to 6 weeks after the inoculation a skin biopsy is performed at that site; in the event of a positive reaction, granulomatous changes will be observed, characteristic of the lesions of sarcoidosis. Positive reactions have been demonstrated in 70 to 80 per cent of patients with sarcoidosis, in contrast with an incidence of less than 5 per cent of positive reactions in patients with diseases other than sarcoidosis or in normal individuals.

Treatment. In the absence of any firm etiologic basis, no specific therapy for sarcoidosis has as yet been devised. Steroid hormones produce remissions in this disease, but relapse invariably follows the omission of these drugs. The prognosis is excellent, to the extent that death rarely can be attributed directly to this disease. On the other hand, the most important factor contributing to the death of many patients with sarcoidosis is cor pulmonale, the sequel to pulmonary fibrosis and the most serious complication of this condition.

CONGENITAL DISORDERS OF THE SKIN

Ichthyosis (fish skin) is a congenital abnormality of the skin which from birth is thick, also harsh and dry, since sweat and oil secretions are deficient, and often covered by platelike scales or nodules. The only subjective symptoms are slight itching and the formation of painful fissures.

In the mildest form of ichthyosis (ichthyosis simplex or xeroderma) the skin over the entire body surface, but particularly on the extensor surfaces of the extremities and the back, is dry, rough and thick, its normal lines accentuated. This condition is worse during cold dry weather; the patient may not notice it during the summer. Often eczema and various keratotic skin diseases develop in association with it.

In the more marked grades of ichthyosis the body is covered with quadrilateral or irregularly shaped thin scales, like those of a fish, and, in extreme cases, by thick, horny plates separated by deep furrows, like those of an alligator.

Congenital ichthyosis explains the so-called *harlequin fetus* covered with armorlike plates. Such children are usually stillborn or soon die.

The treatment is mainly supportive. Soap should be avoided whenever possible. Emollient oils, creams or ointments applied regularly are helpful. Large doses of vitamin A may benefit the patient.

ULCERS AND TUMORS OF THE SKIN

Ulcerations

The superficial loss of surface tissue due to death of the cells is called an *ulceration*. A simple ulcer, such as is found in a small superficial second-degree burn, tends to heal by granulation if kept clean and protected from injury. If exposed to the air, the serum that escapes from it will dry and form a scab, under which the epithelial cells will grow and cover the surface completely.

Special diseases cause characteristic ulcers —thus, there are tuberculous ulcers of the skin and syphilitic punched-out ulcers of the leg.

Ulcers of the skin arise usually either from infection or from an interference with the blood supply. Infectious ulcers are not uncommon. They develop usually from an infection with anaerobic streptococci or from a combination of infections in which hemolytic anaerobic streptococci live in symbiosis with staphylococci. Ulcers of this type tend to progress peripherally and are seen often in the lower extremity or on the abdomen or the chest after operation. They are characterized by an overhanging edge, and culture from them usually shows the type of organism causing the infection. These ulcers tend to resist ordinary forms of treatment, but the application of zinc peroxide, which liberates oxygen over a long period of time, converts the anaerobic portions of the wound into an aerobic area. Penicillin locally or intramuscularly also is highly effective. Healing occurs rapidly due to the inability of the anaerobic streptococci to live in an unfavorable environment.

Ulcers due to a deficient arterial circulation are seen in patients with peripheral vascular disease, arteriosclerosis, Raynaud's disease and frostbite. In these patients, the treatment of the ulceration must be carried out in conjunction with the treatment of the arterial disease. The danger is from secondary infection. Frequently, amputation of the part is the only effective therapy. (See Varicose Ulcers, p. 499.)

Cysts

Sebaceous Cysts. Cysts of the sebaceous glands are seen very frequently on the hairy parts, especially on the scalp. These result from a blockage of the drainage duct, the continued secretion of the gland being dammed up within the dilated duct. The cysts cause relatively few symptoms other than disfigurement, but, occasionally, they become infected and, in older people, may undergo a malignant degeneration. They may be removed easily under local anesthesia without the necessity of hospitalization.

Tumors

Verrucae (warts) are benign skin tumors that appear more commonly in children but are seen also in older people. Occasionally, they are painful, and they may become infected. Usually, they can be cured by irradiation therapy or by destruction by electrocoagulation.

Nevi (birthmarks) are vascular tumors of benign nature affecting the skin and, often, the subcutaneous tissues. They may be simple dilatations of cutaneous vessels, and these are spoken of as *portwine birthmarks*. They may disappear with age, but, usually, they are treated with irradiation or carbon dioxide snow. The *strawberry birthmark* is a true benign tumor of the capillaries. It is raised very slightly above the surface of the skin, and it occurs most often in the upper part of the body or on the face or the neck. Nevi respond very well to irradiation therapy as a rule.

Moles are of various types: flat or raised, smooth or lobulated, always pigmented, some of them containing hair. Generally, they are benign, but those deeply pigmented and raised above the surface of the skin may take on a malignant change suddenly and become melanotic tumors. As a rule, no treatment is necessary unless the mole is disfiguring, but, in cases in which the mole is lobulated, raised above the surface and in a position in which frequent irritation may induce malignant change (as, for instance, under the arm or on the back of the neck), excision is indicated as a prophylactic measure against the development of malignancy.

Keloids. A keloid is an overgrowth of fibrous tissue at the site of a scar. It may occur without warning and is especially prone to develop in scars in the Negro. It causes no particular difficulty, except disfigurement, and frequently responds to irradiation therapy. Excision is advisable occasionally (Fig. 301).

Fibromata of the skin are benign connective tumors, simple or multiple, flat or pedunculated.

The majority of fibromata, if multiple, are neurofibromata, arising from the connective tissue of the nerve trunks of the skin. They are of all sizes, some as small as a pinhead and others huge painless pendulous masses (Fig. 302). The skin may even be covered by these. These may be excised without danger of recurrence.

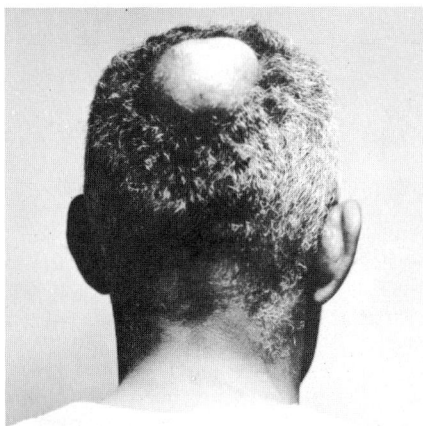

FIG. 300. Large sebaceous cyst of the scalp.

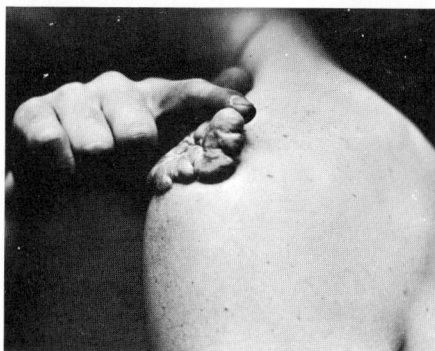

FIG. 301. Keloid of shoulder after minor injury.

Neurofibromata, often single, arise also from the deeper nerves of the skin. These tend to recur if excised.

Malignant Tumors of Skin

A nurse can be most helpful to an individual with a noninvading skin lesion by urging him to see a physician. If the sore or the lump is a cancer, it is the most curable of all cancers if treated early; in spite of this, these lesions are responsible for 6 per cent of all cancer deaths.

Carcinoma of the skin or epithelioma may occur from either the superficial cells of the skin (the so-called prickle-cell epithelioma) or from the deeper cells of the skin (the so-called rodent ulcer or basal-cell carcinoma). The former type occurs at any site on the body, most often on the hands and around the various orifices of the body. The basal-cell carcinoma or rodent ulcer appears on the face, especially on the temples. Of the two, the prickle-cell epithelioma is the more malignant. Both respond very well to local therapy, either irradiation with radium or destruction of the tumor by electrocoagulation.

Basal-cell Carcinoma. The face, especially the cheeks about the nose and the eyes and in front of the ears, is a common site for the development of cancer in patients past middle age. The growth may spring from an old warty or papillomatous tumor, or frequently from areas of hornified skin, a condition spoken of as senile keratosis. Such lesions, therefore, should be regarded as predisposing to cancer and the patient should be referred to a physician for competent treatment. These cancers are of the slow-growing type, called rodent ulcers, and are characterized by invasion and erosion of contiguous tissues but by very late and infrequent metastatic growths.

Metastatic Skin Carcinoma. Metastatic cancers growing in the skin arise most frequently from cancers of the female breast or of the prostate gland. These, the so-called *lenticular* skin carcinomata, start as small nodules in the deep layers of the skin, vary in size from that of a pinhead to a cherry, and are pink or red in color; the dome is generally covered with enlarged capillaries. As a result of their growth and multiplication they become so crowded that they form an extensive hard nodular area which, in extreme cases, covers almost the entire upper chest like an armor plate. These so obstruct

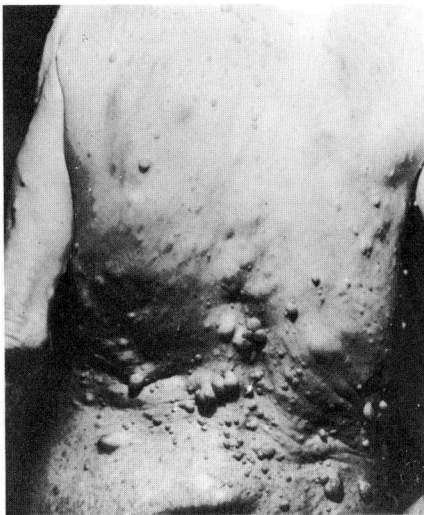

FIG. 302. Multiple neurofibromata (Von Recklinghausen's disease).

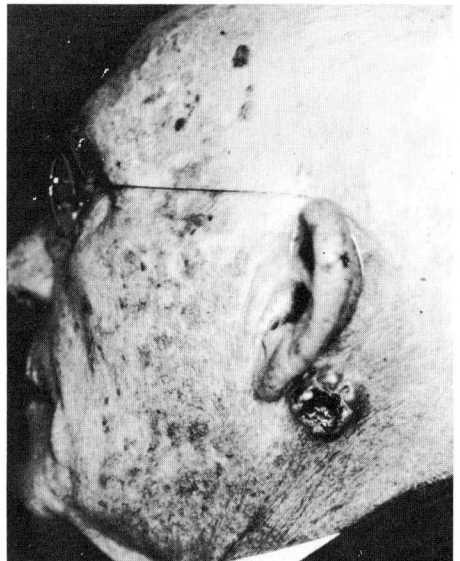

FIG. 303. Basal cell carcinoma (rodent ulcer) originating from one of the numerous senile keratoses observed over the head and the neck. (Ralph E. McDonnell, M.D., New Haven)

the superficial lymphatics and the veins that the arms become considerably swollen.

Melanotic Sarcomata. These start as firm hyperpigmented nodules, from pinhead to pea in size, within the substance of moles which previously had shown signs of malignant changes (crusting, bleeding or increase in size, firmness or depth of color). When further developed, their surface is flat, convex or fungoidal; their color ranges from slate to purplish-black. If fungoidal, they eventually ulcerate. These sarcomata are known for their extreme viciousness and resistance to irradiation. Numerous secondary nodules often cluster around the primary growth, crowding together in patches. Occasionally they metastasize to internal organs. In some cases, the first evidence that the mole has become malignant is metastatic enlargement of the adjacent glands or the appearance of cutaneous metastases involving distant parts. Their invasion of internal organs causes melanemia (free pigment in the blood stream), melanuria (black urine) and cachexia.

The treatment of melanoma is to excise with a wide margin all pigmented moles which, being subject to friction, pressure or other forms of irritation, have shown evidences of growth, tenderness, ulceration or bleeding. Dissection of the regional lymph nodes commonly is combined with radical local removal of the melanoma.

Treatment and Nursing Care. Treatment may be by one of several methods: the excision of the growth (curative only if done early), the application of radium or a combination of both. Skin cancer is benefited and often cured by radiation therapy.

The nursing care consists of the application of sterile dressings to the lesion and careful observation for any signs of hemorrhage. Hemorrhage often occurs after operation, but it may result simply from the erosion of a large vessel without any reference to operation.

The nurse can explain the nature of radiotherapy to the patient receiving this treatment for the first time.

Being alone in a small room with a huge machine will be less frightening when the patient has some understanding of it. Re-

assure the individual who fears that this treatment will cause sterilization, for it will not. Explain to him that he may experience some reddening and perhaps blistering of the treated skin. Lanolin or any soothing lubricant will keep the skin soft after radiation therapy is completed. The patient should know that he always will have delicate skin; therefore, he must protect it from excess exposure to the sun, cold and so forth. The importance of follow-up care must be stressed, for there is always the possibility of recurrence or of a new primary lesion.

Prevention essentially includes the elimination of irritation caused by ill-fitting appliances, broken teeth, repeated injury and friction, as well as prompt attention to erosive or ulcerated lesions which have a hard margin or base, a raised border, a tendency to bleed readily, and which extend to adjacent lymph glands.

DISORDERS INVOLVING THE HAIR

Alopecia

Alopecia (the loss of hair) may be congenital, senile or premature. Temporary alopecia may follow acute fevers, notably typhoid, but in from 75 to 90 per cent of all cases it occurs in association with seborrhea or eczema seborrhoicum. The alopecia of early syphilis seldom produces conspicuous baldness, but rather a thinning of the hair in many small ill-defined areas, giving the scalp a moth-eaten appearance.

Alopecia areata is a condition, its cause unknown, characterized by the appearance on the scalp, rarely on the bearded regions and still more rarely on the eyebrows and the eyelashes, of one or more circumscribed oval or bandlike patches of complete baldness. The exposed skin of these patches usually is quite normal (this excludes ringworm), but occasionally is slightly depressed and anesthetic, especially at the center of the patches. These patches may appear suddenly, the hair falling out within a few hours; but more often they are several weeks in developing, during which time the alopecia is preceded often by such premonitory symptoms as headache, itching, burning or merely a feeling of irritation. For a while these patches tend to spread peripherally, and then remain stationary for weeks or even indefinitely. While seldom more than two or three bald patches appear, and these rarely over 1 or 2 inches in diameter, they may steadily increase in area and, coalescing, finally make most of the scalp bald. In one type, indeed, the end-result is complete baldness, not only of the scalp, but also of the eyebrows, the eyelids, the axillae and, possibly, the entire body surface. In some patients with alopecia areata the nails become white, spotted and brittle.

With recovery, these bald areas first become covered by a temporary growth of fine white (lanugo) hair or of coarse hair, often pigmented but sometimes white, which finally is replaced by normal hair. A condition resembling alopecia areata follows overdoses of thallium.

Treatment. The treatment of baldness (other than that due to lues and ringworm) is unsatisfactory, since nothing is known of its cause. Doubtless the circulation of the scalp should be increased by massage and heat, with correction of any discovered endocrine defect such as hypothyroidism. Ultraviolet-light baths of the closely clipped head certainly are of benefit provided that the hair follicles have not atrophied too far. Nearly all good hair tonics in use are for the seborrhea present.

Hypertrichosis (Excessive Hair)

The conspicuous hair growth on the upper lip of some women is a hereditary trait which, contrary to general belief, is not at all related to ovarian function. Extreme beard growth in women evidently depends on the same factors that also lead to premature sexual development (dysfunctions of the pituitary, the adrenal and other endocrine glands).

Treatment. To remove superfluous hair, some use epilating waxes (made up of beeswax and resin) which merely pull off the hair; others use depilatory applications (containing barium sulfide or calcium sulfide) which erode the hair shafts. The results of these measures are only temporary. Shaving is a satisfactory method; it probably does not make the hair stiffer. For permanent removal of superfluous hair, however, the only safe method is the individual destruction of each hair follicle by the electric needle.

DERMATOLOGIC SURGERY AND PLASTIC RECONSTRUCTIVE SURGERY

Reconstructive surgery is performed to repair defects and malformations, both congenital and acquired, and to restore function as well as to prevent further loss of function. Occasionally, plastic surgery is done primarily for cosmetic improvement. It is applicable to many parts of the body and to numerous structures such as bone, cartilage, muscle, nerve and cutaneous structures. For bone it includes bone inlays and transplants for deformities and nonunion; muscle can be transferred; nerves can be reconstructed and spliced; and cartilage can be replaced. Lastly, but as important as any, is the reconstruction of the cutaneous tissues around the neck and the face; this is referred to as *cosmetic surgery*.

Availability of Facilities. The patient who is in need of plastic or reconstructive surgery may not know that such help is available. In this situation, too, the nurse is in a position to disseminate information. Parents who have a congenitally deformed child often delay in seeking assistance either because of guilt feelings, conviction that they must bear their own burden, false feelings that perhaps the child will outgrow his handicap, or ignorance about what can be done. Scars or portwine stains are not uncommon; their presence may affect adversely an otherwise healthy personality and result in a maladjusted person whose future happiness is jeopardized.

Children and individuals up to the age of 21 with congenital defects are eligible for financial support to meet the costs of plastic or reconstructive surgery. Plans for medical care of crippled children are available in each state; these, in turn, are partially supported by the Crippled Children's Bureau of the U. S. Children's Bureau.

Preparation of the Patient. As in any other form of treatment, it is necessary to evaluate the patient as a whole and the patient's problem in its entirety. What is his problem? Is his defect a threat to his position or security among his daily contacts? Does the defect affect his personality? Are personality changes out of proportion to the size or the nature of his physical problem? What does he expect of surgery? What does the surgeon expect to do for the patient? Does the patient recognize that it may involve succeeding operative procedures? Does he know that perfection cannot be achieved? What are his future hopes and ambitions? These are a few of the questions which the patient and his family, the physician, the social worker, the psychologist and the nurse will need to investigate before a schedule of reparative procedures can be set up. It is important that the tissues concerned be free of infection, and that other conditions, such as syphilis, tuberculosis, and diabetes mellitus, be under control. The general condition of the patient with regard to nutrition, age and morale should be at optimal levels.

The patient should be told that immediate postoperative appearances of a wound are temporary and that it may take days for changes to take place before the site takes on its eventual appearance. Redness, distortion, swelling and unattractive suture lines are characteristics that change with time.

The family needs to be informed of the postoperative appearance, the condition and the recovery plans of the patient. Their genuine encouragement and support can mean a great deal to the apprehensive patient.

Nature of Flaps and Grafts

In all reconstructive work, tissue to fill the defect must be obtained either from a distant site or nearby. This is accomplished by flap or graft. A *flap* is a piece of tissue used to cover or fill a defect. It has been lifted from its bed but still has a partial attachment by a pedicle, from which it receives its blood supply until healed in its new location.

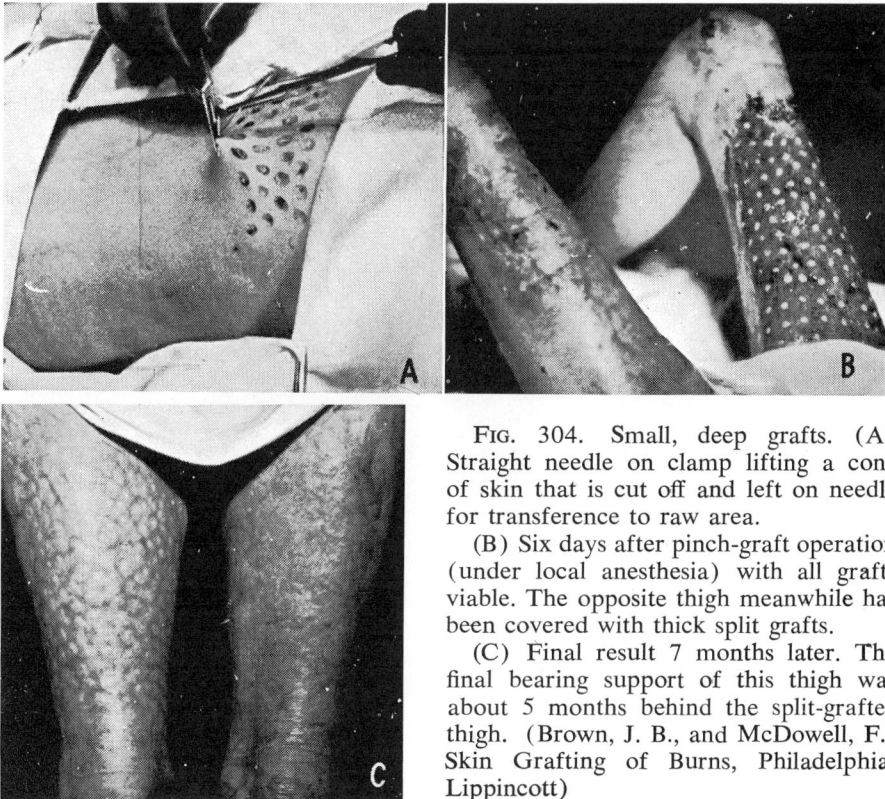

FIG. 304. Small, deep grafts. (A) Straight needle on clamp lifting a cone of skin that is cut off and left on needle for transference to raw area.

(B) Six days after pinch-graft operation (under local anesthesia) with all grafts viable. The opposite thigh meanwhile has been covered with thick split grafts.

(C) Final result 7 months later. The final bearing support of this thigh was about 5 months behind the split-grafted thigh. (Brown, J. B., and McDowell, F.: Skin Grafting of Burns, Philadelphia, Lippincott)

A *graft* is a piece of tissue separated completely from its normal and original position and transferred by one or more stages to correct a distant defect. Transfers or transplants from the same person are termed *autografts;* from a different person *homografts.* The former type is much the better, being safer and more likely to be successful.

Skin Grafting

As this type of reconstructive or plastic surgery most often is found necessary to correct unsightly and embarrassing deformity around the face, the mouth and neck, attention will be given especially to the maxillofacial technic and nursing care.

So that the operation may be a success, the area to be covered with grafts must be free of infection and sloughs, because grafts "take" or grow only on a clean "granulating" surface. Therefore, a period of preparation of the wound usually is necessary before the operation can be undertaken. Warm saline or penicillin dressings often are used, and penicillin usually is given systemically. The donor area most often is the anterior thigh, but, because the nurse cannot tell where it is to be, she should ask for specific instructions. The preparation of the donor area consists of a shave and a thorough cleansing by a germicidal soap and water.

Several types of grafts are in common usage. To cover small surfaces, the *Reverdin* or *pinch graft* often is used. Bits of skin are picked up on the point of a needle or with forceps and cut off with the scissors; these "islands" are applied to the area to be grafted (Fig. 304). This operation may be performed easily under local anesthesia.

The *Ollier-Thiersch graft* is used to cover larger surfaces. Strips of superficial skin are shaved off with a razor and applied to the granulating wound. This type of graft is relatively difficult to handle, because of its tendency to contract and wrinkle. On the other hand, it is the type most likely to grow in areas where the blood supply is poor, e.g., over bony prominences, and its donor site is re-epithelialized rapidly.

Split-thickness grafts are grafts of approximately one half the thickness of the skin, removed by a knife or a dermatome (Fig. 305). These grafts are handled more easily and, as in the case of the Ollier-Thiersch graft, skin at the donor site regenerates quickly.

Wolfe-Krause grafts differ from the previous types in that they consist of the full thickness of the skin. These are taken when

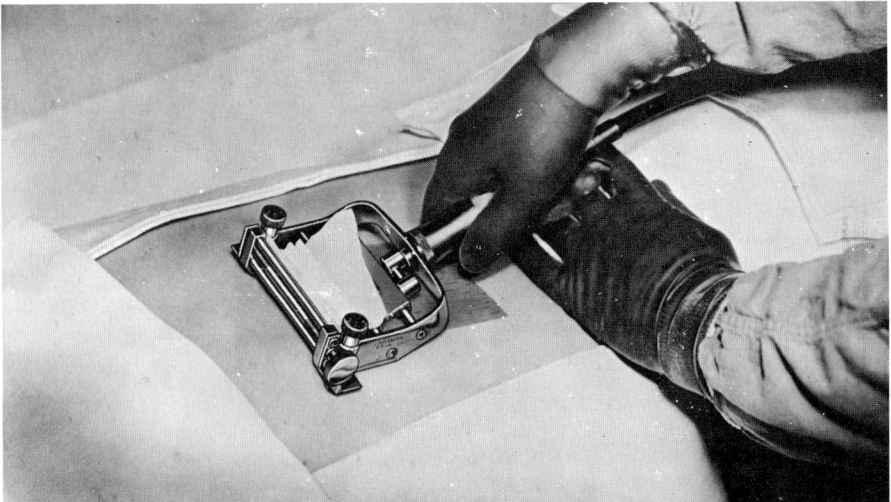

Fig. 305. The Brown-Electro Dermatome is operated electrically to obtain the desired thickness graft in widths from 1¾″ to 3″. Blades are disposable; the apparatus is easily operated. (Zimmer Manufacturing Co., Warsaw, Ind.)

the matching of skin color and texture is important. Obviously, more problems are to be expected with this type of graft, because of the difficulty of establishing a blood supply.

In the treatment of contractures from scars of old burns or injuries, especially those of neck and chin, it is necessary often to excise a large amount of contracted (scar) tissue. The area thus denuded most often is covered with a *pedicle* or *Gillies tube flap*. This flap is so cut that a tube or pedicle may be left attached through which the graft may obtain its blood supply. The flap is applied to the surface to be covered with the pedicle still attached. After the flap is well united to its new location, blood vessels grow into it and the pedicle can be removed (Fig. 306).

Other areas of the body may require plastic work of greater surface magnitude, in patients with extensive burns, mutilated limbs and crippling scar contractures. Here will arise the problem of donor areas for Reverdin, Ollier-Thiersch or sliding grafts. The Thiersch type may be made with a sharp razor blade or by the Padgett dermatome for the larger sheets of skin split of a definite thickness. When a cavity such as the orbit, the mouth or the nostril is to be relined, the graft may be sutured round a previously fashioned mold of dental rubber or plastic material.

In some circumstances, instead of free grafts or pedicle flaps, "sliding" flaps of skin and subcutaneous tissue from the surrounding area can be used. One application of the sliding flap method is the Z-plasty, very

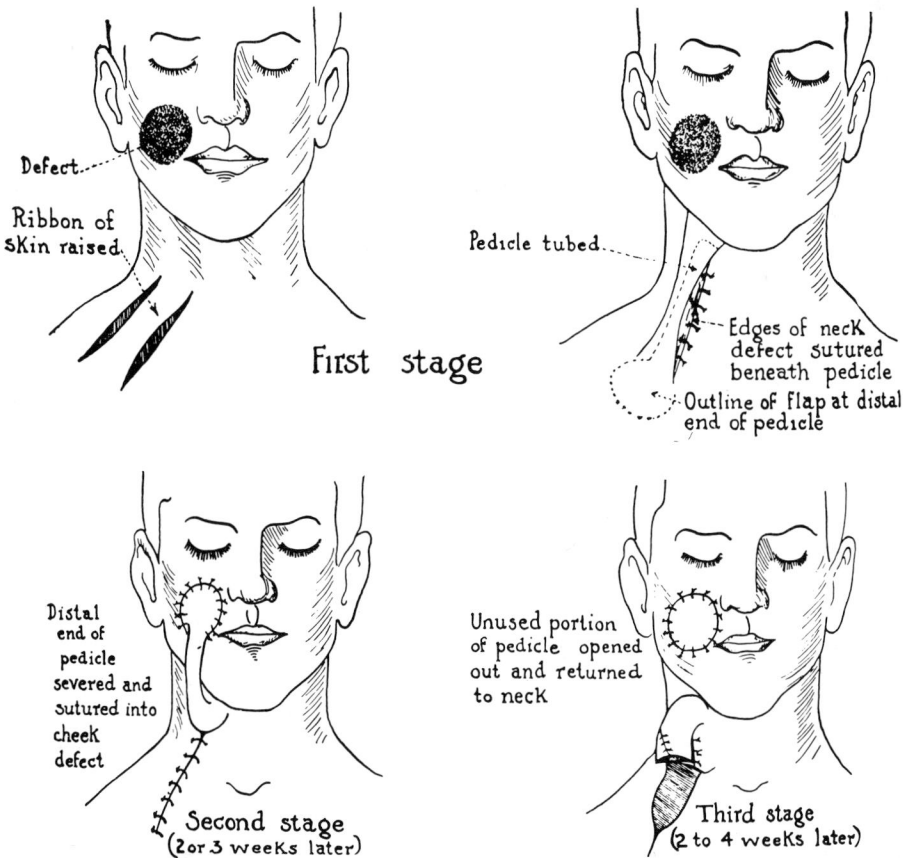

FIG. 306. Diagram showing preparation of tube pedicle flap, after Gillies. (Ivy, R. H.: Plastic and reconstructive surgery of the face, mouth, and jaws *in* Nelson's Loose Leaf Surgery, vol. II, p. 682)

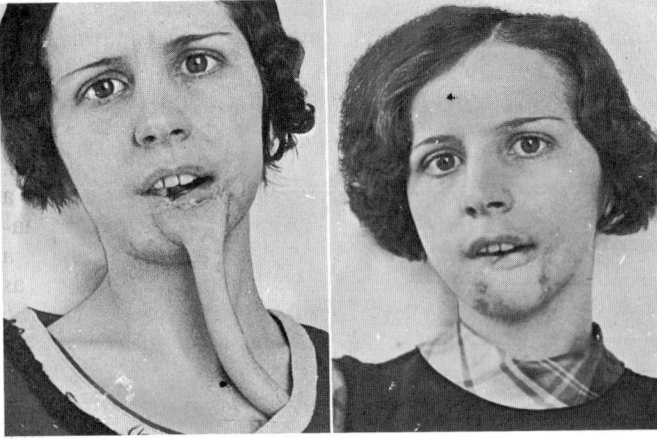

Fig. 307. (*Left*) Showing tube pedicle flap from chest, used for repair of chin defect. (*Right*) After pedicle had been severed. (Robert H. Ivy, M.D.)

useful for relieving comparatively narrow scar contractures about the neck or about joints such as the axilla, the elbow, the knee or the wrist. The application of the Z-plasty to a scar contracture of the axilla is shown in Figure 308.

Fascial transplants have numerous uses. They are obtained generally from the fascia lata of the thigh and are adaptable for use as suture material, for repair of hernia defects and for replacement of tendon loss.

Cartilage transplantation may be immediate and direct, taken from the costal cartilages and transferred to the nose.

Bone grafts demand meticulous aseptic technic and rigid fixation in their new site. They may be taken from the crest of the tibia, the upper border of the iliac bone or a rib.

All donor areas should receive the same careful treatment given any other surgical wound. If possible to close safely by suture, such is done. For the raw, wide area left from the Thiersch method, paraffin mesh, Albolene or petrolatum gauze permits a painless dressing within 8 to 10 days.

The area from which the free graft is to be taken, usually the anterior surface of the

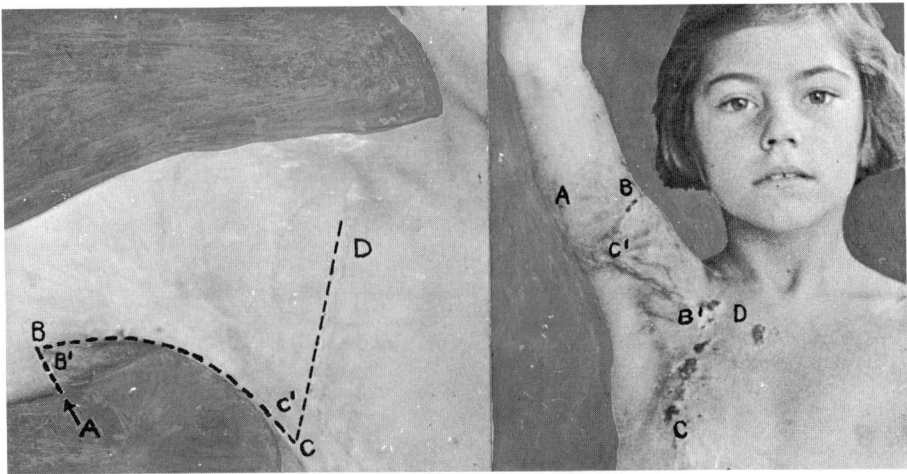

Fig. 308. (*Left*) Scar contracture of axilla, causing restricted elevation of arm, suitable for correction by Z-plasty. Incisions indicated by dotted lines. (*Right*) After operation, showing free elevation of arm. Lettering indicates relocation of flaps. (Robert H. Ivy, M.D.)

thigh or the abdomen, is designated by the surgeon for preparation. The hair should be shaved from it, but generally no antiseptics are used until the patient is taken to the operating room.

After the application of the grafts, a dressing which will effect rapid epithelialization is applied. A perforated plastic or fine-mesh gauze appears to be ideal, particularly if it is impregnated with a thin layer of a dry type of ointment such as paraffin; this acts as a scaffold on which new tissue grows. Frequently, more adequate pressure is maintained by incorporating in the dressings sponge rubber, moist sea sponge or cotton waste. No redressing is necessary for from 3 to 5 days, at which time only the gauze is removed, the paraffin mesh being left in place. Care must be exercised in removing the dressings so as not to disturb the grafts.

Nursing Care of the Maxillofacial Patient

The face is a part of the body which every person desires to keep at its best; many individuals try to improve on nature by various and sundry methods. When the face becomes disfigured, an emotional reaction occurs. Consequently, the victim of an automobile accident, whose face is injured, presents a problem which demands the utmost in understanding by the nurse. The patient's reaction to his problem, to his family and to the medical and the nursing personnel are all indices of his inner feelings which are most significant if appropriate measures are to be taken to help him.

Preoperative Attention. The patient may have a good meal the evening before, and a light breakfast or fluid up to 4 hours before the operation. For the comfort of the patient, operation is done best in the morning.

The mouth should be made as clean as possible to lessen the danger both of lung complications after general anesthesia and of infection in the wound.

Preoperative medication is ordered with specific regard to relaxing the patient and reducing mouth secretions.

If the patient is a man, the skin of the face should be shaved closely and, of course, well cleansed with soap and water. If the operative field extends up toward the scalp, this should also be shaved as far as is necessary.

Postoperative Management. Immediate postoperative care is concentrated on maintaining an adequate airway. Car must be taken to prevent disturbance or soilage of dressings. Observe for impairment of circulation and edema.

Occasionally, after operation within the mouth, the nurse may be alarmed by undue bleeding from the gums. All ordinary hemorrhage of this nature can be controlled by inserting a gauze pad in the mouth against the bleeding part of the jaw and bringing pressure of the opposing teeth to bear against it. If the patient is conscious, he can be made to bite on the pad. This pressure of the jaw often can be applied even when no teeth are present. In case of difficulty, the nurse should make pressure with the pad until the doctor arrives. The gauze pad can be changed as it becomes soaked with blood or saliva. After plastic operations on the face, frequently no dressings are used. If the incisions have been closed accurately with sutures, no dressings are necessary unless it is desired to control oozing of blood by pressure. Particularly near the mouth, dressings tend to become soaked with saliva and food, which may lead to infection of an otherwise clean wound. Slight oozing of blood from the incisions generally occurs for a short time after operation. If this blood is allowed to clot on the wound, infection may occur under the clot and spoil the cosmetic result. For the first hour or so after operation the nurse should wipe the blood that oozes from the incision with an alcohol sponge so that it will not clot on the surface.

In plastic operations the flaps sometimes become blue and congested, due to partial obstruction of the venous circulation. The surgeon sometimes scarifies the surface of the flap, making numerous small openings to relieve the blood congestion and avoid gangrene of the flap. The blood flow from these small incisions then can be kept up by the continuous application for several hours of hot fomentations of 1 per cent sodium citrate. These must be applied in an aseptic manner in order not to infect the flap. Probably the most convenient way is for the nurse to drop some of the warm sodium citrate solution on the dressings from time to time with a syringe.

Pain is more likely to follow operations involving the jaw bones than the soft tissues alone. For postoperative pain, either a hot-water bag or an ice bag may give relief. Whichever works best in the individual patient is employed. Sedatives ranging from aspirin to morphine may be required.

Maxillofacial patients need not be denied fluids for any length of time after operation, as may be the case after abdominal operations. The patient may have cracked ice or water as soon as postanesthetic vomiting is over, and liquid diet may be started as soon as the patient has a desire for food. Very often soft diet is started the day after operation.

When there is a wound of the mouth, the mouth should be cleansed after each feeding. It is not sufficient always for the patient to use a mouthwash. Frequent swabbing of the gums and the teeth with cotton on applicators soaked in hydrogen peroxide will accomplish a great deal in keeping the mouth clean. The mouth, and especially the wounded or diseased part, should be irrigated 3 or 4 times a day with some antiseptic fluid. The syringe should require only one hand to operate it, leaving the other hand free to retract the cheek or hold a light. A very convenient syringe is the one used for irrigating eyes. This consists of a fairly large rubber bulb and a small glass nozzle of the medicine dropper type. An all-rubber ear syringe or a power spray also may be used. When very frequent irrigation is required, a reservoir (bag or douche can) may be suspended over the head of the bed, not more than 2 feet above the patient's head, and the fluid carried to the mouth through a plastic nozzle. Sometimes the patient himself can use this.

Gauze packing frequently is placed in mouth wounds. This should not be allowed to remain longer than 48 hours without change. If no packing is used in the mouth, no treatment other than frequent irrigation is required.

Suppurating superficial wounds can be cleansed with hydrogen peroxide. Granulating surfaces are treated by application of penicillin solution and covered with petrolatum gauze.

Nutrition. The diet for maxillofacial patients is very important. Many of them, particularly those with fractures of the jaws, have to have the upper and the lower teeth fastened together for weeks and, therefore, can take only liquid food. Others are able to take soft food, but are unable to masticate. These patients are not to be classed with the ordinary postoperative patient on liquid diet, to whom the liquid is given in small amounts because he is in no condition to assimilate more, and to whom a soft and, finally, a full diet is given after a short time.

In patients obliged to remain for a long time on liquid diet because of an injury to the jaw, sufficient quantity and quality should be given to maintain them in a state of good nutrition. Under this regimen a loss of weight will be noted at first, but, if properly carried out, it is possible to obtain a gain in weight. Much can be accomplished with the liberal use of stewed fruits and fruit juices, soft cereals, malted milk, cocoa, coffee, tea and so forth. A proper vitamin content must not be overlooked. The soft diet for patients able to manage it also demands careful preparation. The usual routine soft diet in hospitals is not always suitable for patients unable to masticate. All meat, vegetables and cooked fruits should be divided finely or mashed. The patient must be fed often in order to obtain the equivalent of a full diet.

Psychological Support. The nurse is in a unique position to help these patients to accept their many experiences more easily. Rehabilitation is often a combination of both physical and mental aspects. Such rehabilitation depends not only on eradication of a physical scar but also on the correction of psychic trauma which is so markedly influenced by the patient's social and emotional background. An understanding of these factors helps greatly in promoting the progress of this patient to the ends desired.

Many times, the ultimate objective requires a number of operations separated by long intervals of time. Patience is a real

MANAGEMENT OF THE PATIENT WITH A DERMATOSIS: NURSING OBJECTIVES AND PROCEDURES

1. To control itching and relieve pain:
   A. Examine area of involvement.
      a. Attempt to discover the cause of discomfort.
      b. Record observations in detail, using descriptive terminology.
   B. Encourage rest and immobility to reduce stimuli of pain and itching, and to raise the threshold of discomfort.
   C. Eliminate foods and beverages that produce flushing, e.g., condiments, coffee and alcohol.
   D. Employ measures that produce vasoconstriction.
      a. Maintain cool environment.
      b. Reduce excess bedding or personal clothing.
      c. Provide tepid, cooling baths.
      d. Apply cool wet dressings.
   E. Apply anesthetic lotions or ointments.
   F. Supply analgesic and antipruritic medications as indicated.
   G. Administer tranquilizing agents or sedative drugs, as necessary, to control intense pruritus or other discomfort.
   H. Instruct patient to refrain from self-medication with salves or lotions that are commercially advertised.
   I. Assist the anxious patient to improve his insight, identify his problems and find their solution.

2. To treat an inflammatory lesion:
   A. Apply continuous or intermittent wet dressings to reduce intensity of inflammation.
   B. Remove crusts and scales before applying topical medications.
   C. Use topical applications containing corticosteroid drugs, as indicated.
      a. Rub topical medicaments well into skin to enhance penetration.
      b. Observe lesion periodically for changes in response to therapy.

3. To control oozing and prevent crust formation:
   A. Remove medications with mineral oil before reapplying.
   B. Provide tub baths and wet dressings to loosen exudates and scales.
   C. Use mildly astringent solutions to precipitate proteins and decrease oozing.
   D. Supply a high protein diet if oozing is voluminous and serum loss substantial.
   E. Administer antibiotics by topical application or by mouth, as indicated.

4. To avoid damage to skin:
   A. Protect healthy skin from maceration when applying wet dressings.
   B. Remove moisture from skin by blotting gently and avoiding friction.
   C. Guard carefully against risk of thermal trauma from excessively hot wet dressings.

5. To ensure efficacy of topical applications:
   A. Use occlusive dressings, as needed, to retain medication in constant contact with affected skin.
   B. Elicit the patient's cooperation in performing his own dermatologic treatments.
   C. Instruct patient clearly and in detail to ensure that treatments are carried out as prescribed.

factor. Recreational, occupational and spiritual therapies need to be explored fully with the interests of the individual patient kept intact.

Often, the kinds of dressings that have to be worn, the unusual positions that have to be maintained and the temporary incapacities that must be experienced can be very upsetting to the most stable patient. The nurse must be able to offer hope and encouragement and to combine this with a wholesome sense of humor. Tact and patience, and attention to small details will make the nurse an invaluable colleague as the patient regains his self-assurance and more normal usefulness and appearance.

Dermal Abrasion

Dermal abrasion, or surgical planing of the skin, is being done in selected cases of facial disfigurement including traumatic scars, tattoo scars, nevi, freckles and scars resulting from acne, chickenpox or smallpox. Planing is performed either manually with coarse abrasive paper or mechanically, with an abrader or a rapidly rotating wire brush.

Preparation of the Patient. When the entire face area is treated, it is desirable for the patient to have general anesthesia; in addition, the use of a freezing anesthetic for stabilizing and stiffening of the skin may be desirable. The depth of planing can be readily gauged, and the refrigerated area is momentarily bloodless. During and after planing, copious saline irrigations remove debris and allow for inspection.

Postoperative Care. Usually, petrolatum gauze or perforated plastic-faced bandages are applied. During the first postoperative day there are swelling and oozing. After about 48 hours, the dressings are removed, and the sensation is one of severe sunburn. When the crust forms, petroleum jelly, cold cream or cocoa butter relieves the sensation of tightness. Within 14 days, the crusts have separated, and, although the skin will still be red, most of the scars will be gone. Repeat treatments may be necessary. The patient's chief complaint is that the procedure is more a nuisance than discomforting. The effects produced are well worth the inconvenience.

CLINICAL SITUATION

William Sawyer, a 29-year-old clerk, is hospitalized with a painful furuncle on the bridge of his nose.

1. Which of the following terms is synonymous with "furuncle"?
   A. Pompholyx.
   B. Boil.
   C. Carbuncle.
   D. Comedone.

2. The most dangerous complication(s) threatening this patient is (are) extension of his infection with resultant
   A. Carbunculosis.
   B. Exfoliative dermatitis.
   C. Intracranial venous thrombosis.
   D. Rhinophyma.

3. To protect the healthy skin around the furuncle when wet dressings are applied, the nurse should
   A. Apply a lubricant.
   B. Use a drying agent.
   C. Massage the skin gently.
   D. Do none of the above.

4. Which of the following statements is correct?
   A. The infection is presumed to be of streptococcal origin.
   B. The furuncle should be emptied by means of local pressure.
   C. After localization of infection, the furuncle may be incised.
   D. Localization may be hastened by the application of cold compresses.

BIBLIOGRAPHY AND SUGGESTED READING
Books
Brown, J. B., and Pryer, M. P.: Principles of general plastic surgery, pp. 1165-1212 *in* Allen, J. G., *et al.*: Surgery: Principles and Practice, Philadelphia, Lippincott, 1957.

Leider, M.: Practical Pediatric Dermatology, St. Louis, Mosby, 1956.

Lerner, M. R., and Lerner, A. B.: Dermatologic Medications, Chicago, Yr. Bk. Pub., 1960.

Macgregor, F. C., *et al.*: Facial Deformities and Plastic Surgery, A Psychosocial Study, Springfield, Thomas, 1955.

Nordmark, M. T., and Rohweder, A. W.: Science Principles Applied to Nursing, pp. 155-164, Philadelphia, Lippincott, 1959.

Pillsbury, D. M., Shelley, W. B., and Kligman, A. M.: Dermatology, Philadelphia, Saunders, 1956.

————: A Practical Guide to Management of Common Skin Disorders, Philadelphia, Saunders, 1961.

Robinson, H. M., and Robinson, R. C. V.: Clinical Dermatology, Baltimore, Williams & Wilkins, 1959.

Sauer, G. C.: Manual of Skin Diseases, Philadelphia, Lippincott, 1959.

Sulzberger, M. B., *et al.:* Dermatology—Diagnosis and Treatment, Chicago, Yr. Bk. Pub., 1961.

Wilkinson, D. S.: The Nursing Management of Skin Diseases, London, Faber, 1958.

Articles

Burks, J. W.: Hypnosis and dermabrasion, A.M.A. Arch. Dermat. **81:**378-380, Mar., 1960.

CA, A Bulletin of Cancer Progress, Vol. 7, No. 6. Issue devoted to skin cancer, Am. Cancer Soc., Nov., 1957.

Cahn, M. M.: The skin from infancy to old age, Am. J. Nursing **60:**993-996, July, 1960.

Campbell, E. B., Hogsed, C. M., and Bogdonoff, M. D.: Lupus erythematosus, Am. J. Nursing **62:**74-77, June, 1962.

Edwards, E.: Mycosis fungoides, Am. J. Nursing **61:**61-63, Feb., 1961.

Foley, A. J.: More than skin deep, Am. J. Nursing **60:**1266-1267, Sept., 1960.

Hall, J. W.: Drug therapy in infectious diseases, Am. J. Nursing **61:**56-60, Feb., 1961.

Iverson, P. C.: Dermal abrasion, Am. J. Nursing **57:**860-864, July, 1957.

Klauder, J. V.: Some aspects of occupational dermatoses, J.A.M.A. **160:**442-448, 1956.

Noojin, R. O.: Common scalp conditions, Am. J. Nursing **56:**870-872, July, 1956.

————: Local preparations for skin lesions, Am. J. Nursing **58:**387-388, Mar. 1958.

Osment, L. S.: Tinea capitis, Am. J. Nursing **60:** 1264-1265, Sept., 1960.

Shellow, H.: The mouth in certain diseases of the skin, Am. J. Med. Sc. **235:**456-470, 1958.

Staneruck, I. D.: Nursing care after dermal abrasion, Am. J. Nursing **57:**864, July, 1957.

Stewart, W. D., *et al.:* Sun worshippers, beware! Canad. Nurse **57:**626-627, July, 1961.

Underwood, G. B., *et al.:* Overtreatment dermatitis, J.A.M.A. **130:**249, 1946.

Patient-Teaching Aids and Information

Cancer of the Skin. A small 19-page booklet, No. 7 in Cancer Series, Prepared by National Cancer Institute and available from the Supt. of Doc., U. S. Govt. Printing Office.

Haserick, J. R., and Kellum, R. E.: Primer for Patients With Lupus Erythematous, an excellent 32-page booklet from the Dept. of Dermatology, The Cleveland Clinic Foundation, Cleveland, Ohio.

The Skin—Our First Line of Defense. A pocket size booklet, S. M. Edison Chemical Co., 2710 S. Parkway, Chicago 16, Ill.

Scabies. A leaflet, Pub. Health Serv. Pub. No. 79, Washington, D. C., U. S. Dept. of Health, Ed. and Welfare, 1959.

Agencies

Society for the Rehabilitation of the Facially Disfigured

Institute for Reconstructive Plastic Surgery
New York University Medical Center
550 First Avenue
New York 16, New York

35

Patients With Problems of the Breast

THE DEVELOPMENT OF
THE BREAST

Up to the time of puberty it is impossible to find microscopically any difference in the breasts of the two sexes. At puberty, some slight swelling appears in the male breast. At the same time, a pronounced increase in size occurs in the female organ. This begins about the 10th year and increases rapidly up to between the 14th and the 16th years. The development of the mammary gland is a result of hormone action that begins with puberty in the female. At this time, the nipple takes on its natural protruding form. In the male, contrary to some statements, breast tissue always exists and may take on growth.

The breast is a glandular organ with many lobules; its secretion passes via collecting ducts to the nipple. In some women, there is a cyclic engorgement of the breasts, associated with tingling and tenderness. This is due to a hormonal disturbance. The symptoms begin usually in the latter part of the menstrual cycle and disappear when menstruation occurs. About 8 weeks after conception, the breasts enlarge greatly, the nipples become more prominent and sensitive, and the breast is prepared to nourish the infant to come. When pregnancy is over and lactation has ceased, the breast shrinks, loses its excessive fat and often becomes flabby and flattened.

DISEASES OF THE FEMALE BREAST

Fissure of the Nipple

Fissure of the nipple is a longitudinal ulcer that is apt to develop in any woman who is nursing a baby. The ulcer is irritated constantly by the act of suckling and causes the mother considerable pain, often associated with bleeding of the nipple. Prophylactic treatment, cleanliness and washing and drying of the nipple after each nursing usually will prevent the occurrence of this condition. If a fissure develops, it should be washed at frequent intervals with saline solution, and nursing should be permitted only with an artificial nipple. If healing does not occur promptly, or if the case is severe and painful, nursing should be stopped and a breast pump substituted for it. Ulceration that persists suggests carcinoma or a primary luetic lesion.

The Patient With An Inflammation
of the Breast

Acute mastitis may occur at the beginning or the end of lactation. Mastitis may result from the transfer of microorganisms to the breast by the hands of the patient or those of the personnel caring for her. The baby with an oral, eye or skin infection may be a source of infection. Mastitis is also caused by blood-borne organisms. An infection of the ducts results, with stagnation of milk in one or more lobules. The breast becomes tough and doughy, and the patient complains of dull pain in the region affected. A nipple that is discharging pus, serum or blood demands investigation.

TREATMENT consists of taking the baby off the breast temporarily. Heat and cold are used to treat the inflammatory process. A saline cathartic is usually administered. The patient may also be given a broad-spectrum antibiotic.

Progesterone has been found to reduce breast congestion, which, in turn, will relieve the pain. The patient should wear a firm breast support and follow good habits of personal hygiene.

Mammary Abscess. Breast abscess usually develops as a sequela of an acute mastitis, although it may occur independent of lactation. The area affected becomes very tender and dusky red, and pus may be expressed from the nipple. Chemotherapy and antibiotic therapy are being used with success; however, incision and drainage may be indicated. Dressings soaked in hot solution increase the drainage and hasten resolution. The use of the suction cup has proved to be valuable in the treatment of such abscesses.

Chronic cystic mastitis is a disease of the breast in which many small cysts are produced, due to an overgrowth of fibrous tissue about the ducts. The disease occurs most commonly between the ages of 30 and 50 and is characterized by an uncomfortable feeling in the breast, the presence of small nodules that feel like tiny lead shot, and, occasionally, by shooting pains.

Any mass in the breast should raise a suspicion of malignancy, and for that reason surgical advice should be obtained. If the disease occurs before the age of 38, when it is important to preserve the function of the breast, the lesion may be kept under close observation for a time. In older women, or in younger women when any doubt exists as to the diagnosis, it is safer to remove the mass for pathologic examination.

Retention Cysts. There is a continuous secretion from the epithelium of the mammary ducts which is so small in amount that it escapes unnoticed at the nipple under normal conditions. With advancing age and the cyclic changes that occur in the breast with each menstrual period a mammary duct may become obstructed by fibrosis, with the result that the secretion of the duct behind the obstruction collects and dilates the duct to form a retention cyst. These are most prone to appear near the menopause and in women whose breasts have not functioned in lactation and nursing.

These cysts appear as firm, smooth, round masses in the breast and, often, are tender on palpation or pressure. The cyst itself rarely has any malignant potential, although breasts containing cysts may be more prone

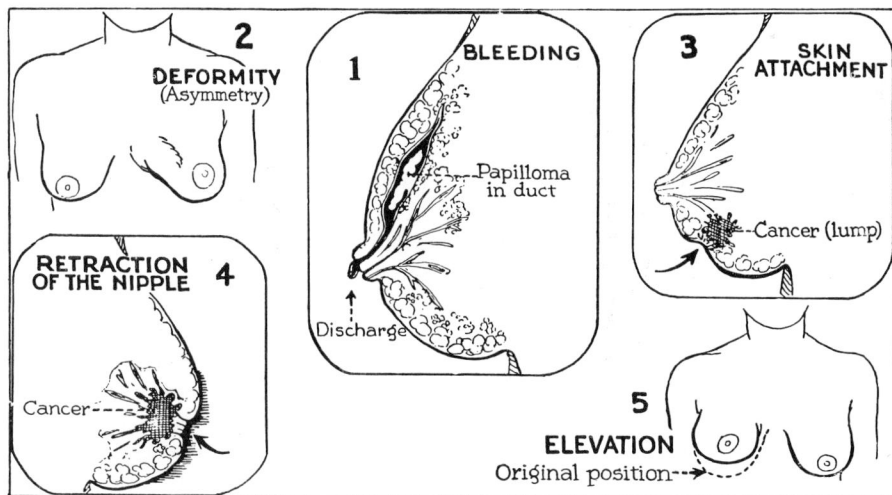

Fig. 309. Signs of cancer of the breast. (1) Bleeding from the nipple arising from a papilloma in the duct. This may be a benign lesion at first, but it is definitely considered to be a premalignant lesion. (2) Deformity or asymmetry of the breast. (3) Skin attachment at the site of a malignant mass. (4) Retraction of the nipple when cancer appears at the center of the breast. (5) Elevation of the breast involved due to contraction and shortening of the fibrous tissue trabeculations brought about by the malignant tumor. (American Cancer Society, New York)

to develop cancer than are normal breasts. Most cysts can be treated by simple aspiration of the fluid under local anesthesia. No surgery is required.

Bleeding or Bloody Discharge From the Nipple. (See Fig. 309–1.) At times, a bloody discharge may be noted on the clothes, and on investigation the discharge is found to be coming from the nipple. Often, there may be one area at the edge of the areola where pressure produces the discharge. Although a bloody nipple discharge may occasionally be due to malignancy, it is most commonly due to a wart-like papilloma growing in one of the larger collecting ducts just at the edge of the areola. This bleeds on trauma and the blood collects in the duct until it is pressed out at the nipple. The duct can be identified in the nipple and traced down so that the duct and the papilloma can be excised through a small periareolar incision.

Tumors

Every tumor of the breast should be viewed with suspicion and should be removed unless there is a contraindication.

Fibroadenomata. These are firm, round, movable, benign tumors of the breast, usually appearing in the breasts of girls in their late teens and early twenties. They cause no pain and are not tender. They can be removed through a small incision and have no malignant potential.

Paget's disease of the nipple is seen most frequently in women over forty, and, usually, it is unilateral. Most often it begins as a mild eczematoid condition of the nipple that may spread over the areola and even part of the breast; later, it may become ulcerated or eroded. In the more advanced stages, there may be retraction of the nipple. This is a true carcinoma of the ducts of the breast that converges at the nipple.

When any lesion of the nipple is not healed in a few weeks under treatment by simple cleansing and protective measures, a suspicion of Paget's disease should be confirmed by biopsy examination. It demands the same treatment; that is, early and total removal of the mammary gland, as does carcinoma of the mammary gland itself.

Carcinoma

The breast is a most frequent site of development of carcinoma in the female. It is so common that one author states that most tumors of the breast in women over 40 years of age are carcinomatous. Of tumors diagnosed as benign before operation, 10 per cent are found after removal to be cancerous.

Course of Disease. The tumor is located most frequently in the upper outer quadrant of the breast. As it grows, it becomes attached to the chest wall or the overlying skin. If no treatment is given, the tumor invades the surrounding tissues and extends to the lymph glands of the adjacent axilla. When the tumor arises in the medial half of the breast, its extension may involve the lymph nodes within the chest along the internal mammary artery.

Metastases may be to the lungs, bone, brain or liver. In untreated cases death usually results in 2 or 3 years.

The situation of the patient with an inoperable cancer of the breast is a most distressing one. It is distressing also to the surgeon, who realizes that there was a time when the tumor was curable, but that the patient through ignorance, neglect or fear appeared for treatment when it was too late. The situation of the inoperable patient also is distressing because the tumor spreads to such areas as the brain, the lungs, the liver and to bone and causes symptoms that are hard to relieve. Pain, cough, ascites, paralyses and fractures are a combination of terminal symptoms for which little can be done. Sedation in increasing doses and sympathetic nursing offer some relief.

Detection. Women now are educated to regard any lump appearing in the breast with suspicion. However, the nurse can do much to improve the chances for early detection. She must recognize that one of the responsibilities of every nurse is to know and disseminate information regarding the earliest signs of cancer. In her contacts she can point out the importance of frequent self-examination of the breasts. Since carcinoma of the breast is one type of malignancy that can be detected early because it is accessible to palpation and observation, every woman should palpate her breasts frequently and examine them carefully before a mirror. Hands lathered with soap and water are more satisfactory than dry hands for breast examination. The nurse should make it clear that any untoward sign or noticeable change should be sufficient reason for her to seek medical advice promptly.

Symptoms. The symptoms of the disease, unfortunately, are insidious. The patient finds a nontender lump, which may be movable, in the breast, usually the upper outer quadrant. Pain usually is absent, except in the very late stages. Eventually, a dimpling or "orange peel" skin may be observed. On examination in the mirror, the patient may note asymmetry and an elevation of the affected breast. Nipple retraction may be evident. Later, she may notice more or less fixation of the breast on the chest wall and nodules in the axilla. Finally, ulceration occurs and cachexia becomes prominent.

Diagnosis and Treatment. There are numerous benign masses, adenofibroma and cysts, that have no serious implication, but a painless mass appearing in a woman past 35 should be looked upon as a carcinoma until this is disproved. In many instances the physician is able to make a positive diagnosis by palpation and inspection, but many times a diagnosis cannot be made with certainty. X-ray photographs of the breast are used by some in the diagnosis of breast masses.

The only safe method is removal of the mass and microscopic examination. In many cases the examination is made immediately by a technic known as a "frozen section." If a positive diagnosis of cancer is received, a radical removal of the breast is performed while the patient still is under anesthesia. If the tumor is benign, the small wound is sutured and only a small scar results.

The treatment of carcinoma of the breast is removal or destruction of the whole tumor. It is evident that complete removal of the tumor can be accomplished most surely when the cancer still is confined to the breast. This is borne out by clinical experience, which shows a rate of cure better than 70 per cent if the tumor is confined to the breast. When it has spread to the nodes of the axilla, the cure rate falls to 40 per cent.

Surgical removal of the breast and the muscles of the chest wall beneath it, as well as of the lymphatic pathways if the cancer has spread to the axilla, is looked upon as the best method of treatment in operable cases. Occasionally, when a breast tumor is inoperable so far as cure is concerned, the surgeon may remove the breast to free the patient from a foul, ulcerating lesion. There are other methods of treatment, however, that are used in addition to surgery or by themselves. X-rays may be used before and after operation. Radium needles may be introduced into the tumor mass in inoperable cases. There is evidence to support the belief that ovarian hormones influence the growth of breast carcinoma. In some instances, surgical or x-ray castration may be performed, especially in menstruating women. Male sex hormone (testosterone) has been found helpful, especially in the treatment of metastasis. In some patients removal of the adrenal glands or the pituitary gland has produced regression of the recurrent growth. There is no reason to believe that any of these measures will produce a cure of breast carcinoma, but they may have a palliative effect for a time.

The patient who is admitted to the hospital with an inoperable carcinoma of the breast calls for the utmost in sympathy and understanding: her physical and mental comfort is the primary goal. Details of care follow the regimen used in terminal carcinoma of any part of the body. (See page 326.)

Hypertrophy of the Breast

Hypertrophy, with the production of unilateral or bilateral pendulous breast, not infrequently is the cause of pain and of psychological trauma that bring the patient to the surgeon. Plastic operations have been devised by which much of the hypertrophic tissue is excised and a breast of normal size is produced.

Diseases of the Male Breast

The male breast may be the site of inflammatory or malignant changes, although this is much less common. The same treatment

Fig. 310A. Radical mastectomy. Area of dissection in intermediate stage. The pectoralis major muscle has been reflexed and the deep pectoral fascia exposed. (Garside, E., and Mella, L.; Radical mastectomy, S. Clin. North Amer. **41**:183)

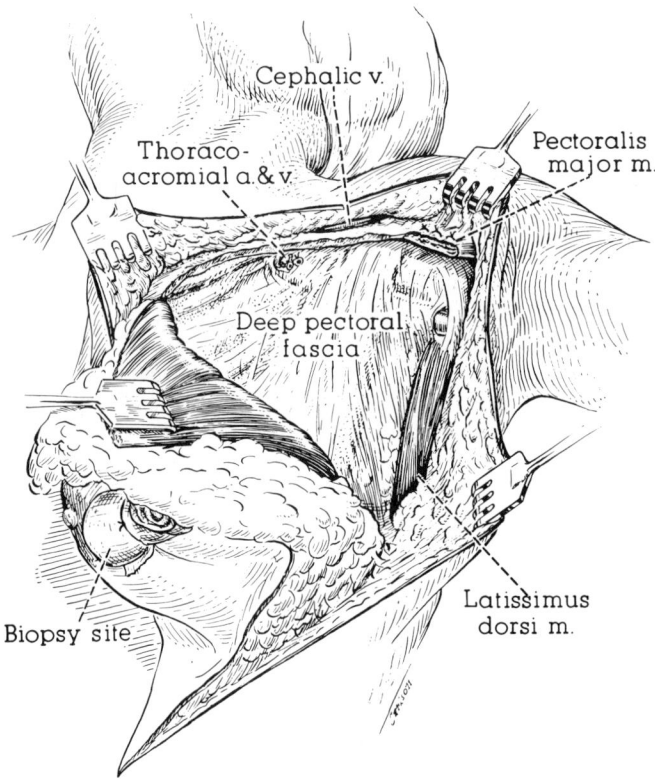

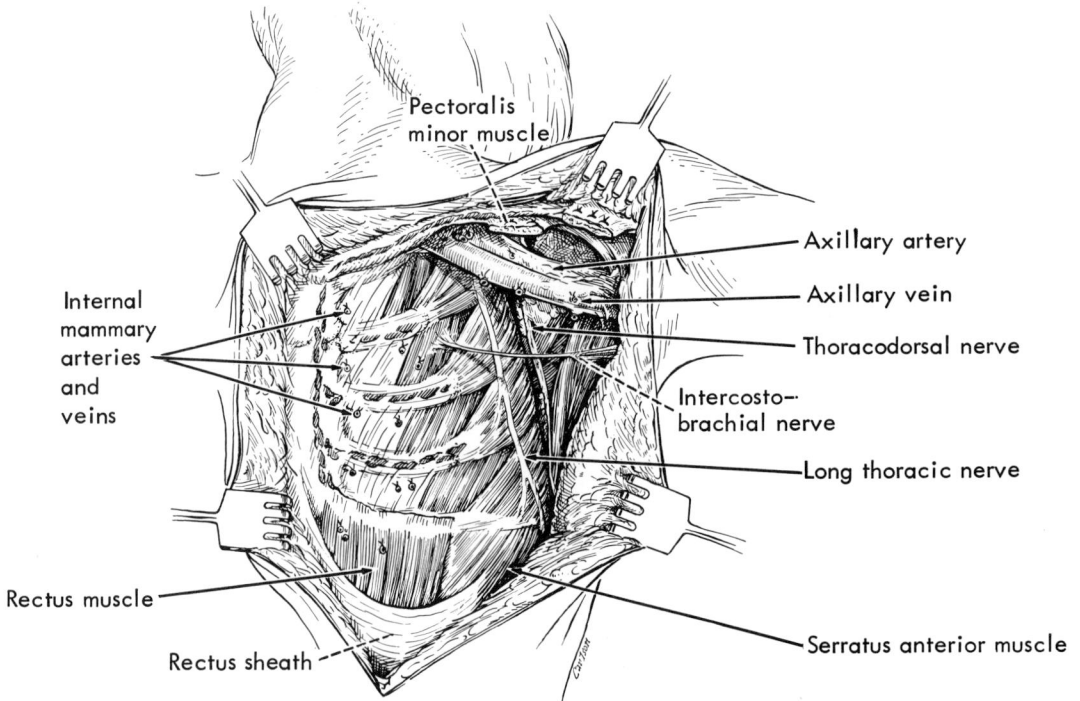

FIG. 310B. Radical mastectomy. Dissection completed. (To the student: [1] Why is the drainage so profuse following a radical mastectomy? [2] Why is the dissection subcutaneously so extensive?) (Garside and Mella, *op. cit.*, p. 184)

Fig. 310C. Radical mastectomy. Wound closure with suction tube in place. (Garside and Mella, *op. cit.,* p. 186)

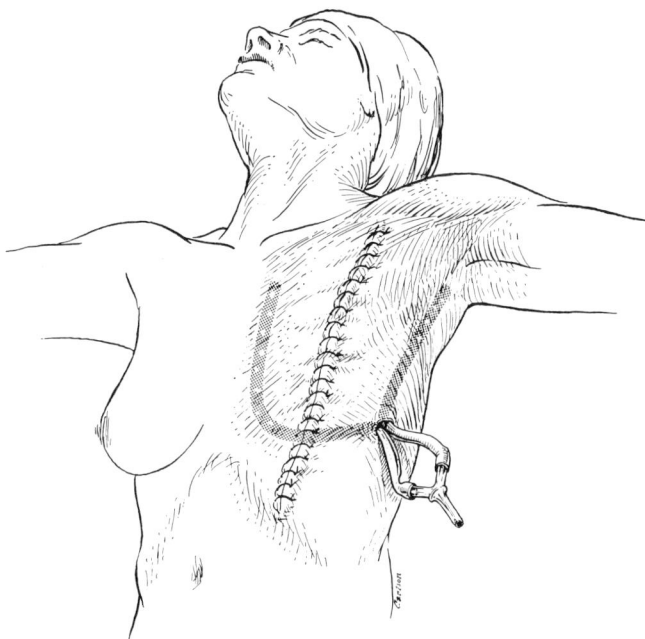

Fig. 310C. Radical mastectomy. Wound closure with suction tube in place. (Garside and Mella, *op. cit.,* p. 186)

as for corresponding lesions of the female breast is indicated.

NURSING CARE OF THE PATIENT HAVING A BREAST OPERATION

Before Operation

Upon admission to a hospital for a questionable tumor of the breast, most women have a real fear of cancer. Unfortunately, many times this fear has made them delay seeking treatment until the tumor has metastasized. Fear also stems from the emotional trauma of knowing that the breast may be removed.

The nurse can help greatly in the psychologic preparation of the patient for breast surgery. She can point out that the breast usually is functionless in most patients with cancer and that loss of the breast as against loss of life is a small price to pay. She may be able to allay the patient's fear of disfigurement by describing artificial appliances that can be used.

The only delay before operation should be that necessary to check the physical and the nutritional needs of the patient. If radical surgery is anticipated, in which there may be fluid and blood loss, blood replacement must be available. The patient is told by the surgeon that there is a possibility of radical surgery if it is indicated. No patient should go to the operating room anticipating a half-inch incision for a tumor excision and return having had a radical mastectomy. Because the emotional factor is a significant one, encouragement and reassurance must be given. A hypnotic is administered and the usual physical preoperative preparation is carried out. Skin preparation should be extensive enough to meet the maximum possible surgery. If it is known that radical surgery, including a skin graft, is to be done, the donor skin area (usually the anterior aspect of the thigh) must be shaved and cleaned.

Operation

The dorsal position is used on the operating table, the arm of the affected side being carried upward to expose the axilla. A radical mastectomy comprises removal of the breast and the underlying muscles down to the chest wall after removal of the nodules and the lymphatics of the axilla (Fig. 310). Such a radical operation is necessary to remove the tumor and the area of lymphatic spread. Bleeding points are ligated and the skin is closed as well as possible over the chest wall. A drainage tube usually is placed in the axilla. A blood transfusion often is given during the operation to compensate for blood loss.

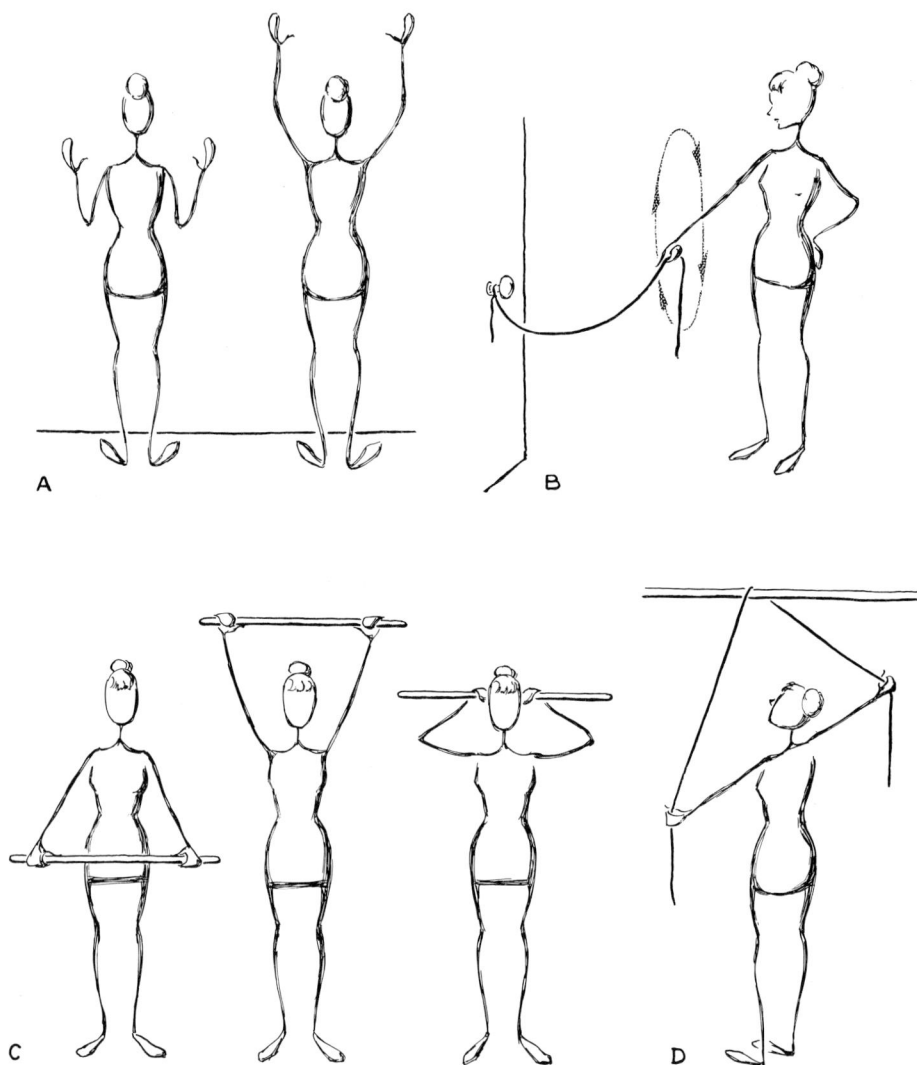

Fig. 311. Muscle-training exercises after mastectomy. The purpose of the exercise program is to secure a complete range of motion of the affected shoulder joint.

A. *Wall hand-climbing*. Stand facing the wall, with the toes as close to the wall as possible—feet apart. With elbows somewhat bent, place the palms on the wall at shoulder level. By flexing the fingers, work hands up the wall until arms are fully extended. Work hands down to starting point.

B. *Rope turning*. Stand facing the door. Take free end of light rope in hand of the operated side. Place other hand on hip. With arm extended and held away from the body—nearly parallel with the floor—turn rope, making as wide swings as possible. Slow at first—speed up later.

C. *Rod or Broom*. Grasp rod with both hands, held about 2 feet apart. With arms straight, raise rod over the head. Bend elbows, lowering rod behind the head. Reverse maneuver, raising rod above head, then to starting position.

D. *Pulley*. Toss rope over shower curtain rod or doorway curtain rod. Stand as nearly under rope as possible. Grasp an end in each hand. Extend arms straight and away from body. Pull left arm up by tugging down with right arm, then right arm up and left down—like a seesaw.

(Adapted from Radler: A Handbook for Your Recovery, New York, The Society of Memorial Centers)

After Operation

The anesthetic of choice usually is general for a radical mastectomy. Postoperative care is given with special attention to pulse and blood pressure, as they are valuable indices in detecting shock and hemorrhage. Dressings must be inspected for bleeding, especially under the axilla and the area on which the patient is lying.

After the patient has recovered from the anesthesia, sedatives are given for the relief of pain, and the patient is encouraged to turn and take deep breaths to avert pulmonary complications. The dressing usually is fairly snug; however, it should not be so tight that lung expansion is restricted. Some surgeons prefer to include the arm (flexed at the elbow) in the dressing to give added pressure. In other instances, gauze fluffs or foam rubber sponge may be added to the dressing within the binder to provide pressure. In many patients a drainage catheter is inserted through a stab wound into the axilla; then this catheter is attached to a suction machine and drained into a trap bottle. By this means serum and blood collected are aspirated rapidly, and the skin flap is held tightly against the chest wall. Thus, serum collections and hematomas are avoided. In many patients pressure dressings may be eliminated early in the postoperative period. Positioning of the patient depends on the dressing; semi-Fowler usually is desirable. The arm, if free, should be elevated with each joint positioned higher than the more proximal joint. Thus, gravity helps to remove the fluid by the lymphatic and the venous pathways. Whether the arm is flexed or extended depends on the orders of the physician. Such elevation helps to prevent lymphedema, which is a common postoperative occurrence due to interference with the circulatory and the lymphatic systems. After 24 hours, the arm on the affected side should have passive exercise. This can be increased each day with the patient doing more herself. By the 10th day she should be able to reach the top of her head and comb her hair. Failure to encourage exercises such as "climbing the wall with the fingers" may prolong the disuse of the arm and promote the development of a contracture. (See Muscle Training Exercises, Fig. 311.) Exercise should not be accompanied by pain; if the patient has plastic reconstruction or the incision was closed with considerable tension, such exercises will be limited greatly and done very gradually.

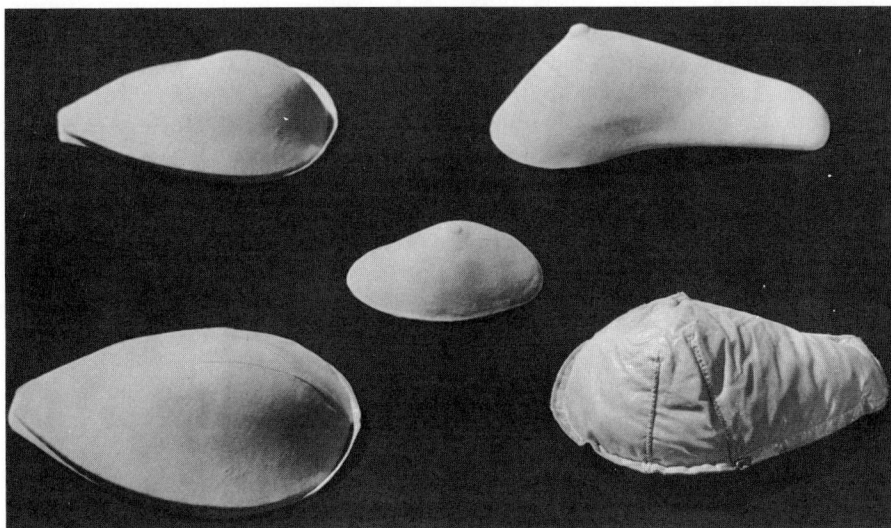

FIG. 312. Various types of prostheses for use after breast amputations. By the use of these appliances, held in place with a suitable brassière, deformity is minimal.

The patient usually is allowed out of bed on the 2nd or the 3rd day after operation; often the arm on the affected side is held in a sling for a time to prevent tension on the wound. A normal diet may be given unless nausea is a symptom. If a drainage tube has been inserted, it is removed usually on the 2nd or the 3rd day. The patient may be advised to have x-ray treatment after operation to lessen the possibility of recurrence. Anorexia, nausea and vomiting are not infrequent symptoms after irradiation; to abstain from eating and drinking 3 hours before and after these treatments often helps.

Follow-up care is important in an effort to detect possible recurrences or metastases. When the wound has healed sufficiently, the surgeon will give instructions concerning when and what kind of prosthesis will be best for each individual patient. There are many types of breast prostheses available. A properly fitted brassiere is essential to a well-fitted prosthesis. The most satisfactory prostheses are those that are filled with a slow flowing thick fluid. The principle which is followed is that the breasts readily follow the law of gravity and change their contour and position with every body motion. Often, when a patient knows that such appliances are available, her fear of disfigurement is eliminated. No prosthesis should be worn until the physician has authorized it.

Although nine out of ten postmastectomy patients escape massive lymphedema, this complication would occur even less frequently if nurses impressed their patients with the importance of elevating and massaging the affected arm for 3 or 4 months postoperatively. Movement increases circulation and thus helps to prevent edema. Other valuable suggestions which the nurse can offer to her patient about lymphedema treatment at home are: Elevate the arm frequently; do exercises and massage ordered by the physician; swing the arm while walking; wear loose or nonconstricting cloththing; keep mastectomy site, underarm and arm scrupulously clean; and wear gloves when gardening.

Psychological Aspects. The woman who has undergone a radical mastectomy cannot help having innumerable questions. The nurse should convey to her patient that she has time to discuss any problems that may be troubling her. Frequent questions are these: Is it normal to drain so much? Will the swelling of my arm go down? How will my husband react to my deformity? Will I be able to wear a regular bathing suit? Will people be aware that I am a cripple? Will I be able to swim, play tennis or golf, drive a car?

After studying this chapter, the nurse should be able to answer these questions intelligently. Her attitude should not be impersonal; this patient needs someone with whom she can share her troubling throughts.

A point that should not be overlooked is the preparation of the husband. An example of this need is illustrated by the husband who thought that he was being kind by not looking at his wife, whereas she interpreted his reaction as one of rejection and repulsion. If time had been taken to tell the husband how he might help his wife in making her adjustment, such an experience would have been avoided.

CLINICAL SITUATION

Mrs. Betty Morrison, a 42-year-old housewife and mother of two children, recently discovered a small hard lump in her left breast on a routine breast self-examination.

1. When should breast self-examination be done?
   A. One day prior to the onset of menses.
   B. Midway during her menstrual cycle.
   C. Immediately after her menstrual period.
   D. On the third day of menstruation.
2. The first symptom of female breast cancer is usually ignored by the patient. This symptom is
   A. Tenderness.
   B. Drainage from nipple.
   C. Puckering of the skin.
   D. Swelling.
3. Mrs. Morrison had a right-sided radical mastectomy which will be followed by radiation therapy. Lymphedema is a complication following a radical

mastectomy; this may be minimized by
A. Elevation of the arm.
B. Active circumduction of the arm.
C. Alternate hot and cold applications to the upper arm.
D. Keeping the arm in a functional position.

4. A most important rehabilitation factor for the nurse to remind Mrs. Morrison of while caring for her postoperatively is the need to
A. Pull the affected shoulder down to balance with the other shoulder.
B. Do active range-of-motion exercise of the affected arm and shoulder on the first postoperative day.
C. Begin gradually to do range-of-motion exercise starting with the fingers, the hand and the wrist and working up gradually.
D. Make sure to be fitted for prosthesis during the immediate postoperative period.

5. The principle underlying radiation therapy is
A. Roentgen rays destroy hyperplasia.
B. Malignant cells are more sensitive to radiation than normal cells.
C. Roentgen rays cause a leukopenia and reduce the patient's susceptibility to x-ray damage.
D. The resistance of normal cells is increased.

BIBLIOGRAPHY AND SUGGESTED READING

Allen, J. G., Breast *in* Allen, J. G., *et al.:* Surgery. Principles and Practice, Chap. 25, pp. 501-536, Philadelphia, Lippincott, 1957.

Alexander, S. E.: Nursing care of a patient after breast surgery, Am. J. Nursing **57:**1571-1572, 1957.

Bernstein, D. E., Biskind, G. R., and Brown, A. L.: Autotransplantation of adrenal cortex to the mesentery combined with adrenalectomy and oophorectomy in the treatment of metastatic carcinoma of the breast, Am. J. Surg. **92:**174-188, 1956.

CA. A Bulletin of Cancer Progress, Vol. 9. Entire issue devoted to Cancer of the Breast, Sept.-Oct., 1959, American Cancer Society.

Carrington, E. R., and Sivak, A. M.: Epidemic puerperal breast abscess, Am. J. Nursing **58:**1683-1686, 1958.

Egan, R. L.: Cancer diagnosis with mammography, Radiology **75:**894-900, 1960.

Farrow, J. H.: Fibroadenoma of the breast, CA, A Cancer Journal for Clinicians **11:** 182-190, Sept.-Oct., 1961.

George, C.: I'm glad I had my breast removed, Today's Health **35:**50-51, 1957.

Hamit, H. F.: Implantation of plastics in the breast, A.M.A. Arch. Surg. **75:**224-229, 1957.

Higginbotham, S.: Arm exercises after mastectomy, Am. J. Nursing **57:**1573-1574, 1957.

Lewison, E. F.: The psychologic aspects of breast cancer, GP **13:**99-105, 1956.

————: The treatment of advanced breast cancer, Am. J. Nursing **62:**107-110, Oct., 1962.

MacDonald, I., and Osman, K.: Post mastectomy lymphedema, Am. J. Surg. **90:**281-286, 1955.

MacDonald, I., and Wilcox, N. E.: Prognosis of mammary carcinoma in young women, Cancer **9:**281-287, 1956.

Self-examination of the breasts, Am. J. Nursing **52:**441, 1952.

Smith, G. W.: When a breast must be removed, Am. J. Nursing **50:**335-339, 1950.

Stephenson, K. L., and Mosely, J. M.: Reconstructive problems of the chest and breast, Am. J. Surg. **92:**26-36, 1956.

Sugarbaker and Wilfley: Cancer of the breast, Am. J. Nursing **50:**332-335, 1950.

The rehabilitation of the mastectomy patient, The Canadian Nurse **51:**390-392, 1955.

Patient-Teaching Aids and Information

Breast Self-Examination, a well illustrated folder, Pub. Health Serv. Pub. No. 48, from Supt. of Documents, U. S. Govt. Print. Office, Washington 25, D. C.

Cancer of the Breast, No. 2 in Cancer Series, Supt. of Doc., U. S. Govt. Printing Office, Washington, D. C.

After Mastectomy and Help Yourself to Recovery, 2 booklets describing activities for the postmastectomy patient, American Cancer Society.

Lasser, T.: Reach to Recovery, a 24-page illustrated booklet for the person who has had a radical mastectomy, Reach to Recovery, 666 Fifth Ave., New York 19, N. Y.

Lewison, E. F.: The total care of your mastectomy patient, pub. 1958. An excellent 40-page brochure available to the nursing profession (when requested on official stationery) from:

    Identical Form, Inc.
    17 West 60th St.
    New York 23, N. Y.

The Nurse and Breast Self-Examination, a pamphlet illustrating self-examination of the breast, American Cancer Society.

Radler, Helen B.: A Handbook for Your Recovery, a 16-page booklet describing and illustrating exercises and activities for the patient who has had a radical mastectomy.

> The above booklet has an insert on Fashion Suggestions from the Leading Pattern Companies.
> An additional supplement is a pamphlet, Man to Man, which physicians find helpful for the husband of the woman who is recovering from a mastectomy.

You have just been through the same ordeal I experienced a few years ago, an excellent pamphlet available from Identical Breast Form, Inc.

Other brochures, instruction sheets and teaching aids are available from Identical Form, Inc.

Information regarding breast prostheses:

> Brochures available from Surgical Supply houses, corsetieres, and prosthetic manufacturers.

Films:

1. Breast Self-Examination (16 mm. sound, color, 15½ min.)
2. Breast Cancer. The Problem of Early Diagnosis (16 mm. sound, color, 34 min.)
3. After Mastectomy (16 mm. sound, color, 20 min.)

These films are available from State Health Dept. or the State Division of the Cancer Society.

36

Patients With Burns

PROBLEMS OF BURNS

Approximately 10,000 persons die of burns each year in the United States. At the First International Congress on Burns held in Washington, D. C. in 1960, the conclusion reached was that further reduction in morbidity and mortality from burns must depend most heavily on prevention of burn accidents. Some authorities estimate that, with reasonable caution and the increased use of well-known safety measures, 75 per cent of all burns could be prevented. Four fifths of all burn accidents in the U. S. occur in the home and are caused primarily by ignorance, carelessness or childhood impulses. By taking advantage of opportunities to teach and promote legislation for safety practices wherever hazards exist, the nurse can play an active part in preventing fires and burns.

The problems of burns can be focused on through 3 main points: (1) prevention; (2) institution of life-saving measures in the severely burned person, and prevention of disability and disfigurement through early specialized, individual treatment, and (3) rehabilitation of the individual through reconstructive plastic surgery and allied rehabilitative procedures.

CAUSATIVE FACTORS

The causative factors of burns include:

Heat, either moist, such as steam or boiling water, or dry, such as a flame, a hot-water bottle, hot metals.

Chemicals, strong acids, such as sulfuric or nitric; strong alkalies—for example, caustic soda (lye)—and other strong chemicals. (In most cases, dilution by flushing the part with water is the best treatment.)

Electricity, the effects of which vary widely, depending on the type, the voltage and the amperage of the current. Accidental burns usually are noted where the current enters and leaves the body. In addition to these local effects, systemic changes that produce respiratory, circulatory and central nervous system disturbances may be noted.

Irradiation, which may be by ultraviolet rays, x-rays and radium. Sunburn and burns from ultraviolet lamps usually are superficial and produce short-lived effects. Those from x-ray and radium are slow to appear, and the most marked effects, such as ulceration, may not occur for years.

Friction. This is caused by a prolonged rubbing of the skin.

CLASSIFICATION OF BURNS: FIRST AID TREATMENT

Burns are classified for purposes of description and identification.

First-degree burns produce a redness of the area with a mild degree of pain. These burns are not serious unless large areas of the body are involved.* Mild ointments are often used in their treatment; occasionally, pain-relieving drugs are necessary.

Second-degree burns are those associated with blisters (vesicles). The superficial layers of skin have been destroyed, but the deeper layers have escaped. Small areas of second-degree burn are extremely painful, but not serious or life threatening, but when large areas (25 to 30% or more of the body surface) are involved, the burn becomes a serious threat to life, especially in children

* Immerse the burned area in cool water if possible. Cold acts as an anodyne and causes vasoconstriction with a decreased loss of tissue fluid.

and older individuals. Small areas of second-degree burn may be treated with mild ointments and protective dressings. Patients with large areas of second-degree burn require hospitalization, and attempts at emergency dressing are useless. Since the entire thickness of the skin has not been destroyed in second-degree burns, skin healing can take place from the deeper skin cells that have escaped destruction. It is difficult to tell the depth of the burn; therefore, at first, many of these burns are treated as burns of third-degree.

A **third-degree burn** implies a destruction of the full thickness of the skin and often of the underlying fat, muscles and, even, bone. It is understandable that third-degree burns of any extent are often lethal wounds. Emergency care is often of little use; the important measure is rapid transport to a hospital where appropriate treatment may be given.

MEDICAL AND NURSING MANAGEMENT OF THE BURN PATIENT

The treatment of the patient with burns must be divided into two parts. One is systemic treatment; the other, local treatment. In extensive burns, the serious part of the difficulty lies in the systemic derangement that occurs as a result of the burn. This begins with shock due to the pain of the burn, and it continues with the loss of fluid into the tissues surrounding the burn area, into the vesicles and from the surface of the burn. This loss of fluid—mostly blood plasma—produces a loss of the circulating fluid in the entire body. The result is a relative increase in the relationship of the blood cells to the blood fluid—in other words, an increase in the hematocrit. This makes for a less efficient circulation, a fall in blood pressure and a seriously ill patient.

The treatment of the primary shock entails the supplying of fluid to the patient, either by mouth if the patient can drink, or intravenously. As much as 3,000 to 4,000 ml. may be given intravenously during this phase of the burn therapy. As a rule, an indwelling catheter is inserted in order to determine the amount of hourly fluid output through the kidneys. Narcotics are given to

these patients carefully in order to relieve their pain, but not enough to depress them.

The course of the vascular derangement is observed by frequent estimates of the hematocrit. As long as the hematocrit is elevated, the fluids are given in large amounts until the hematocrit returns to normal.

In addition to these vascular difficulties, many burn patients have difficulty breathing because they have inhaled flame and fire. This produces the same sort of reaction in the respiratory mucous membranes and epithelium as it does on the surface of the body. The result is a marked interference with the passage of air into and out of the lungs, and, therefore, a tracheotomy is performed on many of these patients.

Many of these life-saving measures demand the utmost in nursing attention. But, in addition to these measures, attention must also be directed toward the local care of the burn.

Local Care of the Burn

There are two methods of burn care which are being used widely today. One of these is the use of a sterile dressing which is applied with gentle pressure so that the edema that occurs with the burns will be less in amount. With the lessened edema, there is less fluid loss in the tissues and, therefore, less systemic reaction. Pressure dressings are applicable to burns on the extremities where bandages can be applied snugly.* For burns around the face and the head, pressure dressings may be secured more effectively with a stockinet. It is almost impossible to apply dressings to the trunk and the perineum.

A second method of treating burns is called the "open air" or exposure method. This is a method which became popular in caring for burns in disasters, when large numbers of people had to be taken care of and dressings could not be applied. These people were placed in bed on sterile sheets with protective cradles over them. The burns

---

* The part must be in proper position to prevent deformities and facilitate resumption of function; likewise, no two skin surfaces are left in contact but should be separated by a thin layer of petrolatum gauze. Signs of impaired circulation must be noted.

FIG. 313. Simple equipment useful in working out postoperative stiffness or even secondary contractures. Even a trapeze hung in a transom of the hospital or at home may suffice. The instillation in the patient of a will to help himself may be more important than the type of equipment. Massage, baking and baths seldom are necessary if restoration has been adequate and the patient is able to exercise. (Brown, J. B., and McDowell, F.: Skin Grafting of Burns, Philadelphia, Lippincott)

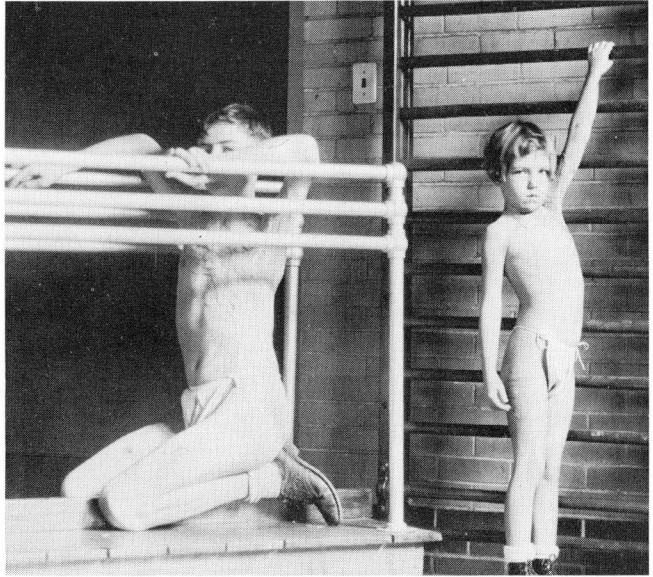

were cleaned up as well as possible, but no dressings were applied. This method has a great advantage in that it can be used in disaster areas and, probably, in wartime. Of course, this does not preclude the systemic care that is necessary in the treatment of burns.*

There is hardly any other patient whose life depends on his nursing care as much as does that of the burn patient. There is a

tendency to give narcotics in relatively larger amounts than would be used in other patients. This may be very dangerous because it may depress an already sick person, with fatal outcome. On the other hand, there is no reason to withhold sedative drugs when the patient is to experience a painful dressing.

After a week or two, the burned tissue tends to separate from the remaining normal

---

* All persons who come in contact with these patients must wear a sterile gown and mask and carry out isolation technic. The room should be kept scrupulously clean with screens to keep out flies. The use of a sterile "burn pack" facilitates the care of this patient and may contain sheets, pillowcases, wash cloth, bath blanket, loin cloth, halter and, perhaps, a gown and a mask.

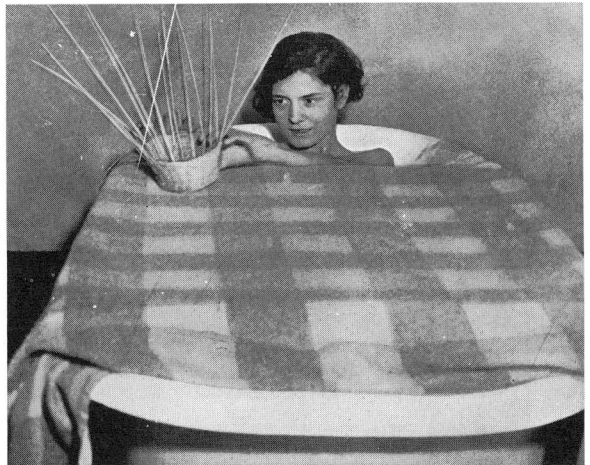

FIG. 314. Patient with severe burn of leg who has started occupational therapy for burned contracted fingers even before operation. (Brown, J. B., and McDowell, F.: Skin Grafting of Burns, Philadelphia, Lippincott)

MANAGEMENT OF THE PATIENT WITH BURNS: MEDICAL AND NURSING OBJECTIVES AND PRINCIPLES

1. To prevent and treat burn shock:
   A. Provide for blood, fluid, electrolyte and colloid replacement immediately.
      a. Weigh the patient on admission (if possible) and daily thereafter.
      b. Insert an indwelling catheter.
         (1) Measure hourly urinary output.
         (2) Describe the appearance and the color of the urine.
      c. Encourage the patient to drink sodium chloride and sodium bicarbonate mixture if ordered.
      d. Prepare the patient for cannulization of vein for continuous I.V. therapy.
      e. Have accessible and labeled the daily ordered I.V. fluids.
      f. Maintain a detailed intake record of oral and I.V. fluids.
      g. Know and be alert for the symptoms of dehydration and overhydration.
      h. Increase and decrease the rate of intravenous fluid flow according to the symptoms of fluid shift and the clinical response of the patient.
      i. Notify the physician immediately if symptoms of overhydration or dehydration occur.
      j. Give I.V. analgesics with caution if patient is in shock.
   B. Maintain careful nursing observation during transfusion therapy.

2. To evaluate the patient's response to the injury:
   A. Watch the patient's systemic reaction and his response to therapy.
      a. Keep sphygmomanometer cuff on accessible artery.
      b. Record vital signs hourly.
      c. Ensure that blood samples are obtained by the laboratory personnel at specified times.
         (1) Watch for rising hematocrit or hemoglobin.
         (2) Report changes in serum protein, blood urea nitrogen and serum electrolyte levels.
      d. Obtain 24-hour urine specimens for 17-ketosteroid and 17-hydroxysteroid tests if requested.
   B. Keep the patient physically comfortable and emotionally supported.
      a. Elevate the burned extremities.
      b. Control the patient's pain.
      c. Maintain the patient in physiologic positions.
      d. Allay the patient's fear and anxiety.

3. To prevent complications:
   A. Guard against infection.
      a. Keep burned areas covered with sterile dressings if indicated.
         (1) Mask, gown and glove personnel during dressing changes.
         (2) Employ rigid aseptic technic during dressing changes.
      b. Keep the environment free of pathogens.
         (1) Use isolation precautions.
         (2) See that room is damp-dusted periodically.
         (3) Restrict visitors.
      c. Obtain wound cultures as ordered.
      d. Maintain optimal personal hygiene for the patient.
         (1) Give frequent oral hygiene.
         (2) Wash unburned areas with hexachlorophene soap or detergent and water.
         (3) Give meticulous attention to the patient's eyes, ears, nares and nails.
         (4) Shave pubic and axillary areas.
         (5) Cleanse area around meatus and catheter at intervals.
      e. Keep the patient's nutritional status at optimal level.
      f. Give antibiotics as ordered.

B. Observe for symptoms of sinus tachycardia.
   a. Watch the patient's pulse rate and volume carefully.
   b. Give digitalis as ordered.
C. Watch for symptoms of respiratory embarrassment.
   a. Evaluate the respiratory rate, chest movements and respiratory symptoms.
   b. Determine whether or not the hair is singed, the pharynx is red, the voice is hoarse, the patient is coughing, or respiratory stridor is present.
   c. Prepare for tracheostomy if needed. (See pp. 389-393).
   d. Keep the room air humidified if respiratory problems become apparent.
   e. Encourage the patient to cough frequently.
   f. Have oxygen equipment accessible.
D. Prevent contractures and deformities.
E. Observe for untoward elevations of body temperature.

4. To promote wound healing:
   A. Maintain the patient in the best condition possible for future surgical procedures.
      a. Assist with local wound care.
         (1) Provide sterile equipment for cleansing and debridement of wound.
         (2) Provide dressing for occlusive therapy or sterile sheets, etc., for exposure method of treatment.
      b. Prepare the patient for grafting procedures when indicated.
      c. Maintain the nutrition of the patient.
         (1) Encourage the intake of a high protein diet.
         (2) Give supplementary protein feedings.
         (3) Record the amount of diet eaten.

5. To promote the rehabilitation of the patient:
   A. Maintain the patient in a correct position.
      a. Use a foot board.
      b. Splint affected hands and utilize hand rolls.
      c. Provide posterior splints for affected legs.
      d. Keep burned extremities elevated and immobilized in a position of function.
      e. Utilize bed cradles.
   B. Employ passive and full range of motion exercises at the earliest possible time as indicated by the surgeon.
      a. Use tilt table to provide for early weight-bearing activity.
      b. Apply elastic bandages to the legs of the ambulatory patient with burns of the lower extremities.
   C. Assist the patient to adjust to his physical limitations.
      a. Provide self-help devices for eating and other activities.
      b. Encourage the patient to participate in his own care.
      c. Assist the patient to develop realistic future goals.
      d. Refer the patient to the proper agencies for follow-up care.

---

tissue. The burned area forms an eschar which is a firm, dark area of tissue destruction. This can be separated from the underlying viable tissue, leaving a granulating, painful, bleeding wound. Many of these wounds which appear to be very deep gradually will be found to have some epithelium still remaining in them, and healing will take place from these islands of skin. In other areas where the skin is completely destroyed, nature must have some help to heal the tremendous wounds left by the burn. It is in these patients that skin grafts are most effective. The split-thickness type of skin graft is most often used to cover the area which is left after removal of the eschar. Nursing care is most important to adjust the part to its most comfortable position and to prevent the skin graft from being dislodged. Skin loss in areas such as the neck, the elbow, etc. produce scars which contract and cause marked deformities. It is in these areas especially that early skin grafting is most efficacious.

Large areas of burn often require a considerable time in the hospital to permit healing. This is a trying time for the patient, and diversional therapy is most helpful. Occupational therapy and other types of therapy which take the patient's mind away from his troubles are very helpful.

The healing of the burn takes place most rapidly in the patient whose nutrition is maintained at a normal level. This means a diet high in calories and protein and, frequently, transfusion to overcome the anemia that is associated with a burn.

Large wounds such as are produced by burns are almost invariably infected. Many of these infective organisms do not produce a marked reaction. On the other hand, it is hardly conceivable that such a wound should heal completely without having some pathogenic bacteria invade it. It is for this reason that antibiotics are often used in the prophylactic care of the infection that invades the burns. The invaders are mostly staphylococcus, streptococcus and pseudomonas and are controlled in most cases by either penicillin or the broad spectrum antibiotics.*

In the preparation of the burned area for skin grafts, warm saline baths are frequently used. The patient may be immersed in such a bath for an hour at a time, while the burned areas are washed gently to remove the debris which is usually attached to them. As soon as the burn wound becomes a red, granulating area without slough, skin grafts may be used. During the care of the patient in the bath, the nurse should wear a cap, a mask and sterile gloves in order not to infect the burned area.

Occupational therapy is started as early as possible in these patients, especially therapy that has to do with finger, hand and leg motions. The idea is to prevent the stiffness of the joints and the contractures which occur if the parts are not used. Physiotherapeutic exercises are also extremely helpful. Many

---

* Odors may be present whether infection exists or not. Frequent changing of soiled bedding, removal of soiled dressings from the room and room deodorizers are helpful.

---

times, the nurse must be instructed in the methods that add to the efficiency of these therapies. (See chapter on Rehabilitation, p. 350.)

CLINICAL SITUATION

Mr. Thomas Robinson, a 45-year-old gas station manager, was brought to the hospital by ambulance with 2nd and 3rd degree burns involving the anterior aspect of both legs, the lower trunk and both hands. While purchasing gasoline, a motorist discarded the cigarette into what appeared to be water. Unfortunately, the "water" was spilled gasoline which ignited and burned Mr. Robinson.

1. Using a 2-column approach, list the complications that could occur in this patient and measures that can be taken to prevent them.

2. Define the occlusive method of treating burns.

   A. Compare the advantages and the disadvantages of this method.

   B. What is the nursing care involved with this type of treatment?

3. Define the exposure method of burn treatment.

   A. Compare the advantages and the disadvantages of this method.

   B. What is the nursing care involved with this type of treatment?

BIBLIOGRAPHY AND SUGGESTED READING

Baker, T. J.: Open technique in the management of burns, Am. J. Nursing **59:**1262-1265, 1959.

Barnett, C.: This, to me, is nursing, Nurs. Outlook **8:**72-75, Feb., 1960.

Brantl, V. M., Brown, B. J., and Nemec, B. M.: Ben was severely burned, Nursing World **132:**13-16, August, 1958.

Collentine, G. E., Jr.: How to calculate fluids for burned patients, Am. J. Nursing **62:**77-79, March, 1962.

Crews, E. R., and Brown, S.: Nursing care of massive burns, Nursing World **131:**9-11, July, 1957.

Eckelberry, N. E.: Electric burns, Am. J. Nursing **55:**836-838, 1955.

Krumanocker, Major J. M.: A master nursing care plan for the burn patient, Tomorrow's Nurse **3:**20-25, June-July, 1962.

Lloyd, E.: Care of a patient with burns, Am. J. Nursing **62:**103-104, Aug., 1962.

Prevention of burn accidents, Abbott's What's New, No. 224, June-July, 1961, pp. 8-11.

Rhodes, V. A., and Shannon, A. M.: Nursing care of the burn patient, Am. J. Nursing **59:** 1265-1268, 1959.

Sarvajic, J.: Principles in the treatment of burns, Nursing World **131:**19-20, May, 1957.

Schumer, W.: Method for removal or debridement of burn wound eschar, A.M.A. Arch. Surg. **79:**630-631, 1959.

Shulman, A. G.: Ice water as primary treatment of burns, J.A.M.A. **173:**1916-1919, 1960.

Stewart, W. D., Danto, J. L., and Madden, S.: Sun worshippers, beware! Canad. Nurse **57:** 626-627, 1961.

Ziffren, S. E.: Management of the burned elderly patient, J. Am. Geriatrics Soc. **3:**36-42, 1955.

National Agencies

National Fire Protection Assn.
60 Batterymarch St.
Boston 10, Mass.

National Safety Council
425 N. Michigan Ave.
Chicago 11, Illinois

Unit XIII. Nursing in Allergic Disorders

ORIENTATION

The term *allergy,* in its broadest sense, refers to any activity occurring in human or animal tissue as the result of an interaction between an antigen and an antibody. An *antigen* is any substance which, in the course of repeated contacts with the body, stimulates the body to produce another substance, a globulin, called an *antibody,* capable of combining with it in a very specific manner (p. 1052). This antibody may be of a type that circulates freely in the blood or one that is "fixed" in the tissues. Antigens likewise differ, and there are corresponding differences between various antigen-antibody reactions with respect to their location, the manner in which they operate and how their operations are manifested.

These reactions, the basis of so-called allergic phenomena, involve the preliminary sensitization of a particular tissue or organ, and this, in turn, implies previous contact with the antigenic substance, or *allergen.* The nurse, from her knowledge of microbiology and immunology, will recall immediately the role played by sensitization and its various sequelae in the defense of the body against infection.

The human body is menaced from the time of its birth by a host of potential invaders—for the most part, living microbial organisms—which are constantly threatening its surface defenses. Having penetrated those defenses, these agents compete with the body for its nutrients and, if allowed to flourish unimpeded, disrupt its enzyme systems and destroy its vital tissues. Against these agents, the body is equipped with an elaborate blockade system. The first line of defense consists of the epithelial cells which coat the skin and compose the lining of the respiratory, the gastrointestinal and the genitourinary tracts. The structure of these surfaces and the effects of their penetration have been discussed in connection with certain specific infections.

One of the most effective of the body's defense mechanisms is its capacity to equip itself rapidly with effective weapons individually designed to meet each new invader, namely, specific protein antibodies. These are capable of reacting with foreign protein materials in a variety of ways: (1) coating their surface, if they are particulate substances; (2) neutralizing them, if they are toxic, or, (3) precipitating them out of solution, if they are dissolved. In any event, the antibodies make the foreign materials safe for handling by the mobile defense units, namely, the phagocytic cells of the blood and the tissues.

Up to this point the implication has been, perhaps, that specific reactions of the type described invariably are protective and beneficial to the body. But this is not the case; in certain instances, their only obvious effect is to cause tissue damage or, at least, considerable discomfort to the individual. Such a reaction apparently serves no useful purpose and should be regarded as an unfortunate by-product of what is otherwise an invaluable defense mechanism, one which permits the development of specific immunity against infection. Under certain circumstances an antibody is produced which reacts not only in response to the presence of some noxious agent but also against materials that are ordinarily harmless, although similar in chemical composition to the material originally responsible for this particular defense reaction.

There is another possible basis for the development of antibodies which react with materials not ordinarily antigenic, namely, an abnormal tendency on the part of certain individuals to become sensitized when exposed to miscellaneous foreign proteins, particularly after repeated exposure in certain areas of the body surface, such as the respiratory mucosa in patients with hay fever, or the gastrointestinal mucosa in some cases of food allergy.

This situation does, in fact, apply in a considerable number of cases: specifically, in about 7 per cent of the population. These individuals apparently are sensitized with unusual ease, producing antibodies against any number of substances that are prevalent in the environment but excite no response in most people. The resulting antigen-antibody reactions are responsible for a number of clinical disorders. Included among these is an important type of dermatitis, featured by the recurrent development of inflammatory lesions on the body surface, which are confined to areas where there has been direct contact with a specific substance to which the patient is "sensitive." Striking examples of this phenomenon are shown in Plate 7. Other disorders which are likewise "allergic," in the immunologic sense, include those types of hay fever and asthma which are due to such airborne allergens as pollens, mold spores, animal danders and house dust. The role of allergy is equally clear cut in cases of urticaria and gastrointestinal disturbances that are associated with the ingestion of particular foods. Allergies such as these are apparently based on a hereditary susceptibility to sensitization, the conditions enumerated above being exhibited often by several members of the patient's family. The term *allergy* is similarly applicable in another group of conditions, including serum disease, dermatitis venenata (for example, poison ivy) and certain drug reactions. Likewise in this category are the local skin lesions that appear following the inoculation of killed bacteria, or bacterial products, for diagnostic purposes, exemplified by the tuberculin reaction.

Many diseases are classed tentatively as allergic disorders, despite the fact that no antigens have been identified in relation to their causation. These include some cases of vasomotor rhinitis and certain cases of asthma, eczema and urticaria. Whereas these conditions may have originated from antigen-antibody reactions, the principal cause, in each instance, appears to be an excessive reactivity on the part of the particular tissue or organ involved. These disorders, and those in which an immunologic mechanism is demonstrable, often are grouped together under the term *atopic disease*.

The importance of the allergic disorders from the standpoint of their statistical frequency, production of disability and threat to life becomes apparent when it is realized that between 10 and 20 per cent of children are afflicted with infantile eczema, hay fever and/or asthma; that more than 24 million persons in the United States suffer from a major allergic disorder; and that one of these disorders, asthma, is responsible for between 6,000 and 7,000 deaths in this country each year.

Special problems complicate the nursing care of the allergic patient. For example, persons with symptomatic allergy are inclined to be apprehensive to a degree that is nearly unique. Their state of mind is likely to be concealed in a manner that belies their anxiety, conveying instead an impression of impatience, lack of consideration, aggressiveness, even frank hostility—or they may display merely the attributes of "high strung" individuals. The nurse must understand her allergic patient, offering her services and lending an interested, friendly ear, but remembering that, so far as her own emotional reactions are concerned, empathy remains the keynote! In the course of her many contacts with her patient, she may garner enough data and impressions to characterize him accurately from the psychological standpoint, to discern with clarity the environment in which he habitually dwells, and therefore to discover what factors are most important from the standpoint of "triggering" attacks.

The nurse also must be prepared to meet the dangerous emergency that allergy creates on occasion in the form of anaphylactic shock or fulminating asthma, when swift and effective countermeasures may spell the difference between life and death.

37

Patients With Allergic Disorders

HAY FEVER

Hay fever (allergic coryza; pollinosis) is a rhinitis induced by airborne pollens and, therefore, characterized by a seasonal occurrence. The spring type, the so-called *rose cold,* apparently stimulated by the pollens of certain trees (oak, elm, poplar and others), occurs from late March to early June; the summer type is induced by the pollens of certain grasses (such as timothy or red top); and the fall type, which develops from the middle of August to the first frost, is stimulated by pollens, particularly those of the ragweed family. Each year the attack begins and ends approximately the same dates. Usually it starts in the mucous membrane of the nose, which may become so edematous and swollen that the nostrils are closed completely. The nasal mucous membrane itches, burns and secretes a thin irritating discharge. Violent paroxysms of sneezing are the rule. The eyes, usually also involved, become red, burn and lacrimate.

Sensitivity Tests. The patient's hypersensitivity to the pollens which induce his attacks often, but not always, may be confirmed by proper skin, conjunctival or intradermal tests. Nevertheless, these reactions, though spectacular, are not necessarily specific, for the dosage of the pollen injected is important, and the majority of patients are hypersensitive not to one but to several pollens (and may not react to the ones which induce their attacks). Ragweed would seem to be the most potent of all.

Treatment. The best treatment of hay fever, if the nasal passages and the paranasal sinuses otherwise are normal and, especially, if the attacks began in childhood, is a seasonal change of climate. When and to what district, however, depends on the experience of the individual case. Nasal sprays containing ephedrine help some persons. Cauterization of the nasal mucous membrane may afford relief for a limited season. However, if sinusitis or another nasal lesion is present, it should be treated thoroughly during the free seasons. Various eyewashes will relieve the conjunctivitis.

Prophylactic injections of extracts of the pollens which seem to be involved in each case (usually, mixed vaccines of nonspecific proteins are used), given once each week, beginning each successive year several months before and continuing during the attacks, will relieve the coryza symptoms in a fair percentage of cases but will not cure the condition. Antihistamine therapy during the active phase is of symptomatic benefit in the majority of patients.

VASOMOTOR RHINITIS

Vasomotor rhinitis, one of the commonest of allergic manifestations, is a form of noninfectious rhinitis which is induced by certain foods (such as milk, eggs, fish or shellfish) and by certain medicines (such as quinine), when these are ingested. In some patients it is caused by the toxins of germs growing within the body, particularly in the paranasal sinuses.

The symptoms of vasomotor rhinitis in many cases are quite similar to those of hay fever; but some persons have paroxysms of sneezing only, while others merely develop temporary nasal obstruction with or without discharge, due to sudden turgescence of the mucous membrane of the nose. However, the rhinitis that follows the ingestion of foods to which the person is hypersensitive is usually a minor part of a general reaction, other features of which are urticaria, asthma and gastrointestinal disturbances. Vasomotor rhinitis is difficult to distinguish from infectious coryza. However, the former has no prodromal period with malaise, and the discharge does not present the same changes as that of the common cold.

BRONCHIAL ASTHMA

Asthma is a form of paroxysmal dyspnea, predominantly expiratory in type, which is characterized by wheezy breathing. Heredity seems to be present in two thirds of all cases. The hay fever attacks of about 50 per cent of all patients end as asthma.

The stimuli of essential asthma may be extrinsic or intrinsic. Of the extrinsic stimuli, pollens and dusts are the most common for adults, and foods (especially egg white, cereals or cow's milk) for children. The stimuli of intrinsic cases are abnormalities in the respiratory tract (such as adenoids, spurs or sinus infections), infected tracheobronchial lymph nodes and pulmonary infections. Adults previously free from asthma have developed it after repeated bronchial infection or long-continued exposure to mildly irritating dusts.

The asthmatic attack starts suddenly with cough and a sensation of tightness in the chest. Then slow, laborious, wheezy breathing begins. Expiration is always much more strenuous and prolonged than inspiration, which forces the patient to sit upright and use every accessory muscle of respiration. He becomes blue from hypoxia and breaks out into a profuse sweat; his pulse is weak; his extremities are cold; there may be fever, and, occasionally, pain, nausea, vomiting and diarrhea. The cough, often absent in extrinsic cases until the attack is almost over, at first is tight and dry, but it soon becomes more violent and raises with difficulty a distinctive sputum of thin mucus in which swim small round gelatinous masses. These are the "pearls of Laënnec," which are molds of the smaller bronchi and contain Curschmann's spirals. The attack may last from one half to several hours. Finally it subsides, and the tired patient can breathe again without undue effort. Such attacks are rarely fatal.

Related Reactions. Among other allergic reactions related to asthma are eczema (present at some time during life in 75% of asthma patients), urticaria and angioneurotic edema (present in 50% of the patients).

Diagnosis. A clear history of hypersensitivity to some known substance which may be inhaled or ingested, such as a pollen, a particular type of food, feather, animal hair, face powder, etc., or a history suggesting the probability of such a sensitivity, is very important in determining the type of asthma presented in any given case. The close association of the attacks with simple hay fever or vasomotor rhinitis, together with the discovery, during the attack, of marked pallor and swelling of the nasal mucous membrane, aids in establishing the case as one of extrinsic allergic asthma. The finding of an abnormally high count of eosinophilic cells in the blood or the sputum tends to confirm this diagnostic impression. However, "all that wheezes is not asthma," and it is important to be able to rule out congestive cardiac failure or bronchial obstruction due to a foreign body or a tumor as the underlying cause or precipitating factor which may explain the attack. Hence the necessity for careful radiologic and, often, bronchoscopic examination in every case of doubtful origin.

Treatment and Nursing Care. It should be remembered that asthma is a syndrome in the production of which many widely different factors may enter. Not the least of these is emotional hyperexcitability and stress, and the importance of mental relaxation in the therapy of the acute attack cannot be overestimated. Often a mere change of environment, such as from home to hospital, is sufficient to halt a severe attack. The patient should be isolated from relatives and friends; he should be placed in a quiet room and surrounded with an atmosphere of calm and encouragement. Mild sedatives—for example, a barbiturate—may be indicated at times, but they should be administered cautiously if the patient is exhausted as a result of prolonged respiratory difficulty, for, in such cases, death may ensue due to respiratory failure. If cyanosis is present, oxygen in high concentration should be administered, preferably with helium. Adrenalin chloride, injected either subcutaneously in 1:1,000 solution or sprayed intratracheally in a strength of 1:100, or Isuprel Hydrochloride administered in the form of a 1:200 to 1:100 solution by means of a nebulizer or by oxygen-aerosolization usually brings prompt relief. The inhalation of steam, unmedicated or with benzoin tincture also may be effective.

The corticosteroids, e.g., predinosone in oral doses of 10 to 30 mg. per day, will terminate dramatically the majority of asthmatic attacks, regardless of their severity. Moreover, the frequency and the severity of recurrent attacks are reduced sharply in most instances by the continued administration of these drugs. Their action, however, is by no means curative, and the dangers inherent in maintenance steroid therapy (see pp. 841-844) so far outweigh its merits in this condition that its use generally is restricted to patients who truly are incapacitated or endangered by their asthma.

Respiratory efficiency may be improved and comfort increased during an acute asthmatic attack by elevating the head of the bed and supporting the pillows in position by strapping. The patient is likely to be most comfortable leaning forward, with arms supported on a pillow-upholstered over-bed table. Every opportunity for sleep and rest should be fostered after an acute asthmatic attack.

These patients are prone to perspire excessively, introducing the need for protection against chilling. Covers made of flannel are to be preferred, and frequent changes of gown should be carried out as needed.

Special dietary orders, for patients on elimination diets, and prescriptions concerning fluid intake are to be observed with care during the acute phases of the illness and precise instructions transmitted to the patient (and his family) with respect to food and fluids permitted after discharge from the hospital. Detailed and accurate instructions are also to be provided in connection with: (1) injections or aerosol inhalations to be administered at home; (2) activities which are permissible and those which are contraindicated; (3) types of contact which are considered potentially provocative of asthmatic attacks and are, therefore, to be avoided; and (4) the scheduling of return visits for check observations during and following convalescence.

The social worker can be of great assistance in securing the best possible environment as regards the type of employment that may be undertaken, if a change of occupation is desirable.

Prognosis. The acute asthmatic attack per se is seldom serious, although occasionally it does prove to be fatal through respiratory exhaustion, which becomes a particularly dangerous possibility if sedatives are administered too freely. Frequent attacks may lead to pulmonary emphysema and chronic asthmatic bronchitis, thereby establishing a vicious cycle wherein the asthma becomes increasingly resistant to all forms of therapy, and, eventually, the patient, afflicted with status asthmaticus, suffering from agonizing and exhausting dyspnea, slowly fails and dies.

Prevention. In every case of recurrent asthma, evidence should be sought which might implicate a foreign protein to which the patient is hypersensitive, and to which exposure, as a possible precipitating cause of his attacks, might be avoided. If attacks chiefly occur at night when the patient is in bed, he should be skin-tested with the material composing his mattress and pillows, and, if hypersensitivity to these becomes evident, the proper changes and substitutions should be carried out. If attacks appear to be associated with the presence of a particular species of animal, such as a horse or a cat, skin tests made with an antigen composed of hair or skin scrapings from the animal concerned may indicate the basis for this association and the attacks may be lessened through avoidance of such contacts. Search is made for foci of bacterial infection—consisting, for example, of chronically infected sinuses or teeth—for, if such are found, in a certain proportion of cases their eradication may be strikingly beneficial. A seasonal incidence of attacks in a patient suggests an air-borne antigen as the chief etiologic agent. In such cases, therapy may be attempted with pollen vaccines. Air conditioning offers possibilities in the prevention of attacks, depending on the extent to which the patient can restrict his life to air-conditioned rooms during the asthma season. A complete change of climatic environment to a locality with different flora during that period is the most satisfactory solution when feasible.

Asthmatic children should be provided with the best available facilities for good mental and physical hygiene, including proper rest, nourishment and any social readjustments that may be indicated.

Psychotherapy Is Important. It is important to remember that asthmatic attacks, once started, may continue as an asthma habit: that in some patients suggestion alone can induce them; that asthma attacks furnish the psychoneurotic person with an avenue of escape from some unpleasant situation and the hysteriac, with a means of gaining desired ends, such as pity or attention. The asthma paroxysms of some adults begin after a period of mental stress and strain, and they cease after the reason for the anxiety has been removed. Children without intent may develop asthma by imitating the attacks of others, and persons who voluntarily practice asthmatic breathing may later suffer from spontaneous attacks whenever they catch cold.

SERUM DISEASE

Serum disease is an acute malady which not uncommonly follows the injection of a serum—usually an antiserum prepared from horse or rabbit blood. Also, it develops occasionally after a course of penicillin injections. Its characteristic features, which appear after an incubation period of from 6 to 12 days, include urticaria, enlargement of the regional lymph nodes, mild fever and pain in the joints—symptoms which disappear entirely in from a few days to 3 weeks. In severe cases the skin rash is purpuric in character, the temperature for a week or 10 days ranges irregularly from 103° to 104°F., the lymphadenitis is general, the spleen is enlarged, and the joints are as red and swollen as in acute rheumatic fever. Other features often present are headache, abdominal pain, vomiting, diarrhea, proteinuria and cylindruria. This is potentially a serious complication, not one to be regarded as a mere annoyance. Not only does it share many of the clinical characteristics

of rheumatic fever and periarteritis nodosa, but it is also known to produce pathologic lesions which are very similar to those found in the two conditions.

One of the rarer consequences of serum sickness, which is important because of the permanent disability it can produce, is peripheral neuritis. The nerves most often involved are components of the brachial plexus. Their damage results in atrophy and weakness of muscles in the shoulder and the upper arm (Erb's palsy). It may affect the muscles of respiration, with potentially fatal results.

Treatment. Serum sickness, with all of its manifestations, including neuritis, if present, responds promptly to the administration of the steroid hormones. The speediest recovery can be anticipated after the parenteral administration of hydrocortisone in doses of 200 to 300 mg. or dexamethasone, 8 to 12 mg., given intravenously over periods of 12 to 24 hours. Mild cases, exhibiting merely urticaria and arthralgia, may respond satisfactorily to one of the antihistaminic drugs, supplemented by aspirin and codeine.

Prevention. Avoidance of allergic phenomena following the administration of horse serum is possible to a large extent if each prospective recipient is questioned closely regarding the possibility of sensitivity to horse dander, and if a skin test is carried out with horse serum. If either yields positive results, it still may be feasible to employ the antiserum if the patient first can be desensitized by a series of small injections.

When contemplating the inoculation of a virus or rickettsial vaccine, it must be borne in mind that the materials incorporate egg yolk and, therefore, are a source of grave danger to individuals who are sensitive to eggs.

ANAPHYLACTIC SHOCK

Anaphylactic shock, one of the so-called *serum accidents,* is the immediate shocklike, and sometimes fatal, reaction which follows the administration of an animal serum to an individual who, because of a previous injection, has become sensitized to that foreign protein.

The onset of serum shock may be immediate, almost before the needle is withdrawn.

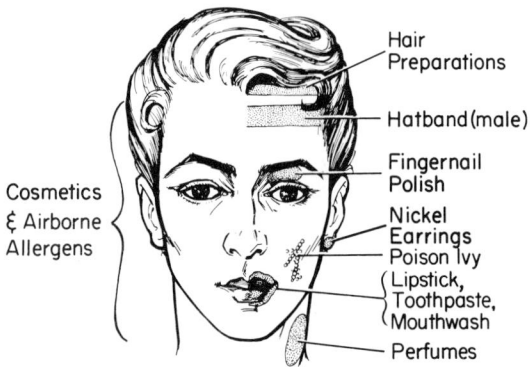

Fig. 315. Contact dermatitis of the face. (Sauer, G. C.: Manual of Skin Diseases, p. 42, Philadelphia, Lippincott)

There are local edema, itching, sneezing and prickling feelings in the throat. Soon there appear edema of the face, hands and even of the whole body, cyanosis, a choking cough and violent asthma. The pupils dilate, the pulse is weak; there may be fever and in some cases, convulsions. Death may follow in from 10 minutes to several hours, or the illness may follow the course of a serious case of serum disease.

No serum ever should be administered without a previous sensitivity test. This applies especially to those patients who have ever had asthma or hay fever, or who recently had received an injection of horse serum. If he is found to be sensitive, the patient should be desensitized by a series of frequently repeated subcutaneous injections, in ascending doses, of the serum to be used, and the use of the serum should be preceded by a 50-mg. to 100-mg. dose of an antihistaminic drug. Epinephrine, in doses of from 0.5 to 1 ml. (1:1,000), is a specific remedy for this type of accident.

ALLERGIC DERMATOSES

Dermatitis Venenata

Dermatitis venenata (poisons), or plant poisoning, is caused by direct exposure of the skin to certain plants. However, the eruptions which result will depend much more on the sensitiveness of the individual's skin than on the plant. They vary from a simple hyperemia to intense inflammations

which may be edematous, erysipeloid, papular, vesicular, bullous, pustular or even gangrenous in character.

Dermatitis venenata appears suddenly, first on exposed surfaces; later, it is often spread to other regions of the body by the fingers in the process of scratching. One or more attacks of dermatitis venenata, in the case of those susceptible, may lead to a true eczema.

Among the 60 or more plants which may cause dermatitis venenata those most commonly encountered and responsible for the severest lesions are poison ivy, poison oak, poison dogwood, poison elder and poison sumac.

Poison ivy usually produces an erythematous area which is more or less swollen and covered with vesicles, bullae and occasionally pustules. The blebs may be confluent, hence the integument soon becomes denuded. The primary lesions are most frequently on the hands, between the fingers especially, on the face or on the buttocks.

Treatment and Nursing Care. The exposed area of skin should be washed thoroughly at once and repeated with strongly alkaline soap and water. The poisonous oil may be present on outer garments that have been in contact with poison ivy. They should be laundered or drycleaned before being worn again. Potassium permanganate (5% solution) may destroy the toxic substance and arrest the development of vesicles. Cold wet packs are helpful when blisters and oozing are present. Antihistaminics frequently will allay the itching. If the condition is severe, corticosteroids may be ordered, as they reduce the inflammation and make the patient more comfortable.

Contact Dermatitis

Contact dermatitis is a local inflammatory lesion of the skin produced by direct exposure of the affected part to a chemical irritant or substance to which the patient has been sensitized. Dermatitis of almost any description, from erythema to gangrene, may follow external applications of arsenic compounds, iodine tincture, chrysarobin, mercurial ointments, tar preparations, mustard, cantharides, carbolic acid, turpentine oil, dyestuffs, petroleum products, alkalies, acids, strong soaps, the aniline and corallin dyes used in socks or veils, pyrogallol and, especially, paraphenylene diamine, much used in hair dyes. Such dermatitis, if severe, may spread far beyond the exposed areas and cause severe constitutional symptoms.

The dermatitis observed in those who work with sugars, flour, polishing material, pastes or tobacco usually is eczematous in nature (for instance, that acquired by bakers —the so-called *bakers' itch*—bookbinders or polishers).

Nurses may develop contact dermatitis in response to antiseptic solutions and drug preparations of various types, such as penicillin.

Drug Reactions (Dermatitis Medicamentosa)

Dermatitis medicamentosa is the term applied to skin rashes that are induced by the internal administration of certain drugs, about 200 in number. While, as a rule, the same drug tends to induce eruptions of similar types, individuals react differently to each of them.

In general, it may be said that drug rashes appear suddenly, have a particularly vivid color, present characteristics that are more spectacular than the somewhat similar eruptions of infectious origin and, with the exception of the bromide and the iodide rashes, disappear rapidly after the drug is withdrawn. Some drug rashes are accompanied by constitutional symptoms. The patient should be warned that he reacts peculiarly to a particular drug and should be advised not to take it again. The nurse has a very important responsibility in relation to drug eruptions, for these lesions offer a warning of serious trouble pending, and she is in a position to detect the signal before anyone else. She must be on the alert for it and report its appearance at once, so that the physician will omit the offending drug without unnecessary delay.

Macular erythematous eruptions follow the administration of animal serums, antipyrine, phenacetin, the salicylates, quinine, belladonna, morphine, some barbiturates, the sulfonamide drugs and a host of others.

Urticarial eruptions may follow any of the above-mentioned drugs, but notably animal serums, arsenic, the iodides, the bromides, penicillin, phenacetin, cinchophen and phenolphthalein. These drugs also may produce eruptions that suggest erythema multiforme.

Vesicular eruptions are caused by arsenic, the bromides, iodides, quinine, antipyrine, antimony, chloral and sodium thiosulfate.

Herpes simplex and herpes zoster may follow the use of arsenic.

Bullous eruptions are produced by the iodides, quinine, antipyrine, phenacetin, barbital, the salicylates, the bromides, chloral and, especially, it is said, the administration of the last two together.

Pustular eruptions follow the use of the bromides and the iodides, antimony, antipyrine, arsenic, chloral, the salicylates and turpentine. These eruptions are usually acneiform; but the bromides and the iodides sometimes produce large vegetating granulomata; and arsenic, chloral, the bromides, the iodides and quinine may produce gangrenous ulcerations.

Hemorrhagic eruptions may follow the use of ergot, the bromides, the iodides, quinine, antipyrine, the salicylates and animal serums.

Pigmentation is caused by silver salts, bismuth and arsenic.

Atopic Dermatitis (Eczema)

Atopic dermatitis is a common, chronic, pruritic disorder of unknown cause, generally regarded as a manifestation of hypersensitivity.

Atopic dermatitis always is inflammatory, producing a definite infiltration of the skin, but this is so superficial that scarring never results. The primary eczematous eruptions may be erythematous, papular or vesicular; the later lesions are exudative, crusted, scaly or thickened patches. The secondary lesions are excoriations and scars as the result of scratching, while secondary infections may produce pyogenic skin lesions and enlargement of regional lymph nodes. Eczematous areas almost without exception shade off imperceptibly into the surrounding unaffected skin. They always itch or burn. In all individuals there is, or has been, a liquid exudate (weeping) which forms crusts. Always, at some time, there is a tendency to cracking or fissuring of the skin, especially about the joints. And finally, the course of each case is marked by exacerbations and remissions.

While no part of the body is exempt, the eczema of infancy and early childhood affects particularly the flexures of the knees and the elbows, the axillae, the face and the scalp; that of youth, the fingers, the hands and the forearms; that of middle life, the skin about the genitalia; and that of elderly persons, most often the face and the lower legs. Due to traumatic scratching and secondary bacterial infection, the lesions may extend to involve an adjacent mucous surface, which becomes indurated and fissured and discharges pus.

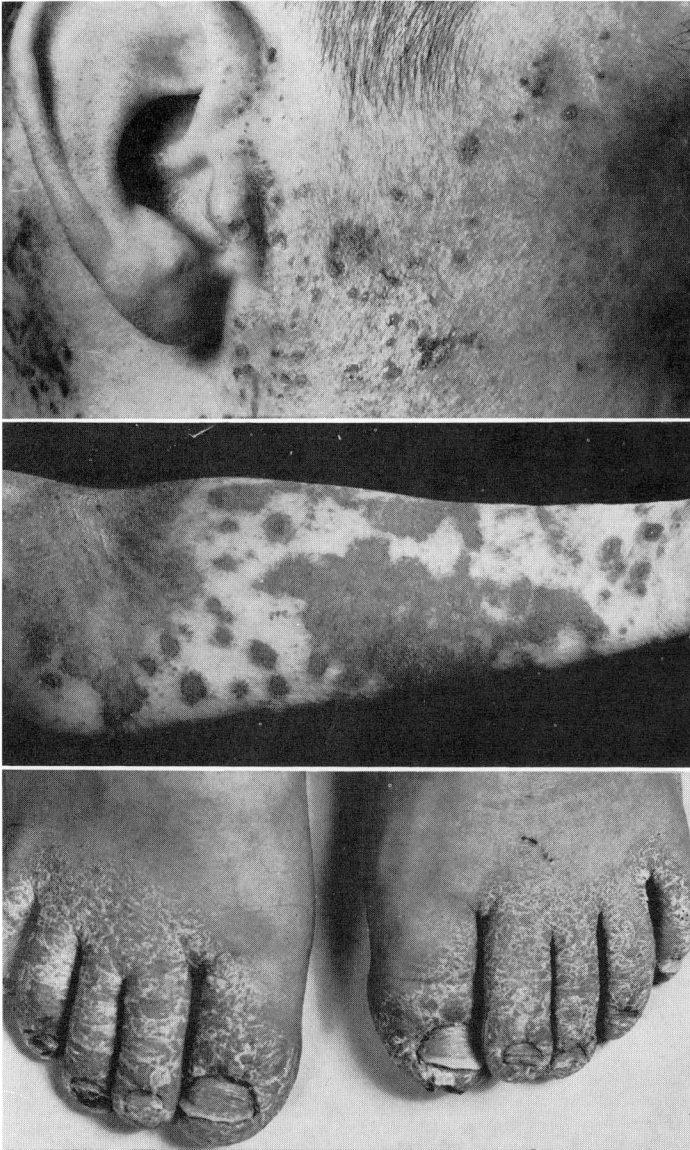

FIG. 316. Atopic eczema. (Sauer, G. C.: Manual of Skin Diseases, p. 50, Philadelphia, Lippincott)

Treatment and Nursing Care. The objectives of treatment are to relieve the itching, guard against superimposed skin infections and heal the skin. Cool applications and bland ointments have a soothing effect. Sedatives, tranquilizers or antihistamines relieve the patient's itching. The patient should be instructed not to wear wool next to his skin. He should be assisted in having insight into his problems, as emotional tensions and conflict can produce exacerbations of this condition. If specific causes are found, such as foods, inhalants, or other environmental factors, they should be avoided.

The condition often persists for weeks despite utmost care in handling the skin lesions and in selecting the diet. This is particularly true in children. Fortunately, as the child matures and approaches adolescence, the attacks tend to abate in severity and frequency, usually disappearing altogether before the second decade of life. Persons who are, or at one time have been, subject to atopic dermatitis are likely to exhibit sooner or later during life other allergic manifestations—such as urticaria, hay fever, asthma or abnormal reactions to particular foods and chemicals.

Some patients have specifically localized areas of atopic dermatitis. Patients with such a condition affecting the hands (housewife's eczema) should be instructed to wear rubber gloves whenever they are doing work that would keep their hands moist or wet or in contact with any type of external irritant (Plate 7).

Urticaria and Angioneurotic Edema

Urticaria (hives) is an allergic affection of the skin characterized by the sudden appearance of pinkish edematous elevations, variable in size and shape, which itch and smart. They may involve any part of the body, including the mucous membranes, especially those of the mouth, the larynx (occasionally with serious results) and the gastrointestinal tract. Each hive remains for from a few minutes to several hours, then disappears. For hours or days crops of these may come, go and return in a most capricious manner. If this sequence continues indefinitely, the condition is called *chronic urticaria;* if the individual lesions themselves persist for several days, it is known as *urticaria perstans.*

Symptoms. The swellings of angioneurotic edema vary in size from a few millimeters in diameter to several centimeters. On occasions, one that covers the entire back is seen. The skin over them may appear normal, but often it has a reddish hue. It does not pit on pressure as ordinary edema does. The regions most often involved are lips, eyelids, cheeks, hands, feet, genitalia and tongue; also, the mucous membranes of the larynx, the bronchi and the gastrointestinal canal, particularly in cases of the hereditary type. An eye may be completely closed; one lip may become so large that eating is impossible; one hand may become so huge that the fingers cannot be flexed. These swellings may appear suddenly in a few seconds or minutes, or slowly, in 1 or 2 hours. In the latter case, their appearance often is preceded by itching or burning sensations. Seldom does more than a single swelling appear at one time, although one may develop while another is disappearing. Only infrequently do they recur in the same region. The individual lesions usually last from 24 to 36 hours. On rare occasions they recur with a remarkable periodicity, at intervals of 3 or 4 weeks.

The swellings of angioneurotic edema along the gastrointestinal canal may cause acute crises of pain with vomiting, which suggest acute appendicitis, acute cholecystitis, renal colic or intussusception; those in the throat, edema of the glottis; those in a primary bronchus, massive pulmonary collapse.

Treatment. Many patients are relieved by antihistamine drugs; others require injections of epinephrine. Tracheotomy becomes necessary if laryngeal edema threatens to obstruct the glottis.

GASTROINTESTINAL ALLERGY

To a few persons, certain common foods are veritable poisons. There are those who cannot eat strawberries or shellfish without an attack of urticaria; or pork, or cheese, no matter how well disguised these foods may be, without vomiting promptly; or, if the food is retained, without diarrhea often accompanied by considerable pain (due, it is

THE PATIENT WITH ASTHMA
Objectives and Principles of Medical and Nursing Management

The Problem: During an acute asthmatic episode, the ventilatory processes are altered due to airway obstruction. The ensuing hypoxia can be life-threatening to the patient.

1. *To treat the patient during the acute asthmatic episode:*
   A. Relieve the airway obstruction.
      a. Give the medications as directed:
         (1) Isoproterenol (0.5 ml. of 1:400 sol. or 0.25 ml. of 1:200 sol.) administered by nebulizer to oropharynx
         (2) Intravenous aminophylline (250 to 500 mg.) administered slowly
         (3) Epinephrine (0.2 to 0.5 ml. of 1:1000 sol.) subcutaneously
      b. Evaluate patient's reaction to medication.
      c. Observe for symptoms of congestive failure.
      d. Prepare for bronchoscopic aspiration to eliminate bronchial obstruction if indicated.
   B. Relieve the hypoxia:
      a. Use intermittent positive pressure breathing (page 435) to assist respirations.
      b. Use oropharyngeal oxygen with caution.
      c. Observe for symptoms of carbon dioxide narcosis.
   C. Liquify the bronchial and the respiratory secretions:
      a. Add sodium iodide (0.5 Gm.) to intravenous solutions as directed.
      b. Humidify the room.
      c. Replace fluid and electrolyte losses.
      d. Encourage oral intake of fluids as soon as possible.
   D. Alleviate the patient's anxiety and exhaustion:
      a. Use mild sedatives cautiously.
      b. Give corticosteroids if needed to combat effects of prolonged stress.
      c. Promote the comfort of the patient:
         (1) Use supportive devices for orthopneic position.
         (2) Keep the environment cool and quiet.
         (3) Restrict visitors.
         (4) Have a positive and calm approach to the patient.
         (5) Ensure that patient sleeps undisturbed following attack.

2. *To individualize the patient's therapy to prevent future attacks:*
   A. Avoid precipitating factors that will trigger an asthmatic attack.
   B. Remove the patient from allergic material.
   C. Carry out program of desensitization.
   D. Conduct the program of maintenance therapy:
      a. Bronchodilators
      b. Sedatives
      c. Corticosteroids
      d. I.P.P.B. treatments
   E. Control secondary infections:
      a. Teach patient to call physician at first symptoms of respiratory infection.
      b. Observe the color of respiratory secretions.
      c. Treat "minor" respiratory infections vigorously.
      d. Avoid persons with colds and infections.
   F. Promote the rehabilitation of the patient:
      a. Teach and supervise breathing exercises.
      b. Teach patient to avoid irritants.
      c. Keep environmental air humidified and filtered when possible.
      d. Refer to state office of vocational rehabilitation when needed.
      e. Institute balanced program of nutrition, rest and exercise.
      f. Encourage the patient to ventilate his anxieties.
      g. Assist the patient to have insight into his situational problems.

surmised, to urticarial lesions along the gastrointestinal mucosa). Often asthma and urticaria result as well.

DESENSITIZATION, ANTIHISTAMINICS AND HORMONES IN ALLERGY

It is of the utmost importance that the nurse become familiar with certain general concepts regarding therapy in allergic diseases, since she is very apt to find herself an active participant in their treatment and will almost certainly be in the position of advisor to patients who are potential candidates for one or another of these procedures.

The commonest method of treatment employs the serial injection of one or more antigens which are selected in each particular case on the basis of *skin tests*. Skin testing entails the simultaneous intradermal inoculation (or superficial application), at separate sites, of several solutions containing individual antigens, comprising an assortment of those allergens deemed most likely to be implicated in the patient's disease. A positive reaction, evidenced by the appearance of an urticarial wheal or by localized erythema in the area of inoculation or contact, is regarded as being evidence of sensitivity to the corresponding antigen. Skin tests lend important weight to other evidence obtained from the patient's history, indicating which of several antigens are most likely to provoke his symptoms and providing some clue as to the intensity of his sensitization. (On the other hand, it should be recognized that the skin test is a test of skin reactivity, and any deduction that might be drawn from it relative to allergic phenomena in other tissues, such as the respiratory or gastrointestinal mucosa, is largely a matter of correlation and conjecture.)

A positive skin test may be regarded as an indication for a series of desensitizing injections, a course involving the repeated inoculation of the suspected allergen in graded doses and at regularly spaced intervals over a period of several weeks or months. The value of such injections has been fairly well established in those cases of hay fever and asthma which are clearly due to sensitivity to one of the common pollens or molds or to house dust. With respect to the treatment

itself, although referred to as a "desensitization" procedure, its effects are very probably attributable to the opposite process, i.e., immunization, for it appears to stimulate the production of a new antibody, one having the capacity of neutralizing the allergy-provoking properties of the responsible antigen.

One approach to the symptomatic treatment of allergic disorders has been by the administration of certain chemical agents called "antihistaminic drugs." These, most of which are derivatives of aminoethanol and ethylenediamine, are capable of neutralizing histamine, a substance that is liberated in the course of tissue antigen-antibody reactions and has been considered to be responsible, in part at least, for the symptoms they provoke. In actual practice, the effectiveness of these drugs is sharply limited, some symptomatic benefit having been observed following their use in certain cases of hay fever, vasomotor rhinitis, urticaria and mild asthma, but rarely in other conditions, or in severe conditions of any sort.

Administration of the steroid hormones eliminates, in dramatic fashion, any allergic phenomena that happen to be in progress at the time. The reason for their effectiveness in allergic disorders, although not completely established as yet, appears to be related to their inhibiting effect on inflammatory reactions in general. In this sense, their beneficial effect in allergic cases must be classed as nonspecific, bearing no relation to any specific antigen-antibody reaction that may be responsible for the disorder. There are certain unusual circumstances which justify the administration of these hormones, but, in the vast majority of cases, their usefulness in the field of allergy is far outweighed by the risks that are inherent in their use, as will be discussed in Chapter 38 on pages 841 to 844.

CLINICAL SITUATIONS

The Patient With Acute Bronchial Asthma

Mary Watson, 16, is admitted to the emergency room with a diagnosis of acute bronchial asthma.

1. Which statement best describes the breathing of a patient during an acute asthmatic attack?

    A. Noisy with paradoxical chest movement.

B. Wheezy, predominantly expiratory.
C. Wheezy, predominantly inspiratory.
D. Noisy with one-sided chest movement.

2. Mary is sensitive to pollen and house dust and has recurrent attacks of hay fever. An allergic individual may manifest his allergic differences by:
A. Dilatation of smooth muscle and vascular constriction.
B. Constriction of smooth muscle and vascular dilatation.
C. Exudation of fluid into bronchi.
D. Becoming hyposensitized to foreign proteins.

3. Asthma may be caused by all of the following *except*:
A. Smoking.
B. Chronic pulmonary disease.
C. Allergic reactions.
D. Infections.

4. It has been said that "all that wheezes is not asthma." A patient who is wheezing requires careful nursing. Which of the following could safely be given a narcotic?
A. Patient with atopic asthma.
B. Patient with cardiac asthma.
C. Patient with infectious asthma.
D. None of the above.

The Patient With Atopic Dermatitis (Eczema)

Miss Jane Meyers is an 18-year-old patient with atopic dermatitis. She has areas of dry, lichenfied plaques on her chest, neck and back.

1. The most characteristic feature of atopic dermatitis is
A. Vesiculation.
B. Pruritus.
C. Paresthesia.
D. Urticaria.

2. Frequently, the patient with atopic dermatitis has a family history of
A. Diabetes mellitus.
B. Peripheral vascular disorders.
C. Addison's disease.
D. Respiratory allergy.

3. The physician advised hospitalization for this patient in order to secure a change

of environment. To alleviate the itching from an overly dry skin, the nurse should place Miss Meyers in a room that
A. Has cross ventilation.
B. Has a low humidity.
C. Is air conditioned.
D. Is dust free.

4. Corticosteroids may be used in patients with atopic dermatitis mainly to
A. Stop the itching.
B. Minimize emotional tension.
C. Correct endocrinologic dysfunction.
D. Reduce inflammation.

BIBLIOGRAPHY AND SUGGESTED READING

Briscoe, W. A., and McLemore, G. A., Jr.: Ventilatory function in bronchial asthma, Thorax **7:**1-124, 1952.

Carryer, H. M.: The management of acute asthma, A.M.A. Arch. Int. Med. **99:**82-92, 1957.

Chobot, R.: Infectious factors in pediatric and adult allergy, J.A.M.A. **150:**1480-1482, 1952.

DeJong, R. N.: The treatment of migraine, Am. J. Nurs. **62:**67-71, July, 1962.

Hackett, A. M.: The care of a patient with contact dermatitis, Am. J. Nursing **58:**84-86, Jan., 1958.

Koelsche, G. A., Carryer, H. M., Peters, G. A., and Henderson, L. L.: Management of the seriously ill asthmatic, J.A.M.A. **166:**1541-1545, 1958.

Lea, W. A., Jr.: Rouges and rashes, Am. J. Nursing **58:**82-84, Jan., 1958.

Lowell, F. C.: Bronchial asthma, Am. J. Med. **20:**778-788, 1956.

Lowell, F. C., and Schiller, I. W.: Significance of changes in the expiratory rate observed during measurement of the vital capacity in asthma, J. Allergy **24:**492-498, 1953.

Michelson, A. L., and Lowell, F. C.: Antihistaminic drugs, New England J. Med. **258:**994-999, 1958.

Mueller, H. L.: Serious allergic reactions to insect stings, Am. J. Nurs. **60:**1110-1112, Aug., 1960.

Pinkerton, H. H., Jr., and Van Metre, T. E., Jr.: Immediate therapy for the acute attack of asthma, New Eng. J. Med. **258:**363-366, 1958.

Rapaport, H. G.: Psychosomatic aspects of allergy in childhood, J.A.M.A. **165:**812-815, 1957.

Rostenberg, A., Jr.: The allergic dermatoses, J.A.M.A. **165:**1118-1125, 1957.

Segal, M. S.: Current status of therapy in bronchial asthma, J.A.M.A. **169:**1063-1071, 1959.

Sherman, W. B.: Diagnostic methods for allergic diseases, Am. J. Med. **20:**603-611, 1957.

Spain, W. C.: The immunologic aspects of allergic conditions, Ann. Int. Med. **38:**188-198, 1953.

Patient-Teaching Aids

Useful pamphlets published by the National Tuberculosis Association:
    Asthma, The Facts. 1962.
    Hay Fever, The Facts. 1962.

Voluntary Organizations

Asthmatic Children's Foundation
Denver U.S. National Center
Denver 17, Colorado

National Foundation for Asthmatic Children
6015 E. Broadway
Tucson, Arizona

ORIENTATION

No organism as complex as the human body could possibly function with any degree of efficiency without precision equipment for the integration and the control of its innumerable metabolic activities. Designed specifically for this purpose is the endocrine system, comprising a series of ingenious regulating devices which are fully automatic and operate in accordance with the most advanced principles of cybernetics. Its functioning components are the endocrine glands. These units can function individually, in series or in parallel, their activities being integrated closely. Communication with each other and with the tissues under their control is established by means of chemical signals, or *hormones,* which they produce, store and release as required, and which are distributed throughout the body by means of a mechanical conveyor, the circulating blood.

The Endocrine Glands

These glands, with but two exceptions, have no means of communicating with other tissues excepting via the blood stream, depending exclusively on chemical signals for their own regulation. In most instances the agent stimulating or inhibiting their activity is the hormone produced by the corresponding target gland, an arrangement calculated to ensure stability of operation.

The two exceptions noted above are the adrenal medulla and the posterior pituitary gland. These are connected with, and are part of, the autonomic nervous system, secreting their hormones in response to electrical stimuli originating in higher centers in the brain and reaching them via the nerve fibers which link them to that system. Stimulation of the posterior pituitary causes the prompt secretion of one or more hormones called *pitressin.* Stimulation of the adrenal medulla results in the immediate release of epinephrine (adrenalin) and l-norepinephrine (l-norepinephrine also is liberated at the terminal ends of all sympathetic nerve fibers in response to electrical stimulation via those fibers).

These hormones, in contrast with all others, have widespread effects that are achieved almost instantaneously and involve many organs. Their net objective is to fortify the body against disaster, when disaster is threatened, and to compensate for bodily injury, when injury has occurred. The effect of epinephrine is to increase the efficiency of the circulatory and respiratory systems; to mobilize quick-energy glucose from storage depots into the circulating blood; to improve the acuity of vision; and to reinforce the clotting mechanism, in anticipation of massive bleeding. It even goes so far as to set into motion a series of reactions that would have the effect, a few hours hence, of lessening the severity of the body's responses to any tissue damage that might be incurred in the interim! Norepinephrine in the circulating blood produces constriction of all arterioles throughout the body, except those within the heart muscle. As a result of this action, the systolic and diastolic arterial pressures are elevated, and blood flow through the myocardium is increased.

Pitressin helps the body to survive despite severe hemorrhage and to correct the resulting deficiency in blood volume. Through its antidiuretic action this hormone prevents further loss of body water through excretion in the urine. By causing smooth muscle everywhere to contract, it forces the evacuation of all hollow viscera, including the pregnant uterus. It also reduces the capacity of the vascular bed and tends to maintain the arterial pressure in the heart and the brain at functional levels until the blood volume can be restored.

The remainder of the endocrine system includes the following secretory tissues: the anterior portion of the pituitary gland, the thyroid, the parathyroids, the adrenal cortex, the pancreas, the ovarian follicles and the interstitial cells of the testes. Their secretions, as a group, are concerned with tissue

814

growth and metabolism, the storage and the utilization of fuel substances, reproductive processes and other phases of the bodily economy. One gland, the anterior pituitary, is charged with the responsibility of integrating the activities of the entire system. This gland, either through its own secretions, or through other glands which are among its targets, exerts a potent influence on every phase of metabolic activity throughout the body. The action of each individual hormone from the anterior pituitary, however, and from all other glands in this group as well, is highly selective and strictly limited, in marked contrast with the effects of adrenalin and pitressin.

Secretions of the anterior pituitary gland number at least six. Its *somatotropic* (or growth) hormone regulates cell division, hence organ and body growth. It also elevates the concentration of glucose in the blood by decreasing the rate at which glucose is consumed by the tissue cells and by preventing its deposition in the liver, effects which may be described as "diabetogenic." The *lactogenic* hormone prepares the breasts for lactation during pregnancy and stimulates milk production after the fetus is delivered.

The remainder have as their targets individual endocrine glands, whose hormones inhibit, in each case, the production of that particular stimulant by the anterior pituitary. The *adrenocorticotropic* hormone (ACTH), for example, stimulates the adrenal cortex to produce hydrocortisone, aldosterone and other steroid hormones, while the rate of ACTH production, in turn, is regulated by the concentration of those hormones in the circulating blood. The *thyrotropic* hormone, by stimulating the enzymatic breakdown of stored thyroglobulin, forces the liberation of thyroxine from the thyroid gland. The resulting level of thyroxine in the blood determines the amount of thyrotropic hormone that is produced by the anterior pituitary at any given time.

There are two *gonadotropic* hormones from the anterior pituitary. One of these, the *follicle-stimulating* hormone, or FSH, is responsible for the development of graafian follicles in the ovary and for the proliferation of spermatozoa by the testis. The other, called the *luteinizing* hormone (LH), causes the follicle to atrophy and to become converted into another type of structure, known as the corpus luteum. In the adolescent and adult male, LH stimulates the interstitial cells of the testis to increase its production of testosterone, the male sex hormone.

Thyroxine and *triiodothyronine,* the hormones of the thyroid gland, speed oxidative reactions which energize all cellular activities. The parathyroids and their product, *parathormone,* regulate the metabolism of calcium and phosphorus and direct the migration of these ions between the bones and the blood. Pancreatic *insulin* enables the glucose that is contained in the circulating blood to penetrate the membranes and to enter the cytoplasm of tissue cells, thus providing these cells with ready access to this vitally needed fuel. Another pancreatic hormone, *glucagon,* speeds the liberation of glucose from its storage form, namely, glycogen, thereby increasing its concentration in the blood. The *hormones of the adrenal cortex* perform a variety of functions, including the conversion of proteins into glucose (gluconeogenesis), the control of lymphocyte production, the development of secondary sex characteristics and the prevention of sodium loss in the urine, causing the cells of the renal tubules to extract this ion from the glomerular filtrate and return it to the blood.

The testes and the ovaries, discussed in Unit 11, are likewise an integral part of the endocrine system. Their secretory functions, controlled by the pituitary through its gonadotropic hormones, are responsible for the formation of the secondary sex characteristics, the functional and anatomic changes that are involved in the process of menstruation and for the changes that occur during pregnancy.

38

Patients With Endocrine Conditions

THE THYROID GLAND

The thyroid gland, as illustrated in Figure 317, sits astride the trachea just below the larynx, its two lobes clasping the trachea on either side and the intermediate portion, or "isthmus," overlying that structure anteriorly. The lobes of the normal gland usually can be felt as they elevate during the act of swallowing. If the thyroid is enlarged significantly it produces a visible swelling in the neck, or *goiter*.

The function of this gland is concerned with the rate at which all tissues metabolize. It regulates the speed of their chemical reactions, the volume of oxygen they consume and the amount of heat they produce. With respect to these activities, the thyroid gland is an "energizer," so to speak, assigned to stimulate the tissue cells to whatever level of activity is required to maintain the total body temperature at a preset level. In the absence of the thyroid gland, metabolism continues, but at an exceedingly retarded pace. (The complications that attend hypometabolism are described on p. 817.)

The thyroid achieves its stimulating effect through the production and distribution of two hormones, one of which is called L-*thyroxine* and the other, *triiodothyronine*. Both compounds contain iodine which is protein-bound. According to present evidence, the function of thyroxine is to maintain the body's metabolism in a steady state, and at a level suitable for an individual who is situated in a stable, normal environment. Whenever there is a sudden need for a substantial increase in heat production, some of the thyroxine is converted into a more active agent, namely, triiodothyronine, which is approximately 5 times as potent as thyroxine.

Tests of Thyroid Function. In the majority of thyroid disorders the most prominent signs and symptoms are those which reflect an excessive or inadequate production of thyroid hormone. These signs provide a useful basis for evaluating the activity of the gland, as will be discussed later in relation to hyperthyroid and hypothyroid states.

A far more reliable and definitive index of thyroid function is the concentration of protein-bound iodine (PBI) in the blood. The usefulness of this determination, however, is seriously impaired by technical difficulties associated with tests for iodine in the quantities contained in blood. Normal values range from 4 to 8 μg. (0.004 to 0.008 mg.) per 100 ml. of plasma. Values above 8 μg. are indicative of thyroid overactivity; conversely, a concentration less than 4 μg. may be interpreted as being evidence of hypothyroidism.

Radioiodine (I^{131}) tests of thyroid function, and the responsibilities of the nurse in connection with these tests, are described on pages 107, 321 and 821.

BASAL METABOLIC RATE. A semiquantitative estimation of thyroid activity is possible from the basal metabolic rate, or B.M.R. The term "basal metabolism" refers to the oxygen consumption of an individual who is at rest, whose body temperature is normal and who has fasted for at least 14 hours in order to escape the stimulating effect of recently ingested food. From the volume of oxygen that is absorbed in a standard period of time under these conditions, it is possible to compute the rate at which heat is produced by the body. An average adult male produces heat at a rate of approximately 1,500 calories, and an average adult female, 1,300 calories, per 24 hours. Expressed in terms of heat production per square meter of surface per hour, the average metabolic rate for a normal individual under basal conditions is approximately 40 calories, depending on sex and age.

The B.M.R. should be determined in the morning, after a fast of at least 14 hours, while the patient is reclining quietly. Ambulatory patients should rest in bed quietly for an hour immediately before the test is performed. The entire procedure, which involves breathing through a rubber tube for several minutes with nostrils clamped shut, should be described fully to the patient in advance, for apprehension and emotional excitement, through stimulation of the sympathetic nervous system, increase the oxygen consumption (that is, metabolism) and the result is a high figure for the B.M.R. not at all indicative of thyroid overactivity (Fig. 318).

Hypothyroidism and Myxedema

If the thyroid gland is removed surgically, is destroyed by disease or becomes inactive for any reason, the metabolism of the patient declines proportionately as the production of thyroid hormone is reduced. Complete extirpation of this organ is followed by a steady drop in the B.M.R., which in approximately 3 months' time stabilizes at a level of about −40 per cent.

Mild grades of hypometabolism are encountered not uncommonly. Such patients exhibit decreased mental and physical vigor; they are lethargic; they doze readily in the daytime; they are forgetful; their skin and hair becomes dry; their sensitivity to cold increases; and headache may become a daily complaint. All of these symptoms improve remarkably upon the institution of thyroid replacement therapy.

With severer grades of this disorder the temperature and the pulse rate become subnormal; the patient begins to gain weight; the skin becomes thickened, for in the subcutaneous tissues there accumulates a mucilaginous substance (the origin of the term *myxedema*). Menorrhagia is apt to develop; the hair thins and falls out; the expression of the face becomes stolid, stupid and masklike. At first the patient may be irritable, but as the condition progresses he becomes com-

pletely complacent, the emotional responses subdued and the mental processes dulled (Fig. 319). The advanced myxedematous state is one of utter bovine placidity, much less distressing to its possessor than to his associates. It is not without its complications, however, for there is an associated tendency to the rapid development of arteriosclerosis, with all the undesirable features of that disease, and also anemia.

Treatment and Nursing Care

One of the most brilliant of all medical discoveries has been the finding that thyroid deficiency can be remedied by giving animal thyroid tissue extracts by mouth. This replacement therapy now is provided in the form of desiccated thyroid extract or synthetic crystalline L-thyroxine by mouth. Preparations of thyroid extract, standardized and of uniform potency, are available in tablet form. It is administered in one daily oral dose of from ¼ to 5 grains (15 to 300 mg.), the usual initial dose for adults being 1 grain (60 mg.) and for children, ½ grain (30 mg.). L-thyroxine (Synthroid) is distributed in tablet form, a 0.1-mg. tablet being equivalent in potency to 1 grain (60 mg.) of the extract. The dosage range for

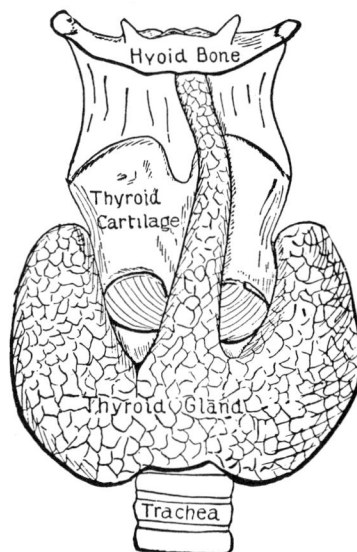

FIG. 317. The organs of the neck. (The thyroid cartilage is the Adam's apple.)

this product is from 0.025 mg. to 0.5 mg. daily.

The dosage for either material is scheduled on the basis of the patient's metabolic response, as ascertained by repeated measurements of the B.M.R. or of the iodine[131] uptake.

If replacement therapy is adequate, the symptoms of myxedema disappear and normal metabolic activity is resumed.

Nursing care in myxedema entails the observation of certain important precautions. The first, which is applicable in severe untreated hypothyroidism, is based on the fact that this disorder is attended by an increased susceptibility to all hypnotic and sedative drugs. These agents, even in small doses, may induce profound somnolence lasting far longer than is anticipated. Moreover, they are prone to cause respiratory depression which could easily prove to be fatal. With this in mind, the dosage of any such drug should be most conservative, e.g., no more than a half or one third of the dosage ordinarily employed in patients of similar age and weight who are not myxedematous. Drugs in this category should not be used at all, unless the indications are very clear cut, and, if they are given, the nurse must be unusually watchful for signs of impending narcosis or respiratory failure.

Myocardial Infarction. Another occasion for anxiety in patients with myxedema is the possibility that myocardial ischemia or infarction may occur in response to therapy. Coronary sclerosis of some degree is almost certain to be present in any patient who has been myxedematous for a long period of

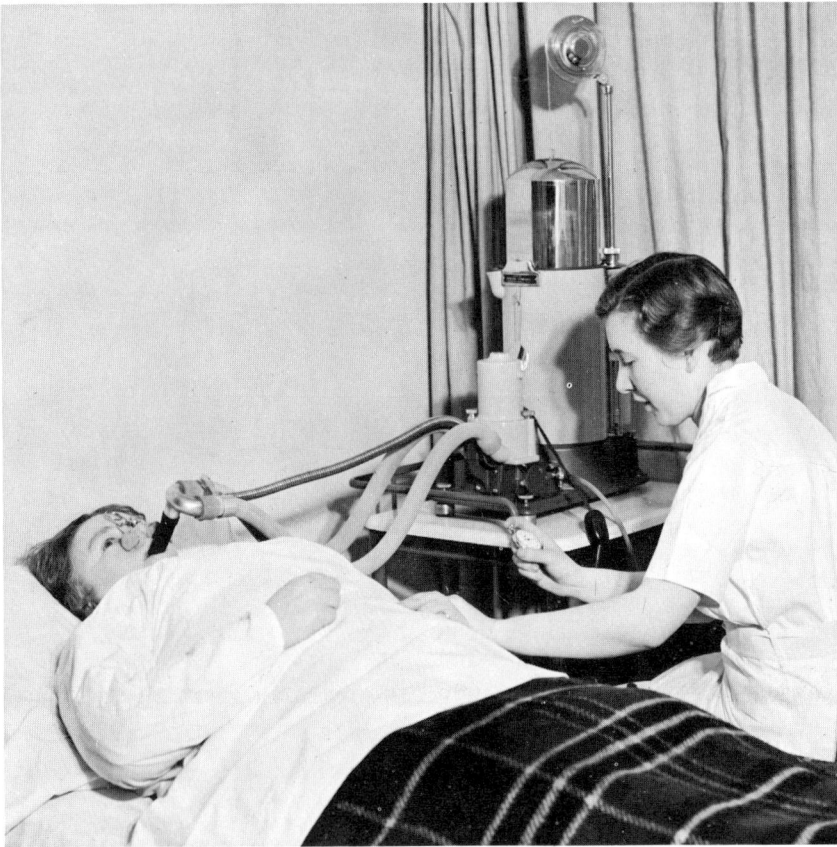

Fig. 318. Determining the basal metabolic rate.

time. As long as metabolism is subnormal and the tissues, including the myocardium, require relatively little oxygen, a reduction in blood supply is tolerated very well. However, when thyroid hormone is given the situation changes: the oxygen requirements are greater, but its delivery cannot be speeded up unless, or until, the arteriosclerosis improves, which will occur very slowly, if at all. The signal that the oxygen needs of the myocardium are outstripping its blood supply is angina pectoris.

The nurse must be unceasingly alert for that signal, especially during the early phase of treatment, and if the signal is detected it must be heeded at once if a fatal myocardial infarction is to be averted. The administration of thyroid hormone obviously must be discontinued immediately, and, later, when it can be resumed safely, substitution therapy should be applied with the utmost caution, at a lower level of dosage and under the close observation of the doctor and the nurse.

Cretinism

This term applies to patients born with thyroid deficiency of mothers likewise deficient. In these patients, prenatal development has not proceeded normally, and the results are irreparable. Cretinism is encountered with frequency only in endemic goiterous districts, notably in parts of Switzerland and in other countries situated in the Alps, where the iodine content of the water, the food and the air is insufficient to meet human requirements for the manufacture of the thyroid hormone. The condition is evident at birth. In the mildest cases the skin merely may be cold, dry, wrinkled, loose and present a faded yellowish color; the face looks senile rather than infantile. Some cretins are incurable idiots from birth; still others are deaf, because of failure to develop. Over 50 per cent have iodine-deficient goiters from birth. In the United States, this disease is relatively rare.

Marked clinical improvement follows the administration of desiccated thyroid, L-thyroxine or L-triiodothyronine. Signs of myxedema disappear promptly; maturation and linear growth of the skeleton proceed rapidly; but mental retardation persists.

Hyperthyroidism

Overactivity of the thyroid gland with overproduction of thyroid hormone is evidenced by weight loss in the presence of an adequate dietary intake, nervousness, tachycardia, fine tremor of the hands, intolerance to heat, excessive perspiration and easy fatigability. The systolic blood pressure and the pulse pressure are increased. The basal

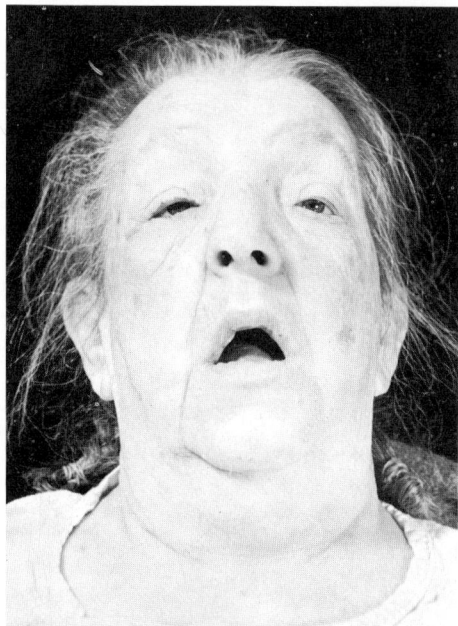

FIG. 319. Myxedema.

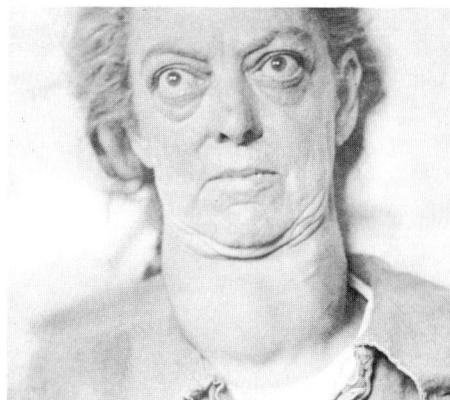

FIG. 320. Exophthalmos.

metabolic rate is persistently above normal. The concentration of protein-bound iodine in the blood is elevated, and the uptake of radioactive iodine (I^{131}), after ingestion of a test dose, is abnormally rapid and complete, as measured by Geiger counts over the site of the gland. All these symptoms and signs can be induced in a normal individual by the administration of excessive amounts of thyroid extract or L-thyroxine, and they are produced even more readily by triiodothyronine.

Spontaneous hyperthyroidism constitutes a well-defined disease entity, variously designated as *Graves' disease, Basedow's disease* and *exophthalmic goiter*. This disease occurs more commonly in women than in men. Its etiology is unknown, but it is believed to represent a dysfunction of the pituitary gland, whereby this gland produces an excess not only of thyrotropic (thyroid-stimulating) hormone but of other hormones as well, accounting for symptoms of this disease not attributable to thyroid over-activity. It may appear after an emotional shock, nervous strain or an infection—particularly one involving the upper respiratory tract—but the exact significance of these relationships is not understood.

Symptoms. Patients with well-developed hyperthyroidism exhibit a group of symptoms and signs which are quite characteristic. Their presenting symptom is often nervousness. They are emotionally hyper-excitable, their state of mind is apt to be irritable and apprehensive; they cannot sit quietly; they suffer from palpitation; and their pulse is abnormally rapid at rest as well as on exertion. They tolerate heat poorly and perspire unusually freely; the skin is flushed continuously, with a characteristic salmon color, and is likely to be warm, soft and moist. A fine tremor of the hands may be observed. Many patients exhibit bulging eyes (exophthalmos), lending a startled expression to the countenance and described as *crystallized fear* (Fig. 320). To some extent, the thyroid gland always is enlarged; it is soft and may pulsate; a thrill often can be felt over the thyroid arteries—a sign of greatly increased blood flow through the organ. Other important symptoms include an increased appetite (unless gastrointestinal

symptoms develop), progressive loss of weight, abnormal muscular fatigability and weakness, amenorrhea and changes in bowel habit, either to constipation or diarrhea. The pulse rate of these patients ranges constantly between 90 and 160; the systolic, but characteristically not the diastolic, blood pressure is elevated; atrial fibrillation may appear and cardiac decompensation is common. In the more advanced cases, the diagnosis is established readily on the basis of the symptoms and the signs described above: an elevated B.M.R., which declines over a period of several days on iodine therapy; an increase in protein-bound iodine in the blood; and an increased iodine[131] uptake by the thyroid.

The course of the disease may be mild, characterized by remissions and exacerbations and terminating with spontaneous recovery in the course of a few months or years. On the other hand, it may progress relentlessly, the patient, unless treated, becoming emaciated, intensely nervous, delirious—even disoriented—and the heart eventually "racing itself to death."

Treatment and Nursing Care

As yet, no treatment for hyperthyroidism has been discovered which combats its basic cause. However, reduction of thyroid hyperactivity provides effective symptomatic relief and removes the principal source of its most important complications.

Three forms of treatment are available for the control of excessive thyroid activity: (1) pharmacologic, employing antithyroid drugs that interfere with the synthesis of thyroid hormones; (2) radiation, involving the administration of the radioisotope iodine[131] for its destructive effect on the thyroid gland; and (3) surgical, accomplishing the removal of most of the thyroid gland.

Antithyroid Drugs. Certain drugs block the utilization of iodine by the thyroid gland and, consequently, prevent the formation of thyroxine. One of these is propylthiouracil, which is very active in this respect, can be administered with relative safety for long periods of time and is readily available.

Propylthiouracil is administered in doses varying from 100 to 600 mg. daily. Therapy is controlled on the basis of clinical criteria, including changes in pulse rate, pulse pressure, body weight, size of the goiter and basal metabolic rate. Toxic complications of propylthiouracil are relatively uncommon; nevertheless, periodic examinations cannot be neglected in view of the possibility that drug sensitization, followed by fever, rash, urticaria or even granulopenia, may develop in its recipients.

Radioactive Iodine. Practically all of the iodine that enters and is retained in the body becomes concentrated within the thyroid gland. This applies to the radioactive isotopes of iodine as well, providing the basis for a very effective device for the selective inhibition of thyroid activity, namely, the administration of radioiodine (I^{131}). The objective of this treatment is the irradiation of the gland, which is accomplished by this technic without jeopardy to other radiosensitive tissues. Radioactive iodine has been used successfully in most varieties of thyrotoxicosis and is especially preferred for the treatment of the older patient.

Subtotal Thyroidectomy. The surgical removal of about five sixths of the thyroid tissue practically assures a prolonged remission in most cases of exophthalmic goiter. Before surgery the patient is given propylthiouracil until signs of hyperthyroidism disappear. Iodine also is prescribed, either before or after a full remission has been achieved with propylthiouracil. The effect of iodine is to reduce the size and the vascularity of the goiter. It may be given in the form of potassium iodide or hydriodic acid. Patients receiving this medication must be watched for evidence of iodine toxicity (iodism), the appearance of which is the signal for immediate withdrawal of the drug. Symptoms of iodism include swelling of the buccal mucosa, excessive salivation, coryza and skin eruptions.

Thyroidectomy usually is scheduled within a few days after the patient's basal metabolic rate has been reduced to normal.

Thyroiditis

Acute inflammation of the thyroid gland, referred to as "acute nonsuppurative thyroiditis," presents as a painful swelling in the anterior neck which lasts 1 or 2 months then disappears without residual. Women in their 50's are affected predominantly. The thyroid enlarges symmetrically and painfully. The overlying skin is often reddened and warm. Swallowing may be difficult and uncomfortable. Irritability, nervousness, insomnia and weight loss—manifestations of hyperthyroidism—are common, and many patients experience chills and fever as well. X-ray irradiation of the thyroid and steroid therapy have been applied with reported benefit.

Chronic thyroiditis, predominantly a disease of women in their 50's and 60's, has been classified as "Hashimoto's struma" or "Riedel's struma," depending on the histologic appearance of the inflamed gland. In contrast with acute thyroiditis, the chronic varieties are unaccompanied by pain, pressure symptoms or fever, and thyroid activity is apt to be normal or low, rather than increased. Steroid therapy likewise has been recommended for these patients.

There is evidence to suggest that thyroiditis, acute and chronic alike, may represent disorders of "auto-immunity" analogous to acquired hemolytic jaundice (see p. 467), as evidenced by the presence of antithyroid antibody in the serum of these patients.

Thyroid Tumors

Tumors of the thyroid gland are classified on the basis of their benign or malignant character, the presence or the absence of thyrotoxicosis associated with them and the diffuse or irregular quality of the glandular enlargement. If the enlargement is sufficient to cause a visible swelling in the neck, the tumor is referred to as a "goiter."

All grades of goiter are encountered, from those which are barely visible to those producing an unsightly disfigurement. Some are symmetrical and diffuse, others nodular. Some are accompanied by hyperthyroidism, in which case they are described as "toxic"; others are associated with a euthyroid state and are called "nontoxic" goiters.

Endemic (Iodine-Deficient) Goiter

The most common type of goiter, encountered chiefly in geographic regions where the natural supply of iodine is deficient (for example, in the Great Lakes area of the United States), is the so-called *simple* or *colloid goiter*. It represents a compensatory hypertrophy on the part of the entire gland, presumably due to stimulation by the pituitary gland. Thus, the pituitary gland produces a hormone controlling thyroid growth, and this production is excessive if there is subnormal thyroid activity, as is the case when insufficient iodine is available for production of the thyroid hormone. Such goiters usually cause no symptoms except for the swelling in the neck, which, however, when excessive, may result in tracheal compression. Many goiters of this type recede after a course of treatment with thyroid extract, which tends to depress the pituitary's thyroid-stimulating activity. The operative removal of very large goiters occasionally is desirable.

Prevention. This is accomplished by providing children in iodine-poor districts with iodine compounds. The effectiveness of this measure is evident from the statistical results of its use by growing girls in certain midwestern cities. Since the administration of iodine to grade-school children has been in progress, the percentage of goiter has decreased to less than 10 per cent; previously, 40 per cent of the young people entering high school had colloid goiters. The amount of iodine required is very small indeed; it is supplied easily as a constituent of table salt.

Nodular Goiter

Certain thyroid glands are nodular because of the presence of one or several areas of hyperplasia (overgrowth) which appear to develop under conditions similar to those responsible for the colloid goiter. No symptoms may arise as a result of this condition, but, not uncommonly, these nodules slowly increase in size, perhaps descending into the thorax and there causing local pressure symptoms. Some become malignant and some become associated with a hyperthyroid state. For these reasons, many nodular thyroids eventually require surgical attention.

Thyroid Cancer

Benign thyroid tumors, or "adenomas," become cancerous in a fair percentage of patients. Thus, between 5 and 15 percent of patients with toxic nodular goiter are discovered to harbor a carcinoma when the gland is removed and examined microscopically. The most vicious form of thyroid cancer is the rapidly growing, widely metastasizing adenocarcinoma, which occurs predominantly in middle-aged and elderly individuals. This type may respond briefly to one course of x-ray irradiation, but is otherwise refractory to treatment, and few patients survive longer than 2 years after its initial appearance. The second group comprises the "papillary cancers" (papillary adenocarcinomas). This variety is encountered with about equal frequency in every decade of life. Its growth is slow, and its spread usually confined to the lymph nodes that drain the thyroid area. The chance of cure is excellent after surgical removal of the thyroid gland, together with these involved nodes.

The rarest, and the most peculiar, type of thyroid cancer is familiarly known as "benign metastasizing goiter" or "metastasizing adenoma." Each metastatic nodule, like the parent gland itself, takes up iodine with great avidity, a property that renders it vulnerable to detection and localization after the administration of iodine[131], by simple scanning for gamma emanation with a Geiger tube. By the same token, the administration of radioactive iodine in large doses offers a practical and effective means of irradiating the tumor therapeutically, a procedure of great value from the palliative, if not the curative, standpoint, especially when carried out in conjunction with total surgical removal of the thyroid gland, i.e., thyroidectomy.

Thyroidectomy

Preoperative Treatment and Nursing Care

Patients suffering with exophthalmic goiter cannot be operated on without requisite preoperative preparation. These extremely nervous individuals must have some considerable period of rest in bed in the most quiet atmosphere possible. They must be protected from disturbing sights and should be placed so that they will not come in contact with very ill patients. For psychological reasons it may be well to place this patient beside one who has made a satisfactory recovery from operation. The nurse should see that he has an abundance of fresh air and an ample amount of carbohydrate and protein foods. Usually this patient is embarrassed about his unusually large appetite and may hesitate to ask for another helping. The nurse should recognize this dietary need, which is due to the increased metabolic activity and the rapid depletion of glycogen reserves. A daily caloric intake of from 4,000 to 5,000 calories is not only desirable but essential. Supplementary vitamins, particularly thiamine and ascorbic acid, are necessary. Tea or coffee is not given without the permission of the physician.

The nurse should gain the complete confidence of her patient and by every method attempt to keep him free from worry and anxiety. Some forms of occupational therapy are quieting and are given at the direction of the surgeon.

The patient with hyperthyroidism often comes to the hospital from a home made tense and unhappy by restlessness, nervousness and loss of efficiency, which are the symptoms of the disease. It is necessary to protect the patient from a continuance of such unpleasantness and unhappiness. Therefore, the nurse should watch carefully the effect of visitors upon the patient. If there is any evidence of nervous upsets by their visits, it may be advisable to limit the visiting privileges during the preoperative period.

Sedatives (bromides and phenobarbital) are administered frequently, and because many older patients with hyperthyroidism have associated cardiac disease, digitalis may also be given.

Operation. The immediate preparation of thyroid patients for surgery includes a good night's rest the preceding night, adequate shaving of the neck (see p. 211), nothing by mouth after midnight and a pre-anesthetic hypodermic about 20 or 30 minutes before surgery. The operation is performed with the patient in the dorsal position, with a sandbag or air pillow under the shoulders and the head low (neck hyperextended) to make the neck more prominent. The patient's hair should be enclosed in a cap. Through a transverse incision in the lower part of the neck the thyroid is exposed and excised, leaving only a small amount of glandular tissue on the posterior capsule of the gland on each side. This small amount of thyroid tissue is all that is necessary for normal function, and an inadequate removal of the gland predisposes to a recurrence of hyperthyroidism. The wound usually is closed with clips and often is drained for a day or two.

Postoperative Nursing Care

The patient should be moved carefully, care being taken to support the head so that no tension is placed on the sutures. The most comfortable position is the semi-Fowler with the head elevated and supported by pillows. The utmost quiet is observed, and morphine is given hypodermically to relieve the painful effects of the operation. Occasionally the patient is placed in an oxygen tent for the first few hours to facilitate breathing. The nurse should anticipate any apprehension in the patient and inform him that by being in the tent his breathing will be easier, and he will be less tired. Fluid may be given by vein, but water may be given by mouth as soon as nausea ceases. The nurse should inspect and reinforce the dressings when necessary, remembering that when the patient is in the dorsal position, evidences of bleeding should be looked for at the sides and the back of the neck as well as anteriorly. In addition to checking the pulse and the blood pressure, it is also important to be on the alert for complaints from the patient of a sensation of pressure or fullness at the incision site. These may be indicative of hemorrhage and should be reported. Ice caps applied over the dressing are routine in many hospitals to help in bleeding control. Usually, there is a little difficulty in swallowing, and in this condition experience has taught that cold fluids, or ice, may be taken better than others. Often a soft diet is preferred by many patients rather than a liquid diet. Occasionally, difficulty in respiration is observed with the development of cyanosis and noisy breathing, due to an edema of the glottis or to an injury to the recurrent laryngeal nerves. Since this complication demands the insertion of a tracheostomy tube, the surgeon in charge should be summoned at once.

Little talking should be permitted, but

when the patient does speak, the nurse should note any voice changes, which might indicate injury to the recurrent laryngeal nerves that lie just behind the thyroid next to the trachea.

When the nurse is not in constant attendance, an overbed table is a great comfort to the patient. On it may be placed the materials which are needed frequently, such as paper wipes, water pitcher and glass, small emesis basin, etc. These are kept within easy reach so that the patient is not required to turn the head in search of them. It is also convenient to use this table when inhalations are given for the relief of excessive mucous secretions.

The patient usually is permitted out of bed on the first postoperative day and has a choice of diet. A well-balanced high-caloric diet is to be prescribed to regain any weight loss. Sutures or skin clips usually are removed on the second day. By the fifth day, the average patient is ready for discharge from the hospital.

Complications. Hemorrhage, edema of the glottis and injury to the recurrent laryngeal nerve are complications which have been reviewed in the preceding section. Occasionally, in operations on the thyroid, the parathyroid glandules may be injured or removed. This produces a disturbance of the calcium metabolism of the body. As the blood calcium falls, there appears a hyperirritability of the nerves, with spasms of the hands and the feet and muscular twitchings. This group of symptoms is termed *tetany,* and its appearance should be called to the attention of the surgeon at once. Tetany of this type usually is relieved by the administration of parathyroid extract or calcium in some form.

Convalescent Care. The patient should not be permitted to resume his former activities or to adopt his former responsibilities in full until thyrotoxicosis has been eliminated. The necessity for rest, relaxation and nutrition is explained, both to the patient and to his family, at the time of discharge. Specific instructions are issued regarding the scheduling of subsequent visits to the physician or the clinic, for repeated studies and check-up examinations are inevitably necessary and invariably important.

Family responsibilities and a variety of factors relating to the home environment engendering emotional tension often have been implicated as precipitating causes of thyrotoxicosis. The patient's hospitalization affords an opportunity for a fair evaluation of these factors. An opportunity also is created for the accomplishment of desirable alterations in the environmental situation. Finally, this is the most favorable time for the establishment of close rapport with the patient and for supplying him with whatever psychological support and assistance in emotional readjustments that he may require.

THE PARATHYROID GLANDS

The parathyroid glands are 4, 6 or even 8 small, bean-sized structures situated on the posterior aspect of the thyroid gland, in the substance of which they are imbedded. These bodies furnish an internal secretion, *parathormone,* which influences the concentrations of calcium and phosphorus in the blood and the migration of these elements between the blood and the bones. Its basic role is to promote the urinary excretion of phosphorus by preventing reabsorption of the phosphate ion by the kidney tubules. If parathormone is inadequate, as in hypoparathyroidism, too much phosphate re-enters the blood from the renal tubules; the blood phosphate level becomes abnormally high. A reciprocal relationship exists between phosphate and calcium levels in the blood; accordingly, in hypoparathyroidism, the blood calcium declines to an abnormally low level, to the extent that the patient may experience muscular hyperirritability and uncontrollable spasms: i.e., hypocalcemic tetany. If there is excess of parathormone, too little phosphorus will be retrieved from the glomerular filtrate and an excessive amount will escape in the urine. The concentration of phosphorus in the blood, therefore, will decline. This has the effect of causing some of the calcium phosphate contained in the bones to dissolve in the blood. This additional phosphorus also is removed with dispatch by the kidneys. However, the added calcium is not cleared with the same rapidity, and an elevated blood calcium results.

In summary, the net effect of parathormone is to depress the concentration of phosphorus and to increase the concentration of calcium in the blood and to decalcify the bones.

Hyperparathyroidism

Hyperparathyroidism (Von Recklinghausen's disease), due to an overgrowth of the parathyroid glands, is characterized by bony decalcification, the development of calcium phosphate stones in both kidneys and a depression of the neuromuscular apparatus. Parathyroid hyperactivity with similar manifestations also occurs in patients with chronic nephritis and so-called "renal rickets," presumably as a result of phosphorus retention. These patients experience symptoms of apathy, fatigue, muscular weakness, nausea, vomiting, constipation and cardiac arrhythmias, all attributable to an increased concentration of calcium in the blood. The formation of stones in both kidneys, related to the increased urinary excretion of calcium and phosphorus, is one of the important complications of hyperparathyroidism. The renal damage that results from the precipitation of calcium phosphate in the renal pelves and parenchyma (nephrocalcinosis) often is responsible for pyelonephritis and uremia and

explains many of its most prominent clinical manifestations. The skeletal changes, however, are the characteristic hallmark of hyperparathyroidism, whether this occurs as a primary disorder or as a secondary complication of calcium and phosphorus retention in patients with chronic renal disease. There are two aspects of this bony involvement to be considered: (1) demineralization of the bones, resulting in skeletal pain and tenderness, pain on weight-bearing, pathologic fractures, deformities, shortening of body structure and the formation of bony cysts; (2) the development of bone tumors, composed of benign giant cells and representing an overgrowth of osteoclasts. This variety of neoplasm is encountered occasionally on dental examination as a tumor of the jaw, in which location it is referred to as an "epulis."

Treatment. The treatment of hyperparathyroidism is surgical removal of enough parathyroid tissue to restore the calcium-phosphorus metabolism to normal.

Hypoparathyroidism

This condition follows the operative removal of too much parathyroid tissue; also, it is encountered in association with idio-

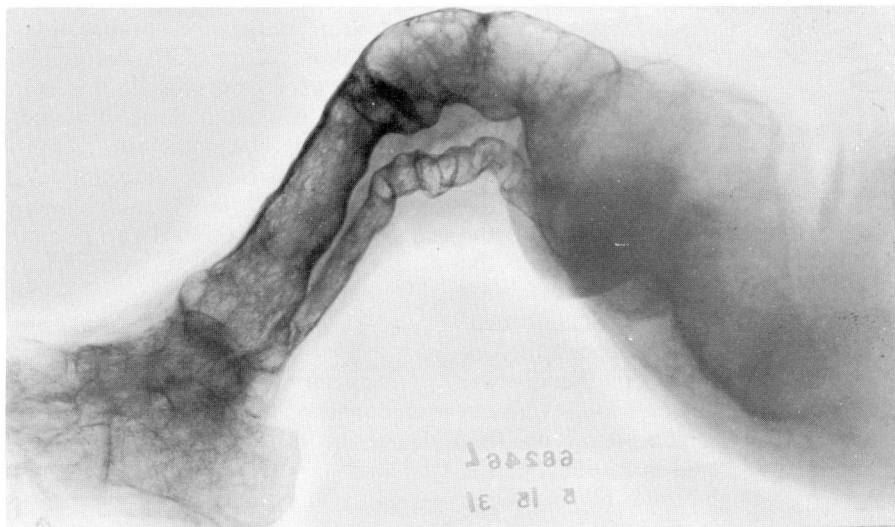

FIG. 321. Roentgenogram of the lower limb of a male patient who had a large adenoma of a parathyroid gland that caused decalcification, multiple fractures, cystic degeneration and skeleton deformities and resulted in a loss of stature. Removal of tumor stopped the loss of calcium and recurrent fractures.

pathic atrophy. Its symptoms and signs are due to a deficiency of parathormone, which results in an accumulation of phosphorus in the blood and a decrease in the concentration of blood calcium.

Tetany. The chief symptom of hypoparathyroid disease is tetany, by which is meant a general muscular hypertonia with tremor and spasmodic or incoordinated contractions following any effort to make a voluntary movement. In typical cases, there is tonic (i.e., steadily tense) flexion of the arms at the elbows, of the wrist and of the fingers at the metacarpophalangeal joints. The muscular irritability is so great that a muscle goes into spasm following pressure on its vessel or a tap on its nerve. Also, there is, at times, spasm of the larynx; even convulsions may occur.

This symptom is due to the low blood calcium and resembles, so far as the nervous system signs are concerned, the phenomenon that occurs in alkalosis due to overbreathing or results from severe acute chloride loss from persistent vomiting.

Treatment. The treatment of hypoparathyroidism consists in elevating to normal the blood-calcium level by the oral or parenteral administration of calcium salts; by injections of parathyroid extract; by supplying vitamin D in massive doses; or, most satisfactorily, by the ingestion of dihydrotachysterol (A. T. 10), a substance that is related chemically to vitamin D.

THE PANCREAS

The pancreas manufactures and secretes into the blood stream two hormones, *insulin* and *glucagon*. Insulin is required for the utilization of glucose by the tissue cells as the principal source of energy for their metabolic activities. Its role apparently is concerned with the transport of glucose through the cell membrane. Glucagon, the other endocrine product of the pancreas, serves to prevent excessive drops in blood glucose concentration (hypoglycemia). Secreted in response to the development of hypoglycemia, this hormone stimulates the rapid conversion of liver glycogen to glucose (glycogenolysis), the effect of which is to elevate promptly the blood sugar. In the absence of insulin, the glucose that is absorbed from the gastrointestinal tract neither is stored nor utilized, but merely accumulates in the circulating blood and escapes in the urine. Every cell in the body, although bathed in glucose—high concentrations of glucose—starves for the lack of it, for the glucose cannot get inside. This is the situation that exists in an extremely important and relatively common disease called *diabetes mellitus*.

Diabetes Mellitus

Diabetes mellitus may be defined as a chronic metabolic disorder, the basis of which is an inability of the cells to utilize glucose. This defect probably is due to a deficiency of insulin production by the islet cells of the pancreas, since it can be corrected by the administration of this hormone. Its cardinal signs are hyperglycemia, or an increased concentration of glucose in the blood, and glycosuria, the spillage of this substance in the urine, when its blood concentration exceeds the renal threshold. Other clinical manifestations can be explained almost entirely on the basis of tissue starvation and the toxic accumulation of abnormal metabolites.

The importance of diabetes mellitus is obvious from its prevalence alone. Based on data extracted from random surveys of the population, the U. S. Public Health Service has estimated that the number of diabetics in the United States exceeds two million. Thus, one out of 80 persons in this country is a diabetic. Almost half of these persons are unaware of their affliction. Approximately 65,000 new cases of diabetes develop each year; about 4,750,000 individuals presently residing in this country who now are free of diabetic symptoms will develop diabetes during their lifetime.

Etiology

Diabetes mellitus is presumably based on an inherited defect of some sort, since at least one third of all patients describe the occurrence of the disease among their relatives. It is estimated that 40 million persons in the United States, i.e., 1 person out of every 4, are diabetic "carriers," transmitting, or capable of transmitting, a tendency to diabetes although not exhibiting this trait themselves. Another factor in its origin is racial susceptibility, as evidenced by its increased incidence among Jewish people. Granting an inherited tendency, the onset of diabetes mellitus, when it occurs in middle life, as it usually does, often is precipitated by the excessive ingestion of carbohydrates by those who exercise too little.

Symptoms and Course

The onset of diabetes mellitus in children is usually acute, with loss of weight and strength, polyuria and glycosuria. In the younger age group the disease is always comparatively severe. Among adults, the onset often is so gradual that the disorder is not noticed for months, or even years; in about 10 per cent of all patients its discovery is the surprise result of routine urine examinations.

The early symptoms most commonly noticed by adults are loss of weight and strength, polyuria, polydipsia (great thirst), polyphagia (voracious appetite) and an itching, dry skin. Other symptoms of well-developed untreated cases include boils and carbuncles; arteriosclerosis with all its sequelae, including gangrene of the feet; cataract; peripheral neuritis; and coma.

Diagnosis

The presence of sugar in the urine does not invariably signify diabetes mellitus, nor do patients with diabetes mellitus invariably excrete sugar in the urine. Nevertheless, patients exhibiting the combination of chronic glycosuria and hyperglycemia are assumed to have diabetes mellitus until proved otherwise.

All patients, irrespective of their presumptive diagnosis, should be examined for glycosuria as a matter of routine. If a positive test is obtained, the blood sugar should be determined when the patient has been fasting for at least 3 to 4 hours. Moreover, in every doubtful case, both the fasting blood sugar and the glucose tolerance should be determined; otherwise, many cases of mild diabetes with sugar-free urine will not be discovered. These tests are described in Chapter 6 (pp. 71, 80, 82).

Complications of Diabetes

Acidosis. Acidosis, the most common and most dreaded of all complications of diabetes mellitus, may begin acutely or insidiously, may be mild or severe, may be temporary or chronic.

CHRONIC ACIDOSIS. If not severe, it may persist for weeks or months without change. The symptoms, which are not necessarily striking, include easy fatigability, anorexia, sporadic headache and general languor. These symptoms usually improve following correction of the acidosis.

ACUTE ACIDOSIS AND COMA. Acidosis may begin suddenly, with nausea, vomiting, epigastric discomfort or pain, subnormal temperature and drowsiness progressing to coma. The patient's face is flushed at first, but soon becomes pale; he breathes rapidly, yet without difficulty (Kussmaul's air hunger); his breath has a fruity odor due to ketone bodies. As a result of his dehydration he looks extremely emaciated; his skin is dry and shrunken; his tongue, throat, mouth and lips are red, glistening and beefy; and his eyeballs feel soft. The temperature is slightly above normal, and the leukocyte count often is elevated to 25,000 per cu. mm., but with a normal differential count. Albuminuria and cylindruria frequently appear; the finely granular casts sometimes are so numerous that they form a sediment filling about one third of the glass. The CO_2 content of the blood is low, and the cations, sodium and potassium are similarly decreased.

The gastrointestinal symptoms are frequently so stormy that patients with acute acidosis often are diagnosed as cases of intestinal obstruction, acute cholecystitis, acute appendicitis, peritonitis or pancreatitis, but the laboratory findings of glycosuria and hyperglycemia correct the error. The treatment of the acidosis and the coma complicating diabetes will be discussed in detail as the therapy of diabetes is considered.

Boils and Carbuncles. Usually on the neck and the back, formerly these were common complications of diabetes, but this complication is less true today, since modern treatment keeps the disease under better control.

Other Complications. These are marked arteriosclerosis, with all its sequelae, including gangrene of the extremities; hemorrhagic lesions of the retinae; cataract of the lens of the eyes; and polyneuritis, which is usually due to thiamin deficiency.

Treatment and Nursing Care of the Diabetic Patient

Modern therapy in this disease is designed to provide the patient with a diet properly proportioned as to constituents and adequate to maintain normal weight, growth and strength. At the same time, enough insulin is supplied to compensate for the deficiency in the patient's own production of this hormone and to permit the metabolism and utilization of these dietary constituents to proceed normally. The principal therapeutic guide in diabetic management, aside from the general condition of the patient, is the degree of glycosuria present, for this is one of the most significant of the readily elicited signs which are indicative of the metabolic state in diabetes mellitus. The aim is to keep the urine sugar-free, not by distortion of the diet, but by the administration of insulin.

THE DIET

In planning the diet, the first problem is the patient's basic caloric requirement, which varies according to age, body weight and degree of activity. Generally, it is granted that the normal adult leading a sedentary existence requires a diet which furnishes 30 Cal. per Kg. of body weight per day; one at light work, a diet which provides from 35 to 40; and the heavy laborer, one which supplies from 40 to 50 (or more). If the patient is obese, the caloric content is reduced sufficiently to effect a slow weight reduction.

The distribution in the diet between carbohydrate, fat and protein should not deviate greatly from the usual normal well-balanced diet. Deviation is required in the carbohydrate intake, which almost always is restricted. The usual protein allowance for the adult patient is from 1.0 to 1.2 Gm. per Kg. of body weight, or from 70 to 100 Gm. daily. During the process of regulation, it is important that the patient eat all, and nothing except, the diet specified for him. Food that is refused should be identified and its quantity evaluated, so that appropriate corrections can be applied in calculating the amount of protein, fat and carbohydrate actually ingested. Vomiting, or the refusal of any significant portion of the diet, should be reported at once to the physician in charge.

As soon as it is practicable, the diabetic patient is offered a systematic course of instruction in dietetics. Participants in this educational program, which is of paramount importance in diabetic care, are the physician, or a dietitian, and the attending nurses, who must be sufficiently well versed in the subject to discuss its problems intelligently with the patient and to furnish his family with whatever instructions they may require relating to his diet. The responsibility for the care of the sick diabetic is not ended until the patient's ability to continue his prescribed diet is assured. If he is incapable of selecting his own meals without supervision, someone who is thoroughly acquainted with his dietary needs must do it for him.

INSULIN THERAPY

Many obese patients with mild, uncomplicated diabetes may be controlled solely by means of a low-caloric diet, without insulin. Many patients who are not obese, whose diabetes is mild and who have experienced the onset of diabetes during their adult years, can be controlled satisfactorily by diet plus one of the oral hypoglycemic drugs, such as Orinase (tolbutamide). However, all diabetic children, all diabetic adults who have lost an excessive amount of weight, all diabetics with acute complications and all individuals with severe diabetes require regular hypodermic injections of insulin.

Forms of Insulin. Six insulin preparations are available for therapeutic administration: regular insulin and crystalline zinc insulin, which act most promptly and briefly, and the biologic properties of which are almost precisely similar; and protamine zinc insulin (PZI), globin insulin, NPH (isophane) insulin and lente insulin, the effects of which are delayed and relatively long sustained.

The preparations most widely used at present are NPH insulin and lente insulin. NPH insulin usually begins to act within a period of 4 to 5 hours after injection; its effects become maximal in 8 to 10 hours and persist up to 20 to 24 hours following its receipt.

Lente insulin, a suspension of large, very slowly absorbed (ultralente) mixed with small, more rapidly absorbed (semilente) insulin crystals, exerts its maximum effect between 8 and 12 hours after injection, some activity persisting for as long as 18 to 24 hours. Regular insulin and crystalline zinc insulin begin to act within a period of about 30 minutes following injection, their effects becoming maximal between 4 and 6 hours and terminating 6 to 8 hours after administration; their principal use is in conjunction with NPH insulin and in the treatment of diabetic acidosis. NPH insulin, in contrast with lente insulin and PZI, can be mixed with regular or crystalline zinc insulin, if desired, without impeding the latter's speedy effects or altering its own rapidity of action.

Injection. As soon as the need for insulin therapy has been established, treatment and patient education should begin. Moreover, from the very beginning, the patient is instructed in the self-administration of insulin. The instructor usually is the nurse. Initially, the patient's participation in this program may take the form of observation, but at the earliest propitious occasion he is given an opportunity to perform his own injection under the direct supervision of the nurse.

Regulation of Dosage. The dosage of insulin is adjusted according to the presence (or absence) and the degree of glycosuria, and also according to the time of the appearance of the glycosuria in relation to insulin injections and meals. The regulation of insulin dosage is aided further by determinations of the blood-sugar level, which should be measured periodically during the period of hospitalization. The results of these tests should be charted routinely and presented at

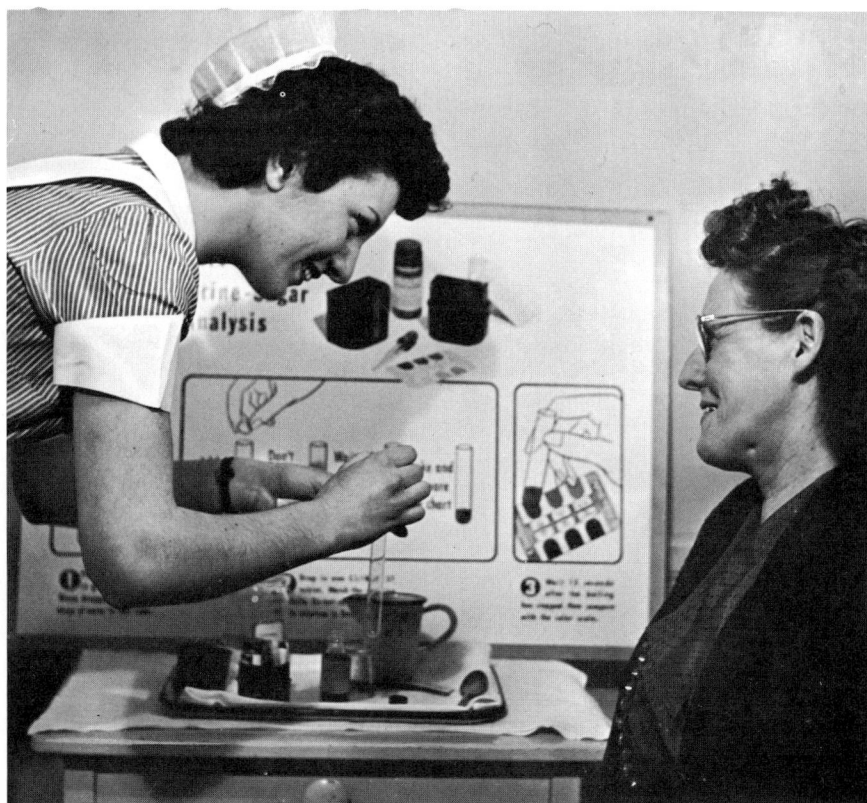

FIG. 322. Hospitalized diabetics should have ample opportunity to observe and rehearse the method of urinalysis that they will use after discharge.

specified intervals to the physician or the clinic. In preparation for this task, hospitalized diabetics should have ample opportunity to observe and rehearse the method of urinalysis that they will use after discharge (Fig. 322). Indeed, it is good practice to conduct these tests, occasionally at least, at the patient's bedside from the very beginning.

In the absence of complications, treatment may be started with 10 to 20 units of NPH insulin, given subcutaneously just before breakfast; this dosage may be increased at 2- to 7-day intervals, if necessary, by additions of 5 to 10 units until glycosuria is absent throughout the day and the night and the fasting blood-sugar level is normal. If the diabetes is obviously severe, larger doses are employed from the outset, and these are increased as rapidly as necessary. Patients receiving NPH insulin who exhibit glycosuria during the daytime only may receive supplementary injections of regular or crystalline zinc insulin. The latter is given in an initial dosage of 4 to 8 units, 2 to 8 units more being administered each day until glycosuria is controlled completely. The dosage of NPH insulin meanwhile is lowered, if necessary, in order to reduce the risk of delayed hypoglycemic reactions, which can be very dangerous, especially if they occur at night while the patient is asleep.

This regimen usually provides adequate control of the diabetes, especially if the carbohydrate intake is distributed appropriately. These patients should receive bedtime nourishment, consisting of 10 to 20 Gm. of carbohydrate, together with whatever fat and protein may be required to make this nourishment palatable. The remainder of the carbohydrate quota is divided as follows: one fifth for breakfast, two fifths for lunch and two fifths for supper. Those patients receiving combinations of NPH and crystalline (or regular) insulin before breakfast may be allotted one third of their carbohydrate quota at breakfast time, one third at lunch and one third at supper time, but a portion of the noon allotment (e.g., one serving of fruit) is prescribed as a midmorning snack, and an equal or larger portion of the evening meal is deferred until bedtime.

Complications of Insulin Treatment

LOCAL ALLERGIC REACTIONS. These consist of erythematous wheals, which usually disappear in the course of a few days. They may follow early injections of insulin. If such reactions continue to occur, crystalline insulin should be tried, for in many cases these allergic manifestations represent a sensitivity on the part of the patient to beef or pig protein present in the regular, but absent in the crystalline, product.

INSULIN LUMPS. These may appear at spots where injections are repeated at too frequent intervals. In these areas, absorption is diminished, and there is an increased susceptibility to local infection.

LOCALIZED FAT-TISSUE AND MUSCLE-TISSUE ATROPHY. This develops on rare occasions at the sites of injection and requires several months for restoration. Trials with other preparations—for example, those prepared from other animals or the crystalline product—are indicated.

HYPOGLYCEMIC REACTIONS. These are likely to occur when for any reason the blood sugar falls below 60 mg. per 100 ml. of blood. They result usually from the omission of a meal or the vomiting of a meal after taking insulin. Some attacks follow undue exertion. The majority of attacks occur in the morning and in the early evening.

These reactions begin in from 5 to 20 minutes following an injection of regular insulin, but not for several hours after NPH insulin is given. *The symptoms and the signs should be familiar to every nurse, and the warning symptoms should be described carefully to every diabetic patient receiving insulin.* If the blood sugar falls to a level between 70 and 50 mg. per 100 ml., general muscular weakness develops, together with mental confusion, restlessness, profuse sweating, vertigo, pallor or flushing of the face, trembling and, occasionally, hunger pangs in the epigastrium. If the level drops rapidly to below 50 or 40 mg. per 100 ml., the patient may become comatose. Some patients experience hypoglycemia so rapidly that the symptoms progress almost without warning to those of epileptiform convulsions. Hypoglycemic reactions exhibited by patients receiving NPH insulin may not follow this

FIG. 323. A sample identification card carried by diabetics on insulin to ensure the correct diagnosis and treatment if found in hypoglycemic shock.

SPECIAL IDENTIFICATION CARD

PLEASE NOTE: I use Insulin and am subject to Insulin reaction. If found bewildered, dazed or unconscious GIVE ME SUGAR IN ANY FORM AVAILABLE (Fruit Juice, Candy, Syrup, etc.) IMMEDIATELY ... then call nearest doctor.

Name_____ Phone_____

Address_____ City_____

My Doctor is _____ Phone_____

Address_____ City_____

FOR THE INFORMATION OF ANY DOCTOR			
MY DAILY DIET IS:	MY DAILY INSULIN DOSE IS:		
_____grms Carbo.	A.M.	NOON	P.M.
_____grms Prot.	_____Units	_____Units	_____Units	Prot.
_____grms. Fat	_____Units	_____Units	_____Units	Reg.

typical pattern; instead of pallor and sweating, the skin may be flushed, hot and dry, the patient disoriented and psychotic, or merely drowsy.

For immediate treatment, when the warning symptoms appear, the patient should take a drink containing sugar or consume a piece of candy. All patients on insulin should carry a chocolate bar, a few lumps of sugar or several crackers in their pockets. Such carbohydrate ingestion checks the reaction within a few minutes. If the patient is unconscious, *glucose* may be injected intravenously. A subcutaneous injection of *epinephrine* (0.3 to 0.5 ml. of a 1:1,000 solution) or *glucagon hydrochloride* (0.5 to 1.0 mg.) may be administered with the object of raising the blood sugar sufficiently to restore the patient to consciousness long enough to accept a sweetened drink, the effect of which will become manifest after perhaps 10 minutes and will terminate the attack.

In order to be assured of a correct diagnosis and prompt treatment, if discovered in a hypoglycemic state, every diabetic receiving insulin always should carry on his person an identification card similar to the type shown in Figure 323.

ORAL HYPOGLYCEMIC AGENTS

Effective control of diabetes solely by means of diet and oral medication has been a goal long sought by metabolic investigators, and material progress toward this objective has been made in recent years through the development of hypoglycemic drugs which share, to some extent, the therapeutic properties of insulin. Of these, the most widely tested to date have been tolbutamide (Orinase), which appears to stimulate the production of insulin by the pancreas and the reduction of glucose output by the liver. It is usually prescribed in a dose of 0.5 to 1.0 Gm. twice daily by mouth. Few complications have attended its use, approximately 3 per cent of patients receiving this drug having experienced digestive disturbances, exhibited skin eruptions and complained of intolerance to alcohol. Therapeutic effectiveness depends on close dietary control.

Orinase has proved to be most useful in the management of patients with stable diabetes which has had its onset in adult life and whose insulin requirement is less than 40 units daily. It is not suitable for patients whose diabetes began in childhood or early adolescence, whose diabetes is severe or of variable severity, who have ever experienced diabetic coma, who are undergoing major surgery or suffering from an acute infection.

Other hypoglycemic agents which may prove to be of value in the management of diabetes include chlorpropamide (Diabinese), administered in a single daily dose of 0.1 to 0.5 Gm., and phenethyldiguanide (DBI), which is ingested with meals or at bedtime in daily doses totaling 50 to 200 mg.

DIABETIC ACIDOSIS AND COMA

One of the most important functions of the nurse engaged in diabetic management is to be on the lookout for symptoms suggesting the onset of coma, the severest complication of diabetes mellitus—a complication to be dreaded, yet one that is entirely preventable and, if treated promptly and energetically, in most patients, curable. The severe cases are constantly faced with its threat. Its onset may be precipitated by many factors, including infections of all types, exposure and dietary indiscretions. The early symptoms include thirst, anorexia, nausea, vomiting, abdominal pain, headache, listlessness, drowsiness, weakness, vertigo, ringing in the ears, visual disturbances, excitement or delirium. Coma is ushered in with symptoms of air hunger (Kussmaul breathing), characterized by very deep, yet not labored, respiratory movements—a symptom of profound acidosis. The breath has a sweetish odor. The patient is drowsy and soon becomes comatose. Examination of the blood at this time reveals a high sugar concentration (and often an elevated N.P.N.), a low CO_2-combining power and increased acidity. The urine output may be diminished, and urinalysis shows marked glycosuria and the presence of ketone bodies (due to incomplete metabolism of carbohydrates, of which these are intermediary products). The situation at this stage is serious, but if therapy is initiated at once and pursued vigorously, improvement in most patients is evident within a few hours, and recovery is complete within from 1 to 3 days.

The patient with incipient coma should be put to bed, kept warm and given insulin, from 25 to 50 units subcutaneously immediately. Thereafter insulin is injected at intervals of from one half to 2 hours in doses of from 15 to 50 units, depending on the degree of glycosuria. Larger doses are safe only if the blood-sugar level can be determined before each injection. If the patient is unable to void, catheterization is advisable in view of the necessity for repeated collections and tests of the urine at this stage of treatment. Parenteral fluids are supplied in liberal amounts and consist of electrolyte repair solutions containing sodium, chloride and potassium ions and dextrose, for death in diabetic coma usually is attributable to dehydration and electrolyte imbalance. Norepinephrine is kept available in anticipation of the advent of vascular collapse.

Complete Diabetic Coma. This necessitates exactly the same procedure, except that all fluids have to be given parenterally, and

the insulin should be given at more frequent intervals (perhaps every hour). Ideally, each dose should depend on a blood-sugar determination, but this is rarely feasible, and, unless there is anuria, quite satisfactory and safe regulation can be accomplished on the basis of hourly urine examination. In any case, but particularly if glycosuria is to be the guide for insulin treatment during coma, the safe policy—and one which permits most vigorous insulin therapy—is to provide in the solution, which is being administered intravenously, enough glucose to "cover" the insulin (approximately 2 Gm. per unit). In this way the patient is protected from the danger of fatal hypoglycemia due to overenthusiastic insulin administration which develops subtly in the comatose patient.

Another immediate need of the patient in diabetic coma is for sodium, which may be injected intravenously in the form of sodium chloride. For the treatment of acidotic patients with renal failure, the physiologically correct proportions of sodium and chloride ions (approximately 3 to 2) are provided in the intravenous solution.

Another dangerous possibility is a deficiency in the concentration of potassium in the blood, giving rise to paralytic complications. This phenomenon is explained by the rapid migration of the potassium ion from the body fluids into the cells. In order to maintain its concentration in the blood, Butler's mixture or another source of potassium is included among the parenteral fluids administered at this stage. Electrolyte solutions are injected continuously until dehydration and acidosis are controlled, the urine output has improved and the patient is no longer comatose. Procrastination in fluid replacement may be responsible for the complication of hemoglobinuric nephrosis (p. 683), the patient perhaps recovering from his stupor, electrolyte imbalance, hyperglycemia and dehydration, only to relapse and finally succumb in terminal uremia.

Nursing Problems. Constant nursing care is an extremely important aspect of treatment in cases of diabetic coma, which is to be regarded in all respects as an emergency situation and treated as such. The patient is protected from excessive cooling by the application of extra blankets, and with the addition of an external heat source if the situation warrants.

The nurse is responsible for seeing that the equipment is assembled and making whatever preparations are necessary for gastric lavage, indicated for gastric dilatation of the stomach; catheterization; collection of venous blood; enemas; intravenous or subcutaneous infusions of saline, glucose and special electrolyte injections of repair solutions; blood transfusions; insulin injections; parenteral stimulants, such as caffeine, Coramine, Neo-Synephrine or norepinephrine. Frequent recordings are made of the blood pressure and the pulse rate, and the total amounts of parenteral fluid and insulin received and the time of their administration are noted. Her nursing notes should provide a concise description of the current situation, including the patient's clinical status and details regarding any change in the latter for better or for worse.

Treatment, unless hopelessly delayed, should be successful in the vast majority of cases, consciousness being restored and all metabolic disturbances corrected within 24 to 48 hours. The problem then becomes one of diabetic regulation, the various aspects of which have been considered. The precipitating cause of the coma and the manner of its onset must be investigated in an effort to discover some underlying condition that requires treatment or the recurrence of which may be prevented.

Education of the Diabetic Patient

Diabetes mellitus is a chronic disease requiring skillful, exacting and continuous care. Controls never can be relaxed; therefore, since professional supervision can be but occasional, the responsibility for carrying out treatment, to a large extent, must rest with the patient himself. As long as the course is uneventful, he serves as his own physician, nurse and laboratory technician, in preparation for which he must be well educated, not alone in the problems of diabetes, but also in matters pertaining to nutrition, preventive medicine, general health and hygiene. This educational program is extended whenever possible to include at least one responsible member of the patient's family.

Patient's Conception of the Disease. The patient must have a clear conception of the general character of diabetes. He must realize that his body metabolism is, and always will be, embarrassed by a deficiency in a chemical required for normal food utilization, but that this defect can be met perfectly satisfactorily by means of certain dietary adjustments, supplemented, if necessary, by injections of the missing material extracted from the pancreatic tissue of animals. He should be made to understand that, provided he follows faithfully the regimen that is prescribed for him, his prospects for a long, happy and effective life are excellent. Optimism along these lines, tempered with caution, is altogether proper, and its effects are highly beneficial as a stimulus to morale and a motive for self-discipline. On the other hand, he should be urged to avoid constructing for himself the concept that he is one of the afflicted: an individual set apart, who cannot identify himself with the normal group.

A completely favorable prognosis, if it is to be interpreted literally, implies that no irreversible damage to the vascular system had occurred before treatment was begun and that future damage can be prevented by perfect regulation of the diabetes. Unfortunately, however, this may not be the case; diabetic patients are unusually subject to the development of arteriosclerotic vascular disease, and in many instances this complication is well established before medical attention is sought. Obviously, irreparable disabilities which are present already should be de-emphasized, for discussion of these merely creates unnecessary anxiety in the patient's mind and serves no useful purpose. On the other hand, the patient must be familiarized with the preventable complications of diabetes in order to understand his own responsibilities in connection with their early recognition and their prevention.

Infection. The dangers associated with infection are important. Febrile illnesses decrease the food tolerance and raise the insulin requirement. Under such conditions, acidosis may develop quickly. Even mild respiratory infections should be treated with the greatest care. In any circumstances, if glycosuria is not controlled by the pre-

COMPARATIVE STUDY OF DIABETIC KETOACIDOSIS AND HYPOGLYCEMIA

The Patient with Diabetic Ketoacidosis

Definition

A lack of insulin resulting in a derangement of carbohydrate, fat and protein metabolism with dehydration and electrolyte imbalance.

Symptoms

Restlessness	Drowsiness
Dry skin	Rapid pulse
Flushed face	Deep respirations
Thirst	Lowered pulse pressure
Vomiting	Coma
Abdominal pain	

Objectives and Principles of Management

1. To restore carbohydrate utilization and correct electrolyte imbalance.
   - A. Secure blood and urine samples immediately.
     - a. Insert indwelling catheter (if so ordered by physician).
     - b. Obtain specimen at prescribed times.
     - c. Report blood glucose, CO_2, pH, electrolyte, acetone, BUN and hematocrit levels.
   - B. Administer rapid acting insulin intravenously.
     - a. Report blood glucose levels to the physician.
     - b. Give doses of insulin as ordered.
   - C. Replace fluids and electrolytes.
     - a. Give isotonic saline/sodium lactate solution I.V. to replace sodium loss.
     - b. Give supplementary potassium if ordered.
     - c. Measure and record intake and output.
     - d. Offer potassium-rich and sweetened fluids as soon as tolerated.
   - D. Treat for circulatory collapse if present.
     - a. Record vital signs every ½ hour.
     - b. Elevate the lower extremities.
     - c. Administer vasopressors as ordered.
   - E. Prepare for gastric lavage if ordered.

The Patient with Hypoglycemia

Definition

Low blood sugar usually due to excessive insulin due either to excessive insulin intake or to absorption from a tumor of an islet of Langerhans.

Symptoms

Headache	Tachycardia
Nervousness	Slurred speech
Hunger	Irrational behavior
Faintness	Convulsion
Sweating	Coma
Tremor	

Objectives and Principles of Management

1. To restore normal cerebral function as quickly as possible.
   - A. Secure blood and urine samples.
   - B. Prepare intravenous injection of 50 per cent glucose.
   - C. Prepare glucagon for subsequent use if necessary.
   - D. Obtain intravenous equipment for glucose infusion.
   - E. Remain with patient until he regains consciousness.
   - F. Have oral carbohydrates available.
   - G. Watch patient closely for evidences of recurrent hypoglycemia.

COMPARATIVE STUDY OF DIABETIC KETOACIDOSIS AND HYPOGLYCEMIA

The Patient with Diabetic Ketoacidosis (continued)

Objectives and Principles of Management

2. To prevent the recurrence of diabetic ketoacidosis:
   A. Avoid infection.
   B. Make insulin and dietary adjustments during the periods of illness.
   C. Teach the patient to:
      a. Accept responsibility for following his plan of care.
      b. Keep in balance his regimen of diet, insulin, and exercise.
      c. Keep his urine sugar free.
      d. Eat prescribed diet regularly.
      e. Increase his food during periods of exercise.
      f. Inform his physician when infection, vomiting, or diarrhea is present.

The Patient with Hypoglycemia (continued)

Objectives and Principles of Management

2. To prevent the recurrence of a hypoglycemic reaction:
   A. Reduce insulin dose.
   B. Test the urine 4 times daily for sugar and ketone.
   C. Adjust the patient's diet according to the patient's clinical response.
   D. Plan exercises according to patient's individual needs.
   E. Teach the patient to:
      a. Understand and develop an awareness of the actions of insulin.
      b. Keep in balance his regimen of diet, insulin, and exercise.
      c. Eat when the symptoms of hypoglycemia *first* occur.
      d. Carry candy or lump sugar in his pocket.
      e. Have available vials of injectable glucagon hydrochloride.

To facilitate recognition and treatment, instruct the patient to carry an identification card on his person at all times (Fig. 323).

scribed regimen, medical advice should be sought; and should any untoward symptoms, such as nausea, vomiting, faintness, etc., develop, the patient should go to bed at once and summon the physician.

Skin Care. It is particularly important to keep the skin clean, warm and free from irritation. If the diabetes has been regulated improperly, the skin is very apt to be dry and rough; it may be the site of intense itching and eczematous involvement, and boils, carbuncles, decubitus ulcers and gangrenous lesions are unusually prone to develop. Prerequisite to improvement of these skin complications is adequate regulation of the diabetes; healing, then, is facilitated by the application of unguents. (Alcohol lotions, which further dehydrate the skin, are to be avoided.)

Scrupulous care of the feet and the toes is of paramount importance. Shoes should fit, and be kept in good repair. The patient is taught to avoid constricting the circulation. Clean socks or stockings should be worn at all times, and these should be woven from cotton or wool thread rather than nonwettable plastic fibers.

The nurse has an opportunity to teach ways of preventing skin breaks. Pressure points, such as corns, calluses, blisters and ingrown toenails, can be eliminated if properly fitting shoes and stockings are worn. The feet should be washed daily and patted dry with a soft towel. No friction should be exerted. Lanolin spread thinly is effective in keeping the skin soft, and the placing of lamb's wool between the toes will help to prevent friction. Nails may be cut straight across.

The patient must be made aware of the

> The American Diabetes Association has prepared the following checklist of nine basic elements of treatment that should be included in the education of every diabetic patient:
>
> 1. Diet
> 2. Urine testing
> 3. Action of insulin and other hypoglycemic agents
> 4. Technic of insulin injection and sites for it
> 5. Care of syringe and of insulin
> 6. Symptoms of hypoglycemia
> 7. Symptoms of uncontrolled diabetes
> 8. Care of the feet
> 9. What to do in case of acute complications
>
> Every member of the health team should see that the diabetic patient has an understanding of these elements of treatment.

dangers of bruises resulting from accidentally bumping into carelessly placed footstools and other furniture. Proper lighting and well-fitting eyeglasses are necessities for these individuals.

In the presence of advanced peripheral arteriosclerosis, so common in diabetes, what appear to be trivial infections about the nails may become gangrenous and lead to the loss of the limb. An appreciation of the great importance of skin care should be inculcated before the patient is discharged from the hospital, and in this part of his education the nurse must participate conscientiously in order that he may be able to carry out a satisfactory hygienic regimen thereafter.

General Regimen. The regimen imposed on the patient is adjusted to conform as closely as possible to his normal habits of life. The necessity for the provision of adequate rest and relaxation should be emphasized. If insomnia becomes a difficulty, mild sedatives are indicated. Moderate, but consistent, muscular activity is advisable to maintain sound health and normal vigor, for the carbohydrate tolerance is, thereby, increased and the insulin requirement is lowered.

Social service departments are usually instrumental in providing the equipment needed for insulin injections and urinalyses, if they cannot be secured otherwise because of economic reasons. The public-health nurse often serves a most important role in the education of the diabetic patient, in-

structing him in hygienic precautions, the interpretation of urine tests and the self-administration of insulin. Group instruction has proved to be an effective method of education, and diabetic clinics, organized on this basis by physicians, hospitals and public health departments, have contributed much to the comfort, welfare and security of these patients.

Prognosis

There is no conclusive evidence that diabetes mellitus is ever cured, although prolonged amelioration of the disorder has been observed—this, however, not as a result of therapy but related to metabolic changes in the individual, associated, for example, with the correction of obesity or the healing of an infection. However, although the underlying metabolic disorder may be expected to persist indefinitely, it can be compensated satisfactorily by means of a proper diet and insulin regimen. These measures, together with those designed to improve the general condition of the patient, restore to the diabetic a metabolic state that is essentially normal. If treatment is begun early, before arteriosclerotic changes have appeared, and is directed skillfully and followed faithfully, there is every reason to anticipate a reasonable life expectancy.

Diabetic patients should no longer die of diabetes; diabetic coma, which formerly was responsible for the death of almost two thirds of all patients, must now be considered to be the result of gross neglect. Of all diabetic complications, arteriosclerosis is the most unfortunate, coronary and peripheral arterial disease constituting a very real hazard in even the mildest cases. It is probable that the incidence of this complication will eventually be reduced among cases treated early and adequately.

Infections are more difficult to treat in the diabetic, both because susceptibility to them may be increased and because the diabetes itself becomes temporarily more severe in the course of infections. Every means must be utilized to prevent them, and their early diagnosis is imperative. Chest roentgenograms should be taken in the course of the diabetic study to rule out tuberculosis; they should be part of the routine examination of all diabetic children, among whom the incidence of tuberculosis is significantly higher than it is among the general population. Its prognosis, however, if both the infection and the carbohydrate metabolism are well controlled, is probably no less favorable than in the absence of diabetes.

Surgery in Diabetes

Surgery is not used to treat diabetes. However, many diabetics require surgery for other conditions, some of them complications of diabetes. In either case, it is generally conceded that a patient with diabetes is a poor operative risk. This is due, in part, to the fact that the majority of such patients are old and are already in a state of general decline or are prematurely "old" because of early arteriosclerosis. The resistance to infection is low, healing is usually delayed, and serious diabetic complications, such as coma, often follow minor infections and even minor operative procedures.

With the advent of insulin and the facilities for chemical analysis of the blood, the prognosis for the diabetic has improved materially. The metabolic problems which previously complicated nearly every surgical operation now can be solved rapidly and often surely by proper pre- and postoperative treatment. Insulin and the administration of glucose, either by mouth (orange juice) or intravenously, are the usual preoperative measures. Fluids should be supplied in abundance. The operation should take place not more than 2 hours after the last prescribed food given in liquid form.

The anesthetics which experience has shown to be best fitted for the diabetic are the gases (nitrous oxide or ethylene) or spinal anesthesia. Postoperatively, food and fluids are given as soon as possible, with sufficient insulin to prevent acidosis. Because postoperative vomiting may often occur, it is the practice in some clinics to pass a nasogastric tube before or immediately after operation. Fluids and liquid foods may be given slowly by this method almost immediately after operation. The operations most commonly performed are amputations for gangrene. The utmost care must be employed in dressing the wounds of diabetics to prevent infection. (See Chap. 42, p. 1014.)

Gangrene of the toes and the foot is the most frequent surgical complication of the diabetic. It occurs due to an early development of arteriosclerosis. Many prophylactic measures have been suggested, the chief of which is cleanliness of the feet. A second is a warning against the promiscuous cutting of corns and calluses. A frequently obtained history is one of the onset of gangrene immediately after cutting a corn on unclean feet. The cold and painful extremities which are the premonitory signs of gangrene are often carelessly treated by heat. Burns which too often occur may mark the onset of gangrene. The treatment of early gangrene has been described elsewhere (p. 497).

Diet for Surgical Diabetics. The preoperative treatment is to store sufficient glycogen in the liver to protect the patient against the anesthetic. This carbohydrate may be given in the form of tea and toast, orange juice, oatmeal, or oatmeal gruel. Insulin must be given in order to metabolize it. After operation, as well as before, hyperglycemia and its threatening acidosis or hypoglycemia due to starvation caused by insufficient food or excess of insulin to burn the food eaten must be guarded against. For the first 24 hours after nausea ceases oatmeal gruel or orange juice, plain or with glucose added, is given. If not tolerated by mouth, glucose is given intravenously. The carbohydrate feedings should be stopped 3 hours prior to the operation and resumed 3 hours after the operation. Insulin should be given before each feeding to ensure the utilization of the food.

When liquid diet may be replaced by soft and light diet, the patient will gradually be put back on his former diet or one that is found to be more suitable.

Nursing Care. Any infection is a source of potential danger because organisms thrive and spread more rapidly when blood sugar content is above normal. Whether the patient with diabetes has had surgery or is to have surgery, the principles of care remain the same. Essentially, trauma to tissues must be minimized if not eliminated, and the metabolic balance must be maintained. If not, the patient risks the hazards of spreading infection with necrosis and experiences the metabolic imbalances of diabetic coma or insulin shock.

A furuncle or corn never should be squeezed or cut; scratches and burns must be prevented. Once a local infection is present, it is difficult to control.

When a wound is present, aseptic technic must be followed in an attempt to prevent infection from spreading.

The nurse is responsible for serving an attractive diet, noting what has not been eaten and reporting it so that a proper substitute may be made to maintain metabolic balance. She is also responsible for the collection of urine and blood specimens and their proper disposition to the laboratory. These two functions are as important as the giving of medications.

The surgical patient may face any one or all three of the following disturbances which interfere with a properly balanced metabolism: (1) Vomiting. This should be inspected for food loss and reported so that essential food value may be replaced intravenously. (2) Starvation. Prior to surgery, a patient is placed on nothing by mouth. Infusions of glucose and injections of insulin are used to maintain balance. (3) Febrile reactions are sufficient to upset carbohydrate metabolism, and appropriate steps must be taken to maintain metabolic balance by increasing insulin. In addition to the above, an adequate protein reserve must be established prior to operation and the salt and water balance must be maintained.

Diabetes with the threat of coma or insulin shock requires close attention and observation on the part of the nurse. She should have insulin and intravenous glucose solution on hand for immediate use in any possible emergency.

Hyperinsulinism

This disorder develops as a result of the overproduction of insulin by the pancreatic islets. Its symptoms resemble those which follow excessive doses of insulin and are attributable to the same mechanism—an abnormal reduction in the concentration of blood sugar. Clinically, it is characterized by attacks, or episodes, in which the patient experiences unusual hunger, nervousness, sweating, headache and faintness; in severe cases, convulsive seizures and episodes of unconsciousness may occur. As in patients with hypoglycemia due to insulin therapy, all of the symptoms that accompany the spontaneous variety are relieved by the oral or parenteral administration of glucose. The findings at the time of operation, or postmortem examination, may indicate hyperplasia (overgrowth) of the islets of Langerhans, or a malignant tumor, i.e., carcinoma, involving the islets and capable of producing large amounts of insulin. This condition is of considerable interest inasmuch as it occasionally is responsible for epileptic seizures, convulsions coinciding with decreases in the blood sugar concentration to levels which are inadequate to sustain normal brain function (i.e., below 30 mg. per cent). Surgical extirpation of the hyperplastic or neoplastic tissue from the pancreas offers the only successful method of treatment. (See Chap. 31, p. 672.)

Hypoglycemic shock, due to injections of insulin, has been discussed as a complication of diabetic management. Its purposeful induction in nondiabetic patients has been employed with some success in treating certain mental diseases, notably schizophrenia, although its therapeutic value in these patients has not been satisfactorily explained.

THE ADRENAL GLAND

Each adrenal gland represents, in fact, two different glands, with different anatomic characteristics and different functions to perform in the endocrine system. In some animals these structures are actually separate in location; in man, however, they are fused together and incorporated in one organ, forming the cortex and medullary portion of each adrenal.

The medulla is the source of epinephrine and produces about one half of the total supply of l-norepinephrine in the body, both hormones being secreted in response to nerve impulses transmitted via the sympathetic nervous system. The cortex of the adrenal, on the other hand, receives its controlling stimuli via the blood stream, delivered in the form of a hormone from the anterior pituitary gland (i.e., the adrenocorticotropic hormone, or ACTH).

The Adrenal Cortex

Four hormones are known to be produced by the adrenal cortex: hydrocortisone, in 10- to 20-mg. quantities each day; aldosterone, 0.2 to 0.4 mg. daily; corticosterone, and 11-oxy-17-ketosteroids, which are delivered in very small quantities. Hydrocortisone is concerned with the transfer of sodium, chloride and other ions through cell membranes, hence, with regulating the volume and the composition of intracellular and extracellular fluids. It enhances the metabolic breakdown of body proteins and fat to form glucose, thereby providing a source of quick energy at times of stress and duress; and it tends to retard reticuloendothelial growth and activity, thus limiting the vigor of immune responses and restricting the intensity of inflammatory reactions. Aldosterone promotes the secretion of potassium and hydrogen ions into the urine, as a result of which sodium is returned to the blood from the glomerular filtrate. This is one of the mechanisms by which the concentrations of these ions are adjusted individually and maintained at physiologic levels. Corticosterone and 11-oxy-17-ketosteroids serve many functions in relation to organic metabolism and to the development of secondary sex characters.

Addison's Disease

Addison's disease, due to a deficiency of cortical hormones, results when the adrenal cortex is destroyed. This is most commonly the result of tuberculous infection of the gland. This hormonal deficiency gives rise to a characteristic clinical picture. The chief signs and symptoms include muscular weakness, anorexia, gastrointestinal symptoms, emaciation, generalized dark pigmentation of the skin and the findings of low blood pressure, low blood sugar, low B.M.R., low blood sodium and high blood potassium. Most of the symptoms arise from the disturbance of sodium and potassium metabolism, the potassium retention enhancing the excretion and, hence, depletion of the sodium, which circumstance results in water loss and severe chronic dehydration.

Diagnosis. The diagnosis of Addison's disease depends on the proper identification of the signs of adrenocortical insufficiency. These include a decrease in the concentrations of blood sugar and sodium (hypoglycemia and hyponatremia), an increased concentration of blood potassium (hyperkalemia) and lymphoid hyperplasia. Particular importance is attached to the finding of a decreased concentration of sodium in the blood.

A valuable contribution to diagnosis is the observation that no change occurs in the number of eosinophils in the blood or in the excretion of uric acid in the urine (which reflects the dissolution of body proteins) following artificial stimulation of the adrenals by an injection of potent pituitary adrenocorticotropic hormone. Unless the adrenal cortex is destroyed or is incapable, for any reason, of responding to this stimulus, a fall in the circulating eosinophils and an increase in uric acid excretion is expected in about 4 hours; in Addison's disease, the response is diminished or absent.

Treatment and Nursing Care. Treatment of Addison's disease consists of an attempt to restore the normal electrolyte balance, first by a high-sodium, low-potassium diet and fluids, and second by the administration of hydrocortisone (17-hydroxycorticosterone). Patients in addisonian crisis should receive this hormone in injectable form (e.g., Solu-Cortef; Hydrocortone Phosphate) by the intravenous route in 50 to 100 mg. doses, as required. Effective replacement therapy may be supplied on a long-term basis by the daily ingestion of hydrocortisone in 30 to 40 mg. doses.

Nursing Precautions. During hospitalization a close watch is kept for changes in the vital signs. Any symptoms such as cyanosis, nausea, vomiting or sudden fall in blood pressure are suggestive of a sudden exacerbation of the disease (addisonian crisis). Even slight overexertion, exposure to cold, acute infections, a decrease in the salt intake or diarrhea from overenthusiastic purgation may lead to circulatory collapse; the systolic pressure falls to 40 or 50 mm. of mercury, the pulse is weak, the skin is cold and clammy, and there is danger of death. In this situation the blood volume must be increased as soon as possible by means of blood transfusions, intravenous injection of sodium chloride solution and by the administration of cortical extract or hydrocortisone. External heat is applied, and circulatory stimulants are injected. Patients frequently recover from these crises of adrenal insuffi-

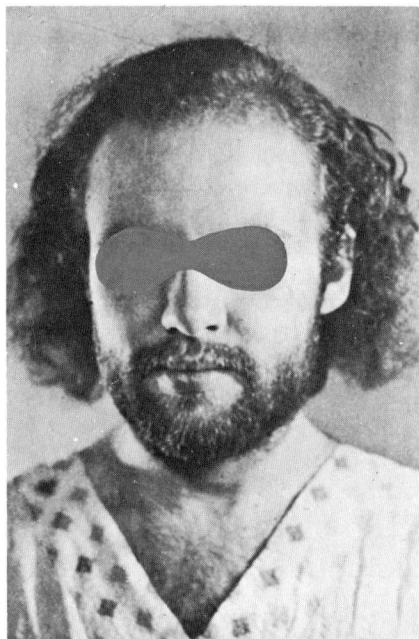

FIG. 324. A 16-year-old girl with developed hirsutism, masculinity and a heavy beard that grew with great strength in childhood. She menstruated 1 day only when she was 16 years old. A large adrenal shadow was demonstrated by roentgenogram after perirenal injection. At operation a large cortical adrenal adenoma was removed.

ciency and may die unexpectedly when apparently quite well.

The nurse has a particular responsibility in the accurate calculation and recording of the salt intake and the urine output. Emphasis is placed on adequate rest, warmth and the avoidance of overexertion, catharsis and exposure to cold. A high salt intake, adequate diet, cortical hormone and care of underlying tuberculosis, if such is present, are of paramount importance. With proper therapy the prognosis is favorable for extended periods of time.

Cushing's Syndrome

Cushing's syndrome is the antithesis of Addison's disease, its clinical characteristics reflecting excessive, rather than deficient, adrenocortical activity. The basic lesion responsible for Cushing's syndrome may be either a tumor arising in the cortex of one of the adrenal glands or a basophilic adenoma of the pituitary gland (see p. 847) involving an overgrowth of pituitary cells producing the adrenocorticotropic hormone (ACTH).

The outstanding features of this syndrome include an increase in blood sodium and blood sugar and a decreased concentration of potassium, a reduction in the number of blood eosinophils and a disappearance of lymphoid tissue. When overproduction of the adrenal cortical hormone occurs in childhood, precocious puberty is observed, and in females of all ages, masculinization, or "virilism," is produced.

Virilism is characterized by the appearance of masculine and the recession of feminine physical and mental traits. There is an excessive growth of hair on the face (hirsutism), the breasts atrophy, the menses cease, the clitoris enlarges, and the patient's voice and habits approach the masculine. Arrhenoblastoma of the ovary will simulate the above symptom complex. When the disease occurs in children, a precocious puberty results. If these changes occur in utero, a true hermaphrodite may be the result. If the change begins in early childhood, pseudohermaphrodism will result.

Primary Aldosteronism

The principal action of aldosterone is to conserve body sodium. This is accomplished at the expense of potassium and hydrogen ions which the kidneys excrete in increased amounts, while the excretion of sodium is lessened, under the influence of this hormone. Excessive production of aldosterone, which occurs in some patients with functioning tumors of the adrenal gland, causes a distinctive pattern of biochemical changes and a corresponding set of clinical signs and symptoms which are diagnostic of this condition. Such patients exhibit a profound decline in the level of potassium (hypokalemia) and in the hydrogen ion concentration in the blood (alkalosis), as demonstrated by an increase in its pH and carbon-dioxide-combining power. The blood sodium is elevated (hypernatremia).

Hypokalemia is responsible for the periodic development of marked muscle weakness in patients with aldosteronism, as well as an inability on the part of their kidneys to concentrate the urine. Accordingly, the urine volume is excessive; these patients complain of polyuria. Their blood sodium, by contrast, becomes abnormally concentrated, which explains their excessive thirst (polydipsia) and may account for arterial hypertension. Tetany and paresthesias are to be expected in such patients, as complications of alkalosis. Cure usually follows surgical removal of the adrenal tumor.

Therapeutic Applications of Corticotropin (ACTH) and the Corticosteroids

Of the many notable achievements of medical science during the past few years, among the most outstanding have been the chemical identification and synthesis and the large-scale production of agents which share the endocrine properties of the adrenal steroid hormones. As a group, these compounds are referred to as the "corticosteroids." They include *cortisone* (17-hydroxy-11-dehydrocorticosterone), *hydrocortisone* (17-desoxycorticosterone), *prednisone* (delta-1-cortisone), *prednisolone* (delta-1-hydrocortisone), *triamcinolone* (9α-fluoro-16α-hydroxyprednisolone) and *dexamethasone* (9α-fluoro-16α-methyl prednisolone). The availability of pituitary extracts with potent corticotrophic activity (ACTH) and the advent of these synthetic corticosteroid drugs represent a therapeutic milestone. These drugs, possessing the endocrine activity of the adrenal cortex, and ACTH, which activates the adrenal cortex, offer remarkable benefits in

many diseases. Their value, as therapeutic agents, is poorly understood but appears to rest on their ability to suppress inflammation. Inflammatory processes, and processes of repair, although basically protective, may be damaging to the patient.

Inflammatory reactions are reduced in severity, or altogether prevented from occurring, whether they are excited in response to chemical irritants, antigenic foreign proteins or micro-organisms. This action on the part of the adrenocortical hormone provides the rationale for its use in such inflammatory disorders as rheumatic fever, rheumatoid arthritis, lupus erythematosus disseminata, periarteritis nodosa, severe allergic reactions involving the skin, the respiratory tract and the gastrointestinal tract or inflammatory lesions within the eye. Depression of antibody production is one of the reasons for its effectiveness in acquired hemolytic jaundice and in idiopathic thrombocytopenic purpura, caused by red cell and platelet antibodies, respectively. Moreover, in purpura of all types, as in all varieties of inflammation, the presence of this hormone appears to improve the stamina and to maintain the integrity of the smaller blood vessels, thus preventing their leakage or their rupture.

The inhibiting effect of the hormone on reparative processes stems from its ability to prevent the congregation of reticulum cells, as well as local accumulations of lymphocytes and fibroblasts. Not only does it impede production, but it also favors disintegration of reticulum and fibrous tissue in areas of inflammation, thereby forestalling their disabling activities in vulnerable regions, such as the joints and the eyes. The "lympholytic" action of the hormone is used to advantage in treating the lymphoid tumors, including lymphatic leukemia, lyphosarcoma and the lymphomas.

Other disorders that are reportedly benefited by the administration of adrenocortical hormone include chronic ulcerative colitis and idiopathic steatorrhea, the granulomatous lung lesions of sarcoid and beryllium poisoning and poisoning by animal venoms. These drugs are also useful in the treatment of some types of malignant tumors. The adrenal hormone also is said to facilitate drug withdrawal in cases of addiction and to speed recovery from delirium tremens.

The biologic products and synthetic drugs that currently are available for corticosteroid therapy are specified below, together with details concerning their administration.

ACTH (corticotropin, Acthar), in contrast with the adrenal hormones, is available not as a pure synthetic compound but as a complex mixture of proteins extracted from animal pituitary glands. Given intramuscularly once or twice daily, its anti-inflammatory effect is approximately equal, milligram for milligram, to that of hydrocortisone. The most efficient, but least convenient, method of giving ACTH is in the form of a constant intravenous infusion.

Cortisone usually is given by mouth in the form of tablets containing cortisone acetate. A microcrystalline suspension of this material in physiologic saline is available for intramuscular injection.

For the topical application of cortisone to the eye, one may utilize a microcrystalline suspension of the acetate, or an ophthalmic ointment consisting of a petrolatum base and containing cortisone acetate.

Hydrocortisone likewise is available in tablet form as the acetate ester (Cortef). This product is twice as potent as cortisone, and its dosage is correspondingly smaller. For purposes of intravenous or intramuscular administration hydrocortisone phosphate (Hydrocortone, Cortiphate) or succinate (Solu-Cortef) may be selected. A microcrystalline suspension of hydrocortisone acetate in saline is available for intra-articular injection in cases of noninfectious inflammatory diseases of the joints. A collyrium for the local treatment of inflammatory lesions in the anterior segment of the eye may be prepared by diluting this suspension with 4 parts of physiologic saline solution, or with a 1:5,000 solution of aqueous Zephiran Chloride.

Prednisone (Meticorten, Deltra, Deltasone) and *prednisolone* (Meticortelone, Meprolone, Cordex) are entirely comparable as regards potency, therapeutic efficacy and side-effects. Their anti-inflammatory and antiallergic actions are approximately 5 times as powerful, but their salt-retaining effect is less pronounced, than that of cortisone. These compounds are absorbed readily and are rapidly effective after oral ingestion.

Aqueous suspensions of prednisolone acetate are available for injection into joint cavities and bursae, and prednisolone sodium hemisuccinate is distributed as a sterile, pyrogen-free soluble powder, ready for solution and intravenous injection.

Triamcinolone (Aristocort, Kenacort), a fluorinated derivative of prednisolone, exhibits 50 per cent more anti-inflammatory, anti-allergic and antirheumatic activity than prednisone or prednisolone. It is approximately 4 times as effective therapeutically as hydrocortisone and 6 times as effective as cortisone. On the other hand, triamcinolone has little or no tendency to cause sodium retention, edema or potassium excretion.

Dexamethasone (Decadron, Deronil) is the most potent anti-inflammatory agent in the pharmacopeia. Another fluorinated derivative of prednisolone, this drug is 4 to 5 times as effective as triamcinolone (30 to 40 times as potent as hydrocortisone), and its dosage is computed accordingly.

Nursing Activities Related to Steroid Therapy

Many potential hazards attend the use of these powerful endocrine agents, each complication being based on one or more of the physiologic properties of the adrenocortical hormone that have been described.

Prolonged administration of the corticoids results in complete suppression of ACTH formation by the pituitary. Too abrupt cessation of steroid therapy, therefore, is dangerous from the standpoint of precipitating adrenocortical failure, i.e., the equivalent of an addisonian crisis.

The suppressive effect of this therapy on inflammatory lesions strips the patient of some very important defenses against bacterial invasion. Moreover, it tends to obscure the presence of an infection. Latent tuberculosis may be reactivated and spread extensively, or a virulent bacterial pneumonia may develop with complications of bacteremia, yet remain entirely unrecognized and unsuspected until death. All candidates for this endocrine therapy should be questioned with care, and have their lungs examined by x-ray before treatment is started, in order to exclude pulmonary tuberculosis. After treatment has begun, each should be scrutinized repeatedly each day by the nurse and the physician in search of any evidence which might suggest the onset of some infectious complication, so that effective antibacterial chemotherapy, if indicated, will not be delayed.

Interference with inflammation implies interference with tissue repair, introducing an important and difficult problem in the care of any patient who has sustained a traumatic wound or who may require surgical treatment. It also favors the reactivation of peptic ulcer as well as the penetration of a peptic ulcer into or through the visceral wall, silently and without warning. With this in mind, patients with a history suggestive of peptic ulcer, in the present or in the past, should receive steroids only if the therapeutic indications are compelling, and provided that appropriate studies have been completed which appear to exclude the presence of a lesion.

The effect of the adrenal cortex on water and electrolyte metabolism constitutes a potential danger in patients with diminished cardiac reserve because of the risk of promoting edema through excessive sodium and water retention. All patients receiving ACTH, cortisone or hydrocortisone should be restricted in their sodium intake. Moreover, such patients should be weighed and examined for edema each day in order to detect any signs of water retention. Because of its effect on potassium metabolism, which is responsible for the wastage of that element in the urine, the patient's diet should be supplemented with potassium in the form of 2 to 3 Gm. of potassium chloride each day. The nurse should determine to her own satisfaction that this supplement has, in fact, been received and ingested; moreover, she should be on the alert for signs of potassium deficiency, notably generalized muscular weakness.

Certain complications may be of less serious import, and yet may be the principal source of anxiety on the part of the patient and demand logical and convincing explanations on the part of the nurse. In the course of steroid therapy the skin is apt to become more darkly pigmented. Moreover, the skin becomes thinned, sometimes to the point of

uncovering pigmented striations in the region of the thighs, the buttocks and the abdomen. Acne may erupt on the face and the trunk. Female patients may be very disturbed by the discovery of an appreciable growth of facial hair and may be further concerned by the appearance of her face, if the typical "moon facies" has become pronounced.

A complication that occurs not uncommonly, and may present unusual difficulties from the nurse's standpoint, is the development of a psychological disturbance following the onset of steroid therapy. There is no uniformity of pattern that is evident in these manifestations, except to the extent that they often appear to represent an exaggeration of some pre-existing aberration of personality.

Psychiatric complications of steroid treatment, like its other complications, are reversible in time, but the length of time that is required for complete return to the pretreatment status may extend to 2 or 3 months, and, meanwhile, the patient may be in serious jeopardy as a potential suicide. Every patient who is placed on steroids or ACTH should be regarded by the nurse in the category of a potential psychiatric casualty, and she should continue to regard each one as such until his response to therapy has become stabilized and he can be evaluated from the standpoint of emotional pattern, degree of activity and excitability, level of mood, coloring of interpretation, relations with other persons in his environment and his integration in general. If these appear to be within normal limits and represent no essential change from his earlier status, he may be given a good prognosis as regards his psychological integrity.

A potential hazard associated with steroid therapy is the chance that treatment may be discontinued abruptly as a result of inadvertent omission of the appropriate orders. This error may be made when a patient, previously on maintenance therapy, is first admitted to the hospital. It also can, and does, occur from time to time when a patient is transferred from one hospital service to another or, in the case of postoperative patients, when a new set of orders is written. Thus, in preparation for surgery, a patient who is on oral steroid therapy will have all oral medications omitted as a matter of hospital routine. Parenteral steroids, for example, in the form of intramuscular hydrocortisone, will be substituted for the oral hormone. Forty-eight hours later all parenteral therapy is discontinued, including parenteral fluids, nutrients, stimulants, sedatives and hydrocortisone. It is not difficult to imagine that the hydrocortisone may be dealt with in the same manner as the other injected drugs and materials, without thought of continuing its administration in another form. When this happens, the patient's postoperative course becomes very stormy indeed. Blood pressure drops to levels that are alarmingly low; he becomes febrile, complains of fever, weakness and abdominal pain, and may experience vomiting, diarrhea or both. The longer the patient has been maintained on steroids and the higher the maintenance dose, the more severe will be the withdrawal symptoms, and before the situation is recognized, he may die in an addisonian crisis. The nurse is in a position to minimize the risk of such tragedies and should be on the alert to the possibility of its occurrence in any case whose preoperative or operative orders have included steroid therapy.

The Adrenal Medulla

The medullary portion of the adrenal gland is the source of two powerful stimulants, *epinephrine* and *norepinephrine,* which are secreted instantly in the event of an emergency, real or threatened, placing the individual in a state of readiness for "fight or flight," as the case may be.

These two hormones function jointly to speed the delivery of fuel to organs whose activities are of immediate importance, and facilitate the removal of wastes, including excess heat, from those organs. Norepinephrine causes all arterioles, excepting those in the heart muscle, to constrict, thereby raising the systolic and diastolic pressures. The effect of epinephrine is to increase the pulse rate and cardiac output. It also counteracts the vasoconstricting action of norepinephrine in crucial areas, such as the brain, the muscles of the trunk and the extremities and the skin, causing all vessels in those organs to dilate. The net effect of both

hormones, therefore, is to increase both the flow rate and the volume of blood flowing through the brain, the muscles, the myocardium and the skin.

Epinephrine causes the liver to unload some of its carbohydrate stores, with the result that the level of blood sugar is increased. It induces sweating, which, together with hyperemia of the skin, permits more rapid cooling of the blood. It also dilates the ocular pupils, assuring maximum acuity of vision. Finally, among its other effects, epinephrine stimulates the anterior pituitary gland to produce adrenocorticotropic hormone (ACTH) and, thereby, forces the release of hydrocortisone and aldosterone from the adrenal cortex. The latter is the basis of the so-called "alarm reaction," which serves to reduce the severity of tissue responses, in general, to injury.

Pheochromocytoma

Functioning tumors of the adrenal medulla, or *pheochromocytoma,* cause arterial hypertension and other cardiovascular disturbances. The nature and severity depend on the relative proportions of epinephrine and norepinephrine in its secretions.

The hypertension may be paroxysmal or chronic. If it is of the chronic, sustained type, it may be difficult to distinguish these cases from those having so-called "essential hypertension," a differential diagnosis which is most important. In addition to hypertension, the symptoms are essentially the same as those encountered after the administration of epinephrine in large doses, namely, tachycardia, excessive perspiration, tremor, nervousness and hyperglycemia.

The clinical picture of pheochromocytoma usually is characterized by acute, unpredictable attacks, lasting several hours or only a few seconds, during which the patient feels excessively anxious, tremulus and weak and suffers from headache, vertigo, blurring of vision, tinnitus and air hunger. Other symptoms include polyuria, nausea, vomiting, diarrhea and abdominal pain.

Diagnosis and Treatment. The diagnosis of pheochromocytoma is suspected if signs of sympathetic overactivity occur in association with marked elevations of blood pressure. Diagnostic proof may require surgical exploration, but a presumptive diagnosis is often possible before operation with the aid of tests which depend on the reaction of the blood pressure to *provocative* drugs and to *adrenergic blocking* drugs. Provocative agents are those which stimulate a sharp rise, and adrenergic blocking drugs a definite fall, in arterial pressure in patients with this disease. The provocative drugs include histamine, tetraethylammonium chloride (or bromide) and methacholine (Mecholyl). The testing agent of choice among the adrenergic blocking agents is phentolamine (Regitine), which neutralizes the action of epinephrine. Injections of this material in patients with epinephrine-secreting tumors cause a precipitous fall in the arterial blood pressure. Determinations of the catecholamines in urine and blood offer the most direct and conclusive test for overactivity of the adrenal medulla. VMA (vinyl mandelic acid) determination in particular is preferable. (Normal urinary values: 2 to 6 mg/24 hrs.)

Patients with pheochromocytoma may be cured by excision of the tumor. In anticipation of surgery, attempts are made to localize the tumor by the injection of air into the retroperitoneal tissues. By this injection the retroperitoneal structures may be outlined on an x-ray film. The pheochromocytoma presents as an enlargement of the shadow of the adrenal on the side of the tumor.

Adrenalectomy

For Adrenal Tumors. All of the endocrine disturbances associated with a functioning tumor of the adrenal cortex or medulla can be relieved completely, and the patient improved dramatically, by surgical removal of the involved gland. Adrenalectomy is performed through an incision in the loin or the abdomen. In general, the postoperative care resembles that given for any abdominal operation. Some patients with adrenal cortical tumors may require the temporary administration of a steroid hormone, such as hydrocortisone, after operation. More serious problems may attend and follow adrenalectomy for pheochromocytoma, manipulation of this tumor at operation often producing extreme fluctuations in arterial pressure that must be counteracted by appropriate drugs. After ligation of the vessels leading from the tumor, an abrupt fall in blood pressure is apt to occur, which may require the administration of large amounts of epinephrine intravenously. Nursing care in the postoperative state often involves frequent estimation of blood pressure and the regulation of vasopressor intravenous drugs for as long as 24 to 48 hours.

For Malignancy of Breast or Prostate. Certain malignancies, notably those of the breast and the prostate, are affected by the hormones produced by endocrine glands. Thus the ovary is known to have an effect on carcinoma of the breast, and the testes on carcinoma of the prostate. In some cases, even after ablation of endocrine stimulation, the hormones are still present, and they have been found to arise from adrenal glands. For this reason bilateral adrenalectomy is often performed in an effort to control or benefit recurrent carcinoma of the breast or the prostate. The adrenals are approached either transabdominally or through the bed of the 12th rib from behind. Postoperatively, adrenal cortical hormone must be administered in appropriate dosage to overcome the sudden deprivation of these hormones by the operation. As time goes on, the dosage of adrenal cortical hormone may be reduced gradually as the body adjusts itself to its new plane of hormone production.

For Hypertension. Since the adrenal is an important organ in the production of epinephrine, which constricts blood vessels and increases blood pressure, the adrenals have been removed in an effort to treat hypertension and sometimes in conjunction with the division of splanchnic and sympathetic nerve trunks. The postoperative care of these patients, in addition to the regulation of blood pressure by administration of vasopressor drugs intravenously, requires that adrenal cortical hormone must be given as substitution therapy until the body adjusts itself to a new plane of blood pressure and hormonal balance.

THE PITUITARY GLAND

The pituitary gland is a small organ, approximately the size of a cherry, situated immediately below the midbrain and just posterior to the plane of the orbits. It is composed of three parts, the most anterior having a glandular structure, and the poste-

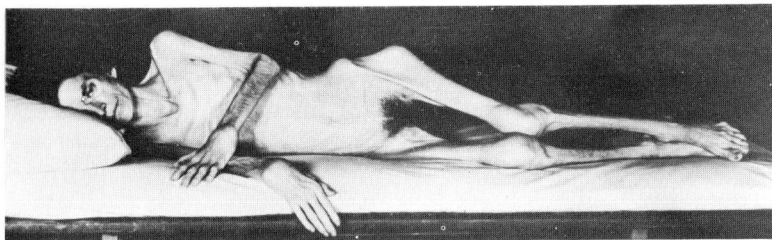

Fig. 325. Extreme cachexia in a patient 68 years of age, comparable with that seen in Simmonds' disease. (Hamblin, E. C.: Endocrinology of Woman, Springfield, Ill., Thomas)

rior one being composed largely of nervous tissue. The central area is best described as a thin sheet of epithelial tissue, the structure and the vascularity of which do not indicate either a secretory or a nervous function. The posterior lobe is the source of an agent called *pituitrin,* the injection of which causes contraction of the smooth muscles and a marked reduction in urine volume. The activity of the anterior lobe is more diverse, furnishing hormones which stimulate growth, the secretion of milk and the activity of the thyroid and the adrenal glands. The development of the ova and the sperm and the production of the ovarian and testicular hormones also are regulated by the anterior portion of the pituitary gland.

Diabetes Insipidus

Diabetes insipidus is a disorder of water metabolism caused by pituitrin deficiency. Its predominant symptom is an enormous daily output of 6, 8 or even 40 L. of very dilute urine, in appearance like water, with a specific gravity from 1.001 to 1.005. The urine contains no abnormal substances, such as sugar and albumin. Some cases of this disease are secondary to lesions of the brain (tumor, fracture of the skull, gumma, etc.) all in the region of the pituitary gland, on which, if possible, the treatment should be centered. Others are called *primary,* since no demonstrable lesion can be found. The theory on which this polyuria is explained ascribes it to circulatory changes in the kidneys, secondary to a deficiency of a posterior lobe hormone or to a lesion in the midbrain.

The primary symptoms may begin at birth. In adults, the polyuria may have an insidious onset, but sometimes it occurs suddenly and may be related in sequence to a fright or an injury. The general health and duration of life are little affected by this disease.

Symptoms. In general it is the polyuria, not the excessive thirst (polydipsia), which is the primary symptom in diabetes insipidus. The disease cannot be controlled by limiting the intake of fluids. Attempt to do this and the patient will suffer extremely from an insatiable craving for fluid. Great embarrassment, inconvenience and interference with daily activities are occasioned by this urgent need to allay thirst and pass urine.

Treatment. The administration of pituitrin (1 ml. three times each day) is the only remedy which controls this polyuria. This drug may be given by subcutaneous injection, by spray or by pledgets of cotton inserted into the nasopharynx. The amount of urine voided daily, as the result of this treatment, will be reduced from 10 to 12 or more liters to perhaps 3, or even less, assuring these unhappy patients of more restful days and nights.

Panhypopituitarism (Simmonds' Disease)

The destruction of the pituitary gland by surgical excision, a tumor or a vascular lesion removes every stimulus that is normally received by the thyroid and the adrenal glands. The resulting endocrinopathy, called Simmonds' disease, is characterized by extreme weight loss, emaciation (Fig. 325), atrophy of all organs, hair loss, impotence, amenorrhea, hypometabolism, hypoglycemia, eventual coma and death.

Hypophysectomy for Metastatic Carcinoma

In an effort to alter the hormonal milieu of the body with the intent of creating a hormonal environment that is hostile to the continued growth of a neoplasm, removal of the pituitary gland is being carried out. This type

Fig. 326. Acromegaly. (*Left*) Patient prior to the onset of the disease. (*Right*) Patient at the age of 36, 4 years after the development of characteristic signs and symptoms. (Hamblin, E. C.: Endocrinology of Woman, Springfield, Ill., Thomas)

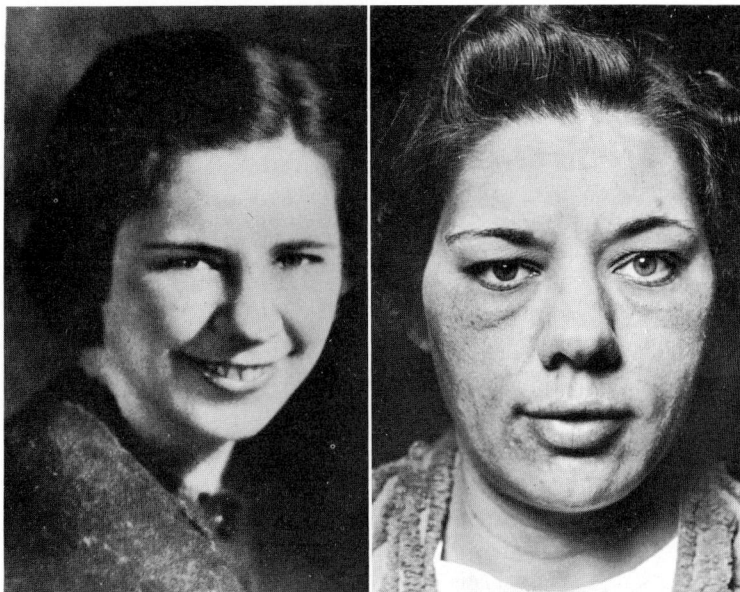

of treatment is useful only in those tumors that are endocrine-dependent, especially carcinoma of the breast, and is used as a palliative measure in patients with metastatic disease.

The rationale of hypophysectomy for carcinoma of the breast is not completely clear, but it is known that certain pituitary hormones have to do with the growth of the normal breast and with the function of the ovaries and the adrenal glands. By hypophysectomy the hormonal influences of these glands are removed. About half of the patients have regression of the tumor and its metastasis for 6 months or longer after operation.

Pituitary Tumors

Tumors of the pituitary gland are of three principal types: those representing an overgrowth of eosinophilic cells, of basophilic cells or of chromophobic cells (i.e., cells with no affinity for either eosinophilic or basophilic stains).

Eosinophilic tumors, if they develop early enough in life, produce gigantism. The individual thus affected may be over 7 feet tall and large in all proportions, yet so feeble that he can hardly stand. If the disorder begins during adult life, the excessive skeletal growth occurs only in certain portions of the body, notably in the feet, the hands, the superciliary ridges, the molar eminences, the nose and the chin, giving rise to the clinical picture called *acromegaly* (Fig. 326). Enlargement, moreover, is not confined to the skeleton, but involves every tissue and organ of the body. Many of these patients suffer from severe headaches and become partially blind due to the pressure of the tumor on the optic nerves. Decalcification of the skeleton, muscular weakness and endocrine disturbances, similar to those occurring in patients with hyperthyroidism, also are associated with tumors of this type.

Basophilic tumors give rise to the so-called *Cushing syndrome* (see p. 840), with features which are largely attributable to hyperadrenalism, including masculinization and amenorrhea in females, girdle obesity, hypertension, osteoporosis and polycythemia. Since this type of tumor rarely enlarges to the extent that is characteristic of eosinophilic adenomas, local pressure symptoms such as headaches and blindness are uncommon.

Chromophobe tumors produce no hormones but destroy the rest of the pituitary gland, causing hypopituitarism. Patients with this disease are inclined to be obese and somnolent, exhibiting fine, scanty hair, dry soft skin, pasty complexion and small bones. They also experience headaches, loss of libido and visual defects progressing to blindness. Other symptoms include polyuria, polyphagia, a lowering of the basal metabolic rate and a subnormal body temperature.

CLINICAL SITUATION

Mrs. Lyons, 46, has been admitted to the hospital for dietary and insulin regulation of diabetes, which was discovered during her yearly physical examination.

1. Mrs. Lyons was given lente insulin daily before breakfast. If she were to have a hypoglycemic reaction, the nurse would expect it to occur at:
   A. 6:00 a.m.
   B. 12:00 noon.
   C. 6:00 p.m.
   D. 12:00 midnight.

2. The nurse caring for Mrs. Lyons is aware that she must also be observed for symptoms of ketoacidosis. Diabetic ketoacidosis may be produced by:
   A. Not enough insulin.
   B. A skipped meal.
   C. Too much insulin.
   D. Increased exercise.

3. In teaching this patient, the nurse should emphasize that the complications of diabetes may be prevented by:
   A. Carefully controlling the disease.
   B. Avoiding excesses in exercise.
   C. Guarding against emotional upsets.
   D. Keeping the meals uniform.

4. Since diabetes is a hereditary disease, Mrs. Lyons' teen-aged son and daughter are counseled to:
   A. Refrain from eating sweets.
   B. Keep their weight at normal levels.
   C. Eat more protein and fats.
   D. Have monthly blood sugar evaluations.

5. Mrs. Lyons is an ardent golfer and wants to continue to participate actively in this sport. Which fact is necessary for her to know in order for her blood sugar to remain in balance during periods of exercise?
   A. Exercise increases the blood sugar.
   B. Exercise decreases the blood sugar.
   C. Insulin should be increased during exercise periods.
   D. Less food should be taken during exercise periods.

BIBLIOGRAPHY AND SUGGESTED READING

Books

Martin, M.: Diabetes Mellitus, Philadelphia, Saunders, 1960.

Articles

Cohen, A. S., *et al.:* Diabetic acidosis: an evaluation of the cause, course and therapy of 73 cases, Ann. Intern. Med. **52:**55-85, 1960.

Cope, O.: Diseases of the thyroid gland, New Eng. J. Med. **246:**368-372, 408-416, 451-457, 1952.

Daughaday, W. H.: Dietary treatment of adults with diabetes mellitus, J.A.M.A. **167:**859-862, 1958.

Dehawter, D. E., and Moss, J. M.: Tolbutamide —orally effective drug for diabetes mellitus, Am. J. Nurs. **58:**1106-1108, 1958.

Frohman, I. P.: The steroids, Am. J. Nurs. **59:**518-521, Apr., 1959.

Gould, G., and Golden, J.: Teaching the diabetic at home, Am. J. Nurs. **57:**1170-1171, Sept., 1957.

Greenblatt, R. B., and Metts, Jr., J. C.: Addison's disease, Am. J. Nurs. **60:**1249-1252, Sept., 1960.

Jay, A. N.: Hypoglycemia, Am. J. Nurs. **62:**77, Jan., 1962.

Lanes, P.: Primary aldosteronism, Am. J. Nurs. **61:**46-47, Aug., 1961.

Martin, M. M.: Detection is your protection, Am. J. Nurs. **60:**1608-1609, Nov., 1960.

———: New trends in diabetes detection, Am. J. Nurs. **63:**101-103, Aug., 1963.

———: The unconscious diabetic patient, Am. J. Nurs. **61:**92-94, Nov., 1961.

Moss, J. M., and Dehawter, D. E.: Oral agents in the management of diabetes mellitus, Am. J. Nurs. **60:**1610-1613, Nov., 1960.

Nelson, T. G., Rumer, G. F., and Nicholas, T. H.: Cricothyroidotomy, Am. J. Nurs. **61:**74-76, Nov., 1961.

Nordyke, R. A.: The overactive and the underactive thyroid, Am. J. Nurs. **63:**66-71, May, 1963.

Pearson, O. H., and Lubic, R. W.: Adrenalectomy and hypophysectomy, Am. J. Nurs. **62:**80-86, Apr., 1962.

Rauen, K. M.: Learning to live with diabetes, Am. J. Nurs. **59:**1290-1291, Sept., 1959.

Reich, B. H., and Ault, L. P.: Nursing care of the patient with Addison's disease, Am. J. Nurs. **60:**1252-1255, Sept., 1960.

Patient Teaching Aids and Information

A Handbook for Diabetics. A 28-page illustrated attractive booklet available from Squibb Pharmaceutical Co.

A Pocket Reference for the Diabetic. A 60-page, useful booklet with blank pages for the insertion of the menu. It also contains food exchange lists, recipes, and the common methods of testing the urine. Eli Lilly Co., Indianapolis 6, Indiana.

A list of patient education materials is available from the American Diabetic Association. Some of their publications are:

ADA Forecast, a bimonthly magazine for diabetics and their families, available on a subscription basis.

A Cookbook for Diabetics. A 176-page, indexed, spirally-bound book of recipes for $1.00.

Facts About Diabetes. A 32-page book of factual information.

Identification cards.

Duncan, G. G.: A Modern Pilgrim's Progress for Diabetics, Philadelphia, Saunders, 1956.

U. S. Department of Health, Education and Welfare, Public Health Service Publications:

Simple Goiter, Health Information Series, No. 56, a pamphlet.

Diabetes Fact Book, No. 890.

Diabetes, Health Information Series, No. 70, a pamphlet.

Diabetes Program Guide, No. 506.

Voluntary Agency

American Diabetes Association, Inc.
1 East 45th Street
New York 17, New York

39

Patients With Problems of the Eye

THE NURSE AND EYE HEALTH

The eye is such an important organ that its care and protection are a major consideration. Care begins at birth and is continued throughout life because, with advancing age and conditions of life, changes occur in the eye, and these can be corrected in various ways. The recognition of the importance of eye care has extended to industry. Protective devices are a necessity in industrial procedures in which there is danger of injury from foreign bodies, dust and so on. The importance of adequate and well-placed light in preventing eyestrain is essentially no longer a medical problem but one of general and social interest.

The nurse, as an important member of the health team, is looked on as a teacher and a practitioner of sound health habits. One of the most vital fields in health education is the care of the eyes and the prevention of eye diseases. Since many problems and habits begin in childhood, sound principles of safe care need to be stressed at this time. Complaints such as these need to be investigated: headaches, dizziness, tiredness after close eye work, "can't see well," letters "jump" or "run together," eyes are scratchy or itch. The appearance of inflamed or watery eyes, red rimmed, encrusted or puffy lids, recurring styes, crossed eyes and unequal pupils may be significant. Unusual behavior also should be noted—such as holding a book too close, frowning, blinking, skipping words, squinting, rubbing the eyes, stumbling, and failing in school work. A combination of these signs may be of short duration and often expected with an upper respiratory infection; however, persistence of these complaints indicates the need for an eye examination.

Faulty diet may account for the onset of many eye difficulties. For instance, deficiencies of vitamins A and B may cause changes in the retina, the conjunctiva and the cornea. Sensible eating habits can correct some problems; however, it must be emphasized that prolonged lack of vitamins A and B may produce irreversible eye damage.

Just as the eyes often reflect a systemic problem, an eye weakness may affect the total well-being of a person. The concept of total health care must be recognized by the nurse. An individual may complain of a minor visual disturbance and pass it off as something that may clear by itself. Such procrastination may have serious consequences.

The National Society for the Prevention of Blindness and other medical groups have been responsible for the dissemination of invaluable information on eye care.* It is important for the nurse to become familiar with them so that she may offer sound advice when a patient asks her such questions as: Will watching television damage my eyes? Are tinted glasses helpful for night driving? What kind of sun glasses are safe to wear?

Eye-Care Specialists

Public misunderstanding of the specific function of eye specialists is widespread. The nurse can clarify their roles and direct individuals intelligently for proper care. Here, the importance of adequate eye examination cannot be emphasized too strongly. Too often we find patients using a pair of glasses that belonged to a relative or was purchased at the dime store.

* See Patient-Teaching Aids at the end of this chapter.

The care of the eye is undertaken by three groups of specialists:

1. The *optician,* not a physician, whose concern it is to grind, mount and dispense lenses.

2. The *optometrist,* who is licensed to examine for refractive errors in the eye by mechanical means and to provide appropriate corrective lenses. He is not a physician, and he does not use drugs in the examination of the eyes.

3. The *oculist,* the *ophthalmologist* or the *ophthalmic physician* is a medical doctor who is skilled in the treatment of all conditions and diseases of the eye. Because of training and experience, he is able to make a more thorough and complete examination of the eye for refractive errors and other changes.

ANATOMY AND PHYSIOLOGY

Anatomy

The eyeball is a spherical organ situated in a bony cavity called the *orbit.* It is rotated easily in all the necessary directions by six muscles attached to its outer surface. These are similar to the reins on a team of horses. However, there are muscles not only on each side of the eye but also on the top and the bottom of the eye. Each of these 4 muscles leads back to the apex of the orbit and turns the eye in or out, up or down; these are the *rectus* muscles. The 2 other muscles of the eye run from the globe toward the medial wall of the orbit; these are the *oblique* muscles.

For the purpose of study, the eyeball may be divided into 3 coats or tunics. The dense white fibrous outer coat is called the *sclera.* Anteriorly it becomes continuous with the *cornea,* the translucent structure that bulges forward slightly from the general contour of the eye. Posteriorly, there is an opening through which the optic nerve passes into the eyeball. The nerve spreads out over the posterior two thirds of the inner surface of globe in a thin layer called the *retina.* In it are situated the tiny nerve endings. These, when properly stimulated, transmit visual impulses to the brain which are interpreted as sight.

Between the sclera and the retina is the pigmented middle coat known as the *uveal tract.* This tract is composed of three parts. The posterior part, the *choroid,* contains most of the blood vessels that nourish the eye. The anterior part is a pigmented muscular organ, the *iris.* It gives the characteristic color to the eye (blue, brown and so forth). The circular opening at its center, the *pupil,* is made smaller or larger, according to the intensity of the light, by its two sets of muscle fibers. The circular fibers by their contraction constrict the pupil; the radial fibers enlarge it. Between the iris and the choroid is the third portion of the uveal tract, a muscular body known as the *ciliary body.* It is composed of radial processes, the ciliary processes arising from a triangular-shaped muscle (ciliary muscle). Between these processes and to them are attached delicate ligaments that pass centrally and become inserted in the capsule of the crystalline lens.

The *lens* is a semisolid body enclosed in a transparent elastic capsule. It is capable of being modified to varying degrees of convexity by the contraction and the relaxation of the ciliary muscle, thus changing the focus of the eye as it looks from one object to another.

The cavity within the eye is divided by the lens into two parts. The posterior part contains a jellylike translucent substance called the *vitreous humor,* which is the chief factor in maintaining the form of the eyeball. The anterior part contains a clear, watery fluid, the *aqueous humor,* which is secreted by the ciliary processes. It bathes the anterior surface of the lens, escapes at the pupil and enters the space between the iris and the cornea known as the *anterior chamber.* Finally it is drained from the eye through lymph channels (the canal of Schlemm) located at the junction of the iris and the sclera.

Appendages. The eyelids are the protective coverings of the eye. Lining the lids and entirely covering the anterior part of the eye is a highly sensitive membrane, the *conjunctiva,* the surface of which is kept moist by a constant flow of lacrimal fluid (tears). This fluid is excreted from the lacrimal gland, which is located in the upper and outer part of the orbit. It flows downward and inward across the eye and drains into tiny channels (lacrimal punctae). By these channels it is conducted to the lacrimal sac and duct, which pass downward, backward and outward and open into the nasal cavity beneath the inferior turbinate bone.

Physiology

Vision is made possible by the passage of rays of light from an object through the cornea, the aqueous humor, the lens and the vitreous humor to the retina. In the normal eye, rays coming from an object 6 meters or more distant will be brought to a focus on the retina by the lens while perfectly at rest. If, under the same conditions, the rays of light are brought to a focus in front of the retina, the condition is spoken of as *myopia,* or nearsightedness; and *hyperopia* (farsightedness) is the condition in which the rays are focused behind the retina (Fig. 328). In such conditions glass lenses are prescribed. These, in association with the lenses of the eye, will correct the fault and restore a normal focus at the retina.

Rays from objects situated at shorter distances (less than 6 meters) require a "stronger" lens to focus them on the retina. This is brought about by a contraction of the ciliary muscle that relaxes the lens capsule and causes the lens to become more convex. This function is called *accommodation,* and by its means objects at different distances from the eye can be seen distinctly. As age approaches, the elasticity of the lens decreases, and accommodation for near vi-

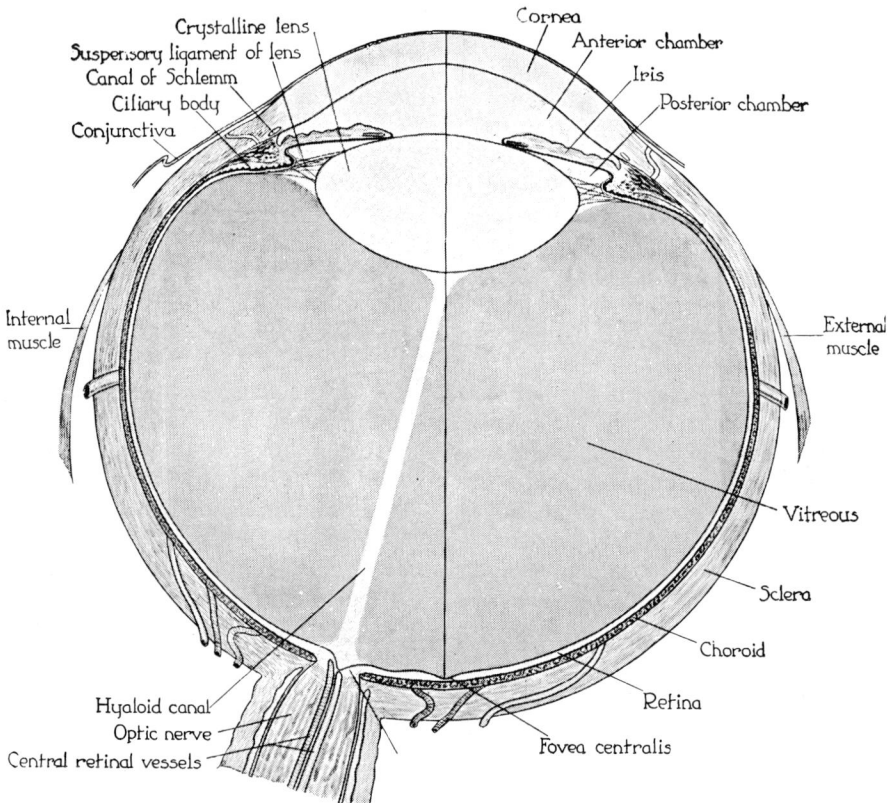

FIG. 327. Diagrammatic horizontal section of right eye (×3½). (Piersol, G.: Human Anatomy, Philadelphia, Lippincott)

FIG. 328. *(Left)* Diagram illustrating rays of light converging in A, normal eye; B, myopic eye; and C, hypermetropic eye. The parallel lines indicate light rays entering the eye; X is the point of convergence or focus. In A, the rays are brought to a focus (X) on the retina. In B they come to a focus in front of the retina. In C they would come to a focus behind the retina. *(Right)*

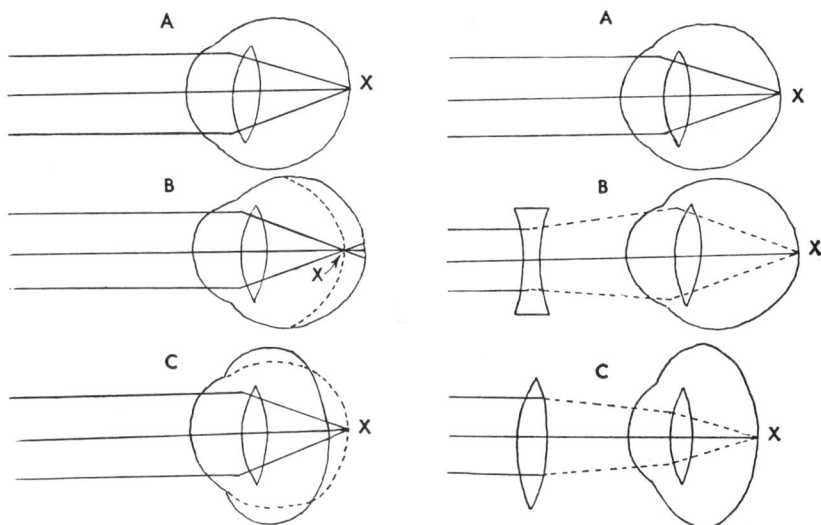

Diagrams illustrating the convergence of the light rays in a normal eye (A) and the effects of concave lens (B) and convex lens (C) on rays of light. (Kimber, D. C., Gray, C. E., Stackpole, C. E., and Leavell, L. C.: Anatomy and Physiology, ed. 14, p. 668, Fig. 384, New York, Macmillan)

sion is not complete. It is common to see older people reading with the paper held at arm's length, an example of this condition, which is called *presbyopia.* Lenses may be given these patients to enable them to focus rays from near objects on the retina—"reading glasses."

Astigmatism results from uneven curvature of the cornea so that the curve instead of being equal in all directions is shaped somewhat like the bowl of a spoon. Two foci thus are given the eye instead of one and, as a consequence, the patient is unable to focus horizontal and vertical rays on the retina at the same time. These defects also may be corrected with appropriate lenses.

EXAMINATIONS AND DIAGNOSTIC PROCEDURES

External Examination

The eye is an organ that can be examined with relative ease both as to its function and its structure. In its functional examinations are included its ability to move in its orbit and the reaction of the pupil to light and accommodation.

The usual function of the eye is tested in several ways. The patient may be asked to identify illuminated letters or objects of varying sizes on what is known as the Snellen chart. Usually each eye is tested alone. Letters or objects are of the size that can be seen by the normal eye at a distance of 20 feet from the chart. Rows of letters of larger sizes are designated as 30, 40 and so on. These really are letters of a size that should be seen by the normal eye at distances of 30 feet, 40 feet and so on. When an eye can identify letters of size 20 at 20 feet, the eye is said to have 20/20 vision. If it can identify only the letters of the number 40 line, it is said to have 20/40 vision. (The figure 6/6 is the same as 20/20 in the metric system. Instead of using 20 feet, this method uses 6 meters which equals 20 feet.) The visual fields are spot tested by a perimeter, an instrument that tests the peripheral or side vision with the eye fixed at a central point. Tests for color vision are made by having the patient identify various colors or wool yarn or figures or letters that can be seen only if the patient can identify colors in a color plate.

Refraction

The normal eye, by reason of its lens apparatus and the cornea, is able to refract parallel rays of light so that they focus on the retina. By this mechanism, we are able to see clearly. Due to abnormalities in the eye structure or in the lens structure, defective vision may occur because objects are not focused correctly on the retina.

The drug atropine paralyzes the nerve endings that function in accommodation, and for this reason "drops" of this drug or homatropine, a short-acting, derivative, are placed in the eye before an examination for "glasses." The ophthalmologist thus is able to ascertain the function of the eye with the lens completely at rest (see p. 856).

By various examinations and tests with trial lenses, the ophthalmologist can determine the strength and the type of lens that will overcome the refractive error. In the case of presbyopia, two different types of lenses may be used—bifocals—one for far distance and one for near vision and reading. Trifocal lenses are also available; these add a third segment which gives sharp focus in the 27-inch to 50-inch range. Most lenses are prescribed for use in "glasses," but in some cases this may be avoided by the application of a lens directly to the surface of the eye (contact lens).

Internal Examination

Examination of the structural part of the eye may be made in several ways. Tension within the eyeball is measured by a tonometer. In certain diseases, especially glaucoma, the tension in the eyeball is increased markedly. (Normal tension is 10 to 25/mm.) The surface of the eyeball and the conjunctiva may be more closely inspected by the magnifying loupe. This also is used in the search for foreign bodies. The slit-lamp is an instrument that projects a beam of light onto the anterior segment of the eye for detection of disease. With the ophthalmoscope, a small beam of light is reflected through the pupil and, through a small opening in the mirror, the examiner may view the interior of the eye. The instrument is fitted with a series of lenses that permit examination of structural changes. Thus, in certain diseases of the brain, the optic nerve may be pushed forward into the eyeball. This is spoken of as *choking of the disk* and, by means of the lenses in the ophthalmoscope, the amount of choking may be estimated and described in diopters; for example, choked disk of 3 diopters. In addition, the blood vessels of the interior of the eye may be visualized and, since this is the only area in the body in which blood vessels can be observed by direct vision, it is an important source of information, not only in diseases of the eye but also in many systemic conditions; for example, hypertension and diabetes.

By means of a contact glass and a magnifying device, the angle of the anterior chamber may be seen (gonioscopy). Such visualization is desirable in congestion, inflammation, tumors, cysts, trauma, glaucoma and congenital anomalies. It is particularly helpful in diagnosis, management and surgery of glaucoma.

"EYE GLASSES" AND CONTACT LENSES

The stigma of wearing glasses has been removed in the past decade with the advent of attractive frames. The shape, the color, and the decorative features of eye glasses are selected by the wearer to enhance his physical features as well as personality. Thus there are glasses for study and business wear and other styles for more formal occasions. They are adapted to the needs of all age groups.

Contact Lenses. About 97 per cent of all contact lenses are plastic corneal lenses. Scleral lenses are larger and used for special medical conditions and some sports. The corneal lens is light-weight, paper-thin plastic about 10 mm. in diameter. When properly fitted, they "float" on the fluid layer of the eyeball and are held loosely in place by capillary attraction and the upper lid.

The popularity of contact lenses has increased in recent years because of better technics for measuring the eye, the discovery of the ideal fluid for lubrication, and better supervision and instruction in the use of the lenses. They are particularly effective in certain occupations; they are desirable for cosmetic reasons in many others. Some medical conditions in which corneal contact lenses are used are absence of lens, absence of iris, congenital absence of pigment, near and farsightedness, cone-shaped deformity of the cornea, and turn-in eyelashes. Contraindications are allergic or chronic blepharoconjunctivitis, corneal infection, severe exophthalmus, glaucoma, iritis, pterygium or local neoplasm.

DRUGS USED FREQUENTLY IN EYE CONDITIONS

In caring for ophthalmic patients, nurses are advised to wash their hands before and after the instillation of drops (see p. 857). To carry any of the solutions to their own eyes would cause serious inconvenience.

Adrenalin Chloride. This drug is used in solutions of 1:1,000 as an astringent and hemostatic. It is of use in preventing hemorrhage during minor operations on the eye, in contracting the blood vessels in inflammatory conditions of the eye and in increasing the rapidity of action of certain other drugs; for example, atropine in iritis.

Adrenalin chloride should be kept in dark bottles, as it undergoes changes when exposed to the light.

Fluorescein Solution. This is a yellowish-green fluid that is used to detect corneal abrasions and ulcers. When a small amount of the solution is placed in the eye and is followed by an irrigation with normal saline solution, the corneal injury appears stained a bright green. The physician thus is enabled to locate the site of the injury and to estimate its exact extent. Fluorescein is now available in autoclaved filter strips (Fluoristrip), which are moistened when touched against the eye to release fluorescein.

Sulfonamides. The various sulfa derivatives may be used in inflammatory diseases of the eye orally, parenterally and locally. Applied locally they may be used in powder form, in a solution of the sodium salts or in an ointment base. The indication for their use is the establishment of the presence of organisms against which the sulfonamides are effective.

Antibiotics. Penicillin is an antibacterial agent that is effective both locally and parenterally. It has been used in eyes and found to be dramatically effective for both superficial and intraocular infections, particularly those caused by gram-positive cocci. The eye usually tolerates a solution containing from 1,000 to 2,000 units per ml.

Bacitracin ointment and neomycin ointment have been found effective in specific infections of the eye.

Steroids. Steroids do not act against the cause of an eye condition; however, they do suppress inflammatory reactions in all types of irritation—chemical and traumatic injury, bacterial infection and allergy. Thus, painful swelling and scar-tissue formation is prevented.

To remove the cause of eye inflammations, steroids are often combined with antihistamines and/or antibacterial agents. Some of the steroids are dexamethasone (Decadron, Deronil, Gammacorten), methylprednisolone (Medrol), and triamcinolone diacetate (Aristocort, Kenacort). Cortisone and hydrocortisone drops or ointment in strength from ½ to 2½ per cent frequently are used to reduce postoperative inflammation of the eye.

Drugs Used For Antiseptic Action

Silver Nitrate. Silver nitrate, in from 1 to 3 per cent solutions, is used as an astringent and antiseptic in acute contagious diseases of the eye, especially those due to the gonococcus. As a rule, it is brushed directly on the everted lids after irrigation. A second irrigation of physiologic saline should follow this application to lessen the pain and the irritation caused by the drug. Silver nitrate solutions must be kept in dark bottles because of the rapid decomposition caused by the access of light.

Boric Acid. Boric acid is used in a 2 per cent solution as a mildly antiseptic, nonirritating lotion. For irrigating the eyes, the solution should be warmed.

Bichloride of Mercury. Bichloride of mercury in 1:10,000 solution often is used as an irrigating fluid.

Yellow Oxide of Mercury. This drug, from 1 to 2 per cent, long has been used in the form of an ointment in the treatment of eye affections, especially affections of the lid margins (blepharitis).

Penicillin G Potassium Ointment. Each gram of this ointment contains from 200 to 2,500 units of penicillin. Many physicians believe that penicillin should be used only for serious infections because of the possibility of developing sensitivity to it.

Drugs to Dilate the Pupil (Mydriatics) and Paralyze Accommodation (Cycloplegics)

Atropine Sulfate. Atropine sulfate, in from 0.5 to 2 per cent solutions, probably is used more commonly than any other drug in ophthalmology. It is used in the treatment of inflammatory diseases of the uveal tract (iritis and cyclitis) and the cornea, to rest the iris and the ciliary body and to prevent adhesions of the iris to the lens (posterior synechia). In refraction of the eyes it sets the lens at rest by causing paralysis of accommodation. Its effects usually are complete in half an hour and last from 7 to 10 days. During this time the pupil is unable to contract; therefore, the eyes should be protected from bright lights by the wearing of dark glasses, and no attempt should be made to use the eyes for near vision, because accommodation for near vision cannot take place.

Toxic symptoms sometimes appear after the use of atropine in the eyes. Blond adults and children develop toxic signs more frequently than brunettes. Swelling of the lids, dryness of the mouth and the throat with difficulty in swallowing, dizziness, flushed skin with pallor around the mouth, rapid full pulse, restlessness and, at times, delirium are symptoms that should warn the nurse of atropine poisoning. The administration of the drug must be discontinued until the doctor can be notified. The use of atropine is contraindicated absolutely in patients with primary glaucoma and in most cases of conjunctival affections.

Homatropine Hydrobromide. This drug, in solutions of from 1 to 4 per cent, acts in a manner similar to atropine, except much weaker. It dilates the pupil and paralyzes accommodation, as does atropine, but its effects disappear within 24 to 48 hours.

A number of new drugs, most notably Cyclogyl, have been introduced in an attempt to give some of the effects of homatropine, but with fewer side-effects and shorter action.

Euphthalmine Hydrochloride. This drug, in 5 per cent solution, is used in examinations of the eye. Its action is short-lived, and it has the advantage of dilating the pupil without affecting accommodation.

Neo-Synephrine (10%) and **Paredrine** (1-3%) are other dilating medications.

Drugs Used to Contract the Pupil (Miotics)

Pilocarpine Hydrochloride. This drug, in from 0.5 to 4 per cent solutions, is one of the principal medications used in diseases of the eye caused by increased tension within the eyeball (glaucoma). By the contraction of the pupil caused by the drug, the aqueous humor is permitted to escape more easily into the lymph channels, which drain it from the eye. Pilocarpine also is used in preventing prolapse of the iris after wounds of the cornea.

Eserine Sulfate. Eserine sulfate, in solutions of from 0.25 to 1 per cent, is more powerful than pilocarpine. This drug must be kept in dark bottles. Exposure to light causes it to turn pink or red and, although in this form it retains its original properties, it is much more irritating than a fresh solution would be. After long-term use, many patients unfortunately become sensitive to it.

Drugs Used to Produce Anesthesia

Pontocaine. This drug, a brand of tetracaine hydrochloride, in 0.5 and 1 per cent solutions, is one of the most popular drugs used for surface anesthesia. The aqueous solution is unaffected by prolonged boiling and can be sterilized easily this way. It exhibits a higher efficiency than cocaine solutions of corresponding strength; usually it is unattended by irritation or tissue injury, and it does not exert any effect on the blood vessels. It is less likely than cocaine to affect the corneal epithelium, and it does not dilate the pupil, disturb accommodation or increase intraocular pressure. The stronger concentrations may produce a sensation of burning. This, however, is transient. It is valuable not only for operations but as an anesthetic for removing sutures and relieving tension and other painful procedures, such as the removal of a foreign body from the eye.

Holocaine. This drug is used in 1 to 2 per cent solutions. Its anesthetic action is rapid and without any effect on the pupil. It is especially useful in operations for glaucoma and in the removal of foreign bodies from the cornea.

Procaine. Procaine, in 1 and 2 per cent solutions, also is used by injection for lid anesthesia, as well as for the O'Brien facial nerve block and the Van Lint block.

Cocaine. Cocaine is employed in 2 and 4 per cent solutions to produce anesthesia of the conjunctiva for short operations on the eye. It may be instilled with a sterile pipette—one drop every 3 minutes to a total of 4 drops in the eye to be operated upon. Besides producing a loss of sensation, it causes a contraction of the capillaries and dilates the pupils. When it is instilled into the eye, the patient often experiences a smarting sensation, but this may be avoided in large measure by dropping the solution on the everted lower lid while the patient is looking upward. Both eyes should be kept closed after the instillation of each drop. Cocaine is not as popular as it once was. Two disadvantages are that it may cause stippling of corneal epithelium and may raise intraocular tension.

Ophthaine (½%) and **Butyn** (1%) also may be used to produce anesthesia. The former rarely produces an allergic response.

PSYCHOLOGICAL AND PHYSICAL NEEDS OF THE EYE PATIENT

It is well to remember that a patient with an eye problem may have other problems as well. Often other physical conditions are primary and affect the eye as a consequence. In some disturbances of other parts of the body, the appearance of the eye can alert the patient and the physician of these difficulties even before other symptoms present themselves. The mental anxiety frequently experienced by the ophthalmic patient requires as much consideration as does his physical condition.

One's dependence on sight is highlighted when there is a temporary or possible permanent loss of this vital sense. Worry, fear and depression are common evidences of a patient's concern. Even tension, resentment, anger and rejection may develop. By encouraging the patient to express his feelings, the nurse may discover the basic problems caused by his blindness—loss of employment, disfigurement, whatever the case may be in the individual patient. When these basic problems are known, assistance in solving them can be secured. Perhaps the physician can handle them best, or the medical social worker, the nurse, or a member of the patient's family.

When permissible, the nurse should use such means as the radio and occupational therapy to keep the patient's mind occupied. She should not be oversolicitous, but she should show interest, empathy and understanding. Because of differences of personality, her approach in overcoming his mental anxiety will vary. When permanent blindness is apparent, re-education may be done by others so afflicted or by specially-trained people. In this way the process of development of a well-adjusted individual will be hastened.

The daily care of ophthalmic patients should be the same as for other bed or ambulatory patients. The patient should be assisted as much as possible; at the same time, he should be encouraged to help himself so that he will not feel that he is a burden. A patient who cannot see should be fed; or, if he is accustomed to feeding himself, he should be supervised. Proper elimination should be promoted by cathartics or enemas, as ordered. Ambulatory patients should have a daily rest period in the afternoon.

Ophthalmic patients should not read, smoke or shave unless given permission by the physician. They must be cautioned against rubbing their eyes or wiping them with a soiled handkerchief. All patients receiving atropine should wear dark glasses.

Light. As light causes pain in many cases of disease of the eye, and as the eyes should be rested as much as possible before and after undergoing operation, it is well to treat the ophthalmic patient in a darkened room. Dimmed artificial lights may be used by the nurse for her own needs.

Eyedrops. Solutions of various drugs are employed in the treatment of nearly every kind of eye disease. The administration of these drops often is the responsibility of the nurse, and often she instructs others.

Before instilling drops the nurse must be sure that she has the prescribed drug and identifies the affected eye. Some drugs (for example, atropine and eserine) act in exactly opposite ways (see page 856). Therefore, if one of these drugs is indicated in the treatment of a certain eye disease, the other is contraindicated. It may seem needless to emphasize this warning, but experience has taught how easy it is in a dimly lighted room to pick up the wrong bottle from a tray containing similar vials.

The nurse then should inspect the solution for color changes or sedimentation. These signs are evidences of decomposition, and, if present, the solution should be discarded and a fresh one ordered and sterilized for use. The importance of using fresh medicines can be stressed with patients who often use drugs that have been in the medicine cabinet at home for months or years.

An eyedropper usually is employed for the instillation of drops. This instrument is composed of a glass pipette fitted with a small rubber or plastic bulb. The glass part is washed and sterilized easily, but the rubber undergoes gradual deterioration, and for this reason only a small amount of solution should be drawn into the pipette. The dropper never should be inverted or filled too full, as there is risk of contaminating the solution by contact with fine particles of rubber found in the bulb. An excess of solution remaining after instilling the drops should be discarded because of the possibility of contamination if it is returned to the bottle. Eye drops may be packaged in single-dose plastic containers, thus eliminating the need for a dropper and a stock bottle of medication.

INSTILLATION. The lids and the lashes are cleansed before instilling the medication. Then the head of the patient should be tilted backward (Fig. 329) and inclined slightly to the side, so that the solution will run away from the tear duct. This latter precaution is especially necessary when poisonous solutions, such as atropine, are employed, because absorption of the excess drug via the the nose and the pharynx may lead to toxic symptoms. In most cases it is well to press the inner angle of the eye after instilling the drops to prevent the excess of the solution from entering the nose. The lower lid is depressed with the fingers of the left hand, the patient is told to look upward, and the solution is dropped on the everted lower lid. Care must be taken that the pipette does not touch any part of the eye or the lids to guard

against contamination of the dropper and injury to the eye. After placing the drops (1 or 2 at most) in the eye, the lid is released and any excess of fluid is sponged gently from the lids and the cheeks with sterile cotton. After the medication is instilled, the nurse can tell her patient to close his eyes gently; this patient often has a tendency to "squeeze" his eyes closed, thereby expelling the medication.

After using the dropper, if contamination has been avoided, it may be replaced in the bottle, but in no circumstances should it be used for other solutions until after it has been cleansed thoroughly.

To instill drops in the eyes of children is often a difficult procedure. Two methods are employed commonly. If there is no discharge, the child may be placed flat on his back in bed and, while the eyes are closed, the prescribed drop may be placed at the inner corner of the eye. As soon as the lids are opened, the fluid enters the eye. The second method requires two persons, who sit facing each other. The child is placed across their laps so that the head can be held between the knees. The lids can be opened easily, and the drops are instilled. In the older patient, it will help the nurse to remember that he is often likely to jump or grab the nurse's hand; therefore, precautions are necessary.

Ocular Irrigations. Ocular irrigations are indicated in various forms of inflammation of the conjunctiva, in the preparation of the eye for operation and in the removal of inflammatory secretions. Also, they are used for their antiseptic effect. The fluid to be employed depends on the condition present. Irrigations should be warmed before using.

The irrigating apparatus is simple, consisting of a sterile eyedropper, an irrigating syringe or an undine, a bottle of warmed fluid and a small curved basin and cotton for catching the fluid and the secretions.

The patient should be flat on his back or sitting with the head tilted backward and inclined slightly toward the side to be treated. The basin may be held by the patient, if sitting, or so placed that when he is lying down it will catch the fluid as it runs from the eye. The nurse stands in front of the patient, in order to see exactly what she is doing.

After carefully cleansing the lids of dust, secretions and crusts, she holds them open with the thumb and the fingers of one hand, and with the other hand she flushes the eye gently, directing the stream away from the nose (Fig. 330). The fluid never should be directed toward the nose, because of the danger of spilling over into the other eye. The procedure should be continued until the eye is entirely free of secretions. It must be remembered that very little force should be used, because of the danger of injury. For the same reason and to prevent contamination, no part of the irrigator should touch the eye, the lids or the lashes. When the irrigation has been completed, the eye and the cheek should be dried gently with cotton.

Hot Compresses. Heat relieves pain and increases the circulation, thereby promoting absorption and reducing tension in the eye. It is especially valuable for the deep-seated inflammations of the eyeball, iritis, acute glaucoma and so forth, as well as for such superficial ones as keratitis and conjunctivitis. It is best applied in the form of compresses of 7 or 8 thicknesses of gauze or cotton, just large enough to cover the eye.

The patient is moved to the side of the bed, and a towel is used to cover the chest. The skin of the lids and the adjacent cheek may be anointed with cold cream or petrolatum. The compresses then are moistened in a basin of water or any other prescribed solution that has been heated by an electric hot plate placed on a table beside the bed. The fluid, which should be kept at a temperature of between 115° and 120° F., should be expressed from the pad and, after being tested for temperature on the back of the hand, the compress is placed gently over the closed lids. The pads should be changed every 30 to 60 seconds for 10 or 15 minutes, and the application should be repeated every 2 or 3 hours. At the completion of the period of application, the lids should be dried gently with cotton. New pads should be used for each application and, if the eyes have a purulent secretion, the compresses should be applied to one eye at a time, the solution and the basin being changed between applications in order not to carry infection from one eye to the other.

Cold Compresses. Cold causes a capillary

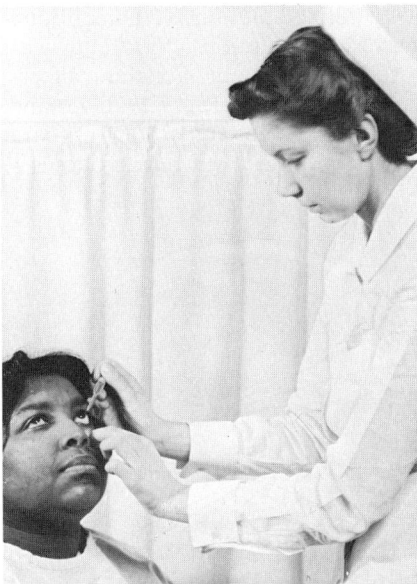

Fig. 329. Instilling drug into the eye. Note that the nurse, in using the dropper, rests her right hand against the patient's forehead and with her left hand depresses the lower lid. The eyedropper is held directly above the sulcus, between the lower lid and the eyeball.

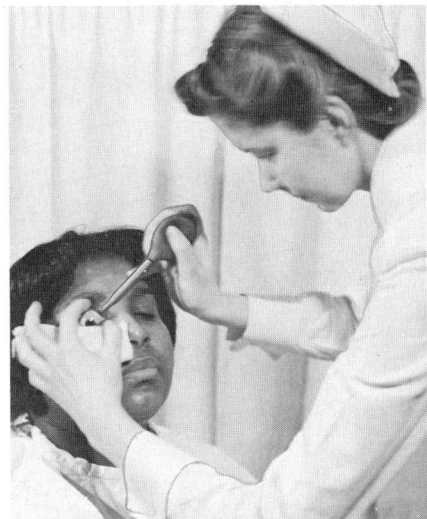

Fig. 330. Eye irrigation with rubber syringe and glass or plastic tip.

constriction that tends to reduce the amount of secretion and relieve pain during the early stages of acute inflammatory conditions of the conjunctiva. It is indicated also in the treatment of injuries or after operations on the eye, as it tends to reduce swelling and to retard bacterial growth. Cold compresses are useful in relieving itching due to allergic conjunctivitis.

The patient is prepared in the same manner as for the application of hot compresses. The pads are moistened in boric-acid solution and placed in rows on a block of ice suspended by a gauze sling over a basin. They are applied to the closed lids and are changed every 15 to 30 seconds. The duration of the application usually is from 5 to 15 minutes each hour. Cold compresses never are used in the treatment of deep-seated inflammations of the eye (iritis, keratitis), because cold, by constricting the capillaries, interferes with the nutrition of the cornea.

Ointments. Ointments of various kinds are used frequently in the treatment of inflammatory diseases of the lids, the conjunctiva and the cornea. Those ordered most commonly are boric acid, penicillin, sulfonamides, bacitracin, neomycin, zinc oxide, bichloride of mercury, yellow oxide of mercury and pontocaine ointments. These are applied best by pulling down gently the lower lid and expressing a small amount of the ointment from the tube to the conjunctiva of the lower lid. Care is taken not to touch the eye or the eyelid with the tube. The lid then may be massaged gently in such a way as to distribute the drug over the eyeball.

THE PATIENT WITH TRAUMA TO THE EYE

The prevention of eye injuries is a phase of child and adult education that cannot be emphasized too strongly. Children need to be reminded frequently of the dangers of sticks, arrows and darts, BB guns, "sparklers," sling shots, rubber bands, and even harmless looking toys. Protection is necessary from very bright lights, sun shining on the snow, fumes of chemicals, flying chips of wood. Elderly folks or those unsure of their footing need to have safeguards where there is a possibility of injury.

General measures to follow in caring for patients with eye injuries: (1) irrigate the eye with saline solution; (2) instill one drop of fluorescein solution—the yellowish-green dye used to detect abrasions and ulcers; (3) irrigate the eye again; (4) evaluate and treat injury; and (5) employ follow-up care.

Foreign Bodies. Foreign bodies (dust,

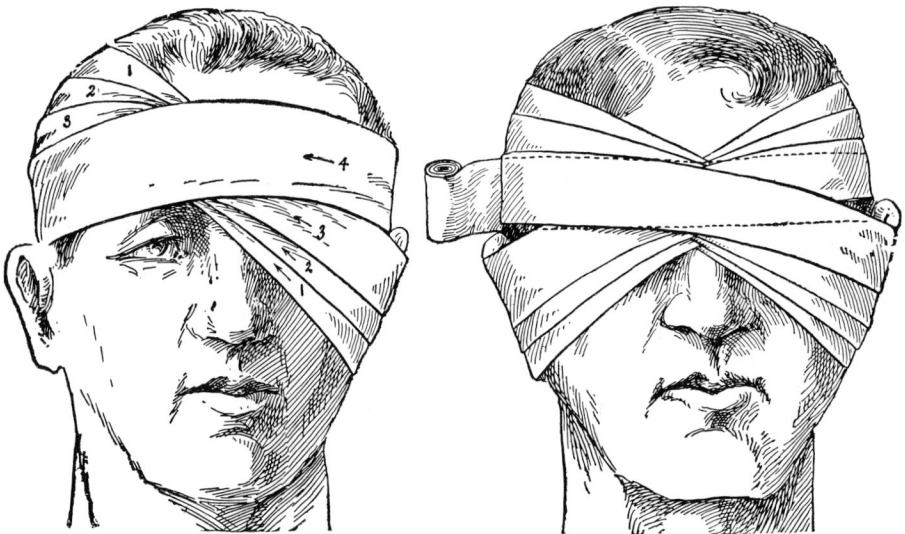

FIG. 331. Crossed bandages of *(left)* one eye and *(right)* both eyes.

cinders and so forth) frequently cause considerable discomfort, due to irritation of the sensitive conjunctiva. If the body has been in the eye only a short time, it may be removed by a nurse. The lower lid should be everted, the patient instructed to look up and the lower half of the conjunctival sac examined. If the body is not found, the upper eye should be examined by everting the upper lid.

In examining the upper eye, the nurse stands in front of the patient and instructs him to look down at his feet. She then takes the lashes between thumb and fingers of one hand and with the other places a matchstick, an applicator or a toothpick across the upper part of the lid. The lashes are pulled downward and forward away from the eye as the applicator is pressed downward gently. The foreign body may be removed by touching it gently with a small applicator tipped with cotton and moistened in saline solution.

If removal by this method is unsuccessful, or if the offending particle has been in the eye for a considerable time, the nurse should not attempt to remove it. It may have become embedded in the cornea and there is considerable danger of serious injury if removal is attempted by unskilled hands. The ophthalmologist usually requires local anesthesia, a hand lens, fluorescein, an eye spud, normal saline for irrigating the eye and, as a prophylaxis against infection, an antibiotic solution to instill after removal of the offending particle. If it is known to be a metal, the doctor may use a magnet to remove it.

Acid and Alkali Burns. Whenever acid or alkali get on the lids or in the eye, an emergency exists in which there is frequently no time to wait for the physician. In such a condition, the lids, the conjunctiva and the cornea must be flushed copiously! The easiest and quickest way for this to be done may be the best, i.e., simply immerse the patient's head in a bucket or a basin of water. More satisfactory is to flush the eye using a syringe, if available, taking care not to contaminate the other eye if it has not already been contaminated. Continuous flushing for at least 15 minutes is desirable. Plain tap water is adequate under such circumstances.

Contusions and Hematoma ("Black Eye"). Hemorrhage into the orbit from trauma is a frequent occurrence. The bleeding that takes place into the loose tissues of the orbit spreads rapidly and produces a discoloration of lids and surrounding skin. In itself the injury is not too serious, but frequently it is frightening to patients because of discoloration and marked swelling in such a prominent site. The bleeding usually stops spontaneously, but it may be reduced in amount and the swelling made less by the application of cold compresses (see above). Absorption of the blood may be hastened after the first 24 hours by the use of hot compresses applied 15 minutes at a time at intervals throughout the day.

Corneal Abrasions. Lacerations of the cornea can be detected after one drop of fluorescein solution is instilled. Usually a local anesthetic and antibacterial drops are administered before an eye patch is applied for 24 to 36 hours. The patient is instructed to keep the eyes at rest for comfort and to facilitate the healing process. A few physicians recommend no eye dressing. The danger to be guarded against with an abrasion is the development of a corneal ulcer.

Lacerations. Lacerations of the eyelids are not serious unless they are accompanied by an injury to the eyeball. Injuries to the lids are treated in the same way as any other wound but, because of his special training, the ophthalmologist usually is requested to care for them. Lacerations of the eyeball are more serious because of the danger of the production of visual defects, and more extensive injuries may even endanger the entire eye. These are referred invariably to the ophthalmologist for appropriate care. They may entail transplantation of conjunctival flaps to prevent leakage of ocular fluids, excision of prolapsed iris and, in severe injuries, even removal of the eye.

Retinal Detachment. This is a separation of the retina from the choroid. It may appear as tears or holes as a result of trauma or arise from degeneration, frequently in myopia. Flashes of light, blurred vision, a sensation of a veil coming across the eye and, finally, loss of vision are the usual symptoms. The suddenness of the incapacity creates confusion in most patients, as well as a fear of blindness. Usually, it means that the man abandons his business or the woman gives up her activity, with little or no time to make plans. The patient may be treated with bed rest and have both eyes bandaged, in the hope that the retina will regain its normal position. Sedation and the tranquilizing drugs keep the patient comfortable and quiet. However, surgery often is required. With a diathermy needle, holes are made in the sclera to allow the subretinal collection of fluids to escape. The retina falls back into place and becomes adherent to the choroid, due to the reaction caused by the diathermy current.

NURSING CARE. When the patient returns from the operating room, he must be reminded of the restrictions on his position. This will depend on the nature of the repair and the specific orders of the ophthalmologist. Small pillows and sandbags are useful. Side rails also will remind him that he must remain in bed. The patient should not brush his teeth or comb his hair until the ophthalmologist gives permission. All comfort measures are instituted which will allow the patient to relax while maintaining a restricted position. He is cautioned about sudden mo-

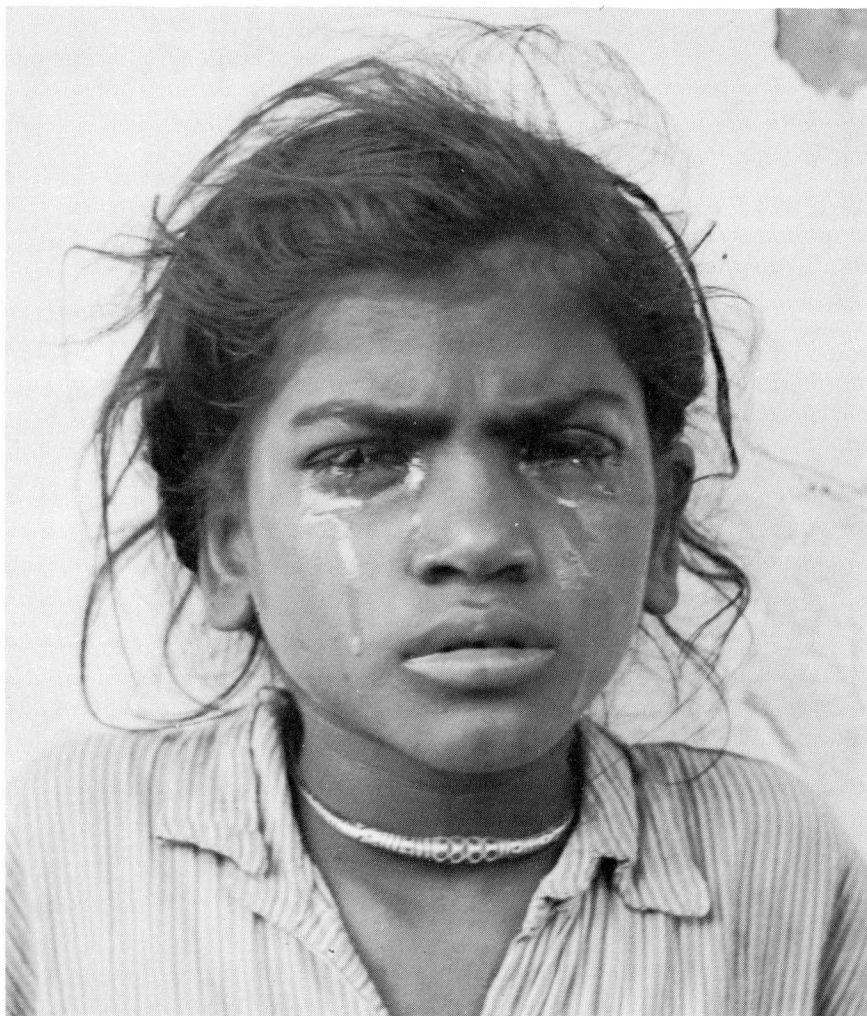

FIG. 332. (A) Tears of trachoma (India). When the eye is infected by the virus of trachoma, the delicate membranes called "conjunctiva" are the site of small granulations that give them a characteristic, roughened appearance. Indeed, the term *trachoma* comes from a Greek word meaning *roughness*. (World Health Organization)

tion, sneezing or coughing; such activity may redetach the retina. After about 7-8 days, peephole glasses are worn, which allow central vision but limit the movement of the eyes. He is allowed out of bed, and physical activity is increased gradually. Because of newer surgical technics, the patient's movements may not be as restricted as they used to be. Early ambulation may not be a detriment to the effects of surgery. Hospitalization may be reduced to 2 weeks.

The psychological nursing care of this pa-

tient is of major importance. Diversion that is relaxing is desirable, such as conversation, listening to music, having someone read a favorite book and so forth.* These individuals become depressed easily; therefore, every attempt should be made to prevent this reaction. The nurse should be sure that the patient understands all instructions for post-hospital care and follow-up visits.

* Recordings of books may be obtained from the public library or local association for the blind.

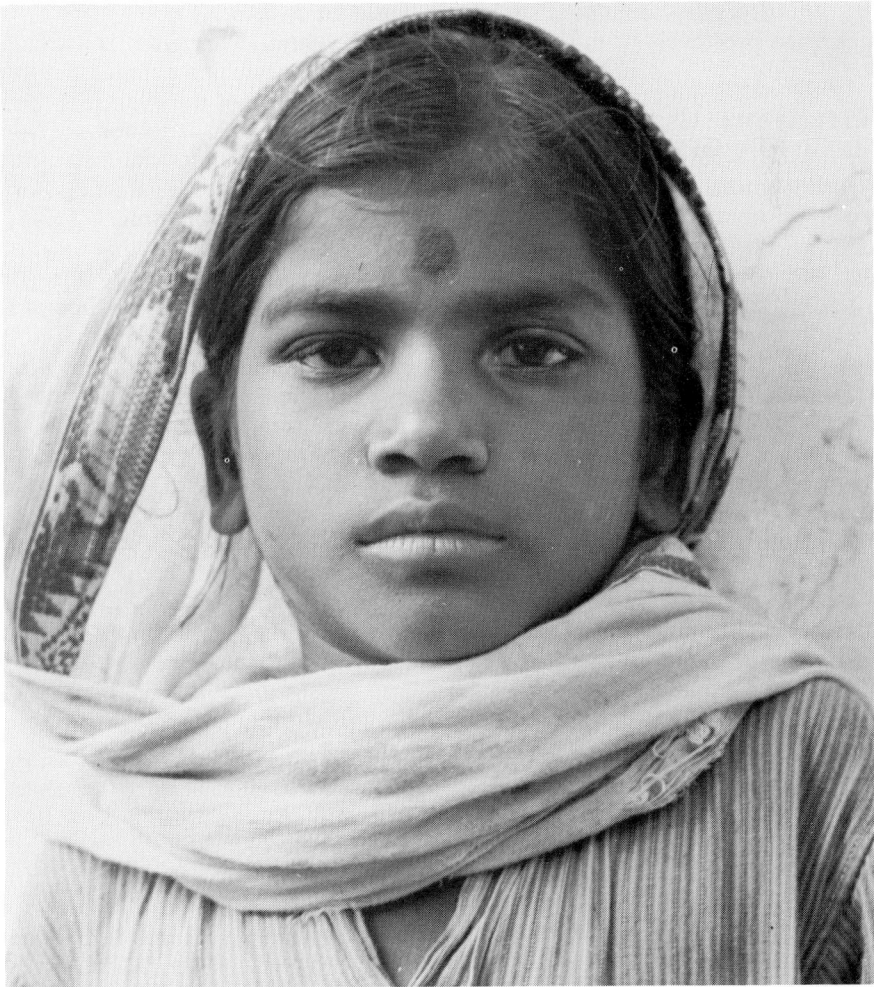

FIG. 332. (B) Ten days later. Treatment with Aureomycin ointment has given back their sparkle to the young patient's eyes. Other common eye inflammations of tropical regions make it easier for trachoma to take root. A large number of countries have launched antitrachoma campaigns with help from WHO. (World Health Organization)

Enucleation. Removal of the eyeball is called *enucleation*. It is necessitated by such trauma that the contents of the globe escape, by infections and by other injuries in which there is a fear of sympathetic ophthalmia—a condition in which the uninjured eye may develop an inflammatory reaction after an injury to the other eye. During the removal of the eye, muscles are cut as close to the globe as possible. By using sutures, these muscles are approximated to a plastic prosthesis, thereby providing the means for co-ordinated motion with the patient's real eye. This prosthesis is colored to match the patient's eye. In successful cases it is difficult to distinguish the prosthesis from the normal eye.

THE PATIENT WITH AN INFLAMMATION OF THE EYE

Stye (Hordeolum). A *stye* is an infection of the tiny glands that empty at the free edge of the eyelid. The area becomes swollen, red, tender and painful. An eyelash will be found in the center of the yellow point that appears. Hot compresses, applied in the early stage, will hasten the pointing of the abscess. Removal of the central lash often is followed by drainage of pus, but incision sometimes is necessary. Antibiotic therapy hastens control of the infection.

Chalazia. A *chalazion* is a cyst of the meibomian glands. It is noted as a small lump, hard and painless, in the lid. Occasionally, such a cyst may become infected. When this occurs, hot compresses are used; it may be necessary to do an incision and a drainage. For the uninfected cyst, massage may help it to be reabsorbed; however, the usual treatment is to make a small incision and express the cyst.

Conjunctivitis. Conjunctivitis may result from (1) bacterial infection, (2) allergy or (3) trauma. Specific therapy depends on the nature of the inflammation. However, the symptoms are similar: redness, pain, swelling and lacrimation. The amount and the nature of discharge depend on the offending organisms; for instance, with the pneumonococcus and the gonococcus, there is abundant purulent discharge. Frequent saline or boric acid irrigations are required to remove the discharge. Precautions must be taken to prevent dissemination of infection.

Trachoma. This chronic, highly communicable disease of the eyelids (Fig. 332) is caused by a virus. After an acute inflammatory process, follicles appear on the conjunctiva. Due to scar formation, the eyelid turns in, which causes the lashes to scratch the cornea, thereby irritating and infecting it. This inflammation often leads to ulceration and blindness. With early antibiotic therapy, the disease may be controlled. This disease is rarely seen in America. Hygienic measures will eventually rid the rest of the world of it also.

Pterygium. Pterygium is a triangular fold of membrane which extends onto the cornea from the white of the eye. It is thought to be caused by chronic irritation, as from dust or wind. Surgical interference prevents its growth and protects against loss of vision.

Gonorrheal Ophthalmia. This is an acute purulent conjunctivitis that occurs in newborn babies and is due to the gonococcus. The infection occurs at the time of birth from the infected birth canal of the mother. It is such a serious disease, often causing blindness, that every child should be given prophylactic treatment. As soon as the baby is born, the lids should be cleansed and 2 drops of a 1 per cent solution of silver nitrate dropped into the outer angle of each eye.*

The acute stage of the disease begins on the third day after birth, with gradually increasing swelling of the lids and severe pain. The discharge, at first only turbid, becomes yellowish and profuse. If untreated, the disease causes ulceration of the cornea and the whole eye may become involved. Recovery

---

* Penicillin vs. silver nitrate. Newborn infants are considered to be immunologically immature and not easily sensitized to foreign proteins. If this is so, one of the major objections to the use of penicillin in prophylaxis may be discarded—namely, the danger of sensitizing a large number of infants to the future use of this drug. However, there are several additional objections to the use of penicillin. (1) Intramuscular injections may bring about a Herxheimer reaction in syphilitic infants. (2) Frequent applications are necessary when penicillin is used topically, a disadvantage when babies are born at home. (3) There is now some evidence that strains of gonococci resistant to penicillin are occurring. (Ormsby, H. L.: Prophylaxis of ophthalmia neonatorum, Am. J. Nurs. **57:**1175, 1957)

TABLE 20. Differential Diagnosis of the Red Eye*

	Acute Conjunctivitis	Acute Iritis	Acute Glaucoma	Corneal Ulcer or Trauma	Scleritis	Episcleritis
Only Superficial Vessels Dilated	YES					
Superficial & Deep Vessels Dilated		Yes	Yes	Yes	Diffuse	Sector
Pupil	Not Affected!!!!!	Small	Lg. Shallow Anterior Chamber	Small if 2° Iritis	Small if 2° Iritis	
Increased Pressure		May have 2° Glaucoma	Marked			
Opacity	Cornea Uninvolved	Iris & Ant. Chamber may be hazy	Steamy Cornea	Corneal Opacity Fluorescein Staining	May encroach on cornea	
Ocular Discharge	YES			YES		
Decreased Vision	No!!!	YES	YES (Rainbows)	YES		
Severe Pain			YES (Vomiting)	YES		
History	Contagious	Often Recurrent	Often Hereditary	Often Trauma	Often Arthritis	
Therapy	Antibiotics	Atropine Cortisone	Pilocarpine Diamox ? Surgery	Antibiotics	Systemic & Topical Cortisone	Topical Cortisone
Prognosis	Self-limited 3–5 Days	MAY BE EXTREMELY SERIOUS WITHOUT PROPER TREATMENT				Self-limited 2–4 Weeks

*Medical Science, 2:31, 1957.

from the advanced stages of the disease is accompanied by varying degrees of blindness. Both eyes usually are affected.

NURSING CARE. After the disease has developed, the treatment falls largely into the hands of the nurse. The patient must be isolated and strict medical aseptic precautions followed.

Treatment in the early stages consists of the application of cold compresses 15 minutes out of every hour to help control chemosis. Pencillin or sulfa drugs are used.

Corneal Ulcers. Inflammation of the cornea is called *keratitis* and, if this process is associated with a loss of substance, a corneal ulcer results. The inflammatory reaction often spreads deeper to the iris (iritis), with the result that pus is formed and collects as a white or yellow deposit behind the cornea (hypopyon). If the ulceration perforates, the iris may prolapse through the cornea, or other serious complications may follow. Because of the importance of the cornea to vision, any ulceration must be considered as a most serious condition. The healing of any but the very superficial ulcers

is attended with some degree of opacity of the cornea and, therefore, with some diminution of vision.

SYMPTOMS. The symptoms of corneal ulceration are pain, marked photophobia and increased lacrimation. The eye usually appears somewhat injected or "bloodshot" (lay term).

TREATMENT. Prevention is much simpler and easier than cure. Therefore, it is important for the nurse to realize that prompt removal of foreign bodies and early treatment of infections may prevent the occurrence of a corneal ulcer.

Dark glasses are provided to relieve the photophobia. Mydriatics are given at frequent intervals. Tetracaine (Pontocaine) may be used to relieve pain. Fluorescein generally is used to outline the ulcers before the application of the healing solutions. Antibiotic solutions are employed in irrigations of the eye several times daily. Warm compresses go far in relieving the pain in this condition. If the ulcer is deep, the ophthalmologist often cauterizes with silver nitrate 2 per cent followed by saline irrigation.

Fever Therapy and Nursing Care. Other methods of treatment of corneal ulcers are small doses of x-rays and fever therapy, a bacterial antigen of typhoid bacilli being used.

After the injection of the antigen, the patient's temperature, pulse, respiration and blood pressure are taken every hour until the temperature reaches 100° F. At this time the readings are made at 15-minute intervals so long as the temperature is elevated. The patient should be placed in bed after the temperature reaches 99° F. If a chill occurs, hot-water bottles should be placed round him and blankets should be added immediately. Hot liquids should be encouraged and other food given as the patient desires it. Codeine often is prescribed for the patient's comfort.

After the fever subsides, an alcohol rub should be given and the patient placed in dry clothing and a clean bed. Wet clothing should be changed p.r.n. during and after dry clothing and a clean bed. Wet clothing should be changed p.r.n. during and after the temperature rise.

Fever therapy is used frequently in many inflammatory diseases of the eye. The temperature should not exceed 104° F. If this occurs the physician should be notified at once.

THE PATIENT HAVING EYE SURGERY

Preoperative Nursing Care

The preparation of the patient for an ophthalmic operation must be carried out with the most scrupulous care. The lower bowel is evacuated in the morning of the day of operation, and only liquid diet is given after that. The hair of female patients should be so arranged that it will remain in place for several days, and bandages may be applied over it. Usually it is recommended that long hair be plaited into two braids that may be pinned up over the head. Before preparing the eyes for operation, the heads of all patients should be covered with a stockinet cap. The male patient should have his face shaved. The eyebrow above the eye to be operated upon is shaved only in special cases ordered by the surgeon. The eyelashes of the eye to undergo operation are cut with blunt scissors covered with petrolatum in order to catch the lashes. Both eyelids, the nose, the forehead and the cheeks are scrubbed thoroughly with pHisohex and then are rinsed with saline solution; sterile cotton sponges and forceps are used. After this procedure both eyes are irrigated with 2 per cent saline solution, followed by drops of an antiseptic or antibiotic solution into the eye to be operated on. This varies in different clinics. A small cross mark then is made with a colored solution on the forehead over the eye to be operated on. Both closed eyes then are covered with eye patches wet with boric acid solution, and the eyes and the forehead are protected with sterile gauze dressings bound in place with a 2-inch bandage. In the preparation of patients for operations on the eye, no adhesive should be used on the skin.

Before the patient is taken to the operating room, precautions as to the removal of artificial eyes, dentures and so forth must be taken. These are the same as those described for any other surgical operation. If the patient is to have local anesthesia, he should be instructed to hold his head still and to look up or down as directed by the ophthalmologist. He should be cautioned not to "squeeze" the eye during or after operation.

Postoperative Nursing Care

After operation the patient is returned to bed to lie in the supine position with a small pillow under the head. Sandbags may be used under the pillow on each side of the head to keep the head quiet. Where possible, the patient should have a call bell and should be instructed to ring when necessary rather than to move or strain in an attempt to be self-sufficient. Inasmuch as the patient often has both eyes covered, it is well for any personnel who enter his unit to announce himself. The application of bed sides to the bed of a patient with bandaged eyes frequently gives him a sense of security.

The ophthalmologist should be notified immediately if the patient is restless, if he coughs, turns, develops a rhinitis, has excessive pains or disturbs the dressing.

The mouth should be swabbed twice daily, but the teeth should not be brushed until permission is given by the ophthalmologist. Female patients should not have their hair combed until they are allowed out of bed.

When the patient complains of abdominal discomfort due to gas, a hot-water bottle to the abdomen and the insertion of a rectal tube often give relief. Catheterization may be necessary when there is difficulty in voiding. Morphine never should be given to ophthalmic patients unless it is certain that vomiting will not injure the eye.

As indicated in the preoperative care of these patients, diversional or recreational therapy is important. This should be of such a nature that the eyes are not fatigued in any way. Even the environment of this patient is an important consideration. The walls and the ceiling should be painted in soft pastel shades. Light should be regulated so that it is not bright and does not produce a glare.

Before the patient leaves the hospital, he must be informed thoroughly by the physician regarding medications, eye aids ("glasses"), the type of work he can do and his follow-up visits.

Corneal Transplantation (Keratoplasty)

All too frequently, the sight in the eyes of patients with corneal ulcers is badly im-

paired, even to complete loss of vision after extensive scars due to trauma or infection. Here the plastic procedure of corneal transplantation is employed, with marvelous success in many cases. Transplants may be taken from the same person or from a donor, or from the eye of a recently deceased person.* Experiments are being done on the value of inert plastic corneas.

Treatment and Nursing Care

The patient's general condition is checked, and attempts are made to attain optimum health. The day before surgery, cultures usually are taken of the conjunctiva, and the flora of organisms is reduced by antibiotic eyedrops. The psychological factor cannot be dismissed; therefore, these patients must be cared for with understanding.

The care after operation is the same as

* The national eye bank (Eye-Bank for Sight Restoration, Inc., 210 E. 64th St., New York, N. Y.) was founded in 1945. Eyes have been donated from persons all over the country and distributed to qualified ophthalmologists throughout the United States.

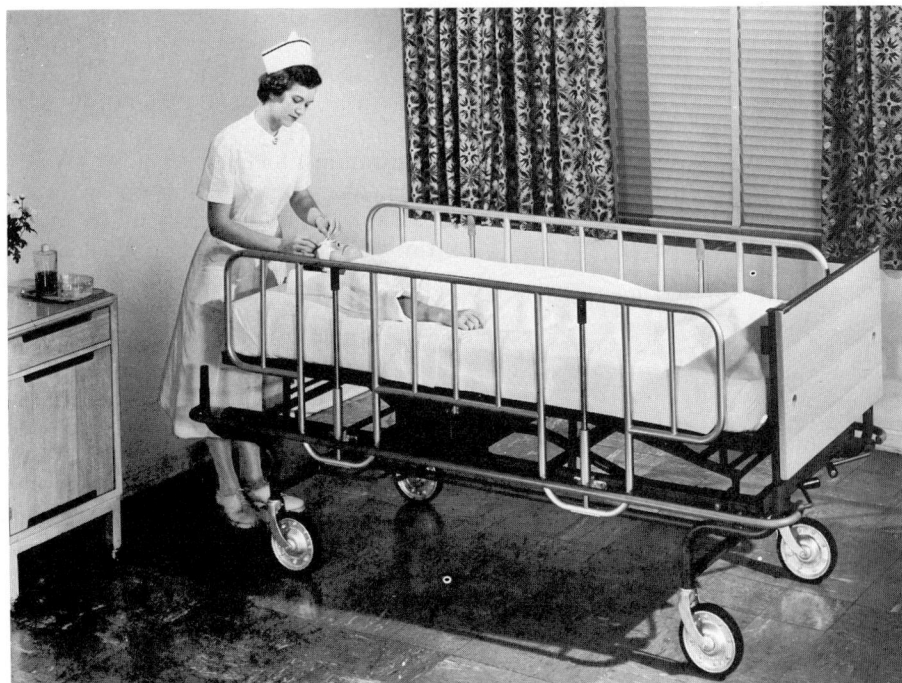

FIG. 333. Postoperative nursing care of the patient following eye surgery. Note the free access to the head and face. (Hill-Romm Co., Batesville, Ind.)

that after operation for cataract (p. 869), except that the duration of bed rest without
head motion is longer, i.e., about a week.
The first dressing then is done, and pressure
dressings are retained from 2 to 4 weeks.
Skin care, mouth care and adequate semi-
soft diet are given during the first week; a
mild cathartic followed by an oil retention
enema will eliminate undue straining on defecation. Every precaution is taken to prevent infection. Home care is directed primarily at avoiding straining of the eyes.
Dark glasses may be worn, reading reduced
to a minimum, and prolonged watching of
television must be avoided. Gradually
strength and vision in the eye are regained.

Glaucoma

*"Glaucoma means sea green, which is the
color of the light reflex from the pupil after
vision has been destroyed. Glaucoma was
known to Socrates four centuries before
Christ. The disease is not hopeless, but the
degree to which treatment for it can be successful depends on how early it is detected
and how cooperative the patient is."*
—Headland, M. F.: I'm winning my
fight against glaucoma, Today's
Health 34:44, Dec. 1956.

Glaucoma is the name given to the disease
characterized by increased tension or pressure within the eye. This disease ordinarily
occurs in individuals past 40 and may be
classified as primary or secondary:

1. *Primary:*
   a. Chronic simple glaucoma (wide-
   angle)
   b. Congestive glaucoma (narrow-
   angle)
      1. Acute
      2. Chronic
2. *Secondary:*
   Under this may be listed many types
   secondary to such conditions as
   trauma, aphakia, iritis, tumor, hemorrhage, etc.

The cause of primary glaucoma is unknown, although it often is associated with
emotional disturbances, endocrine imbalance, allergy or vasomotor disturbance. Secondary glaucoma results as a complication of
some other disturbance within the eye. This

increased intraocular tension may be noted
with the fingers, but more accurately by
means of a *tonometer*. Normally, fluids that
enter the eye globe are balanced by those
that leave the eye. In glaucoma, more fluid
enters the eye than leaves it, which results in
an increased intraocular tension. When this
imbalance occurs gradually, symptoms are
slight; however, when it occurs rapidly, pain
results because of the pressure on the optic
nerve. Peripheral vision is impaired long
before there is any effect on central vision.
Artificial lights appear to have a rainbow
around them. Vision becomes cloudy or
smoky. These symptoms are aggravated after
the patient has been in dim light (e.g., watching movies or television) or after an emotional upset. If untreated, glaucoma leads to
blindness.

Treatment and Nursing Care

The Prevention of Blindness Society estimates that 40,000 Americans have lost their
vision and another 150,000 have become
partly blind from glaucoma. It is estimated
that about 2 per cent of the over-40 population of the United States has glaucoma.

"When the glaucoma was detected in a
late stage, vision continued to fail in 50 per
cent of patients despite treatment. But when
the disease was detected in an early stage
and the patient conscientiously used miotic
eyedrops, 81 per cent showed no visual deterioration in five years."* A California
medical survey† indicated that a test for
tension in the eye, if included in every routine physical examination, could substantially
reduce the incidence of blindness from glaucoma. By the use of miotic drugs the pupil
is contracted and the iris is drawn away from
the cornea, thus allowing the aqueous humor
to drain through the lymph spaces into the
canal of Schlemm. Pilocarpine, eserine or
Carcholin are the drugs employed. Diamox,
a sulfonamide derivative and a diuretic has
proved to be of value in the treatment of the
glaucomas. It may aid in getting some patients in better condition for surgery and, in
others, may control tension to such an ex-

* Reed, H., and Bendor-Samuel, J. E. L.: The
early detection of glaucoma, Canad. M. A. J., Jan.
1, 1958.
† Medical Science, 2:59, 1957.

tent that surgery is not necessary. Recently, many new drugs have been introduced into the medical treatment of glaucoma, such as Humorsol, Phospholine-iodide, and Epitrate.

There are many types of surgery. In acute cases (narrow-angle glaucoma), an incision is made through the cornea so that a portion of the iris may be drawn out and excised (*iridectomy*). This permits drainage of aqueous from the anterior chamber and reduction of intraocular tension. Other operations on the iris (*iridencleisis*) are modifications having the same objective, that is, to permit fluid to escape.

Chronic (wide-angle) glaucoma often is treated by combining miotics with carbonic anhydrous inhibitors. Remissions may occur, but, if there is no improvement, surgery may be done by making a small opening with a circular knife at the junction of the cornea and the sclera. This operation, called *corneoscleral trephining,* leaves a permanent opening through which aqueous humor may drain. Usually it is covered by a flap of conjunctiva. In the preoperative treatment of these patients, irrigations of both eyes are often prescribed, and weaker solutions of pilocarpine are instilled in the unaffected eye.

After operation, the patient is kept flat and relatively quiet for 24 hours in order to prevent prolapse of the iris through the incision. A liquid diet is permitted. Narcotics or sedatives may be given if necessary. After the first dressing is changed, the patient is allowed more freedom. Usually, he is discharged on the fifth day. He is expected to visit the ophthalmologist regularly, since glaucoma is a condition that must be followed periodically.

Teaching Suggestions. Remind the patient of the importance of avoiding worry, fear, anger and excitement. Tight clothing such as a tight belt, collar or corset should not be worn. Suggest that he exercise in moderation to keep the blood circulation active. Coffee as well as tea should be limited to a cup a day. Bowel habits should be regular. He should keep his teeth clean and healthy and take care of acute or chronic colds. He should avoid dark rooms as much as possible; go to movies or watch television only if the ophthalmologist permits. Eye drops or eye washes should be used only with the consent of the eye physician. He must be conscientious about keeping appointments for eye examinations.

Cataract

Cataract is the term applied to an opacity of the crystalline lens or of its capsule. The most common type occurs in adults past middle age, but it may occur in younger individuals as a result of trauma or disease. Occasionally it occurs at birth (congenital cataract). As the rays of light entering the eye must pass through the pupil and the lens to reach the retina, any opacity in the lens behind the pupil will produce alterations in vision. Very often the opacity is not complete at first, so that vision may be improved by an iridectomy (removal of a piece of iris), which allows light to pass through the part of the lens uncovered by the operation. As time goes on, the degenerative processes cause more opacification of the lens, opacity becomes complete and the cataract is said to be ripe or mature and can be cured only by operation.

The preparation for operation has been described. Usually the patient is given a proteolytic enzyme, Alpha-chymotrypsin (Alpha-Chymar), which acts specifically on the lens ligaments, dissolving them so that the cataract can be removed more easily. The nurse should explain to the patient some of the restrictions he will face immediately postoperatively. He will accept these limitations more gracefully at that time. At the operation, an incision is made through the sclera barely outside of the cornea, the lens capsule is excised and the lens is expressed by pressure on the eye from below with a metal spoon. This is called an *extracapsular extraction.*

Another type of cataract operation is known as an *intracapsular extraction*. In this operation, the lens is removed within its capsule. The incision is closed with very fine black silk sutures.

After the extraction of the cataract, both eyes may be covered with sterile eye patches (some surgeons cover the operated eye only) held in place with two pieces of transparent surgical tape, and additional protection is supplied by a metal or plastic eye shield. Occasionally an ocular mask of black buckram is applied to cover the entire dressing.

At present, some eye surgeons are trying plastic lens as a substitute for the real lens when it is removed. The postoperative patient must wear a pair of glasses or contact lenses in order to focus the light rays, inasmuch as the lenses of his eye have been removed. The introduction of the plastic lens into the eye dispenses with this problem.* However, this technic is more complicated and not accepted by all ophthalmologists.

Postoperative Nursing Care

The patient is permitted a low firm pillow immediately after operation and may have the head of the bed slightly raised. Any strain felt by the patient may be relieved somewhat by placing pillows under the knees or the small of the back. Liquid diet is supplemented with custards, junkets, gelatin and so forth. Iced water, fruit juices, milk and other gas-producing foods are avoided. Soft diet or diet of choice usually is resumed on the second day. The patient is allowed out of bed in 24 to 48 hours, depending on his condition and his physician's orders.

If patients wear a face mask which covers both eyes, it helps the patient if anyone who

* For further information on the plastic lens, the reader is referred to Perritt, R. A.: Intraocular acrylic lens in cataract, Medical Science 3:159-161, 1958.

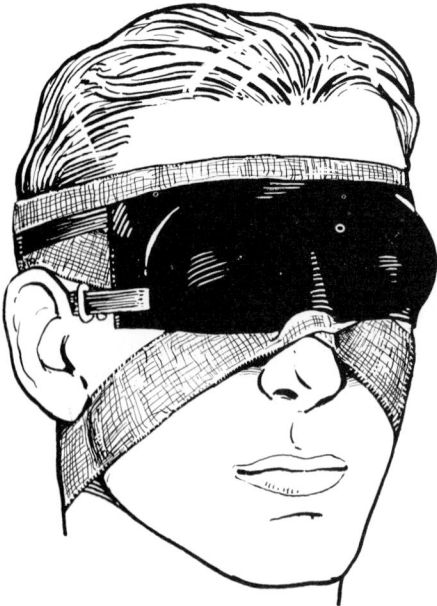

Fig. 334. Ring's ocular mask.

comes near his bed speaks to him. He wonders what is going on about him and is apt to be less apprehensive if he knows. Side rails often give the patient a feeling of security, and they should be used especially at night.

During the first 24 to 48 hours many patients become anxious and worried over the results of the operation. This is not to be wondered at if it is remembered that the patient's mind may be active, even though both eyes are closed. The efficient nurse can do much to reassure her charge and direct his thoughts away from himself toward other and more diverting subjects.

Many of these patients are in the older age group. Psychoses as well as pulmonary and circulatory complications have occurred postoperatively in cataract patients as a result of covering both eyes and restricting their physical activities. Consequently, there is a trend to increase their activities earlier. Some eye surgeons do not cover the unoperated eye. The rule usually followed is that the older the patient, the fewer the restrictions, and often early ambulation is permitted.

Pain usually is slight after cataract extraction but, should it become severe, the surgeon should be notified at once, as this may be the symptom of a serious complication, such as hemorrhage.

The surgeon usually will dress the eye 24 hours after operation and once daily thereafter until the seventh or the eighth day. When the sutures are removed, the eye is anesthetized with 1 per cent pontocaine; sterile eye speculum, forceps and scissors are required. The patient is discharged when his eyes have become accustomed to ordinary daylight.

Six or eight weeks after the removal of the cataract the patient may be fitted with glasses, which in a measure take the place of the crystalline lens. In 6 months' time the eyes will have made their adjustment and permanent glasses may be ordered. However, the power of accommodation is lost, so that two glasses must be used, one for distant and one for near vision (or a bifocal lens).

Strabismus (Squint)

Strabismus or *squint* is a condition in which one eye deviates from the object at

THE PATIENT WITH CATARACT SURGERY
Objectives of Care and Principles of Nursing Management

1. To prepare the patient for cataract surgery:
   A. Orient the patient to his new environment.
      a. Walk with the patient around the unit.
      b. Explain the hospital routine.
      c. Provide side rails on bed if patient is elderly.
   B. Begin rehabilitation measures as soon after admission as possible.
      a. Teach patient to breathe deeply, move extremities and do quadriceps muscle setting without moving his head.
      b. Instruct the patient how to close his eyes slowly without squeezing the lids.
   C. Reduce the conjunctival bacterial count.
      a. Obtain a conjunctival culture.
      b. Use local broad-spectrum antibiotics as ordered.
      c. Use aseptic technic when doing eye treatments and procedures.
   D. Prepare the affected eye for surgery.
      a. Instill local mydriatic if ordered.
      b. Determine whether the pupil is dilated after the instillation of a mydriatic is completed.

2. To give optimum nursing care postoperatively:
   A. Reorient the patient to his surroundings.
   B. Prevent increased intraocular pressure and stress on the suture line.
      a. Instruct the patient not to cough, sneeze, or move too rapidly.
      b. Position the patient on his back and unoperated side.
      c. Elevate the head of the bed 30 to 45 degrees for comfort.
      d. Keep the eye shield on the operated eye to protect it from injury.
   C. Promote the comfort of the patient.
      a. Position him to relieve back pain.
      b. Give mild analgesics to control pain.
      c. Maintain a quiet and relaxed environment.
      d. Inform the patient when you enter the room.
   D. Observe and treat for complications.
      a. Nausea and Vomiting.
         (1). Support the patient's head when he is vomiting.
         (2). Use antiemetic drugs and cold compresses to throat.
      b. Hemorrhage
         (1). Notify physician immediately if patient complains of sudden pain in eye.
         (2). Observe for and try to allay restlessness.

3. To promote the rehabilitation of the patient:
   A. Encourage the patient to become independent.
      a. Teach him to increase his activities gradually.
      b. Walk with him when he first becomes ambulatory.
   B. Instruct the patient and his family about the use of eye drops.
   C. Refer the patient to proper agencies if home assistance is needed.
   D. Assist the patient to participate in a program of diversional activities during the convalescent period.
   E. Inform the patient that:
      a. Dark glasses may be used after the eye dressing is removed.
      b. Temporary corrective lenses may be prescribed during the convalescent period.
      c. Permanent lenses will be prescribed 6 to 8 weeks after surgery.

which the person is looking (lay term "cross-eyed"). The deviating eye may turn in (*eso-tropia*) or out (*exotropia*). It may result from paralysis of the nerves supplying the extraocular muscles, due to injury or disease. Double vision or diplopia results. In children, a strabismus due to ocular defects often develops. It is characterized by single vision usually because the image seen by the divergent eye is suppressed involuntarily.

The strabismus in children often may be corrected by the wearing of properly fitted glasses. Orthopedic training for muscle disturbances, such as strabismus, is successful in occasional instances without operation. It consists of a series of muscle exercises carried out by means of various instruments, cards and test objects. Patients who have a marked degree of squint are operated on usually after having had some training; then, after the eyes are straightened, the exercises are employed again. Early detection and immediate medical consultation are to be encouraged if the defect is to be corrected satisfactorily.

THE NURSE AND THE NEWLY BLIND

There are about 1,000,000 blind persons in America, and each year nearly 40,000 more go blind. Of these newly blind cases, approximately half could be prevented with our present knowledge.

When an individual has marked visual impairment or is newly blind, he needs a great deal of help in making the adjustment so that he will emerge as a confident, happy and useful person. For the most part this care is entrusted to those skilled in this work. However, there are certain practices which a nurse can follow as she cares for such a person.

A blind person always should be treated as a normal human being. Avoid expressions of pity and sympathy. Keep him from becoming discouraged by seeing that he has someone with whom he can talk or some other form of diversion such as a radio. Help him to overcome his feeling of awkwardness as he performs simple activities. If he is allowed out of bed, the blind person should survey his room by walking around and touching the furniture. Thereafter, the nurse should be sure that the furniture remains in

the same position. Never leave a door half open; it should be either open or shut. When walking with a blind person, allow him to follow you by lightly touching your elbow. Do not push him ahead of you. When he walks alone, a lightweight walking stick can be used as an extended hand to warn him of obstacles. It should not be used for tapping the sidewalk or the floor. Electronic guidance devices are still under investigation.

Personal appearance is a significant part of the patient's care. He should be allowed to dress by himself; a woman even can learn to fix her hair and use cosmetics. Table etiquette, smoking, writing and so forth all are activities that can be acquired with practice. The nurse should be familiar with the programs offered by such groups as The Seeing Eye, Inc., Morristown, N. J., where blind persons can learn the value of a dog guide.

CLINICAL SITUATION

Mr. J., 52, a writer, has noticed a gradual decrease in vision. He went to his ophthalmologist, who took a tonometer reading.

1. The tonometer is a device used to:
   A. Record intraocular pressure.
   B. Evaluate lens opacity.
   C. Determine the presence of corneal abrasion.
   D. Remove fluid from the anterior chamber.
2. When the pressure in the eyeball is higher than normal, the condition is called:
   A. Hyperhydrosis.
   B. Iritis.
   C. Trachoma.
   D. Glaucoma.
3. The purpose of instilling pilocarpine eye drops in Mr. J's eyes is to:
   A. Remove the obstruction in the ciliary body.
   B. Increase the production of vitreous humor.
   C. Widen the angle between the iris and cornea.
   D. Relieve the clouding of the cornea.
4. If the patient with glaucoma is not treated early, he will lose his sight due to:
   A. Opacity of the crystalline lens.
   B. Pressure on the optic nerve.
   C. Detachment of the retina.
   D. Recurring secondary conjunctivitis.

BIBLIOGRAPHY AND SUGGESTED READING

Books

Adler, F. H.: Textbook of Ophthalmology, ed. 7, Philadelphia, Saunders, 1962.

Manhattan Eye, Ear and Throat Hospital: Nursing in Diseases of the Eye, Ear, Nose and Throat, Philadelphia, Saunders, 1958.

Articles

Blodi, F. C.: Retrolental fibroplasia, Am. J. Nurs. **53:**718-720, 1953.

Blodi, F. C., and Honn, R. C.: Tumors of the eye, Am. J. Nurs. **56:**1152-1156, 1956.

————: Glaucoma, Am. J. Nurs. **63:**78-83, Mar., 1963.

Brueggen, S. L.: Nurses' opportunities to conserve sight, Nurs. Outlook **10:**658-660, Oct., 1962.

————: Eye health in industry, Am. J. Nurs. **61:**83-85, 1961.

Burian, H. M.: Strabismus, Am. J. Nurs. **60:** 653-656, May, 1960.

Chambers, W. G.: Learning to wear contact lenses, Am. J. Nurs. **61:**82-83, June, 1961.

Crawford, O. E.: Eye injuries in a chemical plant, Nurs. Outlook **3:**447-449, 1955.

Cunningham, F., and O'Neil, J. E.: Eye safety in schools, Nurs. Outlook **5:**522-524, 1957.

Eye conditions, Canad. Nurse **57:**225-247; 255-265, Mar., 1961.

Faye, E. E.: Visual aids for the partially sighted, Nurs. Outlook **8:**320-322, June, 1960.

Gamble, R. C.: The medical eye examination, Am. J. Nurs. **57:**1590-1592, 1957.

Gordon, D. M.: Disease of the eye, Clinical Symposia, vol. 14. Entire issue devoted to this subject, Summitt, N. J., Ciba, Oct.-Nov.-Dec., 1962.

Guiding principles and procedures for industrial nurses in care of eye injuries, Am. J. Nurs. **61:**86-88, Sept., 1961.

Jaeckle, C. W.: Contact lenses and the physician, J.A.M.A. **179:**696-698, 1962.

Jones, I. S., and Bosanko, L.: The cataract extraction operation and nursing care, Am. J. Nurs. **60:**1433-1437, Oct., 1960.

Leopold, I. H. Anti-inflammatory agents in ophthalmology, Am. J. Nurs. **63:**84-87, Mar., 1963.

Pinkerton, G.: Learning to live with blindness, Nurs. Outlook **3:**432-435, 1955.

Problems in adjusting to blindness (Abs.), Am. J. Nurs. **56:**74, 1956.

Reed, H.: Squint or strabismus, Canad. Nurse **55:**16-20, 1959.

Sampson, M. T.: Going blind, Am. J. Nurs. **61:** 55, May, 1961.

Stocker, F. W., and Bell, R.: Corneal transplantation and nursing care, Am. J. Nurs. **62:** 65-70, May, 1962.

Weiss, M. O.: Psychological aspects of nursing care for eye patients, Am. J. Nurs. **50:**218-220, 1950.

Willma, I. R.: As a blind nurse sees, Am. J. Nurs. **55:**205-208, 1955.

Patient-Teaching Aids and Information

Another Eye Saved, The Wise Owl Story. A folder describing the Wise Owl Club of America, The Nat'l Society for the Prevention of Blindness.

Cataract and Glaucoma; Hope Through Research. (U. S. Public Health Service Publication No. 793 and Health Information Series No. 99) 15 pages. 1961.

Eye Cues for Eye Care. An illustrated folder describing eye complaints. From National Medical Foundation for Eye Care, 1961.

Eyes that See and Ears that Hear. A 20-page pocket size booklet. John Hancock Life Insurance Co.

Glaucoma, Pub. No. 13. A 7-page pamphlet, National Society for Prevention of Blindness.

Glaucoma—What It Is—What It Is Not, Pub. No. 6. Illustrated 7-page pamphlet. National Society for the Prevention of Blindness.

Horizontal Section of a Right Eyeball. A labeled line drawing on a single page 8½ x 11, Pub. No. 169. National Society for Prevention of Blindness.

The Newly Blinded. A 17-page booklet prepared by The Seeing Eye, Inc., Morristown, N. J.

The Occupational Health Nurse and Eye Care, Pub. No. 133. A 16-page useful booklet with detailed information by National Society for the Prevention of Blindness.

Ogg, E.: Save Your Sight (Public Affairs Pamphlet No. 215), N. Y. Public Affairs Committee, 1954.

Physiological Effects of Age on the Visual Process, Pub. No. 195. National Society for Prevention of Blindness.

Prevent Retrolental Fibroplasia in Premature Infants with Oxygen Control, Pub. 290. National Society for Prevention of Blindness.

Rules for Glaucoma Patients. A sheet of instructions from the National Society for Prevention of Blindness.

The Sight-Saving Review. A quarterly publication of the National Society for the Prevention of Blindness.

The Treatment of Trachoma, Pub. 293. An 8-page reprint, National Society for Prevention of Blindness.

Veirs, E. R.: So You Have Glaucoma. A 64-page book, New York, Grune, 1958.

What You Should Know About Cataracts. An 8-page pamphlet. National Society for Prevention of Blindness.

Your Eyes after Forty, Pub. No. 28. A folded pamphlet describing normal developments and dangerous possibilities from National Society for Prevention of Blindness.

Additional lists of publications and information available from:

American Foundation for the Blind
15 West 15th St.
New York 11, New York

Braille Institute of America, Inc.
741 N. Vermont Ave.
Los Angeles 29, California

National Council to Combat Blindness
41 West 57th St.
New York 19, New York

National Medical Foundation for Eye Care
250 West 57th St.
New York 19, New York

National Society for the
  Prevention of Blindness
16 East 40th St.
New York 16, New York

Retina Foundation
30 Chambers St.
Boston 14, Massachusetts

40

Patients With Problems of the Ear and the Mastoid

Revised by BERNARD J. RONIS, M.D.*

The ear is a very complex sense organ for hearing and equilibrium. The early detection and the accurate diagnosis of ear disease are important both in children and in adults. The importance of hearing in a child's development in early life and the later adjustments have been stressed in recent years. Among those who take an important part in the diagnosis of patients with auditory disorders are pediatricians, otolaryngologists, psychiatrists, neurologists, psychologists, speech pathologists, educators and audiologists. Before a child can speak, he must first be able to hear, then interpret what he hears, and, last, he must be able to express himself in the development of speech. Diverse occurrences during birth, disorders due to birth injury, bacterial and virus infections in childhood, toxic drug effects, damage to the ear by noisy occupation, changes in the ear as the result of aging are only a few of the problems confronting the otologist in diagnosis, treatment and rehabilitation.

ANATOMY AND PHYSIOLOGY

The ear, with its dual function of hearing and equilibrium, may be divided into 3 portions for study: The external ear, or that part visible, includes also the external canal and the eardrum (tympanic membrane) (Fig. 335). The middle ear, a small cavity adjoining the eardrum contains the 3 ossicles or ear bones (malleus, incus and stapes), which transmit vibrations from the eardrum to the third portion, the inner ear or laby-

rinth. One portion of the labyrinth is the cochlea, containing the organ of Corti, the center of hearing; the other portion comprises the 3 semicircular canals, which contain the nerve centers for the sense of equilibrium.

The auricle or external ear varies in size, shape and position on the head, and it aids in the collection of sound waves and their passage into the external auditory canal. The external auditory canal is a skin-lined tube that ends at a disklike structure, also lined with skin, the eardrum. The skin of the canal contains highly specialized glands that secrete a brown waxylike substance, *cerumen* (earwax). This material serves as a protective for the skin. There are also hair follicles and sweat glands.

The middle ear, with its contained ossicles and attached ligaments and their connection to the eardrum, is vitally concerned in the function of hearing. The middle ear connects with the posterior portion of the nose by means of the eustachian tube. It is by this means that equal air pressure is maintained on both sides of the eardrum. The tube, normally closed, opens by action of the muscles of the palate on yawning or swallowing. The tube serves as a drainage channel for normal and abnormal secretions of the middle ear and equalizes pressures in the middle ear to the atmosphere. When the membrane of this tube is inflamed, it offers an easy passage for infection into the middle ear.

Sound waves transmitted by the drum to the ossicles of the middle ear are transferred to the *cochlea,* the organ of hearing, lodged in the labyrinth or inner ear. An important

* Professor and Chairman, Department of Otorhinology, Temple University Hospital, Philadelphia, Pa.

ossicle is the stapes, which rocks on its posterior portion, not unlike a piston, and sets up vibrations in fluids contained in the labyrinth. These pressure waves, passed through the cochlea, produce sound stimuli by setting into vibration hair cells in the organ of Corti, which in turn are passed along the auditory nerve to the cerebral cortex in the brain, where sound is analyzed and interpreted.

Balance of the body is maintained by the cooperation of muscle, joint, tendon, visceral senses, the eyes and the inner ear or vestibular apparatus. The last is the most important in this function. This inner apparatus informs the individual as to the movements and the position of the head in space, coordinates all body muscles and positions the eyes in rapid motion or head movement. This apparatus consists of the utricle, the saccule and the semicircular canals, of which there are 3 in each ear. Each canal lies in a plane at right angles to each other, and they are grouped in working pairs for this complex function. The mechanism of action of the semicircular canals may be likened to the cochlea or organ of hearing. Here, also, fluids are set in motion by head or body movement which, in turn, are transmitted to extremely delicate nerve fibers which transmit messages as electric impulses along the nerve to centers in the brain related to the function of equilibrium, eye movement and body position.

GENERAL HYGIENE OF THE EAR

Cleansing of the external auditory canal by the introduction of matches, hair pins and other implements is dangerous, since trauma to the skin may result in accidental infection of the skin or damage to the ear drum. Wax deposits may be softened by the instillation of a few drops of warmed glycerine daily, followed by irrigation at body temperature, using a bulb syringe or a special ear syringe. The inner ear is easily stimulated with water temperatures either below or above body temperature, creating annoying vertigo. After irrigation, the canal is dried carefully with a sterile applicator and cotton. The removal of impacted cerumen or earwax may require the skilled attention of the physician. Vigorous blowing of the nose or douching of the nose may be dangerous during acute infection, such as the common cold. Middle ear infection via the eustachian tube is not uncommon. Patients with a history of ear infection, and particularly those with perforations of the drum, should avoid contamination of the ear with water at bathing, swimming or diving. The patient is instructed to plug the ear with cotton or lamb's wool saturated with petrolatum and to wear a rubber cap at time of ocean bathing or swimming.

Certain forms of deafness are due to the damaging effect of work in noisy surroundings. The so-called boilermaker or punch-

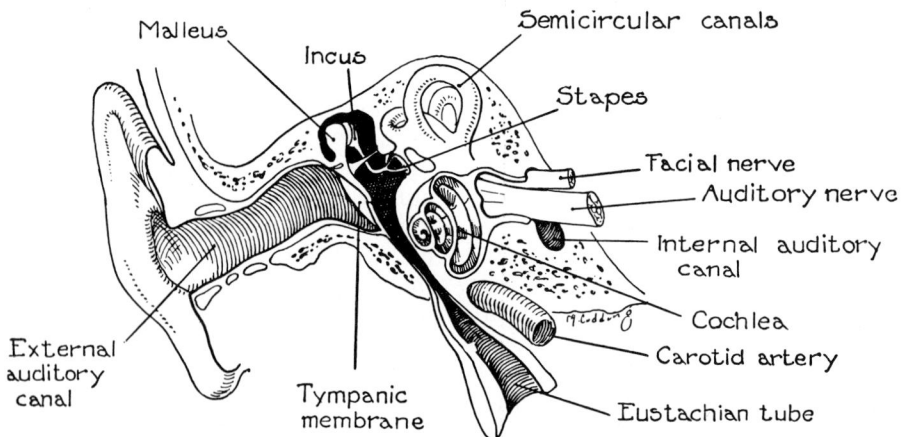

Fig. 335. Semidiagrammatic drawing of the ear to show the relations of the structures of the external and the internal ear. (Wolf, G. D.: Ear, Nose and Throat, Philadelphia, Lippincott)

press operator deafness are examples of this form of impairment. Those susceptible to the damaging effect of noise should avoid these surroundings. The effect of noise can be minimized by wearing protective ear plugs. In modern industry this poses a serious problem to the worker. Sudden changes in atmospheric pressure, such as occur in flying in an airplane, may cause serious middle ear symptoms. No one with acute respiratory infections or allergic disorders of the nose that block the eustachian tube and prevent adequate ventilation of the middle ear should fly. Those flying should be taught to inflate the ears by the so-called Valsalva method. In this technic the nostrils are held tightly, and the ears are inflated by vigorous blowing; thus pressure in the middle ear is equalized to relieve annoying symptoms. Deafness, ear pain or discharge from the ear of any type should make the patient seek the advice of a physician.

HEARING TESTS

Hearing tests not only help to determine the particular type of hearing defect present but also to establish the potential of the patient's hearing.

Tuning Fork. This inexpensive instrument can differentiate between *conductive deafness* (caused by a disorder in the auditory canal, the eardrum or the ossicles) and *perceptive deafness* (due to a disorder of the organ of Corti or the auditory nerve).

In the *Weber test,* the fork is placed on the forehead in order to compare hearing in the two ears. For example, in normal hearing or in deafness that is equal on both sides, the patient will indicate that he hears the vibrations in the middle of his head. Variations will suggest hearing inequality. The next step will be the *Rinne test.* In this test, after striking the tuning fork, the doctor first places the handle against the mastoid process, behind the external auditory opening. Then he holds the tines beside the ear and asks the patient to tell where he heard the sound better or longer.

These two tests do not give quantitative information, which is obtained by audiologic study (audiogram).

Audiogram. In deafness, the audiometer is the single most important diagnostic instrument. Audiometric testing is of two kinds: (1) pure-tone audiometry, in which the sound stimulus consists of a pure or musical tone (the louder the tone before the patient perceives it, the greater the hearing loss; the unit of measure of loudness of sound is the *decibel*); (2) speech audiometry, in which the spoken word is used to determine the ability to understand and discriminate sounds.

For accuracy, audiometric tests should be done in a soundproof room. The patient wears earphones and is instructed to signal when he hears the tone and again when he no longer hears it. When the tone is applied directly over the external auditory opening, air conduction is measured. When the stimulus is applied to the mastoid bone, thereby bypassing the conductive mechanism, nerve conduction is tested.

The normal human ear perceives sounds ranging from about 20 cycles per second to 20,000 cycles per second; however, only the frequencies from 500 to 2,000 are important in understanding everyday speech. Clinically, this range is referred to as *speech range.* The critical level of loudness is around 30 decibels. In treating patients surgically to improve hearing loss, the aim is to improve the hearing level to 30 decibels or better within the speech frequencies.

PATIENTS WITH PROBLEMS OF THE EXTERNAL EAR

Deformities. Deformities of the ear and the external canal occur as congenital malformations and may be manifested as abnormal size or protrusion of the ear, atresia or closure of the external canal. Acquired deformities, such as cauliflower ear in the boxer and loss of a part or all of the ear, result from accident or injury. These disorders can be aided or cured with appropriate plastic surgery.

Furuncle of the External Canal. Here there is an infection of the skin and the subcutaneous tissue of the external canal. There are usually great pain, marked tinnitus, deafness and ear noise in the ear affected. There may be fever, severe headache and enlargement of the local lymph nodes. This disorder may be mistaken for mastoid infection. The early administration of antibiotics is usually followed by definite improvement, but surgical drainage may be necessary, with incision of the furuncle. Wet dressings follow and are important to facilitate drainage and relieve pain.

Foreign Bodies in the External Canal. Small objects are inserted usually by young children. Such objects may be nonirritating and remain for years without symptoms. Vegetable foreign bodies have a tendency to swell, so irrigation is contraindicated. Attempts at removal may be dangerous in unskilled hands, because the body may be pushed completely into the bony portion of the canal, lacerating the skin of the canal and perforating the drum. Serious infections of the middle ear and the mastoid, with ensuing deafness, may result. Instrumental removal should be under general anesthesia in the very young; when skillfully done, there are no sequelae.

Traumatic Perforation of the Drum Membrane. Accidental perforation of the drum may occur from a slap on the ear, by concussion or by the introduction of objects used for scratching the ear or the removal of cerumen. The symptoms may be minimal, with bloody discharge only, but there may be deafness, vertigo, nausea and vomiting. Secondary infection may supervene, with a purulent discharge. Douching and ear drops are to be avoided, and only a sterile piece of cotton is worn in the ear. The patient is cautioned against blowing the nose vigorously, and the ear should not be contaminated by shampooing the hair or bathing. In most instances, with time, the perforation of the drum will heal. When evidence of infection supervenes, the antibiotics are important until healing takes place.

Fungus Infection of the External Canal. Such an infection appears to be more common during swimming season. By wearing a snug fitting bathing cap, and limiting swimming to the surface of the water, this painful ear problem may be prevented. Ear medications and possibly ear irrigations may be prescribed. For the duration of the ear infection, the patient is cautioned not to swim or allow water to enter the ear when shampooing or showering.

Irrigation of the Ear

Various types of equipment may be used to irrigate the ear, but the most acceptable is an irrigating can and tubing with an irrigating tip. Usually up to 500 ml. of solution is used. The purposes may be varied: to clean the ear when discharge is present, to remove a nonvegetable foreign body from the external canal and to apply heat in order to localize infection or to relieve pain. The solutions for irrigating the ear should be used at a temperature of about 105° to 110° F. Solutions that are too hot or too cold or are used with too much force may result in pain or dizziness to the patient. He may sit or lie with his head tilted toward the side of the affected ear. He may support the curved basin under his ear to receive the returning solution. To be effective the fluids must reach the eardrum, and to this end the nurse is advised to pull the auricle upward and backward in order to straighten the external auditory canal. In children this canal may be straightened by pulling the auricle down and back. Extreme gentleness should be used, and care must be taken that the fluid has free exit so that it will not be driven into the middle ear. After the irrigation, the external opening should be plugged lightly with sterile cotton, which is changed when necessary. After the procedure, the patient is instructed to lie on the affected ear so that gravity will facilitate drainage.

With the present-day problem of bacterially resistant organisms despite the commonly employed antibiotics, it is important for the nurse in attendance to maintain close observation of the patient and his presenting clinical picture, which may change from hour to hour. Ominous signs recognized early may be lifesaving, with surgical intervention.

PATIENTS WITH PROBLEMS OF THE MIDDLE EAR

The most common cause of middle ear disease is involvement of the eustachian tube by swelling, with extension from the nose as part of an acute respiratory infection. Swelling also may be present in nasal allergy or in children who show enlargement of the adenoid with encroachment on the orifice of the tube in the nasopharynx. New growths involving the nasopharynx are more uncommon causes of middle ear symptoms. In the early phase of otitis media, with obstruction of the eustachian tube, exudates cannot leave the middle ear and therefore accumulate, causing symptoms of fullness and deafness.

Retention of exudates in the middle ear also can result after acute inflammation that has been treated with antibiotics, and symptoms such as ear pain and fever subside only to have the exudates in the middle ear rendered sterile, and because of tubal inflammation they are not evacuated. Then the child or the adult will persist with deafness and a sense of fullness in the ear caused by the exudates. Simple myringotomy, or incision of the drum, will evacuate the contents of the middle ear, and healing will take place in a few days, with complete resolution and relief of symptoms. This form, secretory otitis media, is commonly seen today in patients treated with wide-spectrum antibiotics. When unrecognized, it can be a common cause of persistent deafness in children and in adults.

Acute Otitis Media (Abscess in the Ear)

The essential cause of acute otitis media is the entrance of pathogenic bacteria into the normally sterile middle ear when the resistance is lowered or the virulence of the organism is great enough to produce inflammation. Bacteria commonly found, in the order of importance, are: the hemolytic streptococcus, the pneumococcus, the staphylococcus and the influenza bacillus. The mode of entry of the bacteria in most cases is by spread via the auditory canal or the eustachian tube during the indiscriminate use of nose drops or nasal douching, forcible blowing of the nose or sneezing; or, in rare cases, infection may enter after fracture of the skull. The symptoms may vary with the severity of the infection and may be either very mild and transient or very severe and fraught with serious complications. Pain is the first symptom in and about the ear. It may be intense and will be relieved after spontaneous perforation of the drum or after myringotomy. Fever varies and in severe cases may range between 104° and 105° F. Deafness, ear noises, headache, loss of appetite, nausea, vomiting and, in infants, convulsions due to the high fever are other symptoms.

The end-results of otitis media depend on the virulence of the bacteria, the efficiency of the therapy and the resistance of the patient. With early and appropriate wide-spectrum antibiotic therapy, otitis media may clear with healing, and no serious sequelae result.

The condition may become subacute, with long-persistent purulent discharge from the ear. Healing may take place with permanent deafness. Perforation as the result of rupture of the ear drum may persist and develop into a chronic form of otitis media. Secondary complications, with involvement of the mastoid, and other serious intracranial complications such as meningitis or brain abscess, may result.

The nurse should be alerted to the problem of symptoms masked by the antibiotic therapy, and to the fact that during the course of treatment of an acute middle ear infection, symptoms such as headache, slow pulse, vomiting and vertigo are all significant and should be recorded carefully for evaluation by the otologist. It goes without saying that the appropriate antibiotic, often determined by culture and sensitivity tests, is all-important in the prognosis for eventual cure. In mild cases treated early, myringotomy may not be necessary. However, if pain persists, this procedure is important for promoting surgical drainage and offers a ready means of identification of the type of organism present for test of its sensitivity to a chemotherapeutic agent in use or proposed.

Chronic Otitis Media and Mastoiditis

Chronic otitis media results from repeated attacks of otitis media causing persistent perforation of the drum, and it is due to particular virulence of the infecting organism or to bacterial resistance to antibiotic therapy. The chronically infected ear is characterized by persistence or recurrence of purulent discharge, with or without pain, and varying degrees of deafness. Most chronic otitis media begins in childhood and may persist to adult life.

The condition is divided into two forms, both of which have entirely different significance: (1) simple chronic otitis media, which is caused by central perforation of the drum with the presence of a mucuslike discharge, this being the so-called nondangerous type of otitis media, and (2) chronic otitis media, with marginal perforation of the drum membrane with cholesteatoma. This last, caused by ingrowth of skin from the perforation in the drum filling the area in the mastoid and the middle ear, by its encroachment may involve vital structures, such as the facial nerve, the labyrinth and the adjoining areas in the brain. The symptoms may be minimal, with mild deafness and the presence of a persistent or intermittent foul-smelling discharge of variable quantity. The diagnosis is corroborated by the physical finding, but, in addition, roentgenograms of the mastoids will usually show pathologic changes. In the nondangerous type of chronic otitis media, treatment often is successful, bringing about cessation of the foul discharge and, in some patients, improvement of hearing.

Local treatment can be effectual, but antibiotics, while often tried, are largely disappointing, because most of the organisms present in this chronic malady are resistant, and it is difficult to get the drug into prolonged contact with infected areas in sufficient concentration. In chronic otitis media of the dangerous type, with cholesteatoma, surgery may be indicated, based on clinical and x-ray findings. There is usually no pain unless complications ensue. Serious complications as a result of chronic disease may be protracted or sudden in onset. Symptoms such as sudden facial paralysis, unusually profound deafness or dizziness, onset of headache with dizziness and stiff neck may intimate beginning meningitis or brain abscess. Surgical intervention is thus elective or may represent a serious emergency.

Simple Mastoidectomy

Mastoid cells, a honeycomb of bone that adjoins the middle ear, must be removed when there are positive signs of disease in the mastoid process. In acute cases there is marked swelling, redness and tenderness behind the ear over the mastoid. The operation is performed when there are recurrent or persistent tenderness, fever, headache, and discharge from the ear.

Preparation of the Patient. The patient is prepared as for any operation. The field is made ready by clipping the hair, then shaving the scalp for 1½ inches about the ear—this for the incision behind the ear (the postauricular approach). In patients in whom the approach to the mastoid is by the endaural route, in which the incision is created from the canal of the ear outward, the shaving of the hair post-auricularly may be omitted. In the operation the infection is removed com-

pletely from the mastoid process, with drainage from the middle ear, thus preventing spread of the infection to surrounding structures. The middle ear can be saved from further damage and the possible resulting permanent hearing loss.

Nursing Care. Sedatives usually are indicated after the operation and during the first post-operative days, to control pain and restlessness. Fluids are given freely when the anesthetic reaction clears. Temperature, pulse and respiration are taken every 4 hours. Prolonged nausea and vomiting may require intravenous fluids. The mastoid is packed with gauze for drainage, and the packing is usually removed at the end of 5 to 7 days. Dressings are done with sterile precautions every day or every other day, as indicated by the surgeon (Fig. 336).

A complication after mastoidectomy is facial paralysis, and the nurse may be the first to note this serious indication of facial nerve inflammation or injury. Here the patient shows immobility of the side affected, so that the eye cannot be closed, and the mouth droops. He is unable to drink without water dripping from the mouth, and he is unable to whistle. On speaking or grimacing, the facial paralysis is more pronounced, due to the immobility of the paralyzed side. The continued use of antibiotic agents is important for combating the infection and aiding healing. When there is evidence of facial paralysis, cortisone derivatives are useful in restoring the nerve to function.

Radical Mastoid Operation

The purpose of this operation is the removal of all disease from the mastoid and the middle ear; and in the surgery, the external canal, the middle ear and the mastoid are merged into one cavity. The operative preparation and the postoperative care are essentially the same as for the simple mastoid operation. Here the surgery is carried out by either the postauricular or the endaural technic, and in some instances the mastoid wound is lined by skin graft. Segments of skin are removed from either the arm or the leg, preceded by the appropriate skin sterilization. Here mention must be made again that with this serious otologic operation the nurse should be on the alert for unusual symptoms that may intimate complications. Persistent headache, unusual rise in temperature, with chills, stiff neck, nausea and vomiting should alert the attending nurse to the possibility of serious sequelae.

Perforations of the Eardrum

Etiology and Pathology

The most frequent cause of permanent perforations of the tympanic membrane is infection. Perforations of the drum membrane that fail to heal are often the end-result of acute or chronic suppurative otitis media.

Before the advent of antibiotics, clinicians often were confronted with the acute otologic complications of the exanthemas in children. In patients with acute fulminating streptococcal infection, spontaneous rupture of the drum followed by necrosis could result in a perforation so large that only the thicker rim portion of the drum remained. In chronic otitis media, infection of the middle ear and the mastoid perpetuates the purulent otorrhea and prevents healing of the perforation.

Second to infections of the middle ear, trauma may be a cause of permanent perforation of the drum. Blast effect of high explosives or intense compression caused by a severe blow on the ear can rupture the drum. Burning of the drum by a welder's spark is no rarity. Less frequent causes are perforation of the drum by foreign objects, water burns of the face that include the external ear and the drum membrane, and postmyringotomy defects.

Medical Management

Most accidental perforations of the drum membrane heal spontaneously. Some will persist due to the growth of scar tissue over the edges of the perforation, thus preventing extension of the epithelial areas across the margins and final healing. Central perforations of the drum lend themselves to medical treatment for eventual closure, except in patients who have only a rim of the drum membrane remaining. In some patients, persistent care consisting of cauterization of the perforation with trichloroacetic acid at frequent intervals and the use of a prosthesis will result in a completely healed drum membrane by scar.

Myringoplasty

Myringoplasty is a plastic surgical procedure designed to close perforations of the

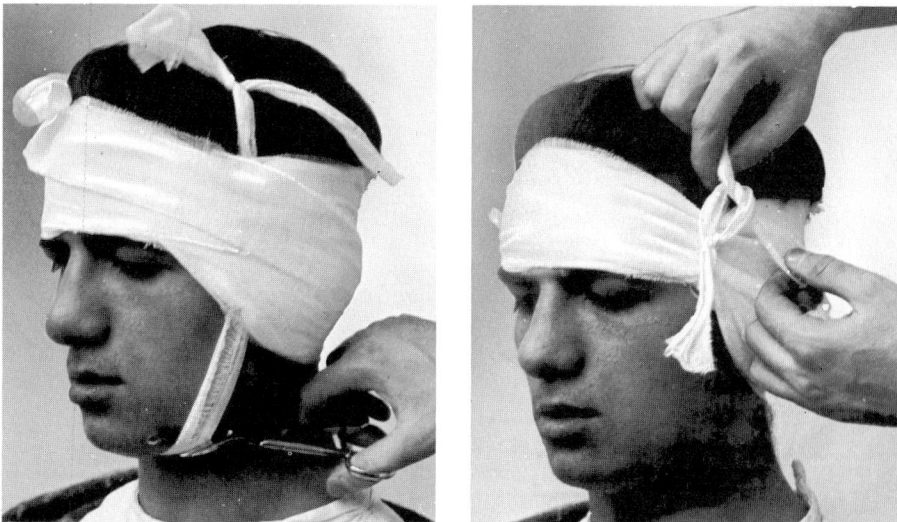

Fig. 336. Improved ear bandage. *(Left)* Extra piece of bandage tied loosely around the head and the chin before bandage is applied. *(Right)* Extra bandage cut in two pieces and tied over each temporal region, the end of the bandage being tied in a knot on one side.

tympanic membrane. The operation has a dual purpose: to create a closed middle ear cavity by graft over the perforation, and to improve hearing.

Indications and Contraindications. The most important advantage of the closed tympanic membrane is the avoidance of the risk of contamination of the middle ear during bathing, swimming or diving. The reactivation of a chronic otitis media and/or mastoiditis thus may be prevented. Dramatic improvement in hearing may result from closure of a perforation if there is no involvement of the ossicles. The probability of improved hearing after closure of the drum membrane can be prognosticated to some degree by an audiometric study with evaluation of the air-bone conduction levels. Preoperative testing, with and without a patch prosthesis over the perforation, usually provides a fairly accurate estimate of the degree of hearing levels. Temporary patching of the defect with glazed paper, latex, or a cotton collodium disk should be a routine maneuver during the preliminary examination of the patient. When the patching of a perforation of the drum is not followed by audiometric improvement, one must consider involvement of the ossicular chain. During the surgical repair of a perforation, a careful inspection of the middle ear contents, with particular attention to the continuity of the ossicles, is important.

Medical or surgical closure of perforations of the drum in the presence of an active infection usually is contraindicated. In chronic disease of the middle ear with malfunction of the eustachian tube, and therefore inadequate drainage from the middle ear (the only avenue for egress of discharges), surgery is contraindicated. Involvement of the nasopharynx because of chronic infectious discharge from sinusitis or allergy, plus a history of acute exacerbations of otitis media, is an obvious contraindication.

Type A Myringoplasty. Surgical technics for myringoplasty may be classified as Type A or Type B. Type A includes those procedures that employ the adjoining skin of the canal wall to repair the defect. Type B includes those in which free grafts are employed, usually from non-hair-bearing areas, after the preparation of a suitable vascular bed over the drum remnants and adjoining skin of the canal.

Type A myringoplasty, with the utilization of pedicle grafts in the canal wall or of the skin of the canal with advancement to close marginal or attic perforations, is more easily carried out now that present-day technics permit the use of the magnification and the illumination of the operating microscope. The technic whereby a defect is created in the bony canal and a free graft is utilized over the bony wall thus created has the advantage that a graft is more likely to take in this area.

Type A myringoplasty is particularly suitable in marginal perforations. In small perforations adjoining the annulus (the bony plate between the canal and the drum), the scarred area of perforation is excised. Then an angular knife or pick is used to elevate the marginal epithelium adjoining the perforation, and then, by means of a small punch, the skin is stripped from the drum membrane. The skin of the canal wall adjoining the marginal perforation is then carried up into the bony portion of the canal. The vertical extension of the incision in the canal is extended to a point where the cartilaginous and bony canals meet, approximately 7 or 8 mm. from the annulus. With elevation of the periosteum and the adjoining skin to avoid tension or tear, the skin is then advanced, and this is continued to 2 mm. over the edge of the perforation, thus covering the previously denuded portion of the drum membrane adjoining the perforation. The exposed bony canal created by the advancement of this flap is then covered by a segment of skin removed from the postauricular area. A small strip of Gelfoam is placed over the graft site, and the canal is lightly packed with ¼-inch gauze moistened with a topical antibiotic ointment dressing. The postauricular area from which the skin graft was taken is covered with a strip of Gelfoam and a dressing.

PEDICLE-FLAP TECHNIC. In this procedure, the skin of the anterior or posterior canal wall is utilized to cover a marginal perforation. In perforations of the anterior quadrant of the drum, the canal usually must be widened to expose the anterior portion of the tympanic annulus. The technic is essentially the same as that for posterior perforations of the drum, including the maneuver for enlarging the canal for better visualization and manipulation.

Postoperative Care and Instructions. An antibiotic is administered routinely for at least 5 days after surgery. The patient remains in the hospital for 3 or 4 days at the most, and the dressing is left undisturbed except for the external bandage, which may be changed if it becomes soiled from bleeding. The gauze strip is removed from the canal on the 7th day; the Gelfoam is left undisturbed. No suction or probing is carried out at this time.

On the 12th day, capillary suction can be used carefully to remove the Gelfoam or crusted debris. Gentle inflation can be carried out with a Politzer bag to test the efficiency of the closure of the perforation by the graft. Ear drops never are used, and the only topical treatment is a dusting powder of Neosporin or Chloromycetin-Boric.

The patient is seen at 5-day intervals and is instructed to avoid contaminating the ear with shampoo or shower. Antibiotics are given for 1 week, but can be continued if there is evidence of complicating respiratory infection. An antihistaminic with an ephedrine derivative is used routinely for 1 month postoperatively. In those patients with known seasonal or perennial rhinologic allergy, an antihistaminic is continued.

Tympanoplasty

Tympanoplasty denotes a number of reconstructive operations on middle ear structures that have become diseased or are congenitally deformed. The procedure entails the construction or the preservation of the conductive mechanism to maintain or improve hearing. The impetus that led to this work in recent years has been due largely to advances in surgical technics with the illuminated binocular microscope. This surgery has been helped by the protection of the antibiotics to insure a sterile procedure in uninfected patients and the use of these drugs in the eradication of chronic otitis media and mastoiditis.

Anatomic and Physiologic Principles. The conductive function of the eardrum and the ossicles transforms sound waves from airborne vibrations to mechanical stimulation of the endolymphatic fluids (see Plate 12). The prevailing physiologic concept holds that the ratio of the large tympanic membrane to the smaller oval window, combined with the lever action of the ossicles, transforms stimuli from the air to the inner ear fluids with great increase in force. It is calculated that the lever ratio for the tympanic membrane to the oval window is 22 times. It is obvious, then, that defects in the tympanic membrane or interruption of the ossicular chain will disturb that mass relationship to the oval window and will cause a loss of what is called the sound-pressure ratio, resulting in hearing loss.

The functional physiology of the round and oval windows plays an important role as well. The oval window is bordered by the annular ligament and the unimpeded motility of the stapes foot-plate receives impulses transmitted by the incus and the malleus from the drum membrane. The round window, opening on the opposite side of the cochlear duct, permits motion of the endolymphatic fluids with sound-wave stimulation. With the normally intact drum membrane, sound waves stimulate the oval window first, and a lag occurs before the terminal effect of the stimulus reaches the round window. This phase lag, normally present with an intact drum, is changed by a perforation of the drum that is large enough to allow sound waves to impinge on both the round and oval windows simultaneously. This effect cancels the lag and prevents the maximum effect in labyrinth fluid motility and its subsequent effect in stimulating the hair cells in the organ of Corti.

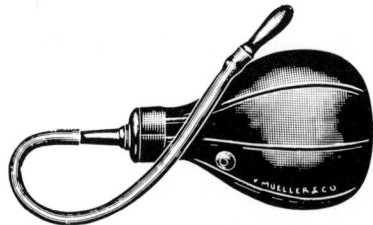

FIG. 337. By gentle inflation the Politzer bag is used to test the efficiency of the closure of the perforation by the graft in myringoplasty. (V. Mueller, Chicago)

In tympanoplasty the physiologic effect of the ossicular transformer action between an intact drum membrane and the oval window must be achieved to be successful. A middle ear cavity that is air-containing with ventilation and pressure equalization of the eustachian tube and an unimpeded round window are essential to normal function and good hearing.

Pathology. Pathologic sequelae vary after otitis media, with minimal or large defects remaining in the tympanic membrane. In protracted or virulent infections, there may be necrotic involvement of the ossicles. Involvement of motility may occur with fibrosis or necrosis of all or part of the ossicular chain. The malleus commonly is involved, the handle lost by osteonecrosis as the perforation in the drum enlarges. The lenticular process of the incus often is involved, because of its tenuous blood supply. Osteonecrosis may involve the entire ossicular chain, so that the stapedial foot-plate is the only remaining portion. The oval and round windows may be impeded functionally by granuloma, polyps, fibrous or bony plaques. Otosclerosis may exist along with the pathologic sequelae of otitis media. Obstruction of the tympanic orifice of the eustachian tube by pathologic tissue deposits or fibrotic stenosis may result in dysfunction of this structure.

The prime goal in tympanoplasty is the eradication of disease in the middle ear and the mastoid and the maintenance or the improvement of hearing.

Prosthetics. A part of the tympanoplastic procedure is the restoration in the continuity of the sound mechanism, when it is involved. Ossicular interruption is most frequent in otitis media, but problems of reconstruction occur with malformations of the middle ear and ossicular dislocations due to head injuries.

Polyethylene tubing, stainless steel wire, bone and cartilage have been used as replacements either to utilize the remaining parts of the ossicles or to create a columella (little column) effect for the transmission of impulses from the tympanic graft to the oval window.

A two-stage procedure may be necessary —the first for the surgical eradication of all pathology and to achieve a healed, dry middle ear, and the second for the reconstructive process. The ear should remain dry for 2 or 3 months before the second stage for the exploration of the window niches and the restoration of a conductive mechanism. Remaining parts of the ossicular chain can be used by repositioning to establish impulse transmission to the oval window.

Clinical Results. Patients with a lengthy history of disease can achieve hearing gains as great as those with less protracted infections. In patients whose otitis media has been healed and the ear dry for a lengthy period, hearing improvement can be marked after tympanoplasty. Younger patients achieve better results than older patients. The simpler the surgery, the better the chance for hearing gain, and, of course, this relates directly to the functional integrity of the ossicular chain and the degree of efficiency of the newly-created tympanic covering.

The bacterial flora should be studied in all patients by culture and sensitivity tests. In those whose treatment is carried out parenterally with the appropriate antibiotic, the postoperative morbidity is less. Infection due to resistant organisms can be treated postoperatively with the use of a catheter placed in the wound with the instillation of the topical antibiotics. This often facilitates healing. Topical and systemic antibiotic treatment should precede the surgery on the frequently recurrent or continuously discharging ear.

It would appear that the tympanoplasty procedure offers the patient the opportunity for complete eradication of disease with a better chance for maintenance or improvement of hearing levels.

Tympanoplasty, utilizing modern technics, can result in a high percentage of healing in the middle ear and the mastoid. In addition, present-day knowledge of the physiology of the conductive mechanism, coupled with the newer microsurgical technics, offers better results in hearing rehabilitation. Despite the limitations created by pathologic destruction of vital structures concerned with the sound conduction mechanism, the ingenious development of the technical and prosthetic procedures by pioneers in this surgery have opened new vistas for the otologic surgeon.

The role of the nurse in the operating room is important. Instruments of microscopic dimension and the intricacy of the steps in the operations call for experienced, dedicated personnel.

Otosclerosis

Otosclerosis is the term applied to a form of progressive deafness caused by the formation of new spongy bone in the labyrinth, fixing the stapes and preventing sound transmission by the vibrating ossicles to the inner ear fluids. The cause of this condition is unknown, but it occurs most commonly in women, beginning after puberty, and it has a hereditary basis. The condition begins with insidious loss of hearing, with ringing or buzzing ear noise, and both ears usually are involved about equally. The patient gives a history of slowly progressive hearing loss without middle ear infection.

The diagnosis is evident from the findings of the audiometer test. Tuning-fork sound transmission by air is markedly reduced, while intensification of sound is noted by placing the tuning-fork handle over the mastoid and recording the marked difference in hearing between air and bone. The bone conduction is far better than air conduction, which is the reverse of normal. There is no known treatment for this form of deafness other than the help offered by amplification with an electric hearing aid, the stapes mobilization operation and the fenestration operation.

Stapes Mobilization Operation

In the 19th century otologists reported their observations on the improvement of hearing in otosclerosis by stapes mobilization. Reports from numerous observers indicate that this procedure will restore hearing in patients deafened by otosclerosis.

The operation is done under local anesthesia with light preoperative sedation. The skin lining the osseous canal is elevated after radical incision, and the middle ear is exposed with dissection of the drum and with the skin of the canal attached. The operation is done through an ear speculum with magnification. With careful instrumentation, the drum is lifted, and the middle ear contents are exposed. The chorda tympani nerve, the tendon of the stapes and the ossicles are important landmarks. With fine probes, the ossicles are palpated, and the tendon of the stapes is used as a factor to determine mobility of the stapes itself. Specially devised instruments are directed toward mobilizing the fixed stapedial foot plate. Hearing improvement is often dramatic in the successfully operated patient, with immediate good hearing. When the manipulative procedure is completed, the drum is replaced, and the skin of the canal is smoothed in its position, with approximation of the skin flap. The ear canal is packed for a few days, and rapid healing takes place without complication. The use of antibiotics prevents secondary infection and facilitates healing. The postoperative course usually is uneventful, and the patient requires little or no treatment after the first dressing.

Stapedectomy

Rosen in 1957 advanced a new technic in the treatment of otosclerosis. In his technic, a portion of the foot plate at its center was extracted by a special hooklike excavator and the defect covered with a strip of Gelfoam. In the performance of this technic, carried out at that time with the use of 2½ magnification of the binocular loop and using the illumination of a head lamp, it is most reasonable to assume that the few lasting hearing improvements that resulted were due to mobilization of the foot plate as a whole or to fragmentation of the thin portion of the foot plate with subsequent motility that persisted. However, in most cases the hearing improvement was short-lived, and in many, the hearing remained acute only in the operating room until the tympanomeatal flap was reflected back in position; the hearing then regressed. Later, John J. Shea, Jr., began his search for a technic to remove the stapes in toto and to fashion a suitable prosthesis to restore this part of the conductive mechanism in otosclerotic patients. Otologic surgeons also have pioneered in the technics of *stapedectomy*—the removal of the otosclerotic lesion at the foot plate of the stapes and the creation of a suitable tissue implant with a prosthesis to replace this portion of the conductive mechanism.

Indications. Stapedectomy at first was reserved for patients with otosclerotic lesions diffuse enough to involve the entire foot plate of the stapes, making it impossible to employ stapes mobilization, and for advanced cases of otosclerosis requiring either a chisel or the motor-driven burr to excavate or fenestrate the oval window. As a consequence of the increasing numbers of regressions that occurred after stapes mobilization, stapedectomy was employed as a secondary operative technic to salvage the failures of initial mobilization attempts. With the initial success of this operation, the indications have extended to all classes of otosclerosis; and in clinics where this technic is carried out, virtually all patients with otosclerosis are treated by a routine stapedectomy.

Technic. After the exposure of the middle ear with adequate removal of the bony annulus to expose the incudostapedial joint, the incus, and its major portion of the lenticular process, the facial canal, and the adjoining foot plate of the stapes should be well delineated. Hemostasis control is important and is achieved by Gelfoam soaked in epinephrine, or by the coagulating current in minute amperage. The removal of the stapes begins with separation of the incudo-stapedial joint, using a fine angular pick. In the technic of Shea, with the use of a polyethylene implant, care must be exercised to preserve the terminal knoblike structure of the lenticular process, this being utilized for insertion into the upper end of the polyethylene tube and serving to fix the prosthesis firmly in the oval window niche. The crura then are fractured and removed by delicate forceps. If the foot plate is thin and blue with only a peripheral otosclerotic lesion,

one must be wary of sudden mobilization of the foot plate or extraction of the foot plate at the time of crural fracture. At this point, the mucosa adjoining the oval window niche over the promontory and the adjacent facial canal is carefully stripped by a fine pick. The mucosa of the foot plate and its margins are left undisturbed. A strip of Gelfoam then is placed over the foot plate, and the prosthesis is fashioned after the distance is measured accurately from the level of the foot plate to the underside of the lenticular process.

At this point the prosthesis is fashioned. Schuknecht's type is the steel wire and fat implant; Kos uses wire and a segment of vein as a plug in the oval window, and Shea advocates a vein graft with polyethylene tubing. In any case, the prosthetic device should be fashioned and ready preliminary to the removal of the stapedial foot plate.

Today stapedectomy is the operation of choice in the surgical treatment of otosclerosis. This operation has largely supplanted the stapes mobilization and fenestration operation.

Nursing Care. The nursing care in this extremely delicate operation is essential for consistently successful end-results. Microscopic instruments and the detailed steps of the operation makes the experienced help of the nurse an important phase of this newer surgery of the deaf.

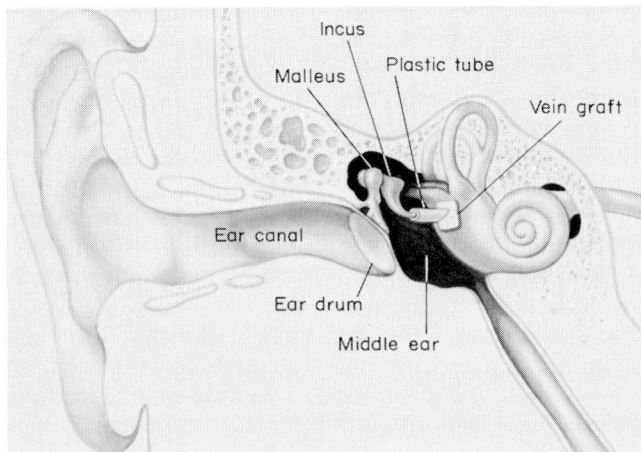

Fig. 338. Stapedectomy. Diagram of ear shows where plastic tube replaces tiny but important bone, the stapes. Abnormal bone growth on the base of the stapes, here cut away and replaced by vein graft, had made it stick fast so it could no longer vibrate.

FIG. 339. A typical hearing aid and how it works. A hearing aid is a miniature sound-amplifying set. It picks up the speaker's voice through a microphone (A), changes the sound into electrical impulses, and sends the impulses along a conducting cord (B) to a speaker or ear button (C). A diaphragm in the button vibrates, creating strong sound waves that enter the ear through a hollow plastic ear mold (D). Some patients wear a bone-conduction button (E) instead of the ear button. This is held firmly against the mastoid process of the temporal bone by a headband.

The aid has an on-off switch, which also controls the volume, and a tone-control switch. A battery (or batteries) is located inside the aid. A wire clip is provided for fastening the aid to the clothing.

Most hearing-aid wearers use an individually fitted plastic ear mold. But some use a standard cone-shaped earpiece. In either case, the ear button snaps into the ear mold or earpiece as shown. The conducting cord has a miniature plug at each end. One plug fits into a socket at the top of the aid and the other fits into a similar socket on the ear button. It's best to leave the cord plugged into the aid and ear button when the aid isn't being worn. This prevents possible damage to the plug. (Thorne, B. C.: When your patient wears a hearing aid, RN **24**:49-55)

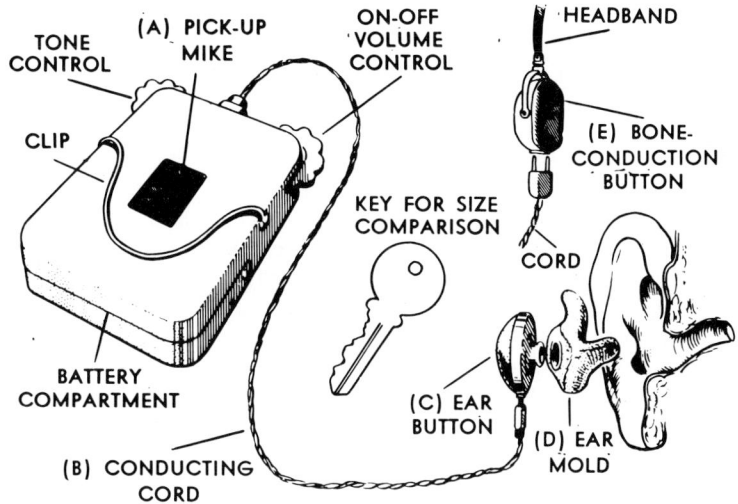

In the postoperative care the nurse should record unusual symptoms such as fever, headache, vertigo or ear pain. External otitis and otitis media have occurred as complications and require treatment with antibiotics. Vertigo initiated by this operation may protract the patient's hospital stay. Although the patient becomes ambulant in 24 hours, the nurse should be alert for the occasional patient who has vertigo and gait disturbance that may mean labyrinthitis or inner ear reaction requiring further observation and treatment. The initial hearing gain at the time of operation is masked by the ear packing and subsequent swelling of the tissues, so reassurance should be offered by the nurse that hearing gain may be noted from one to several weeks after operation. Reports from various observers doing this work indicate that a fair percentage of patients can obtain useful hearing levels by this relatively simple operation.

Fenestration Operation

For over 50 years early pioneers have attempted the surgical treatment of otosclerosis by fenestration of the labyrinth, but only in the past 10 or 15 years has it been brought to a state of perfection. In the present-day operation, a new window for passage of sound waves into the labyrinth is created, after a partial mastoidectomy. The newly created window reroutes sound, and an artificial covering for the newly created window, or fenestra, is made from the skin of the external canal. The surgical procedure is delicate and is performed by those specially trained in the technics. The high-speed, motor-driven dental drill and cutting bur are essential to the operation. Optical aids, such as a loop worn by the operating surgeon or a dissecting binocular microscope, make details of the operation safe. The procedure will restore hearing in those patients afflicted with the disease, and in from 75 to 85 per cent of properly selected patients, good results can be expected.

Nursing Care. In the postoperative care, skillful nursing will aid in the patient's comfort and convalescence. The immediate effect after operation will be extreme nausea and vertigo, lasting from 24 to 48 hours. The patient usually will lie on the operated ear and, because of the annoying vomiting, may require intravenous fluids. The motion sickness remedies, Dramamine, Bonamine, or Marezine, are used to control the vertigo. With vomiting, the drug can be given by intramuscular injection. Antibiotics are important in the postoperative management to aid in healing and to prevent infection of the delicate inner ear structures.

Because of the extreme vertigo, patients should be observed carefully by the nurse in charge when they become ambulant. With gait disturbance, the patient should be supported at the beginning of ambulation. Catheterization may be necessary during the first 24 or 48 hours. The patient leaves the hospital on the 3rd or 4th postoperative day, after daily dressings. It goes without saying that sterile precautions are used during the dressings—with sterile tray, instruments, packing and bandage. Hearing gain is not manifested during the hospital stay after surgery. There is a gradual ascent in hearing in the weeks that follow.

For those handicapped by deafness due to otosclerosis, who do not wish to wear a hearing aid, stapes surgery offers an extremely good chance for hearing restoration to useful levels. With present technics, coupled with the use of antibiotics, healing with convalescence is rapid, and in approximately 2 or 3 weeks the patient can return to his usual duties. The stapedectomy operation is reserved for those patients who have failed to have hearing restoration with the stapes mobilization procedure.

PATIENTS WITH PROBLEMS OF THE INNER EAR

Meniere's Syndrome

Although there is almost general agreement that the symptoms of Meniere's syndrome stem from labyrinthine dysfunction, the cause has not been definitely established. Symptoms are recurring attacks of dizziness, tinnitus, headache, nausea and vomiting, incoordination and reduced hearing. Attacks

are sudden and the patient complains of the room appearing to spin around him. Any sudden motion of the head may induce vomiting. This symptom complex usually occurs in persons who have had previous ear trouble and allergic symptoms, especially vasomotor rhinitis. When vasospasm of the blood vessels occurs, the mucous membrane of the cochlea becomes swollen and congested, the fluid increases in quantity, and the resultant pressure on the labyrinth produces the symptoms of Meniere's syndrome.

The patient's most comfortable position is lying down with probable favoring of one side. He may be irritable and withdrawn and reject food. Every effort must be exerted to prevent noise and sudden jarring. He should be fed; bathing and turning should be done gently.

The *caloric test* may be done to differentiate this syndrome from an intracranial lesion. Fluid of above or below body temperature is instilled into the auditory canal. The normal person will complain of being dizzy; the patient with an acoustic neuroma has no reaction, and a severe attack is produced in the patient with a Meniere's syndrome.

Treatment. Usually the patient is placed on a low sodium diet to aid in edema control. Vasodilators are given to control vasospasm. For this reason also, no smoking may be recommended. Fairly successful symptomatic treatment* is being reported by using a combination (Antivert) of 2 medications: meclizine, which eases vestibular tension, and nicotinic acid, which acts as a vasodilator. Symptoms are relieved, but hearing does not improve.

When medical efforts have failed, surgical severance of the auditory nerve may be done. Ultrasonic surgery† for this disease also has been reported.

HEARING AIDS

Whether an individual would benefit by a hearing aid can best be determined by an otologist. When the hearing loss is more than 30 decibels in the range of 500 to 2,000 cycles per second in the better ear, a patient

---

* Scal, J. C.: Meniere's syndrome: Effective symptomatic treatment. Eye, Ear, Nose and Throat Monthly 38:738-741, Sept. 1959.

† Ariagno, R. P.: Ultrasonic surgery for Meniere's Disease, Am. J. Nurs. 60:1778-1780, Dec. 1960.

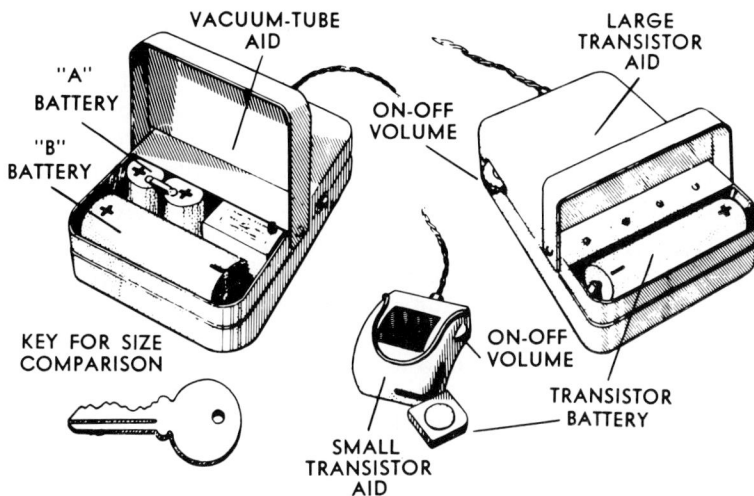

FIG. 340. How to replace the batteries. Hearing aids vary widely in shape and size; but basically they're of two kinds: the vacuum-tube aid and the transistor aid. The vacuum-tube aid requires two batteries; the transistor aid, one. The batteries, too, come in many shapes and sizes.

In some small transistor sets, a slot is provided for the battery (see center sketch). In larger sets, the battery compartment is in the lower half of the aid, opening at the back. Batteries usually are marked with a plus sign (+) at one end and a minus sign (−) at the other. They're inserted to match the same signs printed in the set.

If two batteries are needed (see sketch at far left), they're marked "A" and "B." The "B" battery is always the larger one. The set may be marked to show which battery goes where. Occasionally two "A" batteries are required, as shown. Some aids have a switch marked "Spare." This can be turned on if one of the "A" batteries suddenly goes dead. In that case, of course, the patient (or the nurse) replaces the dead battery as soon as convenient. Then the next time the patient needs to use the spare, it's again available. (Thorne, B. C.: When your patient wears a hearing aid, RN **24**:49-55)

can benefit from a hearing aid used with this ear. A variety of aids are available; the problem is to select the best aid for the individual patient. He or a salesman cannot make the decision alone. It should be made with the advice of an otologist. Even this does not ensure optimum benefit from such an instrument. Psychological factors, such as vanity, may be involved, as well as other types of sensitivity.

The patient needs to know that the aid will not restore his hearing to the level of the person with normal hearing but will improve it in the range of 300 to 3,500 cycles per second (range of primary speech). Fig. 339 shows a typical hearing aid.

In caring for a hearing aid, the ear mold (Fig. 339D) is the only part of the instrument that is washed. It should be washed in soap and water daily and the cannula cleansed with a small applicator or pipe cleaner. Before snapping it into the receiver, the mold must be dry. The transmitter usu-

ally is worn by men in the shirt pocket and by women in a special pocket just under the dress as on the outer side of a slip. Children may wear the transmitter in a cloth pocket as a harness over the outer clothing. A spare battery and cord should be carried by the wearer at all times.

To replace batteries, see Figure 340. When a hearing aid is not working, several steps can be followed: (1) Note whether the on-off switch is on. (2) Check the positioning of the batteries. (3) Try a new battery. (4) Examine the cord for breaks and whether it is plugged in correctly. (5) Examine the ear mold for cleanliness. If the aid still will not work, notify the local service agency. Meanwhile, if the unit requires days to repair, the agency from whom it was purchased may lend an aid, or one may be borrowed from the local Chapter of the American Hearing Society.

A hearing aid makes speech louder but it does not always make it clear enough for the deaf person to understand what is said. Auditory training and speech reading (lip reading) may also be necessary to make the new hearing aid effective.

COMMUNICATING WITH A PERSON WHO HAS A HEARING IMPAIRMENT

Terry *et al.** offer the following suggestions for better communication with deaf persons whose speech is difficult to understand:

1. Devote full attention to what he is saying. Look and listen—do not try to give attention to another task while listening to him.

2. Engage him in conversation where it is possible for you to anticipate his replies. This will enable you to become accustomed to the peculiarities of his pattern of speech.

3. Try to catch the essential context of what he is saying; you can often fill in the details from context.

4. Do not try to appear as if you understand him when you do not.

5. If you cannot understand him at all or have serious doubt about your ability to understand him, have him write his message rather than risk misunderstanding. Having him repeat the message in speech, after you know its content, will also aid you in becoming accustomed to his pattern of speech.

Suggestions for better communication with deaf persons who lip-read:

1. When speaking, always face the person as directly as possible.

2. Make sure your face is as clearly visible as possible; locate yourself so that your face is well-lighted; avoid being silhouetted against strong light; do not obscure that person's view of your mouth in any way; avoid talking with any object held in your mouth.

3. Be sure the patient knows the topic or subject of your verbal expression before going ahead with what you plan to say—this will enable him to use contextual clues in his lip-reading.

4. Speak slowly and distinctly, pausing more frequently than you would normally.

5. If you question whether the patient has understood some important direction or in-

struction, check to be certain that he has the full meaning of your message.

6. If for any reason your mouth must be covered (as with a mask) and you must direct or instruct the patient, there is no alternative but to write the message for him.

CLINICAL SITUATION

Choose the *best* answer.

1. Excessive cerumen in the ear may block the canal and cause an impairment of hearing. The most effective method of removing cerumen is with:
    A. Cotton applicators.
    B. A sharp instrument.
    C. An ear syringe.
    D. None of the above.

2. In most patients with acute otitis media, the infection extends up the eustachian tube from an inflammatory process in the:
    A. Nasopharynx.
    B. Blood stream.
    C. Inner ear.
    D. Sphenoid sinus.

3. The process of incising the ear drum to promote drainage and prevent extension of infection to the mastoid cells is called:
    A. Trephining.
    B. Fenestration.
    C. Mobilization.
    D. Myringotomy.

4. Which of the following medications may have an ototoxic property?
    A. Sulfathiazole.
    B. Dihydrostreptomycin.
    C. Adrenocorticotrophic hormones.
    D. Aureomycin.

BIBLIOGRAPHY AND SUGGESTED READING

Books

Manhattan Eye, Ear, and Throat Hospital: Nursing in Diseases of the Eye, Ear, Nose and Throat, ed. 10, Philadelphia, Saunders, 1958.

Shambaugh, G. E., Jr.: Surgery of the Ear, Philadelphia, Saunders, Philadelphia, 1959.

Articles

Bell, H.: Technique of tympanoplasty, Arch. Otolaryng. **66:**554, 1957.

Dorner, H.: Teaching patients about stapes mobilization, Am. J. Nurs. **60:**819-820, June, 1960.

* Terry, F. J., *et al.:* Rehabilitation Nursing, p. 310, St. Louis, Mosby, 1957.

Farrior, J. B.: Ossicular repositioning and ossicular prosthesis in tympanoplasty, Arch. Otolaryng. **443:**449, 1959.

Goldman, J. L., and Rosenwasser, H.: Current concepts of the management of otitic infection, J.A.M.A. **171:**509-512, 1959.

Guilford, F. R., Wright, W. K., and Draper, W. L.: Tympanic skin grafting and reconstruction of the middle ear sound-conduction mechanism, Arch. Otolaryng. **69:**70, 1959.

House, H. P., and Sheehy, J. L.: Stapes mobilization, Am. J. Nurs. **60:**816-818, June, 1960.

House, H. P.: Surgical repair of the perforated ear drum, Ann. Otol. **62:**1072, 1953.

House, L. R.: Clinical experiences in tympanoplasty; results in 61 cases, Laryngoscope **68:** 1481, 1958.

Jongkees, L. B. W.: Reconstructive surgery of the middle ear in chronic otitis, Pract. Otorhinolaryng. (Basel) **19:**107, 1957.

Markle, D. M.: Hearing aids, Am. J. Nurs. **57:** 592-593, 1957.

Myers, D., Schlosser, W. D., and Winchester, R. A.: Otologic diagnosis and treatment of deafness, Clin. Symposia; **14:** April-June, 1962.

Proctor, B.: Results of tympanoplasty, Laryngoscope **68:**900, 1958.

Quimby, M. A.: Care of patients with labyrinthine dysfunction, Am. J. Nurs. **60:**1780-1781, Dec., 1960.

Riley, E. C.: Preventing deafness from industrial noise, Am. J. Nurs. **63:**80-84, May, 1963.

Ronnei, E. C.: Hearing aids, Am. J. Nurs. **63:** 90-93, May, 1963.

Transistor hearing aids, Nurs. Outlook **3:**251, 1955.

Wright, W. K.: Repair of chronic central perforations of the tympanic membrane by repeated acid cautery by skin grafting, Laryngoscope **66:**1464, 1956.

Patient-Teaching Aids and Information

Carter, H. A.: Noise and what you can do about it. An 8-page pamphlet reprinted by American Medical Association.

Carter, H. A.: What to do when Hearing Fades. A reprint from American Medical Association.

Eichenlaub, J. E.: Hear again, A reprint, American Medical Association.

Eyes that See and Ears that Hear, A 20-page pocket size booklet available from John Hancock Mutual Life Insurance Co.

Hearing Aids—A list of those accepted by the Council on Physical Medicine and Rehabilitation, A.M.A. Available from American Hearing Society.

Hearing News. A monthly periodical published by the American Hearing Society.

National Bureau of Standards. Selection of Hearing Aids. Circular No. 516, Supt. of Documents, U. S. Govt. Printing Office, Washington, D. C.

Seltzer, A. P.: Head Noises, a reprint, American Medical Association.

Additional Information available from:

Alexander Graham Bell Association
for the Deaf
  1537 35th St., N.W.
  Washington, D. C.

American Hearing Society
  919 18th St., N.W.
  Washington 6, D. C.

American Speech and Hearing Association
  101 Connecticut Ave., N.W., Suite 532
  Washington 6, D. C.

ORIENTATION

The care of patients with neurologic disabilities encompasses every phase and facet of professional nursing. It may be said without qualification that no group of patients presents greater opportunities for the exercise of diligence and skill on the part of the nurse, and in no category of disease is therapeutic success more dependent on excellence in nursing care.

As a cause of death and disability, neurologic disease ranks among the most important of all categories of illness. The mortality incidence of cerebrovascular disease is second only to that of heart disease, numbering approximately 175,000 per year in the United States alone and representing over 11 per cent of all deaths.

Recovery from organic disease of the nervous system is not always followed by complete restoration of function. The rehabilitation needs of these patients are unusually complex, their solution requiring occupational therapy and guidance, recreational opportunities, physical therapy and re-education of the most difficult sort. The most important of the neurologic disorders and the principal problems of neurologic nursing are considered in Chapter 41.

The field of neurosurgical nursing is a fascinating one. Within its scope the nurse has an opportunity to utilize all her powers of observation. By her careful charting she is a vital source of information for the surgeon in the making of a diagnosis and in the post-operative care of her patient.

By her optimism, nursing ability and concern for the patient as a person, the nurse can help to ease many of the difficult experiences of her patient and his family. When she realizes that the behavior and the personality of a person can be affected markedly by organic lesions of the brain, she is less inclined to think of an individual as an uncooperative patient with a foul disposition; instead he becomes one who needs help and understanding. His reactions may be beyond his control; the nurse must realize this.

The many interesting diagnostic tests in which the nurse participates are much like solving a puzzle. But the diagnosis is not the end; it is merely a steppingstone to the removal of the cause. Surgery must be done accurately, for otherwise the penalty may be the death of the patient or the reduction of his mental and/or physical abilities to the level of mere existence. Although surgery has many successful cases, there are instances in which the injury is too great to repair, or the tumor too extensive to remove, and the patient's prognosis is hopeless. It is important that even in these instances the nurse exercise as much concern for the comfort and the feelings of her patient as she does in situations in which the prognosis is more encouraging. This kind of care is significant, not only from the point of view of the individual patient but also from that of his family.

The nurse has an opportunity to use many procedures in giving sound, conscientious bedside care. It is important to apply the principles of good body mechanics, since the position of the patient must be changed frequently. From the moment the patient shows response after his operation, the nurse is on the alert to help him in his rehabilitation. Often every activity may have to be relearned, such as using his fingers to hold a spoon, learning to say words and sentences, acquiring the ability to write, etc. In addition, he needs psychological assistance in the form of encouragement. The nurse is a key person in that she is with him day and night and therefore is responsible for much of his future progress.

41

Patients With Neurologic and Neurosurgical Problems

NORMAL AND ABNORMAL ANATOMY AND PHYSIOLOGY

Cerebrospinal Components and Connections

The nervous system comprises the brain and the spinal cord, together with all extensions therefrom and neural connections thereto. Its function is to control and to coordinate cellular activities throughout the body. The signaling device which it employs involves the transmission of electrical impulses, a system which permits each stimulus to be placed accurately in the area that is intended to receive it. These impulses are routed via nerve fibers, pathways that are direct and continuous, and the responses that these elicit are practically instantaneous, for changes in electrical potential transmit the signals.

The Brain. The brain is a soft organ, located in a rigid, bony box—the skull or cranium. At the base of this box is the foramen magnum, an opening through which the spinal cord is continuous with the brain (Fig. 341) and the spinal cord. The brain has 3 coverings. These are (1) the dura, the outer covering of dense fibrous tissue that closely hugs the inner wall of the skull, (2) the arachnoid and (3) the pia mater, which adheres closely to the brain and the spinal-cord surfaces (meninges).

The brain is divided into cerebrum, midbrain, cerebellum, pons varolii and medulla oblongata or brain stem (Fig. 342).

The *cerebrum* is divided into 2 hemispheres and consists of 5 lobes: frontal, parietal, temporal, occipital and insular (Fig. 343, *top*). The cerebrum is the largest part of the brain, and on its surface or cortex are located the "centers" from which motor impulses are carried to the muscles, and to which sensory impulses come from the various sensory nerves.

The *midbrain* connects the pons and the cerebellum with a hemisphere of the cerebrum.

The *cerebellum* or "little brain" is located below and behind the cerebrum. Its function is the control or the coordination of muscles and equilibration.

The *pons varolii* is situated in front of the cerebellum between the midbrain and the medulla and is a bridge of union between the two halves of the cerebellum as well as between the medulla and the cerebrum.

The *medulla oblongata* transmits the fibers from the brain to the spinal cord, motor fibers crossing at this point. It also contains important centers controlling heart, respiration and blood pressure and gives origin to a number of cranial nerves. The 12 cranial nerves find exit from the brain at the base of the skull.

There are two glands present in the brain: the pituitary and the pineal. The pituitary gland is frequently approached surgically. It lies at the base of the brain in a bony fossa termed the sella turcica, just posterior to the optic chasm, upon which it may press when the gland is enlarged.

Spinal Cord. The spinal cord, surrounded by the vertebral column, extends from the foramen magnum of the skull, where it is continuous with the medulla oblongata, to the first lumbar vertebra, where it tapers off into a fine thread of tissue (Fig. 341). The spinal cord is an important center of reflex action for the body and contains the conducting pathways to and from the higher centers in the cord and the brain.

Cerebrospinal Fluid. Within each cerebral hemisphere is a central cavity, the lateral ventricle. This is filled with water-clear *cerebrospinal fluid,* which forms at this site by a process of extraction from the blood as the

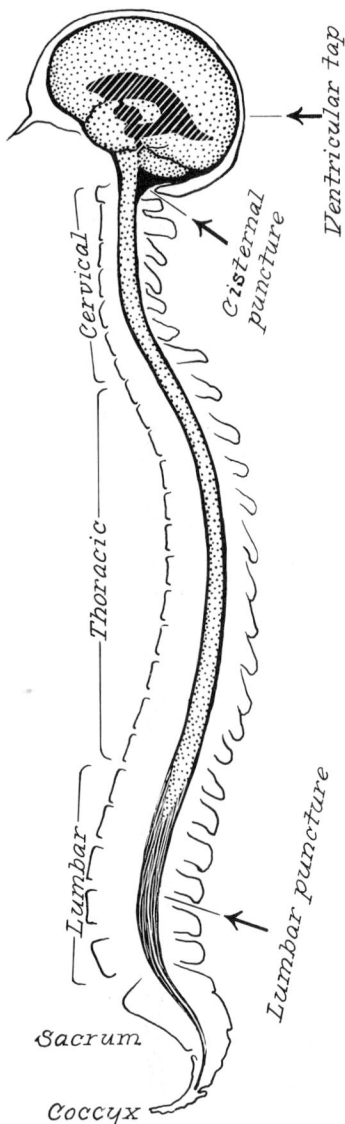

Cervical

Cisternal puncture

Ventricular tap

Thoracic

Lumbar

Lumbar puncture

Sacrum

Coccyx

FIG. 341. Diagrammatic representation of the cerebrospinal system, showing the brain, the cord and the spaces occupied by cerebrospinal fluid, ventricles and dural sac. The sites for the introduction of needles for ventricular tap, cisternal puncture and lumbar puncture are indicated.

systems contain about 150 cc. of this fluid. Inasmuch as the fluid is considered to be a dialysate from the choroid plexuses, its composition includes those substances also present in blood plasma, which is its source.

Disease produces changes in the composition of this fluid. Determinations of the protein content and the quantity of glucose and chloride present constitute the chief chemical examinations. In a state of health there are a minimal number of white cells and no red cells in the spinal fluid; thus the examination for cells is important. Other diagnostic examinations include the Wassermann reaction for syphilis and the colloidal-gold reaction, which is a colloidal precipitation test based on the protein content in the spinal fluid.

By replacing cerebrospinal fluid with air, the radiologist is able to visualize with x-rays (encephalogram and ventriculogram discussed later) the size, the shape and the position of the ventricles. Any interference or distortion may be suggestive of a space-occupying lesion. (See Fig. 351 A.)

Cerebral Cortex. The cells in the cortex are quite similar in appearance; their functions, however, vary widely, depending on their geographic location. Figure 343 depicts the topography of the cortex in relation to certain of its specific functions. The posterior portion of each hemisphere, i.e., the occipital lobe, is devoted to all aspects of visual perception; the lateral region, or temporal lobe, incorporates the hearing center. The mid-central zone, or parietal zone, posterior to the fissure of Rolandi, is concerned with sensation; the anterior portion is concerned with voluntary muscle movements. The large uncharted area beneath the forehead, i.e., the frontal lobes, contain the association pathways that determine emotional attitudes and responses and contribute to the formation of thought processes. Damage to the frontal lobes as a result of trauma or disease is by no means incapacitating from the standpoint of muscular control or coordination but has decided effect on the

latter circulates through the capillaries of the choroid plexus by well-defined channels from the lateral ventricles through narrow tubular openings to the 3rd and the 4th ventricles. From this narrow cavity it escapes to the subarachnoid space to bathe the entire surface of the brain and the spinal cord. The cerebrospinal fluid normally is absorbed by the large venous channels of the skull and along the spinal and the cranial nerves.

The spinal fluid is clear and colorless, having a specific gravity of 1.007. The average patient's ventricular and subarachnoid

personality of the individual, as reflected by his basic attitudes, sense of humor and propriety, self-restraint and motivations. Surgical division of frontal lobe tracts has been carried out as a therapeutic measure in patients with major psychoses.

Internal Capsule, Pons and Medulla. Nerve fibers from all portions of the cortex converge in each hemisphere and make their exit in the form of tight bundles known as the "internal capsule." Having entered the pons and the medulla, each bundle crosses the corresponding bundle from the opposite side. Some of these axons make connections with axons from the cerebellum, basic ganglia, thalamus and hypothalamus; some connect with the cranial nerve cells. Other fibers from the cortex and the subcortical centers are channeled through the pons and the medulla into the spinal cord.

Vision and Cortical Blindness. There is a definite area in the rear of each hemisphere where the fibers of the corresponding optic nerve end. It is by means of these receiving cells that we see. The eyes may be normal and the optic nerve perfect, but if these cells in one hemisphere are diseased, the person is half blind. In such a case he has *cortical blindness.* He cannot see to one side of the midline. He sees only half of any object. This is *hemianopsia* (half blindness).

Cortical blindness of one optic area (that is, of the posterior tip of one cerebral hemisphere) always affects both eyes equally. Total blindness in one eye may be due to disease of that eye itself or to disease of its optic nerve. Just behind the two eyes, however, the two optic nerves become confluent (the chiasm), then again become separate and continue to the brain as the two optic tracts.

In each of these tracts is just half of each

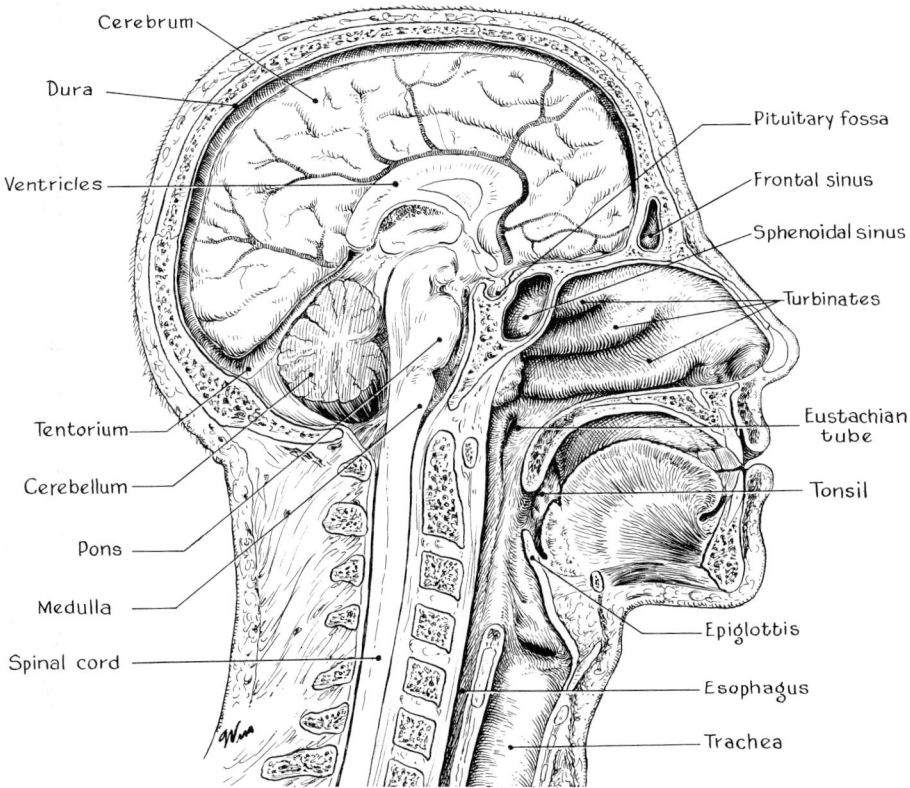

FIG. 342. Cross-sectional view, showing the anatomic position and the relation of structures of the head and the neck.

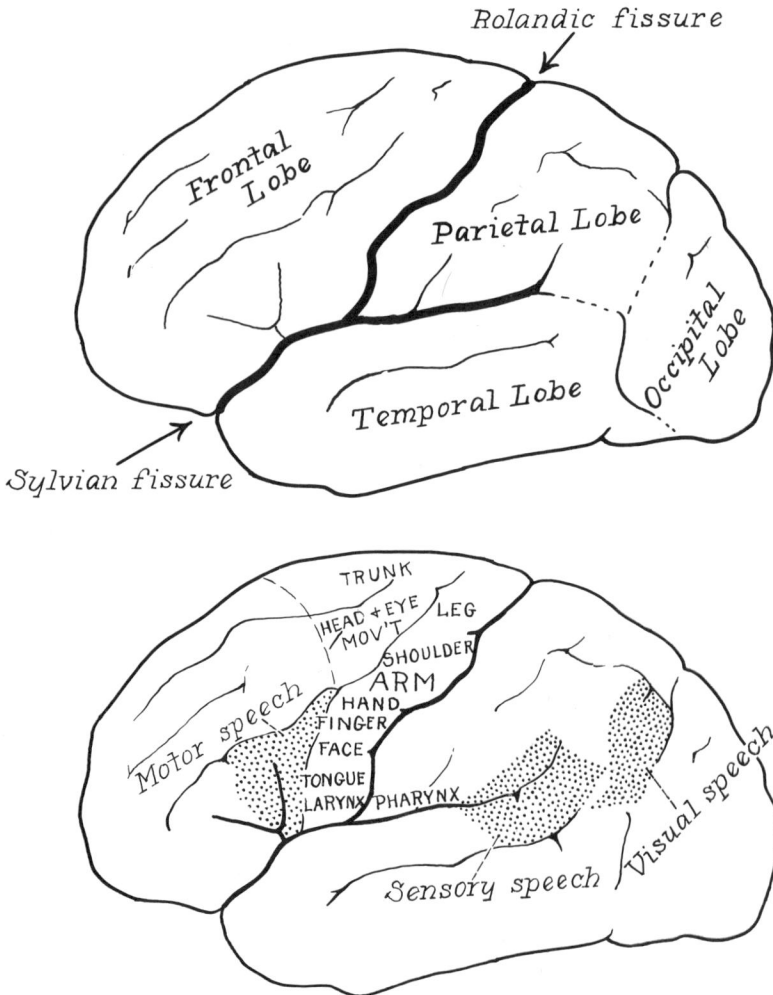

FIG. 343. (*Top*) Diagrammatic representation of the cerebrum, showing relative locations of various lobes of the brain and the principal fissures. (*Bottom*) Diagrammatic representation of cerebral localization for motor movements of various portions of the body.

optic nerve, so that if one tract is injured, there is complete blindness of exactly one half of each retina. For example, if the right tract is injured, the patient is blind on the right half of each retina, so that with either eye he can see nothing to his left but will see perfectly to his right. Destroy the cortical optical area of the hemisphere to which that tract runs and we have this same form of hemianopsia. The pituitary gland is located just beneath the chiasm; a tumor of this gland often disturbs the chiasm and produces blindness of both inner halves of the retinas, since it is only the fibers in the nasal halves of the optic nerves which cross. In many cases of blindness it is thus possible to locate the disorder.

Verbalization and Aphasia. The cortical area that is responsible for integrating the myriad association pathways required for the mere understanding of words and for controlling the countless motor activities that are entailed in the process of verbalizing measures little more than a square inch in extent (marked Motor speech in Fig. 343 *bottom*). This speech center, called *Broca's area*, is located in a convolution adjoining the motor cortex on the left side in the case of right-handed individuals, or on the right in left-handed persons. Here are stored the combinations of muscular movements necessary to speak each word. They are not the cells which govern the muscles of speech; these cells are in the motor area itself. Each

Fig. 344. A cross section of the left hemisphere of the brain through the motor area. The subdural meningeal hemorrhage compresses the brain over the arm-neck area. There is no real destruction of brain substance, but paralysis would result from pressure. (B) Subcortical hemorrhage. This hemorrhage does destroy brain substance. Although a smaller hemorrhage than the subdural, it possibly produces more paralysis, since it cuts fibers that have converged somewhat. (C) Hemorrhage into the internal capsule. This explains the common stroke of paralysis. Although the hemorrhage is small, it causes total paralysis of the right side of the body, since it cuts all the fibers in the internal capsule.

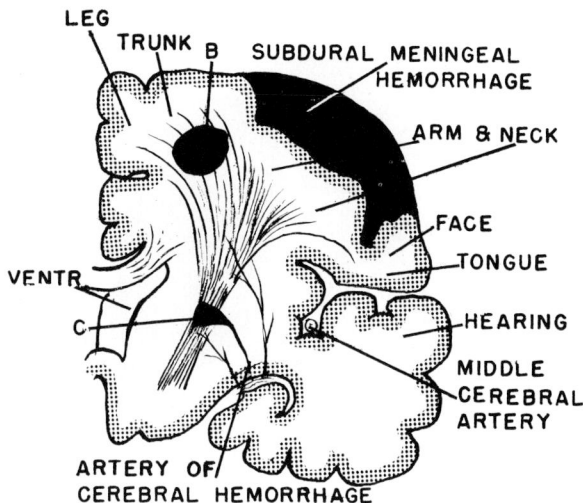

word requires for its utterance a combination or sequence of combinations of muscular contractions. Not only must the muscles of the vocal cords contract, but also those of the throat, the tongue, the soft palate, the lips and the chest wall. In the cells of Broca's convolution these combinations are stored. They direct the cells of the motor area, and these make their muscles contract at the proper time and with the proper force.

Broca's area is so near the left motor area that disease of the latter often affects the former. This is the reason that so many persons who are paralyzed on the right side (due to a lesion of the left hemisphere) are unable to speak, whereas those paralyzed on the left side almost never have speech disturbances. Some patients do, but these usually are left-handed persons whose speech area is on the right hemisphere.

MOTOR APHASIA. The destruction of Broca's convolution by hemorrhage, thrombosis or tumor results in motor aphasia. The patient understands all that is said to him; he knows the words he wants to say; he may be able to write them and read them; but, although he has absolutely no paralysis of the vocal cords, he cannot produce the sequence of movements necessary to utter them, and, if he tries, he makes an unintelligible noise. He is conscious of this defect, and it distresses him. This type also is called *emissive aphasia*. To cause a permanent motor aphasia, however, the lesion must

(and it usually does) affect the white matter beneath this convolution where the fibers are going to and coming from other parts of the brain. When only the gray matter of Broca's convolution is destroyed, the aphasia is transitory. The inability to write (agraphia), often lost in motor aphasia, probably is due to the involvement of the posterior end of the second frontal convolution.

CORTICAL SENSORY APHASIA. Auditory aphasia is the inability of a person to understand and to repeat words spoken to him. Often he talks jargon, but he is unaware that he is not talking correctly. This defect is the result of lesions in the posterior part of the left superior temporal convolution, where the memory of sounds is stored. This type also is called *receptive aphasia*. The patient has difficulty in naming objects set before him, and yet he understands their use. Pure word blindness (*alexia*) is due to lesions in the angular gyrus (marked Visual speech in Fig. 343, *bottom*).

The most common type of aphasia is the result of cerebral hemorrhage which injures the left internal capsule and the surrounding fibers and also produces marked hemiplegia without loss of sensation. This is the mixed type, with loss of voluntary speech, impaired ability to read and difficulty in the comprehension of spoken words.

In some cases it would seem as though another part of the cortex could take over

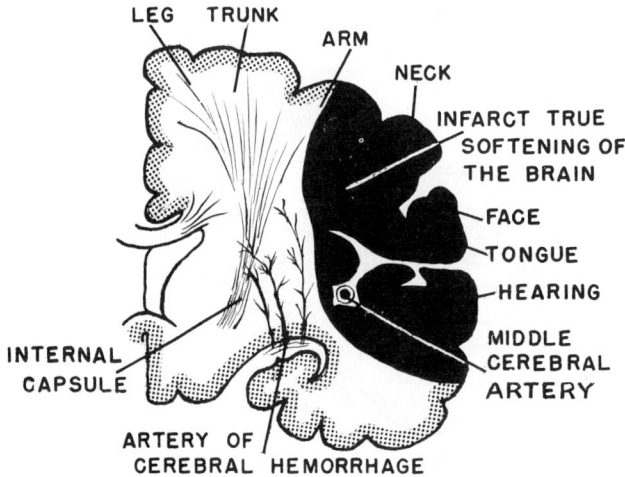

FIG. 345. A cross section of the left hemisphere of the cerebrum through the motor area. The middle cerebral artery is represented as plugged by a thrombus. That part of the brain (black area) supplied with food by this artery has died (infarction or softening). This patient would have paralysis of the right side of the face, the tongue and the neck and part of the right arm; he would be unable to talk or to understand what was said to him.

the work of the destroyed area, for through careful training a man with motor aphasia may learn to talk again.

THE PATIENT WITH APHASIA. In working with the aphasic patient the nurse must remember to *talk* to the patient while she is caring for him. This keeps the patient in a social world. Requests and directions should be simple. When he attempts to communicate, the nurse should make a real effort to understand him. The patient is treated as an intelligent adult. He never should be forced to correct his mistakes, as this merely adds to his tension.

The patient may react with frustration and depression when he is unable to communicate. The nurse accepts his behavior, relieves his embarrassment, and gives support by assuring him that there is nothing wrong with his intelligence, and that she realizes he knows what he wants to say. The environment should be relaxed and permissive, and the socialization of the patient with his family and friends should be encouraged. The language retraining program is carried out by a speech therapist.

The Spinal Cord and Its Connections. The spinal cord, a direct continuation of the medulla oblongata, is that part of the nervous system within the vertebral column. It is a cord about 18 in. long and approximately the thickness of a man's finger. Like the brain, it consists of gray and white matter, but, although in the brain the gray matter is external, and the white internal, in

the cord the gray matter is in the center and is surrounded on all sides by the white fibers, both those of sensory tracts running up to the brain and of motor fibers going down from the brain (Fig. 346).

GRAY MATTER. The gray matter is shaped like two pairs of horns, the anterior horn and the posterior horn. The cord gives off 31 pairs of spinal nerves. Each is formed by the union of two roots, an anterior or motor root and a posterior or sensory root on which is the sensory ganglion. These two roots unite to form one spinal nerve. As a result, all the spinal nerves are mixed. Those leaving the right side of the cord supply the muscles, the skin and the organs on the right side of the body; those of the left side supply the corresponding muscles on that side of the body.

Motor Controls: Paralysis and Dyskinesia

A vertical band of cortex on each cerebral hemisphere governs the voluntary movements of the body. This region, known as the "motor cortex," can be located accurately (Fig. 343).

The exact spot is known where lie the cells in which originate the voluntary movements of the muscles of the face, the thumb, the hands, the arm, the trunk or the leg. Before a person can move a muscle, these particular cells must send the stimulus down along their fibers. If these cells are stimulated with an electric current, the muscles which they control will contract.

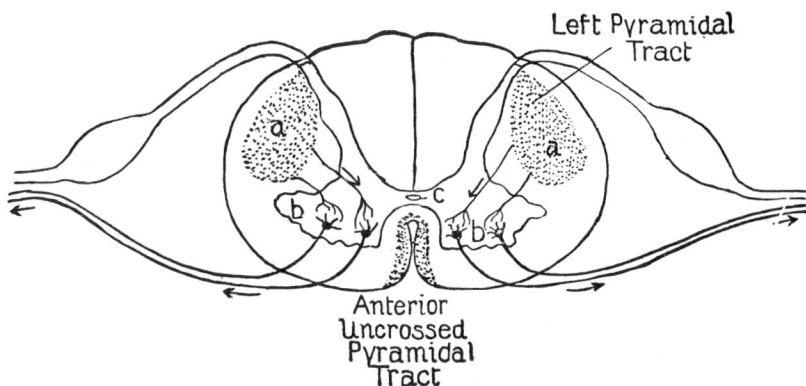

FIG. 346. A cross section of a normal spinal cord. The dotted areas represent the location of the motor fibers that run from the cortex of the brain to the motor nerve cells that control the muscles. (a) Pyramidal tracts of motor fibers. (b) Anterior horn cells, the nerve cells that directly govern the contractions of the muscles.

En route to the pons, as described previously, the motor fibers converge into a tight bundle known as the capsule. A comparatively small injury to this bundle will paralyze more muscles than will a much larger injury to the cortex itself. The brain is like a telephone station, in which one blow of an axe can sever all the wires at the point where they leave the building, but a similar blow on the switchboard would sever only a few.

The ordinary cause of apoplexy, or stroke, followed by paralysis of one half of the body (hemiplegia), is usually a small hemorrhage from a blood vessel in this capsule (see Figs. 344 and 345). A much larger hemorrhage nearer to or in the cortex might paralyze one limb, but hardly half of the body. Hemiplegia may be due to the rupture of a miliary aneurysm of a tiny artery running to the internal capsule or to the plugging of this artery by a thrombus or an embolus, and the subsequent death of the fibers which it supplies with blood.

Immediately after a shock, one half of the body, as a rule, is paralyzed. Then, gradually, the person recovers the use of certain muscles, usually those of the leg, often those of the upper arm, least often those of the hand. The reason for this is that while the hemorrhage actually may destroy the fibers of only a few muscles, yet it injures temporarily all those in its neighborhood, perhaps by the pressure of the escaped blood or by the edema which surrounds it. As the swelling from the hemorrhage diminishes, these latter fibers will resume their function, but those destroyed never will do so.

Within the medulla the motor axons from the cortex form two well-defined bands known as the *corticospinal* or *pyramidal tracts*. Here the majority of these fibers cross (or decussate) to the opposite side, continuing thereafter as the "crossed pyramidal tract" (Fig. 347). The remainder enter the cord on the original side as the "direct pyramidal tract," each fiber in this tract finally crossing to the opposite side of the cord near the point of termination and coming to an end within the gray matter comprising the anterior horn on that side, in close proximity to a motor nerve cell. Fibers of the crossed pyramidal tract terminate within the anterior horn and make connections with anterior horn cells on the same side. All of the motor fibers of the spinal nerves represent extensions of these anterior horn cells (Fig. 348, e), each fiber (f) communicating with one particular muscle fiber (g). Thus each muscle fiber is under voluntary control through a combination of two nerve cells. One is located in the motor cortex, its fiber in the direct or crossed pyramidal tract, and the other is located in the anterior horn of the spinal cord, its fiber running to the muscle. The former is referred to as the upper motor neuron; the latter, as the lower motor neuron. Every motor nerve serving a muscle is a bundle comprised of several thousand lower motor neurons.

Several motor nerve tracts, other than the

corticospinal, are contained in the spinal cord. Some represent the pathways of the so-called "extrapyramidal system," establishing connections between the anterior horn cells and the automatic control centers located in the basal ganglia and the cere- bellum. Others are components of reflex arcs, forming synaptic connections between anterior horn cells and sensory fibers that have entered adjacent or neighboring segments of the cord.

Motor Paralysis. Paralysis of a muscle

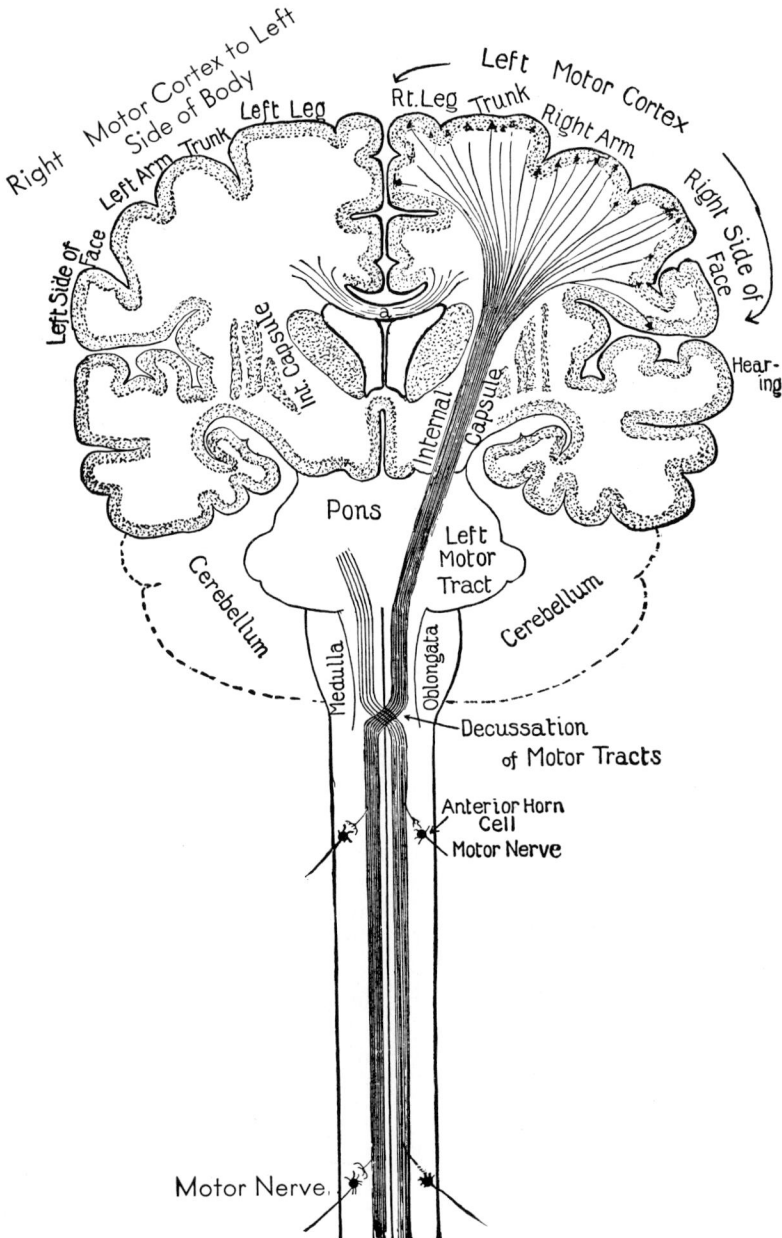

FIG. 347. Diagram of the motor tract.

FIG. 348. Scheme of the motor path. (A) Upper motor neuron. (B) Lower motor neuron. (a) Motor cortex, containing the cells of the upper motor neuron. (b) Fibers of the upper motor neuron which run down the cord and end in the anterior horns (d) in contact with the anterior horn motor cells (e). (f) Fibers of the anterior horn cells (e) which run to muscle fibers (g). (c) Decussation of the pyramidal tracts.

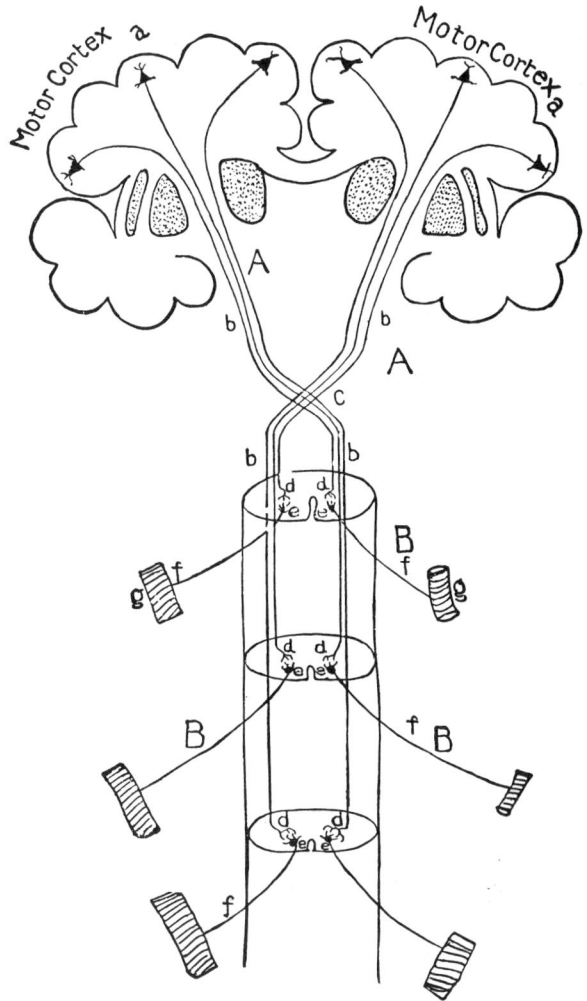

may be due to pathologic changes in either the upper or the lower motor neuron. Suppose the motor nerve is cut somewhere between the muscle and the spinal cord: that muscle will be paralyzed, and the individual will not be able to move it. Furthermore, it will take no part in reflex movements. But that is not all. This muscle becomes limp and wastes away; that is, it atrophies owing to disuse. Possibly, the injury to the spinal nerve trunk will heal, and the patient will regain the use of the muscles that it supplies. But in the event that the anterior horn motor nerve cells are destroyed, then the nerve will not regenerate, and that muscle never will be useful again. In anterior poliomyelitis this is exactly what occurs.

But suppose the upper motor neuron is destroyed: then a different condition exists in the muscle. It will be paralyzed as far as voluntary movement is concerned, but not necessarily for reflex (involuntary) movements, for these originate in the nerve cells in the cord or the medulla. It will not atrophy, and it will not become limp; on the contrary, it will remain permanently more tense than normal. This paralysis seldom affects a part of one muscle, one single muscle or only a few muscles but usually a whole limb, both limbs or an entire half of the body (hemiplegia).

A good illustration of this form of paralysis is the spastic (that is, stiff) paralysis of those infants who during birth receive some mechanical injury which may have caused the rupture of a blood vessel in the meninges of the brain. The long-continued pressure of the escaped blood may injure large areas of cortex; hence these children are usually mentally deficient. Many have convulsions. When such a child begins to walk, it is noted that the legs and the arms are stiff. During life his movements are awkward, stiff and weak. Since those muscles which draw the feet and the knees toward each other (the adductor muscles) are naturally stronger than those which spread those limbs apart (the abductor muscles), these persons walk by crosslegged progression, called also the *scissors gait;* that is, in each step the leg is moved not only forward but is swung round across the front of the other. When both legs and both arms, or both arms only, are paralyzed, the disease is called *diplegia;* when both legs alone, *paraplegia;* and when the arm and the leg on the same side are paralyzed, *hemiplegia.* Paralysis of all four extremities is *quadriplegia.*

A more common illustration of upper motor neuron paralysis is the hemiplegia of adults. If a hemorrhage, an embolus or a thrombus destroys the fibers from the motor area in the internal capsule, the arm and the leg of the opposite side promptly become stiff and more or less paralyzed, and the reflexes are exaggerated. Another illustration of upper neuron disease is seen in adults with spastic paraplegia, a chronic stiffness of both legs due to a gradual degeneration of the fibers in the pyramidal tract. The person so afflicted walks stiffly, as though wading through water, the knees always touching each other, and scarcely raising his feet from the ground (the spastic gait).

Both an upper and a lower motor neuron paralysis may result from an injury which crushes the spinal cord, a type of injury that is all too common. A boy diving into too-shallow water, for example, strikes his head and "breaks" his neck. That is, at one point the vertebrae are no longer in line, and the cord is badly crushed at the point of the dislocation. Knuckling of the backbone due to tuberculosis may do the same thing, only more slowly. The result of such crushing of the cord leads to a rigid paralysis on both sides of all muscles whose nerves leave the cord below the crushed spot, the limp paralysis of the muscles whose motor nerve fibers come from cells in the crushed place. There also will be insensibility of the skin below the crush, since the sensory fibers from below the injury no longer reach the brain. Tumors of the cord ultimately will cause this same picture. At first, only that part of the cord directly involved will be disturbed, but as the tumor grows, it may completely crush the cord.

Extrapyramidal Motor Controls. The smoothness, the accuracy and the strength that characterize the muscular movements of a normal individual are attributable to the influence of the cerebellum and the basal ganglia.

The cerebellum (Fig. 342), nestled beneath the posterior lobe of the cerebrum, chief assistant to the higher motor centers in the cerebral cortex, is responsible for coordinating, balancing, timing and synergizing with precision all muscular movements that originate in those centers. Through the agency of the cerebellum, the contractions of opposing muscle groups are adjusted in relation to each other to maximum mechanical advantage; muscular contractions can be sustained evenly at the desired tension and without significant fluctuation, and reciprocal movements can be reproduced at high and constant speed, in stereotyped fashion and with relatively little effort.

The basal ganglia are masses of gray matter in the midbrain beneath the cerebral hemispheres. These border or project into the lateral ventricles and lie in close apposition to the internal capsule. It is their function to control habitual or automatic acts and to maintain a "postural background" against which voluntary movements are performed. These ganglia, aided by their connections with the organs of special sense, keep the contractile tone of every muscle in the trunk and the extremities in a constant state of adjustment, so that an individual is able to keep his balance regardless of the posture of his body, in darkness as well as in light and irrespective of the status underfoot. Moreover, thanks to this control station, the individual is equipped to react swiftly, appropriately and automatically to any smell, sight or sound that demands an immediate response.

Dyskinesias. Loss of cerebellar function, which may occur as a result of intracranial injury, hemorrhage, abscess or tumor, results in muscular flabbiness, weakness and fatigue. The patient exhibits a coarse involuntary tremor which increases in intensity in association with voluntary movements. He is unable to control his movements accurately or to coordinate his muscles efficiently or smoothly, every act being performed in disjointed fashion, according to stages, or "by the numbers." He is incapable of performing alternating movements with speed or uniformity, a characteristic of cerebellar disease called "adiadochokinesis. When he walks, he staggers, lurching from side to side as though intoxicated, feet wide apart but steps short and not stamping, i.e., with the vertiginous, reeling gait of cerebellar ataxia.

Destruction or dysfunction of the basal ganglia does not lead to paralysis but to muscular rigidity, with consequent disturbances of posture and movement. Such patients are afflicted by a tendency to display involuntary movements. These may take the form of coarse tremors, characterized by approximately six oscillations per second; athetosis, namely, movements of a slow, squirming, writhing, twisting type; or chorea, marked by spasmodic purposeless and grotesque motions of the trunk and the extremities and facial grimacing. Clinical syndromes based on lesions involving the basal ganglia include Parkinsonism (p. 949), Sydenham's chorea, Huntington's chorea (p. 951), Wilson's disease, or "hepatolenticular degeneration," and spasmodic torticollis.

Sensory Pathways and Disturbances

The transmission of sensory impulses from their points of origin to their cerebral destinations involves three neuron relays; more-

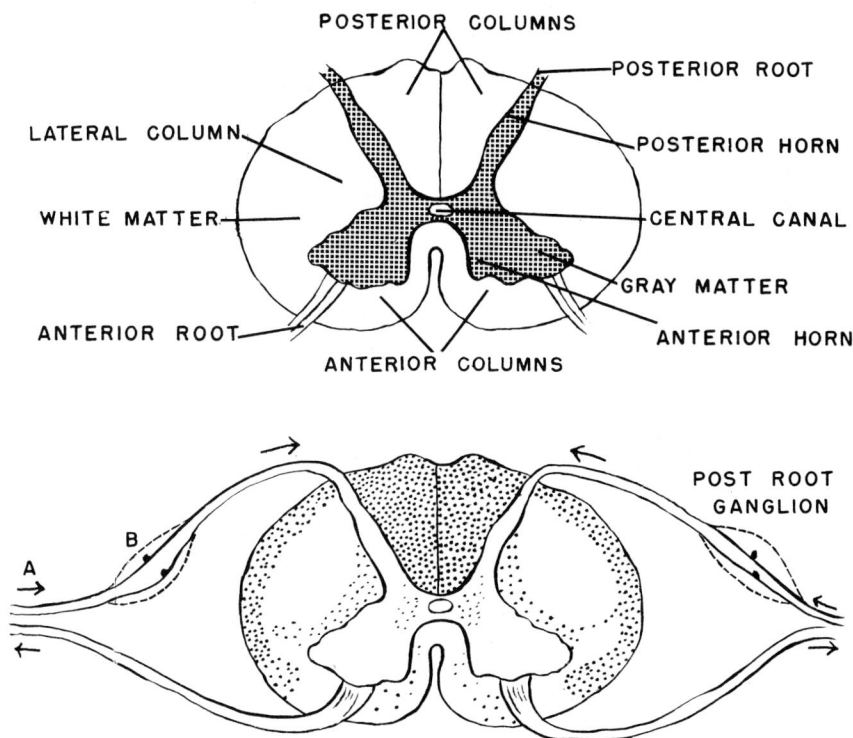

FIG. 349. (*Top*) Cross section of the normal spinal cord. (*Bottom*) The dotted areas show the location of the sensory fibers (A) which run through the posterior root ganglia (B) to the cord and up to the brain.

over, there are three major pathways by which they may be routed, depending on the type of sensation that is registered. Specific knowledge regarding these paths · is of great importance from the standpoint of neurologic diagnoses, being indispensable for the accurate localization of brain and cord lesions in many patients.

The axon of the nerve in which the sensory impulse originates enters the spinal cord via the posterior root. Axons conveying sensations of heat, cold and pain immediately enter the posterior gray column of the cord, where they make connections with the cells of secondary neurons. Pain and temperature fibers cross immediately to the opposite side of the cord and course upward to the thalamus. Fibers carrying sensations of touch, light pressure and localization do not connect immediately with the second neuron but ascend the cord for a variable distance before entering the gray matter and completing this connection. The axon of the secondary neuron crosses the cord and proceeds upward to the thalamus.

The third category of sensation, produced by stimuli arising from muscles, joints and bones, includes position sense and vibratory sense. These stimuli are conveyed, uncrossed, all the way to the brain stem by the axon of the primary neuron. In the medulla, synaptic connections are made with cells of the secondary neurons, whose axons then cross to the opposite side and proceed to the thalamus.

Sensory Losses. Severance of a sensory nerve results in total loss of sensation in its area of distribution. Transection of the spinal cord yields complete anesthesia below the level of injury. Selective destruction or degeneration of the posterior columns (Fig. 349, *bottom*), a characteristic of combined system disease, is responsible for a loss of position sense in segments distal to the lesion, unaccompanied by loss of touch, pain or temperature perception. Such individuals, unless they look, cannot tell where their feet are, or in what direction they are pointing. Moreover, they cannot perceive vibrations in the affected area. A lesion such as a cyst in the center of the cord causes dissociation of sensation, that is, loss of pain at the level of the lesion. This is explainable

on the basis of the fact that the fibers carrying pain and temperature cross the cord immediately upon entering; thus, any lesion that divides the cord longitudinally divides these fibers likewise. Other sensory fibers ascend the cord for variable distances, some even to the medulla itself, before crossing, thereby bypassing the lesion and avoiding destruction.

Dysesthesias. Irritative lesions affecting the posterior spinal nerve roots may cause intermittent severe pains that are referred to their areas of distribution. This phenomenon explains the pains of tabes dorsalis. Finally, the sensation of tingling of the fingers and the toes constitutes a prominent symptom of combined system disease, presumably due to degenerative changes in the sensory fibers that extend to the thalamus, i.e., belonging to the spinothalamic tract.

The thalamus, major receiving and communication center for the afferent sensory nerves, is a large and complicated structure located in the midbrain. It lies in close relation to the 3rd ventricle, forming its lateral wall, and to the lateral ventricle, forming its floor, and is in close proximity to the basal ganglia and adjacent to the internal capsule. To the thalamus may be attributed the vague awareness of sensations described as "feelings" of pleasure, discomfort or pain, as the case may be. Moreover, it is responsible for the routing of all sensory stimuli to their many destinations, including the cerebral cortex, which receives them and translates them automatically into appropriate responses.

Autonomic Systems and Syndromes

The contractions of muscles that are not under voluntary control, including the heart muscle, the secretions of all digestive and sweat glands and the activity of certain endocrine organs as well, are controlled by a major component of the nervous system known as the *autonomic nervous system*. The term "autonomic" refers to the fact that the operations of this system are independent of the desires and the intentions of the individual. It is not subject to his will; i.e., it is in a sense autonomous. To the extent that it is not subject to regulation by the cerebral cortex, the autonomic nervous sys-

TABLE 21. Comparison of Parasympathetic and Sympathetic
Effects on Specific Organs and Tissues*

Organ or Tissue	Parasympathetic Effects	Sympathetic Effects
Vessels:		
Cutaneous	—	Constriction
Muscular	—	Variable
Coronary	Constriction	Dilatation
Salivary gland	Dilatation	Constriction
Buccal mucosa	—	Dilatation
Pulmonary	Variable	Variable
Cerebral	Dilatation	Constriction
Of abdominal and pelvic viscera	—	Constriction
Of external genitalia	Dilatation	Constriction
Heart	Inhibition	Acceleration
Eye:		
Iris	Constriction	Dilatation
Ciliary muscle	Contraction	Relaxation
Smooth muscle of orbit and upper lid	—	Contraction
Bronchi	Constriction	Dilatation
Glands:		
Sweat	—	Secretion
Salivary	Secretion	Secretion
Gastric	Secretion	Inhibition? Secretion of mucus
Pancreatic		
Acini	Secretion	—
Islets	Secretion	—
Liver	—	Glycogenolysis
Adrenal medulla	—	Secretion
Smooth muscle:		
Of skin	—	Contraction
Of stomach wall	Contraction (predominantly)	Inhibition (predominantly)
Of small intestine	Increased tone and motility	Inhibition
Of large intestine	Increased tone and motility	Inhibition
Of bladder wall (detrusor muscle)	Contraction	Inhibition
Of trigone and sphincter	Inhibition	Contraction
Of uterus, pregnant	None	Contraction
Of uterus, nonpregnant	None	Inhibition

* Best, C. H., and Taylor, N. B.: Physiological Basis of Medical Practice, ed. 6, Baltimore, Williams and Wilkins, 1955.

tem resembles the extrapyramidal systems that are centered in the cerebellum and the basal ganglia. However, in other respects it is unique. First, its regulatory effects are exerted not on individual cells but on large expanses of tissue and on entire organs. Second, the responses that it elicits do not appear instantaneously, but only after a lag period, and they are sustained far longer than other neurogenic responses, a type of response that is calculated to ensure maximum functional efficiency on the part of receptor organs, such as the blood vessels and the hollow viscera.

The quality of these responses is explained by the fact that the autonomic nervous sys-tem transmits its impulses only part of the way via nerve pathways, the remainder of the route being serviced by chemical mediators, resembling in this respect the endocrine system. Electrical impulses, conducted through nerve fibers, stimulate the formation of specific chemical agents at strategic locations within the muscle mass, the diffusion of these chemicals being responsible for the contraction.

The autonomic nervous system comprises two divisions that are anatomically and functionally distinct, referred to as the sympathetic and the parasympathetic nervous systems. The majority of the tissues and the organs under autonomic control are innervated by both systems. Sympathetic stimuli are mediated by norepinephrine; parasympathetic impulses, by acetylcholine. These chemicals produce opposing and mutually antagonistic effects, as indicated in Table 21.

Sympathetic Nervous System. Sympathetic neurons are located in the thoracic and the lumbar segments of the spinal cord, their axons, called *preganglionic fibers,* emerging via all anterior nerve roots from the 8th cervical or 1st thoracic segment to the 2nd or 3rd lumbar segment, inclusive. A short distance from the cord these fibers diverge to join a chain composed of 22 linked ganglia which extends the entire length of the spinal column, flanking the vertebral bodies on both sides. Some form multiple synapses with nerve cells within the chain. Others traverse the chain without making connections or losing continuity to join large "prevertebral" ganglia in the thorax, the abdomen or the pelvis, or one of the "terminal" ganglia in the vicinity of an organ, such as the bladder or the rectum. Postganglionic nerve fibers originating in the sympathetic chain rejoin the spinal nerves that supply the extremities and are distributed to blood vessels, sweat glands and smooth muscle tissue in the skin. Postganglionic fibers from the prevertebral plexuses, i.e., the cardiac, the pulmonary splanchnic and the pelvic plexuses, supply structures in the head and the neck, the thorax, the abdomen and the pelvis, respectively, having been joined in these plexuses by fibers from the parasympathetic division.

The adrenals, the kidneys, the liver, the spleen, the stomach and the duodenum are under the control of the giant celiac plexus, familiarly known as the "solar plexus." This receives its sympathetic nerve components via the three splanchnic nerves, composed of preganglionic fibers from nine segments of the spinal cord, i.e., T-4 to L-1, and is joined by the vagus nerve, representing the parasympathetic division. From the celiac plexus, fibers of both divisions travel along the course of blood vessels to their target organs.

Parasympathetic System. The preganglionic nerve cells of the sympathetic division, as described above, are consolidated in consecutive segments of the cord, from C-7 to L-1 or L-2. Those of the parasympathetic system, on the other hand, are located in two sections, one in the brain stem and the other from spinal segments below L-2. On this account the parasympathetic system is referred to as the "craniosacral" division, as distinct from the "thoracolumbar" division of the autonomic nervous system. The cranial parasympathetics arise from the midbrain and the medulla oblongata. Fibers from cells in the midbrain travel with the 3rd oculomotor nerve to the ciliary ganglia, whence postganglionic fibers of this division are joined by those of the sympathetic system. Forming the ciliary nerve, these channel to the ciliary muscles of the eye to control the caliber of the pupil. Parasympathetic fibers from the medulla travel with the 7th (facial), 9th (glossopharyngeal) and 10th (vagus) cranial nerves. Those from the facial nerve end in the sphenopalatine ganglion, whence emanate the fibers that innervate the lacrimal glands, the ciliary muscle and the sphincter of the pupil. Those from the glossopharyngeal nerve innervate the parotid gland. The vagus nerve carries preganglionic parasympathetic fibers without interruption to the organs that it innervates, joining ganglion cells within the myocardium and within the walls of the esophagus, the stomach and the intestine. Preganglionic parasympathetic fibers from the anterior roots of the sacral nerves coalesce to become the pelvic nerves, consolidate and regroup in the pelvic plexus, and terminate around ganglion cells in the musculature of the pelvic organs. These innervate the colon, the rectum and the bladder, inhibiting the muscular tone of the anal and the bladder sphincters and dilating the blood vessels of the bladder, the rectum and the genitalia. The vagus, the splanchnic, pelvic and the other autonomic nerves carry impulses generated in the viscera to the dorsal nucleus of the vagus, where connections are made with efferent parasympathetic neurons, forming a series of reflex arcs. These provide the basis for self-regulation, a cardinal feature of the autonomic nervous system, and one reason for "autonomy."

Autonomic Functions and Dysfunctions. A detailed listing of the effects produced by the two divisions of the autonomic nervous system is supplied in Table 21. Perusal of this listing provides impressive evidence of the scope and the importance of autonomic activity in relation to all bodily functions and from the standpoint of survival itself. Both sympathetic and parasympathetic divisions are in a constant state of activity, the activity of each relative to the other being one of controlled opposition, with a delicate balance maintained between the two at all times.

Overall supervision of the autonomic nervous system is considered to be a function of the hypothalamus. The hypothalamus is a portion of the diencephalon (interbrain) located immediately beneath and lateral to the lower portion of the wall of the 3rd ventricle. It includes among its components the optic chiasm, the tuber cinereum, the pituitary stalk, which originates from the latter, and the pituitary gland itself. Large cell groups in adjacent portions of the hypothalamus have been assigned the role of being the probable centers of autonomic regulation. These centers are richly endowed with connections linking the autonomic systems with the thalamus, the cortex, the olfactory apparatus and the pituitary gland. Here reside the mechanisms for the control of visceral and somatic reactions that were designed originally for defense or attack, but in man these are associated with his emotional states, i.e., his fears, anger, anxiety, etc.; for the control of metabolic processes which include fat, carbohydrate and water metabolism; for the regulation of body temperature, arterial pressure and all muscular and glandular activities of the gastrointestinal tract; the genital functions; and the sleep rhythm. The close proximity, histologic similarity and multiple connections between the pituitary gland, master gland of the endocrines, and this portion of the brain suggest that here may be located the supreme headquarters of the endocrine and autonomic nervous systems, commanding all vital processes.

Sympathetic Syndromes. Certain syndromes are distinctive of diseases of the sympathetic nerve trunks. Among these are dilatation of the pupil of the eye on the same side as a penetrating wound of the neck (evidence of disturbance of the cervical sympathetic cord); temporary paralysis of the bowel (indicated by the absence of peristaltic waves and the distention of the intestine by gas) following fracture of any one of the lower dorsal or upper lumbar vertebrae, with hemorrhage into the base of the mesentery; and the marked variations in pulse rate and rhythm that often follow compression fractures of the upper six thoracic vertebrae. Certain diseases, few in number, including Raynaud's disease, acroparesthesia, erythromelalgia, scleroderma and giant colon, also are considered to be autonomic nervous disturbances.

ASSISTING WITH THE NEUROLOGIC EXAMINATION
Cranial Nerve Tests

In addition to the usual complete physical examination, every patient suspected of having a neurologic disorder and every neurosurgical patient is subjected to a systematic and detailed neurologic examination. This involves the testing of each cranial nerve in the manner specified in Table 22. Maximum cooperation of the patient is essential for the proper conduct of this diagnostic routine and can be elicited only if he understands what he is expected to do. All equipment for these tests should be available in one place.

Examination of the peripheral motor and the sensory systems also is done. Motor tests include observation of posture and gait, reflex tests, coordination observations, etc. Sensory tests determine skin sensation and deeper tissue sensation, as well as the ability to recognize objects by the sense of touch.

The nurse should know the results of the findings of the neurologic and the physical examination, because only then is she able to observe intelligently the symptoms and aberrant reactions of her patient. These deviations must be charted accurately if they are to be meaningful to the physician or the neurosurgeon.

Lumbar and Cisternal Punctures

Frequently it is necessary to insert a needle into the spinal subarachnoid space to determine the pressure of the fluid and to obtain fluid for examination. In the ma-

TABLE 22. Neurologic Examination for Testing Cranial Nerves

Nerve	Equipment	Procedure
1. Olfactory	Four small bottles of volatile oils, such as (1) turpentine, (2) oil of cloves, (3) oil of winter-green, (4) vanilla	Instruct the patient to sniff and to identify the odors. Each nostril is tested separately.
2. Optic	Ophthalmoscope	In darkened room the patient is examined with this instrument. More detailed examination with special equipment is used for accurate determination of visual fields.
3. Oculomotor 4. Trochlear 6. Abducens	Flashlight	Because of close association these nerves are examined collectively. They innervate pupil and upper eyelid and are responsible for extraocular muscle movements.
5. Trigeminal	Test tube of hot water Test tube of ice water Cotton wisp from cotton applicator stick Pin	*Sensory branch*—Vertex to chin tested for sensations of pain, touch and temperature. This includes reflex reaction of cornea to wisp of cotton. *Motor branch*—Ability to bite is tested.
7. Facial	Four small bottles with solutions which are salty, sweet, sour, and bitter (Four clean medicine droppers)	Observe symmetry of face and ability to contract facial muscles. Instruct patient to taste and to identify substance used. He should rinse his mouth well between each drop of solution. This is a test for the anterior ⅔ of tongue.
8. Acoustic	Tuning fork	Tests for hearing, air and bone conduction
9. Glossopharyngeal	Cotton applicator stick	Test for taste posterior ⅓ of tongue and check gag reflex
10. Vagus	Tongue depressor	Checking voice sounds, observing symmetry of soft palate will give suggestion of function of vagus.
11. Spinal Accessory		Since this innervates the sternocleidomastoid and the trapezius muscles, the patient will be instructed to turn and to move his head and to elevate shoulders with and without resistance.
12. Hypoglossal		Observe tongue movements.

jority of patients this is done by inserting the needle into the subarachnoid space between the 3rd and the 4th lumbar spinous processes (*lumbar or spinal puncture*). For technical or other reasons it may be necessary to introduce the needle between the rim of the foramen magnum and the 1st cervical lamina into the cisterna magna (*cisternal puncture*). For both procedures the patient must be relaxed, since straining will produce a false increase in the pressure reading. Normal pressures in the recumbent position range between 80 and 200 mm. of water. Pressures with the patient in the sitting position are much higher and not reliable.

The lumbar puncture tray should contain:

1. Local anesthesia syringe, needle, and 0.5 per cent procaine solution
2. Covers—sterile
3. Skin antiseptics and sterile cotton
4. Spinal puncture needle with stylets to fit
5. Water manometer and rubber tube attachment. (All of these parts must be tested before sterilization to ensure patency of the tubes and accurate fitting of the parts to the manometer and the needles.)
6. Sterile test tubes, 2, with nonabsorbent cotton plugs or corks

The nurse should have a pair of sterile rubber gloves ready for the physician.

Before a lumbar puncture the bladder and

the bowels should be emptied. The patient is placed on his side at the edge of the bed, with his back toward the operator. The thighs and the head are flexed acutely and the body is curved forward as much as possible to increase the space between the spinous processes of the vertebrae. A small pillow is placed under the head, so that the patient's spine is horizontal (Fig. 350). It may be necessary for the nurse to hold the patient in this position, especially in the case of children and nervous adults.

For a cisternal puncture the neck must be shaved up to the external occipital protuberance in the midline. The patient is placed on his side, with his head on a sandbag to keep the head in a straight line with the thoracic spine; at the same time he flexes his head forward on his chest. It is very important that the patient refrain from moving during the procedure.

Queckenstedt Test. This test determines the presence of any obstruction between the cranial cavity and the lumbar puncture needle. Pressure is made firmly upon the jugular vein in the neck for 10 seconds. The increase in intracranial pressure caused by the compression is noted, and if the pressure does not return to its original position in 10 seconds, the pressure is recorded at 10-second intervals until it has returned to its original level. If there is any obstruction in the spinal subarachnoid space, the rise and the fall of pressure will be slow and gradual or none at all. A blood pressure cuff may be used to apply compression about the neck at intervals of 20, 30, 40 and 50 mm. of pressure, the cerebrospinal fluid pressure being measured simultaneously.

Usually, specimens are sent to the laboratory for cell count, culture and chemical analysis. These should be sent immediately, since changes will take place that will alter the result if the specimens are allowed to stand.

Following the lumbar puncture, the patient should lie quietly for several hours.

Postpuncture Headache. Within a period of a few hours or days following a lumbar puncture there frequently develops a throbbing occipital headache that is particularly severe when the patient sits or stands upright, and that tends to disappear when he lies horizontal. The cause of this unpleasant complication is the leakage of spinal fluid at the puncture site, the fluid continuing to escape via the needle tract from the spinal canal into the tissues, whence it is absorbed promptly by the lymphatics, never having accumulated in sufficient volume to be detected. Depletion of cerebrospinal fluid as a result of this leak causes the supply remaining in the cranium to be insufficient for proper

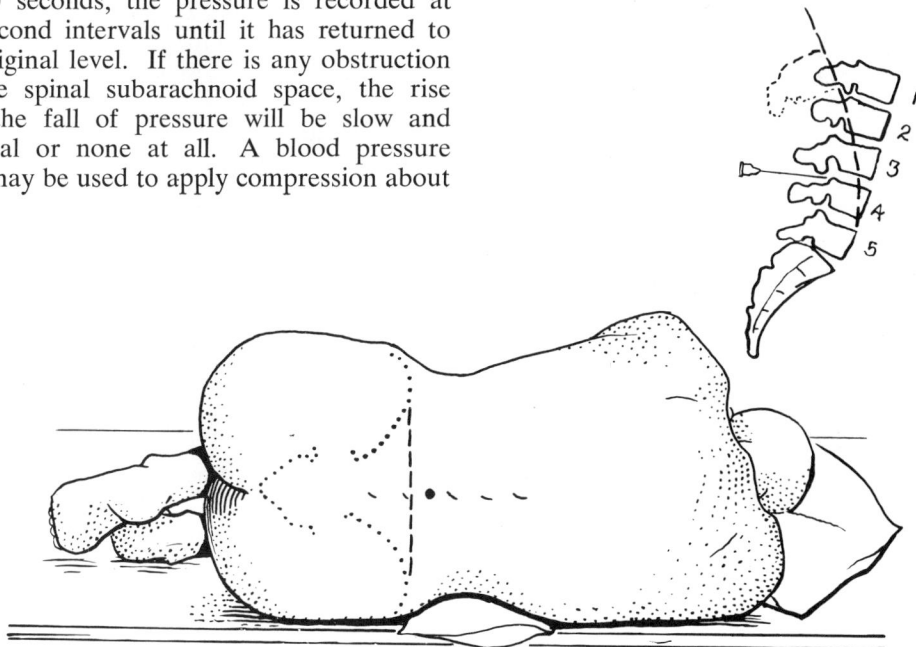

FIG. 350. Lateral position for lumbar puncture.

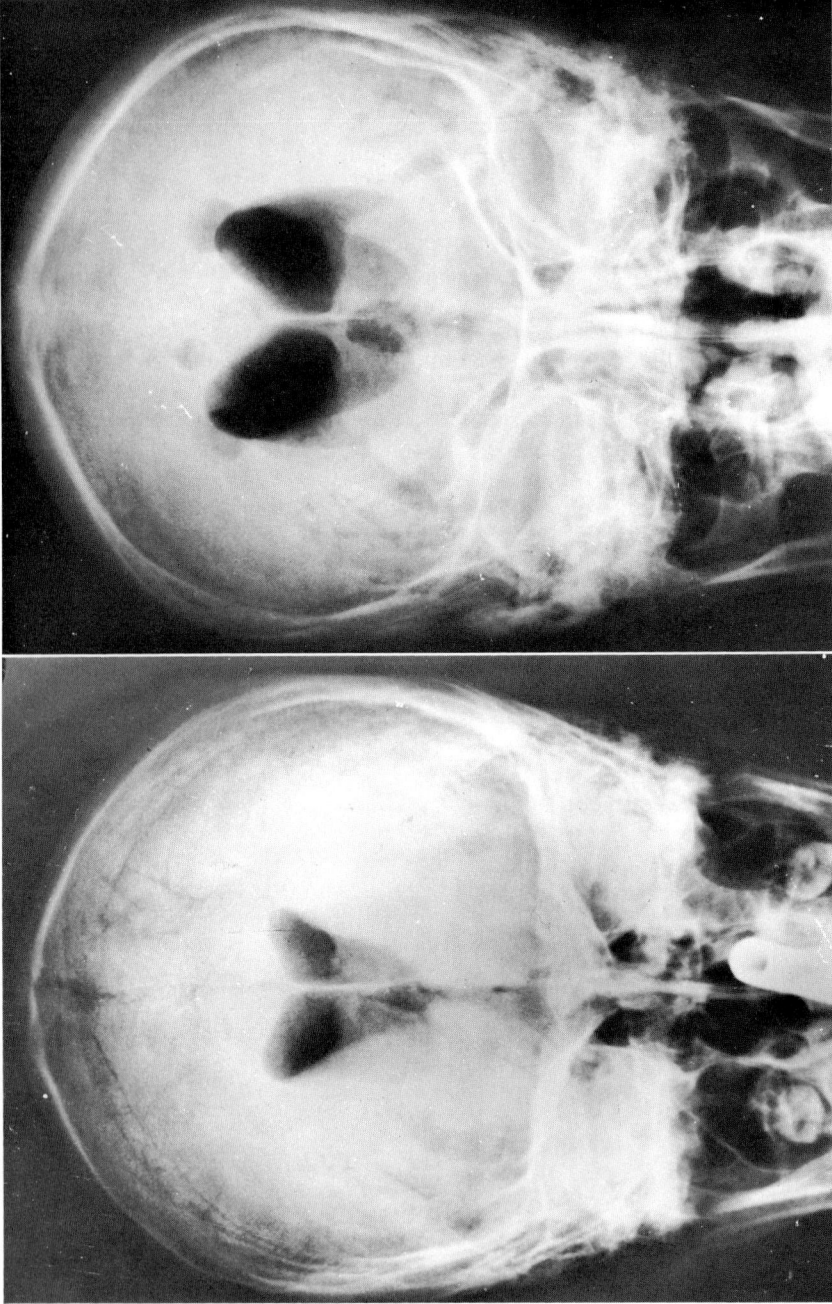

FIG. 351. (A) Anteroposterior view, showing normal lateral and third ventricles as demonstrated by pneumoencephalography. (Compare with B.) (B) Markedly dilated lateral and third ventricle as demonstrated by ventriculography.

mechanical stabilization of the brain. The latter becomes displaced caudally, exerting traction on the dural attachments to the venous sinuses and causing headache. Traction on these pain-sensitive structures is maximal, and the pain is most severe when the patient is in a vertical position; both traction and pain are lessened by recumbency, which also reduces the leak. The lumbar puncture headache is avoidable to a large extent by using the smallest needle practical and by insistence that patients remain recumbent for 12 to 24 hours following lumbar puncture.

Pneumoencephalography and Ventriculography

The cerebrospinal fluid spaces in and around the brain can be seen in x-ray examination when the contained fluid is replaced with a gas. Withdrawal of fluid and injection of a gas directly into the ventricles through openings in the back of the skull is called *ventriculography*. A similar injection made by the spinal subarachnoid route is called *pneumoencephalography*. The latter procedure is done as a general rule in patients without evidence of increased intracranial pressure.

Preparation of Patient. The night before encephalography or ventriculography the patient should have a good rest. On the morning of operation the breakfast is withheld to avoid vomiting. Appropriate sedatives and analgesics should be administered prior to departure for the operating room or X-ray department. The back of the head should be shaved before ventriculography, or all of the head if craniotomy is to follow. All hairpins should be removed, and long hair should not be braided before pneumoencephalography, since braids will cast shadows on the x-ray films. As with other surgical procedures, dentures are removed.

Pneumoencephalography. This is done under local or general anesthesia. Because of the severe reaction of headache, retching, shock and sometimes unconsciousness when done under local anesthesia, general anesthesia is to be preferred. A lumbar puncture is performed with the patient in the sitting position—usually in a special chair with

casters to allow easy movement of the patient while taking x-ray pictures. Ten ml. of fluid is removed, and 10 ml. of air or a gas is injected until all of the fluid has been removed. A nurse may be assigned the duty of checking the vital signs of pulse, respiratory rate and blood pressure throughout the procedure. If the procedure is done under local anesthesia, it is important to have adequate personnel to treat the complications. At no time should the patient be left alone, even when the roentgenograms are being taken.

Ventriculography. This is usually done under local anesthesia with the patient sitting in a special chair. The posterior half of the head is prepared and draped. Through $1\frac{1}{2}$-inch scalp incisions trephines are made, the dura is opened, and blunt brain cannulae are introduced into each ventricle. The fluid is replaced with air, the cannulae are withdrawn, and the scalp wounds are closed. During the procedure the patient develops a mild headache, may become nauseated, may retch and very rarely may have a convulsive seizure. The reaction to this procedure is usually milder than that attending pneumoencephalography (Fig. 351 A, B).

Nursing Care. Following the above procedures the nurse must observe the patient for signs of increased intracranial pressure or shock reaction. Special care must be taken to see that the patient does not aspirate any vomitus. For the first 6 hours vital signs are taken at intervals of a half hour. Parenteral fluids may be necessary for the first 24 hours.

Since headache is the major complaint, an icecap to the head and adequate analgesics must be given for the duration of the headache, which usually lasts for 2 to 4 days, depending on the speed with which the intracranial air is absorbed and replaced once more with fluid. Occasionally, especially following pneumoencephalography, headache persists much longer.

Fractional Pneumoencephalography. In this test small amounts of fluid are withdrawn, and small amounts of air are injected. During the procedure the patient is placed in different positions so that specific areas of the ventricles and the subarachnoid system are filled and visualized. With smaller amounts of air injected into the ventricles, more subtle lesions can be demonstrated, and the attention is directed to the specific area rather than the whole ventricular system. The patient does not have to be under general anesthesia and is able to cooperate in assuming the various positions. There is less incidence of headache following this diagnostic test. Fractional pneumoencephalography is used to diagnose space-occupying lesions and atrophy or blockage of the ventricular system.

Electroencephalography

This procedure is the recording of the electrical activity passing through the surface of the brain by applying electrodes to the unshaved scalp. Tumors, abscesses, brain scars, blood clots and infection may cause electric changes that are different from the normal pattern or rhythm. Thus, this test some-

times helps not only in diagnosis but also in localization.

Arteriography

Following the injection of a radiopaque substance into the common carotid artery or into the vertebral artery, it is possible to visualize by means of x-rays the cerebral arterial system. Through abnormal positions and configurations of the blood vessels it is possible to detect aneurysms, abscesses, tumors and other lesions. The dye is injected through a No. 18 spinal needle that has been inserted into the artery. The procedure can be done under local or general anesthesia and either by the "open" or the "closed" method. In the open method the artery is exposed, whereas in the closed method the artery is palpated, and the needle is inserted through the skin into the artery. As the dye is injected into the artery, roentgenograms are taken (Fig. 352).

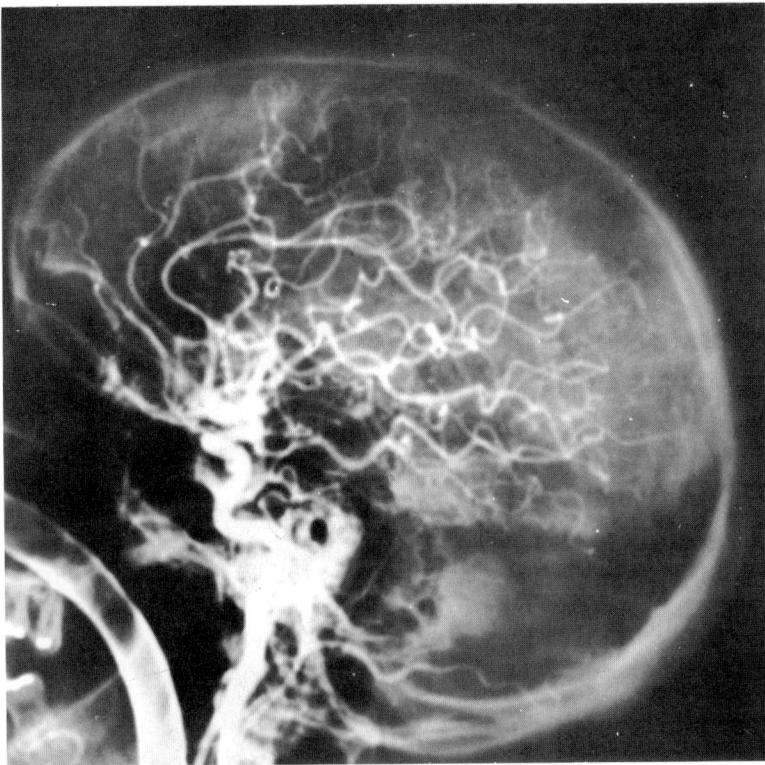

Fig. 352. Normal arteriogram of the brain.

Following the procedure the site of injection must be observed for hematoma formation. The region usually is somewhat swollen, painful and tender. An icecap will help to relieve swelling and discomfort. In a small percentage of patients, either during the actual injection or following the procedure, the irritant dye in the blood vessel. These include alterations in the state of consciousness, weakness on one side and speech disturbances. It is necessary for the nurse to make repeated observations of the patient for these signs and to report them immediately.

Radioisotope Studies

Certain radioactive substances, such as radioactive phosphorus, when injected intravenously, will be absorbed by cerebral tumors in greater amounts then normal brain tissues. A type of Geiger counter is used to locate the tumor. This may be done before or at the time of surgery.

Myelography and Discography

In a *myelogram* a radiopaque oil is injected into the spinal subarachnoid space through a lumbar puncture needle. The subarachnoid space surrounding the spinal cord is visualized by x-ray pictures, and abnormalities of the oil column may indicate spinal cord tumors, herniated intervertebral disks or other lesions (Figs. 353, 354). After the x-ray examination is completed, the oil is withdrawn, because the continued presence of oil can cause inflammation of the arachnoid membrane. To withdraw the oil, the needle has to be manipulated. By this maneuver the needle frequently touches the nerve roots and causes pain. Sedation prior to the procedure and informing the patient just before the pain is initiated will help the patient to better accept a myelogram. Following the procedure the patient should be treated like a patient who has had a lumbar puncture.

Discography is the injection of a radiopaque substance directly into the intervertebral disk. The pathology of the disk then can be seen by taking AP and lateral views of the spine. This study is very useful in patients suspected of having a herniated nucleus pulposus that is undiagnosed by myelography. Discography is confined primarily to the lumbar disks of L-3, -4 and -5.

SPECIAL PROBLEMS OF NEUROLOGIC AND NEUROSURGICAL PATIENTS

General Nursing Care

Nursing Observations. The nurse's observations relative to all systems of the body may be of great assistance in establishing the diagnosis of many neurologic disorders. Of utmost importance are changes in muscle strength and disturbances of sensation. The appearance of pain, its type and location, should be noted with care. Anuria and incontinence should be reported; also any episode of vomiting should be reported, with a full description of it (whether or not accompanied with nausea, its relationship to the preceding meal and the nature of the vomitus). Mental and nervous symptoms should be observed and studied analytically, for their complete description is likely to prove to be of value in the diagnosis and the therapy of the case. The general attitude of the patient may reveal depression or euphoria; the mood swings may run the gamut of irritability, apprehension, anger and elation. Disturbances of vision, hearing, speech, smell, taste, touch, pressure or pain may be elicited in the course of routine care, possibly indicating a new development in the patient's neurologic status. In other words, the nurse should practice observation as she cares for the neurologic patient, for the diagnostic value of her findings, completely and accurately described, can be very significant.

Skin Care. Special nursing problems arise from paralyses, sensory disturbances, psychosis and coma. If hyperesthesia is present, superficial pain may be aroused through slight stimulation of the terminals of the affected nerve branches by simple drafts or gentle friction, causing marked discomfort.

Disturbances in the skin innervation may cause anesthesia, thereby favoring the development of decubitus ulcers. Since pressure is one of the major causes of decubiti, the

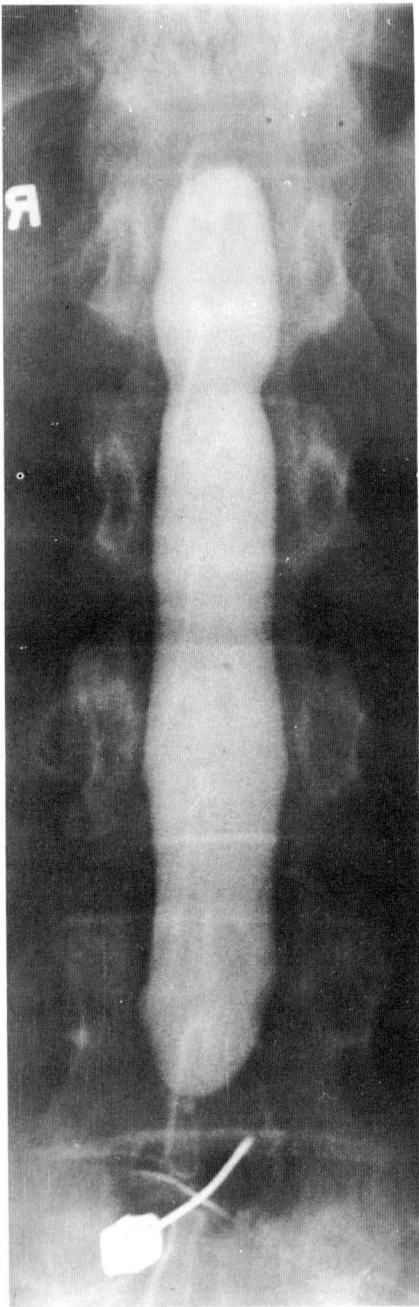

FIG. 353. Normal lumbar myelogram.
(Compare with Fig. 354.)

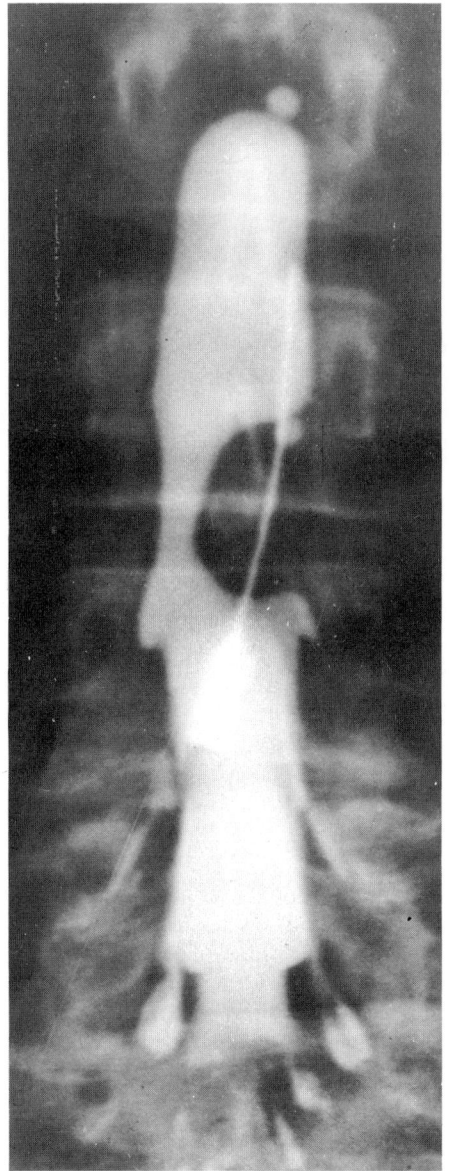

FIG. 354. Abnormal myelogram.
For comparison with normal myelogram, see Figure 353.

patient's position should be changed frequently. Small foam rubber pads under pressure areas are beneficial. The skin must be kept scrupulously clean and dry. Provision should be made on the nursing care plan for frequent nursing inspection of areas susceptible to decubiti. Special skin care (bathing and massage in a circular motion) should be done at specified intervals. Unusual care is indicated in the use of hot-water bottles, the temperature of which should not exceed 115°F. to prevent the development of skin burns. (See pp. 360-361.)

Nutritional Needs. Nutritional problems arise if there is any disturbance connected with the swallowing reflex. They may be overcome by homogenizing the patient's meals in a food blender and feeding him via a tube. Vitamin preparations usually are added to the feeding. The blenderized meal is tolerated well, since the patient's gastrointestinal tract is accustomed to this type of diet, and there is less incidence of diarrhea. Plastic drinking tubes should be used by patients who are subject to convulsions, and dentures, of course are removed from the mouths of such patients, as well as from those in coma.

Oral Hygiene. The condition of the patient's mouth should be checked often, for the buccal structures are prone to become exceedingly dry after a short period of mouth breathing if this process is sustained without interruption, as is likely to be the case. The lips, the tongue and the gums should be lubricated systematically, and the hydration of the patient should be maintained at an adequate level.

Eye Care. Patients with facial palsy on any basis, who are incapable of shutting their eyes, need special eye care in the form of irrigations with sterile saline and lubrication of the outer lids with trace amounts of mineral oil to prevent drying. These procedures should be carried out several times each day, and the eyes should be inspected regularly for signs of inflammation. Should such signs appear, the doctor is to be notified without delay. Patients who are conscious and cooperative can administer their own eye care with proper instruction and supervision.

The Incontinent Patient. Many patients with diseases of the central nervous system initially or eventually, temporarily or permanently, exhibit urinary and fecal incontinence. The hygienic care of patients with incontinence is a grave responsibility, for it is essential that the patient be kept clean and dry.

Urinary incontinence is an indication for a retention catheter or tidal drainage. The latter, much the preferable method, permits continuous rhythmic lavage of the bladder, thereby simulating and stimulating the reflex control of normal bladder activity. The number of catheterizations required is lessened. The bladder is irrigated continuously with a mild antiseptic solution (ordinarily, potassium permanganate in 1:5,000 dilution), and residual urine is eliminated by this technic. Urinary tract infections are thus to a large extent prevented.

Placing the patient on a regular bowel program will avoid the occurrence of spontaneous defecation. A regular routine is developed in which prune juice is given nightly. A glycerine suppository is inserted above the patient's internal sphincter at the same time every morning. The patient is encouraged to wait for an interval before attempting to have a bowel movement. Then he is given the bedpan. If the nurse sees that this routine is carried out regularly every day, the patient will form a habit pattern that is the basis for bowel training.

Prevention of Deformities. Any paralyzed extremity deserves careful attention on the part of the nurse. Care must be taken lest a patient lie on it, or its circulation in any way become impeded. Footboards or cradles prevent pressure from weighty linen.

To prevent contractures, the nurse must see that the patient is positioned correctly, and that the joints are moved, either actively or passively, through their range of motion. When the condition of the patient permits, active exercises (bathing, walking, therapeutic exercises) are desirable. Massage may be instituted and perhaps later supplemented by electrical stimulation. Passive exercises and, as soon as possible, active motions are prescribed for the purpose of developing strength.

Psychological Aspects. Various psychic disturbances appear in neurologic patients and complicate their care in hospital and home; and some patients present diagnostic problems with mild symptoms that strongly suggest neuroses. A sincere attempt should be made to accept the complaints in good faith, and the patient never should be made to feel that he is not believed. The consulting psychiatrist will guide the medical therapy and give suggestions regarding the proper approach for meeting the personality requirements of the individual. The family attitude may be unsympathetic, and a feeling of reserve and tension and a general lack of understanding may develop. The physician must give the family a point of view that will be helpful, and the medical social worker must help to plan for future care.

Occasionally, patients are admitted to the medical wards with a manic psychosis. They obviously require confinement in a mental hospital, where the equipment is adequate for their care, and they should be transferred there as soon as the diagnosis is confirmed, and commitment is arranged. Meanwhile, good nursing practice requires that adequate protection and care be given.

THE PATIENT WITH A HEADACHE

Possibly the commonest of all human afflictions and a symptom that virtually no man is spared wholly is headache or *cephalgia* ("condition of head pain"), as it is known in technical parlance. A clue to its extraordinary prevalence is that the annual expenditure in this country for headache remedies is reported to be in excess of $300,000,000! As a major source of distress and disability this disorder poses an array of therapeutic challenges, problems of prevention, and nursing opportunities that cannot be disregarded.

Headache is in no sense a disease entity; nor does it represent a discrete abnormality. It is a symptom, albeit a symptom that is singularly lacking in uniformity and specificity, and consequently it is difficult to interpret. On the other hand, its presence or absence is extremely important in relation to many diagnoses, and its characteristics as described by patients assist materially in the identification of many major illnesses. Accordingly, its incidence, basic nature and special features in those diseases are of importance to the nurse.

Headache may arise from a variety of sources, through several possible mechanisms and for many different reasons. Its basic cause may reside inside or outside of the skull, originating from without more often than from within. Headaches of extracranial origin include (1) those caused by distension or inflammation of arteries in the scalp; (2) those produced by spastic contraction of the neck muscles that are attached to the cranium and the upper cervical vertebrae, and (3) those originating in the mucosal lining of infected paranasal sinuses or sinuses under low pressure. Headaches of the intracranial type may derive their stimuli from the walls of intracranial arteries and the adjacent perivascular tissue when these vessels are widely dilated and pulsatile; from the meninges; or from the dural walls of the great venous sinuses, the dural septa and/or the dural attachments supporting the brain. These membranes are equipped with nerve fibers and give rise to pain when inflamed or stretched. Described below are the types of headache that are experienced most commonly and certain other headaches that are especially important from the standpoints of diagnosis, treatment and prevention.

Headaches of Extracranial Type

"Tension Headaches." Produced by the spastic contraction of neck muscles, these headaches probably outnumber all other types of headache combined. Sustained contraction of these muscles may be provoked by postural strain, unaccustomed exertion involving the head and the neck, cervical arthritis, or possibly inflammatory processes residing in the muscles themselves, i.e., "myofibrositis." However, most tension headaches occur in the complete absence of arthritis, myositis or any other demonstrable organic lesion, muscle spasm in many of these cases apparently reflecting some emotional or physical stress—for example, stress produced by pain elsewhere. The headache itself may be characterized as a steady, pressing ache, which usually begins in a restricted area, such as the forehead, the temple or the nape of the neck, then spreads to involve one whole side of the head or the entire head. The pain is intensified by changes of posture and by exposure to cold or to a cold draft, which may have precipitated it in the first place. Its severity may be slight or great, and its duration may be a matter of minutes, hours or days.

Relief often is afforded by the application of heat from an electric pad, hot shower or hot tub bath; by gentle massage of the neck muscles; and by the adoption of an optimum, restful posture. Various pharmacologic agents are useful in the treatment of severe tension headache, including analgesics, such as aspirin, phenacetin and codeine; muscle relaxants; tranquillizing agents; and soporifics. Drug combinations with multiple effects of the type desired are exemplified by a product called Equigesic, containing meprobamate (Equanil, Miltown), ethoheptazine (Zactane) and aspirin. Drugs with relaxant, analgesic and sedative effects combined include carisoprodol (Rela, Soma) and phenyramidol (Analexin). If adequate relief is not obtained as a result of the above procedures and drugs, the physician may locate areas of the neck in which spasm and tenderness are principally marked and infiltrate these with procaine or spray them with ethyl chloride, with the expectation of interrupting muscle spasm long enough to break a vicious cycle and terminate the headache.

Eyestrain Headache. Pronounced refractive errors or prolonged use of the eyes under unfavorable lighting conditions may stimulate sustained contractions of the extraocular muscles of the orbit, with spreading of the spasm to the frontal, the temporal and even the occipital muscles and production of a special variant of the tension headache described above. Pain so produced is referred predominantly to the orbit or the temple and may include the occiput. It is a steady, not a throbbing, pain which tends to be worse toward evening, is increased in severity by general fatigue and is aggravated by further use of the eyes. It is experienced more frequently in association with hyperopic (far-sighted) astigmatism than with myopia (near-sightedness). Relief and prevention depend on the acquisition of glasses that compensate for the refractive error and on the improvement of illumination or body posture while the patient is reading. Analgesic medications, such as aspirin, are useful as a temporary expedient.

Sinus Headache. Patients with acute infections of the paranasal sinuses are likely to experience pain and skin tenderness in the periorbital area in the case of frontal sinusitis; or in the vertex, the occiput or elsewhere with involvement of the sphenoidal sinus. Whenever the air pressure within a sinus becomes reduced to a level below that of atmospheric pressure, the mucous membrane lining that sinus becomes edematous, and pain is produced, or, if present, it is intensified. This is the situation that obtains when the small channel connecting the sinus and the nasal cavities becomes obstructed by inflammatory exudate and edema; the sinus effectively is isolated, and the intracavitary pressure drops. During sleep it may remain low for several hours. For this reason the pain of sinusitis tends to be most severe as the patient awakens in the morning, and to improve after he has arisen, is vertical, and the sinus blockade has been relieved. It also explains the exquisite pain that is experienced during an airplane descent by the individual with sinusitis whose sinus remains completely blocked throughout the descent and therefore retains at ground level the lower, high-altitude pressure.

Sinus headache is alleviated by salicylates and similar analgesics, and complete relief is to be anticipated with subsidence of the inflammatory process. Recovery may be hastened by the administration of an appropriate antibiotic drug and is favored by the application of nasal drops or sprays containing a vasoconstrictant, such as Neosynephrine solution, ¼ per cent, which shrinks the edematous nasal musosa and tends to maintain the patency of the channels of communication between the nasal and the sinus cavities.

Temporal Arteritis. The temporal and the occipital arteries and other branches of the carotid arteries for obscure reasons may become involved in an inflammatory process that eventually leads to thrombosis. However, prior to that event and for many weeks or months thereafter, the patient may experience local pain and tenderness in the region of the affected vessels, and in addition he may suffer from more generalized and severe headaches. Visual disturbances and other manifestations of central nervous system dysfunction may develop, including periodic disorientation or even coma, together with constitutional symptoms, such as fever, malaise and anorexia. Arterial pulsations distal to the involved segments are diminished or absent, depending on the presence or the extent of thrombosis within the vessel.

Treatment of the patient with temporal arteritis includes the administration of a corticosteroid drug, such as prednisone, for its anti-inflammatory effect, and analgesic agents for comfort. Anticoagulant therapy may be prescribed on a chronic basis, pending subsidence of the inflammatory process, i.e., until thrombosis or the extension of existing thrombi no longer threatens.

Headaches of Intracranial Origin

Headaches that appear to be produced by stimuli within the skull include those occurring in response to histamine injection, the postlumbar puncture headache and those that are associated with meningitis, subarachnoid hemorrhage and brain tumor. Hypertensive, febrile and migraine headaches are of mixed origin, arising from the walls of arteries within and outside the cranium.

Histamine Headaches. The headache that almost invariably follows the injection of histamine (e.g., for purposes of gastric analysis) is provoked by the stretching of pain-sensitive tissue around the large intracranial arteries, notably the anterior and the middle cerebral arteries. In response to histamine, these vessels become dilated and pulsate widely, producing severe pain that throbs synchronously with the arterial pulse. Located initially in the region of the temples, the headache soon spreads to the vertex and the occiput, and within a period of 8 to 10 minutes it disappears.

The headache is alleviated or terminated prior to that time by maneuvers that lower the cerebral arterial pressure (e.g., carotid compression) or elevate the spinal fluid pressure (e.g., jugular compression), the effect of which in either instance is to reduce the dilatation of the cerebral arteries and to limit the excursion of their pulsations.

Meningeal Headaches. Headache invariably occurs in association with meningitis, usually appearing as one of its cardinal features and often as the initial, presenting symptom. The typical meningeal headache is a generalized headache, one that is extraordinarily severe. It is accompanied by nuchal rigidity (stiff neck) and is markedly aggravated by the slightest movement of the head. The source of pain is the inflamed meninges, in which pain fibers are stimulated by chemical irritants in the inflammatory exudate. By producing mechanical distortion of the meninges, movement serves to reinforce the chemical stimulus and hence augments the pain. The major significance of this headache is not as a problem of therapy but as a diagnostic clue, one which provides an opportunity to treat early—and therefore successfully — a dangerous infection that otherwise might well prove to be fatal. Pending control of the infection by measures described elsewhere (page 1083), which will terminate the headache, analgesic drugs and opiates are employed as required.

Subarachnoid Hemorrhage. Usually caused by rupture of an arterial aneurysm at the base of the brain, this hemorrhage produces a headache very similar to that of meningitis, i.e., one of intense severity. The headache is located occipitally and invariably is attended by nuchal rigidity. It is uncertain whether the factor principally responsible for this headache is irritation of the meninges or sudden stretching and dissection of the perivascular tissues by the escaping blood. Sedatives and opiates constitute the extent of the armamentarium for its relief.

Great caution must be exercised in prescribing and administering the opium alkaloids to patients with elevated cerebrospinal fluid pressure or brain damage of any type, including patients with meningitis and those with subarachnoid hemorrhage, in view of their susceptibility to respiratory depression.

Headache in Brain Tumor. Headache is the cardinal symptom of brain tumor. Initially, it occurs in brief paroxysms, lasting but a few seconds or a few hours, which are precipitated by activities involving changes in the position of the head. With further growth of the tumor these attacks tend to become increasingly severe and prolonged until the pain is nearly incessant and inordinately severe. (It should be pointed out that in some patients with brain tumor, headaches are mild and infrequent or even altogether nonexistent.) The headaches associated with this disease apparently are attributable to two factors: (1) distension of the basilar arteries, which varies in degree, depending on fluctuations in the intracranial pressure; and (2) displacement of the intracranial septa by the space-occupying lesion, with resultant tension on the pain-sensitive tissues surrounding the dural sinuses. These headaches respond in a variable extent to analgesic drugs, but they are less and less responsive as tumor growth proceeds. Of course, complete and sustained relief hinges on the success with which the neoplastic tissue within the cranium can be extirpated surgically or lysed by irradiation or chemotherapy.

Headaches of Mixed Origin

Hypertensive Headaches. Patients with arterial hypertension commonly experience headaches. These may be very severe, and they may be attended even by nausea and vomiting. The characteristic hypertensive headache is occipital in location, is worse on arising in the morning and tends to disappear within an hour or so after its onset. The pain is thought to emanate from overly stretched arteries both outside the cranium and within, but its precise mechanism is uncertain. The symptom often is relieved by a drink of strong coffee or the ingestion of caffeine, e.g., in the form of caffeine sodium benzoate, 200 to 400 mg. Successful elimination of these headaches depends ultimately on effective control of the arterial pressure by such measures as those described in Chapter 26.

Febrile Headaches. The headache of fever presumably is based on a mechanism similar to that responsible for the histamine headache, namely, relaxation, followed by expansion and wide pulsation of the large intracerebral arteries. In patients with febrile headaches, however, an additional component appears to be operative: stimuli from dilated, pulsatile scalp arteries as well. Their pain is of the throbbing type; and its location is chiefly frontal or occipital, although at peak intensity it may become generalized. Relief usually is achieved promptly and completely with aspirin and similar analgesic medication.

Migraine. Of all the forms of headache that have been described thus far, migraine alone may be regarded as a clinical entity, headache being its presenting complaint, cardinal feature and sole source of disability.

Migraine, popularly called *sick headache,* is a relatively common ailment. It is characterized by headache, which occurs periodically and paroxysmally. Between attacks the sufferer is completely symptom-free. The headache often is preceded by prodromal symptoms or an aura; the pain tends to involve half the head. Frequently, there are associated disturbances—nervous, gastrointestinal or psychic—and, following each attack, there may be temporary depression. Few migraine attacks, however, present all these characteristics.

Migraine attacks may recur with remarkable periodicity or at irregular intervals. Usually, they begin in the early morning hours. In some cases they are preceded hours before by some prodromal symptoms, such as drowsiness, mental and physical hyperactivity; in others, immediately by an aura. The most common aura is a cloudy area (scotoma), usually to one side, in the field of vision. This soon becomes a spot of scintillating light, flashing in zigzag fashion, and after 5 to 20 minutes this fades away, ushering in the headache. The pain, seldom bilateral, may remain local or spread over half the head. It varies from a slight soreness to a pounding, bursting or viselike agony. Always, even though mild, it is strikingly incapacitating. Usually, after a few hours to 1 or 2 days it gradually fades away, but it may stop suddenly—in some patients after an attack of vomiting or of complete unconsciousness. Attacks may follow one another in rapid succession (status hemicranicus).

Among motor disturbances which frequently appear as part of migraine attacks are aphasia, diplopia, ptosis, paresis (usually of the ocular muscles alone, but sometimes of half the face and also occasionally of an arm or a leg) and ataxia. Among sensory features are numbness of an arm, cutaneous hypersensitivity and neuralgia of the head. Among vasomotor features are vascular spasm (which explains white migraine, with paleness, dryness and coldness of the skin over half the face or the entire face) and vascular paralysis (which explains red migraine). Some temporary psychic disturbance would seem to be part of every migraine attack: mental sluggishness, psychic depression, amnesia, marked change of personality, a phobia, hallucinations of sight and of hearing and, on rare occasions, a true psychosis. Severe attacks of migraine may be followed by euphoria, polyuria, exhaustion or drowsiness, which often last several days. Migraine attacks are practically always afebrile.

In addition to the above-described severe attacks, there occur those which are mild, incomplete or abortive. These, however, seem to have the same significance as severe ones. A common type of incomplete attack begins with chilliness followed soon by a scotoma, then by a depressed, apprehensive state of mind, but without pain, and ends by a definite feeling of relief.

The mechanism responsible for the migraine attack, including the characteristic headache, the prodromal symptoms and all associated phenomena, appears to reside in the walls of certain major arteries: specifically, the frontal, the temporal and the occipital arteries in the scalp, and the middle meningeal artery coursing through the membranous dura that lines the interior wall of the cranial vault. The initial phase of the attack coincides with the occurrence of marked and sustained contraction of these vessels. During this period the patient remains free of headache but is experiencing the prodromal phenomena that have been described. Next, the constrictive phase having concluded, these arteries dilate widely; their walls, now abnormally relaxed, are stretched excessively by the pressure of arterial blood within, and headache ensues.

The reason for these arterial changes is obscure. Allergy at one time was thought to be implicated in the pathogenesis of migraine, but no substantial evidence has been found to support this thesis. Emotional stress, often regarded as an important precipitating factor if not the major causative factor in the production of migraine attacks, likewise is of questionable etiologic significance. It remains a debatable question whether emotional disturbances predispose to migraine attacks or merely reflect the neurovascular disturbance that precedes an impending attack.

TREATMENT. Mild migraine may require no special treatment other than a full and frank discussion of the situation with the patient, reassuring him that these attacks are basically harmless and entirely without ominous significance. Mild attacks usually respond to aspirin, supplemented perhaps with caffeine. The more severe attacks require the administration of an ergot preparation. Dihydroergotamine methanesulfonate, 1 mg., or ergotamine tartrate, 0.5 mg., injected intramuscularly or intravenously within a period of 1 hour following the onset of an attack, will abort this attack in 80 to 90 per cent of patients. The oral ingestion of ergotamine tartrate, 2 mg., and caffeine sodium benzoate, 200 mg., at the onset of an attack and again a half hour later, if necessary, (ingesting half of the original doses) likewise terminates the majority of migraine attacks. Ergotamine also is available in forms that both promote rapid absorption and facilitate self-administration of the drug: one, an inhalant (Medihaler-Ergotamine) and the other, a liquid preparation for rectal instillation (Rectalad-Migraine). Recurrences of migraine attacks may be reduced in frequency or prevented altogether by the daily ingestion of the drug methysergide.

THE PATIENT WITH INCREASED INTRACRANIAL PRESSURE

The usual causes of increased intracranial pressure are brain tumor, abscess, hemorrhage, infection or head injury. In the majority of patients having cranial surgery, there are varying degrees of cerebral edema or, rarely, bleeding causing increased intracranial pressure. Therefore, it is important to know the following signs:

1. Headache: constant, increasing in intensity and aggravated by movement or straining

2. Vomiting: may be projectile but not necessarily

3. Changes in the level of consciousness: from an alert state to drowsiness, stupor and finally coma

4. Vital signs. During the development of increased intracranial pressure, the pulse rate slows and then becomes more rapid. The pulse pressure—the difference between the systolic and diastolic pressure—widens; the respiratory rate slows gradually, becoming Cheyne-Stokes in character; the temperature usually rises but does not follow a consistent pattern (Fig. 355).

5. Tense bulging decompression. In most patients part or all of the temporal bone is removed during the craniotomy for the purpose of relieving the postoperative brain edema. This area is located in front of the ear on the side of operation, and its tension is an indication of the degree of intracranial pressure. The nurse should palpate the area periodically and note the degree of tension without contaminating the wound.

The treatment of increased intracranial pressure consists of administering steroids and/or intravenous urea (Urevert) and mannitol. With this therapy, urinary output is recorded hourly; vital signs and level of consciousness are evaluated frequently. Fluid intake is maintained up to 2,500 ml., with special consideration given to the proper electrolyte balance.

FEBRILE AND HYPOTHERMIC PATIENTS

Because of severe intracranial infection or damage to the heat-regulating center in the brain, neurologic and neurosurgical patients often will develop very high temperatures. Such temperature elevations must be controlled, and with the persistent use of proper therapy, there is seldom a patient in

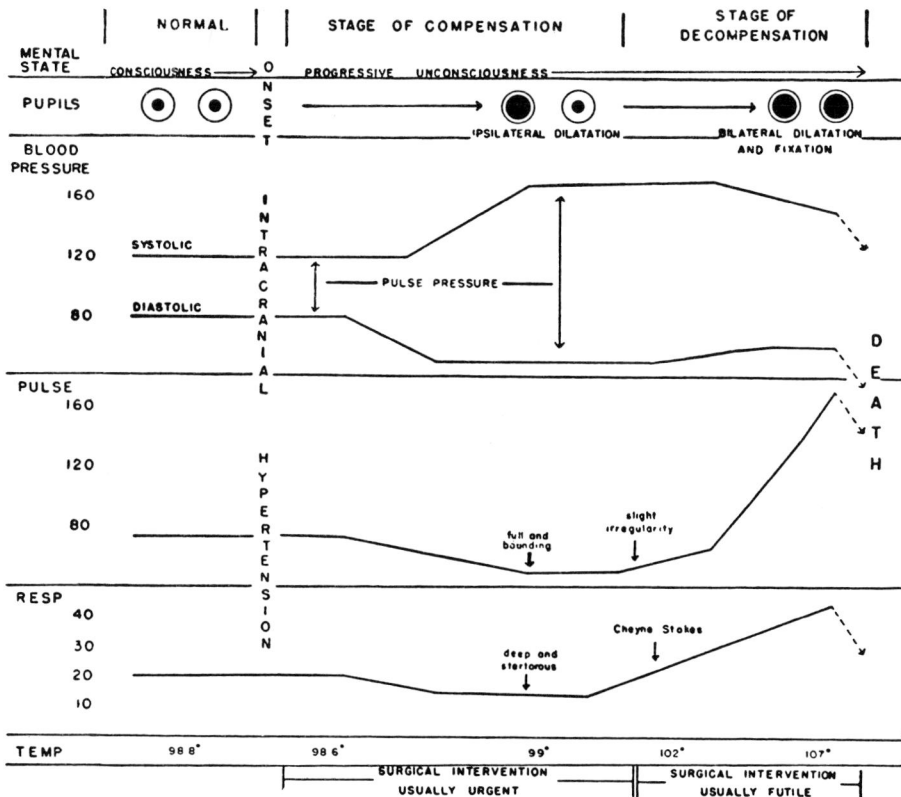

FIG. 355. Chart showing changes in mental state, pupils, blood pressure, pulse rate, respiration rate and temperature before and after the onset of fatal increase of intracranial pressure. (Penfield: Canadian Army Manual of Military Neurosurgery, Ottawa, Government Distribution Office)

whom the temperature cannot be lowered in a matter of 2 or 3 hours. It has been shown that body temperatures well below normal decrease cerebral edema and lower the metabolic rate of the brain. Occasionally, it is desirable to lower the body temperature to a level ranging between 86° and 90° F. The measures in the order of increasing effectiveness are:

1. Aspirin medication and sponging of the trunk and the extremities with alcohol

2. Ice bags applied to groin and axilla

3. Aspirin, alcohol sponging and an electric fan blowing directly on the patient

4. All clothes, except a loin cloth, are removed from the patient. A bath towel saturated with cold water is placed over the trunk. An electric fan, placed at the foot of the bed is directed toward the saturated towel. When the towel becomes almost dry, it is resaturated with cold water. Rectal temperatures should be taken every 15 minutes during this treatment to prevent lowering the temperature too rapidly.

5. The use of a cooling blanket connected to a temperature-regulating apparatus

6. Another method is to suppress the heat-regulating center in the brain by the use of drugs, whether alone or in combination with the above methods. The usual combination is Thorazine, Demerol and Phenergan, commonly called the "lytic cocktail." It is used practically always to reduce temperatures to a below-normal level.

THE UNCONSCIOUS PATIENT

Unconsciousness is a condition in which there is a depression of cerebral function. This may range from stupor to coma. In stupor the patient will show symptoms of annoyance when stimulated by something unpleasant, such as a pinprick, loud clapping of hands, etc., by drawing back, facial grimacing and making unintelligible sounds. In coma there is no response.

Nursing care of this type of patient is more important than the care of a conscious patient. His every need should be attended to, and conversation about him must not take place in his room. Detailed nurses' notes are to be kept, and the physician should be notified of any change in activity, reflex action, vital signs, pupillary variations, etc.

The temperature of his environment will be determined by his condition. If he has a temperature elevation, he should have a sheet or perhaps only a loin cloth covering him. The room may be cooled to 65° F. However, if the patient is older and does not have an elevation of temperature, he needs a warmer atmosphere. Regardless of the temperature, the air should be fresh and free from odors. The body temperature of these patients never is taken by mouth. Rectal temperature is preferred to the less-accurate axillary temperature.

Special attention is given to these patients because they are insensitive to external stimuli. They must be turned frequently and positioned properly (see Fig. 356). To prevent decubiti, attention should be given to those areas where pressure is greatest. Sheets must be free of wrinkles, crumbs and moisture. A lotion with lanolin may be used to keep the skin lubricated.

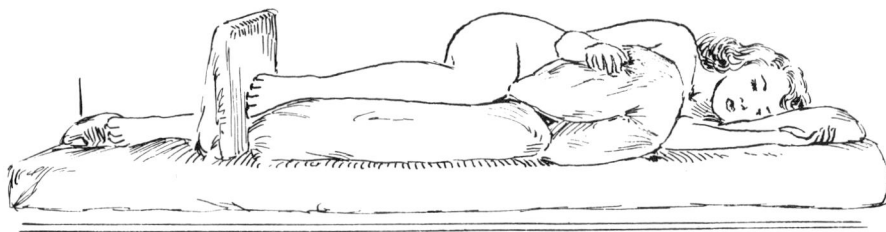

FIG. 356. Posture for nursing an unconscious patient. Note pillows placed at the feet and underneath the upper leg and arm and the head to maintain the patient in correct posture. (Redrawn from Gutiérrez-Mahoney and Carini: Neurological and Neurosurgical Nursing, St. Louis, Mosby)

The mouth of the unconscious patient is an area which also needs conscientious care. The mouth should be swabbed carefully and rinsed thoroughly. The tongue as well as the space underneath must be included. A soothing lubricant within the mouth and on the lips will prevent drying and the formation of encrustations.

Because there are occasions when the corneal reflex is absent, the cornea is likely to become irritated or scratched. It may be necessary to irrigate the eyes with normal saline solution and lubricate them with mineral oil. Often, a patient will have periocular edema following head surgery. Cold compresses may be used, and care must be exerted to avoid contact with the cornea.

If there is ear or nasal bleeding, or oozing of cerebrospinal fluid, the physician should be notified immediately. A small cotton pledget may be placed loosely in the nostril, but no attempt to clean the nose should be made until the physician sees the patient.

The accumulation of secretions in the pharynx presents a serious problem that demands energetic and conscientious treatment. Since the unconscious patient is unable to swallow and lacks pharyngeal reflexes, these secretions must be removed to eliminate the danger of aspiration. Portable electric suction or wall suction with a No. 16 multiholed, soft rubber catheter can be used. Oral and nasal routes both may be tried; by the latter method accumulations deep in the pharynx can be reached more easily. A water-soluble lubricating jelly is the most acceptable lubricant. The force of the suction should not exceed 5 lb./sq. in.; the catheter should be closed while it is being passed through the vestibule of the nose. Gently gliding the catheter back and forth in the hypopharynx is most effective, and occasionally withdrawing the tube completely so that it can be flushed with water will prevent its becoming clogged. The frequency of suctioning is determined by the needs of the patient.

The nutritional needs of this patient are met by giving the required fluids intravenously. Intravenous solutions and blood transfusions for patients with intracranial conditions must run in slowly. If given too rapidly, they may increase the intracranial pressure.

Sixty drops per minute is the average rate of flow. In addition, a nasogastric tube may be passed, and the patient can be given liquid feedings. The procedure is much the same as for gastrostomy feedings (see pp. 608-609). One way of testing to see whether the patient is able to swallow without choking is to give him a swab wet with water to suck. *Never give fluids by mouth to the patient who cannot swallow.*

Urinary incontinence can be taken care of by inserting a retention catheter such as the Foley. This is important if diuretics are used. Clamping the catheter off at intervals will help to prevent contracture of the bladder, as this procedure more closely approximates normal functioning. A full bladder, on the other hand, may be the overlooked cause of incontinence. Colonic irrigations administered every 2nd or 3rd day will eliminate fecal incontinence or reduce the frequency of involuntary stools.

Maintaining good body position is important; equally important is passive exercise of the extremities, so that contractures are prevented. The use of a footboard will aid in the prevention of footdrop and eliminate the pressure of bedding on the toes. Trochanter rolls supporting the hip joints will keep the legs in good position. The arm should be in abduction, the fingers lightly flexed, and the hand in a position of slight supination.

If the patient is restless, side-rails should be provided. If it is possible for him to sustain injury against the side attachments, they should be padded satisfactorily. Every measure that is available and appropriate for the calming and quieting of the disturbed patient should be tested before restraints are applied. Any form of restraint is likely to be countered by rebellion, whether the patient is fully conscious or not, and fury so incited may lead to self-injury or to a dangerous increase in intracranial pressure.

PATIENTS WITH CRANIAL, SPINAL AND PERIPHERAL NEUROPATHIES

First Cranial (Olfactory) Nerve

Disturbances of the olfactory bulbs by intracranial diseases reveal themselves by either loss of smell sensation (anosmia) or alterations in it (perversions).

Anosmia. This follows fractures of the base of the skull which lacerate the olfactory nerves (fine filaments which pass from the bulb to the olfactory mucous membrane through small holes in the cribriform plate of the ethmoid bone). Falls or blows on the back of the head that merely jar the skull by contusing these filaments also may produce temporary anosmia.

Second Cranial (Optic) Nerve

Diseases of and injuries to the optic nerves, whatever their nature, cause reduction in the acuity of vision and contraction of the visual fields, symptoms that may progress to complete blindness.

Choked Disk. Edematous swelling of the head of the optic nerve appears in all conditions that increase the intracranial pressure, such as tumor and abscess of, and acute hemorrhage into, the brain.

Secondary Optic Atrophy. This is the outcome of prolonged severe choking of the disk, neuritis of the optic nerve, closure of its central artery, pressure against it by brain tumors and fractures of the base of the skull that involve the optic foramen (through which the optic nerve leaves the skull). Optic atrophy is an important early sign of multiple sclerosis. It is one of the manifestations of central nervous system syphilis and a product of methanol poisoning.

Third, Fourth and Sixth Cranial (Oculomotor, Trochlear and Abducens) Nerves

The oculomotor nerve supplies all but two of the muscles that move the eyeball. Of these two, one, the superior oblique, is innervated by the 4th cranial (trochlear) nerve; the other, the external rectus muscle, which rotates the eyeball outward, is innervated by the 6th cranial (abducens) nerve. Paralysis of any one of these three nerves produces strabismus (squint), the type of which depends on the muscle paralyzed; but paralysis of the 3rd nerve produces ptosis and dilation of the pupils as well. Such paralyses follow poisoning by alcohol, lead or carbon monoxide; infections, such as those of diphtheria, botulism, measles and encephalitis, but much more often, syphilis and multiple sclerosis, and fractures of the base of the skull and middle ear infections, both most apt to injure the 6th nerve.

Fifth Cranial (Trigeminal) Nerve

The trigeminal nerve supplies all the sensory fibers to the skin of the face (except the angle of the jaw and the anterior half of the scalp), those to the teeth, the conjunctivae, the mucous membranes covering the inside of the mouth, the nose, the paranasal sinuses and the greater part of the tongue. The lowest branch of this nerve also contains the motor fibers which control the muscles of mastication.

One, two or all three branches (the ophthalmic, the maxillary and the mandibular) of this nerve may be affected by diseases and by trauma, and the disturbances that follow always correspond exactly to the areas of distribution of the branch affected. Severe injury to one of these nerves, such as contusions over the supra-orbital notch or the infra-orbital foramen, is followed by anesthesia of the area it supplies; but it is followed by pain if the trauma merely irritates or compresses it. If, however, the trauma causes bleeding into the tissue about the nerve, the scar tissue that forms afterward may so compress its fibers that months later localized pain appears in the forehead or the cheek. This pain may continue indefinitely.

Herpes. The pustular rash and burning neuralgic pains of ocular herpes, one form of herpes zoster, are limited to the area of distribution of the upper branch of one trigeminal nerve and therefore are likely to involve the lid, the conjunctiva and the cornea. The healing of pustules on the cornea may leave it scarred, resulting in impairment of vision. Herpes simplex (cold sores) about the nose and the mouth, also attributed to irritation of the trifacial ganglion, appears in all sorts of acute infections, ranging from common colds to cerebrospinal meningitis.

Symptomatic Trigeminal Neuralgia. This is due both to lesions which directly irritate the trigeminal nerve or its ganglion and to diseases of other organs which refer their pains to its area of distribution. Among such lesions are inflammatory processes and neoplasms in the soft tissues and the bones of the face; paranasal sinus infections; infected teeth; unerupted third molar teeth; tumors and aneurysms about the base of the skull; venous sinus thrombosis; basilar meningitis; tumors of the gasserian ganglion; diseases of the sphenopalatine ganglion, the middle ear and the orbit of the eye; such conditions as eyestrain, migraine and multiple sclerosis; and, occasionally, syphilis, diabetes, nephritis and malaria.

Idiopathic Trigeminal Neuralgia. This is a malady characterized by paroxysms of lancinating or burning pain limited in its radiation to the area of distribution of one, two or all three branches of one trigeminal nerve and separated by periods of complete comfort. Its early attacks, which appear most often during the 5th decade of life, usually are infrequent, mild and brief; but with advancing years they tend to become more and more frequent and agonizing. This, the commonest of all primary neuralgias, is a disease whose cause is unknown. Sclerosis of the vessels and degeneration of the gasserian ganglion may be responsible for a few cases; however, disturbances in the subthalamic vasomotor nuclei now are thought to be more important.

The pain of this neuralgia is felt in the skin, not in the deeper structures, but it is more severe at the periphery of the areas of distribution of the affected nerve, hence, notably over the lip, the chin, the ala nasi and in the teeth. Paroxysms of it are aroused by any stimulation of the terminals of the affected branches, such as washing the face, brushing the hair or the teeth, eating, drinking, a draft of cold air and direct pressure against the nerve trunk. Certain areas are called *trigger points,* since the slightest touch over one of them at once starts a paroxysm. In severe cases of this neuralgia, called *tic douloureux,* the paroxysms are accompanied by quick contractions of some of the facial muscles, such as a sudden closing of the eye or a twitch of the mouth.

TREATMENT. The drug most commonly used in the treatment of trifacial neuralgia is trichlorethylene, administered by inhalation. Injection of the affected nerve branch with alcohol may bring about relief for 6 to 18 months. The operative treatment consists in dividing the nerve paths that carry the painful impulses to the brain. The operation is performed in the sitting position. An opening is made into the skull in the temporal region, and after elevating the dura the nerve is cut as it enters the brain stem. The wound is sutured.

After the operation the patient has a complete loss of sensation in the area supplied by the divided nerves. This "woodeny" feeling may alarm the patient, but the nurse should reassure him. Herpes labialis (fever blister) frequently appears but soon disappears without treatment.

Another operation for trigeminal neuralgia involves sectioning the root of the 5th nerve in the brain stem. This requires a suboccipital approach, similar to that used for tumors of the cerebellum. This operation is termed *tractotomy.* Its advantage lies in the preservation of the sense of touch in the face and the eye.

NURSING CARE. Preoperative care of a patient with trigeminal neuralgia includes a recognition on the part of the nurse that certain factors may aggravate excruciating facial pain. Food which is too hot or too cold may initiate this pain; careless handling, such as jarring a bed, also may precipitate discomfort. Even washing the face, combing the hair or brushing the teeth may produce acute discomfort. The nurse can lessen these discomforts by using cotton pads to wash the face, substituting a blunt-tooth comb to comb the hair, etc.

Among the most serious of the complications that may follow a trigeminal nerve operation is a corneal infection (keratitis). Sensations in and about the eye are mediated by a branch of this nerve. Destruction of the latter renders the cornea insensitive to injury and to the presence of foreign bodies, thus opening the gates to infection. To protect the eye from this danger it should be irrigated three times daily with warm saline solution and sometimes kept covered with an eye shield. The patient later is provided with a special form of protective glasses for a time. He should be instructed to carry a pocket mirror and to inspect his eye for foreign bodies several times a day. He is taught to do his own eye irrigations, using an eye cup. (If sensation of the eye has not been destroyed, these precautions are unnecessary.)

As the patient with trigeminal neuralgia usually is an older individual, every precaution should be taken to prevent pulmonary complications. Turning, deep breathing and early ambulation are the usual preventive measures.

The stay of this patient in the hospital is usually less than a week. His chief adjustment is to become accustomed to the lack of sensation in the area involved and to recognize and to avoid anything that might irritate his face or eyes without his feeling it. A specific point to remember is that he should visit his dentist regularly, since he may not have a toothache in the presence of dental caries.

Seventh Cranial (Facial) Nerve

The facial nerve is the chief motor nerve of the muscles of the face. Its few sensory fibers will be disregarded in this discussion.

Facial Paralysis. There are three types of facial paralysis: the peripheral, the nuclear and the upper motor neuron type. The peripheral type is produced by interruption or dysfunction of the facial nerve due to involvement of its trunk distal to its exit from the skull or within the temporal bone through which it courses. External lesions are usually the result of direct trauma or a suppurative infection of the parotid gland, whereas those occurring within the skull are encountered as complications of mastoiditis, mastoid surgery or fractures of the skull that involve the temporal bone. Peripheral facial neuritis is manifested by complete paralysis of the face on the same side as the lesion. Because of it, the mouth is drawn toward the normal side, whereas on the paralyzed side the wrinkles of the forehead and the nasolabial fold are obliterated, and the eye remains open, its upper lid drooping and its lower lid slightly everted, allowing the tears to escape over the cheek. The patient cannot puff out the cheek, close the mouth or show the teeth on the paralyzed side.

The most common type of peripheral facial paralysis is the so-called Bell's palsy. This has its onset following local chilling of the face and is considered by some physicians to represent a type of pressure palsy, the inflamed, edematous nerve becoming compressed to the point of damage, or its nutrient vessel occluded to the point of producing ischemic necrosis of the nerve within its long canal—a channel in which the fit at best is very snug.

The treatment of peripheral palsies of the facial muscles, including Bell's palsy, is to keep these muscles in as good condition as possible by repeated galvanic stimulation and, eventually, by massage.

The nuclear type of facial palsy is caused by destruction of the nuclei from which the fibers of the 7th nerve originate by luetic, neoplastic, vascular or degenerative lesions in the pons.

In upper motor neuron facial paralysis due to lesions (such as tumors, abscesses, depressed skull fractures, etc.) which injure the motor cortical area governing the face there is paralysis of the muscles of the lower half of the face only (those about the eyes and of the forehead escape), but it is on the side opposite to that of the lesion. Patients with facial palsy of the upper motor neuron type cannot force a smile, no matter how hard they try, but they do smile involuntarily when amused. Their 7th nerve connections to the cortex are severed, but the 7th nerve itself is intact, and the subcortical centers are in sole control.

Eighth Cranial (Auditory-Vestibular) Nerve

Each 8th nerve has two divisions: the auditory (cochlear) and the vestibular portions (the nerve to the semicircular canal system). Disturbances of the auditory nerve impair hearing; disturbances of the vestibular nerve produce vertigo (sensations of turning or falling) and nystagmus.

Ménière's Syndrome. Due usually to infections or hemorrhages that injure the vestibular mechanism, this syndrome is one of sudden brief attacks of buzzing in the ears, vertigo, nystagmus, sweating, vomiting and, occasionally, unconsciousness. Each attack leaves any previous tinnitus and impairment of hearing a little worse than before.

Many patients with Ménière's syndrome respond favorably to conservative measures, such as the use of mild sedation, the administration of ammonium chloride or of potassium salts. For those who fail to respond, a number of surgical procedures are available. Most of the latter involve the sectioning or the avulsion of the 8th nerve, or the destruction of the labyrinth on the affected side, which usually (but not always) halts the vertigo and also, of course, produces complete deafness on the operative side. One operation that does not produce deafness, is far simpler and is reportedly effective from the standpoint of permanent elimination of vertigo entails merely the sectioning of the chorda tympani, either alone or in conjunction with section of the tympani plexus— Jacobson's nerve. If the reputed efficacy of this procedure is confirmed, it will doubtless become the procedure of choice for the treatment of refractory Menière's disease.

Ninth Cranial (Glossopharyngeal) Nerve

Glossopharyngeal Paralysis. This (usually in association with disturbances of the vagus nerve) causes difficulty in swallowing, anesthesia of the upper portion of the pharynx and loss of taste over the posterior one third of the tongue on the same side as the lesion. It most often is due to brain diseases—for example, tumors.

Glossopharyngeal Neuralgia. Due to neuritis of this nerve, this is characterized by severe pain radiating from the base of the tongue to deep in the ear and also by increased salivation. It may be cured by resection of this nerve.

Tenth Cranial (Vagus) Nerve

The vagus nerve is the motor nerve of the voluntary muscles of the throat and the larynx, the one which slows the rate of heartbeat and supplies the parasympathetic nerves to the lungs, the stomach, the esophagus and other abdominal organs.

Neuritis. Neuritis of this nerve occasionally occurs in such acute infectious fever as typhoid, pneumonia, influenza and diphtheria and results from the action of such poisons as alcohol, lead and arsenic. The vagus nerve (usually in association with the glossopharyngeal) frequently becomes injured by lesions of the pons and the base of the skull.

Paralysis. Paralysis of one vagus causes unilateral paralysis of the larynx, with resultant impairment of speech, difficulty in swallowing, temporary changes in the heart rate and rhythm and, occasionally, vomiting, abdominal pain and anorexia. Complete paralysis of both vagi is followed by permanent tachycardia, since the accelerator nerves of the heart (sympathetic fibers) then lack the normal inhibition of the vagi.

The recurrent laryngeal branch of this nerve, because of its position, is injured easily. The result is paralysis of the larynx and, therefore, hoarseness. This may be caused by the pressure of mediastinal tumors, masses of enlarged lymph nodes in the mediastinum or the neck, aneurysms of the aorta or the subclavian artery and malignant growths of the thyroid gland or adjacent structures. This nerve occasionally is cut by wounds and operations on the neck, such as thyroidectomy.

Eleventh Cranial (Spinal Accessory) Nerve

The spinal accessory nerve, entirely motor in nature, supplies the sternomastoid muscle and the upper portion of the trapezius muscles. Injuries to and diseases of this nerve, therefore, weaken the power to rotate the head to the side opposite the lesion and cause a slight drooping of the shoulder on the side of the lesion. Such paralysis may result from penetrating wounds and operations on the neck, fracture of the skull, injuries to and diseases of the cervical vertebrae, rickets, unilateral poliomyelitis and all diseases that involve the upper portion of the cervical cord.

Twelfth Cranial (Hypoglossal) Nerve

The hypoglossal nerves, entirely motor in character, innervate the muscles of the tongue only. It is rarely that one of these nerves is injured, with resultant paralysis of that side of the tongue, by deep penetrating wounds, abscesses and tumors of the neck, and by trauma to and tuberculosis of the 1st cervical vertebra; much more often this paralysis is evidence of brain disease.

The tongue, paralyzed on one side, when protruded, deviates toward the weak side. When both hypoglossal nerves are paralyzed, the tongue cannot be moved; hence, speech, mastication and swallowing cannot be performed properly.

The Brachial Plexus

Paralysis of the brachial plexus and the nerves arising from it occasionally follows violent movements of the shoulder, the head and the arm, which overstretch or even tear the root of this plexus. Erb's palsy of the infant results from dislocation during birth of the humerus, which forcibly pushes the head of the bone against this plexus. The brachial plexus (also its roots) occasionally suffers from the pressure of local tumors, aneurysms and masses of enlarged lymph nodes in the neck or the axilla.

Cervical Ribs. A cervical rib is one or a pair of extra ribs attached usually to the 7th cervical vertebra. If a pair is present, one only may produce symptoms. They are found more frequently in women than in men, occasionally in several members of the same family, and usually in association with other anatomic anomalies.

A cervical rib is a lifelong hazard to the brachial plexus. Because of one, the plexus may be crushed by accidents that suddenly force or pull the shoulder down; this trauma is followed by pain and numbness, felt first in the fingers and gradually extending up the forearm, and later by weakness, followed by atrophy of the muscles of that hand and arm. The continuous pressure of a cervical rib on the brachial plexus (the symptoms of which seldom appear before middle life) affects first its sympathetic nerve fibers, as shown by such vasomotor signs as cyanosis, coldness, paleness and edema (a syndrome that early may suggest Raynaud's disease). Later this pressure causes disturbances of sensation and finally atrophy of the muscles of the arm and the hand.

Since the presence of a cervical rib frequently produces developmental abnormalities in the pattern of the brachial plexus, the findings on physical examinations often are puzzling. Thus, various muscles and skin areas of the arm and the hand seem to be supplied by the wrong nerves; the arteries of the shoulder region may lie in an unusual position or be abnormal in their relative size; and often the pulse volume of the radial artery of that arm is unusually small and the blood pressure low. Cervical ribs are not always visible on x-ray films, since some constitute merely fibrous bands. However, they exert pressures just as serious as those composed of bone.

The Nerves of the Arms

Fleeting Neuralgic Pains. Pains referred to the shoulder and the upper arm are common following exposure to cold, in chronic and often latent general infections, in cases of spondylitis and of chronic subdeltoid bursitis. To this region, particularly on the left side, are referred the pains of aortitis and coronary artery disease (for example, angina pectoris); and to both sides, those of acute pleuritis. More constant pains, with or without accompanying muscular weakness, result from pressure against the roots of the brachial plexus by spinal tumors, a herniated cervical disk and occasionally by the scalenus anticus neck muscles, between which these nerves course. A true toxic neuritis, which affects the radial nerve in particular, is one of the features of lead poisoning.

Radial Nerve Paralysis. This paralysis, causing wristdrop, may be the result of pressure against the trunk of this nerve as it lies in the axilla, as by a crutch, or the back of a bench over which the arm is thrown. It also follows blows against the outer aspect of the upper arm, where this nerve lies in an unprotected position. The same type of paralysis likewise may be caused by a tourniquet applied to the arm too tightly or allowed to remain on for too long a time. Late radial paralysis, appearing in from 3 to 4 weeks following fracture of the humerus, is due to the gradual compression of this nerve by either excessive callus formation or—and more often — by contracting scar tissue formed in tissues infiltrated by blood.

Ulnar Nerve. The ulnar nerve is often traumatized at the elbow, where it lies in an exposed position. "To hit the crazy bone" really is to strike the ulnar nerve. Even the simple act of reclining on the elbow may cause a pressure paralysis of several weeks' duration of the muscles which this nerve supplies. Dislocation of the elbow and fracture of the bones near this joint, by stretching or compressing this nerve, may cause immediate paralysis of the same muscles or weakness due to delayed neuritis.

The Intercostal Nerves

The intercostal nerves may be injured by trauma to the chest wall and fracture of the ribs, causing pain in their areas of distribution. Anesthesia never results if only a single nerve is injured because of the overlapping of the areas supplied by the two adjacent nerves.

Neuritis. Neuritis of the intercostal nerves is often part of a general neuritis; but neuralgic pains referred to but a few nerves occur as symptoms of diseases of the spinal cord, such as tabes dorsalis (the "lightning pains" of this disease occasionally are almost limited to this radiation), thoracic herpes zoster, in which case they may precede as well as accompany the herpetic skin eruption, both precisely limited to the area of distribution of the intercostal nerve; malignant tumors or exostoses of the vertebrae (as in hypertrophic spondylitis); and spinal tuberculosis, all diseases which irritate the roots of these nerves.

The Lumbar Plexus

Tumors of the vertebrae, retroperitoneal neoplasms, enlarged inflamed pelvic lymph nodes and psoas abscesses occasionally press on the lumbar plexus sufficiently to cause weakness or paralysis of the anterior thigh muscles that are supplied by the femoral nerve.

The Sacral Plexus

The sacral plexus may be torn by fractures of the lower lumbar vertebrae and the sacrum, may be pressed on by large fibroid tumors of the uterus and malignant growths within the pelvis, and may be traumatized during difficult labor.

The chief symptom produced is spasmodic or continuous pain, often called *sciatica,* which extends down the back of the leg, even to the ankle. The trunk of the sciatic nerve is subject to all forms of neuritis that affect other nerves, with, if all its fibers are involved, resultant motor and sensory disturbances of the leg.

Sciatica

The term *sciatica* refers to any condition in which the most prominent symptom is pain along the course of the sciatic nerve. Its etiology in the great majority of cases is uncertain. Some patients give a past history of sprain of the lumbosacral or the sacroiliac joints; for other cases, spondylitis, spondylolisthesis or a ruptured intervertebral disk pressing on the cauda equina may be responsible. In some instances primary neuritis is assumed. It is believed that the usual cause of sciatica is mechanical compression or irritation of the 5th lumbar spinal root, the one from which it receives the majority of its fibers. This root not only is the largest trunk that enters into the formation of the sacral plexus, but also it emerges from the spine through the smallest of the foramina accommodating these roots. Therefore, it easily would be compressed by the slightest amount of edema or exudate that might result from minor traumata, such as strains, contusions or arthritis of the lower lumbar spine.

Peripheral Neuropathies

Neuritis. This is the term applied to both demonstrable inflammatory or degenerative changes in peripheral nerves and (less scientifically) to symptoms that suggest these changes. Although, of the latter, pain is often a prominent feature, and such distress may correctly be called *neuralgic,* yet the use of the term *neuralgia,* usually applied to pains referred over normal sensory nerves to normal regions of the body, implies ignorance of their cause.

Neuritis may involve one nerve only (mononeuritis), or many, this condition being called *polyneuritis* or *multiple neuritis.* In all cases of the latter, the same nerves on the two sides of the body are involved similarly. The symptoms of all types of neuritis, according to the character of the nerves involved, are sensory, motor and vasomotor, these always being limited to the structures that the affected nerves supply. Mononeuritis and polyneuritis, however, differ much in their etiology, course and treatment.

Neuritis of a sensory nerve causes pain and disturbances of sensation, provided that the nerve is able to function in some degree, therefore, in mild cases and in severer ones during the stages of development and healing of the neuritis. Anesthesia occurs if the process is severe. In the case of nerves partly or wholly motor, the result of neuritis is either weakness or complete paralysis of the muscles that they control; which it is will depend on the severity.

Mononeuritis. This is neuritis limited to a single peripheral nerve and its branches. It arises when the trunk of the nerve is traumatized, as when it is bruised by a blow; overstretched, as in cases of dislocation of a joint; pressed upon, as by a tumor, a cervical rib, bony exostoses (for example, in that type of arthritis that narrows the apertures between adjacent vertebrae through which the spinal nerves pass) or the use of a crutch; punctured by the needle used to inject a drug or poisoned by the drugs thus injected; or inflamed because of the extension to its trunk of an adjacent infectious process.

One type of mononeuritis appears many months after injuries that caused considerable bleeding into the tissues surrounding a nerve. In tissues thus infiltrated with blood, considerable scar tissue forms, and this, contracting, slowly compresses the nerve. Similarly, delayed nerve paralyses follow the healing of an abscess, the encapsulation of a foreign body or sequestra of bone and the knitting of fractured bone. In this last case, however, the nerve trunk is caught in the callus.

Seldom is pain a conspicuous symptom of mononeuritis due to trauma; but in patients with complicating inflammatory conditions, such as arthritis, this feature is prominent. Such pain is increased by all body movements that tend to stretch, strain or cause pressure on the injured nerve, and by all sudden jars of the body, such as those incident to coughing and sneezing. The skin in the areas supplied by nerves that are injured or diseased may become reddened and glossy; its subcutaneous tissue may become edematous, and the nutrition of the nails and the hair in this area, defective. Chemical injuries to a nerve trunk, as by drugs injected into or near it, often are permanent.

TREATMENT. The treatment of mononeuritis, if possible, is to remove the cause, such as by freeing the enmeshed nerve. The pain may be relieved by aspirin or codeine, and the function of the muscles may be maintained by weak galvanic currents.

Causalgia. This is the term applied to a painful posttraumatic condition which be- gins weeks or months after injury to a nerve trunk. This condition resembles both neuralgia and neuritis, but in fact it is neither. The nerves most often affected, and in order of frequency, are the median, the ulnar, the radial and the internal and the external popliteals.

The chief symptom of causalgia is severe burning pain along the course of the traumatized nerve. This is more or less persistent, but becomes severe following such physical stimuli as the contact of clothes. The skin over the affected limb becomes hot, shiny and, at times, swollen; it shows abnormalities in sweating and, eventually, atrophic changes involving also the nails. The patient holds the limb quiet, since each movement tends to increase the pain.

Polyneuritis. This is a disease which involves many nerves, those of the legs and the arms in particular, but always the same nerves on both sides of the body. Although the symptoms of this disease suggest that the terminal branches of the affected nerves alone are involved, yet multiple peripheral neuritis involves nervous pathways as wholes, that is, terminal branches, trunks, related fibers in the spinal cord and possibly in the brain.

CAUSES. The causes of polyneuritis include poisons and toxins circulating in the blood stream and a dietary deficiency involving the B complex, notably thiamine. Among exogenous poisons important in the causation of this disease are methyl alcohol, lead, bismuth, mercury, arsenic, sulfonamides, carbon disulfide, aniline and other coal-tar products, emetine, apiol, thallium and several less common drugs and poisons. "Jake paralysis" was the popular name of a severe type of peripheral neuritis due to tricresol phosphate, a common constituent of many varnishes and lacquers at one time used in the manufacture of cheap ginger. The paralysis which follows even small doses of this chemical is serious and usually lasts a long time. Peripheral neuritis may occur in the course of various infectious diseases, particularly diphtheria, typhoid fever and lues.

A deficiency of thiamine causes disturbances in the metabolism of nerve tissue, as a result of which this tissue is unable to utilize carbohydrates normally. This inability gives rise to symptoms of muscle pains, tenderness and weakness after use, which clear up rapidly after the oral administration of thiamine.

Anatomic polyneuritis, much slower to heal, which involves reflex changes, skin hyperesthesias, or hypesthesias, motor weakness or diminution or loss of the deep-tendon reflexes, probably is due to deficiencies involving other components of the water-soluble vitamin group. This accounts for the polyneuritis formerly called *alcoholic neuritis,* since it was supposedly due to the direct action of ethyl alcohol on the nerves. The deficient diet of habitual drinkers now is considered to be altogether responsible. Similar are the polyneuritides of beriberi, diabetes, pregnancy and malnutrition (particularly if there is a preponderance of carbohydrate in the diet).

Although in cases of multiple neuritis all the peripheral nerves have an equal opportunity to become affected, yet each poison and toxin attacks certain nerves in particular. Thus, botulinus toxin injures the nerves to the muscles of the eyes and the throat, and lead poisoning, those to the muscles of the hands and the feet.

SYMPTOMS. Polyneuritis, whatever its cause, when well-developed presents a fairly uniform clinical picture. The symptoms may be sensory only, but they are never exclusively motor; sensory changes always accompany any muscular weakness or paralysis that appears. The terminal structures of the extremities (that is, the hands and the feet) are most affected. Sensations of numbness, hyperesthesia and diminution of heat perception and cold perception appear early and may last for weeks. Sometimes there is a slight fever.

The initial symptoms are followed by anesthesia of the fingers and the toes, which gradually extends toward the trunk. Associated with this is marked tenderness of the affected nerve trunks and of the skin overlying their branches. Pain is a marked early feature in some patients. There is more or less loss of the deep sensations; hence the pseudotabetic (ataxic) gait occasionally present, observed particularly in the cases complicating diabetes mellitus and chronic alcoholism.

Muscular weakness then follows, either suddenly or over a period of days. Since the fibers to the extensor muscles of the feet and the hands are more susceptible to the effects of toxins than are those to the flexor muscles, the first motor symptom to appear is an ankledrop or a wristdrop; but after a week or two, paralysis of the entire limb may become complete. Convulsions may occur—they frequently are noted in children—for, as stated above, the pathology is not limited solely to the peripheral nerves.

In the majority of patients the symptoms of polyneuritis are superimposed on those of the more primary disease (diphtheria, for example); but in a few patients they so overshadow all others that it is difficult to determine the cause.

TREATMENT. The treatment of polyneuritis is first to treat the cause—for example, to eliminate all exposure to lead, to supply thiamine in the diet and by parenteral injection, and to treat any infection present. In all cases the patient should rest in bed and receive general supportive treatments. Since the nerves will require months to recover, during which time the muscles they control may become so weak and atrophied as to become permanently useless, the latter should be kept in good condition by daily massage, passive movements, oil rubs or galvanic stimulation, so that later, when the nerves heal, they also will be well. Often splints are indicated to prevent footdrop and wristdrop.

The pain of polyneuritis may be relieved by painting the limbs with menthol and then wrapping them in cotton batting or by hot fomentations. Analgesic drugs often are necessary.

THE PATIENT WITH A CEREBRAL VASCULAR ACCIDENT

Cerebral Hemorrhage, Thrombosis and Embolism (Stroke, Apoplexy)

Cerebral Hemorrhage. Brain hemorrhage, or the rupture of a cerebral artery with the escape of varying amounts of blood into the surrounding brain tissues, which it destroys, is one of the most common of cerebral accidents. It may occur at any age, but it usually occurs after the 40th year of life, and in men more frequently than in women.

Apoplexy is always the result of some disease of a cerebral artery (such as sclerosis, a congenital defect or an acute infection of the intima) which has so weakened its walls at one point that finally it cannot withstand the pressure of the circulating blood. The rupture most often occurs in the middle cerebral artery, and especially in a certain branch of this artery.

A stroke due to hemorrhage (Fig. 344) may come on without warning, although usually the patient remembers later that he did have certain premonitory symptoms: numbness of one side of the body, dizziness, thickening of the tongue (disturbance of speech), anxiety or disturbed vision. With the hemorrhage there usually is sudden and total loss of consciousness, with complete flaccidity of the arms and the legs, loss of the pupillary reactions, anesthesia of the cornea and, sometimes, incontinence of urine. In other patients the loss of consciousness is more gradual, while in still others, the paralysis develops without loss of consciousness.

During the stage of coma the respirations are slow, deep and snoring, or Cheyne-Stokes in character; the cheeks, particularly on the paralyzed side, are blown out at each expiration. One side usually is completely paralyzed (hemiplegia), but this during coma can be recognized only by raising the arms and letting both fall together: the paralyzed arm will fall more limply. At the onset there may be a convulsion; the eyes often are turned to one side—to the side of the brain in which the pathology occurs. (The patient "looks at his lesion.") In a few hours the fever begins. The patient gradually regains consciousness, and then the hemiplegia becomes more apparent.

The paralysis affects the side opposite the trouble. Usually, it is at first a complete hemiplegia, involving one half of the face and the tongue, and the arm and the leg of the same side. The muscles of the thoracic and the abdominal walls escape, since they are supplied by nerves from both sides of the brain. When the paralysis is of the right side, aphasia also usually is present.

When one scratches the sole of the foot forcibly with a sharp metal instrument, starting at the heel and running the scratcher with one sweep along the outer side of the sole to the ball of the foot and then across to the base of the big toe, this toe, if the person is normal, will flex strongly downward toward the sole of the foot. However, if this toe should extend forcibly upward toward the dorsum of the foot, Babinski's test is said to be positive, and this reaction indicates some disturbance within the pyramidal tract. If one draws the back of the thumbnail forcibly down the shin bone, the big toe will behave much as when the sole of the foot is scratched, and its movement will have the same significance (Oppenheim's test).

The paralysis is usually much more complete at first than it is later, since many of the pyramidal fibers are injured only temporarily (by edema pressure) and later recover their function. For the same reason, a paralysis may disappear entirely if the hemorrhage was not in the internal capsule or if the disturbance was only temporary and not due to an actual rupture of a vessel in that location.

The preceding paragraphs have described chiefly the results of the destruction of the motor area of the cortex or its fibers in the pyramidal tract; but, of course, there are other cortical areas, the lesions of which will give just as definite localizing symptoms, such as cortical blindness, involving one half of each field of vision; cortical deafness; abnormalities in smell; inability to distinguish the form of objects; or inability to understand written words. All of these "speaking" areas collectively, however, comprise but a small part of the cortex. The rest of the cortex is called *silent,* although changes in personality have been known to follow lesions of the frontal lobes.

Cerebral Thrombosis and Embolism. Cerebral hypoxia, followed in severe cases by infarction of brain tissue, occurs if the arterial blood supply is cut off by an intravascular clot or embolus, and the cerebral dysfunctions that follow such an occlusion generally are permanent.

THROMBOSIS OF A CEREBRAL ARTERY. This usually is the result of arteriosclerosis. Closure by thrombosis of a small vessel may occur without loss of consciousness, merely with a period of transitory mental confusion, headache or vertigo. Occlusion of a larger vessel often is followed by a convulsion, accompanied by vomiting, prostration, delirium and, occasionally, coma; but this last state is seldom as profound as in cases of cerebral hemorrhage.

CEREBRAL EMBOLISM. The emboli that plug cerebral arteries usually have their origin in vegetations on the endocardium of the left side of the heart, most commonly on the edges of the flaps of the mitral valve. Occasionally, they occur from similar vegetations on the inner wall of the aorta or one of the pulmonary vessels, the pulmonary site being characteristic of patients with chronic sepsis of the lungs.

Cerebral embolism occurs most frequently in young adults with bacteremia arising from an endocarditis. The symptoms of cerebral embolism, as far as the brain is concerned, are identical with those of cerebral thrombosis, except that in the former they begin more suddenly and progress more rapidly. A final differential diagnosis can be made only by finding the source of the embolus.

Carotid Artery Thrombosis

Partial or complete occlusion of an internal carotid artery (Fig. 357) is responsible for one of the well-recognized neurologic syndromes. The usual cause of occlusion is atherosclerosis; it has also been described as a complication of thromboangiitis obliterans (Buerger's disease).

The syndrome is featured by a history of transient, sometimes recurrent signs of cerebral dysfunction, such as numbness or weakness of the face, the arm or the leg, and aphasia. If a portion of the basilar artery is similarly involved, there may be additional symptoms of mental confusion, blindness or unconsciousness.

Confirmation of the diagnosis may be obtained by ophthalmoscopic observation of the retinal arteries on the affected side. If these vessels are now distributing blood from the carotid artery on the opposite side, they usually will show visible narrowing on digital compression of that artery. Diagnostic proof is obtained by x-ray visualization of the carotid artery following the injection of Diodrast into the external carotid on that side.

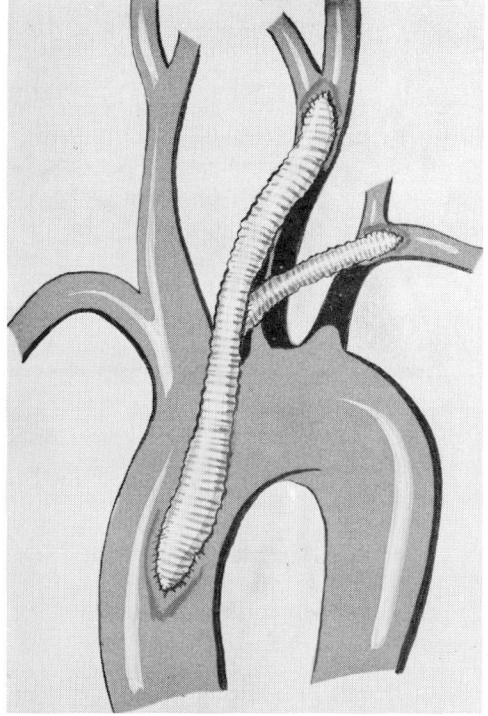

FIG. 357. The use of shunt in the treatment of vascular block of the carotid, used in some types of "strokes."

Carotid Artery Ligation. The treatment of intracranial aneurysms and arteriovenous fistulae often is accomplished by ligation of the common and/or the internal carotid artery in the neck. The purpose is to reduce the pressure in the aneurysm or the fistula and thereby to prevent further rupture. The complications that may follow this procedure are due to a reduction in blood supply to the cerebral hemisphere on the sides of the ligation, with resulting hemiplegia on the opposite side of the body, and if it is the dominant hemisphere (the left in a right-handed individual and the right in a left-handed patient), aphasia or loss of speech; or thrombosis beginning at the side of the ligation and ascending into the vessels of the brain, producing the same neurologic picture.

The operation is done under local anesthesia, and the strength of the opposite side of the body is tested frequently after tempo-

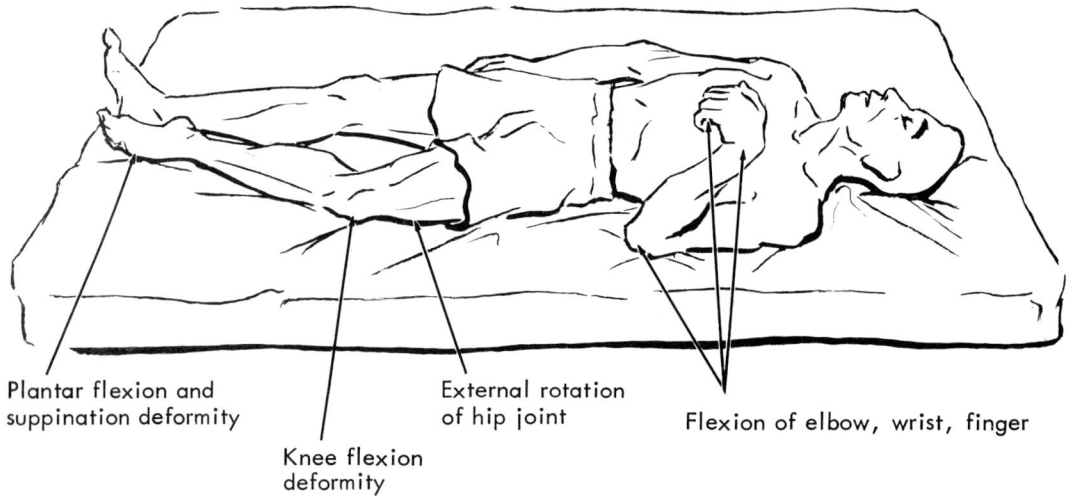

Plantar flexion and
suppination deformity

Knee flexion
deformity

External rotation
of hip joint

Flexion of elbow, wrist, finger

Fig. 358. Hemiplegic deformities. The involved leg immediately falls into external rotation. The knee almost invariably flexes. As soon as knee flexion occurs, abduction of the upper leg follows. The foot falls into plantar flexion, so there is always a footdrop and a shortening of the Achilles tendon. This position of the leg is assumed whether the leg is flaccid or spastic.

The arm on the affected side is held against the body. Often, a flail arm is placed across the body for convenience in handling the patient, but if spastic, the elbow flexes to about 90°. With the arm across the body, the wrist is dropped. If the arm is spastic, the fingers curl into a fist, with the thumb adducted and flexed under the fingers. (Covalt, N. K.: Preventive technics of rehabilitation for hemiplegic patients, G.P. **17:**131)

rary occlusion of the artery for a 15-minute period. If no sign appears, the artery is ligated. Even with this precaution, signs may develop within the next 24 to 72 hours or in a week. The nurse should evaluate the patient frequently for the development of weakness of the opposite side of the body and difficulty with speech where indicated, especially during the first 2 days. Any changes, no matter how small, should be reported to the physician immediately, for it may be necessary to remove the ligature, begin anticoagulant therapy and/or perform stellate ganglion blocks.

The Patient With Hemiplegia

Nursing During the Acute Phase. Skillful nursing is required during the period that the patient is unconscious. One of the primary nursing objectives is the maintenance of the airway. The patient should be placed in a lateral or semiprone position with the bed flat. If stertorous respirations are present, an artificial airway should be inserted. The

negative pressure produced by the stertorous respirations will cause an increased amount of secretions.

If oropharyngeal suctioning is indicated, the nurse should lubricate the catheter with water, "pinch it off," and then pass the catheter through the nose to the epiglottis. This will initiate the cough reflex and serve to make the suctioning procedure more efficient. Repeated irritation to the mucous membrane by suctioning produces an increase of secretions, which is the direct opposite of its purpose. Oxygenation should be provided if there is any indication of a decreased blood flow, insufficient pulmonary ventilation, or impending heart failure.

A rectal temperature should be taken frequently, as a patient with cerebral hemorrhage may readily develop hyperthermia. The temperature of the skin may not necessarily reflect the degree of body heat. If the hypothalamus has lost control, the skin may be cold while the thermometer records a high temperature. To reduce this type of central nervous system fever, warm sponges are administered to "bring the blood to the surface." When this is accomplished, cool sponges are given to promote superficial cooling. The nursing management of hyperthermia is discussed on pages 921 to 922.

Nursing observations are of the utmost importance in diagnosis, and therefore they should be recorded in detail. The following observations are especially significant:

1. A change in the level of consciousness as evidenced by movement, resistance to changes of position, and response to stimulation

2. Presence or absence of voluntary or involuntary movements of the extremities; the tone of the muscles; the body posture and the position of the head

3. Stiffness or flaccidity of the neck

4. The equality and the size of the pupils and pupillary reactions to light

5. The color of the face and the extremities; the temperature and the moisture of the skin

6. The quality and the rates of pulse and respiration; the body temperature and the arterial pressure

7. The volume of fluids ingested or administered, and the volume of urine excreted each 24 hours

While the patient is unconscious, an indwelling catheter is used. The problem of incontinence is resolved by initiating a program that simulates normal bladder functioning as soon as the patient shows that he is aware of his environment. The program should include offering the patient the urinal or bedpan at scheduled short intervals and increasing the time intervals as more control is gained.

When the patient begins to regain consciousness, he will be confused due to the nature of his illness and the change in his environment. If his right side is affected, there probably will be some degree of aphasia present. The patient should be informed that he has "trouble" with his speech, will be taught to communicate, and reassured that he has not lost his mind. (See p. 898.)

Rehabilitation Phase. The patient with hemiplegia has a unilateral paralysis and requires intensive rehabilitation nursing.

When control of the voluntary muscles is lost, the strong flexor muscles will exert control over the extensors. The arm will tend to adduct (adductor muscles are stronger than abductors) and to rotate internally. The elbow and the wrist will tend to flex. The affected leg will tend to rotate externally at the hip joint, flex at the knee, and plantar flex and supinate at the ankle joint (Fig. 358).

Positioning. Correct positioning in bed is of prime importance. By the use of proper positioning the nurse can help to prevent contractures, relieve pressure, and assist in maintaining good body alignment. A bed board under the mattress will give the body firm support. The patient should remain flat in bed except when he is engaged in his activities of daily living. Maintaining the upright position in bed for extended periods of time is one of the greatest contributors to hip flexion deformity. A footboard is used to keep the feet at right angles to the legs when the patient is in a supine (dorsal) position (Fig. 359 A). This prevents footdrop and heel cord shortening, caused by contracture of the gastrocnemius muscle. The footboard also will prevent the weight of the bed linen from pushing the feet into plantar flexion.

Because flexor muscles are stronger than extensor muscles, it may be necessary to apply a posterior splint at night to prevent flexion of the affected extremity. If such a splint is not available, it can be made by applying a cast to the affected extremity and bivalving it. The posterior portion is padded. The heel portion should be well padded with foam rubber or lamb's wool. The leg is positioned in it and wrapped with an Ace or muslin bandage to keep it in an extended position. The posterior splint is used only at night to maintain correct positioning while the patient is sleeping.

To prevent external rotation at the hip joint, a trochanter roll (Fig. 106, p. 359) is used. The trochanter roll should extend from the crest of the ilium to the midthigh, as the hip joint lies between these two points. Sandbags applied laterally to the leg do not prevent external rotation. This motion originates in the ball and the socket joint of the hip. The knee has no such rotating func-

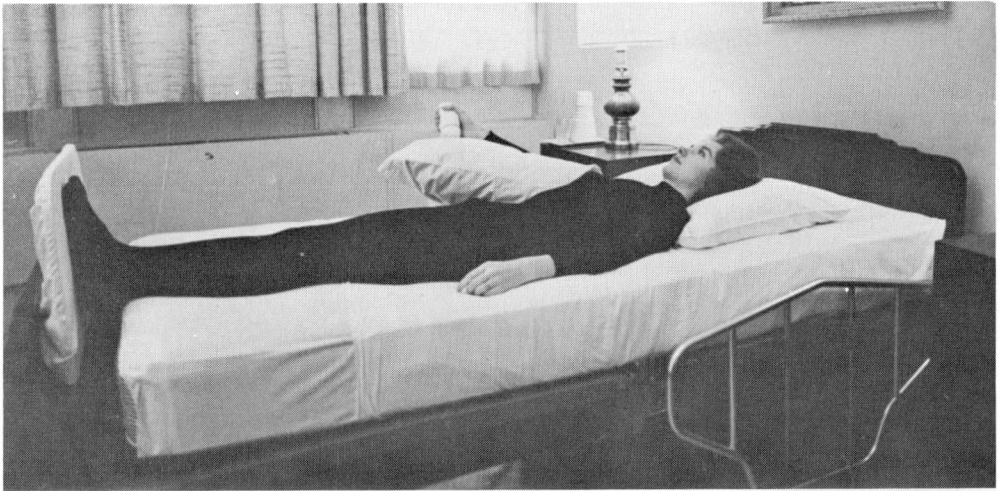

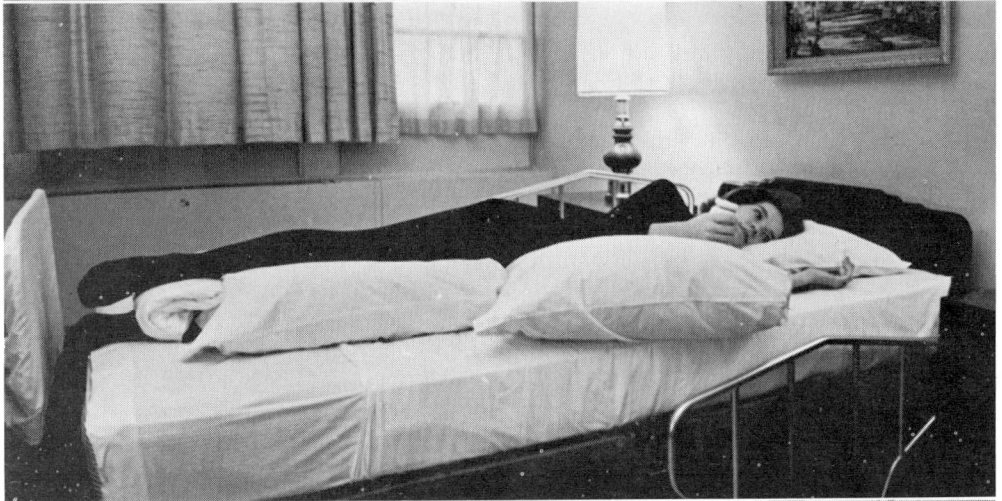

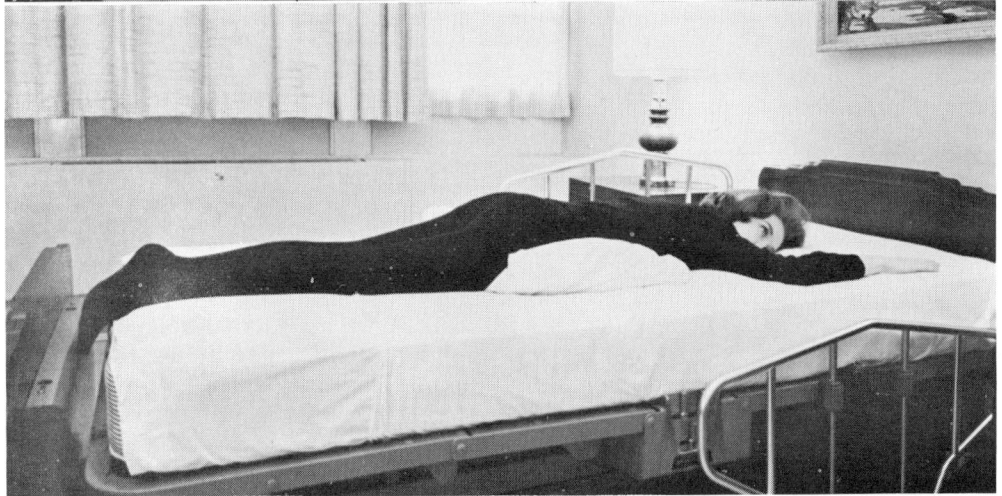

FIG. 359. (*Top*) Dorsal supine position. Note that the heels are suspended in the interspace between the mattress and the footboard. (*Center*) Lateral or side-lying position. (*Bottom*) Prone position.

FIG. 359 (*Continued*). (*Right*) Assisting the patient to a standing position. First, the nurse makes sure that the patient's hands are firmly secured to the back of a chair to prevent slipping when the body weight is supported on them. (*Bottom, left*) Note the nurse stabilizing the patient's knee. (*Bottom, right*) Standing position.

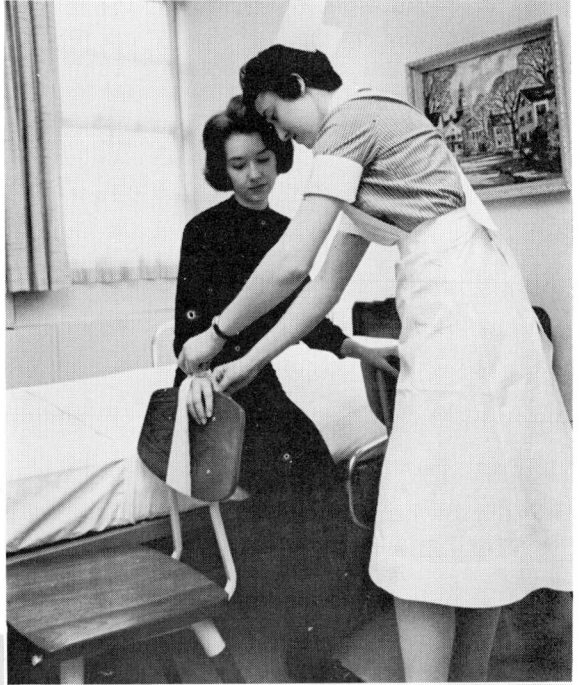

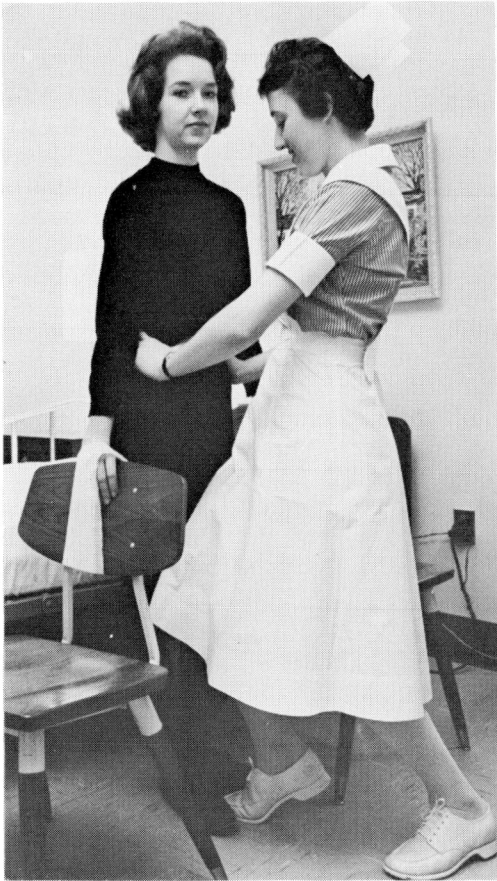

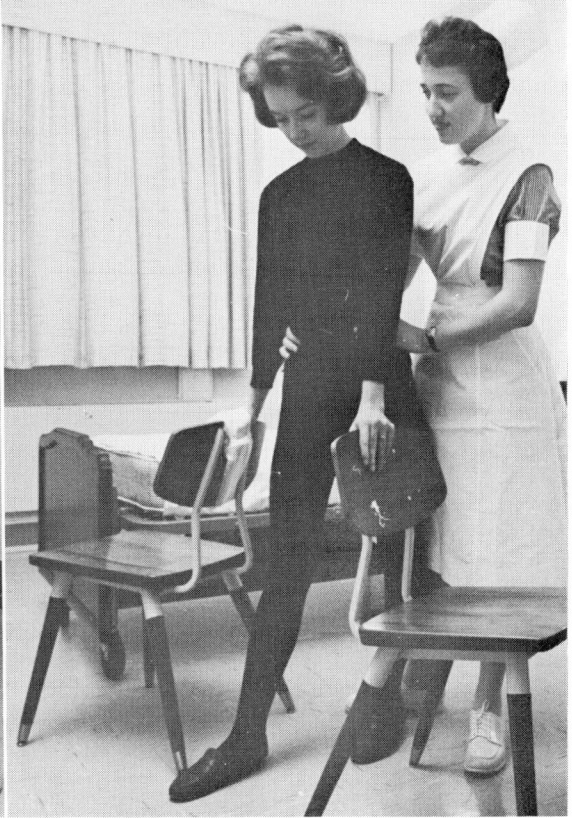

tion. The trochanter roll acts as a mechanical wedge under the projection of the greater trochanter and prevents the femur from rolling.

To prevent adduction of the affected shoulder, a pillow is placed in the axilla. This keeps the arm away from the chest. A pillow is placed under the arm, and the arm is placed in a neutral (slightly flexed) position, with each joint positioned higher than the preceding one. Thus the elbow is higher than the shoulder, and the wrist is higher than the elbow. The elevation of the arm helps to prevent edema and the resultant fibrosis that will prevent future use if control returns. The fingers are positioned so that they are barely flexed. A small hand roll will help to maintain this position and keep the thumb away from the hand in the position of opposition. The hand is placed in slight supination, which is its most functional (i.e., useful) position.

The patient's position should be changed every 2 hours. To place a patient in a lateral (side-lying) position, put a pillow between his legs before turning him. The patient should be turned on his unaffected side. His upper thigh should not be acutely flexed (Fig. 359 B).

It is desirable to assist the patient to a prone position for 15 minutes to a half hour several times a day. Place a small pillow or a support under the pelvis and extend it from the level of the umbilicus to the upper third of the thigh (Fig. 359 C). This helps to promote hyperextension of the hip joints, which is essential for normal gait.

Exercise. The affected extremities are exercised passively and put through a full range of motion 4 to 5 times a day. Frequent short periods of exercise always are preferred to longer periods at infrequent intervals. The patient is encouraged and reminded to exercise his unaffected side at intervals throughout the day. It is well to work out a written time schedule that can be used to remind the patient of his exercise activities. The nurse has the responsibility of supervising and supporting the patient during these activities. The patient can be taught to put his unaffected leg under his affected one to move it when he is turning

and exercising. Bed exercises prepare the patient for ambulation and give the patient a goal. Quadriceps muscle setting and gluteal setting exercises are started early to improve the muscle strength needed for walking. These are done at least 5 times daily for 10 minutes at a time.

QUADRICEPS SETTING. Instruct the patient to contract the quadriceps muscle (on the anterior portion of the thigh) while he raises the heel and attempts to push the popliteal space against the mattress. Hold the muscle contracture until the count of 5. Then relax until the count of 5. Repeat. This exercise is performed by each extremity.

GLUTEAL SETTING. Contract or "pinch" the buttocks together until the count of 5. Then relax until the count of 5. Repeat.

GETTING OUT OF BED. A patient who is hemiplegic from a thrombosis usually is started on an active rehabilitation program as soon as he regains consciousness, whereas a patient who has had a cerebral hemorrhage cannot participate actively until cessation of all evidences of bleeding. If this means waiting a number of weeks or months, as it may, all precautions should be taken to ensure function when the patient is permitted to start activities.

As soon as the physician permits, the patient may be out of bed. A patient with this condition tends to lose his sense of balance rapidly. He will need to learn to balance himself in the sitting position before he can be expected to balance in the standing position. The bed should be in a low position, so that his feet can rest on the floor. (Place a chair under his feet if an adjustable bed is not available.) Extend the patient's unaffected arm with his hand flat on the bed behind him to assist in balancing him. The nurse stands in front of the patient to observe and, if necessary, to help him to maintain this posture. A change in color, shortness of breath, increasing pulse rate or profuse perspiration is an indication that he should be placed flat in bed again. The sitting time is increased as rapidly as the patient's condition permits.

STANDING BALANCE. As soon as he is able to balance while sitting, he is taught standing balance. He should wear walking shoes with a strong shank for all ambulation activities. Seat the patient on the edge of the bed, and place a straight-back chair on each side of him (Fig. 359 D). If the patient lacks strength to grasp and to push the chair with his affected hand, the hand can be tied to the top of the chair. This stabilization gives the patient greater support. The nurse may help the patient to come to a standing position by grasping him around the waist and supporting his affected knee with the side of her knee. This support will prevent the patient's affected knee from buckling (Fig. 359 E). The patient should be reminded to lean forward when he comes from a sitting to a standing position. The patient's arms must be left free for balance and support. The nurse stands behind the patient and stabilizes him at his waist (Fig. 359 F). It is well to put a waistband or a belt (a scultetus binder can serve as a waistband) around the patient's waist, so that the nurse can grasp it for patient support. Dizziness, pallor and an increasing pulse rate indicate that the patient should be permitted to rest in a sitting position, and if the symptoms continue, the patient should be put back in bed. With repeated effort the patient will tolerate this activity for longer periods.

SUPPORTS AND SPECIAL EXERCISES. If the patient has a weakened or absent quadriceps muscle, support for the knee joint with a posterior knee splint may be advisable. Reflex contractures of the muscles of stance are brought into play by putting on a posterior knee brace and standing the patient. Splinting of the extremity and early standing accomplish the following: (1) they keep muscles in good tonus through reflex action, (2) they give the patient a better command of balance, and (3) they prevent loss of position sense. After a period of time has elapsed, the physician will determine if the patient will need to be fitted with a short or a long leg brace. As the patient gains in strength, he can begin to walk alone, using an adjustable aluminum cane. In the beginning a three- or four-prong cane will provide the patient with a more stable support.

If the patient's arm is paralyzed completely, subluxation (incomplete dislocation) can occur. The weight of the paralyzed arm causes the incomplete dislocation at the shoulder. A sling (Fig. 360) will prevent subluxation when the patient is ambulating and a pillow support or an arm chair will aid its prevention when he is seated. Another painful and difficult condition to reverse is frozen shoulder, which comes as a result of lack of motion. The sling must be taken off at intervals to permit the patient to exercise. He may exercise his affected arm by raising and lowering it with his unaffected one. A clothesline may be strung through a pulley attached to a door jamb (or over a shower rod) and tied on the affected hand. The patient pulls the rope up and down with his unaffected hand and so exercises his own affected arm and shoulder. The combination of sling support and range-of-motion exercises will prevent the painful frozen, subluxated shoulder. By changing the position of the chair, other shoulder motions can be achieved. When the patient is seated, the arm should not remain limply in his lap but should be elevated on a support. The patient is instructed to flex his affected

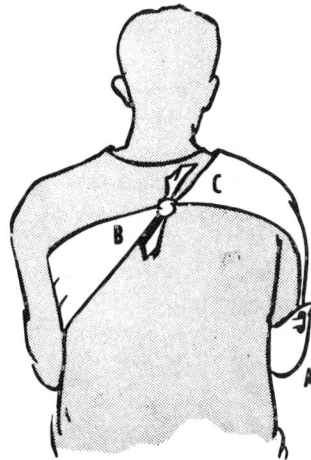

FIG. 360. Sling support to prevent subluxation of the shoulder. The sling should support the wrist and the hand; there should be no pull at the shoulder. (Strike Back at Stroke, Publication No. 596, p. 33, Public Health Service, Washington, D. C., U. S. Dept. Health, Education and Welfare)

wrist at frequent intervals and to move all the joints of his affected fingers.

The patient is taught to assist in his personal hygiene as soon as he is able to sit up. Emphasis is placed on using the unaffected extremity, as many grooming activities can be done with one hand. He should be encouraged to brush his teeth, comb his hair, and bathe and feed himself. The unaffected side is thereby strengthened with use.

Dressing Activities. The morale of the patient will improve if he can do his ambulatory activities while he is fully dressed. The family is instructed to bring in clothing that is preferably a size larger than that normally worn. Clothing fitted with front fasteners is the most suitable. The patient has better balance if he does most of his dressing activities while he is seated. In the early stages the patient will need to be helped or supported by the nurse. He should not be permitted to become overfatigued and discouraged.

The following procedure for dressing has been found to be workable for many patients. However, the nurse must use judgment in assisting the patient to work out individual modifications.

UNDERCLOTHING. Use a flare leg or boxer-type shorts with an elastic waistband. With the unaffected hand bring the affected ankle to rest on the top of the unaffected knee. Place the unaffected hand through the outside opening of the shorts. With the hand through the shorts, grasp the affected foot firmly and shake the garment off the unaffected hand and well over the affected foot. While holding the garment, allow the affected foot to rest on the floor. Draw the shorts up the affected leg. Then put the unaffected extremity into the shorts, and pull them up as far as possible. To complete the procedure of bringing the shorts up over the buttocks, roll to each side, and pull up the shorts on the opposite side.

UNDERSHIRT. Place the undershirt in the lap, back up. Thread the paralyzed arm arm through the appropriate armhole to above the elbow. Introduce the normal arm through its armhole. With the good arm pull the garment on the affected side up to the shoulder and over the head, and adjust the garment with the normal hand.

BRASSIERE. Stabilize one end of the garment with the affected arm while fastening it in the front with the unaffected hand. Slide the garment around the body, so that the fastener is in the back. With the unaffected hand pull the affected arm through the strap and place the strap over the shoulder. Then place the unaffected arm through the other strap.

SHIRT, BLOUSE OR FRONT-FASTENING DRESS. Button the cuff on the normal side. Thread the sleeve over the paralyzed arm to the shoulder. Place the hand and the arm through the other sleeve. Button the sleeve on the affected side. It is wise to wear collars a size larger than normal, because buttoning a tight neckband is difficult. Snap-on ties may be worn, or four-in-hand ties may be loosened and removed over the head without untying.

TROUSERS. The use of suspenders makes it easier to pull up the trousers. Trousers are put on in the same manner as shorts. If the patient prefers, he can pull the shorts and and the trousers up over the buttocks at the same time. When more balance has been achieved, an over-the-head type of garment (dress, slip, sweater) is put on in the same manner as is the undershirt. It is suggested that stretchable clothing be used.

Preparing the Patient and the Family for Discharge. It is desirable for continuity of care that the public health nurse who coordinates the patient's program after discharge become acquainted with the patient and his family while he is still in the hospital. If the public health nurse is aware of the patient's problems, she can help the family to plan modifications of home arrangements that will make the transition to the home easier for all concerned.

The patient is apt to have some brain damage, and he may be emotionally labile. The family should be prepared to expect occasional episodes of emotional instability. The patient may laugh or cry easily, and he is likely to become depressed. The family can help by supporting the patient and praising him for the progress that is being made. The pamphlet *Strike Back At Stroke** has pictorial

---

* Write the Superintendent of Documents, U. S. Government Printing Office, Washington 25, D. C.

and written instruction that may be useful to the patient and his family.

A shower is more convenient than a tub for the hemiplegic patient. Sitting on a stool of medium height with rubber suction tips will permit him to wash with greater ease. A long-handled bath brush with a soap container is helpful to the patient who has only one functional hand. If a shower is not available, a stool can be placed in the tub and a portable shower hose attached to the faucet. Handrails can be attached by the bathtub and the toilet. There are numerous self-help devices on the market that can assist the patient in his activities of daily living.

Where it is feasible, it is best if the patient can return to work or some modification of his former job. The local or the regional branch of the State Office of Vocational Rehabilitation provides individual evaluation and retraining services, depending on the needs of the patient.

All nurses coming in contact with the patient, whether as members of the hospital health team, public health nurses, office or industrial nurses, should encourage the patient to keep active, faithfully adhere to his exercise program, accept his limitations, and yet, confidently continue to remain as self-sufficient as possible.

PATIENTS WITH BRAIN TUMORS AND ANEURYSMS

Tumors of the brain, which appear at all ages of life, originate in the brain (including the roots of the cranial nerves and the meninges) in about 95 per cent of all patients. The remaining 5 per cent are either metastases from primary growths elsewhere in the body (Fig. 361) or malignancies of the skull that have ulcerated through into the cranial cavity.

Classification of Brain Tumors

Brain tumors may be classified into three groups: (1) those arising from the coverings of the brain, such as the dural meningioma; (2) those developing in or on the cranial nerves, best exemplified by the acoustic neurinoma and the optic-nerve spongioblastoma polare and (3) those originating in the brain tissue, such as the various gliomas, sarcoma, tuberculoma, gumma and metastatic lesions. Tumors may be benign or malignant. However, because it may be in a vital area, a benign tumor may have malignant effects.

Cerebellar Tumors. These are the most common brain tumors found in children. The vomiting, the staggering gait and the headaches gradually become very severe unless operation is performed. As tumors in the cerebellum lie very near the medulla oblongata, death may occur very suddenly.

Pituitary Gland Tumors. The pituitary gland is a small olive-shaped body located in a small pocket just below the optic nerves. The functions of this gland—among other things the regulation of the growth and the development of secondary sexual characteristics—may be increased or decreased by the presence of a tumor in it. Increased function (hyperpituitarism) accelerates growth, which in children results in gigantism. In adults the face becomes coarse and the hands large, a condition called *acromegaly* (Chap. 38).

A decrease in function leads to hypopituitarism, characterized by marked adiposity and loss of sexual characteristics. In addition to these disturbances of function, the tumor, by pressure on the optic nerves, causes increasing loss of vision resulting in blindness. Roentgenograms are an important aid in the diagnosis, showing an enlargement or deformity of the bony shell surrounding the pituitary gland.

Angiomas. Brain angiomas, masses composed largely of abnormal blood vessels, are found either in or on the surface of the brain. Some persist throughout life without causing symptoms, others give rise to those of brain tumor. Occasionally, the diagnosis is suggested by the presence of another angioma somewhere on the head or by a bruit audible over the skull. Since the walls of the blood vessels in angiomas are thin, a cerebral vascular accident frequently occurs. In fact, cerebral hemorrhage in persons under 40 years of age always should suggest the possibility of this diagnosis.

The Patient's Symptoms and Treatment. The symptoms of brain and meningeal tumors may be divided into general and local.

General Symptoms. These are caused by a gradual compression of the brain due to the tumor growth. The pressure of the cerebrospinal fluid usually is increased when it is estimated by lumbar puncture. The most common symptoms produced by this increased intracranial pressure are headache, vomiting, choked disk and stupor. Headache is most common in the early morning and increases in severity and frequency. Often it is generalized; but even when the pain is local, it gives no clue to the position of the neoplasm. Vomiting occurs often without preceding nausea and without relation to meals. It is of the forceful type described as "projectile" vomiting. Papilledema or choking of the disk is present in 70 to 75 per cent of the patients.

Localizing Symptoms. These are the neurologic signs produced by the tumor. Because the physician knows the functions of the different parts of the brain, he is able to diagnose the location of the tumor from disturbances of function brought about by its presence. For example, a tumor of the motor cortex manifests itself by causing convulsive movements localized to one side of the body, spoken of as "jacksonian epilepsy." Tumors of the occipital lobe cause blindness of half of each eye (hemianopsia) by involving the centers or the tracts for vision of one side of the brain. Tumors of the cerebellum cause dizziness and a staggering gait, with a tendency to fall toward the side of the lesion, and marked muscle incoordination and nystagmus (rhythmical vibration of the eyeballs). Tumors of the frontal lobe cause a disinterested mental attitude, and the patient often becomes extremely untidy and careless and uses obscene speech.

Tumors of the cerebellopontine angle usually originate in the sheath of the acoustic nerve and give rise to a sequence of symptoms that is the most characteristic of all brain tumors. First, tinnitus and vertigo appear, soon followed by progressive nerve deafness (8th nerve dysfunctions); next, numbness and tingling of the face and the tongue (due to involvement of the 5th nerve); still later, weakness or paralysis of the face (7th nerve involvement); and, finally, since the enlarging tumor presses on the cerebellum, the cerebellar syndrome mentioned above.

Many tumors are not so easily localized, because they lie in the so-called silent areas of the brain (i.e., areas whose functions are not definitely determined).

Since definite localization of the tumor must be ascertained before an operation for its removal can be attempted, the surgeon frequently resorts to encephalography or ventriculography. (See Fig. 351.)

Treatment. "An untreated brain tumor uniformly leads to death." If the increase in intracranial pressure continues without relief, headache and increasing blindness become the most distressing symptoms. If the tumor cannot be localized, or if the condition of the patient does not warrant an attempt at a curative operation, a decompression may be performed. This may restore sight and relieve all symptoms for a time. Often the tumor may be removed later.

If the tumor involves the cerebrum, an attempt to remove it may be made by an operation called a *craniotomy*. A large flap of scalp and bone is turned down, the dura is incised, and the tumor is removed. After bleeding is controlled, the bone flap is replaced, and the muscle and the scalp are sutured.

Tumors in and about the cerebellum are removed by an operation called a *suboccipital craniectomy*. The scalp and the muscles are dissected away from the base of the skull, and the bone is removed by rongeur forceps. After removal of the tumor, the dura is sutured, and the soft tissues are closed over it, leaving a defect in the bone.

Some inoperable tumors respond to x-ray or radio-cobalt irradiation therapy. This response is especially true of radiosensitive metastatic brain tumors of the breast.

Nursing Care

Preoperative Care. The nurse should become familiar with the symptoms of the patient, so that she can make comparisons postoperatively. These should include observations on paralysis, vision, personality, speech and incontinence. Paralysis of the hand can be tested by the hand grip. Observations of leg movement should be specially noted if the patient is not ambulatory.

If there is paralysis of the extremities, the

nurse should apply trochanter rolls to both extremities and position the feet against a footboard. Patients who have speech difficulties, failing vision and hearing loss challenge the nurse's ingenuity. If the patient is aphasic, writing materials or picture and word cards showing the bedpan, glass of water, blanket, etc., may be supplied to help him to communicate. The emotional preparation of the patient is important. Many times he does not realize that he is about to undergo surgery. Even so, encouragement and attention to his needs usually will make his amenable to any form of treatment. The patient is encouraged to ambulate if he is able to do so. The environment should be one that is conducive to rest, and the nurse's approach should be quiet and unhurried. Reassurance and consideration for the family is extremely important, for they recognize the seriousness of a brain operation.

Preparation for Operation. The preparation for an operation on the brain or the skull consists first in shaving the entire scalp. Usually, a shampoo of the scalp on the day before operation is advisable. Any infection found on the scalp should be reported to the surgeon before the operation. All evacuations of the rectum should be made without causing straining by the patient, as death may occur due to the increased intracranial pressure.

Morphine sulfate usually is not given to neurosurgical patients because of its action as a respiratory depressant and its masking of pupillary signs.

Postoperative Care. This is almost as important as the operation itself. While the patient is in the operating room, the bed is made with the head position reversed, so that there will be easy access to the patient's head. A turning sheet, placed from the head to the midthigh level, will facilitate moving the patient.

The equipment which should be available in the room includes the following:

Suction set with catheter for aspiration of the mouth secretions

Padded tongue depressor, to be used during seizures

Ventricular tap set, to be used if there is evidence of increasing intracranial pressure

Emergency drugs, such as stimulants and

hypertonic solutions, with syringes and needles

Lumbar puncture set

Sphygmomanometer, stethoscope and vital sign sheet

It is preferable that a nurse be in attendance for at least the first 24 hours. When the patient is unconscious, the care outlined on pages 922 and 923 is followed.

In order to follow the patient closely, the surgeon requires that the blood pressure, the pulse and the respiration be taken and recorded every 15 minutes for 3 hours, then every half hour for 3 hours, and then every hour for the remaining 24 hours. Thereafter, the taking of vital signs is done as the patient's condition indicates. The temperature should be taken rectally every half hour for 6 hours and every hour for the remaining 24 hours. Any marked changes should be reported at once.

SHOCK. The operations are usually long, and shock is the earliest postoperative complication. The nurse should see that the bed is warm, and that heat is available. If shock develops, the usual treatment is carried out, blood transfusion being particularly effective for these patients. The patient is placed in Trendelenburg position only upon the order of the physician, for this head-low position may increase intracranial pressure, a result that is undesirable.

RESPIRATORY FAILURE. This is more apt to occur in the patient operated on for cerebellar tumor. Removal of the cerebrospinal fluid is usually the treatment that the neurosurgeon carries out at once. This procedure is called a *ventricular tap*. For convenience, a sterile brain cannula is attached to the head of the bed at all times. The treatment for increased intracranial pressure also includes giving intravenous injections of 50 per cent glucose or sucrose (see Treatment, p. 921).

STATE OF CONSCIOUSNESS. The nurse should be particularly observant of the state of consciousness after a local anesthetic or after a reasonable period of time following a general anesthetic. This can be determined by first addressing the patient by his name. If he does not respond, command him to do something, such as showing his tongue or moving his leg. If there is still no response, observe his reaction to painful stimuli, such as a pinprick.

The nurse must remember that the patient may display signs of mental disturbance and confusion following head surgery, particularly if the frontal lobe was involved. Tolerance and a patient attitude must be assumed by all who care for him. Prolonged unconsciousness, cyanosis, or abnormal color changes in the skin should be noted and reported promptly.

TURNING AND POSITIONING PATIENTS. The patient is kept quiet immediately after operation; later, turning is ordered at frequent intervals to prevent respiratory complications and pressure sores. These should be prevented on the scalp and the ears as well as the sacrum, the hips, etc.

In the uncomplicated case, the head may be raised slightly when recovery from anesthesia occurs, and general care is given as for any postoperative patient.

Paralysis of the legs or the arms, the hand or hands, or of the swallowing function, and incontinence or aphasia should be watched for and reported. The extent of these abnormalities should be compared with preoperative observations.

DRESSINGS. Often the dressing is stained with blood shortly following operation. It is important that sterile pads be placed immediately about the dressing by the attending nurse, so that contamination by capillary attraction can be avoided.

The wound usually is dressed on the 3rd to the 5th day. At times, especially in wounds following suboccipital craniectomy, there may be a leak of cerebrospinal fluid through the wound. This complication is dangerous because of the possibility of meningitis. Any sudden discharge of fluid from a cranial or spinal wound should be called to the surgeon's attention at once.

When the dressings are removed, the nurse may notice a piece of silver foil directly over the incision line. This is frequently used to prevent dressings from adhering to the wound. A convenient headrest for a patient receiving a dressing is a piece of sponge rubber (3 in. x 8 in. x 8 in.) covered with a towel. Some surgeons prefer to use gauze dressings to clean the incision rather than cotton balls, because wisps of cotton may cling to short hairs and stitches. Head dressings can be held in place by a gauze roll, Ace bandage, gauze bandage or by a stockinet cap.

On healing of the wound, the scalp should be cleaned thoroughly. Often crusts are removed more easily after the application of warm oil dressings for a few hours.

Suboccipital Craniectomy. Patients with suboccipital craniectomy are dressed with firm adhesive strappings to prevent movement of the head and the neck. These patients must be turned from side to side at frequent intervals to prevent the development of pressure sores at the back of the head. In turning the patient, it is important to turn the body and the head as one piece to prevent any strain on the wound, with resultant tearing of sutures.

Water must not be given to a patient who has had a suboccipital craniectomy until it is ordered by the physician. Due to the operation, the patient temporarily may not be able to swallow. Aspiration of fluids or mucus may cause pneumonia, a complication avoidable by good nursing care.

Rehabilitation and Convalescence. The convalescence of a neurosurgical patient is dependent on the extent of trauma and the success with which treatment was carried out. When a tumor is benign and is removed successfully, it is most gratifying to help the patient to make his recovery. Good nursing will eliminate untoward complications and permit the major emphasis to be placed on regaining function. Gradual exercising of extremities, getting out of bed, learning to feed himself are devices by which the nurse can help the patient to help himself. Doing everything for the patient is a hindrance to his successful rehabilitation. Close cooperation between the nurse and the physical therapist will help the patient to achieve good muscle function. He should be accompanied when he is walking, for sudden attacks of dizziness or unconsciousness may occur. If aphasic, the patient may have to relearn to talk. This is likely to become a long-term and time-consuming project—one demanding great patience and continual encouragement on the part of the nurse. With regard to the appearance of the head in the convalescence following surgery, men usually have no problem because of short hair. Women who still have very short hair can wear attractive turbans, scarfs, or a wig. The family must be aware of the limitations of the patient but should be informed of his progress and how they can help to promote his recovery.

When tumor, injury, or disease is of such a nature that the prognosis is poor, convalescence is geared to making the patient comfortable and as happy as is possible. Perhaps he is left with a paralysis, is blind or suffers from seizures. The family is kept informed of the progress of the patient by the surgeon; however, many times the real expression of their emotions takes place after the physician leaves. It is then that the nurse must help them to accept their responsibility. Often the care of this patient is transferred to some member of the family. Whoever is responsible must have proper instruction regarding the physical and the emotional care of the patient. If some member is not able to give this care, perhaps some adjustment can be made with a visiting nurse to assume

part care as needed. The medical social worker may be called in to assist in making financial arrangements or to help in placing this individual in good hands.

Intracranial Aneurysms

An aneurysm is an outpouching, a "blister or bubble" on the wall of an artery. (See Fig. 362.) Most of them are due to a congenital defect in the arterial structure. Aneurysms produce symptoms by enlarging and compressing nearby cranial nerves or by rupturing and causing intracranial hemorrhage. Diagnosis depends largely upon arteriography. The object of any treatment is to stop or to diminish the flow of the blood in the aneurysmal sac. If there is a stalk connecting the aneurysm to the parent artery, it may be possible to do a craniotomy, isolate the aneurysm and place a small clip on the stalk. This would stop all blood flow to the aneurysm. Occasionally, it is possible to put clips on the parent artery above and below the aneurysm. It may be necessary to ligate the carotid artery in the neck or to wrap muscle around the aneu-

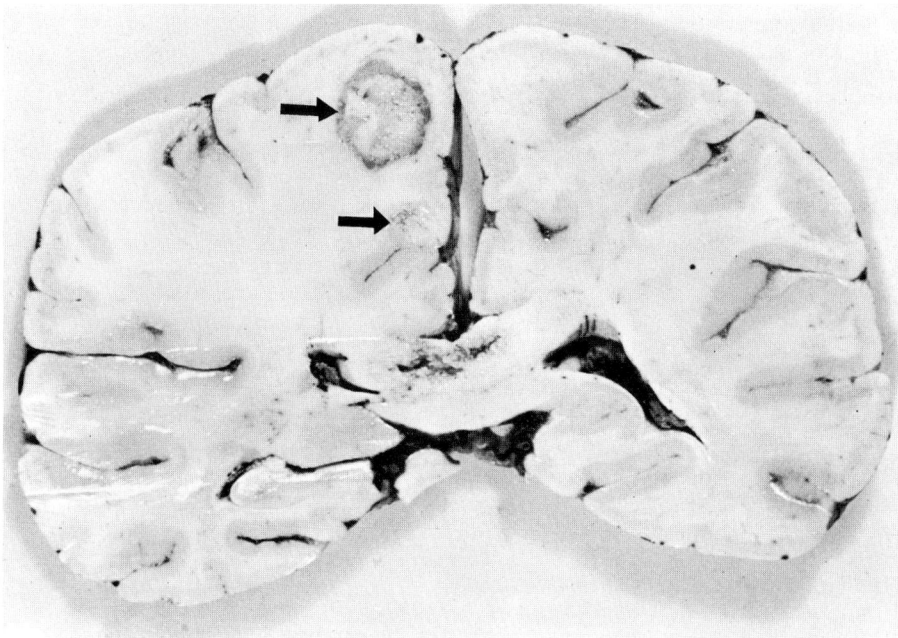

FIG. 361. Twin nodules in the brain, representing cerebral metastases from a carcinoma of the lung. (Rudolph Osgood, M.D., Boston)

rysm. In the latter instance the muscle will form scar tissue on the wall and possibly prevent rupture.

Nursing Care. A patient admitted to the hospital when he is drowsy, stuporous or in coma with a history of the sudden onset of severe headache a few hours or 1 or 2 days previously is suspected of having a leaking aneurysm. The patient in coma is treated like any unconscious patient. The patient who is alert or partially cooperative must be kept in bed, and to prevent fatal bleeding, he must be prevented from doing anything that requires exertion, such as straining during an enema. Periodic observations should be made for decrease in mental alertness, increase in headache and alteration in size of pupils, and any changes should be reported to the physician immediately. These changes usually signify additional bleeding, and speed of action is necessary if a fatal hemorrhage is to be prevented. The crucial time for a second episode is during the 2nd or the 3rd week after the first hemorrhage.

THE PATIENT WITH MULTIPLE SCLEROSIS

Multiple or disseminated sclerosis, one of the most common of all neurologic disorders, is a chronic, progressive disease of unknown cause that appears in early adult life. In this disease, scattered irregularly throughout the central nervous system, degeneration of the myelin nerve axon sheaths occurs; subsequently, the axons themselves degenerate. The areas of involvement are distributed in patches which are without consistency or regularity, so that the resultant symptoms and signs, when nerve conduction along the unsheathed and diseased axons finally is interrupted, are most varied in character.

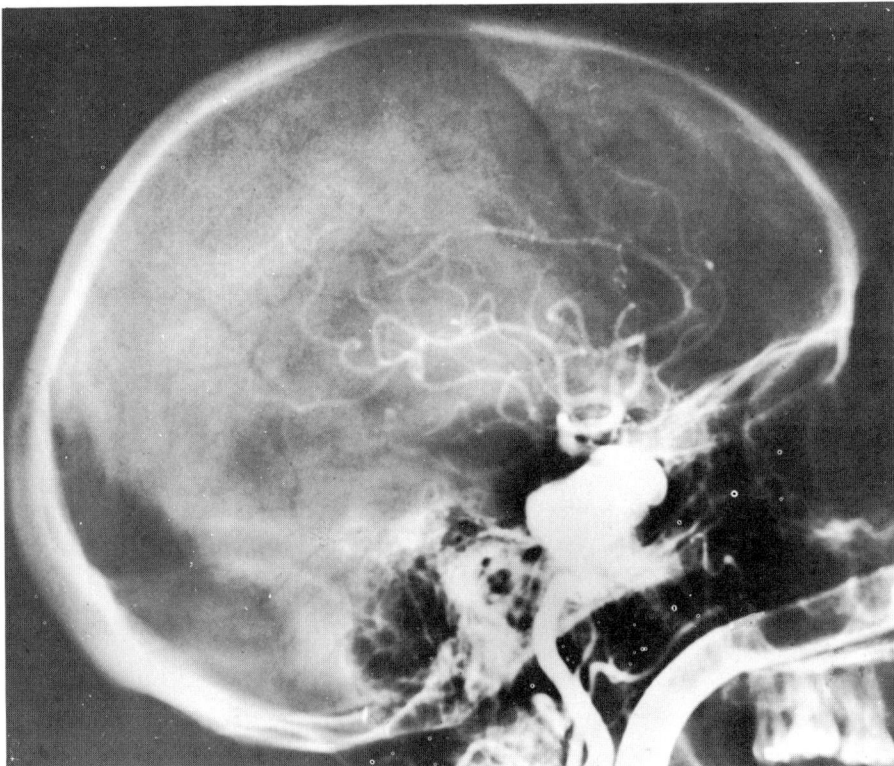

FIG. 362. Arteriogram showing aneurysm of the cerebral artery. (See Fig. 352 for normal arteriogram.)

Symptoms

This disease is marked by long remissions and exacerbations of several neurologic symptoms (Fig. 363). These symptoms are multiple and variable due to the multiple neural lesions. They include visual disturbances, due to lesions in the optic nerves or their connections; nystagmus; "scanning" speech, of slow, monotonous and slurred character; muscular intention tremor and loss of tonicity, due to cerebellar lesions. Spastic weakness of the extremities and loss of the abdominal reflexes are due to involvement of the main motor pathways (pyramidal tracts) of the spinal cord. Euphoria and emotional hyperexcitability result from loss of cortical control connections to the basal ganglia. There may be vertigo, with nausea and vomiting if the vestibular nuclei or their connections are diseased; bladder, rectal and genital disturbances, if the process involves the cord pathways connected with the sacral plexus. The most common group of symptoms includes spastic paraplegia with slight speech disturbance, nystagmus and muscular tremor.

The prognosis for a fairly prolonged life is good. Symptoms abate and recur with increasing frequency and severity each time for many years, death usually resulting from an intercurrent infection, most often of the urinary tract.

Control

Multiple sclerosis is characteristically a disease of cold, damp climates; it is aggravated by exposure to cold, damp weather and improves when and where the climate is mild and dry. Pregnancy, of all predisposing factors in multiple sclerosis, is one of the most potent, the onset of the disease in more than 40 per cent of all female patients having occurred while they were pregnant. Fatigue, malnutrition and acute febrile infections likewise have been shown to predispose to the occurrence of exacerbations, if not the initial onset, of multiple sclerosis.

Treatment

Encouraging results have been reported in cases of multiple sclerosis treated with vaso-

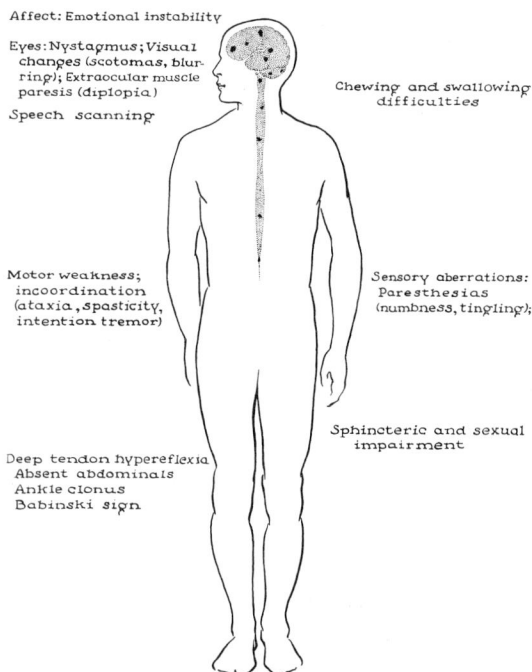

FIG. 363. Characteristic signs and symptoms of multiple sclerosis.

dilator drugs. The basic assumption underlying this form of treatment considers that acute symptoms in these patients are attributable to ischemia of nerve tissue caused by spasm of the arterioles supplying localized areas in the nervous system.

Drugs capable of dilating blood vessels effectively relieve symptoms, provided that they are administered within a few minutes following the initial appearance of those symptoms or of their re-exacerbation. To assure lasting benefit, the dilator drug must be given repeatedly. Carbon dioxide, inhaled in the form of a mixture containing 5 per cent carbon dioxide and 95 per cent oxygen, is easiest to administer and is also the most effective agent that has so far been tested in this connection.

Nursing Management and Rehabilitation of the Patient With Multiple Sclerosis

Although rehabilitation measures will not alter the disease process, it is the aim of the rehabilitation program to bring about functional improvement, so that the patient can perform his activities of daily living whether he is ambulatory, in a wheelchair or confined to bed. If the patient's disease is not progressing too rapidly, the goal is to return the patient to satisfying employment or to keep him happily engaged in his present employment. He is placed on an individualized therapeutic program that is determined after an appraisal has been made of the extent of his disability and muscle strength. Relaxation and coordination exercises promote muscle efficiency, and progressive resistive exercises are used to strengthen weak muscles. The nurse can encourage the patient to work up to the point of fatigue without becoming exhausted. If certain muscle groups are irreversibly affected, other muscles can be trained to take over their action. Warm baths, packs and muscle relaxants may be beneficial if painful muscle spasm is present. Sometimes the patient presents the clinical picture of hemiplegia, although more commonly he may have the same disabilities as does the patient with paraplegia. Any one extremity or combination of extremities may be involved. Therefore, the principles of rehabilitation of these conditions can be used for the patient who has similar problems due to multiple sclerosis. (See pages 935 to 941.)

Occupational therapy is prescribed as part of the muscle education program, and it also serves to keep the patient motivated. Hobbies will help the patient's morale and give him satisfying interests when he reaches the stage in which he is unable to participate in normal activities.

Management of bladder and bowel control are among the patient's most difficult problems, because there may be sphincter impairment. The sensation to void must be heeded immediately, and the bedpan or the urinal should be readily accessible. If urinary incontinence develops, pads and protective pants or a catheter draining into a collecting bag attached to the thigh will help the patient to feel more socially acceptable. A bowel-training program is effective if there is loss of bowel control. (See pp. 370-371.)

As the patient's disease progresses, self-help devices that include feeding devices, handrails, canes, braces, wheelchairs and ramps are utilized to maintain independency as long as possible. When vision begins to fail, painting the cane tip and the shoe tips with fluorescent paint will help.

The National Multiple Sclerosis Society conducts a research and educational program. Local Multiple Sclerosis units give direct services to patients. Through group participation the patient has an opportunity to learn of self-help methods in a social environment.

The nurse has the responsibility of emphasizing to the patient and his family the importance of a regular program of work, exercise and recreation. The patient should stay under constant medical supervision. Reassurance and encouragment by those who come in contact with the patient are neces-

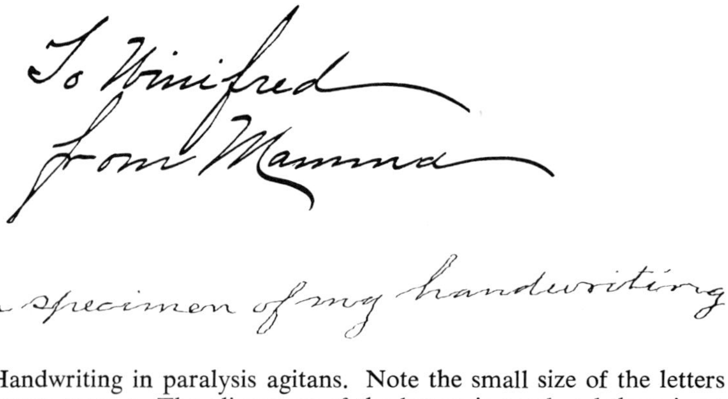

Fig. 364. Handwriting in paralysis agitans. Note the small size of the letters and the continuous tremor. The alignment of the letters is good and there is no ataxia. The upper specimen shows the normal handwriting about 1 year before the onset of the disease. (Stieglitz, E. J.: Geriatric Medicine, ed. 3, Philadelphia, Lippincott)

sary in helping the patient to maintain a good adjustment to his disease, therapeutic program and environment.

PATIENTS WITH EXTRAPYRAMIDAL DISEASE

Parkinsonism

Parkinson's disease is a disease of the basal ganglia, the chief symptoms of which include muscular rigidity, tremor and weakness. The cause of the disease is not always known. It usually is due to cerebral vascular disease, but it also may follow encephalitis, carbon-monoxide or manganese poisoning and electrical shock. The anatomic lesion found at necropsy consists of atrophy and destruction of the cells of the basal ganglia, especially the globus pallidus, at the base of the brain.

Characteristics. In this disease the mental faculties are unimpaired. Early, the patient notices that his limbs are getting stiff, a wax-like rigidity in the performance of all movements develops, and later the tremor begins, often first of one hand and arm (Fig. 364), then of the other and later of the head.

The tremor is characteristic. It is a slow, turning motion (pronation-supination) of the forearm and the hand, and a motion of the thumb against the fingers, as of a man rolling a pill. If the patient gets excited, the tremor becomes worse; when he makes a voluntary motion, it ceases, allowing him to perform the most delicate acts, such as picking up a pin. At the same time the rigid limbs are becoming definitely weaker. His facies, station and gait are characteristic. Since its muscles move but little, the face has so little expression that it is said to be *mask-like,* a feature that can be recognized at a glance. The patient stands with head bent a little forward and walks as if in danger of falling on his face. Push him a little forward, and he tends to go forward faster and faster (propulsion); pull him back, and he tends to run backward faster and faster (retropulsion).

The aim of treatment of the patient with Parkinsonism is to keep the patient functionally useful and productive as long as possible. This is done with appropriate medications, physical therapy and rehabilitation technics, and patient and family education.

Patient Education. It is important that the patient be oriented correctly with respect to the ailment that he is destined to live with. Its nature must be explained to him in detail. The disease may be described as one that affects a small motor control station at the base of the brain—but not the brain itself; one that is neither inherited nor contagious; one that progresses in severity, but very slowly, the periods of progression alternating with periods lasting from 5 to 15 years or more when there is little or no progress; one that does not impair intellect, sight or hearing and does not shorten life; one that causes rigidity and tremor, but does not lead to paralysis and is painful only if neglected.

Medication. Symptomatic improvement is afforded in the majority of patients by the long-term use of an appropriate drug or combination of drugs. These are prescribed on the basis of 3 or 4 doses daily, and the dosage is adjusted primarily in accordance with the patient's age, patients over 50 years of age receiving ½ to ⅔ the amount prescribed for individuals in a younger age group.

As the basic medication for control of the majority of symptoms, including rigidity, tremor, akinesia (muscular weakness) and mental depression, the physician may prescribe Artane or Pagitane. If muscle cramps persist, Cogentin may be prescribed. Severe tremor may yield to Parsidol or hyoscine (1-scopolamine). Nervousness, obsessions, delusion or hallucinations may be controlled by Rauwolfia, lethargy by Dexedrine, and insomnia by Thorazine.

Problems of Patients With Parkinsonism. A patient with Parkinsonism has severe problems with constipation. Among the factors causing this condition are weakness of the muscles used in defecation, lack of saliva (lost from drooling), lack of exercise, and an inadequate fluid intake. Then, too, the drugs used for the treatment of the disease also inhibit normal intestinal secretions. The nurse assists the patient in establishing a bowel routine by seeing that he follows a regular habit time, consciously increases the fluid intake, and eats high-residue foods. A raised toilet seat is a useful device to facilitate toilet activities, since the patient has difficulty in changing from a standing to a sitting position.

The patient also has a problem in maintaining normal weight. He becomes embarrassed by his slowness and untidiness in eating. His mouth is dry from the medications, and he experiences difficulty in chewing. In time he will have a sizable weight loss. Demineralization starts in the bones from malnutrition. Thus he is faced with the added threat of fractures in the event of falling. Supplementary feedings will keep his caloric intake up, and an electrical warming tray will keep food hot and permit him to rest during the prolonged time that he takes to eat.

Rehabilitation. Physical therapy is useful in the treatment of the rigid musculature and in the prevention of contractures that occur when affected muscles are not in use. Warm baths with massage and active and passive motion will help to relax muscles. Stretching exercises will loosen the joint structures. Postural exercises are important, as the patient's head and neck will be drawn forward and downward if measures are not taken to prevent this posture. The gait becomes shuffling and propulsive. The patient also may walk off balance due to the rigidity of the arms. (Arm swinging is necessary in normal walking.) The patient is taught early in the course of the disease to concentrate on walking erect, using a broad base, i.e., walking with the feet widely separated. Instruct him to raise his feet consciously and to walk with a heel-toe, heel-toe gait. He must think while *deliberately* swinging his arms in a reciprocal back and forth motion.

The nurse should seek every way possible to encourage the patient to care for his own daily needs. Placing an adjustable mirror on the lavatory and providing a chair for the patient to be seated will enable a man with Parkinsonism to shave himself. This is just one example of the modifications that can be made by an imaginative nurse.

Faithful adherence to an exercise and walking program will help to delay the progress of the disease. Encouragement and reassurance can be given by all who care for the patient and all those about him by praising him for his perseverance and pointing out that his activities are being maintained through his active participation.

Surgery for Parkinsonism. During recent years it has been discovered that in some cases destruction of the globus pallidus or a specific part of the thalamus will diminish or stop the rigidity and the tremor of the disease. The destruction is accomplished by either electrocoagulation, freezing (*cryosurgery*) or alcohol. It is known as chemosurgery. *Chemopallidectomy* means that the globus pallidus is destroyed, and *chemothalamectomy* that the thalamus is destroyed. An operation not yet generally accepted has been used experimentally in the treatment of Parkinsonism. Its advocates claim relief of tremors.

PROCEDURE. The surgery usually is done under local anesthesia. A previous pneumoencephalogram is done, and then by measurements on the roentgenograms the specific area to be destroyed is determined. An opening is made in the skull, and a cannula or an electrode is inserted into the desired region. The area is destroyed by injecting alcohol through the cannula or by electrocoagulation through the electrode. The cannula may be left in place for several days, during which time additional alcohol may be injected to obtain the desired effect.

Nursing Care. The manifold types of neurologic, psychological, medical and nursing problems demonstrated by victims of Parkinson's disease demand almost a team approach in finding some solutions. Even the careful selection of patients for surgery is done by a group of specialists, with the result that only a portion of Parkinson patients meet the criteria.

Depending on the overall condition of the patient postoperatively, some type of rehabilitation program is initiated. Transient speech difficulties and psychological difficulties often are apparent. The needs of the patient must be evaluated and met on an individual basis.

In addition to observing the vital signs postoperatively, the nurse will note the muscle strength of the upper and the lower extremities, the presence or the absence of tremor, the quality of speech, and the state of consciousness. A catheter usually is in place and must be protected from dislodging. At prescribed intervals, the physician will inject an alcohol-pantopaque solution, as described under the procedure above. The patient continues to be observed for unilateral weakness. The rehabilitation program and follow-up care continue beyond the patient's discharge from the hospital.

Hereditary (Huntington's) Chorea

Huntington's chorea is a chronic, incurable, fatal disease of hereditary origin, the basic pathology of which is unexplained atrophy of the basal ganglia and portions of the cerebral cortex. The most prominent clinical feature of the disease is the onset in early adult life of uncontrolled, spasmodic jerking movements of the extremities and the trunk. These motions are completely devoid of purpose and lacking in direction; their rhythm is totally irregular, their rate, approximately 80 per minute. All of the body musculature is involved. Facial movements produce grimacing of the most grotesque sort. Speech is affected; it is sometimes hesitant and again explosive in character, and eventually it is incoherent. The gait is similarly disorganized, to the point that locomotion becomes impossible. The sensorium likewise is involved, and in particular the special senses. Equanimity gives way to uncontrollable fits of anger; judgment and memory are lost; deterioration of the intellect, marked by delusions and disorientation, finally leads to complete dementia, and death supervenes.

No treatment has yet been discovered that succeeds in halting or reversing the underlying process. Recent evidence, however, suggests that variable degrees of symptomatic improvement may follow the administration of procaine, e.g., in the form of procaine amide (Pronestyl), given orally in doses of approximately 1 Gm. 4 times each day.

PATIENTS WITH CEREBRAL INFECTION

Brain Abscess

True brain abscesses are collections of pus within the substance of the brain itself. From 33 to 50 per cent of them are secondary to middle ear infections. Others are due to septic thrombosis of a dural venous sinus, penetrating wounds and compound fractures of the skull that perforate the dura mater, cerebrospinal meningitis, and infections of the face and the scalp, particularly erysipelas; whereas a few are caused by septic emboli to the brain, often from the lungs and the bones.

Symptoms. The patient has general symptoms similar to those of all mild chronic infections, wherever located: malaise, slight fever, anorexia and loss of weight. The signs of increased intracerebral pressure usually are slight, since a brain abscess is an area of liquefied brain tissue infiltrated by pus which, unlike a tumor, unless surrounded by a zone of edema, adds little to the contents in the cranial cavity. Headache is the patient's most constant symptom; vomiting is common, but seldom is it projectile in type, whereas choked disks appear rather late. Such localizing symptoms as occur are most inconstant and less complete than in cases of brain tumor and, when present, they usually indicate pathology in either a temporal lobe or the cerebellum, since so many abscesses are aural in origin.

Treatment. Brain abscesses, depending on the character of the infection, may subside and heal completely in response to antibacterial chemotherapy, precisely as expected had the infection localized elsewhere in the body. When they fail to give a satisfactory response to conservative measures, surgical drainage, with chemotherapy as an adjunctive measure, then is undertaken.

Postoperative Nursing Care. A single abscess may be cured by incision and drainage. After operation copious dressings should be applied, and the patient should lie with the opening downward to promote drainage. The nurse should watch these patients carefully for retraction of the head, stiffness of the neck, headache, chills, sweats, etc., symptoms suggestive of a postoperative meningitis.

It is important that this type of patient be maintained on a high-caloric diet. Palatable forms of carbohydrates and proteins should be administered at 3-hour intervals in addition to the usual diet.

Central Nervous System Syphilis

During the early dissemination of the spirochete *Treponema pallidum* throughout the body, doubtless within a few weeks after the primary infection, this germ often induces slight lesions in the central nervous system. The majority of these later disappear, but a few develop further.

Since the distribution of the luetic lesions throughout the brain and the cord varies greatly, there arise several syphilitic diseases of this system which are clinically quite dissimilar. The most important of these are meningovascular syphilis, gumma of the brain, meningoencephalitis (general paresis), tabes dorsalis (locomotor ataxia), syphilitic myelitis and various combinations of the above.

Meningovascular Syphilis

This type, some cases of which are predominantly meningeal and others predominantly vascular, may manifest its presence early, but in the majority of cases it appears about 5 years after the primary infection. It always responds to antiluetic treatment.

Meningeal Form. Meningovascular syphilis, localized chiefly in the meninges of the brain, may run an acute or a chronic course. The chief symptoms of acute cases are headache, vomiting and slight rigidity of the neck. Fever generally is present, convulsions may be a prominent feature, and Kernig's sign usually can be obtained. This clinical picture often closely resembles that of acute meningitis due to other germs, except that in the former picture evidences of syphilis can be found elsewhere in the body. The spinal fluid in this disease is bacteria-free; yet it contains an abnormal number of lymphocytes, and generally it gives a positive Wassermann reaction.

Chronic syphilitic meningitis closely resembles tuberculous meningitis. Symptoms common to both conditions are chronic headache, rigidity of the neck, a positive Kernig's sign, low fever and marked loss of weight. Unlike the tuberculous form, chronic syphilitic meningitis is much more common in adults than in children; the spinal fluid is clear, and in it no pellicle forms; and the serologic tests for syphilis generally are positive.

Vascular Form. It is believed that all luetic processes start in the media of the smaller arteries. It is not surprising, therefore, that in meningovascular syphilis the symptoms of vascular disease often long antedate gross arterial lesions. Formerly, it was taught that well-defined arteriosclerosis limited to the cerebral vessels was evidence of lues; today syphilis is thought to explain comparatively few of such cases.

Symptoms. The clinical symptoms, also the pathologic changes, in cases of luetic cerebral vascular disease are almost identical with those of cerebral arteriosclerosis. Features common to both are chronic headache and paralyses which vary in extent from that involving a single muscle to complete hemiplegia. The chief clinical differences between these two types are, first, that in lues, cerebral infarction usually is by thrombosis, seldom by rupture (apoplexy belongs more to the nonluetic type); and, second, that cerebral infarction due to lues occurs at a much earlier age than in the nonluetic type.

Gumma of the Nervous System

The infiltrations of late lues usually are diffuse. Occasionally, however, they assume the form of local tumor masses, the gummas. The majority of these are microscopic, but some may be 2 or 3 in. in diameter. Nevertheless, although cerebral lues is a common disease, of all brain tumors large enough to cause local pressure symptoms, only about 1 per cent are gumma. Gumma of the spinal cord, on the other hand, never is large enough to give rise to the signs of cord tumor. The signs and the symptoms of brain gumma are identical with those of brain tumor, except that in cases of the former the blood and the spinal fluid generally give positive complement-fixation reactions. If gumma of the brain is suspected, vigorous antiluetic therapy is started at once. Prompt cerebral decompression occasionally is performed as well, lest the increased intracerebral pressure blind the patient before the gumma will have become absorbed.

Tabes Dorsalis (Locomotor Ataxia)

The essential lesion of tabes dorsalis is degeneration of the posterior columns of the spinal cord (Fig. 365). Its earliest lesions, however, would seem to be in the meninges of the sensory roots of the spinal nerves (the fibers of which, after entering the cord, form the cord's posterior columns).

Symptoms. Locomotor ataxia appears generally after the patient has had his lues for 5 to 20 years. The first complaints are lightninglike (shooting) pains, followed in the same areas by temporary paresthesia or partial anesthesia, felt usually in the legs, but occasionally in the arms, about the trunk and in the areas supplied by the trigeminal nerve. Soon the patient loses the sense of position of his legs (and occasionally of his arms); hence he becomes ataxic and walks with a stamping gait, his feet wide apart, watching each step, since he increasingly must depend on vision. In the dark he is helpless. When he tries to stand with his feet together and his eyes closed, he sways and even falls (Romberg's sign). There is hypotonia (great flaccidity) of the muscles, especially of those of the legs; the knee jerk is absent; and the Argyll Robertson pupil (one that reacts to accommodation but not to light) is practically always present.

The tabetic patient generally looks ill, is underweight and complains of general physical weakness. He often suffers sudden attacks of extreme visceral dysfunction due to intense muscle spasms, the so-called *tabetic crises,* which may involve the stomach, producing violent vomiting (gastric crises); the urinary bladder; the rectum and even the larynx. Chronic trophic ulcers (perforating ulcers) appear on the soles of the feet, and often a Charcot joint (p. 1121) develops. Atrophy of the olfactory and the optic nerves (causing anosmia and blindness) and paralyses of the 3rd, the 4th and the 6th cranial nerves, leading to eye squints, frequently appear. A certain number of tabetic patients show mental disturbances, but this symptom is evidence not of their tabes but of other concurrent syphilitic manifestations, cerebral arterial disease and general paresis. The condition with the features of tabes and paresis combined is called *taboparesis.*

Diagnosis. Although the simultaneous presence of the ataxic gait, a positive Romberg's sign, absent knee jerks and Argyll Robertson pupils are almost conclusive of the presence of tabes, yet even then the spinal fluid tests (cell count, Wassermann reaction and tabetic colloidal-gold curve) should be found positive before that diagnosis is considered to be proved.

General Paresis

General paresis, the parenchymatous type of cerebral lues, is a disease characterized

clinically by gradual mental deterioration and pathologically by widespread degeneration and atrophy of the brain cortex, to which the thickened pia arachnoid is found to be firmly adherent.

Symptoms. The symptoms of general paresis usually develop insidiously, first appearing from 10 to 20 years after the patient has contracted syphilis. Occasionally, however, the first evidence of paresis in an individual who had enjoyed apparently normal health is a sudden epileptiform convulsion or apoplectic stroke, immediately followed by the full-blown picture of general paresis. It is known that generally for 20 or more years before the patient shows his paresis, degenerative changes have been developing in his brain cortex, and that during these years tests of the spinal fluid would have permitted a correct diagnosis. Also, it is known that from the microscopic examination of the brain at necropsy there is no evident relationship between the grade of the lesions present and the degree of mental disturbance exhibited before death.

In the majority of patients, however, the clinical picture of paresis develops gradually: first with headache, loss of memory, lack of concentration or poor judgment concerning business affairs, features that suggest merely a fatigued condition. As the disease progresses, the patient's faults become so glaring, and he becomes so undependable that it

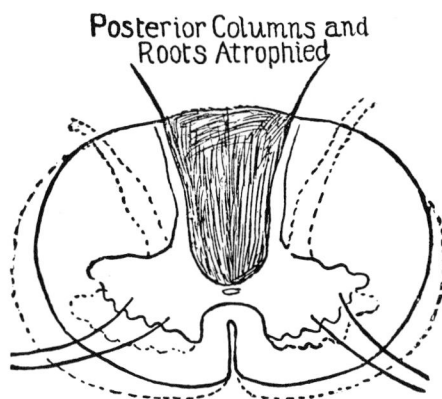

FIG. 365. Cross section of the spinal cord of a patient with tabes dorsalis. The dotted lines show the outline of the normal cord.

is only too evident his trouble is serious. His personality at this stage of his disease may seem to be radically changed; his superior qualities gradually have faded away, whereas his more elementary ones, especially his primitive passions, previously held in restraint, are becoming more and more dominant. Thus some paretics become more and more morose; others overexalted; some unduly benevolent; others mean, suspicious and irritable; and some terrified.

That the patient's malady is an organic disease of the nervous system is made evident early by his pupils, which are unequal in size, irregular in shape and sluggish in reactions, and by his deep reflexes, which usually are hyperactive, but may be normal and occasionally are lost. Early in the disease the paretic may appear to be in excellent physical condition. Gradually, however, all his physical as well as his mental powers weaken progressively until, finally, he becomes physically helpless (hence the older name, *general paralysis of the insane*) and completely demented.

Diagnosis. The diagnosis of general paresis is suggested by the presence of the above-mentioned personality changes and physical signs. However, it should be confirmed by spinal fluid examinations with especial reference to a positive Wassermann reaction and positive paretic colloidal-gold curve.

Treatment of Neurosyphilis

Treatment, if instituted sufficiently early in the course of the disease, offers an excellent chance of complete functional recovery; some degree of remission is expected at even later stages, and complete arrest of the active disease process is possible at any stage.

Penicillin, which is at least as efficacious as any other agent or combination of agents of known value in neurosyphilis, and by far the safest, now is used practically to the exclusion of all others for these patients.

The therapeutic program recommended for all forms of neurosyphilis involves the intramuscular injection of 1.2 million units of penicillin G in oil and aluminum monostearate (PAM) at intervals of 2 to 4 days until a total dose of between 6 and 10 million units has been received. An alternate program, predicted to be equally satisfactory, specifies 3 intramuscular injections, one week apart, of benzathine pencillin G, 2.4 million units each. For patients who prove to be penicillin-resistant, or who demonstrate penicillin sensitivity, carbomycin may be prescribed in 2- to 3-Gm. doses daily by mouth for 15 to 20 days.

THE EPILEPTIC PATIENT

Epilepsy, a disease characterized by attacks of unconsciousness, comes on with or without convulsions. The lay mind can scarcely believe that epilepsy and fits are not synonymous; and yet some of the most pronounced epileptics have few convulsions—possibly none at all—whereas violent epileptiform convulsions, in every way similar to those of epilepsy, may be due to other conditions. The mildest cases of true epilepsy also may have no true convulsions but merely attacks of momentary unconsciousness (petit mal), although actually these have the same significance as the most violent seizures.

Types

Epilepsy is classified as "genetic," or "essential," if it is based on an hereditary defect rather than an organic lesion in the brain, and as "acquired," or "symptomatic," if it is attributable to organic brain pathology. The genetic type, which usually begins in childhood and persists throughout life, is the presumptive diagnosis in all patients with epilepsy without evidence of organic brain disease prior to the onset of convulsive seizures. Symptomatic epilepsy may result from a traumatic injury to the brain before or during birth, or at any time thereafter; it also may appear as a complication of cerebral tumors, vascular lesions or infections of the central nervous system. Convulsive seizures that are not epileptic in origin, and must be distinguished with care from epilepsy, include hysterical convulsions, syncopal or convulsive attacks due to carotid sinus sensitivity, low-calcium and alkalotic tetany, hypoglycemic convulsions and malingering.

The most common problem in differential diagnosis is presented by the epileptiform convulsions of hysteria, which may be characterized as follows. The patient never falls as if shot, but is careful to select a safe spot and to fall in such a manner as to avoid injury. The movements are not truly convulsive but rather struggling in character; or, the whole body is rigid, and the person trying to restrain the patient is definitely aware of resistance to his effort. Indeed, the restrainer must beware lest he be struck or bitten. The hysterical person may scream during the attack; the epileptic never does after the onset. The epileptic seizure is over in a few minutes; the hysterical often not for hours, but it may be terminated by distracting the patient.

Epilepsy to a large extent is a diagnosis of exclusion. As a basis for excluding other possibilities, certain diagnostic procedures are indicated, including a urinalysis, hematologic and chemical examinations of the blood, x-ray examination of the skull, lumbar puncture and complete study of the cerebrospinal fluid. A pneumoencephalogram is performed if the diagnosis of symptomatic epilepsy is suspected, and other tests are done, depending on the nature of the problem.

Of all the tests now available, however, the most illuminating is the electroencephalogram, which furnishes positive diagnostic evidence in a substantial proportion of epileptic patients, aids in their classification and serves as a guide in establishing their prognosis. Abnormalities in the electroencephalogram usually continue to be apparent between attacks, or, if concealed, may be brought out by hyperventilation, by sleep or by the slow intravenous injection of Metrazol.

The Epileptic Seizure

Six major types of convulsive seizure are observed in epileptics: jacksonian, grand mal, focal, psychomotor (psychic equivalent), petit mal and autonomic (diencephalic) types.

Jacksonian Seizures. These are characterized by clonic convulsive movements, or abnormal sensations, which begin in one hand or foot and spread centrally in an orderly "march" to other muscle groups, the manner of progression always being the same. Convulsions may be limited to one limb, and consciousness may be retained, so that the patient may be able to observe the entire episode; or it may be generalized, developing into a grand mal seizure, with complete loss of consciousness.

Grand Mal Seizures. These usually are preceded by an "aura," a sense of dreamy detachment, warning of the impending attack. The signal may be a hallucinatory flash of light or sound. But these warnings are of little or no help to the patient, since the convulsion follows so promptly that he has no time to save himself. Other individuals, however, have no aura, and the first they know of their attack is after it is all over. The convulsion begins with a cry, possibly a scream, and the patient falls as if shot, making no effort whatever to protect himself, and, therefore, he often is injured. At first the body is perfectly rigid, jaws fixed, hands clenched and legs extended (the tonic stage). The muscles of respiration likewise are in spasm; hence the patient becomes cyanotic.

In about 15 seconds the convulsive movements begin. These are slight, at first, then become increasingly severe and soon involve practically every muscle in the body (the clonic stage). Often the tongue is chewed; stools and urine may be passed involuntarily. After 1 or 2 minutes the convulsive movements become less violent, the body relaxes, and the patient lies in deep coma, breathing noisily. The respirations at this point are chiefly abdominal. For a few minutes or even hours the patient cannot be aroused, then he begins by degrees to regain consciousness, and finally he awakens, sometimes alert, but usually confused, suffering from headache, malaise and nausea.

Focal Seizures. The type most often observed in patients with posttraumatic epilepsy, these may be characterized by either motor or sensory phenomena. As in the jacksonian type, the symptoms of focal epilepsy are localized on one side of the body or in one portion of an extremity; the characteristic "march," however, that typifies the former is lacking. These patients may exhibit clonic movements of an extremity, a twitching of the face or a turning of the head and the eyes to one side. Following the seizure, the muscles on the affected side may be very weak for a time. Focal seizures may consist entirely of paroxysmal, unilateral sensations of numbness, tingling or, rarely, pain in the distal portion of an extremity. The patient may experience hallucinations of odor, sound, taste or sight that develop and disappear very suddenly and without warning, whereas others describe merely a sense of unreality.

Psychomotor Seizures. These seizures are marked by periods of amnesia, occasionally accompanied by tonic spasm or contortion of the trunk muscles. These patients sometimes perform movements in automatic fashion, appearing dazed or stupid and quite out of touch with their surroundings. Some sit quietly, muttering or ruminating. Others have "running fits," becoming violent if restrained. Nothing of these events, however, is remembered afterward, the patient being totally unaware of any unusual occurrence.

Petit Mal Seizures. Called also "pyknoepilepsy," these are manifested solely by repeated transient loss or impairment of consciousness. Attacks last only from 5 to 30 seconds and may be scarcely noticeable. The patient, as though momentarily dazed, stops talking, walking or whatever he is doing, and then he resumes, as though no interruption had occurred; to him, the attack was just a blank moment. A rhythmic twitching of the eyelids or the head may be observed during an attack; the patient may jerk his head or make some other automatic motion, sometimes a violent one; a sudden muscular collapse may allow the head to nod, or the patient to crumple, suddenly helpless, to the ground. Whatever its manifestations, petit mal epilepsy is distinguished by its rarity in adults and by the frequency of its attacks, which may recur several times each day.

Autonomic Seizures. An uncommon variant of the disease, these seizures are featured by sudden episodes of extreme flushing or pallor of the skin, sweating, tachycardia, gagging, fluctuations in blood pressure, fever, hyperperistalsis and fear, or some other emotion, which cannot be explained, usually appearing in patients who exhibit other manifestations of epilepsy.

Status Epilepticus

This term denotes a rapid succession of epileptic seizures, which may be grand mal or petit mal in type. If they are of the former type, the patient continues to convulse violently, with only short pauses and without return of consciousness between attacks, heroic sedation occasionally being required to prevent exhaustion. Status epilepticus of the petit mal variety is characterized chiefly by mental confusion, which may persist for many hours.

Treatment. The medical management of epilepsy is planned according to a long-range program, one that will cover a period of many years, and is tailored to meet the special needs of each individual patient. One of the salient features of all such programs is the insistence on regularity: regularity in the matter of the diet, the quantity of fluids ingested, the amount of exercise indulged in, the duration of rest each day, and the timing of all activities, i.e., regularity of schedule. Another aspect of treatment that is shared in common by all epileptic programs is the use of anticonvulsant drugs, such as those discussed below.

DILANTIN SODIUM. Sodium diphenylhydantoin is an effective anticonvulsant drug, without hypnotic action, which is useful in the control of psychomotor and convulsive seizures alike. The average dose prescribed in adults is between 0.3 and 0.5 Gm. daily, or whatever amount is sufficient to control seizures without producing unpleasant side-effects. If tolerance is exceeded, the patient may experience muscular tremor, double vision, unsteadiness of gait and giddiness. Measleslike eruptions occur in 1 or 2 per cent of the cases, the appearance of which is a signal for discontinuance of therapy, reinstatement of the drug being possible in some patients at a later date. Other complications of lesser significance include dyspepsia, hypertrophy of the gums, drowsiness or mental aberrations of a mild sort, requiring a readjustment of dosage. If adequate doses of the drug are barred because of the occurrence of side-effects, another anticonvulsant, such as phenobarbital or Mesantoin, may be prescribed in addition.

PHENOBARBITAL. Phenylethylbarbituric acid is a valuable anticonvulsant, but it also is a hypnotic, the latter effect limiting its usefulness to a certain extent. The dose required to control seizures in adults varies from 0.06

Gm. to as much as 0.60 Gm. daily. Drug rashes, occurring in allergic individuals, are characteristically of the scarlatiniform variety, which disappear almost immediately on the discontinuance of the drug.

MYSOLINE. Primidone, another derivative of barbituric acid, may be prescribed as a supplement to one of the other anticonvulsant drugs, such as Dilantin, which is without sedative effect. For children the dosage of Mysoline ranges from 0.25 to 0.75 Gm. daily; for adults, these values are doubled.

MESANTOIN. Methylphenylethyl hydantoin is an excellent anticonvulsant drug, and as such may be employed as a substitute for Dilantin or phenobarbital. It is valueless, however, in petit mal epilepsy; it also is prone to cause drowsiness and to provoke allergic responses in its recipients. The usual adult dose ranges from 0.3 to 0.9 Gm. daily.

TRIDIONE. Trimethadione is most effective in cases of petit mal and in the treatment of psychomotor seizures when an anticonvulsant effect also is required; the dose, if inadequate, may be reinforced by the adjunctive use of phenobarbital, Dilantin or Mesantoin. Tridione is prescribed for adults in a dosage of from 0.9 to 1.8 Gm. daily. Side-effects include the development of generalized measleslike rashes, photophobia on exposure to sunlight (hemeralopia) and bone marrow changes, reflected by blood pictures of the leukemoid or aplastic type.

PARADIONE. Paramethadione, similar to Tridione in activity, dosage and effectiveness, occasionally is used in preference to the latter on the grounds of lesser toxicity.

MILONTIN. Phensuximide, given in daily doses of from 1.5 to 3.0 Gm., is indicated and likely to be effective in the occasional case of petit mal epilepsy which has not responded satisfactorily to either Tridione or Paradione.

BROMIDES. Sodium or potassium bromide may be prescribed in doses of from 2 to 6 Gm. daily for the occasional patient who fails to respond to other anticonvulsants. Somnolence, acnelike eruptions, which occasionally produce disfiguring scars, and gastrointestinal symptoms may develop as complications of its use.

OTHER MEASURES. Cerebral stimulants, such as caffeine and amphetamine (Benze-drine Sulfate), occasionally are prescribed in the treatment of petit mal or for the purpose of counteracting the soporific effects of sedative anticonvulsants. Surgery may be undertaken in certain cases of symptomatic epilepsy due to tumors or trauma, anticonvulsant medication still being required, however, in many of these patients postoperatively. Dietary considerations are no longer of importance since the advent of modern anticonvulsant therapy.

Treatment of status epilepticus of the grand mal type obviously entails constant observation of the patient and the employment of whatever measures are required to protect him from exhaustion and self-injury. Convulsions, if extremely violent and uncontrolled by other measures, may be treated by rectal instillations of Avertin with amylene hydrate, an effective dosage being 70 mg. per kilogram of body weight, or by intramuscular injections of sodium phenobarbital (0.2 Gm.) or paraldehyde (2 to 8 ml.), given at 8-hour intervals. Failure of the seizures to subside, despite these medications, is an indication for the induction of general anesthesia with ethyl ether and oxygen mixtures, supplemented, perhaps, with injections of curare to produce muscular relaxation.

Nursing Care

Any patient who could have a seizure should have at all times bed sides in place on the bed and a padded tongue depressor taped to the bed. If a seizure develops, the padded tongue depressor or any soft, firm object is placed between the molar teeth to prevent tongue biting. The head should be protected from striking any hard surfaces, but no attempt should be made to restrain the patient. A major responsibility of the nurse is to observe and to record the march of symptoms. Note should be made of:

1. The first thing the patient does in an attack, where the movements or the stiffness starts, and the position of the eyeballs and the head at the beginning. (In recording, always state whether or not the beginning of the attack was observed.)

2. The type of movements of the part involved

3. The parts involved. (Turn back bed covers and expose patient.)

4. The size of both pupils

5. Incontinence of urine or feces

6. Duration of each phase of the attack

7. Unconsciousness, if present, and its duration

8. Any obvious paralyses or weakness of arms of legs after the attack

9. Inability to speak after the attack

10. Whether or not the patient sleeps afterward

Most seizures are controlled by anticonvulsant medication. Status epilepticus is an emergency disorder and may require general anesthesia to control. The focus of uncontrolled jacksonian seizures may be localized by electroencephalography and the area excised with reasonable success. Removal of the anterior part of the temporal lobe is the present therapy for psychomotor seizures. In children with intractable convulsions cerebral hemispherectomy is done occasionally.

Education. The complete cooperation of the patient and his family is of the utmost importance. They must have confidence in the value of the regimen that is prescribed and must be taught that eventual freedom from seizures, with or without the continued use of an anticonvulsant drug, definitely is to be expected. It also should be emphasized to those receiving continuous medication that the medicine they are taking is not a habit-forming "dope," but can be taken without fear for many years, if necessary, no harm resulting from its use when it is supervised by the physician, provided that the latter's instructions are followed faithfully.

Of all the services that are contributed by the nurse to the care of the epileptic, perhaps the most valuable are her efforts to reorient the attitude of the patient and of his family to the disease itself. Concepts still prevail regarding epilepsy, which reflect all of the ignorance and the brutality that might be associated with the Middle Ages. For other patients there are public sympathy and support in abundance; for the epileptic, abhorrence, rejection, ostracism and legal shackles.

For the average person an epileptic seizure is a terrifying or a repulsive spectacle; for the individual who experiences them, every seizure, therefore, is inevitably a source of humiliation and shame, which in turn breed anxiety, depression, hostility, secrecy and deceit, to which the public reacts with abhorrence, etc., and the vicious cycle is complete. The reaction of shame and the recourse to deceit is not confined merely to the epileptics themselves but extend to their families as well, representing a population of well over 4 million persons in this country alone.

In order to escape from this vicious cycle, epileptics, their families and the public at large need facts. These are the facts:

Epilepsy is not a mysterious disease; it does not reflect the supernatural. The usual case is due to a metabolic disorder, like diabetes. It is not a stigma. Epilepsy is no more disgraceful than diabetes, pernicious anemia or hyperthyroidism. It is not a form of insanity. It does not tend to get worse with time. It

SPACES   LAYERS

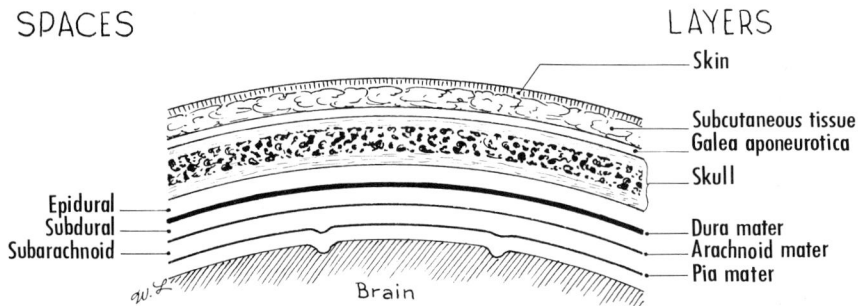

FIG. 366. Diagrammatic drawing showing the various layers from skin to brain. (*Left*) The intracranial spaces are indicated. (*Right*) The various layers of tissue structure.

can be controlled effectively. It should not prevent the child from completing his schooling or keep the adult from work. Activity tends to inhibit, not stimulate, epileptic seizures. Epilepsy is abhorrent to most people because it frightens them; it frightens them because they do not understand it. Understanding of epilepsy is increasing rapidly, and the public is becoming better informed. As knowledge improves, attitudes change, and complete social acceptance of this disease is only a matter of time. Once social acceptance is achieved, epilepsy in the great majority of cases is no barrier to a normal life.*

The nurse should relate this information to the patient and his family in the knowledge that, to whatever extent it is assimilated and believed, their morale as a group and their effectiveness as individuals will be restored.

* Paraphrased from Lennox, W. G., and Markhorn, C. H.: J.A.M.A. 152:1690-1694, 1953.

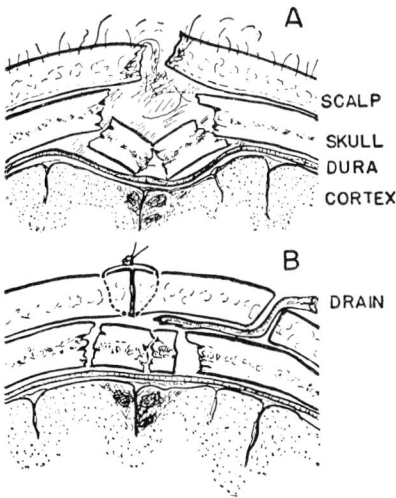

Fig. 367. Diagrammatic drawing showing a depressed fracture of the skull. (A) The fracture has not punctured the dura, but it has caused contusion of the underlying cerebral cortex. (B) Shows the relation of the structures after operation and elevation of the depressed fragment. (Penfield: Canadian Army Manual of Military Neurosurgery, Ottawa, Government Distribution Office)

PATIENTS WITH INJURIES OF THE CENTRAL NERVOUS SYSTEM

Scalp, Skull and Cranial Injuries

Parts of the head which may be injured are the scalp, the skull and the periosteum, the meninges and the blood vessels and the brain itself. (See Fig. 366.)

Scalp Injury. Because of the many blood vessels, the scalp bleeds readily when injured. Trauma may be an abrasion ("brush wound"), contusion, laceration or avulsion. Before such a wound can be cared for properly, an area of about 2 inches should be shaved around the wound. The injection of procaine makes it easier for the surgeon to clean the wound thoroughly and to treat it. If the patient is unconscious, showing evidence of shock, this type of wound is the last to receive attention except for the application of a sterile dressing.

Skull Injury. If there is a depression of cranial bones, the likelihood of increased intracranial pressure is great and must be watched for. When the fracture is compound, the area must be cleansed, débrided and closed as early as possible, because there is the added danger of infection. (See Fig. 367.)

Fracture of the skull is treated as a neurosurgical condition, because the fracture in itself is of less importance than the injury to the brain that may be produced. For this reason every patient with head injury, even though it appears to be slight, should be under the constant observation of a surgeon for several days.

SYMPTOMS. The symptoms, besides those of the local injury, depend on the amount and the distribution of brain injury. Fractures of the vault produce swelling in the region of the fracture, and for this reason an accurate diagnosis cannot be made without a roentgenogram. Fractures of the base of the skull frequently produce hemorrhage from the nose, the pharynx, or the ears, and blood may appear under the conjunctiva. The escape of cerebrospinal fluid from the ears and the nose is a diagnostic sign of importance. Bloody spinal fluid, if present, suggests brain laceration or contusion.

TREATMENT. Depressed skull fractures

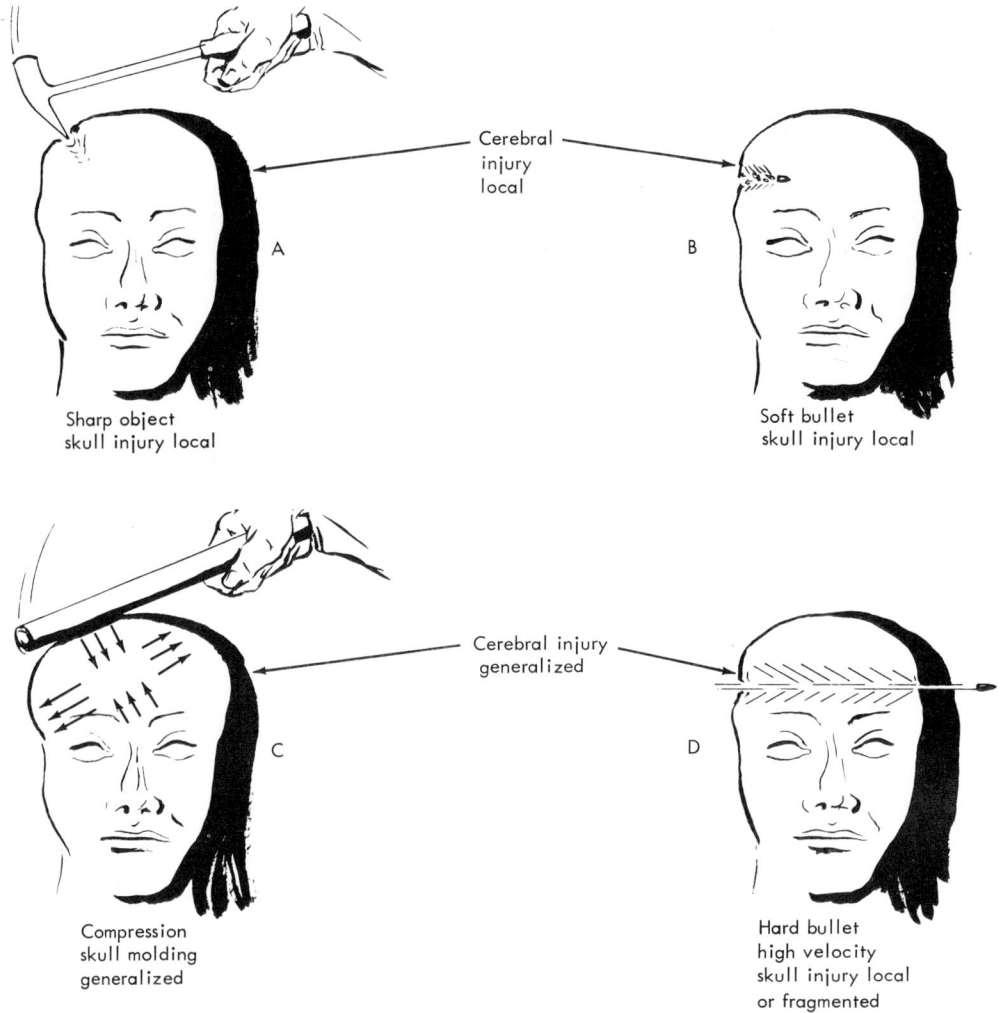

Fig. 368. Compression injury. (A, B) Local cerebral injury—prognosis good. (C, D) Generalized cerebral injury—prognosis grave. (Mullan, S.: Essentials of Neurosurgery, p. 139, New York, Springer)

are treated by operating, after recovery from shock, to reduce the incidence of infection and further brain damage. Foreign bodies and loose pieces of bone are removed.

Bony defects that may result from extensive fractures, from osteomyelitis of the skull or following the removal of tumors involving the skull may be repaired by *cranioplasty*. This consists of the insertion of a substitute material to protect the brain and for cosmetic reasons. Such a substitute may be bone (calf skull), Vitallium, tantalum, acrylate or polyethylene sheeting. There are advantages and disadvantages to each.

Brain Injury. Serious brain injury may occur following blows or injuries to the head, with or without fracture of the skull. When the lesions produced are microscopic, and the immediate symptoms are mild and not of long duration, the condition is spoken of as a *concussion*. The jar of the brain may be so slight as to cause only dizziness and spots before the eyes (spoken of as "seeing stars"), or there may be complete loss of consciousness for a time.

In more marked cerebral injuries (Figs. 368, 370), with bruising of the brain or hemorrhage on its surface, unconsciousness is present for a considerable period. These are spoken of as *cerebral contusions,* and the

Date and Time	Level of Consciousness	Description of Motor and Sensory Involvement	Pupils	Blood Press.	Pulse	Resp.	Temp.	Seizures	Position of Patient	Intake	Output	Other Observations
10/1/6 7 P.M.	SEMICONSCIOUS	MOTOR: No LOCALIZED WEAKNESS. SENSORY: REACTS TO PAINFUL STIMULI.	EQUAL	130/70	70	20	100ᴿ	NONE	SUPINE			
8 P.M.	INCREASING STUPOR	MOTOR: MOVING LEFT EXTREMITIES LESS. SENSORY: UNCHANGED	UNEQUAL WITH RT. SLIGHTLY DILATED	150/90	68	18	101ᴿ	NONE	SUPINE			NEUROSURGEON NOTIFIED
9 P.M.	COMATOSE	MOTOR: PARALYSIS OF LEFT EXTREMITIES. SENSORY: SLIGHT REACTION TO PIN PRICK ON RT. EXTREMITIES.	WIDELY DILATED ON RIGHT. No LIGHT REFLEX.	180/100	54	16	101ᴿ	NONE	SUPINE			TAKEN TO O.R. @ 9:10 P.M.

Name of Patient:	MALLORY, MR JOHN M.	Location of Injury:	LINEAL FRACTURE IN RT. TEMPORAL REGION

FIG. 369. Observation record for patients with neurologic conditions. (Adapted from Sheldon, K. W.: Management of Strokes, Philadelphia, Lippincott)

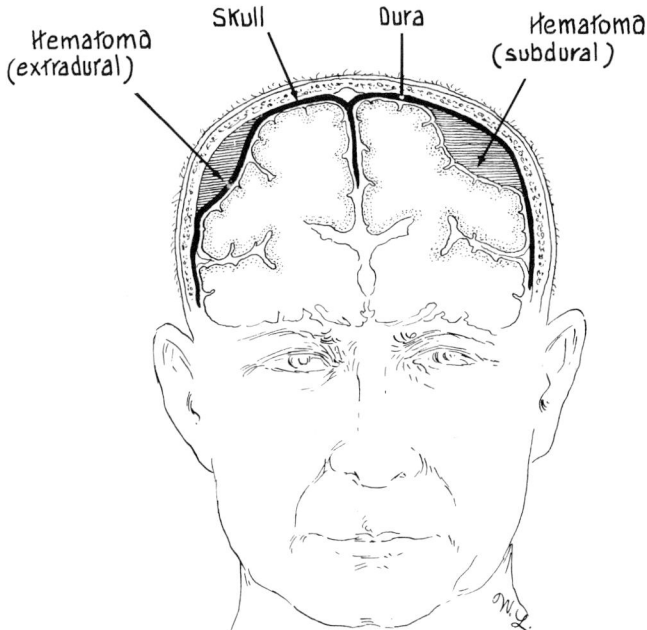

FIG. 370. Diagrammatic views showing the difference in the relations of an extradural hematoma (*left*) and a subdural hematoma (*right*).

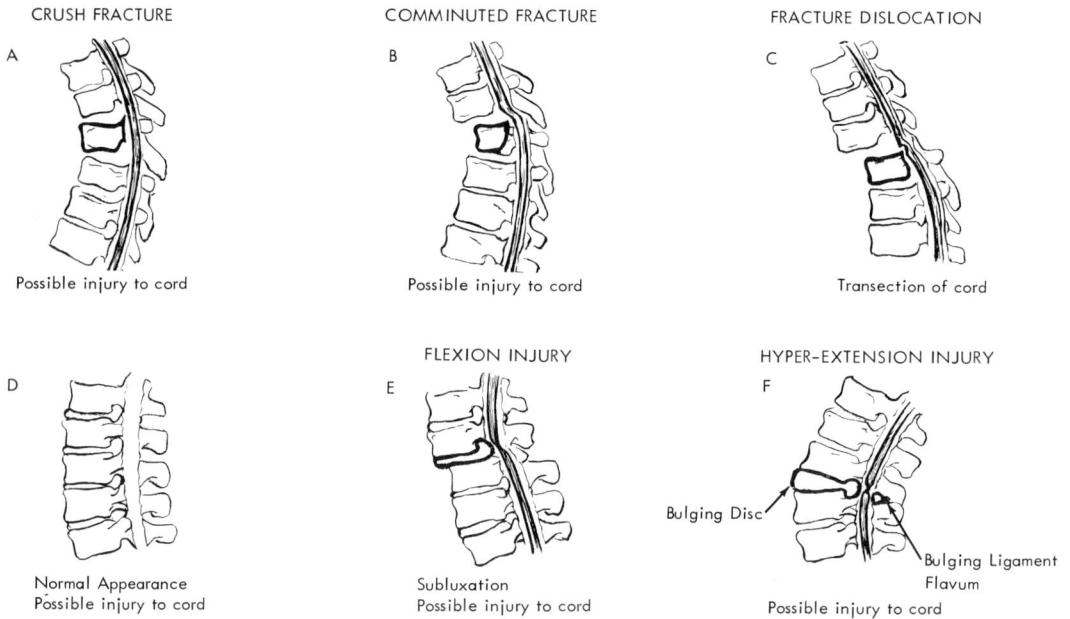

FIG. 371. Vertebral trauma. The radiograph may show: (A) a crush fracture; (B) a comminuted fracture; (C) a fracture dislocation; or (D) a normal appearance. The patient whose radiography looks normal may have had (E) a hyperflexion injury or (F) a hyperextension injury which caused severe cord damage at the moment of the accident. (Mullan, S.: Essentials of Neurosurgery, p. 160, New York, Springer)

symptoms, as would be expected, are more marked. The patient lies motionless with feeble pulse, shallow respiration and pale, cold skin. Often there is involuntary evacuation of the bowels and the bladder. He may be aroused with effort but soon slips back into unconsciousness. The blood pressure and the temperature are subnormal, and the picture is somewhat similar to that of shock. The patient may never recover from this primary state. On the other hand, however, he may recover completely and perhaps pass into a second stage of cerebral irritability. Vomiting is commonly the first symptom indicative of recovery from the stage of primary shock.

In the stage of cerebral irritability the patient is no longer unconscious. On the contrary, he is easily disturbed by any form of stimulation, noises, light and voices, and he may even become maniacal at times. Gradually, the pulse, the respiration, the temperature and the other body functions return to normal. However, recovery is not complete at once. There are commonly residual headache and vertigo and often impaired mentality or epilepsy as a result of irreparable cerebral damage.

Extradural Hemorrhage. In cases of injury to the head, with or without fracture of the skull, rupture of the middle meningeal artery may occur. This artery runs between the dura and the skull, and hemorrhage from it causes pressure on the brain as a clot is formed in this location (Fig. 370, *left*).

The symptoms are characteristic. There is usually a momentary loss of consciousness at the time of injury, followed by an interval of apparent recovery. Then, often suddenly, signs of compression appear, usually with muscular twitchings or convulsions, because the clot presses on the region of the cortex which sends impulses to the muscles (the motor cortex).

TREATMENT. The treatment consists in making an opening through the skull, removing the clot and controlling the bleeding artery.

Subdural Hematoma. Not infrequently, either with or without injury, hemorrhage may take place over the surface of the brain underneath the dura (Fig. 370, *right*). This hemorrhage may give few symptoms at the time that it occurs, but as time goes on, a thick-walled pseudocyst may be formed which causes pressure on the brain surface and may produce very alarming symptoms. This lesion is one that is most amenable to treatment. A simple trephine opening through the skull will permit a puncture of the cystic mass and relief of the pressure that it produces. When this condition occurs in infants, it is possible to do a subdural tap through the coronal suture. The presence of old blood aspirated from this space is diagnostic of hematoma. Subdural hemorrhage may occur at birth due to injury attendant on delivery.

TREATMENT OF SEVERE HEAD INJURIES

1. Place the patient flat in the bed on one side or flat on the abdomen with the head to the side.

2. Oxygen therapy—if rhinorrhea, use oxygen tent; if no rhinorrhea, use oropharyngeal oxygen.

3. Keep nasal and tracheal passageways clear of secretions by aspiration as often as necessary.

4. Turn patient from one side to the other every 2 hours.

5. Temperature (by rectum), blood pressure, pulse and respirations every ½ hour for first 12 hours, and then hourly if signs are stable.

6. For rectal temperatures of 102° or over, start treatment for hyperthermia (see pp. 921-922).

7 Insert indwelling catheter for intermittent bladder drainage.

8. Levin tube feedings (300 ml. every 3 hours).

9. No sedation or morphine derivatives.

10. Frequent neurologic evaluations to be made and recorded. If pupils become unequal, notify neurosurgeon. (See Fig. 369.)

11. For convulsions, give 2 grains of sodium phenobarbital intramuscularly (on physician's order).

Nursing Care. In fractures of the vault an operation always is necessary if the fracture is compound, or if fragments are so depressed as to press upon or be driven into the brain. After shaving the scalp, the wound is cleaned by cutting away the infected and the devitalized tissue. Bone fragments are removed or elevated. A metal or a polyethylene plate can be shaped to fit the opening at a later time.

Fractures of the base are much more serious because of the danger of grave cranial complications and meningitis. The nasopharynx and the external ear should be kept clean, and usually a plug of sterile cotton is placed in the latter channel to absorb discharges. At times repeated lumbar punctures are performed to remove the bloody fluid in an attempt to lessen adhesion formation between the spinal cord and its membranes, which would otherwise occur.

All fractures of the skull should be suspected of brain injury until proved to be otherwise. The nurse must bear in mind that the patient may have other injuries that are masked by his head injury. The successful treatment of this condition falls largely to the nurse. The patient should be placed in bed, often with the head slightly elevated. The initial shock should be treated. Close observation of the patient's temperature, pulse, respirations and blood pressure should be made.

The general treatment consists in absolute mental and physical rest in a cool, darkened room. Absolute quiet should be preserved, including the exclusion of all visitors. During the stage of recovery the patient should be watched very closely for the development of neurologic signs, convulsive movements, spasms or stupor. These symptoms of increased intracranial pressure, including a rise in blood pressure and fall in respiration and pulse, or increasing drowsiness may appear rapidly and should be reported to the neurosurgeon at once.

An icebag may be applied to the head, and sedative drugs may be administered. Every form of stimulation is to be avoided at first, and mental as well as physical rest should be enforced. Reading and even conversation should be resumed very gradually.

Liquid diet should be continued until the danger of complications is past. A limited fluid intake is necessary when signs of increased intracranial pressure are noted. Glucose or sucrose, 25 or 50 per cent, usually is administered intravenously to relieve the pressure, as well as magnesium sulfate by rectal drip.

If the patient is irrational, he should be restrained by physical means only when there is danger that he may injure himself. It is imperative that he be kept quiet, and medications such as Thorazine, chloral hydrate, bromides and barbiturates are given. The nurse should note the urine output; a distended bladder may be the cause for the restlessness.

Following cranial trauma, the patient must be kept constantly in bed for a minimum of 7 to 14 days. The greater the period of rest following the injury the less likely is the occurrence of the so-called posttraumatic syndrome of periodic headache.

Spinal Fractures and Dislocations

Fractures and dislocations of the spine are serious injuries because of the danger of injury to the spinal cord (Fig. 371). They appear most commonly in the neck (cervical region) and the lower back (lumbar region).

Fractures of the Cervical Vertebrae. In fractures of the cervical vertebrae, usually the body is crushed due to hyperflexion of the neck (Fig. 371). Such injuries occur in diving accidents, auto accidents and from being struck on the head by a heavy object. During war gunshot injuries are not uncommon. The danger from cervical vertebral fractures is injury to the spinal cord, which in this area is relatively large, and injury to the spinal cord may produce paralysis of the entire lower body. The injury usually results from crushing the cord by acute hyperflexion of the neck. For this reason the neck must be extended and the head held well back in the position of extension even in the medical emergency mangement of these patients. It is desirable to reduce the fracture as soon as possible to prevent cord damage.

In the treatment of fractures lower down in the spine, hyperextension can be obtained by the use of a Bradford frame or other appliances. In cervical fractures, however, this is not so easy, and some form of weight extension often is used. Leather-covered slings under the chin and the occiput have been used, but they are uncomfortable. More positive traction can be obtained by the use of Crutchfield, Barton or Vinki tongs apparatus. Through small incisions, the short

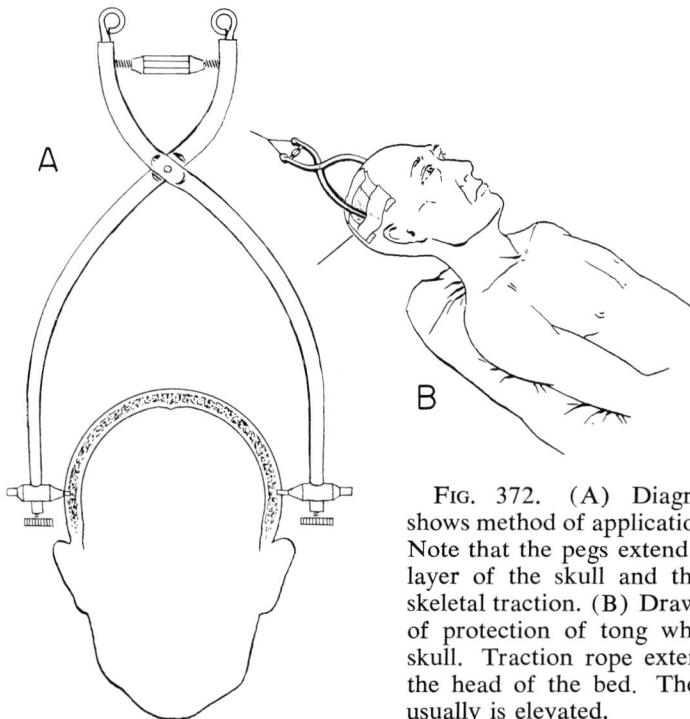

FIG. 372. (A) Diagrammatic drawing shows method of application of skull traction. Note that the pegs extend through the outer layer of the skull and thus produce direct skeletal traction. (B) Drawing shows method of protection of tong when applied to the skull. Traction rope extends over pulley at the head of the bed. The head of the bed usually is elevated.

TURNING A PATIENT WITH CRUTCHFIELD TONGS WHO IS NOT ON A STRYKER FRAME

If a patient has Crutchfield tongs and is not on a Stryker Frame, an order from the physician must be obtained before turning him. The patient's head *never should be flexed,* neither forward or laterally, and at all times should be kept in a direct line with the axis of the cervical spine.

To Turn the Patient:

The nurse supporting the head gives the commands for turning. Place a pillow between the legs of the patient to prevent the upper leg from slipping forward and jarring the patient's head.

Place a pillow longitudinally on the chest, with the patient's upper arm resting on it. The pillow prevents the shoulder from sagging and pulling on the neck as the patient is turned.

Three persons should turn the patient in a log-rolling fashion, making sure that the shoulder turns with the head and the neck. One nurse should support the head; the second nurse or attendant, the shoulders; and the third person, the hips and the legs.

As the patient is turned, the traction should be moved carefully to keep it in direct line with the cervical spine. The patient's position should be adjusted so that the traction, the patient's head and the cervical spine are in correct alignment.

While the nurse still supports the head in the lateral position, a small pillow is placed under the head to maintain cervical alignment.

---

pins of the tongs are inserted through the outer table of the skull (Fig. 372). Traction then can be provided by weight and pulleys. A small longitudinal support is placed between the scapulae, and the head is maintained in a position of extension. With the chest slightly elevated on pillows and the head low, extension can be maintained easily. Extension of the neck is more effective if the head of the bed is raised (countertraction). Usually, 10 pounds of weight are applied at first, and gradually the weights are built up to 30 pounds. The period of traction is about 4 to 6 weeks. Patients with subluxation may have to wear a plaster or a plastic cast for some weeks after the skeletal traction is removed.

Nursing Care of a Patient With a Cervical Vertebral Fracture. In a compression fracture of the vertebral body an attempt is made to restore the normal contour of the spine by a head halter or tongs, to which traction is applied. The head halter is made of heavy canvas or leather and can cause considerable pressure on the skin. Thin, soft padding inside the halter may make it more comfortable for the chin and the ears. For the male patient, it is sometimes possible to obtain the consent of the physician to remove the halter long enough to shave him. (Traction can be maintained by exerting manual pull on the same parts as the halter, e.g., the chin and the occiput.) Care to the back is achieved by pressing down on the mattress with one hand and washing or massaging with the other. Other pressure areas that especially need attention are shoulders, sacrum and heels. Pieces of foam rubber padding placed under the pressure areas will be helpful. If possible, the patient should be turned on his side while he is being fed to minimize the possibility of aspiration of food and fluids. More leeway is permitted in the turning of the patient who has Crutchfield tongs. During this process, the patient must be observed carefully for signs of respiratory impairment.

The foot end of the bed (the patient's head) can be elevated on shock blocks to

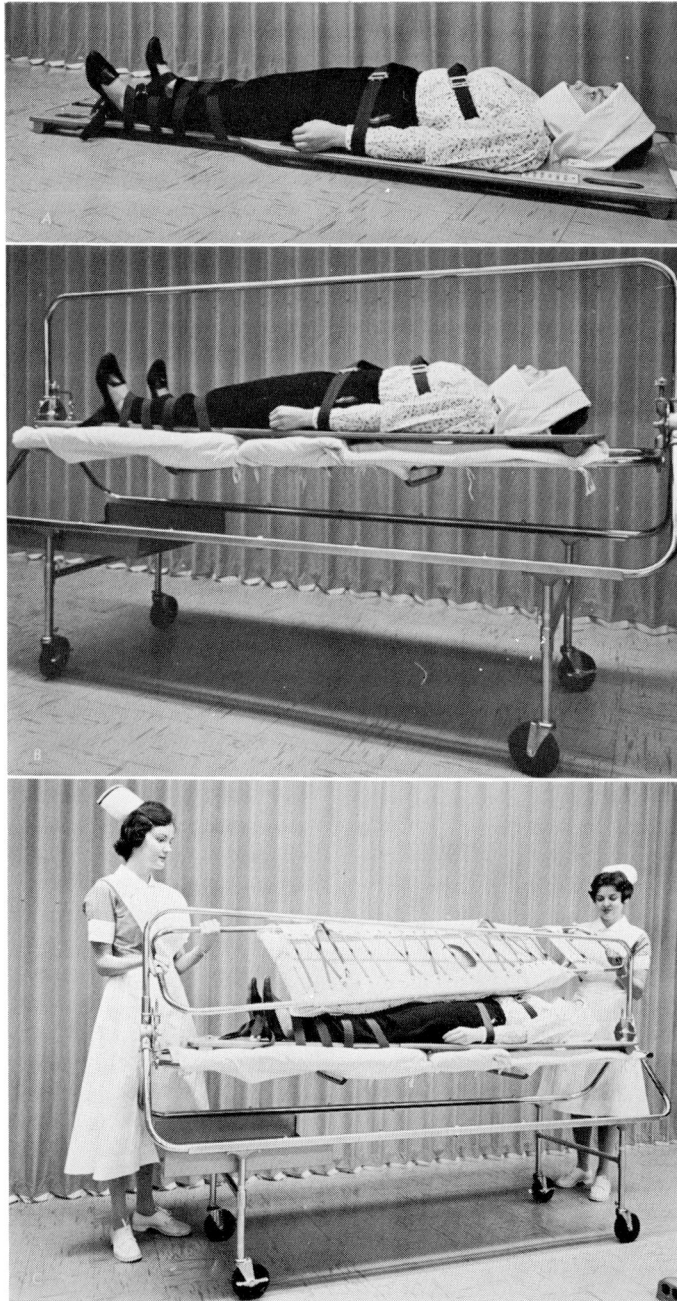

FIG. 373. (A) Position of the patient on a transfer board. Note the bandage that is used to keep the head and the neck in a neutral position. (B) The board is placed on top of the posterior frame. (C) The anterior frame is placed in position. (D) The anterior frame is secured with the frame straps. (E) The frame is turned. Observe the position of the nurses' hands while turning the Stryker frame. (F) The posterior frame is removed; then the transfer board is removed.

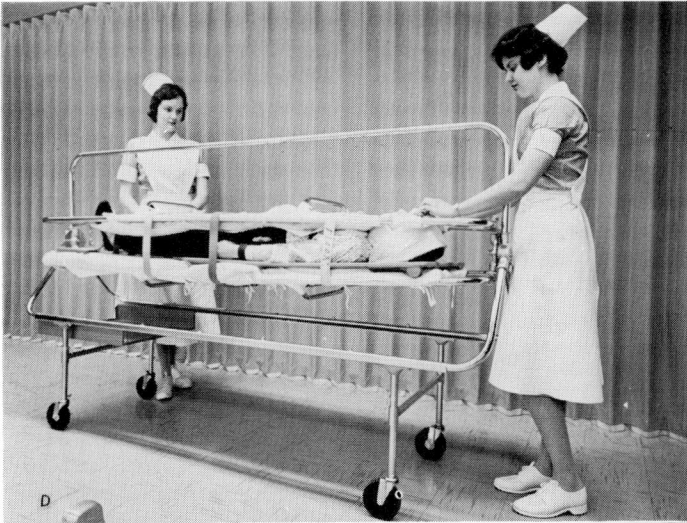

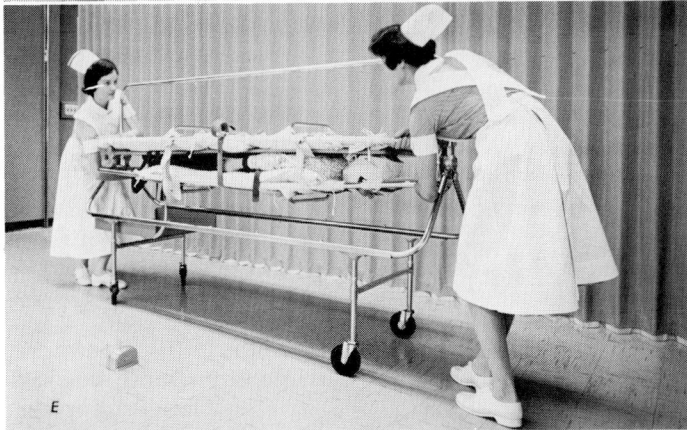

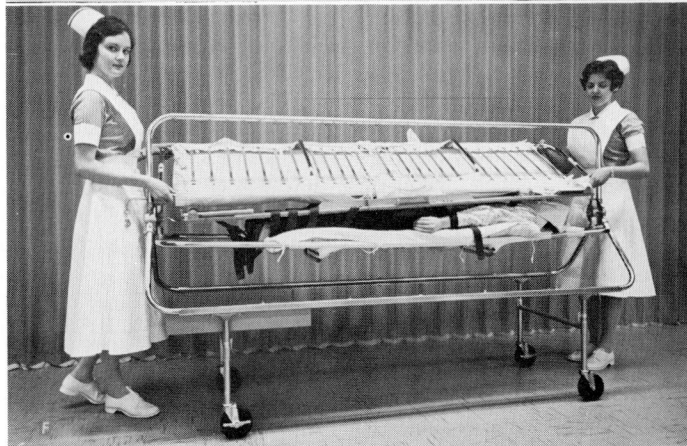

provide countertraction. The nurse must watch for drainage from the stab wounds and for other signs of infection. The back of the head must be checked periodically for signs of pressure; massage will help. All extremities should be put through the normal range of motion several times daily on order of the physician.

The use of the Stryker frame for this patient is an added advantage, inasmuch as the nurse can turn him more easily and administer care more satisfactorily.

Diversional activity provided by the radio, television, visitors, etc., may be helpful. A frame can be made to hold a book conveniently for this kind of patient. Reassurance and patience are essential. The period of time an individual is thus incapacitated varies with the nature of the problem. Often a plastic collar or a Thomas collar is used to replace traction, and greater freedom is permissible.

The Patient With a Spinal Cord Injury.

NURSING DURING THE ACUTE PHASE. *The first aid and later handling of these patients is extremely important, because much damage can be done to the spinal cord by inexpert care.*

At the scene of the accident the patient should be placed in a neutral position (head, back, legs, knees and arms straight). If he is lying in a twisted position, his extremities should be straightened with extreme caution. At least four persons should slide him carefully on a board for transfer to the hospital. Any twisting movement may irreversibly damage the spinal cord by causing a bony fragment of the vertebrae to cut into, crush, or sever the cord completely.

As soon as possible, the patient should be evaluated for motor and sensory changes. Motor ability is tested by requesting the patient to move his toes or to turn his feet. Sensation is evaluated by pinching the skin, starting at the shoulder level and working down both sides of the extremities. He is asked where he feels the pinching sensation. It is necessary to record these findings immediately, so that changes can be evaluated accurately. Edema of the spinal cord can occur with any severe cord injury. The patient must be watched constantly for any indications of motor or sensory loss, and these should be reported immediately.

EMERGENCY MEDICAL MANAGEMENT. During the emergency treatment the patient is kept on the board, and he should remain on it while the x-ray pictures are being taken. The transfer of the patient to a bed presents a definite nursing problem. The patient always must be maintained in an extended position. No part of the body should be twisted or turned; nor should the patient be allowed to assume a sitting position. He should be placed on a Stryker frame when he is ready to be transferred to bed. Later, if it is proved that there is no cord injury, the patient always can be moved to a conventional bed without harm; the reverse, however, is not true. If a Stryker frame is not available, the patient should be placed on a firm mattress (preferably foam rubber) with a bedboard under it.

Figure 373 A to F shows how a patient should be transferred from a board to a Stryker frame. Place the patient who is strapped to the board directly on the posterior frame. Unstrap the patient from the board. Do not remove the head strappings. Place a blanket roll between the legs. Place the anterior frame in position, and secure the frame straps. Turn the frame so that the patient is in the prone position. Remove the frame straps and the posterior frame. Remove the head strapping with care. Then remove the transfer board.

The patient is watched for symptoms of progressive neurologic damage. Symptoms of cord compression depend on the level at which the compression occurs. It may be impossible in the early stages of injury to determine if there has been an anatomic transection of the cord, since the clinical symptoms of cord transection are indistinguishable from those of cord edema. There is a loss of sensation, with complete paralysis of all muscles supplied by the nerves arising from the cord at the level of the lesion and below. Therefore, if the patient has no feeling and is unable to move an extremity, cord compression should be suspected. Some neurosurgeons advocate that a laminectomy be done if this paralysis occurs, as this procedure permits direct exploration and decompression of the cord.

Every patient with a spinal cord injury

must be watched for symptoms of spinal shock. In this condition there is a depression of all the reflexes. The blood pressure falls, and the parts of the body below the level of the cord are paralyzed and without sensation. The reflexes that initiate bladder and bowel function likewise are affected. The patient does not perspire on the paralyzed portions of his body, as sympathetic activity is blocked. Therefore, he must be watched carefully for an abrupt onset of fever. Hyperthermia is treated as outlined on pages 921 to 922. Usually, the acute period of spinal shock is transient, but residual results may linger for a much longer time.

The patient should be watched closely for bladder and bowel distention. Since the patient has no sensation of bladder distention, urinary tract damage can occur at this time. An indwelling catheter is inserted early in the acute phase. The catheter is removed as soon as possible, so that a bladder-training regimen can be started. If the bowel distention is severe, the use of neostigmine methylsulfate (0.5mg.) and intestinal decompression sometimes is indicated.

PREVENTION OF DECUBITUS ULCERS. The patient is very apt to develop decubitus ulcers in areas of local tissue ischemia where there is continuous pressure, and where the peripheral circulation is inadequate as a result of the spinal shock and recumbency. Turning not only aids in the prevention of decubiti but also prevents the pooling of blood and tissue fluid in the dependent areas. The patient should be turned every 2 hours. (If the patient is not on a Stryker frame, a doctor's order is necessary before the patient may be turned.) Every 12 hours the patient's skin should be washed with a mild soap, rinsed well, and *blotted* dry. Sacrum, trochanters, ischia, iliac spines, knees and heels are especially susceptible to pressure. These areas should be kept soft and well-lubricated with an emollient lotion. Massage should be done gently with a circular motion. The linen under the patient must be kept dry. (See pp. 360-361.)

PREVENTION OF DEFORMITIES. The patient must be maintained in proper alignment at all times. It is a nursing function to improvise ways to support paralyzed parts of the body.

The patient is placed in *the dorsal or the supine position* as follows:

The feet are positioned against a padded footboard to prevent footdrop. There should be a space between the end of the mattress and the footboard to allow free suspension of the heels. A wooden block on either end of the mattress will prevent the mattress from pushing against the footboard. Trochanter rolls are applied from the crest of the ilium to the midthigh of both extremities to prevent external rotation of the hip joints.

Due to disuse the patient will undergo atrophy of the extremities. If ordered by the physician, passive range of motion can be started to the affected extremities within 48 to 72 hours after injury. These exercises will preserve joint motion and stimulate circulation. A joint that is immobilized too long will become fixed as a result of tendon and capsule contracture. Toes, metatarsals, ankles, knees and hips should be put through a full range of motion at least 4 and ideally 5 times daily. Range-of-motion exercises can prevent many complications.

If the neurologic examination reveals that the patient has partial cord function, indicating that some nerve units are intact, the patient is not permitted to get up. Activity may produce further injury to the cord. Ambulation activities are scheduled by the neurosurgeon.

Herniation of an Intervertebral Disk (Herniation of the Nucleus Pulposus)

One very distressing complaint is pain in the back. This may arise from various muscular strains or ligamentous sprains, but these usually improve rapidly. Lumbar back pain that persists, is severe, and radiates into the buttock and down the sciatic nerve often is due to pressure on a spinal nerve from a ruptured intervertebral disk.

The intervertebral disk is a cartilaginous plate which forms a cushion between the vertebral bodies. This tough gristlelike material is incorporated in a capsule. A ball-like condensation in the disk is called the *nucleus pulposus*. Incidental to back injury, falls, automobile accidents, lifting strains, etc., the cartilage may be injured. In most cases the

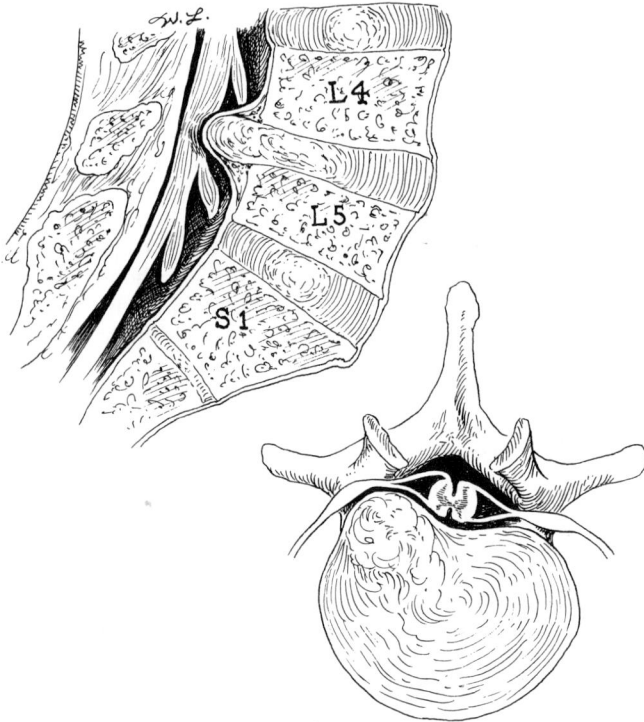

Fig. 374. Diagrammatic drawing shows herniation of the nucleus pulposus. The upper drawing shows how such herniation presses upon the structures of the spinal cord. The lower drawing shows how such herniation may press upon the exit of the spinal nerve and produce pain and other symptoms.

immediate symptoms of trauma are short-lived, and those resulting from the injury to the disk do not appear for months or years. Then with degeneration in the disk, the capsule pushes back into the spinal canal, or it may rupture and allow the nucleus pulposus to be pushed back against the dural sac or against a spinal nerve as it emerges from the spinal column (Fig. 374). This sequence produces pain due to pressure in the area of distribution of the involved nerve. The pain is intensified when the pressure is increased by coughing, sneezing, bending or lifting. Continued pressure may produce degenerative changes in the involved nerve, such as changes in sensation and reflex action. A myelogram will usually demonstrate the area of pressure.

Treatment. This injury may be treated by conservative means, rest in bed, heat and massage, reconditioning exercises, traction, fitted back braces, etc. If this does not give relief, a more direct attack is decided upon, removing the basic pathology. Frequently, an additional stabilizing procedure is added, in which a bone graft from the tibia or the fibula is used to fuse the spinous processes.

The spinal fusion has the purpose of bridging over the defective disk to prevent a recurrence of pain or deformity.

Nursing Care. Preoperative preparation is a shave and a hexachlorophene soap scrub of the back, from the midthorax to the middle of the buttocks. In addition, a leg should be prepared if spinal fusion also is to be done. Most patients possess a fear of surgery of any part of the spine and therefore need assurance and explanations all along the way. The usual preanesthetic drugs are given as ordered.

Postoperatively, the patient's bed is kept flat. There need be no restriction of diet. Frequent turning from side to side relieves pressure, and the change of position is welcomed by the patient (Figs. 375 to 378). He must be reassured that no injury will result from such turning. Sometimes immediately after operation or more often after removal of the sutures, a body cast is applied from the axilla to the groin. This must be inspected for areas of pressure. The patient wears the cast from 6 to 8 weeks and then is fitted for a brace to be worn for an additional 3 to 6 months. Some surgeons keep patients in bed from 6 to 8 weeks in the cast;

others allow them to be up and about, their activities limited only by the cast.

Spinal fusion involves the added danger of a longer procedure carrying the potential of greater shock. The patient has an additional wound and cast of the leg, and it may be several days before he is alert and relatively pain-free. Postoperative care also includes attention to moving the operated leg. Pillows must be adjusted for support and comfort, and care must be taken to avoid sudden flexion and extension at the knee, which cause pain. The recovery period is somewhat slower than in those patients with simple removal of the ruptured portion of the disk, because bony union must take place, which requires 6 to 8 weeks.

Other details of nursing care are similar to those mentioned in the care of patients with spinal cord injuries and tumors.

Spinal Cord Tumors

Tumors within or pressing on the spinal cord cause symptoms that are in effect the same as those caused by fracture of the spine, except that they are slower in development. There is usually sharp pain in the distribution of the spinal roots arising from the cord in the region of the tumor, associated with increasing paralysis below the level of the lesion. The level of the tumor usually may be determined by a neurologic examination; however, myelography is necessary for exact localization.

Operation. The treatment consists in a laminectomy with the removal of the tumor. This operation, in which the spinal cord is exposed, is performed with the patient in the prone position. A median incision is made over the spinous processes, and the soft tissues are separated on each side. These bony projections are removed with large bone-cutting forceps, and the posterior part of the vertebral arch is removed to expose the dura. After obtaining a bloodless field, the dura is incised, and the tumor or clot is removed. The dura then is closed, the soft tissues are sutured over it, and an adhesive dressing is applied.

The Paraplegic Patient

Following injuries or lesions that completely sever the spinal cord, the patient requires extensive rehabilitation which will be less difficult if the preceding nursing measures have been carried out. Nursing care is one of the determining factors in the success of the rehabilitation program.

It is usually some time before the patient comprehends the magnitude of the disability. He may be successively depressed and withdrawn or even hostile and anxious. He is involved in a struggle with himself, and in addition he must meet the strenuous physical demands of the rehabilitation program. Moreover, he may become afflicted with decubitus ulcers, genitourinary infections and calculi, joint pains and muscle spasm. Most of these complications are preventable, and every effort should be made to prevent them, for if they occur, they will delay the patient's rehabilitation.

Weight-bearing Activities. A patient with complete severance of the cord should begin weight-bearing activities early, because no further damage can be incurred. Early standing lessens the opportunity for osteoporotic changes to take place in the long bones. Weight-bearing also diminishes urinary infections and the formation of renal calculi and enhances many other metabolic processes. A tilt table permits the patient to assume this position (Fig. 112). At first the patient may be able to tolerate only an elevation of 45° (or less), but gradually the angle of elevation is increased. The patient should be observed closely for signs of intolerance. These include nausea, perspiration, pallor, dizziness and syncope. The patient's blood pressure is taken before getting him up and as soon as he is positioned on the tilt table, since periods of recumbency favor the development of orthostatic hypotension.

Bladder Training. Immediately after a spinal cord injury the patient is unable to recognize the desire to void because of the interruption of the sensory pathways to the brain. Therefore, the care of the bladder is a major problem to the patient and a challenge to the nurse. There are two major objectives to attain: (1) the prevention of infection of the urinary tract and (2) the preservation of the normal bladder capacity and musculature. There should be meticulous management of the indwelling catheter. Sterile irrigations with an antiseptic solution are done daily to insure patency of the

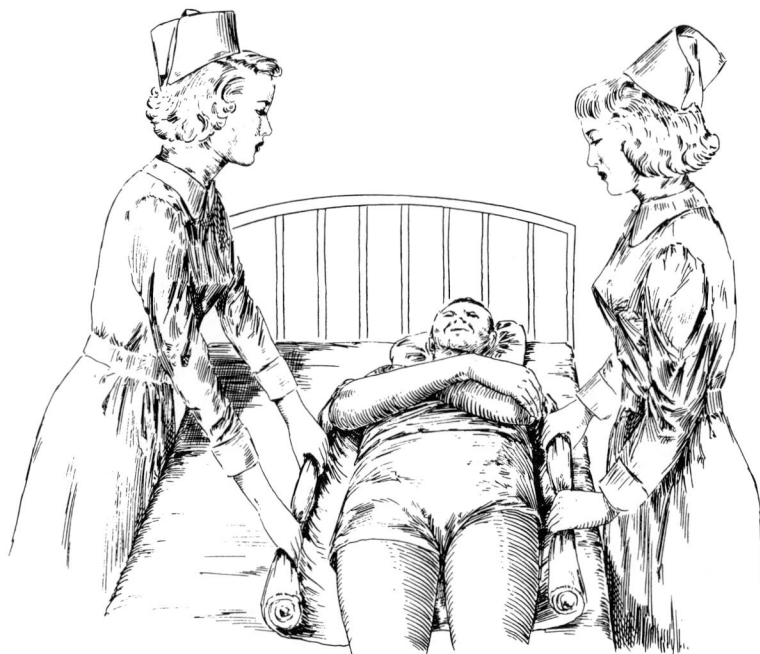

FIG. 375. Method of turning the patient after a laminectomy or a spinal-cord tumor or operation. It is important for the nurse to remember that the patient should be turned as a whole. Two nurses are required to do this. The turning or the draw sheet has been placed on the bed before the patient is put in the bed. Then the patient is positioned in the middle of the turning sheet, with arms folded across his chest. A pillow should be placed between his legs. He should be instructed not to take any part in the turning maneuver. The turning sheet is rolled toward the center from each side by the nurses, and with tension exerted by the nurses' hands on the rolls, the patient is pulled toward the side of the bed. (Redrawn from Gutiérrez-Mahoney and Carini: Neurological and Neurosurgical Nursing, St. Louis, Mosby)

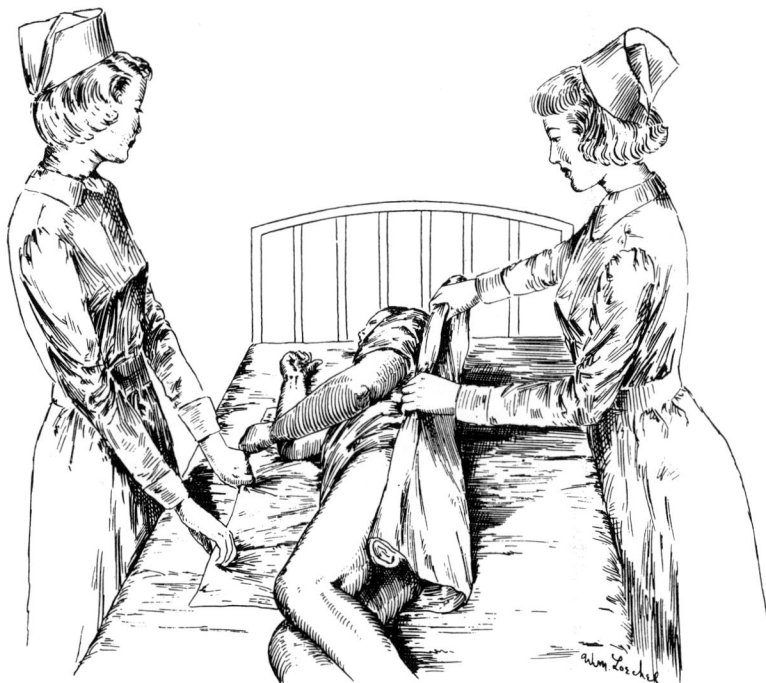

FIG. 376. The patient is rolled on to his right side by the nurse on his left. A pillow should be placed between his legs. The rolling is done by pulling upward on the rolled sheet, rolling the patient over like a log. (Redrawn from Gutiérrez-Mahoney and Carini: Neurological and Neurosurgical Nursing, St. Louis, Mosby)

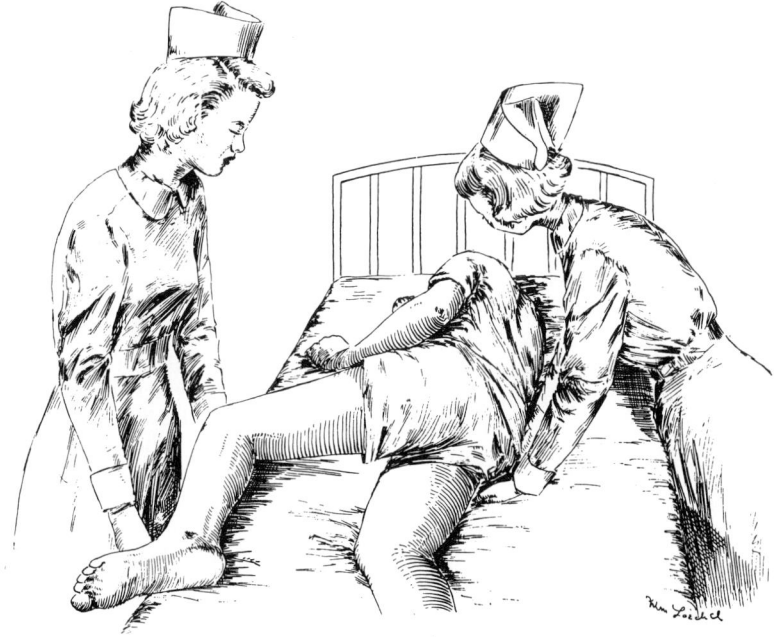

FIG. 377. The patient has been rolled on to his right side, and the nurses are making ready to position him properly in bed. The uppermost leg should be placed on a pillow. (Redrawn from Gutiérrez-Mahoney and Carini: Neurological and Neurosurgical Nursing. St. Louis, Mosby)

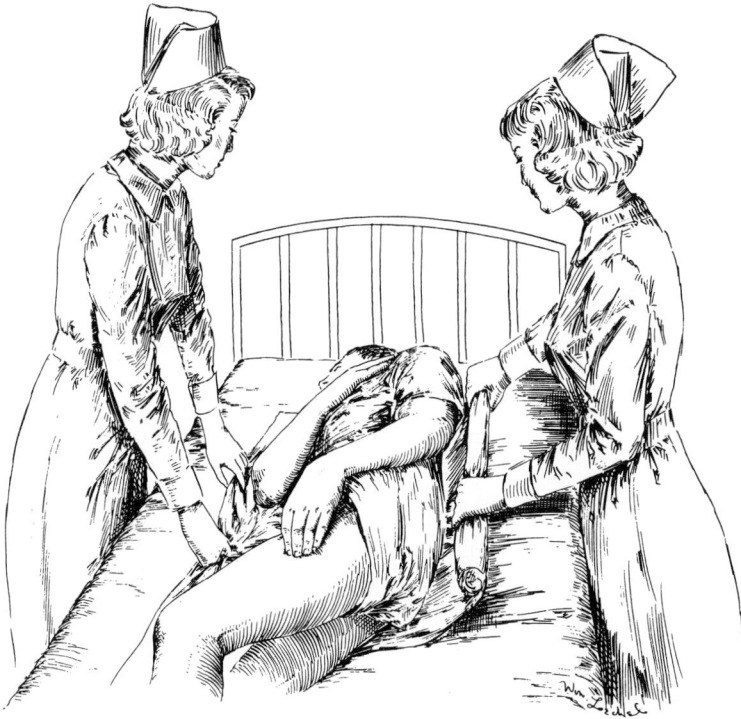

FIG. 378. When it is desired to turn the patient or to place him on his back, the nurse at the patient's back rolls the sheet again and holds it taut while the nurse on the patient's right pulls the sheet so that the patient is rolled again onto his back. (Redrawn from Gutiérrez-Mahoney and Carini: Neurological and Neurosurgical Nursing, St. Louis, Mosby)

drainage system and to minimize bladder infections. Supportive treatment is given with antibiotics or chemotherapy.

It is desirable that a urologic evaluation be obtained before a bladder program is started. Tidal drainage usually is instituted early, as the periodic filling and the emptying of the bladder simulates normal bladder functioning.

This apparatus (Fig. 379) alternately fills the bladder to a predetermined degree of intravesical pressure and then empties it by a combination of siphonage and gravity flow, the siphonage being interrupted when evacuation is complete. Dr. Donald Munro, of Boston, describes this method as follows:

The solution in the 1,000-ml. container flows about 40 to 60 drops per minute into the reservoir. During this filling, air escapes through the air vent. When the reservoir is filled to the level of the horizontal arm of the T tubes, the solution flows through the tubing to the bladder and rises simultaneously in the glass manometer and tubing (a). This continues until the solution, filling both the bladder and tubing, reaches the desired intravesical pressure determined by the height of the curved tubing (a). When the liquid reaches the apex of the curved tube, it begins to flow down into the waste bottle, thereby creating suction, the loop acting as a siphon to empty the reservoir of solution and to drain the bladder of its contents. Since the glass tube in the reservoir is one half the size, or less, of that of the bladder connection, the reservoir empties only one half as rapidly. When the reservoir is emptied, air enters the system through the manometer, thus breaking the siphonage system and starting a new cycle. It will be recognized that the size of the reservoir and the rate of the flow of the solution influence the length of the cycle. The complete cycle is usually regulated to last 2 to 3 hours. The distance of the loop above the bladder determines the maximum pressure to which the bladder is subjected.*

As the patient begins weight-bearing activities, the tidal drainage is clamped off to permit the patient greater freedom. At this time the patient is observed for signs of leakage around the catheter. When the catheter is removed, the patient is cautioned to be alert for any signs that might indicate that his bladder is full, such as perspiration, coldness of hands or feet, feelings of anxiety, a sensation of fullness. He must develop an awareness of this sensation, as it is an indication that he should void. A position that will increase intra-abdominal pressure is necessary to help the patient to void. It is preferable that the patient's feet rest on a flat surface to allow for acute flexion of the hips and the knees. Instruct him to do several "sit-ups" and then to bend forward. This exercise can be followed by light pressure over the bladder. Thinking about the act of voiding while sipping water may be part of the conditioning routine. The bladder should be emptied as completely as possible. This routine should be followed whenever the patient has the sensation to void or according to a schedule set up by the patient. The fluid intake should be at least 3,000 ml.

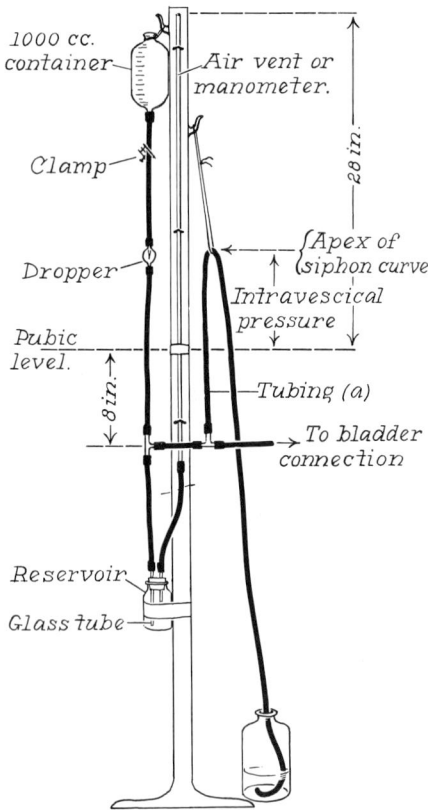

FIG. 379. Munro apparatus for irrigating and emptying the "cord bladder." For instructions as to working of apparatus, see this page.

* Munro, Donald: New Eng. J. Med. **212:**229-239.

daily, and the patient should be instructed to chart his fluid intake and voiding times, so that the pattern of bladder function can be determined. Regularity of routine is the key to the establishment of this habit pattern. The motivation of the patient also determines the success of bladder training. It will be reassuring and encouraging to the patient if the nurse informs him that others have successfully accomplished automatic bladder control.

Gaining Strength for Ambulation. The diet usually is high in protein, vitamins and calories. The unaffected parts of the body are built up to optimum strength, as ambulating with braces and crutches is the ultimate goal for the patient. This requires better-than-normal strength. The muscles of the hands, the arms, the shoulders, the chest, the spine, the abdomen and the neck must be strengthened, since the patient must bear full weight on these muscles. The triceps and the latissimus dorsi are important muscles used in crutch walking. The muscles of the ab-

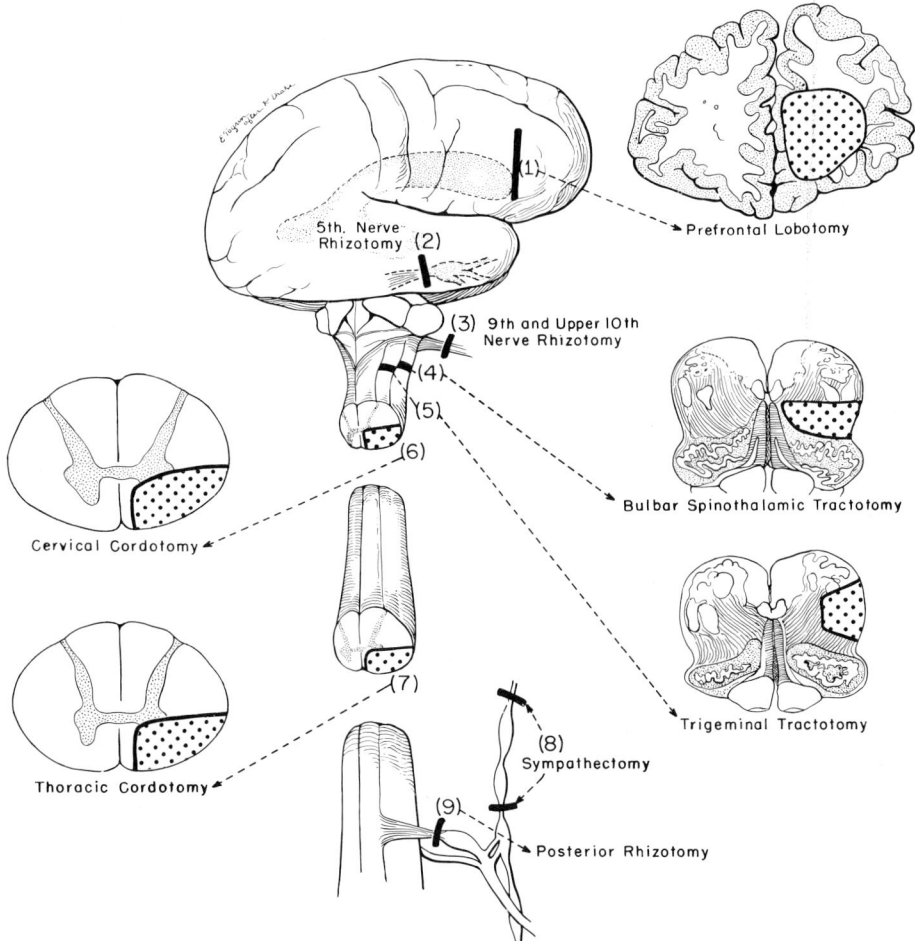

FIG. 380. Sites of standard neurosurgical procedures for relief of pain. The 9th, the 10th and the 11th nerves leave the brain stem along a line dorsal to which lies the descending trigeminal tract (incision 5) and ventral to which lies the crossed pain pathway from the limbs and the torso (incision 4). (Allen, J. G., *et al.:* Surgery: Principles and Practice, p. 1439, Philadelphia, Lippincott)

domen and the back also are necessary for balance and the maintenance of the upright position. To strengthen these muscles, the patient can do "push-ups" when he is in a prone position and "sit-ups" while he is in a sitting position. Extending the arms while he holds weights (traction weights can be used) also will develop muscle strength. Squeezing rubbers balls or crumpling newspaper will promote hand strength. Through the encouragement of all the members of the rehabilitation team, the patient will develop an increased exercise tolerance that is needed for gait training and ambulation activities.

By the application of braces, and with the aide of crutches, these patients can learn to become completely ambulatory and even drive manually operated automobiles. To help the patient to give up his sense of futility and to encourage him in the emotional adjustment that must be made before he is willing to venture into the "outside world" is a role that an intelligent and informed nurse can fill better probably than any other person. She must realize that a too sympathetic attitude may develop a dependence that defeats the purpose of the entire program. She should teach, help when necessary, but not take over activities that the patient can do for himself with a little effort. This type of nursing care more than repays itself in the satisfaction of seeing a completely demoralized and helpless patient begin again to live a happy and a useful life.

THE PATIENT WITH INTRACTABLE PAIN

Intractable pain refers to pain that cannot be relieved satisfactorily by drugs short of drug addiction or incapacitating sedation. Such pain usually is the result of malignancy, but it does occur in many other conditions, such as postherpetic neuralgia, tic douloureux and spinal cord arachnoiditis. Surgery for intractable pain and mental disease involves destroying tissue; therefore, it is resorted to only as a last measure.

Lobotomy

In certain painful states that cannot be relieved by cutting specific nerves or nerve tracts in the spinal cord, it may be necessary to destroy certain pathways in the frontal lobe.

These pathways have to do with the patient's interpretation of the pain. After such a procedure the patient still feels the pain, but the emotional component of pain is eliminated. The pain is there, but it does not bother the patient. The operation is much less popular than it was a decade ago. The problems of rehabilitation are usually very difficult and require almost constant supervision.

The procedure consists of making an opening in the frontal bone and destroying certain areas of the frontal lobe with an instrument, boiling water, or alcohol.

Rhizotomy and Cordotomy

These procedures are used in most instances to relieve intractable pain. In rhizotomy the sensory roots of the spinal nerves are cut before they join the motor root. This procedure is used frequently in controlling the severe chest pain that may be experienced in lung cancer. Cordotomy is the more complicated procedure; the sensory pathway portion of the cord is severed (Fig. 380). This operation is used in controlling severe pain from pelvic cancer. The approach for these operations is the same as for a laminectomy.

Nursing Care. Nursing activities described on page 970 for laminectomy would apply to the postoperative and the rehabilitative requirements of this patient.

It is important for the patient to know what changes in sensation will take place as a result of surgery. The length of the incision for rhizotomy varies directly with the number of nerves to be cut; the incision for cordotomy is relatively small. After operation, the nurse will be on the alert for signs of shock, respiratory distress, bladder disturbances, paralyses and constipation. Since sensations will be limited, the patient may lie in an uncomfortable position and develop pressure sores without realizing it. Those responsible for his care at home must recognize that his sensations are limited. However, this seems to be a small price to pay for freedom from pain.

CLINICAL SITUATIONS
The Patient With a Cerebral Vascular Accident

Mrs. Alice Frazier, an obese 66-year-old woman, was found in an unconscious condition on the street. She was admitted to the hospital with a cerebral vascular accident.

1. Which of the following would be most descriptive of her respirations?
   A. Stertorous.
   B. Cheyne-Stokes.
   C. Rapid and shallow.
   D. Shallow with abdominal retraction.

2. On finding Mrs. Frazier in this condition, the nurse should first
   A. Take her pulse.
   B. Raise her head.
   C. Loosen constricting clothing.
   D. Insure an adequate airway.

3. Mrs. Frazier regained consciousness 12 hours after admission. When should rehabilitation be started on this patient?
   A. On admission.
   B. After she regains consciousness.
   C. When she is ready to ambulate.
   D. On discharge.

4. A fairly common symptom following a lumbar puncture is
   A. Nuchal pain.
   B. Paresthesia of the extremities.
   C. Headache.
   D. Pain in the lumbrosacral area.

5. A lumbar puncture was done on Mrs. Frazier. From which of the following sites is fluid removed in a lumbar puncture?
   A. Dura mater.
   B. Central canal of spinal cord.
   C. Subarachnoid space.
   D. Subperiosteal space.

The Patient With a Craniotomy

When Mr. Rossen became aware that he was listing to one side as he walked, and that he was having visual disturbances, he sought the advice of his physician. The results of a physical and neurologic examination confirmed the suspicion that he had a space-occupying lesion of the brain. After more tests Mr. Rossen submitted to a craniotomy.

1. Mr. Rossen is to have a ventriculogram. This procedure involves
   A. Replacing air in the ventricles with an opaque medium.
   B. Injecting an opaque medium into the main arterial system of the brain.
   C. Replacing fluid in the ventricles with air.

D. Injecting an opaque solution into the spinal canal.

2. Symptoms suggestive of an increasing intracranial pressure are
   A. Increase in blood pressure, increase in pulse pressure, decrease in pulse and respirations.
   B. Falling blood pressure, increase in pulse pressure, increase in pulse and respirations.
   C. Rise in blood pressure, decrease in pulse pressure, slowing of pulse and respirations.
   D. Decrease in blood pressure, increase in pulse pressure, increase in pulse and respirations.

3. Before operation Mr. Rossen had a convulsion. The responsibility of the nurse is to
   A. Try to stop the seizure by slapping him.
   B. Insert a padded tongue depressor between his front teeth.
   C. Cover him with blankets to prevent chilling.
   D. Observe the progression of the seizure and the condition in which it leaves him.

4. The reason that morphine sulfate is contraindicated in this condition is that this drug
   A. Acts as a respiratory depressant.
   B. Relieves apprehension of major surgery.
   C. Masks pupillary signs.
   D. Decreases chances of increased intracranial pressure.

5. Following his craniotomy Mr. Rossen appeared to be going into shock. Without a doctor's order the nurse may
   A. Place him in Trendelenburg position.
   B. Apply hot-water bottles.
   C. Increase the rate of flow of intravenous fluids.
   D. Administer oxygen by mask.

6. While Mr. Rossen is unconscious, desirable body posture can be maintained by
   A. Using a padded footboard to keep each foot in dorsiflexion.
   B. Placing a trochanter roll under the femur of each leg.
   C. Spreading out the fingers and sup-

porting them in this position with a folded bath towel.

  D. Keeping each arm in adduction, using a rolled towel for support if necessary.

7. Psychological rehabilitation is just as important as physical recovery; therefore, it is important to

  A. Remind Mr. Rossen that his persistent bedwetting is unnecessary.

  B. Do everything possible for Mr. Rossen so that his body reserve can be directed toward tissue repair.

  C. Help him to accept slow relearning of walking and talking.

  D. Provide activities for him which are just a step beyond his present abilities.

BIBLIOGRAPHY AND SUGGESTED READING

Books

deGutiérrez-Mahoney, C. G., and Carini, E.: Neurological and Neurosurgical Nursing, ed. 3, St. Louis, Mosby, 1960.

Mullan, S.: Essentials of Neurosurgery, New York, Springer, 1961.

Smith, G. W.: Care of the Patient with a Stroke, New York, Springer, 1960.

Articles

Brain

Baker, E. E., and Sokoloff, M.: Teaching aphasic patients to talk again, Am. J. Nurs. 52:831-832, July, 1952.

Boyce, H. E.: Rehabilitation in multiple sclerosis, Nurs. Outlook 3:549-551, Oct., 1955.

Carini, E., and deGutiérrez-Mahoney, C. G.: Head injuries, Am. J. Nurs. 56:54-58, 1956.

DeJong, R. N.: The treatment of migraine, Am. J. Nurs. 62:67-71, July, 1962.

Dent, D. M.: The nurse and Parkinson's disease, Canad. Nurse 57:40-42, Jan., 1961.

Friedman, A. P., and Merritt, H. H.: Treatment of headache, J.A.M.A. 163:1111-1116, 1957.

Goda, S.: Communicating with the aphasic or dysarthric patient, Am. J. Nurs. 63:80-84, July, 1963.

Hurd, G. G.: Teaching the hemiplegic self-care, Am. J. Nurs. 62:64-68, Sept., 1962.

MacKenzie, M., and Baldwin, M.: Cerebral seizures, Am. J. Nurs. 57:312-316, 1957.

Morgan, M. M., and Denney, M.: Retraining after a prefrontal lobotomy, Am. J. Nurs. 55:59-62, 1955.

————: An understanding approach to the aphasic patient, Am. J. Nurs. 61:51-55, Apr., 1961.

Morrissey, A. B.: Rehabilitation in hemiplegia—major nursing functions, Am. J. Nurs. 62:58-61, Sept. 1962.

Mullan, J. F., and vanSchoick, M. R.: Intractable pain, Am. J. Nurs. 58:228-230, Feb., 1958.

Peszcynski, M.: The rehabilitation potential of the late adult hemiplegic, Am. J. Nurs. 63:111-114, April, 1963.

Pirnie, F. A., and Baldwin, M.: Observing cerebral seizures, Am. J. Nurs. 59:366-369, Mar., 1959.

Potanos, J., Pool, J. L., and Gleason, A. M.: Cerebral edema, Am. J. Nurs. 61:92-94, Mar., 1961.

Raney, R. B.: The minor concussion, Am. J. Nurs. 57:1444-1445, 1957.

Reeves, E. W.: The aphasic patient, Nurs. Outlook 11:522-524, July, 1963.

Rupp, C., Jr.: Management of epilepsy, J.A.M.A. 166:1967-1970, 1958.

Schumacher, G. A., and Palmer, M. E.: Multiple sclerosis, Am. J. Nurs. 57:751-755, 1957.

Smith, G. W.: A stroke is not the end of the world, Am. J. Nurs. 57:303-305, 1957.

Taufic, M.: Rehabilitation after craniotomy, Am. J. Nurs. 58:61-63, 1958.

Tollefsrud, V. E.: When the patient has chemosurgery, Am. J. Nurs. 59:1414-1416, Oct., 1959.

Turner, G. E.: The cerebral vascular accident patient, Nurs. Outlook 8:326-330, 1960.

Waltus, M. E.: Surgical procedures in the x-ray department, Am. J. Nurs. 57:623-624, 1957.

What is stroke? Nurs. Outlook 7:281, May, 1959.

Wylie, C. M.: Delay in seeking rehabilitation after cerebrovascular accidents, J. Chron. Dis. 14:442-451, Oct., 1961.

Spinal Cord

Brave man fights on, pictorial account of rehabilitation of Roy Campanella, fracture of cervical vertebra, Life Magazine, pp. 82-92, July 21, 1958.

Howorth, M. B.: Fracture of the spine, Am. J. Surg. 92:573-593, 1956.

Janes, J. M., and Stifter, R.: Spinal fusion, Am. J. Nurs. 55:1062-1065, 1955.

Martin, J., and Craig, I.: The early care of patients with injury of the spinal cord, Am. J. Nurs. 55:936-939, 1955.

Martin, M. A.: Nursing care in cervical cord injury, Am. J. Nurs. **63**:60-66, March, 1963.

Morrissey, A.B., and Sherman, N.: The tilt board—an aid to rehabilitation, Am. J. Nurs. **56**:1146, 1147, 1956.

Pasternak, S.: The patient with a ruptured disk, Am. J. Nurs. **62**:77-80, Feb., 1962.

Patient-Teaching Aids and Information*

Headache

Headache—Hope Through Research, a comprehensive pamphlet, Pub. Health Service Pub. No. 905, Washington 25, D.C., 1962.

Bladder and Bowel Training

Rehabilitation Monograph III: A Bladder and Bowel Training Program for Patients with Spinal Cord Disease. Edith Buchwald, Margaret McCormack and Emilie Raby, June, 1952; pub. by Institute of Physical Medicine and Rehabilitation, New York University-Bellevue Medical Center, New York, N. Y.

Cerebrovascular Accidents and Strokes

Little Strokes. A 15-page pamphlet, Pub. Health Service Publ. No. 685, Washington 25, D. C., 1959.

Strike Back at Stroke. A 37-page well-illustrated and informative booklet, Pub. Health Service Publ. No. 596, U. S. Dept. of Health, Education, and Welfare, Div. of Chronic Diseases, Washington 25, D. C.

Strokes, A Guide for the Family. Available from the American Heart Association.

Hemiplegia and Paraplegia

California Paralyzed Veterans Association: Paraplegia and You, Long Beach, California, 49 pp. A booklet for the paraplegic or the quadriplegic patient who is living at home and responsible for his own care.

Management of the Patient with Hemiplegia. A 32-page manual for those responsible for the care of hemiplegic patients. Distributed by Health Education Service, P. O. Box 7283, Albany 1, New York. This was produced by the New York State Dept. of Health, 1955.

Patient Publication No. I: Primer for Paraplegics and Quadriplegics. Published by Institute of Physical Medicine and Rehabilitation, New York University-Bellevue Medical Center, New York, N. Y., 1957.

* Complete address given in Appendix. Those publications listed as Public Health Service Publication No. —— are available from the U.S. Government Printing Office, Washington 25, D. C.

Rehabilitation Manual for Hemiplegia, The Kessler Institute for Rehabilitation, West Orange, New Jersey.

Multiple Sclerosis

Multiple Sclerosis Booklet. An informative booklet produced by the National Multiple Sclerosis Society, 1961.

Multiple Sclerosis, Hope through Research, Pub. Health Service Publ. No. 621.

Parkinson's Disease

Exercises for the Parkinson Patient. A pamphlet prepared by Lewis J. Doshay and Samuel B. Feitelberg, National Parkinson's Foundation.

Parkinson's Disease, Hope through Research, Pub. Health Service Publ. No. 811, 1961.

Speechless

Lessing, W. W.: Silent Spokesman—an aid to the speechless, published by Hospital Topics, 30 W. Washington St., Chicago 2, Ill.

Taylor, M. L.: Understanding Aphasia. Available from Institute of Physical Medicine and Rehabilitation, New York University-Bellevue Medical Center, 400 East 34th Street, New York 16, N. Y.

Voluntary Agencies

The Epilepsy League
130 North Wells Street
Chicago, Illinois

National Epilepsy League, Inc.
208 North Wells Street
Chicago 6, Illinois

National Multiple Sclerosis Society
257 Fourth Avenue
New York 10, N. Y.

National Parkinson Foundation, Inc.
135 East 44th Street
New York 17, N. Y.

Parkinson's Disease Foundation
125 East 50th Street
New York 22, N. Y.

United Epilepsy League
226 East 67th Street
New York, N. Y.

United Cerebral Palsy Association
369 Lexington Avenue
New York 17, New York

ORIENTATION

A perusal of this chapter should impress the nurse with the importance of the social and the economic factors that revolve about the disorders of the musculoskeletal system. The crippling effect of these diseases and their chronicity have far-reaching implications from the standpoint of the convalescent care and the rehabilitation of persons who are afflicted.

The word *orthopedia* is derived from two Greek words meaning "straight" and "child." The original scope of this branch of surgery was very narrow, being restricted, as the name implies, to the care of deformed children. With the advent of asepsis, roentgenography and skillful manipulation, orthopedics has become a highly specialized but much broader branch of surgery. Today orthopedics has to do with the cause, the prevention and the correction of deformities of all the apparatus of locomotion, and in some localities it embraces bone and joint diseases, as well as fractures.

42

Patients With Musculoskeletal Problems

MUSCULOSKELETAL STRUCTURES AND FUNCTIONS

The musculoskeletal system, composed of bones, muscles, cartilage, ligaments and fascia, provides the body with its structural framework, its protective casing, its power plant, its power tools, its weapons of combat, its static stability, its means of locomotion and a great deal else besides. It is made up of many bones, attached to each other by strong ligaments at the joints. The ends of the bones are provided with smooth coverings of cartilage where they articulate with each other. At other sites, where flexibility instead of rigidity is desirable, cartilage is found instead of bone. Thus, cartilage is found as part of the framework of the nose and the rib cage and as a cushion between the vertebral bodies.

The bony framework can act as a support and a protective mechanism for body organs; also, it can move, because the bones have attached to them a system of motor muscles that are fastened by strong fibrous cables called *tendons*. The muscles act as motors by reason of their ability to contract (shorten) and to relax (lengthen) under the control of nerve impulses arising in the cerebral cortex. The power of muscles permits the bones to act as levers with the joint as a fulcrum, to rotate with the joint as an axis, or to remain in a fixed position. In most places in the body the muscles are so placed as to have one set acting as antagonist to the other group; thus, the biceps flexes the forearm on the upper arm, whereas the triceps extends it. The muscles are divided and surrounded by strong fibrous envelopes called *fascia*. In the extremities they surround and give support to the main blood vessels and nerves.

The joints have a smooth lining called *synovium;* this secretes a synovial fluid that lubricates the joints to prevent friction. At points where muscles glide over bony prominences, e.g., the greater trochanter of the femur, or where one bone glides under another, as at the shoulder, or where skin glides over a bony point, as at the elbow, nature develops a gliding mechanism called a *bursa,* a closed cavity in the *areolar tissue.*

The smooth working of this complex system is dependent on all parts functioning normally and together.

PATIENT PROBLEMS AND NURSING SOLUTIONS

Psychosocial Problems

The patient with a musculoskeletal condition faces not only physical problems but also psychological and social problems. The nurse must be able to meet the needs and to help to solve the problems of patients who cannot engage in normal activities. Orthopedic patients are of all ages; economic problems usually are present. Protracted periods of disability are especially threatening to the wage earner, and the patient may develop a hopeless attitude toward his illness. Many patients faced with long disability are in need of physical, emotional and spiritual rehabilitation.

To meet the patient's psychological needs, it is desirable to keep him busy. "Action absorbs anxiety" is a rehabilitation axiom that is doubly true in orthopedic nursing. A patient receives security and a sense of purpose when he is participating in a regularly scheduled program of activity. This schedule should be written on the nursing care plan so that all nursing personnel know the patient's program. If possible, the patient should engage in an exercise regimen. Occupational therapy that has been designed with the patient's problems in mind is beneficial. During rest periods the patient may read, watch television or listen to the radio. If the patient is completely immobilized, he still should be consulted about his preferences and encouraged to make some decisions relative to his activities of daily living.

Muscle Spasm

These cramps commonly interrupt the sleep of bedfast patients who are elderly and arteriosclerotic. Pain, often intense, is the result of strong involuntary muscular contractions that may be sustained for several seconds or several minutes. The calf muscles are involved most frequently, the effect of their contraction being a forcible extension and inversion of the foot and the plantar flexion of the toes. There is no certainty regarding the precise mechanism responsible for these abnormal contractions; the phenomenon apparently is attributable to an impairment of the blood supply to the lower extremity due to the mechanical compression of the popliteal or the posterior tibial artery or a major branch of those vessels supplying arterial blood to the affected muscles. As a result of deficient oxygenation, these muscles become abnormally susceptible to nerve stimuli and contract with maximal vigor in response to the weak discharge that is received constantly via the motor nerves, a discharge that normally excites a steady but minimal contractile response described as muscle "tone." If such is the case, the cramp represents a terrifically exaggerated muscle tone.

The development of this complication is favored by any posture that permits pressure to be exerted in the region of the popliteal space, behind, immediately proximal or distal to the knee. The prolonged application of such pressure normally provokes sufficient discomfort in the calf muscles to compel an individual, unless deeply asleep, to shift position and thereby to relieve the compression, but individuals with sensory disturbances may be incapable of perceiving this premonitory discomfort. The patients most susceptible to repeated muscle cramps are those with advanced arteriosclerosis whose leg muscles are weak, flaccid and reduced in volume following prolonged immobilization in bed rest, and in whom ischemia of the calf muscles is produced readily as a result of external compression, particularly following sedation, when ischemic pain is not perceived quickly.

Treatment. Prompt relaxation of a muscle cramp is achieved through "reflex inhibition," i.e., by vigorously contracting the opposing muscle group. If, for example, the cramp involves the muscles of the calf, relief is obtained by forcibly elevating the foot and the toes into a position of dorsiflexion, simultaneously pressing downward on the dorsum of the foot with the heel of the opposite foot, so that the ankle on the affected side is held at an angle of approximately 90°, a procedure that automatically inhibits the transmission of all motor nerve impulses to the spastic muscles. Massage of the cramped muscles helps to restore the circulation of blood to these anoxic tissues; massage should be performed in conjunction with the maneuver just described or as an alternative measure when reflex inhibition is impossible.

Nursing Care and Prevention. Preventive measures to be undertaken for patients exhibiting an abnormal susceptibility to leg cramps include frequent rearrangement of the patient's position and adjustment of the bed in such a manner as to ensure an even distribution of pressure on the undersurface of the leg, compression of the popliteal space being avoided by slight flexion of the knee. Sedatives and soporifics should be curtailed to a minimum, or if their use is necessary, their dosage should be barely sufficient to induce sleep. Protective bed clothing should be adequate to prevent chilling without imposing excessive weight on the legs, a bed cradle being employed, if necessary, to eliminate its pressure and immobilizing effect on the lower extremities.

Benign muscular cramps usually are prevented by the ingestion of 0.2 Gm. of quinine sulfate on retiring. Myanesin, 250 mg. at bedtime, is reportedly as effective as quinine and is without known hazard, whereas sensitivity to quinine is not uncommon. Moreover, quinine is contraindicated during pregnancy when susceptibility to cramps is notoriously great.

The primary objective in preventive therapy, however, is the avoidance of ischemia through the application of appropriate nursing principles and not merely the abolition by chemical means of its manifestations.

Pain

Most patients with diseases and traumatic conditions of muscles, bones and joints experience pain. Bone pain is characteristically described as aching and boring in nature whereas the patient suffering from muscular pain states that he is "sore and aching." Because orthopedic conditions require long periods of treatment, the management of the patient with pain is important.

Prolonged pain consumes energy, and the patient in pain has a tendency to become self-centered and dependent. The patient should sense that he is important as a person, and that his problems are understood by the members of the health team. The nurse should observe the patient carefully to evaluate the effect of the physical, the emotional and the social factors that may be present. What was the patient doing before he complained of pain? Is his body in proper alignment? Is there pressure from traction, bed linen, a cast or other appliances? Is he overly tired from lack of sleep, exciting stimuli or too much activity? Can he localize the pain? How does he describe it?

Regardless of the cause, the presence of pain is exhausting, and every nursing measure should be directed toward its relief. The patient should be positioned skillfully in correct alignment. Painful parts of the body should be supported, and the patient should be moved gently with coordinated movements. Use of a turning sheet can prevent uneven painful pulling on the patient. Care should be exercised not to bump the bed, as this greatly increases discomfort. Provision is to be made for the patient to have regular periods of rest, as this is important in the control of pain.

Heat may prove to be beneficial in relieving muscle spasm, joint and bone pain. Analgesics are given when necessary, but symptoms of physical or psychological tolerance should be watched for and evaluated. Since pain always is worse at night, sedatives, soporifics and ataractic drugs may be of value. Of course, the administration of backrubs and warm drinks, and the presence of a sympathetic, understanding nurse are all adjunctive measures in the management of pain.

Contracture Deformities

It is the aim of orthopedic nursing to prevent contracture deformities and to maintain as much normal function as possible. Pain and muscle spasm produce limitation of motion. Inflammation also limits the motion of a joint and causes the formation of fibrous tissue that in turn may produce fibrous or bony ankylosis. Any weight-bearing joint that has its normal motion restricted will become deformed. Muscle spasm occurring in the strong flexor muscles will cause these muscles to shorten, as flexor muscles are stronger than extensors. The patient is unable to extend his extremities, and thus crippling flexion deformities result.

Positioning. To prevent muscle contractures and loss of joint function the nurse must position the patient in accordance with correct principles of body alignment. His mattress should be firm or placed on a bed board. The bed should be flat, unless otherwise ordered. To keep the patient in a semi-upright position for prolonged periods of time is highly undesirable; this position promotes flexion deformities of the hip. The nurse should exercise ingenuity in the use of supportive devices, such as pillows and sandbags. (Correct positioning in bed is exemplified in Figs. 359 A to 359 C.)

Muscle Exercises

If a patient becomes inactive as a result of trauma, infection, paralysis or any other cause, the musculature loses strength, joint mobility becomes restricted, and deformities are likely to ensue. To avoid these complications the physician prescribes therapeutic exercises that may be performed under the guidance and with the assistance of the physical therapist or the nurse. The nature and the objectives of the exercise program are dictated by the patient's disease and his general condition. Exercises, properly performed, help (1) to maintain or to improve muscle strength, (2) to maintain or to restore optimum joint function, (3) to prevent deformities, (4) to stimulate circulation and (5) to build endurance.

For a detailed treatment of Static, Passive and Active Exercises, Range-of-Motion Exercises, and Passive Range-of-Motion Exercises Adapted for Nursing (Table 14), see pages 352 to 359 of Chapter 21.

PATIENTS WITH MUSCULOSKELETAL TRAUMA

Basic Problems and Objectives

Injury to one part of the system usually produces injury to other parts and to the structures enclosed or supported by them. If the bones are broken, the muscles cannot function; if the nerves do not send impulses to the muscles, as in paralysis, the bones cannot move; if the joint surfaces do not articulate normally, neither the bones nor the muscles can function. Thus, a fracture also produces injury to the muscles surrounding the injured bone and to the blood vessels and the nerves in its vicinity.

Treatment of Injury. In the treatment of injury to the musculoskeletal system, support is provided the injured part until nature has time to heal it. Support may be accomplished by bandages, adhesive strapping, splints or plaster casts, applied externally. In some patients support may be applied directly to bone in the form of pins or plates. In others it may be necessary to correct deformity and to overcome overlapping by weight-traction.

After the immediate and the painful effects of the injury have passed, consideration must be given to the prevention of fibrosis and the resulting stiffness in the injured muscles and the joint structures. Active function, i.e., use of the part by the patient, is the best form of treatment to guard against this disability. In some cases the support applied may permit active function almost from the start. In other cases the nature of the injury may not permit function, and even in those cases in which partial function is possible, we may aid nature in the healing process and hasten recovery of function by various forms of physical therapy.

Contusions, Sprains and Dislocations

Contusions. A *contusion* is an injury to the soft tissues, produced by blunt force (a blow, kick, fall, etc.). There is always some hemorrhage into the injured part (ecchymosis), due to the rupture of many small vessels. This produces the well-known discoloration of the skin (black-and-blue spot), which gradually turns to brown and then to yellow, until it finally disappears as absorption becomes complete. When the hemorrhage is sufficient to cause an appreciable collection of blood, it is called a *hematoma*.

The local symptoms (pain, swelling and discoloration) are easily explained.

Treatment consists of elevating the affected part and applying moist or dry cold for the first 8 or 10 hours. Pressure in the form of an elastic or an elastic adhesive bandage also is of distinct value in reducing hemorrhage and swelling. When the hemorrhage has stopped, moist or dry heat and massage promote absorption, thus hastening the cure.

Sprains. A *sprain* is an injury to the ligamentous structures surrounding a joint, caused by a wrench or a twist. As is the case with contusions, ruptures of blood vessels occur, with a resultant rapid swelling, due to the extravasation of blood within the tissues. The movement of the joint becomes painful. To be certain that there is no bone injury, all these patients should have an x-ray examination.

The treatment is the same as that recommended for contusions. Some physicians reduce the swelling by the immediate application of tight adhesive strappings, which are renewed every few days until the swelling and the pain have disappeared.

Dislocations. A *dislocation* of a joint is a condition in which the articular surfaces of the bones forming the joint are no longer in contact. Dislocations may be (1) congenital (present at birth, due to some maldevelopment, most often noted at the hip); (2) spontaneous or pathologic, due to disease of the articular or the periarticular structures and (3) traumatic, due to injury, such as the application of force in such a manner that the capsule of the joint is torn.

SYMPTOMS. The cardinal symptoms of a dislocation are four in number: (1) change in contour of the joint, (2) change in the length of the extremity, (3) loss of normal mobility, (4) change in the axis of the dis-

FIG. 381. Roentgenogram, showing greenstick fracture of both bones of the forearm.

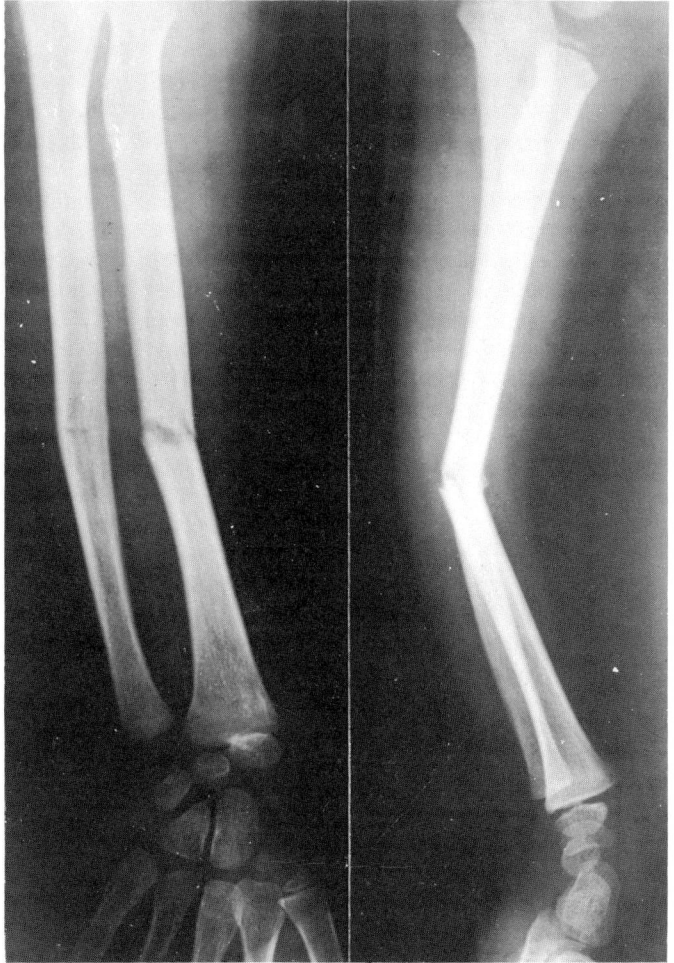

located bone. Roentgenograms will confirm the diagnosis and should be made in every case because not infrequently there is an associated fracture.

TREATMENT AND NURSING CARE. Irreparable damage can result when someone who is not trained attempts to reduce a dislocation. Immobilization of the part is the best first-aid procedure before medical aid is obtained.

Reduction of a dislocation usually is performed under general anesthesia. The head of the dislocated bone is manipulated back into the joint cavity, and the joint is immobilized by bandages and splints for 3 or 4 weeks.

The nursing care following reduction of dislocations is essentially the same as that following the reduction of fractures. The part must be kept immobilized for a sufficient time to permit the ligamentous structures about the joint to heal. Therefore, splints and casts are the usual dressings. The nurse must watch for the complications that are common to such appliances, such as constriction due to tight dressings producing venous and, sometimes, even arterial obstruction. The cyanosis, the pain and the disturbance or the loss of sensation should be familiar to the nurse, who should immediately notify the surgeon. Attention must be paid to the slightest complaint of the patient. The nurse must watch for signs of pressure, both within and outside the immobilization dressing.

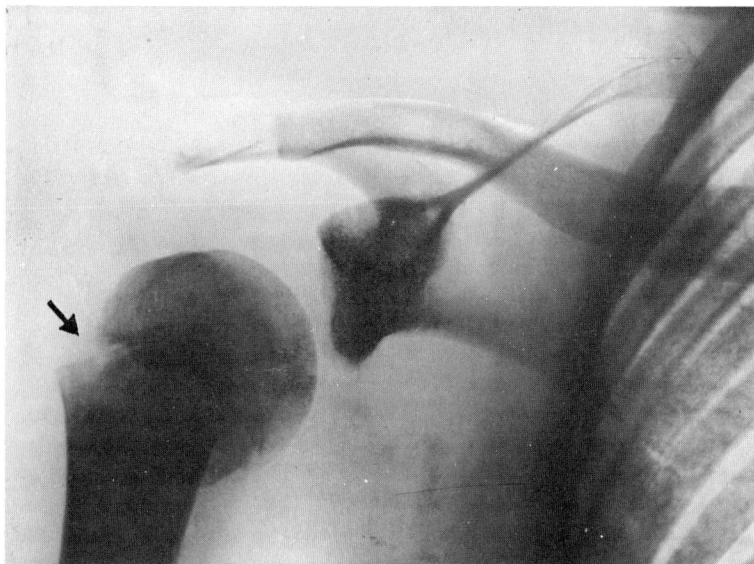

Fractures

Orientation. Any break in the continuity of a bone is called a *fracture*. The break may be *incomplete,* only a line or fissure in the bone, as frequently found in fractures of the skull. It may extend only part way through the bone, splintering the fibers on one side and bending them on the other. This latter form is spoken of as a *greenstick* fracture, and it occurs in children at an age when the bones are soft and pliable. On the other hand, the bone may be *completely* broken, transversely or in a spiral direction, and very frequently it is broken into several (more than two) fragments, when the fracture is said to be *comminuted.*

When the fractured surfaces are protected from contamination with the outside air, that is, when the skin remains intact, it is said to be a *simple* or *closed* fracture; but if a wound occurs at the time of the fracture, so that air and therefore bacteria may be admitted, the fracture is spoken of as being *compound* or *open.* Such a fracture is more difficult to treat than a simple fracture, because the wound and possibility of infection must be considered as well as the fracture itself. At times, soft-tissue injury may be a greater problem than the fractured bone.

Not infrequently other structures such as nerves, blood vessels, joints, lungs, bladder and other organs are injured by the force causing the fracture or by the fracture fragments. When such injuries occur, the fracture is called a *complicated* one.

Growth in long bones in early life takes place from two lines of cartilage, called epiphyseal lines, which separate the main shaft of the bone (the diaphysis) from the articular extremities (the epiphyses). As full growth is attained, these lines of cartilage disappear, being transformed into dense bone.

In childhood and in early youth, an accident frequently occurs which is in effect a fracture, but actually is a separation of the epiphysis from the rest of the bone. These injuries, called *epiphyseal separations,* frequently pass undiagnosed or are called sprains. They are important because an accurate reposition of the epiphysis must be secured and maintained, otherwise the bone may not attain its normal growth. Therefore, such separations are looked upon and treated as fractures.

Most fractures are the result of trauma, but there are some fractures in which the bone itself becomes weakened and cannot bear the weight of the patient's body. This occurs occasionally in older people, due to osteoporosis, but it occurs also in people who are not aged, due to tumors—either primary tumors of the bone or metastatic tumors. When these tumors invade the bone, the bone becomes decalcified to the point that it is no longer strong enough to maintain its integrity under stress and sustains a fracture. Fractures that occur in this type of bone are spoken of as *pathologic fractures*.

Physiology of Fracture Healing. When a fracture occurs, there is a loss of continuity of the bone; in addition, a hematoma forms around the end of the bone. This gradually is absorbed or becomes organized by the ingrowth of cells from the surrounding tissues.

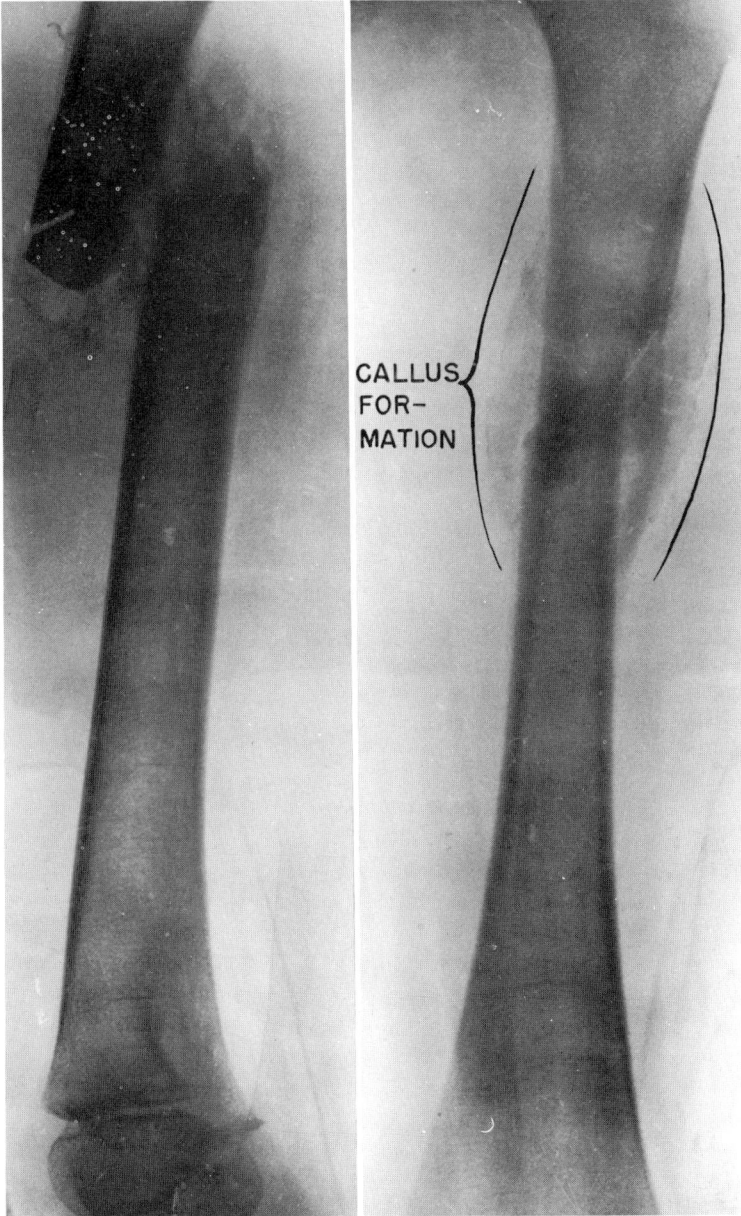

FIG. 383. A fractured femur of 4 weeks' duration. (*Left*) Lateral view. Note overlapping. (*Right*) Anteroposterior view. Note deposition of callus.

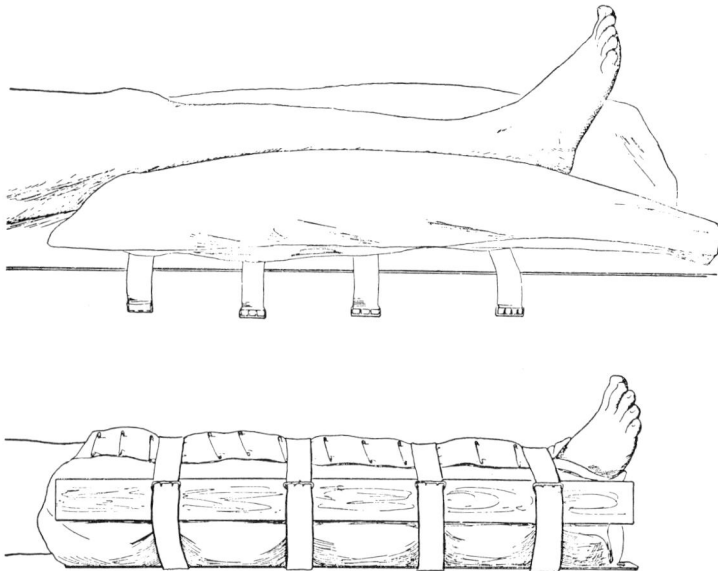

FIG. 384. Emergency pillow splint. (Scudder, C. L.: Treatment of Fractures, Philadelphia, Saunders)

Eventually, a protein framework (*osteoid*) is formed, in which minerals later are deposited. It is believed that an enzyme (alkaline phosphatase) is instrumental in converting organic phosphate ions. These combine with calcium to form *callus*, which is the bony material that forms early at the healing fracture site. This mineral material is deposited also in the osteoid. At first the callus may be much larger than the bone itself, but gradually, as time goes on, this decreases in size until in later years it is very difficult to distinguish the site of a fracture.

Symptoms and Diagnosis. The *symptoms* of a fracture may be learned easily by picturing what happens when a bone is broken.

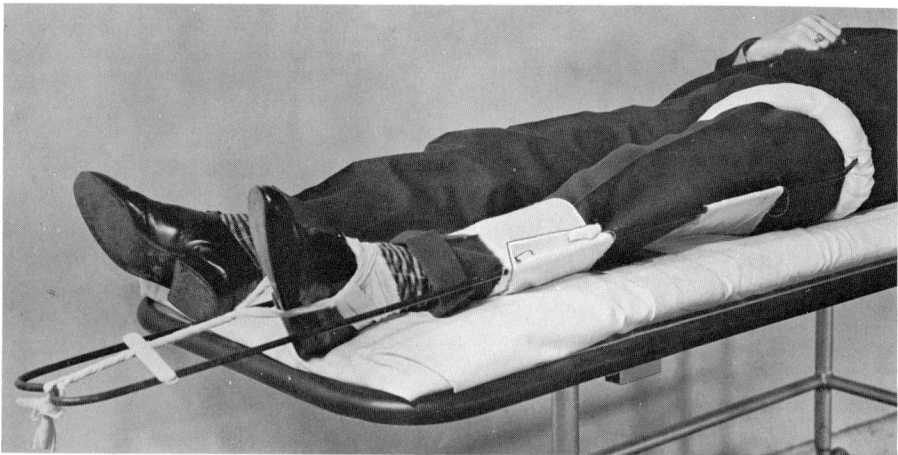

FIG. 385. Emergency splint for a fractured femur; a Thomas splint with traction applied by use of Collin's cinch of muslin bandage. Traction is produced by a windlass twisting of the bandage tied to the end of the splint. Slings of muslin bandage fastened with safety pins support the leg in the splint. A traction fixation never should be attempted by one unskilled in its application, unless under the guidance of a physician.

The break allows unnatural movement in a position which is normally rigid. The displacement of the fragments causes a deformity of the limb when compared with the sound member of the opposite side of the body. The limb cannot function properly because normal function of the muscles is dependent upon the integrity of the bones to which they are attached.

Upon examination of the limb, a grating sensation, called *crepitus,* is imparted to the examining fingers, due to the rubbing of the fragments one upon the other. In fractures of long bones there is actually shortening of the limb, due to the contraction of the muscles which are attached above and below the site of the fracture. The fragments may often overlap as much as an inch or two. Finally, there are pain, tenderness, swelling and discoloration of the skin due to the trauma causing the fracture and the hemorrhage which follows it.

All of these symptoms are not necessarily present in every fracture. When there is a linear or fissure fracture, or in cases where the fractured surfaces are driven together (called *impacted* fractures), many of these symptoms may be lacking.

In modern practice, the *diagnosis* and the treatment of fractures are not thought to be complete without at least one and often many x-ray examinations. By this means the position of the fragments may be determined accurately, and the indications for further treatment confirmed.

The *fluoroscope* is an apparatus by means of which the position of anything opaque to the x-rays may be visualized on a screen. By the aid of this apparatus the bone fragments may be brought into position with considerable ease and accuracy, but a roentgenogram always should follow to serve as a permanent record of the reduction.

Emergency Management. For transportation, the fractured limb should be rendered as immobile as possible by the temporary application of such makeshift splints as well-padded pieces of wood, cane, etc., firmly bandaged over the clothing. Adequate splinting is essential for the prevention of soft tissue damage by bony fragments. It must be remembered that the pain associated with a fractured bone is severe, and the surest way to decrease the discomfort of the patient and the possible shock is by fixing the bone so that the joints above and below the fracture are immobilized. Before transportation is attempted, morphine should be given if available.

In compound fracture the wound should be covered with a clean (sterile) dressing, no attempt being made to reduce the fracture, even if one of the bone fragments is protruding through the wound. Splints should be applied as described above. Immediately following injury, a patient who is in a state of confusion may not be aware of the possibility of a fracture, i.e., he may walk on a fractured extremity. Therefore, it is important to immobilize that part of the body when a fracture is suspected.

IMMEDIATE HOSPITAL TREATMENT AND NURSING CARE. When a patient comes to a hospital suffering from a fracture, at once he should be given morphine or Demerol sufficient to relieve his pain. Then with all care and gentleness his clothes are removed, first from the uninjured side of his body, and then from the injured side. The fractured limb must be moved as little as possible to avoid disturbing it; sometimes the patient's clothing must be cut away on the injured side.

As a rule patients with fractures should not be moved until the injured part has been

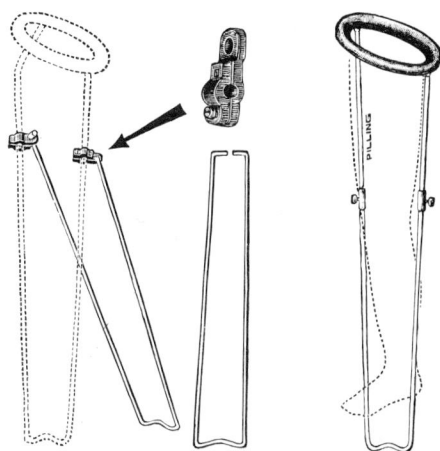

FIG. 386. Splints and fracture appliances in common use. (*Left*) Pearson attachment for Thomas splint. (*Right*) Thomas splint. (See also Fig. 395.)

supported by temporary splints. However, there are times when moving is necessary. In those cases the limb should be supported both above and below the site of the fracture, and traction should be made in the line of the long axis of the bone in order to prevent rotation as well as angular motion.

Fracture Reduction and Immobilization. Before reduction of the fracture, time enough usually elapses for the patient to be undressed, washed and made comfortable. A limb which is to be manipulated and dressed in a splint or a cast must not be dirty.

In treating a fracture, the most important objectives are: (1) to regain correct alignment through reduction, (2) to maintain the alignment, and (3) to regain the function of the involved part.

For most patients anesthesia, either general or local block, is necessary to reduce a fractured bone properly without pain. Anesthesia also produces a relaxation of the muscles and this makes for an easier and quicker reduction. By manipulation and traction, the bone fragments are brought into apposition. Fractures should be reduced usually as soon as possible; swelling is no contraindication. The longer the interval before treatment, the greater is the possibility of complications.

Some fractures, especially those of the femur, may be treated by weight traction. This method gives gradual reduction without an anesthetic.

FRACTURE DRESSINGS. After the fracture has been reduced, the bone fragments must be held in position until union has had time to take place. This immobilization may be accomplished by bandages, adhesive, splints or by extension or traction. If the fragments have been properly reduced and immobilized, the swelling should disappear rapidly, and the part should become less and less painful. If pain persists or increases, the nurse should suspect that something is wrong and call the surgeon at once. Increasing pain usually means an ill-fitting cast or splint. Early remedy is necessary to prevent necrosis.

Bandages, usually of muslin, are used commonly to immobilize certain fractures. The Velpeau bandage dressing is applied by many surgeons for fractures of the clavicle. The Barton bandage is employed occasionally for fractures of the lower jaw.

Splints may be made of any rigid, firm material: wood, plaster of Paris, woven wire, cardboard, wire rods, aluminum, etc.

Wooden splints are useful as temporary dressings for most fractures and occasionally as permanent dressings for many fractures, especially those of the arm. They are manufactured in various sizes and shapes for use as the occasion arises, to accord with a wide

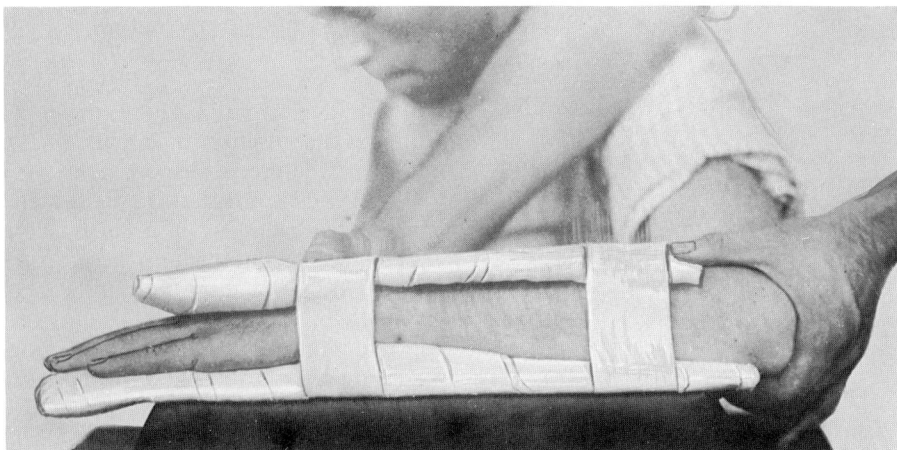

FIG. 387. Forearm splints, showing padding to fit the contour of the part. Note the wrinkles in the straps when the two splints are pressed together, thus illustrating the fact that the straps should retain the splints without undue pressure.

variety of uses. In addition, flexible splints of compressed wood are often incorporated in plaster casts to add stiffness with less plaster.

Wooden splints do not fit the curves of the extremity; hence, they must be well padded with cotton and gauze to avoid pressure points. The padding should be applied only on the side of the splint which lies in contact with the skin; as a rule gauze bandage is used to hold the padding in place on the splint. It is important that the ends of the splint be well covered with padding. Bandages and adhesive strips are used to hold the splints firmly to the limb, but they should not be drawn tight enough to cause constrictions.

Plaster of Paris is perhaps the most valuable of the materials used for fracture dressings. It is usually employed in the form of bandages of crinoline into the meshes of which powdered plaster of Paris has been rubbed. When the bandage has been wet, it becomes soft for a time but soon sets as it dries and hardens, taking the shape to which it has been molded before setting.

Plaster bandages are usually made in several widths (2, 4, 6 and 8 inches wide) and wrapped separately in waxed paper. For use they are stood on end in a bucket of warm water. When bubbles of air cease to rise from the bandage, the nurse will know that the bandage has been wet through. She then takes the bandage so that the palms of the hands cover the ends of the roll and gently squeezes out the excess water (losing as little plaster as possible), and passes the roll to the surgeon in such a way that the roller comes to his right hand and the free end to his left.

Plaster Casts. Before applying a plaster cast, the skin and soft tissue must be protected. Bandages of sheet wadding (cotton batting) usually are employed, and if considerable pressure is likely to result, foam rubber or felt pads are used. If the felt is to be next to the skin, the patient will be more comfortable if it is wrapped with a layer of gauze bandage before it is applied. Elastic tubular jersey sleeving (stockinet) with cotton batting may be applied.

The plaster bandage is then applied turn upon turn, exerting pressure to each layer with the open hand in order to make it unite with the one beneath it. Places where strain will take place, like the groin, back of the knee, etc., must be reinforced in one of these ways: there must be (1) many turns of the bandage at these points (which makes for an extremely heavy cast), (2) a reduplication of plaster bandages may be used.

"Reduplications" are made by rolling the bandage back and forth until a strip is obtained from 8 to 10 layers thick and of the desired length and width, the layers being well rubbed together with the open hand. The reduplication is then molded to fit the desired part of the cast and covered by sev-

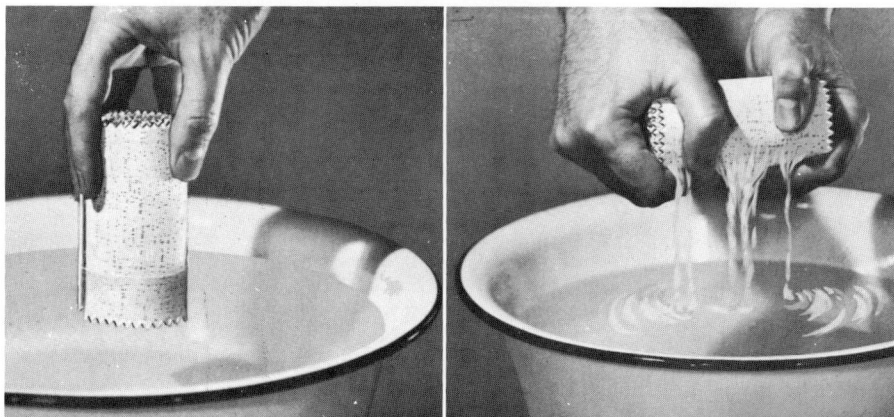

Fig. 388. (*Left*) Plaster bandage is immersed vertically in warm water. (*Right*) Method of squeezing excess water from plaster bandage. (The Scholl Manufacturing Company, Chicago)

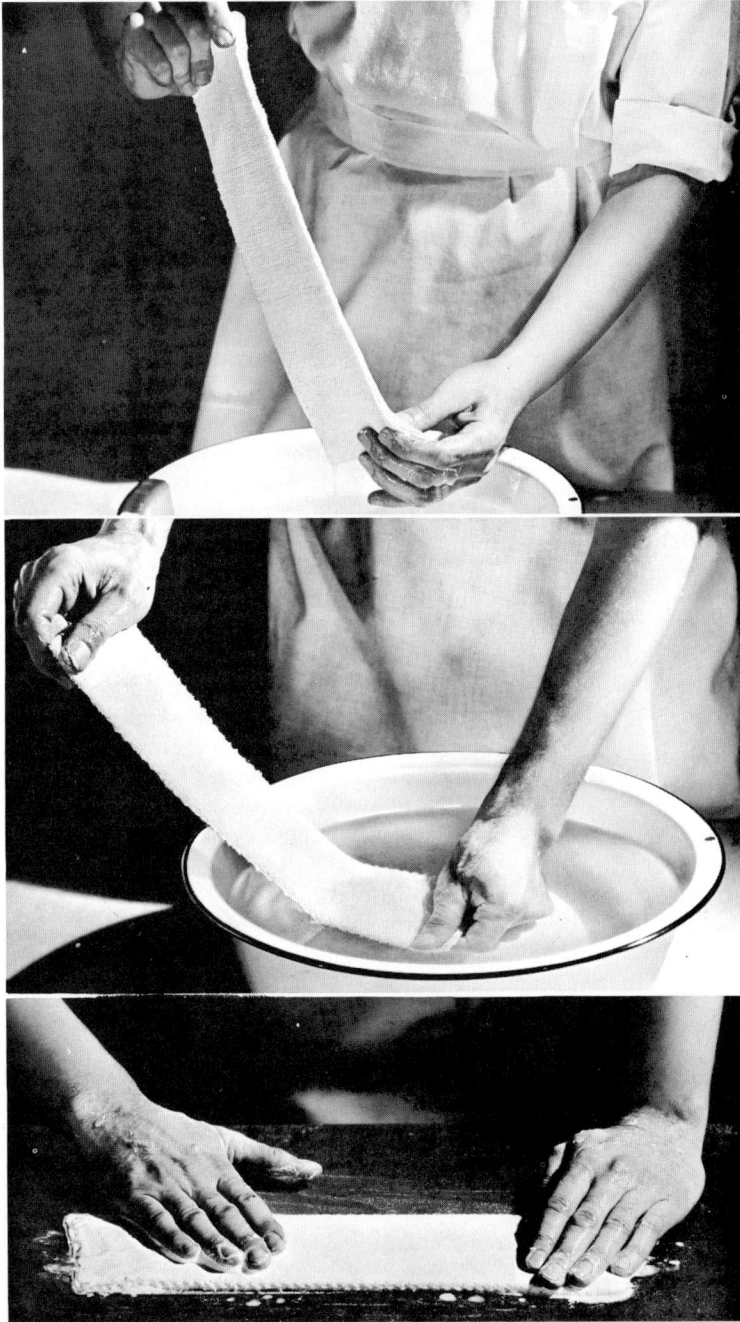

FIG. 389. A, B, C. By dipping several layers of a specially prepared plaster dressing into water, a splint can be made easily and quickly. (Johnson & Johnson)

eral layers of plaster bandage. Such splints or "reduplications" are commerically available in various sizes. (Fig. 389.)

Before the cast is dry the operator should smooth it by rubbing with the open hand, at the same time making sure that it fits the limb. If the first few bandages have been applied firmly and smoothly, the cast usually will be well molded and without wrinkles.

When the plaster has set, but before it is dry, incisions are made with a plaster knife through all the layers of the cast. When such incisions are made on each side of the cast, it may be removed with comparative ease or easily spread to relieve pressure should signs of constriction appear (cyanosis, coldness, or loss of sensation in fingers or toes). Any complaints by the patient of painful areas under the plaster should be reported or investigated.

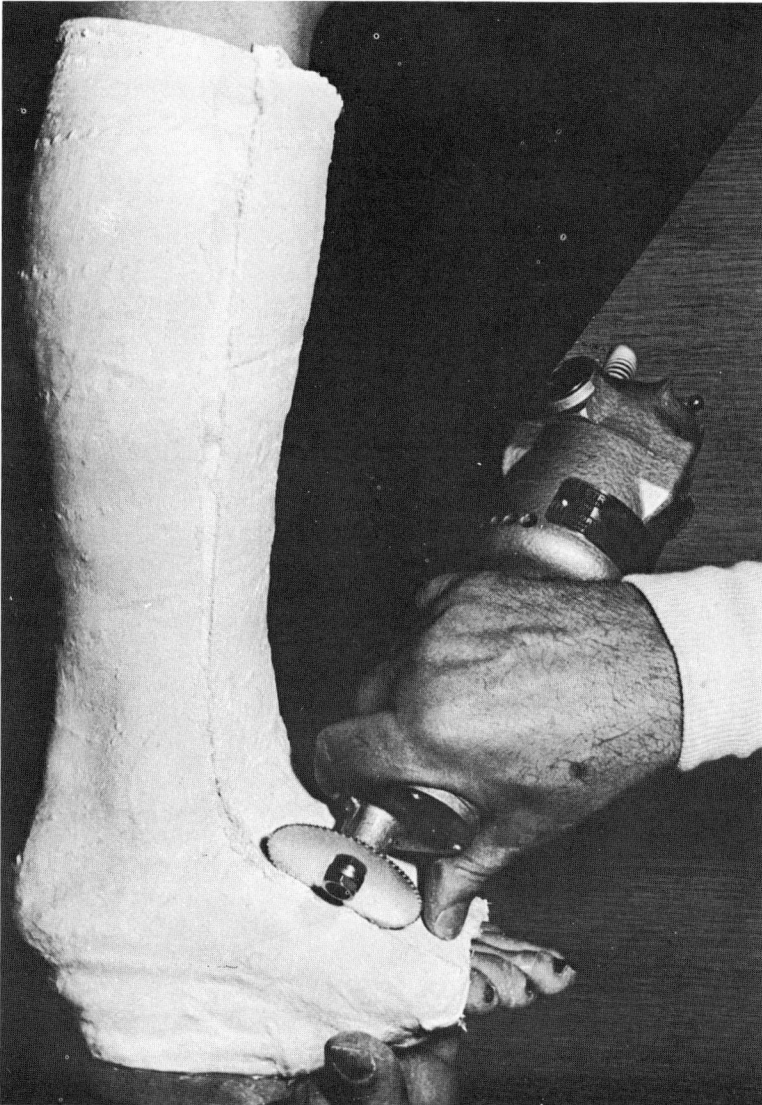

FIG. 390. Stryker electric cast cutter. The blade oscillates, cutting rapidly through rigid plaster with safety. (Orthopedic Frame Co.)

The "hanging" cast can be used for certain fractures of the humerus. It consists of plaster applied from the axillary fold to the wrist with the elbow flexed at right angles. A sling is passed through a ring made with the plaster bandage at the wrist and this is then tied around the neck.

Plaster Splints. Plaster splints are reduplications made upon a pattern of lint. It is well to make the lint pattern about a full inch larger than the size desired. By making the plaster reduplications slightly smaller, enough lint remains to fold over the sharp edges which otherwise have a tendency to cause considerable pressure (see Fig. 404).

As soon as they are made, the plaster splints are bound firmly to the part with gauze bandage. As a general rule, plaster casts or splints are more comfortable if the joints which they enclose are slightly flexed.

APPLICATION OF CAST. When plaster is being used, the hands may be protected by rubber gloves, which are easily cleaned if washed in water before removing. A thin coating of petroleum jelly on the hands may be preferred to rubber gloves. The room in which plaster is applied should be one having a minimum of furnishings to facilitate cleaning. Some form of lubricant applied to the orthopedic table will make it easier to remove plaster and prevent rust formation. Plaster knives and shears are the only instruments needed (Fig. 390). They must be cleaned thoroughly and oiled after use. The

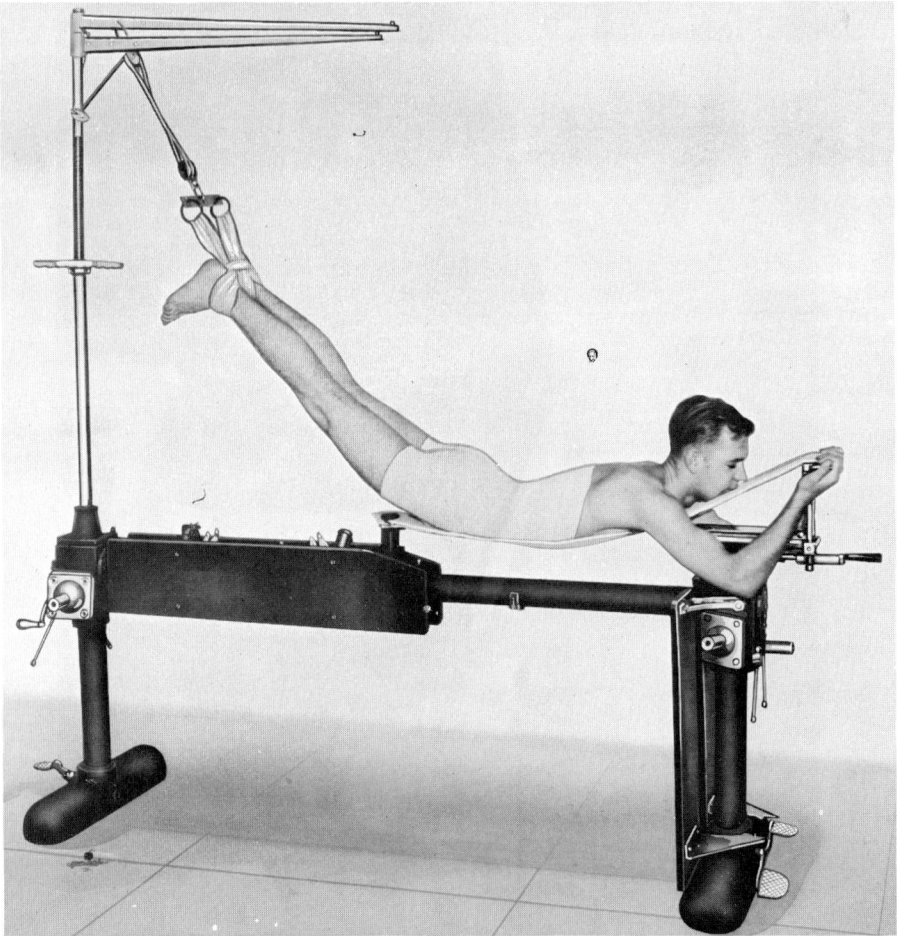

FIG. 391. Orthopedic table with patient arranged for application of body cast.

plaster-laden water in which the bandages are soaked should not be poured into the ordinary drain basin, because a clogged pipe is almost sure to result. It is better to allow the plaster to settle in the bucket, then the water may be poured off, and the remaining plaster emptied into the waste can. In most modern hospitals, plaster traps are installed in the drain pipes of sinks in rooms where plaster is used. The trap will catch most of the plaster poured into the sink, but it must be cleaned frequently if it is to work efficiently.

Newspaper should be spread out so as to protect the furniture (tables, chairs, etc.); since these papers can be discarded after use this makes the cleaning up after plaster application less burdensome. If a marble or board slab is used, this can be placed on newspaper so that plaster drippings are easily caught and discarded. If the bucket in which the plaster is soaked is placed on a table

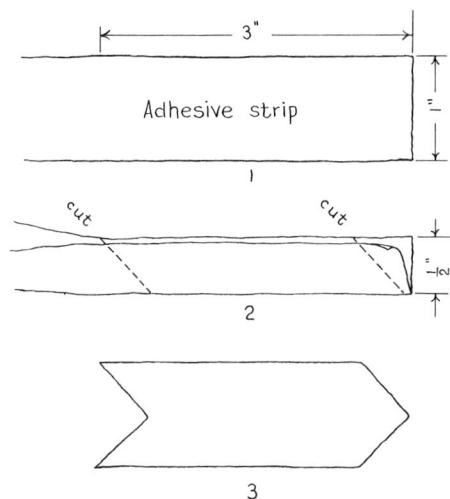

FIG. 392. Drawings to show method of cutting petals for covering edge of the cast. (1) A strip of adhesive is folded so that the adhesive side is out and cut as indicated in the diagram. (2) In cutting several petals from a strip of adhesive, only single cuts are necessary for each petal. (3) A finished petal. The petals are applied to the edge of the cast, as shown in Fig. 393. The length of the petal may be varied to suit the situation in which it is to be used.

protected by newspaper, the plaster drippings that invariably occur when the plaster is taken from the water, and when water is expressed from the bandage, fall on the newspaper, which can be discarded readily. The use of sheets or other drapes to protect furniture from plaster is an expensive protection. Before leaving the cast room, all evidences of extraneous plaster should be cleaned from the patient.

The Patient in a Cast. The purpose of a cast is to immobilize and support the injured part and protect it during the healing process.

A fundamental principle not to be lost sight of is that we are still caring for a patient as well as a cast. Experience has taught that any complaint of discomfort must not go unheeded. Two types of complications occur. One is due to pressure of the cast on tissues, especially on bony points. The pain may be the first indication of local pressure which, if allowed to go untended, may produce necrosis (pressure sores) or paralysis, due to pressure on a nerve which may be over a bony point. The latter is seen most commonly to produce peroneal palsy with footdrop, due to pressure on the peroneal nerve. The second complication is due to swelling underneath the cast which produces a circulatory impairment. Toes and fingers of extremities recently encased in plaster must be inspected frequently to note any signs of circulatory impairment. *This is manifested by swelling, blanching or discoloration, tingling, numbness, inability to move fingers and toes, or temperature change and must be reported immediately,* for serious results such as paralysis and necrosis may occur. Conscientious observations should continue as long as the patient is in the cast; if there is swelling, the cast will seem tighter. Elevation of the part will help to control swelling. If the patient continues to have pain, pressure within the cast on a nerve, a blood vessel, or a bony prominence should be suspected. The cast will have to be bivalved to relieve the pressure. This action does not disturb the alignment of the fracture. Permission from the surgeon should be gained before bivalving the cast.

When a large cast is applied, such as a

body or hip spica, the bed must be prepared before the patient is received. A board under the mattress will give the necessary firmness to the bed. To make allowances for the contour of the cast, 3 plastic-covered pillows placed crosswise on the bed will suffice for the body cast. For a hip spica, 1 pillow placed crosswise at the waist and 2 pillows placed lengthwise for the affected leg are necessary. If both legs are involved, 2 additional pillows are necessary. It is important that the pillows be next to each other, because any spaces in between will allow the damp cast to sag, become weak and possibly break.

In moving a patient from side to side in a large cast, at least 3 people are necessary. Only the palms of the hands are used to lift the cast; fingers make indentations in soft plaster. Support should be given to the entire cast and most particularly at such vulnerable points as the hip and the knee.

The nurse must remember that the patient receives first consideration and his cast is secondary in importance.

DRYING THE CAST. A freshly applied cast should be exposed to circulating air or a blower type drier so that it will dry.

Covers are not necessary for they restrict the escape of moisture. As the moisture evaporates and the cast hardens, heat is gen-erated. In a warm room it may be necessary to use an electric fan to keep the patient comfortable. When a large cast is dried, it is often desirable to use mechanical aids, such as a heat lamp or hair dryer, to facilitate the process. This should not be placed closer than 18 inches, and then it should be moved frequently from one area to another so that drying is achieved evenly. It is to be remembered that burns may occur under the cast from overexposure even though the skin is not exposed directly. If the patient is cold, those parts of the body not encased in plaster should be covered and kept warm. When the patient is in shock, the cast can be exposed piecemeal. It takes about 24 hours for a cast to become dry, depending upon the size of the cast and the moisture in the air; a dry cast is white and shiny, resonant and odorless as well as firm; a wet cast is gray and dull in appearance, dull to percussion, feels damp and has a musty odor.

TURNING THE PATIENT. While the cast is still in the process of drying, the patient should be turned every 6 hours to promote even drying of the cast and to prevent fatigue of the patient (this may vary with the physician or the hospital policy). The initial turning of a large cast is usually done on the evening of the day it is applied so that the posterior surface may be dried. This should

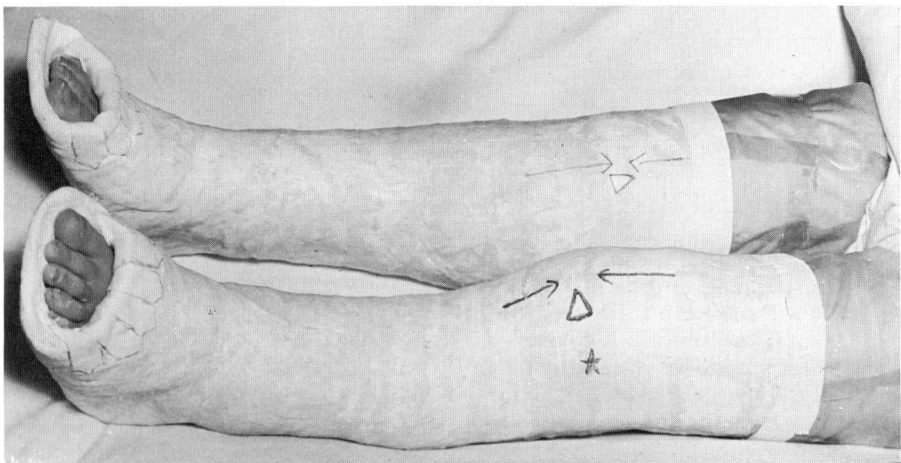

FIG. 393. Photograph showing casts, the edges of which have been covered by petals to protect the foot from the edge of the cast. In this case, the upper ends of the casts have been protected by waterproof plastic material. This type of protection is used frequently in incontinent patients.

be done with sufficient help. The patient is first moved to the side of the bed toward the leg encased in plaster. At this time fresh pillows and sheets can be placed on the vacant side so that it will be ready to receive the turned patient. The patient with a hip spica should be turned as one piece on the leg *not involved* and adequate support must be given to the uppermost leg, which is encased, especially at the groin. His arms may be placed above his head or kept at his sides, whichever is most comfortable. Two persons on the side of the bed to which the patient is closest and one person on the opposite side can turn a patient effectively without lifting him. When he is lying prone, a pillow placed crosswise under the dorsum of the feet will prevent the toes from being forced into the mattress. Sometimes allowing the toes to hang over the edge of the mattress is more comfortable. After the cast is thoroughly dry, pillows are used as necessary to maintain comfort and good body alignment. They are used also to bring the level of the cast up to that of the bed pan when the latter is used. A pillow under the abdomen often adds to the comfort of the patient.

A comfort measure which will be appreciated by the patient in a body cast is the "back scratcher." This can be a length of 3-inch flannel which can be inserted inside the back of the cast by a long alligator forceps. (A thoughtful nurse can suggest this to the surgeon immediately before the application of the cast.) By holding each end of the flannel, the nurse can give the patient a friction rub.

PROTECTION OF THE SKIN AND CARE OF THE CAST. Pressure areas may develop over any bony prominence. A common site of pressure from a large cast is the buttocks. When the patient is turned on his abdomen, the exposed skin can be washed carefully and massaged. The rough edges of the cast here as well as elsewhere must be made smooth. Often pulling stockinet from inside the cast over the rough edge and fixing it to the outside with adhesive will eliminate cast crumbs and make the edge smooth. The nurse should reach up under the cast edges as far as possible with her fingers to remove plaster crumbs and to massage the skin area.

Around the perineal area, it is often necessary to protect the cast against excretions. If the opening is inadequate for hygienic care, the nurse should report this. When the cast is dry, plastic material, cellophane, or waxed paper can be cut in 4-inch strips and tucked under the cast; they can be fastened to the exterior, allowing for adequate coverage of the outside of the cast. These can be pulled out and cleaned or replaced daily.

To clean soiled parts of a cast, it is acceptable to rub the area with a damp cloth. It may be sufficient to apply a piece of plaster bandage ("patch" method) which is cut to cover the soiled area. Another effective method is to use a cloth which has been rubbed over a cake of a cleaning agent such as Bon Ami. The outside of a cast may be shellacked after the cast is thoroughly dry.

FINISHING THE CAST. Cast edges can be molded satisfactorily by "petaling." One-inch or 2-inch adhesive tape can be cut as petals and applied (Figs. 392 and 393). This method is more economical of time and materials than circular petals. Measurements can vary according to need.

The skin around the edges of the cast must be inspected frequently for signs of irritation. All accessible skin should be massaged gently with alcohol. When there is irritation, the area must be treated as a potential decubitus.

STATIC MUSCLE CONTRACTIONS. While the patient is in a cast he should be taught to tense or to contract his muscles without moving the joints. The patient may actually forget how to "will" a motion through the central nervous system pathways to the immobilized muscle. Therefore by static muscle contractions (contracting the muscle without moving the part) atrophy will be prevented, and muscle strength will be maintained.

If the patient is in a leg cast, place your hand under the knee and instruct the patient to "push down." If the patient has an arm cast, instruct him to "make a fist." Static muscle contractions should be done at least hourly while the patient is awake. He is taught to exercise his fingers and his toes frequently and actively.

REMOVAL OF THE PATIENT FROM THE

CAST. A cast is removed by using an electric cast cutter or by making an incision with a plaster knife and cutting the cast with heavy shears. One of the most important things to remember when a cast has been removed is that the part or parts involved have been immobilized for a considerable period of time. When the support and protection of the cast have been removed, there are stresses and strains placed on tissue which has been resting. The patient complains of pain and stiffness, often much different from the original injury, and he is depressed and discouraged, because the early anticipated release from the cast has only added further to his problems.

The responsibility of the nurse is to help make the adjustment of the patient easier. This can be accomplished by supporting the part to maintain the same position as existed in the cast, with small pillow supports under the knee, the lumbar spine, etc., allowing for gradual removal of support. In moving an extremity, the nurse must provide adequate support and move the limb gently. After the cast has been removed, exercises are prescribed to redevelop and to increase strength. If the patient has been doing static muscle contractions, he will not have to relearn to contract his muscles and will progress more rapidly with his rehabilitation program.

The care of the skin is not a pressing problem. Its care is less important than the care to the muscles and the bones; therefore, careful washing with a mild soap, followed by oil or lanolin, is sufficient. The exudate noted on the skin should not be scrubbed with a brush, for it is a good protective agent. If a new cast is to be applied, some surgeons prefer that the skin be powdered only and that there be no washing of the skin which might be traumatizing. Briefly, the skin and the underlying tissues must be handled carefully until gradual restoration of normal function is achieved. Atrophy of the part may be noted, but this will disappear gradually with the return of muscle function. Should the patient go home with a cast, he must be instructed as to the care of his cast. If the cast has been removed, the principles of skin care must be understood. He must know also the signs of impaired circulation and evidence of infection or skin breakdown. The nurse should stress the importance of his returning to his physician or clinic for follow-up care.

TURNBUCKLE CAST. In some instances casts are applied not only for immobilization but also for the purposes of overcoming bony deformities and muscular contractures. Traction with weight pulleys is sometimes used for this purpose, but for many patients casts are applied which can be cut and the contracture overcome gradually by changing the angle of the cast. In such cases a gradual change may be brought about by incorporating a turnbuckle in the cast, usually across a joint. The part may be straightened by gradually turning the turnbuckle. The nurse must be extremely careful in turning the patient that this extra appliance is not pulled on and displaced so as to break the cast and interrupt the patient's treatment. She also must be alert *constantly* for new signs of pressure with each manipulation of the turnbuckle.

The Patient in Traction. Traction is force in two directions, and it is the method of fixation used most often for fractures of the femur. This method is also employed by some surgeons for fractures of the humerus, the tibia and other bones. The traction developed by weights and pulleys is applied to the part by one of two methods: skin traction or skeletal traction with either wire, pins, or tongs.

SKIN TRACTION. By this method traction strips of moleskin or perforated flexafoam bandage are attached to each side of the limb, connected below to weights by a rope passing over a pulley wheel. For a fractured femur the strips should be cut long enough to extend about 4 inches above the knee on each side. In the center of the strip at the sole of the foot should be placed a piece of wood 3 inches high and an inch wider than the greatest distance between the two malleoli. This serves as a spreader and will prevent pressure along the sides of the foot. It should have a hole in the center through which the traction rope may be passed. After the block has been attached, it is held in place by a second strip of moleskin which should extend for 10 or 12 inches on each

NURSING PRINCIPLES AND IMPLICATIONS

The purpose of traction, regardless of how it is achieved, is (1) to reduce and to immobilize a fracture, (2) to lessen or to eliminate muscle spasm, and (3) to prevent fracture deformity. Nursing implications underlying all traction procedures include the following:

1. The patient is placed on a firm mattress with a hinged bed board beneath it.

2. The ropes and the pulleys should be in straight alignment.

3. The pull should be in line with the long axis of the bone.

4. Any factor that might reduce the pull or alter its direction must be eliminated.
   (A) Weights should hang free.
   (B) Ropes should be unobstructed.

5. The amount of weight applied in skin traction must not exceed the tolerance of the skin. The condition of the latter must be inspected frequently.

6. A possibility always to be kept in mind in connection with skeletal traction is the risk of a complicating bone infection. The nurse must be alert to detect odors, signs of local inflammation or other evidence of osteomyelitis.

7. The patient's skin should be examined frequently for evidence of pressure or friction over bony prominences.

8. Provision should be made for supplying additional countertraction by increasing the pull in the opposite direction, i.e., by raising the bed in such a manner that the weight of the patient's body tends to oppose the pull of the traction.

9. Active motion of all unaffected joints should be encouraged.

10. Every complaint of the patient in traction should be investigated.

side of the wood to prevent adhesion to the malleoli. The adhesive is applied and then held in place by gauze or Ace bandage. Shaving the part and painting the skin with benzoin tincture will make the traction strip hold better; benzoin tincture also acts as a skin disinfectant and is said to prevent an itching skin and be more comfortable. The traction may be begun almost immediately. When skin traction (such as Buck's extension) is applied to the leg, pressure not infrequently develops on the Achilles tendon above the heel and should be inspected several times daily.

Skin traction is usually used with the Thomas splint for fractures of the femur. These patients have a tendency to slide down toward the foot of the bed, but this may be counteracted by elevation of the foot of the bed 12 or 15 inches. The pulleys may be of any kind, but the most suitable ones are those attached to the foot of the bed by a clamp (Fig. 394).

Weights may be ordinary traction weights of metal, or bags of shot or sand. Enough weight is applied at first to overcome the shortening tendency of the injured limb but is gradually lessened as the fracture becomes more fixed. *A nurse never should remove weights from a patient with a fracture under any consideration.* Weight and pulley traction is applied to secure constant corrective extension. If, then, the weights are removed to move the patient from one department to

Balanced Suspension Traction

Definition: Balanced suspension traction is a combination of balance and suspension in which the extremity is supported in a suspended position and balanced by an equal force on the opposite side of the traction.

Example: Russell's leg traction for treating fractures of femoral shaft (Fig. 400).

Activities Permitted Patient:

1. The patient may sit, turn slightly and move as desired.
2. The affected heel must remain free of the bed to maintain the traction.

Nursing Implications:

The angle of hip flexion is 20°. (This is the angle between the thigh and the bed.)

A pillow may be used under the thigh to maintain this angle, and a second pillow placed under the calf to support the lower leg.

The ropes and the pulleys should be freely movable, and the traction should be applied securely to the leg.

Observe for skin irritation around the traction bandage.

Check the patient for signs of odor and infection.

Observe for pressure under the sling at the popliteal space.

The patient should have foot supports to prevent foot drop.

Running Traction

Definition: Running traction is a form of traction in which the pull is exerted in one plane. It may utilize skin or skeletal traction, and it may be either unilateral or bilateral.

Example: Buck's extension. (See Fig. 394.)

Activities Permitted Patient:

1. The head of the bed may be elevated to the point of counter traction. (Example: If the counter traction is 8 inches, the head of the bed may be elevated 8 inches.)
2. The patient may not turn from side to side, as the position of the leg on the bed will cause the bony fragments to move against each other.

Nursing Implications:

The foot should be inspected for circulatory difficulties within a few minutes and then periodically after the elastic bandage has been applied.

Special care must be given to the back at regular intervals, as the patient maintains a supine position.

Any complaint or burning sensation under the traction bandage should be reported immediately.

Observe for wrinkling or slipping of the traction bandage.

The patient should have foot supports to prevent footdrop.

another, the whole purpose of their use has been defeated. Many valueless roentgenograms have been made because nurses have removed the weights while taking the patients to the x-ray department. In moving patients with fractures, however, the weights should be steadied and kept from swinging.

SKELETAL OR BONY TRACTION. This method is used by many surgeons in the treatment of fractures of the femur, the humerus and the tibia. The traction is applied directly to the bones by the use of tongs, or a pin is drilled through the bone. Instead of the tongs or pin, many surgeons use the Kirschner steel wire, which is drilled through the bone with a hand- or electric-driven drill. Usually the tongs, pin or Kirschner wire may be inserted through a small opening in the

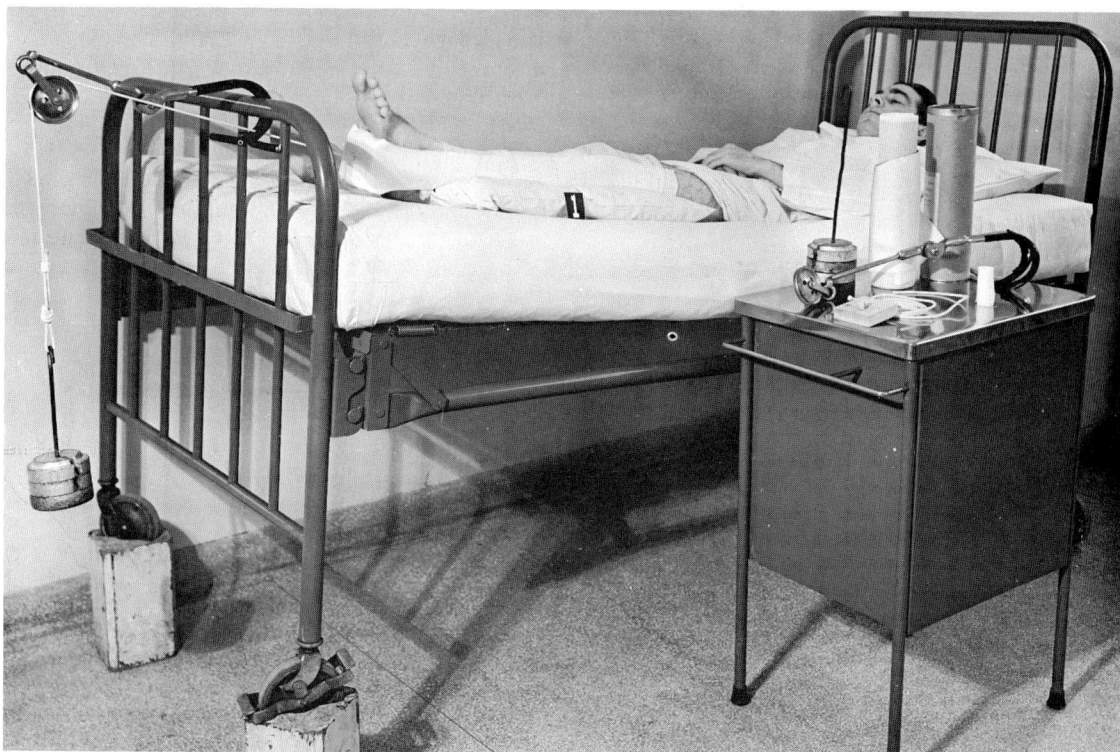

FIG. 394. Buck's extension for skin traction. The leg should be shaved and moleskin cut and applied with bandages as shown. Note (1) the small pillow under the leg. When traction is applied to the lower extremity, it is necessary usually to raise the foot of the bed by the use of bed pins or blocks. Note slots in which bed wheels fit. On the side table are placed materials for the application of a Buck's extension-pulley which may be attached to the bed and weights, moleskin adhesive rope and bandage.

skin made under local anesthesia. They should be sterilized and inserted with all the sterile precautions of an operation. The wound is covered with a small gauze square held in place by adhesive strips. If the wire or pin extends beyond the skin or beyond the caliper, a cork placed over the end of the pin will prevent the tearing of linen and other more serious accidents.

Traction is applied by weights and pulleys as described for skin traction. The Thomas splint with the Pearson attachment is usually used with skeletal traction in fractures of the lower part of the femur (Fig. 386). It may be used with skin traction and other balanced suspension apparatus. Because upward traction is required for these fractures, the patient is placed on a fracture bed.

When the apparatus has been properly adjusted, the fracture should become constantly more comfortable. At times one part of the tongs will slip from its bony anchorage and exert its traction on the soft tissues. As might be expected, considerable pain is caused by this accident. The surgeon should be notified at once.

Inasmuch as fractures occur under varying circumstances and involve individuals of different ages, weights, and body builds, no two fractures are alike, and every fracture patient requires individualized treatment. By the same token, traction procedures may be modified in many ways to meet a variety of special requirements, as exemplified by the so-called "balanced suspension traction," and the "running traction" procedures, which are defined, and the special nursing implications are outlined above. It is to be em-

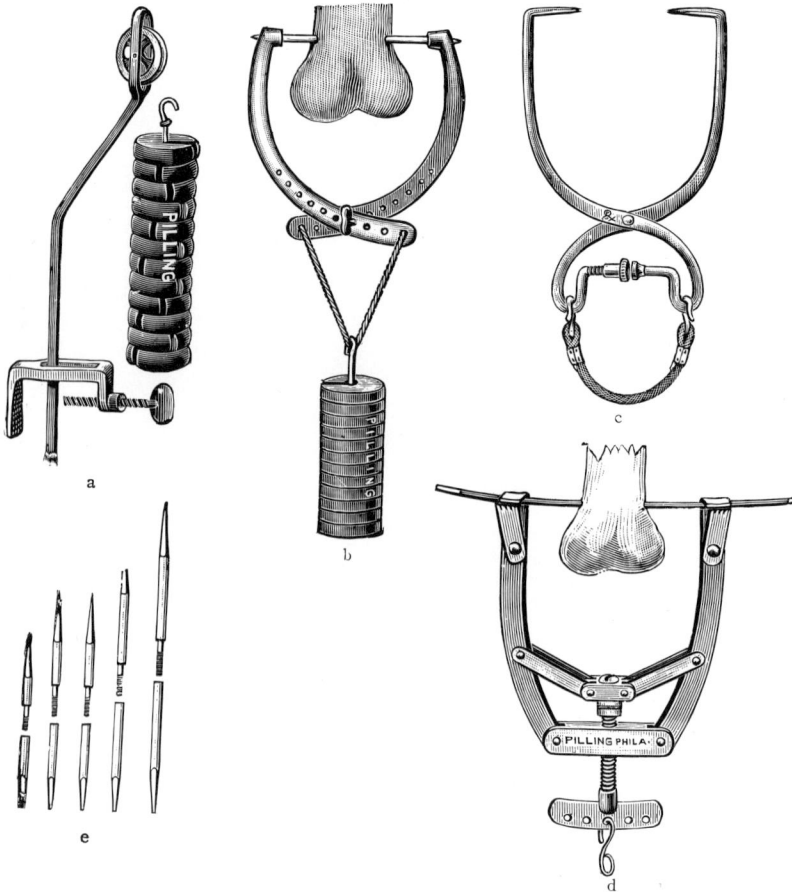

FIG. 395. Fracture Appliances in common use. (a) Weights and pulley. (b) Steinmann pin with attachments. (c) Tongs. (d) Kirschner wire traction. (e) Steinmann pins. (See also Fig. 386.)

phasized that the basic nursing principles for traction procedures in general, as enunciated above, apply equally to these and all other modified forms of traction.

GENERAL NURSING MEASURES. The importance of frequent inspection of the fracture dressing in the first 24 hours after application cannot be impressed too strongly on the nurse responsible for the care of the patient. A bandage that appears sufficiently loose when applied may in a very few hours cause serious constriction which, if not relieved, may lead to gangrene of the extremity.

Dressings always should be applied in such a way as to leave the tips of the fingers and toes exposed. Any cyanosis, loss of temperature, tingling, or loss of sensation in these parts should warn the nurse that the dressings are too tight. If the condition is caused by a single turn of the bandage, the

turn may be divided with the scissors, but it is usually advisable to notify the surgeon who has charge of the patient. After the first 24 hours, the fracture dressing should be inspected by the nurse at least three or four times daily. She should inquire whether there are any painful areas, look for evidences of constriction and see that there are no pressure points, e.g., heel is not on the bed, bedclothes do not rest on toes, there is no pressure on the Achilles tendon, etc. If traction is being used, the apparatus should be inspected to see that the ropes are in the wheel groove of the pulleys, that the weights hang free, that the patient has not slipped down in bed. The foot must be in a natural position; rotation outward or inward should be reported. The rope sometimes frays; therefore, it too must be inspected at least daily. An alert nurse will be sure to examine the skin around the traction for evidence of circulatory impairment.

A comfort measure is to place a firm thin pillow covered with plastic lengthwise under the leg in traction so that the pillow is under the thigh and extends to just above the heel (with permission of the physician). If it is powdered it will eliminate bed friction; the heel will not be resting on the bedclothes and will be free of pressure, which is desirable.

Foot drop may be prevented in several ways: (1) a stockinet boot can be fixed at the ankle with several turns of bandage; the other open end, which is about 2 inches above the toes, is drawn together with stitching as in a purse-string. To this end is attached a metal ring, through which a rope is drawn to the top of the Balkan frame where it meets a pulley. A 1-pound weight is sufficient to keep the foot in proper position. (2) A strip of adhesive attached to the plantar surface of the foot and extending beyond the toes can be attached to the same type of pulley arrangement as described above. A metal eyelet in the adhesive serves as a means of attachment for the rope. (3) Metal or wooden frames, some of which are hinged, can also be secured from instrument companies or can be made in the hospital maintenance department. When fracture beds are used, rings or a trapezelike rod may be suspended overhead within easy reach of the patient. This piece of apparatus is of great help in assisting the patient to move about in bed, on and off bedpans, etc. It is also a help to the nurse in caring for these patients. When a patient is not permitted to turn on one side or the other or on his abdomen, the nurse must make a special effort to give him good back care, keep the bed dry and free of crumbs and wrinkles. This can be accomplished without her straining her back, because the patient may raise his hips from the bed by holding onto the overhead trapeze. Often a patient uses the heel of his good leg to act as a brace when he raises himself. This digging of the heel into the mattress may be injurious to the tissues; hence, it must be massaged with lanolin and inspected for pressure areas. Some physicians wrap both legs of traction patients in elastic bandage in an attempt to decrease the incidence of thrombophlebitis. If the patient is unable to raise himself, the nurse can push down on the mattress with one hand, leaving space for the other hand to massage the skin.

Reduction by Internal Fixation. Methods of fixation applied externally, such as have been described, are suitable for many types of fractures. There are some fractures, however, which are treated by a rigid fixation directly across the fracture line from one fragment to the other. This type of fixation is spoken of as internal, and it may be provided by pins or nails applied through the bones as in fractures of the neck of the femur and in long bone fractures. The use of various types of metal rods (pins) to fix fractures has revolutionized the care of many fracture patients. There is a marked decrease in the length of immobilization and hospitalization.

Open Reduction. In some patients, the fracture may be reduced and internal fixation introduced through a small wound without a formal operation. In many fractures, however, reduction cannot be accomplished because of a separation of the fragments by muscle, fascia, or a detached bone fragment. In others, it may be impossible to hold the fragments in position even though reduction was accomplished by manipulation. Internal fixation may be achieved by the application of a plate to the cortex of the bone across the fracture line. The plate is held in place with screws inserted through holes in the plate into the bone shaft. This necessitates a formal incision and exposure of the fracture site and is called an *open reduction* of the fracture. After closure of the wound, external fixation is often used in addition by the application of splints or casts. The internal fixation may be removed after bony union has taken place, but for many patients it never is removed unless it produces symptoms.

AFTER-CARE. The surgeon in charge of a patient with a reduced fracture will inspect the dressing daily for several days. If the fracture has been accurately reduced and immobilized, the patient should become increasingly more comfortable.

Redressings are required for many fractures dressed with splints, especially those which involve or are near the joints. Fractures complicated by joint involvement, or those treated by the application of a cast, are

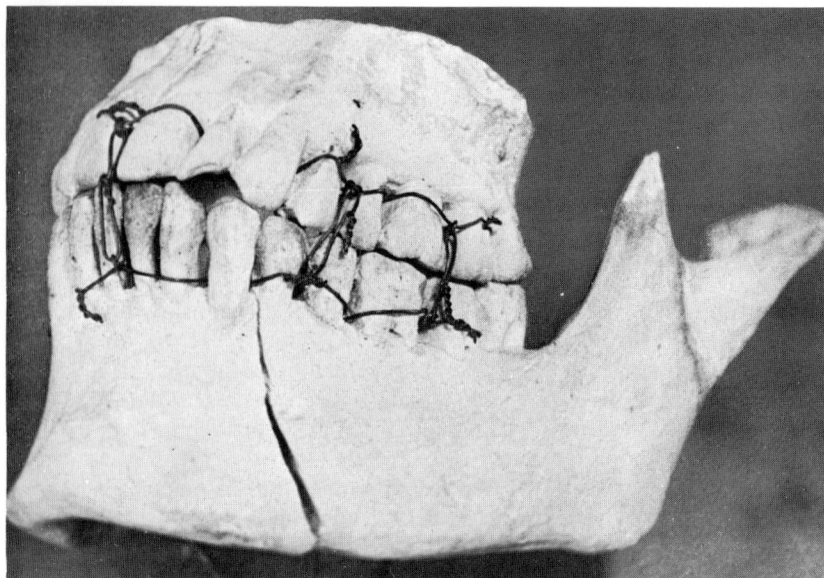

Fig. 396. Fracture of the mandible. Method of wiring teeth in occlusion on each side of the fracture. (Ivy Surg., Gynec. & Obst. **34:**670)

often benefited by a regimen of baking and massage, after union is firm enough for external support to be discontinued. Under ordinary conditions with proper treatment, the fragments of the broken bone unite by the formation of a soft callus in which are deposited calcium salts, so that in time a patch of bone results which is as strong as the original part. (See Fig. 383.)

HEALING PROCESS. The rapidity with which union occurs varies with many factors. For instance, it is well known that fractures that occur during infancy and youth unite much more quickly than those occurring in old age. Fractures of the various bones require different periods of disability before active function can be resumed—thus fractures of the humerus on the average require from 6 to 10 weeks; those of the forearm, from 8 to 10 weeks; those of the femur, 6 months; and those of the lower leg, from 2 to 4 months.

Delayed and Nonunion. Occasionally, because of local causes or systemic disease, union does not take place within the usual period. In many of these cases union occurs if the patient is permitted the use of the limb supported by braces, and appropriate treatment is given the systemic disease which may be present. If union does not result at the end of from 10 to 12 weeks, the fracture is said to be ununited. In these patients the

fragments have between them only fibrous tissue; no bone salts have been deposited. Such patients often develop a false joint (pseudoarthrosis) at the site of the fracture. When such an unfortunate result occurs, braces may be used to give the patient a useful limb, or by an operation the ends of the bone may be freshened, and an attempt made to unite them by means of a graft removed from another bone which is placed in position between the fragments. Fractures of the middle of the humerus, of the neck of the femur in elderly people, and of the lower third of the tibia most frequently result in nonunion.

Compound Fractures. Compound fractures may be associated with so much damage to the soft tissue that amputation of the member is necessary. If it is possible, however, that a useful limb may result, the surgeon will thoroughly débride the wound. After débriding or excising devitalized tissue and removing foreign material, he will place the fragments in position and repair the soft tissues (muscles, nerves and tendons) as well as possible. These wounds may be closed under favorable circumstances, otherwise left open, loosely packed with petrolatum gauze and a compression dressing applied. In these days of antibiotic therapy, compound fractures may be expected to heal primarily with primary closure if they have

FIG. 397. (*Left*) Sayre's dressing, anterior view. Slits for the fingertips and the olecranon are helpful. (*Right*) T splint for immobilization in fracture of clavicle, posterior view. (Magnuson, P. B., and Stack, J. K.: Fractures, ed. 5, Philadelphia, Lippincott)

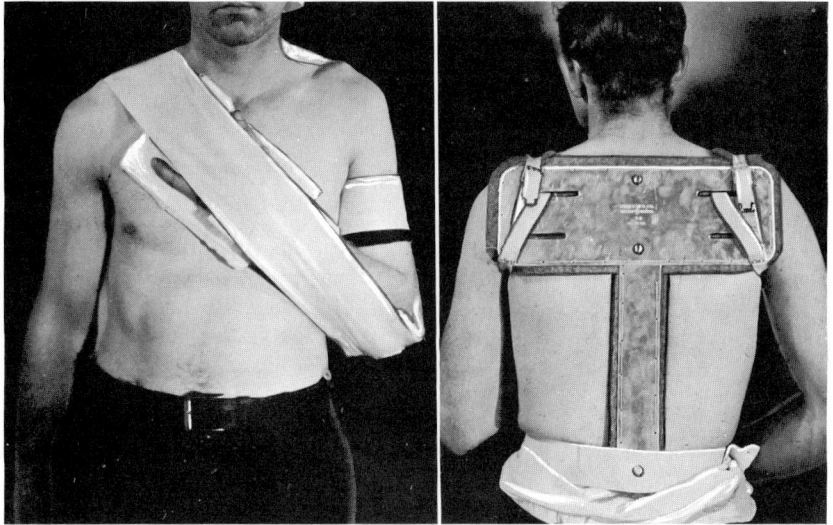

been treated early. When the wounds are grossly contaminated or when there has been delay of treatment, débridement and immobilization are carried out, with secondary closure in 5 to 7 days. When there has been much loss of tissue, skin grafting may be necessary.

Fractures at Specific Sites

SKULL AND SPINE. These have been considered in Chapter 41 on the nursing of neurosurgical diseases.

MANDIBLE (JAW BONE). These fractures are compound, opening into the mouth. They are treated by fixing the lower jaw against the upper by wires placed between the teeth, or by a firm bandage. The problem then is one of treating a fracture compounded into the mouth in a patient who cannot open his jaws. In other instances molded metal bars are wired to the teeth on both sides of the fracture line (Fig. 396).

The nurse should be cognizant of the danger of vomiting in patients having the jaws wired together. She should know that the jaws may be opened by removal of the wire loops if this complication arises. By the use of a simple hemostat the wires which join the loops attached to the upper and the lower teeth may be untwisted. A wire cutter may have to be used if untwisting the wires takes too long. A cutter should be taped to the head of the bed in case of an emergency.

Careful attention to the hygiene of the mouth must be insisted upon, using warm alkaline mouthwashes at least every 2 hours and after each feeding. In addition, the mouth should be inspected at least once or twice daily to ensure thorough cleansing. A flashlight and a tongue blade to retract the cheeks are essential equipment.

The diet must necessarily be liquid, but sufficient caloric and fluid intake can be given easily to these patients. They can be fed through a straw without much difficulty and occasionally soft foods may be given with a spoon. Water should be given after each liquid feeding, followed by a mouth wash.

CLAVICLE (COLLAR BONE). This is one of the most common of fractures and it practically always unites.

A Velpeau or Sayre dressing may be used in ambulatory treatment. For both of these dressings, gauze or lint should be provided for placing in the axilla and between the arm and the chest.

The Velpeau requires muslin bandages 2 or 3 inches in width and a safety pin to secure them.

The Sayre dressing is applied with long adhesive strips cut as wide as the patient's forearm (Fig. 397). A clavicular cross is used as a dressing by many surgeons (Fig. 397). A figure-of-eight strapping or plaster bandage may be used also.

RIBS. Uncomplicated fractures of the ribs are very common and may be treated easily by firm adhesive strapping 2 or 3 inches in width which should reach beyond the midline both front and back. This type of binding is applied as the patient exhales. These patients should be watched carefully for symptoms of pleurisy and other pulmonary complications. Before applying the strips it is well to shave the hairy regions to make removal of the adhesive less painful. Injections of local anesthesia along the intercostal nerves of the injured area and about the fracture site are often given to relieve pain and are used by some surgeons instead of strapping.

HUMERUS. *Surgical Neck*. The commonest fracture in the upper arm and the shoulder is that of the surgical neck of the humerus. It occurs most often in adults, and the patient comes for aid with the affected arm hanging limp at the side, supported with the uninjured hand.

Reduction is best accomplished with the aid of the fluoroscope while the patient is under anesthesia. The dressing applied is the one which will best hold the fragments in position. The simplest dressing is one which employs: (1) A well-padded shoulder cap. This may be made of wood, felt, cardboard or plaster of Paris. (2) An axillary pad. This is a triangular pad of gauze with a base about 4 or 5 inches in width, a perpendicular equal to the distance from the patient's axilla to his elbow, and a little broader than the broadest part of the patient's arm. (3) A wrist sling of 4- to 6-inch muslin bandage. The sling is applied first, and the pad and the shoulder cap are held by bandages about the patient's body, placed so as to hold the arm to the side. The turn about the chest should include the sling in order to draw the hand and the forearm close to the body. This dressing is maintained for from 4 to 6 weeks.

Shaft. These fractures are among the most difficult of all fractures to treat. The bone is surrounded by thick muscles which often become interposed between the fragments and make reduction difficult. The musculospiral nerve lies posterior to the bone, in the musculospiral groove, and not infrequently it is involved in shaft fractures

or in the callus formed by their healing. It is important, therefore, to make frequent inspection for wristdrop, the sign of paralysis of this nerve, both before and after reduction of the fracture.

Many dressings are used for this fracture: the shoulder cap, axillary pad and sling; many forms of traction with splints; the airplane splint.

A form of dressing known as the "hanging cast" is used. A plaster cast is applied to the forearm and the arm, holding the elbow flexed to a right angle. The cast is slung at the wrist, the weight of the cast producing traction upon the lower fragment. Movement of the arm at the shoulder is encouraged. Union occurs without the usual immobilization of the fragments.

Above the Elbow. These fractures are very common in childhood and adolescence. There are many varieties, the most common being the supracondylar type. They are usually attended with considerable swelling, and, because the lower fragment is displaced posteriorly in most cases, the forearm appears to be shortened. The fragments are best maintained in position by holding the arm acutely flexed, and the usual dressings are applied with the arm in this position. A sling from the wrist draws the hand close to the neck.

A very important nursing measure in caring for a patient with an elbow fracture treated by acute flexion of the arm is to observe the hand for swelling and blueness of the nails. These signs may indicate a disturbance of blood supply and should be reported immediately.

FOREARM. *Both Bones of Forearm*. These fractures are most common in the middle third. It is almost impossible to tell which dressings are indicated until the fracture reduction has been completed.

Above the Wrist. These fractures result very often from falls on the out-stretched hand. The Colles (suprastyloid) type is the most common. This is a fracture of the radius from ½ to 1 inch above the wrist, with a posterior displacement of the lower fragment. The hand is deviated to the thumb side. The position is often spoken of as the "silver-fork deformity." These fractures are dressed in many ways, most often by the use of molded plaster splints. Bandage and a sling are always necessary.

PELVIS. Pelvic fractures are commonly found following severe trauma. They are serious injuries, because frequently they are associated with injuries to the intrapelvic structures. The bladder, the urethra, or the intestine may be ruptured and prove to be of more serious import than the fracture itself.

Treatment and Nursing Care. The urine and the stools should be examined daily for several days for evidences of blood, and the patient must be watched carefully for signs of intra-abdominal trouble. The fracture is usually treated by rest in bed, with weight traction applied to one or both legs to immobilize the hips. In some instances the fracture is immobilized by a canvas sling with perpendicular traction. The fracture bed contributes largely to the comfort and the ease of handling these patients (Fig. 403 B). One type of fracture bed is made so that a bedpan may be used without disturbing the position of the patient. This is made possible by mechanical adjustments of the bed. The nurse must frequently inspect all traction apparatus and watch carefully for signs

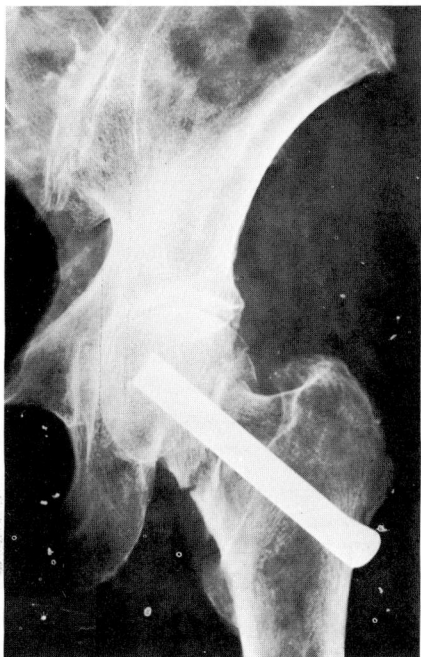

FIG. 398. Smith-Petersen nail inserted for fracture of the neck of the femur.

of pressure. Good care of the skin and gentle handling of the patient do much to prevent complications and to make his difficulties more easily borne.

FEMUR. *Neck.* These fractures occur most frequently in old people, especially in women, and are due often to very insignificant injuries. The patient is unable to move the leg, which lies characteristically with the foot turned outward flat on the bed, knee fully extended. If the limb is compared with its fellow by inspection or by actual measurement, there is found to be considerable shortening. A measuring tape should be at hand in order to estimate and record this finding accurately.

Treatment and Nursing Care. Surgeons usually treat fractures of the neck of the femur by the use of pins or nails (Fig. 398). After reduction of the fracture, the nails are introduced through the trochanter along the neck of the femur into the head. The pins are inserted under local or spinal anesthesia through a very small wound made on the outer side of the thigh. Patients so treated may be up and in a chair within a very few days. As soon as possible, they may be taught to use crutches, bearing weight on the uninjured leg only.

These patients, because of their age, are particularly prone to develop complications which may become more important with regard to treatment than the fracture itself. The shock of the injury may be fatal. Shock also is known to cause bladder incontinence; control is gradually regained later. Other complications are disorientation in the elderly patient, fecal impaction, thrombophlebitis and pulmonary emboli. Because of the necessity for these patients to remain in one position for long periods of time, bedsores frequently develop. The nurse may do much to avert their occurrence by attention to the skin on the back, especially under the hips and the shoulders, and by relieving constant pressure by airfoam pillows, etc. A trapeze suspended from the fracture bed permits the patient to lift himself; this is a great boon to nursing care. Nevertheless, triceps and shoulder exercises should be continued preparatory to ambulatory activities. The patient may be turned on his unaffected extremity. A pillow is placed between the legs to keep the affected leg in an abducted

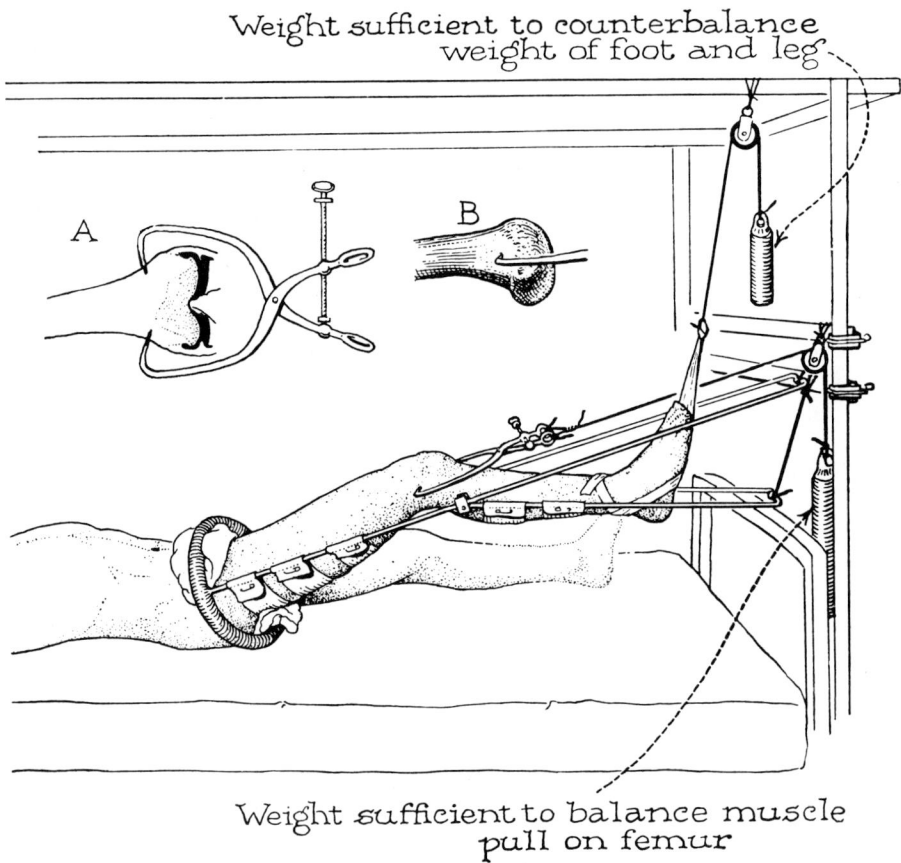

Weight sufficient to counterbalance
weight of foot and leg

A   B

Weight sufficient to balance muscle
pull on femur

FIG. 399. Diagram of the method of use of ice-tong calipers with the Thomas splint and the Pearson attachment in fracture of the femur. (A) Point of application (anteroposterior). (B) Point of application (lateral view). (Magnuson, P.B., and Stack, J. K.: Fractures, ed. 5, Philadelphia, Lippincott)

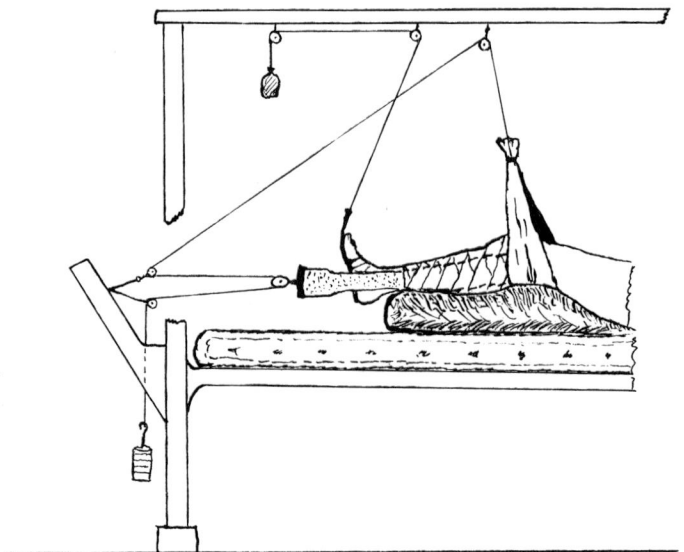

FIG. 400. The Russell method of treating a fracture of the shaft of the femur. A small spring scale sometimes is inserted between the pulley and the traction block so that the amount of traction may be estimated accurately.

position. Then the patient is pulled over gently on his side. After initial soreness has gone, the patient usually may be turned in the same manner on the affected hip.

Renal calculi and other kidney problems may arise. Pulmonary complications such as hypostatic congestion of the lungs and bronchopneumonia can occur and may be fatal. Deep-breathing exercises, change of position at least every 2 hours and protection of the chest with a shoulder blanket are measures which may help to prevent the development of these complications. The nurse should be familiar with the precautions which are to be observed in treating patients with traction or casts.

Shaft. These fractures occur most commonly in youth and middle age. There is marked swelling of the thigh, with shortening. The use of intramedullary pins is becoming increasingly popular. Frequently, reduction is accomplished by traction, using a Thomas splint and Buck's extension, or by the use of a Thomas splint (Fig. 386) with a Pearson (Fig. 386) attachment, applying traction to the lower fragment by means of a Kirschner wire, a Steinmann pin, or tongs (Fig. 399). Some surgeons apply upward as well as horizontal traction on the lower fragment by the Russell method (see Figs. 400 and 401). A spica cast may also be used.

In the treatment of most patients with a fractured femur, a fracture bed is necessary to which the pulleys for traction may be attached. The fracture must be immobilized for 7 to 8 weeks, at the end of which time the patient may be allowed to get up and to walk with the aid of crutches. Full weight bearing must not be allowed for at least 6 months.

Fractures which occur in children under 10 years of age are frequently treated by the Bryant method of vertical suspension. Adhesive traction is applied to both legs equally, sufficient weights being employed just to lift the buttocks off the bed. This dressing is maintained for 6 weeks (Fig. 403).

Medullary Pin. The medullary pin is used in some clinics in approximating fractures of the shaft of the femur (Fig. 402). The patient usually has skeletal traction for a week preoperatively, which allows time for systemic studies and for the reduction of any swelling. The medullary nail may be introduced by the open or the closed method. The chief advantage of such nailing is that the patient can be up and out of bed to begin weight bearing by 3 weeks. Prior to this time, he has opportunity to move his leg, thereby preventing stiffening and muscular atrophy. Disadvantages are (1) there is believed to be some destruction of bone marrow with resultant hemoglobin and red blood cell reduction, (2) there is a possibility of producing bone infection, and (3) there is a chance for the formation of a fat embolism in the closed method. After about a year the stainless steel nail is removed through a small incision.

INTERNAL DERANGEMENT OF THE KNEE. Injury to most joints consists of a tear of its supporting ligaments. In the knee joint, however, there may be also a displacement or tear of the semilunar cartilages. These are two crescent-shaped cartilages attached to the edge of the shallow articulating surface of the head of the tibia. They normally move slightly backward and forward to accommodate for the change in the shape of the condyles of the femur when the leg is in flexion or extension. In sports and falls, the body is often twisted with the foot fixed. Since no torsion movement is normally permitted in the knee joint, an injury results which very

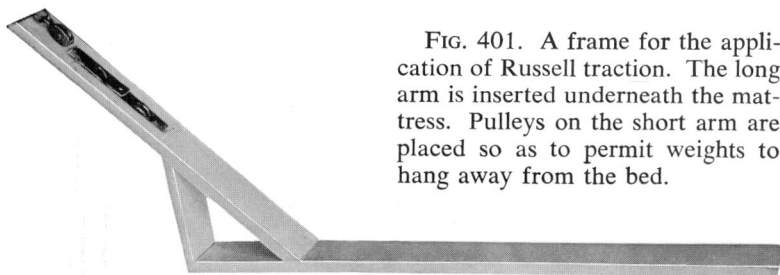

FIG. 401. A frame for the application of Russell traction. The long arm is inserted underneath the mattress. Pulleys on the short arm are placed so as to permit weights to hang away from the bed.

often is either a tear of the cartilage from its attachment to the head of the tibia or an actual tear or fracture of the cartilage itself. These injuries leave a loose cartilage in the knee joint which may slip between the femur and the tibia and so prevent full extension of the leg. If this happens when the patient is walking or running, he often describes his disability as his "leg giving way" under him, and there are times when the cartilage gets

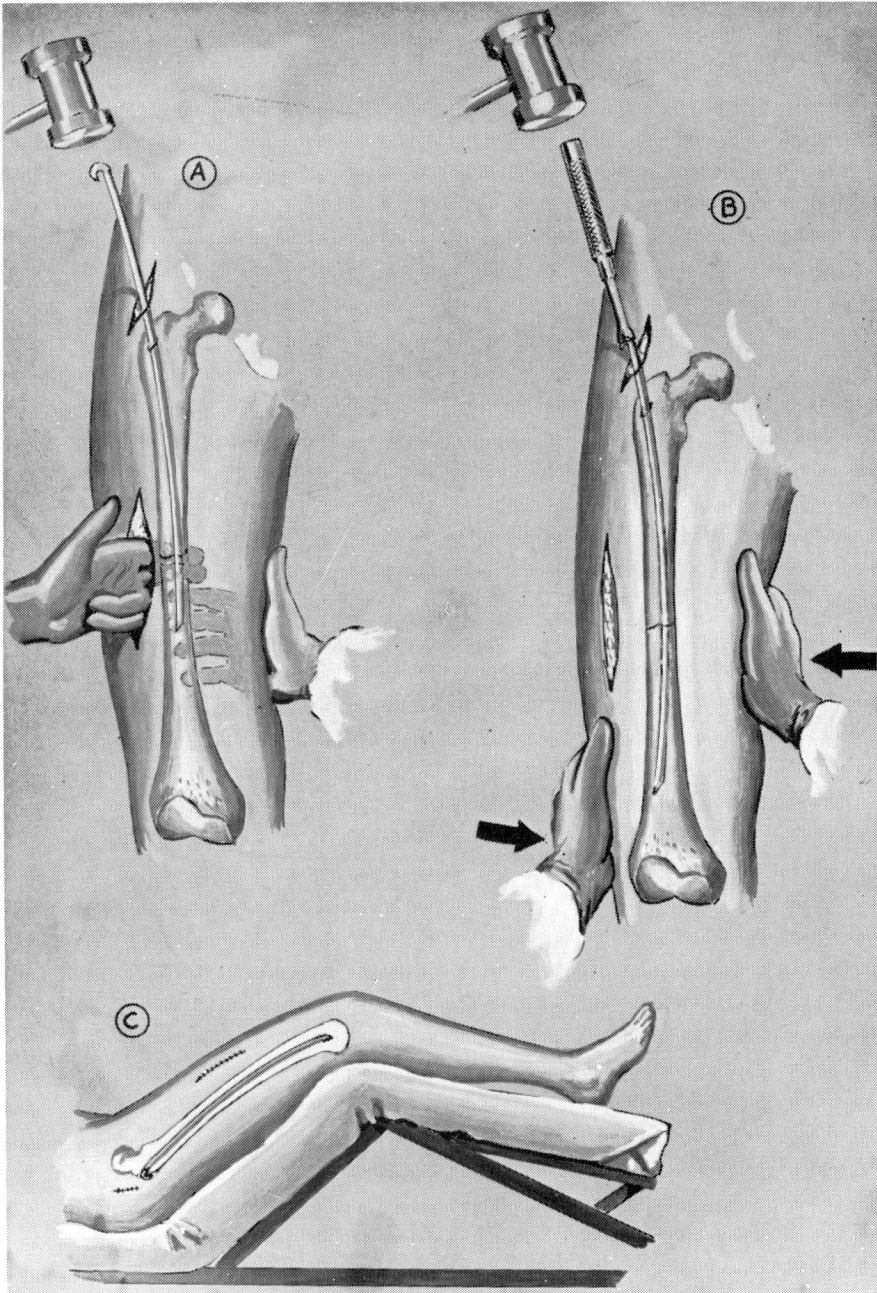

FIG. 402. The Rush medullary pin for fracture of the shaft of the femur. (Berivon Co.)

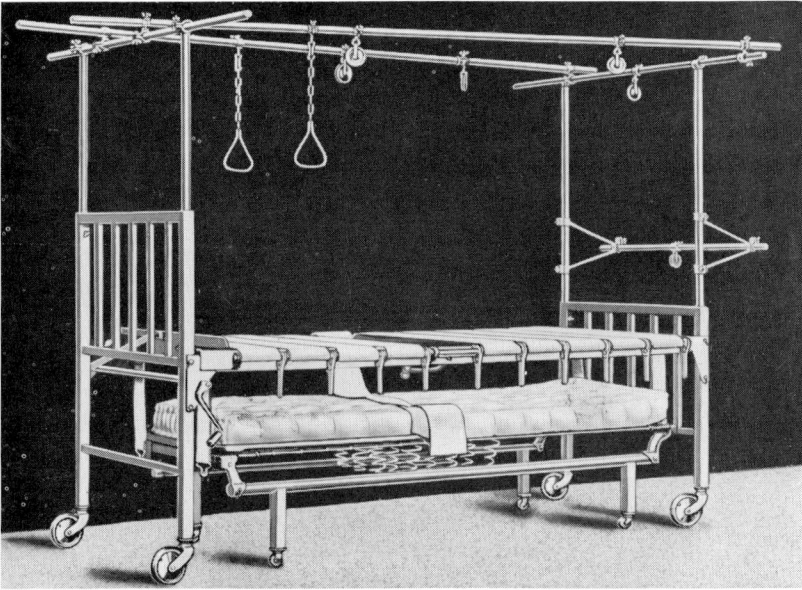

FIG. 403 A. Fracture Bed. Note (1) this bed has an adjustable back rest, (2) the adjustable canvas straps across the bed on which the patient's weight may be maintained while the bed is lowered. One cross strap (as illustrated) or more can be dropped for bed pan use, enema, treatment of pressure areas, and many other nursing activities, and (3) (above) the adjustable pulleys and rings. (Orthopedic Equipment Co.)

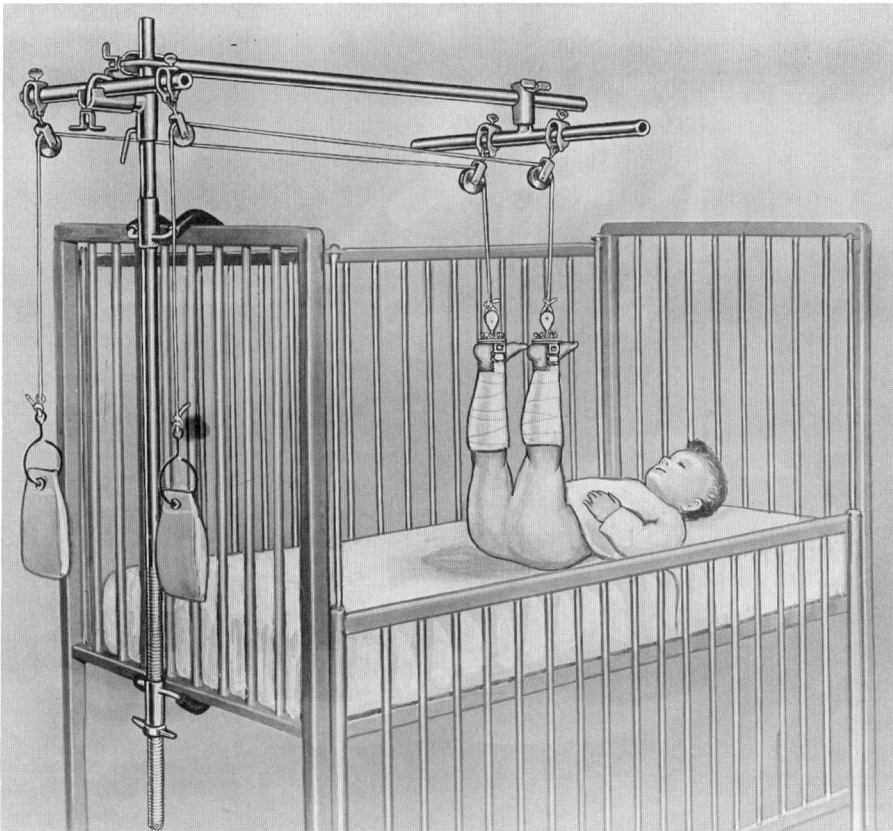

FIG. 403 B. The Bryant method of vertical traction for fractures of the femur in children. Note that both legs are suspended by skin traction with weights sufficient to lift the pelvis from the bed. Bryant's traction may cause ischemia of the feet and the legs. (Gilbert Hyde Chick Co., Oakland, Calif.)

caught between the articulating surfaces so that the knee "locks." The patient may hear or feel a click in his knee when he walks, especially when he extends his leg bearing his weight, as in going upstairs. When the cartilage is attached front and back, but torn loose laterally (bucket-handle tear) it may slide between the bones to lie between the condyles and prevent full flexion or extension.

These various types of injury arising from a common cause are spoken of as an internal derangement of the knee joint, and they produce a disturbing disability because the patient never knows when the knee will give him trouble. The treatment of this disability is removal of the injured cartilage, which can be done with relative ease through an incision into the knee joint. The joint function is thereby returned to normal, and no apparent disability results from the loss of the cartilage.

Preparation for operation consists of a shave of the entire leg. Some surgeons desire a "sterile prep" in addition.

Postoperative Nursing Care. After suture of the wound, a pressure dressing is applied, and at times a posterior splint. The leg should be elevated on pillows with a slight bend at the knee. The most common complication is an effusion into the knee joint which produces marked pain. The physician should be called. Relief can be obtained by cutting the pressure dressing and reapplying it more loosely. Frequently, the joint may be aspirated under local anesthesia and pressure relieved by withdrawing the fluid in the joint. To prevent atrophy of the thigh muscles,

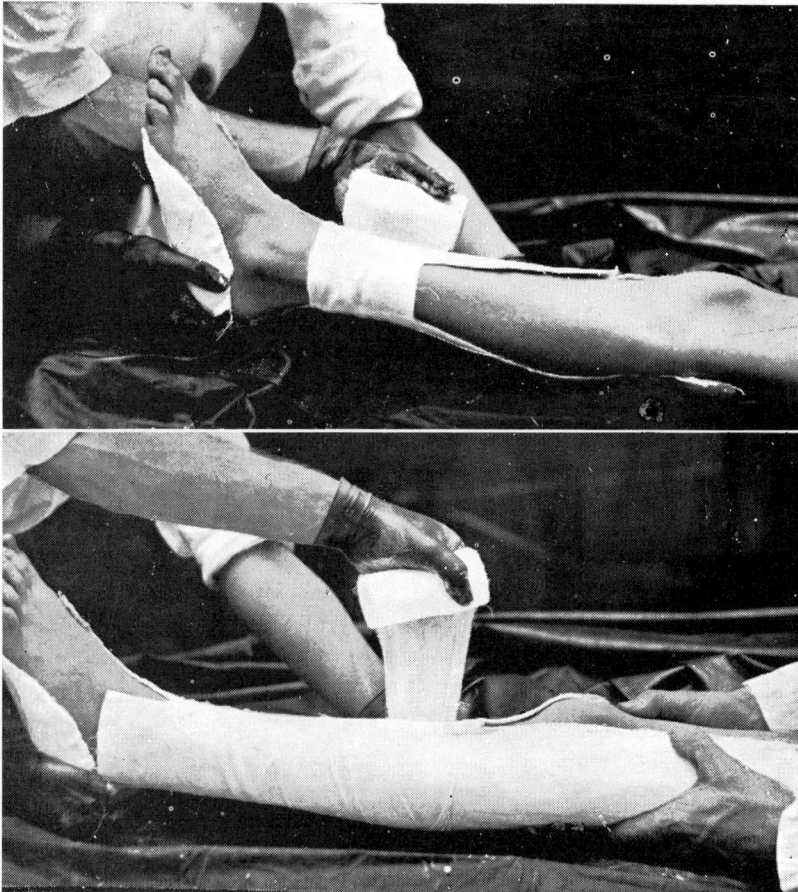

FIG. 404. Plaster splints for leg fractures.

these patients are instructed to "set" their muscles while in bed. After 1 or 2 days the patient may be up with crutches bearing weight by touching only his toes on the operated side. In a short time, 1 to 2 weeks, full weight-bearing is possible, but the knee usually is supported for another few weeks by an elastic bandage. Full and normal function may be looked for in from 6 to 8 weeks from the time of operation.

TIBIA AND FIBULA. Fractures of the shafts of these bones are often associated. There usually is considerable swelling which disappears readily if reduction and immobilization are accomplished early. Reduction is best done under the fluoroscope by traction and manipulation, and the leg dressed in a plaster cast extending from toe to thigh, or better by the use of molded lateral plaster splints, which include the foot and the thigh. Again, an intramedullary pin may be used.

Pott's fracture, the commonest below the knee, is a fracture of lower 2 or 3 inches of the fibula due to "twisting the ankle." There is also a fracture of the internal malleolus and of the posterior portion of the articular surface of the tibia, frequently associated with it. Swelling and discoloration about the ankle are marked.

Fluoroscopic reduction is recommended. The dressing used is a plaster cast, or lateral plaster splints (Fig. 404). Elevation of the leg for several days reduces the swelling very rapidly. Function may be renewed in 4 months.

CRUTCHES. All fractures of the lower extremity require the use of crutches during convalescence. Adjustable crutches should be secured for the patient. They should be about 1 inch longer than the distance from the axilla to the heel and should be fitted with rubber suction tips as well as axillary and hand cushions. (See also Crutches, pp. 364, 1015.)

WALKING IRON. In many clinics these fractures are treated by the application of a cast in which is incorporated a walking iron. This treatment cannot be employed until after the swelling has disappeared. By the use of the walking iron the patient may be able to walk fairly easily without any support or with the aid of a cane (Fig. 405).

THE PATIENT WITH AN AMPUTATION

Amputation of extremities is frequently necessary in the treatment of gangrene, tumors, deformities, septic wounds, compound fractures and severe crushing injuries, gas gangrene, etc. In severe trauma, an amputation is done to save a patient's life. The nurse will be aware that this is a major adjustment for the patient to make. One day he is a perfectly normal individual, and the next day he must accept his loss. For the individual who has a long-standing disease which causes him pain and restricts his ability to get around, the acceptance of an amputation is not as difficult.

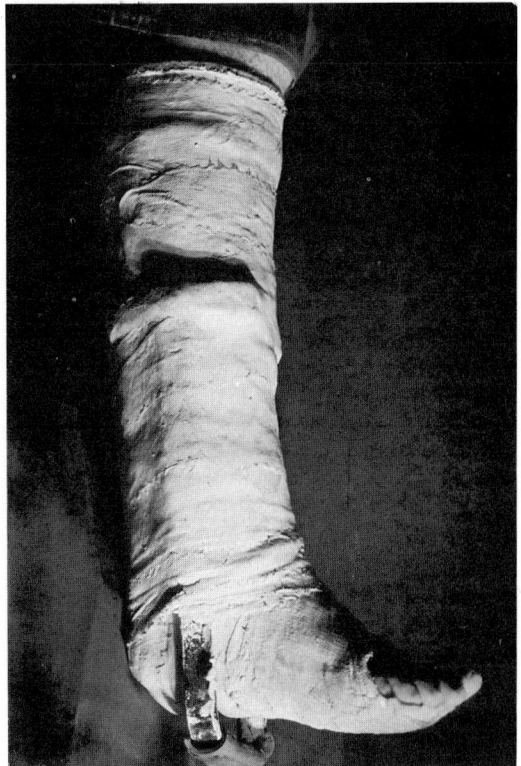

FIG. 405. Fracture of the lower tibia and fibula treated with a cast in which a walking iron is incorporated.

Nursing Care

Preoperative Care. Often before surgery, the physician will perform tests to determine the patency of circulation. These will include surface temperature, color changes when the limb is elevated or dependent, and oscillometric readings. His state of nutrition must be recognized and improved if necessary. Psychological preparation cannot be neglected. The physician and the nurse can help to build a healthy optimism in this patient by making him realize that he can overcome his handicap and be independent. Preparation for the operation when possible should consist in shaving of the part and thorough cleansing with soap and water. Intravenous fluids are administered to combat dehydration; blood is made available. Before the operation the extremity should be elevated continuously for at least 5 minutes to allow the venous blood to drain as completely as possible from the part. This procedure is aided in many clinics by the application of a pneumatic tourniquet or an Esmarch bandage, an elastic bandage of 2-inch rubber applied in the direction of the trunk, to compress the extremity. A tourniquet of heavy rubber then is applied and drawn tight enough to compress the blood vessels.

If the amputation is not an emergency procedure, efforts should be made to strengthen the upper extremities as well as the trunk and the abdominal muscles. It is ideal to teach the patient to crutch walk before the surgical procedure. The patient can be given traction weights and encouraged to flex and to extend his arms while he is holding the weights. Doing push-ups while he is in a prone position and sit-ups while he is seated will strengthen the tricep muscles, which are so important in crutch walking.

Postoperative Care. Amputations are usually performed by making soft-tissue flaps, which are used to cover the bone stump. The site of the amputation is determined by two factors: circulation in the part and the requirements of an artificial limb (prosthesis). In many amputations, especially of the leg, when performed for gangrene of the foot due to vascular impairment,

a high amputation (midthigh) must be done because the circulation of the leg below is insufficient to bring about healing of an amputation site at a lower level.

Experience with artificial limbs has shown that stumps of some certain length function best in these appliances. If the stump is too long, it may be awkward and hard to fit; if it is too short, the adjacent joint cannot function well. When they are made below the knee and the elbow joints, it is well to splint the part for a time to prevent contractures. These patients should be watched carefully for any signs or symptoms of hemorrhage. As a precaution, a tourniquet should be in plain sight at the foot of the bed, and, if bleeding occurs, should be applied to the stump and pulled sufficiently tight to stop the bleeding. It should be left in place until the surgeon can be notified. The stump should be elevated for the first day on a pillow protected with a rubber or plastic pillow case. Such a pillow should support the entire stump from the hip down, in order that knee flexion be prevented. *This pillow is removed as soon as possible by physician's order to avoid hip joint flexion contracture.* In some hospitals it is required that the stump remain uncovered and in full sight for the first 24 to 48 hours, the period in which hemorrhage is most likely to occur. Oozing usually appears at the bottom of the dressing; linen may be spared by placing the stump upon a sterile cellucotton pad. The dressings should be reinforced rather than changed. A footboard should be used to keep the remaining foot in dorsiflexion.

During the first 24 hours, especially in older patients, a shocklike state is frequently present, and the patient does not fully realize that he has had an amputation. Often the realization may come as a shock to him, even though he knew before his operation that an amputation was to be performed. Frequently, these cases are complicated by the production of pulmonary emboli and so must be watched carefully for such findings as cough, chest pain, hemoptysis, severe sudden collapse, cyanosis, or even sudden death. On occasion, especially when the amputation has been done for infection, a guillotine type may be performed without any attempt to suture the skin. In such cases, to prevent the retraction of the skin, traction may be applied and eventual healing brought about. The principles given under Nursing Care of the Patient in Traction (p. 999) apply here.

Rehabilitation. Effective preprosthetic care is important to prosthetic fitting. The major problems that are preventable during this period are (1) flexion deformities, (2) nonshrinkage of the stump, and (3) abduction deformities of the hip. These deformities will delay the prosthetic fitting.

After the first 24 to 48 hours, depending on the physician's orders, the patient should be encouraged to turn from side to side and to be in the prone position to prevent flexion contracture of the hip. A pillow can be placed under the abdomen and the stump; the forefoot can be placed over the edge of the mattress. The legs should remain close together while the patient is in the prone position to prevent an abduction deformity. He must learn to recognize the value of moving the stump so that contractures are avoided. Sometimes patients use an overhead trapeze when changing their position in bed; this will strengthen the biceps. Unfortunately, this set of muscles is not as necessary in crutch walking as are the triceps. These can be strengthened by pressing with the palms against the bed when moving the body and continuing the push-up exercises. Exercises under the supervision of the physical therapist, such as hyperextension of the stump, also will aid in strengthening muscles as well as increasing circulation, reducing edema and preventing atrophy. In getting the patient out of bed, regard must be given to maintaining good posture.

The patient should be fairly adept at balancing himself on one leg and walking with crutches before he leaves the hospital. There may be a time lapse of several weeks or many months before the patient may be fitted with a prosthesis.

Exercises that will assist in developing balance are:

1. Arising from a chair and standing.
2. Standing on toes while holding on to a chair.
3. Bending the knees while holding on to a chair.
4. Balancing on one leg without support.
5. Hopping on one foot while holding on to a chair.

The nurse may stand behind the patient and stabilize him by his waist while he is learning to perform these exercises. While crutch walking, the patient should learn to use a reciprocal gait. The stump should move back and forth while the patient is walking with his crutches. The stump should not be held up in a flexed position to prevent a permanent flexion deformity from occurring.

STUMP CONDITIONING. After the wound has healed, the nurse should learn from the surgeon how he wishes the stump to be bandaged. Thereafter the nurse can teach the patient or some member of his family the correct method of bandaging.

The stump has to be conditioned if a prosthesis is to be fitted properly. (However, the nurse must bear in mind that not every patient can be fitted for a prosthetic device.) To shrink and to shape the stump, the stump must be bandaged correctly (Fig. 406). Bandaging will support the soft tissue and will minimize the formation of edematous fluid while the stump is in a dependent position. The bandage is applied in such a manner that the remaining muscles required to operate the prosthesis are as firm as possible, while those muscles that are no longer useful will atrophy.

The bandage should be laundered frequently in tepid water and placed on a flat surface to dry, so that its elasticity is retained as long as possible.

In order to "toughen" the stump in preparation for using a prosthesis, the doctor usually orders stump conditioning activities. The patient is taught to push his stump into a soft pillow. Progressively he increases the resistance, pushing the stump against a firmer pillow and then against a hard surface.

When amputations of the leg have been performed on elderly, debilitated patients, especially diabetics and arteriosclerotics, particular care should be taken to protect the stump against external infection. Such patients frequently become incontinent of urine and feces, and not infrequently the dressing and the wound of the stump may become soiled. Plastic material secured by a wide adhesive strip about the leg above the dress-

Guide to Bandaging an Above-the-Knee Amputation Stump*

Purpose: The purpose for bandaging a stump is to shrink and to shape the stump for the application of an artificial leg.

Problems: Improper bandaging will produce:

Constriction of the stump

Delayed healing

Skin abrasions

Formation of creases or adipose tissue at distal end

Basic Principles: The bandage is applied before the patient gets out of bed after periods of recumbency. The bandage should be maintained continuously and reapplied when tension is lost. Pressure should be applied under moderate tension to the entire stump, guarding against any tourniquetlike action at the proximal portion of the stump. The stump is kept in *hyperextension* while the bandage is applied.

---

* The material in "Guide to Bandaging an Above-the-Knee Amputation Stump" and all parts of Figure 406 are from Nattern, L. W., Jr.: Orthopedic and Prosthetic Appliance Journal, pp. 51 to 55, June, 1957.

---

ing has proved to be a good prophylactic measure.

Often during the convalescence while the muscle stumps are adjusting themselves, twitchings and spasms occur. Heat, massage, change of position to procure relaxation, a light sandbag on a thigh stump to counteract the psoas action—all will help. During this stage, and often for an indefinite period to follow, the patient may complain as though the pain were in the amputated limb—the "phantom limb" complication so often very difficult to cure.

The complete rehabilitation of an amputee requires a rehabilitation team. The ortho-pedic surgeon, the physiatrist, the limb maker, the physical therapist, and the occu-pational therapist all unite their efforts to condition and to train the patient to make a satisfactory adjustment to his prosthesis. With vocational counseling and job-retrain-ing, where necessary, many of these patients can return to work. If it is not possible for the patient to use a prosthesis, he can be taught to participate in self-care activities in a wheel chair. The pamphlet *Step Into Action*† is a teaching booklet designed for the amputee; it has illustrations and descriptions concerning stump hygiene, bandaging, and other activities that are important to the patient.

Technic of Applying Bandage:

1. Begin the recurrent, vertical turns on the anterior surface of the stump just inferior to the level of the inguinal ligament (Fig. 406 A).

   Pass the bandage over the distal end of the stump posteriorly to the gluteal fold. The patient assists by holding the recurrents in place.

   Make two additional recurrents over the medial and the lateral aspects of the end of the stump.

2. Anchor the recurrents by several horizontal circular turns of the bandage (Fig. 406 B).

† Superintendent of Documents, U. S. Government Printing Office, Washington 25, D. C.

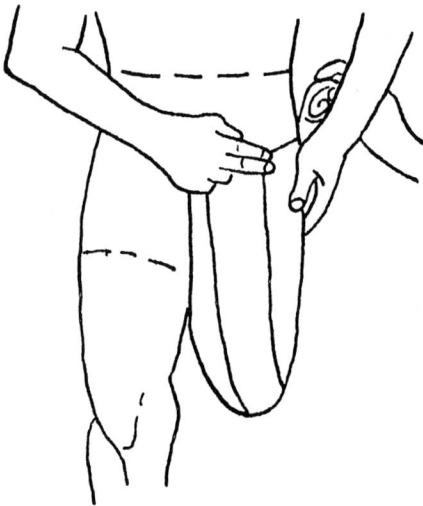

FIGURE 406 A.

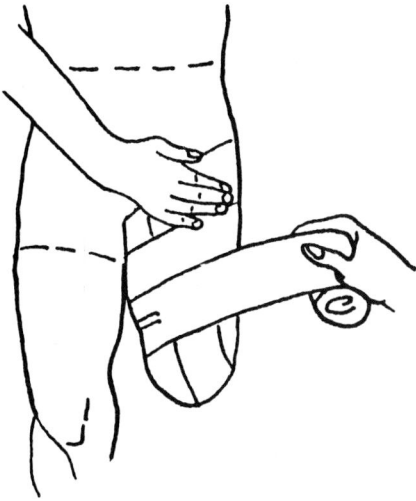

FIGURE 406 B.

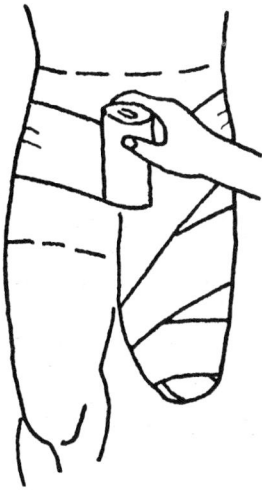

FIGURE 406 C.

When anchoring the recurrents, the circular turns begin at the lateral side and run posteriorly to the medial side.

When the recurrents are firmly secured, bring the bandage down and around the stump and up again using oblique turns or a modified figure-8.

Keep the pressure away, up and out from the distal portion of the stump to eliminate creases. Do not

use circular turns which are not oblique, as they tend to constrict circulation.

3. Start the hip spica from the anterior medial aspect of the stump and bring it laterally across the anterior surface of the stump in the inguinal region (Fig. 406 C). (The hip spica anchors the bandage and covers the tissue high in the groin and the lateral surfaces of the hip, thus eliminating the formation of bulges in this area.)

Bring the bandage around the body on a level with the iliac crest.

4. Return around the stump making a figure-8, and bring the bandage around the pelvis again. Finish the bandage by making oblique turns on the stump.

Anchor the bandage with safety pins at the lateral or the anterior surface of the stump. Fasten where bandage ends and at crossing of spica at the hip (Fig. 406 D).

PATIENTS WITH BONE AND JOINT INFECTIONS
Osteomyelitis

Acute osteomyelitis is an acute infection of the bone marrow that rapidly involves other bony structures. It affects the long

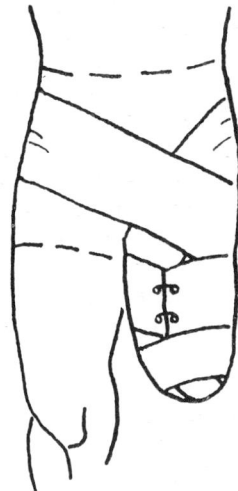

FIGURE 406 D.

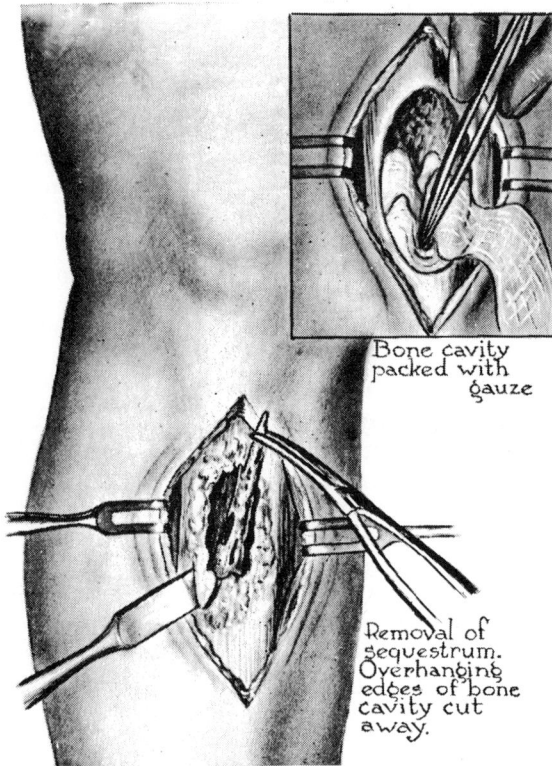

Fig. 407. Method of sequestrectomy and saucerization. Inset shows bone cavity packed with petrolatum gauze. (Steindler, A.: Orthopedic Operations, Springfield, Ill., Thomas)

Bone cavity packed with gauze

Removal of sequestrum. Overhanging edges of bone cavity cut away.

bones most frequently and is caused most commonly by the *Staphylococcus aureus*. The infection usually is blood-borne from other foci of infection, but it may follow slight trauma or exposure to cold and wet. It is essentially a disease of childhood and adolescence. However, osteomyelitis may occur, by direct infection of the bone resulting from compound fractures. The onset of the disease usually is sudden, occurring often with a chill, high fever, rapid pulse and general malaise. In children, in whom the disease usually begins as an acute epiphysitis, these constitutional symptoms at first may overshadow the local signs completely. As the infection extends from the marrow cavity through the cortex of the bone, it involves the periosteum and the soft tissues, and the limb becomes painful, swollen and extremely tender. Thus an abscess of bone is formed. In the natural course of events, the abscess may point and drain but, more often, incision and drainage are done by the surgeon. The resulting abscess cavity has in its walls areas of dead tissue, as in any abscess cavity; however, in this case the dead tissue is bone,

which cannot liquefy easily and be discharged as pus. This dead bone is called a *sequestrum*. Healing in a bone abscess is more difficult than in an abscess in soft tissue, because the cavity cannot collapse and heal. New bone, the *involucrum*, forms in Nature's attempt at repair. Often it grows so as to surround a sequestrum. Thus, even though healing appears to take place, a chronically infected sequestrum remains that is prone to produce recurring abscesses throughout the life of the individual. This is the so-called chronic type of osteomyelitis.

Treatment. Acute osteomyelitis begins as a staphylococcic septicemia, and formerly the acute toxemia frequently was fatal. Since antibiotics became available, early and intensive treatment usually produces a rapid recovery. The development of an abscess of the bone, with the resulting marked and prolonged morbidity, thus can be avoided. In neglected or untreated cases, aspiration or incision and drainage of an abscess may be necessary.

In chronic osteomyelitis, the dead, infected bone must be removed before permanent healing takes place. This operation, called a *sequestrectomy* (Fig. 323), consists of the removal of enough involucrum with mallet and chisel to enable the surgeon to remove the sequestrum. Often sufficient bone is removed to convert a deep cavity into a shallow saucer (saucerization). Muscle sometimes is used to help to obliterate the resulting wound. These operations are becoming increasingly rare since the advent of effective antimicrobial chemotherapy. Primary healing may be obtained frequently by the use of an appropriate antibiotic (e.g., methicillin or oxacillin), if the cavity can be closed and the skin approximated. Sometimes the granulating wound may be covered by a split-thickness skin graft.

When osteomyelitis occurs in a compound fracture by direct implantation of the offending organisms, there is no preceding septicemia, but the treatment is in general as outlined above, except that the fracture must be treated in addition.

Nursing Care. Osteomyelitis is in the group of diseases in which good nursing care is absolutely necessary. The wounds themselves frequently are very painful and require great care and gentleness in their handling. Pillow support to the adjoining joints and maintenance of good alignment are comfort measures. Careful handling also is essential because of the possibilities of cross infection and pathologic fracture. Hot packs may be prescribed for indurated areas. Less pain is experienced if petrolatum gauze is used in the dressing. Scrupulous care of the skin is required to prevent bedsores. Fresh air, sunlight and a high caloric diet rich in vitamins will hasten the convalescence of these patients. They should be watched carefully for any development of painful areas or sudden rises in temperature, as these symptoms usually indicate the formation of a secondary abscess. A frequent problem encountered is an unpleasant odor due to the foul drainage. A deodorizer near the patient's unit may help. Some physicians use a specially prepared charcoal plaster which absorbs the odor. For the most part, to reassure the patient that this is a usual result of bone infection will help. Because of the long period of hospitalization and frequent readmissions sometimes necessary in the treatment of these patients, their morale often is low and they need stimulation and diversion. During their hospital stay the occupational therapy department and the hospital school teacher often are able to find interesting and useful employment suited to their ability.

Acute Pyogenic Arthritis

Acute pyogenic arthritis, or "purulent arthritis," most often is caused by *Staphylococcus aureus* or the hemolytic streptococcus, and less frequently by the pneumococcus, the meningococcus or the gonococcus. Usually, it occurs as a complication of a bacteremia, in the course of which the infecting organism becomes localized in a joint, especially a joint previously damaged by trauma. It also may result from the extension of an osteomyelitis that involves some bone in the vicinity of a joint; and it may be produced by a wound that penetrates the joint.

Symptoms. The symptoms of purulent arthritis are redness, swelling, edema and tenderness of the joint; fluctuation, if the amount of pus is considerable; pain, increased by pressure and by motion; chills, fever, leukocytosis and other general symptoms of sepsis. The pus in joints infected by staphylococci, is thick and creamy; that in streptococcal cases is thin and contains but few pus cells, but the general symptoms of sepsis are severe, out of all proportion to the local signs.

Treatment. Occasionally, it is necessary to drain the joint cavity, either by repeated needle aspiration or by the institution of incision and open drainage, restoration of movement being afforded as soon as possible after subsidence of the infection. The objectives of therapy are to halt the infection by chemotherapy before the joint cartilage is destroyed, and to mobilize the joint before adhesions have formed, and muscle atrophy has progressed too far—i.e., to destroy the organism and to protect the joint.

A bacteriologic diagnosis is established as soon as possible, and chemotherapy is instituted without delay. Instillation of the drug directly into the cavity of the infected joint may prove to be necessary. (For details of antimicrobial chemotherapy as it is applied in specific types of bacterial infection, see Chapter 13.)

Bone and Joint Tuberculosis

Among the commonest forms of nonpulmonary tuberculosis is that involving the bones and the joints. Tuberculous arthritis usually is monarticular, involving most often a vertebra, a hip, a knee or an elbow. It occurs predominantly in children and is characterized by pain of variable severity, wasting of surrounding muscles, weight loss and fever. During its acute stage this disease produces the well-known *cold abscesses,* so-named to distinguish them from the acute inflammatory abscesses that are associated with acute infectious processes, and which are hot or warm to palpation. Sinuses from a tuberculous joint may burrow their way for long distances; those from the spine, for example, opening through the skin of the thigh. Destruction of the joint, with permanent ankylosis and eventual deformity, the logical results, explains hip disease and hunchback. More than one half of these patients show signs of pulmonary tuberculosis.

The diagnosis is suggested by a positive family history of tuberculosis, signs of tuberculosis elsewhere in the body and the monarticular character of the joint involvement, the spine, the hip or the knee joints being most commonly affected.

Tuberculosis of the spine and the hip, tuberculous bursitis and tuberculous tendosynovitis, exemplifying most of the important types of musculoskeletal tuberculosis, are described below.

Tuberculosis of the Spine. Known also as Pott's disease, this is one of the most frequent forms of secondary tuberculosis. It occurs usually in children from 2 to 10 years of age. The thoracic vertebrae are involved most often. The bodies of the vertebrae undergo caseous softening, and, because the weight of the trunk is borne by these parts, a kinking or a knuckling (*gibbus*) of the spine results. This deformity is called *kyphosis* or hunchback by the laity. As the process goes on, cold abscesses form, and often symptoms of the nervous system develop due to injury to the spinal nerves or cord.

SYMPTOMS. The symptoms appear slowly. The child may be listless and fretful. In moving about he tries to protect his back, supporting himself by holding on to chairs and avoiding bending over whenever possible. At night he may be awakened by sharp pains that make him cry out. These are due to the unguarded motion of affected areas. Such "night cries" are a characteristic symptom of tuberculous disease of the bones and the joints. Later, when the body of the vertebrae has undergone caseous necrosis, deformity appears.

TREATMENT AND NURSING CARE. In addition to streptomycin, isoniazid and para-aminosalicylic acid (p. 452), complete rest is an important part of the treatment. By this means the vertebrae may be protected from weight-bearing and, by the aid of proper constitutional treatment, the child is able to overcome the infection. These children are placed on their backs on a Bradford frame or a curved Bradford (Whitman) frame in such a position that the affected vertebrae are directly over the bend in the frame and held in that position by a jacket applied over the chest and the shoulders. This position of hyperextension is maintained to relieve pressure and to prevent possible collapse of vertebrae on the spinal cord structures. The frame should be covered with tightly stretched canvas made in two pieces, leaving a space about 4 inches wide at the buttocks so that the bedpan may be used without disturbing the hips. After removing the bedpan, a canvas strip should be placed under the buttocks and fastened to the frame to prevent sagging. The canvas should be covered with folded sheets. If there is marked kyphosis, pillows or felt should be used in such a way as to remove the weight from the hump.

Because of the prolonged period of treatment, many hospitals have accommodations whereby the schooling of the child is continued.

Extension usually is applied to the legs (Buck's extension) and the head to ensure immobility. Many surgeons employ the arched or inclined frame for treating these patients, applying extension to the legs. The child should remain in one of these two positions for a considerable period of time—at least until all symptoms have disappeared.

The essential part of the treatment is the avoidance of any motion of the spinal column.

The patient should be clothed with a gown that opens in the back and fastens only at the neck. Feeding and drinking may necessitate the aid of a nurse at first, but the child soon learns how to manage his spoon and fork, even though he is lying flat on his back. Fluids are given through a tube or by the use of the "feeding duck."

The daily bath is given with the patient in the same position. When the child must be turned to be bathed and have his back rubbed, the turning must be done in the same manner as rolling a log. This is accomplished best by two nurses. One nurse places one hand on the pelvis and the other hand at the back of the shoulders and rolls the patient toward her. The pillows should be prepared to maintain the same degree of hyperextension. The other nurse, standing on the opposite side of the bed, quickly bathes and rubs the back.

When traction is being used, the nurse must guard against the development of a "pointed-toe deformity." This may occur if the foot is kept constantly in the extended position by the weight of the bedclothes and is not supported. A bed cradle over the feet and a foot board will prevent this complication.

CONVALESCENT CARE. Treatment as described is necessary until all symptoms of the disease have been absent for 2 or 3 months. Often this may take from 6 months to a year. When the child is allowed out of bed, a body brace is applied so that treatment may be continued. If a cast is necessary, it is put on with the patient lying prone on a canvas sling or suspended from the neck and the shoulders. Sufficient padding must be used to prevent pressure over bony prominences, and large windows are cut anteriorly to reduce the weight of the cast and to allow free breathing and feeding. The cast may be worn for from 3 to 6 months without changing, but at frequent intervals it should be inspected thoroughly. The distinctive smell of an excoriated area often is the first indication of pressure. The finding of such signs requires removal of the cast and the application of a new cast or braces. Braces always should be used for a considerable period.

OPERATION. Tuberculosis of the spine may be treated by operation in some cases, the principle of all the types of operation being to fix the spine in one position. In some types, a bone graft, usually from the tibia, may be removed from the leg and transplanted so as to unite the vertebrae. In such cases it is necessary for the nurse to prepare the leg as well as the back for operation. Some bone grafts come from the posterior iliac crest.

After operation, the patient is kept in bed for at least 10 to 12 weeks. The usual precautions against bedsores must be taken. When the patient is allowed out of bed, braces or a plaster jacket should be worn for a time.

This patient needs careful care of the skin area around the gibbus; pressure must be prevented when he lies on his back. In caring for patients with Pott's disease, the nurse should be on the lookout for the appearance of masses (cold abscesses). These usually appear below the groin, but they may develop in the back or the loin and the surgeon's attention should be drawn to them at once. They should be protected from pressure as much as possible. The treatment of cold abscess usually is aspiration and the administration of antibiotics rather than incision and drainage, because of the danger of secondary infection through an open wound.

Tuberculosis of Hip Joint. This is probably the second most common type of tuberculosis involving the bones and joints. It occurs mostly in children under 10 years of age. The first symptoms noticed are stiffness in the hip joint and pain, often referred to the knee, that is due to irritation of the obturator nerve, which often lies in contact with the capsule of the joint but supplies sensation to the knee joint. The stiffness of the hip often is apparent only in the morning when the child gets out of bed. Gradually the limp and pain increase, and "night cries" are common due to pain caused by the relaxation of the muscle spasm while the child sleeps and to the unguarded motion at the affected site. The leg is held in continuous partial flexion, and walking is on the ball of the foot on the side affected. If the condition goes on without treatment—and even at times with treatment—cold abscesses appear, usually on the outside of the thigh or in the gluteal region (buttocks).

TREATMENT. The object of treatment, as for Pott's disease, is to give the part absolute rest. The patient is placed in bed, often on a Bradford frame, and traction is applied to relax muscle spasm and keep the joint surfaces apart. It may be impossible, because of the pain and spasm, to give traction in the horizontal direction. Then, extension is applied with the thigh somewhat flexed, the legs being supported with a series of pads that are reduced gradually in number until the leg reaches the horizontal. The pads should extend for the entire length of the leg.

The care of these patients is similar to that recommended for Pott's disease.

Bed treatment may be continued for from 6 months to 2 years, until all symptoms, pain, fever, limitation of motion and so forth have disappeared. After the patient has remained symptom-free for from 2 to 3 months, a fusion may be done or a brace may be applied from axilla to foot and the patient is permitted to be about with crutches, wearing a high-soled shoe on the unaffected side, so that the diseased limb may swing free. The nurse must watch at all times for any signs that suggest a relapse. Finally, gradual weight-bearing with crutches may be permitted with the brace in place. If, after 8 months or a year, no further joint involvements are evident, crutches are used without a brace until by gradual stages full weight-bearing is proved to be safe.

The healing of tuberculous lesions usually results in a fusion of the bones forming the joint (ankylosis). Experience has shown that more rapid healing can be obtained by operative fusion of the involved bones (arthrodesis). Then the patient is immobilized in a cast until solid union takes place. When there are secondary tuberculous sinuses, the administration of streptomycin is especially valuable.

The treatment of tuberculosis of other bones and joints is carried out in essentially the same manner as has been outlined already for Pott's disease and tuberculosis of the hip.

Tuberculous Tendosynovitis and Bursitis

Tuberculous tendosynovitis most often develops in association with tuberculosis of nearby bones and joints. The tendons most frequently affected are those about the wrists —either the flexor or the extensor group, seldom both. Rarely are those about the ankles similarly affected.

This disease presents both a dry fibrous and a serous type. In cases of the fibrous type, the infected tendons and their sheaths thicken gradually, causing very little pain but marked limitation of joint movements. As the infection progresses, the adhesions between the tendons and their sheaths gradually become firmer, until finally an immobile clawlike hand is the result. This process then may become stationary, progress to caseous degeneration or change to the serous type. In patients with the serous type, the tendon sheaths involved gradually become distended by a clear straw-colored fluid, in which there appear later great numbers of fibrous bodies, the so-called *rice bodies*. This type is practically painless, but it limits greatly the movements of the fingers.

Tuberculous bursitis may be the only demonstrable focus of this infection in the body. This type of bursitis develops very slowly, distending the sac with a serous fluid, in which, later, great numbers of rice bodies appear. Such swelling generally is painless, but it may interfere with the motions of the part which the bursa is intended to aid.

TREATMENT. These periarticular infections, as in the case of other tuberculous lesions, respond quite readily to vigorous chemotherapy conducted as specified earlier. (See p. 197.)

PATIENTS WITH ARTHRITIS
Public Health Aspects of Arthritis

Excluding mental illness, joint disease causes more disability than all other chronic diseases combined. It has been estimated that 1 out of every 10 persons in the United States over the age of 14 years is afflicted with some form of rheumatism. The U.S. Public Health Service reports that each year more than 300,000 individuals are barred from employment because of chronic joint disease, 50 per cent of these persons becoming complete invalids. Thus, rheumatism incapacitates 10 times as many persons as do diabetes and tuberculosis, 7 times as many as all cancers and twice as many as heart disease. Considered from the economic standpoint, rheumatism regularly is responsible for the loss of more than 90 million workdays per year, which is equivalent to a financial loss of half a billion dollars, and is more than is forfeited as a result of any other illness, with the exception of nervous and mental disease. The financial burden alone entailed in providing medical care for rheumatic patients exceeds $100,000,000 every year, a figure which does not take into account the tremendous drain on the productivity of personnel affected with the disease.

It must be recognized, of course, that for every patient who is hospitalized for rheumatism, there are scores of others, equally incapacitated, who are receiving treatment in nursing homes or in their own homes. This being the case, it behooves the nurse to study the application of the therapeutic principles she learns in the hospital to the care of the patient in the home, bearing in mind that her advice will be sought by the families of her arthritic patients regarding the treatment for which they will ultimately be responsible.

Definition and Classification of Arthritis

The term "arthritis" implies joint inflammation, although it frequently is used to describe any disorder involving the joints. "Rheumatism" is used to denote pain, stiffness or deformity of joints, muscles and related structures, while the term "rheumatic diseases" refers to musculoskeletal disorders in which changes take place in the tissues comprising or surrounding the joints. (One can readily understand how these terms have come to be used interchangeably!)

One of the most important varieties of acute arthritis has been described: namely, pyogenic arthritis (p. 1019), the result of bacterial penetration and growth within a joint cavity. Another acute type, one which represents a late response to a hemolytic streptococcus infection, is the arthritis associated with acute rheumatic fever.

Rheumatic Fever

The most prominent clinical manifestations of acute rheumatic fever are fever and arthritis. The latter is an acute nonsuppurative polyarthritis, the onset of which is abrupt and usually is preceded 1 or 2 weeks earlier by a sore throat. It is characterized by excruciating migratory joint pain, accompanied by joint swelling, redness and tenderness, which responds remarkably well to salicylates. The temperature rises rapidly as one or two joints become red, hot, swollen and exquisitely painful; within 24 hours the process is well developed. The pain in the joints typically is excruciating; the slightest weight of the bedclothes and any jolting of the bed are unbearable.

The fever is usually high, the pulse rapid and prostration profound. With the fever there is a polymorphonuclear leukocytosis, elevation of the sedimentation rate and a progressive secondary anemia, often reaching marked grades.

In most cases of rheumatic fever during the acute stage, signs of cardiac involvement may be detected, with findings indicative of acute myocarditis, valvular leakage signifying endocarditis, and occasionally pericarditis. The EKG usually shows signs of delayed conduction of the impulses between the auricle and the ventricle. With clearing of the acute polyarthritis these complications usually terminate. The joints revert to normal, thereafter exhibiting no trace of residual damage. The endocardium, on the other hand, if it has been involved, remains permanently scarred. Moreover, with each successive bout of rheumatic activity more damage is inflicted, with the result that one or more heart valves become deformed to the point of obstruction, leakage, or both, and cardiac function is permanently impaired, as described on page 523 *et. seq.*

Management and Nursing Care. The most important aspects of therapy in cases of acute rheumatic fever include: (1) the eradication of group A streptococcus from the patient's tissues; (2) control of inflammatory reactions throughout the body by the administration of salicylates or corticosteroid drugs; and (3) rest.

Antistreptococcal therapy may take the form of daily injections of crystaline penicillin G for 10 days or a single intramuscular injection of 1.2 million units (720 mg.) of benzathine penicillin G.

Anti-inflammatory treatment can be accomplished with equal efficacy by means of salicylates and corticosteroid drugs, such as prednisone or dexamethasone. Both types of agents may be employed simultaneously. The sore joints may be rubbed gently with oil of wintergreen, wrapped in cotton and, with the aid of pillows or even splints, kept in the most comfortable position possible. The application of hot-water bottles or a heating pad to the affected joints may be welcomed by the patient during the initial phase of therapy before the salicylates have become fully effective.

Rest is mandatory during the acute phase of this illness; i.e., complete and continuous rest is the rule as long as rheumatic activity is apparent. On the other hand, as soon as the patient becomes afebrile, the leukocytosis has disappeared, and the electrocardiographic signs have returned to normal, bed rest is no longer mandatory. Each increase in effort is controlled on the basis of its influence on the pulse rate. The patient's family should be instructed with regard to the patient's medical and nursing requirements at home, and he should be given specific directions concerning his activity. Medical supervision should be exercised for a period of months if signs of heart damage have developed in the course of the illness. The long-range prospects for the patient with rheumatic fever and the preventive aspects of this condition are discussed elsewhere (p. 527).

Next to be described are the prevailing types of chronic arthritis: namely, rheumatoid arthritis, osteoarthritis (hypertrophic or degenerative arthritis), gout, traumatic arthritis and nonarticular rheumatism.

Rheumatoid Arthritis

Rheumatoid arthritis is a chronic systemic disease of unknown cause, characterized most prominently by recurrent inflammation of articular and periarticular structures, joint deformity and loss of joint function. It usually begins acutely as a recurring polyarthritis with fever, the first attacks of which may closely resemble acute rheumatic fever.

Following one attack or, at most, very few such attacks, however, some of the joints involved never quite return to normal, but remain stiff and sore. During subsequent acute exacerbations, other joints likewise become chronically injured, and each attack leaves the joints involved more damaged than before (Fig. 408). The disease affects primarily the joint cartilages and the articular surfaces of the bones, destroying the joint cavity, which becomes filled with adhesions. Marked joint crepitation can be obtained; dislocations are common; ankyloses follow; and muscular contractures may become marked—hence the descriptive name *arthritis deformans*. Atrophic changes appear early, involving the soft tissues about the affected joints. The disease occurs more commonly in females and rarely in children. When it does appear in childhood, it is referred to as *Still's disease* or *Felty's syndrome*.

The clinical picture presented in a well-marked case of this condition is typical. The patient appears chronically ill; the muscles of his extremities, especially of their distal segments, are apt to be wasted; the subcutaneous fat often is greatly decreased. The joints become deformed—some of them dislocated. If the condition is extreme, the patient can scarcely move a single joint in the body. The early immobility of the joints, however, is not due to bony ankylosis, but is the result of tense muscular spasm.

The deformities of the hands are characteristic. The distal phalanges are hyperextended, the proximal flexed, and there is ulnar deviation of the fingers. The skin covering the fingertips is thin, pale, smooth and shiny, the nails are rough and brittle, and the intrinsic muscles of the hand are wasted. The spine may be stiff and the jaw partly fixed. This typifies the most advanced grade of rheumatoid arthritis, the severity of which may vary from this marked degree to a mild stiffening and swelling of the finger joints.

Other clinical phenomena observed in addition to the joint involvement include subcutaneous nodules which are in many respects indistinguishable from those of rheumatic fever; frequent generalized lymphadenopathy and splenomegaly; fever, which may be high and prolonged; anemia, leukocytosis and elevation of the sedimentation rate.

The etiology of rheumatoid arthritis is unknown, and its relation to rheumatic fever is not clear. The disease is coming to be regarded as a disorder of immunity. In support of this concept is the presence in the serum of most of these patients of the so-called "rheumatoid factor," a plasma protein with properties akin to those of an immune antibody which is capable of reacting specifically with human (and/or rabbit) gamma globulin (i.e., conceivably an anti-antibody). However, the origin and the significance of this "factor" remain to be discovered.

The primary objective of treatment in the acute stage of rheumatoid arthritis is the *prevention of crippling deformities*. Other therapeutic goals are to maintain joint mobility and muscle power; to promote comfort; to halt the activity of the disease; to help the patient and his family to adjust to his chronic disability; and to assist the patient to become functionally independent as soon and as completely as possible.

Maintenance of Joint Mobility and Muscle Power. Inflammation, scarring or other mechanical damage to joint structures result in pain and disability. The patient, in an effort to avoid pain, tends to immobilize the affected joints, and muscular spasm further limits their motion. If acutely inflamed, these joints should be rested by the application of splints, sandbags, bivalved casts or any other mechanical device that will maintain them in functional positions. Above all, they should not be permitted to "freeze" in positions of flexion, which is their natural tendency because of the predominant strength of the flexor muscles. While he is in bed, the patient should lie flat on a firm mattress with only one pillow under his head because of the risk of dorsal kyphosis. (At no time should a pillow be placed under his knees, as this promotes flexion contractures of those joints.)

Joints may lose their normal range of motion due to deformity and atrophy. This loss can be prevented to a large extent by systematic range-of-motion exercises. If this activity is painful, the nurse may help the patient (with active-assisted exercises) to perform the required motions. The nurse must emphasize constantly that the daily performance of these therapeutic exercises increases muscle strength, which is essential for the restoration of joint mobility. Rheumatoid arthritis is a long-term disease, and its management is a long-term project, which must include a program of systematic exercises in the home. The pamphlet *Strike Back At Arthritis!** explains and illustrates how these exercises and other therapeutic measures may be carried out.

To promote the patient's comfort, pain must be alleviated. Salicylates are given in doses that are individualized in accordance with the patient's responses. It is desirable that the first dose be given immediately on arising in the morning, and the last at bedtime. The remaining doses should be spaced evenly throughout the day.

Heat relieves muscle spasm and joint soreness. It may be supplied in the form of warm tub baths, hot compresses, homemade bakers, paraffin baths for hands and wrists, and infra-red reflector heat bulbs. Therapeutic exercises can be carried out more comfortably and effectively after heat has been applied.

Rest helps to allay pain. Since arthritis is a systemic disease, the whole patient—not merely his joints—must be treated. Frequent periods of bed rest during the day take the weight off the joints and relieve fatigue. If joint inflammation is severe, the patient should, of course, be placed on complete bed rest. (Nevertheless, range-of-motion exercises should still be carried out.) At bed rest, the patient should lie flat, with his feet propped against a footboard. Trochanter rolls are utilized when he is lying in the dorsal position for prolonged periods. As joint stiffness and tenderness diminish and function improves, the patient is permitted to increase his out-of-bed activities. He may anticipate pain in the knees and hips on arising from a chair. The nurse should select a straight-back chair with a seat that is high enough to permit the patient to keep his feet flat on the floor (or stool) while his hips and shoulders are resting against the back of the chair.

* Superintendent of Documents, U. S. Dept. of Health, Education and Welfare, U. S. Government Printing Office, Washington 25, D. C.

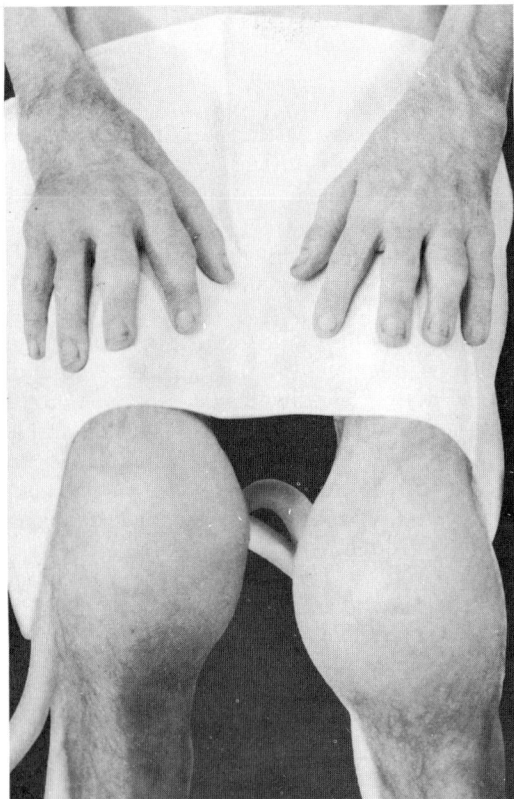

Fig. 408. Rheumatoid arthritis. Fusiform swelling of the fingers and bilateral knee joint effusion.

To halt the disease process, joints that are severely inflamed and fail to respond promptly to the measures outlined above may be treated by the local instillation of 25 to 50 mg. of hydrocortisone acetate. Quiescence of activity may be anticipated almost immediately following this maneuver, and its beneficial effect may be expected to last for several days or even several weeks. Systemic hormonal therapy by the oral administration of one of the corticosteroids, such as prednisone or dexamethasone, while temporarily palliative in effect, is not curative in any sense (see Chap. 38). Steroid chemotherapy carries with it all of the undesirable complications previously described, including sodium and water retention, potassium depletion, hypertension, glycosuria, menstrual irregularities and other features of the Cushing syndrome, and at the same time exposes the patient to a demoralizing dependence on

a treatment that offers no hope of permanent benefit.

To help the patient and his family to adjust satisfactorily to his chronic illness is an important and a challenging responsibility. The nurse must be prepared psychologically to cope with the formidable problems of emotional adjustment that so commonly beset patients with chronic arthritis, reminding herself that a trying personality often is a sign of despair in a person who has had a long and painful illness which has rendered him completely helpless, and to which no end is in sight. For most persons a state of dependency is an unhappy state, especially when they are reduced to it as a result of disease. Fear of being disliked and of becoming an unwanted burden often proceeds to the conviction that such, indeed, actually is the case. In other words, the chronic invalid is highly susceptible to a form of paranoia, manifested by a show of immature hostility toward those who are devoting themselves to his care.

The nurse may assume, as a working hypothesis, that when a patient displays recalcitrance, irritability, inexplicable surliness or unprovoked anger, he is reacting to the imaginary hostility of others toward him. Assuming this to be the case, the role of the nurse in the mental hygiene of her chronic patients is clearly to convince the patient that he is liked, trusted and wanted, and that his care is not an unpleasant necessity but a pleasure. She must educate the family to realize that this sick member is desperately and constantly in need of reassurance, and teach them to reinterpret his show of hostility in terms of anxiety, i.e., viewing it as an indication that he is afraid of their hostility. If they are willing to adopt this interpretation and govern their responsibility accordingly, the prognosis of the patient, from the standpoint of sound mental health, is vastly improved.

The patient must be convinced that, while no quick cure is available, he can stay ahead of his disease and get the better of it by following faithfully his rest and exercise program, by taking the medications and the treatments that have been prescribed, and by continuing to cooperate fully with the physician in whom he has placed his confidence.

To assist him to become functionally independent, the patient should be instructed and trained by the nurse and others of the rehabilitation team in activities of daily living. There are many self-help devices available to assist with dressing, bathing, and eating. Corrective shoes are helpful in treating and preventing foot deformities and will make walking easier. Canes or crutches may be prescribed as assistive devices. As the patient gains more independence, vocational counseling and job placement services may be used to help the patient to secure employment.

To correct pre-existing deformities, progressive resistive exercises that have been individually prescribed for the patient are carried out by the physical therapist.

Should all conservative measures fail, and a particular joint become incapable of function, surgical intervention may be indicated. Occasionally, restoration of joint function may be attempted by an operation called an *arthroplasty.* This consists of removal of the damaged joint surfaces and adjacent bone. In some cases fascia may be used to form a new joint surface, and in others the bone end may be covered with a smooth-shaped surface of Vitallium. Often, a metallic prosthesis may be inserted where the grossly deformed head and neck of the femur have been resected. Fusion of the joint may be done for still other patients. The ankylosis produced may cause a disability that is less than the painful arthritis.

Rheumatoid Spondylitis

Rheumatoid spondylitis is a systemic disease, which, as a result of inflammatory involvement, causes pain and stiffness of the sacroiliac, the intervertebral and the costovertebral joints. If the disease progresses, there is ossification and ankylosis of these joints, and the entire spine and the thorax become extensively ankylosed.

Poker spine, one that is perfectly rigid, may develop slowly without pain, and the patient may be quite unconscious of its presence, or it may appear with severe root pains (Bechterew's type). This disease, which may be akin to rheumatoid arthritis, predominates in males. Its usual starting point is with involvement of the lower thoracic intervertebral joints.

Treatment. The goal of therapy is to help the patient to maintain an erect posture, so that if spinal ankylosis occurs, the patient will be in a functional upright position.

The treatment is similar to that of rheumatoid arthritis, with emphasis on periodically resting on a flat surface, avoidance of strain and fatigue, and the administration of analgesics. The nurse has the responsibility of reinforcing the physician's health teaching and encouraging the patient to carry out his prescribed remedial exercises.

Osteoarthritis

Osteoarthritis, otherwise known as "hypertrophic arthritis" or "degenerative arthritis," is the commonest of all joint diseases, the result of "wearing out" of the articular structures. It is characterized by spur formation at the edges of the joint surfaces and thickening of the capsule and the synovial membrane. The joint cartilages degenerate and atrophy, the bones harden at their articular surfaces, and the ligaments calcify. Nevertheless, the joint spaces themselves remain preserved; no adhesions form in them. Sterile joint effusions not infrequently develop, particularly in the knees.

Osteoarthritis may be limited to the spine, affecting most markedly its cervical and lumbar regions. Minor grades of this condition are so common that many clinicians consider them to be almost normal; but this spinal arthritis is responsible for much of the backache so common in persons of middle age and older. Films of the spine demonstrate spur formation and gross irregularities involving the margins and the articular surfaces of the vertebral bodies, which greatly restrict their freedom of movement. In extreme cases, ossification of the spinal ligaments may be observed.

Heberden's nodes, a manifestation of osteoarthritis, are nodular bony excrescences that grow in pairs, symmetrically placed, on the distal joints of a few, several or all of the fingers. They appear most often among middle-aged women, particularly those who work hard, and whose hands are much exposed to wet and cold. While forming, these nodes may be sore; but when fully developed, they cause no pain and very little limitation of joint motion. No known treatment modifies their development.

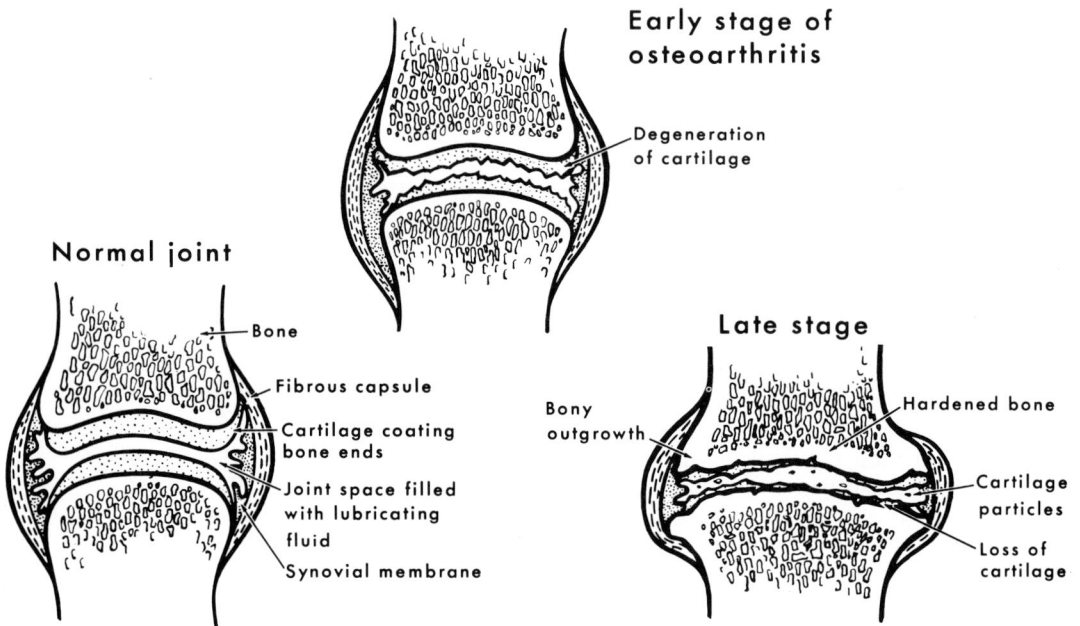

FIG. 409. Osteoarthritis. (R.N. **25**(9): 67)

Nursing Care and Teaching Principles for a Patient With Osteoarthritis

1. Relieve strain on the affected joints.
   A. Rest involved parts with splints, braces, cervical collars, etc.
   B. Avoid pain-precipitating factors.
   C. Relieve stiffness with prescribed forms of physical therapy.
   D. Give analgesics for pain control.
   E. Use correct body mechanics.
   F. Avoid emotional strain, which increases muscle tension and joint strain.
   G. Use crutches or cane, when indicated, to reduce weight on the joints.

2. Avoid trauma and further wearing of the weight-bearing joints.
   A. Use postural exercises to correct poor posture.
   B. Wear corrective shoes for foot disorders.
   C. Carry out weight reduction under medical supervision.
   D. Stop excessive weight-bearing activities, such as lifting, carrying heavy loads, excessive vigorous overhead reaching, etc.

3. Restore function to the maximum extent possible.
   A. Use range-of-motion exercises to prevent capsular and tendon tightening.
   B. Avoid flexion deformities.
   C. Use corrective and graded exercises to improve muscle strength around the involved joint.
   D. Hip arthroplasty, if hip joint motion is seriously restricted.
   E. Orthopedic surgery, when indicated, for severely disabling arthritis of knee joints, etc.

Osteoarthritis is to be regarded essentially as a senescent process—the result of prolonged wear and tear of the joint surfaces which has produced changes, not only in the bony structures but also in the cartilaginous and soft tissue components of the joints. Precipitating factors include repeated traumata, faulty body posture and mechanics, strenuous physical labor and obesity, which subject the weight-bearing joints to unusual strain. Habitual use of vibrating tools, such as pneumatic hammers, predisposes to the development of degenerative arthritis. Another predisposing factor is repeated chilling, which promotes muscle contractions of a type that increases to a considerable extent the contact pressure at opposing joint surfaces and the degree of friction between those surfaces when joints are in motion.

The disease progresses slowly, with early stiffness, and later pain and swelling of the joints. The hips, the knees, the vertebrae and the fingers are the joints particularly affected.

Treatment. The treatment of all types of hypertrophic arthritis is largely symptomatic. Also, it involves measures designed to protect the joints from undue strain and trauma; that is, an obese patient must lose weight, and a physically active patient must learn to adhere to a more sedentary mode of life.

Inasmuch as osteoarthritis in some form or another afflicts almost everyone over the age of 50, opportunities for patient teaching are rife and should not be neglected by the nurse. Irrespective of their basic diagnoses or presenting complaints, many of her patients will be suffering from this condition. Tabulated above is a summary of nursing principles and teaching points that are applicable in relation to osteoarthritis.

Gout

Gout is a metabolic disturbance in which little masses of sodium urate crystals, called *tophi,* become deposited in the vicinity of joints (particularly the great toe), in the ears (Fig. 410) and on the knuckles. Most gouty patients are men beyond middle life.

This disease appears to have its origin in an inherited defect of purine metabolism resulting from the overproduction of uric acid in the gouty subject and, presumably, an inadequate capacity for the excretion of that substance. The patient, therefore, is in a constant state of positive uric acid balance. Uric acid continues to accumulate in greater and greater excess in the body. Its concentration in the blood is almost always high, and, because of its low solubility, it tends to precipitate in the form of deposits at various sites where blood flow is least active, including the cartilaginous tissues.

Symptoms. An attack of acute gout usually begins in the early morning, with agonizing pain in the first joint of the big toe and later in the other joints of the foot. These joints become swollen, red, hot and exquisitely sensitive; the patient feels as if the foot were in a vise. The superficial veins of the foot are swollen. There is fever. Later in the morning the pain abates, may even disappear, and the patient can walk about, although the joints may still appear acutely inflamed. The following night the pain returns, and so on for from 5 to 8 days, its severity gradually diminishing each time. These attacks usually recur, often with intervals of some months. Almost any joint may be involved, but the great toe rarely escapes.

Following repeated acute attacks, some of which may be very mild, the gout may become chronic, leaving certain joints (particularly those of the hands) permanently disabled, much deformed and painful. Tophi

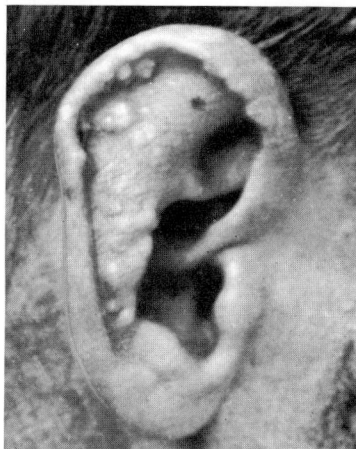

Fig. 410. Tophi of gout.

develop, and the patient suffers from many other symptoms which, possibly, are evidences of gout. Among these are gastrointestinal disturbances with pain, vomiting, diarrhea and constipation; skin diseases, especially eczema; and all the symptoms of chronic nephritis and arteriosclerosis. The deposits of uric acid sometimes form knobs on the knuckles which may ulcerate through the skin (chalk stones).

Tophi. An infallible sign of gout is the presence in the skin of tophi (Fig. 410), from which one may aspirate the typical crystals of sodium urate.

The roentgenograms of the joints likewise may give a positive diagnosis. In the absence of tophi, the presence of gout is indicated when the uric acid in the blood rises to 5 mg. per 100 ml. or over, provided, at the same time, the urea and the creatinine of the plasma are not increased. If they are, one strongly suspects renal decompensation, the occurrence of gout under these circumstances being regarded as a complication of uric acid retention caused by failure of the diseased kidney to excrete this material.

Treatment. An acute attack of gouty arthritis can be terminated, in a high proportion of cases, by the administration of colchicine, 0.5 to 1.0 mg. of the crystalline product being given at 2-hour intervals for a total dose of 6 to 10 mg. The first dose may be administered by intravenous injection. Symptoms of anorexia, nausea, vomiting and diarrhea are common in recipients of colchicine.

The corticosteroid drugs, e.g., prednisone or dexamethasone, speedily reduce the inflammation and eliminate the pain of acute gouty arthritis, and their administration on a short-term basis for this purpose accordingly is beneficial and fully justified. Likewise effective in the relief of acute gout is phenylbutazone (Butazolidin). This drug, ingested in doses of 200 mg. 4 times a day, reduces the fever and eliminates the inflammatory joint changes within a period of 48 hours. Serious complications, including bone marrow depression and reactivation of peptic ulcer, have occurred in patients receiving phenylbutazone for extended periods of time. Its use, therefore, is limited to a small minority of patients who have proved to be both refractory to colchicine (or unusually susceptible to its toxic effects) and also poor candidates for the receipt of a corticosteroid agent, e.g., because of severe arterial hypertension or diabetes.

Nursing Care. During the acute phase of gouty arthritis, the patient is confined by his symptoms to complete bed rest. Bed covers should be raised out of contact with the extremely sensitive joints by means of a bed cradle, and the joints themselves should be positioned in semiflexion, thereby reducing the intra-articular pressure to a minimum and affording the greatest comfort possible to the patient.

Hot or cold applications may alleviate pain to a significant extent, and deserve a cautious trial. Fluids are to be encouraged, in the hope of avoiding the precipitation of urate crystals in the urinary tract. Urinalysis data should be charted promptly.

Following subsidence of the acute attack and as soon as the patient shows a readiness to receive instruction, the points outlined below, bearing on his after-care and on prevention of future attacks, should be presented.

Long-term Management of Gout. Patients with gout should acquire regularity in all habits of living, including habits of eating, exercise and rest. Intake of preformed purine bases should be limited. Foods containing more than 100 mg. of purine bases per 100 Gm. of tissue include meat extracts, glandular meats, roe, shellfish, sardines and brains. Other foods to be especially avoided, or ingested in relatively limited amounts, include kidney, liver, sweetbreads, squab, meats in general, fowl, beans, mushrooms, peas and spinach. A low-purine diet would contain eggs, fat-free milk, cottage cheese, cereals, fruit and vegetables other than those mentioned.

An increase in blood uric acid and the precipitation of acute gouty arthritis in susceptible individuals have been demonstrated as a result of fatty foods, and following the ingestion of ethyl alcohol, the implications of which are obvious.

Drugs of value in the management of chronic gout, tending as they do to prevent the accumulation of uric acid in the body and therefore diminishing the likelihood of acute recurrences, are the so-called "uricosuric agents," drugs that promote the excretion of uric acid in the urine. Such a drug is p-dipropylsulfamyl benzoic acid (Benemid), which is effective in daily doses of 0.5 to 1.5 Gm. by mouth, apparently with no more significant side-reaction than the occasional appearance of a mild gastrointestinal upset and a tendency to constipation. This drug is not to be given in conjunction with aspirin or any other salicylate, each tending to offset the action of the other. Another useful uricosuric drug is sulfinpyrazone (Anturane), which is given orally in daily doses of 200 to 800 mg. Anturane, like Benemid, and the salicylates are mutually antagonistic and must not be administered together.

It is very important to keep in mind that, following the initiation of uricosuric drug therapy, the urinary concentration of urates may rise to such heights that crystals may precipitate out of solution, causing urolithiasis and renal colic. To avoid this complication, the patient should receive fluids in ample quantities and sufficient alkalies to render the urine alkaline during the early phase of treatment.

Traumatic Arthritis

Of all joints, those most susceptible to injury resulting in arthritis are the knee, the lumbosacral and the sacro-iliac joints. Following a sprain, inflammation of the interior joint lining (the synovial membrane) may develop, and, later, in the course of a few weeks, degenerative changes may occur in the cartilaginous articular surfaces and in underlying bones. These changes resemble those found in the hypertrophic arthritis of elderly persons. Joint movements may be limited permanently by scar tissue formed in capsules which have been torn by dislocations, while subluxations (near dislocations) often leave the joints loose and weak. If dislocated pieces of cartilages (for example, the semilunar cartilage of the knee), chipped off into the joint cavity as the result of injury, are not removed by operation, the joint remains painful, and its movements are limited.

Lumbosacral and Sacro-Iliac Strain. Backache due to strain of the lumbosacral joint (the joint which articulates the spine with the pelvis) is a fairly common complaint and often leads to prolonged and painful disability. The only objective finding in cases of this condition may be spasm of the deep muscles of the lower back which hold the spine erect. That the marked abnormalities in the shape of the fifth lumbar vertebra, often seen on roentgenograms (some of them developmental defects and others due to the fusion of one of the transverse processes with the sacrum), ever cause backache is not certain; but in some patients this would seem to be the case.

Sacro-iliac strain, one of the most painful and disabling of conditions, may follow lifting, contusion to the back, a slight misstep or it may appear to develop spontaneously. The wonder is that it is not a more common disorder, since mere standing and walking subject the ligaments of this articulation to great tension. Sacro-iliac strain develops also as the result of inequality in the length of the two legs, ankylosis of one hip and, occasionally, scoliosis of the spine. Relief may be afforded by the wearing of a tight supporting belt or elevation of a heel when inequality of legs is found, but at times it requires surgically induced bone ankylosis of the joint.

Nonarticular Rheumatism

The term *muscular rheumatism* is conveniently applied to all painful conditions of the limbs not definitely localized in the joints. Certain forms, which the laity designate as *lumbago* and *stiff neck,* are due to ruptured intervertebral disks and other abnormalities of the spine which can exert mechanical pressure on the spinal nerve roots, producing pains which radiate to the terminals of the peripheral sensory nerves. The pathology of many cases never is properly elucidated; some are presumed to be due to acute or chronic strain of the supporting muscles of the trunk, as a result of faulty posture or unaccustomed exertion. However, the vast majority of patients in this category can be shown to be suffering from an inflammatory disorder involving one of the periarticular structures—i.e., a structure that is located in close proximity to a joint, although not always an integral part of the joint itself. Three such conditions account for almost the entire group: namely, fibrositis, bursitis and synovitis or tendosynovitis.

Fibrositis. This is a subacute inflammatory disease, usually of unknown etiology, which involves the subcutaneous tissue and other fibrous structures of the extremities (fasciae, sheaths of muscles and nerves, tendons and periosteum).

The onset of this malady follows, within a few hours, exposure to cold and dampness, muscular strain or trauma. Its chief symptom is pain, which is increased by movement, seldom lasts more than 3 or 4 days and is followed by the development in the subcutaneous tissue of brawny inelastic areas. The latter may take the form of nodules varying in size from that of a pea to that of an almond, thick cords of induration or circumscribed tender spots—all due to infiltration of the connective tissue by a serofibrinous exudate rich in small round cells— later replaced by scar tissue. This condition explains the so-called *indurative* or *nodular* headaches, some cases of stiff neck or torticollis, one type of lumbago and some cases of pleurodynia. When chronic, this disease often is called *muscular rheumatism,* since it is characterized by a sense of muscular fatigue, pain in the extremities and stiffness of the joints.

TREATMENT. The affected part should be kept quite warm and immobilized. Salicylates relieve the acute pain. For the more chronic cases, massage is indicated. All chronic infections in the body, of course, should be treated adequately.

Bursitis. A *bursa* is a small space between muscles, tendons and bones. Its function is to promote muscular movement with the least possible amount of friction. These sacs frequently are the seat of inflammation due to trauma, infection or calcareous deposits that form in their walls, and the bursa fills up with fluid, with the result that muscular movement becomes painful. Common examples are those involving the olecranon bursa (which lies over the point of the elbow), which explains miners' elbow, and the prepatellar bursa (superficial to the patella), causing housemaids' knee; hod carriers' shoulder is due to subacromial bursitis. Other bursae often

affected are the tibial (which overlies the tibial tuberosity, to which the patella ligament is attached) and the subdeltoid in the shoulder.

Rest for the part, removal of focal infection and dry heat frequently will effect a cure. If the inflammation becomes acute or is not relieved by conservative treatment, operation with drainage or excision of the bursa will be necessary.

SUBDELTOID BURSITIS. The bursa most commonly giving symptoms is the one which lies between the deltoid muscle and the greater tuberosity of the humerus. This bursa may be injured by falls on the outstretched hand, so that the bursa is pinched between the head of the humerus and the overlying acromium process of the scapula. However, most commonly, the bursa becomes painful as a result of degeneration. Often a calcium deposit appears in the tendons which lie underneath it over the head of the humerus. The calcified area may be the seat of an inflammation producing tension in the dense supraspinatus tendon. This produces acute pain when the shoulder is moved and is spoken of as *acute bursitis.* The chronic form of bursitis often follows repeated use of the arm above the head. There is pain produced by certain abduction movements of the arm, as in putting on a coat, and often pain is noted at night when the patient rolls over on the arm of the affected side. These affections really involve the bursa secondarily but produce marked disability in shoulder motion.

The acute form of bursitis may be relieved by x-ray therapy or by operative removal of calcium deposit. Some forms of the chronic type may respond to conservative therapy, x-ray therapy and injected hydrocortone.

Synovitis and Tendosynovitis

SYNOVITIS. This term is given to an inflammation of the synovial membrane of the joint. It may be due to trauma, traumatic synovitis. It is characterized by a swelling and pain in the affected joint. The knee is the joint injured most commonly, and "water on the knee" is the descriptive term applied to it by the laity. The pain is due in most part to distention of the joint capsule and can be relieved by aspiration of the joint. If the fluid is bloody, an associated fracture or other injury is suspected. As a rule, restriction of motion, pressure bandages and application of heat result in a rapid recovery.

TENDOSYNOVITIS. Inflammatory conditions that involve tendons invariably involve their synovial sheaths as well; therefore, in each case the condition is one of tendosynovitis.

PYOGENIC TENDOSYNOVITIS. This frequently follows infected wounds, develops secondary to infection of adjacent structures, as in cases of osteomyelitis, and, occasionally, is a blood stream infection. The wrists and ankles are peculiarly vulnerable to tendosynovitis of bacteremic origin. The infected structures appear swollen due both to a seropurulent exudate within these sheaths and to edema of the surrounding tissue. The superficial evidences of this condition may be slight, but the pain and the disability it causes are extreme.

The treatment is heat and chemotherapy (Chap. 13).

NONINFECTIOUS TENDOSYNOVITIS. This follows direct blows over the tendons themselves, strains which overstretch them and trauma from overuse. Repeated movements continued over long period of time—for example, those incident to playing the piano or the violin or typing—may give rise to this disorder. Its symptoms are slight swelling and local tenderness on pressure over the injured tendon sheaths and marked pain on motion of the related joints. The proper treatment is rest, change of activities and warmth. This condition arising incidental to a profession often is wrongly named *professional cramp,* which represents quite a different situation.

GANGLION. A ganglion is a round, firm projection usually near the wrist. It is a collection of gelatinouslike material due to degeneration of fibrous tissue near tendon sheaths and joints. It is due to strains, contusions or a series of repeated minor strains, as a result of which the tissues of the sheath or sac involved have gradually become weakened. As a rule, the ganglion is painless, but the affected joint often is weak and moderately painful. It has a tendency to rupture and disappear; it can be made to do

so by a sharp blow purposely delivered; and may be removed by operation but not infrequently it recurs.

THE PATIENT WITH A BONE TUMOR

Tumors involving the skeleton are by no means rare and represent a particularly destructive form of neoplastic disease. Such tumors may be primary, arising from bone tissue cells or bone marrow elements, or they may be secondary, having metastasized from primary sites of malignancy elsewhere in the body. A benign tumor arising from bone cells is known as an osteoma; tumors which are malignant are grouped under the term *osteogenic sarcoma.* To one neoplasm derived from bone marrow tissue, the term *myeloma* is applied.

Osteogenic Sarcoma

The term "osteogenic sarcoma" refers to several varieties of malignant tumors arising from the bone cells. As a rule, they appear in individuals under 30 years of age, and they classically produce signs of local swelling and pain, fever and cachexia. The primary lesion may involve any bone; the most common sites are the femora, the tibiae and the humeri. Metastases very early involve the lungs, whence these abnormal cells are transported by way of the blood stream.

The diagnosis is made on the basis of the clinical features noted above, together with the radiologic findings before and after x-ray irradiation of the site. If the tumor fails to respond to irradiation, amputation is indicated. Only if reasonable doubt as to the diagnosis exists should a biopsy first be taken, for this procedure greatly enhances the opportunity for metastatic spread of this disease. The prognosis is poor despite prompt and radical amputation, so early do these tumors metastasize.

Giant-Cell Tumor

This lesion classically affects the epiphyses of the long bones. Its growth is protracted, but progressive, locally producing much bone destruction with cystic excavation and widening of the bone shaft. Tumors of this type do not metastasize, nor are they likely to recur after irradiation therapy. Therefore, they are to be classed as benign. Many cases, particularly of the multiple type, definitely have been ascribed to hyperparathyroidism.

Clinically, the patient presents signs of swelling and pain at the site of the lesion, but a spontaneous fracture may be the earliest evidence of the disease. The prompt, and usually entirely satisfactory, response to x-ray irradiation is of great diagnostic, as well as therapeutic, value in this condition. Other evidences of hyperparathyroidism

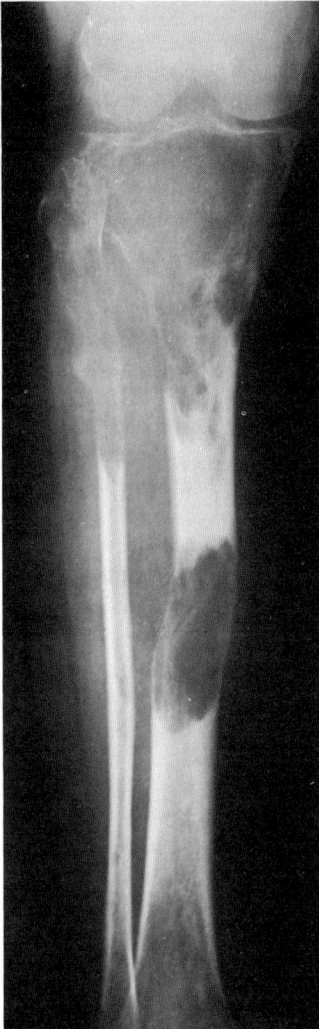

Fig. 411. Roentgenogram showing marked destruction of tibia by metastatic carcinoma. The carcinoma in this case occurred primarily in the breast.

should be sought. If found, cure can be accomplished through the removal of the hyperfunctioning parathyroid tissue. (See p. 825.)

Myeloma

Myeloma (multiple myeloma; myelomatosis; plasma cell leukemia) is a disorder based on a malignant overgrowth of plasma cells. The tissue primarily and predominantly affected is the bone marrow, and the earliest manifestations of the disease usually are those produced by bone destruction. Clinical and radiologic signs of bone involvement, which may be in the form of localized areas of lysis or diffuse osteoporosis, appear almost simultaneously at several sites; the first and the most profoundly affected usually are the "flat" bones, i.e., the ribs, the sternum, the skull, the vertebrae and the pelvic bones. Bone absorption is most pronounced where the proliferation of plasma cells is most active, giving rise to the so-called "punched-out" areas of rarefaction seen on x-ray examination, which are so suggestive of myeloma. Organs and tissues other than the bones and the bone marrow likewise become the site of malignant plasmacytosis, notably the spleen, the liver, the lymph nodes and the kidneys.

The disease occurs most characteristically in middle-aged males, and its presence is revealed clinically through the signs of bone pain, the excretion of Bence Jones protein in the urine and the bone changes seen on x-ray examination. Anemia, splenomegaly, cachexia and pathologic bone fractures (those occurring as a result of apparently trivial trauma) are features commonly observed in the course of this disease.

The plasma globulins (which are manufactured by plasma cells) increase markedly, and if this increase involves a globulin of large molecular size, the patient will exhibit the syndrome of *macroglobulinemia,* of which there are several important complications, including Raynaud's phenomena (p. 498) and excessive bleeding. A pathologic tendency to bleed is characteristic of myeloma for two major reasons: (1) a numerical deficiency of platelets (thrombocytopenia), due to destruction of the megakaryocytes, their parent cells, in the marrow;

FIG. 412. (*Top*) Frog position for congenital hip dislocation. Note child on Bradford frame. (*Bottom*) Bradford frame.

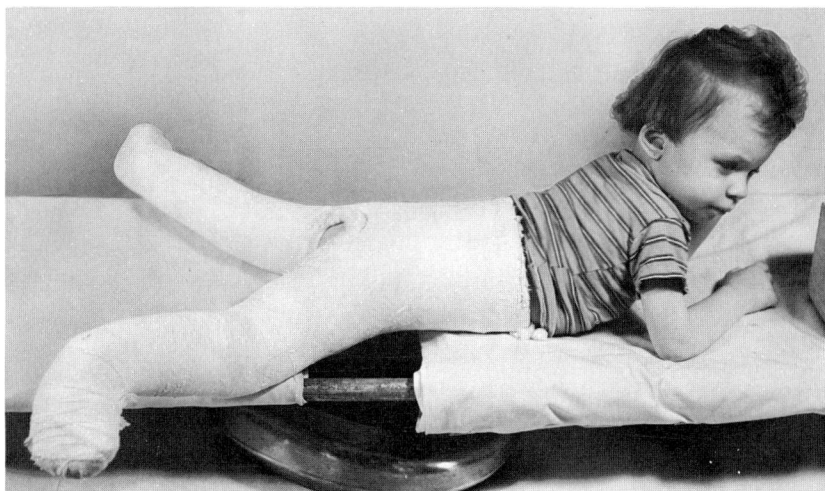

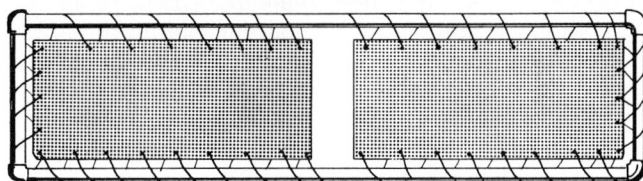

FIG. 412. (*Top*) Frog position for congenital hip dislocation. Note child on Bradford frame. (*Bottom*) Bradford frame.

and (2) platelet dysfunction, the macroglobulins tending to coat these formed elements and to interfere with their hemostatic functions.

The course of myeloma may be prolonged for several years, but a fatal termination still is to be regarded as inevitable. Bone pain may be alleviated by local x-ray irradiation. Distinct, although temporary, benefit may be obtained in some patients as a result of administering radiophosphorus (P^{32}), nitrogen mustard, chlorambucil, corticosteroid drugs and other agents that are applicable to the treatment of the leukemias and the lymphomas, of which myeloma is but a variant.

Metastatic Bone Cancer

Tumors arising from tissues other than the bone may invade the bone, producing localized bone destruction with results that are clinically quite analogous to those occurring in primary bone tumors. Those most frequently metastasizing to bone include carcinomas of the kidney, the prostate, the lung, the breast, the ovary and the thyroid. A sign of diagnostic importance in cases of metastatic carcinoma of the prostate is an elevation of the serum acid phosphatase. The first indication of disease in such cases may be a pathologic bone fracture; in later stages, the peripheral blood may show evidences of bone marrow interference. If the bone marrow becomes seriously crowded by the invading malignancy, a myelophthisic anemia is produced (Fig. 411).

CONGENITAL DEFORMITIES

Congenital Dislocation of the Hip

Congenital dislocation of the hip probably is one of the most frequent congenital deformities. It is due to a malformation of the head of the femur and of the socket in which it rests (the acetabulum). Girls are affected most frequently. Both hips may be dislocated, but more often the deformity is limited to one side.

A partial or a complete displacement of the head of the femur, an extra fold of skin near the gluteal region on one side, unequal leg length and limited movement of one leg are very early signs that suggest a congenital hip dislocation. However, in the usual case, no abnormality is noted until the child begins to walk. Then it is observed that one leg appears shorter than the other and the child walks with a decided limp. If the dislocation is bilateral, a decided waddle is a characteristic symptom. Other deformities (for example, curvature of the spine) develop as the child grows older, so that, unless the dislocation is reduced, the child must face a future of semi-invalidism. Every child who walks with a limp at the hip joint should be examined by x-rays, which will show whether or not the hip is dislocated.

Treatment and Nursing Care. The treatment of this condition is easier and more successful if it is begun as soon as the diagnosis is made. As the child grows older, reduction becomes more and more difficult; often, even with operation, only a partial cure can be effected.

NONOPERATIVE. Two methods of treatment have been employed. In one, the "bloodless" method, by manipulation under anesthesia, an effort is made to place the head of the femur in the acetabulum, holding it there by the application of plaster casts or splints. The leg is dressed in the extreme abducted position, frequently spoken of as the "frog position." This position is maintained for from 4 to 6 months. Smaller children are kept on an elevated frame (Bradford frame) made of small gas piping, between which canvas is stretched. The patient is so placed that the bedpan may be used without moving him. Elevation of the head of the frame will prevent seepage of urine. The plaster cast should be kept dry and clean. The principles outlined on cast care will apply here (see p. 995). In addition, the shellacking of the cast (with the permission of the physician) or the use of tubular stockinet to cover the cast will help the nurse and, later, the mother to keep the cast clean. As with all patients in plaster casts, constant vigilance is necessary to avoid pressure sores at the edge of the cast, and the skin must be kept clean and dry at these points. This is especially important in the perineal region, where urine and feces are apt to cause maceration of the skin. If the area of perineal exposure is not large enough to maintain cleanliness, the nurse should notify the physician. The cast may be supported by pillows or rolled blankets to prevent chafing of the skin from pressure of the cast edges round the extremities.

Older children may be encouraged to walk with support, as use of the legs tends to deepen the socket for the head of the femur. If, at the end of from 4 to 6 months, it is found that the head of the femur will not stay in place, open operation usually is necessary, even in young children. At the end of the 6-month period of immobilization in plaster, the leg is straightened gradually by a succession of plaster casts. After about a year or 18 months, weight-bearing with or without support may be permitted. Normal motion in the hip joint will be impaired for a considerable period, but this disability may be relieved gradually by a period of baking, massage and supervised exercises carried out in an orthopedic gymnasium.

OPERATIVE. In patients over 6 years of age, operation usually is necessary, replacing the femur in the acetabulum or, if this is impossible, forming a new socket ("shelf operation") in which the head of the bone may rest. Casts are applied after operation, including the involved foot, lower extremity and the pelvis, and holding the extremity in extension, abduction and internal rotation. This position is maintained for at least 3 months, after which the extremity is brought down gradually into the normal attitude. The patient then may be permitted to get up without support of any kind, and he is encouraged to use his leg gradually.

After operation, the care of the child is largely in the hands of the nurse. The patient's general condition must be checked carefully. Temperature, pulse, respirations and blood pressure should be taken periodically and recorded on the nurse's chart. Shock should be watched for carefully (see p. 296) and its presence reported at once to the surgeon. Hemorrhage in the region of the operative site may escape detection because of the cast, but periodic examinations should be made of the bottom of the cast, and any increasing blood-staining of the cast should be reported to the surgeon immediately. (See Care of the Patient in a Cast, p. 995.)

Birth Palsy

This is a paralysis of the arm caused by injury to the brachial plexus during birth.

(Erb's paralysis involves the shoulder muscles only.) The nurse may notice the flaccidly hanging arm during the infant's first bath. If only the shoulder is involved, the prognosis is good. By splinting or the application of a cast, the arm can be maintained in abduction and external rotation. The length of treatment varies directly with the severity of the paralysis.

Congenital Torticollis (Wryneck)

Probably due to hemorrhage in the sternocleidomastoid muscle caused by trauma during delivery, the child's head may incline to one side. This is brought about by a shortening of the muscle on the side involved. Palpation of the neck reveals a mass in the muscle, and attempts to straighten the head on the trunk are unsuccessful. This is called *torticollis* or *wryneck*. As healing takes place in the injured muscle, fibrosis and contraction occur and the child keeps the head turned to the opposite side and inclined toward the shoulder on the involved side. If uncorrected, this deformity leads to marked facial asymmetry.

Treatment of torticollis usually is successful if the condition is discovered soon after birth. Heat, massage and carefully regulated stretching as a rule bring a return to normal in a month or two. In untreated cases, the fibrosis and resulting contracture of the muscle result in a deformity that cannot be relieved by conservative means. A cutting of the tendon at its insertion to the clavicle and the sternum is performed. After operation, a plaster cast that includes head, neck and upper chest is applied. The head thus is held in an overcorrected position for a time and brought gradually to its normal position.

Nursing Care. Nursing problems which result from adhesive traction, a brace or a plaster cast applied as a corrective device for torticollis are similar. During the immediate postoperative care, the nurse must be aware of the danger of aspiration because of the restricted movement brought about by one of the above-mentioned devices. Observation of those areas which are in contact with close-fitting apparatus is a necessary nursing function. In addition, cleanliness must be maintained. The use of bibs, water-proofing materials, cleaning agents and deodorants described on p. 995, Cast and Traction Care) should be used. Diversional activity suited to the preferences of the patient will make time pass more quickly. The role of the nurse as teacher here is important. She can help to educate the mother in ways to help the child to help himself; for example, encourage the child to turn his head in the corrected position by the placement of toys or other such devices.

Clubfoot and Other Deformities of the Feet

Clubfoot (congenital talipes; equinovarus) is a deformity thought to be due to arrested growth, a defect in the ovum, familial tendencies or malposition in the uterus. It may involve one foot or both feet. The foot is turned in and, in extreme cases, so deformed that the child walks on the outside of the foot with the heel elevated and the sole turned backward.

Soon after birth the deformity may be recognized, and, if treatment is instituted at that early date, a complete cure usually results. If untreated, the tendons become shortened, the bones and the calf muscles are ill-formed, and a cure is effected with much more difficulty. Treatment may be done in mild cases by means of manipulation and strapping. The nurse can help a great deal by convincing the parents that such treatment must be continuous and adhered to faithfully. Generally this is accomplished best by applying a series of plaster casts to correct the deformity. The forefoot adduction, heel inversion and, finally, the equinus attitude are corrected in that order. The casts are changed weekly at first, and as the condition improves they may be left in place for longer intervals. The casts are made by applying plaster-of-Paris bandages over snugly fitting flannel or cotton wadding that extends from the tips of the toes to just below the knee. The Kite method is the use of a plaster cast that is wedged at intervals as the correction progresses. With this method, the nurse must be on the alert for new pressure areas. During this period of treatment it is of the utmost importance to guard against impairment of circulation and the development of pressure sores, which may require splitting or trimming of the cast and even its removal and the application of a new cast. When the foot has been corrected satisfactorily, as verified by clinical x-ray examinations, the foot may be removed from plaster and manipulated several times daily. The child then may be fitted with clubfoot corrective shoes and allowed to walk. However, it may be necessary to maintain the corrected position at night by means of the appropriate splint.

The Denis-Brown apparatus is another method of treatment, in which the feet are strapped to foot-plates attached to a cross-bar; correction is obtained by the force of the child's kicking in the splint. There are several disadvantages to this method, and when it is used it is usually in treating infants less than 1 year old.

If correction cannot be secured in this manner, especially in older children, anesthesia is administered and the foot is brought into position by forcible manual correction. Casts then are applied as described above to hold the foot in a position of overcorrection. For 24 hours after this operation, the child should be confined to bed with the foot and the leg elevated to prevent undue swelling. After 2 or 3 days, walking is permitted in the plaster cast. After 3 or 4 weeks another dressing similar to the first is applied. Following a series of casts, changed about every 3 weeks, the treatment may be continued with exercises and special shoes. In some cases, elastic traction bands may be used instead of the cast or after cast treatment.

Cutting operations—cutting tendons or ligaments—or operations involving the bones of the foot are reserved for those late cases in which correction cannot be obtained by the above methods. Recurrence of the deformity is not uncommon, and the child should be reexamined by the surgeon periodically for many months.

Hallux valgus is an inward deviation of the great toe at the first metatarsophalangeal joint. This is associated with an exostosis on the head of the first metatarsal and a bursa overlying the exostosis, which is called a *bunion*. Bunions may be acquired or congenital. Properly fitting shoes and support of the metatarsal arch usually relieve pain and discomfort, but in severe cases operative correction of the deformity is required.

Flatfoot deformity in children frequently is found with bowlegs or knock-knees. Usually, prescribed shoes with heel lifts are recommended; these are changed as the child grows. Flat feet are common also as an adult deformity. Supportive arches in shoes usually give relief.

Hammer toes may be congenital or acquired and result from the spasmodic con-

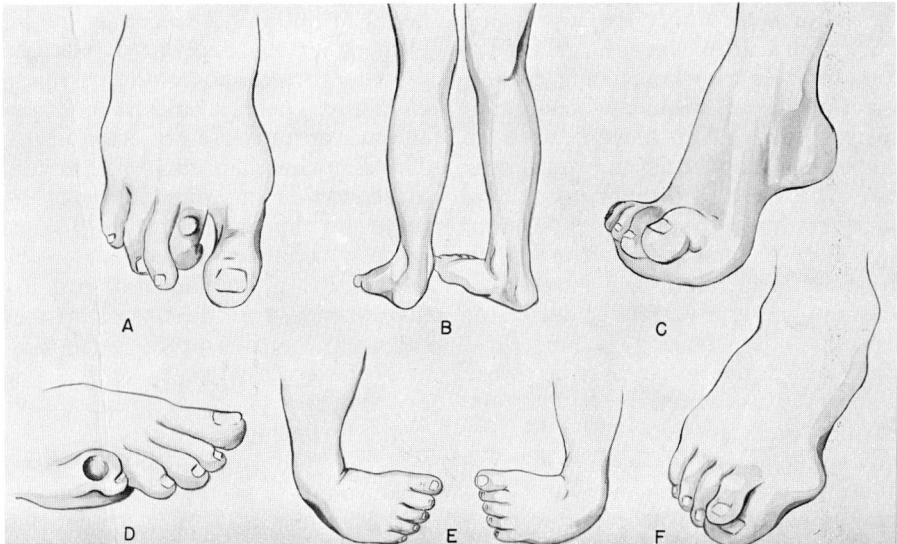

FIG. 413. (A) Second hammer toe. (B) Pronated flatfeet. (C) Clawfoot. (D) Congenital hammer toe. (E) Congenital talipes equinovarus—clubfoot. (F) Hallux valgus.

tracture of the extensors of the toes. The first interphalangeal joint is usually prominent; it is flexed and often has a corn on top. The treatment is any measure to release the contracture of the muscle and often requires operation.

Clawfoot is a contracture of the muscles and the ligaments of the plantar arch and is seen following infantile paralysis. Treatment may involve arch supports and probably a tenotomy of the extensor tendons to the toes.

Nursing responsibility in relation to foot conditions is primarily a teaching one. It is for the nurse to relay important information to her patients regarding foot exercises, the proper selection and care of shoes, the care and the use of foot pads and plates, the care of boot casts and the significance of symptoms of circulatory constriction. The socioeconomic factors must not be ignored.

DEVELOPMENTAL DEFECTS

Spinal Curvatures

Curvatures of the spine may be of three types: (1) *kyphosis,* anteroposterior curvatures, or hunchback, (2) *lordosis,* or exaggerated hollow back and (3) *scoliosis* or lateral curvature.

Kyphosis. Kyphosis, or a general bowing forward of the spine, develops in persons who are physically under par, whose occupations are fatiguing and who wear clothes which are too heavy or too tight. Frequently it develops in consequence of such conditions as chronic bronchitis and asthma, espe-

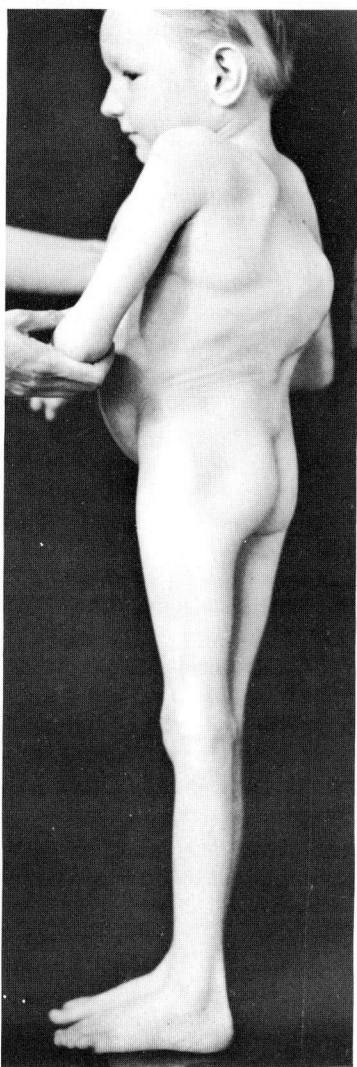

FIG. 414. Kyphosis of the spine —Pott's disease. (Indiana University)

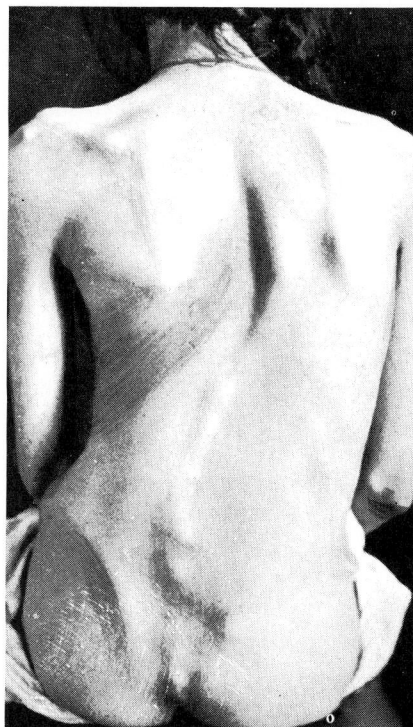

FIG. 415. Scoliosis of the spine. (Indiana University Department of Illustrations)

cially when these occur in childhood. It is a striking feature of pulmonary emphysema (in which condition the kyphosis is due to deformities of the chest) and is the inevitable result of chronic arthritis, Paget's disease, Pott's disease (Fig. 414) and osteomalacia.

Scoliosis (Lateral Curvature of the Spine). This condition may be a secondary result of deformities of other parts—for example, the shortening of one leg, thoracic disease such as empyema, rickets or habitual faulty posture. The last produces what is known as postural or functional scoliosis. It begins merely as a faulty attitude in the decade between 5 and 15 years of age. The spine is curved slightly to one side, and there usually are coexistent round shoulders and round back. Statistics show this minor deformity to be present in from 20 to 25 per cent of schoolchildren. Among the many theories of its origin are heredity; occupation; the posture of the child while sitting; manner of dress; manner of life; general muscular weakness; chronic fatigue; and a timid, apprehensive frame of mind, the physical expression of which is scoliosis (the psychoneurotic stance).

While the condition appears to be of little importance, it should not be neglected, because the tendency is toward an increase in the deformity as growth progresses. The

lateral curvature becomes more noticeable, the shoulder (usually the left) droops, and the right hip becomes prominent. The curve at first is often in one direction only; but sooner or later it becomes S-shaped, since, to maintain body balance, a compensatory curve in the opposite direction develops in the previously normal region of the spine. If the condition goes untreated, structural (bony) changes occur.

TREATMENT. The treatment of this condition often falls to the school nurse, in association with the surgeon. It requires a thorough investigation of the hygienic practices of the patient. Overwork in school and after school should be prevented. An examination of the eyes is indicated if visual error is suspected that would lead to improper posture in reading. The schoolroom desk and chair should be inspected with the child seated at the desk. If the desk is too far from the chair, or if it is too small for the child, habitual faulty posture can hardly be prevented (Fig. 416 A). A patient's family can be taught to help the child in maintaining good posture. Often it is difficult to sell the idea of the need for corrective exercises to the patient. Emphasis on the cosmetic result often is effective. Many orthopedic surgeons relieve weight on the shoulders by having the patient wear clothes that hang from the

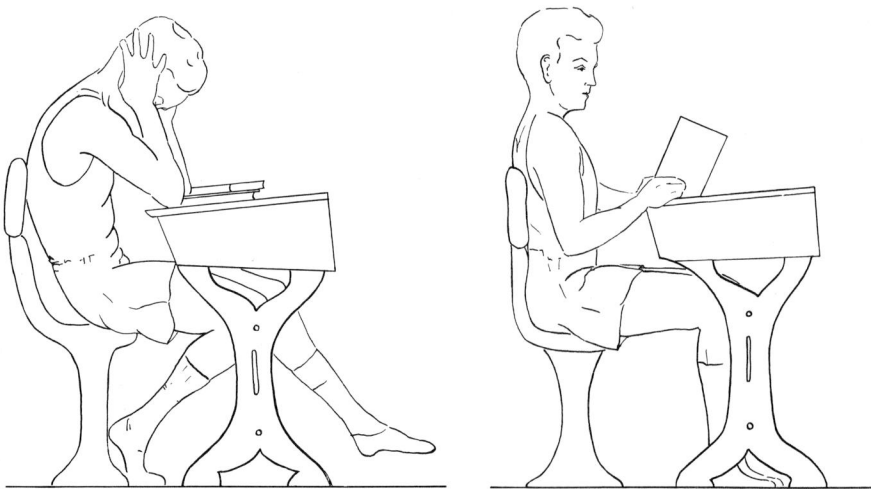

FIG. 416 A. (*Left*) Showing child sitting at desk in improper position. Desk too small for child. (*Right*) Showing child sitting at desk in proper position.

waist as much as possible. Habitual malposture and functional scoliosis may be corrected by spinal gymnastic exercises that are continued for 1 or 2 years.

In those patients in whom there is marked rotation of the ribs associated with the lateral curvature, support often is applied in the form of a plaster jacket having large windows over the compressed portion of the thorax to allow for its expansion. Adequate correction may have to be obtained by applying a cast with wedges cut in either side (Risser jacket), so that the spine may be straightened by the use of hinges and turnbuckles. For many patients, an operation (spinal fusion) may be necessary to hold the spine in the corrected position. When the desired result is obtained, a spinal brace often is employed to maintain the overcorrected position for a time.

Orthopedic Problems
Following Poliomyelitis

Paralytic deformities frequently appear following infantile paralysis. (See p. 1099.) The use of Salk vaccine has reduced greatly the incidence of the paralytic form of poliomyelitis. This disease affects children and adults and results in a destruction of anterior horn cells of the spinal cord. Paralysis appears in the muscle groups innervated by the destroyed cells. It involves most commonly the muscles of the extremities and often is bilateral; but any part may be affected, including the muscles of the spine and the abdomen. The paralysis is of the flaccid type, leaving the limb flail-like. Contractures of the unparalyzed muscles may cause increasing deformities.

As soon as the paralysis becomes evident, it is necessary to prevent, so far as possible, the development of deformity and protect weak musculature. The usual method of accomplishing this is by means of splints or molded plaster casts that maintain the affected extremities in the neutral position; for example, the foot should be at right angles to the leg. The bedclothes are supported with pillows or a cradle.

Sister Kenny's method of treatment consists of the periodic application of hot packs to the affected parts and painstaking re-education of the involved muscles as soon as the patient's condition permits it. For its proper use this treatment requires specially trained nurses and physiotherapists. Physiotherapy measures should be used to maintain the range of motion in the joints.

After the acute symptoms subside, carefully supervised physiotherapy (bathing, massage, electrical treatments, hydrotherapy and exercises) may be beneficial. Swimming exercise in pool or otherwise, still is a most valuable adjunct of the rehabilitation treatment in many cases of paralyses, when muscle action is to be restored. Often some form of supportive brace or appliance is indicated, and the nurse should see to it that these are in the proper position at all times. Considerable improvement may be observed under this treatment. Usually, after the lapse of a year of two, no further improvement will be evident.

Operation is indicated for many of these patients for the relief of deformities that develop from neglect of, or in spite of, proper supporting apparatus and for optimum functional return. Tendons may be transplanted so that functioning muscles may act in place of paralyzed ones or, when paralysis is extensive, the flail-jointed "dangle foot" may be converted into a much more useful member by producing an artificial union of the bones forming the joint. This is done by an operation called an *arthrodesis*. The leg must be encased in a plaster cast for a time (usually 12 weeks) to give the bones a chance to form a solid union.

After operation, the leg should be elevated to prevent undue swelling. Even with this precaution, the toes must be watched carefully for signs of interference with the circulation, i.e., swelling, cyanosis and numbness. Often it is necessary to spread the cast enough to permit an adequate circulation.

Rachitic Deformities

Because of the bony deformities that it produces rickets is important, not only to the nutritionist, the pediatrician and the internist but also to the orthopedic surgeon, and it is of potential concern to all nurses.

Rickets (see p. 153) is a disease of young children (under 3 years of age). It is found most often in children who have been brought up under poor hygienic conditions and have had improper feedings and little sunlight, fresh air or exercise. Research has shown that the lack of vitamin D (found in fish oils, vegetables and certain other types of food) will cause this condition. Exposure of the child to the ultraviolet rays of the sun or a special mercury arc lamp will prevent the condition and benefit it if it has occurred.

Symptoms. The symptoms of the disease usually begin the first or the second year. The mother notices fretfulness, head-sweating and a "backwardness" in walking, crawling and sitting. The ends of the long bones become swollen. This is especially marked at wrist and ankle joints and where the ribs join the sternum. The enlargement at the last-mentioned site often is called the *rachitic rosary*. The bones are soft due to a lack of lime (calcium) deposit that results in various types of deformities. "Bowlegs," "knock knee" and kyphosis are a few of the common types.

Treatment. The treatment of these patients is directed toward the cure of the constitutional disease and the prevention and the relief of disabling deformities. The child should be fed a diet rich in fresh vegetables and vitamins, especially vitamin D, and adequate milk. Open air and direct sunlight are therapeutic agents of more merit than most medicines. Sunlight is of value because of the ultraviolet rays it contains. These rays are lost largely by passage through glass; therefore, the child should be out of doors. Practically the whole body should be exposed. Instead of sunlight, or combined with it, most surgeons use the ultraviolet rays obtained from a mercury arc lamp. The children are exposed to the rays without clothes for increasing periods. Several precautions must be taken in the use of these rays. The eyes of both patient and nurse must be protected by dark glasses or goggles. Overexposure must be avoided to prevent skin burns. A nurse always should be present during the exposure, and a time clock should be set that will ring at the end of the prescribed period.

In the early stages of the disease the treatment is directed toward the prevention of deformities. Braces or plaster-of-Paris splints are used to overcome mild deformities. After the age of 3 years, little improve-

ment can be expected from the brace treatment, and operations have been devised to relieve the deformities. The bones are divided deliberately with a sharp instrument, and the limbs are placed in a plaster cast in an overcorrected position for 6 to 8 weeks. The precautions taken as discussed on page 995 are indicated.

Dupuytren's Contracture

Dupuytren's deformity is an unyielding flexion of the little, ring and, often, middle fingers, rendering them more or less useless. It is a fairly common abnormality, its cause unknown. It starts as a thickening of the palmar fascia. The fibrous thickening extends to involve the skin in the distal palm, and produces a contracture of the fingers to which the palmar fascia is inserted. This condition always starts in one hand, but eventually both become symmetrically deformed. Plastic surgery offers excellent relief; the operation consists of total excision of the involved palmar fascia.

OSTEOMALACIA AND OSTEOPOROSIS

Osteomalacia. This is a disease of the skeleton, the essential feature of which is widespread softening and brittleness of the skeleton due to decalcification of, or failure of calcium salts to become deposited in, the bones. Depending on the age at which this defect occurs, characteristic deformities are produced. The decalcification of the bones is evident from the faint outlines and the absorption from the thinness of their cortex, both observed on roentgenograms. Their softness is shown by the bowing of bones due to body weight and muscle pull; their brittleness by the numerous fractures which occur. Associated with this process are severe pains and tenderness over the affected bones and muscular weakness.

ETIOLOGY. Osteomalacia may occur as a result of inadequate dietary intake of calcium or phosphate ions, failure of these ions to be absorbed from the food or excessive loss of these materials from the body. The juvenile type, or rickets, is attributable to a deficiency of vitamin D and consequent failure of calcium absorption, in addition to a dietary deficiency involving calcium, phosphorus, or both (p. 153). The malnutrition type is apt to occur in destitute populations particularly. The majority of cases among adults, however, occur in women between the ages of 20 and 30 years, two thirds of whom have had frequently repeated pregnancies and lactation, for during pregnancy two factors may operate to produce this disease: one, the fetal demand for calcium and phosphorus, and the other, loss of these minerals in the breast milk.

Gastrointestinal disorders in which fats are inadequately absorbed are prone to produce osteomalacia through loss of vitamin D (among other fat-soluble vitamins) and calcium, the latter being excreted in the feces in combination with fatty acids. Such disorders include sprue, celiac disease, chronic biliary tract obstruction, chronic pancreatitis and small bowel resections or operative shunts involving the small intestine.

Renal disorders causing excessive retention of acids, or which favor the urinary secretion of calcium or phosphorus, are responsible for a type of osteomalacia known as "renal rickets." Finally, hyperparathyroidism, as previously discussed (p. 825), leads to skeletal decalcification, i.e., osteomalacia, through the promotion of phosphorus excretion in the urine.

SYMPTOMS. Osteomalacia in adults may begin so insidiously that bone deformities are the first signs of its presence. Its most common subjective symptom is pain in the affected bones, which may be acutely tender on pressure. Because of body weight and muscle pull, the legs become markedly bowed, the softened vertebrae compressed, thus shortening the patient's trunk and deforming the thorax. The sacrum is forced down and forward, and the pelvis is compressed laterally, these two deformities explaining the characteristic shape of the pelvis which so often makes cesarean section necessary.

TREATMENT. If osteomalacia occurs as a manifestation of calcium or phosphate deficiency, treatment such as is prescribed in classic rickets should be pursued vigorously. This includes a full diet, including milk, eggs, fish and vegetables, supplemented with calcium salts, phosphates and vitamin D.

Osteoporosis. A second large group of bone disorders exists which, like the malacic diseases, is characterized by generalized loss of density and tensile strength throughout the skeleton, and is similarly responsible for an abnormal susceptibility to fractures in response to relatively slight trauma. These represent patients with osteoporosis, the basis of which, however, is not failure of calcium phosphate to become, or to remain, deposited in the bones, but a deficiency of the organic matrix of bone. The matrix either fails to form, atrophies or is destroyed. Familiar examples of osteoporosis are presented by cases of scurvy, due to vitamin C deficiency (p. 153); senile osteoporosis; atrophy of disuse; endocrine disorders, such as Cushing's syndrome, hyperthyroidism and hypothyroidism, acromegaly, Simmond's cachexia, eunuchoidism and estrogen deficiency, as in the postmenopausal state. One type attributable to a congenital defect is called "osteogenesis imperfecta."

OSTEITIS DEFORMANS: PAGET'S DISEASE

Osteitis deformans is a malady which develops slowly and chiefly affects men beyond middle life. Eventually it produces marked hypertrophy and bowing of the long bones and great thickening and irregular deformities of the flat bones. It may start in any part of the skeleton, but usually in the skull, the tibia or the vertebral column. The entire skeleton may become involved—least often the bones of the face, the hands and the feet.

This disease begins insidiously, in many cases with pain and tenderness on pressure in the bones, usually first in the shins. Such pain, which often is attributed to old age, neuritis, rheumatism, etc., may for years precede the gross skeletal changes. In the majority of cases, however, the decreasing height and the increasing size of the head are the first symptoms noticed. For years the disease may seem limited to one bone.

In well-marked cases of Paget's disease the cranium is much enlarged, but not the face, which therefore appears small and triangular in shape. The spine is bent forward and is rigid; the chin rests on the chest. The thorax is compressed and immobile on respiration. The trunk is flexed on the legs to maintain equilibrium; the arms, which are bent outward and forward and appear long in relation to the shortened trunk, give to the patient an apelike appearance; and the legs are greatly bowed, hence the gait is labored and waddling. As a result of the kyphosis and the bowing of the legs, the patient's height may be reduced as much as 12 in. Since the bones involved, though massive, are brittle, fractures occur frequently.

Associated features include general weakness, chronic cardiovascular and pulmonary diseases (such as emphysema and bronchitis) and, occasionally, symptoms indicative of cerebral damage (impairment of sight and hearing, and muscular atrophy or spasticity). Nevertheless, the patient's general health is little disturbed. After advancing for from 20 to 30 or more years, the disease often becomes quiescent. Death usually is due to complications of generalized arteriosclerosis, that is, cerebral accident, cardiac or renal disease. One fatal complication of this disease is the development of bone sarcoma.

Diagnosis

Early cases usually can be recognized on roentgenograms, which will reveal changes developing simultaneously in both the skull and the tibia. Serum alkaline phosphatase, the level of which serves as an index of bone absorption, usually is elevated markedly in this condition, occasionally attaining a figure of 300 Bodansky units (normal, 3 to 5).

Treatment

There is no specific treatment for Paget's disease. Irradiation of the painful extremities has been reported to afford occasional symptomatic relief.

Osteitis fibrosa cystica (Von Recklinghausen's disease) is considered elsewhere (Chap. 38, p. 825).

PRIMARY MUSCULAR DYSTROPHIES

Pseudohypertrophic Muscular Dystrophy

This is a disease characterized by the progressive weakness and final atrophy of groups of muscles. Early the calf muscles, the deltoids and those attached to the scapula may become markedly hypertrophied, yet are very weak. This disease is more common in males and usually appears during childhood.

The first evidences of this disease are the increased size of certain muscles, a marked lordosis and a waddling gait. The patient falls frequently, has difficulty in climbing stairs and is unable to rise from the ground without "climbing up his legs" with the use of the arms. Gradually all the affected muscles atrophy until the patient is helpless.

The juvenile form (Erb's type) of progressive muscular dystrophy, a rare type, is a disease of childhood which starts in the muscles of the shoulder girdle, the back and, occasionally, the pelvic girdle. The muscles of the forearm, the hand, the lower leg and the face long remain normal. The involved muscles may first hypertrophy but later atrophy.

Landouzy-Déjerine Type

In this condition the muscles of the face, the shoulder girdle and the arm become markedly atrophied without preceding hypertrophy. Those of the forearms, the hands, the legs and the back seldom are affected. The atrophy of the facial muscles usually begins early in life, producing the peculiar myopathic facies (the lips are thick, and the lower lip, because of atrophy of the obicularis oris, curves downward, hence the so-called *tapir mouth*).

Summary

The above-mentioned primary myopathies are not different diseases, for patients with any one of them are likely to present features of other types. In none of them can any lesion in the central nervous system be found at autopsy—the primary lesion appears to involve the muscle. Treatment by present means is of no avail; therapy is limited to rest, supportive measures and the prevention of contractures.

MYASTHENIA GRAVIS

Myasthenia gravis is a chronic disease of unknown etiology, affecting young adults particularly. Its one symptom is great muscular fatigue, quickly produced by repeated movements, which soon disappears following rest. Patients with this disease tire on such slight exertion as combing the hair, chewing and talking, and quickly must stop for rest. Symmetrical muscles always are involved, first and foremost those innervated by the cranial nerves. No sensory disturbances are apparent.

Because of the involvement of the ocular muscles, diplopia is a common early symptom. The facies, a sad, sleepy, masklike expression with ptosis of the eyelids, early becomes characteristic (Fig. 416 B). Sudden attacks of dyspnea and collapse frequently occur and are sometimes fatal, but the disease usually runs on, even for years, and some cases improve spontaneously.

No significant lesion is found at autopsy. The muscles show no atrophy and give no reaction of degeneration, but do give the characteristic myasthenic reaction. (When stimulated at intervals of seconds by a faradic current, the muscular contractions become progressively weaker and soon cease, but return after a short rest.)

The diagnosis is confirmed by means of a therapeutic test employing neostigmine: 1.5 mg. of neostigmine methylsulfate, combined with 0.6 mg. of atropine sulfate, are injected intramuscularly, or 1 ml. of a 1:2,000 dilution (0.5 mg.) of neostigmine, intravenously, alone, a positive result being evidenced by a striking increase in muscular strength within a period of 5 to 10 minutes.

The basic abnormality in myasthenia gravis is a defect in the transmission of impulses from nerve to muscle cells. Conduction of these impulses is presumably mediated by acetylcholine. In view of the observation that the intra-arterial injection of acetylcholine corrects the defect, briefly at least, it is quite possible that the principle difficulty in these cases resides in the synthesis, or the release, of acetylcholine at the neuromuscular junction, which is inadequate. Support for this view is provided by the fact that chemicals which delay the enzymatic destruction of acetylcholine in the body (i.e., compounds with anticholinesterase activity), such as neostigmine, tetraethylpyrophosphate (TEPP) or octamethyl pyrophosphoramide (OMPA), produce temporary remissions of the disease, as evidenced by transient gains in muscle strength.

Treatment. Treatment of myasthenia gravis during its acute stages includes rest in bed and, later, the limitation of all unnecessary efforts. Neostigmine bromide, supplied at frequent intervals according to a fixed, permanent schedule, generally is effective in the control of symptoms, at least to the extent that life is protected. Most patients require from 15 to 45 mg. of the drug orally at 2-hour to 4-hour intervals. Severely affected patients must be provided with this agent during their sleeping hours. Those unable to swallow must receive neostigmine by intramuscular injection, the usual dose by this route varying from 1 to 2 mg. every 1 to 3 hours.

Two other anticholinesterase compounds which are equally effective in myasthenia gravis are pyridostigmine (Mestinon) and ambenomium (Mytelase), given orally in 4-hourly doses of 240 and 20 mg., respectively. The action of these agents is sufficiently long to eliminate the necessity of interrupting sleep for medication.

The administration of antibiotic drugs and the application of suction are indicated in the event of an intercurrent pulmonary infection. The use of a respirator and performance of tracheotomy may be life-saving procedures when the muscles of respiration and swallowing become severely involved. Whereas the prognosis is extremely grave for the majority of patients who reach this stage, some have exhibited very gratifying and sustained remissions, enabling them to relinquish the respirator and even to resume normal lives thereafter.

Prognosis. The life expectancy for about one third of all patients with myasthenia gravis is less than 6 years from the onset of symptoms. On the other hand, approximately one quarter of all cases exhibit complete, or nearly complete, remissions in the course of their disease, the average duration of which has been 4 to 5 years.

Precaution. A note of warning is indicated, which the nurse should heed with care, for she may be in a position to prevent a premature and unnecessary death, armed with the following facts.

Morphine, intrinsically a respiratory depressant, is made more potent in its effects by anticholinesterase compounds, such as are customarily received by patients with myasthenia gravis. Its use, therefore, is extremely dangerous in these cases. Even small doses have proved to be fatal. Demerol is tolerated well enough in the average case, but should be given in no more than one half the usual dosage. *No sedative, even the mildest, should be employed in any case of myasthenia gravis in which there is difficulty in breathing or in swallowing; and, to repeat, the use of morphine should be regarded as being strictly contraindicated.*

NURSING CARE OF THE ORTHOPEDIC PATIENT

Nursing Care of Orthopedic Surgical Patients

Preoperative Care. In general, the principles of preoperative care are the same as in the care of any surgical patient. Only the differences will be stressed.

Psychological Care. Many orthopedic patients experience a curious mixture of fear and anticipation before surgery. Will I be able to walk again, or is this too much to hope for? If an individual has been handicapped and dependent for most of his life, he faces reconstructive surgery with added concern. Some patients have faced repeated operations; patience and hope are almost gone. These are the people who need much help from an understanding nurse.

Following surgery, if the patient is to be placed in a different type of bed with special apparatus such as traction or a plaster cast, he should have some preparation for this preoperatively.

Physical Care. Whatever the method used in preparing the skin of the orthopedic patient for surgery, the principles remain the same. The procedure usually is more painstaking because of the difficulty in controlling infection in the bone, should that occur. A meticulous nontraumatizing cleansing of the skin with soap and water, followed by careful shaving, is done first. Then, soap-and-water washing is repeated, and a fat solvent can be used, followed by a mild antiseptic.

Disability can result should infection occur within a bone or a joint. In no instance should one rely on the antibiotics to control infection and thereby justify slipshod preoperative preparation.

It is well to remember that, when a cleansing enema is ordered, it should be given before the skin preparation is begun. Some orthopedic surgeons do not require a preoperative enema for surgery on the extremities.

Adequate hydration is always an essential objective in orthopedic patients, particularly those immobilized for a long period of time. Kidney complications and breakdown of pressure areas will result if this is neglected.

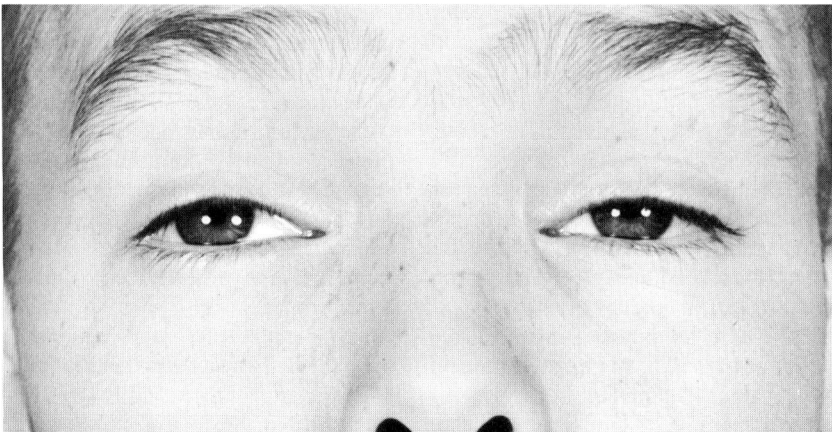

Fig. 416 B. Myasthenia gravis. To elevate the eyelids and keep the eyes open requires considerable effort and cannot be accomplished without raising the eyebrows as well. The combination of droopy lids and furrowed brow, characteristic of the "myasthenic facies," is responsible for the sleepy, saddened expression of the patients.

Postoperative Care. Patients who have bone and joint surgery experience real *pain*. Many times, the person who has had surgery to correct a foot condition is much more uncomfortable than one who has had extensive abdominal surgery. Narcotics and other pain-relieving measures should be administered liberally. However, in the long-term patient it is well to remember that habit-forming possibilities can be a considerable problem. It should be pointed out that even though a patient has had an orthopedic operation, the pain may not necessarily be the result of the wound and of the operative trauma. Swelling frequently follows, and when it occurs under tight bandages or casts, there may be interference with the blood supply, which also produces excruciating pain. This type of pain can be suspected when there is blueness and swelling beyond the limits of the cast, and they can be relieved by cutting the cast or the bandages. Another type of pain occurs in orthopedic patients when there is prolonged pressure over bony prominences such as areas of the heel, the head of the fibula on the lateral side of the leg just below the knee and the tuberosity of the tibia. Even though they have been well padded before the cast has been applied, these areas eventually may become painful. The pain is characteristically of a burning type. It is wise not to treat this with narcotics but to call it to the attention of the surgeon, who may wish to cut away areas of the cast to relieve the pressure. In major orthopedic surgery, *shock* also is a common problem, and the nurse must be on the alert for its symptoms.

Bone does not mend so readily as soft tissues. Therefore, even though the skin incision is well healed, bony structures underneath still need time to repair. This is especially important to remember in surgery of the lower extremities, for in addition to normal movement, bone must be able to bear weight in ambulation.

Other complications which may occur are similar to those of general surgical patients. They are oozing and bleeding, abdominal distention, wound infection and pulmonary and circulatory problems.

Rehabilitation of Orthopedic Patients. In allowing the patient to help himself, he must be taught the best way. The physical therapist working with the physician and the nurse can guide the patient in the proper use of his muscles and joints. Emphasis is placed on activities of daily living so that he will be able to perform those functions which will allow him independence. He will need patience and constant encouragement. He may want to perform a certain activity but fear that self-inflicted injury may result. The extent to which a patient may progress safely must be understood clearly by him as well as all who care for him.

When he goes home, the patient should have explicit instructions which he understands, indicating those activities which he may and may not perform. It is not enough to bid him "good-bye, and take it easy." The patient must know any untoward signs and symptoms which should be reported to his

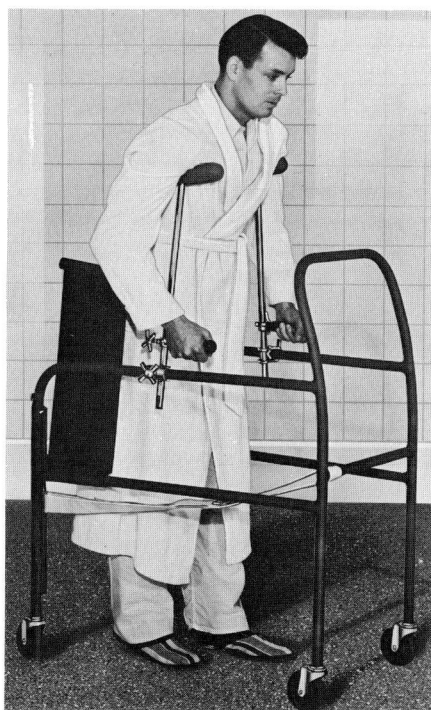

Fig. 417. The Comper Invalid Walker is of clinical and economic value in ambulatory service for orthopedic, fracture, paralytic and postoperative patients. (The Surgical Supervisor, American Sterilizer Co., Erie, Pa.)

physician. He must be aware of the importance of follow-up visits. If he has any difficulties, he ought to know where and how to get help. The nurse has a major part of the responsibility for instructing her patient before he leaves the hospital.

CLINICAL SITUATIONS

Congenital Dislocation of the Hip

Penelope was 15 months old when she began to walk. Her mother noticed an abnormal gait and called it to the attention of the pediatrician. He suggested that "Penny" be hospitalized for the correction of a congenital dislocation of the right hip.

1. Penny's unusual gait could be described best as
   A. A waddle.
   B. A limp on the right side.
   C. A limp on the left side.
   D. Typical of the toddler.
2. Congenital dislocation of the hip might be discovered early if the nurse in the nursery notes
   A. An extra fold of skin near the gluteal region on one side.
   B. A tendency to keep one leg flexed and the other extended.
   C. Limited movement of one leg.
   D. Inversion of the foot and adduction of the forefoot.
3. Congenital hip dislocation probably can be corrected if treatment for Penny is instituted
   A. Immediately.
   B. Between the ages of 2 and 5.
   C. Between the ages of 6 and 10.
4. Following manipulation under anesthesia, the child usually is placed in the following position:
   A. The leg is placed in adduction, 45° to 90°.
   B. The leg is placed in abduction, 45° to 90°.
   C. Any position is permissible; no cast or splint is required.
5. If surgery is done, the objective of the operation is to
   A. Replace the femur in the acetabulum.
   B. Replace the deformed femur with a Vitallium prosthesis.

C. Create a new socket in which the head of the femur may rest.
D. Insert a jointed medullary bar into the femur and the acetabulum.

Fracture of the Femur

Mr. Reilly was admitted to Tompkins East I with a diagnosis of an intertrochanteric fracture of the left femur. Upon admission he was placed in Russell's traction. Two weeks later he was taken to the operating room, where the fracture was reduced; he was encased in a hip spica cast and returned to the floor.

1. Points to be observed in the daily care of Mr. Reilly while he is in traction are as follows:
   A. Be sure that adhesive is secured down over the lateral malleoli.
   B. Remove weights while changing the sheets on the bed.
   C. Be sure that the spreader is in contact with the foot of the bed.
   D. Turn Mr. Reilly frequently to avoid pneumonia.
   E. See to it that the weights are hanging freely.
2. If Mr. Reilly had a comminuted fracture of the femur, it would be one in which the bone
   A. Was broken into many fragments.
   B. Penetrated the skin.
   C. Was fractured on one side and bent on the other.
   D. Was broken across entirely.
3. When Mr. Reilly returned to the ward in his cast, signs which might be indicative of impaired circulation were
   A. Swelling.
   B. Cyanosis of the toes.
   C. Decreased temperature.
   D. Erythema and a feeling of warmth.
   E. Pain.
4. When turning Mr. Reilly in his hip spica cast,
   A. His arms should be at his sides.
   B. He should be moved to the side of the bed closest to his unaffected leg.
   C. Traction should be maintained on the leg that is affected.
   D. His affected leg should be on top.

E. His unaffected leg should be on top.
5. When drying Mr. Reilly's cast, the points to be observed in using an electric dryer are:
   A. Keep the dryer 18 inches from the patient.
   B. Keep the dryer 36 inches from the patient.
   C. Direct the dryer to one area until it is dry and then move to another.
   D. Keep covered with a blanket the part of the cast which is not being dried.
   E. Keep covered the exposed parts of the patient not encased in plaster.

BIBLIOGRAPHY AND SUGGESTED READING

Books

Arthritis and Rheumatism, Med. Clin. N. Am., vol. 45, Philadelphia, Saunders, 1961.
Colonna, P. C.: Regional Orthopedic Surgery, Philadelphia, Saunders, 1950.
Committee on Trauma, American College of Surgeons: The Management of Fractures and Soft Tissues, Philadelphia, Saunders, 1961.
Compere, E. L., Banks, S. W., and Compere, C. L.: Pictorial Handbook of Fracture Treatment, Chicago, Yr. Bk. Pub., 1958.
DePalma, A. F.: The Management of Fractures and Dislocations, Vols. I and II, An Atlas, Philadelphia, Saunders, 1959.
Knocke, F. J., and Knocke, L. S.: Orthopaedic Nursing, Philadelphia, Davis, 1954.
Larson-Gould: Calderwood's Orthopedic Nursing, ed. 4, St. Louis, Mosby, 1957.
Lowman, E. W.: Arthritis, Boston, Little, 1959.
McCombs, R. P.: Internal Medicine, pp. 650-689, Chicago, Yr. Bk. Pub., 1960.
Rusk, H. A.: Rehabilitation Medicine, St. Louis, Mosby, 1958.

Articles

Barckley, V., Bettinger, A., Guenther, L., and Ross, R.: Arthritis and a narrow perspective do not mix, Nurs. Outlook 6:638-639, Nov., 1958.
Bruck, H., and Lambert, C.: Common foot disabilities, Am. J. Nurs. 59:1580-1582, Nov., 1959.
Buck, L. L.: Nursing care during the long rest period (Legg-Calvé-Perthes Disease), Am. J. Nurs. 61:91-92, Oct., 1961.

Dorpat, T. L., and Holmes, T. H.: Psychophysiologic aspects of backache, Postgrad. Med. 25:713-719, June, 1959.
Gould, M. L.: Nursing care of the patient with a fractured hip, Am. J. Nurs. 58:1561-1563, 1958.
Greenwald, W. F., Jr.: Scoliosis, Am. J. Nurs. 59:817-819, June, 1959.
Hughes, J. M.: Nursing care after intramedullary nailing, Am. J. Nurs. 59:239-240, Feb., 1959.
Jordan, V., et al.: Halo body case and spinal fusion, Am. J. Nurs. 63:77-80, Aug., 1963.
Knocke, L.: Crutch walking, Am. J. Nurs. 61:70-73, Oct., 1961.
Lonergan, R.: Osteoporosis of the spine, Am. J. Nurs. 61:79-81, Jan., 1961.
Magee, K.: Myasthenia gravis, Am. J. Nurs. 60:336-339, Mar., 1960.
Mayo, R.: Intermedullary nailing of long bone fractures, Am. J. Nurs. 59:236-239, Feb. 1959.
Mendelson, J.: Sprains and strains, Am. J. Nurs. 61:45-50, June, 1961.
Moser, D.: Nursing care of the myasthenic patient, Am. J. Nurs. 60:340-343, Mar., 1960.
Nagler, J. H.: Immobilizing small joints, G.P. 24:115, Dec., 1961.
Ralston, E. L.: Legg-Calvé-Perthes Disease, Am. J. Nurs. 61:88-91, Oct., 1961.
Talbott, J. H., and Ricketts, A.: Gout and gouty arthritis, Am. J. Nurs. 59:1405-1408, Oct., 1959.

Patient-Teaching Aids and Information

Amputation

Brunnstrom, S., and Kerr, D.: Leg Amputee: Pre-Prosthetic Training (Rehabilitation Series No. 3) From The Kessler Institute for Rehabilitation, West Orange, N. J., 1951. This includes early postoperative care, bed exercises, bandaging the stump, use of crutches and fitting of the prostheses.
Bi-Monthly Courage, $1.00 a year, published by the Fraternity of the Wooden Leg, 600 South Oak St., Sapulpa, Okla.
Levy, S. W., and Barnes, G. H.: Stump Hygiene. An excellent 16-page booklet on problems of the amputee, Biomechanics Lab., Un. of Cal. School of Medicine, Div. of Dermatology, San Francisco, Cal., 1961.
Step into Action. An illustrated booklet to guide the leg amputee, U. S. P. H. S., Pub. No. 980, Supt. of Documents, Washington 25, D. C.

Arthritis

Good handbooks for patients issued by The Arthritis and Rheumatism Foundation are the following:

About Gout, 12 pages, 1959.

Arthritis by Bernard Suman. An excellent illustrated 10-page booklet describing various forms of arthritis, 1959.

Osteoarthritis, 20 pages, 1958.

Rheumatoid Arthritis, 12 pages, 1958.

Arthritis and Related Disorders. A 54-page manual for nurses, physical therapists, etc. Issued by The Arthritis and Rheumatism Foundation.

Arthritis and Rheumatism (clinoptikon). Two excellent colored visual guides to anatomy for patients from The Schering Corp., Bloomfield, New Jersey.

Self-Help Devices for the Arthritic. Lowman, E. W.: Rehabilitation Monograph VI, a 150-page well-illustrated book with very practical information by the Institute of Physical Medicine and Rehabilitation, New York University-Bellevue Medical Center, New York, 1959.

Strike Back at Arthritis. A 45-page illustrated booklet describing exercises, massage, splinting, shoes, canes, and self-help devices, U.S. P.H.S. Pub. No. 747, Supt. of Documents, Washington 25, D. C.

Back

Ishmael and Shorbe: Care of the Back, Philadelphia, Lippincott, 1959.

Kirk, C.: Oh! My Back. An illustrated booklet of helpful hints in prevention of back problems, The Economics Press, Montclair, New Jersey, 1960.

Disabled

American Red Cross, Swimming for the Handicapped, 60 pp., Alexandria, Va., American Red Cross.

Garrett, J. F. (Ed.). Psychological Aspects of Physical Disability. Rehab. Serv. Series No. 210, Department of Health, Education, and Welfare, Washington 25, D.C.

Manual for Training the Disabled Homemaker, Institute of Physical Medicine and Rehabilitation, N. Y. University-Bellevue Medical Center, New York, N. Y.

Feet

Endres, C. L.: Your feet come first, Today's Health pp. 32-33, Sept., 1956. Excellent illustrations.

Muscular Dystrophy

Around the Clock Aids for the Child with Muscular Dystrophy. A 32-page illustrated booklet. Muscular Dystrophy Association of America, 1957.

Voluntary Agencies

Feet

American Podiatry Association
3301 16th St., N.W.
Washington 10, D. C.

Orthopedics

Arthritis and Rheumatism Foundation
10 Columbus Circle
New York 19, N. Y.

Muscular Dystrophy Associations
of America, Inc.
1790 Broadway
New York 19, N. Y.

Myasthenia Gravis Foundation
155 East 23rd Street
New York 10, New York

The National Foundation
800 Second Ave.
New York 17, N. Y.

National Society for
Crippled Children and Adults
2023-55 West Ogden Avenue
Chicago 12, Ill.

ORIENTATION

SCOPE OF NURSING RESPONSIBILITIES

The chapters to follow are concerned with communicable infectious diseases, with particular reference to the role of the nurse in their prevention and eradication. Included are detailed descriptions of nursing situations that are inherent in all communicable diseases and discussions of nursing problems that are peculiar to each category and type of infection. The selection of topics for inclusion in this text and the manner in which they have been presented have been based on the following concepts:

The nurse should be familiar with the typical features and the characteristic course of every common infectious disease entity. She should be informed accurately concerning its pathogenesis and essential pathology, as well as the periods of incubation, prodromata and infectivity that are characteristic, and the type of convalescence that is to be anticipated.

The nurse should be cognizant of the manner in which the common infections are acquired and transmitted. She should know the identity of the micro-organism responsible for each type of infection and understand the nature of this infective agent, understanding its mode of contact with and manner of entry into the human body, its route of excretion and its susceptibility to such factors as sunlight, heat, drying, antiseptic agents and chemotherapeutic drugs—information that is highly pertinent from several standpoints, including the protection of her other patients and her own safety. Finally, she should be aware of any prophylactic measure that may be applicable to each of the common infections and the duration of the immunity so conferred.

The nurse who is in possession of these facts is in the best position to comprehend and to implement the therapeutic program that is prescribed and to discharge with confidence many other important responsibilities in connection with these patients. One such responsibility is that of educating the families of her young patients in methods of controlling communicable diseases, imparting the basic principles of sanitation and emphasizing the value of prophylactic immunization.

Presented in Unit XVIII are clinical descriptions, epidemiologic data, current concepts regarding specific therapy and prophylaxis, descriptions of patient problems and discussions of nursing solutions relating to more than 60 important communicable disease entities. This material is apportioned among 6 chapters, based on the nature of the infective agent responsible for each of these disorders. Chapter 43 describes patients with specific bacterial infections; Chapter 44, those with viral infections; Chapter 45, rickettsial diseases; Chapter 46, protozoan infections; Chapter 47, the patient with a systemic mycosis; and Chapter 48, patients with parasitic infestations. However, discussions of individual diseases will be preceded by a review of the principles and the practice of specific immune prophylaxis, and a description of nursing precautions that are indicated in caring for patients with communicable infections in general.

IMMUNE PROPHYLAXIS

Principles of Active and Passive Immunity

Specific immunity with respect to a particular organism implies that an individual either has been generating the appropriate antibody in his own body or has received this, ready-made, from another source. A child is born temporarily immune to certain infections by virtue of the fact that the mother's antibodies are able to diffuse through the placenta into the fetus. An individual can be rendered temporarily immune by the injection of blood or serum from an immune animal or person, but such "passive immunity" is short-lived and usually effective but a few weeks. It offers a useful method of protecting, for a limited period, persons known to be susceptible to a particular infection, for example, scarlet fever, when they have been exposed to the disease.

For more permanent protection, a person must continuously manufacture his own antibodies, and before his reticuloendothelial cells can be stimulated to undertake this task, they require some immediate experience with the organisms in question—not necessarily the whole live organism, but at any rate some of its characteristic constituent proteins. Having had such contact, they proceed to manufacture the proper antibodies to combat it and continue to do so for some time after the stimulus has departed, often for years or for the duration of that individual's life.

One way of obtaining the necessary contact, of course, is to become infected with the living organism. But, it is precisely to avoid the necessity for such contact, in the case of virulent germs, that preventive immune therapy is used.

Exposure to a living pathogenic organism fortunately is not an obligatory step in the acquisition of a specific, protective immunity: the same immune response can be produced by exposing the reticuloendothelial system to organisms which have been killed by heating (such as typhoid). This mechanism presumably explains the phenomenon of "natural immunity," i.e., resistance to a particular infection on the part of an individual who has never exhibited signs of that infection in the past. Moreover, it is the basis of one of the most important prophylactic measures ever devised for the control of an infectious disease, namely, the induction of a relatively benign infection, "cowpox," in order to stimulate the production of antibodies against a very dangerous infection, "smallpox." This type of vaccination is described in detail below. Other examples of vaccinations include the injection of heat-killed *H. pertussis* to protect against whooping cough; mixtures of killed *E. typhosa* and *S. paratyphi* A and B to prevent typhoid and paratyphoid fevers; chemically inactivated viruses of yellow fever, rabies and poliomyelitis for the prevention of those infections; and the killed *Rickettsia prowazekii* for protection against typhus fever.

These particular immunization technics involve the administration of the infective agent in one form or another, and the type of immunity obtained relates to the organism itself. The nature of the antibodies so produced will be such as to interfere with their growth and spread in the body. But there are some organisms—for example, the diphtheria bacillus—whose toxins are much more dangerous than their invasive qualities. The latter, in fact, may play a very small role as the cause of symptoms or of death in the infected individual. In order to induce the body to produce antibodies against toxins, these must be injected—but before administration they either are altered chemically or mixed with antitoxin prepared from the serum of immunized animals, which lessens, or altogether prevents, their toxic effect when injected. Thus, in the case of tetanus immunization, one may use toxin from the tetanus bacillus after chemically treating it with formaldehyde ("toxoid"). Diphtheria immunization is performed by injecting toxin formed by diphtheria bacilli which was mixed with serum from horses immunized against this organism—a procedure which neutralizes its toxic effect but does not prevent the person injected from manufacturing his own neutralizing antibodies.

By such means, prolonged immunity against organisms and their toxins can be induced artificially, and the body of the immunized individual can be stimulated to protect itself against particular types of infections without having to experience the infection.

Standard Immunization Procedures

Diphtheria-Tetanus-Pertussis Prophylaxis (DTP). Simultaneous immunization against diphtheria, tetanus and pertussis, or "DTP," has become a routine procedure in pediatric practice. This measure involves multiple injections of a mixture containing diphtheria toxin and antitoxin, tetanus toxoid and heat-killed *Hemophilus pertussis,* together with alum which serves to delay the absorption of these antigens. Three or four 0.5-ml. doses are given at monthly intervals, followed by a "booster" injection at a later date. If the first injection is received at the age of 3 months, 4 monthly injections plus 1 booster injection 1 year after the first dose comprise the series. If the first dose is given at 6 months of age, or later, 3 monthly doses are administered in succession, with the first recall dose scheduled several years later.

Children under 3 years of age should receive these injections deep in the gluteal muscles, laterally, on the left and the right sides alternately, starting on the left. Children over 3 years may be injected in the deltoid muscles, the right and the left being selected alternately, the left first. For deltoid injections the needle should be directed distally (toward the hand); after its withdrawal the injection site should be covered with sterile gauze and stroked manually 3 or 4 times in a distal direction. Irrespective of the injection site, the following precautions are applicable:

1. Individual syringes and needles should be employed for each recipient of vaccine, both portions of the equipment being sterilized by autoclaving prior to use; or sterile disposable needles and syringes should be used.

2. Sterile precautions should be observed meticulously in the transfer of vaccine from vial to syringes and in the protection of the injection site after its preparation.

3. The course of the needle should be guided straight, and its direction not changed after its insertion.

4. Approximately 0.1 ml. of air should be injected following the 0.5 ml. of vaccine in order to clear the needle before it is withdrawn.

COMPLICATIONS OF DTP. *Febrile reactions* of mild or moderate severity may follow these injections in a significant percentage of cases. To minimize their severity, mothers of immunized infants should be advised to keep their children as inactive as possible during the 24-hour period after injection, and, if they appear to be restless or feverish, to give them aspirin, increase their fluids, reduce their solid foods, decrease their coverings and protect them from the sun.

Alum cysts are avoided by adhering to the technic outlined above for injecting the vaccine, the objective of which is to avoid tracking the alum-containing material along the course of the puncture wound.

Postinoculation encephalopathy, marked by fever, convulsions and irreversible nervous system changes, occurs rarely after DTP and after other vaccination procedures as well. This phenomenon has been ascribed to the familial occurrence of neurologic disorders, and, by implication, an inherited "instability" of the nervous system. However, a more likely basis for its occurrence is the transmission of virus encephalitis by a contaminated needle or syringe.

Prevention depends on adequate sterilization of injection equipment, i.e., by autoclaving at 120° C. (250° F.) for 20 minutes (the use of sterile disposable equipment is better), and on proper observance of precautions to prevent transmission of infection among vaccine recipients.

NURSING RESPONSIBILITIES IN DTP PROGRAMS. Mass immunization of DTP to preschool children often are located at well-baby clinics, primary schools or mobile units, holding sessions at regular intervals of 1, 2 or 4 weeks. Infants may be referred to the clinic through the public health nurse or some other agency with responsibilities in the area of child welfare.

Ideally, very soon after every birth in the community, a public health nurse should contact the mother, informing her when and where to bring her infant (at age 3 to 4 months) for immunization. Each appointment should be confirmed routinely by a visiting nurse in order to remind the mother of the date on which the first injection is scheduled.

A team of 4 persons, including a registered physician and at least one nurse, can handle 50 children an hour with perfect efficiency and safety. Nursing assistants may keep the records, teach the mothers how to expose the injection sites and hold their infants, give out cards scheduling appointments for second and third injections, etc., and instruct them in procedures to follow in event of febrile reactions. A registered nurse should be responsible for the sterilization and the packaging of syringes and needles, for custody of the antigen and for the activities of the nursing assistants.

The technic of injection is as follows: the physician washes his hands under running water, drying them on clean, individually dispensed towels or tissues, thereafter avoiding all contact with individuals other than the respective recipient until the injection is completed. The infant is held prone on the mother's lap with only the injection site exposed. Her left hand clasps the infant's knees, her right hand pressing downward above the level of the hips to prevent squirming during inoculation. A 0.5-ml. solution of alum-containing DTP (plus 0.1 ml. of air) is loaded into a 1.0- or 2.0-ml. syringe and injected through a 1-in. No. 23 (approx.) gauge needle deep in the lateral aspect of the gluteal region, the injection terminating with the introduction of the air bubble. After a few seconds the needle is quickly withdrawn, and the site, covered with sterile gauze, is massaged gently.

Smallpox Vaccination. *Vaccinia* is the mild, noncontagious, pustular reaction induced by vaccination with lymph from a vesicle of cowpox which protects the individual against smallpox.

TECHNIC OF VACCINATION AND COURSE OF VACCINIA. The region to be vaccinated is scrubbed thoroughly with soap and water, the soap is rinsed off with sterile water, and the area is dried with sterile gauze. The use of antiseptics is likely to prevent a "take." The superficial layers of epidermis are then scratched with a needle or cut with a knife just deeply enough to expose the deeper epithelial cells—but not enough to draw blood. The vaccine is then rubbed in with the instrument, is allowed to dry and the spot covered for a few hours with dry sterilized gauze. Shields should not be used; bunion plasters used for this purpose have transmitted tetanus.

About the 4th day after the vaccination a papule appears, surrounded by a red zone. By the 5th or 6th day this has become an umbilicated vesicle, which on the 10th day has developed into a pustule surrounded by an areola of swollen red skin. Often the arm and the glands in the axilla are sore. On the 11th or the 12th day the areola disappears. On the 14th day, the pustule has dried to a brown scab, which, during the following week, gradually separates and falls off, leaving a superficial pitted scar. (See Plate 9.)

Accelerated reactions are those in which the papule appears on the 4th day, but the pustule reaches its height between the 4th and the 9th days. This indicates that a little immunity, conveyed by a previous vaccina-tion, still persists. An immediate reaction is the macule or papule which appears about 12 hours after vaccination, persists for 48 to 72 hours, then disappears. This signifies a strong immunity.

COMPLICATIONS. *Postvaccinal encephalitis* is an infrequent but dangerous complication of vaccinia. Its development is exceptionally rare during the summer months. It is also rare among children under the age of 2 years and following a revaccination. Therefore, it is recommended that vaccination be performed during the first year of life, and that the child be revaccinated at school age, both inoculations being accomplished during the summer season.

Generalized vaccinia, fortunately rare, follows widespread distribution of the vaccinia virus over the skin, with resultant development of multiple pustular lesions and a profound systemic reaction. It is prone to occur in patients with chronic itching skin disorders, particularly eczema; spread of the virus is accomplished in the process of scratching. In such patients, vaccination should be deferred until any skin disease present has been controlled, and during this period they should be protected from contact with recently vaccinated persons.

Secondary infections may cause ulceration, sloughing, a boil or erysipelas at the vaccinated point.

An attack of vaccinia will protect the patient from smallpox for 14 or 15 years, at the end of which time he should be revaccinated. Vaccinated persons occasionally do contract smallpox, but the attack as a rule is mild (varioloid).

IMMUNE THERAPY

Specific Antisera. A nonimmune patient who has acquired an infection may be aided in his struggle against it, for immune substances prefabricated in other bodies can be furnished to him during the period (usually lasting several days) required for his own antibody production to get under way. Thus, patients with tetanus or diphtheria-bacillus infections are injected with serum from animals immunized against tetanus or diphtheria toxin; patients with pneumococcus pneumonia may be given serum from rabbits or horses immunized against that particular type of pneumococcus, etc. Antitoxins also are available against toxins of the hemolytic streptococcus, *Staphylococcus aureus,* the bacillus of Shiga dysentery, certain anaerobic bacilli causing gas gangrene and one type of food poisoning (botulism) and also snake venoms. These antibodies ordinarily are obtained from serums of animals artificially immunized against the organisms themselves or their toxins.

Gamma Globulin (γ globulin). This is the fraction of plasma that contains most or all, of the antibodies found in the circulating blood. When prepared from vast pools of human plasma obtained from representative groups of adult population, as is the case with Red Cross gamma globulin, the material might be expected to contain, in high concentration, antibodies against most of the infections that are endemic in the population at large, those to which children are principally heir and to which adults generally are immune.

The validity of this assumption has been proved in the case of two viral infections, measles and epidemic hepatitis. Given sufficiently early in the incubation period of measles, i.e., within one week following exposure, and in adequate dosage (0.1 ml. per pound of body weight), gamma globulin prevents this infection altogether. In a lesser amount (0.02 ml. per pound of body weight) it modifies this infection in such a manner that the clinical course is relatively mild, and the incidence of important complications is reduced practically to nil. (Modification, rather than abolition of measles, is the preferable objective unless the exposed individual is in ill health or for some other reason would be seriously jeopardized by virtue of contracting measles, since permanent immunity to the infection is conferred by modified measles, but not, of course, if the disease is prevented completely.)

Gamma globulin is given by intramuscular injection. No complications are anticipated following its administration in the vast majority of cases, since the only ingredient of the material is homologous protein, i.e., globulins of human origin. Exceedingly rare instances of homologous serum jaundice have been reported in recipients of gamma globulin, but the incidence of that complication is so low as to render it of negligible importance as a contraindication to immunization.

COMMUNICABLE DISEASE NURSING

The nurse who is caring for a patient with any of the communicable diseases should be able to answer all of the following questions:

1. What is the nature of the infecting organism?

2. Where is this organism harbored in the host: i.e., the carrier or patient?

3. How is the pathogen disseminated by the host?

4. What is the principal portal of entry for this organism?

5. How does the infective agent survive outside the host; i.e., under what circumstances and how long is it likely to survive?

6. How is immunity to this agent acquired or conferred, and how long is it effective?

7. What communicable disease precautions are indicated in caring for a patient with this infection?

Details regarding the identity and the properties of the causative organism and the epidemiology of each infection are contained in Chapters 43 to 48. (See also Table 23 (pp. 1061-1063). The following paragraphs are concerned with communicable disease precautions that are implicit in the nursing care of infected patients in general.

The basic purpose of communicable disease nursing is to halt all communication between infectious sources and their targets. Varying degrees of isolation are imposed on the infectious patient, depending on the character of the infective organism and the manner of its spread. Direct contact with the patient is limited exclusively to those persons who are responsible for his immediate care, and steps are taken to prevent such a person or any object that has become contaminated through direct contact with the patient from becoming a vehicle for the transmission of the infection.

These objectives can be achieved only through strict adherence to a rigid routine on the part of all who are personally engaged, directly or indirectly, in the care of the patient.

The technical details of isolation nursing will vary from institution to institution, and

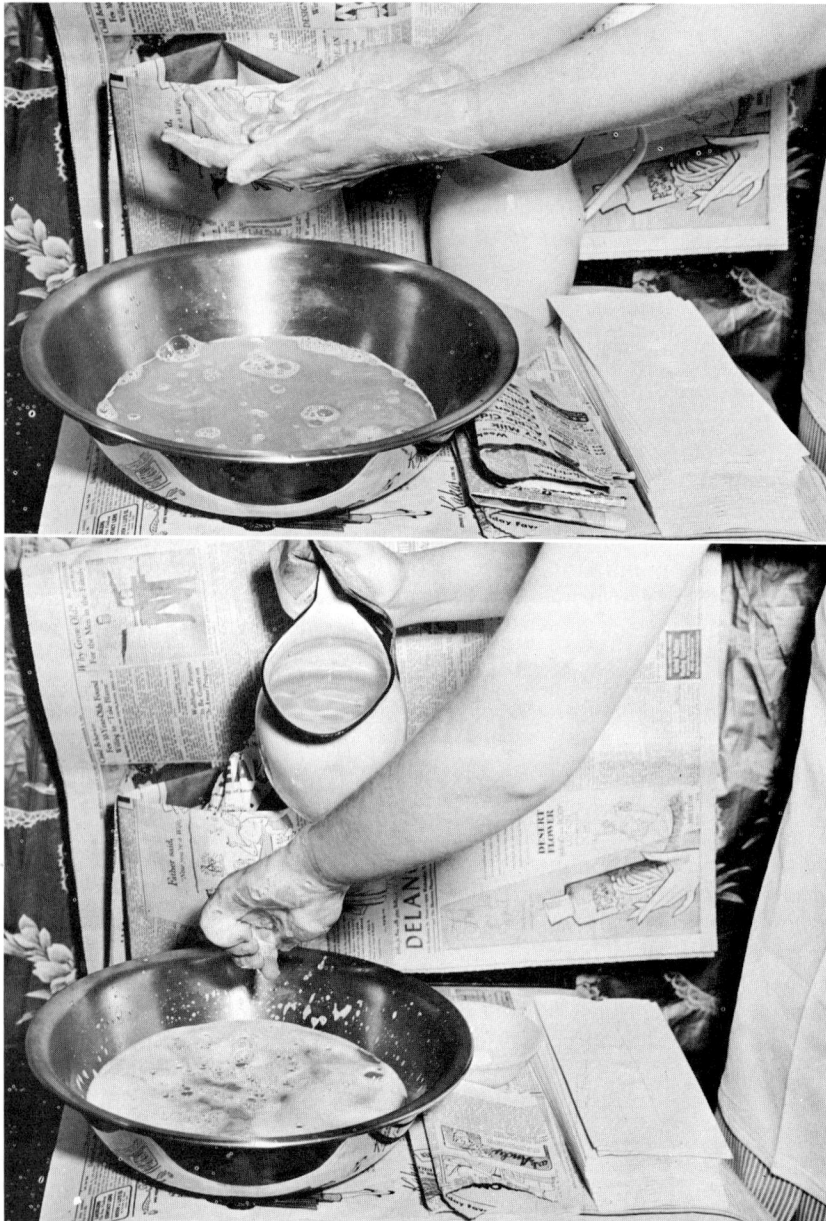

Fig. 418. Communicable disease nursing in the home. One of the most important single steps to avoid spreading and contracting an infection is prompt adequate cleansing of contaminated hands. This can be accomplished satisfactorily without elaborate equipment, provided that a few necessary items have been made ready in advance, are properly located and are used correctly, according to a strict, predetermined, unvarying routine.

will differ from case to case, depending on the nature of the infection. However, the following considerations are generally applicable.

Rooms occupied by infectious patients, including their floors, walls and contents, are considered to be contaminated, as are the interiors of all sinks and hoppers located in that unit of the hospital. On the other hand, corridors, kitchens and service rooms are considered clean and must be kept inviolate.

Gowns should be worn by all persons who are required to make direct contact with the patient who is on complete isolation. In such cases the discard routine should be followed, i.e., each direct contact with the patient involves the donning of a clean gown which then is discarded.

The wearing of a mask is a requirement in some institutions but not in others, there being no general unanimity in opinion concerning the effectiveness of masks. If masks are to be worn, they should be applied in such a manner as to cover the mouth and the nose completely. If contact is to be prolonged, the mask is to be discarded and replaced frequently. A wet mask should not be worn. As soon as a mask is removed it should be discarded into a receptacle that is protected and clearly labeled.

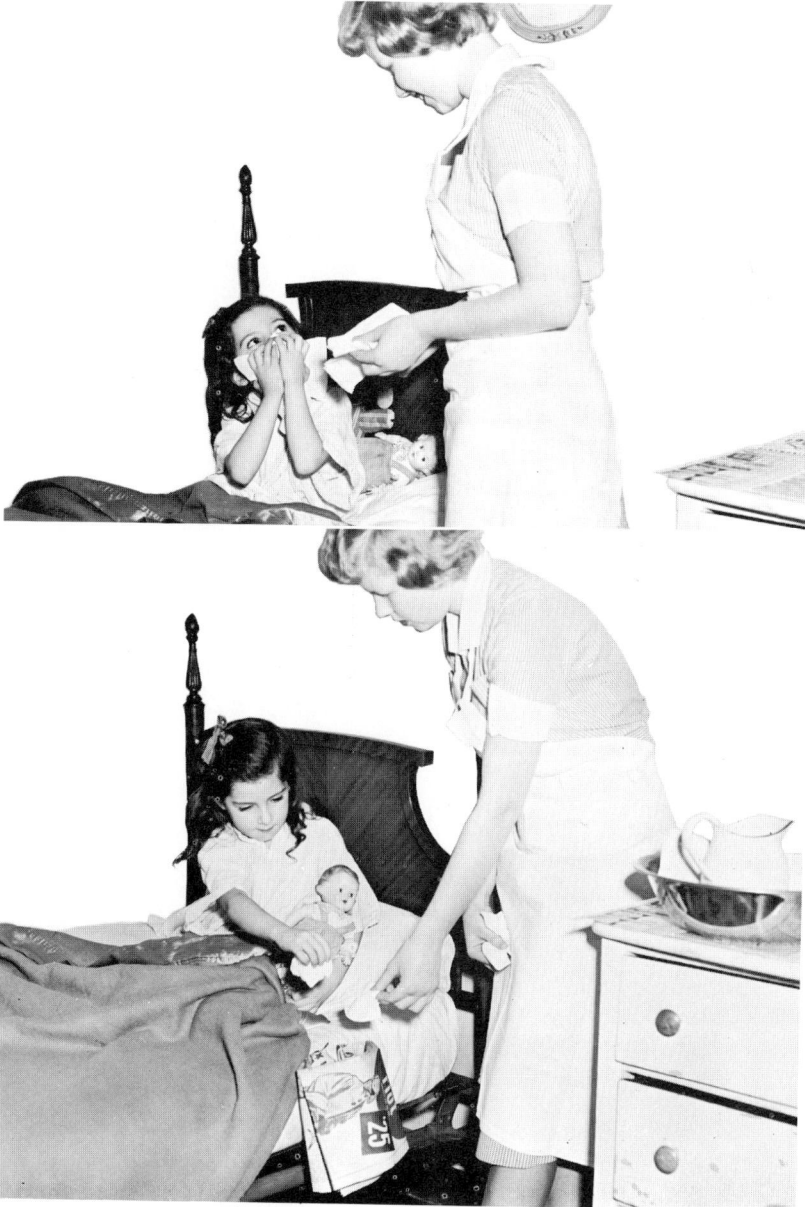

FIG. 419. Communicable disease nursing in the home. Technic of trapping and disposing of nasal secretions and sputum.

The hands should be washed thoroughly after each contact with the patient or with an object that is potentially contaminated (Fig. 418). Ideal facilities for these ablu- tions include a sink with foot or knee con- trols, an adequate supply of hot and cold water, soap solution, a bar of soap or a detergent dispenser, and paper towels. Hand

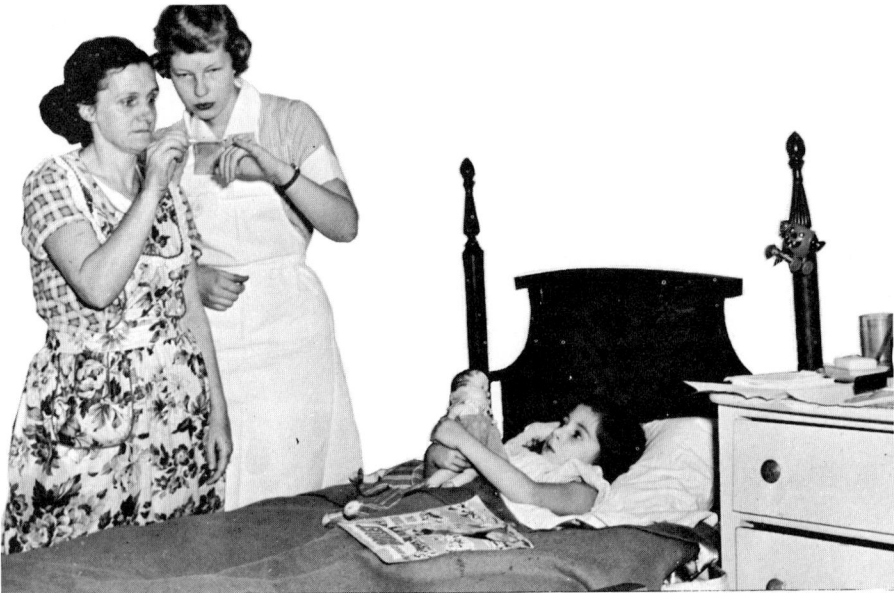

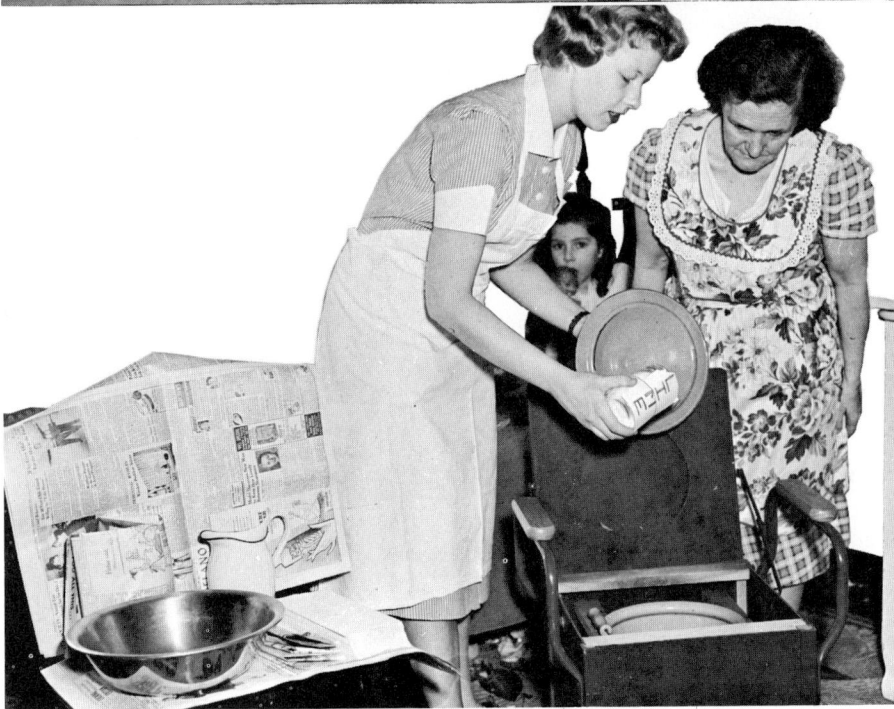

FIG. 420. Communicable disease nursing in the home. The mother learns how to read a thermometer and to set up a commode and decontaminate a stool.

spigots serve adequately and pose no risk from the standpoint of infectious transmission provided that they are washed thoroughly when the hands are first lathered. Detergent dispensers or more liquid soap and soap bars are equally satisfactory. For the protection of her skin, the nurse should take pains to remove all traces of soap or detergent before her hands are allowed to dry.

Decontamination of objects that have been in direct contact with the patient is referred to as *concurrent disinfection*. Items to consider from the standpoint of requiring con-

current disinfection, depending on the nature of the case, include oral and nasal discharges, sputum and drinking cups, urine, vomitus, exudates, contaminated dressings, solid and liquid food wastes, dishes, utensils, trays, water carafes, towels, beddings and other linens, mattresses and pillows, hypodermic needles, syringes, therapeutic instruments and diagnostic equipment, including clinical thermometers.

For the safe disposal of oral and nasal discharges the patient should be supplied with paper tissues and a receptacle in the

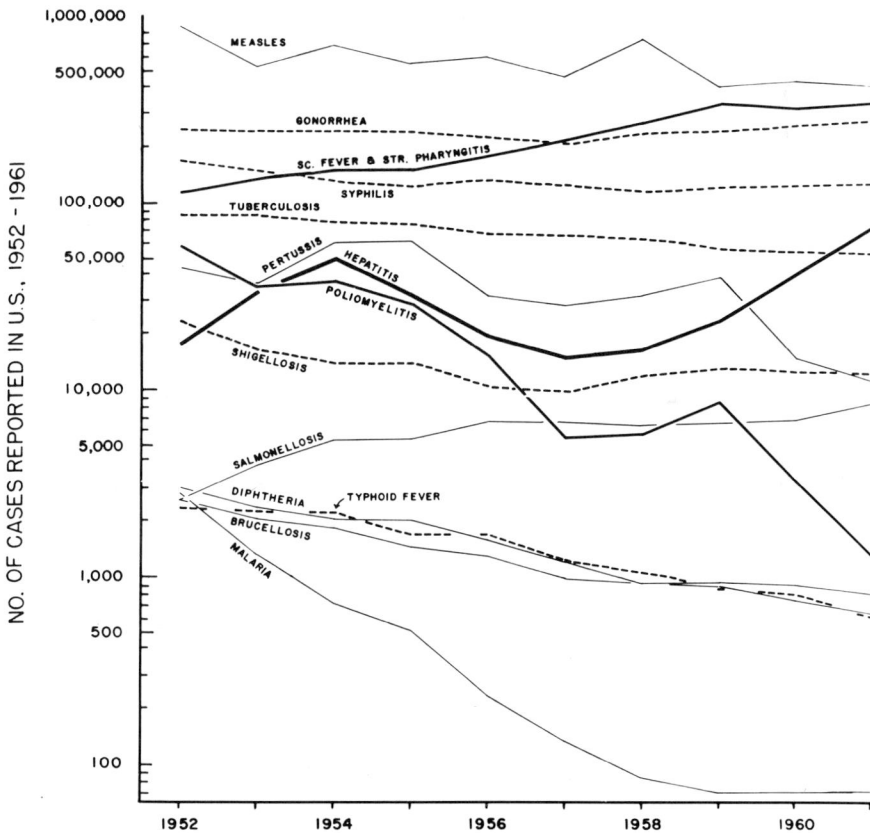

Fig. 421. Annual incidence in the United States of the 14 most prevalent notifiable diseases, 1952-1961. (This chart is based on data from the Morbidity and Mortality Weekly Report of the U. S. Department of Health, Education and Welfare, Vol. 10, No. 53, Annual Supplement, Oct. 31, 1962). Figures for gonorrhea and syphilis are from the Venereal Disease Program, Public Health Service, and refer to civilian cases only. Tuberculosis data are from the Tuberculosis Program, Public Health Service, and include only newly reported active cases. The figures for hepatitis include both the serum [Virus SH] and the epidemic, or infectious [Virus IH] types.)

form of a paper bag of ample capacity, which should be placed in a convenient location near the patient (Fig. 419). Disposable sputum cups should be provided by the bedside and the patient instructed in their proper use. All disposable receptacles, including used tissues, sputum cups and contaminated dressings, together with their paper containers, as well as disposable drinking cups, dishes and utensils, should be collected at frequent intervals and placed in special containers for burning. Liquid food waste may be combined in a special jar and disposed of in a hopper.

In most institutions the sanitary facilities permit disposal of all excreta by the public sewage system that serves the hospital; however, should such facilities not be available, then all stools, urine, vomitus and liquid food waste should be pooled in a covered can containing a disinfectant solution, such as 5 per cent chlorinated lime or 5 per cent creosol, and allowed to stand for 1 hour before they are emptied into the sewage system (Fig. 420). Bedpans, of course, must be sterilized after each use.

Contaminated bed linen from infectious patients should be collected and enclosed securely in special bags. Packaged in this manner, the laundry chute may be used for the transportation of these goods. All contaminated clothing and linens should be sterilized by autoclaving before they are laundered with noninfectious goods.

Instruments and items of equipment used on the patient may be processed safely by thorough scrubbing with soap and water, followed by rinsing and drying. Any article contaminated with a spore organism should be autoclaved at 20-pound steam pressure for 30 minutes or longer. Metallic articles, if thermostable, may be sterilized in a 160° C. (330° F.) oven. Less stable material may be sterilized at 150° C. (300° F.) for 150 minutes, 140° C. (285° F.) for 180 minutes or 121° C. (250° F.) for 16 to 18 hours. Thermometers are rendered safe by soap and water lavage, followed by a prolonged soak in 70 per cent ethyl alcohol, isopropyl alcohol or Zephiran solution.

As soon as the patient is discharged from the hospital, the room in which he was quartered should be subjected to *terminal disinfection*. In most instances this involves merely the thorough scrubbing of the floors, open ventilation and exposure to sunlight, if possible, for 12 to 24 hours. Other aspects of communicable disease control in the hospital will be discussed in the chapters to follow. It is important to emphasize that optimum isolation technic and nursing care in a communicable disease involve much more than merely skill and knowledge; the essential need is a conscientious attitude and a sense of responsibility on the part of the nurse, without which the entire routine of nursing protection becomes a sham and a pretense.

EPIDEMIOLOGY OF THE PREVAILING COMMUNICABLE INFECTIONS

Pertinent epidemiologic data, as well as specific therapy and effective prophylaxis, in relation to 32 important communicable diseases are summarized below, in Table 23.

Figure 421 depicts the incidence in the United States of the 14 communicable infections that were most prevalent during the decade 1952-1961. Apparent in Figure 421, and especially important to note, are:

1. The high incidence of measles, which was consistently greater than that of all other communicable infections before the recent development of measles vaccine (p. 1092)

2. The high and ever-increasing incidence of hemolytic streptococcal infections, despite the possibility of effective control with penicillin (p. 192)

3. The continued high rates of incidence of gonorrhea (p. 1080), syphilis (p. 1118) and tuberculosis (p. 446), which are exceeded only by those of measles and streptococcal infections, despite the availability, the safety, the economy and the certain effectiveness of prophylactic measures

4. The gratifying decline in the incidence of poliomyelitis (p. 1099), diphtheria (p. 1068), pertussis (p. 1071) and typhoid fever (p. 1077) during recent years, attributable in large measure to specific immune prophylaxis

5. The decreasing incidence of brucellosis (p. 1079), a reflection of increasingly effective veterinary controls

The relatively high incidence of malaria in 1952, coincident with our military engagement in Korea, followed by the rapid decline

TABLE 23. Epidemiology, Therapy and Control of Communicable Infections

Disease	Infective Organism	Infectious Sources	Entry Site	Method of Spread	Incubation Period	Specific Treatment	Prophylaxis
Amebiasis	Endamoeba histolytica	Contaminated water and food	Gastrointestinal tract	Patients and carriers; fecal-oral route	Variable	Emetine; chloroquine; diiodohydroxyquin; chlortetracycline	Detection of carriers and their removal from food handling; plumbing safeguards
Bacillary Dysentery	Shigella group	Contaminated water and food	Gastrointestinal tract	Patients and carriers; fecal-oral route	24–48 hours	Sulfadiazine; chloramphenicol; streptomycin	Decontamination of water supplies; detection and control of carriers; inspection of food handlers
Brucellosis	Brucella melitensis & related organisms	Milk or meat from infected cattle, goats & pigs	Gastrointestinal tract	Oral ingestion of infective material	6–14 days	Streptomycin and chlortetracycline; sulfadiazine	Milk pasteurization; safe disposal of infected human excreta; control of infection in animals.
Chancroid	Ducrey bacillus	Human cases and carriers	Genitalia	Sexual intercourse	2–5 days	Sulfadiazine; streptomycin; chloramphenicol; tetracycline	Effective case finding and treatment of infection
Chickenpox (Varicella)	Virus	Human cases	Probably nasopharynx	Probably respiratory droplets	14–16 days	None	Case isolation
Diphtheria	Corynebacterium diphtheriae	Human cases and carriers; food; fomites	Nasopharynx	Nasal & oral secretions; respiratory droplets	2–5 days	Diphtheria antitoxin; penicillin	Active immunization with diphtheria toxoid or toxin-antitoxin mixture; case quarantine; disinfection of carriers
Encephalitis, epidemic (Eastern & Western Equine)	Viruses	Chicken & wild-bird mites; horses; hibernating garter snakes	Skin	Mosquitoes	Variable	None	Formolized virus vaccines
German Measles (Rubella)	Virus	Human cases (early)	Probably nasopharynx	Probably respiratory droplets	10–22 (aver. 18) days	None	Case isolation (?)
Gonorrhea	Neisseria gonorrhoeae	Urethral & vaginal secretions	Urethral or vaginal mucosa	Sexual intercourse	3–8 days	Penicillin; sulfonamide drugs	Chemotherapy of carriers and potential contacts; case finding and treatment of patients
Granuloma Inguinale	Donovan body (bacillus)	Infectious exudate	External genitalia; cervix	Sexual intercourse	3–40 days	Chloramphenicol; tetracyclines; streptomycin	Chemotherapy of carriers and potential contacts; case finding and treatment of patients
Hepatitis, epidemic	Virus (I.H.)	Contaminated food or water; parenteral inoculum	Gastrointestinal tract; skin	Fecal-oral route; parenteral injection	2–6 weeks	None	Enteric precautions applied to infected cases; passive immunization with gamma globulin
Hepatitis, serum	Virus (S.H.)	Infected blood donor; contaminated injection equipment	Skin	Parenteral injection	6 weeks to 6 months	None	Screening of blood donors; avoidance of unnecessary use of blood and blood derivatives; passive immunization of blood recipients with course of gamma globulin injections

TABLE 23. Epidemiology, Therapy and Control of Communicable Infections (Continued)

Disease	Infective Organism	Infectious Sources	Entry Site	Method of Spread	Incubation Period	Specific Treatment	Prophylaxis
Infectious Mononucleosis	Virus	Human cases and carriers	Mouth	Osculation	30–50 days	None	—
Influenza	Virus (types A and B)	Human cases; (?) animal reservoir	Respiratory tract	Respiratory	18–36 hours	None	Specific virus vaccine
Lymphogranuloma Venereum	Virus	Human cases	External genitalia; urethral or vaginal mucosa	Sexual intercourse	2–30 days	Sulfadiazine; chlortetracycline	Case finding and treatment of infection
Malaria	Plasmodium malariae	Human cases	Skin	Mosquitoes (Anopheles)	2 weeks	Chloroquine; primaquine; paludrine	Coordinated measures for wide-scale mosquito control; prompt detection and effective treatment of cases
Measles	Virus	Human cases	Respiratory mucosa	Nasopharyngeal secretions	11–14 days	None	Partial or complete passive immunization with gamma globulin
Meningococcal Meningitis	Neisseria meningitidis	Human cases and carriers	Nasopharynx; tonsils	Respiratory droplets	Variable	Penicillin plus sulfadiazine	Group chemotherapy with sulfadiazine
Mumps	Virus	Human cases (early)	Upper respiratory tract	Respiratory droplets	8–30 (aver. 18) days	None	Convalescent serum during first week following exposure. (Formolized vaccine available.)
Paratyphoid Fever	Salmonella paratyphi A & B; S. typhimurium; S. choleraesuis & related organisms	Contaminated food and water, rectal tubes and barium enemas	Gastrointestinal tract	Infected urine & feces	7–24 days	Chloramphenicol	Control of public water sources, food vendors and food handlers; treatment of carriers; individual vaccination with S. paratyphi A and B vaccine
Pneumococcal Pneumonia	Pneumococcus	Human carriers; patient's own pharynx	Respiratory mucosa	Respiratory droplets	Variable	Penicillin	Control of upper respiratory infections; avoidance of alcoholic intoxication; communicable disease precautions applied to cases
Poliomyelitis	Polioviruses (Types I, II & III)	Human cases and carriers	Gastrointestinal tract	Infected feces & pharyngeal secretions	4–7 days	None	Wide-scale application of parenteral (Salk) and oral poliovirus vaccines; case isolation
Rocky Mountain Spotted Fever	Rickettsia rickettsii	Infected wild rodents, dogs, wood ticks & dog ticks	Skin	Tick bites	3–12 days	Chloramphenicol; tetracyclines	Avoidance of tick-infested areas, or wearing of protective clothing in such areas; frequent search for, and prompt removal of, ticks from body; specific vaccination of exposed persons

TABLE 23. Epidemiology, Therapy and Control of Communicable Infections (Continued)

Disease	Infective Organism	Infectious Sources	Entry Site	Method of Spread	Incubation Period	Specific Treatment	Prophylaxis
Scarlet Fever	Streptococcus hemolyticus	Human cases; infected food	Pharynx	Nasal & oral secretions	3–5 days	Penicillin	Case isolation; prophylactic chemotherapy with penicillin
Syphilis	Treponema pallidum	Infected exudate or blood	External genitalia; cervix, mucosal surfaces; placenta	Sexual intercourse; nonvenereal contact; blood transfusion; transplacental inoculation	10–90 days	Penicillin	Case finding by means of routine serologic testing and other methods, and adequate treatment of infected individuals
Tetanus	Clostridium tetani	Contaminated soil	Penetrating & crush wounds	Horse & cattle feces	5 days to 5 weeks (aver. 10 days)	Tetanus antitoxin; penicillin	Wound debridement; toxoid booster injections for patients previously immunized and tetanus antitoxin plus penicillin for nonimmune
Trichinosis	Trichinella spiralis	Infected pigs	Gastrointestinal tract	Ingestion of infected pork, undercooked	3–7 days	None	Regulation of hog breeders; adequate meat inspection; thorough cooking of pork
Tuberculosis	Mycobacterium tuberculosis	Sputum from human cases; milk from infected cows	Respiratory or gastrointestinal mucosa	Sputum; respiratory droplets; infected milk	Variable	Streptomycin; paraaminosalicylic acid; isoniazid	Early discovery and adequate treatment of active cases; milk pasteurization
Tularemia	Pasteurella tularensis	Wild rodents	Skin; gastrointestinal tract	Insect parasites of infected rodents; ingestion of undercooked infected meat	3–5 days	Streptomycin	Avoidance of contact with potentially infected rodents; adequate cooking of wild rabbit dishes; vaccination of hunters, butchers and laboratory workers risking heavy exposure
Typhoid Fever	Salmonella tyhpi	Contaminated food and water	Gastrointestinal tract	Infected urine and feces	5–14 days	Chloramphenicol	Decontamination of water sources; milk pasteurization; individual vaccination; control of carriers
Typhus, endemic	Rickettsia mooseri	Infected rodents	Skin	Flea bites	5–21 days	Chloramphenicol; chlortetracycline	Delousing procedures; specific vaccination; case quarantine
Whooping Cough (Pertussis)	Hemophilus pertussis	Human cases	Respiratory tract	Infected bronchial secretions	12–20 days	None	Active immunization with H. pertussis (Sauer's) vaccine; passive immunization with hyperimmune pertussis antiserum or immune gamma globulin; case isolation

[1063]

and virtual disappearance (in the U. S.) of this infection with cessation of these operations in 1953

7. The rising incidence of salmonellosis (p. 1064), a type of enteric infection which decidedly is preventable by routine prophylactic measures (pp. 194 and 1078); and

8. A substantial and challenging increase since 1957 of hepatitis (pp. 653 and 654), prophylaxis for which, owing to our limited knowledge, is effective only to a limited extent.

Major accomplishments in infectious disease control during this period and the major challenges in preventive medicine and nursing that still remain are readily identified on inspection of this chart, and will be discussed in detail in the chapters that follow.

43

Patients With Specific Bacterial Infections

TYPES OF BACTERIA

Bacteria include the round *cocci* (berries), and the rodlike *bacilli*. Some cocci exist in pairs, for example, those causing pneumococcal pneumonia, meningococcal meningitis and gonorrhea, and are called *diplococci*. Some, the "staphylococci," grow in clusters and are responsible for skin abscesses, certain abscesses of bone and a variety of other infections. Others, found in chains resembling strings of beads, are the "streptococci," which cause many infections, including scarlet fever, erysipelas and puerperal sepsis. Bacilli are responsible for diphtheria, typhoid fever and gas gangrene, among other diseases. Representative types of cocci and bacilli are illustrated in Figures 422 and 423.

SCARLET FEVER

Scarlet fever is an acute infectious disease caused by *Streptococcus hemolyticus*. It is characterized by a vivid, scarlet skin rash, sore throat, characteristic tongue changes and cervical adenitis. Its incidence attains epidemic proportions during the school months, particularly in the fall. Scarlet fever is spread by the nasal and the mouth secretions, especially after the acute onset of the illness. Its germs remain alive for months in garments or toys and may spread by contaminated food.

The portal of entry in the usual case is the pharynx, but the streptococcus may enter the body through any fresh wound, therefore, surgical patients and women during the puerperium, are quite susceptible to this disease if they have not previously had the infection.

Clinical Course and Symptoms

The prodromal period of scarlet fever lasts from 1 to 11 (usually 3 or 4) days following exposure. Its onset is abrupt, with vomiting, sore throat and often a convulsion in young children. The temperature during the first day rises abruptly to from 104° to 105° F., the throat is sore, there are general weakness and headache, and the body surface is dry and hot. Punctate red spots appear over the hard palate, an early sign of this disease.

During the first 24 hours following the onset of an untreated case, the skin rash appears on the neck, behind the ears and on the chest, and within about 24 hours it covers the entire trunk. The face is least affected, usually not at all. Early, the skin may itch intensely. This rash starts as red points around the hair follicles, which by confluence produce the vivid scarlet color of the skin most characteristic of this disease. This rash, however, is not a true eruption, but an intense vascular congestion. Therefore, it disappears on pressure or during a chill. Nevertheless, always, even in mild cases, there appear a few or many fine petechiae, noticeable at points subjected to pressure or slight injury, which indicate capillary rupture.

With the appearance of the rash, the cervical lymph nodes swell, the tongue assumes the characteristic strawberrylike appearance due to the swollen papillae, and the spleen may become enlarged. (See Plate 10.)

The throat from the first is sore. Sometimes it is merely red and swollen; more often there is follicular tonsillitis, but in severe cases the tonsils and possibly the

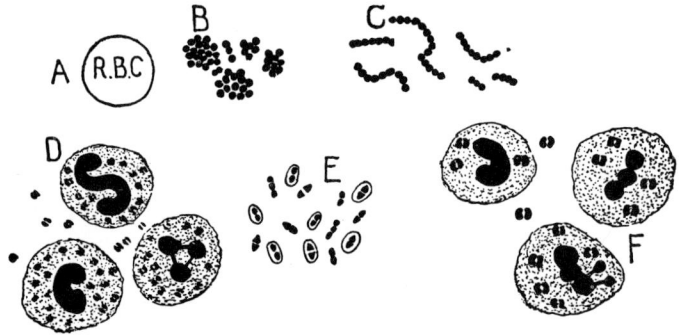

FIG. 422. Bacteria; cocci (all drawn to same scale, × 1,000). (A) A red blood corpuscle, drawn to the same scale for comparison of size. (B) Staphylococci, a common cause of osteomyelitis, boils and carbuncles. (C) Streptococci, the cause of erysipelas, scarlet fever and acute tonsillitis. (D) *Neisseria meningitidis,* or "meningococcus," the cause of epidemic cerebrospinal meningitis. (E) *Diplococcus pneumoniae,* a frequent cause of lobar pneumonia. (F) *Neisseria gonorrhoeae,* the cause of gonorrhea.

pharynx become covered with a membrane which strongly resembles that of diphtheria. The other symptoms are those of all high fevers. There is increased polymorphonuclear leukocytosis, often over 20,000 per cm. Proteinuria is characteristic.

The temperature reaches its maximum in 24 hours from the onset, continues elevated for from 2 to 5 days, then begins to fall. The rash gradually fades, disappearing in about a week, and desquamation at once begins. The latter usually is in the form of fine scales, but following severe cases it may be in large sheets which may carry the hair and the nails with them. The first traces of desquamation are seen under the fingernails before the rash has begun to fade. More visibly, it begins on the neck and the chest and continues until the whole cuticle is shed. This process of desquamation requires from 8 to about 50 days.

Complications and Sequelae

Few diseases have more possible complications and sequelae than has untreated scarlet fever, probably all of them due to *Streptococcus hemolyticus.* These may appear during convalescence, sometimes as late as the 4th week after the temperature reaches normal. Among these are great enlargement and sometimes abscess of the cervical lymph nodes; acute otitis media, formerly the most common cause of deafness; scarlatinal synovitis; purulent streptococcal arthritis; endocarditis and pericarditis; scarlatinal nephritis; occasionally an unusually acute variety of appendicitis; and, very rarely, a fatal purpuric condition presumably due to a generalized increase in capillary permeability (purpura fulminans).

It is to be understood that the complications listed above pose a significant threat only in untreated cases of scarlet fever, not to the patient who receives adequate care.

Chemotherapy and Nursing Care

Scarlet fever, like other streptococcal infections, yields completely and with gratifying speed to penicillin. This antibiotic may be administered in the form of penicillin G (benzathine, crystalline, procaine or potassium) given by intramuscular injection 2 to 4 times daily in doses of 300,000 to 600,000 units, or as potassium phenethicillin (Syncillin) in equivalent doses by mouth (fasting).

Communicable disease precautions must be applied and enforced as long as hemolytic streptococci are recovered from the patient's throat. They may be expected to disappear within a period of 24 to 48 hours.

Symptomatic Relief. The pain associated with the acute pharyngitis and cervical adenitis, which may be exceedingly uncomfortable at the beginning, should abate markedly in intensity in the space of a very few hours and disappear by the 3rd day of treatment. Pending the symptomatic response to penicillin, the application of cold compresses to the neck and irrigation of the throat with hot saline, glucose or Dobell's solution will afford relief. The nares should be kept clear and crusting prevented by the frequent instillation of 0.5 per cent menthol or liquid Albolene. Alcohol sponge baths are indicated

Fig. 423. Bacteria; bacilli. Important disease-producing and harmless bacilli (all drawn to same scale, × 1,000). (A) *Bacillus anthracis,* a very dangerous bacillus, the cause of "anthrax," "malignant pustule," "woolsorters' disease," etc.: 1, a chain of bacilli, each containing a spore; 2, one long bacillus; 3, free spores; 4, a short chain. (B) *Bacillus subtilis,* a harmless ubiquitous bacillus, also called "hay bacillus": 5, a short chain of bacilli without spores; 6, two bacilli containing spores; 7, free spores; 8, two spores "sprouting," that is, developing into bacilli. Note that this bacillus "sprouts" from the side of the spore. (C) *Clostridium tetani,* or the bacillus that causes "lockjaw": 9, a red blood corpuscle drawn to the same scale, introduced for comparison of sizes; 10, the "drumstick-shaped" bacillus containing spores; 11, free spores; 12, a bacillus without a spore on the left. (D) *Hemophilus influenza,* a cause of respiratory infections and meningitis. This germ produces no spores. (E) *Clostridium multifermentans,* a large harmless bacillus: 13, bacilli without spores; 14, bacilli containing spores; 15, a bacillus containing two spores; 16, free spores; 17, a spore "sprouting." Note that this bacillus develops from the end of the spore. (F) *Corynebacterium diphtheriae.* There are no spores formed by this germ. The dots are not spores, but indicate irregularity in staining ("beading"). (G) *Salmonella typhosa,* the cause of typhoid fever. The same picture will do for *Salmonella paratyphi* and *Escherichia coli.* No spores are produced. (H) *Pasteurella pestis,* the cause of bubonic plague. The dots do not represent spores. (I) *Mycobacterium tuberculosis,* the cause of tuberculous lesions. No spores are produced. (J) A leukocyte drawn to the same scale for comparison.

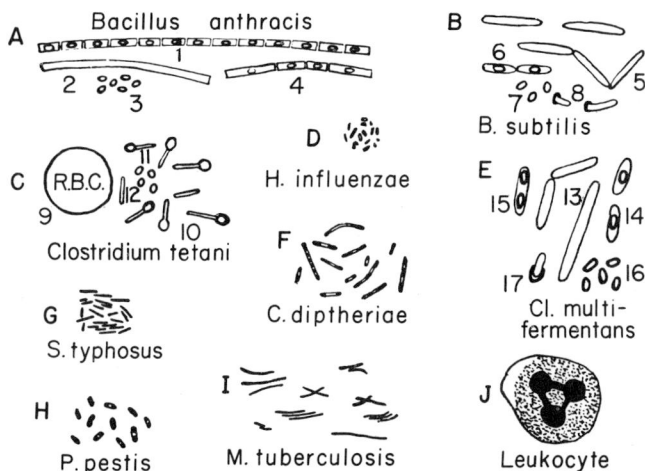

when the patient is delirious or the fever high.

When desquamation begins, the patient should be rubbed daily with liquid petrolatum, and each second day he should be bathed with soap and water.

The diet in scarlet fever depends only on the clinical state of the patient. Food is selected and prepared on the basis of ease of ingestion. Thus, when the temperature is markedly elevated, the throat inflamed and swallowing difficult, cold liquids are most palatable. The fluid and caloric requirements should be met adequately during all stages of the disease. A normal diet is ordered as soon as the patient will tolerate it comfortably.

Prophylaxis

Persons who have been in intimate contact with the patient immediately prior to or coincident with the onset of his acute symptoms should receive a dose of penicillin as a safeguard against a hemolytic streptococcal pharyngitis and against scarlet fever itself in case they are not immune to the exotoxin of that organism. A single injection of benzathine penicillin, 1,200,000 units (720 mg.), will afford protection for as long as 6 weeks.

Dick Test. This test indicates susceptibility to scarlet fever. It is performed by injecting a small amount of streptococcal toxin into the skin of the forearm. When positive, a red tender area appears at the site of injection and persists for from 48 to 72 hours. This indicates that circulating antitoxin is absent, that the patient is not immune to clinical scarlet fever. In other words, it will enable one to state whether or not a rash and other signs of streptococcal toxemia would develop, were the individual to contract a beta-hemolytic streptococcus infection.

ERYSIPELAS

Erysipelas is an acute hemolytic streptococcal infection of the subcutaneous lymph spaces which presents itself as a sharply defined, fiery red, hot, swollen area of skin, with well-defined advancing margin. Blebs often form on the inflamed skin, and, in severe cases, small abscesses appear beneath it. (See Plate 6.)

Erysipelas is most common on the face; yet it may spread centrifugally from minute breaks elsewhere in the skin. Persons particularly susceptible to it are those with fresh surgical wounds, women just after labor (in which case it starts in the uterine tract), newborn infants (vulnerable because of their recently cut umbilical cords), alcoholics and elderly persons with debilitating conditions such as chronic nephritis or cancer.

Symptoms and Course

Facial erysipelas, the most common form, after an incubation period or from 1 to 3 days, begins suddenly with fever which rises abruptly, accompanied by a chill and the appearance of the erysipelas which starts on the bridge of the nose and spreads butterfly fashion over both cheeks. The swollen lids may close the eyes; the lips may become huge. From the time of onset there is headache, often vomiting and sometimes delirium. The prostration is extreme. The temperature usually is high and continuous. There is a marked polymorphonuclear leukocytosis.

The spreading of erysipelas often stops abruptly where the skin is tightly bound to the underlying structures, such as at the hairline or the nape of the neck. However, it may extend over the chest and even the entire body, clearing up behind it as it advances (migratory erysipelas). After from 4 to 8 days the temperature falls, the patch fades, first at its center, and, later, the involved skin desquamates.

Chemotherapy and Nursing Care

Growth and spread of the organisms can be checked and the course of the disease materially shortened by therapeutic doses of penicillin. Cold magnesium sulfate compresses are helpful in hastening the resolution of the local skin lesion. A mask may be made to cover areas involved, that is, the face, the ears and the neck.

Nursing Precautions. It has been emphasized that the responsible germ can cause other types of streptococcal disease in nonimmune persons; that the spread of the organism depends only on the opportunities for distribution of this germ, and the havoc it wreaks, solely on the state of streptococcal immunity possessed by persons whom it infects. Thus, a Dick-positive nurse (see p. 1067) may well develop scarlet fever after exposing herself carelessly to a patient with erysipelas, particularly if this patient harbors the organism in the respiratory tract, as so many do. A Dick-negative nurse will not develop scarlet fever, but may contract a streptococcal sore throat, or, if the organism enters her tissues—through a break in the skin, for example—she can develop erysipelas, a lymphangitis or a streptococcal septicemia.

The patient with erysipelas should be isolated completely, and special care should be exercised by the nurse lest she spread the disease to other patients. Public health nurses visit these patients last, lest they indirectly infect an obstetric patient.

DIPHTHERIA

Diphtheria is an acute infection of the mucous membranes of the throat and the upper respiratory passages by a bacillus, *Corynebacterium diphtheriae* (Fig. 424). It is characterized by a marked toxemia and the presence of a white, leathery, false membrane, the necrotic mucous membrane, infiltrated with a fibrin-rich inflammatory exudate which gives this disease its name (diphtheria means "leather").

The diphtheria bacillus remains and multiplies in the false membrane, while its soluble toxin, absorbed by the blood stream, explains all the constitutional symptoms of diphtheria.

Symptoms and Course

The incubation period of diphtheria lasts usually for from 2 to 5 days, following the exposure. At the onset there are fever, chilly feelings, pains in the back and the limbs, slight general malaise and, soon, a sore throat. At the onset of symptoms, a little patch

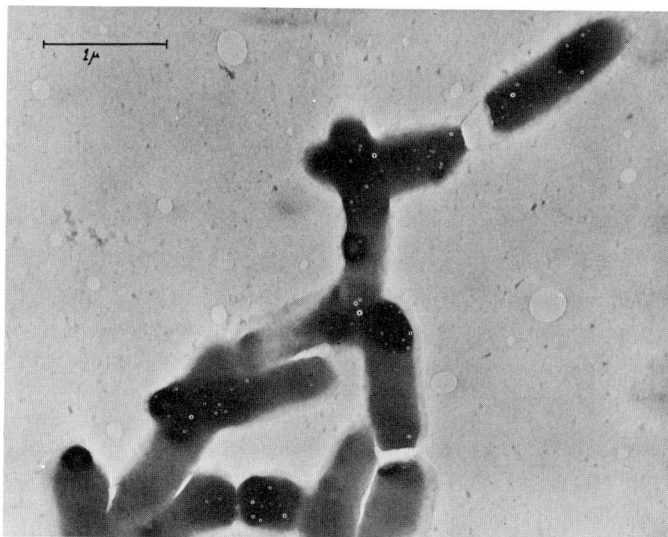

Fig. 424. Diphtheria bacilli, as shown by the electron microscope. Dense granules are seen near the ends of these bacterial cells. ($1\mu = \frac{1}{25,400}$ in.) (Mudd, S., and Anderson, T. F.: J.A.M.A. **126:**561, 632)

of delicate white membrane is visible, usually on one tonsil, and the cervical glands become enlarged. The following day the patch of membrane usually has enlarged and has crept beyond the tonsil, extending over the soft palate to the posterior pharyngeal wall, up the nose and into the nasal sinuses, or down the larynx, the trachea and even into the bronchi.

The severity of the case depends on the toxemia. It never can be judged from the amount of membrane present, for in some fatal cases there is little and in milder cases much. Patients with the severest cases have no fever, with possibly a subnormal temperature until death.

Wound diphtheria, or the formation of a false membrane around recent wounds, occasionally is due to the diphtheria bacillus, but more often it is a streptococcal infection.

Complications and Sequelae

Among the serious complications of diphtheria are toxic myocarditis, which may cause sudden death; acute circulatory failure, due to peripheral vasomotor paralysis; severe nephritis; and bronchopneumonia, due usually to pneumococci and streptococci, a frequent cause of death. Severe cases of laryngeal diphtheria may suffocate unless an airway is established by tracheotomy.

Among the important sequelae of diphtheria are various paralyses due to peripheral neuritis, of the throat and the eye muscles particularly—less often, of the limbs. These paralyses usually develop during the second and third weeks of convalescence. In some cases the diphtheria itself is so slight that it is overlooked until (because of paralysis of the throat) the voice becomes nasal and the patient begins to regurgitate liquid through the nose.

Epidemiology

This disease attacks children for the most part, although adults—nurses and doctors especially—may contract it. Diphtheria is spread not only by mild cases, convalescents and carriers but also by articles such as clothes, to which particles of the membrane cling and in which the organism can live for as long as 5 months. Another potential vector is milk, in which it multiplies without altering the taste.

Throat Culture

Bacteriologic examination is necessary for the diagnosis of diphtheria, since some cases with the membrane entirely on the tonsils really cannot be differentiated by inspection alone from streptococcal tonsillitis.

A throat culture is taken easily. State boards of health provide a box containing two tubes: in one of these is a sterile swab; in the other, Loffler's serum. The nurse carefully removes the swab from the tube and, not allowing it to touch elsewhere, rubs it against the membrane of the throat, then, using the technic of the bacteriologist, rubs it on the media and sends the tube at once to the laboratory.

Prophylaxis

Schick Test. This is a test for susceptibility to diphtheria. A small amount (0.1 ml.) of diphtheria toxin is injected into (not under) the skin of the forearm, about 2 inches below the bend of the elbow. If the child is not immune, a red and slightly raised spot, from 1 to 2 cm. in diameter, appears at the point of injection in from 24 to 48 hours; it reaches its maximum size in 4 days, persists for from 7 to 10 days and then fades, leaving a superficial scaling and a persistent brownish pigmentation. Such is a positive Schick test. This shows that the child's blood contains no diphtheria antitoxin, therefore he is susceptible to the disease and is in danger of contracting it if exposed. In all cases a control test should be made by treating the other arm in exactly the same way, but using a toxin previously heated for 10 minutes at 75° C. (which destroys the toxin).

All children should be tested for susceptibility to diphtheria by means of the Schick test, described above. Children who give a positive Schick test should receive 3 injections, at 1-week intervals, of the toxin-antitoxin mixture or of diphtheria toxoid, one of the ingredients of DTP antigen, which is used on a massive scale for the routine immunization of preschool children against diphtheria, tetanus and pertussis (see pp. 1052-1054). From 75 to 95 per cent of those thus treated will give a negative Schick test after from 6 to 12 weeks and for years will remain immune to diphtheria. To be certain, however, the Schick test is repeated 6 months later. Proof of the effectiveness of diphtheria prophylaxis, as it is currently practiced, is contained in the declining incidence of this infection, the total number of cases reported annually in the U.S. being now approximately 2,000. However, it must be pointed out, that the number of mild, ambulatory and unrecognized cases far exceeds that of the recognized, hence, reported, cases. Moreover, the ambulatory case represents more serious a threat to the community than does the overt case that receives a diagnosis, for, however mild, he is no less a source of infection and the number of contacts which he might establish among the nonimmune is limitless.

Treatment

Since diphtheria antitoxin came into general use, the mortality of diphtheria, formerly a disease fatal in over half of all cases, has fallen below 5 per cent. If its use could be made universal, this mortality would drop almost to zero.

Diphtheria antitoxin may be given intramuscularly, but if the patient is critical, it should be injected intravenously. No time should be lost whenever diphtheria is even suspected; the antitoxin should be given at once, even before the diagnosis has been proved. Total dosage at the onset is better than divided doses. The ordinary case requires about 6,000 units of antitoxin given at once; those moderately severe, from 10,000 to 20,000; severe cases, from 30,000 to 50,000; and those very severe, 100,000 units or more. As much as 10,000 units may be given to a tiny baby in the course of a day. In from 24 to 36 hours the membrane can be seen to shrivel up and loosen. In cases of laryngeal diphtheria, 16,000 units are injected at one dose.

Antitoxin itself does no harm. However, the proteins still remaining in it produce serum disease in about 10 per cent of all cases treated, and especially in persons who have been subject to hay fever, asthma or hives. Such persons first should be tested by injecting intradermally 0.025 ml. of the antitoxin diluted 1:100 with sterile salt solution. If an urticarial wheal rises at the point of injection in 10 minutes, then the antitoxin (concentrated) is injected in ascending doses, one each 20 minutes, the first dose 0.1 ml., until the full amount is given.

Penicillin is effective against the diphtheria bacillus, and always should be used in conjunction with serum therapy. If there is danger of suffocation in a patient with laryngeal diphtheria, intubation or tracheotomy should be performed. Wound diphtheria should be treated with penicillin, administered locally and parenterally, together with intramuscular injections of diphtheria antitoxin.

Quarantine is prescribed for 7 days following infection, or until two successive cultures from the nose and the throat are negative for diphtheria.

Nursing Care

A patient with diphtheria should be cared for in a cool, well-ventilated room. The diet should be liquid, but adequate in caloric and vitamin content. If there is difficulty in breathing, the air should be saturated with moisture, which can be supplied by a steam apparatus designed for that purpose.

If an intubation tube has been fitted into the larynx, the problem of feeding becomes important and presents certain difficulties, since, when the child is being fed, the head should be a little lower than the body. In the meantime, saline and glucose should be given intravenously. If tracheotomy is performed, the nurse must watch the tube, making sure that its two tapes are always in place, keep a piece of gauze moistened with boric acid or saline solution over the shield and frequently remove the inner tube in order to keep it clean. The child should be fed through a nasogastric tube if necessary. Care is taken to avoid aspiration of gauze threads or cotton lint through the tube. The tube is changed at intervals, and the inner tube is removed and cleaned frequently with pipe cleaners and cold water. Suction is applied as often as necessary to remove mucus. A tracheal dilator should be kept at hand to place in the wound to hold the edges apart until the doctor arrives, in the event that the outer tube is coughed out. The patient should be taught to care for his tracheotomy, to suction the tube and even to change the dressing as soon as the doctor thinks he is able. He should always have his signal cord within reach.

Treatment of Carriers. All diphtheria carriers who harbor virulent germs should be isolated, no matter how slight or how long-standing the infection, until at least 3 throat cultures taken on different days are reported negative.

PERTUSSIS

Pertussis (whooping cough) is an acute, highly contagious, specific infection of the upper respiratory passages and the bronchi, due to *Hemophilus pertussis*. It is characterized by severe paroxysms of coughing ending in a whoop. This disease occurs in all seasons and occasionally in definite epidemics, particularly in winter and early spring. Of the patients, 50 per cent are children under 2 years of age and 90 per cent are under 7 years of age.

Symptoms and Course

The period of incubation is about 10 days.

First Stage. The first, or catarrhal, stage, which lasts about one week, resembles an ordinary head cold, with slight fever, weeping eyes and a cough of increasing severity. The only feature then which might suggest pertussis in sporadic cases is the unusually insistent character of the cough. Many cases progress no further. These are most likely to spread the disease.

Second Stage. The second, or paroxysmal, stage dates from the day of the first whoop. Then the diagnosis is no longer in doubt. Paroxysms of coughing due to other infections are brief and interrupted by inspirations after each 2 or 3 coughs; but in this disease the child is obliged to attempt the almost impossible feat of coughing 15 or 20 times on one single expiration. In this attempt the lungs become forcibly compressed by the strong muscles of expiration and at last fill again with one long inspiration, which it draws with a whoop. The product of such paroxysms is the tiny mass of very tenacious mucous sputum, the sticky character of which is responsible for the difficulty in expelling it from the bronchioles and the bronchi. The specific germs readily can be found in this sputum.

During these paroxysms the strain on bronchial tree, heart and blood vessels is severe. The face becomes blue, its veins swell, the eyes bulge, the sclerae become injected, and the child looks as though he might suffocate or rupture a blood vessel. These paroxysms may be stimulated by swallowing, by any irritation of the throat and by the emotions. Some children vomit at the end of each paroxysm, and, if this occurs frequently, the child may also starve.

As mentioned above, some children never whoop; others have only a few paroxysms; and still others, as many as 100 a day. This stage lasts from 3 to 4 weeks, at the end of which time the paroxysms become less and less frequent until they stop. Second attacks are unusual. A child may whoop later with ordinary colds contracted during the year following recovery, but this is not whooping cough.

Diagnosis

In doubtful cases, the pertussis bacillus may be demonstrated in the sputum. Complement-fixation tests and cutaneous reactions to the injection of vaccines now are being used and may prove to be valuable.

Nursing Care

As long as any catarrhal symptoms persist, the child with whooping cough should be isolated from those who have never had this disease. Phenobarbital and Hycodan, or codeine, may be used to quiet the cough and provide much needed rest, but caution must be observed lest these exhausted patients be oversedated.

Early, during the paroxysmal stage, the child should be kept in bed, if possible in the open air, since he will cough much less. Later, children with mild cases are allowed up and about and are handled in groups. All influences which tend to precipitate paroxysms should be avoided. The child should be fed frequently and regularly, and, if the paroxysms cause vomiting, a little food should be given after each.

Convalescence from whooping cough is tedious, and care should be exercised lest the child take cold. It is just at this time that one of its most serious complications is most apt to develop, especially in infants, namely, bronchopneumonia.

Complications

The complications of whooping cough are many. One of the worst of them is broncho-

pneumonia, because of which whooping cough is one of the most fatal of the acute infectious diseases among children under 5 years of age, and is a serious malady for the aged. Blood vessels may burst, and the child may bleed from his eyes, ears or lungs, under the skin or into the brain, causing permanent paralysis. The lungs often are injured; sometimes they become emphysematous; occasionally they actually rupture, giving rise to subcutaneous emphysema. Another of the most serious sequelae is bronchiectasis, which may make the patient a chronic invalid years later. Particularly is this true following whooping cough in adults. Mild tetany not infrequently occurs. Encephalitis is an occasional complication; in rare cases marked degeneration of the cerebral cortex has followed this disease.

Prevention

Protective vaccine (Sauer or Sabin) is recommended. Their value is well established. Although this disease probably is most contagious during its catarrhal stage— that is, during the week before a positive diagnosis can be made—there is danger of transmission even after the acute illness is over, provided that catarrhal symptoms persist. Therefore, the quarantine should be continued until all such symptoms have disappeared.

TYPHOID FEVER

Typhoid fever is due to a bacillus called *Salmonella typhi* (Fig. 425), its characteristic lesions being ulcer formation in the ileum and the colon, and its distinctive clinical features consisting of long-continued fever, rose-spot rash, enlarged spleen, slow pulse and leukopenia.

This bacillus produces no spores. Under suitable conditions, however, it can live for months outside the body, and, since it is eliminated in the stools and the urine of patients, it is very likely to find its way into food and water through sewage, flies and dirty fingers. Unfortunately, the typhoid bacillus changes neither the appearance nor the taste of milk, cream or butter which it contaminates, as harmless saprophytes often do. Today it is spread chiefly by carriers, patients who have recovered from this fever,

FIG. 425. Typhoid bacilli, shown by the electron microscope. The flagella account for the motility of these organisms ($1\mu = \frac{1}{25,400}$ in.) (Mudd, S., and Anderson, T. F.: J.A.M.A. **126**: 561, 632)

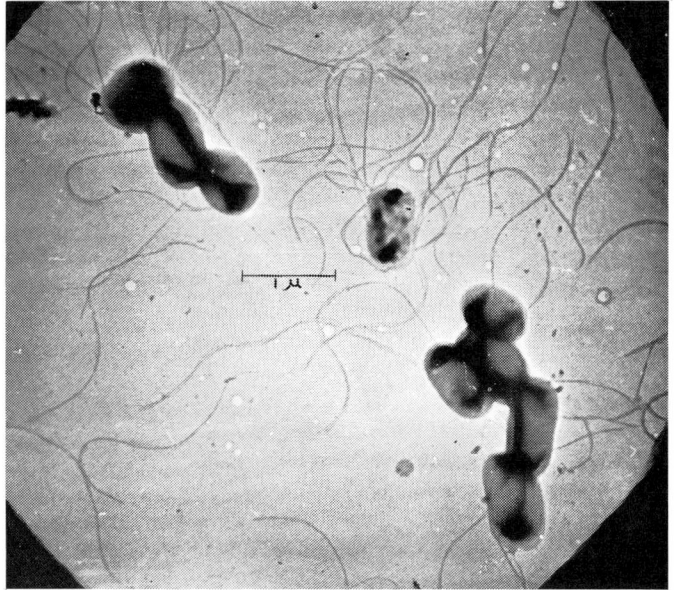

but whose stools, urine or both may for years spread these bacilli. Another common source is the ingestion of oysters and shellfish infected from offshore sewage disposal depots.

Pathology

The organism enters the body by the gastrointestinal tract, the walls of which it invades. There, multiplying rapidly, it gives rise to a massive bacteremia which continues for about 10 days. Its chief localization is in the mesenteric lymph nodes and the masses of lymphatic tissue in the mucous membrane of the intestinal wall, called *Peyer's patches* (Fig. 426), and in small solitary lymph follicles, numerous in the ileum and the colon. The blood vessels of the Peyer's patches become thrombosed, and the swollen mass of lymphatic tissue dies and sloughs away, leaving clean ulcers in the mucous membrane, the floor of which may be the muscularis or even the peritoneum. If the latter, they may perforate, causing peritonitis. The solitary follicles may or may not ulcerate, but they are so tiny that they do little harm. Healing then begins, and soon no trace of these deep ulcers is left.

The spleen is enlarged from the outset, and this provides a very useful diagnostic sign.

Clinical Course

The incubation period of typhoid fever lasts from 5 to 14 days. Then there develop symptoms of generalized malaise, weakness,

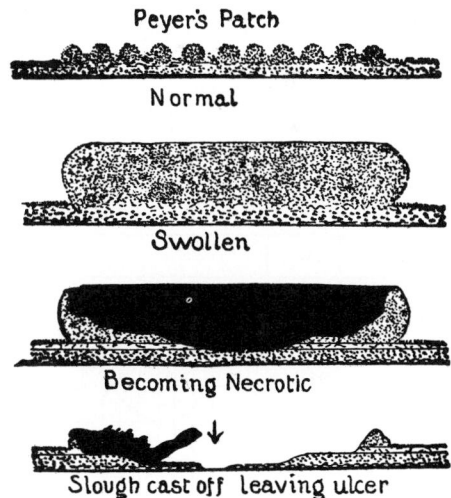

FIG. 426. The characteristic lesion of typhoid fever (magnified slightly). In this fever the Peyer's patches first swell, then this swollen tissue dies and is cast off as a slough, leaving an ulcer. The arrow indicates a point where the bowel wall may perforate and peritonitis result.

headache, muscle pains and fever. Depending on the localization of bacteria during the stage of septicemia, some cases early resemble cerebrospinal meningitis with convulsions, some begin as acute pleurisy, bronchitis or pneumonia and others resemble acute nephritis. Early in the disease, chills and fever may be the predominant symptoms.

Fever. The temperature rises by a stepladder ascent, reaching its highest level (usually from 104° to 106° F.) in from 3 to 7 days. During this period of rising temperature the headache is severe sometimes excruciating.

Usually the patient is constipated. Often the abdomen becomes distended with gas (metorism). As illustrated in Figure 427, during the 2nd week of the fever the temperature remains consistently high. During the 3rd week, however, it becomes more and more remittent, a little lower each morning and not quite so elevated each afternoon, the curve, therefore, resembling a snake fence, until in a week or so the highest record is at or below normal.

Nursing Observations

The pulse in typhoid fever at its height is usually remarkably slow (between 80 and 90). Also, one often feels the dicrotic wave so distinctly that there is danger of mistaking it for a separate beat.

The rose spots characterististic of typhoid fever, few or many in number, usually appear at the end of the first week, often in successive crops. These are low papules, rose-red in color, which disappear entirely on pressure. They are most common over the abdomen.

Laboratory Studies

The white blood cell count usually declines below 5,000, sometimes to a level as low as 1,500 cells per cu. mm. A progressive anemia is characteristic of typhoid fever. During the first week of the fever, the typhoid bacillus can be grown from the blood in practically every case. After the first week, blood cultures occasionally are positive, but more often the germ can be grown from the urine and the stools. The easiest method of diagnosis, then, is the Widal agglutination test, which is negative at first but becomes increasingly positive as the disease progresses.

Complications

Many structures may become infected in the course of typhoid fever. These include the lungs, the pleura, the pericardium, the heart, the kidneys and the bones. However, the commonest of the dangerous complications, are intestinal hemorrhage and perforation of the bowel with resultant peritonitis.

Hemorrhages from the bowel occur in at least 5 per cent of all cases and cause about

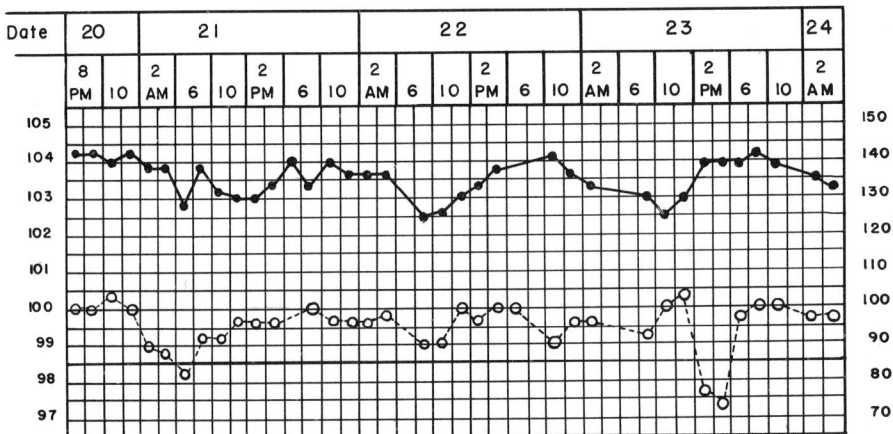

FIG. 427. Typhoid fever, second week, in a young man.

10 per cent of all deaths from typhoid fever. They occur most frequently during the 3rd week. Some patients have many. Evidently, they come from ulcerating Peyer's patches, the slough of which opens a small artery as it separates.

Intestinal perforation, the most dreaded complication of typhoid fever, occurs in 5 per cent of all cases and explains almost a third of all fatalities. It may occur at any time, but most often it happens during the 3rd week. It arises when the ulcer causing the slough involves the entire thickness of the bowel wall. The intestinal contents pour into the abdominal cavity, at once producing peritonitis.

Late complications, appearing from the 3rd to the 6th weeks, are not infrequent. As is liable to happen to severely ill, bedfast patients, phlebitis often develops. This is evidenced by long-continued fever and painful swelling of an extremity, usually a leg, which should be immobilized and protected with a cradle. Cholecystitis, marked by the development of crampy right upper quadrant pain accompanied by tenderness, nausea, vomiting and jaundice, may occur from direct infection of the gallbladder by the typhoid bacillus. This is treated conservatively with sedatives, antispasmodics and parenteral fluids. Urinary tract infection, favored by the enforced bed rest with its attendant feature of mechanically difficult urinary drainage, complicates many a typhoid convalescence. Its treatment depends, of course, on the degree and the bacteriologic type of infection. Typhoid spine, giving rise to severe low back pain, may be due to an arthritic process or to a typhoid abscess in a vertebra. The spine should be immobilized mechanically during the acute stage.

Chemotherapy and Nursing Care

Chemotherapy now available for the treatment of typhoid fever is efficacious in a high proportion of cases. Chloramphenicol (Chloromycetin) is the drug of choice. The recommended dose of Chloromycetin is 50 mg. per Kg. of body weight initially, followed by 0.25-Gm. doses at 2-hour to 3-hour intervals, this schedule being continued for 5 days after complete subsidence of the fever. Defervescence may be expected within

3 to 5 days from the time of the initial dose, paralleled by disappearance of clinical signs and subjective improvement. However, bacteriologic cure is not obtained in all cases, relapses having occurred and positive stool cultures having been obtained after one course and even after repeated courses of antibiotic therapy. Thus, while chloramphenicol has reduced the fatality rate of typhoid fever significantly and has curtailed the excretion of typhoid bacilli during convalescence, it has not reduced the frequency of complications or the incidence of the chronic carrier state following typhoid fever.

Nursing Care. With or without specific chemotherapy, typhoid fever is largely a nursing problem. In planning the care of each patient, certain features of this disease should be borne in mind.

First, typhoid fever is distinctly dangerous from the standpoint of contagion, since both urine and stools from these patients are apt to be heavily laden with typhoid bacilli.

Second, the mental state of the patient during the active febrile stage is one of drowsiness, indifference to his surroundings or physical hypesthesia, accompanied by a partial incontinence of urine and feces. In other words, a patient in a "typhoidal state" is prone to be careless and noncooperative in matters of personal hygiene.

Isolation technic must be carried out in full, and no precaution may be relaxed until the patient's stools are free of *S. typhi.* Wearing of a gown is obligatory. Every necessary step must be taken to exclude flies from the patient's room and its environs. All dejecta from the patient and food wastes on his tray must be disposed of, and their containers sterilized, without delay. His garments, linens, dishes and utensils, as well as his clinical thermometer and any other items with which he has had contact, must be sequestered with great care until they have been disinfected.

The temperature should be taken by rectum, since the patient cannot be trusted to keep his mouth closed while holding the thermometer. At first it should be taken every 2 hours day and night. An alcohol sponge is given at frequent intervals for temperatures of 104° F. or more.

This is one of the few diseases in which it is desirable to arouse the patient for the purpose of recording his body temperature on schedule. Also, it may be necessary to arouse him for each feeding and for the administration of fluids. It is important that he be turned methodically from side to side in order to avoid the formation of decubiti due to prolonged pressure over bony prominences. Many patients are so toxic that they lose the urge to void, with the result that the bladder becomes distended; the nurse should not be deceived by frequent involuntary voidings which often accompany urinary retention and bladder distention, but should measure and record the urinary output daily in order to obtain quantitative data concerning the state of the water balance. Special mouth care is necessary for the avoidance of stomatitis and parotitis, as well as for the comfort of the patient.

Retention of feces, as well as of urine, may pose a problem in patients with typhoid fever. In order to avert constipation, repeated low-saline enemas (500 ml.) may be employed, the fluid reservoir being elevated no higher than the level of the hips, to diminish the chances of intestinal perforation caused by an increase in the pressure or the volume of the fluid within the colon.

Distention may be reduced by turpentine stupes or the insertion, for short intervals (20 minutes), of a rectal tube, the latter arranged so that its free end projects through an opening in the paper top of a specimen bottle. Constipation should be relieved not by drugs but by enemas, as indicated above.

Perforation is the most important of all complications from the standpoint of risk and the necessity for early recognition. Every hour, every minute after the appearance of the first symptom is of great importance, for the earlier the operation the more successful it will be. Therefore, the nurse should know the danger signals and report them at once to the doctor in charge. The initial pain may be located anywhere in the abdomen. It occurs suddenly and is different from any previously experienced by the patient. This pain lasts for a few seconds, then stops, and in a few minutes the patient may be sound asleep. This last point is deceiving,

for the nurse hardly can believe that such a pain can be important.

Decubiti, unless skillful precautions are taken to forestall this complication, can be severe. They occur with the greatest frequency if the patient is not kept clean and dry, or if steady pressure on the back, the sacrum, the buttocks or the heels is not prevented by pillows, pieces of foam rubber, and frequent changes of position.

The mouth should be rinsed repeatedly and swabbed to prevent mouth infections and parotitis. Maintenance of adequate general hydration is most important from this point of view.

When hemorrhage has occurred or is suspected, the foot of the bed is elevated, the patient moved as little as possible, and nothing is given by mouth except sips of water.

The diet is a therapy of major importance. Prescribed is a soft diet (milk, broths, gruels, soft-boiled eggs, milk toast, etc.), and, by adding lactose or glucose to the liquids, the caloric value of these foods is raised to a point which covers the body needs (at least from 2,000 to 2,500 calories per day for an adult man). Some doctors give solid food as soon as it is desired by the patient.

Hydrotherapy (cold sponges, cold packs or alcohol rubs) is useful in reducing the fever and has an excellent tonic effect. As a result, the delirium disappears, the patient feels better, his mind is keener, and the condition of the skin is better.

Convalescence

Typhoid fever is a self-limiting disease; that is, the body cures itself by developing an adequate immunity against the invading organism. In this fever, however, the process is a slow one. The convalescence of typhoid fever, therefore, is long and tedious; it even may take months, and during this time the various sequelae may arise. The temperature often remains continuously subnormal (between 96° and 98° F.) and the pulse rate slow, possibly 50 or less to the minute.

The patient convalescing from typhoid fever must be kept under observation until urine and stool cultures are consistently negative. Approximately 2 per cent of typhoid cases become chronic carriers, continuing to harbor the organism and to excrete it in urine and stools. It may be impossible to cure this carrier state without removing the focus of infection, which most commonly is the gallbladder. For carriers of the younger age group cholecystectomy, although not invariably successful, should be advised.

Prophylaxis

Typhoid fever, also the paratyphoid fevers, in large degree can be prevented by prophylactic vaccination with the dead organisms of these diseases. One milliliter of the triple vaccine usually used contains 1 billion typhoid bacilli and 750 million each of paratyphoid A and paratyphoid B, all killed by heat at 53° C. for 30 minutes and by the 0.5 per cent phenol added to the suspension. The first injection for an adult is one half a milliliter, and the second and third, 1 ml. each. These injections are given subcutaneously, at intervals of one week. This measure should be enforced in hospitals, schools, armies and throughout the community. However, it is no substitute for good sanitation, for the immunity produced can be broken down by massive infection.

In 1910, the annual incidence of typhoid fever in the United States was in the neighborhood of half a million. No fewer than 35,000 persons died every year as a result of this infection. It was the fourth leading cause of death. In 1950, by contrast, typhoid fever cases totaled less than 2,500 and, in 1961, only 841. (See Fig. 241.) The prevalence of typhoid began to decline sharply prior to 1910; by 1920, the disease had been brought under epidemiologic control generally. A very important factor in the success of this achievement was the widespread adoption of typhoid vaccination as a routine prophylactic measure. Of equal, and possibly greater, importance was the decontamination of drinking water, which by then had become standard practice throughout the country.

The infection confers an immunity presumed to last for at least 3 years. After this interval of time, whether after vaccination or after convalescence from the disease itself, revaccination is advisable, and this is certainly true if one contemplates traveling in an area where health standards are uncertain.

PARATYPHOID FEVER

Paratyphoid fever is a name applied to numerous intestinal infections caused by bacilli of the salmonella group, which were not differentiated from the typhoid bacillus, or from each other, until precise bacteriologic technics became available. The organisms most commonly producing salmonella infections include *Salmonella paratyphi, Salmonella schottmülleri, Salmonella typhimurium, Salmonella hirschfeldii* and *Salmonella enteritidis*. The diseases resulting from these infections are quite similar clinically, and the infecting organisms are spread in exactly the same manner as is the typhoid bacillus. They are all food infections.

Symptoms and Course

An occasional case of parathyphoid fever presents throughout its entire course a clinical picture identical with that of typhoid fever. Generally, however, the salmonella infections run a briefer course, their complications are milder and their mortality lower. The incubation period varies from 7 to 24 days, and the duration of the acute disease from 3 to 10 days. The onset is usually more acute than that of typhoid, often with a chill, malaise, generalized aching and marked apathy. The initial headache, bronchitis, vomiting, diarrhea and abdominal cramps are more pronounced than in typhoid fever.

The temperature curve usually reaches its peak, not by a slow, step-ladder climb, but within 48 hours or less. As a rule, it is markedly irregular, the remissions occurring frequently, accompanied by profuse sweating, and the patient is usually afebrile within 2 weeks. The pulse rate, while relatively slow, seldom can be described as a true bradycardia. Petechiae, splenomegaly and leukopenia are features of paratyphoid as well as typhoid fever.

Complications

Intestinal perforation and hemorrhage are unusual complications of salmonella infection, and relapses are rare in this disease.

The mortality rate varies between 1 and 10 per cent.

Diagnosis

Early in the disease, every attempt should be made to recover and identify the infecting organism from stools, blood, vomitus and urine. Later, after subsidence of the acute infection, serologic agglutination tests are useful in establishing the diagnosis.

Treatment and Nursing Care

Patients with salmonella infections of all types present essentially the same problems as those described in typhoid fever (p. 1072) and are managed in the same way. Chloromycetin, as with typhoid fever, is the chemotherapy of choice. The mode of transmission, too, is via the ingestion of food and fluids in most cases, and, to the extent that it is a food infection, its control is a community problem, involving detection and control of carriers, decontamination of water supplies, checking of food handlers, etc. However, there are other possible routes of infection, including infected barium enemas and contaminated rectal tubes, the elimination of which clearly is the responsibility of the nurse and other members of the medical team.

Prophylactic immunization is carried out, in the case of *Salmonella paratyphi* infections, by the incorporation of the killed organisms in typhoid vaccines. It should be pointed out that *S. paratyphi* A and B are responsible for little more than half of the salmonellosis cases currently extant. The remainder, caused by organisms other than types A or B, for which no vaccines are available, are equally dangerous.

BACILLARY DYSENTERY (SHIGELLOSIS)

Bacillary dysentery includes a group of enteric infections caused by bacilli of the shigella group, the most important of which are the Flexner, the shigae, the sonnei, the Newcastle, the Hiss-Y and the Schmitz strains. While encountered in all countries, bacillary dysentery is endemic in the tropics, where serious epidemics are frequent. It was the scourge of armies before proper methods of guarding food and water supplies

became general. That bacillary dysentery continues to pose a very substantial problem for the civilian population of the United States, is apparent from inspection of Figure 422, the number of reported cases in 1961 having been nearly 12,600.

The pathology of shigellosis in severe cases consists of necrosis involving large areas of the intestinal mucous membrane; indeed, the entire colon wall may be destroyed by the invasion of these bacilli. In milder cases, the denuding of epithelium gives rise to superficial ulcers.

Course

The onset of bacillary dysentery is abrupt, with fever, abdominal pain and the passage of small amounts of blood, mucus and pus. At the height of the active infection, the symptoms are severe and the prostration profound. The patient has a constant desire to defecate, and the straining is severe during the attempts. Death in severe cases may ensue in a few days. The mild cases recover in from 8 to 10 days; others last 2 or 3 weeks, and the chronic cases last several months, or even years, unless adequately treated.

Treatment and Nursing Care

It is essential to maintain the fluid and the electrolyte balance of the patient and to prevent profound dehydration owing to an excessively great loss of water and salts in the diarrheic stools. Adequate amounts of physiologic saline solution are administered intravenously, and large doses of paregoric are given to quiet the inflamed bowel. Morphine may be required to control pain and tenesmus.

The chemotherapeutic agent of choice in bacillary dysentery is one of the soluble sulfonamide drugs, e.g., sulfadiazine by intramuscular injection or sulfisoxazole by mouth, given in a dose of 4 Gm. stat, followed by 1 Gm. every 4 hours for 10 to 14 days. One of the tetracyclines is administered in the event of sulfonamide resistance on the part of the infecting organism.

Prevention

Dysentery bacilli are spread by drinking water polluted by infected human excreta and by food handled carelessly by dysentery carriers, some of whom have the active disease, others being entirely asymptomatic. Thus, the same precautions must be observed, and the same control of water sources and food handling enforced, in the prevention of dysentery as of typhoid fever.

If exposure to this infection is unavoidable or is regarded as a likely possibility, the ingestion of 1.0 Gm. of sulfadiazine daily throughout the period of exposure plus 1 week thereafter will give adequate protection against most strains of Shigella.

BRUCELLOSIS

Brucellosis, or undulant fever, a disease caused by *Brucella melitensis* and related organisms, is a long-continued febrile illness marked by frequent remissions and relapses (hence the name *undulant fever*), a painful arthritis, drenching sweats and splenomegaly.

Three closely related organisms are involved: *Brucella melitensis* of goats (discovered as the cause of Malta fever), *Brucella abortus* of cattle and a porcine variety from pigs. These germs usually enter the intestinal tract with the milk or the meat from infected animals. Undulant fever occurs particularly in young adults and most often during the summer. Milk pasteurization effectively controls spread of the milk-borne disease, but infection also occurs as a result of direct contact with diseased animals. Particularly vulnerable are veterinarians, farmers who assist in deliveries of infant cattle, meat handlers and slaughterhouse workers. During 1961, 636 cases of brucellosis were reported in the U.S.—less than one quarter of the number for 1952, as shown in Figure 421.

Clinical Symptoms and Course

After an incubation period of from 6 to 14 days, the illness gradually develops. Often this starts with sharp pains in the back and the limbs, intense headache, insomnia and hysterical manifestations. The temperature curve for months is markedly irregular, periods of fever which last for weeks alternating with brief periods of apyrexia. The arthritis varies from fleeting joint pains to severe attacks of acute polyarthritis, the joints swollen and sore, but not red.

Epistaxes and hemorrhages from intestinal ulcers are not uncommon.

Some patients during the entire illness have so little malaise that they are hardly incapacitated. In the severe cases, pneumonia, pleurisy with effusion and cardiac failure are serious complications.

The mortality of undulant fever in the past has varied from 2 to 15 per cent; however, a substantial reduction of this figure is to be anticipated as a result of the advent of effective chemotherapy.

Diagnosis

Blood cultures taken early may demonstrate the organism. After the 5th day of the disease, agglutination tests are usually positive.

Chemotherapy and Nursing Care

Chemotherapy. On occasion sulfadiazine, streptomycin and chlortetracycline all have proved to be curative in cases of brucellosis, and the combination of the last two appears to be the most promising of the agents so far tested.

Nursing Care. Brucellosis is spread via the fecal-oral route; consequently, the communicable disease precautions that have been specified for patients with typhoid fever are applicable likewise in these cases. Strict precautions must be observed in handling and disposing of all excreta from these patients, for the organism is excreted in the urine and the stools.

The patient, while his temperature is high, should remain in bed and receive abundant food and adequate fluids. Sponges, in part, will control the fever. Heat, supplied by an electric cradle or by hot, wet compresses, often is efficacious for the joint pains.

BOTULISM

Botulism (sausage poisoning), due to the toxin of the anaerobic bacillus *Clostridium botulinum,* is a serious condition, the chief symptoms of which are cranial nerve palsies. The germ itself introduced into the body is not pathogenic; it liberates its toxin while growing under strictly anaerobic conditions in nitrogenous foods. So poisonous is it that death has followed the mere tasting of infected food—it was not swallowed.

Preserved Foods. Home-preserved foods are most dangerous, for this germ is a spore bearer, hence is not killed rapidly at boiling temperature. (Reliable commercial packing houses sterilize their products at 248° F., which kills all the spores.) Preserved foods in which this germ has been growing look soft, contain gas bubbles and give off an odor of decay. Since this toxin is destroyed rapidly by heat (within a few seconds at temperatures over 180° F.), foods containing it are safe if heated to the boiling point before being eaten; but if allowed to cool and stand for a while, the organism will immediately proceed to form more toxin.

Clinical Symptoms and Course

The symptoms of botulism begin in from 4 hours to 6 days, but usually in from 18 to 36 hours, after the ingestion of the contaminated food. Although the toxin enters the body by way of the gastrointestinal canal, nevertheless gastrointestinal symptoms seldom develop. Early, there are malaise, headache, dizziness, a progressive and profound muscular weakness and incoordination which result in an unsteady gait. Incontinence of urine is common. Eye signs, very important in diagnosis, appear early. These include photophobia, ptosis, paralysis of the eye muscles and sometimes blindness. Progressive weakness of the muscles of speech, of swallowing and finally of respiration also appears early. The clinical picture, when fully developed, is quite characteristic. The patient is cyanotic, helplessly weak, his pulse is rapid, he cannot swallow, cannot talk, struggles more and more to breathe and finally dies of asphyxia. The deep reflexes remain normal. There are no sensory disturbances and no pain. The mind remains clear.

Botulism may continue for from 48 hours to 26 days, but the majority of cases terminate fatally before the 5th day. In each of its epidemics some of the cases have been very mild.

Convalescence is slow and tedious, with months of weakness and disturbed vision.

Prognosis

The mortality from botulism in general ranges between 45 and 60 per cent, the total number of cases reported in the United States varying from 6 to 28 annually during the decade prior to 1962.

Treatment

Antitoxins for two pathogenic strains of this organism have been prepared. They are protective and, if injected early, curative. While waiting for the antitoxin to take effect, artificial respiration should be continued as long as the heartbeat can be felt.

GONORRHEA

Gonorrhea is an infection, almost always venereal in origin, which is notable for its chronicity, its latency and multiplicity of localization. Next to measles, it is the most prevalent of all the notifiable communicable diseases. Moreover, as indicated in Figure 421, the incidence of gonorrhea is by no means on the wane; on the contrary, it is increasing steadily. The number of cases reported in 1952, excluding military personnel, was 244,957; in 1961, 264,158. The gonococcus (*Neisseria gonorrhoeae*) causes a surface infection, ascending in almost all cases via the lower genital tract. The primary infection, following an incubation period of from 3 to 8 days, takes place in or near the urethra. If drainage is good, it subsides spontaneously and clears in the course of a few days or weeks. However, infection of the prostatic urethra in the male and also of the female urethral and vaginal glands predisposes to chronic infection, with occasionally very serious sequelae. Females are apt to contract secondarily a mixed infection of the endometrium and, thereafter, of the tubes, constituting *pelvic inflammatory disease,* with resultant pelvic peritonitis. The ascent of infection is precipitated by such factors as menstruation, douches and the trauma associated with sexual intercourse or instrumentation.

Symptoms

The initial symptoms of gonorrhea, in both sexes, are urinary frequency, dysuria and the discharge of a yellowish exudate from the urethra or the vagina. If, in the female, tubal infection (salpingitis) ensues in from 2 to 3 weeks, this usually will be

FIG. 428. A cross section of the spinal cord from a patient with meningococcal meningitis. Note that there is an increased amount of cerebrospinal fluid and that the pus is chiefly posterior. If a hollow needle is stuck through the dura, a cloudy fluid will gush out. (a) Spinal nerve; (b) posterior root ganglion.

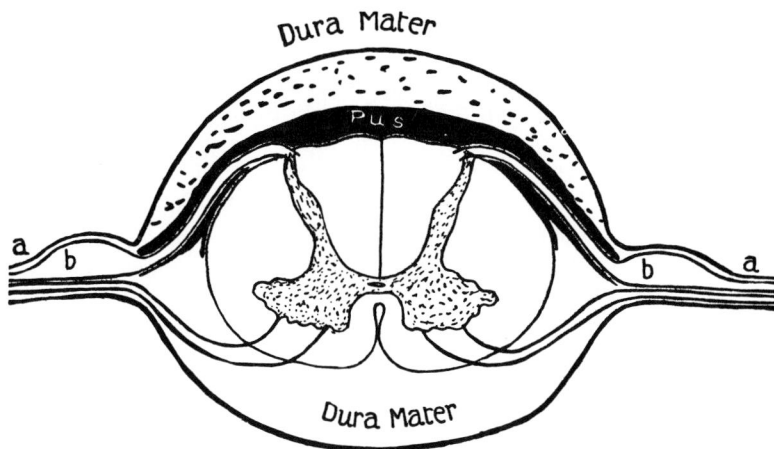

manifested by symptoms of low abdominal and back pain which is aggravated by defecation and dysmenorrhea or menorrhagia. Gonorrheal salpingitis is typically self-limited, and pelvic inflammatory disease of the chronic variety generally is considered to be the result of a mixed infection (that is, due to other organisms in association with the gonococcus) or of recurrent infection from a chronic gonorrheal focus in the lower genital tract.

Complications

The commonest complications of gonorrhea in the female include chronic inflammation of the glands about the urethra and the vagina, chronic cervicitis and salpingitis. Associated with the last named may be severe peritoneal inflammation followed by adhesions about the pelvic organs, including the rectum, and about the liver. Strictures of the cervix and the fallopian tubes are responsible for many cases of sterility.

Chronic gonorrhea in the male usually involves the prostate, constituting a common cause of chronic prostatitis. Occasionally the seminal vesicles likewise are infected. Urethral stricture is a complication of the disease in males particularly. Males and females alike may be victims of gonorrheal arthritis and endocarditis.

Treatment and Nursing Care

The treatment of gonorrhea is accomplished successfully in the vast majority of cases by means of penicillin or sulfonamide chemotherapy. All mechanical manipulations, including douches, urethral washes and prostatic massages, are unnecessary and unwarranted during the acute stages.

Acute pelvic inflammatory disease due to gonococcal infection is treated conservatively, the important elements of therapy being bed rest and the administration of sulfonamide or penicillin chemotherapy, supplemented, if necessary, by a bout of artificial fever, the temperature being maintained at 106° F. for 8 hours. Surgical intervention sometimes is indicated for persistent tubo-ovarian abscesses and other late complications of neglected gonorrhea, such as chronic urethral stricture, which is not amenable to dilatation with sounds, and for some cases of cervicitis or chronic inflammation of the vaginal glands.

The nurse must exercise caution in handling pads or other objects potentially contaminated by drainage from the genital tract. Hand washing is indicated after every contact with the patient. The patient should be instructed thoroughly regarding the importance of protecting the eyes and of maintaining adequate cleanliness in general.

MENINGOCOCCAL MENINGITIS

Meningococcal meningitis is an infectious disease due to the meningococcus (*Neisseria meningitidis*). This malady, if it goes through its entire course, starts as an acute infection of the nasopharynx or the tonsils, followed by a meningococcal septicemia, and ends as a localized infection of the meninges of the brain and the upper regions of the spinal cord.

The meningococcus is a tiny diplococcus, the two cocci of the pair flattened against each other, usually found engulfed in leukocytes. Over 20 types of this organism are recognized.

Widespread epidemics of this disease have occurred. However, the majority of them are limited, occurring notably in cities, crowded institutions, army camps or jails, but also in country regions—in which epidemics children in particular are attacked. Its germ is spread by the droplet method, the portals of entry being the mucous membrane of the nose and the tonsils. Of those exposed to it, the great majority do not develop the infection but become carriers, for months harboring this organism in the nasopharynx. In only a few of them does it enter the blood stream.

Pathology

At autopsy the pia mater (the delicate membrane which immediately covers the brain and the cord and in which are the tiny vessels which provide the cortex with food) is found to be congested and infiltrated with a purulent exudate; the pus is most abundant over the base of the brain and the posterior surface of the cord (Fig. 428). The inflammation spreads also to the membrane lining the cerebral ventricles. In acute cases, however, the patient dies from the toxin of the germ before pus has had time to collect.

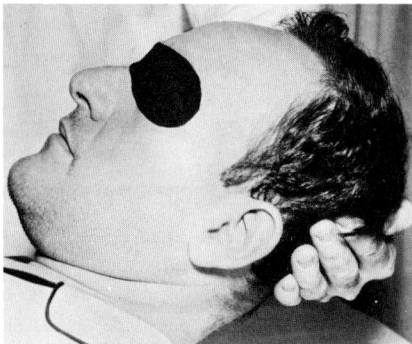

FIG. 429. Nuchal rigidity in a patient with meningococcal meningitis.

Symptoms and Course

During each epidemic some patients are scarcely ill; some, at once overwhelmed by the toxemia, develop high, or sub-normal, temperature, the skin is covered by purpura, and the patient dies within a few hours of the onset (the fulminant type).

The disease, when typical, begins as a cold in the head or an attack of paranasal sinusitis which is soon followed by the stage of septicemia. During the septicemic stage the patient is dull, immobile, refuses to talk, aches all over and desires to be undisturbed. His fever is high and irregular; he may chill. A petechial rash appears on the skin, fever blisters on the lips; joint and lung complications may develop. This stage may last for hours, days or weeks; then the meningeal stage begins. Often, however, there is no definite second stage. In such, the disease begins suddenly with fever, a chill and meningeal symptoms: vomiting, headache, fever, stiffness of the neck and drowsiness.

The meningitis having developed, the patient for most of the time is dull and apathetic, but at intervals he is irritable and restless and, if disturbed, delirious, even maniacal. Later there is stupor, or possibly coma. The headache, which is excruciating, comes in spasms; exquisite pains are felt in the back and the limbs; convulsions are not uncommon. The neck is rigid: try to raise the head and one must lift the shoulders and, occasionally, the entire body from the bed (Fig. 429). In some patients, in infants especially, internal hydrocephalus results, evidenced by severe headaches, cyanosis, engorged veins of the forehead, delirium, vomiting, choked disks and sudden death.

Diagnosis

The diagnosis is made by lumbar puncture, for the cerebrospinal fluid, instead of being perfectly clear, contains so much pus that it looks like thin milk, is under high pressure and the germ can be isolated from it. Blood cultures are likewise often positive for the meningococcus.

Meningococcemia. A certain proportion of patients with meningococcal infection do not develop meningitis, their disease instead being characterized by persistent or transient blood stream invasion by the organism. In these cases the meningococcus spares the meninges but localizes in the skin or in the joint synovia. These patients have fever, which may be of a high, irregular type or a mild, low-grade intermittent affair. A macular rash commonly appears, often the best clue to the clinical diagnosis. Pains in the joints typically are present, and occasionally an acute infection of one of the large joints develops. A leukocytosis may or may not be present. The diagnosis is established by the isolation of the meningococcus from the blood.

Treatment and Nursing Care

In general, the mortality of untreated meningococcal infections is from 50 to 80 per cent. Since the development of the sulfonamides and penicillin, however, it has been possible successfully to control meningococcal meningitis, and other meningococcal infections likewise, with gratifying regularity.

One million units of penicillin should be given intramuscularly at 2-hour intervals, together with sulfadiazine. The dosage of sulfadiazine employed should be sufficient to maintain a blood level of from 10 to 15 mg. per 100 ml. of blood. Patients with meningitis should receive sodium sulfadiazine intravenously in order to be assured of an adequate drug concentration in the blood as promptly as possible. The initial dose of sodium sulfadiazine for adults is in the neighborhood of 6 Gm., followed, from 2 to 4 hours later, by a second dose of 3 Gm. It is essential, when the drug is given intravenously in such large dosage, that the patient be supplied with ample quantities of fluid and alkali, preferably administered intravenously as well—in the form, for example, of physiologic saline and sodium lactate solutions. As soon as vomiting has been controlled and stupor has cleared, and there is every assurance that the patient will be able, thenceforth, to take medication and fluids by mouth, intravenous therapy is abandoned. sulfadiazine, thereafter, being given orally. Its administration is continued in a dosage of from 1 to 2 Gm. for approximately a week following the complete subsidence of signs and symptoms, adequate

hydration and alkalinization meanwhile being maintained. Following the abatement of the symptoms and signs and before the patient is discharged as cured, the spinal fluid examination usually is repeated as a routine laboratory check.

The course of the body temperature must be followed at 2-hour or 4-hour intervals by rectal recordings until the acute phase has subsided. During this period the patient should be protected from injury by the placement of side rails. Of utmost importance is the hydration of the patient, particularly during the administration of sulfadiazine therapy. The intake by all routes, oral and parenteral, must be estimated as accurately as possible and recorded once or twice each day. The urinary output likewise must be measured and volumes recorded for time intervals corresponding to those on which the intake volumes are based.

The patient with meningitis is likely to be uncomfortable for from 3 to 5 days after therapy is begun, complaining of headache, nausea and general malaise. Mouth and skin care should be meticulous. Until full consciousness has returned the patient should be turned frequently. Comfort is afforded by darkening the room, applying tepid sponges and an icecap to the head. Salicylates, codeine and small doses of morphine, if necessary, are used to control headache. Precautions against communicable disease should be taken in caring for patients with meningococcal infection, at least until the acute stage of the illness has passed.

INFLUENZAL MENINGITIS

Hemophilus influenzae is responsible for a type of meningitis that primarily affects children between the ages of 6 months and 6 years—a type that is uniformly fatal, unless treated, and one that cripples permanently unless treatment is prompt, vigorous and correct. Few adults have contracted the disease. Of these, the majority have been individuals with cerebrospinal rhinorrhea, hence unduly vulnerable to bacterial invasion of the central nervous system. (The discharge of spinal fluid through the nose indicates that an individual has previously sustained a fracture of his cribriform plate, the thin bone forming the roof of the nose, as a result of which there is an open communication between his cranial and nasal cavities.)

The prodromal period of influenzal meningitis may be featured by symptoms of an upper respiratory infection, often with additional signs of otitis media or pneumonia. Extension of the infection to the meninges is marked by the appearance of nausea and vomiting, headache and high fever. Convulsions are common, ranging from episodes of generalized twitching to tonic-clonic seizures. The patient may be drowsy, stuporous or deeply comatose. Laboratory studies demonstrate anemia, depressed concentrations of sugar in the spinal fluid and the presence of *H. influenzae* in the blood.

Complications that occur as a consequence of delayed or inadequate therapy and take the form of motor or sensory paralyses, diffuse cerebral dysfunction or a convulsive disorder are attributable to blockage of cerebrospinal fluid circulation or injury to the cranial or spinal nerves at their exit points, by tissue swelling and exudate associated with the infection, or to cerebral hemorrhage or thrombosis caused by direct involvement of the cranial vessels themselves during the acute stages.

Treatment

The treatment which often is the last chance for survival in the absence of complications is one that involves the intrathecal and intramuscular administration of streptomycin and intravenous injections of sulfadiazine or sulfisoxazole (Gantrisin). As the initial step, streptomycin, dissolved in 10 ml. of sterile saline solution, is injected intrathecally in a single dose of 15 mg. for infants less than 1 year old, 25 mg. for children between the ages of 1 and 3 years and 35 mg. for patients older than 3, immediately following the slow withdrawal of 12 to 15 ml. of spinal fluid. In addition, streptomycin is administered by intramuscular injection, 0.5 to 1.0 Gm. (or 30 mg. per Kg. in the case of a young baby) being given in 4 divided doses daily for 2 weeks, together with a sulfonamide, e.g., sulfadiazine or sulfisoxazole, in 4 to 6 Gm. doses daily by intravenous injection or by mouth. As

an alternative to streptomycin, chloramphenicol has been used in daily doses of 50 to 100 mg. per kilogram of body weight.

Nursing problems and details of nursing care are precisely similar to those encountered in meningococcal meningitis.

TULAREMIA

Tularemia, the bubonic plague of wild rodents, particularly rabbits, caused by *Pasteurella tularensis,* is a disease transmitted to man by the insect parasites of infected animals. It also may be contracted as a result of eating the insufficiently cooked meat of such animals. In 1961, 365 cases of tularemia were reported in contrast to a total of 668 patients in 1952.

Symptoms and Course

The period of incubation lasts from 3 to 5 days. The onset is sudden, with headache, vomiting, chills, general aching and fever. In cases contracted through the skin, a papule appears at the point invaded and soon becomes an ulcer; the neighboring lymph glands enlarge. Other cases are contracted through the conjunctiva, which becomes inflamed and ulcerated; others, through the gastrointestinal canal; while in many cases no portal of entry is found. Then follows a long, irregular fever, with marked prostration, loss of weight, sweats and, often, noncharacteristic skin rashes. Not infrequently pharyngitis, pneumonia, both lobar and bronchial, pleurisy, pericarditis and even meningitis, arise as complications. Some cases, however, remain ambulant.

The duration of the disease is usually from 2 to 3 weeks. All but 4 per cent of the patients usually get well. Recovery is slow, without sequelae (in a few conjunctival cases the eye has a residual injury) and is followed by lifelong immunity.

Diagnosis

The diagnosis is best made by the agglutination test, positive in a few days after the onset.

Treatment

Streptomycin is curative in most cases of tularemia and is the drug of choice at present.

ANTHRAX

Anthrax, its specific germ *Bacillus anthracis,* is the most widespread and fatal of all animal plagues. It is most prevalent among sheep and cattle of Asia, the U.S.S.R. and France. This disease is contracted by farmers, butchers, woolsorters and others who handle the meat or the hides of infected animals; also, occasionally it appears in those who use shaving brushes made of nonsterilized horsehair and those who wear infected furs about the neck. Of all the notifiable diseases in the United States, anthrax has become very nearly the rarest; in 1961 only 14 human cases were reported, representing a 75 per cent decline in incidence over a period of one decade.

Malignant pustule, the most common form of anthrax in man, which within 24 hours develops at the point of local infection (usually on the face or the neck), is a large, dark-brown, painless sloughing sore, surrounded by many minute silvery vesicles and resting on extensive areas of edema. There may or may not be an accompanying fever.

The pustule tends to heal spontaneously, leaving a deep scar. It may give rise to septicemia, either with or without visceral lesions. This lesion always appears inflamed, and often the blood is full of anthrax bacilli; yet practically until death the patient is comfortable, mentally clear and shows a characteristic lack of apprehension.

Pulmonary anthrax (woolsorters' disease) is an acute bronchitis due to anthrax spores inhaled from infected hair or wool. Usually it appears in from 18 to 20 hours, rarely in from 1 to 9 days, after exposure, giving rise to a slight tightness in the chest, difficulty in breathing and a mild cough; but more often the patient has practically no respiratory symptoms and is comfortable to within a few hours of death.

Gastrointestinal anthrax, the rarest form, contracted from the ingestion of anthrax germs or developed secondary to malignant pustule, begins with nausea, persistent vomiting, abdominal pain and tenderness and a bloody diarrhea. Areas of necrosis are found along the intestine. The patient often applies for treatment very late, since he feels so well.

Prognosis

If the pustule has not been disturbed, with serum treatment started before the end of the 3rd day the prognosis is good, even in the presence of bacteremia. In both pulmonary and intestinal anthrax the prognosis is grave because of the probable presence of destructive lesions in both the lungs and the bowel wall; but even then the antiserum, if given early, may save life.

Treatment

The pustule requires no local treatment other than a protective covering of sterile gauze. Sulfonamides and penicillin are both effective in the treatment of anthrax, the latter being the drug of choice.

GLANDERS

Glanders, a disease contracted from the nasal secretion of infected horses, a specific infection by the germ *Malleomyces mallei,* is characterized by the appearance of numerous abscesses throughout the body.

The organism, which appears in abundance in the lesions, is identified best through guinea pig inoculation.

Clinical Symptoms and Course

Acute glanders, after an incubation of from 3 to 14 days, starts as an acute fever with malaise, pneumonia or arthritis. Soon or later a multitude of little nodules, called *farcy buds,* appear in the skin. These rapidly ulcerate, discharging abundant, offensive fluid. Similar nodules develop in the muscles and other internal tissues, which become necrotic.

Chronic glanders for months may present as its only symptoms a chronic coryza and one or a few sluggish skin abscesses. Such patients may recover, but the condition suddenly is apt to become fatally acute. Streptomycin is the drug of choice in glanders.

ASIATIC CHOLERA

Asiatic cholera, responsible for the greatest epidemics of the past, is an acute enteritis caused by the specific germ *Vibrio comma.* Its chief feature is a profuse diarrhea causing rapid dehydration, acidosis and toxemia.

Vibrio comma (Fig. 430) is a curved

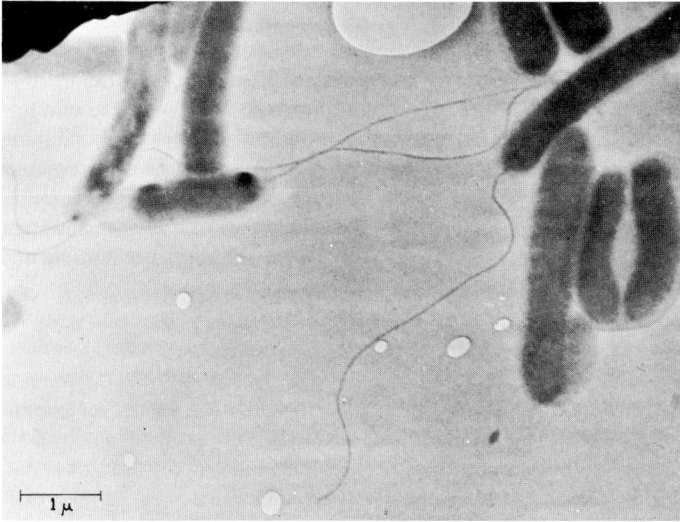

FIG. 430. *Vibrio comma* (the organism of Asiatic cholera), shown by the electron microscope. Note the flagellum attached to the end of each cell. ($1\mu = \frac{1}{25,400}$ in.) (Mudd, S., and Anderson, T. F.: J.A.M.A. **126:** 561, 632)

bacillus pathogenic only to man. It is spread chiefly by drinking water polluted by the stools of persons afflicted with this disease, in which the germs multiply luxuriantly, and possibly also by flies which have access to both these stools and foods. The germ enters the body through the mouth and multiplies enormously in the intestine. The organism itself does not invade the body; its toxin, absorbed through the intestinal wall, causes the disease. It has been epidemic in many countries, including our own, but in most regions has been eliminated by attention to water supplies.

Nursing Observations

The incubation period of cholera lasts from a few hours to several days. The attack usually begins with profuse vomiting, incessant diarrhea, recurrent colic and profound malaise. Then begins the stage of collapse. The blood would seem to pour all its water into the gastrointestinal canal, washing it clean of any fecal matter and bile, for the profuse vomitus and stools consist of water in which are suspended many little white particles of mucus and intestinal epithelium —hence the name *rice-water stools.* The temperature is high. Because of the dehydration, the thirst is excessive and the body visibly shrinks. The cheeks become hollow, the eyeballs sunken; the skin over the body becomes wrinkled, ashen, cold and clammy, and the hands and feet become blue. Urine

secretion stops. The pulse becomes weak, the blood pressure low and the blood count high because of the concentration of the blood. The cramps of the muscles are excruciating.

If the patient is to survive, the diarrhea diminishes, the warmth of the body returns, and the kidneys resume the secretion of urine; but the evidences of acidosis are marked, and all signs of severe renal damage are present.

In each epidemic, cases of all degrees of severity occur: at one extreme are those who for a day or so have merely a mild diarrhea, and, at the other, those who die before the diarrhea even has time to begin (dry cholera).

The mortality of the various cholera epidemics has varied from 30 to 70 per cent.

Prophylaxis

The methods of preventive inoculations in use are safe and fairly efficient.

Even more important are general sanitary measures, including protection of the water supply by chlorination or boiling; avoidance of uncooked salads, fruits and shellfish, if indicated; antifly measures; and detection and isolation of carriers, as well as patients, in danger areas.

Nursing Care

The patient should be isolated; his stools, vomitus and bed linen should be disinfected.

The treatment includes massive intravenous injections of physiologic salt solution and plasma to maintain a normal blood volume and to correct dehydration. Streptomycin is frequently effective and is currently the agent of choice in the treatment of cholera. Warmth and drug stimulation are provided.

BUBONIC PLAGUE

Plague (black death), the most fatal of all acute epidemic diseases, is caused by a specific organism, *Pasteurella pestis.* Its usual host is the rat. Another source of infection in the Western United States is the cottontail rabbit. This horrible epidemic has more than once swept over Europe, killing a quarter of the population. In Asia even today it is killing thousands of persons each year. An occasional case reaches our Western seaports.

In plague of the bubonic type, spread by the rat flea, large masses of swollen lymph nodes, called *buboes,* appear. These, breaking down, cause carbuncles and often a fatal septicemia.

In mild cases (*pestis minor*), after an incubation period of from 2 to 8 days following the fleabite, a fever starts, with headache and malaise. The temperature, often with chilly feelings, rises suddenly, in 2 days reaching about 104° F. Between the 1st and 3rd days buboes as large as a goose's egg may appear, usually in the inguinal region but occasionally in the axilla or the neck, their location depending on the site of the fleabite. In mild cases these buboes may disappear, but as a rule they suppurate and the abscesses break through the skin.

In *pestis major* the symptoms from the onset are much more severe. Subcutaneous hemorrhages, the so-called *plague spots* ("tokens"), appear early. It was this feature which gave the disease its name *black death.* The glandular enlargement becomes general. Often the patient is delirious. The spleen is enlarged, and there is a leukocytosis of even 90,000 per cu. mm. Some severe cases recover, but slowly. Death usually occurs on the 3rd to the 5th day.

In the *septicemic form* of plague (without buboes) the symptoms from the first are severe, with hemorrhages, coma and death occurring on the 1st to 3rd day.

Pneumonic plague, the most fatal form (its mortality is over 96 per cent), is spread by the droplet method, the patient with developing bronchopneumonia expectorating a sputum which is thin, watery, bloody and containing vast numbers of *Pasteurella pestis.* Death usually occurs on the 4th or 5th day.

Diagnosis

The clinical diagnosis of plague is confirmed easily, since the patient's sputum, urine and stools are loaded with plague bacilli, an organism easy to recognize.

Prophylaxis

A plague epizootic among rats always precedes an epidemic. Therefore, the control of this disease involves the destruction of infected rats. One device that has reduced the number of rats belonging to several species has been the use of oats poisoned with Warfarin (akin to Dicumarol), ANTU (alphanaphthyl thiourea) and Compound 1080.

The vaccination measures in use to prevent plague are too severe for general use but promise to be of value. The most rigid isolation of the patient must be preserved. Plague of the bubonic form is not contagious from man to man. So very contagious is pneumonic plague, however, that all persons near the patient should wear masks made of gauze and raw cotton, entirely covering the nose and the mouth, and gowns. All excreta must be destroyed and all clothes disinfected. The dead should be cremated.

Treatment

The patient should be made comfortable, stimulated in every way possible, and the buboes treated locally (by ice compresses or surgical measures). The antiplague serum on the market appears to have reduced the mortality of this disease. The drug of choice in treating plague is sulfadiazine; streptomycin likewise has been reported to be curative in its effects.

LEPROSY

Leprosy is a granulomatous disease due to *Mycobacterium leprae,* the characteristic features of which are its life-long course, waves of acute exacerbations separated by long periods of remission and destructive

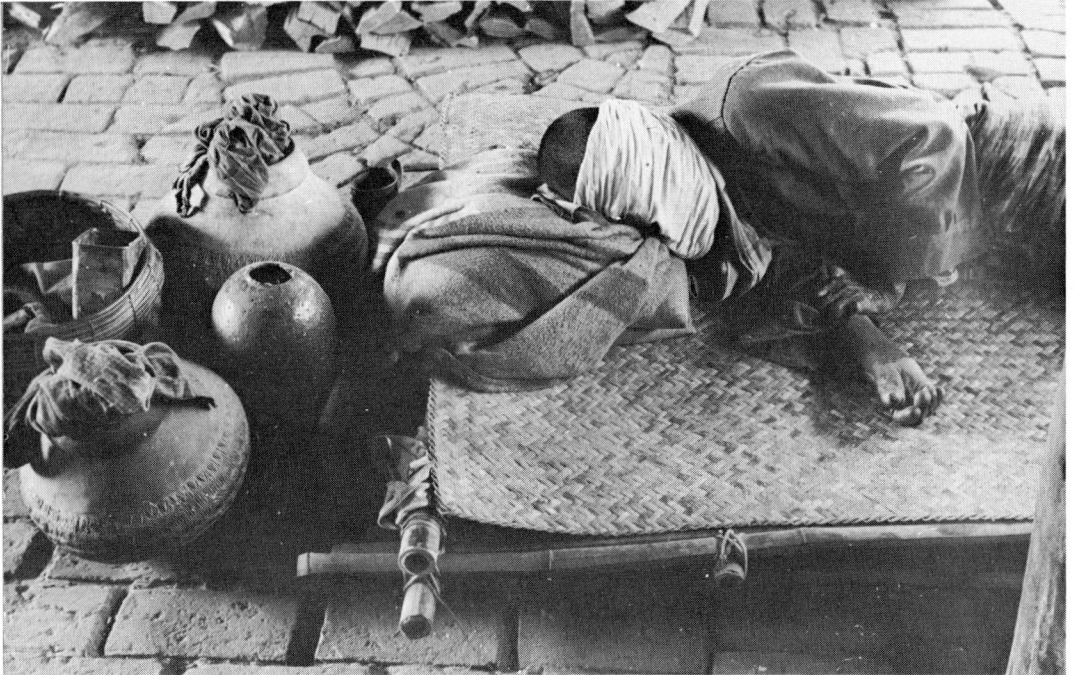

FIG. 431. Leprosy (Burma). Inspired by the new concept that leprosy is "no longer a disease apart," Burma, with an estimated 200,000 leprosy sufferers (over 10 cases per 1,000 population—a prevalence rate twice that of India or Thailand and the highest in Southeast Asia) in 1952 launched a nationwide antileprosy campaign, with the help of the World Health Organization. By mid-June 1957, 42,000 cases had been registered and 33,500 were being treated with sulfone drugs. It was hoped to increase the number of cases under treatment to 50,000 by the end of 1959.

A reminder of a past age: a victim of leprosy, his mutilated face bandaged to hide his sores, sleeps on a mat in the open. To provide shelter and treatment for these people who, in the past, have been driven from home and community on discovery of their disease, is the aim of the Burmese antileprosy campaign. (World Health Organization)

granulomatous lesions which develop in the skin and along the nerves.

Mycobacterium leprae is an organism which, in its appearance and acid-fast staining characteristics, resembles the tubercle bacillus. It differs from the latter, however, in that it does not infect animals and cannot be cultivated. The infectious granulomata of leprosy are larger and more diffuse than those of lues and tuberculosis, are painless, contain surprisingly large numbers of the bacilli and do not caseate.

Incidence

Leprosy is common in Asia, Hawaii, Iceland and Scandinavia; in America there are approximately 500 patients with this disease, between 35 and 75 new cases being reported each year to the U. S. Public Health Service.

Leprosy is transmitted by direct penetration of normal skin (particularly, and perhaps specifically, the skin of a child) by *Mycobacterium leprae*. The invading organism then finds its way into the axis cylinders of nerves via the axon-plasma filaments, i.e., the ultimate terminals of the nerves supplying the skin. Next begins a gradual ascent, organisms breaking out of these nerves at various points in the corium to produce macules and papules. These are painless, of course, since the germs which caused them to form did so after first cutting their communications, i.e., destroying their nerve supply.

Clinical Symptoms and Course

There are two varieties of leprosy, the tubercular and the anesthetic (neural). In the early stages the tubercular variety is characterized by the appearance of crops of dusky-red patches on the skin—the "leper spots." These may either disappear or develop into slightly raised, flat, infiltrated, anesthetic plaques of all sizes. One may cover the entire back. Later, losing their pigment, they may become pale. These nodules appear on the prominences of the body and at points of trauma. Those on the face, together with the loss of the eyebrows and the eyelashes, give the face a typical leonine appearance. These nodules, since anesthetic, easily become infected, ulcerate deeply and heal slowly, leaving deforming scars. This process often dissects fingers and toes, possibly a whole hand or foot. The sight is often lost. Acute exacerbations, characterized by fever and the appearance of a fresh crop of lesions, occur at irregular intervals.

In the anesthetic variety the granulomatous infiltration involves nerve trunks particularly, those under the skin being felt quite easily as nodular cords. As a result of these nerve lesions, anesthetic spots appear in the skin, are red at first but later white, while the muscles and other tissues supplied by these nerves atrophy. The muscular contractures which result may be extreme. Patients with this variety of leprosy may show no conspicuous signs of their disease for years.

Diagnosis

The appearance of the above-described anesthetic lesions is distinctive. Diagnosis often is made first by the discovery of leprosy organisms, usually abundant in the nasal secretion or in a biopsy specimen cut from a nodule.

Treatment

Most promising of all the chemotherapeutic agents presently used in leprosy are the sulfones, exemplified by Promin, Diasone, Promizole and Sulphetrone, all exerting a comparable therapeutic effect. Some subjective improvement often is evident within 6 months, is described by the majority of patients after 1 year and by nearly all after 3 years of sulfone therapy. Mucosal lesions respond most rapidly, oral nodules and infiltrations disappearing within a few months, paralleled with relief of nasal obstruction and clearing of laryngeal lesions. The smaller nodullary lesions in the skin shrink and absorb, leaving only pigment spots, and larger lesions disperse, with eventual scar formation. The recommended dose of Promin, as accepted at the International Leprosy Congress in 1948,* is 5 Gm. intravenously each day for from 1 to 3 months, followed by a rest period of 1 to 2 weeks. Diasone is given by mouth in doses up to 1.8 Gm. daily with a 1-week to 2-week intermission every 2 months, the average dose being 0.9 Gm. daily. Sulphetrone is administered in a daily dosage of from 3 to 6 Gm. orally each day for 6 months, followed by a rest period, determined by individual tolerance to the drug. Toxic complications of sulfone therapy include hemolytic anemia, leukopenia, allergic dermatitis, nausea, vomiting and headache.

The U. S. Public Health Service maintains a leprosarium at Carville, La., where excellent facilities and nursing care are made available to these patients by the Sisters of Charity, and where intensive therapeutic investigations have long been in progress, culminating in the recent developments outlined above, which are the most promising reported to date.

* An International Leprosy Congress Report, 1948, Internat. J. Leprosy 16:209, 1948.

44

Patients With Viral Infections

NATURE OF VIRUSES

In contrast with bacteria, viruses can be visualized only indirectly with the aid of electron microscopes (Fig. 432) and are capable of passing through filters which would hold back the smallest visible bacteria. Therefore, they are known as *ultramicroscopic* or *ultrafiltrable viruses*. Their growth depends on living tissues, apart from which they cannot be cultivated artificially. Strangest of all, while they are under the proper conditions, they obviously propagate themselves. In size they are known to be no larger than some protein molecules—too small, one might believe, to behave as living organisms.

Viruses infect all types of living tissue, plant and animal. There are innumerable varieties of viruses, and they differ greatly in size. Biologic experimentation and clinical observation teach us that they have different specific tissue affinities and "growth" requirements; they damage tissues differently and provoke different immune responses, just as do bacteria. The disorders which they cause are clinical entities and furnish some of our best illustrations of acute communicable disease.

MEASLES

Measles is an acute, contagious disease, caused by a filtrable virus, with conspicuous catarrhal features and a characteristic skin rash. It is so contagious that over half of the cases are in children under 5 years of age, and 97 per cent of the patients are under 15 years of age. It is most highly communicable during the early catarrhal stage through the secretions of the mouth, the throat and the nose, which indicates that

it is spread during the several days before diagnosis is possible. Its infective agent survives long in clothes, bed linen, toys or furniture, and may be carried by a third person. The disease is commonest in late winter and early spring.

Clinical Course

The incubation period of measles—that is, the time interval between exposure and the first appearance of the rash—is from 12 to 14 days. The period of invasion, called the *catarrhal stage,* begins approximately 11 days after exposure. This lasts 3 or 4 days, and during this time the patient has a running nose and eyes and generally feels wretched. In 97 per cent of all cases Koplik's spots, an early and positive sign of this disease, appear in the mouth in from 1 to 3 days before the rash develops. These are little bluish-white dots, pinpoint in size, each with a red areola, the majority of them being on the inner sides of the cheeks opposite the first molar teeth.

Toward the end of this prodromal period, headache, nausea and chilly sensations begin; the temperature rises (Fig. 433) and the coryza (as indicated by coughing, sneezing, redness of the eyes and lids and marked photophobia) increases. Then the measles rash appears; the forehead and the face are affected first, and in less than 3 days the entire body is covered. However, it is always most intense over the face and the back. It starts as little red macules, which, as they increase in number, become tiny papules arranged in groups, often crescentic in shape (see Plate 10). The tongue is furred, and the mucous membrane of the mouth and throat is red. Leukopenia is present.

FIG. 432. Influenza virus (type A), shown by the electron microscope ($1\mu = \frac{1}{25,400}$ in.) (Mudd, S., and Anderson, T. F.: J.A.M.A. **126:**561, 632)

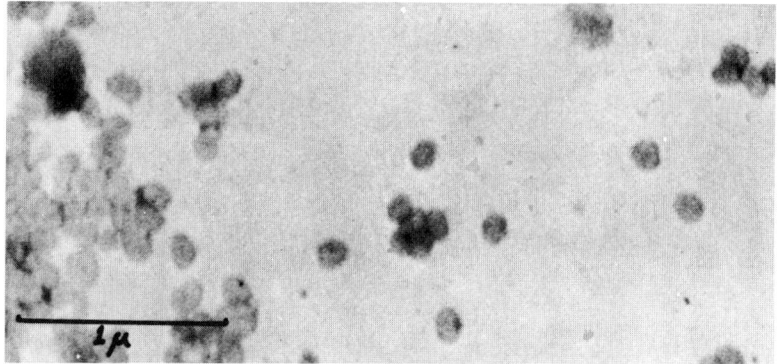

FIG. 432. Influenza virus (type A), shown by the electron microscope ($1\mu = \frac{1}{25,400}$ in.) (Mudd, S., and Anderson, T. F.: J.A.M.A. **126:**561, 632)

On the 5th or 6th day of the fever the symptoms begin to abate, and a fine, brawny desquamation of the skin begins. This usually is complete within a few days, but occasionally it persists for several weeks. In very severe cases the rash, instead of being of the papular variety, consists of numerous minute hemorrhages under the skin, associated with which may be hemorrhages from the gastrointestinal and the urinary tracts (black measles).

Diagnosis

Other diseases to be differentiated include German measles and roseola infantum. The latter does not occur after 2 years of age and is distinguished by the finding of enlarged nodes behind the ear and the delayed appearance of fever on the 4th day of the rash. Drug rashes, especially those due to the barbiturates and quinine, may closely resemble the rash of measles.

Complications

The most important aspect of measles is its predisposition to complications. These include otitis media and cervical adenitis, which no longer are of great concern since the advent of effective antibacterial chemotherapy, plus two others that are very important indeed—namely, encephalitis and bronchopneumonia. Encephalitis, severe enough to be recognized clinically, develops in 1 measles patient in 1,000; i.e., there are over 400 cases of measles encephalitis in the United States every year, and of these patients at least 160, and probably many more, are destined to become afflicted with mental deficiency or a serious personality defect. From the standpoint of mortality, bronchopneumonia is the most serious complication, accounting for the majority of deaths among infants with measles.

Prognosis

The contemporary death rate from measles in the United States is slightly over 0.2 per 100,000 population per year, and the mortality rate (proportion of cases of measles that prove to be fatal) in this country ranges between 0.7 and 1.0 per cent. This rate is not uniform throughout the world, however; in Chile, for example, the mortality rate in 1960 was 2.3 per cent, measles accounting for over half of all deaths from communicable diseases.*

* Ristori, C., *et al.*: Medical Importance of Measles in Chile, Am. J. Dis. Child. 103:236-241, March, 1962.

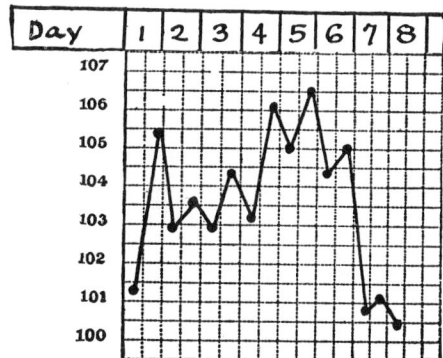

FIG. 433. Temperature chart of a typical case of measles. (von Strümpell's chart redrawn from Sahli)

Nursing Care

The patient with measles should be quarantined carefully for 1 week following the onset of the rash. Treatment is symptomatic and is largely a nursing problem. If the fever is high, fluids should be forced and cooling alcohol sponges applied. The air in the room should be kept fresh and cool. However, great care should be taken lest the patient become exposed to drafts and develop a cold, for secondary bacterial infections of the respiratory tract are prone to occur. Any earache should be reported and local treatment applied. The diet should be simple, abundant fluids supplied and the bowels kept loose by simple laxatives.

The eyes and the nose should be kept clean. Drops of saline or boric acid solution should be used for the eyes. The edges of the lids should be kept moist with petrolatum and the nose with Albolene. All bright light should be avoided, since it may cause intense distress. The room need not be and should not be in complete darkness, however. The catarrh of the nose and the throat is relieved by inhalations of compound of benzoin tincture and by applications of camphorated oil over the chest. Codeine will quiet the cough, and paregoric will loosen it. Starch paste or other mild antipruritics are indicated for severe itching. During desquamation, oil rubs and cleansing baths are indicated.

The physician and the nurse should be on the alert for complications, especially otitis media and bronchopneumonia. Such symptoms as a recurrence of high fever, cough or an increase in the respiratory rate are particularly important in this connection. The patient should be kept quiet in bed as long as there is any fever or any sign of a complication. Quarantine should be continued for at least 2 weeks after the onset.

Prophylaxis

Prevention or modification of measles is possible by the timely administration of gamma globulin, as described on page 1055.

Active immunization against measles has become possible through the development of a live attenuated measles virus vaccine (Enders), which confers a durable immunity without the risks of the serious complications that may attend the natural disease. Febrile reactions to the vaccine, which otherwise are likely to occur and likely to be fairly intense, are reduced in frequency and are ameliorated considerably by the simultaneous administration of immune gamma globulin. It is recommended that 1,000 tissue culture doses of the vaccine be injected subcutaneously into one arm, followed immediately by 0.01 ml. of standard gamma globulin per pound of body weight injected intramuscularly into the opposite arm. Measles vaccination ideally should be carried out between the ages of 9 and 12 months.

GERMAN MEASLES

German measles (Rubella) is a mild, though highly contagious, exanthematous disease of children, caused by a filtrable virus. It is best described as one "having the rash of measles and the throat of scarlet fever," but is not related at all to either. It would seem to be infectious for a day or two before the rash appears, but not later. Direct contact seems to be necessary for its transmission.

Clinical Course

The most distinctive features of this disease are its long periods of incubation (from 10 to 22 days), its short invasive stage (24 hours), with pharyngitis the chief prodromal symptoms, the characteristic skin rash, regional lymphadenitis, its benign course and the absence of complications.

The symptoms at onset are: slight fever (occasionally absent), headache, pain in the back and limbs, coryza and a characteristic swelling of the mastoid, the occipital and the cervical lymph nodes. The skin rash is one of tiny pink raised papules arranged in patches. They appear on the first or second day, first on the face, notably around the mouth and behind the ears, and within 24 hours cover the entire body. After 2 or 3 days this eruption fades, leaving no residue.

Diagnosis

This fever differs from measles by having fewer prodromal symptoms, less fever, a rash that is more diffuse and a little brighter in color, with patches less crescentic in shape.

Nursing Care

The treatment is that of any acute fever. Quarantine may be required for 1 week following the appearance of the rash.

German Measles in Pregnancy

Although it is one of the most benign of all infectious diseases as regards overt complications, German measles is nevertheless serious because of its potential effects on offspring in utero, congenital defects being caused in a significant proportion of patients during the first trimester of pregnancy. Thus, as many as 10 per cent of babies born of mothers who had German measles during the first trimester have exhibited abnormalities. Almost every type of abnormality has been observed, including stillbirths, congenital heart disease, cataracts, deafness, mental deficiency and anatomic defects of the gastrointestinal canal, the eye and the skeleton.

The implications to be drawn are obvious; namely, pending the development of some reliable method of artificial immunization, every female should be supplied an opportunity to acquire German measles before or during adolescence, if she has not already contracted the disease, and the population at large should be instructed regarding the importance of this step as a public health measure.

CHICKENPOX

Chickenpox (varicella) is a mild, acute, contagious disease due to a virus, its one characteristic feature being an eruption of vesicles appearing in crops.

Clinical Course

The period of incubation is from 14 to 16 days. It may, however, range from 4 to 27 days. The onset often is marked by chills, vomiting and headache. Children as a rule do not feel ill; adults, on the other hand, may experience symptoms as severe as those seen in smallpox.

Within 24 hours from the onset of the fever, the rash appears, earliest on the back or the chest, seldom on the face. It is characterized by red papules which rapidly become vesicles full of crystal-clear fluid. These vesicles are dome-shaped and so superficial that they seem to rest on the skin. They vary in number from a dozen, or more, to several hundred. They never coalesce and are without red areolae. Occasionally a few appear in the mouth, rupture and give rise to superficial ulcers. During the 2nd day, these vesicles become pustules, and two days later become dark-brown crusts, which fall off, leaving no scar unless scratched by the patient. Since successive crops of vesicles appear for 2 or 3 days, all stages of vesicle formation are present simultaneously (Plate 10).

Diagnosis

It is helpful in the diagnosis of chickenpox that at least one vesicle will contain a crystal-clear serum which is never seen in smallpox; that the pustules are always discrete and superficial, the skin around and under them not being infiltrated; and that vesicles of all ages are present at the same time.

Treatment is symptomatic. Isolation may

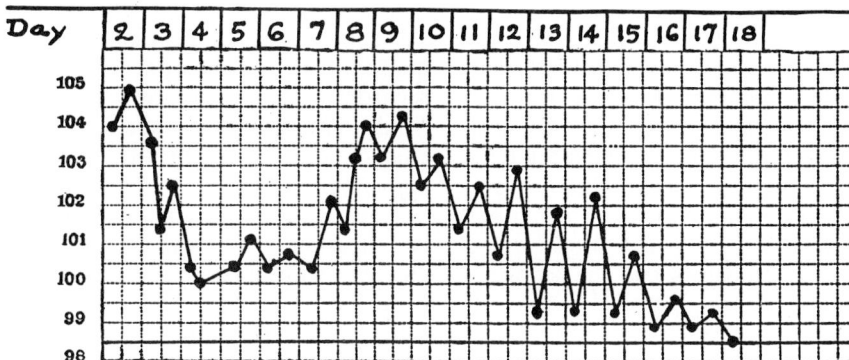

Fig. 434. Temperature chart of a typical case of smallpox. (von Strümpell's curve redrawn from Sahli)

be required until the crusts have desquamated.

SMALLPOX

Smallpox (variola vera) is an acute virus disease with a characteristic skin rash which evolves according to a remarkably regular schedule.

The virus is present in the skin lesions. The disease may be transmitted by direct contact at all stages and, for a long time, by exposed clothes or furniture. Lifelong immunity follows an attack.

Smallpox once was the most dreaded of epidemic diseases, and few exposed persons escaped it; today epidemics arise only in unvaccinated communities.

Clinical Course

The incubation period varies from 5 to 21 days. The onset is sudden—in adults, often with a chill; in children, with a convulsion. Headache and pain in the back and the limbs appear, and the patient vomits; the temperature quickly rises to 104° F. or higher (Fig. 434), the pulse becomes rapid, and sweats are common. At this time a confusing prodromal rash, often slightly petechial, may develop.

On the fourth day of the fever, the typical smallpox rash appears as an eruption of bright red macules from 2 to 3 mm. in diameter, which soon covers the body. These macules within a few hours become shotty papules which develop into vesicles with depressed centers containing pus and blood. These pustules, always most abundant on the face, the hands and the feet, have a characteristic greenish or grayish-yellow color. Each is surrounded by a narrow areola of inflamed skin. With the pustular stage the temperature, which may have subsided temporarily, again rises. This fever abates after 1 or 2 more days, and then the patient usually remains afebrile. The pustules after the 14th day dry down to crusts, which, beginning on the face, gradually drop off, often leaving a slight scar. Pitting, however, is made worse if the pustules and the scabs are scratched or picked.

The rash in severe cases may appear within 3 days after the onset of fever, and the total duration of the acute stage may far exceed the usual 3 weeks. The mortality is high in the severe forms of the disease. In those who recover, all the crusts may not have separated at the end of a month, and in this case the face is always left badly pitted.

Hemorrhagic Smallpox. More severe cases assume hemorrhagic features. On the 2nd or 3rd day of the fever in true hemorrhagic smallpox (black smallpox), subcutaneous hemorrhages cover the entire body, subconjunctival hemorrhages appear, and there is bleeding from the mouth, the nose, the lungs, the rectum and the kidneys. While a few patients recover, the majority die—some even before the smallpox eruption has had time to appear.

Complications

The complications of smallpox include laryngitis with edema of the larynx, bronchitis, bronchopneumonia and acute nephritis.

Prognosis

The general mortality of epidemics formerly was between 25 and 35 per cent. It now is between 6 and 8 per cent. Over 80 per cent of all fatal cases are of children under 10 years of age. In each outbreak, cases of all grades of severity occur, including those so mild that the patient remains up and about with an eruption consisting only of a dozen or so pustules.

Nursing Care

Any patient who has been acutely ill for less than 4 days with severe headache, backache and vomiting who presents papules, vesicles, pustules or crusts on the forehead and the wrists, all eruptions being at about the same stage of development, should be quarantined as a possible case of smallpox, regardless of how comfortable he may feel. Mild ambulatory cases dismissed as cases of chickenpox are responsible for the spread of epidemics.

The patient with smallpox must be cared for in a suitable hospital. The treatment is chiefly symptomatic. The severe pains of onset may be relieved by phenacetin, acetylsalicylate or morphine. Hydrotherapy is the best measure to control the fever. Paregoric will check the diarrhea.

Early in the attack the patient should be kept at bed rest despite the benign character of his symptoms, since complications are most apt to arise during this stage. The room is darkened, for the eruption is less severe if the skin is protected from bright light. During the vesicular and pustular stages the affected areas should be covered with an antibacterial agent such as tyrothricin or penicillin. Later the crusts are kept moist with petrolatum.

The amount of pitting is reduced by relieving the intense itching through use of calamine zinc lotion with phenol (2 per cent), so that the patient will not pick at his skin lesions. The eyes should be irrigated frequently with boric acid solution. If signs of conjunctivitis are detected, an ophthalmic ointment should be applied which contains an antibiotic, such as tetracycline (Achromycin), 1 per cent, and hydrocortisone, 1.5 to 2 per cent. A liquid diet is indicated.

The patient should be kept in isolation until every scab has separated, at which time precautions may be relaxed.

Prevention

A cross-immunity exists between smallpox and another viral infection, which is relatively mild and harmless, called "cowpox." By inducing the latter through the inoculation of the active virus, as described on page 1054, a permanent active immunity against smallpox is conferred (see Plate 9).

MUMPS

Mumps is a contagious disease due to a filtrable virus which causes an acute non-suppurative inflammation of the salivary glands, usually the parotids. Transmission is through the saliva. Its contagiousness is greatest at the onset of the attack. Mumps occurs in epidemic form in schools, armies and other groups. Children between 5 and 15 years of age are particularly susceptible.

Course and Symptoms

Mumps usually appears after an incubation period of about 18 days (the extremes are 8 and 30 days) following exposure. It starts with fever, malaise, chilly feelings and often a sharp pain on ingesting sour substances. A day or two later painful swelling of one or more of the salivary glands appears, most often of one parotid (hence the scientific name *epidemic parotitis*), but sometimes of a submaxillary or a sublingual gland.

Parotid swelling increases for 4 days, during which time other salivary glands usually become involved, although this spread may be delayed for as long as 6 weeks. At the height of the attack the fever is high and prostration is profound. The mouth can scarcely be opened, there is pain on swallowing, and often earache. The skin over the swollen glands is never red. After a fastigium of 1 or 2 days the swelling begins to subside.

Mild cases last but from 4 to 7 days; severe ones, 2 or 3 weeks. While some patients with mumps are scarcely ill, others are quite sick. The latter is particularly true of adults.

Complications

Orchitis and epididymitis in boys, and oophoritis in girls, the former followed by atrophy of the gland, are common complications. Other serious complications, which may prove to be fatal, are pneumonia, edema of the glottis and meningo-encephalitis. This last complication, common in some epidemics, may leave the patient deaf, blind or paralyzed. Involvement of the pancreas apparently is more common than generally regarded. Inflammation of this organ may cause abdominal pain radiating to the the back, together with marked epigastric tenderness. No disturbance of pancreatic function is associated with this form of pancreatitis.

Prophylaxis

It is claimed that the subcutaneous injection of convalescent serum during the first week after exposure to mumps will prevent an attack in an exposed child. The immunity so obtained is short, and the serum has no therapeutic value after symptoms of the disease have appeared.

Nursing Care

Mouth care is of considerable importance in this infection because of the dryness attendant on blockage of salivary secretion. A thick exudate of unpleasant taste is discharged into the mouth, and its removal is a great aid to comfort.

The pain associated with parotitis and orchitis, due to distention of their respective capsules, is lessened by the application of cold packs. If orchitis is severe, early surgical splitting of the testicular capsule may be carried out to relieve pain as well as to prevent pressure necrosis and atrophy of this organ. Should encephalitis develop, lumbar punctures are performed to relieve the increased intracranial pressure.

The patient should be kept quiet in bed, not only until the temperature is normal, but also until all glandular swellings have subsided entirely. This though difficult, is the only safe course, since serious complications possibly may be avoided thereby. Cold sponge baths are agreeable while the fever is high. A liquid diet is indicated. The mouth should be kept scrupulously clean. Hot or cold compresses applied over the inflamed glands may afford comfort. Proper support and an icebag relieve the pain of an orchitis.

Quarantine should be continued until all swelling of the parotid glands has subsided, or for a minimum period of 8 days from the onset of illness.

INFECTIOUS MONONUCLEOSIS

Infectious mononucleosis, or glandular fever, is an acute infectious fever, characterized predominantly by sore throat, painful enlargement of cervical lymph nodes and prostration. This disease is encountered almost exclusively in individuals between the ages of approximately 14 and 30 years. The distribution of incidence between sexes is almost precisely equal. The term "mononucleosis" is derived from the appearance of the blood leukocytes at the height of the infection, when the majority appear to be young histiocytes, which bear a superficial resemblance to monocytes, or hybrid forms, combining the features of monocytes, and lymphocytes (i.e., "atypical lymphocytes").

Epidemiology

Infectious mononucleosis, although very common indeed among individuals in the age group specified above, is not a highly contagious infection. Transmission from one member of a family to another, or from one roommate to another, is rare. Hospital patients with this disease appear to pose no

hazard to other patients on the ward. Neither nurses nor other hospital personnel seem to acquire the infection from these patients. Transmission from blood donor to transfusion recipient, however, probably has occurred. The most satisfactory explanation for the vast majority of cases proposes that the infectious agent is an extremely fragile virus that is excreted in the saliva of patients with the active disease and of individuals who are convalescent following the infection, or whose convalescence is complete, but who are carriers of the virus. Passage of the virus from one individual to another appears to require salivary interchange. The incubation period ranges from 30 to 50 days.

A typical attack begins with fever, chills and sweating, sore throat, cough and abdominal pain. On the second or third day, the lymph nodes begin to swell and become tender, usually the posterior cervical group first, then the anterior groups, later, sometimes, those of the axillae, and, on rare occasions, those over the entire body. These lymph nodes remain firm and later return to normal size. Occasionally the spleen also is enlarged. A morbilliform (measleslike) rash may appear transiently. The fever, which is high and markedly intermittent, continues for 2 or 3 weeks.

The leukocytosis, with an absolute decrease in the number of granular cells, is the most characteristic sign. The morphology of the leukocytes may be so atypical that a diagnosis of acute leukemia may be entertained and an unwarranted bad prognosis tendered. The total white cell count reaches its height (usually from 20,000 to 30,000 per cu. mm.) from the 10th to the 14th day of the fever. A valuable test for diagnosis is the heterophilic antibody agglutination test. It is positive if the serum or the plasma, after preliminary heating, in dilutions of more than 1:16, causes a suspension of sheep erythrocytes to agglutinate.

Complications

The enlarged spleen of infectious mononucleosis is unusually vulnerable to injury and may fracture if subjected to relatively mild trauma. Inasmuch as the consequences of splenic fracture are potentially serious, because of the substantial volume of blood that may be lost into the peritoneal cavity, patients with splenomegaly in the course of infectious mononucleosis must abstain temporarily from all exertional activities. A small percentage of patients (0.7 to 1.0) develop signs of encephalitis; a larger number may acquire the symptoms and signs of viral hepatitis (see p. 653); and rarely there may appear an acquired hemolytic anemia, a thrombocytopenic purpura, a self-limited cardiac complication or evidences of renal inflammation.

Practically all patients recover. The treatment is to keep the patient in bed and as comfortable as possible during the acute, febrile stage of the disease.

INFLUENZA

Influenza is a viral infection which has swept through the entire civilized world approximately every 20 years, attacking as many as 40 per cent of individuals in affected areas. The striking features of these epidemics have been the rapidity of their spread and an extremely high attack rate.

Typical epidemics of influenza have been characterized by 3 successive waves, separated by brief intermissions. The first wave lasts from 3 to 6 weeks, is explosive in outbreak, is widespread, and the majority of cases are mild and with few complications. The second wave also is widespread, but lasts longer; the cases are more severe, and the complications are serious. The third wave lasts still longer (from 8 to 10 weeks), involves fewer persons, but the complications are quite severe. During the years succeeding a major epidemic there follow scattered local waves of decreasing severity, with sporadic cases of influenza occurring during the intervals.

Etiology

The primary factor in the etiology of influenza is a filtrable virus, of which two major strains have been isolated, designated Types A and B. The most recent pandemic, which occurred in 1957, was caused by an antigenic variant of Type A (Asian, or Far East strain). Complications are due to secondary invaders, such as *Hemophilus influenzae,* various streptococci, pneumococci and other organisms.

Symptoms

True influenza, in the majority of cases, after a short incubation period of about 2 or 3 days, begins as an acute coryza, but one which presents several characteristic clinical features; suddenness of onset with high fever, a fiery redness of the upper respiratory mucous membrane, profound prostration, severe aching pains in the back and the extremities, injection of the conjunctivae and leukopenia.

Other cases start as an acute sinusitis, bronchitis, pleurisy or bronchopneumonia. These always are abrupt in onset and prostrating. In another group of cases, nervous features—headache, profound depression and prostration—predominate from the first; in still another group there are gastrointestinal symptoms of nausea, vomiting, abdominal pain, diarrhea, jaundice and collapse ("intestinal flu"); and, finally, in each epidemic, cases develop without local symptoms but with chills almost typical of malaria or with a continuous fever suggesting typhoid. The acute fever of the influenza itself lasts but from 1 to 4 days, and convalescence is rapid.

Influenzal bronchopneumonia, usually due to the pneumococcus, to *Hemophilus influenzae* or to streptococci, is the most common serious complication of influenza. The most dreaded type of this complication is streptococcal or staphylococcal pneumonia, which during severe epidemics develops early and may prove to be fatal within 24 hours from the onset of the influenza.

Late in an epidemic the cases develop serious complications, probably due to organisms for which the influenza virus seems to have prepared the soil. Among these are pericarditis, endocarditis, septicemia, peritonitis, appendicitis, nephritis, chronic bronchitis, bronchiectasis, otitis media and infections of the central nervous system.

The immediate mortality of uncomplicated cases of influenza is only 0.5 per cent, but its complications, such as the acute pneumonias and empyemas, are exceedingly serious. Other sequelae, of a chronic nature, include paranasal sinusitis, bronchitis and pneumonitis.

Prophylaxis

It has been recommended by the Surgeon

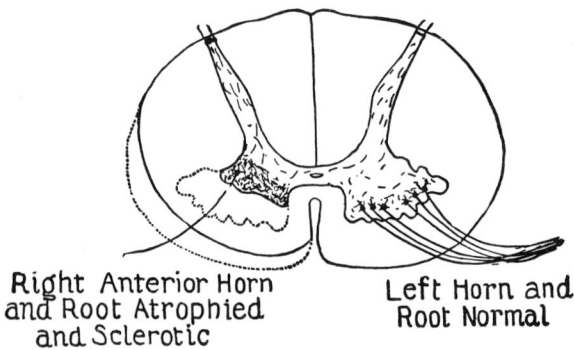

FIG. 435. Cross section of the spinal cord of a patient with anterior poliomyelitis. Note that the right horn has atrophied, its cells have disappeared, and the anterior root of the spinal nerve is shrunken.

Right Anterior Horn and Root Atrophied and Sclerotic

Left Horn and Root Normal

General's Advisory Committee on Influenza that individuals over 65 years of age, pregnant women, and persons who have chronic cardiovascular, pulmonary, renal, or metabolic disease be immunized against influenza.

Vaccines have been prepared from certain strains of influenza A and B. Ample evidence was obtained during the epidemic of Asian influenza in 1957 to indicate that individuals immunized against the Denver strain of Type A were not protected against the Asian strain of the same type. Any vaccine which could be expected to check an epidemic would have to be in readiness and on hand well in advance, long enough, in fact, to have been inoculated into a sizable proportion of the population at least 2 or 3 weeks ahead of the outbreak.

Nursing Care

There is no specific treatment for influenza. Phenacetin or aspirin may relieve the general aching. The nurse should be instructed as to proper local treatments to keep the nasal passages clear. Secondary pulmonary infections with streptococci or pneumococci may be expected to respond to penicillin or sulfonamide therapy. Any empyema which develops should be aspirated, or surgically drained if the effusion is large.

The greatest danger in cases of influenzal bronchopneumonia is that of vasomotor collapse for which vasopressor drugs are indicated. Dehydration must be combated by the intravenous administration of saline solutions and blood, as indicated.

The patient with influenza should be kept in bed until convalescence is well estab-

lished, in hope of preventing complications and sequelae. It is doubtful whether there is any virtue in isolating him or in disinfecting his sputum, since this disease would seem to be communicated to others immediately before its onset. The patient should receive from 3,000 to 5,000 ml. of fluid daily and the fullest diet that can be retained. Because of his great physical and mental depression, he should receive every encouragement and his surroundings should be made as pleasant and comfortable as possible.

Because of the frequency with which paranasal sinusitis complicates this disease, the nurse should see that medications in the

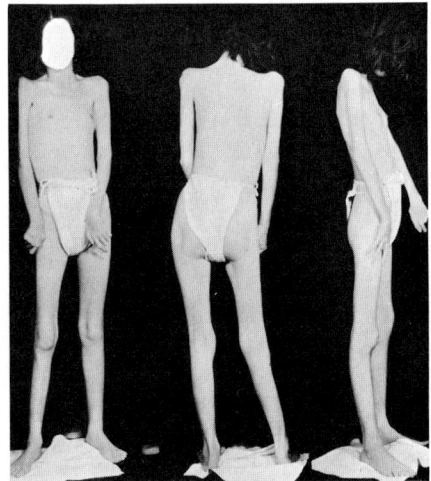

FIG. 436. Muscular wasting and postural deformities following severe poliomyelitis. (Louis Weinstein, M.D., Boston)

form of nose drops or inhalants, prescribed to keep the nasal passages clear, are applied regularly.

The patient with influenzal pneumonia demands particularly careful attention. The nurse should assist him in every movement of his body. Should the slightest cyanosis appear, she should report this to the physician at once and be prepared to administer oxygen.

Weeks or months may pass after an attack of influenza before the patient is truly well. For many patients a change in climate, when possible, is of great aid.

POLIOMYELITIS

Acute anterior poliomyelitis, or epidemic infantile paralysis (*polio* means gray, and *myelitis,* inflammation of the spinal cord) is an acute viral disease which, beginning as a general infection, gives rise to scattered foci of degeneration in the central nervous system. This occurs particularly in the anterior horns of the spinal cord, with a resulting flaccid paralysis of few or many muscles (Fig. 435). Other parts of the nervous system, however, may be affected similarly.

Anatomic Considerations

It is in the anterior horns of the cord that the nerve cells lie, the fibers of which form the peripheral motor nerves. If a motor nerve fiber is injured, a new one will grow from the cell to takes its place; but if the motor cell dies, its function never is restored. The nerve fiber and the muscle cell which it controls likewise die. This injury is permanent.

Epidemiology and Etiology

Acute anterior poliomyelitis attacks children during the second year of life most frequently, those between the ages of 3 and 7 years commonly, and adults rarely. Poliomyelitis is caused by a virus known as the poliovirus, of which 3 strains are known to exist. The polioviruses, in turn, belong to a group labeled enteroviruses, since they reside in the gastrointestinal tract. The Coxsackie viruses and the ECHO viruses, described on page 1104, also are enteroviruses. The portal of entry of the poliovirus is the oropharynx; its principal route of excretion is via the stools. The virus appears to be spread first by persons who become infected but develop no paralysis (the abortive type), and also by those who harbor the virus in the stools without showing any symptoms.

The disease occurs sporadically and also in scattered epidemics, which usually appear during the summer and the early autumn.

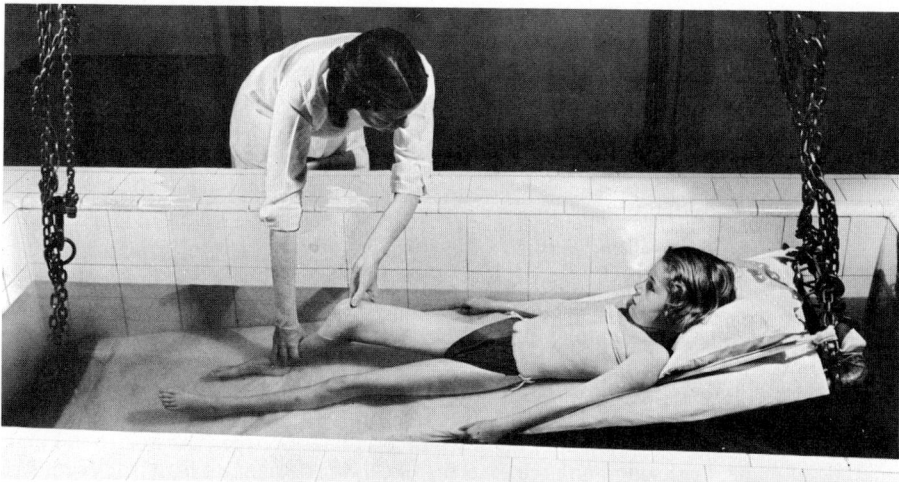

Fig. 437. The use of hydrotherapy for exercise and restoration of muscles paralyzed as a result of poliomyelitis. (Albert B. Street, New Haven Hospital)

Symptoms and Course

After an incubation period of from 4 to 7 days, acute anterior poliomyelitis may begin acutely as a head cold, with general toxemia and fever, or as malaise with such gastro-intestinal symptoms as marked diarrhea and vomiting. The fever lasts only a day or two, during which time the child is restless and somnolent by turns and always irritable. The disease may progress no further (the abortive cases). Frequently, moreover, the symptoms of this acute stage are so mild that they pass unnoticed. However, for many patients this is the preparalytic stage, often followed by a remission of apparent recovery lasting from one to several days. Then, suddenly, the child again becomes ill with headache, constipation and paralysis, and at the end of the first day the illness is at its height. In cases without a definite preparalytic stage, the mother suddenly discovers that the child does not move one or more of the limbs normally.

The *paralysis* at first would seem to be extensive, but gradual improvement begins at once, since the nerve cells that are not badly injured soon regain their function. Those actually destroyed, however, never do. There is seldom any sensory disturbance, for, as a rule, motor cells alone are affected.

At the onset of the paralysis the cell count in the spinal fluid rises; yet this fluid remains clear and no pellicle forms in it. There is a polymorphonuclear leukocytosis in the blood and general enlargement of the lymph nodes throughout the body.

The permanent paralysis may be exten-

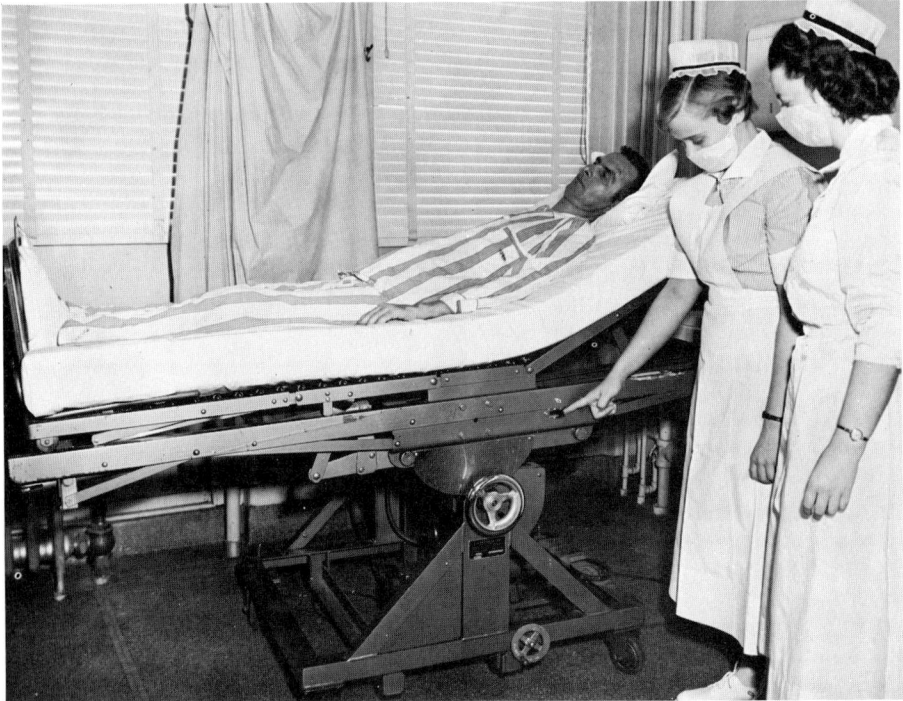

FIG. 438. A patient with partial respiratory paralysis, due to epidemic poliomyelitis, is about to enjoy a period of passive breathing on the rocking bed, a motor-driven, swivel device on which the Gatch frame oscillates between the horizontal and an inclined plane, or through an arc centering about the horizontal plane. This causes the abdominal contents to shift up and down in reciprocal fashion, alternately displacing the diaphragm upward, expelling air from the lungs, then allowing it to descend, aspirating air into the lungs.

sive, possibly limited to a few muscles of one or more limbs, and sometimes to only parts of muscles. This paralysis shows few characteristics in common with other types. It may involve the face, the diaphragm or the intercostal muscles. If the lesions are at the upper-motor-neuron level, the paralyzed muscles are spastic. If all the muscles of an extremity are paralyzed, this extremity, as the child grows, fails to develop normally and remains throughout life shorter and more shrunken than its mate—weak, limp and flaccid (flaillike) (Fig. 436). If a muscle is affected while its antagonist is not, the unopposed pull of the latter bends the joint and may cause serious deformity. This explains the development of one type of clubfoot. One attack of this disease confers an immunity which is permanent.

Nursing Care

During the acute paralytic stage the patient should be confined at complete bed rest. Hot, moist packs are applied for the relief of muscle spasm, and massage and passive exercises are instituted as soon as possible in order to avoid contractures and maintain muscle viability (Fig 437). Graduated active exercises soon are added to the schedule of physiotherapy. This program is pursued as intensively as possible during the early stages, for after 12 months have passed, little benefit is apt to be forthcoming except for the correction of static deformities by orthopedic surgery.

The first need of patients with poliomyelitis is an atmosphere of optimism, for nearly all of them, regardless of age, are plagued with fear. The nurse must provide the necessary explanations with patience, tact and kindness. In addition to establishing a sound relationship with the patient, she also must help the family to overcome tensions and anxieties. Both the patient and his family should have careful instruction from the doctor and the nurse regarding the

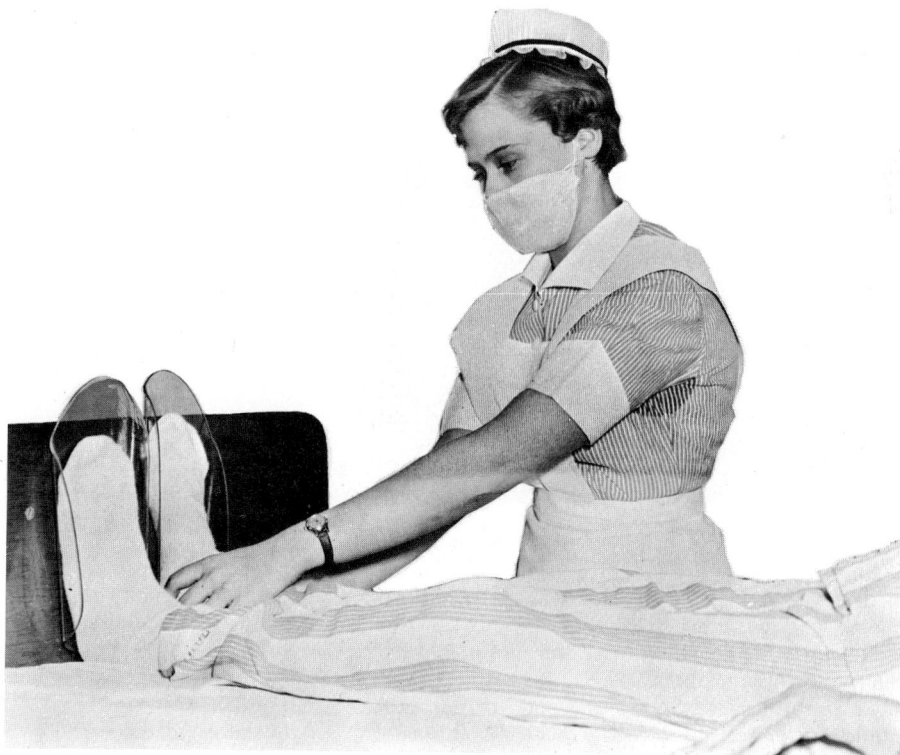

Fig. 439. A close-up view of the feet of the patient in Fig. 438 illustrating the manner in which these are held in correct alignment while the bed is rocking.

diagnosis, prognosis, treatment, isolation regulation and visiting hours and should be informed concerning the other members of the medical team who will participate in the patient's care.

The patient will be isolated, either separately or in a group, during the acute stage and then will be transferred to a convalescent unit. Those caring for the patient during the acute stage will wear a gown and use the hand-washing facilities which must be available to the unit. Concurrent disinfection will include the burning of nose and throat discharges, boiling of dishes and disposal of gastrointestinal tract discharges according to state health rules.

A regular hospital bed with a firm mattress protected by waterproof material is used; a full-length bedboard should be placed under the mattress, hinged to adjust to the Gatch frame. The use of the bedboard in connection with the firm mattress is an aid to the prevention of orthopedic deformities. A footboard is an essential addition to the regular hospital bed, the board being separated from the mattress by 4-inch blocks to prevent pressure of bedclothes, to provide a firm surface against which the patient may press his feet and to prevent pressure by allowing space for the heels.

The bed may be made with blankets with a sheet under the head. The blankets are

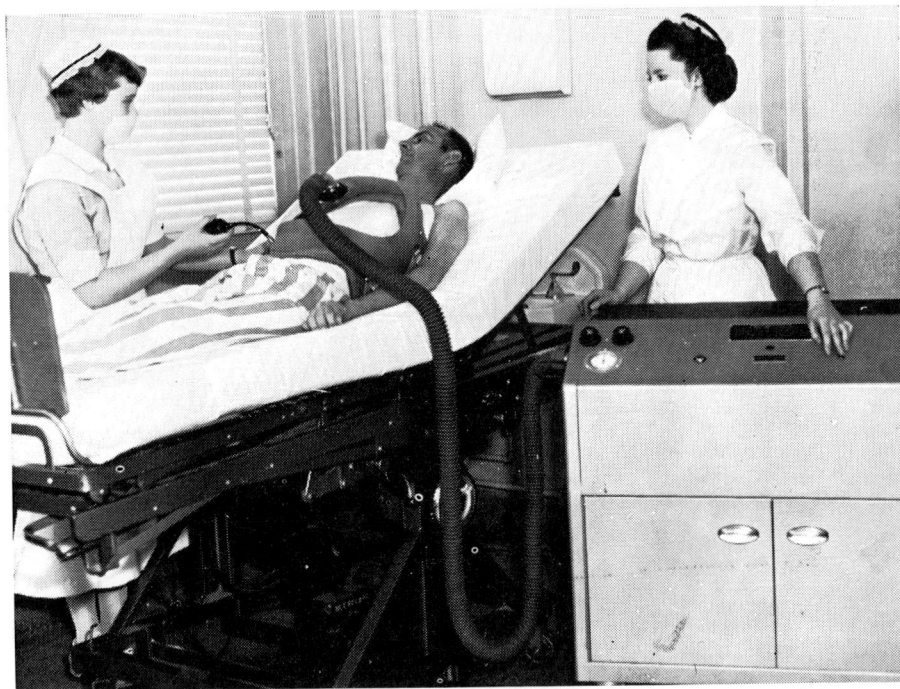

FIG. 440. A chest respirator has been placed on the patient (Fig. 438), and the nurse is sealing it airtight to the skin by inflating a rubber tube incorporated within the wall of the device. The cabinet at the right contains an air pump which alternately injects and withdraws air from the closed space surrounding the patient's chest, thereby producing rhythmic contraction and expansion of the thorax and passive ventilation of the lungs. The chest respirator compensates for the paralysis of the intercostal muscles; the rocking bed, for paralysis of the diaphragm. Either may be employed alone, or both together in combination. In the latter instance the two devices must be synchronized in such a manner that the chest is compressed each time the foot of the bed is elevated; otherwise, instead of reinforcing, each will impair the effectiveness of the other.

more absorbent than sheets and help to prevent chilling the patient. A neck roll may be used to support the neck muscles. Because rest is an essential part of the treatment, the environment should be peaceful in so far as possible.

Of paramount importance in preventing deformities is good body alignment. Frequent changes of position are essential, and when the patient is turned he is moved as a unit. The nurse must consider her own body mechanics in this procedure as well as those of the patient. As the patient is turned, gently but firmly, the joints are supported, taking care to avoid the muscle bellies which are acutely tender. While caring for these patients the nurse should become familiar with the variety of positions conducive to his comfort, described on page 352.

Personal hygienic measures should be carried out as usual with gentleness and a minimum of unnecessary handling. The skin, the mouth and the nose all should receive careful daily attention. The diet probably will progress from nourishing liquids to a regular one. The capacity for swallowing may be a factor in the feeding. Elimination should be supervised carefully to prevent constipation and retention. A record of fluid intake and output should be maintained and the doctor consulted regarding the use of laxatives and enemata. The bedpan should always be warm, and the nurse should warm her hands before touching the patient to avoid muscle spasm due to sudden changes of temperature.

Moist heat in the form of packs may be ordered. These help to relieve pain and spasm in the affected muscles and stimulate circulation to the affected part. The frequency of the packs will be determined in relation to pain and muscle tightness. They should be applied as hot as the patient can tolerate, using a team of aide and nurse if possible.

When caring for a patient with bulbar poliomyelitis, there are a few specific nursing responsibilities to be emphasized. The extent of involvement will determine nursing care. If pharyngeal paralysis is present, the primary objective will be to maintain a clear airway, which may be accomplished by suctioning, postural drainage or by a tracheotomy. The nurse must be on the alert for swallowing difficulties and report this immediately. Feedings by mouth should be withheld until ordered by the doctor, and when given the patient must be carefully supervised. Oxygen and a respirator should be kept available for instantaneous use. These patients should never be left alone.

Patients with respiratory muscle paralysis usually need the help of a mechanical aid to respiration. These include the tank respirator, the chest-abdomen respirator, the chest respirator and the rocking bed, all designed to provide the patient with adequate ventilation (Figs 438-440). The selection of the machine will depend on the degree of muscle impairment and on the general condition. When it becomes necessary for the nurse to care for a patient in any of these devices, she should become entirely familiar with all the mechanical parts as well as the technical skills needed to care for the patient. The making of the bed, changing positions, caring for the patient's personal needs, application of packs and the actual operation of the machine all should be reviewed.

Since convalescence for these patients is apt to be prolonged, the nurse should supervise the planning of such aspects of care as diversional therapy and rehabilitation. These will involve other members of the hospital team such as the social worker and the physical and occupational therapists. The need for the use of the public health nurse also should be investigated and plans made for discharge with follow-up care in the home.

Skillful nursing care is essential for all stages of the disease, and details of all phases should be made available to the nurse before she performs the care.

Polio Vaccination

Active immunization against poliomyelitis, which has been carried out on a wide scale since 1957, has resulted in a striking reduction in the incidence of this infection (see Fig. 421) and bids fair to eliminate it altogether as a serious threat to the public health. The initial method of vaccination involved multiple injections of formalin-treated, ultraviolet-light-irradiated, inactivated, tissue-cultured polioviruses (Types 1, 2 and 3), comprising the so-called "Salk-type vaccine." This method has been largely superceded and is likely to be replaced altogether by one that is simpler, safer from the standpoint of potential allergic complications, and equally or more effective—namely, the oral ingestion of attenuated live polioviruses (Sabin vaccine). This may entail, for example, the oral administration of 0.2 ml. of monovalent Type 1 attenuated virus (100,000 tissue culture doses) and, 6 weeks later, 0.2 ml. of bivalent vaccine consisting of Types 2 and 3 viruses mixed, 100,000 tissue culture units each.

OTHER ENTEROVIRAL INFECTIONS

The 3 strains of poliovirus that cause acute poliomyelitis represent one group of enteroviruses, so-named since poliomyelitis patients and carriers harbor the infective virus in their gastrointestinal tracts and the gastrointestinal mucosa is its portal of entry. Other members of the enteroviral family are the Coxsackie and the ECHO viruses, which have been implicated as the cause of several epidemic infections, including cases which are practically indistinguishable from "minor" or "nonparalytic" poliomyelitis.

Coxsackie Viruses

"Coxsackie" viruses are named after the town in New York State where the initial epidemiologic studies were carried out in connection with these agents. Two major types of Coxsackie virus are recognized, designated "A" and "B." Nineteen Type A and 5 Type B Coxsackie viruses have been distinguished so far. Type A has been responsible for aseptic meningitis, such cases having been precisely similar to nonparalytic cases of polioviral infection, or to lymphocytic choriomeningitis (page 1108). Type A also is the cause of a mild infectious illness of children called "herpangina," a disease of summer, which is characterized by the abrupt onset of fever and sore throat, the appearance of a vesicular eruption on the buccal mucosa and the pharynx and gastrointestinal disturbances, all of which subside completely within a period of a week or less. A rather nonspecific summer illness marked by fever, headache, stiff neck or back, an occasional rash and variable muscle aches also has been ascribed to Type A Coxsackie virus. Type B has been known to cause all of the illnesses enumerated above, including aseptic meningitis, which has been complicated by a transient and mild motor weakness comparable with that occurring in mild paralytic poliomyelitis. Type B also has produced a nonspecific febrile illness, with and without skin rash, as well as one variety of epidemic pharyngitis. It is the etiologic agent in epidemic pleurodynia, and it is also responsible for a dangerous type of myocarditis that occurs during the neonatal period and in early childhood and carries a high mortality.

ECHO Viruses

The term "ECHO," designating the third group of enteroviruses, is composed of the first letters of the words "enteric (indicating their intestinal location) cytopathogenic (producing damage to the cells supporting their growth in tissue culture) human orphan." Orphan refers to the fact that this viral species was discovered before it was known with what, if any, disease it might be associated. Approximately 20 strains of ECHO viruses are recognized, some of which have been responsible for an aseptic meningitis comparable with nonparalytic poliomyelitis. Paralytic cases of ECHO viral infection have been reported also. Other forms of ECHO infection include a nonspecific febrile illness, occasionally complicated by a skin rash; febrile illnesses accompanied by upper respiratory and gastrointestinal symptoms; and "summer diarrhea" of infants and young children. Most of the enteroviral infections are confined to the summer months. Two notable exceptions are caused by ECHO Types 10 and 20, both illnesses marked by a combination of respiratory and gastrointestinal symptoms.

Treatment

None of the enteroviruses is susceptible to any chemotherapeutic agent now available. Nursing measures are indicated, depending on the nature and the severity of the symptoms in each individual case.

EPIDEMIC PLEURODYNIA
Symptoms and Course

Epidemic pleurodynia (devils grip), an infection caused by Coxsackie virus, Type B, presents itself as an acute but brief febrile paroxysm of excruciating pleuritic pain referred to the line of attachment of the diaphragm to the chest wall, greatly exaggerated both by deep breathing and by the extension of the trunk. The temperature reaches its maximum (101° to 104° F.) within a few hours after the onset. With the pain there is a marked tachypnea of from 30 to 60 painful shallow respirations per minute. The leukocyte count is normal. The temperature falls with sweating, and the pain ceases usually within less than 24 hours following the onset. Often after 1 or 2 days of relative comfort the condition recurs, but in milder form.

The treatment consists of bed rest and analgesia, afforded by salicylates or, if necessary, morphine. Enthusiastic reports have been made on the use of quinine. In very severe cases the administration of oxygen, to permit adequate aeration with minimal respiratory movement, may be a comforting procedure.

EPIDEMIC ENCEPHALITIS

The epidemic encephalitides comprise a group of acute infections that affect predominantly the central nervous system. Each variety of encephalitis is caused by a specific virus. For each of these viruses there exists a particular animal reservoir, and each finds its access to man through the bite of a particular species of blood-sucking arthropod. Von Economo encephalitis (encephalitis lethargica, or "sleeping sickness"), first of the pandemic encephalitides to be recognized as such, has not recurred since 1926, in other words, since virologic technics have developed to the stage which would permit the identification of its causative organism, its vector or its animal reservoir. With respect to the viruses responsible for other forms of epidemic encephalitis, however, such identification has been possible and these data are available. The name,

common designation, geographic distribution, seasonal incidence, mortality rate, incidence of sequelae, mode of transmission, suspected animal reservoir and susceptible animals are specified for 7 important varieties of encephalitis in Table 24.

The clinical features of epidemic encephalitis are extremely variable and depend less on the type of virus that causes the infection than on the age of the patient who contracts it. Two forms of the disease, namely, the von Economo and the St. Louis types, have been characterized unusually well and are described jointly as being representative of the group as a whole.

Von Economo Encephalitis

This type of encephalitis, commonly known as "sleeping sickness," is characterized by its mild and gradual onset, with headache, insomnia and diplopia due to early paralysis of the eye muscles. Symptoms of meningeal and spinal cord involvement are not prominent. This stage is followed by one of pronounced lethargy. There is a marked tendency to permanent sequelae.

The first (acute) stage, which lasts from 1 to 7 days, often beginning as an upper respiratory infection with slight fever, headache, malaise and general muscle soreness, often is interpreted as influenza, but there also is marked insomnia and often diplopia. Following this stage some patients recover. Others progress to a stage of lethargy, during which, with consciousness clear, they lie motionless in bed or sit for hours staring ahead, incontinent and apparently oblivious to their surroundings. They eat nothing unless it is placed in the mouth; they never speak unless they are asked a question, when they respond briefly but clearly. Many other features, however, may dominate: paralyses, ataxia and symptoms suggesting paresis or dementia praecox. The patient may recover at this point, but usually with one or more permanent sequelae, such as paralysis of one of the cranial nerves, deafness or vertigo.

The second stage of this disease, of variable duration, is characterized by easy fatigability, headaches, insomnia or alterations in character suggesting psychoneurosis.

The third (parkinsonian) stage, almost characteristic of the von Economo type,

TABLE 24. Epidemic Encephalitis, Epidemiology and Prognoses*

Type	Geographic Distribution	Seasonal Incidence	Per Cent		Vector	Suspected Reservoir	Animal Disease
			Mortality	Sequelae			
Von Economo (encephalitis lethragica)	World-wide	Winter; early spring	30	20	?	?	?
St. Louis (SLE)	Central and western U.S.	Spring; early summer	5–30	Infants, 10–40; Adults 5	Mosquitoes	Chicken mite; mosquito (?)	Inapparent infection in many vertebrates
Japanese B (Murray Valley; Russian autumn (?); Australian X (?)	Japan, Java, Philippines, Australia, Korea, Manchuria, East Siberia, Indo-China	Summer; autumn	45–80	Rare	Mosquitoes	Horse (?); chicken (?)	Horse; inapparent infection in many vertebrates
Western equine (WEE)	Central and western U.S., Canada, Argentina	Summer	8–15	Rare	Mosquitoes	Chicken mite; wild bird mites; garter snakes	Equine animals
Eastern equine (EEE)	Eastern and central U.S., Canada, Mexico, Cuba, Panama, Brazil	Summer	65	60	Mosquitoes	Chicken mite	Equine animals; pheasants
Venezuelan (VEE)	Northern South America and Panama	Summer	Low (?)	Rare	Mosquitoes	?	Equine animals; rodents; birds
Russian spring-summer (RSSE; louping ill)	Far East provinces, USSR; Europe	Late spring; summer	30	20	Wood ticks	Ticks	Woodland mammals and birds

* Adapted from Coriell, L., in Harrison, T. R., et al.: Principles of Internal Medicine, ed. 3, New York, McGraw-Hill, 1958.

presents slowness of thought (bradyphrenia), slowness of muscular movements (bradykinesia), tremor resembling that of paralysis agitans and other possible sequelae, including tics, disturbances of sleep and characteristic personality changes. Such patients may become actively aggressive, unruly, destructive, cruel, yet without any sense of responsibility for their occasionally murderous acts, and they are not at all deterred by punishment. Young children may suffer permanent arrest of intellectual development.

St. Louis Encephalitis

This type of encephalitis is characterized at the onset by symptoms which suggest an acute infectious disease much more than do cases of the Economo type. Usually it begins suddenly with high fever, severe headache, a leukocytosis of from 12,000 to 20,000 per cu. mm., mental confusion or a delirium, often with pronounced signs of meningitis and spinal cord irritation, but seldom with paralyses of the eye muscles. The course of this disease usually is stormy. However, after 2 or 3 weeks improvement starts, and this often is the beginning of rapid and complete recovery. A chronic stage seldom develops.

The spinal fluid in all types of epidemic encephalitis is clear, its pressure moderately raised (from 60 to 120 mm.), its cell count fairly high (from 50 to 200 mononuclear cells per cu. mm.); there is only a slight pellicle or none at all, globulin is not increased, and the glucose level is normal.

The prognosis is varied. In outbreaks of epidemic encephalitis recoveries have ranged from 20 to over 60 per cent.

Secondary (Sporadic) Encephalitis

Secondary or "sporadic" encephalitis, clinically somewhat similar to the more primary types, occasionally follows various acute infectious diseases, particularly influenza, smallpox, chickenpox, vaccination, whooping cough, measles and mumps. It appears at a fairly definite period in the course of the primary disease, that is, after the disease has subsided and the patient is ambulatory. In cases following measles and other of the acute exanthemas the meningeal features are quite prominent (hence the term *meningoencephalitis*).

Nursing Care

In general, the treatment of acute encephalitis of all types is unsatisfactory. Elevation of the cerebrospinal fluid pressure is an indication for frequently repeated lumbar punctures and perhaps hypertonic sucrose intravenously. Respiratory paralysis necessitates the use of a mechanical respirator. For high fever, alcohol sponge baths and antipyretics are administered; sedatives are used to advantage for discomfort and restlessness.

Therapy in the chronic stages likewise is symptomatic. Stramonium, atropine and belladonna are of some value in the treatment of the spasticity of parkinsonism. Patients with postencephalitic narcolepsy and myasthenia are benefited by the administration of Prostigmin and amphetamine. Behavior disorders require educational therapy, and if this approach is unsuccessful, commitment to a mental hospital may be the only solution.

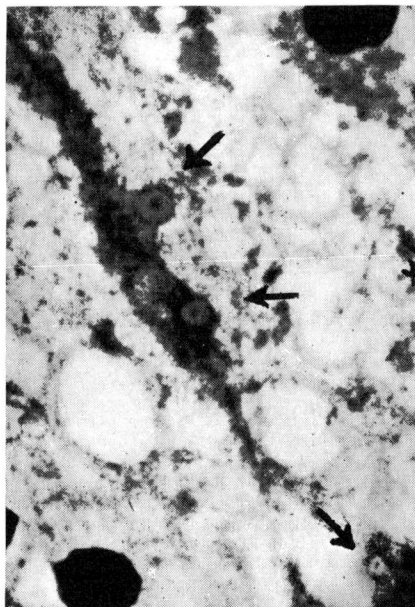

Fig. 441. Rabies. The arrows indicate the Negri bodies seen in a brain film or smear of a rabid animal. (The large black bodies at the corners are the nuclei of cells.) (Noguchi: J. Exper. Med., Rockefeller Institute)

The patient should be isolated, kept quiet in bed in a darkened room, fed an adequate liquid diet, through a nasogastric tube if necessary, and given fluids in abundance. Because of the incontinence so common, the urinary bladder and the rectum should be watched carefully for retention or fecal impaction, and scrupulous attention should be paid to the protection of the skin. To quiet the patient, hydrotherapy, paraldehyde and the barbiturates are recommended; however, if cerebral edema is present, morphine is never given, since this drug will tend to depress the respiratory center further.

LYMPHOCYTIC CHORIOMENINGITIS

Lymphocytic choriomeningitis is a virus infection of the meninges which gives rise to fever and symptoms of meningeal irritation resembling clinically those encountered in any form of meningitis. The epidemiology is not understood clearly. The virus probably enters the body through the respiratory tract, but the gastrointestinal tract, too, may be a site of entrance.

Clinically, the outstanding features include fever and generalized malaise, often developing subsequent to an ordinary upper respiratory infection, headache, vomiting and stiff neck due to meningeal inflammation and increased intracranial pressure. The course is benign, usually terminating without sequelae within 2 weeks.

The diagnosis is suspected when, in an acutely ill febrile patient with meningeal signs, sterile spinal fluid under pressure and containing an abnormal number of mononuclear cells is found.

Treatment is purely symptomatic and is directed toward the patient's comfort. Elevation of the spinal fluid pressure is controlled by means of repeated spinal drainage.

RABIES

Rabies (hydrophobia) is an acute and almost invariably fatal disease communicated to man through the saliva of a rabid animal—usually a dog, and occasionally a bat. Dogs, fortunately, always present evidence of the disease before becoming infective. The etiologic agent is an ultramicroscopic virus present in the saliva and the central nervous system. Negri bodies (round objects about one quarter the size of red blood corpuscles) are found in the brain tissues so constantly in this disease that their presence is sufficient for diagnosis (Fig. 441).

The course of rabies in dogs is characterized by an incubation period of from 20 to 30 days. This is followed by a period of excitement, when the animal becomes vicious. The excitement stage may not be evident at all (dumb rabies) or may be entirely absent. Paralysis then develops, first involving the hind legs and thereafter becoming general. Death occurs within 10 days following the first symptom.

During the year 1952 there were 8,469 cases of rabies reported to the U.S. Public Health Service; 8,445 of these were in animals, and 24 in man. In 1961 there were 3,599 infections in animals, and 3 in man.

Clinical Course in Man

In humans the incubation period varies from 2 weeks to 1 year, depending on the location of the wound and the extent of the bite. After infection from a wound, the average period of incubation is 40 days. This period is shorter following bites on the face.

The attack starts with a premonitory stage, during which the flesh around the point bitten becomes inflamed, and the patient is mentally depressed and irritable. Then follows the stage of excitement, during which even the slightest sensations produce violent spasms, particularly of the throat. The very sight of water induces such spasms that the patient writhes (therefore, the name *hydrophobia*). Maniacal attacks occasionally occur but are rare. This stage lasts from 1 to 3 days and is followed by the paralytic stage, which lasts from 6 to 18 hours, terminating in coma and death.

Diagnosis

If a dog is suspected of being rabid, the animal should not be killed, but instead should be captured and closely watched. If within 2 weeks no signs of disease have developed, rabies is ruled out. If the above-described symptoms develop, the animal is killed at once and the brain is examined for the characteristic Negri bodies. If the dog escapes observation (as is usually the case), should rabies be suspected in the slightest degree, the person bitten must be vaccinated.

Prophylaxis

The bite should be subjected to thorough lavage at once, and as soon as it can be procured, antirabic serum should be infused into, and injected under, the wound. Rabies vaccination (Pasteur treatment) should be started immediately, since, by virtue of the long incubation period in this disease, it may be possible to stimulate an active immunity in the patient before the virus takes effect.

Pasteur found that by inoculating one rabbit after another, each with an emulsion of the spinal cord of the former of the series, the virulence of the rabies virus so increased that its incubation period shortened from 15 or more to only 7 days. Preparations made from spinal cords of rabbits infected with this "7-day virus," attenuated by drying for various periods of time, are injected subcutaneously into the patient in ascending doses for 21 consecutive days. The result of Pasteur treatment, when properly applied, is occasionally satisfactory.

The Semple vaccine now is used most commonly. The virus, obtained as described above, is weakened with formalin. Its injection daily over a period of 2 weeks affords a measure of protection which hopefully lasts for several months.

Nursing Care

If the disease does develop, the patient is placed in a quiet dark room, sedated heavily and given hypnotics, analgesics and antispasmodics without stint. Curare, administered under expert supervision, occasionally is beneficial. Nevertheless, a fatal outcome is to be anticipated in a high proportion of cases.

Nursing Precautions. It is to be borne in mind that the rabies virus is contained in the saliva of patients with this disease, constituting a distinct hazard to nurses and attendants who are responsible for their care. All personnel must be on guard against being bitten by such a patient and, if bitten, must receive the same treatment as the patient, including antirabic serum and rabies vaccine.

LYMPHOGRANULOMA INGUINALE

Lymphogranuloma inguinale is one of the important venereal diseases, although, like syphilis, it may occur also after extragenital contact with an infected individual. It is due to a filtrable virus which produces its effect by attacking the lymphatic structures adjacent to the site of inoculation. As a result, there eventually develops lymphatic obstruction, lymphedema and, finally, scar formation in the tissues so involved.

Course

Clinically, the disease is characterized by the development, a few days following contact, of a small, comparatively innocent-appearing primary papule at the point where the virus has entered the body, usually on the penis or the vulva. This lesion disappears in the course of a few days, and much later, perhaps after several weeks or months, the inguinal nodes enlarge progressively. There is inflammation of other communicating lymph glands as well; in the female those nodes encircling the rectum commonly are involved. Often present at this stage is fever, which may be prolonged for weeks or months.

Secondary to blockage of the lymphatic channels communicating with these inflamed nodes, there is swelling of the soft tissues which they drain. Thus, in the male there is edema of the penis and the scrotum, and in the female, swelling of the labia. Later, scarring of the nodes and the adjacent structures takes place. In women this may produce rectal stricture of high grade, occasionally necessitating complete rectal resection. A significant percentage of infected persons, however, appear to suffer few ill effects from the disease—a circumstance which renders its control a difficult public health problem.

The *diagnosis* of lymphogranuloma inguinale is made on the basis of a positive skin reaction (Frei test) through use of an antigen material from previously unopened infected lymph nodes (buboes). This gives positive results in about 95 per cent of the cases.

Treatment

Favorable results in acute cases of lymphogranuloma inguinale have been obtained with the use of sulfadiazine, and especially chlortetracycline, in response to which buboes usually diminish in size within 4 days, rectal bleeding ceasing and ulcerations healing very promptly thereafter. (Granuloma inguinale, with similar clinical manifestations, but caused by a bacterium rather than a virus, is equally responsive to chlortetracycline.) Rectal strictures developing late in the course of the disease are affected little by chemotherapy, although partial symptomatic relief has been observed in patients receiving chlortetracycline, the use of which, it is hoped, may eliminate, at least, the necessity for radical resection of the rectum.

DENGUE

Dengue is an acute fever which often appears in pandemic form, due to a virus transmitted by the mosquito *Aedes aegypti* (the same one that is responsible for yellow fever), also by the *Aedes albopictus*. Its attack is characterized by suddenness of onset, high temperature and extreme pains. Because of its duration, it is called *seven-day fever,* and because of its pains, *break-bone fever.* The facial expressions it induces suggest the name *pantomime fever,* and the stiff gait of ambulatory cases, *dandy fever.*

Dengue is common in the West Indies, the Pacific islands, in countries about the China Sea and in the vicinity of the Mediterranean. Never is it encountered in temperate climates nor in subtropical regions after the first frost. In the Southern states, epidemics have occurred in association with yellow fever; but dengue is particularly prevalent in India, a country where yellow fever does not appear.

Clinical Symptoms and Course

The incubation period of dengue is from 3 to 9 (usually 7) days. Its onset is sudden, with a rapid rise of temperature as high as 106° F., rapid pulse, intense headache accompanied by nausea and severe pains in the eyeballs, the back and the limbs. In a few hours the patient is prostrated, his headache intense, and he cannot move because of excruciating pains in the limbs on active (but not on passive) movements. This stage lasts from 1 to 3 days. Then the temperature rapidly falls to normal, often with a profuse sweat, and for a period of from 1 to 3 days the patient feels well. The fever may rise again and the pains return, whereupon the specific skin rash appears on the back, the chest and the extremities. This rash consists of a crop of small, bright-red macules which disappear on pressure. They may coalesce, giving the appearance of scarlet fever.

In a few hours the fever may subside, and the rash disappears in from 1 to 3 days. Often during this period there is marked bradycardia, a generalized lymph node enlargement may appear, and leukopenia (to 1,200 cells per cu. mm.) is observed. The urine only rarely contains a trace of albumin. A second, milder attack may soon follow, even a third and fourth, still milder. The complications which may occur include hemorrhages from the nose, the stomach, the bowel and the uterus.

Convalescence usually is speedy and permanent. The mortality of the disease is less than 0.1 per cent.

Nursing Care

Symptomatic treatment alone is possible. The salicylates may be useful in affording relief from the joint pains, but the severity of these pains may be such as to require the use of morphine. Purges should be avoided, so painful are the muscular movements involved. General tonic treatments will be necessary later.

The patient should be made as comfortable as possible, given a liquid diet, cold drinks in abundance and cold sponges for hyperpyrexia.

Prevention

Measures that are important in the prevention of dengue include the use of screening, bed nets and other measures effective against the *Aedes aegypti* mosquito.

YELLOW FEVER

Yellow fever, caused by a virus transmitted by the mosquito *Aedes aegypti,* presents a characteristic triad of symptoms: early jaundice (hence the name); a tendency to hemorrhage, particularly from the stomach (therefore the black vomit); and marked albuminuria.

Yellow fever is endemic in the West Indies, Central and South America and in a limited region of West Africa. During the summer, however, following the migrations of the *Aedes aegypti* mosquito, epidemics have spread to the temperate zone, even to New England. This mosquito becomes infective 12 days after it has bitten a patient with early-stages yellow fever. The control of that mosquito, by the draining or oiling of its breeding places, has eliminated this disease in Panama and Havana.

Clinical Symptoms and Course

The incubation period varies from 2 to 12 days. The onset is sudden, with fever which in 24 hours reaches about 104° F., the pulse rate meanwhile becoming slower and slower. Definite mental excitement, marked injections of the conjunctivae, muscular pains that are most severe in the lower back and the calves of the legs and profound prostration follow. On the 2nd day the specific symptoms appear: jaundice, a petechial skin rash, uncontrollable bloody vomiting, stools which are diarrheal and tarry, profuse epistaxis, bradycardia and marked albuminuria. On the 4th day the case reaches its height, with all the above symptoms most intense.

The outcome of the disease depends to a large extent on the kidneys, for in fatal cases the nephritis progresses until death, which occurs between the 4th and the 7th day. Of the nonfatal cases, the convalescence is usually with perfect recovery. A single attack confers a permanent immunity.

Diagnosis is by specific agglutination tests. Infectious jaundice (Weil's disease) presents practically the same symptoms, only milder.

Yellow-fever vaccine confers an effective immunity lasting several years.

The *mortality* of epidemics of yellow fever has varied from 15 to 85 per cent.

Nursing Care

There is no specific therapy for yellow fever, hence treatment must be symptomatic. Transfusions, parenteral fluids and stimulants often are necessary to combat vascular collapse.

The patient should be given absolute rest in bed. Intravenous glucose and saline solutions are administered until the patient is able to take carbohydrate and fluid in sufficient quantity by mouth. The diet thereafter is prescribed, depending on clinical evidences of liver and renal damage. A long period of convalescence usually is required, activity being resumed by slow degrees.

PSITTACOSIS

Psittacosis is a specific acute virus disease of parrots and birds of the parrot family, highly contagious for exposed persons. The virus may be demonstrated in the droppings of sick birds. It withstands prolonged drying and enters man through the mucous membranes of the upper respiratory tract. It is disseminated from infected persons by way of the excreta and the sputum. However, these patients cough very little, and transmission from man to man, therefore, is not a serious problem.

Symptoms and Course

After an incubation period lasting from 7 to 15 days (it may be as long as 6 weeks in man, 6 months in a parrot), the disease begins abruptly with malaise, headache, photophobia and chills. Its course is characterized by high fever, great weakness, marked depression and delirium, with surprisingly slow pulse and respiration. Typhoidlike rose spots may appear on the skin. The respiratory complications of bronchitis and bronchopneumonia characteristically are present. This pneumonia is central and, therefore, difficult to discover except by x-rays. In cases which recover, the temperature falls by lysis during the 2nd or the 3rd week. Convalescence is slow, and relapses are common.

The *mortality* of psittacosis is approximately 20 per cent, although it has been reported as high as 40 per cent. Among older individuals, death in the early stages is most apt to be due to heart failure; in the late stages, as a result of pneumonia.

Psittacosis responds to antibiotic therapy with penicillin and particularly with chlortetracycline, the administration of which ordinarily is followed by a rapid and uneventful convalescence. Active immunity is acquired as a result of the infection; artificial immunization, therefore, theoretically is possible, but its value has not as yet been demonstrated.

FOOT-AND-MOUTH DISEASE

Foot-and-mouth disease (epidemic stomatitis, aphthous fever) is a contagious virus disease of animals with cloven hooves. It is transmitted to man through the milk of infected animals, as well as by contact with the animals. The features of this disease, which persist for as long as 10 days to 3 weeks, are malaise, fever and an eruption of vesicles in the mouth and the pharynx (rarely on the hands and the feet) which rupture, leaving shallow ulcers.

Its *mortality* is about 8 per cent.

Treatment is symptomatic for the fever, a mouth wash of potassium permanganate and the local application of silver nitrate for the ulcers. The patient should be isolated.

45

Patients With Rickettsial Infections

RICKETTSIAE

The rickettsial diseases, of which the three commonest on this continent are typhus fever (Fig. 442), Rocky Mountain spotted fever (Fig. 443) and trench fever, are named after Dr. H. T. Ricketts who first discovered one of their germs. They are vermin-spread infections caused by tiny organisms shaped like bacilli, found in the patient's tissues and in the bodies of their insect vectors, the latter, for the most part, being ticks and fleas. As in the case of ultramicroscopic viruses, these organisms make their habitat, thrive and produce their effect within the tissue cells, as contrasted with the bacteria whose activities are extracellular. Like viruses, the rickettsiae cannot live apart from animal cells, and their culture, to date, has proved impossible in artificial media other than that containing live tissue. It is obvious from this fact that the survival of these organisms in nature depends on the accessibility of suitable living hosts, called *reservoirs.* Serving as reservoirs of the rickettsiae are rodents, monkeys, dogs, dog ticks and wood ticks. Individuals harboring rickettsiae are likely to exhibit fever and skin eruptions and to be afflicted with disorders of the central nervous system, as will be described in this chapter.

Typical of all rickettsial infections is the appearance in the blood serum of a bacterial agglutinin that has the property of agglutinating bacilli of the Proteus OX group. (The reason for this is obscure, for there is no other relationship known beween Proteus OX and the rickettsiae.) The phenomenon is the basis for a diagnostic test useful in differentiating this group of diseases, as a whole, from other infectious diseases. Fur-

ther differentiation of one rickettsial disease from another is made possible by the use of tissue cultures and protection tests (inoculating suspected material into susceptible animals and into animals previously vaccinated with rickettsiae of known identity).

TYPHUS FEVER

Epidemic typhus fever (camp fever, ship fever, prison fever), one of the most deadly epidemic diseases in history, is an acute infectious fever, world-wide in distribution, caused by *Rickettsia prowazekii.* Its natural reservoir is man himself, and its vector is the body louse, which transmits the infection by inoculating feces, contaminated with the organism, into broken skin. The most prominent characteristics of this disease are its sudden onset, severe headache, marked nervous and mental features and hemorrhagic and gangrenous skin lesions.

Brill's disease is regarded as being a mild variant of epidemic typhus, i.e., a recurrence of the latter following a lapse of many years following the original *prowazekii* infection. This form of the disease has been encountered principally in the United States, Switzerland and Yugoslavia.

Endemic typhus fever (murine typhus), likewise world-wide in distribution, is caused by another organism, namely, *Rickettsia mooseri.* Its reservoir consists of small rodents, whence it is transmitted to man by fleas, which inoculate the skin with infected feces. Scrub typhus, a disease of Asiatics, Australians and Pacific Islanders, is caused by *Rickettsia tsutsugamushi,* which is transmitted from small rodents to man by the bites of mites.

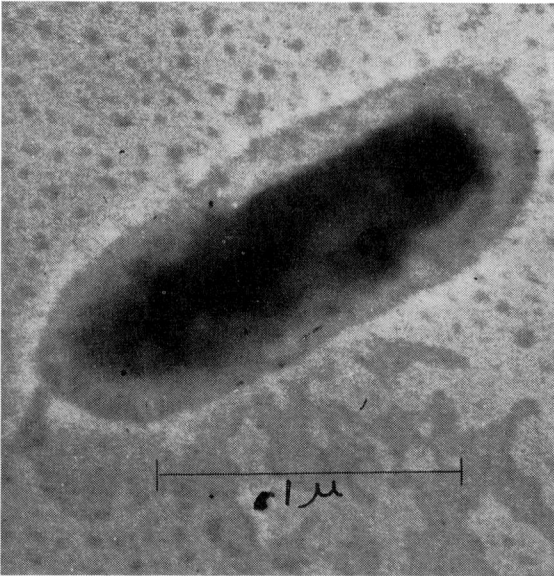

FIG. 442. Rickettsia from a patient with epidemic typhus fever shown by the electron microscope. ($1\mu = \frac{1}{25.400}$ inch.) (Mudd, S., and Anderson, T. F.: J.A.M.A. **126**:561, 632.)

Clinical Symptoms and Course

The period of incubation lasts from 5 to 21 days. The onset is abrupt with rapid rise of temperature, chills, severe headache, pains in the limbs and marked mental depression. The face becomes flushed, its expression tense, excited and anxious. The conjunctivae are deeply congested. Prostration is extreme. Severe headache is the most constant symptom. Delirium is present in all but the mildest cases; in those more severe, a typhoidal state, or the physical signs of meningitis (with clear spinal fluid), may develop.

The typhus skin rash appears on about the 5th day of the disease, first on the shoulders and the trunk, but in time it may cover the entire body surface except the face. At first, it is characterized by erythematous macules from 2 to 5 mm. in diameter, which become increasingly hemorrhagic. Often bleeding occurs from the stomach, the bowel or the kidney. Skin necroses, due to thromboses of the superficial blood vessels, appear over the bony prominences (such as hips, sacrum, elbows and scapulae). Symmetrical gangrene of the extremities is not uncommon.

The temperature for about 12 days is elevated but irregular, the pulse rate is high in proportion to the fever and markedly intermittent, and the blood pressure is low. The spleen is enlarged. There is seldom a leukocytosis. The urine contains albumin.

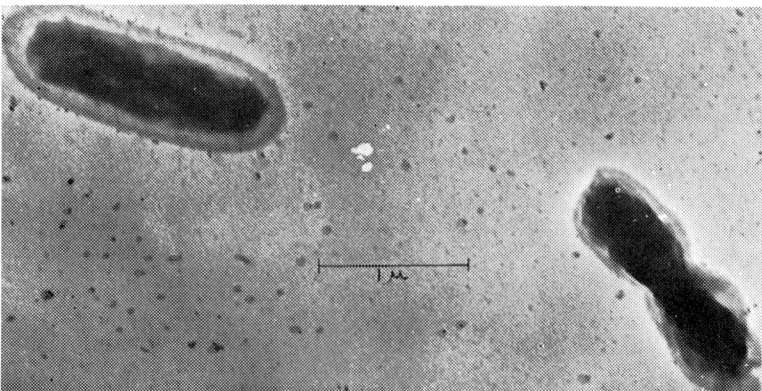

FIG. 443. Rickettsia from a patient with Rocky Mountain spotted fever, shown by the electron microscope. ($1\mu = \frac{1}{25.400}$ inch.) (Mudd, S., and Anderson, T. F.: J.A.M.A. **126**:561, 632.)

The profuseness and hemorrhagic features of the eruption and the severity of the nervous and mental features between the 10th and the 12th days are the best indices of the prognosis. In favorable cases improvement begins anywhere from the 10th to the 12th day, and, unless complications arise, the temperature reaches normal on approximately the 14th day. Even with the temperature normal, however, the delirium may develop into coma. Fatal cases usually survive but a few days and then die of bronchopneumonia.

Prognosis

The mortality in typhus fever epidemics has varied from 5 to 70 per cent; in sporadic cases, from 2 to 3 per cent; in cases of the American type, less than 1 per cent. Few under the age of 20 years die, but the mortality increases with age. An immunity which persists for a number of years follows an attack of typhus fever.

Chemotherapy and Nursing Care

Prompt, specific therapeutic responses have been observed to both chloramphenicol and chlortetracycline, 2 to 3 Gm. daily, in cases of scrub typhus and murine typhus, chlortetracycline being particularly effective in the treatment of epidemic typhus fever. Otherwise, therapy consists of rest, hydrotherapy for the fever, barbiturates or chloral hydrate for the insomnia and codeine or another sedative for the relief of cough.

If the patient is well deloused there is no danger entailed in caring for him. The diet should be soft and ample, with liquids in abundance. An icebag may relieve the headache. The mouth must be kept clean.

The treatment of the convalescent should be continued for a long time because of the persisting nervous and mental exhaustion.

Prevention

Typhus vaccine apparently possesses definite prophylactic value. Other methods of equal importance in endemic areas, when practical, include frequent baths and changes of underclothing, the use of insect repellants containing DDT and frequent inspection of the clothing and the hair. The clothing may be deloused by exposing it to methyl bromide gas (available in ampules), which is effective against eggs and nits as well as the adult lice. Dry heat (135° F.) for 5 minutes is adequate but difficult to obtain throughout an entire mass of clothing; steam, although efficient, is ruinous to clothing. Hair contaminated with head lice may be clipped short, massaged with vinegar and shampooed vigorously with hot soapy water containing kerosene in a concentration of 25 per cent.

All patients with typhus should be segregated in quarantine for a period of 16 days following an attack.

ROCKY MOUNTAIN SPOTTED FEVER

Rocky Mountain spotted fever typically is characterized by a continuous fever of 3-weeks' duration. It begins abruptly with a chill, severe pains in the bones and muscles, headache and a profuse skin eruption, at first macular and later petechial. In severe cases there appear also areas of skin necrosis due to an endarteritis (inflammatory blockage of the arterioles). The disease is prevalent in Montana, Idaho and along the Atlantic seaboard from New York to Georgia.

The organism responsible for Rocky Mountain spotted fever is *Rickettsia rickettsii*. The infection has its reservoirs in small wild rodents and in dogs, and its principal or sole vector is the wood tick. Individuals of all ages have been affected. The majority of patients have resided in rural areas and have engaged in removing ticks from dogs.

Clinical Symptoms and Course

The incubation period of this disorder lasts from 2 to 12 days. The skin rash, consisting of rose-colored macules of variable sizes, usually appears on the 3rd day, first on the wrists, the ankles and the back, but it gradually spreads to cover the entire body and sometimes also the mucous membrane of the mouth and the pharynx. After a few days the macules become petechial. Large subcutaneous hemorrhages also may appear. Restlessness, insomnia and hyperesthesias are among the most distressing symptoms of this disease. Delirium is common at the height of the fever, but convulsions rarely occur. The spleen is large and tender. There are a slight leukocytosis and a slight secondary anemia. Pneumonia, not frequent, is the only serious complication reported, but mental confusion, deafness and visual disturbances are common and may last for weeks.

Fatal cases terminate in coma which usually begins between the 6th and the 12th days. In the cases which recover, the temperature at the end of the 2nd week falls by lysis and reaches normal by the end of the 3rd week. The rash subsides with the fever, leaving the skin pigmented and somewhat scarred. During the 3rd week necrosis may involve ear lobes, fingers, toes and scrotum, areas at the extreme periphery of the vascular system.

Prevention

Those who are apt to be in an area where ticks abound should be immunized against Rocky Mountain spotted fever.

Prognosis

The prognosis of Rocky Mountain spotted fever differs much in different localities. In Idaho the mortality is stated to be 3.5 per cent; in the Bitter Root Valley (Idaho-Montana border), 90 per cent; in eastern Montana, 15 per cent; on the Atlantic Seaboard, 25 per cent.

Chemotherapy and Nursing Care

Chloramphenicol, chlortetracycline or oxytetracycline, all of which have rickettsiostatic properties, are effective in this disease if administered at an early stage in its course, i.e., coincident with the first appearance of the rash. Sedative drugs are indicated for relief of pain, restlessness and exhausting insomnia. In areas where the disease is endemic, annual revaccination has been advised.

The patient's strength should be maintained early in the disease by a liberal and nutritious diet. Liquids should be provided in abundance.

Ticks are removed from the body most easily if they are first incinerated by the touch of a lit cigarette or match.

Q FEVER

Q fever is an acute infectious disease which follows the inhalation of dust particles contaminated with *Rickettsia burnetti* derived from the excreta of sheep, cattle or goats infected with this organism. The distribution of the disease is widespread throughout the United States and other countries in all parts of the world.

Course

After an incubation period which may range from 5 days to 5 weeks, but usually is from 10 to 20 days, the patient experiences an acute onset of headache, chills, fever, joint pains, gastrointestinal complaints and, a few days later, symptoms of pneumonitis. X-ray changes in the lungs may stimulate those of atypical pneumonia. In over 20 per cent of cases, fever persists for 4 weeks or longer; approximately a third of these patients develop clinical jaundice, which is indicative of an acute hepatitis. An important nursing observation in this disease, and one of its characteristics, is a relative bradycardia, the pulse rate rarely exceeding 100 in the face of temperature elevations above 103° F.

Convalescence is apt to be protracted in untreated cases of Q fever, or if treatment is delayed beyond the first stage of active clinical infection. Moreover, relapses are prone to occur, especially in elderly patients. However, eventual recovery without sequelae is the rule in this disease, with or without specific therapy.

Chemotherapy and Nursing Care

Chloramphenicol, chlortetracycline or oxytetracycline, received early in the course of Q fever, tends to reduce the severity of symptoms, eliminate complications and shorten convalescence. Maintenance of an ample carbohydrate and protein intake is important in patients who become jaundiced, as discussed on page 649 in connection with other forms of acute hepatitis.

RICKETTSIALPOX

Rickettsialpox is a relatively mild, self-limited illness caused by the organism *Rickettsia akari* which is transmitted from house mouse to man by means of mite bites. Most of the cases that have been identified to date have been encountered in the Northeastern United States.

Course

Seven to 10 days following the mite bite, a red papule appears at that site, which eventually vesiculates, encrusts and heals slowly, leaving a scar. Three to 7 days following its appearance, the patient becomes febrile, experiencing chills, headache, sweats, muscle pains, photophobia and anorexia. Concomitantly, or soon thereafter, a generalized eruption is observed, which becomes vesicular, as in the case of the original lesion. Scabs form, which scale eventually, but leave no scar. The diagnosis is established on the basis of a specific complement-fixation test.

Chemotherapy and Prophylaxis

Chloramphenicol, chlortetracycline and oxytetracycline are effective in controlling the manifestations of rickettsialpox, all of which start to subside within a period of from 24 to 48 hours. Rapid recovery then ensues. Epidemiologic control of this infection depends on the elimination of house mice, its reservoir, and of the mites which serve as its vector.

TRENCH FEVER

Trench fever (or 5-day fever) is caused by *Rickettsiae quintana,* which is transmitted from man to man by the body louse. It presents itself in the form of recurrent attacks of fever which last from 1 to 5 days. Among its characteristic features are severe pain and tenderness in the muscles and bones (especially the shins, hence the name *shinbone fever*), profound prostration, an enlarged spleen and an early appearing red macular rash.

Incidence

Since 5-day fever is a louse-borne infection, it has occurred largely in armies and among unclean populations.

Clinical Symptoms and Course

The period of incubation averages 21 days. The attack begins abruptly with a chill, accompanied by a sudden rise of temperature and pulse. The skin rash, which is typical (though not always present), appears during the first 12 to 20 hours of the disease as an eruption of a few or many red macules from 2 mm. to 1 cm. in diameter, first on the lower thorax and abdomen. It may persist for from a few hours to several days, but returns with each relapse of the fever. Only one such paroxysm may occur, or there may be others at regular intervals of 5 or 6 days.

No immunity is conferred by an attack of this malady. The one prophylactic measure against the disease is systematic delousing. Since lice have become infected from patients more than a year after an attack of this disease, there is danger of late relapses.

Diagnosis

The clinical symptoms of this disease are distinctive.

Prognosis

Trench fever never is fatal, yet there is a tendency for the disease to recur months or even years later.

Chemotherapy and Nursing Care

Chlortetracycline (Aureomycin) or oxytetracycline (Terramycin) may be prescribed. Heat and salicylates usually are adequate to relieve the pain, but morphine may be required.

Rest, a liberal diet, sunshine and fresh air greatly hasten recovery. During the afebrile periods maintenance of optimum nutrition is important.

Convalescence must be guarded carefully. Mild active and passive exercises, massage and physical therapy then help much, but even moderate exertion or exposure may precipitate a relapse.

46

Patients With Protozoan Infections

PROTOZOA

Protozoa are single-celled animals which, despite their unicellular structure, possess protoplasmic devices adapted for several different functions (Fig. 444). They are considerably more complicated in their make-up than are the bacteria. Most of them possess, to varying degrees, the ability to move about under their own power and are equipped with differential tissue structures which enable them to feed, breathe, eject excreta and attach themselves to other objects.

Spirochaete, one genus of protozoan, is a threadlike, corkscrew-shaped organism which moves about by rotation on its long axis, propelling itself with the aid of flagella.

Leptospira, one species of which causes Weil's disease, curves at one end to form a hook.

Borrelia, the agent causing relapsing fever, has large wavy spirals and a long filamentous end.

Spirilla, responsible for rat-bite fever, has a motile flagellum at each end.

Treponema, which include the organisms causing syphilis and yaws, have flagella and small spirals (Fig. 445).

Other varieties of protozoa include the *Sporozoa,* which are without organs of feeding or locomotion; the *Sarcodina,* which move about by means of pseudopodia (temporary projections of their bodies) and the *Mastigophora,* which are protozoa possessing flagella (whiplike appendages) for purposes of locomotion. The Sporozoa of greatest importance to man is the *Plasmodium,* the genus causing malaria. Of the Sarcodina, the most hazardous for humans is of the genus *Endamoeba,* responsible for amebic dysen-

tery. In this country, the most common Mastigophora infestation producing symptoms is that of *Trichomonas vaginalis,* but in Africa and the Orient are to be found diseases of much more serious consequence caused by protozoa of this group, for example, kala-azar, caused by the *Leishmania,* and African sleeping sickness, a *Trypanosoma* infection. The clinical aspects of certain of the more serious protozoan infections are considered in this chapter.

SPIROCHETAL INFECTIONS

Syphilis

Syphilis, or lues (the "great pox"), is an infectious disease induced by the protozoon *Treponema pallidum,* which, if untreated, runs a characteristic course. There is a single initial lesion at the point where the treponemata entered the body; widespread transistory cutaneous and visceral manifestations then appear and, years later, scattered destructive granulomatous lesions.

Treponema pallidum is a threadlike, actively motile protozoon, from 6 to 20 micra long, twisted into a corkscrew spiral. Always it produces its effects locally—never at a distance, as through toxins. It is killed quickly by a few minutes' exposure to cold or drying.

Community Problems

Lues today is arousing the civilized world to aggressive measures for its control. The incidence of new cases each year in America is estimated as 1 per 1,500 of population. At least one third of all untreated cases are doomed to suffer serious late complications

FIG. 444. Spirochetes and other protozoa. (A) A red blood cell for comparison of size. (B) The organism of Asiatic cholera. (C) The organism of lues or syphilis. (D) The organism of relapsing fever. (E) The organism of sleeping sickness.

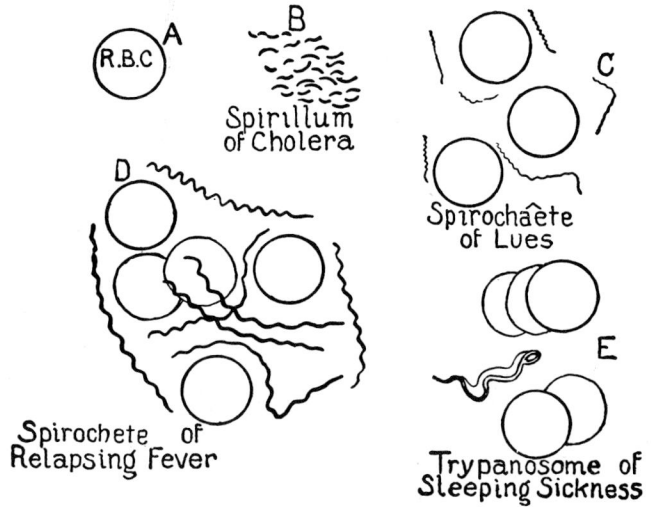

which may involve the central nervous system, the cardiovascular system, the bones, the skin and the viscera.

Transmission. Lues is not entirely a venereal disease. Doctors and nurses occasionally become infected on the hands while examining and caring for luetic patients. It may be transmitted by means of transfusion with blood from a luetic donor. Congenital lues is acquired by the infant from the mother through the placenta. However, the vast majority of cases are acquired through genital contact with a person who has been infected within a year, usually within a few weeks, and has a superficial ulcer teeming with spirochetes.

Course and Symptoms

Some of the manifestations of lues are designated as early and others as late. The time interval between early and late syphilis is about 4 years, during which period the patient has developed a partial immunity and an altered tissue response to the spirochete.

Early Syphilis. The manifestations of early lues include the chancre, generalized

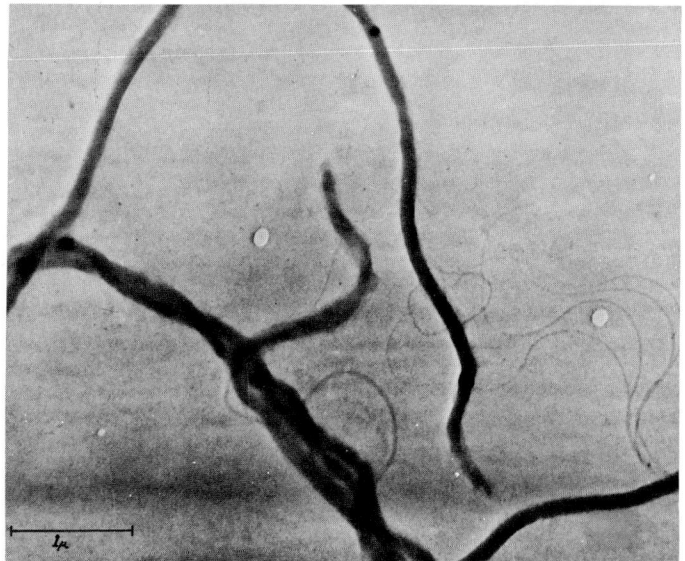

FIG. 445. *Treponema pallidum*. Electron microphotograph showing intertwined spirochetes. One tuft of four flagella is clearly visible; other flagella are shown less distinctly. ($1\mu =$ $\frac{1}{25,400}$ inch.) (Mudd, S., and Anderson, T. F.: J.A.M.A. **126**:561, 632.)

skin eruptions (see Plates 5 and 11), enlargement of the lymph nodes and widespread visceral involvements which are more or less transitory.

THE CHANCRE. The chancre, or primary sore, typically single, usually appears in from 10 to 28 days following the infection and always at the point where the treponemata entered the body—in about 10 per cent of all cases on one lip, the tongue, a finger, an

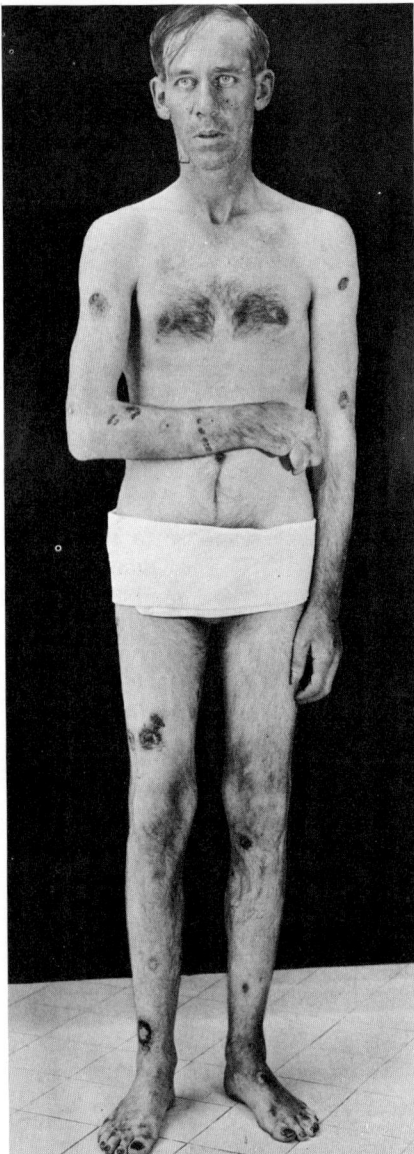

FIG. 446. Multiple gummata of the skin. (Ralph E. McDonnell, M.D.)

eyelid or a nipple. The primary sore usually is painless; although ulcerated, there is no discharge; there is induration of the underlying tissues. Invariably the regional lymph nodes become enlarged. In some cases, however, no primary sore can be found.

Chancres on the lip often appear as a painless crack in the mucous membrane which for weeks refuses to heal; one on the eyelid may be mistaken for a sty; those on the fingertips often constitute an insignificant persistent fissure at the edge of the fingernail.

In untreated cases the chancre disappears in 4 or more weeks, usually leaving a permanent scar.

THE GENERAL INFECTION. Even before the chancre appears, and while it is present, the treponemata have begun to spread throughout the entire body by way of the lymph and the blood stream. In many cases this period of general dissemination is symptomless; in others there are lassitude, a slight fever, loss of weight and anemia, which in some patients is marked.

SECONDARIES. In from 6 weeks to 6 months following the healing of the chancre, the so-called *secondaries* appear. These include the skin eruptions; a general lymphadenitis (enlargement of the epitrochlear and posterior cervical nodes especially characteristic); acute luetic arthritis, which may resemble closely acute rheumatic polyarthritis; pain in the bones, which is worse at night, caused by luetic osteitis and periosteitis; enlargement of the spleen and the liver, sometimes with jaundice; acute iritis, in some cases the first and only symptom of this disease; otitis media, usually bilateral; various neuralgias, neuritis of various nerves, especially of the optic and auditory; and, on rare occasions, an acute luetic meningitis.

EARLY LUETIC SKIN ERUPTIONS. The rashes, which may fail to appear altogether, present so many variations that they may simulate practically every known skin disease. However, certain features are more or less common to them all: their lesions are bilaterally symmetrical in distribution and the distribution is generalized; the eruptions are almost invariably polymorphous (that is, almost never are the skin lesions of any one type only, as macules alone, or papules alone); they cause no itching and no pain;

they persist for weeks; even untreated, they gradually fade entirely, leaving no scars; and, finally, they quickly disappear under treatment. Concomitantly, the hair often drops out, sometimes in patches, giving the scalp a motheaten appearance.

The macular eruption (the roseola), which usually appears early, may cover the entire trunk, sparing the face. It may be merely a diffuse rosy blush, rose-colored spots, or an eruption of slightly elevated copper-colored macules. Papular luetic lesions, covered with scales, may appear on the body surface. These papules are prone to become secondarily infected, and the resultant pustular eruption may resemble acne vulgaris, impetigo or even smallpox. Nodular skin lesions, small, bluish-red or brown in color, also may develop. These nodules may persist for years and, on disappearing, leave areas of pigmentation.

The luetic lesions which develop on moist skin surfaces, for example, about the anus, take the form of broad wartlike plaques (the so-called *condylomata*), which tend to crack and ulcerate. Those which appear on the mucous membranes of the mouth and the tongue are glistening, slightly elevated flat circumscribed patches, usually covered with a white or yellowish exudate. These papules, the so-called *mucous patches,* are the most characteristic, persistent and infectious of all luetic lesions. Other papules, dry and scaly in character, develop on the palms and the soles. Those on the fingertips occasionally destroy the bed of the nails, which become brittle and fissured. This luetic onychia is most refractory to treatment.

Late Syphilis. After the disappearance of the early luetic manifestations in untreated or inadequately treated cases there follows a period of apparent good health; more than half the patients have no further trouble, with or without treatment. But, after about 4 years, those less fortunate begin to show signs of the late (formerly called *tertiary*) luetic lesions. The most distinctive form that these lesions take is the gumma, a discrete tumor (Fig. 446); but the much more common diffuse luetic infiltrations have the same significance. Any organ of the body may be attacked.

LATE LUETIC SKIN LESIONS. No sharp line can be drawn between the skin and the mucous membrane lesions of early and late lues; but those of late lues are few in number, are not symmetrically distributed, contain few treponemata, are more infiltrated, chronic and destructive. Such lesions produce the large, deep punched-out ulcers on the lower legs, which, healing, leave characteristic scars with sinuous borders, pigmented areolae and atrophied bases; the rupia lesions seen round the elbow, with peculiar many-layered crusts; the lesions in the mouth, the throat and the nose, which, ulcerating, perforate the soft palate or the septum and explain the saddle nose; the diffuse thickenings on the tongue which may either ulcerate or become cancerous.

LATE BONE AND JOINT SYPHILIS. Among the important late luetic bone lesions are necrosis of the cranial bones; bony overgrowths or exostoses due to periostitis, which make the shins, the clavicles, the sternum and the cranial bones nodular; and gumma of bone, which is destructive and occasionally causes deformities of the spine and other bones.

Late luetic arthritis, usually monoarticular, is a gummatous thickening of the synovial membrane and the joint capsule, because of which the joint is swollen and fluctuates. This condition is remedied quickly by antiluetic treatment. The Charcot joint, a feature of locomotor ataxia, on the other hand, is a special type of arthritis, notably affecting the knee. It is characterized by the gradual and extensive painless disintegration of all joint tissues, which results in great joint deformity. Because of the tabetic spinal cord changes, all joint pain is lost and traumatic changes become extreme. The patient, therefore, continues to use the disintegrating joint as long as it will support any weight.

LATE VASCULAR OR VISCERAL SYPHILLIS. Lues can affect nearly all the organs of the body. The most marked effects are usually those of the vascular system, but there are hardly any organs or systems of the body that escape.

Congenital Lues

Women with active syphilis give birth to luetic children. Luetic children, born late in the course of the maternal infection, at birth may or may not present evidences of the disease. If they do, the most common symptoms are snuffles, various distinctive skin eruptions, rhagades (scars at the corners of the mouth), fissures of the skin, onychia, alopecia, enlarged liver and spleen and emaciation.

Other infants with congenital lues show no signs of this disease until they are 10 or 12 years old, or even later. Then there may appear: Hutchinson's teeth (the notched and usually peg-shaped upper middle permanent incisors); the luetic lesions of the liver which occasionally result in cirrhosis at puberty; enlarged spleen; tender enlargements of the bones and the epiphyses, particularly of the femur and the tibia; and saber shins. Still later may appear an almost pathognomonic bilateral interstitial keratitis, which, if inadequately treated, results in permanent cloudiness of the cornea, optic neuritis and deafness. The simultaneous presence of Hutchinson's teeth, interstitial keratitis and deafness (Hutchinson's triad) is diagnostic of congenital lues.

Diagnosis of Lues in General

The chancre, if typical, can be recognized without difficulty; in any case, the treponemata should be sought in serum expressed from the suspected sore or aspirated from a neighboring lymph node. Throughout life the presence of the scar of the chancre is of great aid in diagnosis.

Most important to exclude is the chancroidal ulcer (soft sore), a deep, characteristically punched-out ulcer, often multiple, with elevated undermined edges, an inflammatory areola and a dirty, moth-eaten soft floor, which exudes an abundant purulent fluid containing Ducrey's bacillus.

Diagnostic Serum Reactions. The Wassermann reaction is one of the most consistent of laboratory tests for lues, but today most clinics use, in addition, one of several precipitin reactions, such as the Kahn, Klein, Hinton or Kolmer tests.

A positive serologic reaction in the great majority of cases indicates that the patient has, or has had, active syphilis. A falsely positive test may appear in systemic lupus erythematosus, leprosy, infectious mononucleosis, following smallpox vaccination and in other spirochetal diseases such as yaws. A negative Wassermann in the presence of active lues may occur in cardiovascular syphilis and in several varieties of central nervous system syphilis. More specific serologic tests for syphilis now are undergoing world-wide trial. These include the *Treponema pallidum* immobilization test (TPI) of Nelson and Mayer, the *T. pallidum* immune adherence (TPIA) test and the *T. pallidum* complement-fixation (TPCF) test, one or more of which may well be adopted generally as a supplement to the simpler, standard serologic tests in order to identify or exclude biologic false-positive (BFP) reactions.

Chemotherapy

Penicillin alone is effective against all forms of syphilis. Early syphilis, in almost all cases, responds to a single treatment with 2,400,000 units of benzathine penicillin G (Bicillin, Permapen), 4 ml., containing 300,000 units per ml., being injected into each buttock. Alternatively, procaine penicillin G in oil and aluminum monostearate (PAM) may be injected intramuscularly in divided doses of 1,200,000 units at intervals of from 2 to 4 days. Recommended treatment for all forms of late syphilis is intramuscular PAM in a total dose of 6,000,000 to 10,000,000 units, individual doses of 1,200,000 units being given 2 or 3 times a week. The existence of pregnancy does not appear to alter the therapeutic requirements. Congenital syphilis is treated in the same manner as is acquired syphilis, except that smaller doses of penicillin may be administered to children weighing less than 32 Kg. (70 lbs.). The total dose in such cases may be from 75,000 to 100,000 units per Kg. of body weight. This may be administered in the form of procaine penicillin in oil and aluminum monostearate, given intramuscularly in doses of from 0.5 to 1 ml. (150,000 to 300,000 units) every 2 to 4 days until the course is completed.

Penicillin-sensitive individuals, or penicillin-resistant syphilis, require the substitution of another antibiotic. Early syphilis responds satisfactorily to 3 or 4 Gm. of oxy-

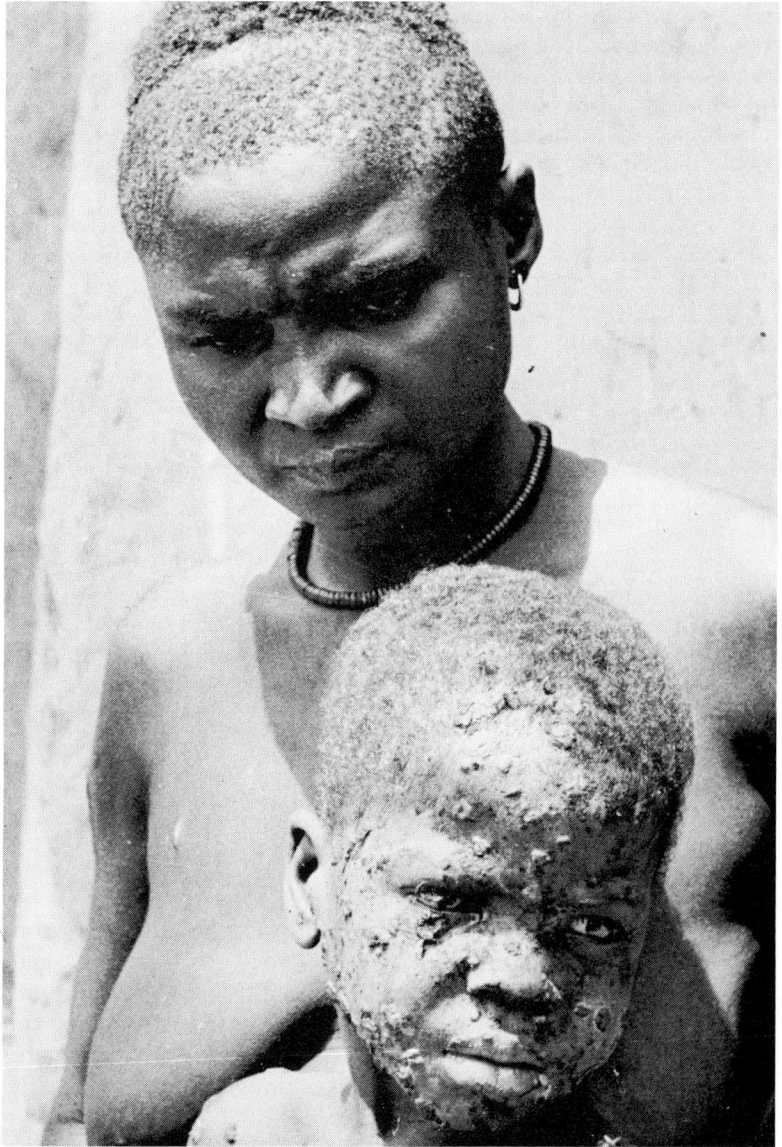

FIG. 447. These ugly sores can mean a lifetime of pain. Yaws is a disease that is widespread throughout tropical areas. In Africa alone, some 25 million suffer from this unsightly and painful disease. Usually contracted in childhood, it can last a lifetime if not treated, destroying the skin and attacking the bones. This little boy, Ede Nwaebgo, is 5 years old. He lives in a bush village in Nigeria. The misery of yaws is clearly reflected in the unsmiling faces of Ede and his mother. That was before the visit of a WHO-assisted yaws team. (World Health Organization)

tetracycline or chlortetracycline, or 2 to 3 Gm. of carbomycin (Magnamycin) daily by mouth for 10 days. For late syphilis, 2 to 3 Gm. of carbomycin daily by mouth for 15 to 20 days is recommended.

Congenital syphilitic interstitial keratitis should be treated with the topical administration of cortisone (5 mg. of cortisone acetate to 1 ml. of isotonic sodium chloride solution), 1 drop instilled every 3 hours, as a supplement to antisyphilitic penicillin therapy.

Public Health Education

Information regarding syphilis should be disseminated widely; education of physicians as well as of the general public must be undertaken. Syphilis must be regarded as a disease, not a stigma. The treatment must be initiated as early as possible. Congenital syphilis can be prevented readily by prenatal blood tests and prompt therapy.

Public funds are available to ensure adequate treatment. Most states finance blood tests and antiluetic medications with the assistance of the U. S. Public Health Service. The public health nurse has a responsibility in interpreting the doctor's instructions to patients and impressing them with the importance of treatment and the value of premarital and prenatal blood tests. Her attitude must be understanding and her approach skillful in order to secure the confidence of her patients, for whose guidance she is in part responsible.

Yaws (Frambesia)

Frambesia (raspberry) is a highly contagious disease of the tropics, due to *Treponema pertenue* (a germ quite similar to that of lues), the two chief features of which are anemia and an eruption of granulomata scattered over the body surface (Fig. 447).

The primary lesions, "mother yaw," which appears at the site of inoculation (most often on the face or the neck) as a tubercle or group of tubercles, grows in size, becomes conical and confluent and discharges a yellow exudate which dries to form a crust.

In from 4 to 6 weeks following the initial lesion *the secondary stage* begins, with fever, mild constitutional symptoms and a rash of minute reddish papules (yaws) which appear in crops, on the face and the extremities especially. These papules grow to become raspberrylike lesions, 1 or 2 cm. in diameter, the majority of which become crusted, the crust covering a red pulpy tubercle which resembles a raspberry and exudes a serum with a disagreeable odor. Those on the moist surfaces become condylomatous; those on the dorsa of the feet, warty; those on the palms and the soles, painful ulcers. After a few weeks those lesions disappear, leaving white areas which later become pigmented.

A tertiary stage may follow, the characteristic lesions of which are indolent deep-skin ulcers which may involve underlying bones also. These, healing, leave disfiguring scars.

The blood serum of patients with yaws almost invariably gives a positive Wassermann reaction. Nevertheless, the organism causing yaws is not *Treponema pallidum:* this disease is extragenital and nonheredi-

tary, the mucous membranes are not involved, and the skin eruption, unlike that of lues, is uniform. Yaws responds readily and rapidly to penicillin therapy.

The tertiary stage of yaws evidently explains *gangosa,* a mutilating nasopharyngitis seen in the West Indies, and *goundou* (of Africa and South America), an ulcerating process which attacks the nose, often entirely destroying it.

Weil's Disease

Weil's disease (Leptospirosis Icterohaemorrhagica) is an acute epidemic malady due to *Leptospira icterohaemorrhagiae,* probably spread by infected rats which excrete the organism in the urine. Individuals most likely to be affected include swimmers who frequent rat-infested waters, sewer workers, fish cutters, poultry dressers, abattoir workers, inhabitants of rat-infested houses, laboratory workers and veterinarians.

The disease is characterized by the sudden onset of chills and fever, ocular injection, muscle aching and tenderness, headache and stiff neck between 4 and 20 days after exposure. During this initial phase, which may last for a period of from 3 to 9 days, the leptospira can be demonstrated in the patient's blood by means of cultures or animal inoculations. The white blood cells are increased, and the spinal fluid contains leukocytes and often leptospira as well. The second stage is marked by variable degrees of jaundice, hemorrhagic phenomena, symptoms of meningitis and signs of renal infection, including hematuria and albuminuria. The liver may enlarge and a skin rash may appear. Leptospira may be recovered from the urine now and for a period of from 2 to 5 weeks hence. Serum agglutinins, specific for leptospiral antigen, can be demonstrated, and muscle biopsy might show characteristic lesions. Fever and symptoms usually begin to subside during the course of the second or third week of the disease. Convalescence is apt to be slow and characterized by depression, weakness and anemia. Relapse may occur. The mortality of the disease has approached 50 per cent in some reports.

Treatment consists in the administration of penicillin, still the drug of choice in all

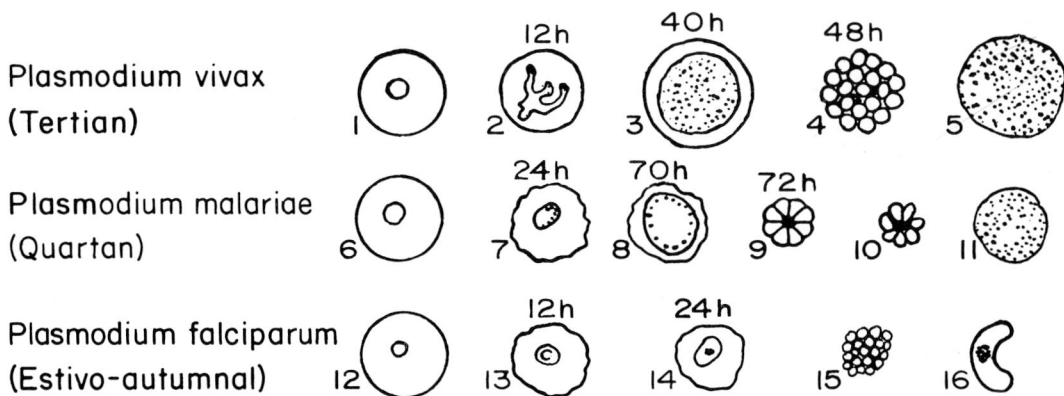

FIG. 448. The malarial parasite ($\times$ 1,000).

(*Top*) *Plasmodium vivax,* the parasite of tertian malaria. (1) A young hyaline which has just entered the red corpuscle. (2) The same, 12 hours later; the parasite is larger, actively ameboid and now contains pigment granules. (3) The same when 40 hours old; the red corpuscle is swollen, the parasite is large and contains much pigment. (4) The same when 48 hours old; the red corpuscle has disappeared. The parasite has divided into 20 small parasites called *segments.* These will separate and make their way into other red corpuscles, as was the case with 1, and start the cycle over again. (5) Some of the parasites, like 3, do not segment but grow to a form which will develop further only in the mosquito's stomach. There the fifth type will grow and divide into thousands of tiny forms, which if injected into a person's blood by the bite of this infected insect will, like 1, start the cycle.

(*Center*) *Plasmodium malariae,* the parasite of quartian malaria. Note the difference in ages, in size, the different effect on the red corpuscles, which shrink, and the coarser granules of pigment. (9) The marguerite form, or presegmenter, which divides to only about 7 segments. 11 is similar to 5.

(*Bottom*) *Plasmodium falciparum,* the parasite of estivo-autumnal malaria. Note the differences in ages, in size, in the effect on the red corpuscles, and the peculiar shape of the parasite, 16, which, like 5 and 11, is designed for the mosquito's stomach.

spirochetal infections. This is one of the very few spirochetal infections that fail to respond to arsenical therapy.

Rat-Bite Fever

Rat-bite fever, due to *Spirillum minus* which is introduced into the body by the bite of an infected rat, is characterized by a series of febrile paroxysms which may continue for months or years; a skin rash of large, sharply defined, red macules; weakness; and polyarthritis. The period of incubation may last for months. Then the original wound which was caused by the rat bite, and perhaps had healed, becomes swollen, red and ulcerated, and the regional lymph nodes are enlarged.

The attack begins with a chill and a fever which last 3 or 4 days. Then the skin eruption appears, with pain in the muscles and joints, and sometimes delirium. Each paroxysm lasts for 7 or 8 days, and each 2 are separated by 1 or 2 weeks of apyrexia.

Treatment consists of cleansing the wound and administering an intensive course of penicillin.

Relapsing Fever

Relapsing fever is a mild epidemic disease due to protozoa of the *Borrelia* group transmitted by lice or ticks. It is characterized by recurring attacks of usually high fever interspersed with periods of apparent recovery.

These treponemata (spirally coiled, threadlike organisms) easily are found in the patient's blood early in the paroxysms. Infected lice and ticks do not transmit this disease by their bites; the organisms in the insect's secretions or body fluids are deposited on the skin when the insect is crushed, and they enter the body through a scratch wound.

Transmission. *The louse-borne disease* occurs notably in the U.S.S.R., the Baltic States, India and China. In these countries it is a disease of the poor, living in overcrowded hovels on the verge of starvation, hence the name *famine fever.*

The tick-borne disease occurs in Africa, in Central America and also in the southern United States.

Clinical Symptoms and Course. The febrile paroxysms of relapsing fever, usually 2 or 3 in number (hence the name *relapsing*), begin suddenly with a chill and rapid temperature rise, nausea, vomiting and pains in the back. The temperature remains continuously elevated for from 2 to 7 days, then suddenly falls by crisis, the attack followed by an intermission of about the same length of time during which the patient seems practically well.

The mortality of this disease is about 4 per cent, but in some epidemics it has reached 40 per cent.

This disease responds promptly to the administration of penicillin.

MALARIA

Malaria is an acute, infectious disease caused by protozoa which strongly resemble leukocytes (except that they are much smaller and multiply differently). Their transmission is by way of an intermediate host, the mosquito. There are three varieties of malarial parasites, grouped under the general name *Plasmodium malariae,* each causing a different type of malaria (Fig. 448).

Each malarial parasite lives within a red blood corpuscle, utilizing the hemoglobin as food. When full grown, it divides (segments) into from 10 to 20 small, young parasites, called *hyalines* (or segments), which burst the cell. Free in the plasma, the majority of these hyalines die, but a few find their way into new red cells, and the process described above is repeated.

The tertian parasite is so named because its life cycle requires just 48 hours, hence the chills occur on alternate days (but if

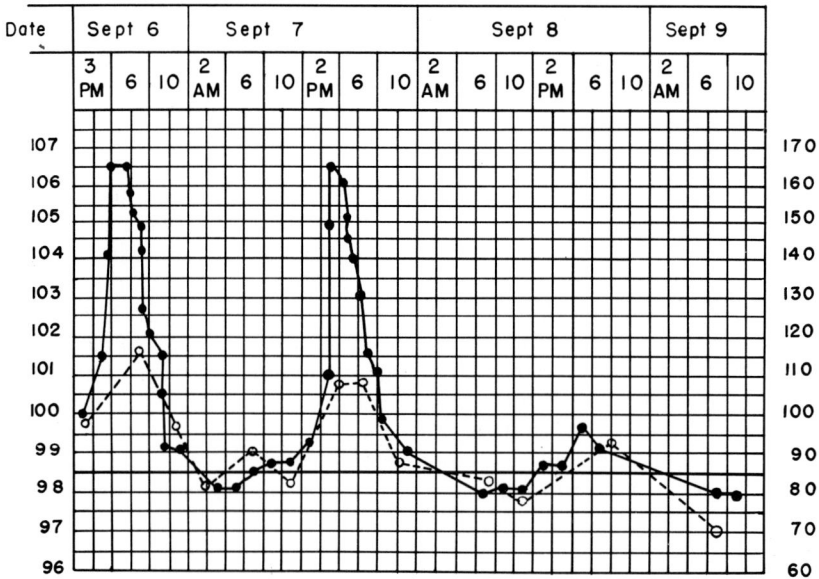

Fig. 449. Temperature and pulse chart of a patient with double tertian malaria.

two broods of this parasite are present, the patient has a chill each day) (Fig. 449).

The quartan is so named because its cycle takes just 72 hours: hence, if one brood is present there is a chill each fourth day; if three, one each day. In cases of tertian and quartan malaria the hundreds of millions of parasites of each group are all of the same age, hence their segments are free in the blood at approximately the same time. It is just then that the chill with sharp temperature rise occurs, and it is at that time also that quinine, if present in the blood, will destroy them.

The estivo-autumnal parasite, so named because the malaria that it causes is worse in the summer and the fall, has a cycle which varies between 24 and 72 hours in duration. This is the most virulent of the malarial parasites and is responsible for the most serious form of malaria. The reason for this is that after the first few days parasites of all ages are present in the blood at the same time. Therefore, some of them are segmenting continually (this taking place in the spleen and the bone marrow, not in the peripheral blood as is the case in the other two types). At first there may be a few chills, but as the case goes on they become less and less acute (dumb chills), until the fever is continuous.

We have spoken thus far only of the parasites of each group which cause fever in man. These are the asexual forms. Some hyalines of each group, however, do not segment. These, the sexual forms, remain in the body unchanged, perhaps for months, doing the patient no harm. However, if any are in the blood which a mosquito sucks from the patient, these mature in the body of the insect, producing myriads of young forms, some of which that mosquito will inject into the blood of its next victim, where as asexual forms they will multiply until, in about 2 weeks, they are numerous enough to produce the symptoms of the type of malaria that they cause.

Only one variety of mosquito, the *Anopheles,* can act as the intermediate host of malarial parasite. This mosquito, resting on a wall, can be recognized at a distance, for, instead of standing hunchbacked, as does the ordinary mosquito (*Culex*), it stands with body, thorax and bill in a straight line, forming with the wall an angle of about 30° (Fig. 450).

Clinical Symptoms and Course. Patients with tertian and quartan malaria feel well on days when they have no chill. The chill, which lasts about 10 minutes, begins suddenly, often with intense headache, nausea and vomiting. During the next 30 minutes to 4 hours the temperature rises rapidly, as high as 107° F., and the patient becomes intensely hot and flushed. Then, suddenly, with a profuse sweat, the temperature falls rapidly to normal, and in a few minutes the patient feels well. The entire paroxysm lasts from 10 to 14 hours.

Patients with severe malaria of any form

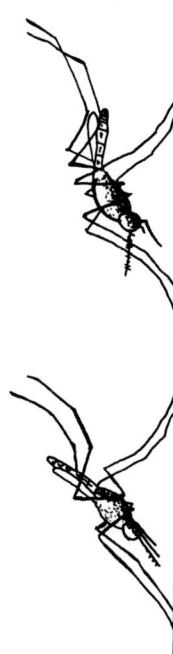

Fig. 450. Two common mosquitoes, recognized by their attitudes of rest on a vertical wall. (*Top*) Culex, which occasionally transmits filaria embryos, the cause of filariasis. (*Bottom*) *Anopheles,* the malaria mosquito. (Park and Williams: Pathogenic Micro-organisms, Philadelphia, Lea & Febiger)

may become comatose and die (pernicious malaria); or they may develop renal failure (due to the precipitation of free hemoglobin in the kidney tubule), a serious gastrointestinal disturbance or cerebral symptoms (due to an accumulation of the parasites in the blood vessels of the affected organ).

To escape malaria one must avoid *Anopheles* mosquitoes which about 3 weeks previously have fed on the blood of patients with malaria. This insect usually bites only after sundown, and never a person in motion. Houses should be well screened, especially the room of a patient ill with malaria, lest *Anopheles* mosquitoes become infected from him. All pools of stagnant water (it is these in which mosquitoes breed) should be eliminated. If this is impossible, these accumulations of water should be treated with oil or a preparation of the insecticide DDT.

Diagnosis. The diagnosis of malaria is established by the finding of the plasmodium in the patient's blood. The most favorable time for the discovery of the parasite is from 12 to 18 hours after a chill.

Chemotherapy. Therapy should be started promptly after the diagnosis is made. The treatment currently recommended for *P. vivax* malaria is chloroquine plus primaquine. A loading dose of 1.0 Gm. of chloroquine diphosphate is given by mouth, followed in 6 hours by 0.5 Gm., then 0.5 Gm. on each of 2 succeeding days. If nausea and vomiting are severe, chloroquine may be given by intramuscular injection, in doses of 0.2 Gm. (of the base), the full course then being completed by the oral route.

Primaquine is given in a dose of 10 to 15 mg. (base) daily for 14 days, starting immediately, or as soon as the acute phase is controlled by chloroquine. Complications of primaquine therapy in "primaquine-sensitive" individuals are discussed on page 199.

P. falciparum malaria should be treated with chloroquine alone, 2.5 Gm. of the phosphate (or 1.5 Gm. of the base) being given in the course of 3 days as outlined above.

Paludrine effectively terminates acute vivax or quartan malaria. Although curing the latter, it is no better than chloroquine as regards a permanent cure of vivax infection. Customarily it is given in a total dosage of 50 to 150 mg., doses as small as 12.5 mg. being effective in some instances. It is highly effective as a prophylactic against falciparum malaria, 0.1 Gm. daily completely preventing the infection of individuals who are heavily exposed under natural conditions; it is equally valuable in suppressing vivax infections, only, however, as long as its administration is continued. Due to an almost complete lack of toxicity, Paludrine may prove to be the most useful of all drugs as a prophylactic and suppressive agent in malaria.

Prognosis. The recurrence rate in malaria undoubtedly is destined to be modified to a considerable extent by modern chemotherapy. By using quinine or quinacrine alone, relapses in cases of vivax malaria were regularly anticipated for 3 or 4 years following the initial attack, and in quartan malaria, repeated attacks over a course of 15 to 20 years. Falciparum malaria, on the other hand, rarely relapses after 6 to 9 months. The chief complications attending chronic malaria are anemia, enlargement of the spleen and cachexia. Treatment is carried out as outlined above and is supplemented with iron therapy, blood transfusions and dietary measures as indicated.

Prevention. The essence of malaria control is the eradication of malaria as an endemic disease, which is accomplished if the number of cases in a given area can be reduced, and maintained, below a certain critical figure for a period of 8 to 10 years. In several areas of the world this goal has been achieved, and in the United States it is being approached. Thus, from 140,000 cases and 4,000 deaths in 1936, and 40,000 cases with 350 deaths in 1946, the morbidity and mortality rates for malaria in the U. S. in 1956 had dropped to about 200 cases and 20 deaths. From a global standpoint, however, malaria remains the number one problem in human health, continuing to attack 200,000,000 and kill 2,000,000 people each year throughout the world.

Effective control of this disease, where it has been accomplished, has relied on two principal measures, employed in combination: (1) the practice of "residual spraying" of dwellings in infested areas with such toxicants as DDT, benzine hexachloride and chlordane, which has been carried out in systematic, coordinated fashion and on a wide scale for a definitive period of time, e.g., 4 years, to the end that all, or nearly all, *Anopheles* mosquitoes infected with malarial parasites have been destroyed, and (2) the institution of a "system of surveillance," which has undertaken to investigate every suspected case of malaria occurring in that area following discontinuance of spraying, from the standpoint of its origin, epidemiology and vector, and to initiate and direct whatever corrective measures might be indicated in each case. This program and its rigid timetable are designed to circumvent one important problem which imposes a serious limitation on the use of insecticides, namely, the development of resistance to these agents on the part of insects generally. However, it has been found that eradication of malaria can be accomplished within a period of from 8 to 10 years, including 4 to 6 years of nation-wide spraying, without inducing insect resistance.

AMEBIASIS

Amebae are protozoa, larger than leukocytes, which move by ameboid action (they project part of their body at one point as a pseudopod and flow into this). Only a few amebae infect man; the most important of these is *Endamoeba histolytica,* the cause of amebic dysentery. This, as seen under the microscope, moves actively, has a small round nucleus and a protoplasm full of leukocytes, red blood cells and bacteria ingested by the parasite. These amebae survive outside the body in resistant encysted forms. From the number of the nuclei of these cysts one may determine the type of ameba.

Amebic Dysentery

Amebic dysentery is a disease of the tropics, especially Egypt, India and the Far East, but is common also in our Northern states. It occurs in epidemics spread by water and also by food handled by amebae carriers—persons who may or may not have had amebic dysentery but who harbor this protozoon in their intestinal wall.

The amebae burrow their way into the mucous membranes of the colon and the lower ileum, and in the submucous tissue form pus pockets with only a small orifice opening into the bowel, from which numerous burrows extend for considerable distances in all directions under the mucous membrane. Here the amebae live, probably for years. Later, the protecting mucous membrane roof of this burrowing abscess sloughs, exposing an underlying ulcer. The large bowel may be so covered by such ulcers that very little normal mucous membrane is left. Usually the floor of these ulcers is the muscle wall of the bowel, but they may perforate its entire wall and cause fatal peritonitis.

Clinical Symptoms and Course. The chief symptoms of a case of acute amebic dysentery are slight fever, weight loss and the passage of frequent small stools containing considerable amounts of blood and mucus, the latter swarming with amebae. The two important features of this disease are its chronicity, one attack of acute dysentery following another, separated by periods of constipation which last for months, and the tendency of the infection to cause liver abscesses through its metastases to that organ by way of the portal vein.

Chemotherapy. Four drugs are especially valuable in the treatment of amebiasis: emetine, chloroquine, diiodohydroxyquin and chlortetracycline. The manner in which they are used, their relative effectiveness in various specific forms of amebiasis and certain toxic complications associated with their use are discussed in Chapter 13.

Amebic Liver Abscess

Amebic liver abscesses differ from those due to bacteria in that they are more often single than multiple, always are large, have little evidence of real inflammation in their walls and give surprisingly few symptoms. They are merely large holes in the liver, full of necrotic and liquified liver tissue, the walls of which contain hosts of amebae. Such abscesses may heal by perforating and draining through the lung, but the outcome in this event is exceedingly precarious. One point to be emphasized is that not infrequently these abscesses are found unexpectedly in patients who have, or have had, few or no symptoms suggesting dysentery.

The treatment is that outlined for amebic dysentery. Needle aspiration of the liver abscess is not advised.

KALA-AZAR

Kala-azar (tropical splenomegaly, Dumdum fever) is a chronic, usually fatal, infectious disease, often lasting for 1 or 2 years. It is due to the protozoon *Leishmania donovani,* and its characteristic features are a huge spleen, emaciation and anemia.

Leishmania donovani is a protozoon which resides in the reticuloendothelial tissue, the cells of which are so overfilled by these parasites that they burst. As seen in these cells, these protozoa are oval bodies containing two chromatin masses; but as grown in cultures, they are motile flagellated organisms closely resembling trypanosomes.

Kala-azar is widespread in certain sharply defined regions of India and China. In less severe forms (such as oriental sore, Aleppo boil or Delhi boil) it is found throughout Mediterranean countries. Children in particular are affected. How the disease is transmitted is not definitely known: one method may be by the sandfly; another, possibly, by the oral route.

Clinical Symptoms and Course. The incubation periods vary from weeks to months. The onset is with fever, sometimes continuous, like that of typhoid, occasionally intermittent and associated with chills, like that of malaria (for years this disease was thought to be a form of malaria resistant to quinine), but peculiar in that the temperature may rise sharply 2 or 3 times each day. Long periods of apyrexia are common. After about 6 months the enormous spleen and the large liver nearly fill the abdomen. Anemia and granulocytopenia progressively develop. Hemorrhagic phenomena are common. Malaise is relatively slight; children, anemic and emaciated, their growth stunted and the abdomen huge, continue at their play. Death usually comes in 2 or 3 years, but as a rule, from complications due to other organisms, such as bronchopneumonia and amebic dysentery.

The organism is demonstrable in material obtained from splenic and bone-marrow biopsy.

Treatment. The intravenous administration of pentavalent antimony preparations, such as Neostibosan or sodium-antimony-gluconate (Solustobosan), is the most common form of therapy. Diamidinostilbene— an aromatic compound, not an antimony preparation—likewise is effective in the treatment of this disease. Inasmuch as it is relatively toxic, the drug usually is reserved for those cases which fail to respond to an antimony preparation.

Treatment has reduced the mortality of kala-azar from 90 to approximately 10 per cent.

AFRICAN SLEEPING SICKNESS

African sleeping sickness (trypanosomiasis (is a severe disease of tropical Africa due to the protozoon *Trypanosoma gambiense* (or the similar *Trypanosoma rhodesiense*). It is characterized early, while the organism is free in the blood stream, by irregular fever, weakness and swelling of the lymph nodes, and after the organism has invaded the central nervous system, when the sleeping-sickness stage begins, by marked emaciation, tremors, paralyses, mental disturbances and drowsiness leading to coma and, finally, death.

These trypanosomes are eel-shaped protozoa, from 10 to 30 micra long, with long flagella. They are transmitted by the bite of the tsetse fly. Various wild animals are the reservoir whence these flies become infected. Cattle cannot survive in regions where the disease is widespread.

Diagnosis. The organism may be found in the blood, but is located more easily in the cervical lymph nodes and later in the spinal fluid.

Treatment. Tartar emetic, administered intramuscularly or subcutaneously, seems to cure some cases if administered early enough. Better, however, are arsenicals, or stilbamidine, given intravenously.

47

Patients With Systemic Mycoses

ACTINOMYCOSIS

Actinomycosis is a chronic granulomatous disease caused by fungi (plant forms higher than protophytes) of the Actinomyces (ray-fungus) group. The characteristic lesions are local masses of fibrous tissue which suppurate, giving rise to multiple abscesses which discharge through manifiold sinuses an exudate containing the characteristic sulfur granules, representing visible masses of the organism. This disease, if untreated, advances indolently, but relentlessly, for years, destroying all the tissues in its way, frequently, however, disturbing the patient's general health but little.

It is a disease of young adult males in particular and is widely distributed over the United States. The source of this fungus is not known; the mouth probably is its portal of entry, since pathogenic actinomyces often are found in carious teeth and tonsillar crypts of otherwise normal persons.

Clinical Symptoms and Course. Actinomycosis of the head and the neck, the most common locations, starts as a swelling about certain teeth. This, by extension, involves the submaxillary region and the neck, producing a flat, hard, painless tumor mass, with smooth regular surface and uniform dense consistency, which is fixed firmly to the jawbone. From this mass a brawny nodular induration extends into the neck, covered by skin which is wrinkled and dusky red in color. Later this granuloma, breaking down, becomes riddled with abscesses which perforate externally. By extension, this process may involve the cheek, the skull and the brain.

In the abdominal type, any viscus may be affected, including the pelvic organs, especially the ovaries and tubes, but most commonly the appendix and the cecum. Here in time an uneven tumor mass develops. This resembles carcinoma, and by extension may involve the abdominal wall, discharging externally through open sinuses.

In the pulmonary form, induced by inhaled actinomyces spores, a condition, usually unilateral, develops. This simulates tuberculosis with cavity formation, except that usually it involves a lower lobe.

Treatment. Actinomycotic lesions respond to sulfonamide drugs and penicillin, the latter being the drug of choice. Large doses, e.g., 1 million units should be given daily, without interruption for several weeks. Chlortetracycline (Aureomycin), streptomycin and chloramphenicol (Chloromycetin) all have been used successfully and should be tried in the event that penicillin fails to achieve a cure. Surgical drainage and excision of localized lesions occasionally are obligatory.

HISTOPLASMOSIS

Histoplasmosis is a chronic systemic fungus infection caused by a spore-bearing mold called *Histoplasma capsulatum*. This disease has been encountered throughout the globe but is especially prevalent in the Eastern Central United States. In its commonest form it presents as a mild, self-limited respiratory illness without distinctive features, manifested solely by low grade fever and cough. In a few instances, however, granulomatous lesions of the proliferative or ulcerative type become disseminated throughout the body, giving rise to all the constitutional symptoms and signs of a severe systemic infection. Such patients face the prospect of a protracted, unpleasant illness, and the very real possibility of a fatal outcome.

Histoplasmosis is predominantly a disease of young infants and older adults, especially males over the age of 40 years. The infective fungus is harbored in chickens and presumably in animal hosts which as yet are unidentified. One method by which humans acquire the infection is by the inhalation of spore-bearing dust.

Clinical Picture. Some of the clinical features of histoplasmosis resemble closely those of pulmonary tuberculosis, including symptoms of fever, night sweats, anorexia, debility, cough which is productive of purulent sputum, and occasionally hemoptysis. The appearance of parenchymal infiltrates, cavities and calcifications on x-ray examination of the lungs often has led to an erroneous diagnosis of tuberculosis. Other patients present findings that are reminiscent of malignant lymphoma, including anemia, thrombocytopenia, splenomegaly, hepatomegaly and x-ray signs of mediastinal enlargement. Nodules may apear in the skin, and osteolytic bone lesions may be demonstrated by x-ray examination. One group of patients seems prone to develop ulcerations at mucocutaneous junctions, for example, at the lip margins and in the perianal region. Gastrointestinal ulcers may be responsible for massive bleeding, and the syndrome of Addison's disease (see p. 839) may appear as the result of destruction of the adrenal glands by histoplasmosis.

Diagnosis. The diagnosis of histoplasmosis is established by culturing *Histoplasma capsulatum* from the sputum or elsewhere, or by identifying this organism morphologically in smears of blood or bone marrow, or in histologic sections of infected tissue obtained by surgical biopsy. Complement fixation tests and histoplasmin skin tests, while not conclusive, are diagnostically helpful. The characteristic radiologic appearance of the lungs, in conjunction with a negative tuberculin skin test, strongly suggests this diagnosis.

Treatment. At present the treatment of choice for histoplasmosis is surgical resection of the infected lesions, when feasible, combined with chemotherapy. The agent

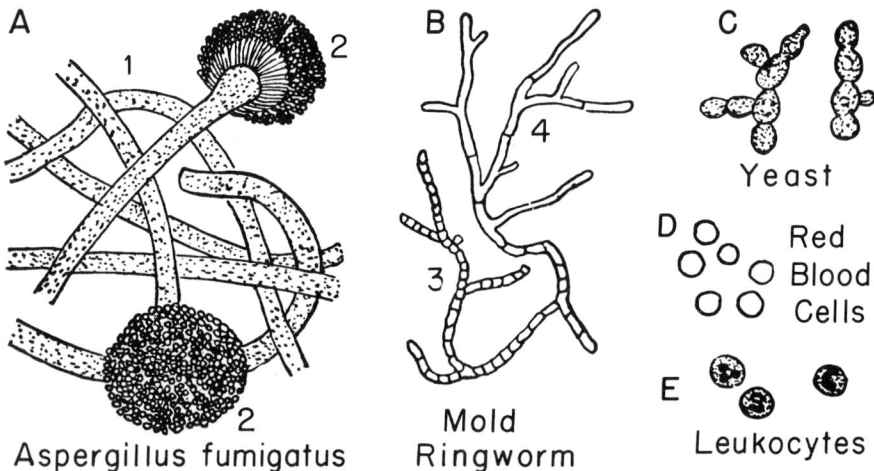

Fig. 451. Important vegetable parasites. (A) A mold: 1, the mycelial threads; 2, the fruit head. (B) The parasite causing ringworm: 3, threads which are dividing into spores, from each of which a new "plant" can grow; 4, threads not sporulating. (C) A common yeast. (D) Red blood corpuscles. (E) Leukocytes, introduced for comparison of size. All are drawn to the same scale ($\times$ 400).

currently preferred for this purpose is amphotericin B, administered intravenously.

Amphotericin B has proved to be effective in the treatment of most of the deep mycoses, including histoplasmosis, North American blastomycosis, sporotrichosis, cryptococcosis and aspergillosis (discussed on this page). The optimum dose of amphotericin B is 1.0 to 1.5 mg. per kilogram of body weight per day. However, because of the frequency with which severe toxic reactions, including nausea, vomiting, chills and fever, follow the institution of therapy with doses in this range, treatment routinely is started at a much lower level. On day 1, for example, 1.0 mg. of the drug dissolved in 250 ml. of 5 per cent dextrose solution is injected intravenously over a 6-hour period; on day 2, the patient receives 5 mg. of amphotericin B in 500 ml., and on day 3, 10 mg. of the drug in 1,000 ml. of dextrose solution. Thereafter, the dose is increased by increments of 5 or 10 mg. each day until the desired level is attained, namely, 1.0 to 1.5 mg. per kilo injected intravenously in concentrations no greater than 1 mg. per 10 ml. dextrose solution. Should toxic reactions ensue nevertheless, they may be ameliorated (or they may be hopefully prevented) by the administration of a salicylate (e.g., aspirin, 0.6 Gm.) and one of the antihistaminic anti-emetic drugs (e.g., promethazine hydrochloride, 25 mg.) by mouth 30 minutes prior to each infusion of amphotericin B.

NORTH AMERICAN BLASTOMYCOSIS

Blastomycosis, in addition to its common skin lesions, sometimes involves the internal organs—the lung in particular and occasionally this organ exclusively.

Treatment. The treatment of this condition includes all measures designed to improve the general nutrition of the patient, together with 2-hydroxystilbamidine (110 to 225 mg. daily, given intravenously in 5 per cent dextrose solution at least 5 days each week for at least 30 days. The majority of patients who fail to respond to 2-hydroxystilamidine may be treated successfully with amphotericin B.

COCCIDIOMYCOSIS

Coccidiomycosis, or coccidioidal granuloma, is similar in many ways to blastomycosis. The infectious agent is the fungus *Coccidioides immitis,* which often produces lesions of the lungs and the bones which suggest tuberculosis.

Treatment. The best treatment is intravenous injections of amphotericin B, which has proved to be curative in at least 50 per cent of patients with the severest forms of coccidiomycosis, resistant to all other chemotherapeutic agents tested.

SPOROTRICHOSIS

Sporotrichosis, due to a spore-bearing fungus which often causes skin lesions, seldom involves the lung. The onset of the general infection is acute, with fever, symptoms of septicemia and the rapid development of multiple lesions throughout the body. This disease can be arrested quickly by the iodides given by mouth or by rectum in ascending doses up to 6 Gm. or more daily and continued for at least 1 month after apparent recovery. Intravenous amphotericin B likewise is effective in this disease.

CRYPTOCOCCOSIS

Cryptococcosis is caused by torula, a yeastlike, budding fungus which seldom attacks the skin but may infect the lungs and, later, the central nervous system, causing a meningitis that may last as long as several years. All forms of cryptococcosis have responded to treatment with amphotericin B. Combined intravenous and intrathecal injections of the drug are indicated in patients with *Cryptococcus meningitis.* Approximately two thirds of these patients have improved or recovered completely on this regimen and very few have survived on any other.

ASPERGILLOSIS

Of the common molds, *Aspergillus fumigatus* alone infests the lung, although the majority of cases of pulmonary aspergillosis are secondary infections of chronic pulmonary tuberculosis.

Acute primary pulmonary aspergillosis, seen rarely among wool-sorters and pigeon feeders (who hold the grain in the mouth), is a bronchopneumonia which leads to a necrosis and softening of lung tissue quite like that of tuberculosis.

Chronic pulmonary aspergillosis produces a chronic pulmonary fibrosis which spreads bushlike from the hilum of the lung. Its symptoms for years are attacks of severe paroxysmal cough, particularly at night, and sputum, scanty or abundant and mucopurulent in type, which contains the spores and mycelial threads of *Aspergillus*. These patients have no loss of weight or strength and no malaise. Often they are diagnosed as cases of advanced pulmonary tuberculosis, although they give no specific tests for that disease and continue for years to live active lives.

Treatment. Recovery from aspergillosis has been reported in response to amphotericin B, but further clinical trial is needed to establish its effectiveness in this mycotic infection.

48

Patients With Parasitic Infestations

FILARIASIS

Filariasis is due to bodily infestation by the adults and the embryos belonging to roundworms of the filaria group.

The most important of these worms is *Wuchereria bancrofti,* a parasite very common in Africa and India. In some regions of India cases of filariasis are as numerous as those of malaria. An occasional case is found in our southern states.

Clinical Course. Its embryos, injected into the skin by the bite of a *Culex* mosquito, which previously has bitten a patient with filariasis, locate and reach maturity in the lymph channels and nodes which drain the part bitten (therefore, most often those of the pelvis and the groin). Here the adults, several inches long, block the lymph flow, causing elephantiasis (that is, the legs become huge from a great thickening of the skin), chyluria or hematochyluria (if the lymphatics in the bladder are obstructed) and hydrocele.

The adult worms produce vast numbers of embryos (about $\frac{1}{75}$ of an inch long) which remain in the blood stream. These seem to do no harm. The embryos of this parasite appear in the peripheral blood at night, during the day remaining in the capillaries of the lungs and other organs. In the case of night laborers, however, the embryos appear only during the day.

In addition to the above-mentioned local symptoms due to lymphostasis, the patient also suffers certain general symptoms, such as irregular fever, headache, generalized malaise, sweating and pruritus.

Treatment. The only possible treatment, if practical (which is rare), consists of removing the adult worm surgically. Antimony administered intravenously relieves the general symptoms but does not reduce the embryo count in the blood.

Other Types

Other types of filarial worms include *Onchocerca volvulus,* the adults of which locate in colonies in the subcutaneous tissue, giving rise to multiple spongy skin nodules, while the embryos are found in the nearby lymph spaces. They are prevalent in certain parts of Africa and Central America. The adults of *Mansonella ozzardi,* a filarial parasite of the West Indies and South America, locate in the mesenteric lymph vessels, while their embryos appear in the blood stream. And, finally, the adults of *Loa loa* (the eye worm), of Africa, travel actively in the subcutaneous and the subconjunctival tissues (whence they are easily removed by operation), while their embryos appear in the blood stream.

TRICHINOSIS

Trichinosis is infestation by a parasitic disease due to *Trichinella spiralis,* one of the roundworms.

Clinical Course. This is a disease of pigs, in the muscle fibers of which these tiny embryos lie encysted. These calcified cysts, barely visible to the naked eye, appear in the meat like tiny grains of sand. If such pork is eaten insufficiently cooked, the embryos are set free by the gastric juice and develop in the intestine during the following week to adult worms from 3 to 4 mm. long. These worms make their way into the mucous membrane and there produce myriads of embryos. The symptoms of this, the period of invasion, which last about 1 week, are diarrhea, a fever suggesting typhoid, nausea, vomiting and occasionally abdominal pain.

The embryos, carried by the blood stream and by their own activity, migrate to all parts of the body. The symptoms during this, the period of migration, which last about 10 days, are pain and soreness in the muscles, edema of the eyelids, scleral hemorrhages, occasionally cardiac irregularities (due to trichinae in the heart muscle, which may be fatal), redness and swelling of the tongue and a marked eosinophilia (even 50 per cent of a total leukocyte count of 30,-000) which continues for months. Very severe cases develop anemia, cachexia, furunculosis and pneumonia. The embryos gradually become encysted, each in a muscle fiber, after which there are no symptoms.

Diagnosis. This is confirmed by the discovery of the embryos themselves in a biopsy specimen of muscle usually removed from the calf of the leg. A skin test using an extract of trichinae as the test antigen becomes positive after from 16 to 20 days and may be positive for years afterward. A precipitin test also may yield information useful in diagnosis.

Prophylaxis. This consists of accurate inspection of the pork when killed and thorough cooking before it is eaten.

Treatment. Piperazine citrate, injected in daily doses of from 2 to 3 Gm. for 7 days, may remove many of the adult worms that are free in the bowel. After they have penetrated into its mucous membrane, nothing can be done.

Prevention. It is estimated that at least 1 of every 7 persons in the United States, i.e., about 25 million persons, harbor this parasite, and that approximately 350,000 individuals acquire new infections each year. Of these, less than 5 per cent experience symptoms, and of those acquiring symptomatic infections about 5 per cent die.

A nationwide program for the control and eventual eradication of trichinosis embodies the following proposals:

1. Establishment of state laws forbidding the feeding of hogs with garbage and offal other than that cooked at licensed establishments.

2. Enforcement of interstate quarantine regulations forbidding the shipping across state lines of uncooked garbage that might be used as swine fodder.

3. The forbidding of movement of swine out of any state that does not have or enforce garbage cooking laws.

4. Education of farmers to remove all uncooked pork scraps and offal from the feed given to his own swine.

5. Public education relative to incineration and alternate methods of garbage disposal.

6. Prohibition by state law of the sale of garbage-fed hogs to slaughter houses that do not operate under Federal inspection or its equivalent.

7. Public education regarding the importance of cooking thoroughly all pork and pork products.

8. Support for continued research on methods of destroying *Trichinella* in pork.

9. Improvement of diagnostic procedures for the identification of trichinosis in hogs and man.

HOOKWORM

Hookworm disease (ancylostomiasis and uncinariasis) is the result of infestation of the upper part of the small intestine by one of two quite similar roundworms about half an inch long: *Uncinaria americana* (the New World hookworm) and *Ancylostoma duodenale* (the Old World form).

Incidence. Hookworm disease is common in rural regions of the tropics, notably of Africa, but also of Europe and of some of our southern states.

Clinical Course. The embryos of this worm, hatched from eggs passed in the stools, live in dirt, sand and clay and easily infest man. They enter by mouth if he eats with dirty hands, or by boring through the skin of bare feet (ground itch). Having gained access to the blood or lymph vessels, they are carried by the blood stream to the lungs, migrate from the pulmonary capillaries into the air cells, reach the pharynx, are swallowed and mature to adult forms in the bowel. The food of these worms is the patient's blood. To obtain this they wound the mucous membrane at many points and leave bleeding all the wounds they make.

The result of these multiple hemorrhages is a severe hypochromic anemia characteristic of chronic blood loss.

The patient, if a child, develops to maturity slowly; he is anemic; his skin has a muddy, pale hue; his eyes are dull and heavy (fish eyes). Later, the skin is edematous, and the patient is weak and short of breath.

The diagnosis of hookworm disease is made easily, since if enough worms are present to cause any symptoms their eggs will be abundant in the stools.

Chemotherapy. Eighty per cent of patients are cured of hookworm disease by a single dose of tetrachlorethylene, the amount given being computed on the basis of 0.12 ml. per Kg. of body weight and not in excess of 5 ml. total at one time. As for the minority of patients whose infestation is not eradicated completely by one dose of the drug, the number of worms that they retain is rarely significant, and this residue can be eliminated completely by repetition of the treatment every 4 or 5 days until the stools are free of eggs.

ROUNDWORM

Ascaris lumbricoides, a roundworm from 4 to 12 inches long, is a common intestinal parasite of children and, as a rule, does no harm. If present in large numbers, however, masses of them may cause intestinal obstruction. This worm may wander up into the stomach, whence it is vomited, or up the esophagus to the pharynx, from which point it may reach the trachea and the bronchi and cause fatal pneumonia. It has been known to enter the nose, or force its way up the eustachian tube, and, having ruptured the drum, appear in the external ear. Also it may enter the common bile duct, causing obstructive jaundice; and occasionally it thrusts its head through a gastric or typhoid ulcer, causing peritonitis.

Chemotherapy. Of the many drugs that are available for the treatment of ascaris infection, one of the most effective is piperazine. This drug may be given by mouth or tube, in cases of intestinal obstruction, without preliminary purgation or preparation of any kind, and may be used safely in infants and children, as well as adult patients. The recommended dose is 75 mg. per Kg. of body weight per day, not to exceed 3 Gm. a day, for each of two successive days, the daily dose being divided into 2 or 3 portions. Almost 100 per cent of patients are cured by this treatment.

PINWORM

Enterobiasis (oxyuriasis) is the commonest helminthic infection in the United States. The pinworm (*Enterobius vermicularis*) is a small white threadlike worm, about a quarter of an inch long, commonly found in the rectum of children. The chief symptom it causes is intense itching, especially at night, when the female crawls out of the skin, depositing eggs about the anus. The fingernails should be examined for eggs, and nail-biting children should be forced to wear gloves until the infection has been controlled, for this is the common mode of reinfection. The worm often resides in the appendix and is said to be responsible for a high proportion of appendicitis cases among young children. Confirmation of diagnosis can be obtained by preparing anal impressions on cellophane adhesive tape. The percentage of anal impressions that prove to be positive, out of a series made on 7 to 10 successive days, provides a rough index as to the severity of infestation and the likelihood of its recurrence after treatment.

Chemotherapy. Most patients with enterobiasis are relieved completely and conveniently of their infestation by a single oral dose of pyrvinium pamoate suspension (Povan Suspension), ingested by the fasting patient in a dose equivalent to 5 mg. of pyrvinium base per Kg. of body weight (or one 5-ml. teaspoonful of the suspension per 22 lbs.). Patients (or their parents) should be alerted to the fact that their stools will acquire a bright red color following medication, a phenomenon to which no ominous significance is attached.

TAPEWORM

Tapeworms are long flat segmented worms, each with a head, a neck and a chain of thin broad segments, or links. These worms live in the intestines.

Beef Tapeworm. *Taenia saginata,* the beef tapeworm, the one most common in America, is acquired by eating insufficiently cooked "measled" beef (that is, beef containing this worm in its larval form). In the bowel of man this worm grows to a length of from 15 to 20 feet. The head, about the size of a common black-headed pin, is provided with suckers only, and the largest links are about a quarter inch broad and a half inch or more long. Broken-off chains of links, full of eggs, often are passed in the stools.

Pork Tapeworm. *Taenia solium,* the pork tapeworm, rare in America, is acquired by eating insufficiently cooked infested pork. It is smaller than the beef tapeworm, being only from 6 to 12 feet long, and has somewhat smaller links. Its head, also smaller, is provided both with suckers and hooks. This worm is much more difficult than the beef worm to expel.

Cysticercus Disease. If, instead of the larval form of the pork tapeworm, man swallows one of its eggs, an embryo will be hatched in the bowel. This penetrates the intestinal mucous membrane and is carried by the blood stream to almost any organ of the body. Wherever it settles, it becomes encysted; and in this larval cyst, about a half inch in diameter, only the head of the tapeworm develops.

The internal organs and the skin of an infested person may contain one or thousands of these cysts. Most of them do no harm; but should one locate in the brain or the eye, its symptoms would be those of any tumor of that size in that location.

No treatment except surgery will remove these cysts.

Fish Tapeworm. *Diphyllobothrium latum,* a tapeworm common in Europe and the Far East, but comparatively rare in America, is acquired by eating uncooked, infested fish. It may grow to a length of from 25 to 30 feet.

Symptoms Caused by Tapeworm. The beef and pork tapeworms cause few if any symptoms, except those suggested by the patient's knowledge that he has the worm. The fish tapeworm, however, occasionally precipitates an anemia which scarcely can be distinguished from pernicious anemia.

Diagnosis. The diagnosis of all large tapeworms is easy, for their links appear in nearly every stool the patient passes, and when seen cannot be mistaken.

Chemotherapy. All forms of intestinal tapeworm infestation respond to quinacrine (Atabrine) chemotherapy. On the day prior to treatment, the patient's intake is restricted to clear soups, rice, cooked cereal and fruit juices; 60 ml. of saturated solution of magnesium sulfate is ingested during the evening. On the following morning, the patient, still fasting, ingests three 0.1-Gm. tablets of quinacrine as the initial dose. This dose is repeated one half hour later and again in 1 hour following the initial dose, a few ounces of orange juice being given with each dose of tablets. Magnesium sulfate solution (60 ml.) is given 1 or 2 hours following the third and final dose of quinacrine. The liquid stools which are likely to follow soon thereafter are collected in a glass jar to permit observation of the tapeworm, which usually is passed, intact, within a period of a few hours. Failure of the head to emerge with the rest of the worm does not imply, necessarily, that the treatment has failed. Under these circumstances, the patient is advised that, if success has not been achieved, segments again will be passed in the stools within a period of from 6 to 12 weeks, and at that time, but not sooner, retreatment can be carried out. The first treatment is successful in about 70 per cent of cases.

HYDATID DISEASE

Hydatid disease, the most serious of all tapeworm infestations, is due to *Taenia echinococcus,* a parasite only about one fifth of an inch long infesting dogs and sheep. Echinococcus disease is common in Australia and Iceland. It is rare in America.

Clinical Course. If an egg of this worm reaches the stomach, it hatches, and the tiny embryo thus set free burrows its way through the intestinal wall and is carried by the blood stream to some distant organ. Wherever it lodges it forms a little cyst, or bladder, the hydatid (drop of water) cyst, which contains the larval head of the worm. Thus far it resembles the cysticercus of the pork tapeworm, but its later development is quite different. This little bladder buds again and again, hundreds of times, each bud producing a new cyst similar to and the same size as the first. These daughter cysts in turn may bud and soon contain many granddaughter cysts. The one original cyst, now of great size, may contain hundreds of these small cysts.

The symptoms of one of these cysts are those of tumor of the organ in which it lies.

Treatment. The treatment is surgical removal of the cysts (always with great care lest it rupture during the operation, setting free one or more tiny embryos, each of which can start a new cyst).

FLUKE INFESTATIONS: DISTOMIASIS

Flukes are parasitic, leaf-shaped flatworms; their infestations of man are called *distomiasis*. The life history of flukes is most complicated, since one, two or three intermediate hosts are necessary for the life cycle of the worm. These cycles include free-swimming larval stages, hence fluke infestations are most common among people who must work in water or eat water plants or raw fish from infested water. Distomiasis, therefore, is endemic only in regions where exactly the right conditions are present; but where it is endemic, it usually affects a large percentage of the population. These infestations must be massive to occasion any symptoms. The diagnosis is always made by finding the fluke eggs (distinctive for each type) in the stools.

Intestinal Flukes

The most important fluke that infests the bowel is the intestinal one, *Fasciolopsis buski* (a flatworm about 1 inch long and a half inch wide), the larvae of which are ingested with aquatic plant foods. If the patient harbors many of these flukes, the symptoms which arise are weakness, a chronic diarrhea of blood-free stools and abdominal pain. After months, an edema, often marked, appears. It starts as an ascites, then involves the lower extremities and, extending upward, the face or even the lungs. In marked cases the temperature is subnormal, and the skin is yellow, harsh and dry; cardiac insufficiency occasionally arises. Death apparently is from malnutrition and dehydration resulting from the continuous diarrhea.

Treatment. After a few days of restricted diet, chloroform, thymol, betanaphthol or carbon tetrachloride is administered; this is followed by a saline laxative. During this treatment the patient should remain in bed. Dead flukes will be passed in about 12 hours, and the patient will begin to improve at once.

Blood Flukes: Bilharziasis

Bilharziasis, or infestation of the blood vessels by one of several types of blood flukes, produces, if a sufficient number of parasites are present, first an initial urticarial and petechial skin rash (due to the invasion of the skin by the larval forms of the fluke) and later hematuria or dysentery, according to the location of the infestation. The liver always is enlarged.

Types. One type of blood fluke, *Schistosoma haematobium* (an elongated fluke about a half inch long and $\frac{1}{25}$ of an inch wide, common in some regions of Africa and Asia Minor), resides in the pelvic veins—especially in those of the bladder and the rectum. Some persons harbor these flukes for years, the only evidence of their presence, if in the bladder wall, being the constant or occasional appearance of small clots of blood in the urine. More serious infestations, however, cause thickening and ulceration of the bladder, hence urinary stasis, bladder calculi or ureteral obstruction. Dysentery with severe tenesmus indicates infestation of the rectal veins. The ova, by embolism, may reach the brain, giving rise to symptoms simulating brain tumor. After persisting for variable lengths of time this parasite often disappears spontaneously.

Another blood fluke, *Schistosoma mansoni,* found in Africa, the West Indies and South America, infests the mesenteric veins, causing emaciation, colic and chronic dysentery. A third blood fluke, *Schistosoma japonicum,* common among the workers of Japan and the Far East, causes a serious disease characterized by diarrhea with or without fever, painful enlargement of the liver and the spleen, edema, anemia and occasionally pulmonary and cerebral symptoms.

All blood flukes seem to develop from their free-swimming larval forms, either those in drinking water or in water in which the person wades, in which circumstance the larvae penetrate the skin.

Chemotherapy. The treatment of choice for *S. haematobium* and *S. mansoni* infestations is the intramuscular injection of stibo-

SUMMARY OF PRINCIPLES AND OBJECTIVES OF COMMUNICABLE DISEASE PRACTICES

1. Assist in identifying the etiologic agent and establishing the diagnosis.
    A. Obtain specimens of blood, urine, stools, sputum, throat swabbings, nasal secretions and pyogenic exudates for bacteriologic study.
    B. Assist in securing smears of blood and other materials for microscopic examination.
    C. Assist with aspirations of spinal fluid, bone marrow and other body fluids or tissues for cytologic, serologic and bacteriologic tests.
    D. Carry out appropriate skin tests for specific diagnostic reactions as directed.

2. Control the infection.
    A. Administer the appropriate antimicrobial agents as ordered.
    B. Assist in administering specific immune therapy, if available, employing immune antiserum, gamma globulin, antitoxin, toxoid, vaccine or an appropriate mixture of antigen and antibody, depending on the circumstances.
    C. Observe patient carefully for evidences of drug or serum sensitivity.

3. Prevent spread of the infection.
    A. Carry out isolation technic as required.
    B. Observe asepsis as indicated.
    C. Use mask technic effectively.
        a. Change mask frequently.
        b. Refrain from handling mask while in use.
    D. Wash hands immediately after each patient contact and after every contact with material that may be contaminated and is potentially infectious.
    E. Disinfect and handle wastes with all due precautions.
    F. Handle bed linens and fomites with care.
    G. Carry out concurrent disinfection of fomites.
    H. Control dissemination of infectious droplets.
        a. Encourage patient to cover nose and mouth when coughing or sneezing.
        b. Wrap contaminated tissues and articles in paper before disposal.
    I. Control dust.
        a. Require damp dusting of furniture and wet vacuum cleaning of floors.
        b. Reduce to a minimum the activity of personnel in the patient's room.
        c. Maintain cleanliness of surroundings.
    J. Ventilate patient's room well.
    K. Keep door to room closed.
    L. Disinfect room air with ultraviolet light, if indicated.

4. Provide physiologic support.
    A. Ensure adequate hydration in the face of excessive fluid loss through vomiting, diarrhea or excessive sweating.
        a. Encourage the ingestion of fluids.
        b. Prepare for the administration of intravenous fluids as required.
    B. Reduce the fever.
        a. Administer antipyretic drugs, as prescribed.
        b. Employ cool sponges cautiously, as indicated.

SUMMARY OF PRINCIPLES AND OBJECTIVES OF COMMUNICABLE DISEASE PRACTICES (Continued)

    C. Measure and record body temperature, pulse and respiratory rates frequently.

    D. Measure arterial pressure at regular intervals if patient exhibits a tendency to vascular collapse.

    E. Weigh patient periodically.

5. Provide symptomatic relief.

    A. Combat generalized aching and malaise.

        a. Utilize warm applications and massage, as indicated.

        b. Apply cold compresses for headache.

        c. Administer analgesic medications as ordered.

        d. Attend to oral hygiene.

        e. Restrict physical activity.

    B. Relieve cough.

        a. Humidify inspired air.

        b. Administer hot gargles and throat irrigations.

        c. Supply expectorants or cough depressants as indicated and prescribed.

    C. Relieve anxiety and depression.

        a. Recognize loneliness of the isolated patient.

        b. Lend strong encouragement to patient faced with prospect of prolonged convalescence.

6. Protect exposed individuals and public at large against infectious illness.

    A. Make available, facilitate or perform whatever vaccination procedures are known to be effective and are indicated for the stimulation of active immunity in exposed and susceptible individuals.

    B. Furnish specific immune serum (heterologous or human convalescent) or human gamma globulin, if indicated, to provide passive immunity and temporary protection to contacts who are particularly vulnerable.

    C. Quarantine patients with communicable infections, as well as known carriers and contacts, when required.

    D. Educate the public with respect to:

        a. The availability and importance of prophylactic immunizations

        b. The manner in which infectious illnesses are spread and methods of avoiding spread

        c. The importance of seeking medical advice in the event of a febrile illness or skin eruption

        d. The importance of environmental cleanliness and personal hygiene

        e. Means of preventing the contamination of food and water supplies

            (1) Discipline, cleanliness and inspection of food handlers

            (2) The dangers of "perishable" foods; the identity of foods that tend to promote bacterial growth; and methods of food preservation

            (3) The significance of milk pasteurization

            (4) The indications for, and methods of, sterilizing foods by means of heat

        f. Knowledge of insect, rodent and other animal vectors and reservoirs of human infections and importance of their elimination

phen (Fuadin), 1 ml. per 13.6 Kg. of body weight, on 20 consecutive days. The maximum dose for any one day should not exceed 5 ml. The rate of administration, but not the total dosage, may be modified in the event of severe vomiting. Dosage schedules entailing the administration of from 90 to 100 ml. of the drug are associated with cure rates approximating 100 per cent. *S. japonicum* infestation is treated most effectively by the intravenous injection of tartar emetic on alternate days until a total dose of 2.5 Gm., or 500 ml. of the 0.5 per cent solution, has been received, the initial dose being 8 ml., and the maximum dose for a single day being 28 ml.

Liver Flukes

Hepatic distomiasis due to tiny liver flukes (*Clonorchis sinensis*) acquired by eating raw fish infested with larvae, is a disease common in the Far East. If a sufficient number of flukes are present (more than 21,000 were found in the liver of one patient), the infestation causes a bloody diarrhea with subsequent ascites, jaundice, marked anemia and fatal cachexia. The liver at first becomes large, but later, small and cirrhotic; the spleen is enlarged.

Treatment. Currently favored as the treatment of choice in cases of liver fluke infestation is chloroquine diphosphate, given in 250-mg. doses twice daily for 7 or 8 weeks.

Lung Fluke: Pulmonary Distomiasis

Pulmonary distomiasis, or infestation of the lung by the lung fluke *Paragonimus westermani* (which has the shape and size of a coffee bean), is a disease common in the Far East and also in Yucatan and Peru. It is acquired by eating raw crabs or crawfish, or by drinking water containing larvae liberated from disintegrating crabs. It is characterized chiefly by thoracic pain, cough and signs of chronic lung infection, with hemoptysis or blood-stained or purulent sputum in which the eggs of this fluke are found easily. This fluke, however, may infest any other organ, with symptoms depending on the organ involved.

Diagnosis. The eggs of the lung fluke may be found in the sputum, the feces and the body fluids obtained by puncture.

Treatment. No therapy is satisfactory.

CLINICAL SITUATION
(Choose the *most nearly correct* answer.)

1. In caring for the patient with a communicable disease, the nurse must maintain strict environmental control. To decrease air-borne organisms, good ventilation is promoted, since:
   A. Air currents neutralize the droplet nuclei.
   B. Ventilation rids the environment of dust.
   C. Air destroys some pathogens by drying.
   D. Ventilation increases the humidity of the room.
2. The nurse's hands may be a major source of contamination. Frequent and thorough hand washing is mandatory to:
   A. Prevent pathogens from becoming part of the skin flora.
   B. Rid the hands of resident bacteria.
   C. Prevent reinfection of the host.
   D. Increase the skin's resistance to pathogenic bacteria.
3. Staphylococcal infections have become a serious problem in hospitals due to several factors. Of the following, all have contributed to this problem with one exception:
   A. Increasing resistance to antibiotics.
   B. Use of germicides for general cleaning.
   C. Development of more carriers.
   D. Rising incidence of different bacterial strains.
4. The mode of transmission of upper respiratory infection is usually through
   A. Eating utensils.
   B. Blood-borne organisms.
   C. Direct contact or droplet spread.
   D. The ingestion of contaminated food.
5. Syphilis is the most dangerous venereal disease and its incidence is rising. One of the major public health problems with this disease is:

A. The paucity of laboratories to support the epidemiologic program.
B. The failure to reach the indigent patient.
C. The high cost of penicillin therapy.
D. The large number of unknown persons with infectious syphilis.

BIBLIOGRAPHY AND SUGGESTED READING

Books

Control of Communicable Diseases in Man, ed. 9, New York, Am. Pub. Health Ass., 1960.

Symposium on Infectious Diseases: Pediat. Clin. N. Am., Vol. 7, Philadelphia, Saunders, Nov., 1960.

Top, F. H.: Communicable and Infectious Diseases, Ed. 4, St. Louis, Mosby, 1960.

Viral and Rickettsial Diseases: Med. Clin. N. Am., Vol. 43, Philadelphia, Saunders, Sept., 1959.

Therapeutic Notes: Special issue on Communicable Diseases, Parke, Davis and Company, Vol. 68, Sept., 1961.

Articles

Defense Against Infection

Ager, E. A.: Immunization as practiced today, Am. J. Nurs. 62:74-79, May, 1962.

Bullough, B.: Where should isolation stop? Am. J. Nurs. 62:86-89, Oct., 1962.

Editorial: Cross-infections from thermometers, J.A.M.A. 164:669, 1957.

Foster, M.: A positive approach to medical asepsis, Am. J. Nurs. 62:76-77, Apr., 1962.

Keck, A.: One dose per syringe, Nurs. Outlook 7:24-25, Jan., 1959.

Kriegel, J.: A coordinated infection control program, Nurs. Outlook 9:152-154, Mar., 1961.

Layton, P.: Adventures with COSTEP, Am. J. Nurs. 60:1270-1272, 1960.

Lester, M. R.: Every nurse an epidemiologist, Am. J. Nurs. 57:1434-1435, 1957.

McCrumb, F. R., Jr.: Immunization (editorial), Ann. Intern. Med. 52:1161-1169, 1960.

Riley, R. L.: Protective measures . . . reasonable or ritualistic, Nurs. Outlook 7:38-39, Jan., 1959.

Sherris, J. C., and Lancaster, L. J.: Physical and chemical means of infection control, J. Chron. Dis. 15:743-755, 1962.

Vesley, D., and Brask, M.: Environmental implications in the control of hospital acquired infections, Nurs. Outlook 9:742-745, 1961.

Bacterial Infections

Calafiore, D. C.: Streptococcal infections, Nurs. Outlook 7:712-715, 1959.

Caswell, H. T.: Staphylococcal infections among hospital personnel, Am. J. Nurs. 58:822-823, 1958.

Chanyo, B., *et al.:* Acute renal failure in Asiatic cholera, Ann. Intern. Med. 52:960-975, 1960.

Coerver, R. M. M.: One man's meat, Am. J. Nurs. 58:690-692, 1958.

Doull, J. A.: Current status of therapy of leprosy, J.A.M.A. 173:363-373, 1960.

Dull, H. B., and Rakich, J. H.: Tetanus today, Nurs. Outlook 7:464-467, 1959.

Edsall, G.: Typhoid fever, Am. J. Nurs. 59:989-992, 1959.

Harder, H. I., and Panuska, M.: A program to control staphylococcal infections, Am. J. Nurs. 58:349-351, 1958.

Hurst, V., *et al.:* Hospital laundry and refuse chutes as source of staphylococcic cross-infection, J.A.M.A. 167:1223, 1958.

Jones, J. M.: Tuberculosis among the aged, Nurs. Outlook 56:675, 1956.

Lester, M. R.: Staphylococcal infections: an annotated bibliography, Am. J. Nurs. 59:1805-1828, 1959.

Levin, B. G.: For more effective shigellosis control, Am. J. Nurs. 61:104-108, Nov., 1961.

Miller, A. L., and McDonald, E.: Staphylococcal infections — a community problem, Nurs. Outlook 7:584-587, 1959.

Pasyotis, F.: Typhoid fever—circa 1958, Nurs. Outlook 7:85-87, 1959.

Perlstein, M. A.: Control of tetanus spasms by administration of meprobamate, J.A.M.A. 170:1902-1908, 1959.

Ravenholt, R. T., and Nixon, M.: The telephone in epidemiology of staphylococcal disease, Am. J. Nurs. 61:60-64, Aug., 1961.

Rogers, D. E.: Staphylococcal disease on general medical services, Am. J. Nurs. 59:842-844, 1959.

Schirger, A., *et al.:* Brucellosis: experiences with 224 patients, Ann. Intern. Med. 52:827-837, 1960.

Southeast Asia Treaty Organization: Conference on Cholera—1960, Pub. Health Rep., Washington, 76:323-334, Apr., 1961.

Spink, W. W.: Current status of therapy of brucellosis in human beings, J.A.M.A. 172:697-698, 1960.

Thompson, L. R.: Staphylococcus aureus, Am. J. Nurs. 58:1098-1100, 1958.

Yow, E. M., *et al.:* The management of hospital-acquired staphylococcal infections, A.M.A. Arch. Int. Med. **102:**948-959, 1958.

Viral and Rickettsial

Benenson, A. S.: Why does smallpox still exist?, Am. J. Nurs. **62:**77-79, Sept., 1962.

Boger, W. P., *et al.:* Asian influenza, New Eng. J. Med. **262:**856-860, 1960.

Bowles, C.: Taking part in smallpox research in India, Am. J. Nurs. **61:**92-93, Dec., 1961.

Cabasso, V. J., *et al.:* Oral poliomyelitis vaccine, Lederle — thirteen years of laboratory and field investigation, New Eng. J. Med. **263:**1321-1330, 1960.

DiSandro, E. H.: Eastern viral encephalitis—nursing experience, Am. J. Nurs. **60:**507-508, 1960.

Dougherty, W. J.: The epidemiology, Am. J. Nurs. **60:**509-510, 1960.

Dougherty, W. J., and Faro, S. N.: Factors affecting the incidence and severity of poliomyelitis, New Eng. J. Med. **261:**934-936, 1959.

Eickhoff, T. C., *et al.:* Observations on excess mortality associated with epidemic influenza, J.A.M.A. **176:**776-782, 1961.

Ferris, B. G., Jr., *et al.:* Life-threatening poliomyelitis, New Eng. J. Med. **262:**370-380, 1960.

Gelfand, H. M., *et al.:* Intrafamilial and interfamilial spread of living vaccine strains of polioviruses, J.A.M.A. **170:**2039-2048, 1959.

Gibbs, F. A., *et al.:* Electroencephalographic abnormality in 'uncomplicated' childhood diseases, J.A.M.A. **171:**1050-1055, 1959.

Gothberg, L. A.: Severe infectious mononucleosis treated with chloroquine phosphate, J.A.M.A. **173:**53-57, 1960.

Hammon, W. M., *et al.:* A study of certain non-poliomyelitis and poliomyelitis enterovirus infections, J.A.M.A. **167:**727-735, 1958.

Jensen, K. E., Woodhour, A. F., and Bailey, A. A.: Considerations involved in immunizations with polyvalent influenza vaccines, J.A.M.A. **172:**1230-1238, 1960.

Langmuir, A. D.: Progress in conquest of paralytic poliomyelitis, J.A.M.A. **171:**271-273, 1959.

————: Asian influenza in the United States, Ann. Intern. Med. **49:**483-501, 1958.

Lennette, E. H., *et al.:* Viral disease of the central nervous system, J.A.M.A. **171:**1456-1464, 1959.

McCrumb, F. R., Jr.: Recent advances in the study of measles virus (editorial), Ann. Intern. Med. **50:**522-526, 1959.

Paul, J. R.: Poliovirus vaccines—killed or live, Am. J. Nurs. **60:**60-62, Jan., 1960.

Riley, R. L.: Air-borne infections, Am. J. Nurs. **60:**1246-1248, 1960.

Romer, M., Heacock, C., and Takacs, V.: An epidemic of swimming pool granuloma, Nurs. Outlook **8:**690-692, 1960.

Smadel, J. E.: Status of the rickettsioses in the United States, Ann. Intern. Med. **51:**421-435, 1959.

Spitznagel, J. K.: Effects of cortisone and ACTH in mumps meningo-encephalitis, Ann. Intern. Med. **49:**61-69, 1958.

Wilson, M. G., *et al.:* Teratogenic effects of Asian influenza, J.A.M.A. **171:**638-641, 1959.

Steele, J. H., and Lester, M. R.: Rabies and rabies control, Am. J. Nurs. **58:**521-536, 1958.

Thompson, L.: Viruses . . . old and new, Am. J. Nurs. **59:**349-351, 1959.

Today's facts about tomorrow's vaccine for measles, Am. J. Nurs. **62:**68-70, June, 1962.

Spirochetal and Protozoan Infections

Brown, W. J.: Venereal disease control, Am. J. Nurs. **61:**94-96, Apr., 1961.

Carpenter, C. M., Miller, J. N., and Boak, R. A.: A 'triplet test plan' for the serologic diagnosis of syphilis, New Eng. J. Med. **263:**1016-1018, 1960.

Cromwell, G. E.: Venereal disease and the teen-ager, Am. J. Nurs. **59:**1738-1739, 1959.

Deschin, C. S.: VD and the adolescent personality, Am. J. Nurs. **63:**59-63, Nov., 1963.

Garson, W.: Recent developments in the laboratory diagnosis of syphilis, Ann. Intern. Med. **51:**748-758, 1959.

Glassberg. B. Y.: Venereal disease among adolescents, Nurs. Outlook **10:**731-732, Nov., 1962.

Lentz, J. W., and Hall, M. N.: Venereal disease control in the twentieth century, Nurs. Outlook **10:**722-729, Nov., 1962.

Maxwell, M.: A careful look at venereal disease nursing, Am. J. Nurs. **61:**94-95, Dec., 1961.

Taylor, S. D.: Clinic for adolescents with venereal disease, Am. J. Nurs. **63:**63-66, Nov., 1963.

The World Health Organization program to rid the world of malaria, Am. J. Nurs. **59:**1402-1404, 1959.

Parasitic Infestations

Most, H.: Current concepts in therapy; anthel-

minthic therapy, I, New Eng. J. Med. **259:**
341-342, and Anthelminthic therapy, II, 441-
443, 1958.

Patient-Teaching Aids and Information

Public Health Service Publication   *Number*

About Syphilis and Gonorrhea	410
Amebiasis	157
Brucellosis	102
Chicken pox	173
Diphtheria	60
Influenza	163
Insects that Carry Disease	594
Leptospirosis	696
Louse Infestation	103
Malaria	166
Measles	303
Meningococcal Meningitis	219
Mumps	61
Pinworms	108
Swine Brucellosis	895
Tapeworm	158
Trichinosis	101
Tuberculosis, the Development of Present Knowledge About	30-A
Tuberculosis	30
Tularemia	135
Typhoid Fever	282
Whooping Cough	220

These may be obtained from:

U. S. Department of Health, Education
and Welfare,
Public Health Service,
Superintendent of Documents,
U. S. Government Printing Office,
Washington 25, D. C.

PART THREE

Nursing Care of Patients Under Emergency and Disaster Conditions

49

Emergency and Disaster Nursing

ORIENTATION

Discussions of nursing principles and practices in preceding portions of this text are predicated generally on the assumption that adequate facilities for patient care would be available automatically. Therapy has been described in ideal terms, according to modern standards, on the implicit assumption that its selection, and the method by which it is conducted, are dictated exclusively by the patient's needs in every case. The fact is, of course, that in certain emergencies it becomes impossible to render ideal medical and nursing care. Circumstances may arise that result in a sudden, unprecedented demand for treatment of a type or on such a scale that the needs cannot possibly be met with the limited facilities and the available personnel.

THE MEANING OF DISASTER

A *disaster* is a catastrophe which is man-made, produced accidentally or by design, i.e., as a hostile enemy act, or which is of natural origin. Disasters caused by war may be thermonuclear, biologic, chemical or psychological. Man-made catastrophes may be train, plane or automobile accidents, or fires and explosions. Examples of natural disasters are epidemics, floods, hurricanes, blizzards, droughts, earthquakes and tornadoes.

Each kind of disaster takes its toll in its own particular way: property is damaged and destroyed; people are injured and killed. A traffic accident involves an automobile and its occupants, a tornado plays havoc with 1 or 2 city blocks, a thermonuclear attack may strike a large metropolitan center; whatever the cause, the product is casualties. The average hospital is able to cope with minor disasters, and the nursing student has valuable learning experiences in the emergency and the operating rooms to prepare her to function adequately and intelligently.

However, a major disaster, such as might occur during thermonuclear warfare, will present additional problems, even though the principles of care are basically the same. When large numbers of casualties need attention, priority must be given to those having the greatest need who yet, with care, are likely to survive; this is determined in large measure by the availability of medical resources. One major factor distinguishing a thermonuclear attack from all other types of catastrophe is the complication of extensive radioactive contamination of terrain, food, water, clothing and all exposed matériel.

Emergency medical care in the broadest sense of the term refers to the care of patients whose needs are urgent and critical, care administered under circumstances that may or may not be optimal, utilizing whatever facilities are at hand in the most effective manner possible. Needless to say, the proper management of the patient requiring emergency care depends on a broad knowledge of nursing principles and intimate acquaintance with a wide variety of nursing technics. So equipped, the nurse is in a position to function effectively in the event of an emergency, whether this is the result of an accident involving a few individuals or a catastrophe involving thousands.

NURSING RESPONSIBILITIES IN RELATION TO WARTIME EMERGENCIES

It is the nurse's responsibility to assume leadership in the planning, the organizing, the directing and the provision of emergency nursing service. Acceptance of this important role assumes a knowledge on her part that must include:

1. An understanding of survival procedures and emergency life-saving measures
2. Familiarity with community plans for emergency action
3. Complete knowledge of warning signals and proper action to be taken in the event of an enemy attack
4. Ability to initiate protective measures against radioactive fallout

The American Nurses Association Committee on Nursing in National Defense has released a publication on *The Role of the Nurse in Disaster.* Our professional organization recognizes that nurses should have additional preparation in applying nursing knowledge and skills "to emergency situations in a disaster environment."

The American Medical Association has developed a list of functions for nurses under mass casualty situations. The functions include:

A. First aid, including but not limited to artificial respiration; emergency treatment of open chest wounds; relief of pain; treatment of shock and the preparation of casualties for movement
B. Control of hemorrhage
C. Attainment and maintenance of patent airway, and intratracheal catheterization, to include emergency tracheotomy
D. Proper and adequate cleansing and treatment of wounds
E. Bandaging and splinting
F. Administration of anesthetics under medical supervision
G. Assisting in surgical procedures
H. Insertion of nasogastric tubes to include lavage and gavage, as directed
I. Administration of whole blood and intravenous solutions, as directed
J. Administration of parenteral medications, as directed
K. Catheterization of males and females
L. Administration of immunizing agents, as directed
M. Management of the psychologically disturbed
N. Management of normal deliveries
O. Operation of treatment and aid stations in reception areas and in communities where physicians are inadequate in number, to include the diagnosis and the treatment of minor illnesses and injuries, institution of life-saving measures and the referral of more serious cases to physicians*

PSYCHOLOGICAL MANAGEMENT OF PATIENTS IN EMERGENCY-DISASTER SITUATIONS

In dealing with patients who are under unusual emotional strain and stress, the nurse must look at her own psychological defenses. Through an understanding of herself the nurse will be able better to cope with and to control her own anxieties in an emergency situation.

Certain patterns of individual reactions are common in disaster. By the application of basic principles the nurse is able to administer emergency medical care to injured individuals. By a similar application of psychological principles the nurse is in a better position to understand herself, her colleagues and casualties.

The American Psychiatric Association Committee on Civil Defense has identified five types of reactions to disaster and offers four basic principles for better understanding of the emotionally disturbed person.

Reactions to Disaster†

1. Normal. Some obvious signs of disturbance are shown, such as trembling, profuse perspiring, feeling weak and even nauseated. Composure is gained fairly soon after the first impact of a trying experience.

2. Individual panic. Judgment seems to disappear and to be supplanted by an unreasoning attempt to flee. This type of reaction occurs in a very few individuals; its danger lies in the fact that it can excite others and may result in mass panic.

3. Depressed reactions. These individuals react as though they were numbed; they are unable to help themselves without guidance.

4. Overly active responses. These re-

* Summary Report on National Emergency Care, American Medical Association, pp. 16-17, Feb., 1962.

† Adapted from the American Psychiatric Association, Committee on Civil Defense. Psychological First Aid in Community Disasters, Washington, The Association, 1954.

sponses are poorly directed, because the individual is easily distracted as he jumps from one task to another. Often he is intolerant of any ideas other than his own and may cause disturbances.

5. Bodily reactions, such as severe nausea and vomiting, hysteria.

Four Basic Principles for Better Understanding of the Emotionally Disturbed Person

1. Accept Every Person's Right to Have His Own Feelings. Remember that each person has had certain unique experiences that can strongly affect his feelings in relation to subsequent events in his life. Years of analysis may often fail to explain fully *why* a person feels as he does. Letting a casualty know that you want to understand *how* he feels can be the first step toward helping him. Establish contact with him; do not overwhelm him with pity nor deprive him of *his* world, which appears to have collapsed.

2. Accept a Casualty's Limitations as Real. Then treat him as a potentially valuable member of the disaster team. He cannot be expected to function normally; therefore, there is no place for such remarks as "Pull yourself together," or "Snap out of it." The nurse should guard against being impatient, which may result from fatigue and resentment.

3. Size up a casualty's potentialities as accurately and as quickly as possible. The person caring for the casualty should act immediately while the patient is still suggestible, as anxiety tends to increase unless the situation is dealt with quickly and decisively. A calm, reassuring person will help the emotionally disturbed individual to mobilize his own psychological resources. Direct the casualty away from the area. Provide for a brief rest period of one or several hours. As soon as possible, give him something to do. The axiom "Action absorbs anxiety" has definite application in the management of frightened individuals.

4. Accept Your Own Limitations in a Relief Role. Know your own weaknesses well enough to handle them in a time of crisis. Are you impulsive, easily angered,

sensitive to criticism, and so forth? By understanding yourself reasonably well, you may hope justifiably to control and even to divert reactions into some more effective channel.

Psychological first aid can help many emotionally disturbed victims to get back into useful activity more quickly. Sedatives never are administered to psychological casualties except as a last resort, and then the administration is done only on the consultation with a physician. Sedation would only add to the casualty's confusion and make him even more inaccessible to more effective treatment.

Special Psychological Problems

Fatigue. It is important to recognize fatigue in one's self and coworkers. This is a common product in a disaster situation and may be heralded by evidence of mounting tension.*

Shelter Living. This presents many unique problems that can complicate the disaster situation. Material is available to assist the nurse in shelter organization and management. She needs to be able to recognize and to manage psychological disturbances that result from confined living.

PRINCIPLES OF EMERGENCY CARE

In this discussion the care of the patient as a whole is to be considered first. Then the care of the patient with injury of component body parts will be presented. The principles of mass casualty management comprise a broad outline of care that involves the exercise of sound clinical judgment and performance that is based on detailed nursing knowledge.

General Considerations

In caring for a patient in an emergency situation there are many crucial decisions to be made. These require sound judgment based on an understanding of the conditions that produced the emergency and their effect on the injured person. (See Appendix: Mobilization of Medical and Nursing Services.)

* The student also is referred to *Disaster Fatigue,* a manual prepared by the American Psychiatric Association, Committee on Civil Defense, 1956.

Certain basic principles are applicable to the emergency management of any patient. These include:

1. Maintaining a patent airway
2. Stopping the bleeding
3. Preventing and treating shock
4. Protecting the wound with a sterile or as clean a dressing as possible
5. Keeping the injured person lying down and covered
6. Allaying anxiety, and keeping him as comfortable as possible
7. Observing and reevaluating the patient at frequent intervals

Maintenance of Respiration: Rescue Breathing; Artificial Respiration

The first requisite in the treatment of any emergency condition is the maintenance of an open airway. If the airway is obstructed, the ensuing hypoxia will produce permanent brain damage or death in 3 to 5 minutes.

To determine if the patient is breathing, place the palm of the hand over his mouth and nose and feel for air movement. *If the patient is not breathing, some form of pulmonary ventilation should be started immediately.*

Mouth-to-Mouth or Mouth-to-Nose Resuscitation. The most practical method of insuring pulmonary ventilation in an emergency situation (if resuscitation equipment is unavailable) is by the mouth-to-mouth or mouth-to-nose technic. The normal expired air contains approximately 16 per cent oxygen and 4 per cent carbon dioxide. Approximately 1,000 ml. or more of air can be expelled with each expiration, and this is blown into the mouth of the patient at the rate of 12 to 20 times a minute. Adequate oxygenation may be maintained, especially if the rescuer breathes more deeply than normally.

The first requirement is that the airway be open. Most of the obstructions to the airway are in the larynx. Therefore, freeing of the larynx by removal of foreign bodies or mucus, etc., with a finger is the first measure to be used. Occasionally, it may be necessary to place the patient on his abdomen and to pat the chest gently to dislodge foreign materials.

The technic of mouth-to-mouth artificial respiration depends on holding the jaw forward so that it "juts out." This pulls the tongue forward and opens the air passage and permits inflation of the lungs. The rescuer's expired air is blown into the mouth or the nose of the patient. In order to do this in mouth artificial respiration, the nose must be held closed to seal the nasopharynx, so that the air may go into the lungs. When mouth-to-nose artificial respiration is given, the mouth is held closed, and the air is blown through the nose into the nasopharynx and the lungs. With either method, it is important that the jaw be held forward in order to open the airway into the lungs. The expired air is blown with a smooth steady action until the chest is observed to rise. This indicates inflation of the lungs with expired air. When the lungs have been inflated, the mouth of the rescuer is removed, and the lungs are allowed to empty. This cycle should be continued at the rate of about 12 to 20 cycles per minute. The rescuer should take a breath about twice the volume of ordinary respiration, and every 20 cycles he should take one deep breath himself. This type of mouth-to-mouth breathing may be maintained for an hour or more without fatigue in indicated cases. If during the active mouth-to-mouth respiration there appears to be a barrier to the flow of the air into the patient's lungs, this usually indicates an obstruction in the larynx or the pharynx which should be removed before continuing with artificial respiration.

SUMMARY

Clear the mouth of mucus and foreign objects.

Lift up the jaw.

Insert the fingers in the corner of the mouth. Grasp the bony portion of the jaw and lift upward *or* push up on the angle of the jaw.

Pinch the nostrils to provide a closed system.

Open the mouth wide and blow until the patient's chest rises.

After blowing, turn the head to the side, and *watch* the patient's chest expansion, and *listen* to hear if air is leaving the lungs. (*Blow, watch, listen!*)

FIG. 452. Technics for mouth-to-mouth and mouth-to-nose resuscitation. (Gordon, Archer S., *et al:* Mouth-to-mouth versus manual artificial respiration for children and adults, J.A.M.A., **167:**326)

Mouth-to-mouth resuscitation
Inspiration   Expiration

Mouth-to-nose resuscitation
Inspiration   Expiration

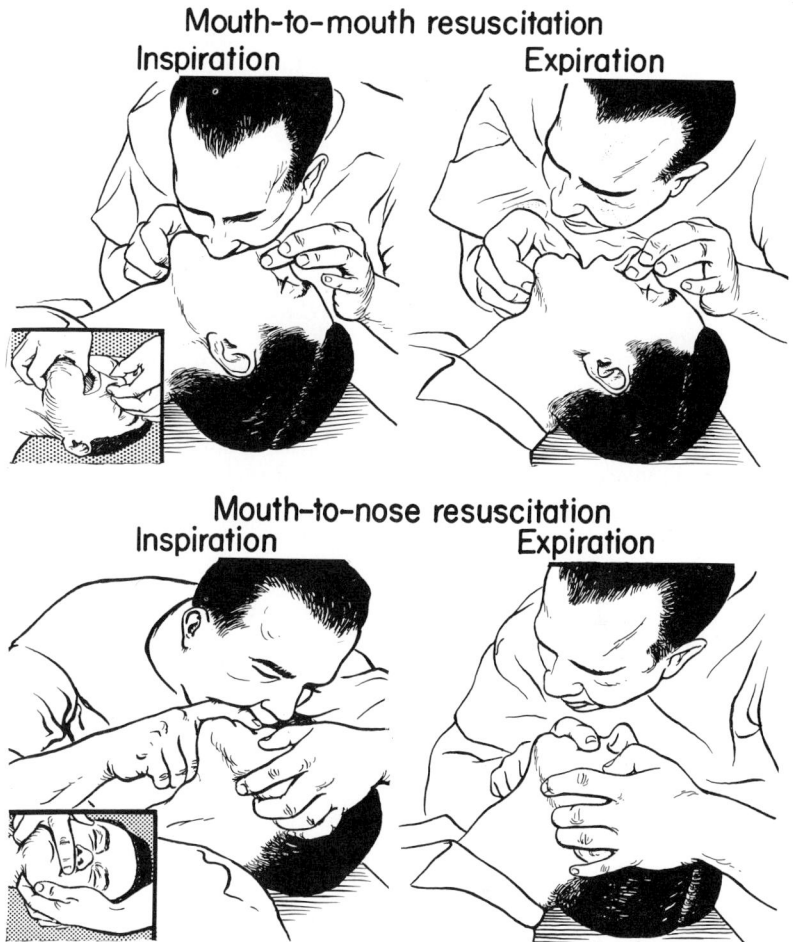

Repeat at the rate of 12 to 20 times per minute.

Prone-Pressure Method of Artificial respiration. If there are poisonous gases in the air, mouth-to-mouth resuscitation procedures will not be effective. Under these circumstances a prone-pressure method of artificial respiration should be used. Of course, the patient must wear a gas mask.

The prone-pressure method of artificial respiration is based on two principles. The first is compression of the chest against the ground by pressure applied to the back (expiration). The second is expansion of the chest by raising the arms and taking the pressure off the chest (inspiration). This method insures good expansion of the lungs and helps to oxygenate the blood reaching the heart muscle. Quick oxygenation of the blood is essential in respiratory arrest.

This method of artificial respiration, which is conducted in cycles, is carried out as follows:

1. The patient is placed face down, with the head turned to one side and the arms bent, so as to keep the mouth and nose free from obstruction.

2. The operator kneels at the casualty's head, with one knee near the head and the other foot alongside the casualty's elbow. From time to time the position of the knee and the foot is alternated.

3. The operator's hands are placed over the casualty's shoulder blades, with the thumbs touching in the midline, the fingers spread out, and the arms straight.

4. The operator bends forward, still keeping the arms straight, and applies pressure over the casualty's chest by the weight of the upper part of his own body. As he executes this movement, he counts steadily and regularly, "One-er, two-er,

and three-er," over a period of 2½ seconds. This maneuver forces out the air (deflation).

5. The operator then gradually releases the pressure on the casualty's chest by lifting the weight of his own body off it. At the same time he slides his hands to just above the casualty's elbows and counts, "Four-er," over a period of 1 second.

6. The operator then raises the casualty's arms and shoulders by bending backward, with his arms straight, until tension and resistance are felt; the chest is not lifted off the ground. While this maneuver, which draws air into the lungs (inflation) is being carried out, he counts, "Five-er, six-er, and seven-er," over a period of 2½ seconds.

7. The operator then lays the casualty's arms down and replaces his own hands on the casual-ty's back, thus returning to the original position, while counting, "Eight-er," over a period of 1 second.

8. This cycle is repeated with rhythmic rocking at the rate of about 9 times per minute until breathing is reestablished. Then the arm-raising and the arm-lowering movements (movements 6 and 7) are carried out 12 times to the minute. The operator counts, "One-er, two-er, and three-er," over a 2½-second period during the inspiratory (arm-raising) phase and counts, "Four-er, five-er, and six-er," during the expiratory (arm-lowering) phase.

9. If there are special regional injuries, the procedure must be modified. If the chest is injured, chest pressure is avoided; the patient lies supine, and only the arm-raising and the arm-lowering movements are executed, at the rate of

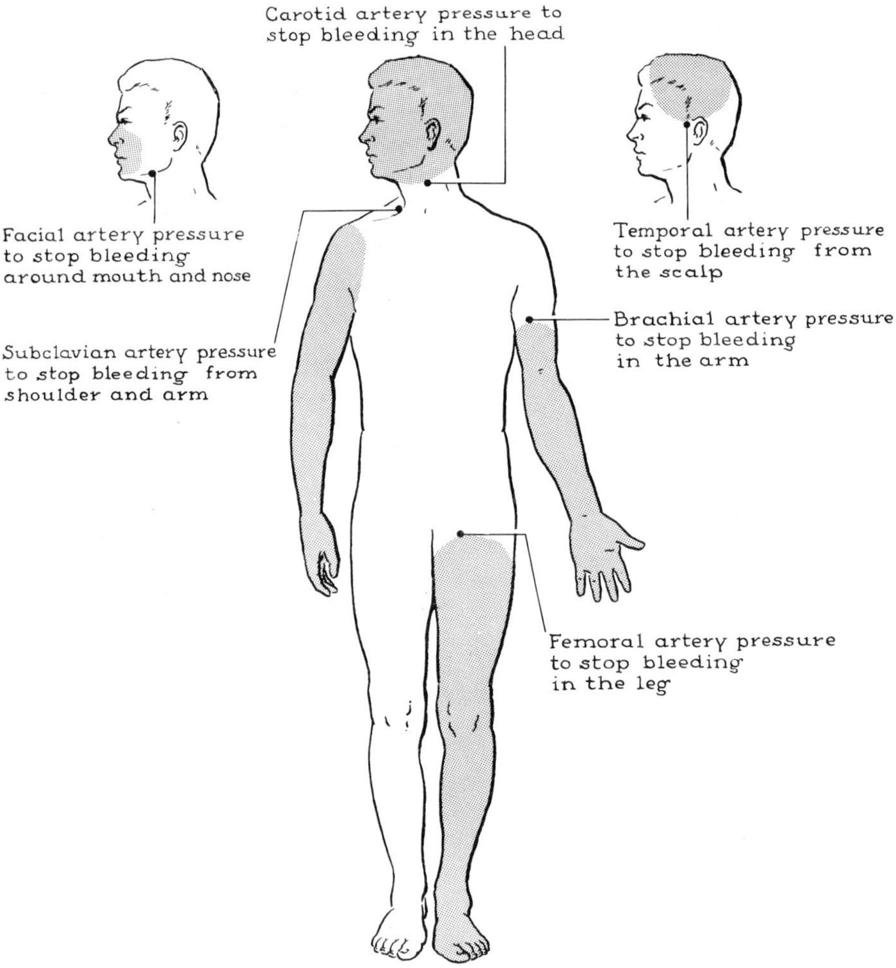

Fig. 453. The 6 principal pressure points for the control of arterial bleeding.

OLIGEMIC SHOCK

HEMATOGENIC OR SECONDARY SHOCK
CAUSED BY LOSS OF FLUID IN ACTIVE CIRCULATION

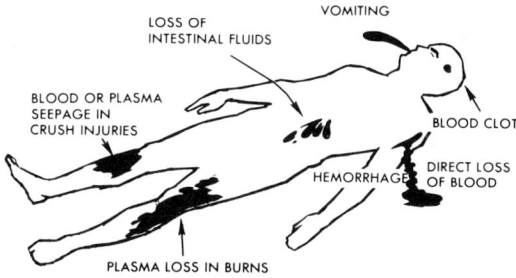

LOSS OF INTESTINAL FLUIDS

VOMITING

BLOOD OR PLASMA SEEPAGE IN CRUSH INJURIES

BLOOD CLOT

HEMORRHAGE

DIRECT LOSS OF BLOOD

PLASMA LOSS IN BURNS

FIGURE 454. (Army War Surgery)

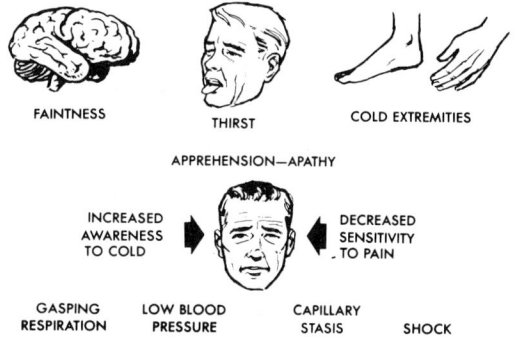

FAINTNESS

THIRST

COLD EXTREMITIES

APPREHENSION—APATHY

INCREASED AWARENESS TO COLD

DECREASED SENSITIVITY TO PAIN

GASPING RESPIRATION

LOW BLOOD PRESSURE

CAPILLARY STASIS

SHOCK

FIG. 455. Symptoms of oligemic shock. (Army War Surgery)

12 times to the minute. If the arms are injured, they are placed by the side of the body, and the complete procedure is carried out as described except that the operator's hands are placed under the hips, and a back-pressure, hip-lift technic is employed. If both the arms and the chest are injured, limited arm-raising and arm-lowering movements are carried out by inserting the hands only under the shoulders.

10. If necessary, artificial respiration can be continued in the vehicle while the patient is evacuated.*

Control of Hemorrhage

One of the primary causes of shock is the reduction in the circulating blood volume. Only a few conditions, such as in obstructed airway or a sucking wound of the chest, take precedence over the immediate control of hemorrhage. "Stop the bleeding" is fundamental to the care and the survival

---

* Emergency War Supply, pp. 187-189, U. S. Department of Defense, 1958.

of patients in an emergency or a disaster situation. (Control of hemorrhage is discussed in detail on page 298.)

The following points are important:

1. Apply firm manual pressure over the wound or the artery involved. Unchecked arterial bleeding produces death.
2. Apply a firm pressure bandage. Do not constrict the circulation.
3. Immobilize an injured extremity to control the blood loss.
4. Elevate the affected part.
5. If the patient is hemorrhaging internally, whole blood or plasma expanders, given at the rate of blood loss, are indicated. The patient who is bleeding internally requires surgery.
6. Apply a tourniquet only as a *last resort* when the hemorrhage cannot be controlled by any other method.

   A. Apply the tourniquet, just above

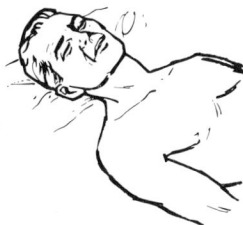

ARREST OF HEMORRHAGE

REMOVE NEUROGENIC CAUSATIVE FACTORS

PREVENTION OF INFECTION AND TOXEMIA

RELIEF OF PAIN

PROTECT PATIENT FROM HEAT, COLD & WET

BALANCE FLUIDS AND ELECTROLYTES

CONSTANT WATCHING OF VITAL SIGNS

PHYSICAL, MENTAL AND NUTRITIONAL COMFORT

FIG. 456. Management of shock. (Army War Surgery)

the wound. Apply it tightly enough to control arterial blood flow.
B. Tag the patient with a notation stating the location of the tourniquet and time applied.
C. Once applied, the tourniquet remains in place until it can be released by a trained medical person who is prepared to control hemorrhage and to replace blood volume as necessary.
D. In the event of a traumatic amputation, apply a tourniquet.

Control of Shock

Any injured patient should be assessed immediately to determine the presence of shock. If shock is present, it must be treated promptly. (Shock is discussed in detail on pp. 296 to 298.)

The following signs and symptoms in varying combinations indicate that the patient is in some degree of shock: cold, moist extremities, pallor, colorless lips, tachycardia, decreased blood pressure, apathy and thirst. Of these, the most dependable criterion is the level of the arterial pressure.

Principles of Management of Shock

1. Remove the cause of shock.
   A. Control the hemorrhage.
   B. Relieve the pain by splinting, supporting, positioning, and proper bandaging.
   C. Treat the wound as soon as possible.
   D. Splint the fracture.
   E. Institute measures to prevent infection.
2. Restore the circulating blood volume.
   A. Control hemorrhage.
   B. Give whole blood or one of the plasma volume expanders.
   C. Give oral fluids to replace volume lost unless contraindicated by abdominal, gastrointestinal injuries or by the patient's condition.
3. Support the defense mechanisms of the body.
   A. Reassure and comfort the patient.
   B. Relieve pain by cautious use of narcotics.

C. Maintain the body temperature. (Do not get the patient too warm, as heat produces vasodilatation, which counteracts the body's compensatory mechanism of vasoconstriction and also increases fluid loss by perspiration.)
D. Protect the patient from cold and dampness.
E. Elevate the feet slightly to improve cerebral circulation. (This position is contraindicated in patients with head injuries.)
F. Give oxygen if indicated.

Emergency Use of Blood Derivatives and Substitutes. Failing access to donor blood in ample supply, other materials may be used in its stead for the restoration of deficient blood volume in cases of oligemic shock. Agents that are suitable for this purpose include human plasma, human albumin (plasma Fraction V) and other plasma fractions containing albumin, now under investigation, as well as a variety of products from sources other than human blood that are referred to as "plasma expanders." Whole plasma, in contrast with certain of its derivatives, cannot be subjected to temperatures that are sufficiently high to achieve sterility, and for that reason its use is attended by the risk of transmitting viral hepatitis. Plasma fractions containing albumin are available, however, that can be pasteurized by exposure to a temperature of 60° C. for 10 hours, can be used with safety as regards infectivity and are eminently suitable for the treatment of shock from every standpoint but one, namely, their failure to supply red cells, a deficiency of relatively minor importance in the early phases of shock. However, it must be emphasized that in an emergency, whatever is available is used, even if some risk is involved.

Plasma expanders include certain materials that possess in common a molecular size such that they are retained in the circulating blood long enough after injection to cause the blood volume to expand, the prime objective of shock therapy. Such agents include dextran, produced by a bacterium; polyvinylpyrrolidone (PVP), a synthetic product; and oxypolygelatin. Attached to dextran is the disadvantage of increased cost and potential antigenicity for persons possessing antibodies against certain strains of pneumococci. Gelatin products exhibit gelation when cool, creating difficulties in the mechanics of injection when the latter must be acomplished in unheated quarters or out-of-doors in cold weather.

Wounds

Wounds will vary from minor lacerations to severe crushing injuries. The aims of emergency treatment are to stop bleeding, relieve shock, maintain an adequate airway and control infection. The principles of emergency care of wounds must be shared jointly by the trained personnel available. The nurse may be called on to carry out some of these procedures as instructed by a physician working with her.

1. Stop bleeding:
   A. Sterile pressure dressing
   B. Elevation of extremity if this is part involved
   C. Application of tourniquet as low on limb of casualty as possible *if hemorrhage is not controllable any other way.* Apply it tightly and do not loosen it at periodic intervals.* A physician should evaluate the situation.
2. Relieve shock (see p. 296).
3. Prevent injuries to respiratory tract.
   A. Maintain adequate airway. Proper positioning—on side or on back with head turned to side to allow drainage of pharyngeal secretions.
   B. Cover gaping chest wounds with an airtight dressing and adhesive.
4. Relieve pain: Sedation not to exceed 10 mgm. morphine.
5. Control infection:
   A. Keep wound covered.
   B. Antibiotic therapy.
   C. Tetanus prophylaxis (see p. 31).
6. Débride wounds;
   A. Open wound for inspection.
   B. Remove devitalized tissue and foreign bodies.
   C. Irrigate gently with saline.
   D. Pack loosely with dry gauze and

* Lindsey, Douglas: The case of the much-maligned tourniquet, Am. J. Nurs. **57**:444-445, 1957.

cover with sterile dressings; immobilize part.
7. Suture of wounds:
   A. Primary. Face, scalp and hand wounds may be cleaned and sutured primarily. Blood supply is abundant, and these parts are suffiiently resistant to infection.
   B. Secondary. Wounds other than the above mentioned may be closed primarily, or if deep and obviously contaminated, left open.
8. Change of dressings: Only for removal of sutures, ischemia, infection or serious hemorrhage.

Mass Management of Wounds. In handling large numbers of injured persons with wounds, it is not possible to carry out ideal wound treatment. However, the objective is to do the best one can for the greatest number of casualties. The following principles serve to accomplish this purpose:
1. Control the hemorrhage.
2. Clean the wounds with soap and water.
3. Dress the wounds with as clean material as is available.

Many wounds will not be closed for several days. Thus the healing will be by secondary intention. Broad spectrum antibiotics if available, will be given to those with the more severe types of contaminated wounds.

Fractures

The basic rule in treating a fracture is to immobilize the joint above and below the fracture. The splint should extend well beyond the joints adjacent to the fracture. Observe the circulation in the affected part by checking for warmth, color and pulsation. Investigate any complaint of pain or pressure. Maintain proper support to the immobilized extremities (see p. 990).

Mass Management of Fractures. With overwhelming numbers of patients, the simple splinting of fractures is done with any material available. Even tying the legs together will serve to splint a broken leg. Hemorrhage has to be controlled, and wounds have to be dressed. The extremity can be elevated to lessen swelling. After 2 or 3 days, sufficient help probably will be available to put more definitive plans of treatment into effect. At this time patients

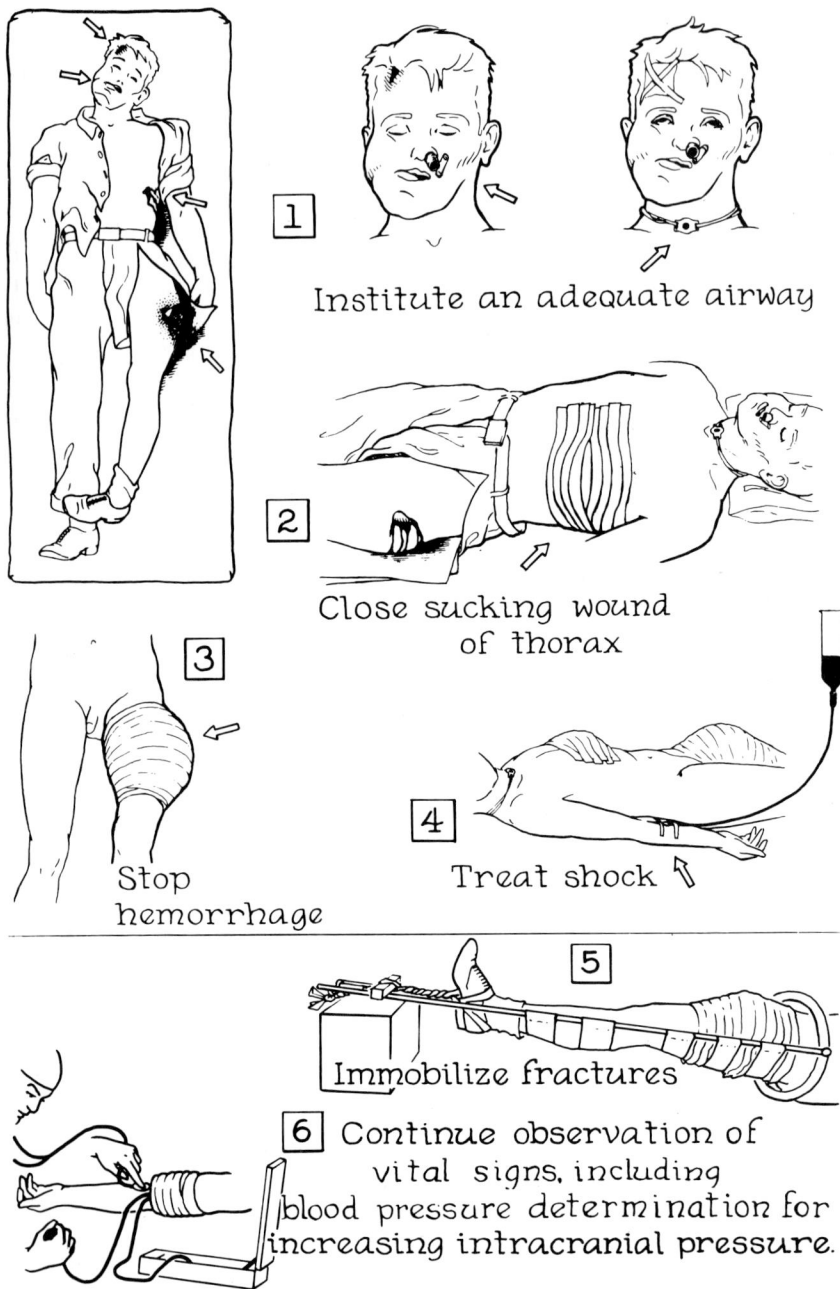

FIG. 457. Treatment of multiple injuries. This is a patient who has a cranial injury (without signs of increased intracranial pressure), a fracture of the mandible with some obstruction of the airway, an open sucking wound of the chest and an open fracture of the femur. The patient has bled considerably and is in shock. Priority treatment would be: Establish adequate airway — endotrachial tube. Close thoracic wound with an occlusive dressing. Start whole blood transfusion as therapy for shock. Sterile dressing to the fracture wound and emergency splinting. Observe for vital and neurologic signs — head injury. Postpone definitive therapy of the fracture of the femur until the life-endangering injuries have been brought under control. (Allen, J. G., et al.: Surgery, Principles and Practice, Lippincott)

with open fractures are among those selected for early treatment.

Crush Injury

An individual who has been crushed beneath debris, or who has been run over, or whose limbs have been compressed in some manner for an hour or more is likely to develop the crush or compression syndrome. Paralysis of the part, erythema, and blistering of the skin may develop as first signs of damage. Shortly after release from compression, swelling due to extravasation of plasma may appear. This initiates oligemic

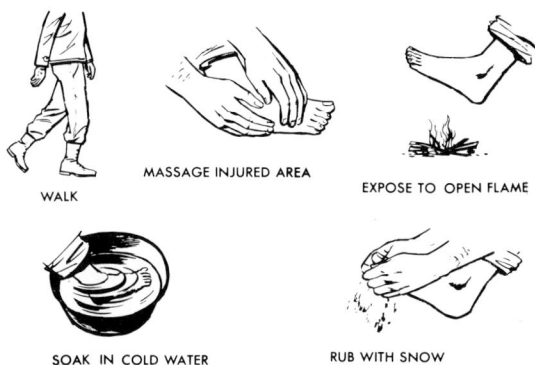

FIG. 458. Don'ts for cold injury. (Army War Surgery)

shock, and the patient's condition worsens. The damaged part, usually an extremity, becomes swollen, tense and hard. Later symptoms include anorexia, hiccoughs, tongue dryness, drowsiness or mental disturbances. Renal dysfunction develops.

Management.

1. Splint early major soft-tissue injuries —to control bleeding and pain, and to reduce shock.
2. Expose limb to air—to reduce tissue metabolism.
3. Incise fascia if blood supply is blocked —to relieve pressure or extravasated fluid.
4. Apply pressure bandages.
5. Administer medication for pain and anxiety.

Cold Injury

When a disaster occurs under freezing-weather conditions, the problem may be complicated even further by cold injury. Casualties, whether seriously traumatized or not, may become injured by cold during evacuation if they are immobilized or inadequately clothed. To prevent injury, armored and insulated boots are available.

Hypothermia. In hypothermia there is a progressive deterioration with ataxia, dysarthria, drowsiness and, eventually, coma. Shivering is suppressed below a temperature of 30° C. Below this temperature the body's self-warming mechanisms become ineffective. The heart beat and the blood pressure may be so weak that the peripheral pulsation becomes undetectable. To deter-

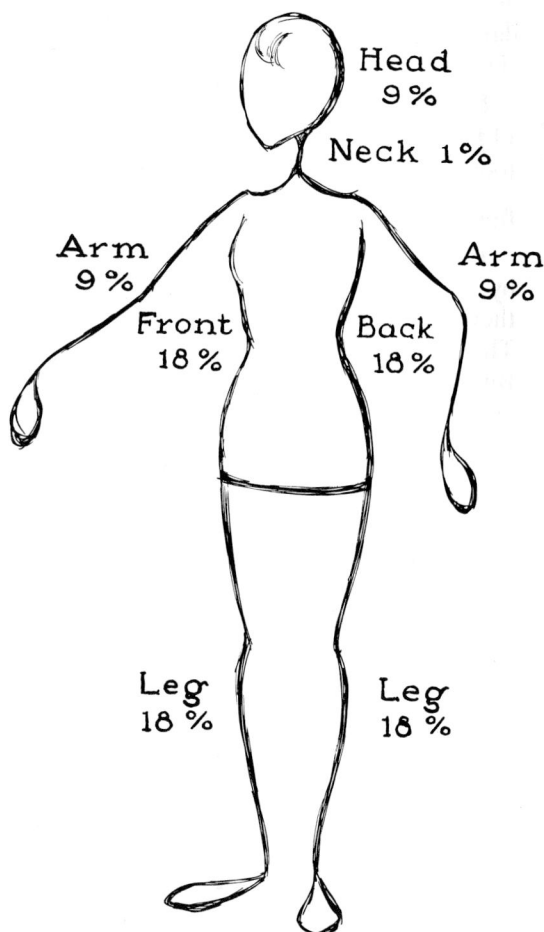

FIG. 459. "Rule of Nine" chart for calculating per cent of body burns. (Actual values have been modified for practical purposes.)

mine whether the victim is still alive, check his pupillary light reflex and tendon reflexes, all of which remain active until shortly before death.

Rewarming. The safest and the best technic for rewarming is still controversial; however, it is generally agreed that artificial ventilation is essential. At temperatures below 30° C. cardiac irregularities may occur; therefore, it seems advisable to raise the temperature to 30° to 32° C. without delay. Thereafter the warming process should be achieved slowly over many hours. Patients who have been severely hypothermic are seriously ill with considerable instability in thermoregulation and vasomotor control; hence they should be observed for 20 or 30 days after restoration to a normothermic state.

Local Cold Injury. This is of two types: (1) nonfreezing cold injury—"immersion foot" or "trench foot"—and (2) frostbite.

Burns

Burns may be caused from fires started by the blast and heat of an explosion, or they may result from intense radiant heat. The latter type are referred to as flash burns. Burns are often associated with other types of injuries that are sometimes more serious

than the burn. Ordinarily, the chief dangers from burns are *shock* and *infection* (p. 796).

Estimation of Extent and Severity of Burns. The extent of the burned area can be quickly calculated by using the "Rule of Nine" chart (Fig. 459).

The severity of burns can be determined as follows:

First degree—Edema; erythema; pain

Second degree—Prompt formation of blisters; pain

Third degree—Deep burns with charring of the skin; pain around the edges of the wound

Conditions	Factors
Chilblains	Above freezing High humidity
Trench foot	Above freezing Damp environment Immobilization
Immersion foot	Exposure of foot Temperature below 50° F.
Frostbite	Freezing temperature Crystallization of tissue fluids Time: minutes to hours
Space frostbite	High altitude Low temperature May be instantaneous

CLINICAL MANIFESTATIONS

1st degree:	Hyperemia Edema Skin peeling Slight swelling Redness Mild cyanosis		3rd degree:	Vesicles Edema Black, hard dry eschar Shrivelling toes
2nd degree:	Redness and slight swelling Vesicles Black eschars		4th degree:	Destruction of entire area involved Gangrene

EMERGENCY MANAGEMENT

1. For involvement of lower extremities do not allow individual to walk but transport otherwise.
2. Remove all constrictive clothing.
3. Rewarm afflicted areas by immersion in water at 90° F. in warm air.

4. Sterile, dry loose dressings should be applied, followed with active physical therapy.
5. Keep body warm and encourage patient to sleep and to rest.

Flash Burns. These also vary in degree; however, they are limited to the exposed area of skin and are sharp in outline, so-called "profile burns." For example, the surface of the ear may be burned, but behind the ear the area may be unharmed. In Japan it was noted that flash burns tended to involve those regions of the body where clothing was tight, such as at the shoulders, the waist and the elbows. White clothing reflects radiant heat, thereby preventing or lessening the severity of flash burns. Dark colors, on the other hand, absorb heat; hence, skin under dark-colored clothing may be burned.

Immediate Treatment. Cover burns with clean dry dressing, such as ironed old sheets or towels. Do not apply ointment or other medication as a first-aid measure. Do not disturb blisters. Evaluate extent of burns; make the casualty as comfortable as possible; loosen constricting clothing and treat for shock.

SORTING FOR TREATMENT. The most experienced person available should classify patients for treatment. Some suggestions which may be helpful are:

Group 1. Patients who can care for themselves

Group 2. Patients having moderately severe burns but in no immediate danger

Group 3. Patients with severe burns who require vigorous therapy

Group 4. Individuals with overwhelming burns

Specific Treatment.

FLUID THERAPY. The purpose of fluid therapy in the burn casualty is to replace the water, the salt and the protein which are lost from the circulation, largely into the burned area, and to restore or to maintain adequate plasma volume and urine output.

DRESSINGS. Use simple sterile dressings for minor burns. The "universal protective dressing"* can be used as a compression dressing for burns as well as for other types of injuries. As a pressure dressing it can be left on for 10 to 12 days. These dressings will be available in an emergency from the

* This cellulose-pad dry dressing was approved by the National Research Council, Subcommittee on Burns, June 8, 1951, and has been adopted by the Department of Defense and FCDA.

State Emergency Medical Service for Civil Defense. For burns of face or the perineum, the trunk or the thorax, the exposure method may be used; obviously, a warm clean environment is essential for this method.

Respiratory Tract Burns. Burn victims may suffer respiratory tract burns from inhalation of hot air, noxious gases or hot particles. This can be an extremely serious injury. Symptoms of mild injury are hoarseness, sore throat and coughing. For severe injury, laryngeal edema progresses to complete obstruction, dyspnea and cyanosis. Emergency treatment for laryngeal obstruction is tracheotomy, employing postural drainage, suction, and oxygen therapy.

Mass Casualty Management of Burns. When there are thousands of casualties, the major emphasis is on supporting the patient systemically. Fluid replacement is given by the oral route. The following solution is an excellent formula for fluid replacement:

½ teaspoon salt
½ teaspoon soda
1 quart of water

Patients who can care for themselves can be given this salt and soda to drink and a supply of antibiotic medications to take. The exposure method of treatment will be the treatment of choice. These individuals can be encouraged to return to work or to help in the care of others.

Patients with moderate burns should be given oral fluids and kept undisturbed in a recumbent position to prevent or to treat shock.

When mass casualties are encountered, local burn therapy may have to be delayed. In patients with moderate or severe burns, the burn is covered with the cleanest available material to protect the area from contamination. The original dressings and the patient's clothing should be left undisturbed, as these offer some protection from infection.

It has been found that even severely burned patients can be evacuated if the evacuation is done within a reasonable length of time after the injury. Patients with severe burns should be evacuated as soon as possible to areas where intravenous therapy and trained teams can institute the treatment that they require.

Summary of Nursing Measures in Caring for Patients with Burns.

1. Relieve pain (with morphine) and attempt to make casualty as comfortable as possible.

2. Estimate carefully or measure intake and output.

3. Safeguard against infection.

4. Observe for shock, pulmonary edema and blood in the urine.

5. Check dressings for signs of constriction.

6. Encourage casualty to take fluids as ordered.

7. Reassure patient and make him as comfortable as possible.

Acute Poisoning

Poisoning from the inhalation and the ingestion of toxic materials, both accidental and by design, constitutes a major health hazard. The problem is one of real magnitude as reflected in the number of cases and the number of deaths at different ages due to specific poisons.

Approximately one half of all poison ingestions involve drugs, other products that are commonly implicated including household preparations, pesticides and petroleum distillates. Preschool-age children have accounted for over 80 per cent of all poison cases and almost one third of all accidental deaths due to poisoning.

Emergency Management of Patients With Poisoning. The following instructions are those proposed by the Committee of Toxicology of the American Medical Association.* These refer to emergency measures to be taken as soon as a poison has been discovered, and they specify the precautions that are indicated for the prevention of poisoning accidents.

The steps listed below are to be taken with all possible speed.

Save the poison container and any contents that may remain. If the identity of the poison is not known, save a sample of vomitus.

1. Swallowed Poisons:

In all cases, *except those indicated below,*

* J.A.M.A. **165**:687-688, 1957.

REMOVE POISON FROM PATIENT'S STOMACH IMMEDIATELY BY INDUCING VOMITING. (See B,2 below.) This cannot be overemphasized, for it is the essence of the treatment and is often a life-saving procedure. Prevent chilling by wrapping patient in blankets if necessary. Do not give alcohol in any form.

A. Do Not Induce Vomiting If:

1. Patient is in coma or unconscious
2. Patient is in convulsions
3. Patient has swallowed petroleum products (i.e., kerosene, gasoline, lighter fluid)
4. patient has swallowed a corrosive poison (symptoms: severe pain, burning sensation in mouth and throat, vomiting)
   CALL PHYSICIAN IMMEDIATELY

   (a) Acid and acidlike corrosives: sodium acid sulfate (toilet bowl cleaners), acetic acid (glacial), sulfuric acid, nitric acid, oxalic acid, hydrofluoric acid (rust removers), iodine, silver nitrate (styptic pencil)

   (b) Alkali corrosives: sodium hydroxide—lye (drain cleaners), sodium carbonate (washing soda), ammonia water, sodium hypochlorite (household bleach)

If the patient can swallow after ingesting a *corrosive poison,* the following substances (and amounts) may be given:

    For acids: milk, water or milk of magnesia (1 tablespoon to 1 cup of water)

    For alkalies: milk, water, any fruit juice or vinegar (1 to 2 cups for patients aged 1 to 5, or up to 1 quart for individuals 5 years old or older)

B. Induce Vomiting When Noncorrosive Substances Have Been Swallowed:

1. Give milk or water (for patient from 1 to 5 years old—1 to 2 cups; for patient over 5 years—up to 1 quart)
2. Induce vomiting by placing the

blunt end of a spoon or your finger at the back of the patient's throat, or by use of this emetic— 2 tablespoons of salt in a glass of warm water

When retching and vomiting begin, place patient face down with head lower than hips. This prevents vomitus from entering the lungs and causing further damage.

2. Inhaled Poisons:
   A. Carry patient (do not let him walk) to fresh air immediately.
   B. Open all doors and windows.
   C. Loosen all tight clothing.
   D. Apply artificial respiration if breathing has stopped or is irregular.
   E. Prevent chilling (wrap patient in blankets).
   F. Keep patient as quiet as possible.
   G. If patient is convulsing, keep him in bed in a semidark room; avoid jarring or noise.
   H. Do not give alcohol in any form.

3. Skin Contamination:
   A. Drench skin with water (shower, hose, faucet).
   B. Apply stream of water on skin while removing clothing.
   C. Cleanse skin thoroughly with water; rapidity in washing is most important in reducing extent of injury.

4. Eye Contamination:
   A. Hold eyelids open, wash eyes with gentle stream of running water *immediately*. Delay of few seconds greatly increases extent of injury.
   B. Wash until physician arrives.
   C. *Do not use chemicals;* they may increase extent of injury.

5. Injected Poisons (scorpion and snake bites):
   A. Make patient lie down as soon as possible.
   B. Do not give alcohol in any form.
   C. Apply tourniquet above injection site (e.g., between arm or leg and heart). The pulse in vessels below the tourniquet should not disappear, nor should the tourniquet produce a throbbing sensation. Tourniquet should be loosened for 1 minute every 15 minutes.
   D. Apply icepack to the site of the bite.
   E. Carry patient to physician or hospital; DO NOT LET HIM WALK.

6. Chemical Burns:
   A. Wash with large quantities of running water (except those caused by phosphorus).
   B. Immediately cover with loosely applied clean cloth.
   C. Avoid use of ointments, greases, powders and other drugs in first-aid treatment of burns.
   D. Treat shock by keeping patient flat, keeping him warm and reassuring him until arrival of physician.

MEASURES TO PREVENT POISONING ACCIDENTS

1. Keep all drugs, poisonous substances and household chemicals out of the reach of children.

2. Do not store nonedible products on shelves used for storing food.

3. Keep all poisonous substances in their original containers; do not transfer to unlabeled containers.

4. When medicines are discarded, destroy them. Do not throw them where they might be reached by children or pets.

5. When giving flavored and/or brightly colored medicine to children, *always* refer to it as medicine—*never* as candy.

6. Do not take or give medicine in the dark.

7. *READ LABELS* before using chemical products.

Barbiturate Poisoning. This accounts for approximately 50 per cent of all deaths caused by drug ingestion. It has been estimated that more than 50,000 such cases are hospitalized each year in this country, a large proportion of these being instances of attempted suicide.

The picture is one of stupor, or coma, and respiratory depression; mental response, if obtained at all, is quite adequate, although slow; the face is flushed, the pupils dilated, the reflexes usually depressed. Death can occur, due to cerebral edema, respiratory failure or pneumonia (not an uncommon sequela). Practically all these patients can be saved, despite a huge dose of the drug—

even 300 grains and more—if the proper measures are instituted within a few hours of the time of ingestion.

TREATMENT. The treatment consists of gastric lavage, to remove any drug still remaining in the stomach, and nervous system stimulation. Gastric lavage may be carried out by stomach tube, using water, or by induced vomiting (see B, p. 1162).

The most important aspect of treatment is supportive therapy, including measures for the stimulation of the depressed respiration, artificial respiration, if necessary, circulatory stimulants, maintenance of fluid and electrolyte balance, close observation and good nursing care. Various analeptic drugs, including picrotoxin, strychnine and bemegride (beta three-ethyl-beta three-methylglutarimide), are effective in counteracting the depressive effects of the barbiturates on the central nervous system. Of these, the latter seems to be least dangerous and is effective in doses of from 50 to 250 mg. increments intravenously at intervals of 3 to 5 minutes to a total of 1,200 mg. Hemodialysis with the artificial kidney clears the blood stream of barbiturates very rapidly and reduces the duration of coma induced by the long-acting preparations.

Morphine Poisoning. Morphine in overdosage may cause death due to respiratory failure. The respiratory rate of a patient receiving morphine therapy must be followed carefully, and the proper measures should be taken if the rate drops below 10 or 12 per minute. Acute morphinism is suspected in all patients in coma with pinpoint pupils and slow respiration.

TREATMENT. A specific antidote for morphine is available in the form of N-allyl-normorphine. Given intravenously in doses of 5 to 20 mg., it counteracts practically every effect of morphine within a period of 1 to 2 minutes. The respiratory rate is restored to normal with great regularity within 10 to 20 seconds after intravenous injection, the respirations thereafter becoming more rapid for a time. Consciousness is restored only partially, if at all, in response to N-allyl-normorphine. The circulatory status is improved to a degree commensurate with the respiratory function.

Mercury Poisoning. This usually is brought about by the willful ingestion of mercuric chloride, an act of suicide that is very often successful. One gram of the material produces serious toxicity and a significant mortality, and the ingestion of 1.5 Gm. is almost always lethal. The earliest response, clinically, in these cases is the precipitous onset of vomiting, which persists. This is soon accompanied by agonizing abdominal pain and diarrhea, which is marked by the frequent passage of liquid, bloody stools. Oliguria is apparent almost at once, the patient thereafter voiding only at infrequent intervals. These specimens of urine, small in volume, are loaded with albumin, red cells and casts. Uremia then develops, with all of its attending complications, progressive in severity and culminating in death, or, in milder cases, terminating abruptly after a brisk, spontaneous diuresis which marks the beginnings of renal recovery.

The prognosis of this nephropathy, if enough mercury is ingested, retained and absorbed to cause any symptoms whatever, is serious; its mortality, no less than 50 per cent. However, if treatment can be initiated within a period of a very few hours, i.e., if conducted as a true emergency, the outlook is favorable.

TREATMENT. BAL, or British anti-Lewisite (2, 3-dimercaptopropanol), is a compound that renders mercury (and arsenic as well) physiologically inert and nontoxic, effectively binding these metals in vivo and rendering them harmless until they are eliminated from the body. Following the injection of this agent into patients with mercurial toxicity, there is an abrupt ending of fresh tissue necrosis, further damage from the metal is forestalled, and the reparative processes may proceed. Tubular tissue can be replaced, fortunately, and this renal lesion, therefore, is reversible, but if there is to be any certainty in its curative action, BAL must be given at the earliest possible moment, before necrosis is extensive, and renal damage is irretrievable.

BAL, administered by intramuscular injection, may be given as follows: 300 mg. stat., followed by 2 or 3 150-mg. doses during the first 12-hour period. The same dose is repeated once or twice during the second 12-hour period and once daily, or every 2nd day thereafter, until no trace of toxicity remains. Gastric lavage is indicated immediately, entirely aspirating the gastric contents, then rinsing the stomach repeatedly with a 4 per cent solution of sodium bicarbonate (1½ oz. of soda per quart of tap water). Colonic flushing also has been recommended. The intravenous infusion of dextrose and electrolyte repair solutions is required throughout the period of oliguria, all parenteral therapy being accomplished with great care and with every precaution taken to prevent overhydration and pulmonary edema, a complication quite as dangerous as the patient's uremia.

With the onset of frank uremic toxicity, evidenced by recurrent nausea, vomiting, neurologic and cerebral disturbances and progressive deterioration of the nitrogen and electrolyte balance, the patient is clearly a suitable subject for peritoneal lavage or for the application of an artificial kidney. The objective of these measures is the elimination by artificial dialysis of diffusible materials that have accumulated to great excess in the blood and the body fluids, utilizing, as a dializing membrane, either the peritoneum or a cellophane tube. They are used in the expectation of bringing about symptomatic relief, a reduction of toxicity and a lengthening of survival, thereby affording additional time for kidney repair and an opportunity for cure that otherwise does not exist.

Carbon Monoxide Poisoning. Occurring as an industrial or a household accident, or by design in attempted suicide, this is of extreme importance. The most common source is atmosphere containing an appreciable concentration of automobile exhaust gases, such as might develop, for example, in a closed garage. A concentration of carbon monoxide as low as 0.03 per cent is potentially dangerous. The effect of carbon monoxide is to render the hemoglobin useless as an oxygen-carrying chemical, because it unites so firmly with the pigment in place of oxygen. One liter of the gas is sufficient to combine with all the blood in the body.

The chief signs and symptoms of this poisoning are due to failure of the body tissues to obtain oxygen, from which lack the nervous system suffers first and most severely. These symptoms include headache, lassitude, drowsiness and coma. The skin color usually is pink. Neuritis, tremor, psychoses, spastic paralyses and visual disturbances may persist following resuscitation.

TREATMENT. This consists in stimulating, as rapidly as possible, the inhalation of atmosphere of high-oxygen concentration, such as with the use of a 95 per cent oxygen-5 per cent carbon dioxide mixture delivered with a closed mask, with the help of artificial respiration (but not a positive-pressure device) if necessary.

Dangers From Fallout: Radiation Sickness

Radiation sickness presents no definite symptoms until several hours or days after exposure, depending on the amount of radiation to which the victim was exposed. In radiation therapy (p. 317) there is a calcu-

---

SMOKING IN BED

To the Patient:

Smoking in bed is never entirely safe. For your own protection and for the safety of other patients, we ask you to follow these suggestions:

1. Be sure you have an ash tray, and be sure to use it—*always.*

2. Do not smoke after the lights are out. If you MUST make an exception notify the nurse before you light up.

3. The risk from smoking will be much less if you will smoke only when you have visitors, and only when you are sitting up.

4. Be certain that all ashes and "butts" are extinguished before the ash tray is emptied.

5. Cooperate with the nurse when she is giving you drugs and treatments which make smoking unsafe. She is required to remove matches and smoking materials at such times.

Never smoke when you or a patient near you is in an oxygen tent.

SAFETY INSTRUCTION CARD
No. H 150
National Safety Council

TABLE 25. Summary of Clinical Symptoms of Radiation Sickness*

Time after exposure	Survival improbable (700 r or more)	Survival possible (550 r to 300 r)	Survival probable (250 r to 100 r)
1st week	Nausea, vomiting and diarrhea in first few hours	Nausea, vomiting and diarrhea in first few hours	Possibly nausea, vomiting and diarrhea on first day
	No definite symptoms in some cases (latent period)		
	Diarrhea Hemorrhage Purpura Inflammation of mouth and throat Fever	No definite symptoms (latent period)	No definite symptoms (latent period)
2nd week	Rapid emaciation Death (mortality probably 100%)	Epilation Loss of appetite and general malaise Fever	
3rd week		Hemorrhage Purpura Petechiae Nosebleeds Pallor Inflammation of mouth and throat Diarrhea Emaciation	Epilation Loss of appetite and malaise Sore throat Hemorrhage Purpura Petechiae Pallor Diarrhea Moderate emaciation
4th week			
		Death in most serious cases (mortality 50% for 450 roentgens)	Recovery likely in about 3 months unless complicated by poor previous health or superimposed injuries or infections

* Glasstone, Samuel: The Effects of Nuclear Weapons, p. 477, United States Atomic Energy Commission, June, 1957.

lated risk and a controlled dosage, but in warfare the dose is completely uncontrolled. Radiation victims have symptoms resembling those of the patient receiving radiation therapy but in more severe degrees.

ACCIDENT PREVENTION

Industrial, vehicular and home accidents occur with such frequency that they now represent the nation's major peril to health and productivity. In both military and civilian populations, accidents are responsible for more deaths and lost working days than any single disease. For persons from 1 to 34 years of age, accidents are the Number 1 cause of death; for those from 35 to 44, they rank 2nd only to heart disease.

The nurse learns, practices and teaches safety principles; she has a unique opportunity to participate in safety programs and to teach accident prevention. Posters, pamphlets and films are available from insurance

TABLE 26. Accidental Deaths Classified According to the International List of Causes of Death

Type of Accident or Manner of Injury	1959*	Change 1958 to 1959
All Accidental Deaths	**92,080**	+ 1.6%
Motor-vehicle accident..	37,910	+ 2.5
Railway accidents (except collision with motor vehicle).................	1,089	− 6.5
Streetcar accident (except collision with train or motor vehicle)...........	19	− 26.9
Other road transport accident (except collision with train or motor vehicle....	230	− 17.3
Water-transport accident..	1,595	− 3.5
Aircraft accident...	1,411	− 6.6
Poisoning by solid and liquid substances...........................	1,661	+ 16.2
Poisoning by gases and vapors..................................	1,141	− 3.9
Falls..	18,774	+ 2.9
Blow from falling or projected object or missile.......................	1,461	+ 5.9
Nontransport vehicle accident...................................	86	+ 11.7
Machinery...	1,970	+ 8.7
Cutting and piercing instruments.................................	100	− 3.9
Electric current..	1,001	+ 5.3
Explosion of pressure vessel....................................	51	+ 8.5
Fire and explosion of combustible material.........................	6,898	− 5.4
Hot substance, corrosive liquid, and steam.........................	391	+ 2.4
Radiation..	4	+ ...
Firearms..	2,258	+ 4.0
Inhalation and ingestion of food.................................	1,782	+ 0.1
Inhalation and ingestion of other object...........................	407	− 1.0
Foreign body entering other orifice...............................	132	+ 6.5
Mechanical suffocation..	1,721	+ 3.8
Lack of care of infants..	41	+105.0
Bites and stings of venomous animals and insects.....................	62	+ 29.2
Other animal accident...	122	− 9.0
Drowning..	5,046	− 0.4
High and low air pressure......................................	3	+ ...
Excessive heat and insulation...................................	267	+ 94.9
Excessive cold...	242	− 21.2
Hunger, thirst, and exposure....................................	187	− 16.5
Cataclysm...	134	− 19.3
Lightning..	183	+ 76.0
Accident in nontherapeutic medical and surgical procedures..............	81	+ 19.1
Accident in therapeutic medical and surgical procedures.................	854	+ 1.4
Late effect of accident (death more than a year after accident)...........	834	+ 6.8
Other and unspecified...	1,932	− 5.4

Source: National Vital Statistics Division.

* Latest official figures available: Accident Facts, Chicago, National Safety Council, 1962.

companies and the National Safety Council.* Helpful aids in patient teaching are the 3 x 5 safety-instruction cards available from the National Safety Council.

The Traffic Accident Problem

Motor vehicle accidents head the list of causes of accidental death, as may be seen in Table 26.

* *Accident Facts* also is published annually by the National Safety Council. This is a detailed analysis of the various types of accidents (425 N. Michigan Ave., Chicago 11, Ill.).

Through automobile accidents, a life is lost every 15 minutes, and an injury occurs every 30 seconds. Furthermore, about 10 per cent of such injuries result in permanent disability. With an annual toll of 38,000 traffic deaths, there is in addition well over a million disabling injuries.

The National Safety Council lists drinking, lack of alertness and fatigue to be important causes of motor vehicle accidents and excessive speed as the most common

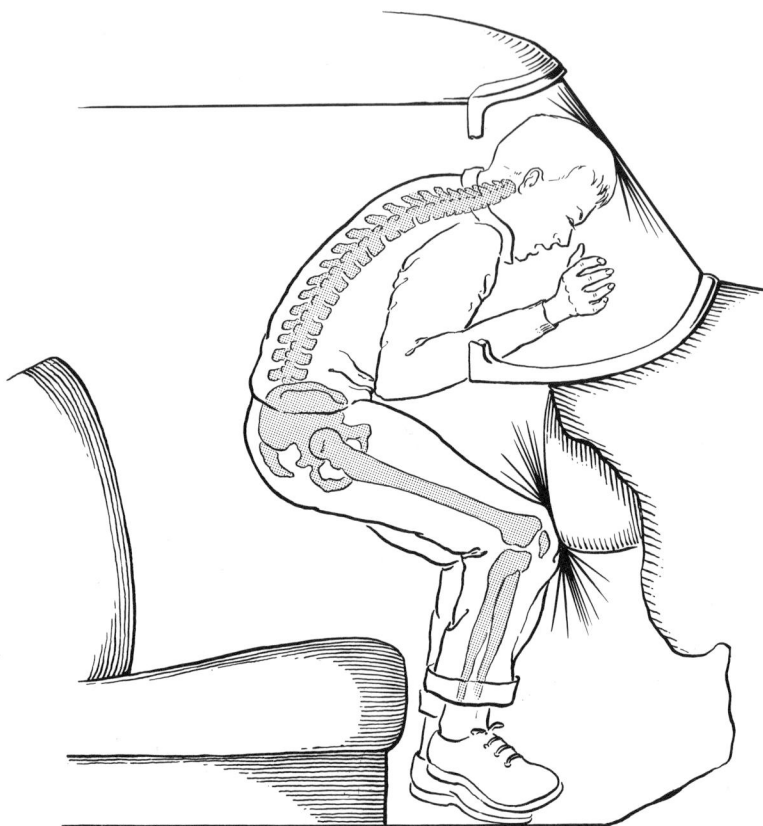

Fig. 460. Diagrammatic drawing to show the mechanism of injury for a front seat passenger when a car strikes an obstructing object. The head hits the windshield, and the knee strikes the dashboard; forces may be dissipated anywhere from the 1st cervical to the 5th lumbar vertebra.

driver violation.* On our high speed highways this often involves several cars and many persons. Almost any type of injury may occur.

The Nature of Injuries. When the car stops suddenly, the occupants continue in motion, and they are killed by blows received when they are flung against the car interior, or they are killed by objects outside the car. One of the most common and most disabling injuries is the so-called *whiplash* (Fig. 460). This has been defined† as "the damage sustained by neck structures when the body, in propulsion, comes to a sudden stop, or when the body is suddenly propelled forward, and the head is thrust forcibly forward and/or backward, and/or

to either side." The parts which may be damaged are the cervical vertebrae, the intervertebral disks and the odontoid process. Emotional and psychological disturbances frequently ensue later on.

The impact of a person against the interior of the automobile is responsible for many serious injuries. The dashboard with its various protuberances accounts for about 40 per cent of injuries, sometimes causing macerations of the liver and resultant hemorrhage, rib fractures, rupture of the spleen, and rupture or laceration of the kidneys. Blows received by the body against the windshield account for another 30 per cent of injuries, which most often consist of extensive lacerations of tissue with possible fractures of the sternum, the ribs, the zygoma, the maxillary sinus, or the frontal bone. Steering-wheel injuries, representing about 10 per cent of the total, most commonly involve a crushing blow to the thorax, with

---

* Other causes of automobile accidents are hidden factors that often are never detected. These have to do with mechanical failures and not enough safety built into the car itself.

† Allen, W. L.: Internat. Rec. Med. 169:1, 1956.

FIG. 461. Home accidents cause more than one quarter of all accidental deaths. (Accidental Injury Statistics, U.S. Department of Health, Education and Welfare)

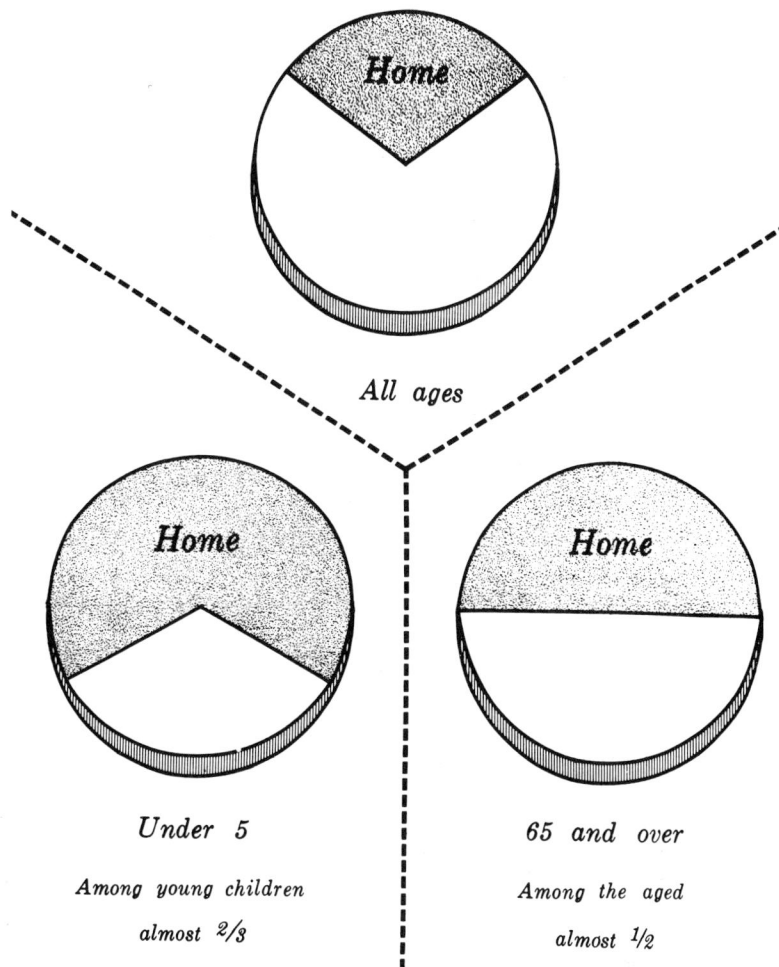

FIG. 461. Home accidents cause more than one quarter of all accidental deaths. (Accidental Injury Statistics, U.S. Department of Health, Education and Welfare)

All ages

Under 5

Among young children almost 2/3

65 and over

Among the aged almost 1/2

possible fractures of the sternum or the ribs and trauma to the heart and the lungs.

On the basis of studies, various safety devices have been suggested. As a member of the health team, the nurse can lend active support to all safety programs which have to do with (1) education of persons in accident and injury protection, (2) construction of safety features in automobiles, especially seat belts and padding, (3) adequate standards for driver licensure, (4) improved state inspections of all cars, and (5) adequate supervision of mechanics to do their job properly.

Care of Injuries from Automobile Accidents. The care of the injured from automobile accidents does not differ from the care of the injured from other civilian acci-

dents except for the recognition of the frequency of cerebral and neck injuries, which demand caution in moving and positioning.

Home Accidents

Falls account for about half the accidents sustained in the home. Poor lighting, loose carpeting, misplaced toys and inadequate bases of support used in reaching articles placed on high shelves are the chief reasons why individuals fall. Home hobbies and repair jobs done by the novice who disregards safety rules contribute to the toll of injuries sustained at home. Fires, burns and poisons are other causes. Inasmuch as mothers, young children and elderly persons are at home most of the time, they are the principal victims, and it is to this group that

NEEDS	IMPROVISED EQUIPMENT*
Making Holes in Rubbers:	Large nails, safety pins, forceps, wire, pen knives, nail files
Cleaning Aids:	Pipe cleaners (clean hollow tubing), soap and water, linen, old clothing and paper, sand abrasion creams and beauty aids
Sealing Bandages:	Cellophane tape, adhesive, putty, wax
Fire:	Wood, paper, waste materials, wood shavings, alcohol lamps, gasoline stoves, glass over paper and sun, fuel oil and kerosene, hair tonics
Refrigeration:	Seal a bottle, place it in cold water, place moistened net over bottle. A hole in ground (9 feet), ice wrapped in newspaper
Marking:	Charred material, ink, pencils, lipstick
Picking up hot materials:	Scissors, tweezers, coat hangers
Restraints:	Canvas, raincoats, plastics, clothing
A bed for a casualty:	6 or 8 straight chairs fastened together. They even have built-in side rails. Chairs might be available from hotels, schools, or an undertaking establishment
A crib for a child:	Arm chairs tied together
An occlusive burn dressing:	Soft, absorbent bath towels encased in an old pillow case. Wash clothes in old muslin will do well for smaller burns
A makeshift autoclave:	A household pressure cooker or a pressure canner. Materials will have to be oven dried after sterilization.

* A hand pump for emergency suctioning is described in Trading Post, Am. J. Nursing 56:1440, 1956. Other ideas on improvisation of equipment may be obtained from Olson, Lyla M.: Improvised Equipment, Philadelphia, Saunders, 1947.

---

educational efforts emphasizing safety and preventive measures must be directed. Continued emphasis by radio, television, newspapers and magazines will help in reaching these persons.

IMPROVISATION AND RESOURCEFULNESS

When the principles of medical emergency management are clearly understood, one does not need hospital equipment in order to function effectively. By using imagination and ingenuity, many commonplace items can be used by the first aider. Sloane* states that in emergency nursing, students are not taught the types of bandages that are seldom used today. Instead, they learn to improvise pressure bandages from bias-cut sheeting, cross-cut T-shirts and old stockings; and they learn to apply triangle, cravat and stocking bandages. A good exercise for the nurse is to take the patient's temperature, pulse and respiration merely by observing him and by touching his skin, then

to take the readings in the conventional way and to compare the results. With practice, the nurse can become quite adept in her evaluations.

Suggested use of materials for improvisation can be found on page 1171.†

CLINICAL SITUATION

A hurricane has caused many hundreds of casualties. A triage (sorting) area has been established, and a nurse is sorting the patients until a physician is available.

1. In the sorting area, where the nurse has only a few seconds to decide the priority of each casualty, the following symptoms would alert the nurse to the need of the victim for immediate care:

    A. Expectoration of pink-tinged sputum.

    B. Cold, clammy skin.

    C. Opisthotonus position.

    D. Bleeding from femoral artery.

2. The patient arrives at the triage area in an unconscious state. The nurse notices

---

* Sloane, Amanda: Disaster nursing in the curriculum, Nursing Outlook 5(2):75-77, Feb., 1957.

† Adapted from FCDA, The Nurse in Civil Defense, TM-11-7, rev. ed., 1954.

Materials	Uses
Cardboard and Cardboard Boxes:	Mattress, beds, baby cribs, tables Oxygen tents Shade, screening Trays, waste containers, bedpans Props and supports, splints
Rubber Tubing:	Tourniquets, holding splints, traction Drinking straws, catheters, rectal and enema tubing, drains, airways, suction, oxygen tubing and infusions
Rubber Stoppers:	Tops for infusion bottles, airtight storage, suction apparatus, enema apparatus (bottle, plus top)
Bottles:	Drinking water, storage, water bottle Urinals, enema apparatus, suction equipment, chest drainage bottles, specimens Bottle filled with sand may be used for traction and weights
Paper:	Warmth, padding, protective covers for heat and cold, splints, plaster casts, protection of surfaces Absorption—towels, toilet paper, diapers Wrapping—sterile dressings, waste Containers—food, drinking cups, waste containers Fire starters
Tin Cans:	Containers for water, storage, cooking, dishes and drinking Containers for specimens, emesis basins, bedpans, enema cans, waste Shovels Bed blocks
Rope and String:	Ties, traction, holding bandages, splints, restraints, and tagging
Plastic Bottles and Bags:	Many of the above uses

dark blood oozing from a scalp laceration. She directs the litter bearers to

    A. Place him in Priority 4 classification.

    B. Position him in the Trendelenburg position.

    C. Turn him on his side.

    D. Stop the bleeding.

3. The casualty has respiratory stridor and is using all accessory muscles of respiration. The indicated treatment is

    A. Mouth-to-mouth resuscitation.

    B. Closed chest cardiac massage.

    C. Tracheal catheterization.

    D. O_2 under pressure if available.

4. Four seriously injured persons are brought simultaneously to the treatment station. To which of the following conditions should the nurse direct her attention *initially?*

    A. Abdominal evisceration.

    B. Protrusion of the brain through scalp laceration.

    C. Sucking wound of the chest.

    D. Compression fracture of the cervical vertebrae.

5. For which of the following conditions could treatment *not* be deferred?

    A. Penetrating abdominal wound.

    B. Fractured femur.

    C. Ventricular fibrillation.

    D. Head injury.

6. Which of the following should receive immediate priority?

    A. Open pneumothorax.

    B. Hemorrhage.

    C. Burn of right leg.

    D. Ruptured bladder.

7. Which of the following casualties would most likely be given Priority 4 classification?

    A. Compound fracture of both arms.

    B. Burns of 20 per cent of body.

    C. Double amputation of lower extremities.

    D. Wounds of both eyes.

8. Which of the following conditions would receive priority for immediate treatment?

    A. Acute pulmonary edema.

    B. Burns of 45 per cent of body.

    C. Penetrating abdominal wound.

    D. Amputation of 3 toes.

9. Which of these symptoms would alert the nurse in the triage area to a potentially serious condition?

    A. Forceful vomiting.

    B. Twitching.

    C. Spasmodic coughing.

    D. Hyperventilation.

10. Which of the following symptoms would place the patient in the "immediate care" category?

    A. Paradoxical chest movements.

    B. Tenderness over the ribs.

    C. Cheyne-Stokes respirations.

    D. Coughing up blood.

BIBLIOGRAPHY AND SUGGESTED READING

Books

American Hospital Association Committee on Disaster Planning: The Principles of Disaster Planning for Hospitals, Chicago, The Association, 1956.

American Medical Association: Summary Report on National Emergency Medical Care, Chicago, The Association, 1959.

American National Red Cross Handbook for Physicians and Nurses, Washington, D. C., Am. Nat. Red Cross, 1959.

American Nurses Association: Emergency Intervention by the Nurse, Monograph No. 1, New York, Am. Nurses' Assoc., 1962.

Cole, W. H., and Puestow, C. B.: First Aid: Diagnosis and Management, ed. 5, New York, Appleton, 1960.

Cullen, S. C., and Gross, E. G.: Manual of Medical Emergencies, ed. 3, Chicago, The Year Book Publishers, Inc., 1958.

Henderson, J.: Emergency Medical Guide, New York, McGraw-Hill, 1963.

Nabbe, F. C.: Disaster Nursing, Paterson, N. J., Littlefield, Adams and Co., 1960.

Report on National Emergency Medical Care, American Medical Assoc., Chicago, 1959.

Sharpe, J. C.: Management of Medical Emergencies, New York, McGraw-Hill, 1961.

Special Committee on Nursing in National Defense: The Role of the Nurse in Disaster, New York, American Nurses' Assoc., 1960.

Symposium on the Management of Medical Emergencies, The Medical Clinics of North America, vol. 46, No. 2, Philadelphia, Saunders, March, 1962.

Articles

Artz, C. P.: Management of patients with multiple injuries, J.A.M.A. **173:**522-526, June 4, 1960.

Beecher, H. K.: Control of suffering in severe trauma, J.A.M.A. **173:**534-536, June 4, 1960.

Bell, H. S.: Nursing service in the emergency department, Nurs. Outlook **10:**392-393, June, 1962.

Bennett, H. J.: Burns—first aid and emergency care, Am. J. Nurs. **62:**96-100, Oct. 1962.

Cameron, B. M.: Whiplash injuries, Am. J. Nurs. **62:**72-75, Nov., 1962.

Dennis, C. L.: Disaster and its aftermath, Am. J. Nurs. **61:**74-76, Aug., 1961.

Elliman, V. B.: The bridge between, Nurs. Outlook **8:**131-133, March, 1960.

Elser, J. R.: Acute barbiturate intoxication, Am. J. Nurs. **60:**1096-1099, Aug., 1960.

Kandel, R. F.: Management of the hospital emergency unit, Nurs. Outlook **10:**390-391, June, 1962.

Kinch, A.: Bellevue responds when disaster strikes in New York City, Am. J. Nurs. **59:**504-509, April, 1959.

King, E. R.: Survival in nuclear warfare, entire volume 14, Clinical Symposia, Ciba, Jan.-Feb.-Mar., 1962.

Linden, M. E.: Some psychological aspects of rescue breathing, Am. J. Nurs. **60:**971-974, July, 1960.

Magnussen, A.: Nursing under the Red Cross today, Nurs. Outlook **9:**158-160, March, 1961.

Management of mass casualties, Part I, What's New **223:**2-6, April-May, 1961; Part II, What's New **224:**20-23, June-July, 1961.

Mueller, H. L.: Serious allergic reactions to insect stings, Am. J. Nurs. **60:**1110-1112, Aug., 1960.

The National League for Nursing and National Defense, Nurs. Outlook **7:**233-234, April, 1959.

Nelson, T. G., Rumer, G. F., and Nicholas, T. H.: Cricothyroidotomy in complete airway obstruction, Am. J. Nurs. **61:**74-76, Nov., 1961.

Nursing in disaster, Am. J. Nurs. **60:**1130-1133, Aug., 1960.

Pearce, M. G.: Emergency service for the poisoned, Am. J. Nurs. **63:**116-119, Mar., 1963.

Price, E. C.: A remote village, a neighborhood nurse and an antidotes chart, Am. J. Nurs. **59:**688-689, May, 1959.

Putt, A. M.: Radiation accidents, Nurs. Outlook **9:**350-351, June, 1961.

Radiation symbol becomes official, Nurs. Outlook **9:**46, Jan., 1961.

Sandick, H.: Emergency care of the injured, Am. J. Nurs. **62:**93-96, Dec., 1962.

Schade, F. F.: Functions of a hospital in a major disaster, J.A.M.A. **170:**1688-1690, Aug. 1, 1959.

Short, P. L.: It **did** happen here [tornado], Am. J. Nurs. **59:**228-229, Feb., 1959.

Soft Tissue Trauma, The Surgical Clinics of North America, Philadelphia, Saunders, Dec., 1958.

Stewart, W. G.: Radiation hazards control, Canad. Nurse **59:**44-48, Jan., 1963.

Sullivan, C. M.: What price survival?, Nurs. Outlook **8:**128-130, March, 1960.

Wilson, W. J.: Heat injury, Am. J. Nurs. **60:** 1124-1125, Aug., 1960.

Without warning [food poisoning disaster], Am. J. Nurs. **60:**984-986, July, 1960.

Worman, L. W., Yount, C. J., and Jacobs, L. E.: The care of patients with gunshot wounds, Am. J. Nurs. **63:**93-96, Feb., 1963.

Zingg, W., and Hildes, J. A.: Cold injury in civil disaster, Canad. Nurse **59:**53-57, Jan., 1963.

National Agencies

Federal and State Civil Defense Administration
Washington 25, D. C.
National Safety Council
425 North Michigan Avenue
Chicago 11, Illinois

Appendix

MOBILIZATION OF MEDICAL AND NURSING SERVICES

The basic plan of operation of medical and nursing services in an emergency is to set up first aid and emergency hospital units and organize professional and auxiliary personnel. Details of such planning should be reviewed as they apply to the local hospital unit, the community and the state.* During

*In the following reference, senior student nurses describe a make-believe disaster which they planned and in which they acted: Cleveland, Laurene, King, Lynelle, and Olson, Mary: Disaster Day, Amer. J. Nursing 56:464-465, 1956.

an emergency there will be increased demand for many of the professions or skills usually regulated by law. The nurse may be called to perform tasks usually done by a physician. Upgrading and regrading of functions often are necessary.

The sorting of casualties (formerly called *triage*) requires clinical judgment of the highest degree. The most responsible and able persons of the medical team should be assigned this difficult operation. Sorting is a continuous process, and it must be borne in mind that trauma can produce profound

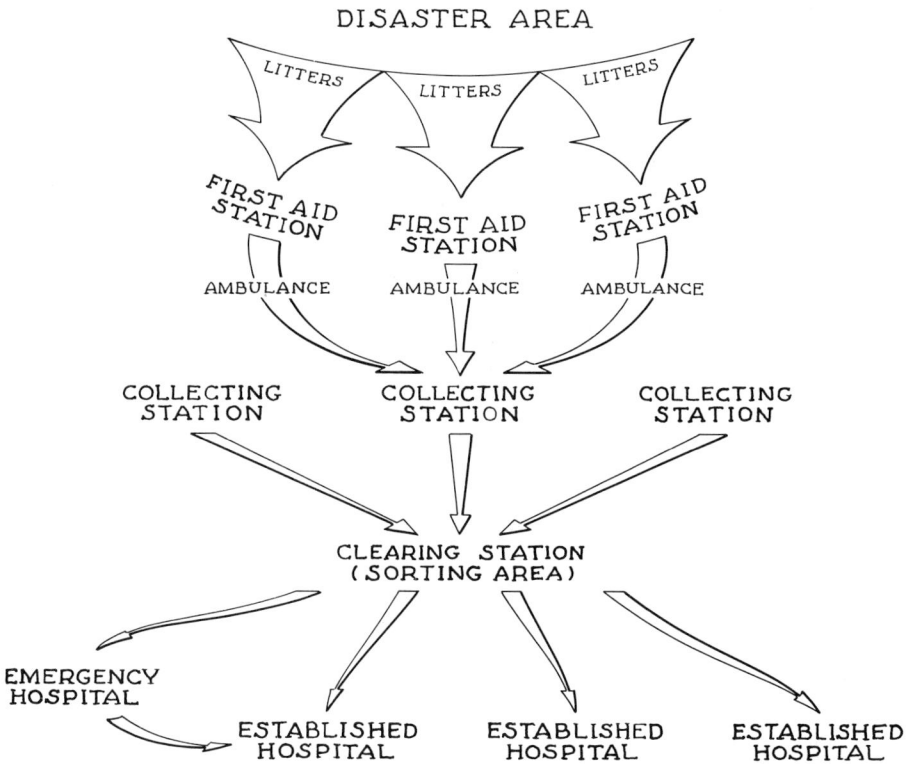

DIAGRAM OF CASUALTY EVACUATION FOR DISASTER

changes in an individual almost minute by minute.

Classification for priority in treatment would be based on the casualties' probability of responding to what is immediately available in the way of medical personnel and supplies.

1. *Minimal Treatment:* Patients who can be returned to effective duty immediately

2. *Immediate Treatment:* Patients for whom the available expedient procedures will save life or limb.

3. *Delayed Treatment:* Patients who, after emergency treatment, will incur little increased risk by having surgery withheld temporarily

4. *Expectant Treatment:* Critically injured patients who will be given treatment if time and facilities are available

The following is a priority schedule which serves as a guide to establish the flow of casualties from the field through the First Aid Station to Forward Treatment Center and Hospital:*

First Priority:

Any wound interfering with airway or causing airway obstruction. (This includes sucking chest wounds, tension pneumothorax and maxillofacial wounds in which asphyxia is present or an impending threat.)

Any wound requiring immediate pressure

Shock due to major hemorrhage, to wounds of any organ system, fractures, etc.

* United States Department of Defense: Emergency War Surgery, p. 172, Washington, D.C., United States Government Printing Office, 1958.

Second Priority:

Visceral injuries, including perforations of the gastrointestinal tract; wounds of the biliary and pancreatic system; wounds of the genitourinary tract; and thoracic wounds without asphyxia

Vascular injuries requiring repair. All injuries in which the use of a tourniquet is necsssary fall into this group.

Closed cerebral injuries with increasing loss of consciousness

Third Priority:

Spinal injuries in which decompression is required

Soft-tissue wounds in which débridement is necessary, but in which muscle damage is less than major

Lesser fractures and dislocations

Injuries of the eyes

Maxillofacial injuries without asphyxia

Identification of casualties is done by an emergency medical tag which should be fastened to a part of the body, preferably the wrist (not to clothing, because the tag may be lost). Details of methods used can be obtained in local and state civil defense manuals. Information about special care or handling of casualties can be noted by a simple initial about 3 inches high printed on the tag:

H—severe hemorrhage

L—litter case

T—tourniquet case (add time of application)

X—person who is definitely dead

COMBINING FORMS AND PREFIXES

These forms, with a prefix or a suffix, or both, are those most commonly used in making medical words. G indicates those from the Greek; L, those from the Latin. Properly, Greek forms should be used only with Greek prefixes and suffixes; Latin, with Latin. Often a vowel, usually a, i, or o, is needed for euphony.

A- or **Ab-** (L) *away, lack of:* abnormal, departing from normal.

A- or **An-** (G) *from, without:* asepsis, without infection.

Acr- (G) *an extremity:* acrodermatitis, a dermatitis of the limbs.

Ad- (L) *to, toward, near:* adrenal, near the kidney.

Aden- (G) *gland:* adenitis, inflammation of a gland.

Alg- (G) *pain:* neuralgia, pain extending along nerves.

Ambi- (L) *both:* ambidextrous, referring to both hands.

Ante- (L) *before:* antenatal, occurring or having been formed before birth.

Anti- (G) *against:* antiseptic, against or preventing sepsis.

Arth- (G) *joint:* arthritis, inflammation of a joint.

Auto- (G) *self:* auto-intoxication, poisoning by toxin generated in the body.

Bi- or **Bin-** (L) *two:* binocular, pertaining to both eyes.

Bio- (G) *life:* biopsy, inspection of living organism (or tissue).

Blast- (G) *bud, a growing thing in early stages:* blastocyte, beginning cell not yet differentiated.

Bleph- (G) *eyelids:* blepharitis, inflammation of an eyelid.

Brachi- (G) *arm:* brachialis, muscle for flexing forearm.

Brachy- (G) *short:* brachydactylia, abnormal shortness of fingers and toes.

Brady- (G) *slow:* bradycardia, abnormal slowness of heartbeat.

Bronch- (G) *windpipe:* bronchiectasis, dilation of bronchial tubes.

Bucc- (L) *cheek:* buccally, toward the cheek.

Carcin- (G) *Cancer:* carcinogenic, producing cancer.

Cardi- (G) *heart:* cardialgia, pain in the heart.

Cephal- (G) *head:* encephalitis, inflammation of brain.

Cheil- (G) *lip:* cheilitis, inflammation of the lip.

Chole- (G) *bile:* cholecyst, the gallbladder.

Chondr- (G) *cartilage:* chondrectomy, removal of a cartilage.

Circum- (L) *around:* circumocular, around the eyes.

Cleid- (G) *clavicle:* cleidocostal, pertaining to clavicle and ribs.

Colp- (G) *vagina:* colporrhagia, vaginal hemorrhage.

Contra- (L) *against, opposed:* contraindication, indication opposing usually indicated treatment.

Cost- (L) *rib:* intercostal, between the ribs.

Counter- (L) *against:* counterirritation, an irritation to relieve some other irritation (e.g., a liniment).

Crani- (L) *skull:* craniotomy, surgical opening in the skull.

Crypt- (G) *hidden:* cryptogenic, of hidden or unknown origin.

Cut- (L) *skin:* subcutaneous, under the skin.

Cyst- (G) *sac or bladder:* cystitis, inflammation of the bladder.

Cyto- (G) *cell:* cytology, scientific study of cells, a device for counting and measuring cells.

Dacry- (G) *lachrymal glands:* dacryocyst, tear-sac.

De- (L) *away:* decompress, relieve pressure.

Derm- or **dermat-** (G) *skin:* dermatoid, skinlike.

Di- (L) *two:* diphasic, incurring in two stages or phases.

Dis- (L) *apart:* disarticulation, taking joint apart.

Dys- (G) *pain or difficulty:* dyspepsia, impairment of digestion.

Ecto- (G) *outside:* ectoretina, outermost layer of retina.

Em- or **En-** (G) *in:* encapsulated, enclosed in a capsule.

Encephal- (G) *brain:* encephalitis, inflammation of the brain.

End- (G) *within:* endothelium, layer of cells lining heart, blood and lymph vessels.

Entero- (G) *intestine:* enterostomy, an opening (mouth) into the intestine.

Epi- (G) *above or upon:* epidermis, outermost layer of skin.

Erythro- (G) *red:* erythrocyte, red blood cell.

Eu- (G) *well:* euphoria, well feeling, feeling of good health.

Ex- or **E-** (L) *out:* excretion, material thrown out of the body or organ.

Exo- (G) *outside:* exocrine, excreting outwardly (opposite of endocrine).

Extra- (G) *outside:* extramural, situated or occurring outside a wall.

Febri- (L) *fever:* febrile, feverish.

Galacto- (G) *milk:* galactose, a milk-sugar.

Gastr- (G) *stomach:* gastrectomy, excision of the stomach.

Gloss- (G) *tongue:* glossectomy, surgical removal of tongue.

Glyco- (G) *sugar:* glycosuria, sugar in the urine.

Gynec- (G) *woman:* gynecology, science of diseases pertaining to women.

Hem- or **Hemat-** (G) *blood:* hemopoiesis, forming blood.

Hemi- (G) *half:* heminephrectomy, excision of half the kidney.

Hepat- (G) *liver:* hepatitis, inflammation of the liver.

Hetero- (G) *other* (opposite of homo-): hetero-transplant, using skin from a member of another species.

Hist- (G) *tissue:* histology, science of minute structure and function of tissues.

Homo- (G) *same:* homotransplant, skin grafting by using skin from a member of the same species.

Hydr- (G) *water:* hydrocephalus, abnormal accumulation of fluid in cranium.

Hyper- (G) *above, excess of:* hyperglycemia, excess of sugar in blood.

Hypo- (G) *under, deficiency of:* hypoglycemia, deficiency of sugar in blood.

Hyster- (G) *uterus:* hysterectomy, excision of uterus.

Idio- (G) *self, or separate:* idiopathic, a disease self-originated (of unknown cause).

Im- or **In-** (L) *in:* infiltration, accumulation in tissue of abnormal substances.

Im- or **In-** (L) *not:* immature, not mature.

Infra- (L) *below:* infra-orbital, below the orbit.

Inter- (L) *between:* intermuscular, between the muscles.

Intra- (L) *within:* intramuscular, within the muscle.

Kerat- (G) *horn, cornea:* keratitis, inflammation of cornea.

Lact- (L) *milk:* lactation, secretion of milk.

Leuk- (G) *white:* leukocyte, white cell.

Macro- (G) *large:* macroblast, abnormally large red cell.

Mast- (G) *breast:* mastectomy, excision of the breast.

Meg- or **Megal-** (G) *great:* megacolon, abnormally large colon.

Ment- (L) *mind:* dementia, deterioration of the mind.

Mer- (G) *part:* merotomy, division into segments.

Mesa- (G) *middle:* mesaortitis, inflammation of middle coat of the aorta.

Meta- (G) *beyond, over, change:* metastasis, change in seat of a disease.

Micro- (G) *small:* microplasia, dwarfism.

My- (G) *muscle:* myoma, tumor made of muscular elements.

Myc- (G) *fungi:* mycology, science and study of fungi.

Necro- (G) *corpse, dead:* necrosis, death of cells adjoining living tissue.

Neo- (G) *new:* neoplasm, any new growth or formation.

Neph- (G) *kidney:* nephrectomy, surgical excision of kidney.

Neuro- (G) *nerve:* neuron, nerve cell.

Odont- (G) *tooth:* odontology, dentistry.

Olig- (G) *little:* oligemia, deficiency in volume of blood.

Oo- (G) *egg:* oocyte, original cell of egg.

Oophor- (G) *ovary:* oophorectomy, removal of an ovary.

Ophthalm- (G) *eye:* ophthalmometer, an instrument for measuring the eye.

Ortho- (G) *straight, normal:* orthograde, walk straight (upright).

Oss- (L) *bone:* osseous, bony.

Oste- (G) *bone:* osteitis, inflammation of bone.

Ot- (G) *ear:* otorrhea, discharge from ear.

Ovar- (G) *ovary:* ovariorrhexis, rupture of an ovary.

Pan- (G) *all:* panhysterectomy, removal of the entire uterus.

Para- (G) *irregular, around, wrong:* paradenitis, inflammation of tissue in the neighborhood of a gland.

Path- (G) *disease:* pathology, science of disease.

Ped-[1] (G) *children:* pediatrician, child specialist.

Ped-[2] (L) *feet:* pedograph, imprint of the foot.

Per- (L) *through, excessively:* percutaneous, through the skin.

Peri- (G) *around, immediately around* (in contradistinction to para-): periapical, surrounding apex of root of tooth.

Phil- (G) *love:* hemophilic, fond of blood (as bacteria that grows well in presence of hemoglobin).

Phleb- (G) *vein:* phlebotomy, opening of vein for bloodletting.

Phob- (G) *fear:* hydrophobic, reluctant to associate with water.

Pneum- or **Pneumon-** (G) *lung* (pneum—air): pneumococcus, organism causing lobar pneumonia.

Polio- (G) *gray:* poliomyelitis, inflammation of gray substance of spinal cord.

[1] **Ped**—from Greek *pais,* child.

[2] **Ped**—from Latin *pes,* foot.

Poly- (G) *many:* polyarthritis, inflammation of several joints.

Post- (L) *after:* postpartum, after delivery.

Pre- (L) *before:* prenatal, occurring before birth.

Pro- (L and G) *before:* prognosis, forecast as to result of disease.

Proct- (G) *rectum:* proctectomy, surgical removal of rectum.

Pseudo- (G) *false:* pseudoangina, false angina.

Psych- (G) *soul or mind:* psychiatry, treatment of mental disorders.

Pyo- (G) *pus:* pyorrhea, discharge of pus.

Pyel- (G) *pelvis:* pyelitis, inflammation of pelvis or kidney.

Rach- (G) *spine:* rachicentesis, puncture into vertebral canal.

Radio- (L) *ray:* radiosensitive, responsive to irradiation.

Ren- (L) *kidney:* adrenal, near the kidney.

Retro- (L) *backward:* retroversion, turned backward (usually of uterus).

Rhin- (G) *nose:* rhinology, knowledge concerning noses.

Salping- (G) *a tube:* salpingitis, inflammation of tube.

Semi- (L) *half:* semicoma, mild coma.

Septic- (L and G) *poison:* septicemia, poisoned condition of blood.

Somat- (G) *body:* psychosomatic, having bodily symptoms of mental origin.

Sta- (G) *make stand:* stasis, stoppage of flow of fluid.

Sten- (G) *narrow:* stenosis, narrowing of duct or canal.

Sub- (L) *under:* subdiaphragmatic, under the diaphragm.

Super- (L) *above, excessively:* superacute, excessively acute.

Supra- (L) *above, upon:* suprarenal, above or upon the kidney.

Sym- or **Syn-** (G) *with, together:* symphysis, a growing together.

Tachy- (G) *fast:* tachycardia, fast-beating heart.

Tens- (L) *stretch:* extensor, a muscle extending or stretching a limb.

Therm- (G) *heat:* diathermy, therapeutic production of heat in tissues.

Tox- or **toxic-** (G) *poison:* toxemia, poisoned condition of blood.

Trache- (G) *trachea:* tracheitis, inflammation of the trachea.

Trans- (L) *across:* transplant, transfer tissue from one place to another.

Tri- (L and G) *three:* trigastric, having three bellies (muscle).

Trich- (G) *hair:* trichosis, any disease of the hair.

Uni- (L) *one:* unilateral, affecting one side.

Vas- (L) *vessel:* vasoconstrictor, nerve or drug that narrows blood vessel.

Zoo- (G) *animal:* zooblast, an animal cell.

SUFFIXES

-algia (G) *pain:* cardialgia, pain in the heart.

-asis or **-osis** (G) *affected with:* leukocytosis, excess number of leukocytes.

-asthenia (G) *weakness:* neurasthenia, nervous weakness.

-blast (G) *germ:* myeloblast, bone-marrow cell.

-cele (G) *tumor, hernia:* enterocele, any hernia of intestine.

-cid (L) *cut, kill:* germicidal, destructive to germs.

-clysis (G) *injection:* hypodermoclysis, injection under the skin.

-coccus (G) *round bacterium:* pneumococcus, bacteria of pneumonia.

-cyte (G) *cell:* leukocyte, white cell.

-ectasis (G) *dilation, stretching:* angiectasis, dilatation of a blood vessel.

-ectomy (G) *excision:* adenectomy, excision of adenoids.

-emia (G) *blood:* glycemia, sugar in blood.

-esthesia (G) *(noun) relating to sensation:* anesthesia, absence of feeling.

-ferent (L) *bear, carry:* efferent, carry out to periphery.

-genic (G) *producing:* pyogenic, producing pus.

-gram (L) and **-graph** (G) *writing* or *written:* electrocardiogram, tracing of electrical activity in heart.

-iatrics (G) *pertaining to a physician or the practice of healing* (medicine): pediatrics, science of medicine for children.

-itis (G) *inflammation:* tonsillitis, inflammation of tonsils.

-logy (G) *science of:* pathology, science of disease.

-lysis (G) *losing, flowing, dissolution:* autolysis, dissolution of tissue cells.

-malacia (G) *softening:* osteomalacia, softening of bone.

-oma (G) *tumor:* myoma, tumor made up of muscle elements.

-osis (-asis) (G) *being affected with:* atherosis, arteriosclerosis.

-(o)stomy (G) *creation of an opening:* gastrostomy, creation of an artificial gastric fistula.

-(o)tomy (G) *cutting into:* laparotomy, surgical incision into abdomen.

-pathy (G) *disease:* myopathy, disease of a muscle.

-penia (G) *lack of:* leukopenia, lack of white blood cells.

-pexy (G) *to fix:* proctopexy, fixation of rectum by suture.

-phagia *eating:* polyphagia, excessive eating.

-phasia (G) *speech:* aphasia, loss of power of speech.

-phobia (G) *fear:* hydrophobia, fear of water.

-plasty (G) *molding:* gastroplasty, molding or re-forming stomach.

-poiesis (G) *making, forming:* hematopoiesis, forming blood.

-pnea (G) *air or breathing:* dyspnea, difficult breathing.

-ptosis (G) *falling:* enteroptosis, falling of intestine.

-rhythmia (G) *rhythm:* arrhythmia, variation from normal rhythm of heart.

-rrhagia (G) *flowing or bursting forth:* otorrhagia, hemorrhage from ear.

-rrhaphy (G) *suture of:* herniorrhaphy, act of repairing hernia by suture.

-rrhea (G) *discharge:* otorrhea, discharge from ear.

-sthen (ia) (ic) (G) *pertaining to strength:* asthenia, loss of strength.

-taxia or **-taxis** (G) *order, arrangement of:* ataxia, failure of muscular co-ordination.

-trophia or **-trophy** (G) *nourishment:* atrophy, wasting, or diminution.

-uria (G) *to do with urine:* polyuria, excessive secretion of urine.

ADDRESSES

Complete addresses for sources of Patient-Teaching Aids as described at the end of each chapter in Part Two:

American Cancer Society
521 West 57th Street
New York 19, New York

American Medical Association
535 North Dearborn Street
Chicago 10, Illinois

American Red Cross
Washington, D.C.

Mental Health Materials Center, Inc.
1790 Broadway, Room 713
New York 19, New York

Metropolitan Life Insurance Co.
1 Madison Avenue
New York 10, New York

National Society for Crippled Children and Adults
11 South LaSalle Street
Chicago 3, Illinois

Public Affairs Committee, Inc.
22 East 38th Street
New York 16, New York

Schering Corporation
Bloomfield, New Jersey

Superintendent of Documents
U.S. Government Printing Office
Washington 25, D.C.

United Surgical Supplies Co.
Port Chester, New York

U.S. Department of Health, Education and Welfare
Washington, D.C.

World Health Organization
Palais des Nations
Geneva, Switzerland

Index

Abdomen, distension, in intestinal
  obstruction, 634
  in paralytic ileus, 633
  in pneumonia, 423
  postoperative, 292, 294
  incisions, 587, Fig. 215
  pain, postoperative, 291
  paracentesis, 100, 658
  topography of, Figs. 200, 201,
    214
  x-ray examination of, 102
Abducens nerve, 924
  testing of, 908
Abrasions, dermal, 780
Abscess(es), alveolar, 572
  appendiceal, 619, Fig. 230
  aural. See Otitis media
  bone, 1018
  brain, 951
  breast, 783
  epidermal, 757
  ischiorectal, 640
  liver, 654, Fig. 250
    amebic, 1129
  lung, 427, Fig. 23
  perinephric, 694
  peritonsillar, 385, Fig. 117
Accidents, fatal, classification of,
    1167
  automobile, mechanisms of
    injury in, Fig. 460
  frequency of, in older age
    groups, 340, Fig. 102
  home, 1169
    incidence of, Fig. 461
  prevention of, 1166
Accidents, traffic, 1167
Acetanilid, 117
Acetest, 72, Plate I
Acetophenetidin, 72
Acetylcholine, 906, 1045
Achalasia, 574, 576, Fig. 205
  hydrostatic dilatation of,
    Fig. 206
  radiologic appearance of,
    Fig. 205
  surgical treatment of, Fig. 207
Achromycin, 193
Achylia, gastric, 463
Acid-base balance, 161
Acid hemolysin, 90, 468
Acidosis, 166
  diabetic, 167, 827, 831
  metabolic, 167, Fig. 31
  respiratory, 400, 436
Acid phosphatase, 82
Acne, rosacea, 753
  vulgaris, 752, Fig. 292
Acromegaly, 847, Fig. 326

ACTH, 842
Actinomycosis, 1131
Activities of Daily Living (A.D.L.)
  Sheet, 362, Fig. 108
Addiction, narcotic, 121
Addison's disease, 839
Adenitis. See Lymphadenitis
Adenoidectomy, 385
Adenoiditis, 384
Adenoids, 377, Fig. 118
Adhesions, postoperative, 633
Adiodochokinesis, 903
Adrenalectomy, 845
Adrenal gland, cortex, 839
  masculinizing tumor of,
    Fig. 324
  medula, 844
Adrenalin. See Epinephrine
Aerophagia, 594
Aerosol therapy, 557, Fig. 144
Afibrinogenemia, 79
Agammaglobulinemia, 79
Age distribution, in population,
  332
Agglutinins, 177
  cold, 468
  red cell, 468
Agglutinogens, 177
Aging, disorders associated with,
    334
  medical aspects of, 333
  nursing aspects of, 334
  relationship of, to chronic
    illness, 333, Fig. 99
Agranulocytosis, 470
  postirradiation, 318
Agraphia, 897
Air, embolism, 485
  encephalogram, 106
  swallowing, 594
Airway, maintenance of, 274
  types of, Figs. 79, 80
Albinism, 750
Albumin, plasma, 78
Albuminuria. See Proteinuria
Aldactone, 656
Aldosterone, 839
Aldosteronism, 840
Alexia, 897
Alkaline phosphatase, 82
Alkalosis, 167, 168
  metabolic, 165, Fig. 30
  respiratory, 400
Alkaptonuria, 69
Alkylating agents, 323, Table 10
Allergens, 800
Allergy, 800, 806
  drug, 807
  gastrointestinal, 809
  insulin, 830

penicillin, 193
  skin, 806
  transfusion, 181
N-Allylnormorphine, 1164
Alopecia, 771
Alveoli, 398
Ambulation, postoperative, 281
  wheelchair, Fig. 109
Amebiasis, 1129
Amebicides, 199
Amenorrhea, 724
Amethopterin. See Methotrexate
Amidopyrine, 470
Amino acid injections, 173
Ammonia, in hepatic coma, 653
Amphotericin B, 196
Ampulla of Vater, Fig. 253
Amputation, 1013
  stump, care of, Fig. 406
Amyl nitrite, 519
Amylase, blood, 81
  pancreatic, 568
Amyloidosis, congo red clearance
  in, 85
Amytal, 125
Analgesics, 116
  urinary tract, 699
Anastomosis, portacaval, 659
Ancylostomiasis. See Hookworm
Anemia(s), 461
  aregenerative, 461
  Cooley's. See Thalassemia
  facies in, 52
  hemolytic, 466
  hypochromic, 462, 468
  iron deficiency, 462
  macrocytic, 463, 466
  Mediterranean. See Thalassemia
  myelophthisic, 462
  osteosclerotic, 462
  pernicious, 463
    nursing care in, 464
  sickle cell, 468
  toxic, 469
Anesthesia, endotracheal, 221,
    222, Fig. 44
  epidural (peridural), 227
  general, 222
  inhalation, 220
  infiltration, local, 228
  in older patients, 341
  intrapharyngeal, 222
  intravenous, 225
  recovery from, 274
  regional block, 228
  spinal, 226, Figs. 45, 46
  stages of, 219, 220, Fig. 43
  types of, 220

Anesthetics, explosive, 260
  flammable, 260
  gaseous, 223
  inhalation, 222
    absorption of, Fig. 42
Aneurysms, 535, Figs. 188, 189
  aortic, 535
    abdominal, 538
    dissecting, 539, Fig. 193
    intracranial, 945, Fig. 362
    mycotic, 535
Angina, agranulocytic, 470
  Ludwig's, 571
  pectoris, 518
  Vincent's, 394, Plate V
Angioaortogram, 537
Angiography, 101
Angiomata, cerebral, 941
Angioplasty, Fig. 190
Anhidrosis, 750
Aniline poisoning, 930
Anorectum, examination, tray for,
    Fig. 217
  surgery, nursing care in, 642
Anorexia, 154
Anoscopy, 589
Anosmia, 924
Anoxia, in shock, 296
Antacids, 598
Anthrax, 1085
Antibiotics, 192. *See also specific
    antibiotic drugs, like* Penicillins,
    Tetracyclines, *etc.*
Antibodies, 19, 800
Anticholinesterase compounds,
    1045
Anticoagulants, blood sample, 77
  therapeutic, 302, 486
Anticonvulsants, 956
Antiemetics, 121
Antifoaming agents, 547
Antigens, 800
Antihistamines, 811
Antimalarials, 198, 1128
Antimetabolites, 323, Table 11
Antimicrobials, 192
Antiseptics, 37, 45
  urinary, 699
Antiserums, 1052
Antispasmodics, 119, 598
Antitoxin(s), 1052
  Botulinus, 1080
  diphtheria, 1070
  gas bacillus, 1055
  hemolytic streptococcal, 1055
  Shiga dysentery, 1055
  snake venum, 1055
  Staphylococcus aureus, 1055
  streptococcal, 1055
  tetanus, 32
Anuria, 686
  calculous, 697
Anus, lesions of, Fig. 244
  pruritus of, 744
Aorta, 484
  aneurysms of, 535, Fig. 191
  coarctation of, 554
  homografts, 538, Fig. 192
  insufficiency, 529, Fig. 183
  stenosis, 529, Fig. 183
  thrombosis, 539
Aortitis, 534
  luetic, 534

Aortograms, 680, Fig. 155
Aphasia, 896, 897
Aphonia, 386
Apnea, 57
Apoplexy, 931
Appendectomy, 620
Appendicitis, 619
  acute, Fig. 230
Appendix, 569, Fig. 229
Appliances, orthotic, 369
Applications, cold, 116
Applicator, Ernst, Fig. 287
ARD (Acute Respiratory Disease),
    394
Area, Broca's, 896
Argyria, Plate VI
Arrhythmias, cardiac, 508
Arsenic, skin reactions to, 807
  toxic hepatitis from, 654
Artane, 949
Arteries, oxygen saturation in,
    397
  pressure measurements, 62
  pressure points, for control of
    bleeding, Fig. 453
  pulse, 59
Arteriogram(s), 484
  abdominal, Fig. 155
  cerebral, 912; Figs. 352 and 362
Arteriosclerosis, 491, Figs. 166,
    167
  aortic, 534
  control of, 522
  coronary, 518
  in diabetes, 827
  in elderly patients, 334
  mortality from, 4, 5
  obliterans, 491
Arteritis, temporal, 917
Arthrodesis, 1041
Arthroplasty, 1027
Ascaris lumbricoides, 1137
Arthritis, 1023
  degenerative, 334
  gonorrheal, 1019
  gouty, 1029
  hemophiliac, 477
  hypertrophic, 1027. *See also*
    Osteoarthritis
  meningococcal, 1083
  posture in, 52
  public health aspects of, 1022
  pyogenic, 1019
  rheumatic, 1023
  rheumatoid, 1024
  traumatic, 1031
  tuberculous, 1021
Ascites, in cardiac failure, 540
  in glomerulonephritis, 689
  in hepatic cirrhosis, 656
Ascorbic acid. *See* Vitamin C
Asepsis, principles of, 36, 237
  surgical, 235
Aspergillosis, 1133
Aspiration, endotracheal, 413,
    Fig. 135
  foreign body, 388, 440
Aspirin. *See* Salicylates
Asthma, bronchial, 803
  cardiac, 59
  management of, 810
  prevention of, 804
  respirations in, 59

Astigmatism, 853
A. T. 10, 826
Ataxia, 54
  cerebellar, 903
  locomotor. *See* Tabes dorsalis
Atelectasis, 406, Figs. 91, 132
  postoperative, 299
Athetosis, 53
Athlete's foot. *See* Epidermophy-
    tosis
Atresia, esophageal, 576
Atrophy, muscle, 901, 997, 1025,
    1098, 1101
  optic, 924
Atropine, 598
Audiogram, 877
Auditory-vestibular nerve, 926
Aura, epileptic, 955
  in migraine, 919
Aural hygiene, 876
Aureomycin. *See* Tetracyclines
Auscultatory gap, 62
Autoagglutination, 90
Autoclave, loading of, Figs. 10, 12
  sterilization, 38, Figs. 9, 10
Autografts, 774
Autonomic dysfunction, 906
Autonomic nervous system, 904
Avitaminoses, 151, 652
Azotemia, 163

Babinski reflex, 932
Bacitracin, 195
Bacteria, types of, 1065, Figs. 422,
    423
Bacteriuria, 74
Bag(s), Bongort, Fig. 232
  colostomy, 639, Fig. 243
  Plummer, 579, Fig. 206
  Politzer, Fig. 337
  Rutzen, Figs. 234, 243
Balanitis, 709
BAL (British Anti-Lewisite), 1164
Bandage, plaster, application of,
    Figs. 388, 389
  T-, Fig. 245
    perineal, Fig. 246
Banthine, 598
Barbiturates, 225
Bartholinitis, 728
Basal metabolic rate (BMR), 816,
    Fig. 318
Basin set, O.R., Figs. 58-60
Baths, 27
  contrast, 501
  sitz, 27
  therapeutic, 747
  whirlpool, 29, Fig. 6
Bed, oscillating, 501
  recovery, Fig. 75
  rocking, 1100, Figs. 438, 439
  tilt (table), Fig. 112
Bedbugs, 762
Bedrails, Fig. 94
Behavior, interpretation of, 130
  mechanisms of, 129
Belladonna, 119
Benemid, 1031
Beriberi, 152
Bicarbonate, blood, 161
Bile, 568, 648
Bilharziasis, 1139

Biliary tract, Fig. 253
  obstruction, 662, 663
  surgery, 665
  x-ray examination of, 103
Bilirubin, 80
Bilirubinuria, 68
Biopsy, tumor, 316
Birth, injury, 901
  palsy, 1036
Birthmarks. *See* Nevi
Blackeye, 861
Blackheads, 752
Bladder, 699
  congenital malformations of, 699
  decompression of, 713
  disorders of, 699
  ileal, 701
  stones, 700, Fig. 270
  training, 370, 971
  traumatic lesions of, 699
  tumors of, 700
Blastomycosis, 1133
  chemotherapy of, 199
Bleeders, 477
Bleeding, disorders, 475
  tests, 91
Blindness, cortical, 895
  night, 151
Blood, chemistry, 77
  circulation, diagram of, 486, Fig. 158
  clotting, 91
  counts, 85
  donors, complications in, 176
  examination of, 174
  flukes, 1139
  gases, 397
    distribution of, Fig. 122
  groups, 177
  pH, 80
  pressure. *See* Arteries, pressure
  Rh types, 178
  sampling of, 77
  substitutes, 1156
  therapeutic components of, 179
  transfusion, 179
    complications of, 181, 184
    incompatible, 182
    nursing role in, 180, 183
  vessels, 483
    disorders of, 485
    structure of, 485
  volume measurements, 90, 108
Blue babies, 548
Body, cast, application of, Figs. 391-393
  position (positioning), following chest surgery, 410
    in coma, 923
    in congestive heart failure, 541
    following cord injury, 969
    dorsal, 280
    lateral, 280
    on operating table, 280
    postoperative, Fig. 82
    for prevention of deformities, 352
    for proctoscopy, Fig. 216
  posture(s), correct and faulty, Fig. 416 A
  weights, optimum, 156

Boils, 755
Bone, demineralization (decalcification), 1042
    in hyperparathyroidism, Fig. 321
    in myelomatosis, Fig. 154
  grafts, 776
  infections, 1017
  marrow, biopsy, 91
    depression, 469
      following irradiation, 318
      toxic, 469
  metastases, 1035, Fig. 411
  pain, 983
  syphilis. *See* Syphilis, bone and joint
  tuberculosis, 1020
  tumors, 1033
Borrelia, 1118
Botulism, 1079
Bowel training, 370
Brachial plexus, 927
  palsy, 927
Bradycardia, 60
Bradykinesia, 1107
Bradyphrenia, 1107
Brain, 893
  abscess, 951
  injury, 960, Fig. 368
  surgery, 943
  tumors, 941, Fig. 361
Breast, 782
  abscess of, 783
  cancer of, 784
    adrenalectomy in, 845
  hypertrophy of, 785
  male, 785
  surgery, nursing care in, 787
  tumors, 784
Breathing, costal, 58
  exercises, 417, 436
  intermittent positive pressure (IPPB), 435
  Kussmaul, 59
  rescue, 1152, Fig. 452
British Anti-Lewisite, 1164
Bromides, 957
Bromidrosis, 751
Bromsulphthalein (BSP) test, 83
Bronchi (-ioles), 398
Bronchiectasis, 430, Fig. 142
Bronchitis, 419
  postoperative, 300
Bronchodilators, 434
Bronchograms, 102, 401
Bronchopneumonia, 421
  postoperative, 299, 300
Bronchoscopy, 401, Fig. 129
Brucellosis, 1079
Bruising, tendency to, 476
BSP (bromsulphalein) test, 83
Buboes, 1109
Buck's extension, 1000, Fig. 394
Bulimia, 154, 595
BUN (Blood urea nitrogen), 80
Bundle of His, 508
Bunions. *See* Hallux valgus
Burn(s), 793
  chemical, 793
  electrical, 793
  injuries, Plate VIII
    evaluation of, 1160, Fig. 459
  mass management of, 1161

nursing management of, 794
  radiation, 793
Bursitis, 1032
  subdeltoid, 1032
  tuberculous, 1022
Busulfan. *See* Myleran
Butazolidin, 117, 1030

Cachexia, facies in, 52
Caffeine, 297
Calcium, blood, 81
  deficiency, 154
    osteomalacia in, 1042
  dietary, 148
  urinary, 75
Calculus (calculi), bladder, 700
  renal, 694, Figs. 268, 269
  salivary, 572
Calories, food, 146
Cancer, 309. *See also* Carcinoma; Sarcoma; Leukemia; Lymphoma; Tumors
  breast, 784, Fig. 309
  cervix, 730
    nursing care in, 736
  chemotherapy, 323, Tables 10-12
    complications of, 325
  colonic, 630
  death rates in, Tables 1, 2, 8, 9; Figs. 95, 96
    analyzed according to sites of involvement, Fig. 145
  detection, 315
  incidence of, 312, 315
  irradiation, 317
  larynx, 386
  lip, 571
  liver, 659
  lung, 439
  metastatic, 310, 659, 1035; Figs. 361, 411
  occupational therapy in, 327
  oral, 573
    nursing care in, 573
  organ, location of, Table 9
  prostate, 711
    adrenalectomy in, 845
  psychologic aspects of, 325
  steroid therapy in, 324
  stomach, 605
  surgery, 316
  terminal, nursing care in, 326
  thyroid, 822
  tongue, 573
Cancer nursing, 315
  psychologic aspects of, 327
Carbohydrates, dietary, 145
  digestion of, 565
  metabolism of, 647
Carbomycin, 194
Carbon dioxide, inhalation, 303
  narcosis, 190
  retention, 399
Carbuncles, 755
  renal, 694
Carcinoid, 630
Carcinoma, basal-cell, 770, Fig. 303
  breast, 784
  bronchiogenic, 439
  colon, 630, Fig. 237

Carcinoma (*Continued*)
  esophageal, 581, Fig. 212
  gastric, 605
  pancreatic, 670
    surgical treatment of, Fig. 258
  penis, 709
  prostatic, 711
  rectum, Fig. 238
  renal, 697
  sigmoid, 630
  skin, 770
  thyroid, 822
  tongue, 573
  uterine, 732
Carcinoma-in-situ, cervical, 732
Cardiac arrest, 515
Cardiac arrhythmias, 508
  nursing in, 517
Cardiac asthma, 59
Cardiac catheterization, 95
Cardiac conduction system, 508
Cardiac defibrillation, 516
Cardiac function, 507
  tests of, 508
Cardiac massage, 515
  closed chest, 515, Fig. 180
  open chest, 516, Fig. 181
Cardiac pacemaker, artificial, 512
  implantation of, 513
  natural, 508
Cardiac pacing, 512
Cardiac resuscitation, 515
Cardiac tamponade, 442
Cardiospasm, 574, 576, Fig. 205.
  See also Achalasia
Cardiovascular deaths, Table 17
Cardiovascular disease, death rates
  in, 459
Cardiovascular surgery, 548
Cardiovascular surgical nursing,
  554
Carotene, 147
Carotid artery, ligation, 933, Fig.
  357
  thrombosis, 933
Caruncle, 705
Caseation, 447
Castration, for prostatic
  carcinoma, 711
Casts, plaster, 991
  urinary, 73
Cataract, 869
  surgical treatment for, 869, 871
Catecholamines, urinary, 76
Catheter, Foley, Fig. 264
Catheterization, cardiac, 95
  nasal, 187
  oropharyngeal, 187, Fig. 34
  tracheal, Fig. 135
  ureteral, 679, Fig. 264
  urinary bladder, 680
Catheters, ureteral, sterilization
  of, 269
Causalgia, 930
Cauterization, 44
Cavernostomy, 453
Cecum, 569, 619, Fig. 229
Cephalgia. *See* Headache
Cerebellum, 902
Cerebral cortex, 894
Cerebral embolism, 933
Cerebral hemorrhage, 931, Fig.
  344

Cerebral infections, 951
Cerebral injuries, Fig. 368
Cerebral thrombosis, 932, Fig. 345
Cerebral vascular accident, 931
Cerumen, 875
Cervicitis. *See* Endocervicitis
Cervix, lacerations of, 731
Chalazion, 864
Chancre, 709, 1120
  oral, Plate V
Chancroid, 709
Charting, intensive care unit, Fig.
  90
  postoperative, 280, Fig. 81
Chemotherapy, antimalarial, 1128
  antimicrobial, 192
  antimitotic, 323
  intrathecal, 1084
  regional perfusion, 324
  tuberculosis, 452
Chest, drainage, 412, 557, Figs.
  133, 134
  open, 427
  water seal, Fig. 134
  fluid, 100
  injuries, 441
  pain, 405
  patients, rehabilitation of, 415
  respirator, 1102, Fig. 440
  surgery, 408
    postoperative nursing in, 409
  tumors, 438
  x-ray examination of, 102
Chickenpox, 1093
  rash, Plate X
Chilblain, 754
Chloasma, 748
Chloral hydrate, 125
Chlorambucil, 323
Chloramphenicol, 194
Chlorides, urinary, 74
Chloromycetin. *See* Chloramphe-
  nicol
Chloroquine, 198
Chlorothiazide, 494
Chlorpromazine, 121
  in hiccup, 303
Chlortetracycline (Aureomycin),
  193, 1129
Cholangiography, 103
Cholangitis, 659
Cholecystectomy, 663
Cholecystitis, 663
Cholecystograms, 103, 662
Cholecystojejunostomy, 672
Cholecystostomy, 663, Fig. 255
Choledochotomy, 663
Cholelithiasis, 662
Cholera, 1085
  Asiatic, 1085
Cholesterol, blood, 80
Choluria. *See* Bilirubinuria
Chorea, Huntingdon's
  (hereditary), 951
  Sydenham's, 53
  tremor in, 53
Choriomeningitis, lymphocytic,
  1108
Chromium⁵¹. *See* Radiochromium
Chyle, 484, 569
Chylothorax, 408
Cigarette smoking, 439
  in emphysema, 432

  in heart disease, 519, 521, 561
  in lung cancer, 439
  in peripheral vascular disease,
    501
Circulating nurse, duties of, 244,
  254, Figs. 55-60
Circulation, portal, 484
  pulmonary, 484
  systemic, 483
  time, pulmonary, 94
Cirrhosis, alcoholic. *See* Cirrhosis,
  portal
  biliary, 659
  hepatic, 655
  portal, 655
    nursing problems in, 660
Cisternal puncture, 99, 907, 908,
  Fig. 341
Claudication, intermittent, 496
Clavicle, fracture of, 1005
Clawfoot, 1039, Fig. 413
Clinistix, 72, Plate I
Clinitest, 72, Plate I
Clonorchis sinensis, infestation.
  See Lung, fluke
Clotting defects, 477
Clotting tests, 91, 92
Clubfoot, 1037, Fig. 413
Clysis, intravenous, 169
Coarctation of aorta, 554, Fig. 199
Cobalt⁶⁰, teletherapy, 320
Cobalt bomb, 320
Cocaine, 229
Coccidiomycosis, 1133
Codeine, 118
Cogentin, 949
Colchicine, 1030
Cold, agglutinins, 468
  applications, 116
  common, 378
  hemolysins, 468
  injury, 754, 1159
  rose, 802
Cold surgery (cryosurgery),
  contraindications in, Fig. 458
Colic, biliary, 662
  intestinal, 612
  renal, 696
  ureteral, 696
Colitis, chronic ulcerative, 623
  ulcerative, roentgenologic
    appearance of, Fig. 233
Collapse, circulatory, 63, 511
  pulmonary, 406, 407
Colon, 569
  disorders of, 612
  resection, abdominoperineal,
    Fig. 238
Colostomy, 625, 631, 635
  bags, 639, Fig. 243
  diet, 638
  irrigation of, Fig. 242
  loop, 635, Fig. 239
  management of, 637
  Mikulicz, Fig. 239
  regulation of, 637
Colporrhaphy, 729
Coma, 922
  epileptic, 955
  diabetic, 827, 832
  hepatic, 652
  hypoglycemic, 830, 838

Coma *(Continued)*
  nursing care in, 922, Fig. 356
  uremic, 685
Comedones, 752
Commissurotomy, mitral, 531,
    Fig. 186
Compazine, 421
Compresses, 26
  cold, 28
  hot, 25, Figs. 5 A, B, C
Concurrent disinfection, 1059
Concussion, 960
Condylomata, 729, 1121
Congenital malformations,
    incidence of, 4
  heart disease, 552
Congestion, pulmonary,
    hypostatic, 301
Conjunctivitis, 864
Constipation, 612
  postoperative, 294
Contracture, Dupuytren's, 1042
Contusions, 984
Convulsions, 53
Cord bladder, 971
  irrigation of, 974, Fig. 379
Cordotomy, 976
Cornea, 851
  inflammation of, 865
  transplantation of, 867
  ulceration of, 865
Corpus luteum, 718
Cortex, cerebral, 894
Corticosteroids, therapeutic
    actions of, 841
Corticosterone, 839
Corticotropin. *See* ACTH
Cortisone, 842
Coryza. *See* Rhinitis
Coughing, 403
Cough routines, preoperative and
    postoperative, Fig. 131
Cough suppressants, 120
Cowpox. *See* Vaccinia
Cramps, 982
Cranial nerves, disorders of, 923
Cranioplasty, 960
Craniotomy, 942
Creatinine, blood, 79
Cretinism, 819
Crosseye. *See* Esotropia and
    Exotropia
Crutches, 1012
Crutch walking, 364, Fig. 111
Crutchfield tongs, 965
Cryoglobulins, 79
Cryosurgery, 950
Cryptococcosis, 1133
Cryptorchism, 708
Crystalluria, 74
Curare, 1109
Cutaneous ureterostomy, 701
Cyanosis, 186
Cycloplegia, 119
Cycloplegics, 856
Cyclopropane, 225
Cylindruria, 73
Cystitis, 699
Cyst(s), 309
  Bartholin's, 728
  bone, 1033
  breast, 783

chocolate. *See* Endometriosis
dermoid, 439
echinococcus, 1138
endometrial. *See* Endometriosis
mediastinal, 439
ovarian, 738
pancreatic, 670
pilonidal, 641
renal, 697
retention, of breast, 783
sebaceous, 768, Fig. 300
Cysteinuria, 74
Cystitis, 699
Cystocele, 729, Fig. 285
Cystograms, 679
Cystoscopes, 269
  disinfection of, 269
Cystoscopy, Fig. 263
Cystostomy, 704
Cystotomy, 696

Deafness, 877
Death rates, cancer, Fig. 95,
    Table 8
  cardiovascular disease, 459
  selected diseases (1900-1950),
    18, Fig. 2
Débridement, 37
Declomycin. *See* Tetracyclines
Decompression, pericardia, 442
Decortication, pulmonary, 427,
    453
Decubiti, 360
  prevention of, 360
  treatment of, 361
Defibrillation, cardiac, 516
Deficiency, states of, 151. *See
    also various specific vitamins,
    minerals and other nutrients*
  G-6-PD (glucose-6-phosphate
    dehydrogenase), 466
  prothrombin, 478
Deformities, contraction, 983
  hemiplegic, Fig. 358
  postparalytic, 1041
  postural, postpoliomyelitis,
    Fig. 436
  prevention of, in neurologic
    patients, 915
  rachitic, 1041
Dehiscence, 308
Dehydration, 162
  facies in, 52
Delirium, 138
  postoperative, 305
Delirium tremens, postoperative,
    305
Demerol, 119
Demethylchlortetracycline, 193
Dengue, 1110
Deodorizers, 37
Dermatalgia, 744
Dermatitis, atopic, 807
  contact, 806, Fig. 315, Plate VII
  exfoliative, 761, 763, Fig. 298
  factitious, 754
  herpetiformis, 764
  irradiation, 320
  medicamentosa, 807
  radiation, 320, 754
  venenata, 806

Dermatologic patients, nursing
    management of, 779
Dermatologic therapy, general
    principles of, 745
  surgical, 772
Dermatology, nursing responsibil-
    ities in, 745
Dermatome(s), 774, Fig. 305
  Brown-Electro, Fig. 305
  Padgett, 775
Dermatomyositis, 765
Dermatoses, allergic, 806
  seborrheic, 752
  traumatic, 753
Desensitization, allergic, 811
Dexamethasone, 842
Dexedrine, 949
Dextran, 1156
Dextrose, parenteral, 169
Diabetes insipidus, 846
Diabetes mellitus, 826
  acidosis in, 167, 831
  coma in, 832
  complications of, 827
  diets in, 837
  gangrene in, Fig. 168
  nursing care in, 828
  surgical nursing in, 838
Diagnosis, x-ray, 100
Dialysis, 684
  peritoneal. *See* Dialysis
Diarrhea, 614
  infectious, 615
  pancreatica, 670
  postoperative, 295
  summer, 1104
Diasone. *See* Sulfones
Diathermy, 26, 116
Diet(s), 150, Table 5
  allowances in, 144
  biliary tract disease, 666
  bland, 150
  colostomy, 638
  congestive heart failure, 542
  diabetic, 828, 837
  gout, 1030
  myocardial infarction, 521
  obesity, 155
  postoperative, 282
  renal disease, 687
  restricted sodium, 150
Diethylstilbestrol, 725
Digestion, 565
Digitalis, 542
Digitalization, 542
Dihydrotachysterol, 826
Diiodohydroxyquin, 199
Dilantin, 956
Dilatation and curettage (D and
    C), 721
Dilaudid, 118
Diphtheria, 1068
  antitoxin, 1070
  bacilli, Fig. 424
  prophylaxis, 1070
  wound, 1069
Diphtheria-Tetanus-Pertussis
    (DTP) immunization, 1052
Diplegia, 902
Diplopia, 872, 1044
Disaster nursing, 1149
Discography, 913

Disease(s), autoimmune hemolytic. *See* Jaundice, acquired hemolytic
Bright's. *See* Glomerulonephritis
Brill's, 1113
Buerger's, 496
celiac, 614
cerebrovascular, mortality from, 4, 5
combined system, 463
communicable, epidemiology, treatment and prevention of, 1061-1063, Table 23
incidence of, 1059, Fig. 421
nursing, precautions in, 1055, Fig. 419
adaptation of, for home care, Figs. 419, 420
in pneumonia, 423
principles of, 1051, 1140
coronary artery, 518
cysticercus, 1138
endocardial, 523
foot-and-mouth, 1112
Graves', 820
Hansen's. *See* Leprosy
hemoglobin S. *See* Anemia, sickle cell
hemorrhagic, 475
of the newborn, 478
Hodgkin's, 473
hydatid, 1138
hypertensive vascular, 493
liver, 650
Paget's, of bone, 1043
of breast, 784
Parkinson's (Parkinsonism), 949
gait in, 54
tremor in, 53, Fig. 364
pelvic inflammatory (P.I.D.), 738, 1080
peripheral arterial, 498
peripheral vascular, nursing problems in, 500, 502
Pott's, 1020
Raynaud's, 496, 498, Fig. 170
serum, 805
von Recklinghausen's, 770, 825, 1044, Fig. 302
Simmonds', 846, Fig. 325
Still's, 1024
tricuspid valvular, 532
valvular heart, 529
Weil's, 1124
Woolsorter's. *See* Anthrax
Disinfectants, 46
antibiotic, 48
Disinfection, 37
chemical, 45
concurrent, 1059
formaldehyde, 47
hydrogen peroxide, 47
potassium permanganate, 47
terminal, 1060
Disk, choked, 924
intervertebral, herniation of, 969, Fig. 374
optic, choking of, 854
Dislocation(s), 984
hip, congenital, 1035

Disorders, atopic, 801
cranial nerves, 923
extrapyramidal, 949
hemolytic, 466
intestinal, 612
laryngeal, 386
pigmentary, 747
rectal, 640
renal, 683. *See also* Kidney
nursing in, 681
secretory, 750
urogenital, male, Fig. 273
Disseminated lupus erythematosus (D.L.E.), 765
Distension, abdominal. *See* Abdomen, distension
Distomiasis. *See* Infestations, fluke
Diuretic drugs, 543
Diuretic therapy, cirrhosis, 656
congestive heart failure, 543
Diuril, 543
Diverticulitis, 621
Diverticulosis, 620
Diverticulum (diverticula), colonic, 620
esophageal, 581, Figs. 210, 211
Meckel's, 621
Douches, 27, 727
Drainage, bronchial, 434
chest. *See* Chest, drainage
duodenal, 662
materials, 257, Fig. 70
pleural, 412
postural, 428, 429, 430, Figs. 141, 142
tidal, 370, 917, Fig. 379
urinary, 682, 974, Fig. 379
Wangensteen. *See* Gastrointestinal tract, nasosuction
Draping, surgical, 242
Dressing(s), adhesive, application of, Fig. 86
removal of, Fig. 84
Montgomery tape, Fig. 87
occlusive, Fig. 291
plastic film, 747
routines, following CVA, 940
Sayre's, Fig. 397
wet, 746
Drug(s). *See also specific names*
addiction, 121
adrenergic blocking, 845
amphetamine, 156
antileukemic, 323
antisecretory, 598
antithyroid, 820
ataractic, 135
diuretic, 543
hypnotic, 124
hypoglycemic, 831
reactions to, 807
sedative, 125
steroid, in cancer, Table 12
tranquilizing, 135
uricosuric, 1031
Ductus arteriosus, open, 552, Fig. 198
Duodenum, 568
Dysentery, amebic, 1129
bacillary, 1078
Dysesthesias, 904
Dyskinesias, 903

Dysmenorrhea, 724
Dyspepsia, functional, 594
Dysphagia, 578
Dyspnea, 58, 404
paroxysmal nocturnal, 540
Dysproteinemias, 79
Dystrophy(ies), muscular, 1044
pseudohypertrophic muscular, 1044
Dysuria, 681

Ear, anatomy and physiology, 875, Fig. 335
bandaging, Fig. 336
fungus infection, 878
irrigation, 878
Eardrum, 875
perforation, 878, 881
Earwax. *See* Cerumen
Ecchymoses, 476
Economo encephalitis, 1107
Eczema, 807, Fig. 316
Edema, angioneurotic, 809
cerebral, 920
dependent, 540
laryngeal, 386
pitting, 689
pulmonary, 545
renal, 689
Effusion, pericardial, 533
pleural, 426, Fig. 140
Elastic stockings, 437, 490, 525, Fig. 164
Electrocardiography, 95
Electroencephalography, 912
Electrolysis, 753
Electrolyte(s), blood, 80, 161
balance, 161
patterns, 162
repair solutions, 167, 169
urinary, 74
Electrophoresis, hemoglobin, 88
serum (plasma), 78
Elephantiasis, 505, Fig. 174
Elimination problems, in elderly, 338
postoperative, 279
Embolism, 485, 487, Fig. 160
air, 485
cerebral, 933
fat, 485
pulmonary, 436
postoperative, 301
Emergency situations, 1149
Emetine, 199
Empathy, 141
Emphysema, pulmonary, 432, Fig. 143
subcutaneous, 391, 443
Empyema, thoracic, 426
gallbladder, 663
paranasal sinus, 381
Encephalitis, epidemic, 1105
measles, 1091
postvaccinal, 1054
St. Louis, 1107
Encephalogram, 106
Endocarditis, 523, Fig. 182
bacterial, 527
rheumatic, 526, Fig. 187
subacute bacterial, 527
Endocervicitis, 731

Endocrine glands, 814
Endocrinopathies, 816
Endometriosis, 738
Enema, barium, 105
Enteric precautions, 616
Enteritis, 615
  regional, 618
Enterobiasis. *See* Pinworm
Enterocolostomy, 631
Enteroviruses, 1104
Enucleation, 864
Enzymes, blood, 81
  gastric, 567
  pancreatic, 568
Eosinophilia, 86, 1136
Ephebiatrics, 330
Encephalitis, epidemic, 1105
  epidemiology and prognosis
    of, Table 24
Epidermophytosis, 759
Epididymitis, 709
Epiglottis, 377
Epilepsy, 954
  autonomic, 956
  focal, 955
  genetic (idiopathic), 955
  Jacksonian, 955
  petit mal, 956
  psychomotor, 956
  symptomatic (acquired), 954
Epinephrine, 814, 844
Epiphyseal separation, 986
  humerus, Fig. 382
Epispadias, 699, 708
Epistaxis, 377
Epithelioma, 571, 770
Epulis, 825
Equinovarus. *See* Clubfoot
Ergotamine, 920
Erysipelas, 1068
Erythema, hyperaemicum, 753
  intertrigo, 753
  multiforme, 762
  nodosum, 762
  traumaticum, 753
  venenatum, 753
Erythremia, 471
Erythroblast, 460
Erythroblastosis, 87
  fetalis, 179, 466
Erythrocytes, 460, Fig. 22. *See
  also* Red cells
Erythromycin, 194
Esophagomyotomy, 579, Fig. 207
Esophagoscopy, 402, 581
Esophagus, 567
  carcinoma of, 581
  conditions of, 576
  dilatation of, 579, Fig. 206
  diverticulum of, 581, Figs. 210,
    211
  resection of, Fig. 212
  strictures of, 576
Esotropia, 872
Essential hypertension, 493
Ether, anesthetic, 222
  divinyl (Vinethene), 223
Ethyl chloride, 223
Ethylene, 224
Ethylene oxide sterilization, 45,
  Fig. 13
Eustachian tubes, 875
Evisceration, 308

Examination, gynecologic, 719
  neurologic, 907
  optic nerve, 908
  pelvic, 719
  rectal, 589
  spinal fluid, 99
  stool, 95
Exenteration, pelvic, 740
Exercises, bed, 282
  breathing, 417
  Buerger-Allen, 501
  convalescent, 282
  leg, 438
  postoperative, 558
  range-of-motion, Table 14
  skeletal, 418
  therapeutic, 353
Exophthalmos, 820, Fig. 320
Exotropia, 872
Expectorants, 120
Expirogram, 94
Extrasystoles. *See* Heart, beats,
  ectopic
Exstrophy, bladder, 699
Eye, anatomy of, Fig. 327
  appendages of, 851
  bandaging of, Fig. 331
  care, 857, 915
  components of, 851
  examination of, 853
  glasses, 854
  injuries, 860
  irrigations, Fig. 330
  medications, 855
    instillation of, Fig. 329
  optical characteristics of, Fig.
    328
  physiology of, 852
  surgery, 866
  treatments, 857

Facies, moon, 843
  types of, 52
Faints, 176
Fallopian tubes, conditions of, 738
Fallout, potential hazards of, 1165
Familial hemorrhagic telangiectasia, 476
Fat(s), dietary, 145
  digestion of, 565
  metabolism, 647
  necrosis, 668
  parenteral, 169
Favism, 466
Fecalith, appendiceal, Fig. 231
Feet, care of, in peripheral
  vascular disease, 500
  congenital deformities of, Fig.
    413
Felon, 757
Femur, fractures of, 1007
Fenestration operation, 887
Fever, 55
  dandy, 1110
  factitious, 56
  interpretation of, 56
  Malta. *See* Brucellosis
  paratyphoid, 1077
  pharyngoconjunctival, 394
  Q, 1116
  rat-bite, 1125
  relapsing, 1125

  rheumatic, 1023
  Rocky Mountain spotted, 1115
  scarlet, 1065
  symptomatology of, 56
  trench, 1117
  undulant. *See* Brucellosis
  yellow, 1110
Fibrillation, atrial, 510
Fibrinogen, 78
  deficiency, 479
  measurement of, 94
Fibrinolysis, 479
Fibromata, cutaneous, 769
Fibrositis, 1032
Fibula, fracture of, 1012
Filariasis, 1135
Fingers, clubbed, 427
Fissure, in ano, 641
  of nipple, 782
Fistula in ano, 640
Flatfeet, 1038
Fluid, balance, 159
  cerebrospinal, 893
  intake, regulation of, in
    congestive heart failure, 543
  intravenous, 169
    injection sites for, Fig. 32
    reactions to, 171
  parenteral, 169
Flukes, intestinal, 1139
Fluorine, dietary, 149
Fluoroscopy, 101
5-Fluorouracil (5-FU), 323
Fluothane. *See* Halothane
Flutter, mediastinal, 441, Fig. 148
Folic acid, 152
  antagonists of, 324
  deficiency, 152, 466
Follicle-stimulating hormone
  (FSH), 815
Food(s), acnegenic, 753
  components, 143
  guide, 143
  poisoning, 1079
Footdrop, prevention of, 360
Forearm, fractures of, 1006
  splints, Fig. 387
Foreign bodies, aspirated, 440,
  Fig. 23
  in ear, 878
  ocular, 860
Fracture(s), 986
  appliances, 1002, Fig. 395
  Colles, 1006
  compound, 1004
  dressings, 990
  emergency treatment of, 989
  femoral, Fig. 383
    in child, Fig. 403
  femoral neck, Fig. 398
  femoral shaft, Fig. 402
  greenstick, Fig. 381
  humerus, 1006
  mandibular, wiring of, Fig. 396
  mass management of, 1157
  nasal, 380
  pathologic, 987
  pelvis, 1007
  Pott's, 1012
  radius and ulna, Fig. 381
  reduction and immobilization
    of, 990, 1003
  rehabilitation following, 1015

Fracture(s) (*Continued*)
skull, 959, Fig. 367
tibia, 1012
tibia and fibula, Fig. 405
ununited, 1004
vertebral, 964, Fig. 371
Fragility, erythrocyte osmotic, 90
Frambesia. *See* Yaws
Frame, Bradford, 1035, 1036,
Fig. 412
Frequency, urinary, 681
Frostbite, 754, 1159
FSH (follicle-stimulating hormone), 815
Fungicides, 196
Furadantin. *See* Furan
derivatives
Furan derivatives, 197
Furuncles, 755

Gait(s), abnormal, 54
in Parkinson's disease, 54
scissors, 902
Gallbladder, diseases of, 662
x-ray study of, 103, 662
Gallstones, 662, Fig. 254
Gammagram, 108
Ganglia, basal, 902
Ganglion, 1033
Ganglionectomy, sympathetic, 498
Gangrene, 491, 497, 498
diabetic, 837, Fig. 168
Gantrisin. *See* Sulfonamides
Gas gangrene, 32
nursing in, 33
Gastrectomy, 601, 607
Gastric disorders, analysis, 96
cancer, 605, Fig. 226
x-ray appearance of, Fig. 227
Gastric juice, 567, 568
Gastric surgery, Fig. 224
complications of, 609
illustrations of, 601
nursing care in, 610, 611
resection, subtotal, Fig. 224
Gastrin, 568, 599
Gastritis, 595
Gastrointestinal tract, allergy, 809
anatomy and function, 565,
Figs. 200, 201
diagnosis of conditions in,
nursing role in, 588
intubation, 591
nasosuction, 558
x-ray examination of, 104
Gastrojejunostomy, 600, 601,
Fig. 224
Gastrostomy, 607, 608, Fig. 228
Gelatin boots, 499
Gelfilm, 252
Gelfoam, 252
Genitourinary tract, components
of, Fig. 262
Geriatrics, 331
physical state of patients, Fig.
100
surgery, 340
Ghon complex, 447
Glanders, 1085
Glaucoma, 868
Gliadin, 614
Globulins, plasma, 78

Glomerulonephritis, 686, 688
acute, 686
Glossectomy, 573
Glossitis, 152, 465
Gloves, sterilization of, 269
Gloving, 239, 241, Figs. 51-54
Glucagon, 815, 826
Glucose, blood, 80
metabolism, 646
parenteral, 169
Tm, 85
urine, 71
Gluten, 614
Glycosuria, 71
Goiter, 816
colloid, 822
endemic, 821
exophthalmic. *See* Hyperthyroidism
Gold, radioactive, 320
Gonadotropin, chorionic, 75
Gonioscopy, 854
Gonorrhea, 1080
Goundou, 1124
Gout, 1029
tophi in, Fig. 410
Gowning, 239, 240
Grafts, bypass, aortic, Fig. 190
vascular, Fig. 190
Ollier-Thiersch, 774
pinch, 774
split-thickness, 774
tube pedicle, 775, Fig. 306
flap, 776
vascular, Fig. 163
Wolfe-Krause, 774
Granuloma, inguinale, 1109
tuberculous, 447
Granulopenia, 469
Griseofulvin, 196, 759
Gumma(ta), 1121
central nervous system, 952,
1121
cutaneous, Fig. 446
Gynecology, examination, 719
problems, 725
Gynogram, 721

Hair, disorders of, 771
Hallux valgus, 1038, Fig. 413
Halothane, 223
Hammer toes, 1038, Fig. 413
Harelip, 570
Harlequin fetus, 768
Hashimoto's struma.
See Thyroiditis
Hay fever, 802
Headache(s), 916
in brain tumor, 918
histamine, 918
hypertensive, 919
lumbar puncture, 909
Health, environmental, 17
Hearing, aids to, 887, 888, Figs.
339, 340
physiologic basis of, 883
tests, 877
Heart, 507. *See also* Cardiac
anatomy of, Fig. 175
atrium, fibrillation, 510
flutter, 510, Fig. 176
septal defects, 553

beats, ectopic, 509
block, 511
diseases of the, 507
mortality from, 4, 5
prevention of, 561
failure, 540
congestive, 540
management of, 541
posture in, 52
function of, 507
mitral insufficiency, 531, Fig.
185
mitral stenosis, 530, Fig. 185
surgery, Fig. 197
Heartburn, 595
Heart-lung machines. *See* Pump
oxygenators
Heat, cabinet, Fig. 4
dry, application of, 25, 116,
Fig. 4
moist, application of, Figs. 5 A,
B, C
sterilization, 37
therapy, 25
Hedulin. *See* Phenindione
Hematemesis, 597
in cirrhosis, 658
in peptic ulcer, 597
Hematocrit readings, 89
Hematoma, 477, 984
postoperative, 307
subdural, 962, Fig. 370
Hematuria, 68, 72, 681
Hemianopsia, 895
Hemiplegia, 899, 934
nursing problems in, 934
Hemodialysis, 684, 1164, 1165
Hemoglobin, 460
electrophoresis, 88
fetal, 88
types, 88
Hemoglobinemia, 88
Hemoglobinometry, 88
Hemoglobinopathies, 468
Hemoglobinuria(s), 68, 467
paroxysmal cold, 468
paroxysmal nocturnal, 468
Hemolysins, 90
Hemolytic streptococcus
infections, 1065, 1068
complications of, 1066
Hemopericardium, 534
Hemophilia, 477
Hemoptysis, 405, 447
nursing in, 452
Hemorrhage, cerebral, 931
control of, 1155
emergency measures for, 1155
extradural, 962, Fig. 370
postoperative, 298
pulmonary, 405
subarachnoid, 918
Hemorrhoids, 641
Hemosiderinuria, 68
Hemostasis, surgical, 251
Hemothorax, 408
Hepatitis, epidemic, 653
posttransfusion, 181
toxic, 654
viral, 653
Herald patch, 764
Hernia, abdominal, 627
diaphragmatic, 577, 579

Hernia, hiatal, 577, 579, Fig. 209
  incisional, 627, Fig. 236
  inguinal, 627, Fig. 235
  umbilical, 627
  vaginal, Fig. 289
  ventral, 627, Fig. 236
Herniation, intervertebral disk, 969
Herniorrhaphy, 628
Herpes labialis. *See* Herpes simplex
Herpes simplex, 385, 924, Plate V
  ocular, 924
  penile, 709
  zoster, 929
Hexachloraphene, 47
Hiatus (hiatal) hernia, 577, 579, Fig. 209
Hiccup, 302
Hip, dislocation of, congenital, 1035, Fig. 412
  tuberculosis of, 1021
Histoplasmosis, 1131
Hives. *See* Urticaria
Home nursing, 1055, 1140
Homografts, 774
Hordeolum. *See* Stye
Hormones, 814. *See also specific endocrine glands*
  adrenocortical, 815
  adrenotropic (ACTH), 815
  gonadotropic, 75, 815
  growth, 815
  urinary, 75
    assays of, 75
Humerus, fracture of, 1006
Hycodan, 120
Hydralazine, 494
Hydrocele, 710
Hydrocephalus, internal, 1082
Hydrochloric acid, gastric, 567
Hydrocortisone, 839, 842
Hydronephrosis, 692, Fig. 266
Hydrophobia. *See* Rabies
Hydropneumothorax, Fig. 132
Hydrotherapy, in poliomyelitis, Fig. 437
Hydrothorax, 408
Hyoscine. *See* Scopolamine
Hyperacidity, 595
Hyperglobulinemia, 473
Hyperglycemia, 826
Hyperhidrosis, 751
Hyperinsulinism, 838
Hyperkalemia, 164
Hypernephroma, 697
Hyperopia, 852
Hyperparathyroidism, 825
  bone tumors in, 1034
Hyperpnea, 57
Hyperpyrexia, 296
Hypertension. *See* Hypertension, arterial
Hypertension, arterial, 62, 493
  adrenalectomy in, 845
  essential, 493
    malignant, 494
  in pheochromocytoma, 844
  treatment of, 494
    malignant, 494
  portal, 650
Hyperthermia, 921

Hyperthyroidism, 819, 820
Hypertrichosis, 772
Hypertrophy, prostatic, 711
Hyperventilation, 400
Hypocalcemia, 826
Hypochromia, 89
Hypofibrinogenemia, 479
Hypokalemia, 149, 167
Hyponatremia, 163, 167
Hypoparathyroidism, 825
Hypophysectomy, 846
Hypopituitarism, 846
Hypoprothrombinemia, 153, 478
  in biliary obstruction, 664
Hypopyon, 865
Hypospadias, 708
Hypotension, arterial, 63
  induced, 231
  postural, 63
Hypothalamus, 907
Hypothermia, 54, 921, 1159
  induced, 230
  in open heart surgery, 550
Hypothyroidism, 817
Hypoxemia, 186
Hypoxia, 186
Hysterectomy, 737
Hysteromyomectomy, 737
Hysterosalpingogram, 721

Ichthyosis, 768
Icterus index, 111
Ictotest, Plate I
Ileal conduit, 704
Ileostomy, 625, 701
  use of bags for, 624, Fig. 232
Ileum, 569
Ileus, paralytic, 633
Immunity, 19, 30
Impaction, fecal, 295
Impetigo, 756, Plate VI
Incision, McBurney, 620
Incontinence, 305, 681
  correction of, 370
Indigestion, 594
  functional, 594
Infarction, myocardial, 520, 524, 525
  in myxedema, 818
  pulmonary, 436
Infarcts, Fig. 162
Infection(s), adenovirus, 394
  ARD, 394
  bacterial, 1065
  bone and joint, 1017
  communicable, 1051
  defenses against, 18, 30
  in diabetic patients, 833, 837
  enteric, 615
    prevention of, 616
  fingernail, Fig. 296
  fungus, chemotherapy of, 199
    cutaneous, 759
  of ear, 878
  fingernail, Fig. 296
  gas bacillus, 32
  hand, 756
  meningococcal, 1081, 1082
  mycotic, 1131
  oral, 571
  protozoan, 1118
    chemotherapy of, 199

pulmonary, 419
rickettsial, 1113
Salmonella, 1077
spirochetal, 1118
Staphylococcus, 33
  chemotherapy of, 34
streptococcal, 392, 1023, 1065, 1068
transmission of, by donor blood, 181
tendon sheath, 758
urinary tract, 692
vaginal, 728, Table 19
Vincent's, 394, Plate V
virus, 1090
  Coxsackie, 1104
  ECHO, 1104
wound, 31
  postoperative, 307
Infertility, 739
Infestation(s), fluke, 1139
  liver, 1142
  lung, 1142
  hookworm, 1136
  parasitic, 1135
    cutaneous, 760
  pinworm, 1137
  roundworm, 1137
  tapeworm, 1137
Inflammation, 20
  complications of, 23
  nursing in, 24, 29
Influenza, 1097
  virus, Fig. 432
Injections, intramedullary, 171
  intrathecal, 1084
  intravenous, 169
Injuries, crush, 1158
  head, 959
  multiple, management of, Fig. 457
  skin, 753
  spinal, 964, Fig. 371
  steering wheel, 1168
  whiplash, 1168
Insomnia, 293
Instrument(s), setups, 263
  sterile, passing of, 257
  sterilization of, 261, 262
Intensive care unit, 271
Intertrigo, 753
Intestines, 569
  obstruction, 632, Fig. 239
    postoperative, 303
  perforation, 1075
  tuberculosis, 623
  tumors, 630
Intubation, of common bile duct, Fig. 256
  gastrointestinal, 591, Fig. 93
  nasogastric, 592
  oropharyngeal, 187, Fig. 34
  tracheal, Fig. 135
Intussusception, 632, Fig. 241
Invalid walker (Comper), Fig. 417
Iodine, blood, 816
  deficiency, 154, 819
  dietary, 149
  disinfection, 47
  protein-bound, in blood, 816
Iridectomy, 869
Iridencleisis, 869

Iritis, 865
Iron, absorption, 462
  deficiency, 154, 462
  dietary, 149
  requirements, 462
  therapy, 463
Irradiation, internal, 320
  therapy, 318
Irrigations, eye, 858
  vulvar, 727
Isolation nursing. *See* Disease, communicable, nursing, precautions
Isoniazid (INH), 197, 452, 454
Isuprel, 804
Itch, Baker's, 807
  Barber's. *See Tinea sycosis*

Jaundice, 649
  acquired hemolytic, 467
  hemolytic, 649
  hepatocellular, 649
  homologous serum, 181, 654
  obstructive, 650
Jejunum, 569, Fig. 202
Joint(s), Charcot, 953, 1121
  hemorrhage, 477
  infections, 1017
  tuberculosis, 1020
Juice, pancreatic, 568

Kala-azar, 1130
Kanamycin, 195
Keloids, 308, 769, Fig. 301
Keratitis, 865
  syphilitic, 1123
Keratoplasty, 867
Keratosis, 754
  labialis, 573
Ketonuria, 72
Ketosis, 831
17-Ketosteroids, urinary, 76
Ketostix, 72
Kidney(s), 676. *See also* Disorders, renal
  alkalotic, 168
  artificial, 684
  congenital anomalies of, 697
  polycystic, 697
  revascularizing of, 495, Fig. 169
  structure and function of, 259, 676
  trauma, 697
Kimograms, 102
Kirschner wire, Fig. 395
Knee, internal derangements of, 1009
Knee-chest position, Fig. 216
Knife blades, handling of, Figs. 61-63
Koplik spots, 1090
Kraurosis, 729
Kyphosis, 1020, 1039, Fig. 414

Laboratory tests, 65-113
  normal values for, 110-112
Lacerations, perineal, 730
Lactogenic hormone, 815
Laminectomy, 971
Laminograms, 101

LAP (Leucine Aminopeptidase), blood, 82
Laparatomy pack, 247
Laryngectomy, 387
Laryngitis, 386
Laryngofissure, 387
Larynx, 377
  cancer of, 386
  disorders of, 386
  spasm of, 386
  tuberculosis of, 386
LDH (Lactic Dehydrogenase), blood, 82
Leg, postphlebitic, 489
Leishmania, 1118
Leishmaniasis, 1130
Lenses, contact, 854
Leprosy, 1087, Fig. 431
Leptospira, 1118
Leptospirosis icterohemorrhagica. *See* Disease, Weil's
Leukemia, 471
  acute, 472
  chemotherapy of, 323
  lymphatic, 472
  monocytic, 472
  myelogenous, 472
Leukoagglutinins, 181
Leukocyte(s), 461
  counts, 85
  differential, 86
Leukocytosis, 85
Leukoderma, 750
Leukopenia, 86, 470
Leukoplakia, buccalis, 573, Fig. 204
  vaginalis, 729
Leukorrhea, 729
Lice, 1113
Lichen planus, 764, Plate VI
Ligation, femoral vein, 302
  venous, 499
Ligatures, 249
Limbs, artificial, 1014
Lipase, blood, 81
  pancreatic, 568
Lipids, blood, 80
Lips, conditions of, 570
Litholapaxy, 696, Fig. 270
Liver, abscesses of, 654
  amebic, 1129
  anatomy and physiology of, 647
  biopsy, 651
  cirrhosis of, 655
  disease, 650
  failure, tremor in, 53
  flap, 53
  fluke infestation, 1142
  function, 647
    tests of, 83
  lobule, Figs. 248, 249
Loa loa, 1135
Lobectomy, 409, 438, 439, 976, Fig. 146
Lockjaw. *See* Tetanus
Lordosis, 1039
Lues. *See* Syphilis
Lumbago, 1031
Lumbar puncture, 98, 907, Fig. 341
  headache, 909
  tray, 908

Lungs, anatomy of, 398, Figs. 123-126
  abscess, 427
  cancer, incidence of, 437
  fluke infestation, 1142
  segmental, resection, 409, 431, 453
  tumors, 439
Lupus erythematosus, 765, Plate VI
Lupus vulgaris, 758
Luteinizing hormone (LH), 815
Lye ingestion, 576, 1162
Lymphadenitis, 504
  tuberculous, 503, Fig. 173
Lymphangiography, 106
Lymphangitis, 503
Lymphatic system, 484
Lymphedema, 505
  postmastectomy, 790
Lymphocytic choriomeningitis, 1108
Lymphogranuloma inguinale, 1109
Lymphoma(s), 473
  chemotherapy of, 323

Macrocytosis, 87
Macroglobulins, 79
Macules, 745
Malabsorption states, 614
Malaria, 1126
  chemotherapy of, 198
  tertian, temperature chart in, Fig. 449
Malingering, 141
Mandible, fracture of, 1005
Mannitol, 183
Marrow. *See* Bone, marrow
Masks, oxygen, 189
Mass casualties, care of, 1156
Mastectomy, 786, 787
  radical, Fig. 310
Mastitis, acute, 782
  chronic cystic, 783
Mastoidectomy, 880
Mastoiditis, 879
Measles, 1090
  German, 1092
  rash, Plate X
  temperature chart in, Fig. 433
  vaccination, 1092
Mecholyl, 845
Medication, antipyretic, 117
  antitussive, 120, 422
  preanesthetic, 212
  soporific, 125
Megakaryocytes, 461
Melaninuria, 69
Melanocarcinomata, 771
Melanoderma, 750
Melanoma, 771, Plate VI
Melasma, 748
Melena, 96
Meningitis, influenzal, 1083
  meningococcal, 1081
  syphilitic, 952
Meningococcemia, 1082
Meningoencephalitis, mumps, 1095
Menopause, 719, 724

Menorrhagia, 724
Menstruation, 718
  disturbances of, 724
Mephyton. *See* Vitamin K₁
Meprobamate, 135
6-Mercaptopurine (6-MP), 323
Mercuhydrin, 543
Meringoplasty, 881
Mesantoin, 957
Metaplasia, myeloid, 462
Metastasis, 310
Methemoglobin, 88
Methicillin. *See* Staphcillin
Methotrexate, 323
Meticorten. *See* Prednisone
Metopon, 118
Metrorrhagia, 724
Microcytosis, 87
Migraine, 919
Milia, 752
Miliaria, 751
Mineral(s), dietary, 148
  deficiencies, 153
  trace, 150
Miotics, 856
Mitosis inhibitors, 324
Mole(s), 769
  warty, Plate VI
Mononucleosis, infectious, 1096
Morphine, 118
  idiosyncrasy, 293
  poisoning, 1164
Mortality statistics, 18
  in cardiovascular disease, 459
Mosquito(es), 1127
  control, 1128
  Culex and Anopheles types,
    Fig. 450
Motion sickness, 121
Mouth, care, 404
  in cardiovascular surgical
    cases, 555
  following gastric surgery, 610
  in oral cancer, 573
  in pulmonary infections, 404,
    423
  conditions of, 571
  infections of, 571
Myasthenia gravis, 1044
Mycoses, 1131
Mucolytic agents, 557
Mucous patches, 1121
Multiple myeloma. *See* Myeloma
Multiple sclerosis, 946
  signs and symptoms of, Fig. 363
  tremor in, 53
Mumps, 1095
Muscle(s), atrophy, 901, 997,
    1025, 1098, 1101
  in poliomyelitis, Fig. 436
  biopsy, 1136
  cramps, 982
  exercises, 983
    in neurologic cases, 938
    postmastectomy, 788, Fig.
      311
    in rheumatoid arthritis, 1025
    setting, 353
  relaxants, 225
  spasm, 982
Muscular rheumatism, 1031

Mutations, genetic, radiation
  induced, 318
Myasthenia gravis, Fig. 416 B
Mycosis fungoides, 475
Mycostatin. *See* Nystatin
Mydriasis, 119
Mydriatics, 856
Myelogram, 913, Figs. 353, 354
Myelography, 913
Myeloma, 473
Myleran, 471
Myocarditis, 532
Myoglobinuria, 69
Myomata, uterine. *See* Uterus,
  fibroid
Myomectomy, 737
Myopia, 852
Mysoline, 957
Myxedema, 817, Fig. 319

Nail(s), 757
  Smith-Petersen, Fig. 398
Nausea, control of, 121
Needles, suture, 267
Negri bodies, in rabies, Fig. 441
Nembutal, 125
Neomycin, 195
Neostibosan, 1130
Neostigmine, 1045
Nephrectomy, 697
Nephritis, 686. *See also*
    Glomerulonephritis
  nursing care in, 687, 690
Nephrocalcinosis, 825
Nephrolithiasis, 694
Nephroptosis, 692
Nephrosclerosis, 691, Fig. 265
Nephrosis, hemoglobinuric, 182
  toxic, 1164
Nephrotomy, 696
Nerve(s). *See specific nerves and
    nerve plexi*
  block, 228, 297, 925
Nervous system, 892
  autonomic, 904
  x-ray examination of, 106
Neuralgia, intercostal, 929
  trigeminal, 924
Neuritis, 929
  intercostal, 929
  optic, 924
Neurodermatitis, 764
Neurofibromata, 770, Fig. 302
Neurology, 893
Neuropathies, 923
Neurosurgical nursing, 913
Neurosyphilis, 951
Nevi, 769
Niacin. *See* Nicotinic acid
Nicotinic acid, 148
Nitrogen mustard (HN₂), 323
Nitrous oxide, 223
Nits, 760
Nodes, Heberden's, 1027
  lymph, 18
    diseases of, 503
  Osler's, 528
  sino-atrial, 508
Nor-epinephrine, 814, 844
Nose, 377
Novatropine, 119

NPN (non-protein nitrogen), 80
Nutritional problems, 151
  in elderly patients, 337
  in maxillofacial patients, 778
  in neurosurgical patients, 915
  in unconscious patients, 923
Nystatin, 196

Obesity, 155
  as operative risk, 208
Obstruction, nasal, 378
  pyloric, 597
  vena cava, 63
Occultest, 68, Plate I
Occupational therapy, 138, 350,
    795, Fig. 314
  in cancer, 327
Ointments, eye, 860
Oleandomycin, 194
Oligophrenia phenylpyruvica, 72
Oligopnea, 57
Oliguria, 182, 296, 684, 686
OMPA (octamethylpyrophos-
    phoramide), 1045
Oophorectomy, 739
Oophoritis, mumps, 1095
Operating room nursing, 234
  safety practices in, 260
Operating table, positioning
    patient on, 231, Figs. 47, 48
  preparation of, 247
Operation, fenestration, 887
  Hofmeister, Fig. 224
  principles of procedures in, 251
  Ramstedt, Fig. 225
Ophthalmia, gonorrheal, 864
Opiates, 119
Opisthotonos, 31, Fig. 7
Orchidopexy, 709
Orchitis, 709
  mumps, 1095
Orinase, 828
Orthopedic nursing, 1046
  postoperative care in, 1047
  psychologic problems in, 1046
  rehabilitation practices in, 1047
Orthopedic table, Fig. 391
Orthopnea, 52
Osteitis deformans. *See* Disease,
    Paget's
Osteoarthritis, 1027, Fig. 409
Osteoarthropathy, hypertrophic
    pulmonary, 427
Osteomalacia, 153, 1042
Osteomyelitis, 1017
  surgical treatment of, Fig. 406
Osteoporosis, 1043
  in hyperparathyroidism, 825
  senile, 334
Osteosclerosis, 462
Otitis media, 879
Otosclerosis, 885
Ovaries, 717
Overnutrition. *See* Obesity
Oxacillin. *See* Prostaphlin
Oxycel, 252
Oxygen, blood, 397
  absorption, 397
  administration, 187
  deficiency, 399
  masks, 189

Oxygen (*Continued*)
saturation, arterial, 95
tents, 189
11-Oxy-17-ketosteroids, 839
Oxyuriasis. *See* Pinworm
Ozena, 378

P³². *See* Radiophosphorus
Pacemaker, electronic, intra-
ventricular type, Fig. 177
permanent implanation of,
Figs. 178, 179
Pagitane, 949
PAH (para-aminohippurate)
clearance test, 84
Pain, abdominal, postoperative,
291
chest, 405
coronary, 521
intractable, neurosurgical
procedures for, 976, Fig. 380
medication, 116
nursing measures for, 125
relief, 115
Palate, cleft, 570
Palsy, Bell's, 926
Erb's, 928, 1036
facial, 926
eye care in, 915
radial nerve, 928
ulnar nerve, 928
Paludrine, 1128
Pancreas, digestive functions of,
668
disorders of, 668
endocrine functions of, 826
tumors of, 670
islet, 672
Pancreatitis, 668
mumps, 1095
Panhypopituitarism, 846
Pantopon, 118
Papules, 745
Para-aminosalicylic acid (PAS),
452
in tuberculosis, 454
Paracentesis, abdominal, 100
Paradione, 957
Paradoxical chest motion, 414,
440, Figs. 136, 147
Paraldehyde, 125
Paralysis, 898, 900
extraocular, 924, 1080
glossopharyngeal, 927
intestinal, 293
jake, 930
pharyngeal, 927, 1103
in poliomyelitis, 1100
sensory, 904
spastic, 901, 902
vagal, 927
vocal cord, 927
Paralysis agitans. *See* Disease,
Parkinson's
Paraplegia, 902, 971
Parasite, malarial, Fig. 448
vegetable, Fig. 451
Parasympathetic nervous system,
906
Parathormone, 815, 824
Parathyroid glands, 824

Paresis, general, 953
Paronychia, 756, Fig. 294
Parotitis, 572
epidemic. *See* Mumps
Parsidol, 949
PAS (para-aminosalicylic acid),
197, 198, 452
Pasteur treatment, 1109
Patches, Peyer's, 1073, Fig. 426
Patent ductus arteriosus, surgery
in, 552
Pediculosis, 760
Pellagra, 152
Pelvis, fractures of, 1007
Pemphigus, 763
Penicillins, 192
Penicillin sensitivity, 193
Penis, 708
disorders of, 708
ulceration, 709
Pentothal, 225
Pepsin, 567
Periarteritis nodosa, 766
Pericarditis, 533
constrictive, 534
Perinephritis, 694
Periostitis, 1121
Peristalsis, 569, Fig. 203
Peritonitis, 622
tuberculous, 623
Perphenazine, 135
Pertussis, 1071
Petechiae, 92, 476
Petechiometer, 92
Petit mal, 954, 956
Pharyngitis, 382
acute, 392
streptococcal, 392
Pharynx, 377
anatomy of, Fig. 117
Phenacetin, 117
Phenindione, 487
Phenistix, for phenylketonuria,
Plate I
Phenobarbital, 125
Phenostix, 72
Phentolamine, 493
Phenylalanine, 72
Phenylbutazone, 117
Phenylketonuria, 72
Phenylpyruvic acid excretion, 72
Pheochromocytoma, 493, 844
urine tests in, 76
Phimosis, 709
pHisoderm, 238
pHisohex, 239
Phlebitis, 485
postoperative, 302
Phlebothrombosis, postoperative,
302
Phlebotomy, blood donor, 175,
Fig. 33
therapeutic, 546
Phosphatases, blood, 82
Phosphorus, deficiency, 154
dietary, 148
serum, 81
Photofluorograms, 101
Physiatry, 350
Physiotherapy, postoperative,
Fig. 313
Picrotoxin, 1164

Pigmenturia, 67
Piles. *See* Hemorrhoids
Pillrolling, 53
Pin, medullary, Fig. 402
Steinmann, Fig. 395
Piparazine, 1137
Pitressin, 814
Pituitary gland, 845, 907
Pituitrin, 846
Pityriasis rosea, 764
Plague, 1087
bubonic, 1087
Plasma, expanders of, 1156
fractions, therapeutic use of,
1156
freshly frozen, 179
volume, 90
Plasmin, 479
Plasmodia, 1118, 1125
Platelet(s), 461
counts of, 86
deficiency, 476
Platform stairs, Fig. 110
Pleura, 399
Pleurisy, 425
postoperative, 292, 301
tuberculous, 449
Pleurodynia, epidemic, 1105
Pneumoencephalogram, 911, Fig.
351 A
Pneumonectomy, 409, 438, 439,
453, Fig. 146
Pneumonia, 420
bacterial, 421
complications, 424
Friedlander's, 194
lobar, 421, Figs. 138, 139
postoperative, 301
primary atypical, 424
tuberculous, 448
viral. *See* Pneumonia, primary
atypical
Pneumoperitoneum, pelvic, 721
Pneumothorax, 408, Fig. 148
tension, 442, Fig. 149
Poikilocytosis, 87
Poisoning, 1162
accidental, 1162
barbiturate, 1163
beryllium, 841
botulinus, 1079
carbon dioxide, 190
carbon monoxide, 1165
carbon tetrachloride, 654
emergency management of,
1162
lead, 470
mercury, 1164
morphine, 1164
Poliomyelitis, 1099
bulbar, 1103
Pollinosis. *See* Hay fever
Polya anastomosis, Fig. 224
Polyarthritis, rheumatic, 1023
Polycythemia, 471
Polydipsia, 827, 841, 846
Polyethylene gloves, 747
Polymyxin B, 195
Polyneuritis, 930
alcoholic, 931
toxic, 930
Polyphagia, 827

Polypnea, 57
Polyps, intestinal, 630
  nasal, 379
Polyuria, 827, 841, 846
Polyvinylpyrrolidone (PVP),
  1156
Pompholyx, 751
Pontocaine (Tetracaine), 229
Porphyria, 69
Porphyrinuria, 69
Position, Fowler's, 281, Fig. 83
  knee-chest, Fig. 216
  semi-Fowler, 281
  sense, 904
  Sims's, 280, Fig. 216
  Trendelenburg, 280
Positioning. *See* Body, positioning
Postoperative care, 271
  complications in, 273, 291, 295
    in elderly patients, 341
    pulmonary, 298
  of elderly patients, 341
  after eye surgery, Fig. 333
Postoperative status, 277
Postoperative symptoms, 276
Posture, types of, 42
Potassium, dietary, 149
  infusions, 172
  replacement, 168
  serum, 81
  solutions, 168
  urinary, 75
Prednisolone, 842
Pregnancy, ectopic, 739
  German measles in, 1093
  tests, 76
Premature beats. *See* Heart, beats,
  ectopic
Preoperative care, 204
  psychologic factors in, 205
Pressure, diastolic, 61
  systolic, 61
  venous, 63
Primaquine, 199
  sensitivity, 199
Procaine (Novocaine), 229
Procaine amide, 514
Prochlorperazine, 135
Procidentia, 737
  uteri, Fig. 289
Proctoscopy, 589
Prolapse, uterine, 737
Promazine, 121
Promin, 1089
Promizole. *See* Sulfones
Prophylaxis, immune, 1051
Propylthiouracil, 820
Prostaphlin, 193
Prostate, 708
  carcinoma of, 711
  disorders of, 711
Prostatectomy, 713
  alternative methods of, 713
  perineal, Fig. 275
  transurethral, Fig. 276
Prostatitis, 705, 1081
Prostheses, 369, 1014
  arm, Fig. 113
  breast, 790, Fig. 312
  vascular bypass, Fig. 163
Protamine, 487
Proteins, blood, 78

  dietary, 146
  digestion, 566
  M, 79
  metabolism, 647
Protein-bound iodine (PBI), 816
Proteinuria, 71
  Bence-Jones, 71
Prothrombin measurements, 92
Protozoa, Fig. 444
Pruritus, 744
  genital, 744
Pseudoarthrosis, 1004
Psittacosis, 1111
Psoriasis, 761, 762, Fig. 297
Psychic energizers, 136
Psychology, adolescent, 330
  aspects of, in disability, 351
    in neurologic disorders, 915
  disturbances of, in steroid
    recipients, 843
  factors of, in nursing, 128
  support of, postoperative, 279
Psychopharmacology, 134
Psychotherapy, 138
  in asthma, 805
  in chronic illnesses, 345
  in geriatrics, 332, 335
Pterygium, 864
Ptosis, 1046
  in myasthenia, Fig. 416 B
Ptyalin, 566
Pulmonary atelectasis, 406
  postoperative, 407
Pulse, arteries, 59
  apical-radial, 547
  bigeminal, 511, 542
  Corrigan, 60, 529, Fig. 184
  deficit, 60
  dicrotic, 60
  examination of, 59
  paradoxical, 534
  pressure, 61
Puncture, cisternal, 99, 907, 908,
  Fig. 341
Puncture, spinal. *See* Lumbar
  puncture
  ventricular, 943, Fig. 341
Pump oxygenator(s), 549, 550,
  Fig. 196
Pupils, Argyll Robertson, 953
Purine antagonists, 324
Purinethol. *See* 6-Mercapto-
  purine
Purpura(s), 476
  anaphylactoid, 476
  thrombocytopenic, 476
  toxic, 476
  vascular, 476
Pus, 755
Pustule(s), 745
  malignant, 1085
PVP (polyvinylpyrrolidone), 1156
Pyelitis, 692
Pyelogram, intravenous (IVP),
  Fig. 267
Pyelography, 105, 678, 691
Pyelonephritis, 692
Pyelotomy, 696
Pyemia, 24
Pylorospasm, 595
Pyridium, 699

Pyridoxine, 148
  in radiation recipients, 320
Pyuria, 73

Quadriplegia, 902
Quinidine, 510, 514
Quinine, 982
Quinsy. *See* Abscess, peritonsillar

Rabies, 1108
Rachitic rosary, 1042
Radiation, detection, 317
  electromagnetic, types of, 317
  hazards, 318
  nursing, 321
  precautions, 319
  protection, 321
  sickness, 1165
  therapy, nursing care in, 319
    in uterine cancer, 733
Radiocobalt, 320
Radioiodine, 322
Radium, therapy of, in cervical
    cancer, 733
  in uterine cancer, Fig. 287
  tubes, sterilization of, 269
Range-of-motion exercises, 358,
  Table 14
  in arthritis, 1025
Rash(es), 745
  chickenpox, 1093
  of Coxsackie infections, 1104
  dengue, 1110
  diaper, 745
  drug, 807
  German measles, 1092
  measles, 1090
  meningococcal, 1083
  psittacosis, 1111
  Rocky Mountain spotted fever,
    1115
  scarlet fever, 1065
  smallpox, 1094
  syphilitic, 1121
  trench fever, 1117
  typhus fever, 1114
  yellow fever, 1111
Rauwolfia, 949
Reactions, anxiety, 137
  drug, 807
  hemolytic transfusion, 182
  hypoglycemic, 830
  intravenous, 171
  post-vaccinal, 1053
  psychoneurotic, 138
  psychotic, 140
  pyrogenic, 171, 181
  transfusion, 181, 182
Records, clinical, 288
Recovery room, 271, Fig. 76
Rectocele, 286, 730
Red cell(s), 85, 460
  agglutination, 177, 468
  counts, 85
  indices, 89
  mass, 108
  osmotic fragility, 90
  survival, 109
Refraction, 853
Regitine, 493

Rehabilitation, 349
  following cerebral vascular
    accident, 935
  following myocardial
    infarction, 523
  in neurosurgical patients, 944
  philosophy of, 349
  post-fracture, 1015
  teams, 350
Rehabilitation nursing, 350
  principles of, 351
Renal failure, 683, 685
  function, 676
  rickets, 1043
  studies, 678
  surgery, 697
Renin, 493
Reproductive system, female, 717,
  Fig. 279
  male, 706, Fig. 252
Resection, abdominoperineal, 631
  submucous, 379
  wedge lung, 409
Reserpine, 135
Respiration, 397
  artificial, 1152
  asthmatic, 59
  Cheyne-Stokes, 57, 932
  external, Fig. 127
  internal, Fig. 122
  Kussmaul, 59
  movements in, 58
  obstruction of, 274, 390
    handling in, Fig. 78
    obstructive, Fig. 77
    postoperative, Fig. 77
  paralysis of, treatment of, Fig.
    438
  physiology of, 397
  rates, 57
  stertorous, 59
  types of, 58
  upper tract of, 376
Respirator, chest, 1102
Rest, therapeutic, 123
Restraints, limb, application of,
  307
  use of, in agitated patients, 8
  in epileptic seizures, 957
  in neurologic cases, 923
Resuscitation technics, 1152
Retention, urinary, 304, 680
Reticulocytes, 87, 460
Reticulocytosis, 87
Reticuloendothelial system, 18
Retina, 851
  detachment, 861
Rhabdomyolysis, 69
Rheumatism. See Arthritis
Rheumatoid arthritis, 1024, Fig.
  408
Rheumatoid spondylitis, 1027
Rhinitis, 377
Rhinophyma, 753, Fig. 293
Rhizotomy, 976
Ribs, cervical, 928
  fractures, 1006
Riboflavine, 148
Rice bodies, 1086
Rickets, 153
  deformities in, 1041
Rickettsia, Figs. 442, 443

Rickettsial diseases, 1113
Rickettsialpox, 1116
Rigidity, nuchal, 1082, Fig. 429
Ring's ocular mask, Fig. 334
Ringworm, 759
Rocky Mountain spotted fever,
  1115
Roentgenology, diagnostic, 100
Roseola infantum, 1091
Rouleaux, 79, 87, Fig. 22
Rubber goods, surgical, care of,
  268
Rubella, 1092
Rubeola. See Measles
Runaround. See Paronychia
Rupture, appendiceal, 303
  myocardial, 522

Sacral plexus, 929
St. Vitus' dance. See Chorea
Salicylates, 116
Saliva, 566
Salivary glands, abnormalities of,
  572
Salmonella carriers, 1075, 1078
Salpingectomy, 739
Salpingitis, 738
Salpingogram, 740
Salpingo-oophorectomy, 739
Salt depletion, 165, Fig. 28
Sarcoid. See Sarcoidosis
Sarcoidosis, 767
Sarcoma, osteogenic, 1033
Saucerization, Fig. 406
Scabies, 761
Scanogram, 108
Scarlet fever, 1065
  strawberry tongue and
    exanthema of, Plate X
  prophylaxis, 1067
Schistosomiasis, 1139
Sciatica, 929
Scleroderma, 766, Fig. 299
Sclerosis, multiple, 946
Scoliosis, 1040, Fig. 415
Scopolamine, 949
Scorpion bites, 1163
Scotoma, 919
Scrofula, 503
Scrofuloderma, 759
Scrubbing, preoperative, 236
Scrub nurse, responsibilities of,
  251, 255
Scultetus binder, 287, Fig. 89
Scurvy, 152
Seborrhea, 752
Sebum, 753
Secretin, 668
Sedimentation rate, erythrocyte,
  79
Seizure(s), autonomic, 956
  epileptic, 954
  febrile, 56
  focal, 955
  grand mal, 955
  Jacksonian, 955
  psychomotor, 956
  states, 954
  tetanic, 31
Senility, 334

Sense, position, 904
  vibratory, 904
Sensory disturbances, 903
Septal defects, 553
Septicemia, 23
Sequestrectomy, Fig. 406
Shigellosis. See Dysentery,
  bacillary
Shock, 296
  anaphylactic, 805
  cardiogenic, 520
  hematogenic, 296, 297, 1155
  hypoglycemic, 830
  management of, Fig. 456
  nursing care in, 297
  oligemic, 1155
    symptoms of, Fig. 455
  in pneumonia, 424
  postoperative, 296
  toxic, 296
  traumatic, 1155, 1156
    emergency treatment of, 1156
Shunt, splenorenal, 659
Sialolithiasis. See Calculus,
  salivary
Siderocytes, 87
Sigmoidoscopy, 589
Sign, Homans', 488
  Romberg's, 953
Singultus. See Hiccup
Sinuses, paranasal, 376, Fig. 115
Sinusitis, 379, 381
Skeleton, x-ray examination of,
  103
Skin, applications, Fig. 290
  bacterial infections of, 755
  care, 745
    in diabetics, 835
  disorders of, congenital, 768
    psychologic aspects of, 744
  eruptions, syphilitic, 1120
  flap, 773
  grafts, 773, 774, Fig. 304
  injuries, 753
  pigment, 747
  preoperative preparation of,
    211, Fig. 39
  structure of, 743
  tests, allergic, 811
  traction, 998, Fig. 394
  tuberculosis, 758
  ulcerations of, 768
Sleep, 124
Sleeping sickness, African, 1130.
  See also Encephalitis, epidemic
Smallpox, 1094
  temperature chart in, Fig. 434
  vaccination, 1054
Smell, 908, 923
Snake bites, 1163
Snake venum antitoxin, 1055
Sodium, dietary, 149
  replacement, 168
  restriction, in cirrhosis, 658
  serum, 81
  urinary, 74
Solutions, hypertonic, 172
  nutrient, 169
Somatotropic (growth) hormone,
  815
Sparine. See Promazine
Spasmophilia, 386

Speech, 896
 esophageal, 388
 scanning, 947
Spermatozoa, 708
Spherocytes, 87
Spherocytosis, 90
 hereditary, 467
Sphygmomanometry, 62
Spinal cord, 893, 898, Figs. 346, 349
 injury, 969
 in meningococcal meningitis, Fig. 428
 tumors, 971
Spinal puncture. *See* Lumbar puncture
Spine, curvature of, 1039
 poker, 1027
 tuberculosis of, 1020
Spiramycin, 194
Spironolactone. *See* Aldactone
Spleen, 19
 rupture, in infectious mononucleosis, 1096
Splenectomy, 479
Splint, nasal, Fig. 116
 pillow, Fig. 384
 plaster, 994, Fig. 404
 T-, Fig. 397
 Thomas, Fig. 385
  with Pearson attachment, Fig. 386
Spondylitis, rheumatoid, 1027
Sponge counting, 257, Fig. 69
Sporotrichosis, 1133
Sprains, 984
Sprue, 614
Sputum, collection, 423
 examination, 423
 studies, 403
Squint. *See* Strabismus
Stapedectomy, 885
Stapes mobilization, 886
Staphcillin, 193
Staphylococcosus, 33
Starvation, electrolyte pattern in, 164
Status asthmaticus, 804
Status epilepticus, 956
Steam inhalations, Fig. 92
Steatorrhea, 96, 614
 in pancreatitis, 670
Stenosis, pulmonary, surgery in, 552
 hypertrophic, Fig. 225
 congenital, 602
Sterile equipment, handling of, 244, Figs. 55-57
Sterile instruments, passing of, Fig. 68
Sterile sutures, passing of, Fig. 68
Sterile transfer technic, Fig. 55
Sterility. *See* Infertility
 maintenance of, 237
 tests for, 44
Sterilization, 268
 applications of, 237
 ethylene oxide, 45, Fig. 13
 gaseous, 45
 heat, 37
 indicators of, 44
 instrument, 43, 261

principles of, 37
 radiation, 45
 steam, 39
 steam pressure, 38, Figs. 9, 10
 ultraviolet light, 45
Stilbamidine, 199
Stockings, elastic, 437, 489, 490, 525
Stokes-Adams attack (syndrome), 511
Stomach, 567
Stomatitis, epidemic, 1112
 Vincent's, 394
Stones. *See* Bladder, stones, and Gallstones
Stool examination, 95
Stool precautions, 616
Strabismus, 870
Strain, lumbosacral, 1031
 sacroiliac, 1031
Streptomycin, 194
 in tuberculosis, 454
Stricture, esophageal, 576
 rectal, 630, 1109
 urethral, 705
Stridor, 59
Stroke. *See* Apoplexy
Struma, Hashimoto's. *See* Thyroiditis
 Riedel's. *See* Thyroiditis
Stryker cast cutter, Fig. 390
Stye, 864
Suction, gastric, 593
 drainage (Gerlinger), Fig. 222
Suctioning, oropharyngeal, 934
Sudamina, 751
Sugar, blood, 80
 urine, 71
Sulfhemoglobin, 88
Sulfonamide compounds, 196
Sulfones, 198
Sulphetrone, 1089
Sunstroke, 162
Surgery, cardiovascular, 548
 chest, 408
 cosmetic, 772
 in diabetics, 837
 maxillofacial, nursing care in, 777
  psychological support of patients in, 778
 open-heart, 549
 perineal, postoperative care in, 730
 plastic, 772
 nasal, 380
 vascular, 488, Fig. 197
Surgical procedures, by-pass, 659
 dressings in, 283, Fig. 88
 technic used in, 283
 gut used in, handling of, Fig. 71
 types of, Fig. 72
 instruments used in as related to hemostasis, 252
 handling of specimens from, 259
Suture(s), 250
 absorbable, 263
 handling of, Figs. 64-66
 materials, 263
 needles, 267
 types of, Figs. 73, 74

nonabsorbable, 265
 passing of, Fig. 68
 types of, Fig. 67
Swallowing, difficulties in, 927, 1103
Sweating, disturbances of, 750
Sympathetic nervous system, 906
Sympathectomy, 493
Symptoms, evaluation of, 50
 postoperative, 276
Syndrome(s), autonomic, 904
 Banti's, 656
 Cushing's, 840, 847
 dumping, 609
 Felty's, 1024
 Leriche's, 539
 Meniere's, 888, 926
 Plummer-Vinson, 463
 Stokes-Adams, 511
 sympathetic, 907
 wet lung, 442
Synovitis, 1032
Syntropan, 119
Syphilis, 1118
 bone and joint, 1121
 cardiovascular, 534
 central nervous system, 951
 congenital, 1121
 early, maculopapular rash in, Plate XI
 late, 1121
 meningovascular, 951
 oral and dermal complications of, Plate V
 primary, 709
 vascular, 1121
Syphilitic meningitis, 952

Tabes dorsalis, 952, Fig. 365
Tabetic crises, 953
Tachycardia, 60
 paroxysmal atrial, 509
Tantalum, radioactive, 320
Tapeworm, beef, 1137
 fish, 1138
 infestation, 1137
Teaching, patient, 11
Team(s), intravenous, 173
 nursing, 8
Teeth, Hutchinson's, 1122
Telangiectasia, familial hemorrhagic, 476
 postirradiation, 754
 spider, 657
TEM (triethylene melamine), 323
Temperature, body, 54
 regulation of, 54
Tendosynovitis, 1033
 tuberculous, 1022
Tenesmus, postoperative, 295
Tenosynovitis, 758
Tension pneumothorax, 442, Fig. 149
Tents, oxygen, 189
Terramycin. *See* Tetracyclines
Test(s), 65-113
 acid hemolysis, 90
 allergy, skin, 802, 805
 antiglobulin, 90
 basal metabolism, 816
 bentonite flocculation, 79

Test(s) (*Continued*)
  benzidine, 68, 96
  for bilirubinuria, 68, Plate I
  bromsulphthalein (BSP), 83
  butter fat tolerance, 83
  caloric, 888
  capillary fragility, 92
  cardiac function, 94
  cephalin flocculation, 79
  choluria, 68
  clot retraction, 92
  cold agglutinin, 90
  cold hemolysis, 90
  colloidal gold, 79, 99, 894
  congo red, 85
  Coombs, 90
  cranial nerve, 907
  cytologic, for cancer, 721
  decholin circulation, 94
  diagnostic, nursing role in, 65
  Dick, 1067
  facial nerve, 908
  fibrinogen, 78
  Frei, 1109
  galactose clearance, 83
  gastrointestinal absorption, 83
  glossopharyngeal nerve, 908
  glucose tolerance, 82
  glycosuria, 71
  Graham-Cole, 103, 662
  guaiac, 96
  hematologic, 85
  hemolytic, 90
  hemosiderin, 68
  heterophile antibody
    agglutination, 1096
  hippuric acid conversion, 83
  hypoglossal nerve, 908
  immunity, diphtheria, 1070
    scarlet fever, 1067
    smallpox, 1054
  intestinal absorption, 83
  inulin clearance, 84
  ketonuria, 72
  17-ketosteroid, 76
  Kveim, 767
  latex fixation, 79
  L.E., 765
  liver function, 83
  melanin, 69
  for melena, 96
  neostigmine response, 1045
  oculomotor nerve, 908
  ophthalmic nerve, 908
  Oppenheim's, 932
  Papanicolaou, 721
  para-aminohippurate (PAH)
    clearance, 84
  phenolsulfonphthalein (PSP),
    76
  pregnancy, 76
  protein flocculation, 79
  proteinuria, 71
  prothrombin consumption, 93
  PSP (phenolsulphonphthalein),
    76
  pulmonary function, 94, 401
  Queckenstedt, 909
  radiochromium, 108
  radioiodine, 107, Fig. 24
  radioisotope, 106
  red cell osmotic fragility, 90
  red cell sedimentation rate, 79
  renal function, 84, 94, 109
  Rubin, 740
  Rumpel-Leeds, 92
  Schick, 1070
  sensitivity, 802
  serodiagnostic, for brucellosis,
    1079
    for infectious mononucleosis,
      1096
    for rickettsial infections, 1113
    for rickettsialpox, 1117
    for syphilis, 1122
    for tularemia, 1084
    for typhoid fever, 1074
    for Weil's disease, 1124
    for yaws, 1124
  Sia water, 79
  sickle cell, 89
  sickling, 89
  skin, allergic, 811
    diagnostic, in histoplasmosis,
      1132
    in lymphogranuloma
      inguinale, 1109
    trichinae, 1136
    tuberculin, 450
  spinal accessory nerve, 908
  spinal fluid, 199, 894
  spleen sequestration, 108
  for sterility, 44
  thromboplastin generation, 93
  thymol turbidity, 79
  thyroid function, 816
  Trendelenburg, Fig. 171
  trigeminal nerve, 908
  trochlear nerve, 908
  tuberculin, 450, Fig. 152
  urea clearance, 84
  urinary calcium, 75
  urinary chlorides, 74
  urine, 66
    acidity, 69
    calcium, 75
    concentration, 70
    foam, 68
    2-glass, 66
    urobilinogen, 75
  vagus nerve, 908
  vitamin A tolerance, 83
  vitamin B$_{12}$ absorption, 109
  Widal, 1074
  xylose (d-xylose) tolerance, 83
Testes, 707
  abnormalities of, 709
  undescended, 709
Testosterone, 785
Tetanus, 31
  antitoxin, 32
  nursing in, 32
  toxoid, 32
Tetany, hypocalcemic, 824, 826
Tetracyclines, 193. *See also*
  specific tetracyclines, like
  Aureomycin, Achromycin, *etc.*
Tetralogy of Fallot, 552
Thalamus, 904
Thalassemia, 468
Therapy, antidistension, 423
  antiemetic, 293
  antihypertensive, 494
  Dicumarol, 486
  fracture, use of ice-tong calipers
    in, Fig. 399
gamma globulin, 1055
  heparin, 487
  immune, 1054
  insulin, 828
    complications of, 830
  iron, 463
  oxygen, 186
    complications of, 190
    precautions in, 186
    in pulmonary edema, 547
  parenteral fluid, 169
    nursing supervision of, 172
  radiation, nursing care in, 319
    in uterine cancer, 733, Fig.
      287
  radioiodine (I^{131}), 821
  radioisotope, 320
  steroid, 841
    in cancer, 324
    complications of, 843
    nursing responsibilities in,
      842
  transfusion, 179
  vitamin B$_{12}$
  x-ray, 317
Thiamine, 148
  deficiency, 930
Thirst, postoperative, 294
Thoracentesis, 100, 403, Fig. 130
Thoracoplasty, 453
Thoracotomy incisions, 409
  muscles affected by, Fig. 137
  open, 427
Thorazine, 949
Throat culture, 382, 1069
Thrombi, Figs. 159, 161
Thromboangiitis obliterans, 496
Thrombocytes. *See* Platelets
Thromboembolism, 485
Thrombophlebitis, 485, 486
Thrombosis, 485
  carotid, 933
  carotid artery, 933
  cerebral, 932
  coronary, 520
  mesenteric, 627
  venous, 437
  venous sinus, 925, 951
Thrush, 394
Thyroid cancer, 822
Thyroid disease, facies in, 52
Thyroidectomy, 821, 822
  nursing care in, 823
Thyroid function tests, 816
Thyroid gland, 816
Thyroiditis, 821
Thyroid tumors, 821
Thyrotomy. *See* Laryngofissure
Thyrotropic hormone, 815
Thyroxin, 815, 816
Tibia, fractures of, 1012
Tic(s), 53
Tic douloureux. *See* Neuralgia,
  trigeminal
Ticks, 1115
Tinea capitis, 759
Tinea circinata, 759, Fig. 295
Tinea sycosis, 760
Tolbutamide. *See* Orinase
Tolserol, 135
Tongue, cancer of, 573
  paralysis of, 927
  sore, 464

Tonsil(s), 377
Tonsillectomy, 384, 385
  body position following, Fig. 119
Tonsillitis, 384, Fig. 117
Tophi, 1030
Torticollis, 53
  congenital, 1037
Tourniquet, application, 547
  test, 92
  therapy, rotation routine in, Fig. 195
Toxemia, 23
Toxicity, Dicumarol, 478
Toxoid, tetanus, 32
Tracheobronchitis, 419
Tracheostomy, 389
Tracheotomy, 389
  postoperative complications of, 389
  set, Fig. 121
  tubes, Figs. 120, 121
Trachoma, 864, Fig. 332
Traction, 998
  cervical, 965
  leg, Fig. 394
    Russell's, 1000
  running, 1000
  Russell, 1009, Figs. 400, 401
  skeletal, 1000
  skin, 998, Fig. 394
  vertical (Bryant), Fig. 403
Tractotomy, 925
Transaminase, blood, 82
Transfusion complications, 180
Transfusion reactions, allergic, 181
  hemolytic, 182
  pyrogenic, 181
  therapy, 179
Transplants, fascia, 776
Trasentine, 119
Trauma, central nervous system, 959
  vertebral, 962, Fig. 371
Tremor(s), 53
  cerebellar, 903
  in hyperthyroidism, 820
  intention, 53
  in multiple sclerosis, 53, 947
  Parkinsonian, 53, 949
  pillrolling, 53
Trench fever, 1117
Trench foot, 1159
Trench mouth. *See* Infection, Vincent's
Trephining, corneoscleral, 869
Treponema pallidum, Figs. 444, 445
Triamcinolone, 842
Trichinosis, 1135
Trichlorethylene, 223
Trichomonas vaginalis, 729
Tridione, 957
Trigeminal neuralgia, 924
Triiodothyronine, 815, 816
Trilafon, 135
Trismus, 31
Trochanter roll, 359, Fig. 106
Trypanosomiasis, 1130
Trypsin, 568
Tsetse fly, 1130

Tube, Blakemore, 582
  Cantor, Fig. 220
  feedings, 608
  Magill, Fig. 44
  Miller-Abbott, Figs. 93, 221
  Sengstaken-Blakemore, 584, Fig. 213
Tuberculosis, 446
  bladder, 700
  bone and joint, 1020
  chemotherapy, 452
  cutaneous, 758
  disseminated, 447
  fever in, Fig. 151
  genitourinary, 694
  hip joint, 1021
  intestinal, 623
  laryngeal, 386
  lymph node, 503, Fig. 173
  miliary, 447
  mortality, 456, Fig. 153
  nursing, 452
  prevention, 456
  pulmonary, 447
    convalescent care in, 455
    management of, 450
    pathology of, Fig. 150
    surgery in, 453
  renal, 694
  skin, 758
  spine, 1020
Tuberculous lesions, oral mucosa and gums, Plate V
Tularemia, 1084
Tumor, acoustic nerve, 942
  adrenal, 840
  bladder, 700
  bone, 1033
  brain, 941, 1033
  breast, 784
  cerebellar, 941
  cerebellopontine angle, 942
  chest, 438
  classification of, Table 7
  gastric, 605
  giant-cell, 1033
  hepatic, 659
  intestinal, 630
  lung, 439
  mediastinal, 439
  nerve, 770
  pancreatic, 670
  pancreatic islet, 672, 838
  parotid, 573
  pituitary, 847, 941
  renal, 697
    radioisotopic localization of, 113
  salivary gland, 573
  skin, 769
  spinal cord, 971
  testicular, 710
  thyroid, 821
  ulcerogenic, 672
Tumor cells, classification of, 310
Turbinates, 377
Tympanites, 623
Tympanoplasty, 883
Typhoid bacilli, Fig. 425
Typhoid fever, 1072
  fever in, Fig. 427
Typhoid vaccination, 1077
Typhus fever, 1113

Ulcers, corneal, 865
  decubitis, 360, Fig. 107, Plate II
  duodenal, 596
  gastric, 596, Fig. 223
    benign, 596
    malignant, 600, 605
    treatment, freezing, 602
  peptic, 596
    diet, 598
    management, 597
    nursing care in, 597
    perforation of, 597
    in steroid recipients, 843
    surgery in, 599
  rodent, 770, Fig. 303
  stasis, Plate II
  thrombophlebitic, Fig. 165
  varicose, 498, 499, Fig. 172
Unconsciousness, 922
Undulant fever. *See* Brucellosis
Unna's paste, 499
Upper respiratory tract, anatomy of, Fig. 114
  infection, 392
  obstruction of, 393

Urea, blood, 80
Uremia, 684
Uremic frost, 685
Ureter, 678, 692, 696
Ureterosigmoidostomy, 701
Ureterostomy, 701
Ureterotomy, 696
Urethra, disorders of, 705
Urethritis, 705
  gonorrheal, 705, 708
Urethrotomy, 706
Uric acid, blood, 80
  in gout, 1030
Urinalysis, 65
  tape and tablet tests for, Plate I
Urinary tract, drainage, 682
  infection, 692
    female, 700
Urine, acidity, 69
  casts, 73, Fig. 21
  collection, 66
  color, 67
  concentration, 70
  diversion of, 700

  hormones, 75
  incontinence of, 305, 681
    in neurologic disease, 915
  preservatives, 66
  radioisotopic measurement of, 113

  retention of, 680
    postoperative, 304
  sediment, 72
  specific gravity, 70
  tests, 66
  urobilinogen, 75
Urinometer, 70, Fig. 20
Uristix, for proteinuria and glycosuria, Plate I
Urobilin, 68
Urobilinogen, urine, 75
Urogenital disorders, male, Fig. 273

Urostix, 72
Urticaria, 809

Uterus, cancer of, 732
  displacements of, 736
  fibroid, 737
  prolapse of, 737

Vaccination, 1052, 1054
  DPT, 1052
  influenza, 1098
  mumps, 1095
  pertussis, 1072
  plague, 1087
  poliomyelitis, 1103
  rabies, 1109
  smallpox, 1054
  technic of, 1053
  typhoid fever, 1077
  typhus, 1115
Vaccine, Sabin, 1104
  Salk, 1104
  Sauer, 1072
  Semple, 1109
  yellow fever, 1111
Vaccinia, 1054
  evolution of, Plate IX
Vagectomy, 599
Vaginal douches, 727
Vaginal infections, 728
  types and treatment of, Table 19
Vaginitis, 729
Vagotomy, 601
Valve, ileocecal, Fig. 229
  pulmonic, lesions, 532
Vaporizer, 300
  Colson, Fig. 92
Varicella. *See* Chickenpox
Varices, esophageal, 584, 656, 657, Fig. 213
  bleeding, 584
    compression treatment of, Fig. 213
  formation of, in cirrhosis, Figs. 251, 252
  surgical treatment of, 584
Varicocele, 711
Varicosities, venous, 490
Variola vera. *See* Smallpox

Vasomotor rhinitis, 802
Vegetations, valvular, Fig. 182
Vein(s), 483
  stasis of, in leg, 490
  stripping of, 499
  thrombosis, leg, 437
  varicose, 490, 497, 498, Fig. 171
Vena cava obstruction, 63
Venesection. *See* Phlebotomy
Venography, 101
Ventricles, cardiac, 507
  cerebral, 894
Ventricular septal defects, 553
Ventriculography, 911
Vermifuges, 1137, 1138
Verrucae, 769
Vertigo, 926
Vesicles, 745
Vibrio comma, Fig. 430
Vinethene. *See* Ether, divinyl
Virilism, 840
Vision, 852
Vital capacity, 94, 401
Vitamin(s), 147
  A, 147
    deficiency, 151
    tolerance test, 83
  B, complex, 147
    deficiencies, 151
  B$_6$. *See* Pyridoxine
  B$_{12}$, 148
    absorption test, 109
    deficiency, 152, 463
      postgastrectomy, 610
    therapy, 464
  C, 148
    deficiency, 152
  D, 147
    deficiency, 153
  E, 147
  folic acid deficiency, 466
  K, 147
    deficiency, 153, 478
  K$_1$, 488
Vitiligo, 750
Volvulus, 632, Fig. 239

Vomiting, cerebral, 942
  fecal, 633
  in peptic ulcer, 597
  postoperative, 292
  projectile, 942
  psychic, 594
Vomitus, aspiration of, Fig. 91
  coffee-ground, 606
Vulvitis, 727
  gonorrheal, 727
Vulvovaginitis, gonorrheal, 729

Walking iron, Fig. 405
Warfarin, 1087
Warts. *See* Verrucae
Water, body, 159
  intoxication, 163
  requirements, 159
  retention, 843
Wheals, 745
Whirlpool baths, 29, Fig. 6
Whitlow. *See* Tenosynovitis
Whooping cough. *See* Pertussis
Wound(s), diphtheria, 1069
  draining, dressing of, 285
  emergency management of, 1157
  healing, 23, 307
  infections, 31
    postoperative, 307
  operative, care of, 283
  sucking, 442
Wristdrop, 928
Wryneck. *See* Torticollis

Xanthochromia, 99
Xerophthalmia, 151
Xylocaine (Lidocaine), 229

Yaws, 1124, Fig. 447
Yellow fever, 1110

Z-plasty, 775, Fig. 308